D1405104

SECOND EDITION
GYNECOLOGY AND OBSTETRICS
THE HEALTH CARE OF WOMEN

SEYMOUR L. ROMNEY, M.D.
Professor, Department of Gynecology and Obstetrics and
Director, Gynecological Cancer Research
Albert Einstein College of Medicine
Bronx, New York

MARY JANE GRAY, M.D.
Adjunct Professor, Department of Obstetrics and Gynecology
School of Medicine and
Gynecologist, Student Health Service
University of North Carolina
Chapel Hill, North Carolina

A. BRIAN LITTLE, M.D.
Arthur H. Bill Professor and
Director, Department of Reproductive Biology
School of Medicine
Case Western Reserve University
Cleveland, Ohio

JAMES A. MERRILL, M.D.
Professor and Head, Department of Gynecology and Obstetrics and
Professor, Department of Pathology
College of Medicine
University of Oklahoma
Oklahoma City, Oklahoma

E. J. QUILLIGAN, M.D.
Professor, Department of Obstetrics and Gynecology
University of California College of Medicine
Irvine, California

RICHARD W. STANDER, M.D.
Professor, Department of Obstetrics and Gynecology
University of New Mexico School of Medicine
Albuquerque, New Mexico

McGRAW-HILL BOOK COMPANY
New York St. Louis San Francisco Auckland Bogotá Hamburg
Johannesburg London Madrid Mexico Montreal New Delhi
Panama Paris São Paulo Singapore Sydney Tokyo Toronto

NOTICE

Medicine is an ever-changing science. As new research and clinical experience broaden our knowledge, changes in treatment and drug therapy are required. The editors and the publisher of this work have made every effort to ensure that the drug dosage schedules herein are accurate and in accord with the standards accepted at the time of publication. Readers are advised, however, to check the product information sheet included in the package of each drug they plan to administer to be certain that changes have not been made in the recommended dose or in the contraindications for administration. This recommendation is of particular importance in regard to new or infrequently used drugs.

GYNECOLOGY AND OBSTETRICS: THE HEALTH CARE OF WOMEN

Copyright © 1981, 1975 by McGraw-Hill, Inc. All rights reserved. Printed in the United States of America. No part of this publication may be reproduced, stored in a retrieval system, or transmitted, in any form or by any means, electronic, mechanical, photocopying, recording, or otherwise, without the prior written permission of the publisher.

1234567890HDHD89876543210

This book was set in Helvetica Light by The Clarinda Company.
The editors were Richard W. Mixter, Stuart D. Boynton, Bob Leap, and John J. Fitzpatrick; the designer was Charles A. Carson;
the production supervisor was Jeanne Skahan.
The drawings were done by J & R Services, Inc.
Halliday Lithograph Corporation was printer and binder.

Library of Congress Cataloging in Publication Data

Main entry under title:

Gynecology and obstetrics.

    Includes index.
    1. Gynecology. 2. Obstetrics. I. Romney, Seymour L.
RG101.G94   1980   618   79-26470
ISBN 0-07-053582-5

Contents

List of Contributors

TOM P. BARDEN M.D.
Professor, Department of Obstetrics and Gynecology, and Associate Professor, Department of Pediatrics, College of Medicine, University of Cincinnati, Cincinnati

MICHAEL L. BERMAN, M.D.
Assistant Professor, Department of Obstetrics and Gynecology, University of Pittsburgh School of Medicine, Pittsburgh

R. B. BILLIAR, Ph.D.
Associate Professor, Department of Reproductive Biology, School of Medicine, Case Western Reserve University, Cleveland

ERIC BLOCH, Ph.D.
Associate Professor, Department of Gynecology and Obstetrics and Department of Biochemistry, and Investigator, Rose F. Kennedy Center for Research in Mental Retardation and Human Development, Albert Einstein College of Medicine, New York

PAUL F. BRENNER, M.D.
Associate Professor, Department of Obstetrics and Gynecology, University of Southern California School of Medicine, Los Angeles

LARRY BUMPASS, M.D.
Director, Center for Demography and Ecology, and Professor, Department of Sociology, University of Wisconsin, Madison

ALEXANDER M. CAPRON
Professor of Law and Professor of Human Genetics, University of Pennsylvania, Philadelphia

DENIS CAVANAGH, M.D.
Professor, Department of Obstetrics and Gynecology, University of South Florida College of Medicine, Tampa

RONALD A. CHEZ, M.D.
Professor and Chairman, Department of Obstetrics and Gynecology, Milton S. Hershey Medical Center, Pennsylvania State Medical School, Hershey

MANUEL R. COMAS, M.D.
Associate Professor, Department of Gynecology and Obstetrics, Saint Louis University School of Medicine, Saint Louis

RHONDA COPELON, LL.B.
Staff Attorney, Center for Constitutional Rights, New York

ALICE T. DAY, Ph.D.
Professor, Department of Sociology, Australian National University Research School of Social Sciences, Canberra

PHILIP J. DiSAIA, M.D.
Professor and Chairman, Department of Obstetrics and Gynecology, California College of Medicine, University of California, Irvine

MARTIN FARBER, M.D.
Associate Professor, Department of Obstetrics and Gynecology, Tufts University School of Medicine; Gynecologist, Department of Obstetrics and Gynecology, New England Medical Center Hospital, Boston

MORRIS B. FIDDLER, M.D.
Assistant Professor, Department of Pediatrics, Northwestern University Medical School; Research Associate, Division of Genetics, Children's Memorial Hospital, Chicago

GILBERT H. FLETCHER, M.D.
Professor and Head, Department of Radiotherapy, The University of Texas System Cancer Center, M. D. Anderson Hospital and Tumor Institute, Houston

DIANE S. FORDNEY, M.D.
Associate Professor, Department of Obstetrics and Gynecology, University of Arizona College of Medicine, Tuscon

HERMAN L. GARDNER, M.D.
Clinical Professor, Department of Obstetrics and Gynecology, Baylor College of Medicine; Honorary Chief, Obstetrics and Gynecology Department, Saint Luke's Episcopal Hospital, Houston

ALBERT B. GERBIE, M.D.
Professor, Department of Obstetrics and Gynecology, Northwestern University School of Medicine; Attending Obstetrician and Gynecologist, Prentice Women's Hospital and Maternity Center, Chicago

RONALD S. GIBBS, M.D.
Associate Professor, Department of Obstetrics and Gynecology, University of Texas School of Medicine at San Antonio, San Antonio

MARY JANE GRAY, M.D.
Adjunct Professor, Department of Obstetrics and Gynecology, School of Medicine, and Gynecologist, Student Health Service, University of North Carolina, Chapel Hill

DAVID A. GRIMES, M.D.
Assistant Professor, Department of Obstetrics and Gynecology, Emory University School of Medicine, Atlanta; Bureau of Epidemiology, Center for Disease Control

WILLIAM R. HART, M.D.
Professor, Department of Pathology, University of Michigan Medical School, Ann Arbor

TERRY HAYASHI, M.D.
Professor and Chairman, Department of Obstetrics and Gynecology, University of Pittsburgh School of Medicine, Pittsburgh

ANDRE E. HELLEGERS, M.D. (deceased)
The Kennedy Institute for the Study of Human Reproduction and Bioethics, Georgetown University, Washington, D.C.

LAWRENCE S. JACKMAN, M.D.
Assistant Clinical Professor, Department of Obstetrics and Gynecology, Albert Einstein College of Medicine, New York

GORDON K. JIMERSON, M.D.
Associate Professor, Department of Gynecology and Obstetrics, College of Medicine, University of Oklahoma, Oklahoma City

HOWARD L. JUDD, M.D.
Professor, Department of Obstetrics and Gynecology, School of Medicine, University of California at Los Angeles, Los Angeles

IRWIN H. KAISER, M.D., Ph.D.
Professor, Department of Gynecology and Obstetrics, Albert Einstein College of Medicine, New York

RAYMOND H. KAUFMAN, M.D.
Ernst W. Bertner Chairman and Professor, Department of Obstetrics and Gynecology, and Professor, Department of Pathology, Baylor College of Medicine, Texas Medical Center, Houston

ZEEV KOREN, M.D.
Professor, Department of Gynecology and Obstetrics, Albert Einstein College of Medicine, New York

WILLIAM J. LEDGER, M.D.
Professor and Chairman, Department of Obstetrics and Gynecology, The New York Hospital–Cornell Medical Center; Obstetrician and Gynecologist-in-Chief, The New York Hospital, New York

JOHN L. LEWIS, JR., M.D.
Professor of Obstetrics and Gynecology, Cornell University Medical College; Chief, Gynecology Service, Memorial Sloan-Kettering Cancer Center, New York

HAROLD I. LIEF, M.D.
Professor of Psychiatry, School of Medicine, University of Pennsylvania; Director, Division of Family Study and of Marriage Council of Philadelphia, Philadelphia

A. BRIAN LITTLE, M.D.
Arthur H. Bill Professor and Director, Department of Reproductive Biology, School of Medicine, Case Western Reserve University, Cleveland

JOHN VAN S. MAECK, M.D.
Professor Emeritus, Department of Obstetrics and Gynecology, University of Vermont College of Medicine, Burlington

LUIGI MASTROIANNI, JR., M.D.
Professor and Chairman, Department of Obstetrics and Gynecology, University of Pennsylvania Hospital and Medical School, Philadelphia

JAMES L. MATHIS, M.D.
Professor and Chairman, Department of Psychiatry, East Carolina University School of Medicine, Greenville, North Carolina

PAUL G. McDONOUGH, M.D.
Professor, Department of Obstetrics and Gynecology, and Chief, Reproductive Endocrine Unit, Medical College of Georgia, Augusta

AUDREY J. McMASTER, M.D.
Associate Professor, Department of Gynecology and Obstetrics, School of Medicine, University of Oklahoma, Oklahoma City

DAVID R. MELDRUM, M.D.
Assistant Professor, Department of Obstetrics and Gynecology, School of Medicine, University of California at Los Angeles, Los Angeles

JAMES A. MERRILL, M.D.
Professor and Head, Department of Gynecology and Obstetrics, and Professor, Department of Pathology, College of Medicine, University of Oklahoma, Oklahoma City

GEORGE W. MITCHELL, Jr., M.D.
Professor and Chairman, Department of Obstetrics and Gynecology, Tufts University School of Medicine; Gynecologist-in-Chief, Department of Obstetrics and Gynecology, New England Medical Center Hospital, Boston

C. PAUL MORROW, M.D.
Professor, Department of Obstetrics and Gynecology, and Director, Gynecologic Oncology, University of Southern California School of Medicine, Los Angeles

HENRY L. NADLER, M.D.
Given Research Professor and Chairman, Department of Pediatrics, Northwestern University Medical School; Chief of Staff, Children's Memorial Hospital, Chicago

WILLIAM B. OBER, M.D.
Director of Laboratories, Hackensack Hospital, Hackensack; Visiting Professor of Pathology, New Jersey College of Medicine and Dentistry

CARL J. PAUERSTEIN, M.D.
Professor and Chairman, Department of Obstetrics and Gynecology, Medical School, University of Texas, San Antonio

M. WALSH PLATT, Ph.D.
Research Associate, Division of Genetics, Children's Memorial Hospital, Chicago

E. J. QUILLIGAN, M.D.
Professor, Department of Obstetrics and Gynecology, College of Medicine, University of California, Irvine

SEYMOUR L. ROMNEY, M.D.
Professor, Department of Gynecology and Obstetrics, and Director, Gynecological Cancer Research, Albert Einstein College of Medicine, New York

JOSEPH J. ROVINSKY, M.D.
Professor, Department of Obstetrics and Gynecology, School of Medicine, State University of New York at Stony Brook; Chairman, Department of Obstetrics and Gynecology, Long Island Jewish–Hillside Medical Center, New Hyde Park

FELIX RUTLEDGE, M.D.
Professor of Gynecology, Department of Gynecology-Oncology, M. D. Anderson Research and Tumor Institute, Houston

JOHN A. SCHILLING, M.D.
Professor and Chairman of Surgery, School of Medicine, University of Washington, Seattle

HAROLD SCHULMAN, M.D.
Professor and Chairman, Department of Gynecology and Obstetrics, Albert Einstein College of Medicine, New York

LESTER SILBERMAN, M.D.
Professor, Department of Obstetrics and Gynecology, College of Medicine, University of Vermont, Burlington

MICHAEL A. SIMMONS, M.D.
Associate Professor, Department of Pediatrics, and Chief of Neonatology, Johns Hopkins University Medical College, Baltimore

SHELDON C. SOMMERS, M.D.
Director of Laboratories, Lenox Hill Hospital; Clinical Professor of Pathology, Columbia College of Physicians and Surgeons, New York

RICHARD W. STANDER, M.D.
Professor, Department of Obstetrics and Gynecology, University of New Mexico School of Medicine, Albuquerque

NANCY STEARNS, LL.B.
Staff Attorney, Center for Constitutional Rights, New York

STEVEN E. VOGL, M.D.
Assistant Professor, Department of Medicine, Albert Einstein College of Medicine, New York

JAMES C. WARREN, M.D., Ph.D.
Professor and Head, Department of Obstetrics and Gynecology, Washington University School of Medicine; Obstetrician and Gynecologist-in-Chief, Barnes and Allied Hospitals, Saint Louis

PAUL C. WEINBERG, M.D.
Professor of Obstetrics and Gynecology, Department of Obstetrics and Gynecology, University of Texas Health Science Center, San Antonio

J. TAYLOR WHARTON, M.D.
Professor of Gynecology, Department of Gynecology-Oncology, University of Texas M. D. Anderson Hospital Research and Tumor Institute, Houston

Preface

The original justification for this text was our conviction that the discipline of gynecology and obstetrics has a major responsibility for the comprehensive health care of women in our present era of rapid social, scientific, and technological change. A nontraditional book evolved. This second edition is intended to refocus, reconfirm, and further meet that responsibility.

As a text and reference, primarily written for the practitioner-clinician providing health care for women, the book is intended to be a source of information rather than a "how-to-do" manual. Consistent with the changing nature of our society and with its search for more effective health care delivery, the content and presentation of this edition have been updated. The text is designed to be useful both to physicians in training and to those engaged in continuing education. Students will find this book uniquely organized for their needs and more than adequately comprehensive.

Instead of gynecology and obstetrics appearing as separate entities, the presentation involves five separate but interrelated parts. Subjects may be addressed in more than one section; thus, different approaches to a subject are offered the reader. The various parts have been carefully cross-referenced.

In the first part, Care of Women, we present an overview of the specialty and its multidisciplinary involvement in current social, economic, political, bioethical, and legal controversies as they influence evaluation and care of the patient and her problems.

The second part, Mechanisms, concentrates on the etiology and mechanism(s) of major disease categories. It offers a broad understanding of alterations in major systems and of processes involving more than one system. The emphasis is on identification of pathophysiologic factors essential to a basic understanding of specific diseases.

In the third part, Approach to the Patient, the woman as a person and her medical problems are considered in relation to age. Infancy, childhood, adolescence, adulthood, and the older years are seen in this perspective. The fetus is treated as a patient within the scope of comprehensive health care.

The fourth part, Manifestations of Disease, is organized around signs and symptoms, such as pain, bleeding, discharge, and psychosexual dysfunction. Here are the logical bases for differential diagnosis and selection of appropriate tests to supplement the history and physical examination. This approach should help users of the problem-oriented medical record, with its insistence that all significant problems, medical and social, be recognized and used as the framework to which data are related and around which plans are formulated.

Part five, Specific Problems, deals with special problems. Essentially, it is a section detailing much of the material presented in traditional texts.

We continue to be indebted to an outstanding group of contributors, who offer many different viewpoints. We encourage the discourse of conflicting views as long as they are responsible and documented. We oppose dogmatism because of our conviction that the study and the practice of medicine involve a flexible blend of art and science in proportions which are difficult to define.

We remain indebted to the many colleagues, residents, and students who have provided words of encouragement or constructive critical suggestions. The sustained support of the McGraw-Hill organization is gratefully acknowledged. Stuart Boynton has seen us through two editions; his personal and professional efforts have been indispensable.

SEYMOUR L. ROMNEY
MARY JANE GRAY
A. BRIAN LITTLE
JAMES A. MERRILL
E. J. QUILLIGAN
RICHARD W. STANDER

GYNECOLOGY AND OBSTETRICS

THE HEALTH CARE OF WOMEN

PART ONE

Care of Women

1

The Physician's Responsibility

JAMES A. MERRILL

The continued success of our society is inextricably bound to the health of succeeding generations, which is linked to the quality of human reproduction.

CHANGING CONCEPTS OF HEALTH CARE

Gynecology and obstetrics is that special field of medicine which deals with the health care of women, with particular focus upon sexual and reproductive function and disorders. The discipline is greatly concerned with the factors which influence the quality as well as the quantity of human reproduction. The scope of this branch of medicine is changing rapidly, just as all of medicine is changing. The primary concern of the gynecologist and obstetrician today is certainly not that which was the primary concern in the past, and predictably the primary concerns of the gynecologist-obstetrician of the future will differ. Although much of this change has been the result of the extension of medical knowledge and the perfection of techniques, much of it reflects increasing societal and individual health care expectations. The very change in terminology from *medical* care to *health* care indicates a basic change in the concept of the role of the physician. Preventive care rather than acute crisis care has become the objective.

CONSUMER UNITS

The increasing demand for adequate health care and the expanding role of government in the health field have stimulated numerous studies of medical education and the systems for delivery of health care. The traditional consumer unit is the *individual,* who seeks the services of a physician for a specific illness or problem. The physician may remain the same, or different physicians may be chosen as different illnesses or problems arise. Increasingly, medical or health care has become *family oriented.* Federal legislation has been promulgated to encourage an emphasis on family practice. There is now increasing interest in population-centered or *community-centered systems* for the delivery of health care. This will assume greater importance as the concepts of preventive medicine and health maintenance are accepted and encouraged. Furthermore, there is increasing pressure to insure effective and readily available health care for the economically deprived segments of our population.

NATURE OF CARE

Initially physician practice and the nature of medical care were general. With the explosion of scientific knowledge in the past half-century, there has been increasing specialization. Physicians have found it essential to limit their activities to increasingly specialized areas. Unfortunately, as specialization has increased, medical care for the individual has become fragmented. The patient or the "consumer" is often trapped between specialty groups; the specialties became independent rather than interdependent, and care became depersonalized when combined with medical fragmentation. Dissatisfaction with the availability of health care has appeared. As personal values have been examined, primary care has been encouraged. The effectiveness of consumer demand for primary health care as opposed to specialized medical care for specific illnesses is enhanced by the greater ability of people to pay for the care they want and the increasing participation of government in the health field. It has been estimated that more than 75 percent of the people in America today are covered by some form of health insurance. It is anticipated that some form of national health insurance will cover everyone. Legislation to accomplish this is not far off. In 1976, 57.8 percent of total health expenditures were paid with private funds, down from 74.3 percent in 1966.

Traditional medicine has involved the diagnosis and treatment of *disease,* and the services of the physician have been sought only after the patient developed complaints. The degree to which attention has been directed to the prevention of disease has varied. Crisis care has characterized the medical care for the

poor, and prevention of disease or care between crises has been uncommon. This tradition has now changed drastically and will change even further. Maintenance of health is a national goal and essentially all of the health care planning is being directed to this end. In the care of women, this is especially apparent. Preventive medicine has long been an essential part of gynecology and obstetrics, as best exemplified by prenatal care—designed to prevent, identify, and treat obstetric complications. Periodic examination to screen for pelvic cancer is widely advocated. Many of the health care needs of women do not involve disease or illness, but involve an educational component consisting of support and counsel concerning normal phenomena such as the menarche, puberty, adolescence, sexuality, fertility control, sexual relationships, pregnancy, and the menopause. Essential to maintenance of health in the female is patient education and information. The effectiveness of health care for women is frequently determined by an openness on the part of her physician to understand the woman's goals and a willingness and interest in educating her to achieve and maintain good health and well-being, both physical and mental. This education should include the early signs and symptoms of cancer, self-examination of the breasts, the importance of periodic examination, the purpose of preconceptional and antepartum examination, and practical aspects of reproductive biology and human sexuality. Moreover, the physicians should explain the health delivery system and the methods of gaining entry for all problems. In the absence of effective patient information and education, unnecessary resentment may develop between the woman and her physician.

HEALTH CARE DELIVERY SYSTEMS

Although individual or "solo" practice is still the most common system of health care delivery, group practice has become a significant form of practice for many physicians. There are essentially three types of groups: (1) single-specialty groups composed exclusively of physicians in one specialty; (2) practice groups composed of general practitioners or family physicians; and (3) multispecialty groups composed of physicians of two or more major specialties. In 1976, almost 50 percent of practicing physicians in the United States were in some type of group practice. In the delivery of obstetric care, groups of two or more obstetricians practicing together provide a far more efficient system of pregnancy care than can be accomplished by individual practice and this type of practice is becoming increasingly common. Furthermore, there is increasing interest in the development and utilization of well-trained nonphysician health personnel working cooperatively with physicians to provide comprehensive gynecologic and obstetric health care. In addition, there is evidence that the consolidation of hospital gynecology and obstetrics services remarkably enhances the efficiency and the economic operation of the facility.

FINANCING HEALTH CARE

The financing of health care in this country is undergoing rapid change. The concept of fee for service for those patients who can afford to pay and charity for those who cannot has given way to the concept of prepaid health care insurance for all. The cost of catastrophic illness has become a problem for all but the most affluent. For example, the average adjusted expenses per inpatient day in community hospitals in 1976 was $151.28. This represents a 13.6 percent increase over 1975, and a 105.2 percent increase over 1970. Another critical problem has been the difficulty in finding entry into the health care system even when means were available to pay for the services. Pressure from consumer groups as well as federal and state health participation are resulting in plans to eliminate this serious deficiency in our health care delivery system.

THE ROLE OF WOMEN

Of particular significance in the contemporary practice of gynecology and obstetrics is the changing role of women in our society (see Chaps. 2 and 5). Much of this has been brought into focus by the women's health movement and the women's liberation movement. Women are no longer willing to accept a stereotype which totally submerges them in family and child rearing. There are an increasing number of options open to women in the 1980s. With new goals and life styles, women want to play a more decisive part in their own health care. Pregnancy has become a voluntary experience as a result of the increased availability of effective methods of birth control and of abortion for unwanted pregnancies. An increasing number of women will choose a role which will not restrict them to the home nor limit their options re-

garding the use of their own sexuality, and hence there is a change in the nature of the gynecologic and obstetric health care they desire. The women's health movement has focused attention upon what some women consider to be demeaning in gynecologic care. This requires an attitudinal change on the part of physicians if they are to keep abreast of the changes that have occurred rapidly in our society (see Chaps. 2 and 5).

GYNECOLOGY AND OBSTETRICS AS A SPECIALTY

Obstetrics arose as an offshoot of midwifery. Since ancient times, midwives, who were self-styled specialists of the obstetric art, have supervised the labor and delivery of women. Not until the end of the eighteenth century did physicians become involved in this practice. There is currently a renewed interest in the training and practice of nurse-midwives, largely as a result of efforts to improve the overall availability of individual care to patients. When nurse-midwifery is appropriately supervised, it has proved to be advantageous. When improperly supervised, it has proved disastrous. Gynecology arose as a surgical specialty and originally was concerned largely with the extirpation of pelvic tumors and the surgical repair of obstetric injuries. As knowledge concerning reproduction increased, the overlap of these two fields became apparent and the unification of gynecology and obstetrics into a single area of specialized medical care was a logical accomplishment. Probably as much as any discipline, gynecology and obstetrics touches upon many fields of medicine. A knowledge of the biology of reproduction, including an understanding of internal medicine, surgery, psychiatry, pediatrics, and preventive medicine, is necessary for the management of patient problems.

Increasingly, the gynecologist-obstetrician is the physician to whom women turn for their ongoing health care and medical supervision, to identify health problems as they arise and make appropriate referral when indicated. There are some who suggest that the gynecologist-obstetrician should be recognized as the primary physician of women, in addition to the role as specialist consultant. Furthermore, the gynecologist-obstetrician may be heavily involved in counseling patients concerning regulation of fertility, pregnancy spacing, and marital problems. Because of its specific concern with human reproduction and human sexuality, the discipline of gynecology and obstetrics is involved, at its very core, in some of the most pressing problems existing in our contemporary society. Gynecologic therapy is intimately involved in social and emotional as well as moral and cultural factors. While the primary objective may, at times, be to treat or remove disease, this must be planned with a full understanding of the impact of such therapy upon the actual or perceived female role of the individual. In addition to the effect the therapy may have upon the anatomy and function of the female organs, there necessarily will be an impact upon the femininity and sexuality of the patient. Thus gynecologic care has an additional dimension not usually present in other types of medical treatment. The interruption or restoration of fertility, the emphasis or deemphasis of perceived femininity, and the alteration of sexuality are frequent concerns of the woman which must be considered in a frank and open manner. The patient should be given sufficient information to understand the nature of her problem, the indications for and nature of recommended therapy and the impact of this therapy upon her life, now and in the future. She should also be educated to maintain her good health or to cope with certain limitations in her activities, plans, or life-style. None of this can be left to common knowledge. Only in this way can unnecessary anguish be avoided.

As scientific advances have increased the knowledge of human reproduction, the practice of gynecology and obstetrics has become more complex. An increasing number of gynecologist-obstetricians have limited their activity to areas of special competence. At present, there are three areas of specialization recognized by certification within gynecology and obstetrics and others are developing. The presently defined areas are (1) *oncology*, which includes the diagnosis and management of female pelvic malignancy; (2) *fetal and maternal medicine*, which includes the specialized care of complicated pregnancies; and (3) *reproductive endocrinology*, which includes the management of patients with the various endocrinopathies which influence the female reproductive process.

TRADITIONAL CONCERNS

The traditional concerns of the practicing gynecologist-obstetrician were to minimize mortality and injury of mothers and infants, to treat by medical and surgical means women with pelvic complaints, to diag-

nose and treat pelvic neoplasm and, through periodic examination, to prevent disease or initiate early and curative therapy. In order to assess the quality of care, statistics concerning operative, cancer, maternal, fetal, and newborn death rates have been studied and reviewed by peer committees with a view toward identifying and correcting the causes.

GYNECOLOGIC THERAPY

In the nonpregnant patient, the usual role of the gynecologist-obstetrician has been the treatment of diseases related to pathology of pelvic structures. This includes medical and surgical treatment of pelvic infections, the management of abnormalities of menstruation, the removal of diseased pelvic organs, and the correction of injuries of the pelvic supporting tissues, usually the aftermath of obstetric delivery. Historically, the modern era of gynecologic surgery (indeed abdominal surgery) began in 1809 when Dr. Ephraim McDowell successfully removed a huge ovarian cyst from Jane Crawford. In addition to surgical extirpation and operative repair, gynecologic therapy increasingly has included the regulation of reproductive function with the use of hormone medication.

Pelvic cancer is one of the most significant gynecologic diseases. The probability that a woman will develop cancer is greater now than it was a decade ago. The American Cancer Society estimated over 383,000 new cases of cancer in females in the United States in 1977. Of these cases, 108,200, or 28 percent, were in the reproductive tract. Cancer of the uterus is the most common, but deaths from this disease have fallen steadily as the result of effective methods of diagnosing it in the early curable stages. Investigation of uterine cancer led to the development of exfoliative cytology as an effective means of cancer screening. Detailed investigation of cancer of the uterine cervix, beginning with exfoliative cytology, has led to an increased understanding of the biology, etiology, and natural history of human malignancy. The effectiveness of cancer screening through cervical cytology has been largely responsible for patient acceptance of periodic health examinations. The details of the cost effectiveness of such screening programs are discussed in detail in Chap. 14. Like prenatal care, periodic pelvic examination for cancer screening is an example of effective preventive medicine which has characterized the practice of gynecology and obstetrics for many years.

MATERNAL MORTALITY

The *maternal mortality rate* is usually defined as death during pregnancy or as a result of pregnancy or its complications. It is customarily calculated as the rate per 100,000 live births. The maternal mortality rate in the United States has shown a sharp decrease over the years. There were 390 women who died in 1976 in the United States as a result of complications of pregnancy, childbirth, and the puerperium; there were 3,171,000 live births, giving a maternal mortality rate of 12.3 per 100,000 live births. This represents a significant decrease from the rates of 29.1 in 1966 and 83.3 in 1950. Over the years the majority of maternal deaths have been caused by hemorrhage, toxemias of pregnancy, and infection; this triad still accounts for the majority of deaths. Although the actual numbers are decreasing, hemorrhage as a cause of death has shown a relative increase. Furthermore, in some reports, deaths due to hemorrhage have been judged to be preventable in as many as 50 percent of cases. With improvement in the management of these common obstetric complications, deaths are reported with a relative increased frequency from such causes as thromboembolism, anesthesia, cardiac disease, and transfusion reaction.

Maternal mortality rates are dependent upon social and economic factors which affect the quality of health care delivery. Thus, in 1976, when the maternal mortality rate was 12.3 per 100,000 live births, the rate for white women was 9.0 and for nonwhite 26.5. The average maternal mortality rate for the 3 years, 1971 to 1973, was 9.7 in the New England states and 29.0 in the East South Central states. Advanced age and high parity both increase the risk of maternal mortality. In 1973, the mortality rate for women age 20 to 24 was 9.3, and for women age 40 to 44, 78.5.

There are many reasons for the striking improvement in the safety of childbirth. Among them is the training of specialists in gynecology and obstetrics. The American Board of Obstetrics and Gynecology was established in 1930; in 1978, there were 15,853 physicians holding a specialty certificate from this board. The development of specialty certification has not only improved the quality of those physicians who are certified but also has had a beneficial impact on the entire practice of gynecology and obstetrics in the community. Coincident with the training of gynecologists and obstetricians has been an effective program of teaching, research, and investigation in the area of human reproduction and reproductive biology.

The development of effective prenatal care together with the increase in hospital delivery are of extreme importance. Federal support for maternal and infant care has made prenatal care and hospital delivery available to large numbers of economically deprived women. The result has been a substantial increase in the overall safety and quality of reproduction. However, there is room for more improvement. In some parts of the country one-half to three-fourths of the deaths are avoidable. While the solution certainly involves physician education, there is clear need for patient education as well. Often the underlying cause of maternal death can be attributed to apparent patient irresponsibility which can be corrected by proper education. This must begin early and be ongoing.

INFANT AND PERINATAL MORTALITY

The *infant mortality rate* is the number of infant deaths under 1 year of age per 1000 live births. Infant deaths rank tenth among all causes of death in the United States and equal all other deaths during the subsequent five decades of life. Thus the intervals of intrauterine existence and the event of birth represent some of the most hazardous periods of life. The 1976 infant mortality rate for the United States was 15.2 per 1000 live births for the lowest annual rate ever recorded here, a decrease of 48.3 percent from 1950. The 1976 decrease in infant mortality over 1975 was 6.3 percent for whites and 2.9 percent for nonwhites.

Another measure of the quality of obstetric care is the *perinatal mortality rate* and its component parts. *Fetal death* is usually defined as death in utero of a fetus weighing 500 g or more, or a fetus of 20 weeks or more gestational age. The *fetal death rate* is the number of fetal deaths per 1000 births. *Neonatal death* is the death of a newborn infant within the first 28 days of life, and the rate is expressed as the number of neonatal deaths per 1000 live births. The *perinatal mortality rate* is the sum of *fetal* and *neonatal* death rates. Although there has been a gradual improvement over the years, the trend of improvement in perinatal death rates is not as great as the decrease in infant deaths. The perinatal death rate in 1975 was 22.4 per 1000 births. Fetal death rate was 10.8 and neonatal death rate was 11.6. The neonatal death rate was 10.4 for whites and 16.8 for nonwhites. The majority of perinatal losses are associated with maternal illness and complications of pregnancy, not with delivery alone. Therefore, the reasons for the decrease in infant and perinatal mortality rates are similar to those for maternal mortality rates. Out-of-hospital births pose a two to five times greater risk to the baby's life than hospital births. This is equally true for those regions currently advocating a return to home births.

Athough statistics are not as readily available, it is important to recognize that the incidence of birth defects and mental retardation parallels that of perinatal mortality. Further, perinatal mortality and mental retardation are both greatly influenced by the rate of premature births. The development of special care facilities for patients with high-risk pregnancies and the development of intensive-care nurseries for sick and premature infants have not only decreased the perinatal mortality rates, but also have diminished the incidence of mental retardation. Not only are more infants surviving in the nursery, but they are surviving to grow up as healthy children. Social and economic factors have a substantial impact upon the perinatal mortality rates. Eight percent of the deliveries, occurring to an identifiable high-risk group, contribute 20 percent of the infant deaths. The higher rates are among patients who receive inadequate prenatal and preconceptional care; who are of young or old age; high parity; who have complicating medical illnesses; who live in crowded, depressed parts of the city; and, in general, who suffer from medical and social stress.

In recent years, the United States infant mortality rate has received considerable attention as one of the key indicators of the level of health of the United States population and, thus, a rough measure of the effectiveness of the nation's health care delivery system. Much of this discussion is centered around the position of the United States in the international ranking of nations according to infant mortality rates. There are so many factors which contribute to differences in infant mortality rates that this is a poor measure of the quality of the total health system. Among the Western countries, the United States has about the lowest rate of stillbirths or fetal deaths. This is due in large part to the effort of the medical profession in this country to prolong gestation for those pregnancies which give evidence of terminating prematurely. Consequently, the number of live-born but premature infants has been increased and this has contributed to an increase in the early infant mortality. Also, the criteria for defining a live birth differ from one country to another, resulting in different allocations of live births and fetal deaths.

The United States also has a remarkably higher proportion of births to mothers under the age of 20 than other Western countries. Young mothers have more premature births, and prematurely born infants

or infants of low birth weight account for two-thirds of the death among the newborn. Rates of infant mortality are affected not only by social and economic levels, but also by differences of cultural background and mode of living. A major problem in respect to infant mortality in the United States has been the high death rates among nonwhite infants. The infant mortality among white infants recently has been at about the same level as among infants in Northwestern Europe. High per capita income and availability of specialized maternal care and social services have a favorable impact on the infant mortality rate. Thus our statistics largely reflect social problems rather than purely medical problems (see Chap. 2).

CONTEMPORARY CONCERNS

The management of normal pregnancy, labor, and delivery and the therapy of benign and malignant pelvic disease continue to be important. Indeed, the sophistication of medicine permits a greater range of therapeutic procedures, and application of surgery, for example, to women of more advanced age and with more serious disease. However, in recent years, the gynecologist-obstetrician has become proportionately less concerned with mechanical techniques and disease therapy and more concerned with the basic biology of femaleness, reproduction health maintenance, and the prevention of disease. The scope of the physician's interests and areas of activity has broadened substantially.

NEUROENDOCRINE PHYSIOLOGY

Rapid advances in the neuroendocrinology of reproduction have provided an opportunity to alter, regulate, and control human fertility and to evaluate the status and well-being of the fetus in utero. The development of oral steroid contraception not only has expanded our knowledge of reproductive endocrinology but has made impact upon the moral and social attitudes of our society. Some believe that certain aspects of the so-called "sexual revolution" are explained indirectly by the availability of this highly reliable method of contraception. Endocrinopathies may be accurately diagnosed and successfully treated. Infertile couples may now have fertility restored by new methods for initiating ovulation in the anovulatory woman. Measurement of hormones of placental origin can accurately reflect not only placental function, but also the metabolic status of the fetus.

FETAL AND MATERNAL MEDICINE

The obstetrician must now approach the fetus as a patient, to be examined, evaluated, and treated, and not considered as an unknown entity until the moment of delivery. Methods are at hand to evaluate the fetus in utero; predict congenital abnormalities; assess changes in growth, development and well-being; and provide therapy while still in utero. Through the technique of aspiration of amniotic fluid and subsequent biochemical, cell culture, and cytologic studies, it is possible to detect fetal biochemical and chromosomal abnormalities as early as the twelfth week of pregnancy, and to determine fetal sex. The latter may be important in dealing with sex-linked inherited diseases such as hemophilia. Amniotic fluid analysis also permits accurate assessment of fetal anemia in cases of Rh isoimmunization with erythroblastosis. In this situation it has been possible to identify accurately those fetuses in distress and to salvage healthy infants by means of intrauterine blood transfusion. The possibility of modifying biochemical defects through administration of specific agents to the fetus is at hand. Measurement of maternal levels of estrogens has proved effective in assessment of the function of the fetoplacental endocrine unit and thus an indirect assessment of fetal well-being. Placental biosynthesis of estriol depends on the availability of precursors of fetal origin and initial metabolic steps occurring in the fetus. In pregnancies complicated with maternal diabetes, for example, falling levels of maternal estriol excretion correlate with fetal death and neonatal morbidity (see Chaps. 9, 15, 3l). Measurements of creatinine and lipids (lecithin and spyngomyelin) in amniotic fluid permit assessment of fetal size and maturity and fetal lung maturity. Using such techniques, it is possible to determine more accurately an appropriate time to terminate complicated pregnancies with the greatest chance of life for the infant. Physiologic monitoring of uterine contractions, fetal electrocardiogram, and fetal electroencephalogram yield objective data and have advantages over palpation and auscultation of the pregnant abdomen in labor. Especially in patients with recognized complications of pregnancy or labor, such close observation permits the obstetrician to detect the earliest signs of fetal distress and to choose the appropriate time and method of delivery consistent with increased fetal survival. The *routine* use of physiologic monitoring of the mother and fetus in labor is practiced in many hospitals. Thus, the obstetrician now assumes a new role as primary physician to the fetus, providing intrauterine health maintenance care, essential diagnosis, and therapy prior to actual birth.

Increased scientific knowledge and improved medical therapy have resulted in higher pregnancy rates among women who have coexisting exotic diseases. Thus, today one may be faced with the management of a pregnant patient with congenital adrenal hyperplasia or a patient pregnant after a successful renal transplant, conditions never encountered in the recent past. The successful management of such patients requires close cooperation of physicians from various disciplines plus the use of modern methods for evaluating fetal growth and development.

ADOLESCENT GYNECOLOGY

The need for sex education and sexual counseling in the teenage population is emphasized in Chaps. 13, 17, and 34. Such counseling activities are assuming increasing emphasis and importance in the practice of gynecology and obstetrics. Education and counseling of the adolescent are important to her general health as well as to help her avoid a first unwanted pregnancy. There are increasing numbers of adolescents in our society with an estimated 40 percent of the population under 20 years of age. The gynecologist thus can expect to see more teenage girls with problems concerning sexuality and fertility and must be prepared to give them sympathetic help.

PSYCHOSOMATIC AND EMOTIONAL PROBLEMS

Many problems are presented to the gynecologist-obstetrician for which no organic cause is apparent. Thorough evaluation of patients with such complaints requires as much time and skill as the patients with uterine fibroids or toxemia of pregnancy. Indeed it has become apparent that emotional factors play a major role in such conditions as menstrual disorders, infertility, repeated abortion, lactation, and chronic pelvic pain. Therefore, the contemporary gynecologist-obstetrician increasingly is evaluating patients' emotional problems and offering help in the form of short-term psychotherapy. Often this is a matter of helping the patient to understand her life situation. Sometimes it involves only being an interested listener. Similarly, an increasing amount of the gynecologist-obstetrician's practice involves counseling patients with marital problems and sexual dysfunction. It is essential that the physician become comfortable and knowledgeable in these areas.

POPULATION CONTROL

In the minds of many, rapid growth of population has become second only to nuclear warfare as civilization's greatest menace. The gynecologist-obstetrician has assumed a leadership role and has recognized the necessity of controlling human fertility not only because of the obvious effect on population growth, but also because of the positive influence of fertility control on the quality of human reproduction. Efforts to make available acceptable methods of birth control, abortion, and sterilization are directed toward improving the quality of life and ensuring as much as possible that each pregnancy is a result of a voluntary, deliberate, and informed personal decision. The goal of each pregnancy is the delivery of a healthy and wanted child.

Illegitimacy rates had been increasing each year for more than a decade until 1972. Then the availability of effective methods of birth control plus more liberal attitudes concerning voluntary sterilization along with removal of laws regulating early abortion, resulted not only in a decrease in birthrate and maternal death from sepsis following illegal abortion, but also a decrease in the rate of illegitimate births (see Chap. 32). But in 1975 the United States recorded a record high proportion of out-of-wedlock births (14.2% of all births). The birthrate in 1977 was 15.3 per 1000 population. Demographers predict that the population will stop growing in about 50 years at approximately 250 million and may even decline. However, the multiple factors influencing fertility rates make predictions hazardous. Some suggest that the American birthrate may have bottomed out and that the country is likely to see a rise in reproduction.

Birth control is not synonymous with population control. Family planning is only a part of an effective population control program. Indeed, there are thoughtful scientists who suggest that the things that make family planning acceptable to couples are the very things that make it ineffective for population control. Specifically, current family-planning programs and methods permit each individual or couple to make an individual decision regarding reproduction, based upon his or her own conscience or desire. The parents have the right to determine *their* family size and time. The individual decision may or may not be in the best interest of the national or global program for population control. It has been suggested that the right to parenthood is a privilege and should be exercised only by individuals capable of meeting the responsiblity of parenthood. Offering only the means for *couples* to control fertility may neglect the means for *societies* to do so. Social and cultural attitudes must change if the pressures of uncontrolled population growth and the many health, social, educational, economic, and other disadvantages of this are to be avoided. The issues related to regulation of human reproduction and the overriding issue of population control are not as likely to be solved by advances in biology as by a greater understanding of behavior and social attitude.

SOCIAL-MORAL ISSUES

Advances in scientific knowledge and changes in sociocultural attitudes raise social and moral issues for the physician who cares for women. Indeed, new bioethical considerations associated with scientific advances, and the second- and third-order consequences of these require the thoughtful consideration of the entire medical profession. The morality as well as the legality of counseling minors about matters of sexuality, contraception, and abortion has not been resolved to everyone's satisfaction. It is evident that young women are in great need of education, information, and help in these areas. Who should assume responsibility for this counsel, and under what circumstances? Totally acceptable answers are not available.

The entire area of "genetic engineering"—encompassing prediction of fetal abnormality, genetic counseling, pregnancy termination, sperm banking, germinal choice, artificial insemination, and in vitro fertilization for certain kinds of female sterility—is new. The gynecologist-obstetrician is expected to play a major role in these activities but the moral, social, and ethical guidelines for such activity have yet to be drawn clearly. They are all new areas of responsibility for the physician who cares for women. (See Chap. 4.)

FUTURE NEEDS AND DIRECTION

CURRENT RECORD

We have a long way to go before we can achieve optimum health care for women. Those women who are most in need of health care are the ones who receive the least and vice versa. For example, the marked increase in vaginal cytology smears received by the laboratories of this country indicates not only that more women are being screened for cancer but that the same women are having more and more smears taken. Despite impressive expansion of organized family-planning services, it was estimated that in 1976 there were almost 10 million low-income women in need of the services and only 59 percent were served. Too many fetuses die in utero or in the immediate neonatal period or are born with deficits which prohibit them from making a meaningful contribution to themselves or to society. Despite the reasons for the differences between perinatal mortality in this country and other countries of the Western world, fetal wastage can be improved. There were over 48,000 infant deaths in 1976. In the United States, the perinatal mortality rate among nonwhites is 1½ times that of whites. Many women in this country receive inadequate care with respect to reproduction. This problem is compounded by the inhumanity of overcrowded clinics and busy office practice. Solo private practice has been criticized as a grossly inefficient system for the delivery of health services to women. Few women currently press the practicing gynecologist-obstetrician for better health care, but in the near future they will do so in rapidly increasing numbers following the lead of a small but vocal group of women who are currently seeking self-help and complaining bitterly about the nature of gynecologic care.

MANPOWER

To bring maternal care to all, with an emphasis on quality to the individual and responsibility to the community requires an enormous effort. There is a need to provide marital, psychosexual, contraceptive, and genetic counseling to those who seek it and to provide therapy for the endocrine, neoplastic, and inflammatory diseases of the female reproductive system in a dignified and empathetic manner. Women need early and ongoing education regarding their reproductive biology with methods of self-assessment to prevent disease and maintain health. Physicians must accept responsibility for those social problems related to health care. All this will involve a reassessment and efficient use of traditional and new types of health manpower personnel, significant alteration in the systems of health care delivery and reorientation of the attitudes of many in the health care professions.

In recent years, the threat of medical manpower shortage has been emphasized by the federal government. There is some question as to whether the manpower shortage is real or contrived. As of December 31, 1976, there were 409,446 physicians in the United States and its possessions. Between 1963 and 1977 the number of physicians in the United States increased by nearly 120,000 with 91 percent of all active physicians involved in the direct care of patients as their primary activity. Maldistribution of physicians including gynecologist-obstetricians is a more serious problem than manpower shortage. The ratio of physicians to population varies enormously in different locations of the country. Rural communities and the crowded inner-city areas of our large metropolitan communities suffer from a low density of physicians and other health manpower. There are few effective incentives currently available to alter this manpower maldistribution.

In 1978, there were 15,853 physicians holding specialty certification in gynecology and obstetrics and over 23,000 physicians who indicated that obstetrics and gynecology was their major professional activity. If 3.2 million births were handled solely by such specialists, this would mean that each physician delivered 139 babies during the year. But of course not all of the babies were delivered by specialists nor need be. Even so, a physician-patient ratio near this figure would leave the obstetrician little time for patients with major problems and little time for reeducation to take advantage of the many advances in medical diagnosis and therapy.

POSSIBLE SOLUTION

The possible solution to an effective system for the delivery of quality health care to women must begin with better appreciation of the attitudes and needs of the human female at all ages in our present society. This need not require embracing the women's liberation movement, but it does require that health professionals caring for women recognize the realities—

that social and cultural attitudes are altering the role of women; and that different women perceive the priorities of their health care needs differently, one woman from the other and, in some instances, differently from the established medical attitude (see Chaps. 2 and 5).

While there may be a need for an increase in number of physicians and an increase in gynecologists and obstetricians, there is a more pressing need to improve the overall efficiency and cost effectiveness of our health care delivery system and to redistribute the medical manpower in gynecology and obstetrics. Concurrently, a variety of nonphysician health personnel should be cooperatively coordinated into the health care team for more effective care. Two or more obstetricians working together as a unit to care for a population of patients can provide more efficient and effective care for women than a solo practitioner. Such a mutually supporting professional experience is also more satisfying to the physician. Time away from routine activity is necessary for the optimum management of problem cases. An extension of this to the "team approach" of medical practice involves not only physicians but specially trained nurses, midwives, nutritionists, social workers, psychologists, and family-planning counselors. Many of the duties performed by the obstetrician can be accomplished by someone with less education acting under the obstetrician's direct supervision. Such a person might be a nurse-midwife or a physician's associate. Availability of such assistants would permit the obstetrician to spend more time with those patients who have complications while providing overall supervision to the many activities of the delivery room, thus improving the quality of care. In order to effectively utilize new health personnel, the team approach to gynecologic-obstetric practice must be implemented. In addition to the nurse-midwife, other types of personnel must be developed. The type, education and duties of the team personnel will vary markedly, depending upon local circumstances. This does not imply different standards of health services for different populations but different needs.

There is a need for centralization and regionalization of health facilities with special facilities for cancer patients, for patients with the complex problems of endocrine disorders and infertility and high-risk pregnancy. Hospital inpatient facilities and ambulatory facilities should be related to population density. Patients with unusual gynecologic conditions such as pelvic cancer and some endocrinologic

problems should be referred to regional centers. Data obtained by the American College of Obstetricians and Gynecologists indicate that full hospital obstetric services, in terms of bed use, organization of essential personnel and cost-effective utilization of facilities for the care of all obstetric complications can only be provided efficiently when more than 1500 deliveries occur per year. Hospital gynecologic-obstetric services should be consolidated in large communities so that at least 1500 deliveries occur annually in each unit. In small communities, services can be provided with reasonable efficiency when at least 500 patients are delivered per year. High-risk obstetric patients should be identified early in pregnancy and there should be an opportunity for them to obtain care in regional centers which are suitably staffed and equipped to deal with their particular problems. Hospitals can be identified as primary, secondary, or tertiary. Regionalization and centralization can involve the development of more efficient methods of communication and transportation of patients from one facility to another. Regionalized perinatal facilities, including transportation, have cut perinatal mortality rates where they have been introduced.

There must be basic reorientation of thinking in regard to the priorities in our health care delivery system. If maintenance of health among women and improvement in the quality of reproduction are to be achievable goals, then adequate funding for the facilities and the mapower required to accomplish these goals must be provided. If priorities are considered, then such questions as "What contributes more to the common good, a heart transplant or expert care for 100 mothers with a high-risk pregnancy?" must be asked.

An orientation toward the prevention and early detection of curable problems suffers from lack of efficient ambulatory care centers. Furthermore, the high cost of hospital medical care makes it mandatory that more and better ambulatory care be made available. Although much care is now provided in physicians' offices or hospital clinics, it is often not accessible to many patients who need it. Simple surgical procedures which can be performed on an ambulatory basis are now performed in a hospital. New ambulatory gynecologic-obstetric facilities should be developed either as separate units or as part of comprehensive health centers and should be accessible to local residents, in inner cities or rural areas. Facilities in which surgical procedures may be performed on ambulatory patients could be developed under hospital guidelines.

The continued success of our society is inextricably bound to the health of succeeding generations which is linked to the quality of human reproduction.

REFERENCES

Barnes AC (ed.): *The Social Responsibility of Gynecology and Obstetrics,* Baltimore: Johns Hopkins University Press, 1965.

Blake Judith: Population policy for Americans-Is the government being misled? *Science* 165:522, 1969.

_____: The teenage birth control dilemma and public opinion. *Science* l80:708,1973.

Bumpass LL, Presser HB: Contraceptive sterilization in the U. S. 1965 and 1970. *Demography* 9:531, 1972.

Callahan D: Ethics and population limitation. *Science,* 175:487, 1972.

Clifford SH: High-risk pregnancy I. Prevention of prematurity the *sine qua non* for reduction of mental retardation and other neurologic disorders. *N Engl J Med* 271:243, 1964.

Davis K: Population policy-will current programs succeed? *Science* 158:730, 1967.

Fam Plan Perspect 10:1978.

Harris TR, Isaman J, Giles HR: Improved neonatal survival through maternal transport. *Obstet Gynecol* 52:294, 1978.

Jacobson HN, Reid DE: High-risk pregnancy II. A pattern of comprehensive maternal and child care. *N Engl J Med* 271:302, 1964.

Jaffe FS et al.: Organized family planning programs in the United States: 1968-1972. *Fam Plan Perspect* 5:73, 1973.

Moore TD (ed.): *Ethical Dilemmas in Current Obstetric and Newborn Care,* Columbus: Ross Laboratories, 1973.

Packard V: *The Sexual Wilderness. The Contemporary Upheaval in Male-Female Relationships,* New York: David McKay, 1968.

Ramsey P: Shall we reproduce? I. The medical ethics of in vitro fertilization. *JAMA* 220:1346, 1972.

Randall C et al.: National health care for women. *Obstet Gynecol* 39:603, l972.

Reference Data on Profile of Medical Practice, Chicago: American Medical Association, 1978.

Reference Data on Socio-Economic Issues of Health, Chicago: American Medical Association, l978.

Sklar J, Berkov B: The American Birth Rate. *Science* 189: 693, 1975.

Toward Improving The Outcome of Pregnancy, National Foundation, 1976.

United States Commission on Population Growth and the American Future, Washington, 1972.

Vital Statistics of the United States U.S. Department of Health, Education, and Welfare, vol II, part B, 1973, vol II, part A,1975.

Vital Statistics Report: U.S. Department of Health, Education, and Welfare, National Center for Health Statistics, vol. 26, no. 12, 1978.

2

Women and Their Gynecologists: Changing Expectations in the 1980s

ALICE T. DAY

INTRODUCTION

RISE OF THE DEMAND FOR GREATER CLIENT AUTONOMY

SOURCES OF STRAIN IN THE GYNECOLOGIST/PATIENT RELATION
Asymmetry in objectives and expectations
    Incompatibility in objectives
    Inconsistencies in the expected behavior
Demographic and social change
    Diversification of roles
    Sense of community among women
    Nature and duration of family roles
    Living arrangements and patterns of residence
    Rising levels of education
    New perspectives on female sexuality and male-female relations
    New perspectives in population and ecology
Changing attitudes of women toward members of their own sex

IMPLICATIONS OF WOMEN'S CHANGING ROLES AND ATTITUDES FOR GYNECOLOGIC PRACTICE
    Expectations about care
    Respect for dignity and individual difference
    Impersonality and inadequate communication
    Power over the childbearing function

SUMMARY AND CONCLUSION

INTRODUCTION

Increasing numbers of women are expressing discontent concerning their experiences with gynecologists. For many American women, the gynecologist/patient relation has become the focus of a conviction that their values and preferences—particularly with regard to their own health and well-being—are not being sufficiently taken into account. The greater involvement of women in positions of responsibility outside the home, and the idea fostered by the women's movement that women should have control over their own bodies precipitated a chorus of complaints by women against their doctors. Women are expecting to play a more active role in their own health care and refusing to receive passively the services of their doctors. It is increasingly recognized that these predominantly male professionals occupy a unique position to influence women's social and biological destinies. The gynecologist's area of specialization gives him or her a wide range of authority not only with respect to the lives of individual patients but also with respect to broader social issues, such as relations between the sexes, family life-styles, the employment of married women, and access to birth control, including abortion. Yet the training many physicians receive in the care of women, rather than increasing understanding of women's changing position and needs, perpetuates orientations toward women's choices that tend to be narrow and traditional. In private conversations, in books and magazine articles, on radio and TV panels, women are saying that they would like things to be different.

Gynecology is not the only target of this kind. The health care professions, in general, have been attracting criticism for the sexist orientations that are purported to permeate the system from professional training to on-the-job practice (Gross). A major theme of the 1978 best seller *Coma,* in fact, concerns a female medical student's confrontation with the sexist attitudes of both her fellow students and her superiors (Cook).

Because it deals with the treatment of disorders associated with the female reproductive organs and includes the delivery of babies, gynecology and obstetrics is particularly vulnerable to stereotyped orientations toward women and their appropriate social roles. The potential for abrasive relations between women and their gynecologists is underlined by the growing extent to which the latter are being called upon to assume a counseling role (Chap. 1). Women in greater numbers are turning to their doctors for advice and guidance in matters that go beyond strict physical and health issues, e.g., whether or not to place an illegitimate child for adoption, what kind of arrangements an employed woman should make for her children, or what to do about unsatisfactory marital relations. The doctor's greater involvement in these issues increases the possibility of a conflict of values. Some women claim that if their life-style is unconventional according to their doctor's lights, they are often made to feel demeaned and humiliated. Rather than presenting the alternatives in an objective manner, they charge, the doctor infuses them with his or her own perspectives about what a woman should be and do. Thus, today's gynecologists may often find themselves in a paradoxical situation: their advice is solicited, as if expert, on issues that not only may lie outside their area of expertise, but may involve personal values that conflict with those of the client seeking guidance.

Many of the grievances against gynecologists cited here would apply with equal if not greater force to women who are poor and black. These women are likely to be the least well informed about medical care, the least secure about their position in society, and consequently, the most anxious about even routine medical procedures. However, the women who have been most vocal about the quality of their medical care are white, middle-class, well-educated—those with enough social confidence to question

ways of treating women that have been accepted as legitimate in the past. It is hoped that raising the gynecologist's awareness of the changing expectations articulated by this growing segment of health-conscious women will serve to deepen understanding of the individual and increase appreciation for the varied values and life-styles of his or her clients—whatever their race or social position.

RISE OF THE DEMAND FOR GREATER CLIENT AUTONOMY

Far from being an isolated phenomenon, the strain between gynecologists and their patients appears to be but one instance of a more general conflict developing between professionals and their clients, not only in medicine, but also, for example, in law, teaching, and city planning. Clients are demanding more individual attention, more consideration of personal needs, more of a say in matters of vital concern to themselves. Overall, in recent decades American society has witnessed a dramatic rise in the dissemination of knowledge, which has meant that when they turn to experts, people are now equipped with a more varied amount of information, and also with the feeling that they have a right to a greater involvement in the decision-making process (Lopata, 1976). Among the social developments that have combined to foster skepticism about professionals' claims to authority are rising levels of education, familiarity with social issues acquired by exposure to the mass media, and a growing sense of the limits of technological approaches to problems that may require basic changes in human behavior and cultural values. A major example in the health field is the increasing emphasis on the importance of preventive health care as distinct from reliance on drugs and medical expertise (Boyden and Diesendorf), implying that individual discretion *before the fact* rather than medical intervention *after the fact* offers the best formula for health and longevity. Responsibility for health maintenance (e.g., a balanced diet, regular sleep and exercise, light consumption of drugs—including alcohol and nicotine) is thus lodged squarely with the lay person rather than with the expert.

The women's movement has both reflected and pioneered this trend toward greater client autonomy. It has disseminated information to women about their bodies (Boston Women's Health Book Collective), and provided the impetus for women to reject "the humiliation of being a patient" (Frankfort). A burgeoning number of journals (e.g., *Women and Health*) and women's self-help organizations (e.g., The Fremont Women's Birth Collective, Seattle, Washington; The Childbearing Center, New York, N.Y.) are not only informing women about all aspects of their sex organs and reproductive system, they are encouraging them to take the initiative in caring for themselves, urging them not to leave the determination of their biological affairs to others, however well qualified professionally. Women's health organizations argue that because the gynecologist-patient relation typically involves a female-patient, male-doctor situation, it exacerbates the tendency to channel women into the socially approved role of passive submission to male authority. Yet many of the conditions which prompt women to consult doctors are not even in the category of "disorders." Menstruation and menopause, sexual relations, contraception, pregnancy, and childbirth, for example, can be defined as "natural conditions" rather than medical crises (Romano). As such they require explanation, assistance, support, and counsel rather than complicated procedures that the average woman cannot comprehend and apply to herself. The women's health movement is making a concerted effort to demystify events such as menstruation and menopause, and by breaking the veil of silence that has surrounded such events, to give women the confidence to make basic decisions concerning their physical and mental well-being (Weideger).

SOURCES OF STRAIN IN THE GYNECOLOGIST-PATIENT RELATION

Specifically, strains in the gynecologist-patient relation are traceable to two general sources: (1) asymmetry of values and objectives between doctor and patient, and (2) changes in the demographic and social setting that have altered women's position in society and consequently the way they view themselves. The two, of course, are closely related. Changes in women's roles and self-images have increased the asymmetry in women's relations with this group of professionals who can play such a profound role in the determination of their future options—for example, deciding whether or not they will bear a child.

ASYMMETRY IN OBJECTIVES AND EXPECTATIONS

Within the gynecologist-patient relation itself, changes in the social position of women have aggravated two potential sources of conflict; (1) incompatibility in objectives and (2) inconsistencies in the behavior expected.

INCOMPATIBILITY IN OBJECTIVES

The priorities and objectives of the patient and the doctor are not necessarily compatible. In general, the patient seeks gynecologic-obstetric care to enable her to make her body responsive to a variety of individual goals, e.g., sexual satisfaction; healthy reproduction and childbirth, or comfortable means to avoid conception; safe termination of unwanted pregnancy; and freedom from physical discomfort or any sort of devitalizing symptoms, mental or physical. The significance attached to these various objectives, however, is not uniform: it varies widely among individual women according to their age, stage in the life cycle, education, marital and employment status, and preferred life-style. For a growing number of women there is, in addition to these fairly specific objectives, the more general objective of gaining understanding of their physiology and of the relationship between physical and mental well-being so that they can maintain their own health without having to depend on professional consultation.

The doctor's objectives in dispensing medical services may or may not coincide with the patient's priorities. As a professionally trained expert, the gynecologist is called upon to exercise judgment and make recommendations concerning biological matters. These judgments can hardly avoid being influenced by the doctor's own moral and ethical values. Sex and reproduction are not only among the most value-laden of all human functions, but decisions made for the individual with respect to these functions can have far-reaching consequences. The doctor's convictions on these issues may conflict with those of the patient. In such cases, contrary to fulfilling the goals the patient has for herself, the doctor's objective may be to bring the patient into line with his or her own expectations concerning the feminine role and social values. Into this potentially volatile relationship, another sort of strain has been introduced; the substantial change in the views of a growing number of women about their own needs, about alternatives in life-styles, sexual choices, social responsibilities, and roles as patients. One result of this change has been to make the "consciousness-raised" patient less willing to accept the consequences of the doctor's normative attitudes where the doctor's judgment may conflict with choices that she feels are hers. Friction ensues because the gynecologist often continues to behave in traditional terms that are no longer appropriate. The patient is upset; the doctor is affronted; and communication breaks down.

INCONSISTENCIES IN THE EXPECTED BEHAVIOR

To the physician any particular patient is one among many seen in the course of a day's work—a person whose physical, psychological, and social problems, although unique, have many elements in common with those of other patients. From the patient's point of view, the doctor who does not provide the full, personalized care she feels is her due has failed. For the doctor, rising expectations for individualized services and "in-depth" communication may pose formidable demands on time, energy, good will, and professional capacities. In the past decade, the strain caused by the inconsistencies in these positions has deepened; women are asking for greater attention to their personal needs; yet doctors have more patients, more techniques to master, more forms to fill out, and less time to devote to discovering the unique qualities of each individual patient.

DEMOGRAPHIC AND SOCIAL CHANGE

> Historically tied to the family, and isolated from their own kind, women are perhaps the most organizationally under-developed social category in Western civilization. (Freeman)

In many ways, the ending of their total submergence in the family and the rising sense of community among women have been among the key factors altering the attitudes and expectations of women over the past decade. It is to these two changes, therefore, that the gynecologist must look for an understanding of the forces that are changing the demands upon the profession.

DIVERSIFICATION OF ROLES

The declining preoccupation of women exclusively with roles within the family is indicated by, among

other things, their increasing participation in the labor force. In the decade 1965 to 1975, the number of women in the American labor force grew by 11 million. During the following year, 1975 to 1976, the increment of female workers was 1.6 million (twice the number of new male workers). Women now comprise two-fifths of the United States work force; nearly half of the female population age 16 and older is employed or seeking employment (U.S. Bureau of the Census, 1976). Not only do these trends alter women's priorities for themselves, but they create a new concern for the gynecologist: the health status of the female worker. For example, in 1977, some 1 million infants were born to women who were employed during pregnancy (Hunt). To an increasing extent, gynecologists will be making decisions concerning the pregnant worker— the potential hazards of her job or her partner's job; the legal and ethical aspects of maximizing safety in the work place; recommendations for placement in a particular job, for continuing work as the pregnancy develops, and for returning to work following delivery. Policy deliberations in the area of women's employment will confront the gynecologist with basic issues concerning women's rights as employees: the right to work, to have conditions of employment and opportunity equivalent to those of men, to earn a supporting wage (American College of Obstetricians and Gynecologists).

SENSE OF COMMUNITY AMONG WOMEN

The rising sense of community among women, though equally significant to the gynecologist-patient relation, is more difficult to quantify. Certainly, the rise of both formal and informal women's groups has been a prominent development of the present decade (Freeman). But it is not something that can be measured by simply adding the number of women who support the Equal Rights Amendment. Whether or not the amendment passes this time around, the debate surrounding it has made women on both sides more conscious of common concerns and has politicized many who heretofore were indifferent (Bennetts).

These two factors (i.e., diversification of roles and a rising sense of community) can be viewed as collective responses to five social trends that have extensively altered the position of women in society: (1) changes in the nature and duration of family roles; (2) rising levels of education; (3) changes in the character of living arrangements and community residential patterns; (4) new perspectives on female sexuality and male-female relations; (5) shifting perspectives on population and environment.

NATURE AND DURATION OF FAMILY ROLES

Taken together, these trends imply a marked shrinkage in the proportion of her lifetime that a woman is likely to be fully occupied with children and family responsibilities. Current population reports show these comparisons with earlier decades: The typical American woman is now considerably more likely to attend college, hold a job before and after her children leave home, become divorced or separated, and she is likely to outlive her husband by 7 years (U.S. Bureau of the Census, 1977). Underlying these trends is the increasing probability that the American woman will have to depend on her own resources for financial and emotional support. This is true not only for the single career woman, the divorced or separated woman, and the older woman who has outlived her husband. It is also increasingly true for the married woman whose husband and children are still living at home.

Since the turn of the century, changes in the patterns of marriage and childbearing, such as an earlier age at marriage, a smaller family size, and the concentration of childbearing within the early years of marriage, have shortened the period during which women are heavily involved in caring for dependent children (Ridley). The average American woman is now about 27 when she bears her last child. By the time she is in her early thirties, her children may all be going to school. At the same time, the decline in household size and the growing tendency for parents to live apart from children have meant that even in their middle thirties, many women find themselves alone at home for long periods during the day. Despite the popular belief that technological change in household appliances means that women have less work to do in the home, time-budget studies show that, on average, women not in the labor force spend as much time at housework as their mothers did (Vanek). Much of this work is solitary, dull, and repetitious.

LIVING ARRANGEMENTS AND PATTERNS OF RESIDENCE

The loneliness of the housewife can be intensified by suburban residential patterns that necessitate commuting between home and work, and hence create even greater physical separation between husband and wife. The mobility among Americans exposes wives to long periods of separation from husbands and their older children, as well as friends and former neighbors (Michelson). Finally, decentralization and the spread of low-density, pseudourban communities further accentuate the housewife's separateness by reducing opportunities for informal neighboring, and fostering dependence on the automobile. These factors pose formidable obstacles to the woman who wants to work or prepare herself for work (Rossi). Erratic school hours and a paucity of child care facilities, the decline of access to domestic help, the distance from urban centers, and the scarcity of public transportation all conspire to keep the suburban housewife at home, sometimes without giving her enough to keep her fully occupied and personally fulfilled.

How the individual housewife deals with the conflicts possible in this situation will vary according to her upbringing, income, education, degree of self-confidence, and orientation (Lopata). Some housewives merely hang on and develop physical symptoms including fatigue and backache (Cushner). Some get through the childrearing years only to break down when their children leave home (Bart; Gove). Others manage to surmount the restrictions of their family roles and become creatively involved on many levels, both within the family and in the community. But even those women who manage to achieve full personal satisfaction within their family may feel stigmatized by the low esteem in which the role of housewife is generally held in American society (Chafe). Thus, there are strong pressures on women to supplant or to supplement their family roles with employment, volunteer work, or other social activities. This is true because a role that once was regarded as a woman's chief contribution, important to the very survival of society, is now defined as routine, restrictive, and less worthy of social recognition than paid employment.

RISING LEVELS OF EDUCATION

Higher levels of education and increased work experience prior to marriage have raised many women's aspirations for independence and creativity. At the same time, ambivalent social attitudes about how women should spend their lives frequently leave them inadequately equipped to choose intelligently or to perform skillfully. Though women attend classes with men, compete with them for academic grades and honors, and in the process, learn to think of themselves as intellectual equals, they are discouraged from thinking about long-range alternatives to marriage and childbearing. One result is that they progressively curtail their opportunities for occupational training. Certain courses and careers are considered inappropriate for women. Fewer women than men do graduate work; still fewer women are found in high academic or professional positions, and relatively little is done to adapt educational programs to the varying needs of women at different stages of life. The skills learned at school and work are largely irrelevant to the tasks that occupy a woman at home. She moves from lab to kitchen; from independence to complete submersion in the lives of others; from the center of a network of close relationships to the solitariness of her later years (Harbeson). This lack of coherence between the various phases of her life accounts for one of the central dilemmas of modern woman: how to determine where her obligations to others end and her duties to herself, as a growing, developing person, begin.

Society reflects ambivalence as well about a woman's participation in occupational roles by relegating to her the dullest jobs and rewarding her work with lower pay. Despite legal and social gains in the 1970s, income differentials of women and men remain substantial. In 1974, the median income for women who had worked year-round full time was 57 percent of the median income of men who had worked year-round full time (U.S. Bureau of the Census, 1976). Some feminists, in fact, attribute the rise of the women's movement to the perception of salary discrimination on the part of the women participating in the labor force since World War II.

NEW PERSPECTIVES ON FEMALE SEXUALITY AND MALE-FEMALE RELATIONS

The monopoly of the family as the unit through which women must satisfy all their needs has been eroded by the increasing separation of sexual activity from reproduction, changing attitudes and values regarding male-female relations, and new perspectives on the nature of female sexuality. Closer contact with men in school and at work, readier access to effective means of birth control, and liberalization of attitudes toward premarital sexual experience may open opportunities to deepen understanding between the sexes (Safilios-Rothschild) as well as reduce the pressure to rush into marriage. Sherfey has hypothesized that throughout history the "inordinate" sexuality of women has been suppressed coercively in order to ensure the continuity of family life. This view may foster a new respect in women for their sexuality and increase their demand to be treated as persons with their own sexual needs and capacities (de Beauvoir). Increasing familiarity with

Masters and Johnson's findings about the female capacity for orgasm may also make women less willing to be used sexually and more willing to wait for a relationship that combines mutual physical attraction with a sharing of values and outlooks. The sale of 2.5 million copies of the *The Hite Report,* a national study of 3000 American women's perspectives on their sexuality (Hite), seems indicative of the widespread interest in women's own definitions of their sexual norms and preferences, rather than norms defined for them by men.

In the context of a lowering of restrictions on their behavior in sexual encounters, however, women may be trading some of the protection they possessed in the past for the ostensibly greater autonomy they have now. To the extent that they engage in sexual relations ouside of marriage, women expose themselves to the risks of unwanted pregnancy and venereal disease. During the last decade, the incidence of these conditions has increased sharply, particularly among younger girls, who tend to be poorly informed about sexual matters, unsure of themselves and their values, and less confident about using effective forms of contraception. For a discussion of the factors associated with contraceptive failure among adolescents, and the gynecologist's role in dealing with the phenomenon of pregnancy among nonmarried teenage women, the reader is referred to Chap. 17. Here it can be pointed out that among the many factors involved, failure to engage in adequate contraceptive protection may be related to stereotyped expectations about the male and female role in sexual relations (Reiss). The norm that females should be sexually submissive and males sexually dominant, and yet that women should take the initiative in contraceptive planning, presents both sexes with conflicting demands. While many young men feel that their partners should protect themselves with oral contraceptives, studies of unplanned pregnancy among college students show that many young women still defer to their partners when it comes to initiating the use of contraceptives (Pool and Pool; Day).

Davis has noted, "The single woman, pregnant with an unwanted child, is a concrete manifestation of her own self-neglect and male dominance." As part of women's demand for sexual equality, the idea is gaining currency that men as well as women are deeply implicated in the process of reproductive planning. Assumptions about women's primary responsibility for the avoidance of conception are now being challenged. If this shift in orientation has the consequence of distributing to men some of the responsibility for contraception and care of the unplanned, illegitimate child, it could lower the frequency with which women find themselves pregnant involuntarily.

NEW PERSPECTIVES IN POPULATION AND ECOLOGY

Over the past two decades, debate about woman's role has been taking place against a background of changing perspectives toward population and ecology. In 1973, the U.S. Commission on Population and the American Future concluded that American society would be better off if women limited their families to an average of two children. Meanwhile, though advertising continues to play upon women as consumers for their families, environmentalists are saying that human survival requires radical changes in the resources consumed by middle- and upper-class American households. Women are not immune to such social schizophrenia. A British sociologist bluntly sums up the incongruity in their position:

> In a world in which for those in the West, over-nutrition is one of the greatest threats to health and in which children are pollution, woman as full-time cook and mother is now redundant. (Kitzinger)

Clearly, the persons most affected by these new perspectives are those women who can afford to raise children comfortably with all the material resources necessary to ensure them the "good" life. Though few women choose as a matter of social principle to have no children, or only one or two, more and more women, attuned to public issues, are beginning to see childbearing as a personal choice, rather than a social necessity. This is a profound change in perspectives about what was once regarded as woman's primary function.

CHANGING ATTITUDES OF WOMEN TOWARD MEMBERS OF THEIR OWN SEX

In history and literature, women have been written about by men, and seen mainly in their relation to men: their fathers, husband, sons, lovers (Woolf). Until as recently as the 1960s, American scholars, with the exception of a few social scientists, neglected systematic study either of woman's place or of her biological and psychological nature. A study of 32 gynecology textbooks published since 1943 found them to reveal "a persistent bias toward and greater concern with

the patient's husband than with the patient herself" (Scully and Bart). Such a male orientation both reflects and perpetuates the barriers preventing women from thinking of themselves as a cohesive social category.

The emergence in the late 1960s and early 1970s of a new level of collective thinking and acting among many American women is something of an enigma, for it cannot be attributed to any marked social change at that particular time (Ferriss), but it has had two dramatic consequences for women: first, they are learning to think of themselves not as solitary individuals with problems peculiar to their own situation, but as members of a community with common problems and common interests; second, in their "rap" groups they are finding a reservoir of human companionship from which they can derive emotional support and the strength to pursue their own interests. The pendulum has swung so far away from the exclusive preoccupation of women with men that "...women for the first time feel free to admit that their friendship with some woman (or women) is as rewarding or sometimes even more so than their marriage or their love affair" (Safilios-Rothschild).

IMPLICATIONS OF WOMEN'S CHANGING ROLES AND ATTITUDES FOR GYNECOLOGIC PRACTICE

The changes sketched above impinge upon the practice of gynecology and obstetrics in two important ways: (1) by changing what women expect from their doctors, and (2) by broadening the areas of responsibility of the practitioner with respect to preventive measures in the health care of women.

EXPECTATIONS ABOUT CARE

Many of the qualities that women now look for in their gynecologists are socially defined as "feminine" traits: tenderness, compassion, empathy, and a willingness to listen without judging. Newly "aware" women are particularly sensitive to directness in human relationships whether between persons of the same or opposite sex. These women presume that the gynecologist, who has unusually intimate access to the minds and bodies of women, will understand their desire for candid communication stripped of moralizing and condescension. Instead, they complain, doctors often patronize them, treat them like children, and cloak themselves in professional impersonality at moments when the patient is experiencing acute distress. Specific charges against practitioners of this specialty fall into three general categories: (1) lack of respect for human dignity and individual difference, especially in sexual matters and life-styles; (2) impersonality and inadequate communication, particularly concerning the birth process; and (3) excessive power over decisions that vitally affect women's lives. Overall, these criticisms represent anguish associated with the kinds of experiences that women have as patients for which there is no equivalent among men.

RESPECT FOR DIGNITY AND INDIVIDUAL DIFFERENCE

Women complain that doctors are insensitive during gynecologic examinations, that they subject women to such indignities as introducing them to colleagues while they are lying down, inviting students to observe without obtaining permission, and allowing people to walk in and out of the examining room unannounced (Women's Community Health Center, Inc.). Women with new life-styles feel, moreover, that their gynecologists not only adhere to family-oriented values, but that they actually abhor new modes of female sexual behavior. Single women report that doctors often make them feel unclean if they seek contraceptive information or relief from vaginitis. Women, single or married, claim that their doctors—unless pressed—ignore their sexuality altogether; that for most doctors, birth control is "family planning" (Luker). Lesbians resent being regarded as "sick," while the woman who chooses chastity objects to being labeled "abnormal." Younger women who deviate from the norm of married-mother-living-with-husband fear that an unsympathetic doctor may subject them to humiliation and pain in examinations, unnecessary suffering in childbirth, or a greater-than-average risk of post-abortion infection and uterine perforations (Graham). This fear, whether justified or not, escalates anger and resentment toward the doctor because it compels the woman to choose between mental or physical anguish and the demoralizing alternative of suppressing her staunch belief in her own right to choose the way she uses her body. In their attitudes toward abortion and birth control, women perceive gynecologists, as a group, to be supporters of a system that penalizes women, while simultaneously exempting men from sharing the responsibilities of heterosexual relationships.

IMPERSONALITY AND INADEQUATE COMMUNICATION

As women pool their experience, there is growing discontent with the present child-delivery system. Their desire is to be treated as individuals with the right to know what is being done and why, and the right to share in whatever regimen is undertaken. A woman in labor wants to be regarded as an intelligent adult with a legitimate interest in her body. The crowded conditions, impersonality, and lack of sustained attention to the woman in labor have made hospital deliveries "often a terrifying and inhumane experience" (Arms). The fact that emotional, human aspects of childbirth have been slighted is interpreted by many women as another example of the way male values dominate the conduct of daily life in Western society.

The expanding interest in natural childbirth, home deliveries, self-examinations, and self-help clinics reflects women's desires not only to be active participants in their own health care, but also to have a wider range of alternatives in the delivery of medical services (Mehl). An increasing minority of women refuses to be cared for in established medical institutions, and by standard gynecologic and obstetric procedures. If the self-help movement continues to grow, the specialty will be confronted more and more with the question of whether to cooperate with the demand for alternative patterns of care, or to hold out for a monopoly of its own standards and thus force dissatisfied clients to go outside the system to meet their desires for a different orientation and a different set of options, particularly with respect to maternity care.

POWER OVER THE CHILDBEARING FUNCTION

A new appreciation of the meaning and importance of the mother-child relationship, both to themselves as individuals and to a world of increasing crowding and scarcity, has emboldened many women to demand the right to decide for themselves whether or not to undertake motherhood. Transferring the right to decide to the woman gives rise to a new set of rights and obligations for both patient and doctor. If women demand self-determination, they must, in turn, accept greater responsibility for the prevention of unwanted conceptions or for the consequences of sexual activity. At present, however, despite substantial research in the area of reproductive control, the capacity to exercise power over the childbearing function still seems inadequately achieved by large segments of American women. As mentioned above, in the United

States—as in other parts of the Western world—social forces underlying women's changing roles have combined to produce an unprecedented incidence of pregnancy among very young women (Ruzicka; Alan Guttmacher Institute). The general effort to increase women's capacity to control their reproduction will surely be an area of major concern to gynecologists in the coming years. At one level, the doctor will be involved in cooperating to make birth control available to all persons who are sexually active, regardless of age, marital status, or race. Some decision about conception and childbirth exists at each sexual encounter a woman has. That this decision is usually implicit rather than explicit does not make it any less real or significant (Luker). Clearly, an understanding of the contraceptive decision-making process is a vital prelude to devising policies to influence the cultural, social, and technological factors that bear on the etiology and outcome of unwanted pregnancy. Whether or not qualified, gynecologists are called upon to act as counselors and educators in the areas of sex and reproduction control. This role in particular, among the many mentioned throughout this text, invests gynecology with a special social significance and emphasizes the importance of establishing candid communication, understanding, and mutual trust in the relationship between women and their doctors.

SUMMARY AND CONCLUSION

For a long time laws and social attitudes have pressured women into bearing more children than they desired; the time is approaching when these may have to influence women and men in a reverse direction. The women's movement is a broad-based effort on the part of both women and men to initiate a new definition of woman in keeping with her altered demographic and social position. Many women will expect that their gynecologists will be understanding allies in the search for new images, new grounds for self-respect, and new life goals. At the most basic level, women with this new consciousness will want their gynecologists to help them make choices for themselves.

Changes in women's attitudes toward themselves that have generated dissatisfaction with the doctor-patient relationship are not fleeting or reversible; they are closely tied in with demographic and social changes that have altered the complexion of life in the twentieth century. The implications extend not only to the doctor-patient relationship but also to the gynecologist's involvement in social issues that will affect the quality of life over the next decades: birth control, abortion, sexual relations, sex education, alternative life-styles, and population growth.

REFERENCES

Alan Guttmacher Institute: *11 Million Teenagers: What Can Be Done About the Epidemic of Adolescent Pregnancies in the U.S.,* New York: Alan Guttmacher Institute, 1977.

American College of Obstetricians and Gynecologists: *Guidelines on Pregnancy and Work,* Chicago: ACOG, 1977.

Arms S: *Immaculate Deception,* Boston: Houghton Mifflin, 1975.

Barnes AC (ed.): *The Social Responsibility of Gynecology and Obstetrics,* Baltimore: Johns Hopkins University Press, 1965.

Bart PB: Depression in middle-aged women, in *Woman in Sexist Society,* V. Gornick, BK Moran, eds., New York: Basic Books, 1971.

_____: Social structure and vocabularies of discomfort: What happened to female hysteria? *J Health Soc Behav* 9:188, 1968.

Bennetts L: Feminist drive is likely to persist even if Rights Amendment fails, *New York Times,* May 31, 1978, p.1.

Boston Women's Health Book Collective: *Our Bodies—Ourselves.* A Course by and for Women, Boston: New England Free Press, 1976.

Boyden S, Diesendorf M: Environment and health, in *The Magic Bullet,* eds. Boyden, Diesendorf, Canberra, Australia: Society for Social Responsibility in Science, 131, 1976.

Chafe WH: *The American Woman,* London: Oxford University Press, 1972.

Cook R: *Coma,* London: Macmillan, 1978.

Cushner IM: The psychologic and family impact of the diseases peculiar to women, in *The Social Responsibility of Gynecology and Obstetrics,* ed. AC Barnes, Baltimore: Johns Hopkins University Press, 1965.

Davis K: The American family in relation to demographic change, in *Research Reports,* vol. 1, *Demographic and Social Aspects of Population Growth,* Commission on Population Growth and the American Future, Washington, 1973.

Day AT: Unplanned pregnancies in the 1970s—an Australian paradox? in *Women's Health in a Changing Society,* Canberra, Australia: Commonwealth Dept. of Health, 1978.

de Beauvoir S: *The Second Sex,* New York: Knopf, 1952.

Ferriss AL: *Indicators of Trends in the Status of American Women,* New York: Russell Sage Foundation, 1971.

Frankfort E: *Vaginal Politics,* New York: Quadrangle Books, 1972.

Freeman, J: The origins of the women's liberation movement. *Am J Sociol* 78:4, 1973.

Gove WR, Tudor JF: Adult sex roles and mental illness. *Am J Sociol* 78:4, 1973.

Graham C: Women and doctors. *Nation Rev* (Australia) June 8–14, 1973.

Gross HE: Women's changing roles—the gynecologists' view. *Women & Health* 2:10, 1977.

Harbeson GE: *Choice and Challenge for the American Woman,* Cambridge, Mass.: Schenkman, 1971.

Hite S: *The Hite Report,* New York: Macmillan, 1976.

Hunt VR: *The Health of Women at Work,* Evanston, Ill.: Northwestern University Program on Women, 1977.

Kitzinger S: Review, *New Society* 23: April 26, 1973.

Lopata HZ: *Occupation Housewife,* New York: Oxford, 1971.

———: Expertization of everyone and the revolt of the client. *Sociol* 117:435, 1976.

Luker K: *Taking Chances: Abortion and the Decision Not to Contracept,* Berkeley: University of California Press, 1975.

Masters WH, Johnson VE: *Human Sexual Response,* Boston: Little, Brown, 1966.

McCance C, Hall DJ: Sexual behavior and contraceptive practice of unmarried female undergraduates at Aberdeen University. *Br Med J* 2:694, 1972.

Mehl LE: Options in maternity care. *Women & Health* 2:29, 1977.

Michelson W: *Man and His Urban Environment,* Reading, Mass.: Addison-Wesley, 1970.

Pool JS, Pool DI: *Contraception and Health Care among Young Canadian Women,* Ottawa: Carleton University Department of Sociology and Anthropology, 1978.

Population and the American Future, *The Report of the Commission on Population Growth and the American Future,* Washington, 1972, pp. 106–107.

Reiss I: *The Social Context of Premarital Sexual Permissiveness,* New York: Holt, 1967.

Ridley JC: The effects of population change on the roles and status of women: Perspective and speculation, in *Toward a Sociology of Women,* ed., C Safilios-Rothschild, Lexington, Mass.: Xerox Publishing Co., 1972.

Romano J: Educating the physician for his role, in *The Social Responsibility of Gynecology and Obstetrics,* ed. AC Barnes, Baltimore: Johns Hopkins University Press, 1965.

Rossi AS: Equality between the sexes: An immodest proposal. *Daedalus* 93, Spring 1964.

Ruzicka LT: Non-marital pregnancies in Australia since 1947. *J Biosoc Sci* 7:113, 1975.

Safilios-Rothschild C (ed.): *Toward a Sociology of Women,* Lexington, Mass.: Xerox Publishing Co., 1972.

Scully D, Bart P: A funny thing happened on the way to the orifice: Women in gynecology textbooks. *Am J Sociol* 78:4, 1973.

Sherfey MJ: *The Nature and Evaluation of Female Sexuality,* New York: Vintage Books, 1973.

Szasz TS, Hollender MH: A contribution to the philosophy of medicine: The basic models of the doctor-patient relationship. *Arch Int Med* 97:585, 1956.

United States Bureau of the Census: *A Statistical Portrait of Women in the United States, Current Population Reports,* ser. P-23, 58, 1976.

———: *Statistical Abstract of the U.S.: 1977.*

Vanek J: Time spent in housework. *Sci Am,* 231:116, 1974.

Weideger P: *Menstruation & Menopause,* New York: Knopf, 1976.

Women's Community Health Center, Inc. *Women & Health* 2:29, 1977.

Woolf V: *A Room of One's Own,* New York: Harcourt, Brace, World, 1929.

3

Fertility and Family Planning

LARRY BUMPASS

This chapter surveys, from a social science perspective, some of the major issues relating to fertility and family planning in the United States. Whole areas of importance are omitted, such as population growth and family-planning programs in developing countries. The objective is to provide the reader with an introduction to some of the trends and issues most relevant to the practice of medicine in low fertility societies.

AGGREGATE FERTILITY TRENDS

The most common and readily available measure of fertility is the Crude Birth Rate (CBR). This measure is simply the number of births occurring in a given year divided by the total population at midyear times 1000. It ranges from highs in the range of 50 or more per 1000 population to lows in the low teens. The CBR is a "crude" measure because it includes population not at risk of childbearing, i.e., males, older women, and young children. (There are more sophisticated and more appropriate measures for fertility analysis; see, for example, Shryock and Siegel, 1973.) Nevertheless, the trend in this rate as seen in Fig. 3-1 provides a general picture of the course of fertility in the United States.

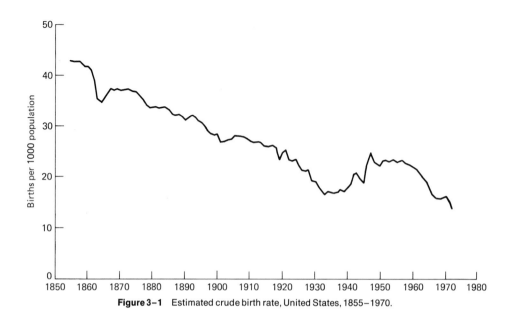

Figure 3-1   Estimated crude birth rate, United States, 1855–1970.

THE LONG-TERM DECLINE

Fertility in colonial America was exceedingly high, estimated at a crude rate of 55. This figure is as high as currently exists almost anywhere in the developing world and corresponds to an average lifetime fertility of 8 children per woman. Predecline rates were considerably lower throughout most of Western Europe, in large part because of later ages of marriage (Hajnal). On the other hand, the secular decline in fertility began much earlier in the United States than in Western Europe. With the exception of France, which also experienced an early decline in fertility, fertility declines in most of Western Europe did not begin until after about 1870.

Intensive research on the timing and correlates of fertility decline, the so-called demographic transition has resulted in no simple explanation (Coale). It is a history shared by every developed country, and the sociologic opinion remains strong that this decline is intimately linked with the changing value of children, resulting from social changes associated with industrialization and urbanization. Such changes are illustrated by the transition of children from economic assets on the farm to economic liabilities in an urban setting with compulsory education, as well as by the reduction in adult dependence upon children as the major source of economic security in old age. Nevertheless, no simple relationship has been found between any measure of urbanization, literacy, or industrialization and the onset of fertility decline.

Indeed, fertility declined in the United States over a long period when the vast majority of the population was rural.

By the 1920s, the CBR had reached a low of 18. High proportions of women who reached childbearing age in the 1920s and 1930s remained childless, and the level of their fertility during these years implied a lifetime fertility at or below that needed for population stability in the long run. This subreplacement fertility was generally understood in terms of the interpretive scheme of the demographic transition, and concern was expressed on numerous fronts about the consequences of low fertility for "national vitality" (Hansen). Indeed a number of European countries instituted various family support schemes to motivate women to bear children (Myrdal).

It may be worth noting that rapid fertility decline preceded the Great Depression and that low fertility is not necessarily an unusual state of affairs deriving from severe economic deprivation. The Depression undoubtedly had important effects on the fertility of some groups in the population, but it probably was not the primary cause of low fertility that was on a long-term trend line. Indeed, that long-term trend bottomed out during the Depression.

The interpretation that low fertility is intrinsic to industrial society led demographers and family sociologists to predict continued declines or, at best, stable low fertility. Some temporary postwar increase was expected as a consequence of making up for delayed marriages and childbearing, but the sustained "baby boom" that followed the war was wholly unanticipated. As we shall see later, the interpretation of low fertility may have been correct, although predictions for the postwar period were drastically in error because important factors were ignored.

THE POSTWAR "BABY BOOM" AND SUBSEQUENT FERTILITY DECLINE

Immediately after World War II there was the expected rapid increase in fertility associated with demobilization. However, this was followed by a sustained period of increase in the birthrate which we now know as the baby boom. We will return at the end of this chapter to consider the prospects for another such baby boom in the United States. It will be essential for that consideration to know more precisely what the baby boom was, or was not. From a low of 18 during the 1930s, the CBR increased to over 25 at the peak of the baby boom in 1957. Associated with this was a 50 percent increase in average family size from just over two for women who entered the childbearing years in the 1930s to over three children for women whose childbearing centered during the 1950s.

There are two essential demographic facts that must be understood about the baby boom. The first is that much of the amplitude of the increase in the birthrate was the result of an acceleration in the pace of childbearing (Ryder, 1970), as women married at earlier ages and had their first births earlier after marriage. Such changes in the pace of childbearing can radically affect the birthrate even if there are no changes in the average number of children that women bear over their lifetime.

The second major point with respect to the baby boom is that it was not primarily a return to large families. The 50 percent increase in average family size noted was overwhelmingly the consequence of increases in the proportion of women who had at least two children (Ryder, 1970). Relatively little was contributed by increases in the proportion having three or four children, and the likelihood of going on to have even larger families continued to decline over the period when the baby boom was occurring. Of the married women who were of childbearing age during the 1930s, 16 percent remained childless, and 24 percent bore only one child. The comparable proportions for married women who reached childbearing age during the peak of the baby boom are 4 and 10 percent, respectively. Following its peak in 1960, the CBR began a period of sustained decline that bottomed out after 1973 at an all-time low of about 15 per 1000. The rate at which women were bearing children

in the early 1970s implies an average family size of fewer than two children per woman—a level below that required for replacement. While this low fertility appears similar to that of the 1920s and 1930s, it is different in very important ways. As we noted, the low fertility of the 1930s was characterized by a high proportion of women who bore no children at all. In contrast, current low fertility results from a very high concentration of small families. Few women expect to remain childless, most expect to bear two children, but very few indeed expect to have four or more children.

	Number of lifetime births expected among wives aged 22 to 24, 1976					
	0	1	2	3	4	5+
percent:	5	12	56	20	5	2

Much as the CBR was inflated during the baby boom by an acceleration in the pace of childbearing, the current low level of the CBR may be depressed somewhat by a deceleration in the pace of childbearing. During this period, women are marrying at later ages and are delaying their first births longer. We will return to a consideration of the prospects for the future after we examine the changes that have occurred in patterns of fertility control.

TRENDS AND PATTERNS OF FERTILITY CONTROL

THE DIFFUSION OF APPROVAL AND USE OF CONTRACEPTION

We know from historical studies that contraception was used prior to the long-term fertility decline, particularly by the elite classes, and that the historical decline in fertility was associated with the increasing use of contraception by successively lower social classes (Coale; Glass and Grebenik). The principal method was withdrawal. It is important at this juncture to emphasize that the diffusion of use of contraception should not be regarded as a primary cause of the decline in fertility, but rather as the means by which changing evaluations of fertility were effected.

By the time of the first national fertility study in 1955, only a small minority of the population (about one-fifth) expressed disapproval of the use of contraception to regulate family size. Such disapproval was much more likely among Catholics than among non-

Catholics, a difference which effectively disappeared over the succeeding period (Freedman et al., 1959; Westoff and Jones, 1977b). The use of contraception is now virtually universal among nonsterile couples.

Two major observations should be noted about lifetime patterns and trends in the use of contraception. The first is that contraceptive use increases in both prevalence and diligence as women approach and then reach the point beyond which they do not want to have more children. Contraceptive use has tended to be less frequent and less effective early in marriage than later in marriage (Ryder and Westoff, 1973). The second major point is that contraceptive use early in marriage has increased. About three-fifths of women who reached marriage age in the early 1950s did not use any contraception prior to their first birth, but this proportion was reduced to about two-fifths among women reaching marriage age in the late 1960s and has undoubtedly declined further since then (Rindfuss and Westoff).

FAMILY PLANNING SUCCESS

The success with which a woman uses contraception can usefully be divided into two components reflecting the period during which she is trying to plan the timing of the births that she wants to have and the period during which she wants to prevent any additional births. Accidental pregnancies that occur during the first interval we refer to as "timing failures"; those during the latter period are "number failures" or "unwanted births."

We are able to estimate the extent of contraceptive failure in actual practice on the basis of questions asked in the National Fertility Surveys (Ryder and Westoff, 1971; Westoff and Ryder, 1977). In these surveys, women were asked a series of questions about their practices and attitudes prior to the occurrence of each pregnancy. If contraception was used and deliberately stopped for the purpose of conceiving, or if contraception was not used because the woman wanted to conceive as soon as possible, the birth was considered a planned birth. If it was unplanned, the woman was asked whether it was a birth that she eventually wanted that simply occurred too soon, or whether at that time she did not wish to become pregnant ever again.

There are obviously a number of difficulties in gathering such data retrospectively. We know from longitudinal research that there is strong bias against reporting a birth that has subsequently become a loved and wanted child as a birth that the mother never wanted to have. Nevertheless, the data indicate that contraceptive failure was the experience of the vast majority of American women during the late 1950s and early 1960s. Of women who had had all the children they wanted at the time of the 1965 National Fertility Study, only one-quarter had managed to reach that point in their reproductive careers without experiencing either a timing failure or a number failure (Ryder and Westoff, 1971). One-third of these women reported that they had an unwanted birth—a birth after they thought they were through bearing children. Of the remainder, two-thirds had experienced at least one timing failure.

How is it possible that a modern, well-educated population using methods known to have high technical efficacy could experience such levels of failure? The answer lies in two very important demographic observations. The first is the distinction between what is called *technical efficacy* and *use efficacy* of contraception. The former term applies to the levels of protection against conception that would be expected on the basis of the technical characteristics of a method. It is common to think of contraceptive methods in terms of this characteristic. Use efficacy, on the other hand, refers to the levels of protection experienced by actual populations using the methods in question. The difference reflects characteristics of methods that affect the care and consistency with which they are used. Methods that require attention to contraception at the time of sexual intercourse, as did virtually all the traditional methods, are very likely to be skipped, especially during periods that are perceived to be relatively safe from conception. Among women in the 1965 National Fertility Study who had used either the condom or diaphragm and jelly in the attempt to prevent an unwanted birth, accidental pregnancies were experienced at a rate that would leave nearly one-half with an accidental pregnancy within 5 years of the birth of their last wanted child (Ryder and Westoff, 1971).

The effectiveness of traditional methods is thus highly responsive to the levels of motivation with which they are used. All methods have higher failure rates during periods in which births are being spaced than during periods in which the attempt is to prevent an unwanted birth.

The second major component to an understanding of the high levels of failure, particularly the high levels of unwanted fertility, is the relationship between long periods of exposure and the likelihood of failure. Even with very high levels of protection, long periods of exposure will cause high proportions of couples to experience the event at risk at least once.

For example, the technical efficacy associated with the condom or diaphragm of about 95 percent would leave only 5 per 100 women pregnant after 1 year, but about a quarter pregnant after 5 years, and over half would experience an accidental pregnancy over a 15-year period. It is important to note in this regard that most women have their last wanted child before the age of 30 and face over 15 years of exposure to the risk of an unwanted birth.

Thus, the common experience of ill-timed and unwanted births reported by women in the mid-1960s was consistent with the levels and methods of contraception reported. The importance of the diffusion of the pill and subsequent trends can only be fully understood in this context.

THE REVOLUTION IN FERTILITY CONTROL—THE INTRODUCTION OF MODERN CONTRACEPTIVES

Contraceptive protection in the United States in the late 1950s was based primarily on the use of three methods in approximately equal proportions—the diaphragm, the condom, and rhythm. The licensing of the pill in July of 1960 set in motion a true revolution in fertility control. Use of the pill diffused rapidly throughout the population, with its initial acceptance most rapid among the young and the most educated (Ryder, 1972). Just 5 years after its introduction, over one-third of women of childbearing age in the United States had already tried the pill. Within a decade this proportion had reached two-thirds. This experience with the pill has had an impact on fertility control far beyond expectations based on the proportion of women using the pill. This is because the pill brought with it a new set of expectations about fertility control.

First, in contrast to preceding fertility control methods, the level of protection afforded by the pill was of an entirely different magnitude. The long-run odds, once clearly against the user, changed to a situation in which at least the expectation was of complete fertility control. The second revolutionary characteristic of the pill was its sexual unobtrusiveness. In contrast to all of the preceding methods, the pill separated concern with contraception from coitus. The importance of this characteristic ought not to be underestimated. Indeed, it probably played as large a role in the rapid diffusion of the pill as did its greater efficacy. The intrauterine device (IUD) shares these aspects of high contraceptive protection and sexual unobtrusiveness; following its introduction in 1965,

increasing numbers of women used the IUD. However, both the pill and the IUD have characteristics that make their use undesirable for some women and medically contraindicated for others. Because of physiologic complications in use or anxiety about such complications, both methods have had rather high discontinuation rates.

Over the 1960s, rates of discontinuation of the pill first declined and then increased as concern about long-term safety began to be raised in the so-called "Nelson Hearings." Around 1970, about one-third of all first users of the pill discontinued use within a year, either because they had physical complications or feared problems. IUD discontinuation rates were somewhat lower, about one-fifth within the first year (Westoff and Jones, 1975). Average levels of discontinuation such as these are hard to interpret and can be very misleading. Discontinuation rates depend heavily upon factors such as age, parity, and available alternatives. For example, while the proportion of currently married women using the pill did not increase between 1970 and 1975, there was a continued increase in pill use among couples in the early years of marriage. There is little indication of a turning away from the pill as a major method of delaying fertility in the younger years, but use of the pill is becoming increasingly specialized toward this objective as concerns grow about the risks of pill use among older women.

It is important that the risks of pill use be evaluated in proper comparative perspective. The alternative to maternal risk associated with the pill is not "zero risk" but rather risks associated with the lower efficacy of most alternatives (Tietze, 1977b). Among younger women, pill use involves no greater risk to life than the use of traditional methods when the joint risks of pregnancy and maternal mortality are included. (This leaves open, of course, the question of any lagged effects of early use.) It is also important that risks taken be evaluated in the context of their absolute as well as relative level, and in terms of the social meaning of competing risks. Risk-taking is essential to social life and small risks are commonly taken in the face of either serious or trivial costs to avoiding risk. For example, smoking, the nonuse of seat belts, eating habits, and an array of sports all involve risks that a substantial number of people judge worth the benefits. In this sense, it is not unreasonable for a woman to decide that the prevention of an unwanted pregnancy is worth some real but relatively low risk. Nevertheless, among older women and especially among older women who smoke, pill use seems ill-advised.

Recent findings on the interaction between smoking and pill use among older women have sharply emphasized a more general question raised by experience with the pill and IUD. Once couples have become accustomed to the expectation of highly effective, sexually unobtrusive contraception, what do they do when use of either of these methods seems undesirable? Do they return to the much higher risk and greater nuisance associated with traditional methods, or is there an alternative that retains the freedom from worry about pregnancy and contraception to which they have become accustomed? This issue has increasingly been resolved by contraceptive sterilization.

CONTRACEPTIVE STERILIZATION

Recent changes with respect to contraceptive sterilization represent a revolution in attitudes and practices. National fertility studies since 1965 have asked explicitly about contraceptive sterilization. A little over a decade ago, a two-thirds majority of the population disapproved of the use of sterilization for fertility control and few couples had chosen to be sterilized (Bumpass and Presser). By 1975, almost half of the couples who intended no more children had been sterilized (Westoff and Jones, 1977a). (The wife had been sterilized in a little over half of these couples.)

It is important to appreciate how significant a change this was. A substantial complex of attitudes and myths had buttressed the commonly held negative evaluation of sterilization. After the turn of the century there were several faddish movements advocating sterilization for purposes as disparate as rejuvenation on the one hand, and the repression of sexual activity among inmates of institutions on the other (Wolfers and Wolfers). Further, the advocacy of sterilization of eugenic purposes had left a particularly negative connotation to the word.

Such undesirable connotations were reinforced by a great deal of confusion about the consequences of sterilization for sexuality. For example, one-quarter of the married women of childbearing age in the United States in 1965 believed that a vasectomy would impair a male's sexual ability. (Among some subgroups this proportion was almost half.) A study in 1970 revealed substantial misinformation on this point even among doctors and medical students (Presser and Bumpass).

As a part of this cultural setting, hospitals maintained very paternalistic procedures controlling access to sterilizing operations. Until 1969, the official manual of the American College of Obstetricians and Gynecologists suggested that before contraceptive female sterilization was performed, a woman should be at least 25 years of age and have five living children, 30 years of age with four living children, or 35 years of age with three living children. Similar standards and prior consultations were common for male sterilization (Presser and Bumpass).

This is not a setting in which rapid change would normally be expected. Yet in a 5-year period, 1965 to 1970, there was a tremendous shift in attitudes (from two-thirds disapproval to two-thirds approval) supported by marked increases in the proportion of individuals sterilized. By 1970, 20 percent of the couples who intended no more children had been sterilized, and two-thirds of all couples were saying that they would give serious consideration to the method at some later time (Presser and Bumpass). These statements were regarded very cautiously at that time. But the proportion sterilized among those intending no more children increased to 32 percent by 1973 and 44 percent by 1975. Sterilization is now the most popular method of contraception for couples married 10 years or more (Westoff and Jones, 1977a). There is reason to believe that this trend will continue.

The trend has been facilitated by advances in the techniques of female sterilization which have made interval operations possible on an outpatient basis and have substantially reduced risks. However, increases in vasectomies have paralleled those in female operations, supporting the more general contraceptive explanation for the increases, rather than the notion that these were a simple response to improved procedures.

Most women face 15 to 20 years of continued risk after they give birth to their last wanted child. Contraceptive sterilization now appears to most to be preferable to the use of any alternative methods over this long period of exposure. A major drawback is the irreversibility of the decision to be sterilized, particularly in light of the high and increasing rate of divorce. Claims of reversibility are now being made, following developments in microsurgery. Such developments would complete the fertility control revolution by shifting fertility control from constant vigilance not to become pregnant, to significant action (surgery) *to* become pregnant.

ABORTION

By the mid-1970s, over two-thirds of all couples were protected by the pill, the IUD, or sterilization, with legal abortion available as a backup in the case of contraceptive failure (Westoff and Jones, 1977a). It is important to understand that the trend toward the legalization of abortion was well underway at the time of the 1973 Supreme Court decision. The basis for the legal termination of pregnancy expanded in 17 states between 1967 and 1972. The number of legal abortions increased from 6000 in 1966 to 500,000 in 1971. The majority of these were occurring in a few states, in particular in California and New York.

The Court ruled in January of 1973 that, on the basis of the concept of personal liberty and the 14th Amendment, the decision to have an abortion may be made solely by the pregnant woman and her doctor up until the end of the first trimester of pregnancy. During the second trimester, state regulation is permissible to the extent that such regulation relates to the "preservation and protection of maternal health." Finally, the Court's ruling permitted states to prohibit abortion during the third trimester of pregnancy. While this decision undoubtedly contributed to the continued increase in legal abortion, its most immediate and dramatic effect was to reduce the distances that women traveled in order to obtain an abortion. Indeed, the number of abortions was actually reduced in states such as California and New York where large numbers of women had been traveling from other states to obtain abortions. The increased accessibility to abortion made possible by the Supreme Court's decision was far from uniform across states; most states saw a growth of clinics providing abortion but relatively little change in the extent to which state hospitals provided abortions (Sullivan et al.). Contrary to expectations at the time, the Supreme Court decision had relatively little effect on trends in attitudes toward abortion. Over the late 1960s and into the 1970s, there was a gradual reduction in the number of people responding to public opinion polls who said they were opposed to abortion.

Attitudes toward abortion are very difficult to measure because such attitudes are contingent upon a whole array of potential conditions that are usually left unspecified. As early as 1965, about 90 percent of women of childbearing age in the United States approved of abortion if it was necessary for the mother's health, about half approved in the case of rape or probable deformity, but only about one-tenth approved if the woman was unmarried, was married and could not afford another child, or did not want another child (Jones and Westoff).

Furthermore, the proportion of those approving of abortion varied markedly depending upon whether the question was interpreted as referring to the moral or legal circumstances surrounding abortion. In 1970 about a quarter of the population approved of abortion on demand when this was interpreted in roughly

moral terms—that is, is it "all right" for the woman to do this?—but about half said that they thought that the decision ought to be "up to the woman and her doctor." For many, attitudes toward abortion are strongly held and rapid changes in these attitudes are not likely to occur. As a consequence, abortion policy will probably continue to be heavily dependent on the outcome of political struggle. (The current prohibition of the use of federal funds to pay for abortions for poor women is a case in point.) Nonetheless, abortion has become a major method of fertility control in the United States.

In the current setting, with high dependence on modern methods of fertility control, one-quarter of all pregnancies are terminated by legal abortion. In 1975, there were approximately 1 million legal abortions, and 3 million live births. About two-thirds of the abortions were performed on unmarried women, about one-third on teenage women (Pakter et al.; Tietze, 1977a). This level of abortion demonstrably affects both the level of fertility and the health status of women. While we have no reliable data on the preexisting or continuing levels of illegal abortions, reasonable estimates suggest that perhaps 70 percent of the current legal abortions would have previously occurred illegally (Tietze, 1975). This shift from the illegal to legal abortion market has very clear implications for the health and emotional well-being of the women involved—effects that are indexed in the component of the maternal mortality rate that is attributable to abortion-related complications. For example, in New York City following the liberalization of its law in 1971, the maternal mortality rate dropped dramatically from previous years as a consequence of the elimination of high mortality associated with illegal abortions (Pakter and Nelson). Yet, even if the majority of current legal abortions would have occurred in any event, the minority number is still a large enough increment to the total number of abortions to have a substantial effect on our birthrate.

The increase in access to legal abortion has a number of roots, deriving in part from concern with the health and safety of women who obtain abortions, in part from the concern with equality of opportunity for women because unplanned births inhibit such equal opportunity, and in part from the development of safer outpatient procedures (in particular, the development of vacuum aspiration abortion procedures). By the mid-1970s, over three-quarters of all abortions were performed by this procedure with a very low complication and death rate (Cates et al.).

It is possible that the use of early vacuum aspiration, the so-called "menstrual regulation" procedure, may play an increasing role in supplementing abortion. By leaving unresolved the question of actual pregnancy this process may be attractive to many who are ambivalent on the moral issues surrounding abortion. If positive pregnancy tests are obtained beforehand, it is, of course, explicitly early abortion *(Studies in Family Planning)*.

However, in addition to other factors facilitating abortion, the revolutionary forces set in motion by experience with the pill have very likely also played a significant role in abortion trends. The ill-timed and unwanted pregnancies that were the normal experience of women under the old fertility regime, and which were easily rationalized within the popular culture, are no longer tolerable. Given expectations of the right to complete fertility control, the costs of an unwanted pregnancy are more salient, and many of the social supports for continuation of such a pregnancy are much less intense.

Given the increasing concern about the long-run safety of the pill, it is an open question whether the proportion of the population protected by such highly effective methods will increase. But it is important to note that there is an implied significant demand for abortion, even given the levels of protection provided by the pill. This follows from the earlier discussion of the implications of a long exposure to risk even with high levels of protection. Given the levels of efficacy of the pill, and a generous allowance for declining fecundity with age, it would be expected that one out of every ten women protected at the level of the pill would experience an unwanted pregnancy over the 15 years of exposure to risk.

It is undeniable that there has been a revolution in fertility control since the introduction of the pill in the 1960s. For the vast majority of the population, fertility control is very effective, sexually unobtrusive, and relatively safe. However, significant problem areas remain, to some extent as a consequence of the lesser appropriateness of existing technology for some groups of the population. In particular, teenage fertility and fertility outside of marriage have been slower to decline. In the mid-1970s, 15 percent of all births occurred to a mother who had not yet married (U.S. National Center for Health Statistics) and one out of every four women was pregnant at the time of marriage (U.S. Bureau of Census, 1975). These relatively high figures not only reflect the very rapid declines in fertility that have occurred among married women, but the changed social conditions under which children are born.

National sample surveys of unmarried teenage girls revealed marked increases between 1971 and 1976 in both early sexual activity and contraceptive use. Among teenagers in 1976, one-sixth reported that they had their first sexual intercourse by age 15; 55 percent reported intercourse by age 19 (Zelnik and Kantner). Taking this increase in exposure into account, the illegitimacy rate of the sexually active unmarried population showed a clear decline in the early 1970s. This decline reflects the increases in contraceptive protection for the unmarried population that occurred in the early 1970s. Use of contraception at the time of last intercourse was reported by only one-half of the unmarried teenagers in 1971, but by almost two-thirds in 1976. This increase was accompanied by an increased tendency for teenagers who used contraception to be using the pill. Nevertheless, contraceptive use remains much less extensive and less effective among teenagers, especially among young teenagers, than among the rest of the population.

A number of explanations have been suggested for these facts. The first has to do with issues of access to contraception for unmarried teenagers. While significant gains may have been made in this respect with the establishment of teenage contraceptive clinics, most of the population is still not served by such clinics (Jaffee and Dryfoos), and the attitudes of private physicians and pharmacists may still constitute significant barriers to contraceptive access for a large proportion of the teenage population.

Interconnected with this problem is the problem of self-definition involved in becoming a regular, though unmarried, contraceptive user. For example, for a young girl to go on the pill is to openly acknowledge to herself, and at least some significant others, that she is or intends to be sexually active. This may be most difficult for those who hold values against premarital sexual intercourse, and is further complicated by the fact that the need for contraceptive protection may vary markedly depending on the fluctuating nature of teenage relationships. There is a real question as to whether pill use is the most appropriate form of protection against indefinite and infrequent exposure, and yet the risks of pregnancy are considerably higher in the absence of either pill or IUD use, both because of the lower technical efficacy of alternative methods and because of the sexual cumbersomeness of these methods. Effective use of traditional methods is highly dependent upon motivation, an undesirable characteristic for teenage protection.

Another factor frequently cited in connection with teenage contraceptive use has to do with the emotional maturity of teenagers. They may be more prone to take risks in the first place, and in risk taking may be more likely to discount long-term costs against immediate gains in the calculation of risk. Luker has outlined the self-defeating cycle that evolves when young teenagers begin taking contraceptive risks under the perception that they are too young to conceive, or that infrequent exposure will not lead to pregnancy. These perceptions can be reinforced by a slowness to conceive associated with teenage subfecundity, but pregnancy is almost inevitable with continued exposure and physical maturation.

A second problem area that has much in common with unmarried teenage pregnancy concerns births to women who are between marriages. One-quarter of twice-married women in the United States in 1970 had experienced a birth after separation and before remarriage (Rindfuss and Bumpass, 1977). This phenomenon is strongly related to the problems of teenage fertility control since the experience was even more prevalent among women who were quite young when their marriages disrupted. While other explanations are possible, such as the use of pregnancy as a last attempt to keep a disintegrating marriage intact, the contraceptive needs of previously married women seem inadequately met in the current setting of generally effective protection. Many of the problems and ambivalence about contraceptive use discussed in the context of unmarried teenage contraception are relevant here as well. Existing fertility control methods are least appropriate for many unmarried and previously married women, as the continued high accidental fertility of these women attests. Until better solutions can be found, this is an area that particularly requires sensitive attention on the part of the physician.

PROSPECTS FOR THE FUTURE

Demographers are of very sharply divided opinions on the question of whether current low fertility is likely to continue into the future. The issue usually is couched in terms of whether or not we are likely to experience another baby boom of the proportions of the one in the 1950s. Following our earlier discussion of the postwar baby boom, it is important to separate this question into timing and number components. The "number" question is whether successive generations of women will return to bearing larger families. Much of the postwar boom was associated with a movement to the two-child family from a previous period in which many women had remained childless or had only one child. Since most women now expect to

have two children, there seems to be little room for this component in a new baby boom. It is possible that there will be a major increase in three- or four-child families, but these increases would have to be much greater than in the previous boom to contribute a comparable number effect.

However, even if average family size were to remain at or below replacement levels, the annual birthrate may follow upward and downward cycles as a consequence of accelerations and decelerations in the pace of childbearing. Such cycles are expected to respond in particular to the economic circumstances of young couples. Richard Easterlin is foremost among those who expect another baby boom of the scale of the last as a consequence of future improvements in such circumstances (Easterlin). He foresees both number and timing responses. Greatly simplified, his theory notes three factors that may coincide to produce such an increase: (1) the relative size of the cohort of young people, (2) general economic conditions, and (3) the relative economic well-being of young people compared with circumstances of their parental families. Persons born during periods of low fertility will enter the labor market with relatively few competitors, contrasting sharply with the experience of those born during a period of high fertility. The postwar baby boom was seen as a consequence of the conjunction of small cohort size for those born during the 1920s and 1930s and reaching marriage age in the 1940s and 1950s, the relative deprivation of their parents' economic circumstances, and the expanding postwar economy. Conversely, the baby boom babies experienced difficulties due to their numbers at all points in growing up, from school class sizes to labor market entrance. Current low fertility is interpreted as a consequence of these factors, in conjunction with a sluggish economy. Those born in the current low fertility period are likely to experience comparatively favorable circumstances, and thus the expectation of another baby boom.

This Easterlin hypothesis calls attention to a set of forces that will tend to generate cycles in fertility. However, the amplitude of such cycles depends heavily on changes in other parts of the total field of forces that affect fertility. It is the conviction of this observer that the revolution in fertility control described earlier in this chapter will serve to markedly dampen future fertility swings. Unquestionably, there will be fluctuations in the annual birthrate. What remains open is how large these fluctuations will be and to what extent average family size will fluctuate as well.

In the context of modern industrial society, the

fertility control revolution has served to strongly reinforce pressures toward low fertility. The potential for complete fertility control makes childbearing—when and if—a matter of choice in an ultimate sense that never before existed. For the first time, motherhood itself is fully a matter for rational evaluation. Since it need not be rationalized because it is inevitable, costs as well as virtues must be weighed. These costs have not just been discovered; the literature is replete with the psychological and emotional costs of motherhood. They have, however, become more relevant to fertility decisions and, in addition, increasingly salient in the context of growing concern with equality of opportunity for women. As nonfamilial opportunities are more equalized, the opportunity costs of childbearing escalate.

Obviously, childbearing roles offer much that is rewarding, but these rewards are not likely to be experienced equally by all women. Motherhood has been the last major vestige of ascribed status in modern industrial society. A primary consequence of complete fertility control is that motherhood is placed more squarely in competition with other social roles. As fertility becomes more a matter for *decision,* the decision progressively focuses on the planning of pregnancy rather than its prevention. The decision to have a child must be weighed not only against the direct social, psychological, and economic costs of children, but also against the loss of the wife's earnings and intrinsic satisfaction with her job. The wife's earnings play an important role in family life-styles. In a majority of the families in which both the husband and wife have incomes, the wife's income represents over a fifth of the total family income (Sweet).

Of course, deeply seated values associating motherhood with all women will not disappear overnight. What is most remarkable is that we have experienced our recent rapid declines in fertility under the influence of strong pronatalist values, suggesting that the staffing of parental roles may become problematic for a society in which young girls are less socialized to expect motherhood (Davis).

There may be two major facets of declines in fertility during this transitional period: (1) Succeeding generations of young women may be expected to hold progressively less to traditional values of motherhood. As they are socialized in a modern fertility control society with an awareness of alternatives to motherhood, their aggregate fertility goals will be lower—perhaps with many women remaining childless. Fertility expectations among young white women under 24 ranged from 3.2 to 3.1 over the years 1955 to 1965, but had dropped to 2.2 by 1972. (U.S.

Bureau of the Census, 1972). (2) Fertility of those socialized under the old fertility regime also may be expected to be lower than intended; that is, the experience of fertility control should lead to smaller family sizes than the women themselves have said that they want. The extension of birth intervals through the reduction of accidental pregnancy should reduce total fertility by increasing the "risk" time available for the reduction of intentions (Freedman et al., 1965). Many women, finding increasing gratification in their jobs and freedom from the intensive demands of infant childcare, will become reluctant to return to childbearing. Others will simply discover that they have passed an age, or age of youngest child, beyond which they no longer wish to become reinvolved in infant care—even if ideally they would "like another" (Rindfuss and Bumpass, 1978). The same process may result in many of those in the younger cohorts remaining childless, though few such women now indicate that they desire to do so.

In summary, average family sizes are likely to remain near or below replacement levels but annual birthrates may fluctuate considerably as births are delayed or made up in response to changing conditions. With increasing role options for women, the control of fertility to permit pregnancy only when it is desired has become a matter of central importance. At stake are not only the life chances and well-being of the women involved, but also those of their children.

REFERENCES

Bumpass L: Is low fertility here to stay? *Fam Plann Perspect* 5:67, 1973.

_____, **Presser H:** Contraceptive sterilization in the U.S.: 1965 and 1970. *Demography* 9:531,1972.

Cates W et al.: The effect of delay and method choice on the risk of abortion morbidity. *Fam Plann Perspect* 9:266, 1977.

Coale AJ: The decline of fertility in Europe from the French Revolution to World War II, in *Fertility and Family Planning,* eds. SJ Behrman et al., Ann Arbor: Univ. of Michigan Press, 1970.

Davis JB: *Coercive pronatalism and American population policy.* Preliminary paper no. 2, Berkeley: International Population and Urban Research, Univ. of California, 1972.

Easterlin R: What will 1984 be like? Presidential address to the annual meeting of the Population Association of America, April 1978. *Demography,* 15:397, 1978..

Freedman R et al.: Stability and change in expectations about family size: A longitudinal study. *Demography* 2:250, 1965.

_____ et al.: *Family Planning, Sterility, and Population Growth,* New York: McGraw-Hill, 1959.

Glass DV, Grebenik E: *The Trend and Patterns of Fertility in Great Britain,* London: 1954.

Hajnal J: European marriage patterns in perspective, in *Population in History,* eds. DV Glass and DEC Eversley, London: Arnold, 1964.

Hansen AH: Economic progress and declining population growth. *Amer Econ Rev* 29:1,1939.

Jaffee F, Dryfoos J: Fertility control services for adolescents: Access and utilization. *Fam Plann Perspect* 8:166, 1976.

Jones EF, Westoff C: Attitudes toward abortion in the United States in 1970 and the trend since 1965, in *Demographic and Social Aspects of Population Growth,* vol. I, eds. CF Westoff and R Parke, Jr., Washington: U.S. Govt Printing Office, 1972.

Luker, K: *Taking Chances: Abortion and the Decision Not to Contracept,* Berkeley: Univ. of California Press, 1975.

Myrdal A *Nation and Family,* New York: Harper, 1941.

Pakter J, Nelson F: Abortion in New York City: The first nine months. *Fam Plann Perspect* 3:5, 1971.

_____ et al.: Legal abortion: A half-decade of experience. *Fam Plann Perspect* 7:248, 1975.

Presser H, Bumpass L: Demographic and social aspects of contraceptive sterilization in the U.S.: 1965–70, in *Demographic and Social Aspects of Population Growth,* vol. I, eds. CF Westoff and R Parke, Jr., Washington: U.S. Govt Printing Office, 1972.

Rindfuss R, Bumpass L: Fertility during marital disruption. *J Marr Fam* (August):517, 1977.

_____, _____: Age and the sociology of fertility: How old is too old? in *Social Demography: Research and Prospects,* eds. KE Taeuber et al., New York: Academic Press, 1978.

_____, Westoff CF: The initiation of contraception. *Demography* 11:75, 1974.

Ryder NB: The emergence of a modern fertility pattern: United States, 1917–66, in *Fertility and Family Planning,* eds. SJ Behrman et al., Ann Arbor: Univ. of Michigan Press, 1970.

_____: Time series of pill and IUD use: United States, 1961–1970. *Stud Fam Plann* 3:233, 1972.

_____, Westoff CF: Contraceptive failure in the United States. *Fam Plann Perspect* 5:133, 1973.

_____, _____: *Reproduction in the United States,* Princeton: Princeton Univ. Press, 1971.

Shryock HS, Siegel JS: *The Methods and Materials of Demography,* vol. 2, Washington: U.S. Govt Printing Office, 1973.

Studies in Family Planning: Menstrual regulation: The method and the issues. *Stud in Fam Plann* 3:249, 1977.

Sullivan E et al.: Legal abortion in the United States, 1975–76. *Fam Plann Perspect* 9:116, 1977.

Sweet JA: *The Employment and Earnings of Married Women,* New York: Seminar, 1973.

Tietze C: Legal abortions in the United States: Rates and ratios by race and age, 1972–74. *Fam Plann Perspect* 9:12, 1977.

_____: New estimates of mortality associated with fertility control. *Fam Plann Perspect* 9:74, 1977.

_____: The effect of legalization of abortion on population growth and public health. *Fam Plann Perspect* 7:123, 1975.

U.S. Bureau of the Census: *Birth expectations and fertility: June 1972. Current Population Reports,* ser. P–20, no. 240, Sept. 1972.

_____: *Fertility history and prospects of American women: June 1975. Current Population Reports,* ser. P–20, no. 288, 1975.

_____: *Fertility of American women, June 1976. Current Population Reports,* ser. P–20, no. 308, 1977.

U.S. National Center for Health Statistics: *Final Natality Statistics, 1976,* 26, no. 12, 1978.

Westoff CF, Jones EF: Contraception and sterilization in the United States, 1965–75. *Fam Plann Perspect* 9:153, 1977.

_____, _____: Discontinuation of the pill and IUD in the United States: 1960–70. *Mt Sinai J Med NY* 42:384, 1975.

_____, _____: The secularization of U.S. Catholic birth control practices. *Fam Plann Perspect* 9:203, 1977.

_____, Ryder NB: *The Contraceptive Revolution,* Princeton: Princeton Univ. Press, 1977.

Wolfers D, Wolfers H: Vasectomania. *Fam Plann Perspect* 5:196, 1973.

Zelnik M, Kantner JF: Sexual and contraceptive experience of young unmarried women in the United States, 1976 and 1971. *Fam Plann Perspect* 9:55, 1977.

4

Bioethical Considerations

ANDRE E. HELLEGERS[1]

GENERAL CONSIDERATIONS

The present surge of interest in bioethical questions stems from the fact that such potent technologies are being developed that they are bound to have societal consequences. This interest runs parallel to certain other trends which have led to an increasing awareness that some acquaintance with ethical methodology forms part of the education of the general public, as well as of the medical specialist.

The issues treated in this chapter are current matters of public interest. They relate to the interface between technological development and its assessment in terms of consequences for society, both economic and value- or disvalue-oriented.

They pose a problem for the medical profession as a whole and, with respect to the subjects treated here, for gynecology and obstetrics in particular. The earnest physician wishes the problem would go away and that the public at large would simply trust the judgment so amply demonstrated in the doctor's devotion to the common medical good. Yet in the increasingly public debate, the question is precisely who can define the good to be pursued in medicine and specifically in gynecology and obstetrics.

Inevitably the debate sooner or later is translated into a question of who shall be allowed to practice the specialty. Willingness or unwillingness to bear allegiance to a specific definition of "the good" becomes

[1]Deceased.

an issue in enrolling the putative candidate into the specialty. Should the specialty tolerate in its midst those who will not sterilize or who insist on sterilizing; those who genetically screen; those who abort for reasons of wrong sex of fetus; those who refuse to inform parents of contraception provided to their minor children, or those indeed who insist on informing parents? Who shall decide? Should one who tolerates the presence of such individuals in the specialty be allowed to refuse to train them? Shall the specialty decide, or the individual trainer? Whom shall we allow into medical school, let alone the specialty?

It can reasonably be foreseen that the issues raised may lead to great tolerance or great intolerance for diversity in medical practice. The notion that "malpractice" is based on community standards may factually shift the focus of decision making from the profession and the specialty to the courts. It would be tragic if the specialty itself had no input into the public debate simply because it does not know the issues or the various modes by which they are reasoned out. It is for these reasons that the American College of Obstetricians and Gynecologists now has a standing Committee on Bioethics. It is for these reasons also that this chapter finds a place in a book which otherwise focuses largely on matters subject to scientific methodology. The fundamental question is precisely whether scientific methodology can suitably be brought to bear on matters which are only subjectively perceived.

The movement called "consumerism," embodied in such notions as "truth in lending" and "truth in packaging," and the protection of the ignorant in matters of law, is now beginning to focus on medicine. Primarily this is expressed in a requirement for informed consent giving by patients prior to their undergoing therapeutic or experimental procedures.

The scientific method usually focuses on the *ends* achieved by procedures. Such an approach, in the parlance of ethical methodology, is called *teleological*. It may run counter to an approach, called *deontological,* in which correctness of the *means* takes priority. In such a construct, certain means, such as the invasion of privacy, may not be employed even if the ends obtained are thought good. A debate can arise around the notion that medical procedures may be done on individuals without their voluntary consent if they are thought necessary for the national "health security." It is increasingly realized that there is an infinity of health needs (infinite, if death is to be warded off indefinitely) with only finite resources, in budgetary terms, to attend to those needs. In debates on how to allocate finite resources to a seemingly in-finite set of problems, theories are evolved on how to do so fairly, as exemplified by John Rawls's theory of "distributive justice" (Rawls).

The difficulty in analyzing the enterprise of medicine in such a context is compounded when the very notions of "health" and "disease" are undergoing change. At least four major concepts of health may be entertained. To the extent that the word disease connotes the obverse of the word health, such attempts at definition must also look at the definition of disease. A first concept of disease—perhaps the most classically held view—would have it that it is a condition which, if not combated, leads to further degeneration and death.

A second concept of disease is based more directly on statistical predictions of mortality and morbidity, even in the absence of presenting complaints by patients. Such diagnoses as hypotension, hypertension, or indeed any other diagnoses which carry the terms "hypo" or "hyper" imply the existence of a "normal" (presumably "healthy") condition, often denoted by the prefix *eu.* Thus "euthyroid" is the healthy condition compared with which hypo- and hyperthyroidism are diseases or entities which at least require follow-up by health care personnel, even if the patient is not yet symptomatic.

A third concept of disease does not restrict itself to the somatically quantifiable body alterations implied in the previous two definitions. Rather it holds that man is diseased if unable to adapt to his environment. Such a notion begs the question of whether it is the person who is "sick" or the environment. A perfectly healthy Jewish nose, superb at inhaling oxygen and exhaling carbon dioxide, could be a life-threatening condition in Nazi Germany. How should a rhinoplasty be considered under such conditions? Would it be therapy? Sagging breasts, facial wrinkles, flaccid buttocks can be surgically "corrected" in societies which have qualms about aging, as in the United States. Are these conditions diseases—and if so, why?

Aberrant behavior is increasingly thought of as the proper province for the medical profession's ministrations. Those deviating from acceptable political tenets in Soviet Russia have been assigned to psychiatric institutions. In the United States many criminals are examined medically. In 1964 hundreds of United States physicians attested, in writing, to the conclusion that Senator Barry Goldwater was unfit for the Presidency, in spite of never having examined "the patient" in person. Millions of Americans, depressed at the nature of their lives, are given stimulants; others are given tranquilizers. It is tacitly accepted and overtly acted upon that, where disharmony exists between human desires and the human environment, it is as legitimate to alter bodily function to fit the environment as vice versa.

This rather recent development is interesting in the light of past medical theory. It was widely held that patients' symptoms should not be treated until the underlying disease, which caused the symptoms, had been identified. To do so was described as "masking the disease." Where the definitions of the words disease and health extend beyond physical well-being into mental well-being, the issue arises whether to treat the mental symptoms without taking action about the environmental factors which cause them. Is this a proper function for a medical profession? Should psychopharmacologic agents be used on patients to make them adapt to social circumstances they cannot stand? Put another way, is it the proper function of the medical profession to mask social problems through medication?

The fourth and broadest definition of health is contained in the World Health Organizations's definition which holds that health is not the mere absence of disease but the presence of total physical, mental, and social well-being. Clearly, adoption of this definition assigns to the health professions tasks which extend much beyond those contained in the first definition which focuses on inflammation, degeneration, injury, and the more traditional concerns of the profession.

This enlargement of the scope of medicine from physical to mental and social well-being is at the heart of many bioethical debates, as we shall see. The reader will have noticed the profusion of quotation marks in the foregoing paragraphs. These do not appear by chance. They represent the fact that the terms are controverted. We shall now examine how these concepts affect the practice of obstetrics and gynecology.

SPECIFIC PROBLEM AREAS

ABORTION

In the continuing debates about the ethics of abortion, several lines of reasoning are used.

In general, there are two schools of thought about the nature of the fetus (Engelhardt; Hellegers, 1973). The first school holds that new human life occurs at conception. This school seeks to protect that life as

invaluable or inalienable in the same way as a child's or an adult's life. It therefore only tolerates fetal destruction in terms analogous to those used for extrauterine life, i.e., "just killing" as in war, capital punishment, self-protection, etc. In brief, it founds its justification for abortion on the presence in the mother of conditions which would ethically permit the killing of the already-born for protection of a greater good than life itself. Such "goods" might include national survival or the prevention of other deaths.

Another school of thought holds that human life is not sufficiently defined by biological terms and requires some other quality in order to be described as "having value," "having dignity," "worthy to be protected under the Constitution," or "having a soul." At which point these qualities are to be conferred and under what conditions becomes the focus of the debate.

The possible ability of two fertilized eggs (or life, dignity, value, worthiness of protection under the Constitution, or soul) to be recombined into one individual to produce a chimera raises the question of whether the point at which irreversible individuality is attained should be seen as a key stage (Hellegers, 1970). The occurrence of a spontaneous heartbeat at 3 weeks is of interest, since it is used in definitions of life and death in adults. Yet in recent definitions of life for adults, an allegedly spontaneous heartbeat is thought not necessarily spontaneous if it is maintained through an artificial respirator. The question then becomes whether the placenta is a fetal organ of spontaneous respiration, or a respirator. Is respiration to be defined in terms of chest expansion and contraction or in terms of O_2 uptake and CO_2 release into an environment other than one's own? In adults, examination of the EEG (electroencephalogram) has been incorporated into definitions of life and death. Yet in the fetus (in whom brain waves appear at around 8 weeks), the EEG carries quite a different connotation than in extrauterine existence. In the adult, a flat EEG has a high statistical coefficient of correlation with nonrecurrence of spontaneous respiration and spontaneous heartbeat in the future. In the fetus the statistical correlations are reversed. Are test findings the masters or servants of physicians in making diagnoses and prognoses?

Perceived spontaneous movement (i.e., quickening) has traditionally been held to be of significance in diagnosing the possible value of fetal life, although such movements are not considered critical in the adult. Moreover, quickening is a perception of the mother rather than a description of the fetus. Some women think they feel quickening when they are factually not pregnant. Some deliver without ever having felt quickening, indeed sometimes without knowing they were pregnant.

The notion that prior to 12 or 13 weeks abortion is safer than childbirth in terms of maternal mortality statistics is a questionable means of assessing the value of fetal life, since it assigns a zero value to the child. In other words, it is methodologically questionable whether the value of a biologic entity can be assessed by an analysis of the safety of a technical procedure. Yet others would assign little or no value to any fetus or child unless it was capable of certain functions such as thought, interpersonal relationships, the giving and receiving of love, or some other putative criterion of humanity. Similar debates and arguments occur about the quality of life or the nature of "meaningful life" at its end as at its beginning. In brief, the debate is between biologic and relational definitions of life.

Quite separate from these debates is the question of how one is to act when one does not know the answers to the questions under discussion? Who makes the final decisions? Here, separate ethical issues are raised. When in doubt, how should one act? Presumptively in favor of life for the fetus? Presumptively in favor of maternal (and/or paternal) decision making? In favor of physician decision making? Suffice it to say that expertise in ethical decision making is not based on what are commonly asserted to be professional insights but rather on value assessments. Hence, the controversial nature of the debate. Suffice it also to say that some see the issue as inherent in the nature of the fetus, while others see it as a conflict between continuation of fetal existence and present, pressing maternal (and/or paternal) interests.

This notion of conflict of interest is key to an understanding of new and future ethical problems of abortion. Is abortion factually and ethically based on separating two parties with a conflict of interest (mother and fetus) or is it the guaranteed destruction of one of the parties (the fetus)? This philosophical issue was at the heart of both the Edelin and the Waddell cases, although their outcomes did not settle the issue.

In the Edelin case, it was alleged that Dr. Edelin, by separating the placenta in utero at hysterotomy, had factually produced the death of a fetus which might have lived had it been delivered. The weight of the fetus was alleged to have been sufficient for survival. The legal decision rode on the issue of whether the fetus had in fact ever been alive outside of the mother. If not, then it never had been a "person" and hence worthy of the protection of the law. Therefore, it would be impossible to speak of murder or homicide. The court decided in favor of Dr. Edelin.

In the so-called "Waddell case," it was alleged that Dr. Waddell induced an abortion by saline induction and that the fetus was born alive. He was then alleged to have strangled it in the nursery. It was never proved that he did so. But, more interestingly, the defense contended that the fetus in the nursery was already dead, or so damaged that to resuscitate it at that point would have constituted "extraordinary means of therapy" (see Death and Dying, this chapter).

In neither case was the philosophical or legal issue really resolved. Is there an affirmative moral or legal obligation to maximize the chances of fetal survival in abortions? Or, to put it as above, are the ethics of abortion grounded in separating the conflicting parties or in the guaranteed destruction, whenever possible, of one of the parties?

The question is of more than passing interest. Suppose that with the passage of time it becomes possible to save smaller and smaller fetuses in extrauterine incubators. Should one then save all aborted fetuses by, say, doing only prostaglandin abortions and saving all the live-born ones? In several states laws have been proposed to ensure exactly this. The question is interesting not only in the context of clinical practice. It can be postulated as a research question. Assume that it becomes possible to produce a child from fertilization onward entirely in vitro. What then becomes the entity of abortion? Presumably such a fetus cannot be in conflict with any maternal interest. May it then be decanted or destroyed at any stage and, if so, on what grounds?

When one analyzes the role of the scientist in these debates one can see how limited the role is. He or she can, unanimously, it is hoped, describe with great accuracy what the products of conception look like. Let us describe the result of the description in the following terms:

$$F_1, F_2, F_3, \ldots, F_{266}$$

Where F_1 to F_{266} is a series of precise daily descriptions of the fetus from conception to term.

The ethical question then becomes: What value is to be ascribed to the fetus on each day between F_1 and F_{266}? Let us describe this value range in the following terms:

$$V_A, V_B, V_C, \ldots, V_Z$$

For the sake of clarity let us say

$$V_A = \text{absolute value}$$
$$V_Z = \text{zero value}$$

It will be clear from abortion debates that some would almost equate F_1 with V_A, assigning absolute value to the fetus on day 1. Others, who see the start of life at the first extrauterine breath, might tend to equate F_{266} with V_Z, assigning zero value to the fetus on day 266 in utero. They would assign absolute value only to the extrauterine fetus which has drawn a breath, and then only for a fetus which has reached viability, say an F_{140} (20 weeks) or an F_{196} (28 weeks).

Obviously, most people fall somewhere in between these extremes. And not all view fetal age as the crucial factor. Some would assign a lower V value to an *abnormal* F_{82} than to a *normal* F_{82} or even to a *normal* F_{59}. These are the value judgments being made and it should be clear that in this exercise the true expertise of the physician is limited to *describing* the fetus. The problem is that it is methodologically impossible to go from *de*scription to *pre*scription or *pro*scription. There, scientific methodology becomes inapplicable, and we enter the field of value judgments.

It should be clear that this intellectual conundrum is not limited to the unborn. It has been part of human history throughout the ages in other forms. At various times values from A to Z have been placed upon organisms of various kinds. Protestants have been judged from age P_1 to P_{100}, so have Catholics, Negroes, Jews, and "infidels," and so have cows in India and, depending upon the values attached to the various descriptions of such individuals, they have been protected or not—and in varying degrees.

How are such conundrums resolved? Usually they are not—and cannot be—unless the issue is moot, and to render it moot only resolves the practical problems, not the philosophical ones. For good or ill, it is society which decides. That means that decisions are usually based on political and legal bases, rather than ethical ones.

In the United States, the Supreme Court decided only that individual states may not interfere with a woman's obtaining an abortion in the first trimester of pregnancy if she can find a physician willing to perform one. It has not forced an individual physician to perform an abortion or a woman to undergo one. This decision is described as permitting "abortion on request," rather than abortion on demand.

In the second trimester, states may not prevent abortions from being performed, but they may regulate where they can be performed in order to safeguard the health of the woman. This distinction simply recognizes the fact that abortion becomes more dangerous to the woman as pregnancy advances.

In the third trimester, the state can take an affirmative interest in the fetus, but not if, in so doing, it places an increased hazard on the woman. In other words, it may not interfere with an abortion necessary to preserve the health of the woman. It is of paramount interest, given the various possible definitions of disease and health described in the introduction to this chapter, that the Supreme Court has clearly adopted the World Health Organization definition of health, stated earlier in this chapter. This, in fact, means that the physical, mental or social well-being of the woman governs whether the pregnancy is deemed to interfere with her health.

Where the courts are the ultimate arbiters of whether, constitutionally, an abortion may or may not be performed, it is the legislatures (subject to their decisions being constitutional) who decide how abortions are to be financed. Will any financial support be given to pay for the abortion?

Clearly there are many semantic debates on this issue, too, and they are debated almost yearly in the Congress.

Some see the issue as one of equity: if the rich can afford to have abortions, so should the poor. Others argue that the government has never financed for the poor all those things which the rich can afford. On this the Supreme Court has ruled that states *may* finance abortions for the poor, but are not obliged to do so.

The result has been that the Congress and individual state legislatures have argued in detail which abortions should be funded and which not. Such debates factually constitute the collective establishment of V values for a variety of F's, in accordance with the individual perceptions of the legislators or the collective judgments of the people they represent. What is of great interest is that such debates are obviously subject to all the difficulties of establishing definitions for the words health and disease described in the introduction to this chapter. In recent years the House of Representatives has tended to suggest the financing of such abortions only when necessary to save maternal lives. The Senate has tended to advocate greater latitude in funding, and senators have often suggested the funding of all those abortions which are "necessary to preserve maternal life or health" or which are "medically necessary." Such a formulation suggests that the medical profession has a uniform definition for health or what is medically necessary. As we have seen, this depends on whether one views the scope of the medical profession to include only physical health, or physical and mental health, or physical, mental, and social health. In other words, legislatures and professions can no more free themselves from semantic considerations than can ethicists.

The American College of Obstetricians and Gynecologists, in a statement on abortion, has attempted to provide at least some guidelines. The pertinent section of its statement reads as follows:

> The College recognizes that situations of conflict may arise between a pregnant woman's health interests and the welfare of her fetus. Both legally and ethically this conflict can lead to a justification for inducing abortion. The College affirms that the resolution of such conflict by inducing abortion in no way implies that the physician has an adversary relationship towards the fetus and therefore, the physician does not view the destruction of the fetus as the primary purpose of abortion. The College consequently recognizes a continuing obligation on the part of the physician towards the survival of a possibly viable fetus where this can be discharged without additional hazard to the health of the mother.

From this statement we may conclude that the college supports the concept that abortion should be a separation of conflicting parties, rather than guaranteed fetal death, provided it does not further endanger maternal life to preserve fetal life. Clearly, also, the college has not, in this statement, tried to define the words disease and health. Neither does it assign a particular value V to a particular fetus F. It is clear, however, that it does not value a fetus at V_z or zero value.

One final issue should be clarified. It is often said that it should be a matter of maternal choice whether to abort, or not. To say otherwise is to force one's ethics on another. Opponents of the argument say that the decision to abort invariably forces one's ethics on the fetus. Such slogans do little to help bring clarity to the ethical issue at hand. As we have seen, it is *inevitable* that abortion involve an ethical decision, since it involves placing more or less value on fetal life. Only if zero value is placed on all intrauterine fetuses is there no ethical problem. Few, if any, adhere to the placing of zero value on the fetus. At least, few would indiscriminately administer thalidomide to pregnant women.

About the only ethical conclusion in the abortion debate on which there is considerable agreement is that abortions should not be performed on women against *their* will. As we shall see, however, even this issue of giving informed consent for medical intervention is not as simple as it looks and can best be clarified in the issues that follow later in this chapter.

FETAL EXPERIMENTATION

The various theories about values in fetal and adult life recur in the ethical issues involved in fetal experimentation. Those who assign a zero value to fetal life obviously have no ethical problem. Ethical issues overwhelmingly arise where a certain value *is* attached to fetal life. At that point, several issues may be considered.

THE DEAD FETUS

The very diagnosis of death eliminates many ethical problems of fetal use for many. Yet even this notion is sometimes questioned. If the aborted fetus is considered to be a killed human being, removal of its body parts may be considered as questionable as the use of body parts from homicide victims.

Put in the singular, would one take kidneys from such a victim for transplantation? Would one do it if the homicide were the result of a societal practice? Some would assert that to derive systematic advantages from an unethical practice makes one an accessory to the practice by obscuring its true nature.

Use of the dead fetus can raise other problems, and some are appearing in the courts. These problems again depend on certain notions of the ethical. If the fetus is viewed as if it is a child, and is dead, then who, if anyone, must give consent for removal of organs, or for autopsy? Usually, consent giving depends for its ethical validity on the consent giver's having the interests of the subject at heart. How far are parents who have consented to have the fetus aborted suitable consent givers? (Congressional Record.) And if either legally or ethically they are to be considered disqualified from consent giving, then can anyone else be considered qualified? Here interesting legal issues may arise. Some might consider such fetuses abandoned corpses. In many jurisdictions abandoned corpses may be used for such medical practices as dissection. In other jurisdictions, there are uniform anatomical gift acts (Sadler et al.; Haney and Allen).

This issue may be viewed as follows. When organs such as corneas, kidneys, etc., are needed for transplantation purposes, various principles may reign, although the principles do not depend on the need itself. Under one set of principles no organ may be used or examined unless it has been willed in advance, or at death by proxy consent. Under another set of principles, all organs are deemed to belong to the community unless refusal to donate has been established in advance, or by proxy refusal. Whether one set of legal and ethical principles is accepted over the other obviously has important consequences for the use of the dead fetus (if the fetus is to be treated as a member of human society). Depending on which societal modus operandi is in effect, almost any dead fetus could be used, or almost none.

Another consideration has been brought to bear on fetal experimentation: timing. Some hold that no drug, at least no drug harmful to the fetus, may be administered to mothers prior to abortion for the purpose of studying its effect in the fetus. Here the rationale is that a woman's option to undergo or not to undergo abortion must be kept open as long as possible. Therefore if an agent damaging to the intrauterine fetus is administered, the freedom of the mother to change her mind about undergoing the abortion may be impinged upon by knowing the fetus is damaged. This has been one of the major reasons for prohibiting experimentation on the fetus in utero in Britain (Peel).

THE LIVE PREVIABLE FETUS

If the fetus is not considered a member of the human race to be protected like any other, there are no more ethical problems than with the use of other tissues.

If it is considered a live human being, the ethical analysis of such fetal use obviously changes. Its impending death, due to nonviability, is considered by some sufficient warranty for its experimental use. This contention however, has never been made in terms of other stages of human life. Neither is it clear what the *legal* status of the "live" extrauterine fetus is. It can neither invade maternal privacy nor interfere with maternal health, the two major reasons given by the Supreme Court to enjoin states from prohibiting abortions *(Roe* v. *Wade; Doe* v. *Bolton).* Does that mean it should be held inviolate?

Another interesting consideration arises in connection with the extrauterine live previable fetus: how to diagnose its death. We have said above that a flat EEG in utero cannot be equated with death since its prognostic significance is different. Once outside the uterus, however, the prognostic import of the flat EEG radically changes and is analogous to that of the adult. The question, then, is whether spontaneous heartbeat, without assisted respiration and with a flat EEG, is possible. (No data are available on the matter.) The question becomes whether the extrauterine

fetus with flat EEG, like his adult counterpart, may be pronounced dead, yet perfused for purposes of, say, thymus transplantation. Such an analysis would be based on the ethical problems of transplantation and the definition of death, rather than on ethical problems of fetal experimentation. Neither would the issue of "immoral procurement," raised about the dead fetus above, be the same, since the issue of thymus transplantation arises so rarely as to fall outside the notion of a *systematic* policy of taking advantage of an allegedly immoral practice. It is more like using corneas obtained from an occasional adult victim of homicide—in which case no one suggests approval of the murder or approval of systematically taking advantage of the process of murder.

THE VIABLE FETUS

One presumes that few ethical problems are specific to the viable fetus, since it is considered a premature infant in obstetrics, and therefore no different from other newborn infants in ethical terms.

It should be realized that those who might argue for the wrongness of fetal experimentation in a given case would not necessarily prohibit all fetal experimentation. If it were shown that for some good of humankind such as survival, fetal experimentation was an absolute requirement, such ethicists might argue for measures like those taken in war. Then, consent giving in fighting a common enemy is abrogated and a draft system instituted. The ethical question becomes how drafting is to be done ethically. In recent times the lottery system has been used precisely because it does not choose *against* individuals on the basis of their social worth (Ramsey). It is sometimes argued that bugging of individuals without obtaining their consent can be ethically defended if the defense security of the nation (some greater good than privacy) is seen to be at stake. Similarly, it may be argued that fetal experimentation would be justified without consent if some greater good were at stake. The issue would become which fetus to "bug," since presumably no particular fetus would be in that critical position of the individual bugged for defense reasons. Granted the premise, a lottery system might logically be suggested.

Given all these considerations pertaining to the ethics of abortion and fetal research, it should come as no surprise that, as each legislature has enlarged the conditions under which abortion may be performed, ethical issues concerning fetal experimentation have been raised. The early 1970s saw public protests against such experiments (Ramsey).

In general, those most opposed to abortion also protest most against fetal experimentation. In one way this link seems obvious. If it is held that fetuses would and could not consent to be killed in utero, one could plausibly argue that they might not consent to be experimented upon either. On the other hand, it can be confidently said that not all protesters against fetal research on the grounds that they were opposed to abortion thought the issues through consistently. As has been seen in the discussion of abortion, above, opposition to abortion is largely based on the premise that the fetus is in a sense already a child, albeit in utero. If the fetus is already a child is one opposed to fetal research because one is opposed to *pediatric* research? So put, the issues appear more clearly. Several conclusions are possible: (1) I am opposed to both; (2) I am opposed to neither; (3) I am opposed to one, but not the other. And under each of these headings it is possible, for specific reasons, to differentiate among conditions which would have to be met, ethically, in order to be in favor of either, neither, or both.

In the United States this analysis was a task given to the National Commission for the Protection of Human Subjects in Biomedical and Behavioral Research. The Commission was asked to establish guidelines under which fetal, infant, and other research might appropriately be carried out. Let us now consider the conclusions reached by this Commission.

The Commission adopted the general principle that fetal research could be done if it was (1) important; (2) if sufficient animal research had preceded the human research; (3) if consent had been obtained from the mother, and (4) if the father did not dissent. With these preconditions, the Commission set the following rules for specific categories of fetuses:

1. So-called therapeutic or beneficial research (i.e., research from which *that specific fetus* could benefit) can be done on the pregnant woman, provided the fetus is placed at minimum risk consistent with meeting the health needs of the mother.
2. Nontherapeutic research (i.e., research from which *that specific fetus* cannot possibly benefit) may be done on pregnant women, provided minimal or no risk accrues to the well-being of the fetus.
3. Nontherapeutic research of the fetus in utero who is *not* to be aborted may be done, provided there is minimal or no risk to the well-being of the fetus.

4. Nontherapeutic research on the fetus in utero who *is* to be aborted should follow the same rules as under number 3 above, but if there is difficulty in interpreting the rule, the Secretary of the U.S. Department of Health, Education, and Welfare may approve the research if it has been approved by a national ethical review board.
5. Nontherapeutic research on the fetus *during* the abortion procedure or on the *live nonviable fetus outside* the womb may be performed if:
   (a) the fetus is less than 20 weeks old
   (b) the abortion procedure is not changed for purposes of the research
   (c) the duration of fetal life is not altered by the research
6. Nontherapeutic research on the *possibly* viable fetus may be performed if no additional risk is imposed on the well-being of the fetus.
7. Research on dead fetuses or their tissues may be done if consistent with local laws and with commonly held respect for dead bodies.
8. The advisability, timing, and method of abortion should not be altered for research purposes.
9. There should be no monetary transactions in fetal research.
10. Fetal research, funded by the United States government outside the United States, should apply the same principles as within the country.

In summary, it is expected of us in fetal research that we shall treat the dead fetus like a dead human being; that we shall not damage fetuses who have a chance of survival, either because they are likely to survive outside of the uterus or because, if they are still in utero, their mothers may change their minds about the abortion. If they are surely going to die, we are asked not to shorten or lengthen their life-span for purposes of experimentation—a reasonable request to which we would surely adhere for other dying patients. It may be argued by some (e.g., Ramsey) that no competents can ever enroll incompetents in any experiment from which they cannot possibly benefit. It may also be argued that mothers who are about to abort their fetuses are unfit consent givers for experimentation upon fetuses whom they are already prepared to see dead. But that assumes that abortion is always a preparedness to see the fetus dead and begs the question, asked above, whether abortion is at heart an issue of separating parties in conflict or assuring the death of one. It also begs the question whether any children (intra- or extrauterine) can ever be the subjects of nontherapeutic research. Eminent ethicists (like Richard McCormick) have argued that they can be if it can be deduced that they would be cause they morally should.

Suffice it here to say that national commissions cannot be expected to do normative ethics. By their very political composition they arrive at compromises among competing claims as to what constitutes the right and the wrong. It is not the purpose of this chapter to adjudicate among the claims, but rather to elucidate them.

CONTRACEPTION

Clearly, contraception and its permanent form, sterilization, differ conceptually from abortion in that no ethical issues surrounding the nature of the conceptus can arise. Nevertheless, many ethical debates still involve the subject of contraception. These debates largely surround two issues.

1. What method of contraception is being discussed: Is it so-called natural family planning, so-called artificial contraception, or a so-called abortifacient agent?
2. Who can give consent to the use and provision of contraceptive methods?

MODE OF ACTION

Debates surrounding the use of natural versus artificial methods of family planning have greatly abated in recent years. Nevertheless, the official teaching of a major religious body, the Roman Catholic Church, still holds that the use of artificial contraceptives is wrong.

This teaching is grounded on two principles:

1. It is wrong to turn oneself wittingly and willingly against the consequences of acts voluntarily entered into.
2. By observing nature it is patently obvious that the act of intercourse is, by its nature, designed for the procreation of children (natural law).

The latter argument does not deny that intercourse serves other purposes, such as the expression of love (sometimes called the *unitive* rather than the procreative purpose of intercourse). Neither does the argument assert that no intercourse may be had unless procreation results, for the Catholic tradition has long permitted intercourse postmenopausally. Rather, the tradition holds that the unitive and procreative purposes of intercourse may not be artificially separated. Thus this tradition would not only condemn artificial contraception (seeking to retain the unitive—called in secular terms the "recreational" aspects of intercourse—while separating it by artifice from the procreative) but it would also condemn artificial insemination, in vitro fertilization, embryo transfer, and cloning as procreation separated from intercourse.

The tradition does permit intercourse where the person is infertile, whether postmenopausally, during infertile parts of the menstrual cycle, following surgical sterility performed for purposes other than inducing the sterility, or in the presence of sterility resulting from conditions beyond the individual's control, e.g., azospermia. The studied use of intercourse for unitive purposes (or the expression of love) during the infertile phase of the menstrual cycle is therefore not frowned upon. The argument proceeds from the notion that nature is a given, both in its fertile and infertile aspects, but that the infertile state may not be willfully induced.

Where the mode of action of a family-planning method is based on an effect occurring after fertilization, the method is called "abortificient." Commonly it is held that such methods include the IUD (intrauterine device), minipills, and morning-after agents. Clearly this analysis is based on the notion that almost absolute value attaches to nascent life from the moment of conception (see the preceding section, Abortion). Quite clearly if the full value of fetal life (value A) is not assigned to a fetus on day 1 (F_1), then there is a grey area between biological fertilization and the point in fetal development where near-absolute value is assigned to fetal life. Such a grey area would constitute a neutral zone in which an agent would be deemed to be biologically not preventing fertilization, but morally not constituting abortion. For instance, some authors (Hellegers; Ramsey) have argued that the possibility that two products of conception can be combined into one (total body chimerism) means that irreversible human individuality does not occur until some time after fertilization. Therefore, prior to the time that this phenomenon of total body chimerism takes place, they would hold the conceptus to be less than fully "ensouled," "dignified," "protection worthy," or endowed with those qualities of individual human life which are at the core of the abortion debate.

Lest the lines of reasoning be deemed esoteric, it is worth remembering that throughout history forms of human life (whether fetal, newborn, Negro, Jewish, Protestant, Catholic, etc.) have been cheapened on the basis of all sorts of intellectual and socioeconomic reasons, with history usually taking a dim view of such trends, at least in retrospect.

CONSENT

The issue of consent giving to contraception is a subspecies of all issues affecting the giving of free and informed consent by individuals. The consent issue involves gynecology and obstetrics in such areas as contraception, sterilization, abortion, fetal experimentation, and the prolongation of life. in general, it is assumed that adults are capable of giving free and informed consent provided they are not incarcerated and provided proper procedures are followed to accurately transmit the information upon which they are to give consent. Whether this involves transmitting information about all complications which might possibly, rather than probably, occur is not yet clear. The greatest difficulty with the issue of consent lies in the area of proxy consent giving, i.e., giving consent on behalf of another, whether a minor or an incompetent. The question is largely one of knowing who may give consent and for what consent may be given. Certain rights are deemed basic, and among these the right to life and the right to procreate are usually thought the most fundamental.

With respect to the right to procreate, or even to have intercourse, certain problems clearly arise. Most countries, societies, or churches demand a certain maturity, usually expressed as a minimum age, to permit entry into the marriage contract, whose subject matter is intercourse. Anyone engaging in intercourse with a minor or with an incompetent may be accused of statutory rape. Throughout the ages, debates have been held on what the appropriate age should be. It varies from country to country and from state to state. In former centuries, the age of 7 was held to be sufficient, that being the age when children were thought to enter into the age of reason and to be capable of distinguishing right from wrong (Sanchez). Although in the recently proposed guidelines of the Department of Health, Education, and Welfare the age of 7 is not considered sufficient to *consent* to medical procedures, it is considered sufficient to *refuse* to consent in spite of parental opinion (Department of Health, Education, and Welfare).

In more recent centuries, the age of 14 has been proposed as minimal for marriage, on the assumption that greater maturity is required for intercourse and marriage than simply being able to distinguish right acts from wrong (Aquinas). In canon law cases, it has been held that where the menarche has occurred, the

presumption should be that the woman has sufficient advertence to understand the purposes of intercourse (Van Ommeren). It is alleged that the age of onset of the menarche has been decreasing at a rate of about 4 months per decade (Tanner) and in the United States now averages about 12.7 years. Thus, without change in the minimum legal marital age, the physical capability and desire for intercourse may exist, but its exercise may fall under statutory rape laws. In most ethical systems, the provision of a contraceptive agent to an adult woman to protect her against the consequences of involuntary rape would be accepted. The Roman Catholic Church (Palazzini; Hurth; Lambruschini) held the use of such agents proper for religious sisters in imminent danger of being raped during the 1960 insurrection in the former Belgian Congo. An attempt has been made to extend the analysis from involuntary to statutory rape, since in both cases the ethical underpinnings might be the same, namely that no *human* act is involved in such biological intercourse (Hellegers, 1965). Human acts, in such analyses, are defined as acts performed with full knowledge and advertence of their purposes and consequences, and are usually analyzed in terms of the mental age of the person performing the act. What is obviously unclear is who could give consent for the contraceptive agent but not for the intercourse, or vice versa, since both depend on free will and knowledge for their ethical justification. Clearly, the ethics of the situation for minors is as controverted as it is in the law.

The conundrum can best be explained in terms of the recent legal case involving movie director Roman Polanski. Few today would have hesitated to provide a contraceptive agent to the 13-year-old girl with whom he engaged in his sexual practices. Yet Polanski was condemned for those practices. What ethical role would a physician play who might have provided the girl with contraceptive agents? In a society in which contraceptives may be dispensed upon request to minors without parental consent, the legal and philosophical entity of statutory rape cannot long persist. It is therefore not surprising that, in spite of massive sexual activity by young teenagers, it is now extremely rare for prosecutors to take statutory rape cases to court.

STERILIZATION

The considerations pertaining to contraception apply even more to sterilization. Not only is there the issue of giving consent to surgery, but, since the procedure is designed to be irreversible, the decision made is irrevocable. This is what most differentiates sterilization from contraception.

As a consequence, recent city ordinances (New York) and federal guidelines (D.H.E.W.) have sought to establish procedures to ensure true consent giving to sterilization procedures. The mechanism proposed insists on a "cooling off" period between the signing of the sterilization papers and the performance of the actual procedure. The established waiting period is 30 days. This waiting period inevitably means that many women will have to undergo two separate operations where one would have sufficed, e.g., an unforeseen cesarean section or hysterotomy. Moreover, it may call for the administration of more than one anesthetic. In cases of abortion, the waiting period may delay performance of that procedure with attendant risks of fetal survival. (If that is considered a disvalue, see previous section, on Abortion.) It is also likely to induce physicians to bring up the issue of sterilization in every pregnancy in order "to have the papers ready, just in case" where previously many physicians never discussed sterilization unless the patient broached the subject. Whether the broaching of the subject by physicians during pregnancy is, in the aggregate, the best way to maximize consent giving is, at the least, problematic. It is also proposed that no one can give consent to be sterilized who has not reached the age of 18, regardless of parity or state of health. Thus, what were once known as therapeutic sterilizations, e.g., for Eisenmenger's complex, may no longer be performed, in spite of the fact that such diseases are no respecters of age.

These regulations raise interesting theoretical questions. First, the lack of exceptions to the cooling-off or age provisions of the regulations assumes the ethical principle that the well-being of a minority may be abrogated for that of a majority. This principle is widely accepted in ethical theory. It does, however, beg the question of whether better rules could not have been written which would have allowed exceptions to the general rules under given circumstances. Admittedly, the language of exception would have led to some untoward effects, but so does the language of no exception. Granted two potential evils, the ethical question asks which is the lesser. The language of no exception will lead to some increase in mortality and morbidity; the language of exception will lead to some unwanted loss of fertility. The ultimate question is: How much wanted fertility is worth how much mortality or morbidity?

The regulations have an interest for ethical theory in another aspect. Clearly we are now in a paradoxical situation with respect to consent giving in gynecology and obstetrics. Minors may now theoretically give consent for contraception and abortion, but not for intercourse or sterilization. Were this approach to be grounded in ethical theory, it would tell us clearly that consent giving is not dependent on achieving a certain all-round ability of mind, but rather on the nature of that to which consent is to be given. The latter approach clearly connotes a value assessment by a public at large. For instance, certain states now permit men or women to get married whom they will not permit to get sterilized.

Nowhere is the ethical theory surrounding contraception or sterilization more controversial than in the subject of mental retardation. A recent court decision forbids the use of federal funding for sterilization of the retarded (*Relf* v. *Weinberger*). It would be interesting to know who, if abortion postimpregnation were to be funded, would be thought the appropriate consent giver in such a case. In a recent case, on appeal, a minor was allowed to refuse to undergo an abortion, although in a lower court her parents' insistence on its performance had been granted (*in re Smith*). No case has yet been adjudicated where a mentally retarded girl has requested or refused an abortion, based on her own consent giving. In other words, it is not yet clear whether minors and incompetents are to be treated totally analogously in law.

Quite apart from the ethical analysis of contraception or sterilization for a given minor or incompetent, there is a need for social-ethical analysis. Although the ethical analysis might well say that, in a given case, contraception or sterilization would be ethical, such action might still be prohibited on social-ethical grounds as containing too great a danger that states or communities might introduce unethical policies. Mental retardation caused by purely genetic factors is usually accompanied by infertility. Hence, almost all sterilization involves women who are retarded on an environmental or social basis. The danger exists that social, rather than medical, notions could begin to determine who was sufficiently bright to procreate. Moreover, it is not clear why breeding for brightness should, for instance, take precedence over breeding for honesty, or morality, or fidelity, unless certain value systems are presumed. For these reasons, many might therefore legally or ethically prohibit sterilization of a given retardate on the basis of a *social*-ethical rather than an *act*-ethical analysis. Left unanswered is whether a given set of parents could give consent for contraception or sterilization for a given retarded child in order to protect it from the consequences of statutory rape.

Where the alternative is institutionalization of the retardate in personality-destroying circumstances, it may be argued that the personal interests of the retardate may best be served by contraception or sterilization. Such an analysis might hold that parentally proposed sterilization or contraception does not carry the social-ethical dangers existing when the *state* becomes the consent giver. Such a parental consent-giving case has not yet gone before the Supreme Court.

These facts should be analyzed against a background of data which show that the retarded have, if anything, a lesser tendency towards promiscuity and infidelity than college graduates.

At bottom, all the above considerations stem from one fundamental fact in societal perception. It is that intercourse and procreation are no longer perceived as directly linked in nature. Over a prolonged period of time, at least in Western culture, the so-called recreational aspects of sex have overtaken the procreational aspects.

SEX THERAPY

The separation of procreational and recreational aspects of sex nowhere comes out more clearly than in ethical problems in sex therapy. Where the purpose of intercourse is deemed to be procreational and where, through impotence or infertility, the procreational end cannot be achieved, it can be plausibly argued that correction of these conditions deals with the corrections of physical defects. Less clearly, but still plausibly, the same can be said in cases of dyspareunia or anorgasmy. It can be argued that insofar as intercourse without pain and with orgasm is a normal condition (even though unnecessary for procreation), interfering physical conditions should be treated so that normalcy can be attained.

Obviously, arguments of this nature become considerably blurred when it is held that it is a medical function to make *any* sexual practice more pleasurable. Ultimately, such arguments say that homosexuality, lesbianism, etc., are "normal" conditions, not to be "corrected." The question then is what disease is the therapist treating? As the psychiatrist Redlich has put it: It is not clear whether we should speak of the practitioners of sex therapy as therapists, educators, or instructors, or their subjects as patients, clients, or students.

Perhaps the dilemma is best put in question form: Suppose that by the swallowing of a single pill, total homosexuality could instantaneously be turned into heterosexuality, how should the patient and the therapist act? It becomes apparent that just as, at one end of a spectrum, there are those who advocate a primary stress on the procreational aspects of sex, there are, at the other end, those who advocate a primary stress on the recreational. The achievement of perfect hedonism (in the nonpejorative sense of that word) can thus be seen as one of the purposes of medicine. It asks the fundamental question: To what end should we biologize?

The perplexing nature of the question can perhaps also be illustrated in the age-old consent question, already alluded to in previous sections of this chapter. At what age can consent to sexual activity legitimately be given? With very few exceptions, even the strongest advocates of the recreational aspects of sex have qualms about permitting sexual activity between adults and children. The question is: Why? No such qualms exist about children engaging in other forms of recreation such as softball, cycling, soccer, etc.

All that can be said conclusively at this point is that there is as yet no coherent ethic of sex therapy in medicine, although laudatory initial attempts to arrive at a systematized ethic are beginning to be made (Masters, Johnson; Kolodny).

DEATH AND DYING

Up to now we have dealt with issues mostly of concern to obstetricians. The dying of adults is more likely to be of concern to gynecologists, and especially to oncologists. There is little doubt that the issue of euthanasia is being discussed today with the interest that abortion was, say, two decades ago. Again, the specialist should be conversant with the common analyses proffered.

The most important principle to keep in mind in discussions of the subject is that no physician has an innate right to treat a patient without that patient's consent. Like all other citizens, physicians have the right and perhaps the duty to prevent people from killing themselves, but, if this is so, the right or duty does not derive from one's diploma; it derives from being a member of the human race.

A second principle, but an ethical rather than a legal one, is that there is no ethical duty to prolong a patient's *dying* (Pius XII). Analytical difficulties arise because the converse of dying is thought of as living, and all living must end in death. The question then becomes: At what point does dying commence?

A third, key, principle used in many debates on

death and dying is that there *is* a difference between omission and commission of acts. This is ethically controverted, but the reason for the controversy on this point can be clarified somewhat. Where the consequences of acting or not acting are unknown, people have little difficulty in understanding the difference. Thus, if sitting on a chair at home at night seems to have no direct consequences, people can easily accept that it is different from getting up to pick up a newspaper. The difficulty seems to arise when, whether one acts or does not act, an identical foreseeable result occurs which is extraneous to one's acting or not. This is the problem for the physician who knows a patient will die whether the physician acts or does not. Many would then see no moral difference between inducing the death and letting it occur, even though they might realize that the former involves positing an act, and the latter does not. Therefore, it is not the difference between omission and commission of acts which is not understood, rather it is the *moral* difference between these entities which is the key issue.

To follow debates on this issue, one must understand the linguistics of the debate. Several terms are frequently used:

1. *Negative or passive euthanasia* is here defined as the *non*administration of an agent, without which the occurrence of death, and perhaps its time of occurrence, is reasonably foreseeable, whether it is preventable or not.
2. *Positive or active euthanasia* here is described as positive, or active, if a person other than the dying one administers an agent (like a bullet or product) which induces the death as a direct, intended result of the administration of the agent. Euthanasia here means "good death."
3. *Facilitated suicide* is the induction of one's own death after someone else has purposely made available the agent with which the death can be induced.
4. *Suicide* is the induction of one's death by administration of a lethal agent, not intentionally procured by someone else.

Within the framework of this terminology, issues in the euthanasia debate are presented in a reverse order to the list shown above.

SUICIDE

In general, society seems to hold the view that suicide is not a rational act to which one can give free and

informed consent. On the basis of this assumed lack of consent, individual and societal interference with suicide is accepted. On this assumption also, many jurisdictions automatically proclaim suicide to have been committed "while of unsound mind." Yet this notion of "unsound mind" is not totally accepted, for instance in suicide following the taking out of a large insurance policy. Therefore, while generally accepted medically as a "disease," suicide is not necessarily so seen commercially.

FACILITATED SUICIDE

Since a large part of the euthanasia debate hinges around notions of whether the patient really wishes to die and consents to it freely and knowingly, it may be argued that the best way to assure this consent is to make the means for suicide available. The means will then be used or not by the patient, revealing the degree of true consent. This, of course, concedes that suicide can be rational, a notion not readily held by physicians.

POSITIVE EUTHANASIA

Apart from the ethics of positively inducing death in another, the issue of free and informed consent again arises. Obviously, facilitated suicide gives proof positive of the intent to die by the taking of the lethal agent, assuming that suicide is ever rational.

Less clear is the situation where the person to whom "the good death" is to be administered cannot give consent because unconscious, non compos mentis, a minor, or an incompetent. If it is thought that next of kin are legally and ethically capable of providing such proxy consent for relatives, the issue still remains whether they do so freely and with informed judgment. If the physician is convinced they do not intend to kill for other than altruistic motives, an initial logical analogy to arguments for facilitated suicide might say that facilitated positive euthanasia would be the most rigid test of the consent of the relatives. The physician could then supply the agent and the next of kin administer it.

These issues are raised because they may help to clarify a question. How full and informed is the consent for death to be? There is a theoretical problem with the "humane" suggestion that euthanasia should be provided by the physician while the patient is unaware of it and no kin is looking on. This procedure, suggested for its humanity, seems at odds with an ultimate test of the consent postulated as underlying its justification. "Euthanasia in the dark" suggests only "sufficient" consent rather than free and fully informed consent.

NEGATIVE EUTHANASIA

The ethical justification for negative euthanasia rests on the notion that humans have no absolute moral obligation to survive, at all costs, for as long as possible. Taken from the point of view of the physician, the justification rests on the notion that no physician may impose ministrations on patients without their consent. If this principle is accepted, then the issue of consent to negative euthanasia is largely resolved and starkly different from that in positive euthanasia. The physician is no longer expected to cure; he or she is only asked, perhaps, to care. The issue becomes solely one of the patient's ethics rather than the physician's. What are the patient's moral duties to survive at all cost, rather than the physician's duties to minister?

It is generally held in all ethical systems of analysis that there can be no moral duty to prolong one's dying. This principle is sometimes expressed by saying that no individual is required to undergo "extraordinary means" or "heroic measures" to sustain a continuation of living or dying. Many misunderstand the terms.

The adjective "extraordinary" does not just qualify the means. It also describes the situation of the patient. Certainly morphine and oxygen are commonly used in medicine, and are not considered extraordinary means or heroic measures in therapy for, say, a myocardial infarction. If, however, a patient is in the terminal phase of life with a generalized carcinomatosis, a myocardial infarction might well be viewed as a godsend, and it would make little medical or ethical sense to resuscitate the patient from the effects of the infarction to permit her to die from the carcinomatosis. Thus the words extraordinary and heroic refer to the patient as much as to the means. All means which are useless in preventing death in the condition in which the patient is can be called extraordinary.

The key question, however, remains for what condition of one's body or mind one may forfeit therapy. We have noted that it is widely held that having started one's dying, one may forgo further therapy. Some ethical systems, particularly the Roman Catholic, have extended the principle much further (Kelly). If the therapy will leave one with intolerable pain or in a totally repugnant state, or will totally ruin one's dependents financially, the individual may refuse further therapy. The reason for the principle or an adequate delineation of its limits has never been fully explained. It remains one of the great areas of study for bioethics. In part, the principle is founded on the religious notion of a purpose in life—to love and serve God and be forever happily united with Him in the hereafter. Where the conditions of loving and serving God are no longer present, a part of the reason for living has disappeared. This would not be lightly assumed since even suffering is, under that system, assumed to have a good purpose (McCormick).

Under this same system, pain-killing drugs may be given in sufficient quantity to overcome the pain even though life may be shortened as a consequence (O'Donnell).

Under another analysis, once the dying has started, the physician's duty changes from a primary one of curing to one of caring. Should the patient then reach a point where she is no longer capable of receiving care, the theoretical possibility of positive euthanasia is contemplated (Ramsey).

What seems common to all analyses is that the patient has no inherent moral duty to undergo, or the physician to administer, therapy once death is inevitable. Only ordinary care such as food and drink may not be purposely withheld.

DEATH-WITH-DIGNITY LAWS AND LIVING WILLS

At present such proposals base themselves ethically on the acceptability of negative euthanasia, or the withholding of extraordinary means of treatment to terminally ill patients. On the basis of anecdotal, rather than empirical, data, it is alleged that doctors today tend not to be willing to let terminally ill patients die. There are really no hard data to prove that it takes longer to die today than heretofore. One difference may be that dying is done more in hospitals than in homes, as in the past, and is therefore more expensive and perceived to last longer. The classic instance in which fracture of the femur of an elderly person was followed by prolonged immobilization in bed, orthostatic pneumonia, and death is now in the past; this is no longer a classical way of dying and therefore scarcely remembered. Nor is the prolonged, slow death due to cardiovascular disease from valvular lesions incident to rheumatic fever. Another possible difference with the past may be that although death is ultimately as inevitable a concomitant of life as in the past, the actual process of dying is no longer as acceptable. It is perhaps the dying which is today more feared than the death. It may be part of what has been called a quest for a "discomfort-free society" (Cooke).

Be that as it may, several considerations arise. There is nothing which prevents anyone from carrying around a document which describes how he or she wishes to be treated if dying. Indeed, anyone can carry around the neck a medallion with medical information, as is already done by those with allergies, blood groups, Rh, etc. What is newly proposed is that such instructions be embodied in law (*death with dignity*). Laws must have teeth in them to be worthwhile. What is to be enforced? By whom? At present, the general premise is that physicians may impose no therapy unless requested or agreed to with full and informed consent by the patient. Proposals for living wills imply that patients must protect themselves against the undesired ministrations of physicians by warding them off in advance. Additionally, the living-will system deaccentuates input from families. In part this results from the perception that families, under stress from the impending death of a relative, may not act in her best behalf, but rather on their own behalf, to reduce guilt feelings by assuring that "all that could be done was done." This same attitude may govern physicians' actions. If present alleged practices are considered unacceptable, the premise of their unacceptability is that the guilt feelings and grieving of relatives should not form part of how the dying patient is to be treated. The premise assigns first priority to the dying patient, who is not to be used as a means by grieving families or physicians with feelings of medical impotence.

Possible ethical problems arise from the proposals. First, they are often based on actions to be taken, or not taken, by physicians under certain circumstances which can be only vaguely described, i.e., if there is a "significant chance," if there is a "substantial risk," if there is "serious reason to believe," etc. Such entities are hardly quantifiable in acute emergencies. If, in future, excessive therapy is to be punishable by law, it may well lead to undertreatment, just as present punishment of deficient therapy may lead to excessive testing and nonessential procedures.

Conversely, the absence of a "living will" may carry certain implications of assumptions to be made about patients' wishes. To be intestate in a world of wills has always carried its own risks. Is the absence of a living will an indication that this patient wishes extraordinary means to be administered? And what then would be the role of family desires?

In brief, the predicament of the medical profession is that its function is to oppose death with dignity with an option of life with dignity. Conversely, no one can advocate the other alternative to death with dignity, which would be death with *indignity*. The problem is to know how the teeth in death-with-dignity laws would work out in practice. Perhaps a more viable and wiser alternative to laws is to educate physicians that death is inevitable, that it is part of the physician's function to accompany the patient through the process, that at such times the family is as much a part of the process as the patient, and that it is unethical for the physician to relieve his own anxieties and frustrations at his powerlessness in the face of death at the expense of those for whom he is to be a servant rather than a master. If it is clear to the physician that a patient is intent on harming himself without cause, the physician, like any other citizen, has recourse to the courts to demand therapy. It should, however, be an uncommon occurrence, if doctors are not to be depicted as believing that they own patients or are protectors of life through some function other than a skill given on request. If this lesson is not learned, criteria may someday be written into law which will remove the freedom to treat or not to treat presently arrived at by free contract.

Two recent cases best illustrate the problems in trying to legislate the dying process. The first case is that of Karen Ann Quinlan, who was in a coma for several months from unknown causes. The overwhelming opinion of the medical profession was that she would never emerge from that coma. Her EEG showed she was not dead. Her adoptive parents pleaded that she be removed from the respirator and allowed to die. Her physicians refused. It is not clear whether they were motivated by fear of being accused of homicide or malpractice, or because they felt obligated to continue treating her as long as technically possible. A first judge (Muir) held that it was solely up to the physicians to decide whether treatment should be continued. The Supreme Court of New Jersey reversed that judgment. The court followed the reasoning above, which justifies a refusal to undergo extraordinary means of therapy. It said in essence that, were Karen Quinlan to have a lucid moment and know that she would be on a respirator, never again to emerge from her coma, she might well decide not to continue the therapy indefinitely. The court held that the family, together with the physicians and a hospital ethics committee, could decide to disconnect the respirator. The role assigned to the ethics committee was more that of a prognosis committee than a therapy-deciding one.

More recently, the Supreme Court of Massachusetts issued a judgment in the case of Joseph Saikewicz. The patient, a 67-year-old, severely retarded person with an IQ of 10, had lived for several years in a home for the mentally retarded. He developed acute myeloblastic monocytic leukemia, and it was proposed to administer chemotherapy, even though it was felt that this would only prolong the patient's life (or dying) by several months. The court held that Mr. Saikewicz would not understand the pain, nausea, and other side effects caused by the chemotherapy, which others would tolerate in the hope of prolonging their life. Then, totally unasked, the court proceeded to criticize the New Jersey court's opinion on how a final decision could be taken. It ordered that in all terminal cases involving incompetents, any decision to start or end life-sustaining therapy should be referred to the courts. Clearly the court had no idea how often such decisions have to be taken.

What emerges is a picture of great confusion in the law. What also emerges is that doctors are divided on these issues. Most of all, however, there emerges the clear picture that unless physicians become capable of clearly articulating the ethical principles by which they act, these principles will be set for them by others. That would turn professionals into mere technicians.

REFERENCES

American College of Obstetricians and Gynecologists: *Further Ethical Considerations in Induced Abortion,* Chicago: ACOG, 1977.

Aquinas T: Commentaria praeclarissima in IV libros sententiarum petri lombardi. Disp. XXVII, q 2, art. 2, ad. 2, Paris, 1659.

Branson R, et al.: A Preliminary Analysis of the Draft DHEW Guidelines for the Protection of Special Subjects in Biomedical Research, Washington, D.C.: The Joseph and Rose Kennedy Institute for the Study of Human Reproduction and Bioethics, Georgetown University, January 4, 1974. *Congressional Record* September 11, 1973, S16350.

Cooke RE: *The Terrible Choice: The Abortion Dilemma,* New York: Bantam Books, 1968.

_____: Whose suffering? *J Pediatr* 80(5):906, 1972.

Death with Dignity, Hearings before the Special Committee on the Aging, U.S. Senate, August 7, 1972, p 33.

Engelhardt HT Jr: The beginnings of personhood: philosophical considerations. *Perkins School of Theology Journal* 27(1):20, Fall 1973.

Gilbert v. General Electric Co., 375 F. Supp. 367 (E.D. Va. 1974), *aff'd.* 519 F. 2d 661 (4th Cir. 1975), *rev'd.* 429 U.S. 125, 97 S. Ct. 401, 50 LEd 2d 343 (1976).

Haney CA: Issues and considerations in requesting an anatomical gift. *Soc Sci Med* 7(8):635, 1973.

Hellegers AE: Some aspects of the use of contraceptive agents in the mentally retarded. *The Jurist* 25(1):106, 1965.

_____: Fetal development. *Theological Studies* 31(1):3, 1970.

_____: The beginnings of personhood: medical considerations. *Perkins School of Theology Journal* 27(1):11, Fall 1973.

_____: Biological origins of bioethical problems, in *Obstetrics and Gynecology Annual,* New York: Appleton-Century-Crofts, 1977, vol 6, pp 1-9.

Hurth F: Il premunirsi nel diritto della legittima difesa. *Studi Cattolici* 27:64, 1961.

Jonsen A, Hellegers, AE: Conceptual foundations for an ethics of medical care, in *Ethics of Health Care,* ed. LR Tancredi, Washington, D.C.: National Academy of Sciences, 1974, pp 3-20. Also appeared in: Veatch RM, Branson R (eds.): *Ethics and Health Policy,* Cambridge, Mass.: Ballinger, 1976, pp 17-33.

Kass, L: New beginnings in life, in *The New Genetics and the Future of Man,* ed. MP Hamilton, Grand Rapids, Mich.: Zerdsman Publishing Co., 1971.

Kelly G: Preserving Life in his *Medico-Moral Problems,* St. Louis: The Catholic Hospital Association, 1957.

Lambruschini F: E legitimo evitare le consequenze dell-agressione. *Studi Cattolici* 27:68, 1961.

Masters W, Johnson V, Kolodny R (eds.): *Ethical Issues in Sex Therapy and Research,* Boston: Little, Brown, 1977.

McCormick RA: Genetic medicine. Notes on the moral literature. *Theological Studies* 33(3):531, 1972.

_____: To save or let die. *JAMA* 229(2):172, 1974. Also appeared in: *America* 130(26):6, 1974.

_____: Proxy consent in the experimentation situation. *Perspect Biol Med* 18(1):2, Autumn 1974.

O'Donnell TJ: *Morals in Medicine,* Westminster, Md.: Newman Press, 1960.

Palazzini P: Si puo e si dere proteggere l'equillibrio della persona. *Studi Cattolici* 27:63, 1961.

Paul VI: Humanae vitae. *Acta Apostolica Sedis* 60, 1968.

Peel Sir J et al.: The use of fetuses and fetal material for research. Report of the Advisory Group, Department of Health and Social Security, Scottish Home and Health Department, Welsh Office, London: Her Majesty's Stationery Office, 1972.

Pius XII: An address by his holiness to the Italian catholic union of midwives, October 29, 1951. *Catholic Mind* 50:49, 1952.

_____: Discourse to doctors. *Acta Apostolica Sedis* 49:1029, 1957.

Quinlan, In the Matter of, 348 A. 2d 801 (N.J. Super. Ct. 1975).

Quinlan, In the Matter of, 355 A 2d 647 (N.J. 1976).

Ramsey P: Choosing how to choose: patients and sparse medical resources, in his *The Patient as Person,* New Haven: Yale University Press, 1970.

_____: Consent as a canon of loyalty with special reference to children in medical investigation, in his *The Patient as Person,* New Haven: Yale University Press, 1970.

_____: On (only) caring for the dying, in his *The Patient as Person,* New Haven: Yale University Press, 1970.

_____: Genetic therapy: a theologian's response, in *The New Genetics and the Future of Man,* ed. MP Hamilton, Grand Rapids, Mich.: Zerdsman Publishing Co., 1971.

_____: *The Ethics of Fetal Research,* New Haven: Yale University Press, 1975.

_____: *Ethics at the Edges of Life: Medical and Legal Intersections,* New Haven: Yale University Press, 1978.

Rawls J: *A Theory of Justice,* Cambridge, Mass.: Belknap Press, 1971.

Redlich F: The ethics of sex therapy, in *Ethical Issues in Sex Therapy and Research,* ed. W Masters et al., Boston: Little, Brown, 1977, pp 143-182.

Relf v. Weinberger, 372 F. Supp. 1196-1205 (1974).

Roe v. Wade, 410 U.S. 113-178 (1973) and *Doe v. Bolton,* 410 U.S. 179-223 (1973).

Sadler BL, Sadler AM Jr: Providing cadaver organs: three legal alternatives. *Hastings Center Studies* 1(1):14, 1973.

Sanchez R: De sancto matrimonii sacramento. Lib. 1, Disp. VIII, no. 5, Antwerp, 1626.

Smith, In re. 295 A, 2d 238 (Med. Court of Special Appeals, 5 October 1972).

Superintendent of Belchertown State School v. Saikewicz, 37ONE 2d 417 (Mass. 1977).

Tanner JM: The trend toward earlier physical maturation, in *Biological Aspects of Social Problems,* eds. JE Meade, AS Parkes, New York: Plenum Press, 1965.

U.S. Department of Health, Education, and Welfare: Protection of human subjects: policies and procedures. *Federal Register* 38(221):31738, 1973.

_____: Protection of human subjects: proposed amendments concerning fetuses, pregnant women, and in vitro fertilization, *Federal Register* 42(9):2792, 1977.

_____: Sterilizations and abortions: federal financial participation, *Federal Register* 42(217):52146, 1978.

_____: Sterilizations and abortions: federal financial participation, *Federal Register* 42(217):52146, 1978.

Van Ommeren WM: *Mental Illness Affecting Matrimonial Consent,* Ph.D. Dissertation, Canon Law Studies No. 415, Washington, D.C.: The Catholic University of America Press, 1961.

World Health Organization: Minutes of the technical preparatory committee for the international health conference, held in Paris from March 18 to April 5, 1946. *Official Records of the World Health Organization* No. 1, 1946.

5

Legal Considerations

ISSUES OF REPRODUCTIVE FREEDOM

NANCY STERNS   RHONDA COPELON

The decision to carry and bear a child has extraordinary ramifications for a woman. Pregnancy entails profound physical changes. Childbirth presents some danger to life and health. Bearing and raising a child demands difficult psychological and social adjustments. The working or student mother frequently must curtail or end her employment or educational opportunities. The mother with an unwanted child may find that it overtaxes her and her family's financial or emotional resources. The unmarried mother will suffer the stigma of having an illegitimate child. Thus, determining whether or not to bear a child is of fundamental importance to a woman.[1]

THE RIGHT TO ABORTION

The gynecologist-obstetrician plays an indispensable role in women's ability to control reproductive function. From the mid-1800s, when restrictive abortion laws were first enacted, to nearly the present, the medical profession supported restrictive abortion laws, even though they had long outlived any health considerations underlying their enactment.

Restrictive abortion statutes fell into three basic categories: those which permitted abortion only when necessary to preserve the life of the woman (Texas);

[1] *Abele v. Markle,* 324 F.Supp. 800, 801–802 (D. Conn., 1972).

those where necessary to preserve life or health; and the "liberalized" or A.L.I.-type statute which also permitted abortion where the pregnancy resulted from rape or incest or where there was a likelihood of fetal deformity (Georgia). The A.L.I. statute normally carried with it a variety of conditions such as obtaining the sanction of hospital committees. Although this so-called liberalized statute was seen as a great breakthrough in the late 1960s, it resulted in a negligible increase in the performance of abortions. This situation changed dramatically when, following a series of favorable decisions in the lower federal and state courts, the United States Supreme Court, in *Roe v. Wade* and *Doe v. Bolton,*[1] extended its earlier decisions recognizing the right to birth control[2] and held that implicit in the liberty and privacy guaranteed by the Constitution is the woman's right to determine whether or not to terminate her pregnancy.

In striking down the restrictive criminal abortion statutes of Texas and Georgia, the Supreme Court set down very specific limits on state power to regulate abortion beyond the standards generally applied to medical services. Moreover, the Court treats such regulation as permissive only, and therefore allows total repeal of any special conditions or limitations on abortion as a constitutional matter.

In articulating the principles that should govern regulation of abortion, the Court developed the "trimester trilogy." During the first trimester, no restrictions may be placed on the performance of abortions. Thus, for example, a state or city may not restrict first-trimester abortions to hospitals or clinics, nor may they establish special more stringent administrative requirements for such clinics. During the second trimester the only constitutionally accepted restrictions are those which are necessary for the health of the woman. Requirements, such as special accreditation for hospitals in which abortions are performed, abortion committees to approve performance of the abortion, and the confirmation of the physician's judgment by two independent doctors, were struck down in *Doe v. Bolton*. In the third trimester, the state may, if it chooses, restrict the performance of abortion except that it must be available where necessary to preserve the life or health, including mental health, of the pregnant woman.

Neither the woman nor the doctor may be required by the state to justify the abortion decision as therapeutic or "medically" indicated in the first two trimesters. The role of the doctor in the abortion decision is basically to facilitate the desired abortion, assuring that the abortion is performed under appropriate precautionary conditions and at an appropriate time in gestation, consistent with technological developments (see Chap. 32). While the Court indicated that the states may limit the performance of abortion to licensed physicians, it did not so require. Therefore, a state could permit the performance of abortions by midwives or other health professionals working under the direction of a licensed physician.

The decriminalization of abortion has had an enormous impact not only on women's liberty and health, but also on the practice of gynecology and obstetrics. Emergency admissions of women and girls suffering from complications of illegal or self-induced abortions has been largely eliminated. Prenatal care is enhanced and labor and delivery are eased by the fact that more pregnancies are wanted.

Since the 1973 decisions, however, efforts have multiplied on all levels of government to restrict the woman's right to obtain and the physician's right and ability to provide appropriate and desired abortion services. None of these restrictions is based on medical considerations. The principal justification is rather that from the moment of fertilization the conceptus is equivalent to fully developed human life, which makes abortion tantamount to murder. This "right to life" claim overrides all other considerations bearing on the life of the pregnant woman, her health and well-being, and the health and well-being of her family or any future child.

Laws founded on the personhood of the conceptus are under challenge in the courts as violating the principle of separation of church and state as well as the privacy of women and physicians. The claim that abortion is immoral and tantamount to murder has been described by legal commentators as "purely religious"[1] and as the product of the "thought . . . of organized religious doctrine."[2] Though its adherents contend that the personhood of the fetus is based on universal moral principles, their viewpoint is not universally shared, even in the religious community. Most Protestant and Jewish denominations, emphasizing individual decision, responsible parenthood, and the primacy of the well-being of the pregnant woman, consider the right to choose abortion a matter of religious liberty, and abortion, in some circumstances, the moral and religiously required choice.

The ultimate goal of the antiabortion forces is a constitutional amendment prohibiting all abortion. At

---

[1]*Doe v. Bolton,* 410 U.S. 113, 410 U.S. 179(1973).
[2]In 1965, in *Griswold v. Connecticut,* 381 U.S. 479 (1965), the Court held that states could not interfere with the right of married couples to use contraceptives. This right was extended to single women and men in *Eisenstadt v. Baird,* 405 U.S. 438 (1972).

[1]Calabresi G: Birth, death and the law. *The Pharas,* April 1974, p.10.
[2]Tribe LH: The Supreme Court, 1972 term—Forward. *87 Howard Law Review* 20,1973.

present, they seek to restrict abortions in every way possible, including, for example, attacking the practice of amniocentesis because one of its consequences may be a decision to abort a seriously defective fetus. Their successes in the legislatures and the courts fall heaviest on the most vulnerable—the young and the poor. Many issues are still unresolved. The outcome of these battles in the courts and legislatures will have a tremendous impact on the scope and quality of care physicians will be able to provide.

PATIENT'S CONSENT

Laws requiring consent which are designed to assure that a woman is informed of the procedure and its consequences and is choosing abortion without coercion are unobjectionable as a constitutional matter.[2]

Constitutional issues of substantial proportions arise, however, when the consent procedure is used as a means to obstruct abortion. A so-called "informed consent" ordinance adopted in some anti-abortion strongholds is constitutionally suspect for two reasons. First, it is completely one-sided, requiring doctors to communicate a list of statistically infrequent and, in many cases, spurious risks associated with abortion, with no mention of its benefits or of the statistically more significant risks associated with its alternative, childbearing. Second, by requiring doctors to advise the woman that the fetus is "human life" from the moment of conception, it compels doctors to profess and women to be subjected to one religious view on the personhood of the fetus, in violation of the First Amendment.

HUSBAND/FATHER CONSENT

In 1976 the Supreme Court declared unconstitutional a statute which required the consent of husband or putative father before an abortion could be performed.[2] Until recently it was not uncommon for doctors and hospitals to require written consent of the husband as a condition to performing an abortion or sterilization. By contrast, the wife's consent has generally not been required for vasectomies. The consent requirement, though based in a few states on statutes, appears for the most part to have been motivated by doctors' fear of lawsuits by angered spouses. Since a husband has no legal right to impede the abortion de-

cision, the fear of liability is unrealistic. The Court also rejected as a constitutional matter the paternalism that often underlay these consent requirements:

> The obvious fact is that when the wife and the husband disagree on this decision, the view of only one of the two marriage partners can prevail. Since it is the woman who physically bears the child and who is more directly and immediately affected by the pregnancy, as between the two, the balance weighs in her favor.

Thus, if a man and woman disagree regarding her insistence upon having an abortion or sterilization, that is a matter for them to settle between themselves. The conflict is frequently resolved by estrangement and/or divorce; neither the doctor nor the law may seek to resolve it by withholding the necessary medical treatment.

RIGHTS OF MINORS

It is also not uncommon for doctors and hospitals to condition the performance of an abortion for a minor upon her obtaining the written consent of her parents. This practice appears to derive mainly from the general common-law notion (embodied in statutes in a few states) that any medical treatment of a minor without parental permission constitutes a battery.[1] Though the battery concept has acted as a strong deterrent, there is not one reported case in which a doctor was successfully sued for battery after treating a minor where the treatment was for the minor's benefit. Nor is there a case reported which has held a doctor liable for providing medical examinations, abortion or family planning services to a minor.[2]

Special statutes requiring parental consent for abortion have been struck down by the U.S. Supreme Court.[3] The question is yet undecided whether a state could condition abortion on parental notification or a prior judicial proceeding. On the other hand, it is generally recognized, and one court has ruled, that parents may not force their minor daughter to have an abortion.[4]

---

[1] Some hospitals utilize the concept of the "emancipated minor" as exceptions to a parental consent requirement. Normally the courts will find that a minor is emancipated if she lives away from home, is employed or self-supporting, or is married (then, of course, the minor may run afoul of a husband's-consent requirement). The doctrine of the "mature minor," capable of giving an intelligent and knowing consent, is also developing in the courts.

[2] Pilpel and Zuckerman, Abortion and the rights of minors. *Case Western Reserve L. Rev.* 23:779, 785 (Summer, 1972).

[3] Ibid.

[4] In re Smith, 16 Md. App. 209, 295A. 2d 23 (1972).

---

[1] Planned Parenthood of Missouri v. Danforth. 428 U.S. 52(1976).

[2] Ibid.

Since nature does not respect the legal definition of adulthood, in many states abortion and birth control matters constitute a special exception to the normal rules requiring parental consent. Given the fundamental nature of the woman's right to control her procreative capacity, she should be able to consent to medical treatment in this area when she reaches childbearing age. The federal government recognizes this principle by defining any female of childbearing age as eligible for family-planning services provided through social service or Medicaid programs. What is more, with respect to abortion, there is a danger that a conflict of interest between parent and child will impede treatment in the best interests of the child. Parents may withhold permission for abortion because of their personal religious beliefs or their anger at learning of their daughter's sexual involvement. Moreover, it may be in the best interests of the child that the parent not be informed of the pregnancy itself.

Of equal importance is assuring the availability of birth control information and services without parental consent. Opponents urge naively that if birth control is not readily available, the teenager will not engage in sexual activity. The Supreme Court rejected this claim and has struck down a statute which prohibited the sale of nonprescription contraceptives to minors under age 16 by anyone other than a duly licensed physician.[1] The question of whether parental notification or consent can be required by statute before birth control counseling or devices can be made available to minors has not yet been decided.

About one-quarter of the states have recognized the special problem of requiring parental consent to pregnancy-related treatment and have legislated a special exception. However, nearly all the states have excepted venereal-disease treatment from the parental-consent requirement. While this is probably because of the communicable nature of the venereal disease, the exceptional treatment recognizes that forcing a minor to inform parents of a condition arising from sexual activity of which the parents disapprove might deter the youth from securing appropriate and necessary treatment.

VIABILITY

States may (and most of them do) proscribe abortion in the third trimester unless necessary to preserve the life or health of the pregnant woman. The constitu-

tional permissibility of restricting abortion in the third trimester turns on the presence of a viable fetus. How the courts define viability and the doctor's responsibility in this regard is essential to a doctor's right and willingness to perform late second-trimester abortions which comprise a small but essential percentage of abortions in the United States.

The Supreme Court used the term "viable" to signify the point when the fetus is potentially capable of meaningful life outside the womb, albeit with artificial aid, noting that this point "is usually placed about 7 months or 28 weeks, but may occur earlier, even at 24 weeks." The Court has recognized that viability is very difficult to assess and emphasized that the decision is one which must be left to the reasonable good-faith judgment of the doctor. The Court has also invalidated a provision which punished as manslaughter the failure to exercise care to preserve a fetus aborted prior to viability, making clear that the manslaughter provisions of criminal law are appropriately invoked only after a viable infant is actually born.[1]

Sensitive to the chilling effect on doctors of the threat of prosecution, the Court's most recent decision stresses that a doctor cannot be held liable for a good faith *subjective* judgment of nonviability—i.e. one based on his or her individual skill and ability—even if a cross-section of the medical community would disagree. It invalidated a statute requiring that if a doctor believes the fetus "may be viable," he or she must use an abortion technique which maximizes the possibility of a live birth so long as a different technique is not necessary to preserve the life or health of the pregnant woman. In ruling that both the "may be viable" standard and the duty to use alternative methods were too vague, the Court emphasized that the physician must be free to give the woman's health and welfare precedence over the fetus. The opinion states that "serious" ethical and constitutional difficulties . . . [would be present if the law required] a 'trade-off' between the woman's health and the additional percentage points of fetal survival."[2]

ACCESS PROBLEMS

A trilogy of Supreme Court decisions in 1977 abandoned settled constitutional principles and stripped the poor of their right to access, through Medicaid or public hospitals, to elective abortion. The scope and

[1]*Carey v. Population Services International,* 431 U.S. 678 (1977).

[1]*Planned Parenthood of Missouri v. Danforth,* 428 U.S. 52(1976).
[2]*Colautti v. Franklin,* (Jan. 7, 1979).

impact of these decisions will be determined within the next few years.

HOSPITALS

In most communities, hospitals are essential to obtaining abortions in the second trimester of gestation, and in the first trimester in communities too small to sustain clinics. Nonetheless, the Supreme Court has also permitted public hospitals to exclude elective abortion services.[1] Questions left open by the Court's decision are whether a public or private hospital which is the only provider of medical care in the community may restrict the provision of abortions; whether the power to deny hospital abortion services applies to paying as well as indigent patients; and whether medically necessary abortions must be provided regardless of wealth or the particular political and moral climate of the community. Doctors with hospital privileges may have a right under their state law or constitution to perform abortions at a public or private hospital regardless of hospital policy to the contrary.

In light of the Supreme Courts's refusal to require hospitals to furnish abortions, it is essential to develop alternatives for second-trimester abortions, as well as to expand first-trimester services. Regulations prohibiting the performance of second-trimester abortions in clinics are under attack as not reasonably necessary to the safety of the pregnant woman undergoing abortion.

A federal statute, known as the Church amendment, enables hospitals receiving federal funds to refuse to perform abortions as a matter of moral or religious belief. The Church amendment also prohibits hospitals from penalizing members of their medical staffs who either refuse or are willing to perform abortions. This latter provision is both constitutional and fair. Likewise, efforts to deny hospital privileges to a doctor who performs abortions at another facility are being challenged as unconstitutional.

PUBLIC FUNDING

For poor women, state or federal reimbursement is an essential in obtaining safe, legal abortions. Thus, restrictions on Medicaid reimbursement are a key objective of the antiabortion forces.

Reacting to their pressure, the Supreme Court

has undermined poor women's right to abortion by allowing states to eliminate "elective" abortion from their Medicaid or other medical assistance programs. The Court has not yet decided, however, whether funding may be denied for therapeutic or medically necessary abortions which it defined broadly in *Doe v. Bolton* as

> a professional judgment that . . . may be exercised in light of all factors—physical, emotional, psychological, familial, and the women's age—relevant to the well being of the patient. All these factors may relate to health. This allows the attending physician the room he [or she] needs to make his [or her] best medical judgment.

Many states have nonetheless eliminated coverage of medically necessary abortions. Congress has also cut off federal funding of abortions except where the doctor certifies that a woman's life would be endangered or severe and long-lasting damage to health would result if the pregnancy were carried to term, or where the pregnancy results from statutory or forced rape or incest promptly reported to a law-enforcement or public health agency.

The only rationale for these restrictions is the claimed personhood of the conceptus. These restrictions are therefore being challenged as establishing and interfering with religious belief as well as denying women needed medical care and interfering with safe, decent medical practice. Doctors testifying in court have criticized the conditions placed on funding as encouraging unethical medical practice at odds with the entire preventive thrust of modern medicine.[1]

The evidence also shows that to avoid bureaucratic review, doctors are generally unwilling to certify eligible cases. Where the funding is restricted, Medicaid-reimbursed abortions have been virtually wiped out even though eminent doctors have testified that the life-endangering exception—broader than the former life-saving exception—should encompass a substantial percentage of the prior Medicaid abortions.[2] Medical experts emphasize the dangers of forcing a poor woman through an unwanted pregnancy. They cite the likelihood that she will resort to self-induced or illegal abortion, as well as the risk that minor health problems will explode into major ones when she is under the stress of an unwanted preg-

---

[1]*Poelker v. Doe,* 432 U.S. (1977).

[1]*McRae v. Califano,* 76 Civ. 1804 (E.O. 'N.Y.).
[2]The chief of OB/GYN Emeritus at New York's St. Vincent's Hospital, which does not perform abortions, estimated that 15% of pregnancies among the poor are life-endangering; Dr. Seymour Romney, an editor of this book, estimated the proportion to be over 50%. *McRae v. Califano.*

nancy and is incapable of observing routine prenatal precautions. Thus, if any restrictions on funding survive court challenge, it is essential that doctors exercise their right to interpret and apply the exceptions to benefit their poor patients. Otherwise, the timidity of doctors will produce restrictions in practice which the legislatures could not have imposed by law.

Except where required by state law, private health insurance frequently does not cover elective abortion and sterilization. Because private insurers are strictly regulated by the state, and often provide employment-related benefits, it is foreseeable that abortion coverage will be limited to the minimum required for the poor.

A more subtle form of discrimination, that between men and women, also permeates governmental funding programs designed to assist reproductive control. Women must have affirmative access to all the means of reproductive control, but to limit the provision of such services to women violates the constitutional guarantee that women and men should be equally burdened and equally benefitted.

The design and attitudes underlying governmental funding programs have contributed to the fact that women today bear virtually all the health risks and the responsibility of birth control. At the core, perhaps, is the fact that far more research and development grants have been devoted to contraceptive measures for women. Also, at the level of delivery of services, federal funds available for family planning are primarily linked to Aid to Families with Dependent Children (AFDC) and therefore limited, in many states, to women. These are sex-discriminatory allocations subject to constitutional challenge.

STERILIZATION

NANCY STEARNS   RHONDA COPELON

We have discussed the problem of conditioning the availability of abortion, sterilization, or birth control on the consent of a third party. Any legal discussion of women's health care would be incomplete without a discussion of the converse problem, involuntary abortion, sterilization, and birth control. Access to abortion, sterilization, and birth control are only one-half of the fundamental liberty protected by the Constitution. Equally sheltered against infringement is the right to procreate. Assuring truly informed consent in regard to such treatment is thus a critical safeguard of constitutional liberty.

The area in which significant abuses are coming to light is that of sterilization of poor and minority women. It is indeed ironic that whereas middle class women have had to go to court to obtain voluntary sterilization, poor women are in danger of the procedure being performed without their consent.

There have been cases where women have awakened from what they thought was minor surgery to learn for the first time that they had been sterilized. The problem, however, is far more subtle than the surprise sterilization. For example, there is a widespread myth that the operation is not permanent and that the tubes will later become "untied." Therefore, even written consent may be neither voluntary nor informed.

Under federally funded programs designed to be voluntary, between 100,000 to 150,000 low-income persons have been sterilized annually over the past few years. In 1974, federal court, reviewing the adequacy of the federal regulation authorizing voluntary sterilization, documented some of the abuses for which both doctors and welfare officers were to be found responsible:

> Although Congress has been insistent that all family planning programs function on a purely voluntary basis, there is incontroverted evidence in the record that minors and other incompetents have been sterilized with federal funds and that an indefinite number of poor people have been improperly coerced into accepting a sterilization operation under the threat that various federally supported welfare benefits would be withdrawn unless they submitted to irreversible sterilization. Patients receiving Medicaid assistance at childbirth are evidently the most frequent targets of this pressure . . . Mrs. Waters was actually refused medical assistance by her attending physician unless she submitted to a tubal ligation.[1]

To redress this situation, the Court ruled that individuals seeking sterilization must be orally informed at the very outset that no federal benefits can be withdrawn if they refuse the sterilization and that this assurance must be prominently displayed on the consent form.

As a result of reports that persons were being sterilized without fully informed or voluntary consent, in November, 1978, the Department of Health, Education, and Welfare issued new guidelines governing federally funded sterilizations.[2] Under those guidelines, the patient must be informed of the

---

[1] *Relf v. Weinburger*, Civil Action 73-1557, U.S. Dist. Ct., District of Columbia (decided March 15, 1974).
[2] 43 Fed. Reg. No. 217, pp. 52146–52175, Nov. 8, 1978.

risks, benefits, and alternatives to sterilization. The consent form must be in the primary language of the patient, or an interpreter must be provided to assist the patient. In addition, 30 days must elapse between the giving of informed consent and the sterilization operation in order to ensure that the sterilization decision is not a precipitous one and is made in a noncoercive atmosphere after the patient has had an opportunity to seek advice of family members, friends, or other doctors.

These guidelines will not prevent all involuntary sterilizations, but they offer one method to ensure that a woman really understands what she is consenting to.

Because hysterectomies are significantly more dangerous than tubal sterilizations, the new guidelines prohibit federal funding of hysterectomies for sterilization purposes. The performance of hysterectomies has been scrutinized more closely in recent years not only because they result in sterilization, but also because studies have shown them frequently to be unnecessary surgery, done for teaching purposes on public patients. Special consent forms have been developed to ensure that the woman understands the risks of and alternatives to the procedure in an effort to minimize unnecessary hysterectomies. These new consent forms may become a model for all surgical consent forms.

Government regulations are only one aspect of the legal protections in this area. Involuntary sterilization also gives rise to the traditional civil damage action for assault or malpractice, and to actions for violation of civil rights, the right to procreate being prominent among them. Since, however, meaningful recourse to the courts for redress of involuntary sterilization is very rare for poor people, the most effective safeguard lies in the sensitivity and conscientiousness of the doctor.

Birth control raises similar problems concerning consent. Doctors often assume that they are better suited to make the decision regarding which form of birth control the woman should use, with scant attention to her preferences or the health hazards involved.[1] Thus it has not been uncommon for doctors and birth control clinics to respond to women's requests for birth control with a package of pills (or in recent years, the insertion of an IUD) without ex-

plaining either the alternatives or the possible dangers of the method selected.

In conclusion, the gynecologist must be supportive in practice and attitude if women are to make and carry out intelligent decisions about their reproductive lives. It is not surprising that many women have seen themselves as the victim, rather than the beneficiary, of such services (Howell). The emerging insistence among women upon self-determination in these matters and the concomitant judicial and legal recognition of their fundamental importance should be recognized—and welcomed—by the profession, to the end of ensuring that these newly won rights will be readily available.

ISSUES OF DYING AND DEATH

ALEXANDER M. CAPRON

The question of euthanasia may not arise often for gynecologists but it may present itself in the treatment of a woman with cancer or where the gynecologist is called in to consult on a patient with another terminal illness. Although physicians have more familiarity with death than most people, it remains a highly charged subject and one which some find difficult to confront. Thus, the best means of caring for the dying patient will have to be worked out according to each doctor's own personality and experience. There are, however, some basic legal rules which should be kept in mind, Although the law has created some confusion, perhaps unnecessarily, in this area, good medical care is consistent with the law with one caveat

ACTIVE EUTHANASIA

The basic constraint on medical decision making about the treatment of the dying patient is the group of laws which prohibit the intentional taking of human life. Traditionally, it makes no difference to the law whether the deceased person was killed voluntarily or unvoluntarily. The consent of the victim is no defense to a homicide charge and, in common law, suicide was also a crime. A change in attitude about the function of the criminal law has led to a revision in suicide laws but not in the basic prohibition on the taking of human life. Suicide is no longer a felony in any state, but three continue to prohibit attempted suicide and most have statutes making it a crime to aid, advise, or

---

[1]This attitude that doctors, not women, should make these basic decisions was exemplified in 1970 by the pressure exerted by the organized medical profession (together with drug companies) against the inclusion in all packages of birth control pills of a detailed warning regarding possible side effects. As a result of that pressure, the Food and Drug Administration was forced to draft what it considered an incomplete "compromise" warning. (Officials Say Millions Get Pill Illegally, *The New York Times*, June 10, 1970).

encourge suicide, or they consider such conduct to be equivalent to murder.

Thus were a gynecologist to administer a poison, such as potassium chloride, to "put the patient out of her misery," he would be exposing himself to prosecution for murder. The good intentions of the physician—to ease the suffering of the patient with no prospect of recovery—would not under current law erase the "malice aforethought," which is the legal term for the willful premeditation that characterizes first-degree murder. Moreover, neither the imminence of death nor the patient's suffering would be a legally effective excuse. Although the time of death may be very near, courts have held the commission of acts intended to accelerate it constitutes murder.[1] Similarly, although jurors may be sympathetic to a physician who has acted out of a desire to end untreatable suffering, such a motive supplies no excuse in a strict view of the law.

Despite the law's apparent stringency, which come into play in a number of "mercy killing" prosecutions of laymen (usually family members), only twice have American physicians been tried for active euthanasia, and in both instances the jury acquitted the accused. The paucity of prosecutions is attributed, by the English legal authority Glanville Wiliams, to such factors as the likelihood that juries will be reluctant to convict a professional person and that executive clemency would be forthcoming if conviction did occur. Furthermore, the prosecutor may be reluctant to try a reputable doctor who has acted in good faith and who will engender support in the medical community. It may also be difficult to prove that a physician's act was responsible for his patient's death; the absence of causation was the central point in the defense of the two physicians who have gone to trial. Moreover, the administration of a drug to ease pain, such as morphine, would not be viewed as "mercy killing" even though the drug has the "double effect" of accelerating the termination of life; if the use of the drug on such a patient is an accepted medical practice for the primary purpose of ameliorating suffering, it would not be equated with a poison, where the law presumes a willful intent to kill.

PASSIVE EUTHANASIA

While the law on the subject of active euthanasia is thus clear, if perhaps not completely congruent with the consensus of the lay community, the law concerning passive euthanasia, which will probably be of more frequent concern to the average physician, is less precise. Passive euthanasia—the bringing about of death through the cessation of further medical interventions—has become a topic of concern to lay people who do not want their final days unduly extended in such a way as to deprive them of a "dignified death." A physician who agrees with the patient, and the latter's family and advisors, that further treatment promises only pain and not recovery and should therefore be ceased, will not find in the law any barrier to executing this decision. Should the patient be unable to participate in the decision or should the physician or family disagree, however, the legal picture becomes clouded.

The treatment of any patient depends on the existence of a physician-patient contract, through which (with greater or lesser formality, depending on the circumstances) the physician indicates the proposed therapeutic options and the patient decides which course to follow. Except in an emergency, when immediate treatment is necessary and it is presumed that the patient would want it if she were capable of giving consent, a medical intervention may not proceed without the explicit or implicit approval of the person being treated or, if she is incompetent, the patient's guardian.

The same principles apply in the case of life-preserving treatment for a dying person. Thus, the physician who concurs with the patient that the appropriate time has arrived to cease battling with terminal illness will face two major legal issues. First, the physician should be assured that the patient understands the significance and consequences of the choice, and that the patient is generally alert and coherent. Where doubt arises, it may be advisable to have another physician, such as a psychiatrist, consult. Second the physician will want to make sure that the patient's family is aware of, and if possible concurs in, the decision to end treatment. Although family members do not have the legal authority to countermand decisions made by a competent patient,[1] their opposition may not only cause a patient to change her mind suddenly but also greatly increases the likelihood that the physician will be sued after the patient's death for improperly ceasing treatment. Consequently, discussions and counseling may be needed with the family that opposes the decision to cease treatment. But the physician's fundamental obligation is to follow the patient's wishes and not to impose unwanted treatments; indeed, continuing to treat

[1]*Commonwealth v. Bowen,* 13 Mass. 356 (1816)

[1]*Lane v. Candura,* Mass. App. Ct. Adv. Sh. 588 (1978).

in the absence of permission to do so amounts to battery, for which the patient or, after death, the patient's legal representative may sue.

If a physician thinks that further treatment would be hopeless, but the patient insists that it be continued, the physician is obliged to see that ordinary medical care is continued; to do otherwise would be to abandon the patient. If the physician is unwilling to continue extraordinary therapies, which promise only to prolong dying and not restore normal functioning, he or she should arrange to transfer the case to physicians who are willing to render care on the patient's terms.

When it is the patient who wishes to cease treatment and the physician who thinks it should continue, the physician should carefully rethink his or her conclusion before acting. Of course, a physician has no authority to force a patient to accept therapy, and the courts generally decline to mandate treatment because "it is the individual who is the subject of a medical decision who has the final say [which] must necessarily be so in a system of goverment which gives the greatest possible protection to the indivdual in the furtherance of his own desires."[1] The only cases in which courts have ordered treatment have been those in which it claimed that: (1) a fairly simple treatment could preserve the life of a patient with minor children dependent for financial or emotional support on their parent;[2] (2) the patient did not want to die but only to refuse a treatment that was unacceptable for religious reasons (e.g., a Jehovah's Witness refusing blood transfusion needed in course of operation for nonterminal illness);[3] or (3) the state has an interest in a healthy citizenry, which would be violated by allowing people to refuse treatment, akin to suicide.[4] None of these rationales stands up to close scrutiny, and all have come under attack recently. Moreover, they have never been upheld by the highest court of any state in the case of a competent adult, and there is no precedent in the law for ordering such a patient to undergo a life-saving treatment against his or her wishes.

INCOMPETENT PATIENTS

The most difficult decisions, both legally and ethically, are those relating to the care of the patient who is rendered unable by a disease or its treatment to communicate and make decisions. There are two means of dealing with this situation. The first is for the patient to reach an advance agreement with the physician about what treatments will and will not be undertaken if certain eventualities occur. This is the approach promoted by the Euthanasia Educational Foundation, which has prepared a "living will" addressed not only to physicians but to the signer's family as well. The major difficulties here are that such a document may not anticipate the patient's own situation exactly enough to give the physician adequate guidance on what course to follow, and that these documents have no binding legal effect. Beginning with the "Natural Death Act" adopted by California in 1976,[1] a handful of states have enacted legislation aimed at overcoming the latter problem. These acts specify the conditions under which a person may execute a "directive to physicians" which will determine the extent of treatment after the patient's condition renders her unable to participate in treatment decisions. Unfortunately, the drafters of these statutes, particularly the California prototype, were attempting to respond to so many conflicting interests that the resulting legislation falls far short of its straightforward objectives. Nonetheless, as problematic as these statutes may be, they indicate that a social consensus in favor of allowing people to limit their care even after incompetence may slowly be emerging.

The second avenue which may be followed in the case of an apparently incompetent patient is to seek judicial guidance. In close cases, the judge may be willing to uphold a patient's refusal to accept further treatment, particularly where the medical staff concurs in this judgment; although the patient is only marginally competent, the nature of the proposed operation (e.g., amputation) or its small likelihood of success may convince the judge that the declination is correct.[2] When a guardian is appointed by the court to make the decisions for an incompetent, the premise is that the guardian will choose whatever course he or she deems in the patient's best interest. Although recent cases have shown that a guardian may be upheld in refusing additional treatment that was viewed as needlessly prolonging dying in a undignified fashion,[3] there seeems to be a great deal of insti-

[1]*Erickson v. Dilgard* 44 Misc. 2d 27, 252 N.Y.S. 2d 705 (Sup. Ct. 1962).

[2]*Raleigh Fitkin-Paul Morgan Memorial Hospital v. Anderson,* 42 N.J. 421, 201 A. 2d 537, cert. denied, 377 U.S. 985 (1964).

[3]Application of the President and Directors of Georgetown College, Inc., 331 F 2d 1010 (D.C. Cir. 1964).

[4]*John F. Kennedy Hospital v. Heston,* 58 N.J. 576, 279 A. 2d 670 (1971).

[1]California Health & Safety Code §§7185-7195 (1978 Supp.).

[2]In re Brooks Estate, 32 Ill. 2d 631, 205 N.E. 2d 435 (1965); in re Raasch (Jan. 21, 1972. No. 455–996. Prob. Div. Milwauke Co. Ct); In re Quackenbush, 383 A.2d 785 (Morris Cty Ct., N.J. 1978); Satz v. Perlmutter, 362 So. 2d 160 (D.C. App. Fla. 1978).

[3]*Palm Springs General Hospital v. Martinez* (July 1971, No. 71-12687, Miami Cir. Court).

tutional pressure for the guardian to consent to whatever treatment the physicians believe is indicated. Thus, the decision to pursue further treatment in the comatose and hopelessly terminal patient is an especially weighty one for a physician, and must be made with attention not only to the obligations to preserve life but also to ease suffering.

REFERENCES

Bok S: Personal directions for care at the end of life. *N Engl J Med* 295:367, 1976.

Cantor N: A patient's decision to decline life-saving medical treatment. *Rutgers Law Rev* 26:228, 1973.

Capron A: Development of law on human death. *Ann NY Acad Sci* 315:45, 1978.

———: Right to refuse medical care, in Encyclopedia of Bioethics, ed. WT Reich, New York: Free Press, 1978.

Doe v. Bolton, 93 U.S. 739 (1973).

Fletcher G: Legal aspects of the decision not to prolong life. *JAMA* 203:65, 1968.

Howell MG: What medical schools teach about women. *N Engl J Med* 291:304, 1974.

Morris A: Voluntary euthanasia. *Washington Law Rev* 45:239, 1970.

Roe v. Wade, 93 U.S. 739 (1973).

Williams G: *The Sanctity of Life and the Criminal Law,* New York: Knopf, 1957.

PART TWO

Mechanisms

6

Genetics

ALBERT B. GERBIE   HENRY L. NADLER   A. WALSH PLATT

The understanding of the genetic contribution to human diseases is in an era of rapid growth. Over 2000 genetic abnormalities have been described; some result from chromosomal abnormalities; others result either from an altered (mutant) gene or multiple interacting factors, among which may exist a genetic component. Included in this era of rapid advances in the field of medical genetics is the ability to diagnose a number of genetic diseases prenatally, to detect carriers of certain chromosomal and single-gene defects, and to successfully alter the course of specific metabolic disorders by medical management.

CHROMOSOMES—BASIC CONCEPTS

Chromosomes are composed of an association of deoxyribonucleic acid (DNA) and certain lysine and arginine-rich proteins (histones). Lengths of DNA which encode a polypeptide sequence are called genes. Genes, then, are the units of heredity which comprise and are linearly located along the length of the chromosome.

The normal chromosome complement in humans consists of 46 chromosomes, including 44 autosomes and two sex chromosomes, an X and a Y chromosome

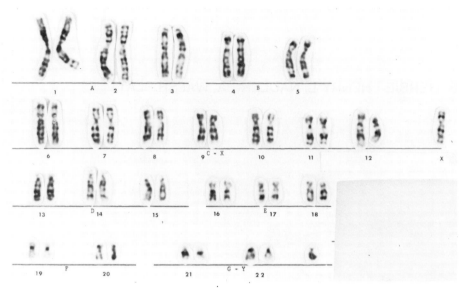

FIGURE 6–1   Karyotype of a normal male, 46XY. *(Courtesy of D. Meeker, Children's Memorial Hospital)*

in males and two X chromosomes in females. The chromosomes are found in homologous pairs 23 paternally derived and 23 maternally derived. Their morphologic characteristics, including position of the centromere (primary constriction), secondary constrictions, banding patterns, and length allow them to be divided into seven groups: group A, 1 to 3; group B, 4 to 5; group C, 6 to 12; group D, 13 to 15; group E, 16 to 18; group F, 19 to 20; and group G, 21 to 22. The X chromosome is similar to group C and the Y chromosome resembles group G. Pairs of chromosomes (homologues) arranged into groups according to size and morphology comprise the karyotype (Fig. 6-1).

A number of chromosomal abnormalities have been described in which the structure and/or number of chromosomes have been altered. In order to understand the pathogenesis of conditions associated with chromosomal aberrations, an understanding of the processes of mitosis (somatic cell division) and meiosis (gametogenesis) is necessary.

Mitosis

Mitosis, or somatic cell division, is a process by which the genetic constancy of an organism is maintained and upon which the growth and normal development of all organisms depend. The result of mitosis is two identical daughter cells. Through a continuous process, mitosis is divided into five stages: interphase, prophase, metaphase, anaphase, and telophase (Fig. 6-2).

Interphase. Though interphase is often referred to as the "resting stage," chromosomal material is replicated during this stage. The diploid number of chromosomes is maintained ($2N = 46$) but the DNA material is doubled ($2C \rightarrow 4C$). At this stage, each homologous chromosome has replicated and consists of two genetically identical chromatids, the two threads of a doubled chromosome.

Prophase. This event is marked by the condensation of the chromatic material into recognizably doubled chromosomes sharing a common centromere. Different chromosomes have centromeres at various locations along their length; recognition of this characteristic, as well as differences in length, makes it possible to distinguish chromosomes from one another (Fig. 6-1). The centromere is the point of attachment of the sister chromatids to the mitotic spindle, a group of filaments that stretch between and connect the two sets of centrioles, and it largely determines the movement of the chromosomes during division. Formation of the spindle gives the cell an orientation; the centrioles form the poles and a plane bisecting the spindle forms the equator, which marks the plane of eventual cell cleavage. Prophase ends as the chromosomes migrate toward the equator and the nuclear membrane and nucleoli disappear.

Metaphase. The sister chromatids align along the equatorial plane and attach to a spindle fiber by the centromere in a random manner. The centromere doubles and splits longitudinally.

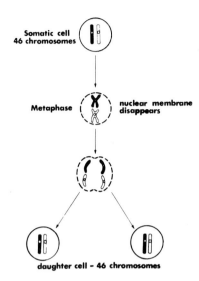

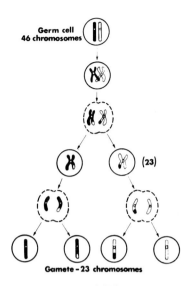

MITOSIS

MEIOSIS

FIGURE 6–2 Mitosis and meiosis in a cell with a pair of homologous chromosomes. The schematic of meiosis shows the exchange of genetic material (crossover leading to genetic recombination) that occurs through chance contact between homologous chromosomes before disjunction. For a detailed description, see text.

Anaphase. The spindle fibers appear to contract toward the poles, accompanied by centromere separation and movement of the sister chromatids to opposite poles. Because they are now single threads, each with its own centromere, the chromatids are now referred to as chromosomes.

Telophase. In telophase, the last stage of mitosis, the chromosomes continue to their respective poles. Two clusters of chromosomes are characteristic of telophase. Moreover, each cluster is identical, each one having received one sister chromatid from each original chromosome. A contraction of the cell appears in the plane of the equator, and separation of the cytoplasm occurs with the formation of two identical cells. The nuclear membrane and nucleoli reform; the chromosomes attenuate to form chromatin.

At this final stage, the diploid number is $2N$, but the DNA content has been reduced to $2C$. A somatic cell is thus $2N$, $2C$.

Meiosis

Meiosis is a process by which the diploid number of chromosomes ($2N = 46$) is reduced to haploid ($N = 23$). This is a two-division process (meiosis I and II) which occurs during the maturation of germ cells. While mitosis assures genetic constancy in the organism, meiosis allows for genetic variation through the independent (random) assortment and disjunction of homologous chromosomes. For example, if an individual is heterozygous for only one gene pair on each pair of chromosomes, the genetic combinations that could be found in his gametes is 2^{23}, or over 8 million. Meiosis I and II have been divided into the same five stages as was mitosis (Fig. 6-2). The two processes differ, however, in that meiosis involves two divisions but only one replication of genetic material.

In the first stage of meiosis, each chromosome replicates ($2C \rightarrow 4C$) and, unlike mitosis, pairs with its homologue. These bivalents, consisting of four chromatid strands (each pair connected by a single unduplicated centromere) then align their centromeres along the equatorial plate. The bivalents segregate by independent assortment during anaphase I, resulting in two clusters of univalents at opposite ends of the cell. The diploid number of chromosomes has been halved during this reductional division ($2N \rightarrow 1N$) as has the chromosomal content ($4C \rightarrow 2C$), with one representative of each of the original pairs in each cluster. Meiosis II is very similar to mitosis in that the univalents align themselves along the equatorial plate, the centromeres divide, and the chromosomes move to opposite poles. As a result of this equational division ($1N$, $2C \rightarrow 1C$), the daughter cells thus produced are genetically identical. This second division does not change the number of chromosomes, although the quantity of genetic material is halved.

Failure of proper bivalent segregation in meiosis I or univalent segregation in meiosis II is termed nondisjunction. In the male, meiosis in the spermatocyte leads to the formation of four mature sperm cells. In the female, however, meiosis in the oocyte leads to the formation of one mature egg cell and three polar bodies because of unequal distribution of the cytoplasm upon cell division.

ABNORMAL HUMAN KARYOTYPES

There is a delicate balance in the amount and kind of chromosome material which is compatible with normal development in humans. Deviations from the diploid (euploid) number, either by changes in the number of chromosomes or certain structural aberrations, lead to abnormal karyotypes that may be related to pathological states.

The normal number of chromosomes in a human somatic cell is termed diploid ($2N = 46$). Gametes, on the other hand, exist with a haploid number of 23 chromosomes ($1N$) until fertilization. Any multiple of the haploid number is known as polyploidy. Numerical aberrations of chromosomes may involve the entire set (triploidy, $3N = 69$; tetraploidy, $4N = 92$), or individual chromosomes, called aneuploidy (45,47,48).

The presence of three homologues of an autosome is referred to as trisomy; the absence of one of a pair of homologues is termed monosomy.

The chief mechanisms leading to abnormalities of chromosome number or structure are nondisjunction, translocation, and deletion.

NONDISJUNCTION

The segregation of chromosomes during mitosis or meiosis is termed disjunction. Failure of chromosomes to sort themselves in equal numbers into daughter cells, thus, is nondisjunction.

In nondisjunction, one cell receives one chromosome too many and the other cell receives one too few. The former condition is trisomic, the latter monosomic.

A lack of material is generally more harmful than an excess of it, so nondisjunction at the first mitotic cell division following zygote formation most likely will result in a trisomic individual, the monosomic cell probably not surviving. Nondisjunction at a later cell division may result in mosaicism in which a population of normal, trisomic, and even some monosomic cells exist in a single individual.

Most often nondisjunction occurs not in mitosis, but in the first stage of meiosis (Fig. 6-2). In this first division, nondisjunction at anaphase I results in one trisomic and one monosomic daughter cell. The monosomic cell from the first stage produces two gametes, each lacking one chromosome. The trisomic cell produces two trisomic gametes. If they are male gametes, all four are capable of becoming spermatozoa. If they are female gametes, only one will be a viable ovum, the others becoming nonfunctional polar bodies.

AUTOSOMAL TRISOMY SYNDROMES

Down's syndrome or trisomy 21 (Fig. 6-3; 47XX, 21+) is the most common autosomal trisomy, occurring in approximately 1 per 600 live births. Trisomy of chromosome 21 accounts for about 95 percent of the cases, the remainder caused by translocation and mosaicism. The flat face, upward-slanting eyes, epicanthic folds, curved little fingers, and mental retardation make up the well-known clinical picture. Congenital heart disease is common, as are anomalies of the gastrointestinal tract. This syndrome probably results from nondisjunction of chromosome 21 at meiosis I of oogenesis and is related to maternal age. In women under 30, the incidence of the syndrome is about 0.6 per 1000 births; this increases to 20 to 30 per 1000 for mothers age 45 and over. Nondisjunction is a phenomenon related to maternal age, but not to paternal age. This becomes easier to understand when it is recalled that the woman's gametes are formed in fetal life and arrested in meiosis I until the time of ovulation (12 to 50 years). The long meiotic prophase in females may thus be related to the increasing risk of meiotic nondisjunction with increasing maternal age. Over the years, environmental influences may also exert an effect on the ability of the immature gametes (oocytes) to complete the meiotic process.

Trisomy of other small autosomes is not uncommon (Table 6-1). The best-known examples are Edward's syndrome (trisomy 18), Patau's syndrome

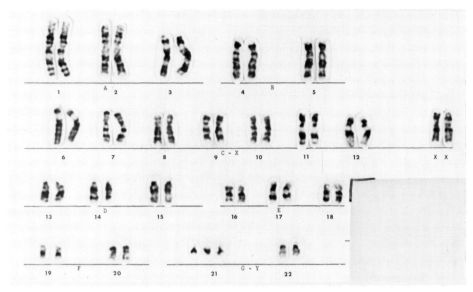

FIGURE 6-3 Karyotype of a female with Down's syndrome or trisomy 21, 47XX, 21 +. *(Courtesy of D. Meeker, Children's Memorial Hospital)*

(trisomy 13), and trisomy 8 (usually a mosaic 46/47 as full trisomy 8 leads to early fetal death).

Monosomy of autosomes almost always causes early intrauterine death or makes the gamete nonviable.

AUTOSOMAL ABERRATIONS

TRANSLOCATION

A translocation most commonly involves the transfer of a segment of the chromosome to another chromosome, leading to an imbalance of chromosome material. Chromosome breaks are not uncommon and can result in a number of anomalies. When two non-homologous chromosomes simultaneously break near their ends and then join with each other to form a single chromosome, for example 15^{21} (also called D/G), the resultant cell contains essentially the normal amount of material from both of these chromosomes (apart from a little lost at the time of the break). These new chromosomes are easily detected by karyotyping since they cannot pair. As no genes are actually lost, this is called a balanced translocation. The person is usually clinically unaffected and is capable of producing children.

Approximately 3 percent of patients with Down's syndrome are translocation trisomics with a karyotype consisting of 45 chromosomes, the G chromosome having been translocated to a D group or another G group chromosome. The risk that a balanced translocation carrier, though phenotypically normal, will have an affected child is significantly greater (but independent of maternal age) than the risk that a karyotypically normal individual will have a child with Down's syndrome. Depending on how this chromosome in her gametes has paired with her normal 21 or D chromosome in meiosis, the ovum she produces on fertilization by a normal sperm may result in a fetus that is normal, that is a normal carrier, that is nonviable, or that has Down's syndrome. Translocation Down's syndrome is clinically indistinguishable from trisomy 21 Down's syndrome.

DELETION

A deletion is a loss of chromosome material following a break or breaks in a chromosome arm; it results in a partial monosomy. Loss of a major portion of the short arm of chromosomes is responsible for a clinical syndrome termed cri-du-chat, or cat-cry. These infants fail to thrive and have a characteristic moon face, microcephaly, and severe mental retardation. Their most dramatic feature is a weak, high-pitched cry resembling that of a cat or kitten. Although cases seem to occur sporadically, there are reports of mul-

Table 6-1 Some Diseases Due to Chromosomal Abnormalities

Disorder		Incidence	Significance to individual	Genetic significance
Aneuploidy				
Autosomal disorders	Down's syndrome (trisomy 21)	1 per 600	Mental retardation, associated congenital anomalies, high risk of leukemia; with antibiotics, may live to adult	Related to advanced maternal age
	Patau's syndrome (trisomy 13)	1 per 5000–6000	69% die in 6 months; more are malformed; cleft lip and palate, small cranium; eye defects; major CNS (central nervous system) and heart defects	Related to advanced maternal age; may also be result of translocation chromosome received from phenotypically normal parent
	Edward's syndrome (trisomy 18)	1 per 3300	85% die in 6 months; 78% females; multiple severe malformations	Related to advanced maternal age
	Trisomy 8 (C trisomy)	Extremely rare	Mild to moderate growth deficiency; mild to severe mental retardation; nonspecific skeleto-anomalies, primarily bone dysplasias	Most are mosaics (46/47); full trisomy 8 appears to be an early lethal
Sex-linked disorders	Klinefelter's syndrome (XXY, other variants)	1 per 500	Sterility; mentally normal or subnormal; alteration in habitus (eunochoidism)	Generally sporadic; increased maternal age a factor
	Turner syndrome (XO, several variants)	1 per 2500	Most XO pregnancies abort; viable individuals show congenital malformations, infantile genitalia, short stature, sterility, ovarian agenesis	Generally sporadic; maternal age seems not to be a factor
	Polysomy X (XXX, other variants)	1 per 1600	Most XXX individuals probably normal; some show mental retardation, infertility	Generally sporadic occurrence; offspring of XXX females usually chromosomally normal; occasional son has Klinefelter's syndrome (XXY)
	XYY syndrome	1 per 700	Tall stature; dull mentality common	Generally sporadic occurrence
Structural aberrations				
Translocation	Translocation Down's syndrome (D/G translocation)	3.5% of all Down's	Mental retardation, associated congenital anomalies; high risk of leukemia; with antibiotics, may live to adult	D/G—30% risk; 21/21—100% risk

Table 6–1   Some Diseases Due to Chromosomal Abnormalities (*Continued*)

Disorder		Incidence	Significance to individual	Genetic significance
Deletions	Cri-du-chat syndrome (partial deletion of short arm of B group—chromosome 5)	Rare	Mental retardation; small larynx; death may occur in childhood due to associated anomalies; may survive to adulthood	Sporadic cases; seem unrelated to parental age
	Partial deletion of long arm of chromosome 18	Rare	Psychomotor retardation; microcephaly; retraction of middle part of face	Sporadic occurrence
	Partial deletion of long arm of chromosome 21 (antimongolism syndrome)	Rare	Mild to severe growth deficiency; severe mental retardation; variable phenotypic expression	Generally sporadic; deletion amounts of long arm different in reported cases; mosaics reported

tiple affected sibs born to a balanced translocation carrier parent.

Partial deletions of the short arm of chromosome 4 (4p⁻) and long arms of chromosome 18 (18q⁻) and 21 (21q⁻) have been described, and are usually sporadic in occurrence. Each of these deletions results in very serious pathophysiologic abnormalities (Table 6-1).

SEX CHROMOSOME ABERRATIONS

The sex chromosomes undergo the same abnormalities as the autosomes. However, because these disorders are less than lethal in outcome, they become clinically very important (Table 6-1). Klinefelter's syndrome is the most common sex-chromosome aberration, with an incidence of over 2 per 1000 live births. The usual karyotype is 47XXY, but many cases with more than two X chromosomes, as well as mosaics, have been described. It is believed that the extra X chromosome is caused by meiotic nondisjunction in either the sperm or ovum.

Sex-chromosome monosomy, as occurs with Turner's syndrome, 45XO, is compatible with life, although it is often found in spontaneous abortion material. Similarly, trisomy of the sex chromosomes is much less damaging than trisomy of the autosomes. The reason for this may be that only one X chromosome is genetically active (the Lyon hypothesis). Other trisomy syndromes involving the sex chromosomes include poly-X syndrome (47XXX, and

47XXX/46XX mosaics) and the XYY syndrome.

Table 6-1 summarizes a number of major chromosomal abnormalities.

OTHER CHROMOSOME DISORDERS

The hypothesis that chromosome damage causes certain neoplasms has received support recently. Carcinogenic agents such as radiation and drugs are known to induce neoplastic disease and also to damage chromosomes, and chromosome damage or abnormality has been detected in some forms of cancer, particularly the leukemias. Translocation of chromosomal material from chromosome 22 (22q⁻; Philadelphia chromosome) usually to chromosome 9 (22⁹) is the specific anomaly detected in patients with chronic myelogenous leukemia; it appears in about 90 percent of such cases.

GENES—BASIC CONCEPTS

A gene is a length of DNA whose function is to direct the synthesis of a polypeptide. This polypeptide may join with others to produce a protein such as an enzyme. Furthermore, the DNA makes duplicates of itself for cell division, ensuring that the descendant cells carry the same genetic information as the parent cell.

DNA is in the form of a double helix, two spiraling strands of nucleotides joined by hydrogen bonds across the space between them. A DNA nucleotide consists of a base, a deoxyribose, and a phosphate. The deoxyribose and phosphate molecules are linked to form the backbone of each strand. Anchoring into each deoxyribose is a base oriented toward the base emerging from the other strand of the double helix. The bases in DNA are thymine, adenine, guanine, and cytosine. Their bonds are such that adenine on one strand is always joined to thymine on the other, and guanine on one is always joined to cytosine on the other.

In protein synthesis, the nucleotide (identified by its base member) is the basic "letter" and a triplet of nucleotides the basic "word" (codon) of the code. For instance, a triplet of adenine nucleotides (abbreviated AAA) specifies the manufacture of phenylalanine, while AAT (T for thymine) leads to production of leucine.

The specificity of the links between bases of the double helix enables the exact copying that takes place before chromosomes themselves divide in cell division. During DNA synthesis, the strands separate and unwind; as this happens, the bases of each strand attract to themselves nucleotides necessary to recreate their former partner. Thus, the genetic information, that is, the order of nucleotides, is exactly reproduced in the second-generation DNA.

Human genomes are estimated to be composed of 50,000 to 100,000 genes. Genotype refers to an individual's genetic constitution, and phenotype to the physical expression (biochemical, physiologic, and anatomic traits) of these genes. An allele is an alternative form of a gene. Homozygous refers to a trait for which an allelic pair are apparently identical. Heterozygous indicates the presence of different alleles (or gene forms) at the two loci (gene sites) of the homologous chromosomes. Alleles interact to determine a particular trait. When one allele in a heterozygote masks the trait determined by its partner allele, the trait expressed is said to be dominant. The one that is masked or not phenotypically expressed is recessive, and the individual is said to be a carrier of the recessive allele. An allele (usually dominant alleles) can vary its phenotypic expression, i.e., show variable expressivity. This is a common occurrence in polydactyly, neurofibromatosis, and Ehlers-Danlos syndrome.

MUTANT GENES AND THEIR EFFECTS

Biochemical and immunologic studies have shown that there are two or more different alleles at approximately a third of the chromosomal loci. Most of these genetic variants, or mutant genes, have little if any effect on the phenotype; that is, they do not influence embryonic development, physiologic functions, or resistance to disease. Some mutant genes, on the other hand, have a moderate or even profound effect on the phenotype.

Gene abnormalities are of two main types: single-gene defects and multifactorial disorders. Single-gene defects are caused by a single mutant gene inherited from one parent or by mutant alleles, one from each parent. (Fresh mutations can also occur in gametic cells, in which case neither or only one of the parents would be carriers.) The gene on an autosome is called autosomal, and on the X chromosome is called X-linked. The criteria in Table 6-2 must be met to fit a genetic disorder within a specific pattern of inheritance. The patterns of inheritance such disorders follow are summarized in Fig. 6–4.

Multifactorial disorders (polygenic) probably result from the interactions of a number of different gene pairs (alleles at different loci) with environmental influences. They are among the most common conditions encountered and include atherosclerosis, hypertension, diabetes mellitus, and peptic ulcer.

SINGLE-GENE DISORDERS[1]

The mechanism by which such mutant genes exert their effect can be thought of in terms of the one-gene–one-polypeptide model of gene function. We know most about disorders which are the result of a mutant gene at a single locus.

ENZYME DEFICIENCY DISORDERS: INBORN ERRORS OF METABOLISM

The prototype of the single-gene disorder is the inborn error of metabolism. Each disorder is the result of a metabolic block caused by either the deficiency or absence of an enzyme (Table 6–3).

[1]The authors acknowledge the contribution of O. J. Miller to this section.

Table 6-2 Criteria for Inheritance Pattern

Autosomal dominant, e.g., Marfan's syndrome, achondroplasia
1. The phenotypic expression of the gene (trait) appears in every generation with no skipping.
2. Half of the children of an affected person on the average have the trait.
3. The trait is not transmitted by unaffected persons to their children.
4. Male and female are equally likely to transmit or to have the trait.

Autosomal recessive, e.g., sickle-cell anemia, Tay-Sachs disease
1. The trait most commonly appears only in sibs, not in their parents or offspring.
2. One-fourth of the sibs of the index case (propositus, proband) on the average are affected.
3. Males and females are equally likely to be affected.
4. The parents of the affected person may be consanguineous; consanguinity also increases the likelihood of bearing children with autosomal-recessive diseases.

X-linked recessive inheritance, e.g., hemophilia, Lesch-Nyhan syndrome
1. The incidence of the trait is higher in males than in females.
2. The trait is passed through all the daughters of an affected man to half of these daughters' sons.
3. The trait is not transmitted from father to son.

X-linked dominant, e.g., vitamin D–resistant rickets with hypophosphatemia, Goltz's syndrome
1. The trait is transmitted from affected males to all their daughters and none of their sons.
2. If the affected female is heterozygous, she will transmit the condition to half her children.
3. Affected homozygous females will transmit the trait to all of their children (similar to transmission of autosomal dominant).
4. Affected females are twice as common as affected males but express the condition in a milder form in rare X-linked dominant disorders.

Source: Modified from JS Thompson, MW Thompson.

Since each individual carries two complete sets of chromosomes, and the genes carried by one set function independently of those on the other set (except for those on the X chromosome, which show "Lyonization"), it follows that an enzyme deficiency due to a mutant gene will occur only if both normal copies of the gene are replaced by a mutant form which does not generate a functional enzyme molecule. One can envision other changes in protein molecules that might produce a phenotypic effect even when the mutant gene in question is present in single doses, as has been described for enzymes comprised of two subunits (dimers). When one of the subunits (monomers) is encoded by a mutant gene, the stability or enzymic capabilities of the potential dimer formed between the mutant and normal monomer can be affected because of the presence of the altered subunit.

In general, inborn errors of metabolism follow a pattern of autosomal-recessive inheritance. Thus, the risk of occurrence of an affected child to two carriers (heterozygotes) for a given disorder is 1:4 at each pregnancy.

Enzyme Deficiencies Affecting Steroid Metabolism: Congenital Adrenal Hyperplasia

There are at least four main types of enzyme defects which interfere with the biosynthesis of adrenal steroids and thus lead to adrenal hyperplasia. All show an autosomal-recessive mode of inheritance.

C21-Hydroxylase Deficiency. This is the most common cause of virilizing adrenal hyperplasia. This enzyme catalyzes three reactions: (1) progesterone → desoxycorticosterone; (2) 17α-hydroxyprogesterone → 11-desoxycortisol (compound S); (3) 21-desoxycortisol → cortisol (compound F). A deficiency of the enzyme leads to decreased production of cortisol, corticosterone, and aldosterone. In the majority of cases, the enzyme defect is partial so that enough cortisol and aldosterone are produced to maintain mineral balance. With a more severe deficiency this is not the case, and a severe salt-losing syndrome occurs which can lead to rapid demise of the newborn infant if not promptly diagnosed and treated.

The metabolic block leads to the accumulation of progesterone and 17α-hydroxyprogesterone, which is converted to the adrenal androgens, Δ^4-androstenedione and its 11-oxygenated derivatives. These lead to virilizing changes in utero with some degree of fusion of the labioscrotal folds, even proceeding so far as to approximate a persistent urogenital sinus. Clitoral enlargement also occurs, and progressive and precocious maturation proceeds, unless replace-

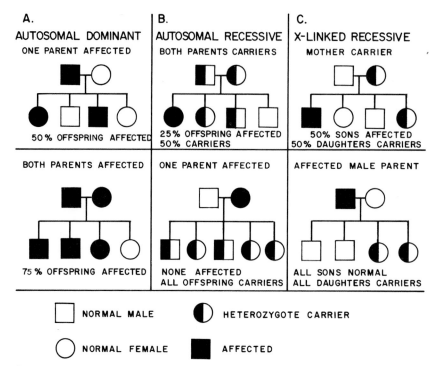

FIGURE 6-4 Mendalian patterns of inheritance. *A* Autosomal dominant: Only a single mutant gene is necessary to produce the altered phenotype. An affected person with one normal parent is presumably heterozygous. If neither parent is affected, an affected child probably represents a new mutation. *B* Autosomal recessive: The trait is expressed only in homozygous individuals. An unaffected parent is presumed to be heterozygous. *C* X-linked recessive: The mutant gene, located on the X chromosome, is expressed by all males who carry the gene. A female offspring who inherits a mutant X-linked gene from her mother will usually receive a normal X-linked gene from her father and so will be clinically normal, though a carrier.

ment therapy with adrenal steroids is initiated to suppress the excessive production of ACTH and overproduction of adrenal androgens.

C11-Hydroxylase Deficiency. Some patients with virilizing adrenal hyperplasia also have hypertension. They have been shown to have a different enzymatic defect, involving C11-hydroxylase. This enzyme catalyzes the following reactions: (1) desoxycorticosterone → corticosterone; (2) 17α-hydroxyprogesterone → 21-desoxycortisol; (3) 11-desoxycortisol (compound S) → cortisol (compound F). A deficiency of this enzyme, therefore, leads to a decrease in the amount of corticosterone, aldosterone, and cortisol; a resultant increase in ACTH production; and overproduction of desoxycorticosterone, which probably accounts for the hypertension, as well as 17α-hydroxyprogesterone, which is routed to the production of adrenal androgens with resultant virilization.

3β-Hydroxysteroid Dehydrogenase Deficiency. This enzyme catalyzes the following three reactions: (1) Δ⁵-pregnenolone → progesterone; (2) 17α-hydroxy-Δ⁵-pregnenolone → 17α-hydroxyprogesterone; and (3) dehydroepiandrosterone → Δ⁴-androstenedione.

A deficiency of this enzyme partially blocks the production of all adrenal steroids, including the androgens. The block may even lead to intersexual development of the external genitalia, leading to male pseudohermaphroditism. A small number of families are known to have a complete enzymatic block at this step, or an even earlier one, in the series of reactions involved in steroid biosynthesis. Males with this block have totally feminized external genitalia, presumably reflecting absence of testicular as well as adrenal androgens. Females with this condition, which appears as a congenital lipoid adrenal hyperplasia, have normal sexual development. The condition is lethal in both sexes.

Table 6–3 Inborn Errors of Metabolism in the Neonatal Period

Disorders of carbohydrate metabolism
1. Galactosemia (galactose-1-phosphate uridyl transferase deficiency)
2. Hereditary fructose intolerance (fructose-1-phosphate aldolase deficiency)
3. Fructose-1,6-diphosphatase deficiency
4. Glycogen storage disease, type I (von Gierke's disease, glucose 6-phosphate deficiency)
5. Glycogen storage disease, type II (Pompe's disease, α-1,4-glucosidase deficiency)
6. Glycogen storage disease, type III (limit dextrinosis, brancher deficiency)
7. Glycogen storage disease, type IV (amylopectinosis, brancher deficiency)

Disorders of lipid metabolism
8. GM$_1$-gangliosidosis, type I (generalized gangliosidosis, β-galactosidase deficiency)
9. GM$_3$-gangliosidosis
10. Wolman's disease (acid lipase deficiency)
11. Niemann-Pick disease, types A and B (sphingomyelinase deficiency)

Disorders of mucopolysaccharide metabolism
12. Hurler syndrome (mucopolysaccharidosis I, α-L-iduronidase deficiency)
13. Hunter syndrome (mucopolysaccharidosis II, iduronosulfate sulfatase deficiency)
14. β-Glucuronidase deficiency

Urea cycle defects
15. Carbamoylphosphate synthetase deficiency (hyperammonemia type I)
16. Ornithine transcarbamoylase deficiency (hyperammonemia type II)
17. Citrullinemia
18. Argininosuccinic aciduria
19. Arginase deficiency

Disorders of amino acid metabolism or transport
20. Maple syrup urine disease
21. Hypervalinemia
22. Hyperlysinemia
23. Hyper-β-alaninemia
24. Nonketotic hyperglycinemia
25. Phenylketonuria
26. Oasthouse urine disease (methionine malabsorption)
27. Tyrosinemia
28. Hypermethioninemia
29. Homocystinuria
30. Hartnup disease
31. Hypersarcosinemia
32. Pyroglutamic acidemia

Disorders of organic acid metabolism
33. Methylmalonic acidemia
34. Propionic acidemia (ketotic hyperglycinemia)
35. Isovaleric acidemia
36. Butyric and hexanoic acidemia (green acyl dehydrogenase deficiency)
37. β-Methylcrotonyl-CoA carboxylase deficiency

Miscellaneous disorders
38. Adrenogenital syndrome
39. Lysosomal acid phosphatase deficiency
40. Renal tubular acidosis
41. Nephrogenic diabetes insipidus
42. Menke's kinky-hair syndrome
43. Orotic aciduria
44. Congenital lactic acidosis
45. Cystic fibrosis
46. Hypophosphatasia
47. Fucosidosis
48. Crigler-Najjar syndrome
49. α_1-Antitrypsin deficiency
50. I-cell disease (mucolipidosis II)
51. Albinism
52. Lesch-Nyhan syndrome

Source: BK Burton, HL Nadler.

Enzyme Deficiencies Affecting Lipid Metabolism: Tay-Sachs Disease

Tay-Sachs disease is a progressive neurological disorder in which a deficiency of the enzyme hexosaminidase A leads to enhanced storage of GM$_2$-ganglioside in neurons and interference with neurological function. The affected individual is usually normal at birth and for several months thereafter. Then hypo-tonia, poor head control, and failure to continue psychomotor development become apparent. Blindness may occur by 1 year of age, and a characteristic cherry-red spot is present at the macula. Hypersensitivity to sounds may be present for a time. Severe seizures frequently occur and are sometimes refractory to anticonvulsive drugs. Death usually occurs by the age of 2 or 2½ years. Like most enzyme deficiencies, Tay-Sachs is inherited as an autosomal-recessive disorder. The mutant gene occurs rarely in non-Jews and reaches its highest frequency in Ashkenazi Jews, where 1 in 30 individuals is a heterozygous carrier of the gene. The frequency of a carrier marrying another carrier in this population is thus 1 in 30^2 or 1 in 900, and the incidence of children with Tay-Sachs disease would be 1 in 3600 if nothing were done to reduce this figure.

Normal carriers of the gene for Tay-Sachs disease have decreased serum levels of hexosaminidase A. When two carriers of this gene have children, their risk of having a child with Tay-Sachs is 1:4 at each pregnancy. Fortunately, carriers can be detected biochemically and, furthermore, the enzyme deficiency can be diagnosed prenatally (cultured amniotic fluid cells)'in time for the affected fetus to be aborted (Chap. 33).

There are many other genetic disorders of lipid metabolism, but many of them are not yet as well understood as Tay-Sachs disease. It seems likely that the obstetrician will be called on to advise a growing number of patients who are found with this kind of problem. Initially, genetic counseling and prenatal diagnosis may be all that can be offered to these individuals. In time, early diagnosis and initiation of treatment will probably be possible.

Other examples of lipidoses include Sandhoff's disease and Niemann-Pick, types A, B, and C.

Enzyme Deficiencies Affecting Carbohydrate Metabolism: Galactosemia

Galactosemia is an autosomal disorder that strikes infants who were normal at birth. Not long after milk feedings begin, i.e., within a few days, they develop vomiting, jaundice, diarrhea, lethargy, and hypotonia. Death may occur quickly. If not, anorexia, hepatomegaly, cataracts, and mental retardation without specific neurologic abnormalities are usual.

Affected individuals have a marked deficiency of galactose-1-phosphate uridyl transferase and are therefore unable to metabolize the galactose derived from milk. Galactose and galactose-1-phosphate accumulate and appear to be toxic to hepatic cells and neurons. Exclusion of milk from the diet can prevent the development of the clinical course of this disorder. The problem, then, is the early detection of infants homozygous for the mutant gene in time to initiate this simple therapy. Screening involves measuring the level of galactose-1-phosphate uridyl transferase in red blood cells.

Prenatal diagnosis of this disorder is now possible, although the diagnosis may be unreliable. Alternatively, later-born children in a family who have had an affected child should be screened for this disorder within a few days following birth. Since carriers of the trait have only about 50 percent of the normal enzyme level in their red cells, it is possible to screen for marriages where there is risk of producing an affected child. The frequency of the gene is so low—perhaps only 1 in 200 people carry it; thus only about 1 in 40,000 marriages between nonrelatives is at risk—that one might question the need for such screening when alert pediatric care can, with early diagnosis, lead to proper medical (therapeutic) management.

Other examples of carbohydrate metabolic disorders include hereditary fructose intolerance and glycogen storage diseases, types I to IV.

Disorders of Mucopolysaccharide (MPS) Metabolism

The mucopolysaccharidoses are a group of at least six rare genetic disorders which have certain features in common. The affected individual stores large quantities of mucopolysaccharides in various tissues and organs and excretes large quantities of related compounds such as dermatan or heparan sulfate or, less commonly, keratan sulfate. Even in the most severe variants, the affected individual appears normal at birth. The progressive storage of mucopolysaccharides begins after birth and leads to coarsening of facial features, corneal clouding, hepatosplenomegaly, joint stiffness, kyphosis, inguinal or umbilical hernia, enlarged head, tongue, and lips, noisy breathing, growth retardation, and, in most variants, mental retardation.

Mucopolysaccharidosis II (*Hunter syndrome*) is inherited as an X-linked recessive disorder. All the other forms of mucopolysaccharidosis are inherited as autosomal recessives. The underlying defect in each case is a deficiency of a lysosomal enzyme involved in degrading mucopolysaccharides.

Mucopolysaccharidosis IH (*Hurler syndrome*) is associated with a severe deficiency of α-L-iduronidase, which cleaves iduronic acid residues, a major constituent of dermatan sulfate and a minor component of heparan sulfate. The clinically milder mucopolysaccharidosis IS (the Scheie syndrome) is associated with a lesser deficiency of the same enzyme and presumably is the result of a different mutation in the same gene which has led to a different change in the enzyme molecule. Type IH differs from IS in its pathophysiological findings, type IH being much more severe. In mucopolysaccharidosis II, there is a deficiency of sulfoiduronate sulfatase; in mucopoly-saccharidosis IIIA (Sanfilippo A), there is a deficiency of HS*N*-sulfatase which removes sulfate groups from heparan sulfate; and in type IIIB (Sanfilippo B), *N*-acetyl-α-glucosaminidase is deficient. Type V (Morquio) has very severe physical stigmata, but no mental retardation. The deficient enzyme is chondroitin-6-sulfate *N*-acetyl glucosamine-4-sulfate sulfatase. In both forms of type VI (Maroteaux-Lamy A and B), distinguished by the severity of the clinical findings, arylsulfatase B is deficient. Type VII is thought to result in the storage of chondroitin-4-sulfate and the deficient enzyme is β-glucosamine.

These storage diseases are expressed in fibroblastic cells cultured from affected individuals. The cells show metachromatic storage granules and also accumulate mucopolysaccharides more rapidly, as measured by the incorporation of ^{35}S. Surprisingly, this rate of accumulation falls to normal when cells of patients with two different forms of the disease are cultured together. That is, each of these metabolic disorders is correctable by cocultivation with normal cells or with cells from a patient with a deficiency of a different enzyme in the pathway of degradation of the acid mucopolysaccharides. This is not the usual finding in the inborn errors of metabolism, but is explicable when one considers the nature of the enzymes in question; i.e., they are confined within cell organelles called lysosomes. Proteins in the medium are known to enter cells by pinocytosis which produces a membrane-lined vesicle (phagosome) which can then merge with a lysosome. As a result, the mucopolysaccharidoses, and presumably any other genetic disorders due to a deficiency of lysosomal enzyme, may be amenable to enzyme replacement therapy. However, this form of therapy would be ineffective for the great bulk of genetic disorders in which the replacement enzyme would be degraded before reaching its intracellular site of action.

The bright prospects for successful treatment of these disorders in the not-too-distant future should not blind the obstetrician to their immediate poor prognosis. Early diagnosis and counseling, with a view to prevention, are quite important. Prenatal diagnosis is possible for the mucopolysaccharidosis disorders (Chap. 33).

Disorders of Amino Acid Metabolism: Phenylketonuria

Phenylketonuria is a rare autosomal recessive disorder affecting about 1 in 20,000 newborns, though fewer in black or Jewish populations. The defect is a deficiency in the liver enzyme, phenylalanine hydroxylase, which catalyzes the conversion of phenylalanine to tyrosine. As a result of the enzyme deficiency, phenylalanine reaches very high levels in the serum and undergoes conversion into a series of products which, perhaps like phenylalanine, are toxic to the developing brain. Within a few weeks of birth, irritability, vomiting, and seizures may be noted, and, if untreated, severe mental retardation usually occurs, with an IQ averaging about 20.

The deleterious effects of phenylketonuria can be largely prevented by early diagnosis and prompt dietary restriction of phenylalanine. Consequently, most states require that every newborn infant have its blood phenylalanine level checked within a few days of birth. It may take a few days for the elevated level to make itself manifest, so testing umbilical cord blood would not pick up the infants who will develop hyperphenylalaninemia on a regular diet. Prompt institution of a low-phenylalanine diet and its maintenance for the early years of life hold out the promise of normal intellectual development for the affected child. After about age 6, the special diet may no longer be necessary.

The obstetrician has an additional worry in dealing with this disorder. When phenylketonuric women become pregnant, they have a very high incidence of children with cardiac defects, microcephaly, and mental retardation. Presumably, these have occurred because of the teratogenic effects of a high blood level of phenylalanine or some of its metabolic by-products, and the genotype of the fetus is irrelevant to these effects. If so, then such patients should be placed back on a low-phenylalanine diet during each pregnancy. No information is yet available to suggest whether such management is effective, and the obstetrician, in counseling the patient, might want to discuss other alternatives, including abortion.

Other examples of disorders of amino acid metabolism include maple syrup urine disease and homocystinuria.

Disorders of Organic Acid Metabolism: Methylmalonic Acidemia (MMA)

Methylmalonic acidemia, which is a very rare metabolic disorder, is transmitted as an autosomal recessive trait. Symptoms begin early in life, and if untreated, the patients usually die in infancy. The clinical manifestations include vomiting, lethargy, hepatomegaly, and failure to grow. Many of the affected children have neutropenia, thrombocytopenia, hypoglycemia, and osteoporosis. The disorder results in ketoacidosis, intermittent hyperglycinemia, and methylmalonic aciduria without vitamin B_{12} deficiency.

Four variants of methylmalonic acidemia have been described; two of which represent defects in vitamin B_{12} metabolism rather than defects in the synthesis of the apoenzyme concerned with methylmalonyl-CoA metabolism. Injection of B_{12} lowers the methylmalonate excretion and prevents ketoacidosis.

Protein restriction and synthetic diets may aid in long-term management of all four variants of methylmalonic acidemia. This disorder can be prenatally diagnosed; however, carrier detection is not readily available at this time.

Other disorders of organic acid metabolism include propionic acidemia and isovaleric acidemia.

OTHER GENE DISORDERS

Membrane Transport Abnormalities

Mutant genes are known which affect membrane transport of water, electrolytes, sugars, amino acids, and proteins. The underlying enzyme defect or other genetic change is not yet well understood in most of these disorders.

Protein Transport: α_1-Antitrypsin Deficiency. Human serum has long been known to contain substances that inhibit proteolytic enzymes such as trypsin, chymotrypsin, elastase, collagenase, and various bacterial proteases. Most of this activity is present in the α_1-globulin fraction in a low-molecular-weight glycoprotein called α_1-antitrypsin. The presence of this chemical in serum is under simple genetic control with a single-locus Pi (protease inhibitor) exercising a major effect. About 1 in 20 individuals is heterozygous for 1 of 11 or more recognized mutant forms of the gene, having an intermediate enzyme level 50 to 60 percent of normal. About 1 in 1600 persons is homozygous and deficient in serum α_1-antitrypsin with <10 percent of the normal level, making this disorder nearly as common as cystic fibrosis. The most important allele is PiZ.

There are two chief clinical effects of α_1-antitrypsin deficiency. The more severe, though less common, is hepatic cirrhosis, which is already manifest in childhood. The genotype of the affected children appears to be always PiZZ. The antitrypsin deficiency can be detected soon after birth, and the clinical disorder is apparent within the first year of life, with hep-

atomegaly and obstructive jaundice leading in time to such complications as esophageal varices, portal hypertension, ascites, and death from liver failure, infection, or other complications.

Examination of the livers of affected children has led to the discovery that the rough endoplasmic reticulum is greatly distended with material which by immunofluorescence appears to be α_1-antitrypsin. The defect in this disorder thus appears to be a failure of the intracellular transport of this protein to the Golgi apparatus and thence to the extracellular space of the serum. The pathogenesis of hepatitis in individuals with serum antitrypsin deficiency remains unclear.

A more common clinical finding in individuals with serum α_1-antitrypsin deficiency is pulmonary emphysema. This occurs at an early age (fifth decade), and more females are affected than with other types of emphysema. In some families, both hepatitis and emphysema have been observed, but this is rather uncommon. The pathogenesis of the pulmonary changes is unclear but may be related to the unopposed action of proteases and a speeding up of aging changes.

Recently, evidence has been accumulating to suggest that α_1-antitrypsin deficiency may be implicated in some cases of the respiratory distress syndrome in newborns.

Water Transport. Diabetes insipidus is a disorder in which the renal tubule has a diminished ability to reabsorb water. The result is polyuria, polydipsia, and dehydration. One form is resistant to treatment with antidiuretic factor (vasopressin) and is discussed further in the section on target tissue insensitivity.

Ion Transport. Phosphate transport in the kidney and intestine is abnormal in familial hypophosphatemic rickets. This disorder shows an X-linked dominant pattern of inheritance with more females affected than males. The defective renal reabsorption of phosphate can be corrected by administration of massive doses of vitamin D (calciferol) i.e., 100 to 400 times the normal requirement.

Calcium transport in the intestine is disturbed in vitamin D–dependent rickets, an autosomal recessive disorder. The result is hypocalcemia, hypophosphatemia, and aminoaciduria starting in infancy. This disorder, too, can be treated by massive doses of vitamin D.

Sodium transport in the red cell is abnormal in hereditary spherocytosis, an autosomal dominant trait. The result is spherocytosis, chronic hemolytic anemia, and hyperbilirubinemia.

Amino Acid Transport. Transport of the amino acid tryptophan by the intestine is reduced in the blue diaper syndrome, named for the positive ferric chloride test seen in some infants who fail to thrive and who show hypercalcemia and nephropathy. This appears to be an autosomal recessive condition.

Vitamin Transport. Myeloblastic anemia in infancy can be due to intestinal malabsorption of vitamin B_{12} in the presence of normal intrinsic factor. This occurs as an autosomal recessive trait.

Multiple Transport Deficiencies

Patients with the X-linked recessive disorder called oculocerebrorenal syndrome (buphthalmos, hyporeflexia, mental retardation, and renal tubular acidosis) show abnormal renal and intestinal transport of water, electrolytes, monosaccharides, and amino acids; i.e., they have a very general transport deficiency.

Disorders Responsive to Vitamin Therapy

At least a dozen genetic diseases are known in which the clinical effects can be ameliorated or completely corrected by the administration of a specific vitamin in doses far larger than the normal requirement. For example, one type of infantile convulsion responds to vitamin B_6 (pyridoxine) in doses 10 to 20 times normal.

Hartnup disease, manifested by mental retardation and cerebellar ataxia, caused by defective intestinal absorption of tryptophan, responds to doses of nicotinamide 8 to 20 times normal.

Two vitamin D–dependent forms of rickets are discussed under Ion Transport, above.

Disorders Affecting Drug Metabolism

Idiosyncratic reactions to drugs frequently have a simple genetic basis, depending upon the presence of a mutant gene at a single locus. Thus barbiturates, which are well tolerated by most adults, may precipitate an acute crisis in an individual with congenital porphyria, an autosomal-dominant condition which can rather easily lead to the misdiagnosis of an acute abdomen with unnecessary operative intervention. Another example is provided by the muscle relaxant succinylcholine. This is metabolized quite well by most individuals and has become an extremely useful drug for the anesthesiologist. But for the rare individual who lacks serum cholinesterase, an autosomal-recessive disorder, succinylcholine is metabolized extremely slowly, and the individual, highly

sensitive to it, shows prolonged apnea. A growing number of examples of hereditary drug sensitivities or, more generally, genetic factors markedly influencing the body's response to a drug, have been found in recent years, giving rise to a new subspecialty, pharmacogenetics. Pharmacogenetics is concerned with genetic factors that influence the effectiveness of antibiotics, and it pinpoints mutant genes which alter an individual's response to other drugs. For example, some individuals do not respond to the usual dose of warfarin used in anticoagulation therapy, but require as much as 20 times the normal dose to produce the desired increase in prothrombin time. This trait is inherited as an autosomal dominant and is associated with a greatly increased sensitivity to vitamin K. The probable explanation of these findings is that the enzyme involved in the synthesis of clotting factors II, VII, IX, and X has undergone a molecular change as a result of mutation so that its binding site has an increased affinity for vitamin K and a decreased affinity for warfarin.

Disorders Resulting from Altered Structural Proteins (the Hemoglobinopathies)

Unquestionably, human hemoglobin is the best-studied of the mammalian proteins. The hemoglobin molecule is two pairs of polypeptide chains (tetramer). Autosomal alleles control the amino acid sequence of the chains. Alterations in these genes bring about changes in the molecule and, often, in the physical properties of hemoglobin. These changes lead to clinical abnormalities.

The major hemoglobins are the adult form, HbA, and fetal hemoglobin, HbF. HbA contains two alpha polypeptide chains and two beta chains ($\alpha_2\beta_2$). HbF contains two alpha chains and two gamma chains ($\alpha_2\gamma_2$). A minor hemoglobin, HbA_2, is found in parallel to HbA. It contains two alpha chains and two delta chains ($\alpha_2\delta_2$). Production of HbF is high in the fetus but declines soon after birth, while the production of HbA and A_2, which are low in the fetus, rises sharply not long after birth.

The genes for alpha and beta chains are thought to be on separate chromosomes; the genes for beta, delta, and gamma chains on the same chromosome.

Alpha chains contain 141 amino acids; beta chains consist of 146 amino acids. The most common inherited abnormalities of hemoglobin arise from replacement of a single amino acid with another kind in either the alpha or beta chain. For example, in sickle-cell hemoglobin, HbS, valine has replaced glutamic acid in position 6 (numbering from the *N*-terminal end of the beta chain). In hemoglobin C, lysine has replaced glutamic acid in the same position. Each of these substitutions is caused by a mutation in the gene controlling that portion of the chain. For example, the RNA nucleotide triplet GAA coding for glutamic acid may have been altered to GUA, which codes for valine, as a result of the HbS mutation.

Alternately, the mutation may involve a deletion rather than a substitution. In hemoglobin Gun Hill, for example, the beta chain is 141 amino acids long instead of 146 because of a deletion of five consecutive amino acids in the chain. Presumably, the genetic event was the deletion of the corresponding nucleotide sequence of 15 bases from the beta gene.

The clinical effect of such a mutation arises from a molecular change in the hemoglobin molecule. If the altered molecule becomes unstable, the result is hemolytic anemia even in heterozygotes. An example is Hb Hammersmith in which serine has replaced phenylalanine in position 42 of the beta chain. In many cases, hemolytic anemia is present even in the newborn child. In the case of Hb Zurich, on the other hand, in which arginine has replaced histidine in position 63 of the beta chain, hemolysis occurs only in response to some exogenous agent. Again, both homozygotes and heterozygotes are affected.

A contrast is provided by hemoglobin C, in which lysine has replaced glutamic acid in position 6 of the beta chain. Only the homozygotes show hemolytic anemia, which appears to be related to the lower solubility of HbC. An even more marked reduction in solubility occurs in HbS in which valine replaces glutamic acid in position 6 of the beta chain. When oxygen tension is reduced, as it is to some extent in capillary and venous blood, the molecules may form aggregates, reducing the volume of the red cell and producing the characteristic sickle shape (see discussion of sickle-cell trait below).

In another type of hemoglobinopathy, the methemoglobinemias, an amino acid substitution (frequently tyrosine for histidine) adjacent to the iron in the heme portion of the hemoglobin molecule interferes with the reduction of iron from the ferric state to the ferrous form after the hemoglobin picks up oxygen, thus interfering with normal physiology. An example is provided by HbM Boston in which tyrosine replaces histidine in position 58 in the alpha chain. The phenol side chain of tyrosine bonds to ferric iron forming a stable complex which is not easily reduced by methemoglobin reductase to give the ferrous form of iron. Increased oxygen affinity without methemoglobinemia can also occur. For example, Hb Yakima involves the substitution of histidine for aspartate in position 99 of the beta chain. Decreased tissue oxy-

genation occurs as a result of the increased oxygen affinity of the abnormal hemoglobin, with a compensatory increase in red blood cells brought about by stimulation of erythropoietin production.

A few examples are known of the opposite change in the hemoglobin molecule i.e., a reduced affinity for oxygen. This is seen in Hb Seattle in which glutamic acid has replaced alanine in position 76 of the beta chain. The total red cell mass is reduced in these individuals because they lack the usual stimulus to red cell production. They thus appear anemic.

Dozens of mutations involving the beta chain and a somewhat smaller number involving the alpha chain have been described. Alpha chain variants are potentially more serious because even the fetal and embryonic hemoglobins require alpha chains; the beta chain only becomes important some time after birth.

Although a tremendous variety of hemoglobinopathies are known, only a few are so common that the obstetrician can reasonably expect to see them in practice. The most common is the sickle-cell trait, the heterozygous HbS condition. This occurs in nearly 1 in 10 American blacks. Rarely is it a cause of disease in the heterozygous carrier, except under conditions of unusual hypoxia—which might occur at high altitude, in a patient with cyanotic heart disease, or under narcosis or anesthesia. Tissue anoxia in localized regions could trigger sickling in these areas, giving rise to blockage of small blood vessels and producing infarcts. These effects are, of course, far more common in the homozygous sickle cell patient and are probably never a medical problem in most heterozygotes.

The major problem of these "carriers" is that they have a fairly high probability of marrying other carriers, in which case the risk in each pregnancy of producing a homozygous sickle cell infant is 1 in 4. Many blacks view this as a public health problem, and large-scale screening programs have been set up in several areas in order to detect carriers as well as homozygotes. Others have objected to this approach because the heterozygotes may be stigmatized or even lose a job because of lack of understanding or unauthorized disclosures of information without the patient's permission. If it becomes possible to distinguish the sickle-cell homozygote from the heterozygote fairly early in pregnancy, every pregnant patient could be offered routine hemoglobin screening at the time of the first prenatal visit, with prenatal diagnosis offered to all carriers. At present, the only way to prevent the birth of an affected child is for known carriers to avoid reproduction with other carriers.

Pregnancy represents a threat to the sickle-cell homozygotes. About 1 in 400 American blacks is an HbS homozygote. The obstetrician should not be lulled into a false sense of security by the mistaken belief that since sickle-cell disease is such a serious disorder, those who have it will not be likely to become pregnant. Both genetic and environmental factors can influence how well the sickle-cell homozygotes compete. Several homozygotes with very mild disease were found to be heterozygotes for hemoglobin Memphis. Thus, an amino acid substitution (glutamine for glutamic acid in position 23) in the alpha chain of hemoglobin lessens the phenotypic effect of the amino acid substitution in the beta chain in sickle-cell disease.

Other Hemoglobinopathies: Thalassemias. The thalassemias are hemoglobinopathies in which there is a markedly reduced production of one or another (usually alpha or beta) globin chain. Beta thalassemia was the first to be recognized; in the homozygote, this is expressed as Cooley's or Mediterranean anemia, a very severe disorder with profound anemia caused by the depressed production of beta chains and the interaction of the excess alpha chains which tend to precipitate in the red blood cells. Family studies indicate that the gene for beta thalassemia is closely linked to, or identical with, the beta chain gene, and has no suppressive effect on the homologous gene on the other chromosome.

Disorders of Binding Proteins

The role of specific binding proteins in the activation of a wide range of metabolic reactions is becoming increasingly clear. The steroid binding proteins are probably as well understood as any. Estrogenic hormones (E) exert their effect by combining with a cytoplasmic protein (P). The protein $(P \rightarrow P^1)$ undergoes a conformational change and the EP^1 complex enters the nucleus and combines with protein of the nuclear chromatin, in this way activating specific portions of the genome and initiating the estrogenic effects. Androgens and adrenal steroid hormones appear to act in a similar manner, involving other specific binding proteins.

Androgen-insensitive male pseudohermaphroditism has been known for many years. Evidence is growing that individuals with this disorder cannot respond to testosterone or dihydrotestosterone. A mutation involving one androgen-binding protein is believed responsible. Despite the mutation in the structural gene for this binding protein, the molecule can still bind testosterone, but it can no longer bind

to chromatin, and its action is thus blocked. The effect is expressed even in heterozygotes. The typical individual has normal female external genitalia at birth, but may have inguinal hernias in which the testes can be palpated. At puberty, feminizing changes occur with breast development and development of mature feminine contours and voice. Usually, axillary and pubic hair are absent or scant; there is no beard, and the body hair is feminine. The vagina is very short, ending as a blind pouch. Uterus and tubes are absent. The Wolffian duct derivatives are incompletely developed, so the epididymides and vasa deferentia are abnormal. The gonads are testes, which have the usual appearance of cryptorchid testes, with absent spermatogenesis despite fairly well differentiated Leydig cells in adults. Fairly normal hormone production by the testes is indicated by measurement of the various steroids and gonadotrophic hormones. The inability of the tissues to respond to androgenic hormones has been confirmed by direct administration of testosterone and dihydrotestosterone.

Disorders of Bilirubin and Heme Metabolism

Hyperbilirubinemia with an elevated level of unconjugated bilirubin occurs to some extent in almost every infant within a few days of birth, producing physiologic jaundice. This is not because of an inherited enzyme defect, but of a delay either in the maturation of the enzyme glucuronyl transferase, which conjugates bilirubin to the glucuronide form in which it is excreted via the biliary system, or in the maturation of uridine diphosphoglucose dehydrogenase, which leads by steps to the glucuronic acid residue which binds to bilirubin.

The inability to conjugate bilirubin, believed to result from a deficiency of glucuronyl transferase activity, is the most consistent biochemical finding in the Crigler-Najjar syndrome, an autosomal recessive disorder. The most severely affected patients have no conjugated bilirubin in their bile and are said to have the type I disorder. The type II disorder is milder, and patients have a small amount of conjugated bilirubin in their bile. Different genes are involved (the two types do not occur in the same family, for example), and the response to barbiturates is different. Type I patients are not helped, but in type II patients, phenobarbital induces a rapid reduction of serum bilirubin from 15 to 20 mg per 100 mL down to 2 to 3 mg per 100 mL. Phenobarbital has been shown to induce an increase in the level of one of the two basic liver proteins that combine with bilirubin and presumably play a role in its metabolism. The level of this protein

Table 6–4 Empiric Risk for Common Malformations Not Showing Simple Mendelian Inheritance

Type of malformation	Incidence among live-born, %	Incidence of same or related malformations, %	
		Siblings	Children
Anencephaly	~0.14	5.0 for anencephaly and spina bifida	
Spina bifida	~0.1	5.1	
Anencephaly, spina bifida and/or hydrocephaly, combined	~0.29		
If one child is affected		4.0	
If two children are affected		10.0	
Isolated cleft palate*	~0.02–0.05	1.8–2.3 (higher for siblings of males)	7.0
If parent is affected		17.0	
Harelip and cleft palate (cheilognathopalatoschisis)	~0.1–0.18		
If one child is affected		3.5–4.4 (higher for siblings of females)	2.0–3.5
If two children are affected		9.0	
If parent is affected		14.0	
Congenital heart disease (CHD) in general (if not part of syndrome with known transmission)	~0.8	2–5	2–4
If two children are affected		5.5–8.0	
Ventral septal defect	~0.2	4.3	1–4
Atrial septal defect [exclusive of autosomal dominant form(s)]	~0.03	3.2	1–4
Fallot's tetralogy	~0.06	2.2	
Pulmonary stenosis	~0.06	2.9	
Patent ductus arteriosus	~0.08	3.2	2–4
Transposition of great vessels (TGV)	~0.08	4–5 for CHD in general 1–2 for TGV	
Valvular aortic stenosis (subvalvular and supravalvular stenosis excluded)	~0.02–0.04	2.6	
Coarctation of aorta	0.02–0.04	1–3	1–3
Congenital intestinal aganglionosis (Hirschsprung's disease)	0.02	0.6–18	
Congenital dislocation of the hip	0.3		
If one child and one parent are affected		36	
Clubfoot	0.1	2.9–3.1 (5.97) (1.95)	

*Single families with apparently monogenic inheritance have been reported.
†In boys with hydrocephalus, the X-chromosomal type must be excluded.
Source: Modified from W Fuhrmann, F Vogel.

is regulated in part by the pituitary-thyroid axis, with thyroxin reducing the level.

Target-Tissue Insensitivity: Diabetes Insipidus

Vasopressin-resistant diabetes insipidus appears to be due to a defect in the distal convoluted tubules and collecting ducts of the kidney. Normally, these reabsorb water from the tubule when vasopressin is present. In its absence, larger amounts of hypotonic urine are excreted; the same happens in vasopressin-resistant diabetes insipidus despite the administration of vasopressin.

This disorder is inherited as an X-linked recessive trait and is present from birth or soon thereafter. The molecular defect is unknown but may reside in the protein to which vasopressin normally binds; thus the defect may reduce the capacity of the protein to bind vasopressin. If this is so, then the administration of massive amounts of vasopressin might correct the disorder, as with vitamin-dependent genetic disorders. Side effects such as abdominal cramping have prevented an adequate test of this idea.

Androgen-insensitive male pseudohermaphroditism, or testicular feminization, is another target-organ insensitivity disorder, one in which a defective binding protein has been implicated.

MULTIFACTORIAL DISORDERS

For genetic traits outside the simple modes of inheritance, it is frequently true that their phenotypic expression is dependent upon a number of genes (polygenic inheritance), each of which may contribute relatively little to the total variation. The contribution of each gene is nonspecific; only the total effect is finally visible. Since each gene contributing to the final phenotypic pattern is inherited via independent assortment and segregation, the more numerous the genes involved, the greater the continuum of variation in trait expressivity. For counseling in cases of malformations outside the simple modes of inheritance, empiric risk figures are most commonly used; i.e., figures based on statistical data gained from research into a sufficiently large random series of the relatives of patients with a particular anomaly (Table 6–4).

ANENCEPHALY AND SPINA BIFIDA

The primary defect in this polygenic malformation is failure of neural groove closure to form an intact neural tube. Anencephaly results from failure to close at the anterior portion of the groove, while failure of mid- or posterior closure results in spina bifida. This congenital malformation can be found to range in expression from the very severely affected (absence of brain) to rather mildly affected (small, surgically reparable). The incidence is 2 to 3 per 1000 live births and the risk of recurrence in a family with one affected member is approximately 5 percent. Anencephaly can be detected with approximately 99 percent accuracy with a combination of ultrasound and amniotic fluid α-fetoprotein determination. Significant neural tube defects can be detected prenatally with about 90 percent accuracy by biochemical testing of α-fetoprotein levels, which are markedly increased in the amniotic fluids of fetuses with this malformation.

Other types of malformations not showing simple modes of inheritance include pyloric stenosis, isolated cleft palate, congenital dislocation of the hip, and congenital heart diseases in general.

REFERENCES

Burton BK, Nadler HL: Clinical diagnosis of the inborn errors of metabolism in the neonatal period. *Pediatrics* 61:3, 1978.

Fuhrmann W, Vogel F: *Genetic Counseling*, 2d ed., New York: Springer-Verlag, 1976.

deGrouchy J, Turleau C: *Clinical Atlas of Human Chromosomes*, New York: John Wiley, 1977.

Harris H: *The Principles of Human Biochemical Genetics*, New York: American Elsevier, 1970.

McKusick VA: Genetics and human disease, in *Harrison's Principles of Internal Medicine*, 7th ed., eds. MM Wintrobe et al., New York: McGraw-Hill, 1974.

_____: *Mendelian Inheritance in Man. Catalogs of Autosomal Dominant, Autosomal Recessive, and X-linked Phenotypes*, 4th ed., Baltimore: Johns Hopkins University Press, 1975.

_____, Claiborne R. (eds.): *Medical Genetics*, New York: HP Pub. Co, 1973.

Smith DW: *Recognizable Patterns of Human Malformation. Genetic, Embryologic, and Clinical Aspects*, 2d ed., Philadelphia: Saunders, 1976.

Stanbury JB et al. (eds.): *The Metabolic Basis of Inherited Disease*, New York: McGraw-Hill 1978.

Thompson JS, Thompson MW: *Genetics in Medicine*, Philadelphia: Saunders, 1973.

Watson JD: *Molecular Biology of the Gene*, 3d ed., New York: WA Benjamin, 1977.

Yunis JJ (ed.): *New Chromosomal Syndromes*, New York: Academic Press, 1977.

7

Endocrinology

A. BRIAN LITTLE R. B. BILLIAR

NORMAL REPRODUCTION IN THE FEMALE

The basis of all reproduction is the reproductive or ovarian cycle. Recently, with the advent of radioimmunoassay, the details of the control of the menstrual cycle have been examined and reviewed by Ross and by Vande Wiele and colleagues in considerable detail. Vande Wiele et al. have also accumulated the variables that presently are known to influence the menstrual cycle and have created a computer program which simulates the hormonal controls described in the human being. This model has been recently modified by Feng et al.

THE MENSTRUAL CYCLE

It has been shown that FSH (follicle-stimulating hormone) increases as estrogen decreases at the end of the menstrual cycle. By the first day of the menstrual period FSH has already risen to a point where it is beginning the stimulus of the primordial follicles (Figs. 7–1 and 7–2). The level of FSH appears to reach a maximum at the time of the onset of flow of the previous period, providing the stimulus for new

FIGURE 7–1 Plasma levels of gonadotropins and gonadal steroids during the human menstrual cycle. The cycle is centered on day 0, the day of the midcycle LH peak. *(From Speroff et al.)*

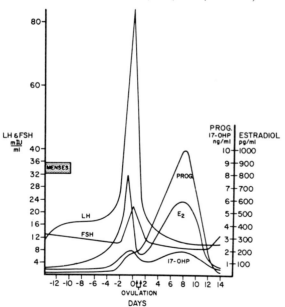

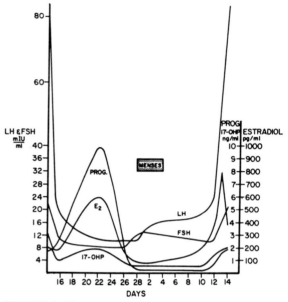

FIGURE 7–2 Plasma levels of gonadotropins and gonadal steroids during the human menstrual cycle. The changes during menses are emphasized by centering the cycle on day 28 and the beginning of menses. *(From Speroff et al.)*

ovarian follicles to grow. At the outset there is little secretion of estrogen by the developing follicle. Six or seven days later estrogens begin to be secreted slowly and then more rapidly. Just prior to ovulation, there appears to be a sharp rise in estradiol, which is responsible for the release of LH (luteinizing hormone) from the pituitary. The timing appears to be that the estradiol rise is followed in 12 to 24 hours by the LH surge and 24 to 36 hours later by ovulation. Circulating 17-hydroxyprogesterone increases at approximately the same time that estrogen increases.

Three factors are required for the normal ovulatory menstrual cycle. (1) Estradiol and progesterone must fall at the end of the cycle and allow FSH to increase and stimulate a new crop of follicles. This is the estradiol tonic gonadotropin inhibition, or negative feedback. (2) There must be a midcycle surge of estradiol which stimulates the LH surge. This is the estradiol cyclic stimulation, or positive feedback. (3) There must be present a normal corpus luteum with its inherent life span.

ESTROGENS

Estrogens are substances associated with those changes which go to make "femaleness." In biologic terms these changes are vaginal cornification (estimated in vaginal cytograms to define the state of endocrine secretion in the menstrual cycle), growth of the uterus in pregnancy, estrous behavior in animals and probably also human beings, and the development of proliferative endometrium. In addition, estrogens have other responses which include the female body habitus, breast development, female hair distribution, and some specific physiologic responses such as the stimulation of the synthesis of circulating binding globulins including transcortin, thyroxine-binding globulin, and transferrin. Estrogen, progesterone, and intrauteral pressure are responsible for the dilatation of the ureters in pregnancy, and the hormones have similar effects on all smooth muscle, including that of blood vessels and the gut. The model of estrogen effect is best illustrated by its influence on the uterus, which has been studied in the rat. The first result of estrogen administration is the inhibition of fluid; this is followed by the increase in synthesis of various proteins until hypertrophy of the muscle itself results.

Three classical estrogens are primarily responsible for the major estrogenic effects and are measured in the various clinical conditions in which estrogen evaluation is called for. These are estrone (E_1), estradiol (E_2), and estriol (E_3). The most estrogenic of these three is estradiol. Estriol is called the estrogen of pregnancy as it is increased the most during gestation. Of considerable importance is the fact that estriol is synthesized from precursors that primarily come from the fetal adrenal in pregnancy. It is used as an indication of fetal wellbeing during the latter months of pregnancy and will drop markedly in the blood and urine following fetal death in utero.

Sites of Secretion

Estrogens are secreted by the ovary and by the placenta in pregnancy and also added to the maternal circulation following the peripheral conversion of precursors which come from the adrenal and the liver of both fetus and mother. During the menstrual cycle the production rate of estradiol during the proliferative phase is 80 μg per day and of estrone, 110 μg per day. In the luteal phase E_2 rises to 270 μg per day and E_2 to 240 μg per day, and at ovulation E_2 reaches 400 μg per day and E_1 reaches 250 μg per day (Tagatz, Gurpide). The rise at the time of ovulation with the reversal of the E_1/E_2 ratio is apparently the stimulus for the LH surge which results in ovulation. In pregnancy the production rate of 17β-estradiol rises to 16 mg per day and total E reaches about 200 mg per day at term (Fishman et al.). In the postmenopausal woman the circulating E_2 production rate is less than

6 μg per day and E_1 is 40 μg per day. However, as has recently been observed, the major circulating estrogen postmenopausally is estrone; it is primarily derived from the peripheral conversion of androstenedione which is largely secreted from the adrenal (Siiteri, MacDonald). During normal cycles the estrogen is primarily secreted by the theca and granulosa cells of the ovarian follicle when it develops from a primary follicle to a graafian follicle just prior to ovulation under the influence of FSH. In the management of cases in which artificial ovulation is stimulated by the administration of gonadotropins (see Chap. 27), the blood or urinary excretion levels of estrogen are closely monitored to determine the development of the follicles so that the ovulatory stimulus of LH [or its biologic equivalent, human chorionic gonadotropin, (HCG), used clinically] may be given at the appropriate time. The understanding of this physiologic sequence allows the HCG to be given at an appropriate time to prevent overstimulation of the ovary, which may be very dangerous. Correct timing has also minimized the ovulation of multiple follicles and the resulting multiple pregnancies which patients fear are associated with "fertility pill(s)."

Physiologic Effects of Estrogens

Estrogens rely for their effects on their interaction with specific tissues and processes in the body. A description of these responses may be helpful in understanding the signs and symptoms of estrogen lack or excess.

During intrauterine development the male hormones are necessary for the development of the male genital system, but this is not the case for the female genital tract, which rather develops in the absence of male hormones. However, the placenta secretes an excess of estrogens during pregnancy, and a most important function of fetal metabolism appears to be to inactivate the strong estrogenic compounds by converting them to the less active metabolites. At birth the female genital system has identifiable estrogen activity in the histologic appearance of cervix and endometrium, although not of an adult type. Following birth there may actually be vaginal spotting or bleeding, and breast tissues may secrete small amounts of "witch's milk."

After birth estrogen activity usually does not occur until puberty. At this time the secondary sex characteristics develop. These include breast development, axillary and pubic hair growth with their specific female patterns, and the development of the female body habitus. With the maturation of the genital tract, enlargement of the uterus, beginning secretion of the endometrial and cervical glands, and the start of normal tubal function, the menstrual cycle begins its rhythm.

Estrogen has effects on other endocrine glands. It exerts its inhibitory and stimulatory effects on the pituitary which either modifies tonic gonadotropic secretion, or at certain times of the cycle, releases an LH surge which results in ovulation. Estrogen effects a change in the circulating binding globulins of many hormones and other carrier proteins. Thyroxine-binding globulin (TBG) is elevated both in pregnancy and following the administration of estrogen. Transcortin [corticosteroid-binding globulin (CBG)], transferrin, estradiol, and testosterone-binding globulin [gonadal steroid-binding globulin (GBG)], and others are similarly increased. This accounts for increased protein-bound iodine (PBI) and other protein-bound substances in pregnancy and also in patients who are being cycled on oral steroid contraceptive pills which contain estrogens.

Estrogens affect salt and water metabolism. There appears to be an effect on sodium and water resorption at the kidney tubule level. It may be a direct effect but may also be mediated through the renin-aldosterone system. Estrogens also affect calcium metabolism and bone growth. The early administration of estrogens in children will lead to premature closure of the long-bone epiphyses. This treatment has been sought by mothers eager to keep their tall daughters at a marriageable "height." Postmenopausally, osteoporosis may be relieved by estrogen administration, but certainly osteoporosis is not solely due to estrogen lack, for such treatment is only symptomatically effective for a short period of time.

Women are less prone to coronary disease up to menopause than are men if the women have no associated diabetes or hypertension. The decline in sex advantage at the menopause relates to the slower increment in the rate of male death than female after that age. Natural menopause does not place women at greater risk. The use of estrogens to reduce this risk is thus not justified. Estrogen alters lipoprotein and triglyceride metabolism and may be partly the reason for this difference. Because of this hypothesis males have been treated with large doses of estrogen to prevent heart disease. The benefits were outweighed by the problems created. Moreover, this hypothesis is also used to advocate estrogens forever in the postmenopausal woman, the advantages of which have yet to be proved.

Cholesterol and triglycerides are higher in young men and reach at-risk levels in the 40 to 55 age range. Estrogen administration will increase triglyceride levels to at-risk values. Steroids do have an effect on lipoprotein fractions: high-density lipoprotein (HDL), low-density lipoprotein (LDL), and very low density lipoprotein (VLDL). Males have higher LDL and lower HDL than women; androgens shift the concentration in the male direction and estrogens in the female direction (lower LDL and higher HDL). Estrogen effects are variable and probably dose-dependent; therefore, there is no sound basis for estrogen administration to control hyperlipemia and thus reduce the risk of coronary heart disease (Ryan, 1976).

Estrogen in Blood and Urine

During the menstrual cycle estrogens increase just prior to ovulation, diminish, then go through a more gentle rise in the luteal phase. Just prior to ovulation urinary estradiol reaches a peak of 5 to 7 μg per day with estrone 15 to 20 μg per day and estriol 20 to 25 μg per day or a total of 40 to 50 μg per day (Fig. 7–3). In the luteal phase there is a rise with a corresponding distribution at about day 17 to 20 with a total of 30 to 40 μg per day in the urine (Brown, 1955).

FIGURE 7–3 Urinary estrogen excretion in a normal nulliparous woman, age 34. *(From Brown, 1955.)*

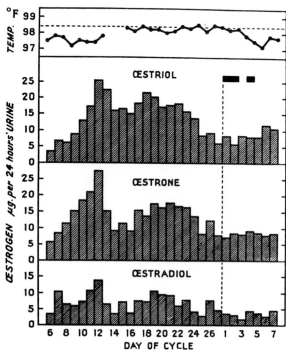

In pregnancy, values rise gradually to term with total estrogens of 40 to 50 mg per day; the major part is estriol at 35 to 45 mg per day; about 1.5 mg is estrone, and about 0.5 mg is estradiol (Brown, 1956). About 20 different estrogens have been identified in pregnancy urine, but other than the three classical estrogens they are excreted in small amounts only and are not known presently to be of clinical significance (Diczfalusy, Mancuso).

Blood estrogens have been examined in the menstrual cycle and parallel the urinary excretion (Fig. 7–4). The singular phenomenon is the striking peak of estradiol concentration prior to the LH surge, rising to 50 ng per 100 mL and reversing the E_1/E_2 ratio as in the urine. Estrone similarly rises to a peak of 20 ng per 100 mL prior to ovulation (Baird et al.). Blood estrogens in pregnancy rise as does the urinary excretion. Concentrations of about 20 μg per 100 mL are observed at term.

Postmenopausally, when the production rate re-

verts to 40 μg per day, the blood value for estradiol is about 3 ng per 100 mL, and urinary excretion of total estrogens is as low as 10 μg per day (Siiteri, Mac-Donald).

Metabolic Clearance, Production, and Secretion Rates of Estrogens

Estrogens can be synthesized de novo from acetate. This occurs, as described below through either the Δ^4 or Δ^5 pathway of steroid synthesis from either pregnenolone through dehydroepiandrosterone (DHA), or progesterone through androstenedione. The DHA is converted to androstenedione (A), and the androstenedione is converted to testosterone (T). Both T and A are aromatized to estradiol and estrone, respectively (Ryan, Smith, 1965). Estrogens can also be converted by peripheral conversion from precursors, particularly in pregnancy by the placenta and in the postmenopausal period by extraglandular tissues. In pregnancy the two major sources of estrogen are the result of the conversion of DHA sulfate (DHS) to DHA to estrone by the placenta, and of 16-hydroxydehydroepiandrosterone sulfate to 16-OHDHA to 16-hydroxyestrone and then to estriol, all by the placenta (Diczfalusy, Mancuso). The precursors are produced by the adrenals of either the mother or the fetus; the latter source is of greater importance as the major amount of urinary estriol disappears following fetal death in utero. In addition to this, there is a large amount of 17-hydroxysteroid dehydrogenase in the placenta which will interconvert estrone and estradiol.

The estrogens are metabolized by hydroxylation, oxidation, and reduction at various points on the carbon molecule and by conjugation with sulfate or glucuronic acid and excreted through the kidneys as a water-soluble product. Estradiol is bound to plasma globulin (GBG) in the circulation, which influences its metabolic clearance rate. The rate at which any steroid is cleared irrevocably from the blood is its metabolic clearance rate (MCR). The overall MCR is the sum of the individual clearance rates of tissues and organs that remove the steroid from the blood. For example, MCR equals the hepatic clearance plus the renal clearance plus the brain clearance plus the utero-ovarian clearance plus all other clearances. MCR is expressed as volume of blood cleared of steroid per unit time (e.g., liters per day). The simplest expression of MCR is that it is composed of hepatic clearance (a major site of steroid metabolism) and extrahepatic clearance (all other sites). Hepatic

FIGURE 7–4 Concentration of luteinizing hormone (LH), unconjugated estrone, and 17β-estradiol in peripheral plasma of women during the menstrual cycle (n = 51). Day 0 in the graph is the day of estimated ovulation. *(From Baird et al., 1969.)*

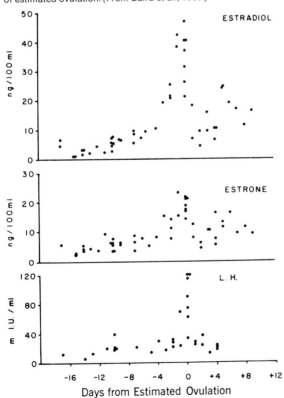

clearance is the product of liver blood flow and hepatic extraction (Baird et al.).

The production rate (PR) of a steroid is the rate at which that steroid appears in the bloodstream from whatever site by whatever means. The PR therefore is the sum of all secretion rates of that steroid from its glands of origin plus that portion of its production which results from the secretion of precursor steroids and subsequent peripheral conversion to the steroid being measured. PR is the product of MCR and the circulating concentration of the steroid. The measurement of MCR is made by either the single injection or continuous infusion of a radioactive steroid and by measuring either the disappearance of the radioactive steroid or its constant level in the blood, in both instances assuming the steady state.

The MCR of estradiol during the menstrual cycle is 1350 L per day, of estrone 2210 L per day, and of estriol 2100 L per day (Table 7–1). The PR of estradiol varies from 80 μg per day in the proliferative phase to as high as 900 μg per day at midcycle and 270 μg per day in midluteal phase. The PR of estrone is 110 μg per day in the early follicular cycle, over 600 μg per day at midcylce, and 240 μg per day in the secretory phase. The PR of estriol is 14 μg per day in the proliferative phase and 23 μg per day in the luteal phase. The secretion rate of the ovary accounts for 85 to 95 percent of estradiol production, but only 70 to 80 percent of estrone production is by direct ovarian secretion (Longcope et al.). About 1 percent of secreted androstenedione is converted to estrone peripherally, which accounts for 20 to 40 μg per day of estrone, almost the entire postmenopausal produc-

tion. This conversion increases with age, body weight, at menopause, and in the presence of cirrhosis. There is apparently a circadian rhythm to circulating estrone concentration but not estradiol. The circadian rhythm of estrone may represent the contribution to its production from androstenedione secretion from the adrenal, which is known to have a circadian cycle.

In pregnancy the production of estrogen, particularly by the placenta, is increased manyfold with about 200 mg per day produced at term, but the definitive values of the MCR and PR are not yet available.

Steroid Biosynthesis

It is now reasonably well established that cholesterol is the obligatory intermediate for most steroid hormones, the possible exception being those estrogens with ring-B unsaturation, i.e., the equilins and equilenins. In the steroid-secreting endocrine glands cholesterol is either synthesized de novo from acetate or is obtained from the blood (Fig. 7–5). The source of cholesterol for steroid biosynthesis in the adrenal and placenta is blood-borne cholesterol. However, there is a greater contribution of de novo synthesis from blood-borne cholesterol for steroid synthesis in the human ovary.

The first step in the conversion of cholesterol, which has 27 carbons, to the steroid hormones is the cleavage of the side chain of cholesterol which results in the formation of the 21-carbon steroid pregnenolone (preg-5-en-3β-ol-20-one) and a six-carbon

TABLE 7–1 Metabolic Clearance Rates (MCR), Plasma Concentrations *(i)*, Production Rates (PR), and Ovarian Secretion (SR) of Steroids in Blood in the Menstrual Cycle (PR = MCR × *i*)

	Phase of menstrual cycle	MCR plasma, L/day	Plasma concentration *(i)*, μg/100mL	PR, mg/day	SR (ovaries), mg/day	References
17β-Estradiol	Early	1350	0.006	0.081	0.07	Baird et al., 1968, 1969
	Midcycle		0.033–0.070	0.445–0.945	0.4 –0.8	
	Luteal		0.020	0.270	0.25	
Estrone	Early	2210	0.005	0.110	0.08	Baird et al., 1968, 1969
	Midcycle		0.015–0.030	0.331–0.662	0.25–0.50	MacDonald et al.
	Luteal		0.011	0.243	0.16	
Estriol	Early	2100	0.0007	0.014	0.018	Flood et al.
	Luteal	2100	0.0010	0.023		
Progesterone	Follicular	2510	0.03–0.10	0.75–2.5	1.5	Little, Billiar, 1969
	Luteal		0.06–2.0	15.0–50.0	24	
20α-Dihydro-	Follicular	2000	0.05	1.0	0.8	Little, Billiar, 1969
progesterone	Luteal		0.25	5.0	3.2	Van der Molen

Source: Tagatz, Gurpide.

aldehyde. This conversion, which requires molecular oxygen and the cofactor nicotinamide-adenine dinucleotide phosphate (NADPH), takes place in the mitochondria of the cell. Only the mitochondria of the adrenal cortex, testes (interstitial cells), ovary, and placenta have the enzymatic capacity to catalyze this complex conversion of cholesterol to pregnenolone. This conversion is irreversible and rate-limiting in steroidogenesis. Trophic hormones affect the rate of steroid synthesis and secretion by increasing, in a manner unknown, the rate of conversion of cholesterol to pregnenolone.

Pregnenolone is converted to androgens in either the testis or ovary by the same pathways. These are oxidation reactions which result in the cleavage of the 2-carbon side chains of the 21-carbon steroid nucleus to a 19-carbon nucleus, resulting in the formation of androstenedione. The two possible pathways from pregnenolone to androstenedione are the so-called Δ^5 (delta-5) pathway and the Δ^4 (delta-4) pathways. *Delta* is used to represent the site of the double bond, Δ^4 being a double bond between carbons 4 and 5 in ring A of the steroid nucleus and Δ^5 being a double bond between carbons 5 and 6 of the B ring of the steroid nucleus. At the present time there are not good quantitative data to indicate whether the Δ^4 or Δ^5 pathway is the more important in either the human ovary or testis. Generally it is believed that the Δ^4 pathway is the more significant one for testicular testosterone synthesis and the Δ^5 pathway for ovarian estrogen biosynthesis.

The conversion of the 19-carbon androgens to the 18-carbon estrogens involves oxidation reactions and the cleavage of a carbon-carbon bond. This conversion actually consists of several enzymatic steps, but the precise details are not known.

A significant feature of the overall conversion of cholesterol to the different biologically active steroids secreted by the endocrine glands is that common pathways and intermediates are used whether the resulting steroids are glucocorticoids, androgens, or estrogens. Unique pathways for the synthesis of each class of biologically active steroid hormones are not used by the different tissues. The quantitative presence of key enzymatic reactions at branch points, therefore, is important in determining the secretion pattern of an endocrine gland once the conversion of cholesterol to pregnenolone has occurred; the secretion pattern for an endocrine gland is primarily determined by quantitative aspects of the enzymology of steroidogenesis rather than qualitative features. For example, if in the adrenal there is a deficiency in the conversion of 17α-hydroxyprogesterone to 11-desoxycortisol, as is common in the adrenogenital syndrome, more substrate becomes available for androgen formation and secretion. Similarly if there is a block in the ovary in the conversion of androgen to estrogen, proportionally more androgen will be secreted by the ovary.

Control of Estrogen Secretion

During the normal menstrual cycle estrogen is secreted predominantly by the ovary and largely by the cells of the graafian follicle and corpus luteum (Ryan, Petro). Follicular development is under control of FSH, at least initially, followed by a gradual increase in LH, and therefore estrogen depends primarily on follicle stimulation, then subsequent follicle growth; later, the formation of a normal corpus luteum and its maintenance are controlled by LH. Estradiol secreted by the ovary suppresses gonadotropin, and as estradiol rises, FSH falls *pari passu*.

Postmenopausally estrogen secretion is presumably controlled by androstenedione production which will fluctuate according to cortisol production under adrenocorticotropic hormone (ACTH) control (Siiteri, MacDonald).

During pregnancy a major component of estrogen production arises from the placental conversion of fetal adrenal precursors. Therefore fetal adrenal control is responsible for estrogen levels in blood and urine—particularly estriol. Cortisol or similar ACTH-suppressing adrenocorticoids administered to a pregnant woman will cross the placenta and suppress the fetal pituitary and thereby the fetal adrenal, resulting in a considerable reduction in maternal estriol excretion (Simmer et al.).

ANDROGENS

By definition, *androgens* are those substances which possess masculinizing activities such as the testis hormone. Major endogenous steroid androgens are testosterone, androstenedione, and dehydroepiandrosterone. These steroids are secreted by the testis, the ovary, and the adrenal and are the products of specific enzymes in each gland acting on precursors from either the Δ^5 of Δ^4 pathways of steroid metabolism which are common to these endocrine glands. Cleavage of the C-21 side chain of either 17α-hydroxypregnenolone (17α-hydroxypregn-5-en-3β-ol-20-one) or 17α-hydroxyprogesterone (17α-hydroxypregn-4-en-3,20-dione) results in the Δ^5 compound DHA or the Δ^4 compound androstenedione (androst-4-en-3,17-dione). Androstenedione is readily con-

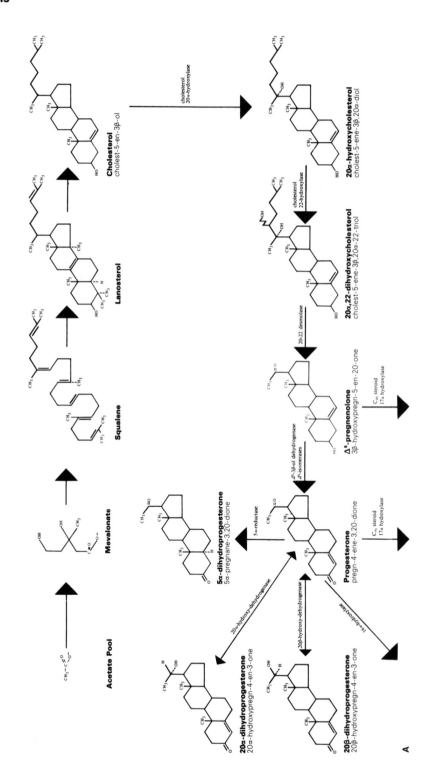

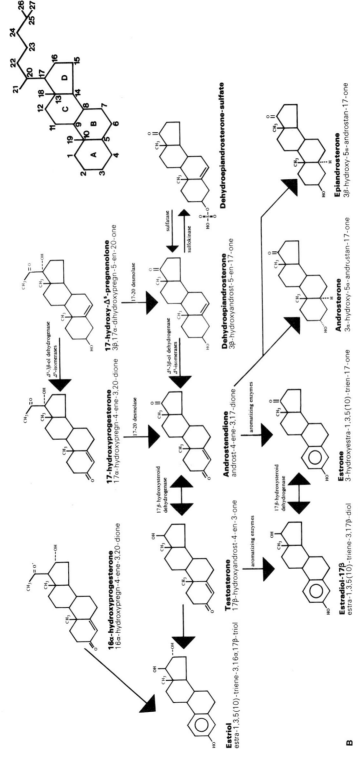

FIGURE 7–5A and B Metabolic pathways of steroid hormones.

verted by endocrine glands and also peripherally as in the liver to testosterone (17β-hydroxyandrost-4-en-3-one) by the 17β-dehydrogenase enzyme. Also, although DHA can be converted to A and testosterone, A and T can be interconverted but have not been shown to convert back to DHA. A, T, DHA, and additional metabolites of theirs (e.g., reduced derivatives androsterone and etiocholanolone) are all 17-ketosteroids. Therefore the demonstration of elevated urinary 17-ketosteroids does not indicate the gland or possible precursor source of abnormal androgen secretion.

Of all androgens testosterone is by far the most androgenic. It might therefore be assumed that a measure of circulating testosterone could delineate androgenic syndromes. However, this is not the case; for example, testosterone levels cannot be used by themselves to differentiate abnormal testosterone metabolism in polycystic ovarian disease or patients with hirsutism. This is so because in these situations the MCR is frequently altered, and as the testosterone production rate is the product of its MCR and its circulating concentration, the production rate may be increased in the presence of normal circulating levels (Kirschner, Bardin). A clinical measure of testosterone metabolism is the determination of free and plasma protein-bound testosterone. In the presence of normal circulatory concentration of total steroid, an increased free testosterone concentration reflects increased clearance and, therefore, an overall increased production.

Sites of Androgen Secretion

In the female both the ovary and the adrenal secrete testosterone. In addition there is a component of overall testosterone production which is the result of peripheral conversion of testosterone precursors (A and DHA) to circulating testosterone.

Of the circulating testosterone in normal women, 5 to 20 percent is secreted by the ovary and 0 to 30 percent by the adrenal, while the largest component is a result of peripheral conversion of androstenedione to testosterone (50 to 70 percent) and DHA to testosterone (15 percent) (Kirschner, Bardin).

Control of Androgen Secretion

DHA is secreted primarily by the adrenal and parallels cortisol secretion. Therefore ACTH will stimulate an increase in both cortisol and DHA. As far as androstenedione is concerned, although a component of its secretion comes from the adrenal and is thought to respond to ACTH as DHA, its ovarian component se-

cretion may be controlled through its conversion to estrone either peripherally or in the hypothalamus. In turn, its circulating levels control gonadotropin secretion, and gonadotropins regulate estrogen secretion by the ovarian follicle, of which a biosynthetic component is androstenedione. Indirect evidence supports the concept that androgens are secreted by the ovary in response to gonadotropins, particularly LH. LH is the same as interstitial-cell stimulating hormone (ICSH) in the male which stimulates the secretion of testosterone by the interstitial cells.

Synthesis, and Metabolic Clearance, Production, and Secretion Rates of Androgens

The MCRs for androstenedione, testosterone, and dehydroepiandrosterone, their concentrations, and production rates are shown in Table 7–2. Testosterone, 5α-dihydrotestosterone, and androstenedione concentrations show cyclical variations, with highest values in the periovulatory period and lowest values in the early follicular and late luteal phases (Vermeulen and Verdonck). The MCR is influenced both by the metabolism of the steroid by peripheral tissues (i.e., peripheral to the gland secreting it) and also by the extent to which the steroid is bound to circulating plasma proteins or the blood cells themselves. The strongest and therefore most influential binding is that to plasma globulins. For example, testosterone is bound to testosterone-binding globulin (TeBG). (Because it also binds estrogen, it is called gonadal steroid-binding globulin or GBG.) In some pathophysiologic states MCR increases and binding decreases, in others MCR decreases and binding increases (Table 7–3). In either event metabolism by the tissues themselves may be influenced. In normal subjects (men and women) hepatic extraction of testosterone is 40 percent, and in virilized women extraction is no different (44 percent) (Fig. 7–6). Therefore as MCR of testosterone in women, virilized women, and men ranges from 600 to 1240 L per day and the hepatic clearance remains the same at between 500 and 600 L per day, extrahepatic clearance varies between close to 0 in normal women, 32 percent in virilized women, and 50 percent in men (Fig. 7–6).

Recently dihydrotestosterone (DHT) has been shown to be a definitive biologically active androgen in some tissues. However, the PR for DHT is only 75 μg per day, of which testosterone contributes 10 μg (15 percent of T production) and androstenedione 65 μg (2 percent of A production). Therefore DHT is probably not secreted primarily by endocrine glands

TABLE 7–2 Metabolic Clearance Rates (MCR), Plasma Concentrations *(i)*, Production Rates (PR), and Ovarian Secretion of Androgens (PR = MCR × *i*)

	MCR (plasma) L/day	Plasma concentration, μg/100 mL	PR, mg/day	SR (ovaries), mg/day	References
Androstenedione	2010	0.159	3.2	0.8–1.6	Baird et al., 1968
Testosterone	690	0.038	0.26		Baird et al., 1968
Dehydroepiandrosterone	1640	0.490	8.0	0.3–3.0	Baird et al., 1968 Mickhail, Allen

in the female. The androstanediols (3α,17β-dihydroxy-5α-androstane and 3β,17β-dihydroxy-5α-androstane) and androstenediol (3β,17β-dihydroxy-androst-5-ene) have androgenic effects, but the contribution of DHA, A or T to their production, secretion, and metabolism is not known (Baird et al., 1969).

PROGESTERONE

Progesterone is the hormone of the luteal phase of the menstrual cycle and of pregnancy. It is primarily secreted by the corpus luteum from which it was originally isolated by Corner and Allen. It was first called *progestin,* and it was described as the hormone which produced a special state of the uterine mu-

cosa, progestational proliferation. The name *progesterone* was coined in a London pub by Willard Allen, Alan Parkes, and Guy Marrian just prior to the Special Conference of the Health Organization of the League of Nations in 1935. It was at this conference that the words *progesterone, estrone, estradiol, estriol,* and *androsterone* were agreed upon as names for com-

FIGURE 7–6 Metabolic clearance rate of testosterone in normal and virilized women. Shaded area: hepatic clearance rate of testosterone. Solid area: clearance of testosterone at extrahepatic sites. *(From Kirschner, Bardin.)*

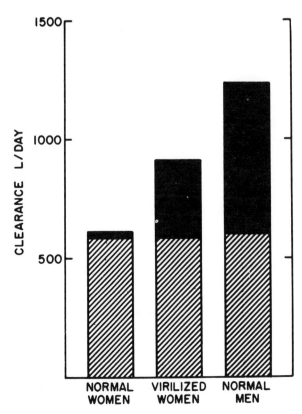

TABLE 7–3 Conditions Altering Testosterone Metabolic Clearance Rates and Testosterone Binding in Blood

	Metabolic clearance rate	Plasma binding
Hypothyroidism	Increased	Decreased
Virilization	Increased	Decreased
Androgen treatment	Increased	Decreased
Dexamethasone treatment	Increased	Decreased
Large adrenal ovarian and testicular tumors	Increased	
Progestins	Increased	Decreased
Obesity		Decreased
Hyperthyroidism	Decreased	Increased
Aging	Decreased	
Pregnancy		Increased
Estrogen treatment	Decreased	Increased
Barbiturate treatment	Decreased	
Erect posture	Decreased	
Hypogonadism	Decreased	Increased
Cirrhosis		Increased

Source: Kirschner, Bardin.

mon use in scientific literature. Fels and Slotta, Butenandt and Westphal, Hartman and Wettstein, and Hisaw and Fevold all were in the race for the isolation of the hormone. It was in this same era that Edgar Allen and E. A. Doisy discovered estrin. The discovery and isolation of these two major hormones of reproduction have had a tremendous influence on the understanding of pregnancy physiology and on the endocrine evaluation of gynecologic problems (Allen).

Sites of Secretion

Progesterone is primarily secreted by the corpus luteum. It appears that the granulosa cells have to be luteinized for the proper secretion of progesterone. The major precursor of progesterone is cholesterol. The cholesterol in the cell first has its side chain cleaved from a C-27 to a C-21 compound, which is pregnenolone. Pregnenolone has the same Δ^5-3β-ol configuration as cholesterol. This is rapidly converted by the 3β-ol steroid dehydrogenase and isomerase to progesterone, which has a Δ^4-3-keto configuration.

In the proliferative phase of the menstrual cycle and postmenopause, there is a small but measurable amount of progesterone in the blood which probably comes from the adrenal.

In pregnancy the trophoblast cells of the placenta secrete progesterone. The placenta appears to take over from the corpus luteum in the secretion of progesterone and estrogen as early as the eighth week of gestation. For this reason, the removal of a corpus luteum in the latter half of the first trimester does not usually lead to spontaneous abortion. The precursor for the biosynthesis of progesterone in the placenta is cholesterol, as in the ovary.

Although a number of progestins which are endogenous in the human being have been identified, including 20α- and 20β-dihydroprogesterone and 17α-hydroxyprogesterone, none of them has significant progestational activity.

Physiologic Effects

The classical experiment of Ludwig Frankel in 1903, in which he removed the corpus luteum of the rabbit a few days after mating and no pregnancy resulted, was the first indication that the ovary contributed a specific substance to pregnancy. It was subsequently shown that the corpus luteum secreted a substance which was necessary for the development of decidua and the progestational changes in the endometrium. Early in this century the cyclic changes in the endometrium were described, and as recently as the 1940s Hertig described the characteristic pattern of each phase of the cycle, including the appearance of the glands and stroma on specific days.

In addition to effects on the endometrium, progesterone has effects on the cervix, vagina, and fallopian tubes. The cervical mucus under the influence of estrogen is viscous and contains high concentrations of salt; these characteristics are used in the tests of spinnbarkeit and ferning (see Chap. 27) in the evaluation of infertility. Progesterone modifies the viscosity and reduces the salt content to a minimum. The vagina undergoes a cycle similar to the endometrium. The influence of progesterone on an already estrogen-stimulated vagina is to change the appearance of a cytologic smear from that of cornified superficial cells to intermediate- and basal-cell predominance. In the fallopian tube estrogen and progesterone have an influence both on the contractility of the tubal muscularis and the activity of the ciliated epithelium. Estrogen leads to increased activity of tubal contraction, and progesterone leads to its inhibition. Similarly, in rabbits it has been shown that estrogen activates the cilia of the tubal epithelium while progesterone inactivates their motion. These features are responsible for the transport and fertilization function of the egg and spermatozoa in the distal third of the tube and the ultimate transport of the fertilized ovum to the uterus.

Progesterone also has a number of systemic effects which have been known for years but whose importance is not entirely understood. A major result of the administration of exogenous progesterone, or the increased secretion of endogenous hormone as in the secretory phase of the menstrual cycle, is a rise in basal body temperature. This change in basal temperature is used as a fertility test to indicate potential ovulation. The breasts require progesterone for lobule-alveolar growth, particularly during pregnancy in preparation for lactation. Large doses of progesterone are known in animals to lead to sleep, and a progesterone fall has been proposed as a possible etiology of postpartum depression; a few cases have been treated with large doses of progesterone with varying results.

In a complete review, Landau has summarized the metabolic influences of progesterone. These include its effect on the regulation of salt and water metabolism, its influence on protein, carbohydrate, and fat metabolism, and its respiratory and thermogenic effects. Progesterone in the nonpregnant subject has a natriuretic effect and acts as an aldosterone antagonist in the kidney tubule. The therapeutic potential of progesterone as an aldosterone antagonist has been developed by pharmacologists into the synthesis of steroidal spironolactones which have similar effects on the kidney and are widely used. Progesterone has to be given intramuscularly, and is therefore not as useful as the spironolactones, in spite of the fact that 200 mg of progesterone has the same effect as 400 mg of spironolactone. In protein metabolism there is a distinctive effect of progesterone: its administration to animals results in a nonspecific weight gain. This may be a part of the mechanism in pregnancy in which progesterone, along with a number of other hormones, contributes to a positive nitrogen balance and an overall weight gain. In human beings there appears to be a net catabolic effect of progesterone in nonpregnant subjects. The administration of progesterone or the stimulus of endogenous secretion by the corpus luteum (after administration of HCG) leads to urinary nitrogen excretion and amino acidemia. In tissues that respond to progesterone, it has also been shown that there is a specific protein synthesis. O'Malley and Strott have done classical studies in the oviduct of the chick to demonstrate the action of progesterone in stimulating an increase in ribonucleic acid (RNA), presumably through its action on transcription. Progesterone effects on protein metabolism are apparently elicited through a specific cytosol and nuclear steroid-binding protein. Such progesterone-binding proteins have also been demonstrated in the endometrium and are being sought in other tissues which are presumed to be the sites of action of progesterone (see Mechanism of Hormone Action below).

Progesterone apparently also has an influence on carbohydrate metabolism. In rhesus monkeys, for example, the administration of progesterone leads to a mild resistance to the hypoglycemic effect of insulin and a slight increase in plasma insulin response to a glucose load (Beck). There is also mild suggestive evidence that progesterone may play a role in fat deposition in women. Fat actually does have the capacity to metabolize progesterone to its 20α-dihydro derivative.

Progesterone also has a significant physiologic effect on respiration and appears to play a part in the changed respiratory dynamics of pregnancy. The administration of progesterone leads to a reduction in arterial P_{CO_2}, and the stimulus-response curve for inspired CO_2 becomes a steeper slope at a lower threshold. These changes may be in part responsible for the reduced P_{CO_2} and altered respiratory dynamics observed during pregnancy (Prowse, Gaensler).

Progesterone Concentration in Blood and Urine

The major metabolite of progesterone which is excreted in the urine is pregnanediol (5β-pregnane-3α-

20α-diol). Pregnanediol glucuronide is present in the urine in concentrations less than 1.0 mg per day before ovulation; it then rises to a peak during the luteal phase of 3.0 to 6.0 mg per day, which drops 2 days prior to the onset of menstruation. Pregnanediol excretion was the classical method of measuring the metabolism of progesterone and still has some value where the more complex measurements of blood progesterone concentration or production rates are not available. It may be used, for example, at the time of midsecretory phase to confirm the fact that ovulation has taken place.

Blood concentration of progesterone goes through the same cycle as that of urinary pregnanediol. In the early follicular phase, a reasonable estimate of plasma progesterone is 0.03 to 0.10 μg per 100 mL, and in the luteal phase it is 0.6 to 2.0 μg per 100 mL (Van der Molen) (Fig. 7–7). In oophorectomized women the concentration is 0.038 μg per 100 mL, which is in the same range as that for males and that in the early proliferative phase (Riondel et al.). 20α-Hydroxypregn-4-en-3-one is a major metabolite of progesterone and appears in less concentration in

FIGURE 7–7 Daily plasma progesterone and 20α-OHP determinations in the luteal phases of three women and the percent contribution of progesterone to the production rate of 20α-OHP in the same phase of the menstrual cycle. *(From B Little et al., Endocrinology, Proc 4th Int Congress of Endocrinology, 1972, Amsterdam, Excerpta Medica, 1973.)*

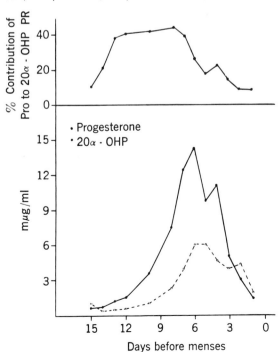

the blood 5α-pregnane-3,20-dione (5α-dihydroprogesterone) concentration is 0.11 ng per mL in the proliferative phase and 1.4 to 2.8 ng per mL in the luteal phase and appears to be present in proportion to the availability of progesterone as substrate for the 5α-reductase enzyme system (Milewich et al.). The contribution of the adrenal to progesterone production in the proliferative phase is major in comparison with the luteal phase (Fig. 7–8).

FIGURE 7–8 The production rates of progesterone in the proliferative and luteal phases and the component contributions from ovarian and adrenal secretion, and from the peripheral conversion of pregnenolone and 20α-OHP.

S_{Ov}	= Ovarian secretion of progesterone
PR	= Production rate of progesterone
S_{Ad}	= Adrenal secretion of progesterone
$[\rho]_B^{Pre} {}_B^{Pro}$	= Transfer constant of precursor to product
S_B^{Pre}	= Secretion rate of precursor
$[\rho]_B^{20\alpha P} {}_B^{Prog}$	= Transfer constant of 20α-dihydroprogesterone to progesterone
S_B^{Pre}	= Secretion rate of 20α-dihydroprogesterone
$[\rho]_B^{Preg} {}_B^{Prog}$	= Transfer constant of pregnenolone to progesterone
S^{Preg}	= Secretion rate of pregnenolone
■	= Contribution of 20α-dihydroprogesterone production to progesterone production rate
$[\rho]_B^{Preg} {}_B^{Prog} \times S^{Preg}$	= Contribution of pregnenolone production to progesterone production rate which is zero

(From B Little et al., Endocrinology, Proc 4th Int Congress of Endocrinology, 1972, Amsterdam, Excerpta Medica, 1973.)

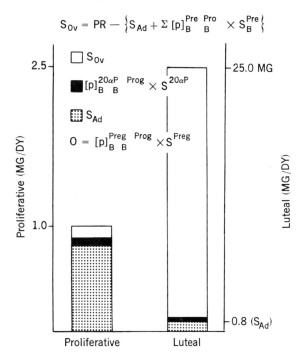

Progesterone secretion

$$S_{Ov} = PR - \left\{ S_{Ad} + \Sigma\, [\rho]_B^{Pre}{}_B^{Pro} \times S_B^{Pre} \right\}$$

Synthesis and Metabolic Clearance, Production, and Secretion Rates of Progesterone

Progesterone is synthesized primarily in the corpus luteum from cholesterol. The side chain of cholesterol is cleaved to pregnenolone followed by conversion by 3β-ol-dehydrogenase and the isomerase to progesterone.

The MCR of progesterone in the menstrual cycle is the same in the proliferative and luteal phases and is 2510 L per day or 1510 L/m² per day. This is different from males and ovariectomized females who have an MCR of 2100 L per day or 1270 L/m² per day (Little, Billiar, 1969) (see Table 7–1).

The calculated PR is 0.75 to 2.5 mg per day in the proliferative phase of the menstrual cycle and 15.0 to 50.0 mg per day in the luteal phase. In males and oophorectomized females the PR is about 0.5 to 0.75 mg per day.

Progesterone secretion begins 16 to 40 hours before the LH peak. Such a progesterone rise is always followed by an LH peak. Progesterone also appears to limit the LH peak to one single surge (Laborde et al.).

Progesterone is excreted both through the bile into the gut and also, following reduction and conjugation with glucuronide, into the urine. About 15 percent of administered progesterone is excreted as pregnanediol glucuronide into the urine. When labeled progesterone (using ¹⁴C or ³H) is administered, more than 95 percent of the anticipated labeled pregnanediol is excreted in 4 days. During the same time more than 50 percent of the radioactivity is excreted as other metabolites of progesterone in the urine. Most of the residual activity is excreted in the feces. If progesterone is labeled at C-21, the label appears in expired air, accounting for about 20 percent of the activity, indicating that part of the administered progesterone is excreted after having its side chain cleaved (Sandberg et al.; Davis, Plotz).

Control of Progesterone Secretion

In the corpus luteum, where the major secretion of progesterone occurs except in pregnancy, the luteinized granulosa cells, which are the major cells of its secretion, are under the control of LH from the pituitary. In amenorrheal patients who require stimulation of the ovaries with exogenous gonadotropins, LH is required following FSH stimulation of the ovary to obtain ovulation. Once ovulation has taken place after a single LH injection, an additional injection of LH is required to maintain the corpus luteum. In patients who have the luteal phase defect (see below), it can be shown that the short secretory phase is due to a diminishing LH secretion with resultant decline in progesterone production. The latter may be due to abnormal follicular development, as circulating estradiol and FSH may be lower than normal and/or out of phase prior to ovulation. Progesterone, on the other hand, is responsible at high levels for the suppression of LH secretion and thereby permissive for luteolysis which occurs in the absence of LH (Vande Wiele et al.).

In pregnancy early in the first trimester, the secretion of progesterone is maintained by HCG secretion from the developing trophoblast, which stimulates the corpus luteum to continue its secretion of progesterone and 17α-hydroxyprogesterone. Once the placenta is established, the trophoblast begins to secrete estrogens and progesterone from maternal and fetal steroid precursors. Progesterone is largely the product of the conversion of maternal cholesterol to pregnenolone and then to progesterone in the placenta.

As there is an excess of circulating cholesterol in pregnancy, there is no lack of substrate. What controls are exerted by the presence and absence of cofactors and enzymes have not been established as yet for clinical disease, but the range of normal progesterone secretion is wide.

The adrenal secretes progesterone, and control appears to be exerted through ACTH, for following ACTH administration there is a resulting rise in the excretion of pregnanediol. Postmenopause, when estrogen production is almost entirely the result of androstenedione production and conversion peripherally to estrone, there is more importance to the secretion by the adrenal, particularly under the stimulus of ACTH. ACTH stimulus can lead to normal ovulatory estrogen levels and will also lead to increased progesterone secretion. This is probably the reason for bleeding following an ACTH test in amenorrheal subjects and for occasional periods occurring in the perimenopausal years associated with stress.

REGULATION OF THE MENSTRUAL CYCLE

Pituitary Gonadotropins

The primary stimulus for the ovary comes from the secretion of two pituitary hormones, FSH and LH (also termed ICSH because of its stimulus of the interstitial cells of the testis). Gonadotropins are secreted by the basophilic cells of the pituitary which stain with periodic acid Schiff (PAS) reagent which reflects their glycoprotein content. Apparently, in the mouse, LH-producing cells are small, polygonal, and adjacent to sinusoids. They contain secretory granules of 100 to 300 nm in size. On the other hand, FSH-secreting cells are larger, rounded, and contain secretory granules of 150 to 300 nm. The granules of FSH are less electron-dense than those of LH. Other data show that LH and FSH are secreted by the same cell (Benoit, DeLage).

Both LH and FSH have a molecular weight of about 30,000 and are glycoproteins. LH, FSH, and HCG are composed of two polypeptide chains, designated α or β. The α chains are either identical or very similar, but the β chains are specific to each hormone. The carbohydrate portions of the molecules include sialic acid, mannose, galactose, and glucosamine. The removal of the sialic-acid portion of the molecule alters the half-time disappearance from the blood ($t_{\frac{1}{2}}$) of both LH and FSH, but they remain active in vitro. Highly purified FSH and LH have been prepared from extracts of human pituitaries, and preliminary characterizations have been made, but neither hormone has been synthesized. In clinical use at present, frequently FSH and LH are replaced by human menopausal gonadotropin (HMG) isolated from the urine of menopausal women, which contains high concentrations of FSH, and HCG extracted from human placentae, which cross-reacts biologically and immunologically with LH.

Biologic Effects of Gonadotropins

In the female the FSH is responsible for the follicle growth in the ovary. The follicle grows to some extent by itself and is then given a stimulus for growth by FSH. FSH stimulates the follicle to produce estrogen, thus making it more sensitive to FSH. Thereafter it grows and at an appropriate time ovulates as a result of the LH surge. Ovulation will not take place in the absence of LH. In the male, FSH is important for certain stages of spermatogenesis. LH is also necessary to the testis for the stimulus of the interstitial cells which produce testosterone. Testosterone is necessary for the normal function of the testis and seminiferous tubules. LH in the female, apart from initiating ovulation, is responsible for the luteinization of the ovary which follows ovulation and which consists of specific changes in the granulosa and theca cells. These changes are associated with the cells' altered function in the luteal phase, i.e., secreting progesterone (Odell, Moyer).

Puberty

LH has been observed in prepubertal girls at low levels. The first sign of increased circulating concentration occurs at night in bursts, until finally the cyclic circadian rhythm is established throughout the entire 24-hour day.

A progressive rise not only of LH but of FSH, estradiol, dehydroepiandrosterone, and androstenedione occurs during puberty to the onset of menarche. A concomitant rise with the onset of puberty occurs for estrone, DHA and DHS, and 17-hydroxyprogesterone. Prolactin and progesterone don't change until after menarche. LH, progesterone, and estradiol levels are generally lower than normal adult concentrations for several months after menarche, suggesting anovulation in most girls immediately after menarche (Lee et al.).

Metabolic Clearance Rate, Production Rate, and Control of Gonadotropin Secretion

The MCR of FSH and LH has been studied in normal cycling women and in postmenopausal women and found to be no different. The MCR for FSH is 20 L per day (14 mL per minute) and for LH is 35 L per day (24 mL per minute) (Ross et al.) (Table 7–4). FSH concentration in blood increases from about 2 to 4 mIU/mL in childhood to 8 mIU/mL as puberty approaches. During the normal menstrual cycle values rise and fall between 8 and 15 mIU/mL except at the time of ovulation, when the peak is 20 mIU/mL. In

pregnancy FSH recedes to very low levels; postmenopausal values increase to levels several times higher than those during the normal cycle. In general, as for FSH values, LH concentrations are low in early childhood (4 to 6 mIU/mL) and rise with the onset of puberty. The values for both FSH and LH rise earlier for girls than they do for boys (Yen et al., 1968; Yen, Vicic). The MCR of LH is unchanged by physiologic changes such as menopause and remains at 35 L per day (25 mL per minute). LH patterns of secretion during the normal menstrual cycle range between 10 and 20 mIU/mL and reach a peak during the LH surge at the time of ovulation of about 80 mIU/mL. Premature menopause or ovarian failure can be diagnosed by elevated LH (over 50 mIU/mL) and FSH (over 40 mIU/mL) in most cases (Goldenberg et al.).

The production rate of FSH is therefore about 60 IU per day in early life and rises to about 240 IU per day in the menstrual cycle with ovulation burst of up to 400 IU per day. During the postmenopausal period this would rise to several thousand (2000 to 3000 per day). The PR of LH is 175 IU per day in childhood and increases to 525 IU per day during the menstrual cycles with surges at ovulation to 1750 IU per day and postmenopausally to 3000 IU per day with a wide range.

The $t_{\frac{1}{2}}$ of FSH disappearance from serum has an initial rate of 4 hours followed by a longer component of 70 hours. The $t_{\frac{1}{2}}$ is much less for LH, being 21 minutes with a record component of about 4 to 6 hours. There appear to be clinical benefits from using HCG instead of LH in the stimulation of ovulation and main-

TABLE 7–4 Metabolic Clearance Rates (MCR), Blood Concentrations *(i)*, and Production Rates (PR) of FSH and LH (PR = MCR × *i*)

	$t_{\frac{1}{2}}$,* hours	MCR		Concentration (i), mIU/mL	PR, IU/day
		L/day	(mL/min)		
FSH					
Premenopausal	4–10	20.4	(14.2)		
Prepuberty				2–4	60
Menstrual range				8–15	240
Ovulatory peak				20	
Postmenopausal		18.1	(12.6)	100	2000
LH					
Premenopausal	6	35.1	(24.4)		
Prepuberty				4–6	175
Menstrual range				10–20	525
Ovulatory peak				40–60	1750
Postmenopausal		36.8	(25.6)	80	3000

*$t_{\frac{1}{2}}$ denotes half-time disappearance from blood.

Source: Ross et al.

tenance of the corpus luteum. At present this advantage is believed to be the result of the longer $t_\frac{1}{2}$ of HCG which is the order of 25 hours; thus only one dose is required rather than repetitive dosage during the luteal phase to maintain the corpus luteum (see Chap. 27).

FSH and LH are released from the pituitary as a result of the stimulus of a releasing factor which reaches the pituitary from the hypothalamus by way of the hypophyseal portal circulation. This latter is a plexus of vessels which surround the pituitary stalk, arising in the vicinity of the hypothalamus and ending in the anterior pituitary before entering the general circulation. The hypothalamus-pituitary system is influenced by the circulating levels of steroids, particularly reproductive steroids such as estrogens, progesterone, and androgen (e.g., androstenedione). There is additional control of the hypothalamus from the higher centers of the brain through nerve impulses controlled either on the basis of nervous response or the release of specific brain amines. In the absence of estrogen or androstenedione, there is a continuous release of FSH as in postmenopausal or oophorectomized women. The administration of estrogen in these cases inhibits the release of FSH-releasing factor and reduces the peripheral concentration of FSH. This is called the *negative feedback effect* of estrogen. LH responds in much the same way to LH-releasing factor, which may be the same as FSH-releasing factor.

However, there are enough differences in the response of LH and FSH to releasing factors to suspect either that FSH- and LH-releasing factors are not the same or that, if they are the same, the releasing factor's action on the pituitary is different with respect to the release of each gonadotropin. LH responds to the administration of LH-releasing factor (LHRF*) more quickly than does FSH. The LH surge which occurs as the result of a sharp increase in the output of estradiol by the ovary apparently results from the action of the estradiol on a different center in the hypothalamus from that which controls the tonic release of LH, leading to an actual release of LH-releasing factor and subsequent response by secretion of LH by the pituitary. This surge of LH following estrogen increase in the circulation is known as the *positive feedback of estrogen*. At the same time as the LH surge takes place there is a concomitant rise in FSH but to a much smaller degree. Progesterone, on the other hand, appears to reduce the level of LH either by its influence directly on the pituitary or by its influence on the release of LHRF. There also may be significant neural

factors which act on LH secretion and presumably on the LH surge which can result in ovulation. For example, it is well known that environmental factors such as sound and light or emotional state will influence the normal secretion of gonadotropins and their influence on ovulation and the menstrual cycle. Recent studies have been directed toward follicular nonsteroidal substance(s) which may decrease FSH secretion ("inhibin").

NEUROENDOCRINE CONTROL OF OVARIAN CYCLE

The control of the ovarian cycle is a complex function which is shared by the ovary, the pituitary, and hypothalamus. In addition, as the influences on the hypothalamus and pituitary have been unraveled, the rest of the brain has been found to exert significant inhibitory or permissive controls on the mechanisms of gonadotropin release. There are essentially three parts which interact in this regulation; they are the ovary with its secretion of gonadal steroids, the pituitary with its secretion of gonadotropins, and the hypothalamus with its secretion of releasing factors (Fig. 7–9). At present it is known that the gonadotropins are secreted with a pulsation every 90 minutes. This pulsatile secretion is maintained both at low levels of secretion and at the time of high secretion, either in the menopause or when the ovaries are removed. In the postmenopausal state the pulsations of release are actually increased, although the periodicity remains the same (Yen et al., 1972a). The tonic secretion, from animal studies, appears to be centered in the ventromedial-arcuate area with neurons terminating in the vicinity of the portal capillaries leading to the pituitary (Fig. 7–10). The cyclic center may be in the preoptic area (rats) or medial basal hypothalamus (primates) from which neurons enter the tonic center. However, whether the influence of these areas is exerted through the final common pathway of LH-releasing factor or two releasing factors (LH and FSH) through the portal system to the pituitary is not clearly defined at present. LHRF releases both FSH and LH but at different rates. There is also evidence that the gonadal steroids, particularly estrogen, act directly on the pituitary. For example, early in the follicular phase at low circulating concentrations of estrogen the administration of LHRF leads to a small response of the pituitary to the secretion of LH, whereas at the expected time of ovulation there is a much higher response of circulating LH to the releasing factor. The pituitary responsiveness therefore appears at present to be the result of estrogen or ovarian steroid

---

*LH-releasing factor is abbreviated LHRF, GnRH, and LRF.

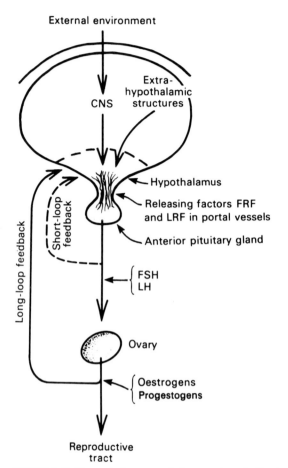

FIGURE 7–9 The central-nervous-pituitary-ovarian axis. Ovarian function is regulated by the blood concentration of anterior pituitary–gonadotropic hormones (follicle-stimulating hormone, FSH; luteinizing hormone, LH). The secretion of FSH and LH is in turn dependent on the transportation of releasing factors (follicle-stimulating hormone-releasing factor, FRF; luteinizing hormone-releasing factor, LRF) from hypothalamic nerve terminals to the anterior pituitary gland by the hypophyseal portal vessels. The hypothalamus itself appears to act as a major integrative center. It appears to have some autonomous function in maintaining anterior pituitary activity. This in turn is modulated by (1) neural inputs from extrahypothalamic brain structures (such as the amygdaloid nuclei), some of which mediate environmental influences, and (2) hormonal feedback through the long-loop system (solid line), and possibly (and therefore denoted by an interrupted line) short-loop system. *(From F Naftolin, GW Harris: Brit Med Bull 26:3, 1970.)*

action directly on the pituitary. This is consistent with the findings of other investigators who have infused labeled estrogen into subhuman primates and demonstrated the highest concentrations of steroid in the pituitary.

Catecholamines are known to participate in the

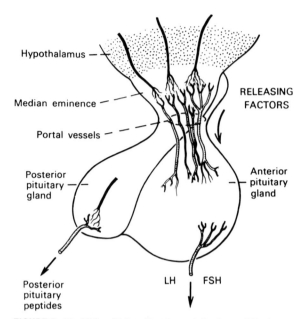

FIGURE 7–10 Midsagittal section through the base of the hypothalamus and pituitary gland to show the structures concerned in the regulation of anterior pituitary activity. Nerve fibers from the hypothalamus enter the median eminence of the tuber cinereum to end on the primary plexus of the hypophyseal portal vessels. It is postulated that releasing factors pass from these nerve terminals into the portal vessels and are carried to the anterior pituitary gland to regulate its secretory activity. This is probably a mechanism similar to that obtaining in the posterior pituitary gland, where peptides are discharged from nerve endings into the general circulation. *(From F Naftolin, GW Harris: Brit Med Bull 26:3, 1970; adapted from CP Fawcett et al.: Biochem J 106:229, 1968.)*

process of LHRF-LH release. Circulating norepinephrine is known to rise preceding or concomitant with LH surge. Within 6 minutes of a single injection of LHRF, there is a significant rise in norepinephrine prior to LH peak (Rosner et al.).

Negative-Feedback Control of Gonadotropins by Estrogens

If the ovaries are removed, there is a resultant rise of both FSH and LH within 2 days and a plateau at about 3 weeks at a level of 10 times the normal concentration. The administration of 17β-estradiol, which is the most important estrogen in feedback, results in a fall in both LH and FSH, although the resultant fall and loss of cyclicity is greater for LH than FSH. The 17β-estradiol appears to inhibit the hypothalamic release of LHRF and also to reduce the sensitivity of the pituitary to LHRF. Following the cessation of estradiol administration, there is a rapid return to the higher circulating levels, and at the same time the pulsatile cycles of secretion are higher than during either the period of control or of estrogen suppression. This has been interpreted by Yen as a combination of positive and negative feedback. Small dosages of estrogen for 1 week (ethinyl estradiol 1.0 μg/kg per day) lead initially to an increased responsiveness to LHRF (150 μg IV), but after prolonged periods of time the response is reduced, until at about 4 weeks the response is minimal. These results emphasize the complex interrelationship between the ovarian secretion, FSH, and LH (Yen et al., 1972b).

Postive Feedback Control of Gonadotropins by Estrogens

The administration of estrogen at midcycle is known to act as a stimulus for the surge in LH, which compares with the one that can be demonstrated in normal cycles. This presumably is the stimulus for ovulation. However, the administration of similar dosages of estrogen which would be expected to lead to this response at other times than midcycle will also produce a surge. In early follicular phase, estrogen administration will result in a lesser surge of LH, but not FSH; no ovulation will result when the developing follicle in the ovary has not been appropriately prepared. The FSH response in concert with the LH response at midcycle also indicates that the hypothalamus and pituitary are responding to the increasing secretion of estrogen. The preparation of the hypothalamus and pituitary to respond in the appropriate manner at the specific time at midcycle has been labeled the "window" of maximal responsiveness (Yen et al., 1972b).

In patients in whom there is primary amenorrhea with elevated gonadotropins, a suppression of these values can be demonstrated with estradiol benzoate injections (1.0 mg per day), and this may be followed by a positive feedback-like effect in which ethinyl estradiol (200 μg per day) results in an LH surge (Yen et al., 1972a).

Progesterone has a similar negative-feedback effect on LH and can be shown to have a positive-feedback effect in a postmenopausal woman on estrogen suppression. However, although the negative feedback is operative in the luteal phase of the cycle, the positive feedback at present is not understood in relation to the cycle, but may play a part in abnormal cycles or infertility. The negative

feedback is also controversial to many investigators.

Effects of Contraceptive Steroid on Hypothalamic Pituitary Function

Contraceptive steroids exert their effects by preventing ovulation through the suppression of FSH and LH. Most synthetic steroids are absorbed and circulate in high enough concentrations to suppress gonadotropin release and surge during the usual 7-day respite in any 28-day cycle. Pituitary function tests by stimulation of growth hormone (HGH), thyroid-stimulating hormone (TSH), prolactin (PRL), and LH and FSH release by hypoglycemia, thyrotropin-releasing hormone (TRF), and LHRF demonstrate that GH and TSH release are unaffected but PRL release is increased by combination pill and progestin alone. In short-term users (newly started), and in most long-term users (many months), LH and FSH release is reduced, but in some long-term users, release of LH and FSH is not affected (Mishell et al.).

PROSTAGLANDINS

Prostaglandins (PGs), as their name implies, are extracts of secretions thought to emanate from the prostate, as the first identified PGs were extracted from semen. Later, it was found that, rather than the prostate, the seminal vesicles are responsible for the presence of PGs in semen. Since then, they have been identified as ubiquitous carboxylic acids formed enzymatically from polyunsaturated fatty acids. Initially, prostaglandin E and F were identified. The E meant ether extract and F, *fosphat* (Swedish, "phosphate") extract.

The 20-carbon structures contain a cyclopentane ring. The basic molecule is prostanoic acid and the carbon atoms are numbered accordingly, the first being adjacent to the carboxyl group and 8 through 12 identifying the cyclopentane ring. PGE (prostaglandin E) contains a ketone group at C-9, while F an hydroxyl group. Additional prostaglandins have been identified, including A, B, C, D, G, H, and I, as well as thromboxanes. The subscript after each letter indicates the number of double bonds in the molecule. The subscript 2, for example, in PGF_2 indicates a double bond at C-13,14 and C-5,6. The α, as in $PGF_{2\alpha}$, denotes the hydroxyl group on C-9 is in the α plane, or below the ring. All naturally occurring PGs have an hydroxyl group at C-15.

In reproduction, PGE_2 and $PGF_{2\alpha}$ are those which have been identified as playing significant roles. Both have been synthesized and used primarily as uterine ecbolic agents in therapeutic abortion or for the induction of labor. However, they are important in endogenous uterine muscular contraction, the onset of labor, in the follicle and at ovulation, possibly as an intermediate in dysmenorrhea, and related to implantation of the ovum.

Arachidonic acid, the precursor of prostaglandins, is released from phospholipids by phospholipase A_2. The rate-limiting step to the synthesis of prostaglandins is then prostaglandin synthetase or cyto-oxidase which converts arachidonic acid to the PG endoperoxides, PGG_2 and PGH_2, which are transient intermediates; thereafter, PGE_2, $PGF_{2\alpha}$, thromboxanes, or prostacyclin (PGI_2) are made, depending on the specific enzyme available in the tissue of action. Prostacyclin and thromboxanes regulate platelet activity. PGE and A are potent vasodilators, while PGF has functions in muscle contraction, ovulation, and vasoconstriction.

Prostaglandin E plays a role in uteroplacental blood flow, both normally and, apparently, in toxemia of pregnancy. $PGF_{2\alpha}$ levels increase with labor, are identifiable in amniotic fluid, and have been identified in the chain of events leading to the onset of labor. It has been suggested that the withdrawal of progesterone in the fetal membranes leads to instability of the lysomes with release of phospholipase A_2. The resultant increase of local available arachidonic acid is converted by prostaglandin synthetase (cyto-oxidase) to $PGF_{2\alpha}$ in decidua and fetal membranes, then acts on the previously prepared myometrium to result in labor. $PGF_{2\alpha}$ is known to sensitize myometrium to oxytocin. The pregnant uterus is 50 times more sensitive to PG. PG receptors have been identified in uterine smooth muscle and PG may be released by oxytocin. PGE has also been shown to be responsible for keeping open the ductus arteriosus in the fetus (which closes after birth, as do the umbilical arteries) by the presence of oxygen, altered flow, and possibly a $PGF_{2\alpha}$-mediated action.

In most studies, the measurement of $PGF_{2\alpha}$ is complicated by its rapid appearance in traumatized tissue, leading to falsely high rates; therefore, a major metabolite, 15-keto-13,14-dihydro-$PGF_{2\alpha}$ which turns over much more slowly, is a more valid measurement.

Blood PGE_2 concentration is less than 50 pg/mL and $PGF_{2\alpha}$ less than 10 pg/mL. In urine, PGE_2 ranges from 23 to 48 μg per 24 hours in women (109 to 225 μg per 24 hours in the male) and $PGF_{2\alpha}$ 40 to 60 μg per 24 hours (40 to 230 μg per 24 hours in the male).

MECHANISM OF HORMONE ACTION

Although the details of the precise mechanism(s) by which a hormone modifies the metabolic activities of a cell and promotes the growth and development of a tissue are not known, studies during the past 15 to 20 years have brought us much closer to understanding the mechanism of hormone action. Hormone actions can be considered as causing either irreversible or reversible changes. An example of an irreversible change is the differentiation of the Wolffian-duct system by androgen into the prostate. The irreversible actions of hormones are seen in the process of differentiation in embryo and fetal development.

Reversible responses by tissues to hormones can be subdivided into tissue responses which are dependent upon the presence of a hormone and tissue activities which are sensitive to, but not dependent on, a hormone. For growth and development of the uterus, estrogen must be present. Removal of the estrogen causes atrophy of the uterus. This is an example of a tissue being dependent for its development upon the presence of a hormone(s). The liver is not dependent upon estrogen for growth and development nor for the specific synthesis and secretion of transcortin. The liver cell is, however, sensitive to the increased circulating concentration of estrogen, as during pregnancy, which results in an increased liver synthesis and secretion of transcortin in the human being.

After the administration of a hormone, target tissues can take up the hormone against a blood tissue gradient and concentrate and retain the hormone. The subcellular distribution of many hormones has now been determined by a combination of autoradiographic and biochemical methods. The polypeptide hormones such as LH and ACTH appear to interact and bind to the cell membrane of their target tissues. The steroid hormones enter the cell by passive diffusion and are concentrated in the nucleus of their target tissue by a complex subcellular transfer mechanism.

The cell surface of a cell such as the corpus luteum contains binding sites for the trophic hormone, in this case LH. This binding site is specific for LH; other polypeptide hormones such as ACTH, TSH, and FSH cannot interact with the LH binding site, although HCG can. Although there is a firm binding of the hormone to the cell membrane, the binding is noncovalent and reversible.

The cellular responses to the polypeptide hormone are believed to be dependent upon the specific interaction of the hormone with the cell membrane. The interaction of the hormone with the cell membrane binding sites changes some properties of the cell membrane in a manner not yet well understood. For example, the catalytic activity of the enzyme adenyl cyclase, which is located in the cell membrane, is increased. This enzyme catalyzes the conversion of adenosine triphosphate (ATP) to cyclic adenosine monophosphate (cyclic AMP), and LH causes the intracellular concentration of cyclic AMP to increase. The increase of cyclic AMP concentrations then results in an increased rate of secretion of steroid hormone. The mechanism by which cyclic AMP increases the rate of steroidogenesis is not known, but activation of the synthesis of a specific protein(s) appears to be necessary for the increased rate of synthesis of steroid to occur in response to LH.

Although an increasing number of reports indicate that a polypeptide hormone does not need to enter the cell to exert its hormonal activities, recent evidence suggests that some of the hormone is internalized. This probably results in proteolytic catabolism of the polypeptide hormone, but it is not known if this is part of its hormonal effect.

Steroid hormones apparently do not bind in a specific interaction with the cell membrane of their target tissues and can pass into the cell by passive diffusion (Fig. 7–11). In the cytosol of the target cell the steroid binds to a specific "receptor" protein. This binding is strong but noncovalent and reversible. In a process still to be completely defined, the steroid-

"receptors" complex of the cytosol is transferred into the nucleus and associates with a nuclear component(s), perhaps the chromatin. Thus there is a two-step mechanism for the transfer and accumulation of the steroid hormone into the nucleus: the steroid interacts and binds with a cytosol protein, and the cytosol steroid-receptor complex is then transferred into and bound in the nucleus.

Evidence which supports the physiologic significance of the steroid-receptor interaction is the observation that nonsteroidal, hormonally active compounds such as diethylstilbesterol also bind to the (uterine) cytosol receptors, and antihormones, such as antiestrogens, compete with the steroid hormones in the target tissues.

An increased rate of deoxyribonucleic acid synthesis and mitosis may be stimulated by a steroid hormone and may be part of the full expression of the hormone action, but this does not appear to be the initial event mediating the action of the hormone since many other cellular activities are changed before an increased rate mitosis is observed. In a tissue such as the uterus, hypertrophy precedes hyperplasia after exposure to estrogen. By the use of inhibitors it has been established that the steroid hormones increase the rate of RNA and protein synthesis, and these increased rates of RNA and protein synthesis are necessary for expression of many of the hormone effects. These observations are in keeping with the major site of cell accumulation of the hormone, i.e., the nucleus, the site of RNA synthesis. Inhibitors of RNA and protein synthesis do not inhibit the interaction of the steroid hormone with the cytosol receptor and translocation of the steroid-receptor complex into the nucleus. This supports the viewpoint that accumulation of hormone in the nucleus is one of the earliest events in the sequel of steroid hormone action.

Steroid hormones can also change the permeability properties of cells. This aspect of hormone action is also poorly understood, but these effects do not appear to be mediated by a direct action of the steroid hormones on the cell membrane, at least not with physiologic concentrations of the hormones. Changes in cell permeability alter the amount of substrates available for RNA, protein, and carbohydrate metabolism and are undoubtedly important in the hormonal effects. Although steroid hormones can alter the cellular concentrations of cyclic AMP, cyclic AMP is not an important mediator of steroid hormone action as it apparently is for polypeptide hormone action.

In summary, steroid hormones are taken up into and retained by their target tissues. The steroids in-

FIGURE 7–11 Sequence of intracellular events before steroid hormone stimulation of RNA synthesis. The steroid hormone (e.g., progesterone), S, enters the cell by simple diffusion and combines with a specific receptor, R_c, in the cytoplasm. This complex is then transferred to the nucleus, $S:R_n$, where it then binds to specific acceptor sites, A_c, on the nuclear chromatin. *(From O'Malley, Strott.)*

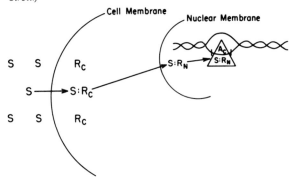

teract with specific cytosol receptors, and the cytosol receptor complex is translocated into the nucleus. It is believed that the nuclear steroid-receptor complex increases, in a manner as yet not understood, the rate of RNA synthesis by the nucleus, which in turn leads to an increased rate of cytoplasmic protein synthesis. Cell permeability is also changed. The primary biochemical changes are amplified to result in changes in the growth and development of the target tissue (O'Malley, Strott; Gorski).

PREGNANCY

The pituitary in pregnancy enlarges, and the histologic appearance changes as a predominance of pregnancy cells develops; these are large chromophobe cells with vesicular nuclei and relatively scant vacuolated cytoplasm. The function of these cells may be the secretion of prolactin, and they involute immediately postpartum. They are responsible for the enlargement of the pituitary during pregnancy. The pituitary blood supply, which is increased during pregnancy, may be compromised by maternal hemorrhage following delivery and lead to infarction with resulting hypopituitarism. The pituitary is not necessary for the normal completion of pregnancy, as patients have continued through pregnancy following hypophysectomy for breast cancer and have been maintained on thyroid and cortisone treatment. Such patients have required vasopressin to relieve their diabetes insipidus. Urine excretion of 10 L daily may be controlled by Pitressin snuff or its equivalent. Postpartum, such patients may no longer require antidiuretic treatment, which emphasizes the change in water metabolism that occurs during pregnancy, and also the fact that in the usual stalk sections performed during hypophysectomy there still is a release from the pituitary stalk of antidiuretic hormone synthesized in the hypothalamus (Little et al.).

Growth hormone blood values are not increased during pregnancy, and both FSH and LH are reduced to low levels. Only recently has it been possible to determine LH in pregnancy because LH and HCG cross-react in bioassay and also in radioimmunoassay. Very recently with the demonstration of alpha and beta subunits of LH, antibodies to the beta subunit have been made, and it has been demonstrated that LH follows the same pattern as FSH and falls to a low level even as the HCG is rising to pregnancy values.

The thyroid and adrenal glands show evidence of increased activity, and both glands increase in size during gestation. Although there are no conclusive data on an increase in ACTH, a chorionic thyrotropin has been demonstrated which may be responsible for some of the increased activity of the thyroid during pregnancy. It has been known for many years that in pregnancy the basal metabolic rate (BMR) increases about 25 percent and also that the PBI increases 25 to 50 percent. This latter increase is the result of more circulating thyroxine-binding globulin, a result of the stimulus of added estrogen secretion during pregnancy; exogenous estrogen, as in birth control pills, will at certain concentrations increase thyroxine-binding globulins and other binding globulins (e.g., transcortin CBG which binds cortisol and progesterone). The rises in the binding globulins of both thyroid and adrenal hormones are probably more responsible for change in their metabolism during pregnancy than increased production of the hormone per se. However, in both cases there results a small increase in the circulating free hormone. The best clinical example of the altered thyroid and possibly adrenal function as a result of the presence of the placenta is in hydatidiform mole; in this condition there is generally no fetus but an overgrowth of placental trophoblast, and hypertension and hyperthyroidism develop with thyrotoxic measurements of thyroid hormone activity, including a marked increase in the gland uptake of [131]I (Odell et al.).

Since the discovery that extracts of the posterior pituitary would stimulate uterine contractions and more recently the synthesis of oxytocin, efforts have been made to measure oxytocin during labor both peripherally and in the uterine vein effluent. These efforts have met with conflicting results. Patients following hypophysectomy during pregnancy go through relatively normal labors. Although oxytocin might be secreted from the pituitary stalk, maternal oxytocin from the pituitary does not seem to be necessary for the onset of labor. Nonetheless, in obstetrics a major drug for the management of desultory labor or dystocia is oxytocin. Over the years there have also been attempts to incriminate vasopressin in the etiology of toxemia of pregnancy. However, this has never been proved.

Following formation of the corpus luteum after ovulation, it is maintained by LH until the time it begins to involute in the normal cycle. This usually occurs after the maximum secretion of progesterone. If pregnancy intervenes and implantation takes place, thereafter HCG is secreted and acts directly on the corpus luteum to maintain its function. However, progesterone secretion is not immediately maintained, for peripheral levels of progesterone fall before they begin to rise again after the placenta is developed and the trophoblast begins to secrete the hormone. HCG is not the only factor that leads to the persistence of the corpus luteum because the administration of HCG will not prolong the life of the corpus luteum indefinitely. In addition, when larger amounts of HCG are secreted, as in the case of trophoblast tumors, there are actually changes in the ovary which include the development of polycystic ovaries with luteinized theca cysts, large, multilobed cysts with high concentrations of HCG. Such ovaries respond to the removal of the trophoblast and will resolve to normal size without excision.

THE FETOPLACENTAL UNIT

During pregnancy the uterus is stimulated to enlarge as the result of an estrogen and progesterone stimulus. Pregnancy is maintained in utero as the result of progesterone secretion. The inhibition of myometrial contraction by progesterone has been studied extensively by Csapo and called the "progesterone block" (see Chap. 9). These hormones are secreted from the uterus, from the trophoblast of its developing conceptus. The placenta was originally thought to be the site of such secretion, but it is now recognized that the fetoplacental unit is a complex functioning unit in which the placenta is only one part, with many active hormone precursors secreted by the mother and the fetus and converted in the placenta (Fig. 7–12). Progesterone is secreted by the placenta, both into the fetus and the mother. It is synthesized primarily from maternal cholesterol. Although the placenta does have the capacity to synthesize cholesterol from acetate, it does so in only small amounts.

PROGESTERONE SYNTHESIS, SECRETION, AND METABOLISM IN PREGNANCY

The corpus luteum is the site of early secretion of progesterone following conception and is the major source of progesterone during the first 12 weeks of pregnancy. It contains progesterone throughout pregnancy, but after 12 weeks' gestation it is no longer the major source of progesterone, nor is the corpus luteum required thereafter for the maintenance of pregnancy. Excision of the corpus luteum has been carried out surgically earlier than 10 weeks of pregnancy without subsequent loss of the fetus. Progesterone and 17α-hydroxyprogesterone reach a peak in the blood 3 to 4 weeks following ovulation and, thereafter, both fall until 6 to 8 weeks' ovulation age, at which time progesterone rises once again, presumably as a result of the increasing secretion from the developing

FIGURE 7–12 A scheme for the metabolism of pregnenolone and progesterone in the human placenta and fetus at midpregnancy. Δ⁵ P = pregnenolone; Δ⁵ PS = pregnenolone sulfate; 17α OH Δ⁵ PS = 17α-hydroxypregnenolone sulfate; DHAS = dehydroepiandrosterone sulfate; DHA = dehydroepiandrosterone; 16αOH Δ⁵ P = 16-hydroxypregnenolone; 20αOH Δ⁵ PS = 20α-dihydropregnenolone sulfate; 16αOH Δ⁴ P = 16α-hydroxyprogesterone; 17αOH Δ⁴ P = 17α-hydroxyprogesterone; 6βOH Δ⁴ P = 6β-hydroxyprogesterone; 20αOH Δ⁴ P = 20α-dihydroprogesterone; DOC = deoxycorticosterone. (From EV Younglai and S Solomon, in Foetus and Placenta, eds. A Klopper and E Diczfalusy, London, Blackwell, 1969.)

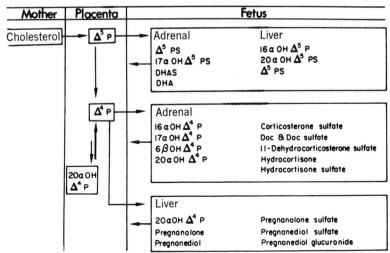

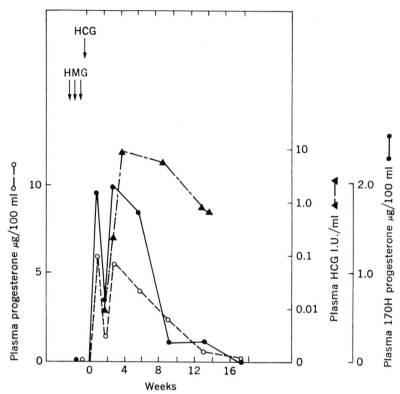

FIGURE 7–13 Plasma levels of progesterone, 17α-hydroxyprogesterone, and HCG in a woman who aborted 17 weeks after induction of ovulation with HMG-HCG. (Note the fall in progesterone prior to the abortion and the nadir prior to HCG appearance.) *(From T Yoshimi et al.: J Clin Endocrinol Metab 29:225, 1969.)*

placenta (Fig. 7–13). The placenta has a limited capacity to convert progesterone to 17α-hydroxyprogesterone, and 17α-OHP is a reflection of the early pregnancy state of the corpus luteum. Following the fall of 17α-OHP at about 6 to 8 weeks' gestation, the corpus luteum plays only a minimal role during the rest of gestation. Although HCG is necessary for the maintenance of the corpus luteum early in pregnancy, it cannot sustain the corpus luteum by prolonged administration, and early in pregnancy, between the fifth and eighth to tenth week of menstrual age, progesterone peripheral levels are actually falling at a time when the secretion of HCG is increasing.

Progesterone is secreted at rates of 50 mg per day in early pregnancy to 250 mg per day at term with a fairly wide range (Table 7–5). Many methods of estimating the amounts of progesterone being secreted at term have been examined. The results are about the same whether the urinary excretion of a metabolite is measured, whether progesterone is measured in the uterine vein effluent, or whether the more precise

blood production rate is determined (Figs. 7–14 and 7–15). The amount going to the fetus has also been estimated to be 50 to 75 mg per day in late pregnancy (Billiar et al.), though it may be less (Escarcena et al.). Progesterone is secreted into the fetus where it is reduced primarily to 20α-hydroxypregn-4-en-3-one (20α-OHP), and it is then returned to the placenta where it is reconverted to progesterone (Zander). This appears to be the way in which the fetal unit conserves progesterone to act at the uterus. The enzyme which interconverts 20α-OHP and progesterone may be the same as that which interconverts estrone and estradiol in the placenta. The proper balance of cofactors, enzyme, and active hormone of the pairs (20α-progesterone–17β-OHP; estrone-estradiol), may be maintained by converting reduced progesterone to the oxidized product and the oxidized estrogen to the reduced member of the pair. Following the administration of labeled progesterone to the fetus, almost all organs examined have shown one or more metabolites of progesterone (Fig. 7–12). These include preg-

TABLE 7–5 Metabolic Clearance Rates (MCR), Plasma Concentrations *(i)*, and Production Rates (PR) of Estrogen, Progesterone, Aldosterone, and Cortisol in Pregnancy

	MCR, L/day	Plasma concentration (i), ng/mL	PR, mg/day	References
Estradiol	1350 ± 40*			Longcope et al.
Early		1.5	2.0	
Mid		8.0	10.8	
Late		28.0	37.8	
Estrone	2210 ± 120*			Longcope et al.
Early		1.0	2.2	
Mid		4.0	8.8	
Late		12.0	26.5	
Estriol	1040			Longcope et al.
Early				
Mid				
Late		29.0	30.0	

	MCR, L/day	Plasma concentration (i), μg/100mL	PR, mg/day	References
Progesterone	2100 ± 638			Little, Billiar
Early		4.3 ± 0.7	90	
Mid		5.5 ± 0.6	115	
Late		10.4 ± 4.27	210 ± 77.8	
Aldosterone, third trimester	1600	0.02–0.17†	0.39–2.6	Tait et al.; Jones et al.
Cortisol, third trimester	130	25	33‡	Gemzell; Migeon et al.

* Estimated values.
† Calculated values.
‡ Based on A.M. values. Because of diurnal variation and episodic secretion of cortisol, this value should only be considered approximate.

nanediol, 20α-OHP, pregnenolone (5β-pregnan-3α-ol-20-one), and 3β-hydroxy-5α-pregnan-20-one as reduced metabolites. Hydroxylated metabolites include 6β-hydroxyprogesterone, 16α-hydroxyprogesterone, 17α-hydroxyprogesterone, and, minimally, cortisol. Conjugated metabolites are also found; conjugates are either glucuronides or sulfates of reduced compounds (Solomon, Fuchs).

No 3β-hydroxysteroid dehydrogenase appears to be present in the fetus, and little 17α-oxidase appears to be in the placenta. For this reason pregnenolone and pregnenolone sulfate (sulfatase is also known to be in high concentration in the placenta) are rapidly converted by the placenta to progesterone and its derivatives, and 17α-OHP appears to be a result of conversion in the fetus. The further conversion of 17α-OHP to androstenedione and testosterone also takes place in the fetus, as its desmolase (lyase) is only in minimal amounts in the placenta. Both 15α- and 16α-hydroxy derivatives of progesterone have been identified in maternal urine and are presumably a reflection of the fetal metabolism.

ESTROGEN SYNTHESIS, SECRETION, AND METABOLISM IN PREGNANCY

Experimental procedures have been carried out to identify the contribution of the fetus and placenta to estrogen metabolism in pregnancy. These include in vitro incubations, placental and fetal perfusions, and studies of the intact fetoplacental unit at midgestation. The placenta has been found to be unable to convert progesterone to 17α-hydroxyprogesterone to estrogens, although it is well understood that the precursors for estrogens in pregnancy are acetate with the intermediates of cholesterol and pregnenolone.

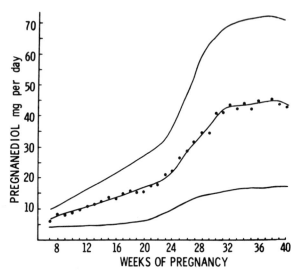

FIGURE 7–14 Pregnanediol excretion in normal pregnancy. The dots represent observed means, the central line fitted means. The upper and lower lines show the 95 percent probability limits. *(From Solomon, Fuchs.)*

The major function of the placenta is the aromatase and sulfatase activity on precursors resulting from secretions by mother and fetus (Diczfalusy, Troen).

In both the mother and the fetus there are secretions of DHA and DHS which reach the placenta through the circulation and are converted to estradiol and estrone (Fig. 7–16). This has been demonstrated by the fact that following the administration of radioactive DHA or DHS to a pregnant woman, labeled estrone, estradiol, and estriol appear in the urine. In contrast, the administration of the same labeled hormones to a nonpregnant woman produces labeled excretory products that are all neutral metabolites. Also, the perfusion of the placenta in situ with either radioactive DHA or DHS will result in the effluent containing labeled estrone and estradiol. From these studies and others, a scheme of estrogen synthesis by the fetoplacental unit has been proposed.

The fetal adrenal secretes 16α-hydroxy-DHS and DHS, which is converted to 16α-hydroxy-DHS in the fetal liver and reaches the placenta through the circulation, where it is converted to estriol by sulfatase and aromatizing enzymes. At the same time, DHA and DHS also reach the placenta and are converted to estrone, which is interconverted to estradiol by the 17β-hydroxysteroid dehydrogenase which is contained in the placenta in large amounts. The interaction of the fetal adrenal secretion with the peripheral conversion of DHA or DHS to 16-OHDHS or 16-OHDHA in the fetal liver, with subsequent removal of the sulfate and aromatization to estrogens, is the major source of estrogen secretion in pregnancy. This pattern of synthesis confirms a well-known fact: At the time of fetal

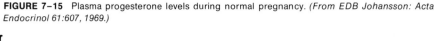

FIGURE 7–15 Plasma progesterone levels during normal pregnancy. *(From EDB Johansson: Acta Endocrinol 61:607, 1969.)*

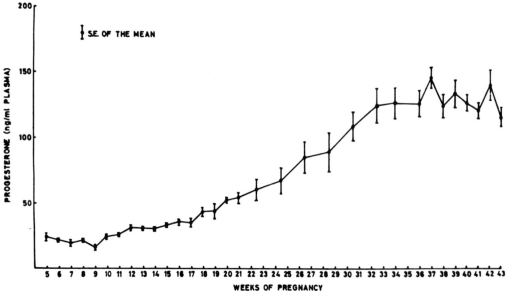

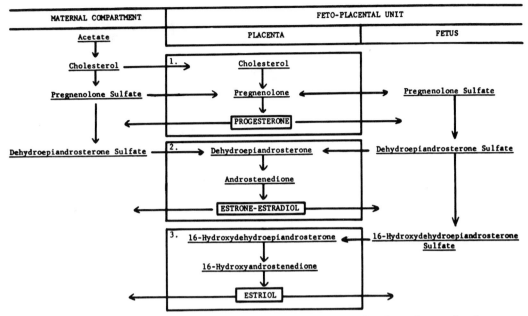

FIGURE 7-16 Major endocrine biosynthetic pathways in maternal and fetoplacental compartments. *(From KJ Ryan, in The Foeto-Placental Unit, eds. A Pecile, C Finzi, Amsterdam, Excerpta Medica, 1969.)*

death in utero the maternal urinary excretion of total estrogens and particularly estriol drops precipitously. This is the basis for the use of estriol excretion as a measure of fetal well-being in late pregnancy (Fig. 7–17). An additional source of precursors for estrogen synthesis is contributed by the maternal adrenals. The maternal adrenals secrete both DHA and DHS in increased amounts during pregnancy. The maternal liver metabolism of steroids is altered during pregnancy so that a considerable component of this secretion is converted to 16-OHDHA and 16-OHDHS by the maternal liver and further aromatized by the placenta. For this reason, patients who have anencephalic fetuses or fetuses in whom the adrenal is abnormal or absent excrete a small amount of estriol. It should also be noted that it is not possible to reduce the excretion of estriol to zero by the administration of large doses of cortisol in pregnancy.

PROTEIN HORMONES OF THE PLACENTA

The first protein identified as secreted by the placenta was HCG. Since that time many other protein hormones have been tentatively identified as being secreted by the placenta. Claims have been made for ACTH, melanocyte-stimulating hormone (MSH), vasopressin, HGH, and lipid-metabolizing hormones. A careful critical review of these claims was made in 1961, and evidence for other placental protein hormones was found to be unconvincing (Diczfalusy, Troen). Since then, human placental lactogen (HPL), now called *human chorionic somatomammotropin* (HCS), has been identified and carefully characterized as to metabolism and physiology. There is also a placental thyroid-stimulating hormone which has been relatively newly identified (human chorionic thyrotropin).

HUMAN CHORIONIC GONADOTROPIN

HCG has been known since Ascheim and Zondek in 1927 observed that blood and urine from pregnant women contained a substance which caused corpus luteum formation in immature mice. The appearance of these so-called hemorrhagic follicles in the ovaries of immature mice following the injection of pregnant urine, or a variant of such a procedure, was used as a pregnancy test (the AZ test) for many years.

Chemistry

HCG is generally purified by selective absorption and desorption on benzoic acid or Permutit, then ethanol fractionation or batch adsorption on an ion exchange,

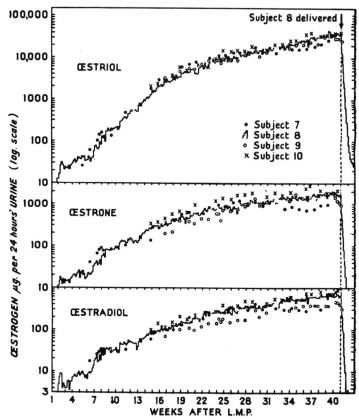

FIGURE 7–17 Urinary estrogen excretion during pregnancy. *(From Brown, 1956.)*

followed by gel filtration and ion exchange chromatography. Such purification steps lead to compounds with 13,000 to 15,000 IU/mg potency when assayed by the rat ventral prostate method (Friesen).

HCG is a glycoprotein with a high content of proline and cystine. The carbohydrate component is about 30 percent of the molecule and contains mannose, galactose, fucose, glucosamine, galactosamine, and sialic acid. The molecular weight calculated from its linear amino acid sequence is 36,000.

HCG contains two nonidentical subunits, which can be prepared by acidifying native HCG. These are called the α and β subunits, the α subunit being eluted off the diethylaminoethyl (DEAE) Sephadex column first. The HCG α subunit can combine with the bovine LH β subunit to give gonadotropic activity and with TSH β subunit to give thyrotropic activity, which indicates a close similarity of the α subunits of these hormones. There is a marked homology between the amino acid sequences of HCG α subunit and those of LH and FSH, and the latter two α subunits are in fact identical.

Placental HCG and urinary HCG may be different, and the electrophoretic patterns of HCG from choriocarcinoma and pregnancy are also said to differ. However, the biologic activity appears to be similar in all three cases, and the differences may be in either polypeptide or carbohydrate components. Modification of structure can affect the activity of HCG. There may be a relationship between the concentration of sialic acid in the molecule of HCG and its longer half-life in blood when compared with its pituitary counterpart, LH.

Cell of Origin

In earlier studies by light microscopy, HCG was thought to be secreted by the cytotrophoblast. More recently ultrastructural localization by immunocytochemical methods has shown HCG on the maternal surface of the apical membrane and in the cisternae of the rough endoplasmic reticulum of the syncytiotrophoblast. Cytotrophoblastic cells in tissue culture from choriocarcinoma have been shown to have the capacity to secrete HCG, but normally secretion is done by the syncytiotrophoblast.

Control of HCG Secretion and Secretion Rates

Other than the fact that HCG is secreted by trophoblast, little is known of its secretion or its control of secretion. In the third month of gestation at peak excretion, production has been estimated at 500,000 to 1 million IU per day; at term this is reduced to about 80,000 to 120,000 IU per day.

Evidence for placental origin of HCG is based on the facts that it can be extracted from the placenta, it is present in the blood and urine during pregnancy, it persists in the maternal circulation following clamping of the fetal cord with the placenta in situ, it is present following maternal hypophysectomy, it is produced by placental transplants to the anterior chamber of the eye and in tissue culture, immunofluorescent techniques localize HCG to placental syncytiotrophoblast, and trophoblastic tumors produce HCG.

The disappearance of HCG from the blood follows a double exponential curve, with the first component having a $t_{\frac{1}{2}}$ of 11 hours and the second, a $t_{\frac{1}{2}}$ of 23 hours, this compares with 21 minutes and 4 hours for LH. HCG thus disappears within 4 to 5 days postpartum as measured by the usual pregnancy tests. However, in practice it may take up to 6 weeks without being feared as indicating trophoblastic tumor because the persistent secretion of residual pieces of the placenta postpartum is biologically variable.

Concentration in Tissue, Blood, and Urine of HCG (Table 7–6)

The placental concentration curve of HCG appears to parallel the curves of urinary and blood HCG during pregnancy. Maximum HCG concentrations of 100 to 150 IU per gram of weight in placental tissue occur by the third month, and diminish to 10 to 20 IU/g at term. Assays of blood and urine reach a peak at about 60 days' gestation and then decrease and remain low until a slight rise occurs prior to term. Blood serum levels rise to 50 to 100 IU/mL, then decrease to 10 to 20 IU/mL to term. Peak values of HCG in the urine are from 20,000 to 100,000 IU per day, and decrease to later pregnancy values of 4000 to 11,000 IU per day. There is a parallel between urine and blood concen-

TABLE 7–6 Half-time of Disappearance from the Circulation $(t_{\frac{1}{2}})$, Blood Concentrations, and Secretion Rates (SR) of HCG and HPL

	$t_{\frac{1}{2}}$, hour	Blood concentration, IU/mL	Urine concentration IU/day	SR, IU/day
HCG*	23			
10 wk		50–100	20,000–100,000	500,000–1,000,000
14 wk to term		10–20	4,000–11,000	80,000–100,000
Cord artery		0.252		
Vein		0.388		

	$t_{\frac{1}{2}}$, hour	Plasma concentration, μg/mL		SR, mg/day
HPL (HCS)†	40			
10–14 wk gestation		0.3		0.10
36–42 wk gestation		5.4 ± 0.5		0.5–3.5
Fetal cord		0.015 ± 0.003		
Amniotic fluid		0.55 ± 0.06		
Placenta		10–20 mg/100 g		
Maternal concentration	1 μg/mL per 100 g placenta			

* From Brody.
† From Josimovich.

trations in the mother. In the fetus the concentration of HCG is 0.252 IU/mL in the umbilical artery and 0.388 IU/mL in the umbilical vein (Brody).

Depending on the pregnancy test used, HCG values may be too low to show a positive test following 14 weeks' gestation. There appears to be no diurnal variation in HCG concentration, but higher values are reported in twin pregnancies, and higher levels are reported in the presence of female fetuses than in males for unknown reasons.

HCG concentrations in patients with diabetes in pregnancy, toxemia, and Rh-isoimmunized pregnancies have been studied with variable results. HCG assays in these conditions are not helpful clinically. However, patients with a diagnosis of threatened abortion who have low HCG values have been shown to go on to complete abortion. In the presence of trophoblastic tumors HCG values are of great help in patient management. In cases of hydatidiform mole urinary HCG titers rise to over 300,000 IU/L. Following molar evacuation these values drop rapidly within 1 month, and in about 90 percent of cases HCG is not detectable by urinary assay after 3 months. In complicated cases with retention of tissue, as in chorioadenoma destruens or choriocarcinoma, values remain elevated, and serial assays are of great value in determining the results of treatment, usually chemotherapy. Blood serum assays of HCG or its β subunit are now being used to follow the course of trophoblastic tumors in most patients.

Physiologic Role of HCG

The major defined role of HCG is the maintenance of the corpus luteum in early pregnancy. This continues until the trophoblast develops to the point where it secretes sufficient estrogen and progesterone to maintain the pregnancy. HCG appears in the urine as early as a few days before the first missed menstrual period. The response of the corpus luteum to HCG appears to be limited, and in spite of the increasing concentrations of HCG being secreted, progesterone concentration in the blood actually falls before it begins to rise again at about 8 to 10 weeks' gestation, presumably the result of progesterone secretion by the developing placenta. This paradox of falling progesterone in the face of rising HCG concentrations is added to by the fact that HCG will prolong the corpus luteum only 9 days in the absence of pregnancy, whereas the corpus luteum of pregnancy functions considerably longer. HCG may require both HPL and PRL to synergize with it in this response, but this remains to be proved.

HCG is selectively removed from the blood-stream by the ovary, as is the case for LH. Both HCG and LH cause hypertrophy and luteinization of interstitial and thecal cells, and both will synergize with FSH to lead to ovulation. However, the precise mechanism of action of LH and HCG on steroidogenesis by the ovary and/or the placenta remains to be fully delineated, in spite of experiments showing increased progesterone synthesis from acetate in corpus luteum slices in vitro due to LH addition, and in some studies a stimulatory effect on aromatization of neutral steroids in vitro.

HCG acts to stimulate the interstitial cells of the testis, leading to the increased secretion of androgens. HCG is occasionally used in the therapy of male infertility. The effects of HCG on the fetus are poorly understood, although there is some evidence that HCG stimulates the fetal adrenal. Some additional evidence indicates that HCG inhibits uterine motility and possibly the motility of the gut. Most recently some evidence shows that HCG may have an immunosuppressive effect on maternal T lymphocytes to render them less likely to reject heterologous transplants such as the fetus, but this is still to be confirmed in humans.

HUMAN PLACENTAL LACTOGEN (HPL) OR HUMAN CHORIONIC SOMATOMAMMOTROPIN (HCS)

In 1962 Josimovich and MacLaren identified a substance in the crude extract of term placenta that cross-reacted with antisera to HGH. This substance also had a marked lactogenic effect when tested in the pigeon crop sac. As the lactogenic component was so great in comparison with its growth hormone effect, it was called human placental lactogen (HPL). Subsequently it was also identified as chorionic growth hormone prolactin (CGP) and purified placental protein hormone (PPH); now, to combine its known functions, it has been named human chorionic somatomammotropin (HCS). Whether the term HPL or HCS survives in the jargon of science and clinical medicine remains to be seen.

Purification and Chemistry of HPL

Although fresh placental tissue may be used for the preparation of HPL as originally described, presently large amounts are obtained during the purification of gamma globulin from large batches of placentas. Recently the National Institutes of Health made available a reference preparation for use to compare all preparations and assay results (see Friesen).

HPL is a single-chain polypeptide similar to HGH

in molecular weight (20,000) and amino acid sequence. There may be a prohormone or "big" HPL which is observed in the placenta at 12 weeks' gestation. There are 188 to 190 amino acids in each hormone. At present 12 of the 20 tryptic peptides of HPL and HGH are identical. Homologies between prolactin (HPr) and HPL and HGH have also been identified. These similarities suggest the possibility of a common primordial peptide. In evolution prolactin is found throughout the vertebrates, whereas HGH and HPL appeared at a later stage in the evolution of viviparity.

Site of Secretion of HPL

Immunofluorescent localization of HPL has shown fluorescence in the syncytial cytoplasm but not syncytial nuclei nor cytotrophoblast and not in the stroma of the chorionic villi. HPL has also been measured in patients with trophoblastic disease. In choriocarcinoma HCG is secreted in considerably higher amounts than HPL, whereas the reverse is true in pregnancy. HPL and HCG have also been identified in patients with nontrophoblastic cancers including carcinoma of the lung, hepatoma, lymphoma, and malignant pheochromocytoma.

Biologic Effects of HPL

HPL produces up to about 50 percent of the activity of the National Institutes of Health (NIH) sheep prolactin standard in the pigeon crop assay but is equal to prolactin in the stimulation of the rabbit breast development. Mammary-gland explants have been shown to be stimulated by HPL as by prolactin. HPL in the presence of insulin and hydrocortisone causes histologic development of breast alveoli and stimulates casein synthesis. Apparently HPL and prolactin are both responsible for mammary-gland development in pregnancy, but whereas HPL and prolactin progressively increase in concentration to term, HPL then disappears while prolactin falls at delivery, then actively increases with the onset of nursing, and subsequently falls as nursing becomes autonomous. Prolactin levels rise from 20 ng/mL in the first trimester to as high as 50 ng/mL at term, then, up to 100 to 200 ng/mL, and finally down to normal nonpregnant values with prolonged nursing.

Luteotropic Activity of HPL. HPL is luteotropic in the rat and has been proposed as being synergistic with HCG in maintaining the corpus luteum in early pregnancy.

Growth-Promoting Effects of HPL. HPL has been shown to stimulate the growth of hypopituitary dwarfs.

To achieve a similar growth effect, the comparable dosage of HPL is very large (400 to 1000 mg per day, i.e., pregnancy levels) when compared with HGH (2.0 mg three times per week). There also may be an augmentation of HGH activity by HPL even at doses of HPL which by themselves produce no growth effect. There is also some suggestion that the HPL monomer produces growth effects but that the dimer does not.

Metabolic Effects of HPL. Some of the metabolic changes occurring during pregnancy may be mediated by HPL. These include an increase in circulating free fatty acids and in mobilization of fat stores. There is also a lack of sensitivity to insulin in pregnancy associated with elevated plasma insulin response to a glucose stimulus and islet cell hypertrophy which may be partly due to HPL. For example, HPL administered to diabetics leads to hyperglycemia and ketosis. HPL alone may not be responsible for these changes as the insulin production by islet cells has been shown to be stimulated by an interaction between HPL and progesterone. The postulated role for HPL has been one of glucose and protein sparing through the stimulation of lipolysis and the resulting increase in serum free fatty acids. The glucose and amino acids are thus conserved for transport to the fetus for its growth and development. Starvation in pregnant women leads to hypoglycemia and hypoinsulinemia more rapidly than in nonpregnant women. With starvation there is a resultant 30 percent rise in circulating HPL, which suggests a direct role for HPL in the metabolism of fuels in pregnancy, presumably for the fetus.

Mammary-Gland Effects of HPL. In animals, in in vivo and in vitro organ culture, HPL has been shown to stimulate breast development and casein synthesis. Its effect appears to be primarily on the cell membrane and leads to a lactogenic response. Two other responses to HPL administration have been noted: one, the stimulus of erythropoiesis; the other, the stimulation of the excretion of aldosterone.

Secretion and Concentration of HPL (Table 7–6)

The disappearance of HPL from the blood serum in studies following delivery and the infusion of labeled HPL has a half-time ($t_{\frac{1}{2}}$) of 13 minutes in the first phase and 40 minutes in the second phase. By use of a calculated distribution volume of 7.2 percent of body weight (± 10 L) and a term plasma concentration of 1.0 to 5.0 μg/mL, the daily secretion at term was calculated to be 0.5 to 3.0 g per day. However, it has been shown that plasma concentrations correlate with

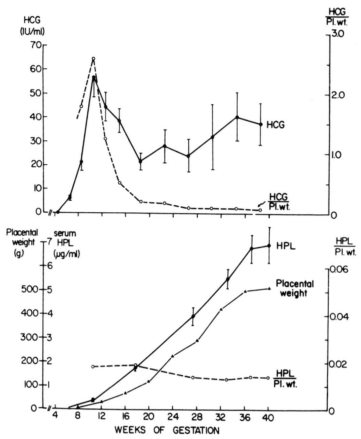

FIGURE 7–18 Secretion patterns of HCG and HPL during normal pregnancy. The upper graph compares the serum levels of HCG with the same levels per gram of placental weight. The lower graph illustrates changes in serum HPL during pregnancy with actual placental weights and the serum HPL per gram placental weight. *(From HA Selenkrow et al., in The Foeto-Placental Unit, eds. A Pecile, C Finzi, Amsterdam, Excerpta Medica, 1969.)*

placental weight and that secretion of HPL is maintained to achieve circulating levels of 1 μg/mL per 100 g placenta (Fig. 7–18).

The larger amount of HPL is found in the mother (15 to 20 mg) compared with the fetus (0.5 mg). The content in maternal plasma increases from 0.3 μg/mL in the first trimester to 5.4 μg/mL at term. The maternal urine and amniotic fluid have considerably lower concentrations. Only 300 μg per 24 hours is excreted in the urine at term, and the cord contains 0.55 μg/mL. The amniotic fluid concentration parallels the maternal concentration as it increases toward term; however, the fetal concentration remains relatively stable in the last trimester. The concentration in the fetal serum is 0.3 percent that of maternal concentration of HPL, whereas for HGH the fetal serum concentration is about 3 percent. What determines the secretion of HPL to the maternal or fetal side of the placenta is not

known. HCG, for example, is found in relatively higher concentrations in the fetus than is HPL.

HPL is presently being used as a measure of the state of the fetus in utero, particularly as it measures placental function. It is not entirely satisfactory as a clinical measurement because there is a large range of normal values as gestation progresses. However, in careful hands the test may be useful to do along with other measurements of fetal well-being to add to the confidence of overall evaluation. This is true for toxemia of pregnancy, chronic hypertensive patients, and small-for-date babies. HPL is not used to follow metastatic trophoblastic disease, because there is little HPL in comparison to the larger concentrations of HCG. In a case where there is confusion about the presence of a mole and no x-ray or ultrasound is available, the ratio between HCG and HPL may be helpful in the diagnosis. At present HPL is not used for its growth hormone activity because its activity is so low that very large quantities are required for effective results.

LABOR AND DELIVERY

The onset of labor has always been a very important area for examining cause and mechanisms, because much perinatal morbidity and mortality result from prematurity. Also the opposite complication is experienced by many patients for whom immediate delivery is essential but for whom the onset of labor is difficult or impossible to achieve. When to these patients are added those who wish to undergo elective abortion, the problem can be seen to be of rather large proportions.

In the past, labor and delivery were considered, in simplest terms to be the result of the opposing uterine forces of the *facultas retentrix* (cervix) and the *facultas expultrix* (myometrium). The complex mechanisms known today, although more sophisticated, are essentially no different. First the cervix must become favorable for dilatation, and at the same time the milieu of the uterine muscle must be changed so that it will lead to the spontaneous onset of contractions. These elements should be easy to define, but they are not, and over the years there have been different theories to explain the onset of labor. Most such theories are not completely applicable and therefore have been rejected for one reason or another.

Presently there is a resurgence of interest in labor, and although all the details have not been worked out in the human being, in sheep there appears to have been a reasonable series of observations which, when linked together, make an acceptable basis for the understanding of labor onset. Liggins et al. showed that if fetal lambs were either adrenalectomized or hypophysectomized and replaced in utero, labor onset would be significantly delayed. To this was added the observation that in human pregnancy in the presence of an anencephalic, the onset of labor was sometimes delayed. It was presumed, therefore, that adrenal secretion or the lack of it either directly or indirectly was required for the normal process of labor to occur. Further studies were done in which the administration of either cortisol or ACTH to the fetal lamb was shown to hasten the onset of labor. It was also shown that the endogenous production of cortisol increased just prior to labor. The questions were then what was the result of the increasing cortisol secretion and concentration, and also what caused the increase in the cortisol production. Neither of these questions has been completely

answered. However, it has been observed that following the increased cortisol secretion there occurs in the mother a fall in progesterone, a rise in free estrogens, and a rise in prostaglandin $F_{2\alpha}$ ($PGF_{2\alpha}$). Labor, which usually begins after the administration of cortisol to the fetal lamb, may be stopped by the administration of large doses of progesterone to the mother. The doses given have to be larger (200 mg per day) than usually considered equivalent to endogenous production for this gestational age, because it is necessary to achieve an appropriate concentration at the myometrium, rather than merely reaching peripheral circulating concentrations expected for the gestational age. The etiology of prostaglandin production in the onset of labor and its usefulness in the achievement of abortion in early pregnancy have made prostaglandins a focus for study. The administration of $PGF_{2\alpha}$ is associated with an increase in free estrogens and a decrease in progesterone as with cortisol and also the onset of labor. The site of the prostaglandin synthesis and secretion in the uterus is not entirely known, but there has been a renewed interest in the decidua as an important site of origin. The stimulation of the membranes and the separation of the choriodecidual membrane are often followed by the onset of labor, as in membrane stripping. Actual rupture of the membranes leads to some decidual necrosis with prostaglandin release, and intrauterine administration of saline is accompanied by prostaglandin release, particularly following decidual necrosis. These endocrine factors are all interrelated with the onset of labor, although one factor alone is probably insufficient to lead to labor and delivery.

The resultant model for the sheep has therefore been proposed (Fig. 7–19). The stimulus for the onset of labor may reside in the fetus as the result of a stimulus originating in the fetal hypothalamus. This leads to pituitary activity and secretion of ACTH. The resulting increased rate of cortisol secretion is due to adrenocortical growth and development, the activation of 11β-hydroxylase in the definitive fetal adrenal cortex, and its increased responsiveness to ACTH. The increased cortisol acts on the placenta in some unknown way to reduce the secretion of progesterone and to increase the secretion of estrogen and $PGF_{2\alpha}$. Progesterone ordinarily inhibits the synthesis and release of $PGF_{2\alpha}$, and therefore the falling progesterone augments the $PGF_{2\alpha}$ effect. The myometrium responds to $PGF_{2\alpha}$ with heightened sensitivity to oxytocin, which may lead to the onset of contractions without changing levels of oxytocin. The changes that occur in the cervix, including a softening, effacement, and dilatation, await further direct observations of the

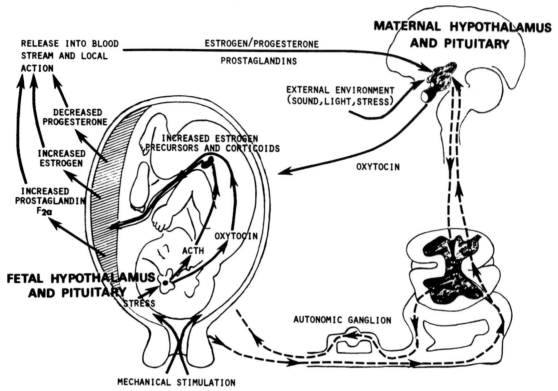

FIGURE 7–19 The control of parturition, based mainly on data obtained in the sheep and human being. *(Adapted from a chart prepared by ALR Findlay for Research in Reproduction, vol. 4, no. 5, 1972.)*

influence of the changing concentrations of estrogen, progesterone, and prostaglandin on the connective-tissue matrix of the cervix.

It must be emphasized that these changes have all been observed in the ewe and lamb and await application to the human. However, in the human, recent additional observations by MacDonald et al., Schultz et al., and Schwarz et al. suggest that as pregnancy progresses there is a diminution of metabolism of progesterone by the fetal membranes which renders cellular lysomes unstable and results in the release of phospholipase A_2. This enzyme acts to increase the availability of the prostaglandin precursor, arachidonic acid. Arachidonic acid availability as a precursor for the enzyme prostaglandin synthetase (cytooxidase) is a limiting factor for the availability of PG and, in large amounts, is known to stimulate labor. PGs are known to be an active intermediate in the onset of experimental uterine contraction and labor. The mechanism of the initiation of parturition is thus becoming clearer.

POSTPARTUM LACTATION

During pregnancy, as previously described, there appears in the pituitary a specific type of large, clear cell whose function has not been made clear. However, an effort has been made to identify these cells by special stains, including immunofluorescence, as prolactin-secreting. In view of the increased secretion of PRL in pregnancy, the appearance of these special cells, their identification with special stains including antibodies to prolactin, and the tenfold increased content of pregnant monkey pituitary glands of PRL, it is believed that these cells do in fact secrete prolactin (Friesen).

Elevated prolactin is measurably increased in the blood at about 8 weeks of gestation and increases to concentrations of 200 ng/mL at term. If there is no subsequent breast-feeding, the values drop to normal low levels 2 to 3 weeks postpartum. In the puerperium during nursing there are three phases. In the first week basal levels of PRL are elevated, and only a modest increase occurs with suckling. During the second and third weeks, to 2 to 3 months postpartum, basal levels are lower, being about twice the values in nonpregnant women, and suckling produces a ten- to twentyfold increase in the circulating concentration of PRL. After 3 to 4 months of nursing, the basal levels of prolactin are reached, and suckling produces no rise in PRL levels. This is consistent with the observations of nursing women who report engorgement at the onset of nursing and some difficulty in nursing in the first week, a time when they may become discouraged. During the next phase they settle down and become comfortable, hardly noting the nursing activity. The final phase is not often carried out in our society, so there is little information at present; however, it is known from past experience that during the latter phase milk is still abundant and normal ovulation may occur. Women may nurse through a subsequent pregnancy and have sufficient milk at the delivery of their child to breast-feed immediately after giving birth.

The onset of lactation appears to be a combination of elevated PRL levels, a fall in steroid concentration, particularly estrogen, and the onset of suckling. Lactation is blocked by the administration of estrogens; however, this is not accompanied by a fall in PRL levels, and it is well known that patients whose milk is suppressed with estrogens may have a subsequent engorgement of the breasts in the puerperium. If patients are given ergocryptine, PRL levels will fall and there will be no lactation. Similarly, there is no engorgement or lactation in patients with Sheehan's disease or those who have had a surgical hypophysectomy.

In the first trimester at a time when the maternal levels of PRL are 20 to 50 ng/mL, the amniotic fluid concentration has been shown to be as high as 10,000 ng/mL; it gradually reduces at term to about 1000 ng/mL, which is four times the maternal concentration at that time. This PRL is apparently produced by the chorion. Reflecting on the viviparity of PRL and its actions in fish that come from salt water to fresh water, in which it acts on the gills to retain sodium, some interesting speculations may be made as to the presence of PRL in the amniotic fluid and survival of the fetus. In patients with hydramnios, the PRL levels may go as low as 50 ng/mL. Prolactin levels are maintained elevated in the newborn and may be responsible, along with the concentrations of steroids, for the small amount of milk that may be secreted from the newborn's nipple.

At least six pituitary hormones play a role in lactation and mammary development; these include PRL, ACTH, HGH, TSH, FSH, and LH. In addition, HCS and steroid hormones secreted by the adrenal, ovary, and placenta play a part. In in vitro experiments PRL, insulin, and cortisol have been shown to be required in the development of and secretion by mammary tissue. The development of the lobule-alveolar structure is influenced by insulin. Differentiation of the cells is brought about by a combination of all three hormones, and hydrocortisone is required for the ultrastructural development of the rough endoplasmic reticulum and paranuclear Golgi apparatus which are essential for protein synthesis and secretion.

HUMAN PITUITARY PROLACTIN (HPRL)

Recently an increasing interest in prolactin has appeared because a radioimmunoassay for human prolactin (HPRL) has been developed through the isolation of the protein hormone from the pituitary which is free of growth hormone. Pharmacologic agents have also been identified which can increase and decrease the secretion of HPRL (e.g., diphenylhydantoin and bromoergocryptine).

BIOLOGIC EFFECTS OF HPRL

As shown by its very name, the focus of attention on prolactin is on its lactogenic function; however, 82 actions of prolactin have been identified, and they can be categorized under the following headings: growth, osmoregulation, reproduction, integumentary effects, and synergism with steroids. Birds and mammals given prolactin will develop brooding and nesting behavior, and other manifestations of maternal instinct. Prolactin is not only mammotropic and lactogenic, but also stimulates growth of the seminal vesicles and prostate in the male.

SECRETION AND BLOOD LEVELS OF HPRL

The levels of HPRL in males and in females are the same until puberty, at which time the concentrations in the female are slightly increased by the stimulus of the increasing estrogen. There is, however, considerable overlap between male and female values. The value throughout the menstrual cycle in the female is 10 ng/mL. At the menopause these values do not change, although there have been suggestions that at a later age the values may increase (i.e., in women older than 75 years). A diurnal variation in HPRL levels has also been shown, with the peak about 4 to 5 hours after the onset of sleep.

Anesthesia, exercise, and surgery will lead to increases in prolactin, with higher levels noted in women than in men. Following surgery, breast engorgement and galactorrhea may even develop. Nipple stimulation and sexual intercourse have been shown to be associated with increased levels of PRL, and cervical or vaginal stimulation in rats is similarly accompanied by a rise in circulating values.

In the hypothalamus a prolactin-inhibiting factor (PIF) has been identified which is controlled by catecholamine levels. A decrease in catecholamines is accompanied by a decrease in PIF and a release of HPRL. The PIF is transported through the portal circulation of the pituitary stalk to the anterior pituitary where it acts on the anterior pituitary to stimulate the secretion of PRL. Increased dopamine levels in the hypothalamus are followed by the opposite effect, in which there is increased PIF and less secretion of PRL. Phenothiazines, reserpines, and alpha methyldopa, by decreasing catecholamine effects, increase the secretion of PRL; L-dopa has the opposite effect. Ergot drugs have the effect of inhibiting the secretion of PRL. A recent drug which has had promising effects in this regard is 2α-bromoergocryptine; acting at the pituitary level, it has been successful in reducing circulating PRL in the presence of elevated levels and galactorrhea. The thyrotropin-releasing factor (TRF) has been shown to not only release TSH but also PRL. As little as 3 μg of TRF causes a significant release of both TSH and PRL, and females respond with a threefold greater release of PRL than do males. Although most hypothyroid patients do not have a concomitant increase of PRL with TSH, there is an increased responsiveness of myxedematous patients to PRL, and some hypothyroid patients do have myxedema, elevated PRL, and galactorrhea.

DISORDERS OF REPRODUCTION

MENOPAUSE

The term *menopause* is used to denote the cessation of menstrual flow only and is not associated, as usually implied, with all the signs and symptoms ascribed to it, which are better called *menopausal syndrome*. There is no characteristic menopause. It can

occur in a number of different patterns. Some women will reach the age of menopause, now averaging 51 years, which is generally a little later than their mothers' and may be as late as 55, and the menstrual periods may suddenly stop. Other women may experience a halt in their periods, then have what to them is a characteristic period, often in the summer, and then have a complete stop in their periods. Other women will begin to skip or miss periods and then stop. It is usual for women as they approach the menopause to become less fertile; at the same time their cycles may become anovulatory. Whether they develop cystic and adenomatous hyperplasia of the endometrium or whether they develop cystic or "Swiss cheese"-type hyperplasia depends on the level and constancy of circulating estrogen. Unopposed estrogen stimulation for prolonged periods of time during the productive years can lead to abnormal endometrium and even adenocarcinoma of the endometrium. At the menopause it is important to distinguish between the somewhat abnormal bleeding that may occur normally at that time and the possible development of abnormal endometrium. For this reason a dilatation and curettage is always recommended at menopause or postmenopause when there is any question of abnormal vaginal bleeding (Kaufman).

It is well recognized that as menopause approaches, the cycle length is shorter and mean estradiol concentrations are lower than in younger women. There is also a striking increase in FSH concentration. The variable cycle length may be due to either irregular maturation of ovarian follicles with reduced responsiveness to FSH, or anovulatory bleeding may follow estrogen withdrawal without progesterone opposition in the face of absent corpus luteum secretion. There has been a suggestion of reduced nonsteroidal inhibinlike material from the follicle as menopause approaches [also called FSH release-inhibiting substance (FRIS)].

Postmenopausally, it has been shown that peripheral conversion of androstenedione to estrone is the major source of estrone and estrogen production. This conversion is increased with age, in the presence of increased weight, and with liver disease.

The adrenal cortex has been shown to be the almost exclusive source of plasma estradiol, progesterone, and 17-hydroxyprogesterone, as well as the most important source of plasma dehydroepiandrosterone, postmenopause. The postmenopausal ovary, however, is responsible for 50 percent of plasma testosterone and 30 percent of the androstenedione levels (Vermeulen).

At the time of natural or surgical menopause the

questions arise as to whether estrogens should or should not be given, and whether they should be given intermittently, cyclically, or with progestins. At the menopause when hormones are not given, a number of women develop hot flushes associated with estrogen lack. These flushes occur over the head and neck and down over the shoulders, may produce sweating, and are very uncomfortable. They may awaken the woman at night and remind her of her diminished ovarian function and make her tired and irritable the next day. This fatigue is usually remarked upon carefully by the family, who remind her gently that she is not as young as she used to be. This, of course, does not help. The administration of estrogen in the latter event is of great therapeutic benefit. The circulating estrogen postmenopausally is the result of the peripheral conversion of androstenedione to estrone. The androstenedione (70 percent) is secreted by the adrenal, and there may be no requirement for additional estrogen. The controversy arises in relation to whether the administered estrogen prevents osteoporosis, atrophy of the vagina, or arteriosclerosis with its accompanying coronary disease. There are proponents of giving estrogens cyclically forever in the belief that to do so is physiologic. Thus estrogen may be prescribed for 21 days followed by a week off, and so on. The amount of estrogen is varied by some physicians according to the patient's need, while other physicians will give the same dose to all patients. Usually given are conjugated estrogens; among them are estrone and its sulfate and the various sulfates and glucuronides of other estrogens including equilin and equilenin, which are estrogens peculiar to the pregnant mare from whose urine the conjugated estrogens are generally obtained. Dosage varies according to the type of estrogen given, but the dose is usually equivalent to that of synthetic estrogens of 0.25 to 0.5 mg of diethylstilbestrol or 0.02 to 0.05 mg of ethinyl estradiol (0.625 to 1.25 mg of conjugated estrogens).

It has not been proved to everyone's satisfaction that the administration of estrogens after menopause prevents the onset of osteoporosis, atherosclerosis, or atrophic vaginas in all cases, for other factors are involved. Certainly estrogens neither perpetuate nor create postmenopausal beauty or youthful libido. It appears to be quite sufficient in most women to administer estrogen as indicated by the symptoms and signs of estrogen lack, which include those discussed above; a vaginal cytogram as an estrogen index may be helpful when in doubt.

The administration of estrogens to relieve menopausal symptoms has recently come into question as a cause of endometrial cancer. Two groups have been studied among those who have endometrial cancer, and more cancers occurred among estrogen users than among controls who did not. The risk was shown to be seven- or eightfold more among estrogen users. However, this has been criticized as an accident of sampling because estrogen may cause bleeding for which dilatation and curettage will be done, thus identifying more abnormal endometria in the estrogen-user group. Whatever the result of this dispute, the result has been a more cautious use of estrogen by menopausal women, plus a mandatory warning, issued as a result of FDA action, which is included with every package of estrogen filled by a pharmacist.

In contrast, recent radiographic studies have demonstrated the long-term effect of estrogen administration, postmenopausally (either natural or surgical), on the calcification of bones, particularly of the hand. Less demineralization of the bone is visible following estrogen treatment.

It would appear, therefore, that judicious estrogen treatment is important, postmenopausally.

Factors other than estrogen relating to calcium and bone metabolism are inherent in the appearance of osteoporosis; it is true that treatment with estrogens may alleviate the disease symptoms. The characteristic symptoms are like those of arthritis with pain mostly in the back. When this is coupled with the x-ray appearance of the typically osteoporotic bone lesions of the spine, the diagnosis may be made. The bone pain is relieved by treatment with sodium estrone sulfate 1.25 mg daily (4 weeks on and 1 week off), but the x-ray appearance does not usually change, and the estrogen often will lose its effectiveness after a period of time. Estrogens primarily affect bone resorption. Calcium and vitamin D therapy are frequently added. Their primary effects are to decrease bone turnover, probably by partial inhibition of parathormone (see also Chap. 27).

AMENORRHEA—GALACTORRHEA

To the classical states of amenorrhea has been added that of amenorrhea following oral contraceptive therapy. The Chiari-Frommel syndrome is amenorrhea and persistent galactorrhea in postpartum women. Ahumada-Del Castillo syndrome, sometimes called Ahumada-Argonz-Del Castillo syndrome, refers to amenorrhea and galactorrhea in nulliparous women. Finally, the Forbes-Albright syndrome denotes the presence of a pituitary tumor with amenorrhea and galactorrhea. As in the evolution of all clinical medicine, these eponyms for diseases are gradually being replaced as we understand the nature of the diseases involved. With the recent development of radioimmunoassays for gonadotropins and most recently for prolactin, some of the confusion surrounding the clinical manifestations of these diseases is being resolved, and they are being reclassified by the identification of the specific pathophysiologic mechanisms (Archer et al.).

Incidence

As in most other complications of oral contraceptive pills, the incidence of postpill amenorrhea is extremely low. The definition of amenorrhea is frequently expressed as absence of menses for 1 year; however, in postpill studies the time limit has been reduced to 3 or 4 months without menses. The return of normal ovulation can be expected in 98 percent of all women within the first three cycles after stopping oral contraceptives. Return of ovulation is not related to length of treatment or type of preparation used including whether it be given in combination dosage or sequentially.

The incidence of postpill amenorrhea is not clearly known, but is quoted as 0 to 4 percent. Whether amenorrhea and/or galactorrhea has increased is even harder to ascertain. However, in a Nova Scotian study, the incidence was shown to increase fivefold after the beginning use of oral contraceptives. This was not true in Sweden, but the former study appears to correspond with clinical experience (S. Clair MacLeod, personal communication).

Although cause and effect have not been demonstrated absolutely, there is a statistical association between the administration of the pill and amenorrhea following its cessation. In a retrospective study Shearman and Smith demonstrated that 42 percent of a group with amenorrhea with and without galactorrhea developed their signs following treatment with oral contraceptives (Table 7–7). A similar percentage of those with amenorrhea alone (41 percent) and those with amenorrhea-galactorrhea (42 percent) had a history of taking oral contraceptives. The incidence of galactorrhea associated with amenorrhea overall was 20 percent and was not different in those who had taken oral contraceptives and those who had not. There are a larger number of those patients with preexisting irregular menstrual cycles who develop amenorrhea than would be expected, and oral contraceptives should be avoided where possible for such

Table 7–7 Causes of Amenorrhea-Galactorrhea

	Number of patients	Percentage
Oral contraception	20	40.8
Phenothiazine	3	6.1
Postpartum	5	10.2
Acromegaly	1	2.0
Cushing's syndrome	1	2.0
Pituitary tumor	6	12.2
No apparent cause*	13*	26.5

*For additional evaluation of patients with no apparent cause, see Archer et al.
Source: Shearman, Smith.

women. From Table 7–7 it can be seen that in Shearman's experience of amenorrhea-galactorrhea 40 percent occurred postoral contraception, 10 percent postpartum, and 12 percent in association with pituitary tumors, with the remainder distributed between adrenal disease, acromegaly, and phenothiazine administration, and a large group with no apparent cause; some in the last group may in the future turn out to be related to an abnormal pituitary or hypothalamic response with resultant inappropriate secretion of prolactin (see Archer et al.).

Urinary gonadotropins, estrogens, 17-hydroxycorticosteroids, and 17-ketosteroids have been measured in a small number of patients with postpill amenorrhea. Gonadotropins are generally low, as are estrogens, but 17-hydroxycorticosteroids and 17-ketosteroids are normal. Varying HGH responses have been reported following arginine infusion and glucose administration. Elevated circulating values of prolactin have been demonstrated in a few cases, and some abnormally high levels have been observed in response to thyroid-releasing factor, which is known to stimulate the release of prolactin under normal circumstances.

The management of patients with postpill amenorrhea depends on the initial establishment of a goal for therapy. For example, patients may wish to conceive or not, or they may wish to cycle "normally." The initial evaluation of a patient with postpill amenorrhea or galactorrhea-amenorrhea will depend on whether the condition is indeed primary or postpill. If primary or at a significant time after stopping the pill (i.e., 6 months), the first test to be carried out is a determination of the circulating prolactin level. In the first instance, to achieve ovulation, either clomiphene citrate or gonadotropin administration is the treatment of choice (see Chap. 27). In the second, cycling a patient with a combination estrogen-progestin pill, although it will not resolve the problem, will provide regular monthly bleeding which may be enough to relieve the patient's anxieties. This latter treatment is obviously not usually acceptable because it compounds the problem; however, it may rarely be appropriate.

HYPOPITUITARISM (SHEEHAN'S DISEASE)

In general, hypopituitary states due to causes other than tumor have been reduced almost to rarities because obstetrics has been improved and, increasingly, blood banks are available in obstetric hospitals to prevent maternal shock. It is hard to define Sheehan's or Simmonds' disease, because they have changed over time. For example, Simmonds' disease was originally described as postpartum cases in which it was thought that pituitary necrosis took place following the lodging of minute bacterial emboli in the sinuses of the gland. Sheehan, on the other hand, believes that there is a reduction of blood flow to the pituitary at the time of normal delivery; if, to this, is added the severe circulatory collapse associated with maternal hemorrhage, it is possible that the blood flow to the anterior lobe is so reduced that thrombosis with resulting infarction occurs.

Simmonds', and to some extent Sheehan's, diseases have been used to include all types of pituitary cachexia, including cachexia resulting from anorexia nervosa, cysts, and fibrosis following infection such as tuberculosis. Sheehan's disease has also been used indiscriminately to include all those cases of amenorrhea which occur postpartum and may wrongfully include cases of uterine synechiae (Asherman's syndrome). Both these diseases were originally described pathologically postmortem in cases where extensive pituitary necrosis was found. Both syndromes, once suspected, may now be defined endocrinologically with much more precision by pituitary hormone tests.

Sheehan's original observation was that pituitary necrosis was not an uncommon finding in women who died postpartum. Animal experiments suggested that at least two-thirds of the anterior pituitary must be destroyed before there were demonstrable symptoms. Subsequently Sheehan showed that about 15 percent of survivors of moderate hemorrhage or 40 percent of survivors of severe hemorrhage had subsequent hypopituitarism. He had to diligently seek out patients with hypopituitarism because one of their main symptoms was severe apathy to the point where not only were they unwilling to find medical help, but they had so alienated their husbands that they refused to seek care for them. In the past there was a direct correlation between the severity of the maternal hemorrhage and the extent of the disease. This is no longer the case, as blood administration at delivery is common, and it is most difficult to tell from a history of bleeding whether the disease is likely to be present or not (Sheehan).

Most frequently, however, Sheehan's disease is suspected by the history of hemorrhage during delivery followed by amenorrhea. The signs and symptoms of pituitary deficiency may take 6 months to several years to be fully developed. The onset of the symptoms is so gradual that often the patient and her family are unaware of the dramatic change that has taken place. There is usually weight loss, a failure of lactation postpartum, persistent amenorrhea, weakness, sensitivity to cold, lethargy, apathy, and loss of libido. In cases in which there is some regeneration of pituitary function, some women have become pregnant again. In one such case the patient died at a subsequent cesarean section as her disease had gone undiagnosed and the stress of the operation was too much for her. In extremes there is wasting and atrophy of the breasts and genitalia, loss of pubic hair, anemia, and myxedema.

In any consideration of differential diagnoses, the question whether the disease is primarily in the pituitary or in the end organ must be asked; for example, is the disease in the thyroid or adrenal rather than pituitary? Anorexia nervosa must also be considered; in this psychiatric disease the patient has severe anorexia, and pituitary function tests are normal. A most important differential is whether the pituitary deficiency is a result of necrosis or tumor. Radiologic air contrast studies can now be done in which the sella turcica can be well visualized. In addition, very sophisticated radioimmunoassays of pituitary trophic hormones can be obtained to define very precisely which functional component of the anterior lobe is compromised. Once defined, treatment is the restoration of normal endocrine activity through the use of replacement doses of thyroid and adrenal hormones. If pregnancy is desired, the use of gonadotropins to produce ovulation is possible. In some women the need for normal menstrual cycles is such that cycling with estrogen and progesterone is appropriate, using the oral contraceptive pills. In other instances a small dose of estrogen may be sufficient to prevent genital atrophy and relieve the hot flushes of estrogen lack.

ANOREXIA NERVOSA

Anorexia nervosa is a syndrome in which hypothalamic hypogonadotropic amenorrhea appears. It is characterized by self-induced starvation and emaciation in the absence of organic disease. It occurs from prepuberty to mid-adult life and is only rarely seen in males.

Diagnosis is made by onset before age 25 and loss of appetite to a 25 percent loss of body weight. This is associated with a distorted attitude to food, hunger, and body image. There may be bradycardia, episodes of physical overactivity, abnormal hunger, nausea, and vomiting. Hypotension and constipation, with excess use of laxatives, are also observed. Although FSH may be in normal circulating concentrations, LH is selectively reduced along with thyroxine (T_4).

Differential diagnosis includes panhypopituitarism, malabsorption syndrome, unusual metabolic disorders, and affective disorders including adolescent behavioral problems. Mortality may be as high as 10 percent, usually due to sepsis, electrolyte imbalance, atonic myocardial failure, or suicide. Major areas of psychologic dysfunction include being unaware of extreme emaciation, a loss of perception of hunger and fatigue, a sense of inactivity, and lack of autonomy.

Treatment involves collaboration with a psychiatrist and endocrinologist. The major goals of treatment are to restore normal nutrition, to relieve the psychologic disorder, and to manage specific somatic problems. The restoration of a normal body weight and gonadotropin levels is an important feature of the treatment of amenorrhea. Restoration of normal body weight is a prerequisite for the resumption of normal menstruation, but other factors may be involved (Beumont et al.).

DISORDERS OF OVULATION AND RELATED FUNCTIONS

LUTEAL PHASE DEFECT

The luteal phase defect (Jones, 1968) by theoretical definition refers to a failure of the normal luteal phase to maintain the endometrium sufficiently to support the implantation of the fertilized egg. In practice it has been assumed to be the inadequacy of progesterone production caused by abnormal ovarian function. This has been defined as valid only when present in repeated cycles, resulting in repeated abortions in the first trimester; less frequently, it is associated with infertility. Both insufficient ovarian response and inadequate LH secretion are possible causes of luteal defect, although it has been considered to be largely the result of psychogenic or neurogenic factors mediating the hypothalamic control of the secretion of LH. With the newer methods of hypothalamus and pituitary evaluation, deficiencies will undoubtedly be shown at each of the theoretically possible areas involved, e.g., the ovary, the hypothalamus, the pituitary, and the corpus luteum itself. In the past this defect has been treated primarily by the administration of progesterone, as this was the simplest hypothetical way in which it could be overcome. However, there is at least a theoretical reason for the use of gonadotropin, as LH has been shown to prolong the life of the corpus luteum when otherwise it was short-lived (Vande Wiele et al.). On the other hand, the use of HCG is more practical as it has a longer half-life and produces the same biologic result.

Incidence

The incidence of luteal defect is about 3.5 percent of infertile patients. It is higher, 19 percent, in those patients who have been demonstrated to have an inadequate endometrial response on one endometrial biopsy (at least a 2-day discrepancy between histologic dating and cycle day by basal body temperature), and is as high as 35 percent on a group of patients who have had repeated abortions of apparently normal fetuses.

Biologic Considerations

The corpus luteum, including both the functions of estrogen and progesterone secretion, may be affected, thereby influencing maturity of endometrium, decidual formation, tubal motility, and the effects on the myometrium of limiting growth and myometrial "block." The results are either occult abortion, which can be identified by basal body temperature charts, or the early abortion of normal conceptuses.

Confirmation of endometrial inadequacy can be made by endometrial biopsy on day 21 at a time when secretory epithelial glands and edema of the stroma would be expected and only subnuclear vacuolization or dense stroma is seen. There may also be an inappropriate association of glands and stroma, indicative of abnormal estrogen and progesterone balance or response.

A urinary pregnanediol excretion of less than 2.0

mg per day between days 19 and 25 is also diagnostic, and more recently blood progesterone values that are similarly low may be diagnostic.

The basal body temperature may also be used to demonstrate short cycles, but these are not appropriate for quantitative evaluation of the progesterone secretion. More recently, with the advent of LH determinations, daily values may be obtained in the secretory phase which show levels inadequate to maintain the corpus luteum (Ross et al.) (Fig. 7–20). In addition to low LH, a failure of FSH to fall from early proliferative phase to a nadir prior to midcycle surge and a corresponding reduced circulating estradiol concentration focus on the follicle as a possible preovulatory inadequate precursor of the short luteal phase. The FSH/LH ratio similarly does not decrease in the preovulatory phase, there may be no FSH surge, and the FSH and LH surges may not coincide with their peaks as normally expected. This has been studied in detail in subhuman primates (Wilks et al.).

Vaginal cytology and cervical mucus examinations may be used to add to the confirmation of the

FIGURE 7–20 Mean (bold line) and 95 percent confidence limits of mean (shaded areas) daily plasma concentrations of LH and FSH during seven cycles with post-LH peak intervals of 8 days or less (short luteal phase cycles). All cycles are synchronized on day of LH peak. *(From Ross et al.)*

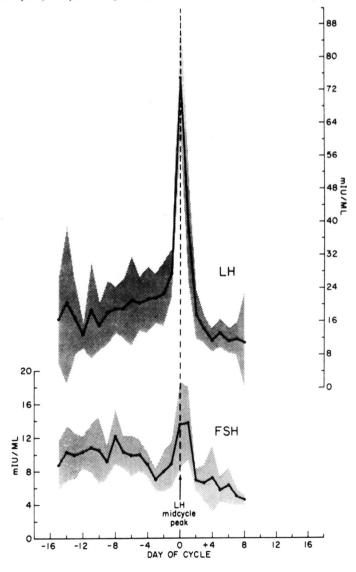

diagnosis, but by themselves they are inadequate. This is because of the well-known limitations of these diagnostic methods, particularly as the result of infections in the vagina which may be asymptomatic.

Management

A good menstrual and fertility history supplemented by basal body temperatures and appropriately obtained endometrial biopsy is important for making the diagnosis. This presupposes the careful instruction of the patient in how to take the basal temperatures, which should be taken at the same time each morning under basal conditions (after 6 hours of rest or sleep) preferably by a rectal basal thermometer (which is calibrated between 96 and 99°F) and not by the usual fever thermometer. It is important to note that the usual endometrial biopsy at the time of the onset of menses will be inadequate to make the diagnosis.

The administration of clomiphene citrate is associated with the release of gonadotropins, but results in only about 25 percent pregnancies, of which there are an increased number of abortions. When the endometrium is examined following clomiphene administration, abnormal endometrial responses can be observed, confirming the necessity of a normal estrogen and progesterone stimulus of the endometrium to result in a normal pregnancy. For this reason it may be necessary to add a small dose of estrogen to such cases as well as progesterone. This can be achieved with stilbestrol 0.1 mg per day, or 0.005 mg per day of ethinyl estradiol. Some patients on clomiphene treatment may develop a short luteal phase which requires treatment.

In extreme cases there may also be aluteal cycles in menstrual cycles which appear clinically to be normal. In such instances the administration of HCG at midcycle or clomiphene citrate at the end of the menses may lead to normal ovulation. The HCG may have to be repeated once during the luteal phase.

Most cases will respond to progesterone given daily following ovulation. This has been suggested to be best achieved by the administration of 12.5 mg of progesterone in oil daily, or 50 mg progesterone given nightly by vaginal suppository. About 50 percent of such patients may respond within five cycles (Soules et al.).

Jones has reported 21 cases of luteal defect in 555 primary infertility patients. Twelve of fifteen patients were investigated and treated and became pregnant with only progesterone treatment. The remaining three were treated with HCG and did not become pregnant. They were all over 35 years of age, a fact thought to be significant. Of 120 women with repeated pregnancy loss, 34 were found to have luteal defect. Thirty-one patients conceived and delivered normally following progesterone therapy. One child was born prematurely and although it left the hospital well, it died at 1 month of age.

ESTROGENIC STATES

HYPOESTROGEN STATES

Abnormal estrogen secretion will usually result in either hyper- or hypoestrogenic states. In hypoestrogenic states the extreme is amenorrhea in women who would cycle normally. The absence of estrogen can be observed by no menstrual periods, no vaginal secretions, incomplete uptake of iodine by the cervix (as in Schiller's test), low karyopyknotic index on cytograms, and low estrogen blood levels or urinary excretion. Low or absent estrogen denotes ovarian failure to form follicles, which may be inherent either to the ovary or the pituitary. In primary ovarian failure the ovary does not respond to pituitary gonadotropins, and FSH and LH may be measured and found to be elevated. This may be the result of conditions which include ovarian agenesis and natural menopause. Premature menopause or ovarian failure in which there are no further oocytes left to develop in the ovary as a result of follicular atresia may also occur. In the management of patients producing low amounts of estrogen, the major decision to be made is whether the ovary is at fault or there is pituitary failure. This can be very simply resolved by gonadotropin assay. Urinary biologic assays are still being done and are reliable in these extreme situations. Precise radioimmunoassays of serum gonadotropins can also now be made in most communities. In patients without ovarian follicles, FSH is greater than 40 mIU/mL and LH generally greater than 50 mIU/mL (Goldenberg et al.). Apart from pathophysiologic effects on the normal secretion of the pituitary, tumor must also be considered.

HYPERESTROGEN STATES

In cases of hyperestrogen states, symptomatology is most frequently bleeding from hyperstimulated proliferative endometrium, unrelieved by ovulation with its subsequent progesterone secretion. Prolonged estrogen stimulation can lead to cystic and adenomatous hyperplasia of the endometrium. Atrophic endometrium may appear following pharmacologic doses of exogenously administered estrogens, as may occur with some vitamin and hormone pills. Prolonged estrogen stimulation occurs primarily as a result of anovulation or tumor secretion. In anovulation, for example that which is associated with polycystic ovarian disease, continued gonadotropin stimulation results in the formation of a number of graafian follicles that do not ovulate. These will continue to secrete estradiol and estrone. In addition, it has been shown that the pattern of hormone secretion changes as the follicle cysts increase in size. This change is primarily one in which the androgens are added in increasing amounts to the ovarian secretion. Androstenedione is converted peripherally to estrone and adds additional estrogen to the estrogen production rate. In this situation the peripheral estrogen levels fail to fall to the low levels required for the positive stimulus of the negative feedback to occur in the hypothalamus leading to the increasing tonic release of FSH. Under these circumstances the ovarian cycling mechanism remains in a state of suspended animation which has been referred to euphoniously, but incorrectly, as "persistent estrus" (Speroff et al.) (Fig. 7–21). In some women, particularly in the years following menarche and just prior to the menopause, there will be changes in the gonadotropin secretion which will result in anovulation and persistent estrogen secretion. These also result in hyperestrogen states. The complexities of the menstrual cycle and its control make it possible, as demonstrated by Vande Wiele and his colleagues (Bogumil et al., 1972a, 1972b), who developed a computer program of the menstrual cycle, for a small change to occur in any one of the 30 to 40 variables presently identified. These may lead to one or more prolonged periods of estrogen stimulation unrelieved by ovulation.

ESTROGEN-SECRETING TUMORS

There are tumors which result in continuous excessive estrogen secretion. They can be of the ovary, adrenal, or pituitary. Usually they are of the ovary. The commonest of these tumors are the thecoma and the granulosa-cell tumor (see Chap. 45). They are formed of theca cells or granulosa cells which usually secrete hormones that result in either abnormal bleeding or amenorrhea. Other tumors of the ovary are associated with abnormal uterine bleeding, but at present their secretions have not been well identified. In cases of adenocarcinoma of the endometrium, there appears to be an association between estrogen stimulation and the development of the cancer itself. This was identified by the demonstration that the cancer was often preceded by the presence of cystic and adenomatous hyperplasia of the endometrium. In addition, some of those young women who begin their menstrual life with irregularities of bleeding and con-

FIGURE 7–21 Contrasting the "steady state" of tonic gonadotropin and estrogen function associated with persistent anovulation and that of the normal menstrual cycle. *(From Speroff et al.)*

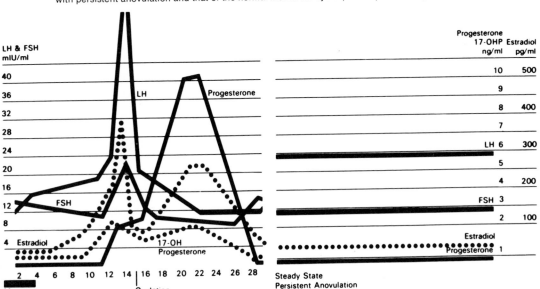

tinue with anovulation and dysfunctional flow are the ones who will develop endometrial cancer at an early age. Postmenopausally, circulating estrone is largely the result of the increased peripheral conversion of androstenedione secreted by the adrenal. In cases who develop carcinoma of the endometrium, it has been shown that there is an even greater increase in the peripheral conversion of the androstenedione to estrone (from 1.2 to 6.8 percent) (Siiteri, MacDonald). These patients demonstrate estrogen effect in their vaginal cytograms and generally show other evidence of increased estrogen secretion, such as increased iodine uptake by the cervix (as in Schiller's test). Excess estrogen secretion by adrenal tumors is usually the result of increased secretion of estrogen precursors with peripheral conversion to estrogens. Ectopic and, rarely, pituitary tumors similarly may produce estrogen effects indirectly through their stimulation of the secretion of intermediate hormones by the adrenal and ovary.

ANDROGENIC SYNDROMES

The clinical manifestations of androgenic states are those of virilization (Kirschner, Bardin). Most commonly they include hirsutism but also in extremes hair changes such as baldness, deepened voice, severe acne, and clitoral enlargement. Usually these changes occur with increased endogenous androgen production from the ovary or adrenal as a result of hyperplasia or tumor, but the exogenous administration of testosterone or its precursors must not be overlooked. These syndromes are summarized in Fig.

7–22. Those enzyme defects of the fetus, as in congenital adrenal hyperplasia, may give rise to intersex problems, which are considered in Chap. 6.

Adrenal Hyperplasia

Congenital adrenal hyperplasia may occur commonly as a result of deficiencies of either 21- or 11β-hydroxylase in the adrenal. In women or girls with 21-hydroxylase deficiency, plasma testosterone levels reach those of adult males. Also, androstenedione production may contribute as much as 90 percent to this elevated testosterone level through peripheral conversion. Similarly in a study of 11β-hydroxylase deficiency, adrenal androstenedione secretion has been suggested as a significant precursor for peripheral testosterone production.

Cushing's Disease

In the presence of increased ACTH production the resulting hyperadrenocorticism leads to hirsutism. Androstenedione production is increased following ACTH, and probably this contributes to the testosterone production in these cases.

Adrenal Tumors

Many adrenal tumors are associated with virilization. Adrenal venous effluents have been measured and found to have extremely high concentrations of both testosterone and androstenedione. In women testosterone production may be increased per se, or the contribution from androstenedione may be the major component of increased testosterone levels. The

FIGURE 7–22 A classification scheme based on the origin of excess androgens from the ovary or the adrenal as a result of either hyperplasia or neoplasia. *(From Yannone.)*

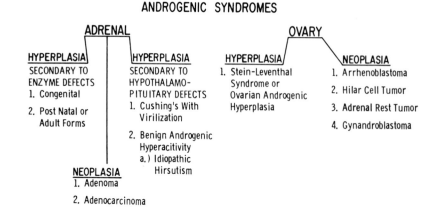

management of adrenal diseases has been well established by the demonstration of the accumulation of specific precursors at the site of the enzyme defect as in congenital adrenal hyperplasia (11-deoxycortisol or 17-hydroxyprogesterone), elevated cortisol production in Cushing's disease, and actual adrenal enlargement and distortion observed by x-ray in the presence of adrenal tumors.

Ovarian Hyperplasia

Ovarian hyperplasia has been variously classified according to its pathology or functional activities. Stromal thecosis (hyperthecosis) and hilar-cell hyperplasia (or Leydig-cell hyperplasia) have both been described as associated with elevated testosterone levels. In several studies of patients in this category, testosterone production has been between 1.0 and 3.0 mg per day (normal females 0.2 mg per day). As much as 95 percent of the testosterone has been secreted by the ovaries. On the other hand, even in the presence of hilar-cell hypertrophy the ovaries secreted only 30 percent as testosterone, while 30 percent came from androstenedione, and another 40 percent came from the adrenal secretion of another precursor.

Ovarian Tumors

Arrhenoblastomas and hilar-cell tumors have resulted in an increase in circulating testosterone. In ovarian carcinoma, testosterone and androstenedione may be high. In the few dermoid cysts of the ovary which have been studied, androstenedione, DHA, and DHS have all been increased without direct secretion of testosterone. Lipoid tumors of the ovary may lead to high blood testosterone levels which may be the result of peripheral conversion of steroid precursors.

POLYCYSTIC OVARIAN DISEASE

Under the heading polycystic ovarian disease (Goldzieher) is included most frequently the entity described by Stein and Leventhal and called the Stein-Leventhal syndrome. However, polycystic ovaries are not limited to the cases described by Stein and Leventhal, and the symptoms and signs ascribed to polycystic ovaries are not necessarily always associated with polycystic ovaries; in some cases there may be normal-looking or even atrophic-appearing ovaries (Yahia, Taymor). In fact, polycystic ovarian disease may not be inherent in the ovary itself but may be the result of gonadotropin dysfunction. Patients with varying signs and symptoms including amenorrhea, obesity, and hirsutism sometimes are said to have the Stein-Leventhal syndrome without definitive evaluation of endocrine function, and so it is not surprising that polycystic ovarian disease is still a rather confused gynecologic diagnosis which frequently makes use of the eponyms because precise diagnosis may be expensive and time-consuming and the specific tests to define the diagnosis are just now becoming available to clinical practice.

History

For years polycystic ovaries have been observed including the sclerocystic changes that are classically associated with the Stein-Leventhal syndrome. Occasional reports of this disorder go back to before the turn of the century. However, interest was focused on these patients when a group was studied whose symptoms included menstrual irregularity including amenorrhea, a history of sterility, masculine-type hirsutism, and, less consistently, retarded breast development and obesity. These patients were studied by gynecography in which x-ray films were taken of the pelvis following the injection of carbon dioxide into the peritoneal cavity. The resulting films revealed enlarged bilateral structures presumed to be ovaries equal in size to the shadow formed by the uterus. The patients were then operated upon to make a diagnosis. Bilateral enlarged shiny sclerocystic ovaries were found, and wedge resections were taken for pathologic diagnosis. The pathology revealed capsular thickening, large graafian follicles, absent corpora lutea, theca luteinization, and hyperplasia of the stroma. Also observed was a lining up of the primary oocytes beneath the ovarian capsule, often described as ova "trying to get out." This description referred to the anovulation and infertility associated with the disease and the apparent inability of the ova to ovulate through the thickened capsule. Since then others have shown that many ovaries in such clinical conditions are normal sized and many have no thickening of the capsule. Special studies of the theca luteinization and stromal hyperplasia have shown that there are no unique diagnostic histologic features to distinguish the polycystic ovary; such ovaries merely contain a wide variation of follicular stages of development. The ovary has the appearance of being chronically stimulated, presumably by gonadotropin. The thickened capsule has been suggested as being similar to the tunica albuginea of the testis, possibly a result of high local concentration of androgens. It should also be pointed out that ovaries of prepubertal girls have many of the characteristics of polycystic ovaries. When it is remembered that the FSH/LH ratio before menarche is reversed, it is tempting to compare this association with the polycystic ovary that develops in young women; for example, polycystic ovaries may be associated with excess tonic LH secretion.

Symptomatology and Natural History

Women who develop polycystic ovarian disease apparently have normal growth and development and pass through puberty uneventfully. A tendency to hirsutism may develop before menarche. Thereafter, periods may commence entirely in a normal fashion for a variable period of time, or irregular cycles may occur right from the start. The pattern may be one of "skips or misses." If a period is skipped, a normal period will follow at the expected time 1 month later. In a missed period, bleeding may occur at any time after the flow is expected. The flow is usually prolonged, and frequently evidence of anovulation is associated. Following such skips and misses, amenorrhea often sets in, and most cases (as in the experience of Stein) usually occur before the age of 23. Anovulation and amenorrhea are most frequent accompaniments of this syndrome, but spontaneous ovulation may occur from time to time, and some patients have been known to become pregnant after prolonged periods of anovulation and even amenorrhea. Hirsutism is common, usually remains stable, and is limited to the face. In fewer cases virilism is also a problem. Rarely patients develop polycystic ovarian disease following one or two normal pregnancies.

Although the "classical" onset of the disease is described above, summaries of a large number of case histories have a very variable incidence of the disease and its symptomatology. The overall incidence of polycystic ovarian disease varies from 0.6 to 4.3 percent in unselected patients; in women at laparotomies it is 1.4 percent; in infertile women it is up to 4.3 percent; at consecutive autopsies in women of all ages it is 3.5 percent. On the basis of a large number of accumulated studies, Goldzieher and Green have reported the relative incidence of symptoms as infertility (74 percent), hirsutism (69 percent), amenorrhea (51 percent), and obesity (41 percent) (Table 7–8). The wide variation of symptomatology has led some researchers to doubt the entity of a syndrome. However, the breadth of response is attractive to the student of pathophysiology who can theorize variations in hormone secretion and end-organ response

Table 7–8 Polycystic Ovaries: Symptomatology of Proved Published Cases*

Symptom	Frequency,%	
	Mean	Range
Obesity	41	16–49
Hirsutism	69	17–83
Virilization	21	0–28
Amenorrhea	51	15–77
Infertility	74	35–94
Functional bleeding	29	6–65
Dysmenorrhea	23	
Biphasic basal temperature	15	12–40
Corpus luteum at operation	22	0–71

*Total number of cases, 1079.
Source: Goldzieher.

which could account for almost all variations of symptoms described.

Associated Hormonal Changes

Estrogens. Before the more complex determinations of estrogens were available, evidence of estrogen secretion was obtained by identification of the endometrium following either biopsy or curettage. Normal, proliferative, hyperplastic, and atrophic (or resting) endometrium have all been observed. Endometrium will reflect not only estrogen secretion, but in some instances an altered responsiveness to estrogen in the presence of androgen. Speroff and Kase have recently proposed that with failure of ovulation ovarian follicles develop to a stage in which they are putting out a constant rather than fluctuating level of estrogen. Whereas in the normal cycle the reduced negative feedback of estrogen at the end of the menstrual cycle is required for the *pari passu* rise in FSH secretion, this does not occur in the presence of polycystic ovaries, and a constant, nonfluctuating level of estrogen is maintained. This state is contributed to by the abnormal androgen metabolism. When it is remembered that circulating androstenedione is converted to estrone, the increased production rate of androstenedione in this condition adds to the pool of estrone, maintaining its constant, unremitting level. The alterations in LH and FSH secretion also contribute to the androgen pool, for as estrogen develops a persistent inhibitory effect, it also loses its stimulatory surge just prior to ovulation, and the gonadotropins maintain similar nonfluctuating levels. There is a failure of release of the ovulatory surge of LH from the pituitary leaving the patient in an anovulatory state. A level of

LH stimulation also persists which promotes androgen (estrogen precursor) secretion by the ovary without follicle development. The circulating androstenedione is also converted to testosterone. In patients with polycystic ovarian disease, peripheral testosterone concentrations may be elevated, which accounts for the hirsutism and virilism encountered.

This considered hypothesis of the hormone control mechanism alteration in polycystic ovarian disease is supported by peripheral concentration measurements of steroids and gonadotropin in such patients. LH is higher, 35 mIU/mL (12.7 mIU/mL normal); FSH is unchanged; estrone is higher, 92 pg/mL (52 pg/mL normal); estradiol is unchanged; testosterone (468 versus 325 pg/mL), androstenedione (2.1 versus 1.1 ng/mL), and dehydroepiandrosterone sulfate (3.4 versus 2.0 μg/mL) were all higher. (Note the different magnitudes of concentration of picograms, nanograms, and micrograms per milliliter.)

The use of clomiphene citrate in the management of polycystic ovarian disease is based on its antiestrogen properties, presumably by acting in competition with the endogenous estrogens for the sites of activity in the hypothalamus which control the gonadotropin secretion. During clomiphene citrate administration there is an immediate rise of LH and FSH, then LH drops and the peripheral estrogen drops; this is generally followed by a rise in FSH, a surge of estradiol with its positive-feedback effect on the hypothalamus, and the release of the LH burst which results in ovulation. Following 5 days' treatment with clomiphene citrate, about 9 days are required to ovulate.

Gonadotropins. Although there were reports of elevated urinary gonadotropins in polycystic ovarian disease in the past, more recently blood levels of FSH and LH have been measured. In some cases LH is elevated, in others both LH and FSH are normal. Whether those with normal values have compensated or whether there are variants in etiology among those with polycystic ovarian disease has not been clarified. In either event with elevated LH or normal values, both types of patients are known to respond to clomiphene citrate. FSH is unaltered. Recent data have shown that abnormalities of hypothalamic-pituitary regulation of gonadotropin secretion are not inherent but are the result of inappropriate estrogen feedback leading to anovulation and inappropriate gonadotropin secretion (Reber et al.; Baird et al.).

17-Ketosteroids. The urinary 17-ketosteroids are measures of those metabolites in the urine which are neutral steroids and have a ketone function at position C-17. They are usually metabolites of androgens and corticoids whose side chains have been cleaved. The urinary levels in polycystic ovarian disease are usually normal or slightly elevated (23 percent), but there is a marked overlap with normal values (Fig. 7–23) (Goldzieher).

The interpretation of an elevated 17-ketosteroid level may be that it comes from the ovary or the adrenal. A little history related to the disease is important, for at the time that endocrinology was making great advances in the physiology of the adrenal gland, it was thought that all corticoids and ketosteroids had their origin in the adrenal. Since then it has been

FIGURE 7–23 Urinary ketosteroid and corticoid excretion in polycystic ovarian disease. *(From Goldzieher.)*

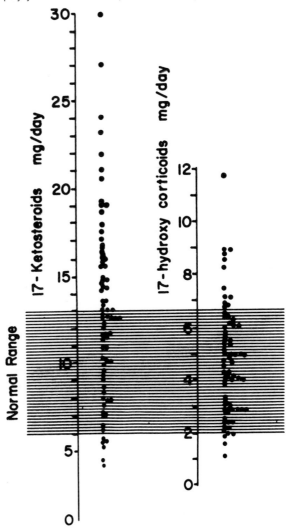

demonstrated that the ovary makes a large contribution to this pool. Also, with the glandular and peripheral interconversion of androgens, it has become important to evaluate overall androgen metabolism. Nonetheless, in the past it was possible to get some patients to ovulate and become pregnant by giving them small daily doses of cortisone (5 to 15 mg per day). From this experience tests evolved to distinguish between the ovarian or adrenal origin of the elevated or high normal excretion of 17-ketosteroids. For adrenal suppression by the administration of dexamethasone, 8 mg is given daily in divided dosage. It would be expected following this suppression that the 17-ketosteroids would fall to levels of less than 3 mg per day. If the values persist above that level, the ovary may be considered to be a major contributing source. To confirm the contribution of the ovary, either HCG or stilbestrol may be given. HCG will act to augment the output of 17-ketosteroids through LH-like stimulation of the ovarian stroma. Stilbestrol will act to suppress the gonadotropins and thereby lead to a further reduction of 17-ketosteroids in the urine. These tests have been used definitively by Lloyd et al. (Fig. 7–24), but others have been less successful, and it appears that there are cases in which the suppression tests may not be diagnostic.

Ovarian Steroidogenesis

The enzymatic changes which have been demonstrated in the polycystic ovary may be helpful in un-

derstanding the urinary and blood hormone values that may be observed. Such observed deficiencies are of the aromatization system and of the 3β-ol-dehydrogenase enzymes. The 3β-ol-dehydrogenase is responsible for the conversion of the steroids of the Δ^5 pathway to the Δ^4 pathway and therefore the pregnenolones to the progesterones. As a result of this defect, accumulation of pregnanetriol in the urine has been demonstrated and has been used in the past to aid in the diagnosis of polycystic ovarian disease. Pregnanetriol (pregnane-3α,17α,20α-triol) is the reduced 17α-hydroxyprogesterone resulting from its metabolism and excretion. The block of aromatization will lead to the accumulation of androstenedione which will be peripherally converted to estrone, resulting in the tonic circulation of estrogens and presumably in the failure of gonadotropin surge and ovulation (the state described above by Speroff and Kase).

Hypothalamic Factors

The control of the ovarian cycle is apparently mediated by the hypothalamus, where the feedback of ovarian steroids determines the release of gonadotropins. There is an area of tonic release of gonadotropins, possibly in the ventromedial and arcuate nuclei in the anterior basal hypothalamus, which is affected by the circulating concentrations of estradiol. Androgens may also play a role in this action, as it has been recently shown that androgens, particularly andro-

FIGURE 7–24 Change in urinary 17-ketosteroids following ACTH, dexamethasone, and dexamethasone plus HCG administration. N = normal; IH = idiopathic hirsutism; PCO = polycystic ovarian disease. *(From Lloyd et al.)*

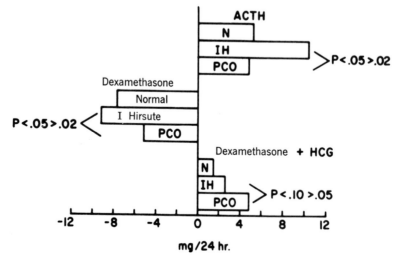

stenedione, may be converted to estrone in the hypothalamus. The tonic secretion of gonadotropins waxes and wanes, therefore, with the rise and fall of estrogens. This action is apparently mediated through the release of gonadotropin-releasing hormone (GnRH, LRF, or LHRF) which acts on the pituitary to release both FSH and LH. These releasing hormones may reach the pituitary by way of the pituitary portal venous system.

At the same time in another area of the hypothalamus, the preoptic area which is the site of the positive feedback of estrogens, the spurt of estrogens from the mature follicle stimulates the release of GnRH followed by the LH surge, which leads to ovulation. The GnRH has been identified as a decapeptide and has been synthesized. In addition to these factors, there are exteroceptive factors that also must play a part, such as the influence of the higher brain centers, because specific brain amines may exert an effect on these releasing substances, or inhibit the classical feedback effects. Animal models of polycystic ovarian disease have been created in which lesions have been placed in the hypothalamic areas described. However, the syndrome that we presently label the polycystic ovarian disease syndrome probably has a number of different etiologies which result from deficiencies at any one of these complex areas of functions. The involvement of the adrenal gland and ACTH can also be understood when it is remembered that the adrenal androgen, androstenedione, is converted to estrogens, which may be one way that adrenal secretion can influence the ovarian cycle.

Clinical Management

The management of this syndrome takes into consideration these possible etiologies. Historically at a time when the ovary was biopsied and the histology was described, it was found that many of these women subsequently reverted to normal cycles and required no further treatment. To try to take advantage of this success, a whole series of operations developed. Wedge resections were usually carried out; however, decortication of the ovary was designed to remove the androgen-secreting cells, and the ovary was also peeled in an attempt to "let the ova out." The reason that wedge resection works is not entirely clear, but probably relates to the trauma done to the ovaries with the subsequent fall in estrogen and testosterone (or precursors) secretion and a change in the continuous stimulus to the tonic areas of the hypothalamus (Judd et al.). Thereafter, there is a renewal of normal cycles of secretion with stimulation

TABLE 7–9 Polycystic Ovaries: Published Results of Wedge Resection*

Result	Frequency, %	
	Mean	Range
Regular cycles	80	6–95
Pregnancy	63	13–89
Decreased hirsutism	16	0–18

* Total number of cases, 1079; number of references, 187.
Source: Goldzieher.

of a new follicle growth, followed by the estrogen and LH surges with ovulation and normal cycling.

Presently, although wedge resection is resorted to from time to time, the usual course of treatment is with clomiphene citrate. Following its administration there is a fall in estrogen, and this is followed by a rise in the output of FSH, a new crop of follicles, an ovulatory surge of estrogen, and a normal cycle. Goldzieher, who has studied this syndrome in depth, records the results of treatment with wedge resection as not completely satisfactory (Table 7–9). He also discusses the use of small doses of corticoid which have been successful; although clomiphene citrate brings on ovulation in 75 percent and pregnancy in 35 percent of cases, a combination of this drug and gonadotropins, either by themselves or added to the clomiphene, may be helpful. Even when wedge resections have failed, gonadotropins or clomiphene may be successful. This is probably the result of the complex etiology of the syndrome.

DISORDERS OF ORGAN RESPONSE

The endometrium goes through its characteristic cycle of 28 days which corresponds to the ovarian cycle. The most consistent part of the ovarian cycle is the luteal phase which is 14 or 15 days in length. The endometrium can be microscopically described as early, mid, and late proliferative endometrium, followed by specific patterns which can be identified for actual days of the cycle in the secretory phase (for example, 17 day, 19 to 20 day, 26 day). In the evaluation of infertile couples, variations from normal can be observed in which there is a failure of the endometrium to correspond to other data available for the dating of a menstrual cycle, such as basal body temperature and mittelschmerz (the pain associated with ovulation). Sometimes such a pattern is associated with irregular shedding of the endometrium, in which case the patient bleeds excessively as in dysfunctional flow, but curettage shows secretory endometrium (as opposed to proliferative or hyperplastic in dysfunctional flow associated with anovulation) and some regeneration of the endometrium. In other cases there may be only a failure of the endometrium to complete its full cycle. There have been attempts to show that this failure of appropriate cycling of the endometrium is associated with a deficiency of thyroid and estrogen secretion, and thyroid extract and estrogen have been given in the past with what were described as good results; however, this is far from confirmed. Hyper- and hypothyroid states are generally associated with anovulation and abnormal gonadotropin secretion.

In other cases there may be amenorrhea in which the endometrium will be absent, as in Asherman's syndrome. In this syndrome curettage, particularly postpartum or postabortal, has shown uterine synechiae or bands of tissue which form across the endometrial cavity and obliterate the lumen. Only small amounts of endometrium may be left; these can be encouraged to cycle once again by carefully dilating the cervix, severing the bands, reestablishing the uterine cavity, and maintaining it with an intra-uterine device (shield).

ANDROGEN INSENSITIVITY (TESTICULAR FEMINIZATION)

A patient with testicular feminization is a genetic male with XY chromosomes, a male pseudohermaphrodite, and is discussed in Chap. 6; the condition is mentioned here as a cause for failure of end-organ response. In these patients the usual hormone-sensitive tissues do not respond to testosterone, and consequently the patients become feminized with breast development. The external genitalia are those of a female, and there are undescended testes in the inguinal canal. It was thought that these patients failed to develop the normal enzyme which converts testosterone to dihydrotestosterone. However, some cases have been identified in which there is absence of the testosterone-binding protein in the normally responsive tissue cells. These patients, who have usually been brought up as girls, should continue as females, and the testes should be removed from the inguinal canals, as there is a high incidence of malignant degeneration when they are left in situ. It is best not to tell the patient all the details about the organs that have been removed, as they can cause an identity crisis. Although such patients are sterile, they are able to enjoy sex.

There now appears to be a whole spectrum of cases with impaired testosterone action from phenotypic males with azoospermia and gynecomastia to phenotypic females with complete testicular feminization. Included are cases with all levels of receptor deficiency and 5α reductase deficiency (the enzyme responsible for conversion of testosterone to dihydrotestosterone) (Wilson et al.; Griffin and Wilson).

PRECOCIOUS PUBERTY

Precocious puberty may result from either constitutional or physiologically premature events, or as a result of organic causes such as cerebral lesions and postencephalitis, postmeningitis, and postcerebral traumata. The signs and symptoms are primarily those of precocious progress through the stages of breast development, the early appearance of axillary and pubic hair, and the premature onset of normal menstrual periods. These cycles are known to be ovulatory, and the girls are known to be fertile as there have been cases of girls less than 8 years old who have conceived and delivered (usually by cesarean section).

The reasons for such premature maturation are not known. It is probable that the hypothalamus, which is less sensitive to estrogens in adolescence as shown by the lack of positive feedback, becomes prematurely responsive, and this leads to normal adult feedback. However, a stimulus from the ovary may also be required, and the interrelation between the ovary and the hypothalamic-pituitary axis in precocious puberty has not been studied in great detail. The onset of menses may occur as early as 6 months of age or less; however, the majority of cases occur between the ages of 5 and 8 years. The developmental steps that usually occur in puberty are accelerated, and breast development, the appearance of hair, and the onset of menses occur in rapid progression. In some children the isolated development of breasts, or the early appearance of pubic hair, occurs. There is a wide range of normal, and these isolated observations are not abnormal, as is the rapid progression through all maturation stages of puberty which occurs with true precocious puberty.

A major problem of the premature onset of menses and the associated higher levels of estrogen secretion is the premature closure of the long-bone epiphyses. Almost all such patients, whether treated or not, are of a smaller stature as adults, although initially they may be taller than their peers at school. This short stature is even more prominent if the disease has persisted for any length of time. X-rays of the carpal bones and the long bones of the hips and arms should be made to determine the extent of the premature closure of the epiphyses.

The differential diagnosis rests mainly between precocious onset of normal development and the presence of a hormone-secreting tumor, such as a granulosa tumor, which will produce the same signs and symptoms. The presence of a pelvic tumor on physical examination is of help in making the diagnosis. The lack of regular menstrual bleeding may be a clue, as is the absence of advanced epiphyseal closure. These may occur as a result of the more rapid appearance of estrogen in the circulation and its higher concentration in the presence of a tumor, rather than the lower, more cyclic, stimulus of the normal cycle which may not be immediately apparent.

Diagnostic steps include examination for tumors and the careful evaluation of circulating concentrations of gonadotropins, estrogen, and progesterone. Diagnosis may also be made by the administration of a progestin (without estrogen) following x-rays of the sella turcica to rule out pituitary tumor. A vaginal cytogram is then examined. If the smear changes from an estrogen-stimulated vaginal smear to that of a progesterone-dominated smear (noted by the disappearance of cornified cells and the appearance of more intermediate and basal cells), the diagnosis is precocious puberty on a constitutional or physiologic basis. If the estrogen smear persists (eosinophilic cornified superficial cells with pyknotic nuclei) as a result of the high level of estrogen secretion, then the source of estrogen is likely to be a tumor, and its site must be sought. The two common tumor sites are the ovary and the adrenal, but the ovary is a more common site of tumor at this age.

The management of patients with precocious puberty is to remove the cause, such as a tumor. If none is present, a course of depot progestin is administered. The progestin is injected intramuscularly in a vehicle which is absorbed slowly. The progestin is usually a conjugate of a progesterone derivative which has a prolonged action. Such a compound is medroxyprogesterone acetate (Depo-Provera), which is given in large enough amounts by weekly or biweekly injection to suppress the gonadotropins and prevent menstruation. Unfortunately, such treatment does not always alter the rate of closure of the epiphyses. In such cases the administration of phenothi-

azine derivatives has been reported to be beneficial (e.g., chlorpromazine).

Lesions of the posterior hypothalamus, pineal tumors, or calcification of the pineal gland are known to be associated with precocious puberty clinically and experimentally. Granulomas, hamartomas, and degenerative lesions of the midbrain and hypothalamus have been identified and are very difficult to distinguish from constitutional precocious puberty. However, with the advent of the tests for pituitary function using the newer hypothalamic-releasing factors, this may now be possible. Whether as a result of granuloma or not, frequently following meningitis, particularly tuberculous meningitis, there may be a resultant spurt in puberty, or the stimulation of breast tissue. Also 4 to 8 weeks after trauma to the head in youngsters, the onset of thelarche may appear, followed by pubertal development. The management of these problems in the absence of a tumor is the same as it is for constitutional precocious puberty with progestins.

DELAYED OR ABSENT PUBERTY

In certain young patients there is a failure or absence of pubertal development which generally implies the lack of estrogens. One of the commonest forms of this problem is gonadal dysgenesis, or Turner's syndrome, in which the ovaries fail to develop and gonadal streaks are left in their place. This is associated with a characteristic chromosomal pattern of 46XO. These patients are short and have web necks, increased cubital valgus, broad shieldlike chest, short fourth metacarpal, and renal abnormalities. These problems are discussed in detail in Chap. 6.

Another rare form of hypogonadotropic hypogonadism is Kallman's syndrome, which is characteristically associated with anosmia (the inability to perceive odors such as coffee or perfume). In this condition, the young women have primary amenorrhea, infantile sex development, low serum LH, a normal 46XX karyotype, and anosmia. The gonads will respond to gonadotropins but not to clomiphene citrate.

HERMAPHRODITISM AND PSEUDOHERMAPHRODITISM

True hermaphroditism is rare and denotes the presence of an ovary and testis in the same patient. They may be combined in the same gonad as ovotestis, or there may be a testis on one side and an ovary on the other. The internal genitalia correspond to the adjacent gonad. Most such cases have ambiguous genitalia. Half of the patients are 46XX, some are 46XY, and the rest are mosaics of which one component is XX.

Female pseudohermaphrodites are masculinized females and are genetically 46XX with ovaries and varying degrees of masculinization of the external genitalia. Of all infants with ambiguous genitalia, almost 50 percent will have congenital adrenal hyperplasia.

Congenital Adrenal Hyperplasia

The adrenogenital syndrome is diagnosed by the presence of masculinized external genitalia and demonstration of excess androgen production by the adrenal either by tumor or hyperplasia. If present at birth, it is due to adrenal virilizing hyperplasia, but if it appears in later life, it is most frequently associated with adrenal tumor.

At birth there may be varying degrees of masculinization of the external genitalia, including fusion of the labial scrotal folds and hypertrophy of the clitoris. The urethra and vagina may share a common sinu. The degree of masculinization of the external genitalia depends on the time in utero at which the androgen influence became dominant. Untreated at birth, the signs will increase so that pubic and axillary hair will appear and even a beard in early infancy. This is associated with an enlarged clitoris, and even a deepening of the voice. The epiphyses will close prematurely, and such children will remain of short stature. In some cases, the hormonal imbalance may lead to salt-losing hypertension and hyperglycemia. This happens in a small proportion of the total group and depends on the site of the enzyme defect in the adrenal.

Enzyme defects in adrenal corticosteroid synthesis may occur at any one of several sites. The most common site of abnormal or absent enzyme activity is that of 21-hydroxylation. The hypertensive form is due to the absence of 11β-hydroxylation. Both these anomalies lead to the absence of sufficient cortisol to control the ACTH secretion by the pituitary. Therefore, there is an excess secretion of ACTH, followed by hyperplasia of the adrenal, and excess secretion of adrenal androgens and other precursors of cortisol, depending on the level of the block. The salt loss is generally dependent on the completeness of the 21-hydroxylase deficiency and relates to the synthesis of aldosterone. In two other types of adrenogenital syndrome, either the 3β-steroid hydrogenase or rarely the 20,22-hydroxylase (cholesterol side chain desmolase) is deficient. In the latter case, the infant does not survive after birth; in the former case, pregnanetriol is absent, the 17-ketosteroids consist mainly of dehydroepiandrosterone, and the infant usually dies in early life.

The treatment in the survivors is to administer the deficient hormone, cortisol. A salt-retaining hormone is also usually necessary. Surgical treatment of the external genitalia may be carried out early in life before gender identity is established. Normal reproduction is possible in such cases, although cesarean section may be necessary for delivery. Following the administration of extra cortisol in labor, the newborn must be carefully evaluated for cortisol suppression and hypoadrenal state. As in patients on replacement doses of cortisol, there is a need for additional dosage at the time of stress, including intercurrent disease and surgery.

Male Pseudohermaphrodites

This term is applied to incompletely masculinized males, who possess testicles but whose external genitalia are not male. The group includes patients with testicular feminization (described above), the Reifenstein syndrome, pseudovaginal perineoscrotal hypospadias, congenital adrenal hyperplasia in the male, the Swyer syndrome, anorchia, and the uterine hernia syndrome.

The Reifenstein syndrome is incomplete testicular feminization, in which there is hypogonadism, feminization, gynecomastia, and sterility. The karyotype is 46XY. These patients should be treated with androgen.

Pseudovaginal perineoscrotal hypospadias is similar to incomplete testicular feminization at birth, but at puberty masculinization occurs. The cleft in the scrotum is often mistaken for a vagina. The condition appears to be the result of a temporary loss of androgen. The karyotype is 46XY. The infant should be modified surgically and reared as a girl if there is an inadequate phallus.

Congenital adrenal hyperplasia in the male is a result of the absence of adrenal 3β-steroid dehydrogenase, 17α-hydrozylase, or 20,22-hydroxylase. As indicated previously, absence of 3β-dehydrogenase or 20,22-hydroxylase results in death in early infancy.

The Swyer syndrome is characterized by a 46XY chromosome pattern with female external and internal genitalia. Apparently both the androgen stimulus and the müllerian inhibition factor are absent or lost in development. Streak gonads may be present, but testicular remnants may also be present; they should be removed as they frequently undergo malignant degeneration.

Anorchia, or the vanishing-testis syndrome, is characterized by the presence of normal male external genitalia but no testicles. It is believed that the testes form long enough to produce the masculine development and Müllerian inhibition, then undergo degeneration.

Infants with hernia uteri inguinale are normal males (XY) in whom Müllerian-duct structures are found in the inguinal canals. This apparently results from the isolated failure of the müllerian inhibition factor. Such males are fertile and normal once the extra genitalia are removed.

HORMONAL AND RELATED FORMS OF TREATMENT OF DISORDERS OF REPRODUCTION

STEROIDS

The major steroid therapy used in reproduction disorders is the prescription of estrogens and progestogens. Endogenous compounds such as 17β-estradiol and progesterone are not effective when given orally as they are either destroyed in the gut or reduced in the splanchnic circulation. Therefore, the pharmaceutical industry has developed various conjugates and compounds with estrogenic and progestational activity which are generally employed. It is important to remember that such compounds do not always have the same endogenous biologic activity as the endogenous steroids themselves. For example, progestins have been developed which have specific known biologic activity in certain tests of progestational function, but they may not produce other metabolic effects of progesterone; e.g., a progestin may show effects on the endometrium but may not have similar effects as an aldosterone antagonist. Usually progestins do not have the same excretory metabolites, and their effects may be difficult to measure objectively.

Estrogens and progesterone are generally used in an attempt to reproduce the normal cyclicity of the reproductive cycle, or to augment what is considered to be a less than optimal response of the patient's own endocrine system. It is important to gain experience with a few selected drugs in each category and to appreciate their anticipated effects and side effects.

The estrogens in general use consist of ethinyl estradiol, mestranol (17α-ethynylestradiol 3-methyl ether), and conjugated estrogens (which contain estrone, equilin, and 17α-hydroxyequilin with additional small amounts of 17β-estradiol, equilenin, and 17α-hydroxyequilnin as salts of their sulfate esters). When estrogens are used alone, as at the time of the menopause, and when there is specific indication, conjugated estrogens may be given and are best tolerated by mouth. The usual replacement dose at the menopause to prevent symptoms is 0.625 mg of conjugated estrogens. Stilbestrol, which is a synthetic estrogen, has been extensively used but is used guardedly at present because of its associated teratogenic effects in the female offspring of women who received it during pregnancy; it may also be given for menopausal symptoms. Comparative dosages of estrogens are ethinyl estradiol 0.05 mg and mestranol 0.75 mg which are equivalent to 1.0 mg of stilbestrol and 2.5 mg of conjugated estrogens. Comparable doses at the menopause are therefore 0.625 to 1.25 mg conjugated estrogen, 0.25 to 0.50 mg stilbestrol, and 0.02 to 0.05 mg of ethinyl estradiol.

Occasionally estrogens in small doses are used to improve cervical mucus in infertility patients and to suppress the effects of androgen stimulation on the skin. Estrogens do relieve acne to a small degree. Estrogen replacement is also given in hypoestrogenic situations such as gonadal dysgenesis.

Most commonly estrogens are used as components of oral contraceptive pills. In this instance the low-dose estrogen is either 0.05 mg ethinyl estradiol or 0.08 mg mestranol. These estrogens form the basis for most contraceptive pills. As many of the side effects associated with such pills are the result of estrogen, it is important to have knowledge of more than one estrogen and be able to use them interchangeably because patients have individual idiosyncrasies which may make it possible for them to tolerate one but not another. Conjugated estrogen preparations are usually tolerated well.

Progesterone derivatives or progesterone itself may be used when appropriate. Progesterone must be given intramuscularly in oil and is therefore somewhat restricted in use but is recommended for some specific problems such as luteal phase defect. Longer acting progestins which are used in pregnancy to support, stimulate, or replace endogenous secretion, and in cases of metastatic adenocarcinoma of the endometrium as a chemotherapeutic agent, are derivatives of progesterone itself. The two main compounds used are medroxyprogesterone acetate and hydroxy-progesterone caproate. Medroxyprogesterone acetate may be given by mouth or intramuscularly. The usual dose is 10 mg per day (per os) to mimic the secretion of progesterone in the menstrual cycle. This dose is given between days 16 and 21 of the cycle, with added estrogen as required. Long-acting medroxyprogesterone acetate is supplied in intramuscular dosage of 100 mg/mL of diluent; dosage varies depending on circumstances. It is known to persist in its effect for a long time, and it should not be given to patients who wish to have normal cycles or conceive shortly after its use. Long-acting medroxyprogesterone acetate is also being used in some difficult cases in which prolonged suppression of menses is required (e.g., hematologic bleeding problems). Hydroxyprogesterone caproate is used in similar situations but must be given intramuscularly.

Progestins used in contraceptives are discussed fully in Chap. 33. A major consideration should be to prescribe a progestin which is either estrogenic in its action such as norethynodrel, androgenic such as norethindrone, or progestogenic such as norgestrel [19-nor-17α-pregna-1,3,5 (10)-trien-20-yne-3,17-diol]. These drugs are available with added estrogens as combined contraceptive pills. For women who may have characteristics that would suggest symptoms of excess androgenicity, an estrogenic progestin may be appropriate; for a patient with estrogenic characteristics, an androgenic compound may be chosen. Thus oral contraceptive combinations can be selected to be most effective and free of side effects for individual patients (see Chap. 33). Recently with availability of low-dose (35 mg) estrogen combination pills, choice is much less critical.

Androgens are used primarily in combination with estrogens for the suppression of lactation and in the menopause, although by themselves they are also of use in relief of symptoms associated with chronic cystic disease of the breast. Although estrogen is still used frequently by itself postpartum for the suppression of lactation, commonly the combination of estrogen and testosterone in the form of estradiol valerate and testosterone enanthate is given. (Deladumone contains 4 mg estradiol valerate and 90 mg testosterone enanthate per milliliter. One 2-mL dose is given IM postpartum.) Postmenopause, an injection of estradiol valerate and testosterone enanthate every 4 weeks may be given (1 mL); or, more simply, when oral doses are tolerated and the androgen is indicated, methyl testosterone may be added to the conjugated estrogen therapy. Care must be taken to choose a dose which will not produce virilizing symptoms or signs. Methyl testosterone may be given in small doses (2.5 mg daily for 60 days) to relieve breast discomfort in those patients who have cystic disease of the breast with menstrual breast discomfort. At low dosage there is little chance of virilization, and considerable relief may be obtained.

Corticoids are given for infertility problems and in cases of amenorrhea, where there may be excess adrenal secretion of androgens. Corticoids are also given for replacement therapy in cases of congenital adrenal hyperplasia. In polycystic ovarian disease, they are also used in the adrenal suppression test for the diagnosis of the adrenal contribution to such problems.

A recent weak anabolic androgen, danazol, has been given for the prolonged treatment of endometriosis. In doses of 800 mg per day in divided dosage over 6 months, gonadotropin suppression and dissolution of endometrial implants occur. The metabolic side effects lead to acne, weight gain, edema, and altered carbohydrate tolerance, which possibly aggravates diabetes. The symptoms of endometriosis, including dysmenorrhea, pelvic pain and dyspareunia, as well as palpable pelvic induration, are reduced. A corrected pregnancy rate in such patients is about 50 percent, following treatment.

GONADOTROPINS

FSH and LH have been purified but not as yet synthesized. For this reason preparations that are presently in use for the induction of ovulation are extracts of postmenopausal urine (Pergonal) and extracts of placental HCG. The HCG cross-reacts biologically with LH and has the same biologic effect. It has a longer $t_{\frac{1}{2}}$ and therefore is actually a better drug to use therapeutically as it does not have to be repeated. FSH and LH are used in the induction of ovulation (see Chap. 27). HCG is used also in some cases of luteal phase defect. In patients who are given these drugs it is important to know that if the ovary is stimulated to excess by the FSH preparation, as can be determined by the excretion or blood concentration of estrogen, the addition of HCG (HCG is given to produce ovulation) will lead to the ovarian hyperstimulation syndrome. HCG should not be given if estrogen excretion is greater than 100 μg per day. In such instances of hyperstimulation, there are major derangements of fluid balance, and severe pain and ascites may take place, or in the milder instances multiple follicles may ovulate, with the accompanying problems of multiple pregnancy. As many as septuplets have occurred (without survival) following such treatment.

Nonetheless, the advent of relatively pure preparation of FSH and LH or HCG has made it possible for patients to have babies who could not do so before, including patients who have had hypophysectomy.

CLOMIPHENE CITRATE

Although clomiphene is discussed in Chap. 27, it is included briefly here. It has been used for patients with demonstrable gonadotropin secretion but who, for some reason that is not presently clear, are unable to ovulate or cycle normally. Such patients include those with polycystic ovarian syndrome. The structure of clomiphene is similar to that of a synthetic estrogen, chlorotrianisene. Current belief is that it acts at the molecular level either in the ovary or the hypothalamic-pituitary level to alter the local effect of estrogen stimulation or inhibition, thus resulting in a normal gonadotropin secretion or release.

LHRF (GnRH)

In normal reproductive cycles FSH ranges from 5 to 15 mIU/mL and LH ranges from 10 to 20 mIU/mL. In amenorrhea three types of gonadotropin secretion are encountered. If LH is high and FSH is normal, the patient either is pregnant, has the Stein-Leventhal syndrome, or has a rare gonadotropin-secreting tumor of the gastrointestinal system or lung. When secondary amenorrhea is accompanied by elevated FSH and LH levels, the causes for ovarian failure must be determined. These could include genetic abnormalities which can be delineated by laparoscopy and chromosomal analysis. Patients with secondary amenorrhea and low levels of FSH and LH should be examined for hypothalamic or pituitary causes for this failure. LHRF has been used to delineate the difference between ovarian, pituitary, and hypothalamic causes of amenorrhea and menstrual dysfunction including polycystic ovarian disease; however, in the individual case the results cannot be interpreted without caution or the use of other tests because there is so much overlap in the values. The complexity of the action of LHRF, its rapid disappearance from the plasma, and the fact that it acts locally and the test involves a peripheral intravenous infusion or repeated intramuscular injections make it at present an investigational drug. However, there is no doubt that some

patients have ovulated and become pregnant following its use, and there are situations that have been clarified by its administration as a test dose. In the future, analogues of the decapeptide LHRF may be used for more precise administration or longer effects, and antibodies to LHRF may be formed which may be useful as a contraceptive. In another usage LHRF has been administered with arginine and TRF for the evaluation of abnormal secretion or possible pituitary tumors which secrete HGH, HPRL, TSH, and LH-FSH. This integrated pituitary function test has been used to some clinical advantage in differentiating functional disease from tumors and may be used more in the future. It has been pointed out that in men HGH response to arginine requires the administration of estrogen, and therefore the sequence of the test should be different, as the estrogen would affect the LH-FSH response.

PROSTAGLANDINS

Prostaglandins are complex lipids containing 20 carbon atoms and are synthesized from arachidonic acid. They are found in many tissues including brain and lung; in reproductive tissues they are found in endometrium, decidua, membranes, amniotic fluid, and umbilical cord. Many prostaglandins and metabolites have now been described; however, each has a different action which may be opposite to that of a structurally similar-appearing compound. For example, prostaglandin $F_{2\alpha}$ ($PGF_{2\alpha}$) has an arterial and uterine muscle contraction effect, while PGE_1 relaxes smooth muscle and dilates blood vessels.

The thrust for study of prostaglandins in reproduction came as a result of their action in stimulating the onset of labor. At the same time, with the upsurge of interest in abortion throughout the Western world, prostaglandins became useful in causing abortion early in pregnancy when oxytocin was less effective and had to be given over a prolonged period of time. In the initial experiments with prostaglandin $F_{2\alpha}$, it was injected intravenously in large dosages. This produced marked systemic effects which included severe nausea and vomiting. Subsequent practice has led to the administration of prostaglandins into either the uterus or the vagina. When they are placed in the uterus, a small bolus or infusion of drug may be put either directly into the amniotic sac or extraovularly between the membranes and the decidua. When prostaglandins are used this way, a smaller dosage is required, and the symptoms of toxicity are greatly diminished or even absent.

Prostaglandins are finding an increasing role in a number of reproductive physiologic and pathophysiologic processes. In addition to affecting the uterine muscle, presumably both by dilating the cervix (or rendering it favorable to dilate) and contracting the myometrium, prostaglandins sensitize the uterus to oxytocin. Experiments have also demonstrated, following the administration of large doses of estrogen as in the "morning-after pill" (to achieve contraception), a rise in $PGF_{2\alpha}$ followed by a fall in progesterone, corpus luteum lysis, and early menstruation.

PGE_1 has also been examined in relation to the presence or absence of hypertension and toxemia of pregnancy. PGE has been shown to be reduced in the kidney in essential hypertension. Early experiments with PGE_1 have also shown that it may be reduced in the presence of toxemia of pregnancy. The possible effects of prostaglandins on the corpus luteum in vitro have been examined, and the presence and absence of $PGF_{2\alpha}$ have been associated with the action of LH on the corpus luteum. The administration of indomethacin has prevented ovulation in animals. The mediation of the ovulatory effect of LH by prostaglandin has led to the proposal that prostaglandin may be a third messenger in the cell, as is the case for cyclic AMP. Prostaglandins may also be part of the mechanism by which intrauterine devices exert their effect of preventing implantation.

Prostaglandins will be increasingly used in abortion, and with the unraveling of the physiology surrounding the onset of labor they may be used in labor as well. Whether antagonists to their action or variants of indomethacin will be created to counteract their peripheral effects remains to be seen.

Certain compounds have antiprostaglandin effects and are being increasingly used as therapy to inhibit the effects of PG. Such are indomethacin, aspirin, and methylxanthines. Known for their relief of pain, arthritis aspirin and indomethacin have been used as specific therapy to relieve dysmenorrhea. Indomethacin has been used to inhibit ovulation, experimentally.

PSYCHOTHERAPY

The psychiatrist has come to recognize that the absence of demonstrable organic changes in the so-called "functional" illnesses does not exclude the possibility of somatic disorders (Deutsch). The gynecologist, on the other hand, has learned that even in cases with organic changes, the etiologic factors and resolution of persistent symptoms might have to be sought for in the psyche (Menzer-Benaron, Sturgis). For this reason, the management of functional dysmenorrhea, premenstrual tension, amenorrhea, infertility, and dysfunctional bleeding, including cases in which endocrine abnormality may be demonstrable, may include psychiatric evaluation and psychotherapy.

REFERENCES

Normal Reproduction in the Female

Feng L-J et al.: Computer simulation of the human pituitary-ovarian cycle: Studies of follicular phase estradiol infusions and the midcycle peak. *J Clin Endocrinol Metab* 45:775, 1977.

Ross GT et al.: Pituitary and gonadal hormones in women during spontaneous and induced ovulatory cycles. *Recent Prog Horm Res* 26:1, 1970.

Vande Wiele RL et al.: Mechanisms regulating the menstrual cycle in women. *Recent Prog Horm Res* 26:63, 1970.

Estrogens

Baird DT et al.: Steroid prehormones. *Perspect Biol Med* 3:384, 1968.

———, **Guevera A:** Concentration of unconjugated estrone and estradiol in peripheral plasma in nonpregnant women throughout the menstrual cycle, castrate and postmenopausal women and in men. *J Clin Endocrinol Metab* 29:149, 1969.

Brown JB: Urinary excretion of oestrogens during the menstrual cycle. *Lancet* 1:320, 1955.

———: Urinary excretion of oestrogens during pregnancy, lactation and the re-establishment of menstruation. *Lancet* 1:704, 1956.

Diczfalusy E, Mancuso S: Oestrogen metabolism in pregnancy, in *Foetus and Placenta,* eds. A Klopper, E. Diczfalusy, London: Blackwell, 1969, pl 191.

Fishman J et al.: Estrogen metabolism in normal and pregnant women. *J Biol Chem* 237:1489, 1962.

Flood C et al.: Metabolic clearance and blood production rate of estriol in normal non-pregnant women. *J Clin Endocrinol Metab* 42:1, 1976.

Longcope C et al.: Metabolic clearance rates and interconversions of estrone and 17β-estradiol in normal males and females. *J Clin Invest* 47:93, 1968.

MacDonald PC et al.: The ultilization of plasma androstenedione for estrone production in women, in *Progress in Endocrinology,* ed. C Gual, Amsterdam:

Excerpta Medica Foundation, 1969, p. 770.

Ryan KJ: Estrogens and atherosclerosis. *Clin Obstet Gynecol* 19:805, 1976.

_____, Petro Z: Steroid biosynthesis by human ovarian granulosa and theca cells. *J Clin Endocrinol Metab* 26:46, 1968.

_____, Smith OW: Biogenesis of estrogens by the human ovary. *J Biol Chem* 236:705, 710, 2204, 2207, 1961.

_____:Biogenesis of steroid hormones in the human ovary. *Recent Prog Horm Res* 21:367, 1965.

Siiteri PK, MacDonald PC: Role of extraglandular estrogen in human endocrinology, in *Handbook of Physiology,* sec. 7: *Endocrinology,* vol. II: *Female Reproductive System,* pt. 1, exec. ed. SR Geiger, Washington: American Physiological Society, 1973, p. 615.

Simmer H et al.: On the regulation of estrogen production of cortisol and ACTH in human pregnancy at term. *Am J Obstet Gynecol* 119:283, 1974.

Tagatz GE, Gurpide E: Hormone secretion by the human ovary, in *Handbook of Physiology,* sec. 7: *Endocrinology,* vol. II: *Female Reproductive System* pt. I, exec. ed. JR Geiger, Washington: American Physiological Society, 1973, p. 603.

Androgens

Baird DT et al.: Steroid dynamics under steady-state conditions. *Recent Prog Horm Res* 25:611, 1969.

Kirschner MA, Bardin CW: Androgen production and metabolism in normal and virilized women. *Metabolism* 21:667, 1972.

Vermeulen A, Verdonck L: Plasma androgen levels during the menstrual cycle. *Am J Obstet Gynecol* 125:491, 1976.

Progesterone

Allen WA: Progesterone: How did the name originate? *South Med J* 63:1151, 1970.

Beck P: Progestin enhancement of the plasma insulin response to glucose in Rhesus monkeys. *Diabetes* 18:146, 1969.

Davis ME, Plotz EJ: Metabolism of progesterone and its clinical use in pregnancy. *Recent Prog Horm Res* 13:347, 1957.

Hertig AT: Diagnosing the endometrial biopsy. *Proceedings of the Conference on Diagnosis in Sterility, 1945,* ed. ET Engle, Springfield, Ill.: Charles C Thomas, 1946, p. 93.

Laborde N et al: The secretion of progesterone during the periovulatory period in women with certified ovulation. *J Clin Endocrinol Metab* 43:1157, 1976.

Landau RL: The metabolic influence of progesterone, in *Handbook of Physiology,* sec. 7: *Endocrinology,* vol. II: *Female Reproductive System,* pt. I, exec. ed. SR Geiger, Washington: American Physiological Society, 1973, p. 573.

Lin TJ et al.: Metabolic clearance rate of progesterone in the menstrual cycle. *J Clin Endocrinol Metab* 35:879, 1972.

Little B, Billiar RB: Progesterone production, in *Progress in Endocrinology,* ed. C Gual, Amsterdam: Excerpta Medica Foundation, 1969, p. 871.

_____, _____: The metabolic clearance rate of progesterone in the menstrual cycle and per cent interconversion to 20α-dihydroprogesterone, Amersterdam: Excerpta Medica Foundation, vol. 210, 1970, p. 451.

Milewich L et al.: Progesterone and 5α-pregnane-3,20-dione in peripheral blood of normal young women. Daily measurements throughout the menstrual cycle. *J Clin Endocrinol Metab* 45:617, 1977.

O'Malley BW, Strott CA: The mechanism of action of progesterone, in *Handbook of Physiology,* sec. 7: *Endocrinology,* vol. II: *Female Reproductive System,* pt. I, exec. ed. SR Geiger, Washington: American Physiological Society, 1973, p. 591.

Prowse CM, Gaensler EA: Respiratory and acid-base changes during pregnancy. *Anesthesiology* 26:381, 1965.

Riondel A et al.: Estimation of progesterone in human peripheral blood using ³⁵S-thiosemicarbazide. *J Clin Endocrinol Metab* 25:229, 1965.

Sandberg AA et al.: Metabolic conjugation and hydrolysis of estrogens and progesterone in the enterohepatic circulation, in *Metabolic Conjugation and Metabolic Hydrolysis,* vol II, ed. WH Fishman, New York: Academic, 1970, p. 123.

Van der Molen HJ: Patterns of gonadal steroids in the normal human female, in *Progress in Endocrinology,* ed. C Gual, Amsterdam: Excerpta Medica Foundation, 1969, p. 894.

Vande Wiele RL et al.: Mechanisms regulating the menstrual cycle in women. *Recent Prog Horm Res* 26:63, 1970.

Regulation of the Menstrual Cycle; Pituitary Gonadotropins

Benoit J, DeLage C (eds.): *Cytologie de L'Adenohypophyse,* Paris: Editions de Centre National de Recherche Scientifique, 1963.

Goldenberg RL et al.: Gonadotropins in women with amenorrhea. *Am J Obstet Gynecol* 116:1003, 1973.

Lee P et al.: Puberty in girls: Correlations of serum levels of gonadotropins, prolactin, androgens, estrogens, and progestins with physical changes. *J Clin Endocrinol Metab* 43:775, 1976.

Mishell D et al.: The effect of contraceptive steroids on hypothalamic-pituitary function. *Am J Obstet Gynecol* 128:60, 1977.

Odell WD et al.: Endocrine aspects of trophoblastic neoplasms. *Clin Obstet Gynecol* 10:290, 1967.

——, Moyer DL: Dynamic relationship of the ovary to the whole woman, and Dynamic relationship of the testis to the whole man, in *The Physiology of Reproduction,* St. Louis: Mosby, 1971, pp. 64, 82.

Rosner JM et al.: Plasma levels of norepinephrine (NE) during the periovulatory period and after LH-RH stimulation in women. *J Obstet Gynecol* 124:567, 1976.

Ross GT et al.: Pituitary and gonadal hormones in women during spontaneous and induced ovulatory cycles. *Recent Prog Horm Res* 26:1, 1970.

Yen SSC et al.: Gonadotropin levels in puberty: I. Serum luteinizing hormone. *J Clin Endocrinol Metab* 29:382, 1968.

—— et al.: Gonadotropin dynamics in patients with gonadal dysgenesis: A model for the study of gonadotropin regulation. *J Clin Endocrinol Metab* 35:897, 1972a.

—— et al.: Variation of pituitary responsiveness to synthetic LRF during different phases of the menstrual cycle. *J Clin Endocrinol Metab* 35:931, 1972b.

——, Vicic WJ: Serum follicle stimulating hormone levels and puberty. *Am J Obstet Gynecol* 106:134, 1970.

Prostaglandins

Demers LM, Gabbe SG: Placental prostaglandin levels in pre-eclampsia. *Am J Obstet Gynecol* 126:137, 1976.

Dray F, Frydman R: Primary prostaglandins in amniotic fluid in pregnancy and spontaneous labor. *Am J Obstet Gynecol* 126:13, 1976.

Gustavii B: Release of lysosomal acid phosphatase into the cytoplasm of decidual cells before the onset of labor in human. *Brit J Obstet Gynaec* 82:177, 1975.

MacDonald PC et al.: Initiation of human parturition: I. Mechanism of action of arachidonic acid. *Obstet Gynecol* 44:629, 1974.

Rao CH V et al.: Prostaglandin F_2 binding sites in human corpora lutea. *J Clin Endocrinol Metab* 44:1032, 1977.

Schwarz BE et al.: Initiation of human parturition: III. Fetal membrane content of prostaglandin E_2 and $F2_\alpha$ precursor. *Obstet Gynecol* 46:564, 1975.

Terragno NA et al.: Prostaglandins and the regulation of uterine blood flow in pregnancy. *Nature* 249:57, 1974.

Venuto RC et al.: Uterine prostaglandin E secretion and uterine blood flow in the pregnant rabbit. *J Clin Invest* 55:193, 1975.

Mechanism of Hormone Action

Gorski J: Estrogen binding and control of gene expression in the uterus, in *Handbook of Physiology,* sec. 7: *Endocrinology,* vol. II: *Female Reproductive System,* pt. I, exec. ed. SR Geiger, Washington: American Physiological Society, 1973, p. 525.

O'Malley BW, Strott CA: The mechanism of action of progesterone, in *Handbook of Physiology,* sec. 7, *Endocrinology,* vol. II: *Female Reproductive System,* pt. I, exec. ed. SR Geiger, Washington: American Physiological Society, 1973, p. 591.

Pregnancy

Gemzell CA: Blood levels of 17-hydroxycorticosteroids in normal pregnancy. *J Clin Endocrinol Metab* 13:898, 1953.

Jones KM et al.: Aldosterone secretion and metabolism in normal men and women in pregnancy. *Acta Endocrinol* 30:321, 1959.

Little B et al.: Hypophysectomy during pregnancy in a patient with cancer of the breast: Case report with hormone studies. *J Clin Endocrinol Metab* 18:425, 1958.

Migeon CJ et al.: Cortisol production rate: VIII. Pregnancy. *J Clin Endocrinol Metab* 28:661, 1968.

Mikhail G, Allen WM: Ovarian function in human pregnancy. *Am J Obstet Gynecol* 99:308, 1967.

Odell Wd et al.: Endocrine aspects of trophoblastic neoplasms. *Clin Obstet Gynecol* 10:290, 1967.

Tait JF et al.: The metabolic clearance rate of aldosterone in pregnant and nonpregnant subjects estimated by both single-injection and constant-infusion methods. *J Clin Invest* 41:2093, 1962.

The Fetoplacental Unit

Csapo A: The defense mechanism of pregnancy, in *Progesterone and the Defense Mechanism of Pregnancy,* Ciba Foundation Study Group no. 9, eds.

GEW Wolstenholme, MP Cameron, Boston: Little, Brown, 1961, p. 3.

Progesterone Synthesis, Secretion and Metabolism in Pregnancy

Billiar RB et al.: Pregnenolone and pregnenolone sulfate metabolism in vivo and uterine extraction at midgestation. *J Clin Endocrinol Metab* 39:27, 1974.

Escarcena L. et al.: Contribution of maternal circulation to blood borne progesterone in the fetus: I. Studies on human subjects. *Am J Obstet Gynecol* 130:462–465, 1978.

Solomon S. Fuchs F: Progesterone and related steroids, in *Endocrinology of Pregnancy*, eds. F. Fuchs, A Klopper, New York: Harper & Row, 1971, p. 66.

Zander J: Progesterone and its metabolites in the placental-foetal unit, in *Proceedings of the Second International Congress of Endocrinology, 1964*, ed. S Taylor, International Congress Series no. 83, Amsterdam: Excerpta Medica Foundation, 1965, p. 715.

Estrogen Synthesis, Secretion and Metabolism

Diczfalusy E, Troen P: Endocrine functions of the human placenta. *Vitam Horm* 19:229, 1961.

Protein Hormones of the Placenta

Brody S: Protein hormones and hormonal peptides, in *Foetus and Placenta*, eds. A Klopper, E Diczfalusy, London: Blackwell, 1969, p. 299.

Diczfalusy E, Troen P: Endocrine functions of the human placenta. *Vitam Horm* 19:229, 1961.

Friesen HG: Placental protein and polypeptide hormones, in *Handbook of Physiology*, sec. 7: *Endocrinology*, vol. II: *Female Reproductive System*, pt. II, exec. ed. SR Geiger, Washington: American Physiological Society, 1973, p. 295

Josimovich JB: Placental lactogenic hormone, in *Endocrinology of Pregnancy*, eds. F Fuchs, A Klopper, New York: Harper & Row, 1971, p. 184.

Human Placental Lactogen (HPL) or Human Chorionic Somatomammotropin (HCS)

Archer DF et al.: Serum prolactin in patients with inappropriate lactation. *Am J Obstet Gynecol* 119:466, 1974.

Friesen HG: Placental protein and polypeptide hor-

mones, in *Handbook of Physiology*, sec. 7, Endocrinology, vol II, Female Reproductive System, pt. II, exec. ed. SR Geiger, Washington: American Physiological Society, 1973, p. 295.

Josimovich JB: Placental lactogenic hormone, in *Endocrinology of Pregnancy*, eds. F Fuchs, A Klopper, New York: Harper & Row, 1971, p. 184.

————, MacLaren JA: Presence in the human placenta and term serum of a highly lactogenic substance immunologically related to pituitary growth hormone. *Endocrinology* 71:209, 1962.

Labor and Delivery

Liggins CG et al.: The mechanism of initiation of parturition in the ewe. *Recent Prog Horm Res* 29:111, 1973.

MacDonald PC et al.: Initiation of human parturition: I. Mechanism of action of arachidonic acid. *J Ob Gynecol* 44:629, 1974.

Schultz FM et al.: Initiation of human parturition: II. Identification of phospholipase A_2 in fetal chorioamnion and uterine decidua. *Am J Obstet Gynecol* 123:650, 1975.

Schwarz BE et al.: Initiation of human parturition: III. Fetal membrane content of prostaglandin E_2 and $F_{2\alpha}$ precursor. *Ob Gynecol* 46:564, 1975.

Postpartum Lactation

Friesen HG: Placental protein and polypeptide hormones, in *Handbook of Physiology*, sec. 7: *Endocrinology*, vol. II: *Female Reproductive System*, pt. II, exec. ed. SR Geiger, Washington: American Physiological Society, 1973, p. 295.

Disorders of Reproduction; Menopause

Kaufman S: Menopause, in *Progress in Gynecology*, vol. V, eds JV Meigs, SH Sturgis, New York: Grune & Stratton, 1970, p. 172.

Riggs BL et al.: Effects of oral therapy with calcium and vitamin D in primary osteoporosis. *J Clin Endocrinol Metab* 42:1139, 1976.

Sherman B et al.: The menopausal transition: Analysis of LH, FSH, estradiol, and progesterone concentrations during menstrual cycles of older women. *J Clin Endocrinol Metab* 42:629, 1976.

Vermeulen A: The hormonal activity of the postmenopausal ovary. *J Clin Endocrinol Metab* 42:247, 1976.

Amenorrhea-Galactorrhea

Archer DF et al.: Serum prolactin in patients with inappropriate lactation. *Am J Obstet Gynecol* 119:466, 1974.

Shearman RP, Smith ID: Statistical analysis of relationship between oral contraceptives, secondary amenorrhoea and galactorrhoea. *J Obstet Gynaecol Br Commonw* 79:654, 1972.

Hypopituitarism (Sheehan's Disease)

Sheehan HL: The incidence of postpartum hypopituitarism. *Am J Obstet Gynecol* 68:202, 1954.

Anorexia Nervosa

Beumont PFV et al.: Body weight and the pituitary response to hypothalamic releasing hormones in patients with anorexia nervosa. *J Clin Endocrinol Metab* 43:487, 1976.

Bruch H: Perils of behavior modification in treatment of anorexia nervosa. *JAMA* 230:1429, 1974.

————: Management of anorexia nervosa. *Resident and Staff Physician* August, 1976, p. 61.

Hart R et al.: Induction of ovulation and pregnancy in patients with anorexia nervosa. *Am J Obstet Gynecol* 108:580, 1970.

Warren MP, Vande Wiele RL: Clinical and metabolic features of anorexia nervosa. *Am J Obstet Gynecol* 117:435, 1973.

Waxmen, JS, et al.: Anorexia nervosa, practical initial management in a general hospital. *JAMA* 229:801, 1974.

Luteal Phase Defect

Jones GS: Luteal phase defects, in *Progress in Infertility*, eds. SJ Behrman, RW Kistner, Boston: Little, Brown, 1968, p. 299.

Ross GT et al.: Pituitary and gonadal hormones in women during spontaneous and induced ovulatory cycles. *Recent Prog Horm Res* 26:1, 1970.

Soules MR et al.: The diagnosis and therapy of luteal phase deficiency. *Fertil Steril* 28:1033, 1977.

Vande Wiele RL et al.: Mechanisms regulating the menstrual cycle in women. *Recent Prog Horm Res* 26:63, 1970.

Wilks JW et al.: Luteal phase defects in the rhesus monkey: The significance of serum FSH:LH ratios. *J Clin Endocrinol Metab* 43:1261, 1976.

Estrogenic States

Bogumil RJ et al.: Mathematical studies of the human menstrual cycle: I. Formulation of a mathematical model. *J Clin Endocrinol Metab* 35:126, 1972a.

————et al.: Mathematical studies of the human menstrual cycle: II. Simulation performance of a model of the human menstrual cycle. *J Clin Endocrinol Metab* 35:144, 1972b.

Goldenberg RL et al.: Gonadotropins in women with amenorrhea. *Am J Obstet Gynecol* 116:1003, 1973

Siiteri PK, MacDonald PC: Role of extraglandular estrogen in human endocrinology, in *Handbook of Physiology*, sec. 7: *Endocrinology*, vol. II: *Female Reproductive System*, pt. 1, exec. ed. SR Geiger, Washington: American Physiological Society, 1973, p. 615.

Speroff L et al.: Anovulation and hirsutism, in *Clinical Gynecologic Endocrinology and Infertility*, Baltimore: Williams & Wilkins, 1973, p. 57.

Androgenic Syndromes

Kirschner MA, Bardin CW: Androgen production and metabolism in normal and virilized women. *Metabolism* 21:667, 1972.

Yannone ME: Androgenic disorders of the female. *J Iowa Med Soc* 56:572, 1966.

Polycystic Ovarian Disease

Baird DT et al.: Pituitary-ovarian relationships in polycystic ovary syndrome. *J Clin Endocrinol Metab* 45:798, 1977.

DeVane GW et al.: Circulating gonadotropins, estrogens, and androgens in polycystic ovarian disease. *Am J Obstet Gynecol* 121:496, 1975.

Goldzieher JW: Polycystic ovarian disease, in *Advances in Obstetrics and Gynecology*, vol. 1, eds SL Marcus, CC Marcus, Baltimore: Williams & Wilkins, 1967, p. 354.

————, **Green JA:** The polycystic ovary: I. Clinical and histologic features. *J Clin Endocrinol Metab* 22:325, 1962.

Judd HL et al.: The effects of ovarian wedge resection on circulating gonadotropin and ovarian steroid levels in patients with polycystic ovary syndrome. *J Clin Endocrinol Metab* 43:347, 1976.

Lloyd CW et al.: Plasma testosterone and urinary 17-ketosteroids in women with hirsutism and polycystic ovaries. *J Clin Endocrinol Metab* 36:314, 1966.

Rebar R et al.: Characterization of the inappropriate

gonadotropin secretion in polycystic ovary syndrome. *J Clin Invest* 57:1320, 1976.

Speroff L et al.: Anovulation and hirsutism, in *Clinical Gynecologic Endocrinology and Infertility,* Baltimore: Williams & Wilkins, 1973, p. 57.

Stein IF: Duration of fertility following ovarian wedge. *West J Surg* 72:237, 1964.

Yahia C, Taymor ML: Variants of the polycystic ovarian syndrome, in *Progress in Gynecology*, vol. V, eds. JV Meigs, SH Sturgis, New York: Grune & Stratton, 1970, p. 163.

Disorders of Organ Response—Androgen Insensitivity

Boyar RM et al.: Studies of gonadotropin-gonadal dynamics in patients with androgen insensitivity. *J Clin Endocrinol Metab* 47:1116, 1978.

Griffin JE, Wilson JD: The clinical spectrum associated with deficiency of the androgen receptor. *Clin Res* 26:306, 1978 (Abstract).

————, ————: Studies on the pathogenesis of the incomplete forms of androgen resistance in man. *J Clin Endocrinol Metab* 45:1137, 1977.

Murphy JE, Murphy P (eds.): Symposium on Danol (danazol). *J Inter Med Res* 5:Suppl. 3, 1977.

Wilson JD et al.: Familial incomplete male pseudo-hermaphroditism, type 1. Evidence of androgen resistance and variable clinical manifestations in a family with Reifenstein's syndrome. *N Engl J Med* 290:1097, 1974.

Psychotherapy

Deutsch H: *Psychology of Women,* vols. 1 and 2, New York: Grune & Stratton, 1944 and 1945.

Menzer-Benaron D, Sturgis SH: Relationship between emotional and somatic factors in gynecologic disease, in *Progress in Gynecology,* vol. III, eds. JV Meigs, SH Sturgis, New York: Grune & Stratton, 1957, p. 235.

8

Reproductive Physiology

LUIGI MASTROIANNI, JR.

A thorough understanding of human reproductive physiology is an essential requisite to successful treatment of reproductive disorders. Ability to control fertility and to treat infertility has been enhanced by availability of information from the laboratory. The purpose of this chapter is to place in perspective certain aspects of human reproductive function, with emphasis on the nonendocrine events associated with procreation. It is hoped that this chapter will provide a scientific basis for selection of the clinical modalities useful in the management of both contraception and reproductive failure.

PHYSIOLOGY OF MALE REPRODUCTION

SPERMATOGENESIS

Spermatogenesis in the adult male is a continuing process. It is initiated at about the time of puberty and continues well into senescence, even if somewhat less efficiently in later reproductive years. The testes provide a steady supply of spermatozoa which, on release, are transported and stored in the accessory male reproductive tract.

Spermatogenesis is initiated and maintained in the seminiferous tubules of the testes. Therein the spermatogonium matures and the sperm-forming elements acquire a tail. Meiosis occurs, and as a result, the spermatozoa which are released are endowed with a haploid number of chromosomes. Thus the testicular spermatozoon is being prepared for its exclusive function, fertilization.

Spermatogenesis is a heat-sensitive process. There is a 2 to 3° C difference between scrotal and abdominal temperatures, allowing spermatogenesis to proceed normally in the cooler environment of the scrotum. Testosterone production is not affected by temperature. When there is failure of the testes to descend into the scrotum (cryptorchidism), spermatogenesis is severely impaired, but testosterone production remains unaffected.

The maturation of human spermatozoa from initiation to completion occupies an interval of 60 days. Recognition of this time interval is important in terms of both male contraceptive development and infertility treatment. Noxious influences, which may impair spermatogenesis, may have exercised their effect long before the damaged spermatazoa appear in the ejaculate. Agents designed as male contraceptives, which influence the early stages of spermatogenesis, do not affect the ejaculate until many days after treatment has been instituted. When a deficient specimen is uncovered in the infertile male, one must consider the possibility that the etiology of the deficiency occurred days earlier. Evaluation of the male is not complete until repeated specimens are studied over time, and the physician should never base a prognosis on examination of a single specimen. Furthermore, when there are abnormalities in spermatogenesis, prompt response to treatment should not be expected.

RELEASE OF SPERMATOZOA FROM THE TESTES

Recent work has established the importance of the anatomic arrangement within the seminiferous tubules to explain the mechanism of sperm release. The developing spermatozoa and the Sertoli cells, which together constitute the cellular makeup of the seminiferous tubules, exhibit a constantly changing relationship. As sperm-forming elements differentiate, they move toward the lumen of the seminiferous tubules along the sides of the supporting Sertoli cells. The location of the Sertoli cells is fixed, in contrast to the changing populations of spermatozoa. Unlike the usual arrangement within epithelium, there are no anatomic connections such as desmosomes and gap

junctions between the spermatozoa and the Sertoli cells. If such cell-to-cell connections were present, they would prevent the movement of sperm-forming elements. There are, however, specialized junctions between adjacent Sertoli cells. These occluding junctions create a barrier separating the epithelium into a basal compartment and an adlumenal compartment. The basal compartment contains the early sperm-forming structures, the spermatogonia, and the preleptotene spermatocytes. The adlumenal compartment contains meiotic and postmeiotic stages of sperm development. Thus the Sertoli cells with their occluding junctions provide an anatomic basis for a blood-testis permeability barrier (Fig. 8–1). This structural arrangement isolates the differentiating germ cells from the general extracellular fluid compartment. Substances reaching the germ cells via the bloodstream must traverse the barrier created by the Sertoli cells. This arrangement provides protection during the sensitive process of early meiotic differentiation.

The Sertoli cells also play an active role in sperm release. It is, of course, necessary that the tight junctions between Sertoli cells break down transiently to permit upward movement of preleptotene spermato-

FIGURE 8–1 Drawing illustrating the manner in which the occluding junctions between Sertoli cells divide the seminiferous epithelium into a basal compartment occupied by the spermatogonia and preleptotene spermatocytes and an adlumenal compartment containing more advanced stages of the germ cell population. The occluding Sertoli-Sertoli junctions are the principal component of the blood-testis barrier. *(From DW Fawcett: In Handbook of Physiology, Sec. V: Endocrinology, Washington, D.C.: Amer. Physiological Society, 1975, Chap 2.)*

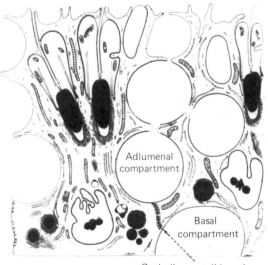

Adlumenal compartment

Basal compartment

Occluding sertoli junction

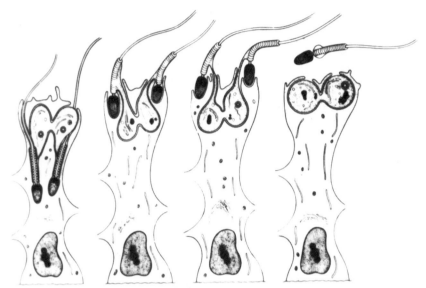

FIGURE 8-2 Diagram of the stages of sperm release. The conjoined cell bodies of the advanced spermatids are retained in the epithelium while the nucleus, neck region, and tail are gradually extruded into the lumen. The narrow stalk connecting the neck region with the cell body becomes increasingly attenuated and finally gives way. Individual spermatozoa are thus separated from the syncytial cell bodies. *(From DW Fawcett: in Regulation of Reproduction, eds., SJ Segal et al., Springfield, Ill.: Charles C Thomas, 1973.)*

cytes into the compartment adjacent to the lumen. As they are being released, the spermatids are drawn into the epithelium of the Sertoli cells. Thereafter the spermatids are moved upward toward the surface of the cell, and are finally extruded, leaving behind some globules of excess cytoplasm (Fig. 8–2). This movement toward the lumen of the seminiferous tubules is brought about by contractions of the cytoplasm at the apex of the Sertoli cells.

Over and above creating a sperm-testis barrier and actively transporting spermatozoa within the seminiferous tubules, Sertoli cells serve yet another function. They are the most likely source of anti-Müllerian substance. This agent is responsible for the inhibition of development of the Müllerian ducts during embryogenesis. It also acts positively to maintain the Wolffian ducts. Thus the anti-Müllerian substance of the Sertoli cells plays a pivotal role in evolving the normal male phenotype. Sertoli cells also produce androgen-binding protein (ABP). ABP has a high affinity for testosterone and dehydrotestosterone. Its synthesis by the Sertoli cells is stimulated by follicle-stimulating hormone (FSH). High concentrations of ABP within seminiferous tubules produce high intratubular levels of androgen. The latter is essential for spermatogenesis and explains the high concentration of androgen in testes fluid, which is five to ten times that of peripheral blood.

TESTICULAR ANDROGEN PRODUCTION

The interstitial connective tissue which surrounds and supports the seminiferous tubules is endowed with testosterone-producing cells, the interstitial or Leydig cells. Leydig cells are the major source of testicular androgen. They act under the influence of luteinizing hormone (LH), and a reciprocal relationship between LH release from the pituitary gland and testosterone production by the Leydig cells is maintained. In addition to establishing and maintaining secondary sex characteristics of the male, testosterone directly affects spermatogenesis. Indeed, the primary function of Leydig cells in reproduction is the secretion of the testosterone required to sustain spermatogenesis. Spermatogenesis will not proceed normally in the absence of very high concentrations of testosterone, and high local androgen concentrations are maintained by the presence of ABP. The sequential relationship among the Leydig cells, Sertoli cells, and sperm-forming elements as influenced by LH, FSH, and testosterone is summarized in Fig. 8–3.

TRANSPORT OF SPERMATOZOA

Leading from the testes are the transporting ducts of the male reproductive tract. They consist of the epididymis, which is connected to the vas deferens,

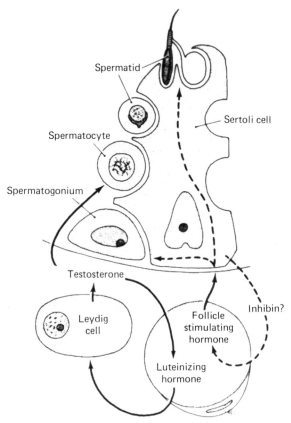

Spermatid

Sertoli cell

Spermatocyte

Spermatogonium

Testosterone

Leydig cell

Follicle stimulating hormone

Inhibin?

Luteinizing hormone

FIGURE 8–3 LH action on the Leydig cells of the interstitial tissue and FSH action on the seminiferous tubules. *(From WB Neaves: In Greep, Koblinsky, Chap. 29.)*

the epididymis exhibit swimming motions which are circular and nondirective; those recovered from the caudal portion of the epididymis are capable of the progressive movement which characterizes ejaculated spermatozoa.

CONTRIBUTIONS OF THE ACCESSORY ORGANS TO THE EJACULATE

Spermatozoa are transported from the caudal portion of the epididymis along the vas deferens to the base of the penis. During ejaculation, semen receives a contribution from the seminal vesicles and prostate gland. The seminal vesicles are paired glands located dorsal to the trigonal area of the urinary bladder (Fig. 8–4). They deliver secretions to the urethra via the ejaculatory ducts, discharging a fructose-rich product. The prostate is located around the base of the urethra and transmits its contents into the urethra during ejaculation via a number of small ducts. It secretes a clear fluid with a slightly acid pH, which is rich in acid phosphatase, citric acid, zinc, and a number of proteolytic enzymes.

It is well established that testicular androgens are responsible for maintaining the function of the accessory sex organs. The principal role of seminal vesicular and prostatic secretions is that of transport of spermatozoa at the time of ejaculation, but they may also contribute briefly to the metabolism of spermatozoa.

SPERM TRANSPORT IN THE VAGINA

The normal ejaculatory process is preceded by sexual excitation and penile erection. Thus, in contrast to the female, the male must experience sexual arousal in order to complete his procreative role. In the absence of erection, penetration is all but impossible, and if erection is lost intravaginally, ejaculation is most unlikely. Thus, for purposes of reproduction, sexual arousal plays a pivotal role in the male. In contrast, the female need not be sexually aroused either to receive spermatozoa intravaginally or to transmit them into the reproductive tract. Sexual satisfaction and procreation are separable in women, a point which is best illustrated by the fact that pregnancies occur following artificial insemination. A healthy sexual response on the part of the female does, however, clearly influence procreation, if only indirectly. Certainly fertility in general can be related to the frequency of intercourse, and when coitus occurs infrequently in association with infertility, responsibility must be shared by both marital partners. Frequency

which in turn leads to the ejaculatory ducts. These ducts enter the urethra (Fig. 8–4). The seminiferous tubules, which if stretched out would traverse a distance of about 10 m, coalesce at the rete testes, which in turn lead into the epididymis. The function of the epididymis is storage of spermatozoa; at the same time, it exerts a substantial influence on the posttesticular maturation of spermatozoa.

During their sojourn in the duct system, spermatozoa are transformed into more mature cells. Maturation within the epididymis requires an interaction of a number of elements, including the spermatozoon itself, the fluid contained within the epididymal lumen, the epithelium of the epididymis, and contributions from the blood and lymphovascular compartments. Within the epididymis, the acrosome, an enzyme-containing envelope located at the head of the spermatozoon, is modified. As spermatozoa move along the epididymis, they develop the capacity for progressive motility. Spermatozoa in the caput (head) of

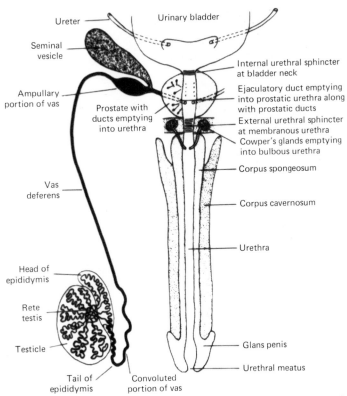

Ureter

Urinary bladder

Seminal vesicle

Internal urethral sphincter at bladder neck

Ejaculatory duct emptying into prostatic urethra along with prostatic ducts

Ampullary portion of vas

External urethral sphincter at membranous urethra

Prostate with ducts emptying into urethra

Cowper's glands emptying into bulbous urethra

Corpus spongeosum

Corpus cavernosum

Vas deferens

Urethra

Head of epididymis

Rete testis

Testicle

Glans penis

Urethral meatus

Tail of epididymis

Convoluted portion of vas

FIGURE 8–4 Schematic representation of the male genital organs, illustrating the relation of the prostate and ejaculatory ducts to the internal and external sphincters, bladder, and urethra. *(From RD Amelar: Infertility in Men, Philadelphia, F. A. Davis., 1966.)*

of coitus is very definitely influenced by sexual adjustment, although there is no evidence to suggest a relationship between female orgasm per se and conception.

SPERM TRANSPORT IN THE CERVICAL MUCUS

On ejaculation, spermatozoa migrate almost immediately into the cervical mucus. The ability of the cervical mucus to accept spermatozoa and support their motility varies with the quality of that mucus, which is modified during the menstrual cycle. The mucus is most receptive immediately prior to ovulation. At that time spermatozoa have been observed in cervical mucus within minutes of ejaculation. This rapid transport explains the futility of the postcoital douche for contraception, and serves as a basis for the use of precoital barrier methods (condom and diaphragm). The spermicidal creams and jellies used in association with the diaphragm are essential to prevent mucus penetration by spermatozoa.

CERVICAL MUCUS

The secretions in the endocervical canal reflect contributions from peritoneal fluid, tubal fluid, and endometrium, but in large measure they are the product of the glandular crypts lining the endocervix. The secretions themselves are composed of strands of mucin arranged in a matrix in an electrolyte-containing fluid, the characteristics of which are altered by hormonal influence. Early in the menstrual cycle, the cervical secretions are scanty, viscous, and cellular; they contain leucocytes in relatively large numbers. This amalgam constitutes a barrier at the cervix against ascending infection. Under the influence of increasing levels of estrogen, the secretions become more abundant and are most copious at the time of the preovulatory estrogen surge. Immediately prior to ovulation, the cervical mucus is copious, clear, and acellular. It can be stretched out for a distance of from 10 to as much as 20 cm into a continuous thread, a characteristic referred to as *spinnbarkheit*. Spinnbarkheit is evaluated by stretching the mucus which has been recovered from the cervix until the thin, continuous

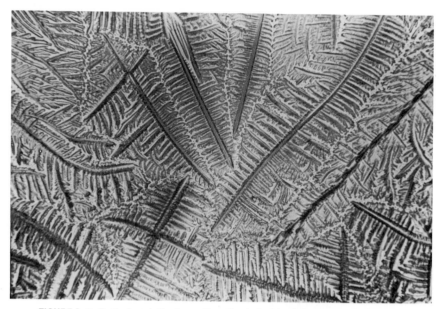

FIGURE 8–5 Typical crystallization pattern (fern) of midcycle human cervical mucus.

thread breaks. A thread of 10 cm or more suggests ovulatory mucus. When dried on a slide, such mucus crystallizes in a fern pattern, as noted on microscopic examination (Fig. 8–5). Mucus displaying these characteristics is usually favorable to sperm penetration.

Following ovulation, under the influence of progesterone, the mucus again becomes opaque, tenacious, and cellular. Spinnbarkheit is decreased and the mucus no longer crystallizes into a fern pattern. Because of these cyclic variations in the quality of the cervical secretions, postcoital tests are best performed within a day or two of the estimated time of ovulation: 14 to 16 days before the next expected menstrual period, when the cervical secretions are most receptive to spermatozoa. The strands of mucopolysaccharides which earlier in the menstrual cycle were arranged in a meshwork pattern are now lined up in parallel bundles, or micelles; channels are created along which spermatozoa may traverse upward into the endometrial cavity (Fig. 8–6).

SPERM TRANSPORT IN THE FEMALE REPRODUCTIVE TRACT

Having traversed the favorable preovulatory cervical mucus, spermatozoa are transported rapidly to the fallopian tube, the site of fertilization. Spermatozoa have been observed to reach the fallopian tube in as short a time as 5 minutes following insemination. At any given time only a few spermatozoa are present within the tube. The lower reproductive tract, the cervix, and the endometrial cavity serve as a reservoir for spermatozoa, and there is a steady upward progression of spermatozoa along the fallopian tube and out into the peritoneal cavity. In time, those spermatozoa located within the uterus or endometrial cavity are phagocytized.

The spermatozoa could not possibly reach the fallopian tube in such a short time by their power of locomotion alone. They are assisted in their upward progression by contractions of the uterus, which are probably stimulated by the large amounts of prostaglandin present in seminal plasma. As they are propelled upward, they traverse the uterotubal junction into the fallopian tube. The exact mechanism by which spermatozoa enter the human tube is not yet known, but the fact that only a few spermatozoa enter at a given time is easily explained by the action of the cilia lining the tube, which beat in the direction of the uterus. It is likely that countercurrents are established within the tubal lumen which allow some spermatozoa to enter and to progress along the tube into the peritoneal cavity. The muscular contractions of the tube may also play an important role in sperm transport.

SPERM CAPACITATION

In most mammalian species exposure to the female reproductive tract is required while the spermatozoa acquire the capacity to fertilize. This phenomenon is

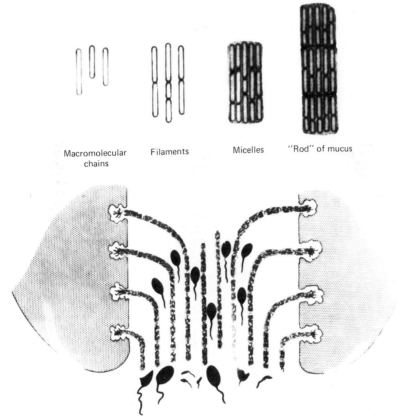

Macromolecular chains   Filaments   Micelles   "Rod" of mucus

FIGURE 8-6 Ascent of sperm through micellar channels formed in cervical mucus at midcycle. *(From L Blasco: Sperm-cervical mucus interactions. Fertil Steril 28:1133, 1978.)*

referred to as *capacitation*. The time requirement for capacitation varies among species; in the rabbit, for example, several hours of exposure to the reproductive tract are necessary. Capacitation appears to be a much less complicated process in the human, and it occurs much more rapidly. The biochemical and biophysical aspects of capacitation are still incompletely worked out. There does, however, appear to be an association between capacitation and some structural alterations in the spermatozoon which precede penetration and which, collectively, are referred to as the *acrosome reaction*.

Spermatozoa are covered distally by a specialized enzyme-containing structure, the acrosome. After the penetration of cumulus layers of the ovum, changes occur in the acrosomal envelope, and the outer acrosomal membrane fuses with the plasma membrane, creating pores or openings (Fig. 8–7). The enzyme-rich contents of the acrosome escape through these openings. As this process continues, the cell membrane which overlies the anterior head of

the sperm head is gradually lost. This exposes the inner acrosomal membrane, which continues to release enzymes during penetration of the zona pellucida of the oocyte. It is likely that capacitation involves biophysical changes in sperm membrane, and in fact it can be produced in vitro in the rabbit by exposing spermatozoa to slightly hypertonic solutions. Human spermatozoa seem to be similar to hamster spermatozoa in that their capacitation can be brought about in vitro by follicular fluid. The fact that human spermatozoa are capacitated in vitro has been confirmed by the successful demonstration of human in vitro fertilization.

RETENTION OF FERTILIZING ABILITY

The duration of fertilizing capability within the female reproductive tract has been explored in a number of laboratory animals. The intervals during which spermatozoa remain motile range from 12 to 15 hours postsemination (in rodents) to 11 days (in dogs). Mo-

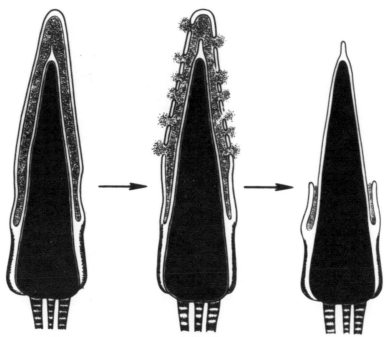

FIGURE 8–7 Depicting successive stages of the acrosome reaction. The outer acrosomal membrane fuses with the cell membrane at the multiple sites creating openings through which the enzyme-rich contents of the acrosome escape. This process leads ultimately to complete loss of the cell membrane over the anterior half of the head. Thereafter the inner acrosomal membrane is the limiting membrane of the sperm head over its anterior portion. The equatorial segment of the acrosome persists. Its function is poorly understood. *(From DW Fawcett, Dev Biol, 44:394–436, 1975.)*

tile human spermatozoa have been recovered from the cervix 6 days following isolated coitus or insemination. Although in general it is felt that the fertile life of human spermatozoa is something on the order of 48 hours, conception has been reported when an isolated insemination has been carried out as long as 5 days preceding ovulation. This remarkable capacity of the human spermatozoon to retain its fertilizing ability may well explain the high rate of failure of the rhythm method of family planning. When prescribing rhythm, one should recognize the possibility that spermatozoa deposited several days prior to ovulation may retain their fertilizing ability.

OOGENESIS AND OVULATION

PHYSIOLOGIC ASPECTS OF OVUM RELEASE

The exact mechanism by which the human oocyte is finally extruded from the ovary is the subject of continuing investigation. In a given menstrual cycle several follicles become competent, i.e., they attain an ability to respond to the gonadotropins, FSH and LH. Under gonadotropin influence, further follicular maturation is stimulated. In a final burst of development, one or occasionally two follicles release an ovum. The remaining follicles which were maturing in that cycle undergo atresia, retaining their oocytes as they proceed through regressive changes. The dominant follicle which is destined to release an oocyte exhibits a rapid accumulation of additional fluid, becoming a mature graafian follicle. It exhibits a markedly thinned-out follicular wall and just prior to ovulation protrudes beyond the surface of the ovary. Ovulation does not appear to be preceded by a sudden increase in intrafollicular pressure. Smooth muscle elements are present in the theca layer surrounding the follicle, and it is reasoned that contractions of these fibers bring about ovum extrusion. The increased contractility of the ovary at the time of ovulation is probably brought about by the prostaglandins, substances which are capable of enhancing muscular contractions and which appear in significant amounts in and near the follicle at the time of ovulation. The endocrine events associated with ovulation have been covered in detail in Chap. 7.

INTRAFOLLICULAR OVUM DEVELOPMENT

At birth, the human ovary is endowed with between 400,000 and 500,000 oocytes. The meiotic process has been initiated but has been arrested in early prophase. The oocytes remain inactive until meiosis is reinitiated about 36 hours prior to ovulation. At that time oocytes contained by those follicles capable of responding to the gonadotropins exhibit a resumption of meiosis; they proceed through metaphase of the second maturation division with release of the first polar body. The ovum is extruded, along with its first polar body, surrounded by a mass of cumulus and corona cells, and on release this aggregate structure is available for pickup by the fimbrian end of the fallopian tube.

Intraovarian oocytes are prevented from proceeding through maturation by an intrafollicular inhibiting substance. This substance, which has been partially characterized, has the capability of inhibiting meiosis in vitro. Its effect is obviated in vivo by the influence of gonadotropins on competent follicles in the hours preceding ovulation. Oocytes which are removed from the developing human follicle are not affected by the meiosis-inhibiting substance, and proceed through nuclear maturation and polar body release in vitro. If removed from the follicle too soon, such oocytes, although they exhibit nuclear maturation, are not fertilizable. If in vitro fertilization is to be successful, ovum recovery must be carried out just prior to the expected time of ovulation. Failure of ova which are removed too early from their follicles to be fertilizable, in spite of completion of nuclear maturation and polar body release, suggests that there must be other intrafollicular mechanisms which influence ovum maturation. It is likely that cytoplasmic as well as nuclear maturation is a requisite for normal fertilization.

TUBAL PHYSIOLOGY

The fallopian tube is a dynamic structure with two basic functions: transport of gametes and the provision of a suitable environment for the reproductive processes which occur at the tubal level. Since under normal conditions the fallopian tube is the site of fertilization, conception is necessarily preceded by efficient transport of spermatozoa into and along the tubal lumen and successful transfer of the ovulated ovum from the point of follicle rupture into the tubal ostium to a level within the ampullary portion of the tube. Subsequent to fertilization, the conceptus is retained within the tubal lumen for a discretely timed interval of approximately 3 days before it is delivered to the uterus. The 3-day residence of the ovum in the human fallopian tube has now been confirmed through elegant studies of Croxatto et al., who used ovum and embryo recovery techniques in patients. It has been shown in several mammalian species that if the embryo is transferred to the uterus prematurely, implantation is less likely.

The environmental factors presented by the tubal lumen are also important. The fluid contained within the oviductal lumen constitutes the milieu in which spermatozoa, ova, and the recently fertilized ovum survive and function. Thus, in addition to transporting gametes, the oviduct provides an appropriate environment for the gametes for the fertilization process, and for the fertilized ovum during the early stages of development. Both tubal transport mechanisms and the environmental influences within the tube have not as yet been adequately assessed in the laboratory. Especially in the primate, including both the monkey and the human, there are deficiencies in our knowledge.

TUBAL TRANSPORT MECHANISMS

The clinical approach to tubal disease in the infertile patient is confined to assessment of the normalcy of the tubal and peritubal anatomy. Efforts are directed principally at evaluation of tubal transport mechanisms. If one is to assess and treat patients with presumed deficiencies in transport mechanisms and if, ultimately, useful techniques are to be developed to evaluate the secretory function of the fallopian tube, better understanding of tubal function in the laboratory animal is pertinent. Although it is clearly inappropriate to transfer information from one species to another, knowledge of tubal physiology from the laboratory has suggested approaches which some day may be useful.

The human fallopian tube is a conduit which provides a passage between the ovary and the uterine cavity. It is surrounded by three layers of smooth musculature. The lining of the tube, the endosalpinx, contains both secretory and ciliated cells. At the distal extremity of the tube, the fimbria consists of fingerlike projections lined with cilia. The anatomic relationship between the fimbria and the ovary is important for understanding the tubal pickup mechanisms during ovulation (Fig. 8–8). One projection from the fimbria, the fimbria ovarica, is longer than the remainder. This contains muscular elements which course from the

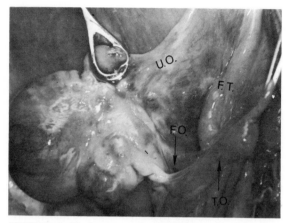

FIGURE 8-8 The human ovary and fallopian tube. The ovary is on the left, the tube (FT) on the right. The tubal ostium (TO) is visible. The clamp is on the uteroovarian ligament (UO). The fimbria ovarica (FO) is attached to one pole of the ovary.

tubal ostium and are attached to one pole of the ovary. In addition, there are some muscular elements in the parovarium, beneath the ovary. Based on observations in the monkey and rabbit, it is suggested that these muscles contract at the time of ovulation and there is a realignment of fimbria over the rupturing follicle. The ovum, surrounded by an entourage of sticky cumulus cells, is picked up by the fimbria as it is released and, by virtue of the action of the cilia lining the fimbria, is transported into the tubal lumen. The cumulus cells surrounding the egg are important in this regard, as the sticky mass of cells allows a forward progression, the result of ciliary action, into the tubal ostium. Once within the lumen, the recently ovulated ovum is transported relatively rapidly to a point well within the widest portion of the tube, the ampulla, where fertilization occurs. The ampullary cilia beat in the direction of the uterus and provide an efficient transport mechanism. Recent rabbit experiments suggest that tubal transport can occur efficiently as a result of ciliary action alone, in the absence of tubal peristalsis resulting from a muscular contraction. Human tubal smooth muscle contractility varies in the menstrual cycle. As the time of ovulation approaches, there is a dramatic increase in the amplitude and frequency of contraction. The tube becomes relatively quiescent in the luteal phase.

During the course of early cleavage, the ovum is retained within the tubal lumen near the junction between the ampulla and the most proximal portion of the tube, the isthmus.

Overall, a number of factors influence the ability of the tube to transport the ovum. These include mus-

cular contractions or tubal peristalsis, ciliary action, and flux of fluid along the oviductal lumen.

Observations in the rhesus monkey have established the fact that there is regeneration of cilia at the fimbriated extremity in each menstrual cycle. Under the influence of estrogen, fimbrial cilia regenerate, reaching full development during the estrogen surge which occurs just prior to ovulation. The cilia then recede, regressing during the luteal phase. The cyclic regression and regeneration of cilia do not occur as dramatically in the human oviduct, although there are alterations in ciliary height during the cycle. The capacity of ciliated cells of the fimbria to regenerate is a source of comfort to the surgeon who is called upon to reconstruct fimbriae when they have been severely damaged.

The mechanism behind the 3-day retention of the ovum in the human fallopian tube is still a matter of speculation. Smooth muscle elements surround the tube at its attachment to the uterus, the uterotubal junction. These constitute a functional sphincter in that area. It is not established that this muscular arrangement is important in ovum transport mechanisms.

For the clinician called upon to treat anatomic tubal disease surgically, a thorough understanding of tubal anatomy is crucial. For example, in the approach to the tube which has been damaged by disease at the fimbriated extremity, the surgeon must be aware of the normal anatomic relationships if the tube is to be reconstructed properly.

An important aspect of fimbrial anatomy is its vascularity. There are large plexuses of vessels at the fimbriated end. These are accompanied by muscular elements. The function of this vascular arrangement is not understood, but the vascularity of the fimbriae is of great importance to the surgeon. The fimbriae constitute the most delicate portion of the tube, and great care must be exercised during the fimbrial reconstruction to avoid unnecessary damage to fimbrial vasculature. The uterotubal junction is treacherous in terms of diagnosis. Spasm of the sphincter in that area may create the false impression that the fallopian tube is anatomically closed near the uterus. If anatomic closure at the uterotubal junction is suspected, intense effort is called for in order to establish this diagnosis before considering surgical correction.

THE TUBAL ENVIRONMENT

A number of approaches have been used to assess the secretory function of the mammalian oviduct. Microscopic techniques including ultrastructural studies and histochemistry have been employed in a number of species, including monkey and man. Elegant studies have been published using scanning electron microscopy (Fig. 8–9). All point to the fact that the human fallopian tube changes in response to the hormonal variations in the menstrual cycle and support the conclusion that there is active secretory process.

Systems have been developed in the laboratory to obtain samples of fluid for analysis. At present, however, there is no completely satisfactory method of fluid collection. Indeed it is unlikely that systems can be developed which will not in some way interfere with physiologic processes. In the rhesus monkey dramatic cyclic fluctuations in fluid volume have been observed (Fig. 8–10). During the menstrual cycle, the rate is low initially and increases abruptly within a day or two of ovulation. It remains relatively high for 2 to 5 days and then decreases to preovulatory levels. The increase in accumulation of tubal fluid has been shown to be brought about by estrogen, and the preovulatory rise coincides with the cyclic surge in estrogen levels. Progesterone causes a decrease

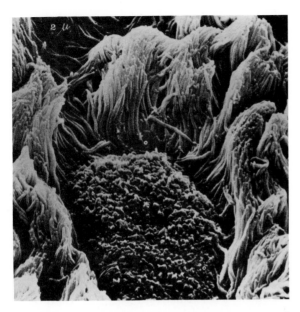

FIGURE 8–9 The human fallopian tube, showing ciliated cells surrounding a nonciliated cell in the midproliferative phase of the menstrual cycle. (*From E Patek et al.: Fertil Steril 23:459, 1972.*)

FIGURE 8–10 Cyclic changes in the rate of tubal secretion in the rhesus monkey. Oviduct fluid accumulation (milliliters per 24 hours) observed in one monkey through 4 menstrual cycles. (*From L Mastroianni et al.: Fertil Steril 12:417, 1961.*)

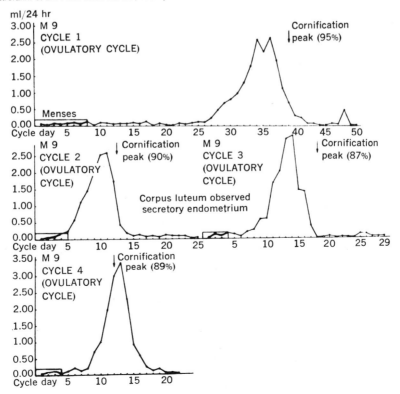

in fluid production. In a system involving cannulation, the greatest quantity of fluid is obtained near the time of ovulation, substantiating cyclic changes in tubal fluid volume in homo sapiens.

The contents of tubal fluid have been studied in several laboratory animals, including the rabbit and rhesus monkey. An externally placed refrigerated system has been used to collect tubal fluid continuously. This allows assessment of the relationship between fluid content and the hormonal status of the animal. Of the metabolic substrates which might be important, lactate and pyruvate appear in significant amounts. Lactate concentration increases following ovulation, and pyruvate probably has physiologic significance, as it has been shown in in vitro ovum culture studies to be an important substrate during early cleavage.

The bicarbonate ion is another important constituent of tubal fluid. The endosalpinx is rich in carbonic anhydrase, and bicarbonate is apparently secreted into the tubal lumen. Bicarbonate is capable of initiating dispersion of the corona radiata cells, a densely packed layer adjacent to the zona pellucida, the protein layer which covers the oocyte. The bicarbonate ion brings about a change in the relationship between the corona cells and the zona pellucida to allow penetration by the spermatozoon to the level of the zona. Although some in vitro fertilized eggs have not been exposed to the tubal environment, every successful system of in vitro fertilization has involved the presence of bicarbonate, and ovum culture is carried out with lactate or pyruvate in the culture medium.

At the very least, the fallopian tube provides exciting avenues for the investigator. It is especially important to consider the myriad approaches which could be used to influence tubal function in order to develop systems of contraception at the tubal level.

TUBAL ABNORMALITIES WHICH AFFECT REPRODUCTION

Anatomic abnormalities of the fallopian tube are the subject of concentrated diagnostic attention. Fertility is certainly impaired when the tubal lumen is occluded bilaterally. Peritubal adhesions which modify the relationship between the ovary and the fimbria may also cause infertility through interference with ovum transport. Gonorrhea, puerperal or postabortal sepsis, and tuberculosis may produce salpingitis and pelvic peritonitis with subsequent tubal occlusion.

The role of extratubal disease is more subtle. A ruptured appendix, especially during childhood when the adnexa and the appendix are relatively

close to each other, endometriosis, pelvic surgery, and diverticulitis may cause pelvic peritoneal adhesions which distort pelvic architecture and occasionally occlude the tube. Endometriosis has assumed an increasingly prominent role in the etiology of tubal involvement in recent years. This is perhaps the result of a trend toward delay of the first pregnancy until late reproductive years when pelvic endometriosis is more common. The location of ectopic sites of endometrium upon the pelvic-peritoneal surfaces is associated with the formation of pelvic adhesions. Each month, there is a "minimenstruation" and the body's reaction to the presence of ectopic endometrium is the formation of fibrous tissue. The net result is the formation of adhesions which often distort the relation between the tube and the ovary. Infertility results from interference with normal transport mechanisms. Conditions capable of involving the fallopian tubes should be accorded special emphasis in the management of infertility.

FERTILIZATION

Fertilization represents a continuum of events. Maturation of the ovum, as described above, has already occurred within the follicle, and the ovum has passed through metaphase of the second meiotic division and polar body release. Thus, at the time of ovulation, the ovum is ready for the final process of maturation which occurs in association with fertilization.

SEQUENCE OF EVENTS

The fertilization process culminates in the union of male and female gametes to form a zygote. In most mammalian species, the process is preceded by capacitation; it begins when the spermatozoon contacts the investments surrounding the oocyte. The process involves penetration through the cumulus oophorus, the corona radiata, the zona pellucida, and finally the egg membrane (Fig. 8–11).

The most extensive studies of mammalian fertilization have been carried out in the rabbit. The loosely arranged outermost layer, cumulus oophorus, can be dispersed with hyaluronidase, presumably released from the acrosomes of spermatozoa. The inner layer of surrounding cells, the corona radiata, is arranged in a radiate fashion around the zona

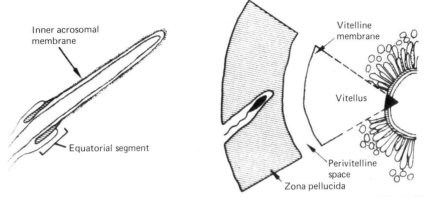

FIGURE 8-11 Status of reacted sperm *(left)* as it penetrates zona *(right)*. *(From RA McRorie, WL Williams: Biochemistry of mammalian fertilization. Annu Rev Biochem 43:777–803, 1974.)*

pellucida. The corona cells next to the zona have pseudopods which project through the zona and establish contact with the egg membrane. Separation of the cells of the corona layer occurs under the influence of the bicarbonate ion, which is present in oviductal secretions.

The zona pellucida is an acellular protein layer which immediately surrounds the ovum. The zona can be dissolved with trypsin. Both hyaluronidase- and trypsinlike activity are found in the acrosomal portion of the sperm head. Release of these enzymes is thought to play an integral role in sperm penetration. Inhibition of fertilization has been demonstrated in vitro with trypsin inhibitors, suggesting that the trypsinlike component of the acrosome is important for sperm penetration through the zona.

Once within the cytoplasm the sperm head enlarges to form the male pronucleus. The chromatin of the ovum condenses into the female pronucleus. As the male and female pronuclei develop and come into apposition, the pronuclear membranes break down; the chromosomes from each pronucleus intermix. The first mitotic division is initiated, and the two-cell stage appears shortly thereafter. Fertilization requires approximately 12 hours in the rabbit, 16 to 21 hours in the sheep, 20 to 24 hours in the cow, and approximately 36 hours in the human.

in the past, does not constitute proof of fertilization. Parthenogenetic cleavage, division in the absence of spermatozoa, has been observed frequently. The presence of chromatin in the individual cells has been observed in parthenogenetically cleaved specimens, and therefore does not rule out parthenogenesis. Furthermore, unfertilized mammalian ova often exhibit degenerative changes which resemble cleavage. In the single cell, appearance of two characteristic pronuclei associated with the presence of clearly identifiable sperm products in the cytoplasm constitutes an acceptable criterion for sperm penetration, but not proof of completion of the fertilization process. The ultimate proof that an ovum has been fertilized in vitro is successful transfer of the in vitro fertilized specimen to a host reproductive tract for continued development and delivery of young.

Since in vivo fertilization within the fallopian tube is inaccessible, in vitro fertilization studies have been essential to understanding mammalian fertilization. Recent successful transfer of in vitro fertilized human embryos, resulting in the birth of normal offspring, has provided proof that this laboratory exercise has been successful and has raised the possibility of use of in vitro fertilization and embryo transfer in the treatment of infertile patients with damaged or absent fallopian tubes.

IN VITRO FERTILIZATION

For nearly a century, efforts have been made to fertilize the mammalian ovum in vitro. Success has been claimed in the rabbit, guinea pig, rat, hamster, mouse, and human. Cleavage, a criterion used widely

IMPLANTATION

The human embryo proceeds from the fallopian tube into the uterine cavity between the 8- and 16-cell stage. Development into a blastocyst continues within the uterine fluid. As a blastocyst develops, specialized trophoblastic cells appear at its periphery, and these cells play an important role in implantation. Meanwhile, the endometrium undergoes dramatic morphologic alterations. In the days prior to ovulation, under the influence of estrogen, the endometrium has proliferated, its cells exhibit marked mitotic activity. Following ovulation, under the continued influence of estrogen, combined with progesterone produced in increasing quantities by the corpus luteum, the endometrial stroma and glands change rapidly. The glands display a secretory pattern, and in time the products of their secretions are discharged. The day-to-day changes in endometrial morphology which occur after ovulation are progressive and predictable. Microscopic examination of the endometrium is useful, therefore, for retrospective diagnosis of ovulation. This endometrial development which occurs in preparation for implantation is easily assessed by endometrial biopsy.

Ultrastructural changes have been observed which are useful in understanding the implantation process. Early, under the influence of estrogen, the microvilli increase in length and number. In addition there is evidence of protein synthesis, indicated by an increase in the number of ribosomes, reflecting increased activity of a number of enzyme systems. The stromal cells of the endometrium take on characteristics classified as a *decidual reaction,* thought to be important in the implantation process. Increases in endometrial histamine, deoxyribonucleic acid (DNA), glycogen, and water content are observed during this deciduation process. Blastocyst implantation can occur only at a discretely timed interval following ovulation, when the endometrium is conditioned to receive the embryo. In the human, implantation occurs between the 5th and 8th postovulatory day. The implantation process itself is preceded by attachment of the trophoblast to the epithelial lining of the endometrium. In the human, the majority of implantations occur in the middle of the posterior wall of the fundus, but they can occur in other places in the uterus. What it is that finally triggers implantation in the human is still unknown. One possibility is that the uterine epithelium produces a substance that activates the blastocyst to implant. Conversely, the endometrium may cease to synthesize a substance that prevents nidation. Another possibility is that the blastocyst somehow promotes a receptivity in the endometrium. The exact sequence of events is not known, but once it is better understood, the clinician will be in a more favorable position to control it. Nearly one-third of postimplantation human embryos exhibit abnormalities which suggest that they were destined to abort, perhaps even before the skipped menstrual period. Such embryonal defects could have occurred as a result of faulty implantation, but they may have been caused earlier in development. A significant number of preimplantation embryos also exhibit abnormalities, and the overall pregnancy wastage is in excess of 50 percent. Such factors as delayed fertilization, which results in the penetration of an ovum that is "overripe," or genetically induced defects in the ovum or spermatozoa have been pointed to to explain the high rate of pregnancy wastage. Continued laboratory studies, coupled with careful clinical observations, will in time lead to a better understanding of these vitally important processes.

REFERENCES

Amerlar RD et al.: *Male Infertility,* Philadelphia: Saunders, 1977.

Croxatto et al.: Studies on the duration of egg transport by the human oviduct: II. Ovum location at various intervals following luteinizing hormone peak. *Amer J Obstet Gynecol* 132:629, 1978.

Greep RO, Koblinsky MA: *Frontiers in Reproduction and Fertility Control, part 2,* Cambridge, Mass.: Ford Foundation, MIT Press, 1977.

_____ et al.: *Reproduction and Human Welfare: A Challenge to Research,* Cambridge, Mass.: Ford Foundation, MIT Press, 1976.

Wallach EW, Kempers RD: *Modern Trends in Infertility and Conception Control,* vol. 1, Baltimore: Williams & Wilkins, 1979.

9

Maternal and Fetal Physiology

PHYSIOLOGIC CHANGES IN THE PREGNANT WOMAN[1]

IRWIN H. KAISER

Pregnancy creates unavoidable requirements for the movement of energy from the environment to the new individual. The mother must transfer the necessary

[1]The authors acknowledge contributions to this chapter by E. F. Greenwald and T. H. Kirschbaum.

metabolites for growth and development to the fetus through the placenta. Women of unusually large size could theoretically mobilize these materials from their own body stores and so conclude pregnancy without an increase in weight. However, for a woman of ordinary stature, weight gain must take place in pregnancy, and there is therefore an increase in caloric requirements.

NUTRITION AND WEIGHT GAIN

It is by no means certain that there is an ideal weight gain for pregnancy. Too many variables are involved. For example, it is known that larger women gain more weight than smaller ones; they also tend to have larger babies. There is increasing evidence that, within limits, the quality of the newborn is related to its size and therefore related to maternal weight gain. This effect is more than the relationship between the duration of pregnancy and the maturity or the weight of the fetus. Several studies have demonstrated that the neonate who is mature both by weight and by dates has a better prognosis than the neonate who is mature by dates alone or by weight alone.

With newborn weight constant, there is a large scatter of weight gains observed among mothers. In an individual woman, the scatter of weight gain from one pregnancy to the next can be greater than the scatter of newborn weights. For a given weight gain there is a scatter of newborn weights. For all these reasons, it is probably fruitless to attempt to state an ideal weight gain in pregnancy. The National Research Council, in its most recent publication on the subject, has suggested approximately 24 pounds. It would be more helpful if recommendations could be worked out for weight gain per unit of prepregnant body weight.

The lifetime nutrition of the mother is also of importance. The studies of Baird and his coworkers in Aberdeen make clear that pregnancy prognosis is related to social class of the woman and also to that of her mother at the time of the mother's pregnancy. Nutrition in childhood and adolescence is presumably also of considerable importance. This is difficult to study in view of the limited social mobility of patients. They tend to be pregnant while remaining in the same social class in which they were brought up. Women in the deprived segments of society have smaller weight gains, smaller babies with a poorer prognosis, and an overall unfavorable prognosis for pregnancy as compared with their advantaged sisters. Nutrition is a major factor. There is, unfortunately, no strong evidence

at the moment that a correction of nutrition will completely undo these effects, although improved diet in pregnancy is probably the most important single item in prenatal care for the general population. In the light of present knowledge, it is wise to recommend a maximal protein diet for all pregnant women, regardless of weight gain.

IRON METABOLISM

Only two items of diet are frequently in short supply in the course of pregnancy; the more important of these is dietary iron (Holly). Normally the losses of iron from the body, other than through bleeding and pregnancy, are trivial. Iron-deficiency anemia is rarely seen in men. Among women the menstrual loss of iron is less than the capacity of the gastrointestinal tract to absorb it from the normal diet by only a small amount. Consequently, any episode of menorrhagia or unusual bleeding at the time of abortion or delivery results in a deficiency state which takes months to correct, if indeed it is corrected at all before the next stress on iron metabolism. Although iron is preferentially transferred to hemoglobin by the bone marrow so long as there is any iron in storage, it is not uncommon for women in the reproductive epoch to remain in a state of chronic iron deficiency and therefore chronic anemia.

The total amount of iron required in pregnancy is about 1.5 g. This requirement includes 500 mg incorporated into the expanded red blood cell mass of the mother, 800 mg principally for fetal blood formation, and 200 mg for normal iron loss in the absence of bleeding. Thus a net absorption of about 6 mg a day is needed for the duration of pregnancy. The requirement is, of course, actually greatest in the third trimester.

Iron is moved across the placenta by active transport into the fetus, which normally is born at term with a hematocrit higher than that of the mother. In addition, the fetus has ample iron stores. If the mother receives no iron during pregnancy, at the end she will have given to the fetus her storage iron and also some of the iron that was in her red cells at the initiation of pregnancy. These facts account for the common observation that the hematocrit and iron storage of pregnant women toward term tends to be substantially lower than it was at the beginning of pregnancy.

The other dietary factor commonly observed to be deficient is folic acid. This deficiency rarely, if ever, occurs among people with normal diets and is also most uncommon outside pregnancy. However, the pregnant state increases the body demand for folic acid, and, with a marginal diet, will result in deficiency. The consequence is megaloblastic anemia of pregnancy, which may coexist in an individual patient with iron-deficiency anemia. It is therefore common practice to administer both folic acid and iron to all pregnant women.

CARDIOVASCULAR CHANGES

It is also necessary for the mother to excrete the waste products from the fetus. This means for the mother a steadily increasing burden of pumping the blood which is the sole transport system for excretion from the fetus across the placenta. The ultimate pathways for all these are the excretory systems of the mother. The metabolic burden consists of the increased mass of the placenta and the uterus and the metabolic activities of these structures and of the fetus.

The most profound maternal changes in pregnancy, other than those related to weight gain of the pregnancy itself, are those which occur in the cardiovascular system (Fig. 9–1). These alter with the increasing size of the pregnancy and the metabolic load imposed for nutrition and excretion.

The blood volume of the mother expands during pregnancy by 30 to 40 percent, with a wide scatter from one woman to the next. In general the increase is proportional to the size of the pregnancy, although there is a greater increase with multiple gestation and with large babies compared with small ones.

The primary increase is that which occurs in plasma volume, a change mediated in large part by hormonal effects. Increases in electrolytes, solutes, and colloids, with the exception of the plasma proteins, tend to be proportional to the expansion of plasma volume. Late in pregnancy, in the absence of any abnormalities of protein synthesis, the proteins are slightly reduced in concentration. There is also a substantial expansion of extracellular, extravascular water, but the concentration of electrolytes and other crystalloid solutes in this water is in full equilibrium with that of intravascular water. Because of these effects, there is a substantial expansion, for example, of exchangeable sodium space, and a marked increase in total body water.

In many of the studies of plasma volume in pregnancy, Evans blue dye (T 1824) has been used. This does not cross the placenta. Since the results were corrected for total body weight, it was noted that plasma volume dropped in the third trimester. Since the T 1824 is not distributed to amniotic fluid or the fetus, this is probably an artifact of the correction fac-

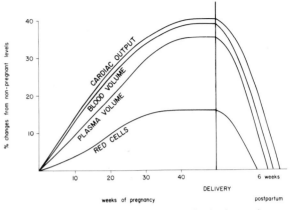

FIGURE 9–1 Changes in cardiac output, blood volume, plasma volume, and red blood cell mass in the course of pregnancy and the puerperium. These are composite curves and represent a consensus of the literature. *(From NS Assali, CR Brinkman: In Pathophysiology of Gestation, vol. 1, ed. NS Assali, by permission of CR Brinkman III and Academic Press.)*

tor. It is more likely that beyond the twenty-eighth week, plasma volume remains about constant. There is a rapid fall in the early puerperium when diuresis takes place. At the same time, there is an increase in red cell mass if iron and protein are available.

ERYTHROPOIETIN

There is an increased concentration of erythropoietin in pregnancy, but it is not certain whether this is a specific effect of pregnancy or a response to a fall in hematocrit. Although the kidney is not the only locus of erythropoietic factor production, the release of an erythrocyte-stimulating factor (ESF) by the kidney in response to a variety of stressful stimuli has been clearly demonstrated. The renal ESF contribution to control of erythropoietic activity is called the renal erythropoietic factor (REF), or erythrogenin. Apparently the major stimulus to the physiologically mandatory increase in red blood cell production during pregnancy, however, is an increased output of REF. There is some evidence that the expansion of red cell mass may also be a response to human chorionic gonadotropin (HCG) and human placental lactogen (HPL). With a very rapid expansion of red cell mass, there is an increase in the proportion of red cells containing hemoglobin F. This must be kept in mind in evaluating smears of maternal blood which are being studied for the presence of fetal red cells due to transfusion from fetus to mother. The highest proportions of red blood cells containing fetal hemoglobin have been observed in patients with hydatidiform mole, where there is no possibility of fetal hemopoiesis.

Hemodilution secondary to volume expansion probably stimulates the release of erythropoietin, much of which is of renal origin. In response to this, red blood cell precursors are committed to maturation and hemoglobin accumulation, with compensatory increase in production and release of mature erythrocytes. During this phase, an elevated reticulocyte count is noted. There has been no documented increase in half-life of erythrocytes during pregnancy. Placental somatomammotropin (HPL) appears to increase the rate of iron incorporation into erythrocytes and may contribute to the rapidity of red blood cell production and hematologic adaptation to the pregnancy state.

Although plasma volume expansion is usually in the range of 50 to 65 percent above nonpregnant values, red blood cell volume increase approximates 33 percent (450 mL). Accordingly, there is a progressive decrease in hemoglobin from a normal in the nonpregnant state of 13.3 g per 100 mL to the average normal in the pregnant state of 12.1 g per 100 mL, reaching its nadir at 32 to 34 weeks. The reason for this incomplete compensation to a nonpregnant hemoglobin level is not clearly understood.

VENOUS PRESSURE

With the movement of the uterus out of the pelvis and up into the abdomen, there is an increase in venous pressure in the lower extremities. This is most marked with the patient supine and the uterus resting against the vena cava. In this position the pressure rise is about 20 cmH$_2$O. It is also present to a considerable degree at any time when the patient is in the erect position. In the lateral recumbent position, this pressure effect vanishes, and venous pressure is equal in the upper and lower extremities. However, pregnant women spend the greatest portion of their time in postures in which the venous pressure in the lower extremity is markedly increased.

Because of the increased venous pressure in the lower extremities, varicose veins already present are likely to become markedly aggravated by pregnancy, and indeed during pregnancy they may become symptomatic and noticeable for the first time in a woman's life. Since an increase in venous pressure in the legs is an inevitable consequence of pregnancy, it is likely that in an individual who is prone to varicose veins, repeated pregnancies will increase symptomatology and actual physical damage.

In addition, it has been well demonstrated that in pregnancy there is an expansion in total volume in both the arms and legs which is principally due to increase in intravascular contents. The increase in the vascular pool is principally venous. This in turn is probably due to an estrogen effect.

When all these effects are combined, accumulation of extracellular water in the lower extremities is almost inevitable. Each leg may accumulate 1 L or more of water during the day, and in many cases in late pregnancy this is identifiable as visible edema. If the patient lies down during the day, and certainly while the patient is recumbent at night, this water is readily mobilized, accounting for a greater urinary volume during the night than during the day. It is also common experience that merely restricting a pregnant woman to bed rest in the last trimester will result in a loss of weight, ordinarily in the vicinity of 2 kg, without the use of any diuretic agents.

CARDIOVASCULAR FUNCTION

There is a slow but steady increase in cardiac output, starting by the fourteenth week, until the maximum value is reached, somewhere between the twenty-eighth and thirty-second week of pregnancy. The increase in cardiac output equals approximately 1.5 L at its maximum; this volume is distributed principally to the uterus but in part to the kidneys. There is a trivial increase in blood flow through the other organs of the pelvis as well.

The increase in cardiac output is accomplished by an increase in pulse rate of approximately 15 beats per minute and an increase in stroke volume of similar degree. The diastolic volume of the heart increases by about 75 mL, equal to the increase in stroke volume.

With the increase in cardiac output and rate, and the rotation of the heart due to elevation of the diaphragm, cardiac murmurs are not uncommon. These usually vary with respiration and are systolic in timing. If it is known that they were not present prior to or early in pregnancy, they can be confidently regarded as transitory and benign.

With the onset of labor, the contractions of the uterus empty the uterine veins into the general circulation, producing an internal transfusion. This results in a rise in cardiac output of a further 30 percent and may be accompanied by modest rises in blood pressure. During the Valsalva maneuvers of the second stage, the cardiac output may rise to 50 percent of resting values.

The maternal blood pressure drops during the second trimester, with a widening of the pulse pressure as well as a lowered systolic. As term approaches, the blood pressure returns toward normal. In labor, with uterine contractions there may be a rise in both pulse rate and blood pressure. Postpartum the blood pressure returns to normal values despite the sudden return of most of the uterine blood content to the general circulation. In labor, with more intense uterine contractions, the cardiac output rises as mentioned. The blood pressure rises as much as 30 mmHg with a contraction, and the pulse rate may increase 10 beats per minute. Supine hypotension is less likely to be noted during active labor.

The circulation time does not change in pregnancy. The electrocardiogram shows changes consistent with deviation of electrical axis to the left by approximately 15°, returning to normal immediately postpartum. No conduction defects are noted.

It has been remarked that several of the changes in cardiovascular function in pregnancy are similar to those experienced with arteriovenous fistulas. This observation has led to the thought that the intervillous space might function as such a communication. Despite the attractiveness of the concept, the intervillous space is not a hollow chamber between arteries and veins. It is solidly packed with villi. Only at the very openings of the endometrial arteries, and in the subchorionic venous lake, are there areas without villi. The mean resistance of the hemochorial placenta is less than that offered by a capillary bed, but nowhere nearly as low as that of an arteriovenous shunt.

PULMONARY FUNCTION

Early in pregnancy there are no significant changes in pulmonary function except that, with the increased basal body temperature, there is a decreased P_{CO_2}, without any change in the pH of pulmonary venous blood.

As the pregnancy enlarges, there is upward movement of the diaphragm and a corresponding change in the axis of the heart. The base of the heart is relatively fixed, but the apex of the ventricles moves to the left and out further toward the midclavicular line. The ribs flare outward, and the thorax tends to increase in its transverse diameter.

All these anatomic changes make possible an increase in tidal volume, partly by a decrease in the inspiratory reserve and in the expiratory reserve, without alteration of the vital capacity (Fig. 9–2). Pulmo-

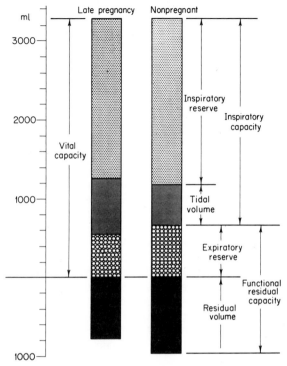

FIGURE 9–2 The components of pulmonary capacity in late pregnancy compared with those of the nonpregnant subject. *(From Hytten and Leitch, by permission of the authors and Blackwell.)*

nary resistance is decreased and airway conductance rises, possibly because of an increased mobility of the thorax. Clearly this set of adjustments helps to provide for the increased oxygen consumption in pregnancy. It may in part be mediated by a direct effect of progesterone on the respiratory center.

Since cardiac output has also risen, there is increased pulmonary blood flow. The time during which the blood is in the pulmonary capillaries is nevertheless sufficient to saturate it fully. The pulmonary venous P_{O_2} remains unchanged with advancing pregnancy.

The maintenance of oxygenation is aided by a small rise in respiratory rate in late pregnancy, perhaps to 22 breaths per minute. This, with the increased tidal volume, increases the minute volume but may also account for the sensation of dyspnea experienced by many pregnant women.

With delivery, these changes reverse rather rapidly. The loss of the uterine mass actually results in a decrease in vital capacity and increased residual volume immediately postpartum, but there is a return to normal within 24 hours.

The basal body temperature returns to normal at about the twentieth week. Since the respiratory changes persist, the P_{CO_2} of the blood remains somewhat reduced.

OROPHARYNX

In the absence of preexisting disease, few oropharyngeal changes are noted that can be considered physiologic. There is, as in many other areas of the body, a generalized hyperemia. Proliferation of interdental papillary blood vessels may be associated with stromal edema and, in the presence of local inflammation, hyperplasia. This results in the commonly noted pregnancy gingivitis, appearing in the second month of gestation and resolving by the ninth month. If a source of localized irritation exists, there may be focal exaggeration of this hypertrophic process with development of a pedunculated or sessile mass, a *pregnancy epulis*. Symptoms related to these disorders include gingival swelling and bleeding, either spontaneous or induced by mastication. An epulis of significant proportions may mechanically interfere with mastication.

Similarly, there may be a vasodilatation in Kiesselbach's area in the nostril, with associated increase in the frequency of nosebleeds in pregnancy.

GASTROINTESTINAL FUNCTION

One of the early signs of pregnancy is nausea and vomiting. Although critical proof is lacking, this is probably a central effect of the elevated estrogen levels of early pregnancy. As pregnancy advances and the uterus rises into the upper abdomen, the incidence of demonstrable hiatus hernia related to the elevation of the diaphragm increases. When pregnant women are subject to esophagoscopy, there is observed an increased incidence of reflux of contents into the lower portion of the esophagus. None of these effects has been correlated in any satisfactory way with the known increase in the incidence of the symptom of heartburn in pregnant women. At present there is no simple treatment, although the complaint is alleviated in most women by the use of an antacid.

As the uterus rises out of the pelvis, the small intestine moves into a more cephalad position in the abdomen. The cecum also rises in the right lateral gutter, and the uterus gradually intrudes between it and the anterior parietal peritoneum. These changes alter the physical findings in acute appendicitis and also the location of the appendix at operation. The sigmoid colon and rectum are not altered in position.

Under the influence of progesterone, the motility of the intestines is slightly reduced, with an increased gastric emptying time and intestinal transit time. There is, however, no symptomatology due to this, except possibly constipation. The gallbladder also loses some motility, and pregnancy therefore increases the likelihood of stone formation. There is no difficulty with defecation, but the increased venous pressure is manifested by an increased protrusion of hemorrhoids.

There are significant alterations in gastrointestinal function and absorption of nutrients in pregnancy, but presently they are not well worked out. With the increase, for example, in transferrin, a response to increased estrogen concentrations, there is an increase in the uptake of iron.

With the onset of labor, there is a relative decrease in bowel function followed by a distention of the gastrointestinal tract immediately postpartum, although this is quite without pathologic significance. Contrariwise, acute gastrointestinal infections which cause markedly increased bowel motility are almost always accompanied by increases in uterine activity, but these episodes do not precipitate labor. For this reason such formerly used techniques for induction of labor as the administration of castor oil and repeated enemas have largely been abandoned.

Liver function is normal in pregnancy. However, a relative decrease in concentration of serum albumin and gamma globulin in the last trimester results in changes in the thymol turbidity and cephalin flocculation tests. The large quantities of steroids of placental origin may complete with hepatic excretion of Bromsulphalein, bile acids, and bilirubin. Bile functions are unchanged, as are those of hepatic alkaline phosphatase, serum glutamic oxaloacetic transaminase (SGOT), and lactate dehydrogenase (DH).

Carbohydrate metabolism is affected by the large amounts of HPL, which raise the free fatty acids and interfere with peripheral utilization of glucose. The plasma insulin rises in response to these stimulating effects on the cells of the islets of Langerhans, and also perhaps to an ability of the placenta to degrade insulin. About 50 percent of fetal energy needs are met by glucose transfer while fasting glucose concentration is slightly depressed. Under these conditions, pregnancy is a stress, and trivial limitations on insulin production may become manifest, premonitory of later clinical diabetes.

GALLBLADDER

The generalized smooth muscle relaxation is probably responsible for the gallbladder hypotonicity often noted during pregnancy. Bile contained within these dilated gallbladders is usually viscous, implying prolonged retention because of delayed emptying of the gallbladder. This and the estrogen-induced alteration in hepatic enzyme activity noted above probably contribute to the propensity for cholelithiasis among women who have experienced several pregnancies.

RENAL SYSTEM

ANATOMIC CHANGES

Hydroureter and some degree of calycectasis are consistently noted in normal pregnancy. The ureter undergoes not only dilatation, almost exclusively above the pelvic brim, but elongation. Because of this increased ureteral length, the pathway of the ureter may be somewhat tortuous. This produces a radiographic appearance of kinks, representing the ureters visualized on end as they bend. There is also frequently some degree of lateral displacement of the ureters by the expanding pelvic organs.

Hydronephrosis of normal pregnancy is related in some degree to the endocrinologic milieu affecting smooth muscle contractility. It is likely that compression of the ureter against the pelvic brim by the expanding uterus also has an effect. Dextrorotation of the uterus may explain the increased incidence of pyelonephritis in the right ureterocalyceal system, which is disproportionately dilated.

Because of ureteral and calyceal dilatation, there is a considerable increase in the dead space of the urinary collecting system. The ureterocalyceal capacity is estimated to be, by the end of gestation, twice that of a nonpregnant female.

URINARY TRACT INFECTIONS

It is likely that the above factors contribute significantly to the relatively high frequency of asymptomatic bacteriuria and pyelonephritis noted in pregnancy. The presence of urinary tract infection may be totally asymptomatic. Indeed, 5 to 6 percent of pregnant women are found to have asymptomatic bacteriuria. About 20 percent of women with asymptomatic bacteriuria will have urinary tract abnormalities demonstrable on intravenous pyelogram. This is probably the same percentage as would be found among any group of patients with symptomatic urinary tract infections. An important point is that the presence of asymptomatic bacteriuria during pregnancy is probably an indication for investigation of the urinary tract by intravenous pyelography after completion of pregnancy. Further, its presence justifies antibiotic administration in an attempt to prevent acute pyelonephritis, to which it predisposes.

All described changes, if benign and totally related to gestation, resolve within 4 to 6 weeks of delivery.

RENAL FUNCTION TESTS

Serum BUN (blood urea nitrogen) and creatinine levels frequently diminish during the latter months of pregnancy. This must be recalled when evaluating renal function in those who are suspected of having renal pathology. A BUN or creatinine value within the upper limits of the nonpregnant norm may represent an elevated value and indicate diminished renal function. Creatinine clearance similarly increases in pregnancy; thus, normal levels may actually represent decreased renal function in pregnancy.

Renin-Angiotensin Mechanism

Clinically, the administration of mercurial and thiazide diuretics initially produces increased glomerular filtration rate (GFR), increased rate of delivery of sodium to the macula densa, and natriuresis. As a result of increased rate of sodium delivery to the macula densa, renin output initially decreases with the use of these diuretics. However, with continued use without repletion of fluid loss, renin levels will subsequently increase because of the renal baroreceptor response to the resulting hypovolemia.

Furosemide and ethacrynic acid consistently produce a rise in renin levels. This apparent contradiction in comparison to thiazide and mercurial effects probably results from the ability of ethacrynic acid and furosemide to inhibit sodium transport across cell membranes, most likely including the membranes of the cells of the macula densa. It is likely that the sodium content of the interstitial fluid surrounding the juxtaglomerular cells actually influences the rate of renin output by these cells. This interstitial fluid arises from the distal convoluted tubular fluid by filtration through the macula densa. Accordingly, if the sodium delivered to the distal convoluted tubule cannot cross the macula densa because of the action of furosemide and ethacrynic acid, the sodium concentration of the interstitial fluid thus produced will be low, resulting in a deceptively low sodium signal to the juxtaglomerular cells. Renin output would thereby be increased in response to therapy with both of these diuretics.

Adrenergic drugs such as epinephrine and levarterenol consistently increase renin release, and this response is enhanced by a state of sodium depletion. Beta-adrenergic stimulation of renin release appears to be mediated by some extrarenal mechanism, possibly by the hemodynamic changes which occur in response to injection of the substances.

The renin-angiotensin mechanism is apparently involved in normal physiologic adjustments in pregnancy and in the pathophysiology of many hypertensive disorders. The initial change in pregnancy is probably related to elevated progesterone levels, which have two effects: (1) natriuresis, producing a mild hyponatremia, and (2) arteriolar vasodilatation, with increased vascular capacity. The hyponatremia results in a decreased rate of sodium delivery to the macula densa, and hypovolemia is detected by the renal baroreceptors. These two factors present potent stimuli for renin production and release to the juxtaglomerular cells. Renin facilitates the conversion of renin substrate to angiotensin I, with subsequent conversion to angiotensin II. In response to angiotensin II, there is an increase in vascular tone, an outpouring of aldosterone from the adrenal cortex, and increased output of antidiuretic hormone from the posterior pituitary. Antidiuretic hormone favors water retention, and salt and water resorption is facilitated by the increased quantities of aldosterone.

The physiologic effects of progesterone, natriuresis, and vasodilatation are compensated by increased vascular tone and retention of salt and water. The net effect is an expanded blood volume and vascular capacity and elevated renin, angiotensin II, aldosterone, and antidiuretic hormone levels (Fig. 9–3).

It is of interest that, in normal pregnancy, in the presence of elevated angiotensin II and aldosterone, there is actually still a state of relative vasodilatation. This reflects a resistance to angiotensin II among pregnant women in that a greater dose is required to achieve an increment in blood pressure than would be effective in the nonpregnant state. The response of the arterioles to the vasoconstrictive effects of epinephrine and norepinephrine is unchanged however. This hyporeactivity to angiotensin II is also observed in other conditions associated with increased renin-angiotensin activity.

KIDNEY FUNCTION

Overall kidney function in pregnancy is considerably altered. There is an increase in renal plasma flow of

FIGURE 9–3 Mechanism of vascular compensation mediated by endocrinologic changes in pregnancy.

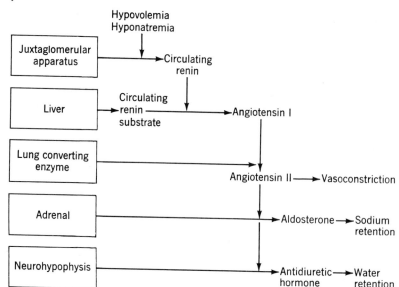

as much as 50 percent by the second trimester. The increase probably persists until term, but is markedly reduced in the dorsal recumbent and erect positions. The GFR increases even more, so that the volume of glomerular filtrate is markedly increased. The efficiency of the tubules, however, is maintained in regard to electrolytes, although there is no increase in Tm for most substances. This fact probably accounts in part for the glycosuria seen in up to 30 percent of women in pregnancy.

The capacity of the system to retain and excrete sodium is maintained, and the kidney responds to diuretic and natriuretic agents in pregnancy. In spite of the high concentration of circulating steroids toward the end of pregnancy, the kidney remains responsive to alterations in aldosterone secretion.

Although most pregnant women have asymptomatic edema at some time during pregnancy, it is remarkable that problems related to disturbed sodium homeostasis do not occur more often in view of the complexity of mechanisms involved in the many humoral and hemodynamic changes that occur. With increased or decreased intake of salt in pregnancy, compensatory adjustments are usually prompt and adequate, although there are some women who tolerate sodium excess or restriction poorly. Because proof of benefit from diuretic therapy is still lacking and risks associated with the use of diuretic agents are many, there are few indications for their use in pregnancy.

As mentioned above, restricting activity of pregnant women toward term results in diuresis and will also result in an increase in the daily excretion of estrogens and other substances which are uniformly distributed in body water.

NEUROLOGIC SYSTEM

Little definitive data is available describing the changes in pregnancy in the central or peripheral nervous system or the supporting structures. No consistent electroencephalographic abnormalities appear in the absence of pathologic conditions, such as toxemia of pregnancy.

Numerous neurologic problems do, however, arise during gestation and have been attributed to any one or a combination of several factors. These factors include (1) fluid accumulation in the central and/or peripheral nervous system or in the supporting structures; (2) nerve-root compression caused by changes in spinal curvature; (3) hypocalcemia result-

ing from the additive effects of multiple factors during pregnancy favoring decreases in serum calcium; and (4) pressure by the enlarging uterus and its contents on pelvic nerves.

FLUID ACCUMULATION

Fluid accumulates in the central nervous system during uncomplicated pregnancy. Numerous complaints of pregnancy are attributed to this phenomenon, including headaches, chorea gravidarum, and the carpal tunnel syndrome. It is felt that carpal tunnel syndrome results from compression of the median nerve in its passage through the carpal tunnel because of fluid accumulation in the transverse carpal ligament.

NERVE-ROOT COMPRESSION

Cervical nerve-root compression theoretically occurs because of exaggerated cervical lordosis and dorsal kyphosis. The increased thoracic kyphotic curvature results from downward traction by the markedly enlarged breasts and in compensation for lumbar lordosis. This, in turn, results from anterior and downward traction of the expanding uterine contents with anterior pelvic rotation. Cervical lordosis compensates for increased thoracic curvature.

Shoulder and arm pain with dysesthesia, exacerbated by head or shoulder movement, usually in the absence of reflex changes, are relatively common complaints. These are attributed to traction or pressure on the brachial plexus nerve roots by the spinal changes noted above.

PELVIC NERVE COMPRESSION

A variety of neurologic changes in the legs are attributed to nerve compression. Dysesthesia in the distribution of the lateral femoral cutaneous nerve is theoretically due to compression of that nerve as it passes beneath the inguinal ligament. Medial thigh sensory deficits with weakness of thigh adduction have been described, starting before or during delivery, probably related to compression of the obturator nerve against the pelvic side wall by the enlarged uterus near term, and occasionally exacerbated by the forces of parturition.

Popliteal nerve injury with foot drop (weakness of dorsiflexion of the toes) is frequently noted 1 or 2 days postpartum. Most are thought to result from compression of this nerve against the head of the fibula by the obstetric stirrups at time of delivery.

HYPOCALCEMIA

True tetany secondary to hypocalcemia is an uncommon phenomenon during pregnancy in the absence of hypoparathyroidism. Serum calcium is noted to decrease somewhat during pregnancy. Essentially, the minimal decrease in serum calcium noted is probably related to the decrease in calcium-binding albumin during pregnancy.

Free, physiologically active calcium is probably present in normal concentrations. Tetany suggests the presence of true pathologic imbalance in calcium metabolism, unrelated to physiologic changes associated with pregnancy.

Correlation between calcium levels and muscular cramps is not reliable. Uncontrolled studies have indicated that ingestion of large quantities of cow's milk (relatively high in phosphorous) may increase the incidence of muscular cramps, which can, subsequently, be relieved by administration of exogenous calcium.

GENERAL CHANGES

SKIN

There is a striking increase in pigmentation of the skin during pregnancy, which does not affect mucous membranes. However, there is a blotchy deposition of brownish pigment over the malar eminences and forehead and over the bridge of the nose, known collectively as *chloasma* (Fig. 9–4). This is clearly a hormonal effect since it can be simulated with oral contraceptives. As noted above, there is an increase in pigmentation of the mammary areolae and the appearance in many women of a darkened line, the linea nigra, which runs from the xiphisternum through the umbilicus and down to the midpoint of the symphysis pubis. It can be quite marked in some patients and barely visible in others. Scars of recent vintage and those incurred during pregnancy become more heavily pigmented, and nevi may increase in pigmentation.

Stretch marks (striae) are also a characteristic of pregnancy. They look like disruptions of the connective tissue of the skin. In some cases the stretch marks have a purplish discoloration. The common sites for these marks are the breasts, buttocks, lower abdomen, and upper thighs. The stretch marks are in part

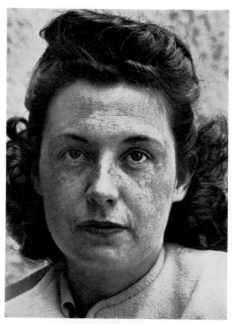

FIGURE 9–4 The characteristic facial pigmentation of pregnancy, known as chloasma, or the mask of pregnancy. It is found prominently on the forehead, the malar eminences, and the bridge of the nose. *(From M Bookmiller and GL Bowen, III; In Textbook of Obstetrics and Obstetric Nursing, Philadelphia: Saunders, 1967, by permission of M. Bookmiller and Saunders.)*

a response to increased deposition of fat in the areas where they occur and concomitant rapid stretching of the skin. They are also clearly hormonal in etiology since almost identical marks are characteristic of Cushing's disease. However, they are not observed when stretching of the abdominal skin occurs with tumors that are not producing hormones. They are more extensive with multiple pregnancies and hydramnios.

In pregnancy there is an increased incidence of spider angiomata, and the clusters of thin-walled, dilated capillaries which are frequently observed on the skin and lower extremities in the absence of pregnancy tend to become more extensive and deeper in color. They regress postpartum but do not disappear entirely.

HAIR GROWTH

In pregnancy there is a tendency to decreased loss of body hair, and in an occasional woman this may mimic hypertrichosis. However, postpartum hair loss is increased for a few months and then reverses once more. The patient can be assured that the hair loss is self limited.

SKELETON

For practical purposes, there are no changes in bony skeleton in pregnancy. It is true that in a woman with repeated pregnancies on a diet strikingly deficient in minerals, the obligatory transfer of calcium and phosphorus to the fetus will eventually result in softening of the bones and the syndrome known as *osteomalacia*. This disease, like severe childhood rickets which can also deform the body pelvis, has now become a medical curiosity.

There is, however, an effect of the bulk of the pregnancy on posture. In most pregnant women it is necessary for the spinal column to assume an increased curvature in the lumbar regions in order to maintain balance. This thrusts the shoulders relatively backwards as compared with the pelvis and accounts for what is called *pregnancy lordosis*. The change, however, is entirely temporary. Although there are trivial changes in the connective tissue structures of the pelvis, the body pelvis does not "soften" in pregnancy nor does it develop any capacity to open. Indeed, full growth of the pelvis in females is ordinarily accomplished and fixed by the time of onset of active menstrual life. The epiphyseal centers on the ischia and ilia, which are not fully closed until the patient is 20 or 21 years old, are nevertheless concerned only with the outside of the pelvis and not with its capacity for childbearing.

HEMATOLOGIC SYSTEM

As was mentioned earlier, there are material changes in the red cell mass in pregnancy. If the supply of iron and protein is sufficient, bone marrow function remains entirely normal, and therefore there are no changes in the morphology of the red blood cells. The familiar indices of size and hemoglobin content remain within normal limits. There is a tendency in pregnancy to a modest increase in the number of white blood cells per cubic millimeter of blood. The reason is not entirely understood, and there is a wide range of variation. However, in the second half of pregnancy the normal white blood cell count of blood is approximately 12,000 per cubic millimeter and may range as high as 15,000 per cubic millimeter. The relative proportion of polymorphonuclear leukocytes and young forms is not changed. This fact can be used to distinguish this gestational change from a genuine leukocytosis. A modest lymphocytopenia may be noted. There are no changes in the relative concentration of platelets despite the changes in blood volume.

The increased concentration of estrogens in pregnancy induces an increase in virtually all the specific transport proteins with a consequent increase in the extent of binding. For example, the concentration of transcortin is substantially increased in pregnancy so that total blood corticoids are materially increased. However, there is only a slight increase in the concentration of free cortisol. The concentration of ceruloplasmin is also markedly increased so that blood plasma of pregnancy ordinarily has a blue to blue-green color when compared with the plasma of nonpregnant women and of men. Interestingly enough, there is sufficient estrogen in the oral contraceptives which were in common use in the 1960s to induce the same blue color in plasma. Transferrin is also increased sufficiently to account for an increase in the uptake of iron from the gastrointestinal tract in pregnancy. This is commonly expressed as plasma iron-binding capacity, and, if an adequate amount of iron in the ferrous state is available in the small bowel, the net absorption of iron per day is thereby increased. It is not unusual to observe an increase in the serum iron concentration during pregnancy, despite the fact that there is active transport of the iron to the fetus across the placenta.

The overall concentration of total plasma proteins does not change materially in normal pregnancy, and there is no noteworthy change in total osmotic pressure. Albumin and gamma globulin fall, while alpha and beta globulins rise. There is an increase in the concentration of specific immune globulins in some patients so that the titer observed in laboratory tests against such antigens as rubella or Rh may undergo an increase in the absence of a specific antigenic stimulus. For this reason, increases in the Coombs titers of Rh antibodies may occur even though the fetus in the pregnancy is Rh-negative. All these antibodies are capable of crossing the placenta, and modest increases in their concentration result in modest increases in the passive immunity conferred upon the fetus by placental transfer.

Fibrinogen increases markedly during pregnancy from the normal nonpregnant concentration of about 350 mg per 100 mL to levels of 650 mg per 100 mL at term. There has been much speculation as to whether this is in any way related to an increased likelihood of thromboembolism in pregnancy or in the puerperium. Factor VII increases from the outset of pregnancy, factors VIII and X rise during the second and third trimesters. Factors IX and II rise in somewhat less than half the pregnant women. Factors V and XII show no change, and factor XIII decreases. The increase in fibrinogen is thought to bring about the marked increase in erythrocyte sedimentation rate.

There are no significant alterations of plasma electrolytes in the course of pregnancy. Concomitant with the elevated temperature of the first half of pregnancy, there is a slight drop in P_{CO_2}, and a corresponding small rise in plasma pH, accompanied by a slight drop in bicarbonate. The latter is compensated for by an equal and slight increase in plasma chloride with no change in the total anions.

In the second half of pregnancy, there is a return of body temperature to normal and continued increase in ventilation which also produces a slight diminution of P_{CO_2} and bicarbonate. However, there are no other changes in the concentration of plasma electrolytes. Since there are accumulations of extracellular water, the amount of exchangeable sodium is increased toward term. This, however, is readily mobilized by changes in posture as mentioned above, and a marked loss of cations, particularly sodium, can readily be induced with the use of saluretics.

REPRODUCTIVE SYSTEM

ALTERATIONS OF REPRODUCTIVE TRACT

The uterus itself undergoes striking enlargement in pregnancy, from nonpregnant weight of less than 100 g to a size between 1.2 and 2 kg in the immediate postpartum state. In the first half of pregnancy, this enlargement is accomplished by an increase in the number of myometrial cells. After the twentieth week, the formation of new cells ceases, and the cells that are present thereafter elongate and hypertrophy, and the thickness of the uterine wall decreases. At term, prior to the onset of labor, the uterine wall is between 4 and 6 mm in thickness, being somewhat thicker at the placental site than elsewhere in the uterus. This growth is only in part occasioned by the distention of the uterus due to the presence of the pregnancy within it since the empty uterus, in the presence of an abdominal pregnancy, also undergoes both growth and hypertrophy. The blood supply of the uterus expands, and the vessels which supply it grow and elongate so that as pregnancy advances, they tend to be somewhat less coiled than in the nonpregnant state. This has the effect of reducing mean peripheral resistance.

Total blood flow to the uterus is 50 mL per minute at 10 weeks, 125 mL per minute at 28 weeks, and 650 mL per minute at term. As stated, there is a great increase in uterine size, so that the flow remains about 12 mL per minute per 100 g of uterus. The maintenance of uterine and hence placental blood flow is critical to the growth and development of the fetus. As mentioned elsewhere, the essential respiratory and excretory substances move by diffusion and hence are flow-limited. Oxygen consumption holds steady at about 1 mL per minute per gram of uterus. With delivery, there is a precipitous drop in oxygen consumption.

The cervix enlarges in pregnancy and has a markedly increased blood supply. Its growth is not nearly as great as that of the muscular portion of the uterus. However, as term approaches and the limits of uterine expansion are approached, the pregnancy tends to expand into the cervix, accomplishing what is ordinarily referred to as *effacement*. The cervical canal becomes shorter, and the connective tissue portion of the cervix blends now indistinguishably into the muscular portion of the wall of the fundus of the uterus above, forming the lower uterine segment. At the same time, the diameter of the cervical canal increases in what is referred to as *dilatation*. With the onset of labor these processes are markedly accelerated. In many patients, effacement of the cervix is completed even before labor begins and only dilatation remains to be accomplished.

The circulatory needs of the cervix are minimal, and there are few, if any, major blood vessels present, particularly in the portion within the vagina which undergoes dilatation in the process of labor. This is in contrast to the active muscle of the body of the uterus which produces the force necessary to dilate the cervix and which has a large blood supply.

The vagina, partly under the influence of increased hormone concentration, undergoes a marked increase in the thickness of the cornified layer of cells and increased activity of the parabasal cells. There is also an increased blood supply so that the vagina toward term tends to have a cyanotic appearance. These changes give the vagina an increased capacity to stretch to accommodate the fetus in its passage from the uterus to the outside without undergoing a laceration. Tears of the vagina, at delivery, ordinarily occur near the introitus where the connective tissue of the urogenital diaphragm and the muscles of the introitus, unchanged for practical purposes by the pregnant state, keep the introitus too small to allow the passage of the term infant without some disruption. This disruption may take place entirely within the levator ani muscles and the endopelvic fascia without involving the mucosa of the vagina or the skin of the introitus. These changes have no important effect on the sphincters of either the urethra or the anus.

OVARIES

In early pregnancy, the ovary is enlarged by the presence of the corpus luteum. When this involutes after the first trimester, the ovaries diminish in size and the corpus luteum may be difficult to find. Since there are no recent follicles, the ovaries appear inactive. They do produce relaxin, whose function is presently unknown.

The surface of the ovaries, and indeed serosal surfaces elsewhere, especially over pelvic viscera, may exhibit friable vascular papillary excrescences. These are the decidual reaction of pregnancy, found either in areas of prior endometriosis or differentiation de novo of serosal cells.

The infundibulopelvic ligaments which include the ovarian vessels enlarge greatly because of the substantial proportion of uterine blood supply which the ovarian vessels supply in the third trimester.

FALLOPIAN TUBES

The fallopian tubes similarly undergo no noteworthy changes during pregnancy. However, the blood vessels of the broad ligament increase immensely in size since they constitute the major portion of the venous drainage of the uterus. Ordinarily this venous drainage goes through the uterine veins into the hypogastric and thence into the internal iliac and common iliac. There may, however, be a substantial increase in the blood vessels of the infundibulopelvic ligament.

BREASTS

The breasts also undergo growth and differentiation during pregnancy, although this varies widely in amount from patient to patient. There is a slow but steady growth in the size and pigmentation of the areolae, and in early pregnancy a substantial growth in the amount of glandular tissue. As the relative amount of progesterone increases, this glandular tissue differentiates, and colostrum begins to be formed. Occasionally the colostrum may leak, and the ability to express some colostrum from the nipple is one of the confirmatory signs of pregnancy. With delivery and the sudden withdrawal of the hormones produced by the placenta, there is a release of prolactin and the beginning of lactation. If sex hormones are administered in adequate amounts, this release is inhibited and lactation is very much reduced in amount. How-

ever, if measures to prevent lactation are not taken and suckling is initiated, as the ducts are emptied, milk formation begins and is ordinarily well established in 2 to 5 days. It is unlikely that the various procedures to prepare the breasts and nipples for lactation are of value.

ASPECTS OF FETAL PHYSIOLOGY

EXCHANGE BETWEEN MOTHER AND FETUS

The substances which undergo transfer across the placenta between fetus and mother can be considered under five major headings, each of which has its particular physical and biological characteristics.

(1) Materials concerned with rapid biochemical homeostasis, i.e., the blood gases and electrolytes, cross the placenta with extraordinary speed. For practical purposes they are not bound by colloids and at the exact site of exchange probably approach equilibrium by diffusion, with the gradient being accounted for entirely by the distance for diffusion between maternal blood in the intervillous space and fetal blood in fetal capillaries. It is not practical to obtain specimens at these points and prove that this close approach to equality exists. However, from observations made in other species with different types of placentas and from occasional experiments which can be carried out in human beings, this appears to be a reasonable explanation for exchange of these materials.

(2) Substances concerned with fetal nutrition probably also move with considerable rapidity. Some proteins are small enough to cross the placenta easily, but the major sources for the fetus are carbohydrates and amino acids. These are large molecules, and active or facilitated transfer is involved for some. Vitamin C is routinely observed to be materially higher in fetal blood than in maternal.

(3) The endocrine status of the fetus is dealt with in detail in a later section of this chapter. However, most hormones are effectively present in the placenta only in bound form, and movement is therefore not particularly rapid. Small amounts of estrogen can be effectively introduced from the placenta into the fetus so that minor hyperplastic changes in the breasts are observed in male and female newborn. On the other hand, this kind of transfer is not sufficient to block the

activity of the inducing substances responsible for male differentiation of the urogenital sinus or the descent of the testes.

A most interesting problem of hormonal transfer is observed in the occasional mother who goes through pregnancy with a parathyroid adenoma. Because there is a tendency in pregnancy to more ready mobilization of exchangeable calcium, the presence of a parathyroid adenoma may be extraordinarily difficult to prove in the pregnant state. However, minor excesses of levels of parathyroid hormone may suppress the activity of the fetal parathyroid. In the immediate newborn state this may result in hypocalcemic tetany at the end of the first week of life. Some cases of parathyroid adenoma in the mother have been detected as a result of the investigation of this alteration of calcium metabolism in the newborn.

The prolongation of pregnancy with anencephalic fetuses who are lacking a hypothalamus and pituitary suggests that fetal hormonal production may contribute to the initiation of labor. Much work is needed in this field.

(4) Antigens and antibodies cross the placenta in a number of forms. Most of them do so relatively slowly because they are relatively large molecules. The smaller immune globulins, for example, are close to equality in the steady state. As is mentioned below, a substantial number of potentially toxic substances also cross the placenta. Many of them, particularly the small unchanged molecules, move with great rapidity. Examples of the latter are many of the drugs that are used for pain relief in labor.

(5) Finally, it is now known that both viruses and bacteria can cross the placenta, although the mechanism is not the same. Some of the virus particles are sufficiently small to pass the placenta without, in the strict sense, infecting the placenta itself. Newborns have been observed with poliomyelitis, rubella, variola, varicella, herpes, and cytomegalic inclusion disease, among others.

It is not absolutely clear whether bacteria can pass the placenta without first infecting it. This is not, however, transfer in the strict sense. Protozoan infestations and malignant disease are effectively filtered out by the placenta. When the placenta itself becomes the site of disease, secondary spread into the fetus can take place. Rare as it is, this has been observed most frequently with malignant melanoma.

Occasional instances of fetal malaria have been demonstrated, and toxoplasma can also pass the barrier.

BLOOD FLOW AT THE PLACENTA

Blood arrives at the maternal intervillous space of the placenta through branches of the uterine artery (Fig. 9–5). These penetrate the muscular wall of the uterus in a somewhat undulating but not coiled manner and then penetrate at the placental site where they open directly into the intervillous space without any intervening capillary bed. There are radial branches to the myometrium which provide myometrial perfusion, but the major flow to the uterus proceeds to the intervillous space. This is entirely lined by endothelium of fetal origin. There is evidence that these cells can also enter the maternal blood vessels at the placental site and line these vessels for short distances.

Blood flow leaves the open ends of the endometrial arteries in spurts or fountains directed by the force of maternal blood pressure which has a mean value of about 70 mmHg at the tips of the arteries. The blood is forced in the direction of the chorionic plate through the complex baffle provided by the presence of numerous branching villi in the intervillous space. Injection studies have demonstrated that the blood, coming out initially as a spurt, diffuses rapidly and peripherally through this space. Small volumes accumulate directly under the chorion where there is a relative deficiency of villi and therefore more actual space. Flow is then in the direction of the distended mouths of the uterine veins emptying through the uterine wall into the larger collecting uterine veins. These drain into the internal hypogastric vein and thence into the iliacs, and a fraction of the venous drainage goes through the ovarian veins directly into the vena cava and left renal vein.

Since this placental circulation is within the uterus, it is subject to alterations in a flow related to uterine contractions. With the initiation of a contraction, there is interference of venous drainage, and the placenta acts somewhat like an erectile structure, since arterial inflow persists after venous drainage is cut off. Studies of this have been carried out most extensively in the macaque, but there is corroborative evidence from placental angiograms obtained in the human being. When intrauterine pressures exceed arterial, afferent flow is interfered with and circulation may cease. Simultaneously, the veins in the myometrium are likely to empty into the maternal circulation so that even though there may be some entrapment of blood at the placental site, there is a net emptying of blood from the uterus into the mother's general circulation. The net increase of maternal blood flow through the uterus at term is probably of the order of 650 mL per minute, and the greatest bulk of this,

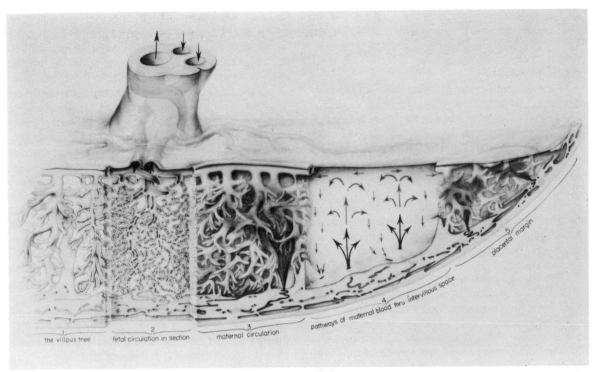

FIGURE 9-5 A composite, idealized drawing of the placenta at term to illustrate fetal and maternal circulations. Fetal blood enters through the umbilical arteries (small arrows at the transverse section of the umbilical cord). These arteries spread on the fetal surface of the placenta and are then distributed to and into each cotyledon. As shown in 1 and 2, they branch into the villous tree and then traverse the capillaries of the villi. The veins then eventually coalesce to form the single umbilical vein which returns blood to the fetus. The maternal placental circulation (3, 4, and 5) begins in the arterial jets of blood which leave the endometrial arteries at the base of each cotyledon. The blood diffuses into the space among the villi and then returns to the veins at the placental site, having traversed the intervillous space rather than a capillary bed. Exchange takes place across the villous tissues between the blood in the intervillous space and that in the villous capillaries. *(Drawing by Ranice W. Crosby, prepared for Elizabeth M. Ramsey, reproduced with their permission and that of the Carnegie Institution of Washington.)*

probably 500 mL per minute, is directed to the intervillous space. However, the volume of any intervillous space at any given moment is probably no more than 250 or 300 mL. Thus, when a uterine contraction occurs, there can be an internal transfusion of approximately 400 mL of blood from the uterus into the general circulation, most of it from myometrial vessels. This transfusion is reflected by a transient increase in cardiac output and blood pressure. Such increases in blood pressure and cardiac output also occur as part of the response to the pain of uterine contraction.

Many efforts have been made to analyze the factors which control maternal blood flow to the placenta, and the present state of our knowledge is somewhat unsatisfactory. It is quite clear that the larger the placenta, the greater the flow—and the larger the baby, the larger the placenta. It is, however, not apparent which is cause and which is effect. It is also clear that multiple pregnancies are associated with materially larger flows and of course, larger volumes of fetus and placenta. Conversely, chronic vascular disease, malnutrition, both acute and chronic, and advanced renal insufficiency are known to be associated with retarded intrauterine development of both the fetus and the placenta. In some diabetic pregnancies, it is possible to correlate growth retardation with evidence of arteriosclerosis of the uterine artery. There are then evidently both fetal and maternal effects and some alterations unquestionably related to nutrition. The evidence is clear that babies born to cigarette smokers are smaller than babies born to women who do not smoke. It is apparent that environmental effects can indirectly or directly have an effect on uterine flow.

During the supine hypotensive syndrome, blood flow through the uterus is diminished. Indeed, some anesthesiologists now recommend a 10 to 15° rotation out of the dorsal recumbent position at the time of abdominal delivery.

Another acute cardiovascular effect which is occasionally observed in the dorsal recumbent position is a marked drop in blood pressure in the femoral arteries coincident with uterine contractions. This is believed to be due to the fact that the contracted uterus interferes with flow in the aorta. Presumably this same interference is taking place in the uterine arteries. Change in position will alter this effect.

Intense vasodilators and other substances which are strikingly inhibitory of uterine contractility, such as halogenated hydrocarbons, can produce an increase in uterine flow, probably by reducing uterine tone.

The basic functional unit of the placenta is the cotyledon which consists of the vascular structures found in the field of distribution of blood from a single endometrial artery. The number of such cotyledons from a functional standpoint in the human placenta has been studied only with difficulty because of the necessity of using radiographic techniques that administer relatively high radiation doses to the fetus. It is, however, thought that for the normal-term pregnancy the number of cotyledons varies from 30 to 45. Because of the way in which the placenta develops, this number probably does not increase during pregnancy and may in fact decrease somewhat through the loss of individual cotyledonary units by intervillous fibrin deposition. All the units are not functioning at any given time. Nothing is known about the local control of this phenomenon, but it is possible to demonstrate in laboratory primates that individual cotyledons come in and out of function. This has been referred to as the *shunting effect* and is consistent with what is known about the rather considerable reserve capacity for placental function of the primate placenta.

FETAL CIRCULATION IN THE PLACENTA

Fetal placental circulation is schematically much simpler than that on the maternal side (Fig. 9–6). Blood leaves the fetus through the umbilical arteries in the umbilical cord and reaches the surface of the placenta, where the arteries divide until at least one main branch goes to each cotyledon. Within the coty-

ledonary units there are further branchings into each of the main stem villi. Within the villous substance the arteries divide into villous capillaries. These capillaries course through the villi, reaching the surface of the villi where they are covered by the very thin layer of cells of the syncytiotrophoblast and its basement membrane. The diffusion distance between maternal and fetal circulations is quite small. The capillaries then return up the villous trunks to form the fetal placental veins which gradually unite into the single umbilical vein returning to the fetus.

It has been thought for many years that there are arteriovenous shunts in the fetal circulation. Unfortunately, although the anatomic evidence for these shunts is reasonably good, there is no physiologic evidence of their existence nor any obvious system whereby they might be controlled. There has also been argument about the presence of nerves which might regulate the caliber of vessels in the umbilical cord, but no one has gone so far as to suggest the presence of any nervous control of the branching vessels on the surface of the placenta or in the villi. At present, it can only be stated that if arteriovenous shunts are present, and if they are endowed with intrinsic chemo- or baroreceptors, they might have something to do with the regulation of flow through the cotyledons or through individual main stem villi.

There is also no evidence of intermittent functioning of cotyledons on the fetal side of the placenta of the sort that has been observed on the maternal side.

It seems clear that another potential mechanism for increasing flow through villi is vasodilatation. However, direct physiologic evidence is not at hand. It appears that in the present state of our knowledge, the only way the fetus can increase flow through the placenta is to increase its cardiac rate while maintaining stroke volume. Unless there is some system for reducing mean resistance across the placenta, this necessarily invokes a considerable increase in the work of the heart.

PLACENTAL GAS EXCHANGE

Fetal hemopoiesis begins on about the 22d day after fertilization. The earliest fetal red cells carry Gower hemoglobin, which is present only for a short period of time. The primitive centers of hemopoiesis which are associated with the earliest developing blood vessel eventually vanish except for those located in the liver and the bone marrow. Once a recognizable fetus is present, the fetal red cells come to contain

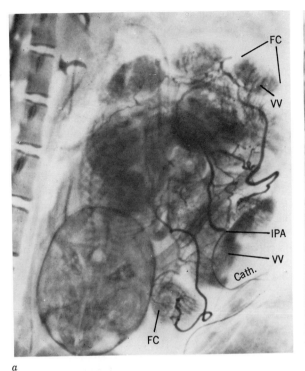
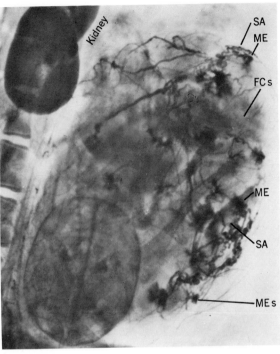

a   *b*

FIGURE 9–6 Spot films made during a combined fetal and maternal injection study in *Macaca mulatta*, to illustrate blood vessel patterns. The animal is 152 days pregnant (term being about 167 days). *A* was obtained 3 s after injection into an interplacental (fetal) artery. *B* was obtained 2 s after injection into the mother. *FC*, fetal cotyledon. *FCs*, fetal cotyledon without corresponding maternal artery. *IPA*, interplacental artery. *ME*, maternal arterial entry spurt. *MEs*, maternal entry with associated cotyledon; *SA*, endometrial spiral artery. *VV*, villous vessels. *(Courtesy of Elizabeth M. Ramsey.)*

hemoglobin F, and this fetal hemoglobin, of course, begins to be replaced as term approaches by adult hemoglobin.

Fetal blood, however, at all times manifests greater affinity for oxygen than adult blood at equal pH and P_{CO_2}. This results, under physiologic conditions, in a more acutely inflected hemoglobin dissociation curve (Fig. 9–7). The consequence is that, at the placenta where pH rises and carbon dioxide pressure drops rapidly, affinity of the fetal blood for oxygen increases rather strikingly; at the tissues where the pH is substantially lower than it is in the adult, oxygen unloading and carbon dioxide uptake are correspondingly enhanced. At the placenta itself, at the precise point of exchange of gases, the differences in the partial pressures of the gases between the bloods are probably minimal. The experience with intrauterine transfusion in babies suffering from erythroblastosis has conclusively demonstrated that hemoglobin F is not essential to fetal life. In some of these babies there has been 96 percent replacement of fetal blood with donor blood. Aside from the severely adverse in-

fluences of the hemolytic process itself, the fact that the fetus has adult red cells does not seem to affect its capacity to survive. There do not seem to be any special biochemical mechanisms operating in utero to achieve fetal oxygenation.

The hemoglobin content of fetal blood in the human being at term is ordinarily substantially higher than that of the mother so that the oxygen capacity per milliliter is strikingly increased. Under these circumstances, although the oxygen saturation of fetal blood, even in the umbilical vein, probably never exceeds 70 percent and probably never has an oxygen pressure of higher than 45 mmHg, the oxygen content of umbilical vein blood is quite sufficient to meet the metabolic needs of the fetus. The blood itself is cyanotic since there is ordinarily more than 6 g of unsaturated hemoglobin.

The P_{CO_2} of umbilical vein blood is ordinarily above 44 mmHg, and the pH is 7.32. This is descriptive of respiratory acidosis, but since exchange at the placenta is adequate, it imposes no stress on the fetus. However, when there is interference with ex-

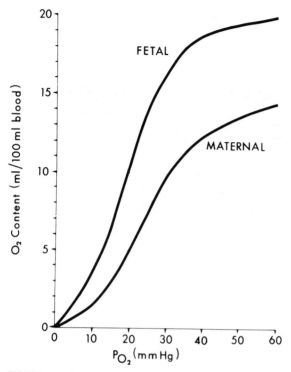

FIGURE 9–7 Relationship of oxygen content in milliliters per 100 milliliters of blood to the partial pressure of oxygen, for maternal and fetal blood. Oxygen capacities of 12 and 16 g/mL, respectively, are assumed. *(From LD Longo: In Pathophysiology of Gestation, vol. 2, ed. WS Assali, by permission of LD Longo and Academic Press.)*

change, as in pathologic states, or with abnormalities of labor, metabolic acidosis may be added, and the fetus has only limited capacity to compensate for this. As has been stated, we do not know that the fetus can achieve any sizable increase in placental flow, nor is there evidence of a feedback from the distressed fetus which would cause an improvement of flow on the maternal side.

The buffer systems of the fetus are not unique. The high hemoglobin is a major asset, and it appears that the P_{co_2} can rise very high without poisoning respiratory exchange at the placenta. Fetal red cells are deficient in carbonic anhydrase, but this is evidently not physiologically significant.

Gross water exchange between the products of conception and the mother exceeds 4 L per hour at term, while the net exchange is about 1.5 mL per hour (Fig. 9–8). The largest proportion moves across the placenta. There is some exchange of water directly between the amniotic fluid and the fetus itself and the mother. Fetal urine makes a small contribution, and it is now established that fluid indeed moves in and out

of the fetal respiratory tract. There is also evidence of movement of amniotic fluid directly from the umbilical cord.

The relationships among these compartments is necessarily complex, and the known facts are limited. Renal agenesis always is associated with marked reduction in fluid volume. Severe erythroblastosis and hypoproteinemia, and other rare causes of fetal cardiac failure, are accompanied by increased volume. Obstructions of the upper gastrointestinal tract also result in polyhydramnios, as do anomalies such as anencephaly which restrict fetal swallowing. Polyhydramnios is more common in diabetic and multiple pregnancy. It must be remembered that only small net increases in water movement can rapidly result in significant extremes of fluid volume. Polyhydramnios is considered to be present when volume exceeds 2 L. Occasionally it is present without any demonstrable explanation.

FETAL NUTRITION

As was stated above, glucose and amino acids cross the placenta with considerable efficiency. Free fatty acids and some proteins cross the placenta more slowly. However, since these substances all pass, for practical purposes, by diffusion and since they are present in ample amounts in the mother's blood except in the presence of advanced maternal disease, the fetus receives enough of what it needs for protein synthesis and the formation of complex organic molecules such as fats and steroids.

Certain substances move across the placenta preferentially. Among these are iron and ascorbic acid. Once again, it appears that the limiting factor on fetal nutrition, except in extremely pathologic circumstances, is placental blood flow.

THE PHYSIOLOGY OF PARTURITION

HAROLD SCHULMAN

When the question is asked, "What initiates labor?" the natural response is to think in terms of a substance which starts the event. The onset of labor, however, should be viewed in quite another perspective. The pregnant uterus has the ability to expel its contents at any time because it is a contractile organ, but

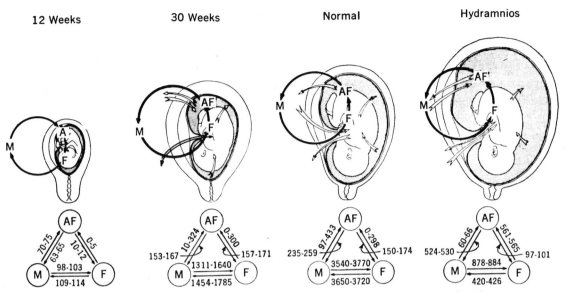

FIGURE 9–8 Schematic representation of the water exchange among mother, *M*, fetus, *F*, and amniotic fluid, *AF*, in normal and pathologic pregnancy. The arrows in the lower, triangular diagrams indicate the direction; the values are in mL per hour. The heavy circles in the upper diagrams designate the net transfer or the circulation of the water. *(From DL Hutchinson et al.: J Clin Invest, 38:971, by permission of the authors and Rockefeller University Press.)*

it is suppressed or inhibited from performing at its effective working potential. The onset of labor should be perceived as a process in which there is a gradual release of inhibition rather than the appearance of a new substance or a new process which triggers the event.

THE UTERUS

The uterus is a hollow organ whose wall contains smooth muscle fibers arranged into an external longitudinal layer and an inner circular layer. No clear structural division exists between these two layers since they interlace to form a meshwork. The arrangement of the smooth muscle bundles in the uterus is similar to that seen in other visceral smooth muscle such as intestine and ureter. A vascular layer lies between the two layers, creating a situation in which the muscle fibers can function as tourniquets around the blood vessels and produce hemostasis without the need for coagulation.

Individual myometrial cells are embedded in a collagen matrix. During pregnancy myometrial fibers increase markedly in number, and in the corpus the smooth muscle content increases three times as much as collagen. The cervix contains less than 10 percent of the muscle fibers, and is composed primarily of collagen and connective tissue.

During the first half of pregnancy the uterus undergoes muscular hyperplasia, but during the second half the principal change is that of hypertrophy. The individual myometrial fiber length increases from 50 to 100 μm to 500 to 800 μm. On the basis of an estimated uterine mass of 880 g at term, there are approximately 200 billion muscle cells. The average pregnant myometrial cell diameter is only 5 to 10 μm, making it difficult to prepare for electrophysiologic studies.

SMOOTH MUSCLE—NATURE AND BEHAVIOR

Muscle fibers are composed of four major proteins: myosin, actin, tropomyosin, and troponin. These proteins have a specific spatial arrangement common to all muscle cells. Myosin molecules are arranged into large bundles which are thick filaments. Each myosin molecule is a long rod with a blunt double head at one end which protrudes perpendicular to the long axis of the bundle of rods (Murray, Weber).

Thin filaments are strands of actin, which are spheroidal molecules linked to form a double helix. Tropomyosin is a long, thin molecule that sits on the string of actins alongside each groove of the double helix. A globular troponin molecule is attached to one end of the tropomyosin strand. Each tropomyosin-troponin complex covers eight actin molecules. Shortening of a muscle fiber occurs when thin filaments are propelled past thick filaments. This occurs when activated myosin complexes attach to activated thin filaments via the troponin molecule and move the entire filament about 100 Å. This process requires calcium and chemical energy, provided by adenosine triphosphate (ATP). Smooth muscle differs from striated muscle in that protein structures called Z lines are lacking. Thin filaments attached to Z lines cause the striated appearance and produce an orderly arrangement of thin and thick filaments. Smooth muscle lacks such regimentation. The filaments are regularly spaced from side to side, but they do not lie in columns. The ends are staggered.

In order for the contractile process to be turned on, depolarization of the myometrial cell membrane must occur. Depolarization is characterized by an influx of sodium and an efflux of potassium from the cell. The resultant depolarization (negative to positive) triggers the release of calcium from sacs within the sarcoplasmic reticulum, which activates the thin filaments; if ATP is present, myosin heads will attach to troponin and produce muscle shortening.

The primary stimulus for uterine growth is 17β-estradiol, but stretch in itself will also create myometrial hypertrophy. The uterine concentration of actin and myosin is similar to other smooth muscle and therefore less than that seen in skeletal muscle.

Electrophysiology

The electromechanical behavior of smooth muscle differs from that of skeletal and cardiac muscle. In skeletal muscle a sharp action potential, created by acetylcholine release at the myoneural junction, leads to muscle tension. Cardiac muscle differs in that there is a prolonged repolarization phase of the action potential, but tension occurs with one spike. Smooth muscle electrical activity is unique in that there are spontaneous recurrent action potentials, and tension occurs only when these discharges are bunched together or synchronous (Csapo, 1973).

Methodology for smooth muscle investigation is more difficult because of the small diameter of the cell. Further, there is no agreement regarding the myometrial changes induced by pregnancy. It would appear, however, from data obtained in the rabbit and cat uterus that electrical activity is suppressed, localized, and asynchronic. This suppression seems most pronounced in the myometrium overlying the placenta, and the different uterine regions do not function in concert (Daniel, Renner). Mechanical activity is negligible when the electrical activity is random and nonsynchronous. As labor approaches, there is a spontaneous evolution of electrical and mechanical activity. The action potentials are grouped together, creating an increase in the amplitude of uterine contractions. However, until labor begins, this procession of action potentials remains nonpropagating, and different portions of the uterus show asynchronous activity. When labor begins, the electrical activity becomes synchronous and propagating, leading to smooth, frequent, large intrauterine pressure cycles.

The resting potential of a muscle cell is of interest as an estimate of the energy requirements needed to depolarize the cell. The membrane potential of skeletal and cardiac muscle is −90 mV, while in the nonpregnant uterus it is approximately −40 mV. In the pregnant uterus, the potential changes to approximately −60 mV, thereby making it less responsive to external stimuli. In general, the estrogen-dominated myometrium has a lower membrane potential than does the progesterone-dominated. Estrogen creates an excitatory state, but progesterone produces inhibition. In the rabbit, measurements of resting potential over placental and nonplacental myometrium demonstrate that the former has a higher level, implying a direct inhibitory effect of the placenta.

Current membrane theory holds that the transmembrane potential is primarily dependent upon the intracellular and extracellular concentrations of potassium, sodium, and chloride. Depolarization is characterized by a change from a negative to positive potential, an efflux of potassium, and an influx of sodium. General agreement is lacking concerning intra- and extracellular concentrations of Na^+, K^+, and Cl^- in pregnant and nonpregnant myometrium, nor is there agreement regarding the effects of progesterone on the movement of potassium in myometrium.

It has been estimated that a propagated impulse travels across the uterus at a velocity of 5 to 60 mm per second. There is not complete understanding of how electrical excitation is transmitted between smooth muscle cells. Some believe that transmission is carried out through gap junctions, areas of the cell where membranes come in contact with adjacent cells. It is possible that these junctions offer low resistance to current flow. Others believe that the extracellular fluid plays a key role. Progesterone-dominated myometrium has a higher stimulation threshold and does not propagate impulses freely throughout a muscle bundle. Uterine contractions which are ineffective show nonsynchronous, nonpropagating electrical activity, and this may be etiologic in some cases of dysfunctional labors.

Mechanical Properties

The work of A. V. Hill suggests that a muscle fiber contains elastic elements in series and in parallel to the contractile elements, and that there are also viscous damping factors. When a fiber is stimulated, the contractile elements must first stretch the elastic elements. Their actions combined with the damping effect of the viscous elements are so large that the peak tension in a contraction is considerably less than the force actually developed in the fiber. If the fiber is quickly stretched before stimulation, a higher tension will be achieved. Myometrial cells underlying the placenta can be viewed as elastic elements which dissipate the contractile forces of the remainder of the uterus. As pregnancy progresses, there is hypertrophy and stretch of the uterus and the relative proportion of nonplacental myometrium increases to the point that it can overcome the resistance provided by placental myometrium. Smooth muscle is unique in that with stretch, the increased tension is transient and followed by an active relaxation or accommodation process. Prostaglandin $F_{2\alpha}$ can prevent active relaxation, the only known substance to do this.

Pregnancy increases the distensibility of the myometrium. Maximum tension is reached over a wider range of lengths expressed as a percentage of resting lengths. The latter relates optimal lengths and maximum tension. In midpregnancy the myometrium is 80 percent of the resting or optimal length, but as pregnancy advances, it approaches the resting length. Smooth muscle also obeys Starling's law in that tension decreases if the muscle is stretched beyond an optimal length. Experimental evidence suggests that these myometrial changes are produced by estrogen, progesterone, and myometrial hypertrophy induced by increasing uterine volume.

Increasing uterine size during the second half of pregnancy is characterized primarily by hypertrophy or stretch of the myometrial muscle fibers. Increase in uterine volume is secondary to the growth of fetus and placenta and the secretion of amniotic fluid. Both fetal growth and amniotic fluid volume increase at a linear rate in the second half of pregnancy, but placental growth occurs at a much slower rate. Therefore, as pregnancy progresses, there is proportionately less myometrium overlying the placenta, which is the area of the uterus demonstrating the least amount of electrical activity. Experimental increase of uterine volume leads to increasing uterine active pressure, and

a point can be reached when the activity will diminish, thereby obeying the length-tension behavior of in vitro muscle bundles. Stretch is a potent stimulus to smooth muscle activity, as we commonly note in bladder and bowel function.

Other physical principles are involved and determine the ability to observe and study clinical labor. Measurement of intrauterine pressure during pregnancy can be carried out in several ways. One is to insert an open-ended fluid-filled catheter into the uterus via a transabdominal needle puncture. The open end of the catheter then is in free contact with the fluid in a closed amniotic sac, and Pascal's principle can be invoked: pressure is transmitted equally in all directions. The hub of the catheter is attached to a pressure-sensitive device such as electronic transducer, and a continuous recording of intrauterine pressure can be carried out (Schulman, Romney). During labor, catheters are frequently inserted through the cervix around the fetal head for an estimate of uterine activity. These measurements and observations are useful, but since the amniotic sac must be ruptured to insert the catheter, we are no longer dealing with a closed fluid-filled space. Frequently, good recordings can be obtained by this method because the fetal head effectively seals off the cervical opening, thereby producing a closed intrauterine space. Clinical situations in which there is poor application of the fetal presenting part to the cervix, such as in breeches or twins, will in general yield poor contraction tracings by the transcervical technique. Another method which works very well is the insertion of a small balloon-tipped catheter through the cervix and between the membranes and the uterine wall. This is called the extraovular technique, and it produces tracings indistinguishable from the transabdominal method with intact membranes.

Intrauterine pressure is dependent upon the myometrial tension and thickness and inversely related to the radius. These equations are derived from surface tension principles in which force (or pressure) times length (or volume) equals tension. When discussed in terms of a sphere, it is often credited to Laplace, and it can be written $P = Tw/R$, where P = pressure, T = tension, w = wall thickness, and R = radius. This equation states that if wall tension is increased either by increasing the thickness or changing the composition, for example, with more collagen elements than elastic, the pressure should be increased. When the active pressures are increased with oxytocin (all muscle fibers being mobilized) and in grand multiparity (more relative collagen), they exemplify changing wall tension without change in radius. Midtrimester

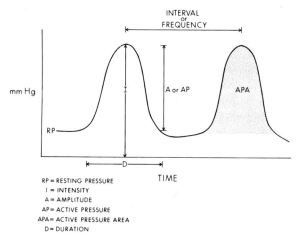

RP = RESTING PRESSURE
I = INTENSITY
A = AMPLITUDE
AP = ACTIVE PRESSURE
APA = ACTIVE PRESSURE AREA
D = DURATION

FIGURE 9–9 Idealized graph of uterine contractile waves and commonly used nomenclature to describe and measure these curves.

uteri (therefore smaller radius) during labor generate higher maximum active pressures than term-pregnant uteri, thereby demonstrating the effect of R on P.

Various methods and nomenclature have been devised to describe uterine contractions, and as yet there is no agreement. Several parameters of the pressure curve can be described (Fig. 9–9). Resting pressure implies the tension of the uterus between contractions. Many authors refer to this as *tonus* which has no specific physiologic meaning or definition. Most quantitative studies have been carried out by measuring (1) all contractions for intensity or amplitude, duration, and frequency; (2) Montevideo units which equal amplitude times frequency per 10-min area; and (3) active pressure area under each pressure curve per 30-min period. When contractions are recorded on magnetic tape, a computer can perform the above computations. The computer and hand measurements agree closely for intensity, frequency, and amplitude but not for active pressure area. Mathematically, active pressure area should be more accurate than Montevideo units (Vasicka, Kretchmer).

Clinical labor is characterized by 100 to 250 Montevideo units, or 8 to 15.6 cm² per 30-minute active pressure area. The latter measurements are made with a paper speed of 1 cm per minute.

THE CERVIX

Since the ultimate effect of uterine contractions is to dilate the cervix, the mechanical behavior of this structure should be analyzed. The cervix is composed primarily of collagen and elastic tissue. To-

ward the end of pregnancy, the cervix softens, usually dilates, and becomes thinner. The causes of these changes are presumed to be hormonal, and possibly mechanical. When labor begins, the woman experiences irregular intermittent painful contractions which produce progressive thinning of the cervix but little additional dilatation of the cervix. When the dilatation reaches 3 to 4 cm in diameter, the cervix abruptly begins to dilate at a rate of 2 to 3 cm per hour until complete dilatation is reached at 10 cm. Length-tension relationships have not been investigated directly, but they have been measured in aorta which is primarily elastic and collagen tissue. These curves very closely resemble cervical dilatation curves during normal labor. For example, as the tissue is being stretched, the tension increases slowly until a small increase in length produces a large increase in tension. Further increase in length produces a blowout phenomenon, e.g., the tension decreases despite increasing length. It has been observed that the cervix feels tense or relatively rigid in the latent phase of labor, but is relatively flexible in the active phase. It can be postulated that the cervix becomes so thin during latent-phase labor that it reaches maximum tension, and then simply gives way as the uterus continues its relentless contractions. Studies in the monkey demonstrated that the primary phenomenon in cervical dilatation was progressive thinning and dilatation rather than cervical retraction.

PHARMACOLOGY

It is generally agreed that the autonomic nervous system does not play a role in the initiation of labor, but uterine activity can be modified by autonomic drugs.

The uterus reacts to both alpha- and beta-adrenergic stimulants, and there are species variations. Beta-adrenergic drugs promote inhibition of uterine contractions. Epinephrine (Adrenalin) acts primarily upon myometrial beta receptors. Isoxsuprine stimulates beta receptors only and has been used clinically in doses of 50 to 250 μg per minute intravenously in an effort to stop premature labor. Propranolol, an inhibitor of beta-adrenergic receptors, leads to increased uterine contractility, and chronic ingestion may lead to reduced uterine blood flow and fetal growth retardation.

Many drugs and gases have a direct inhibitory effect on myometrium. In this category are magnesium sulfate, ethyl alcohol, halothane, chloroform, ether, papaverine, diazoxide, ritodrine, bile salts, and progesterone. Sedatives such as morphine, meperidine, and phenobarbital may decrease uterine activity (but not labor) via a central-nervous-system mechanism in which anxiety is allayed and endogenous secretion of norepinephrine and acetylcholine is diminished.

Uterine activity is stimulated by oxytocin, vasopressin, prostaglandins, amine alkaloids such as ergonovine, sparteine sulfate, norepinephrine, acetylcholine, and estrogen. The intravenous administration of fat emulsion will initiate abortion or labor, but its mechanism of action is unknown. The active product in the fat emulsion is a phospholipid. Another drug, pargyline hydrochloride, a monoamine oxidase inhibitor, when injected into the amniotic sac produces fetal death and abortion.

Oxytocin and prostaglandins are of unique importance and interest in uterine physiology. Oxytocin is produced in the supraopticohypophyseal and paraventricular nuclei, and stored in the posterior pituitary. Among the stimuli which release oxytocin are suckling, coitus, emotions, thirst, increased osmolarity of blood, acetylcholine, nicotine, morphine, anesthetics, fever, cervical dilatation (controversial), and the termination of the first stage of labor (Caldeyro-Barcia, Poseiro). There are some who believe that oxytocin plays a role in the initiation of labor. However, the weight of evidence would seem to foreclose this conjecture in human parturition. Radioimmunoassay has conclusively demonstrated a massive release of oxytocin during the expulsive phase of labor, but relatively little during the earlier stages. Of interest and unknown significance is the fact that there are high levels of oxytocin in fetal arterial cord blood at delivery.

The placenta produces an enzyme, oxytocinase, which progressively rises throughout pregnancy and does not decrease until parturition is completed.

An important and useful observation is that the human pregnant uterus is relatively refractory to oxytocin throughout pregnancy but becomes more sensitive as term approaches. Even massive infusions of oxytocin will not terminate most midtrimester pregnancies. Oxytocin acts on the cell membrane to produce depolarization and regulate the train of action potentials. It does not alter the transmembrane potential, nor does it have a direct effect on actin-myosin complexes.

PROSTAGLANDINS

Prostaglandins are cyclical 20-carbon fatty acids which are ubiquitous in nearly all animal cells. The compounds are derived from polyunsaturated fatty acids in the cells where they act. These phospholipids reside on the membranes, from which arachidonic acid is released by phospholipase A_2, an enzyme residing in the lysosomes (Gustavii). Chemical synthesis of these compounds has stirred an avalanche of investigational activity to elucidate their mechanism of action. The principal prostaglandins in reproduction are prostaglandin E (PGE) and prostaglandin F (PGF). Both PGE and PGF stimulate nonvascular smooth muscle activity, but PGE also acts as a vasodilator, inhibits gastric acid secretion, and inhibits hormone-induced lipolysis.

Prostaglandins play a basic regulatory role in cells. PGE increases synthesis of cyclic adenosine monophosphate (AMP), and a binding protein has been identified in a number of cells including fat cells and luteal cell membranes. Most likely this receptor is in the cell membrane. Studies with different tissues suggest that PGE may affect any of the three parameters of cyclic AMP levels—synthesis, degradation, and substrate levels of ATP. Hence in some circumstances PGE has the net effect of depressing cyclic AMP levels. The excitatory effect on smooth muscle is partially explained by the release of intracellular calcium.

Prostaglandins appear to play an important role as an intracellular regulator in hormone action, and are synthesized at a large number of autonomic nervous system effector sites. PGE and PGF play distinctly different roles in cell regulation, and in many ways can be viewed as the opposing forces in the regulatory process.

PGF differs in action from PGE in that it produces luteolysis in sheep and rats and produces contraction of all smooth muscle. PGF expresses its intracellular action by raising the level of cyclic GMP (cyclic guanosine 3′,5′-monophosphate), another intracellular regulator.

Prostaglandins E and F have a profound stimulatory effect on uterine smooth muscle. The action is immediate, and if there is a sufficient quantity, the response is sustained over a long period of time. Prostaglandins are the only known substances which will maintain a sustained uterine pressure or tension so that accommodation or active relaxation does not occur. When delivered in sufficient concentrations to the pregnant uterus, prostaglandins can initiate labor at any time, from early to advanced pregnancy. Either, therefore, is used as an abortifacient drug, as well as for the induction of labor at term (Saldana, Schulman, Yang). Prostaglandin synthesis occurs in response to smooth muscle stretch, progesterone withdrawal, or estrogen increase, and is believed to be the endogenous effector of normal parturition (Csapo, 1973). Amniotic fluid measurements reveal insignificant amounts of prostaglandin until the 36th week of gestation, after which there is a steady rise in concentration, but not enough to explain the onset of labor. Once labor begins, rapid accumulation of PG metabolites is seen in the amniotic fluid, probably a secondary phenomenon from repeated contractions. Measurement of PGs in rabbit myometrium does not show an increase prior to the onset of labor (Csapo 1976).

UTERINE BLOOD FLOW

Throughout pregnancy uterine blood flow progressively increases to reach a level of 500 to 700 mL per minute in the last month of gestation. 17β-Estradiol is the primary stimulus to increasing uterine blood flow. The action of estradiol is not direct, but it exerts its effect by activating intracellular protein synthesis; the effect on flow is not apparent for 30 minutes, and it can be blocked by cycloheximide. Blood flow is distributed to three areas of the uterus: placenta, decidua, and myometrium. In the sheep in late pregnancy, placental flow constitutes 84 percent of total uterine flow, and the myometrium receives 3 percent. The two principal clinical circumstances in which uterine blood flow is reduced are the various hypertensive states and during uterine contractions. However, in view of the magnitude of blood flow distribution mentioned above, the principal redistribution is for placental flow, not myometrial.

Uterine blood flow is at a maximum at all times. Drugs or blood gases cannot enhance flow. However, drugs and posture, such as standing or lying supine, may reduce uterine blood flow. It is of interest that when a fetus dies, there is no effect on uterine blood flow in the first hour, but a diminution of 30 percent occurs over the next 24 hours.

Angiographic studies in human beings demonstrate that one-half to two-thirds of the intervillous space of the placenta does not fill during a uterine contraction induced by oxytocin. If repetitive vigorous uterine contractions are produced over a period of time, the net effect would be to significantly reduce placental blood flow. This relative ischemia could have the effect of altering placental function and myometrial inhibition, which would lead to breakage of decidual lysosomes and prostaglandin synthesis.

FETUS

The fetus may participate in the initiation of labor in several ways. As mentioned earlier, during the second half of pregnancy fetal growth is significantly greater than placental growth. Since myometrial hyperplasia has also ceased, this means that the increasing uterine volume will be characterized by stretch hypertrophy and progressively less myometrium directly overlying the placenta. The net effect is for a larger amount of myometrium to escape from placental control, and to induce stretch irritability and contractions.

Fetal size, like adult size, appears to be genetically determined. Gestational length in eutherian mammals correlates with size; larger mammals have longer gestational periods. An interesting example of genetic influence is seen in the mating of horses and donkeys. The stallion-mare gestational period is 340 days, and the jackass-jenny gestation is 365 days. However, when intermating occurs, the gestational period is altered toward the male's direction, e.g., the jenny-stallion gestation becomes shorter than the jenny-jackass, and the jackass-mare's period is longer than it is when a mare mates with a stallion. The controlling factors of growth rate and size in the fetus are poorly understood, but for that matter little is known about this in children and adults.

ENDOCRINOLOGY

The endocrinology of parturition is tripartite, mother-placenta-fetus (Ryan). Early in human pregnancy the gestation is maintained by the corpus luteum which manufactures estrogen and progesterone. If luteectomy is performed before the 49th gestational day (Naegele), uterine activity begins promptly and abortion occurs within 1 to 2 days. If luteectomy is performed after 61 gestational days, the pregnancy continues, implying that the maternal-placental-fetal unit is now capable of producing sufficient estrogen and progesterone to maintain the pregnancy. With acute fetal death, progesterone production diminishes only slightly, thereby demonstrating that the human fetus does not play a significant role in the production of this hormone. In contrast, the fetus is significantly involved in the total estrogen production, because fetal death results in a precipitous decline in these hormones, making their measurement of value as an index of fetal health. Evolution provides a spectrum of variations involving the roles of mother, placenta, and fetus and their interplay in the production of estrogen and progesterone. Unfortunately, the absence of an experimental animal with an endocrine profile identical to man's impedes our understanding human parturition more completely. Fundamental and universal is the fact that estrogen is excitatory and progesterone is inhibitory on the myometrium. Progesterone withdrawal would tip the balance to an excitatory state, or progesterone could be impaired from effecting its end action by a surge of a competing compound such as estrogen or cortisone. Finally, progesterone effect can be acutely eliminated by prostaglandin.

The sheep provides a beautiful pure model of these influences (Liggins, 1973). Several days prior to the onset of labor, maternal plasma progesterone begins to decline, and 1 to 2 days before labor there is an acute rise in 17β-estradiol and a slower rise in prostaglandin $F_{2\alpha}$. Of special interest is the decline in maternal progesterone levels which are associated with the initiation of fetal cortisone production. Premature labor can be initiated in the sheep by infusion of cortisone or adrenocorticotropic hormone (ACTH)

into the fetus, and parturition can be delayed by fetal hypophysectomy or adrenalectomy (Fig. 9–10). In the human fetus, the foal, and calf, a cortisol surge has not been observed prior to the onset of labor.

A WORKING CONCEPT OF PARTURITION

Currently there is debate whether the fetus or the placenta is master of the parturitional switchboard. Liggins champions the fetal viewpoint and is primarily responsible for the elucidation of the portrait of sheep parturition.

Csapo postulates that the placenta is in the central position (Csapo, 1965). He has steadfastly investigated the role of the placenta in parturition for the past 25 years, and has advanced the progesterone block theory. The essence of this concept is that the placenta's endocrine action inhibits the uterus from its maximum working capacity, but as the volume of the uterus increases, the muscle slowly escapes from placental control. At some point progesterone influ-

FIGURE 9–10 The Liggins concept of labor's onset. Experimental data derived from the sheep can be interpreted as showing the key modifying role of fetal adrenal in the onset of parturition. *(From GC Liggins, 1973, courtesy of the author.)*

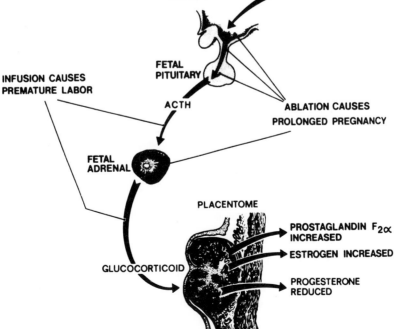

ence diminishes, estrogen prevails to activate intra-uterine prostaglandin synthesis, and labor begins.

Is the fetus escaping from maternal progesterone control? Does the fetus, having attained a given size, exercise its control of estrogen biosynthesis via its adrenal glands and eventually "decide" that the time has come for it to assert its autonomy? Most damaging to the fetal theory is the fact that fetal death is often associated with continuing pregnancy, and the onset of parturition occurs at a much later date, clearly free of fetal influence. In contrast, placental dislocation results in immediate onset of vigorous uterine activity. Figure 9–11 summarizes the Csapo concept. The uterus shows maximal contractile activity during menstruation (estrogen-progesterone withdrawal) and during parturition. When conception occurs, the myometrium is inhibited from expelling its contents, first by the corpus luteum and later by the endocrine interplay of mother-placenta-fetus. The principal force for overcoming the inhibition is the increasing uterine volume. Progesterone production and placental inhibition do not keep pace with uterine volume in the last month of pregnancy. There is a slight fall in plasma progesterone as term approaches, but perhaps more important is the appearance in the last month of a placenta globulin which binds progesterone (Schwarz et al.). This supporting symbiotic relationship is eventually disrupted, and vigorous uterine muscle activity ensues. The mediator of this disruption is probably prostaglandin; it has the capacity to initiate labor at any time. Prostaglandins apparently play a subtle but key role. The release of inhibition allows enough prostaglandin to be formed to sensitize the myometrium to other influences, such as endogenous oxytocin. The resulting contractions bring about greater prostaglandin production and a self-energizing process is created.

CLINICAL APPLICATIONS

The Csapo concept of volume/placental (V/P) inhibition ratio is valuable in explaining many clinical situations in which labor begins too early. For example, in polyhydramnios, labor usually begins before the expected date of confinement, V increasing disproportionately. Premature labor is common in twin pregnancies, and is seen more often in monozygotic (monochorionic placenta) gestations in which the placental area is smaller than in dizygotic or dichorionic placentas.

Next we may look at the denominator of the ratio V/P. If the placenta is located over the cervix, it is not

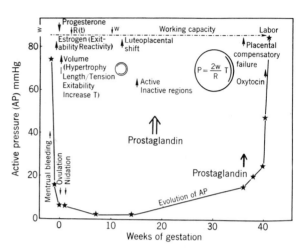

FIGURE 9–11 Csapo concept of the initiation of labor. The dotted line represents the maximum working capacity of the uterus. The solid line, representing uterine activity throughout the menstrual cycle and pregnancy, demonstrates that working capacity is achieved only during menstruation and labor. Therefore the uterus during pregnancy is in an inhibited state, and the onset of labor can be viewed as released inhibition. The arrows pointing upward represent forces contributing to overcoming inhibition; the ones pointing downward, factors attempting to maintain inhibition.

Multiple factors contribute to the evolution of uterine active pressure *(AP)*. Estrogen increases the excitability and reactivity of the myometrium. Increase in uterine volume affects the length, tension, and excitability of smooth muscle. Corpus luteum failure or excision before 60 gestational days can lead to abortion. The circle represents the uterus, the semicircle within represents the placenta. As pregnancy progresses, the nonplacental (active) regions begin to overcome the placental (inactive) regions. Uterine pressure *(P)* is dependent on wall tension *(T)* and inversely related to radius *(R)*; disproportionate increases in volume (tension) can lead to increased pressures.

The principal inhibitory factor is progesterone from the corpus luteum and placenta. *R* and wall tension can maintain a low pressure by being in balance.

Only prostaglandins can disrupt inhibition at any time. Oxytocin can initiate labor at term when inhibition is being released and there is compensatory failure of the placenta. Endogenous prostaglandins probably act as the mediator in normal parturition. *(Modified from Csapo, 1970.)*

inhibiting myometrium. Therefore, one-third of women with placenta previa enter labor at an early date. Acute disruption of the placenta should lead to immediate labor, and it does in abruptio placentae. If the placenta does not receive adequate nourishment, as for example when there is diminished blood flow, labor might begin prematurely or before the expected date. This occurs in toxemia and other hypertensive disorders. Uterine blood flow is diminished with repetitive uterine contractions, hence the probable mechanism of initiation of labor near term with intravenous oxytocin. Finally, placental destruction or poisoning by intraamniotic hypertonic saline instillation has been used as a method of second-trimester abortion.

Prolongation of pregnancy is seen in the anencephalic fetus in which there is no associated polyhydramnios. The average prolongation is 327 days. Although the fetus does weigh less than the average-term fetus, it is believed that the pathophysiology is related to altered fetal endocrine function. With an anencephalic fetus, there is altered estrogen metabolism, and urinary estriol levels are less than 5 mg per 24 hours. The role of fetal cortisone in human parturition is unknown. Missed abortion can be explained by fetal death without placental death; therefore with continued progesterone secretion in the presence of diminished estrogen, the net effect is inhibition of myometrium. When fetal death is secondary to placental death, parturition occurs in approximately 1 week. This may be seen in chronic hypertension. With pure fetal death, such as Rh sensitization, the onset of labor averages closer to 2 weeks.

Within 72 hours of rupture of the membranes, 90 percent of women will begin labor. Some will begin within an hour. It is difficult to fit the V/P theory into this observation, although prostaglandin synthesis can initiate labor without alteration in V, and can counteract the effect of P. Preliminary studies have shown a surge of blood prostaglandins following amniotomy or sweeping of the membranes (Mitchell et al., 1977).

Prostaglandins have the unique ability to activate the myometrial cell and initiate labor at any time. Up to the present time premature labor has not been successfully inhibited with progesterone therapy, but the use of prostaglandin inhibitors offers considerable promise in this area. Unfortunately, fetal effects are of serious concern since it has been clearly shown that prostaglandins are necessary for the maintenance of flow through the ductus arteriosus. Prostaglandin inhibitors have been used successfully to close the ductus arteriosus in small premature infants (Heymann et al.).

FETAL ENDOCRINOLOGY

ERIC BLOCH

This section is concerned with fetal hormone production and catabolism, and the regulatory role of hormones in the fetus. Placental and maternal endocrine activities, and placental transfer of hormones, are considered only as they pertain to the fetal endo-

crine milieu. First, some general principles of fetal-placental-maternal endocrine interrelationships may be stated.

(1) The formation and organization of endocrine glands and tissues are autonomous events, and occur during and are a particular example of general organogenesis. The primordia of the endocrine glands become recognizable during the fifth through seventh weeks of human gestation. Further differentiation and morphologic organization into definitive structures are generally completed by the end of the first trimester of pregnancy. Biosynthetic and secretory capacity is usually established concurrently with morphologic development. The initiation of biosynthetic capacity seems to be independent of trophic hormones or factors, although cellular responsivity to specific regulatory agents appears to be established during or soon after cytodifferentiation. Regulation of hormone production is established somewhat later in development; a period of more or less autonomous function seems generally to precede the establishment of positive- or negative-feedback controls. Several organs do not reach their definitive organization or functional activity until relatively late in pregnancy or after birth.

(2) The fetal endocrine organs secrete the same hormones as the adult, but the amounts secreted and the responsivity to stimulation frequently differ. These tend to be a function of the stage of development, and, depending upon the species, may even at term differ from that of the adult.

(3) The metabolic actions of hormones produced by the fetus are the same as those of the adult. In addition, fetal hormones regulate certain processes associated with differentiation and development, and not found in the adult. This hormonal control of functional and structural differentiation at certain critical periods is part of the continuum of vertebrate development and, in mammals, extends variably into the postnatal and preadult periods. However, fetal survival, unlike that of the adult, does not seem to require a functional endocrine system. There is increasing evidence that in some species fetal endocrine activity is involved in the onset of parturition.

Certain hormones induce the initial synthesis of particular enzymes during development. Such inductive effects may result in cytologic and structural consequences, initiate further molecular differentiation, or determine later expression of genetic information content. Hence, such inductive effects are irreversible and are to be distinguished from hormonal regulation of enzymatic activity, which is reversible and proceeds either by enzyme activation or the synthesis of new enzyme protein. The absence, or delay in the induction, of key enzymes leads to profound disturbances in developmental processes.

(4) The regulatory activity of fetal hormones is a function of a number of independent developmental processes. For activity to be expressed, the mechanisms of glandular secretory activity, plasma transport, and target-cell response must have differentiated.

(5) The maternal endocrine system only indirectly influences fetal endocrine activity. Hormones of maternal origin generally do not reach the fetus in physiologically significant quantities. Maternal polypeptide and protein hormones within physiologic concentration limits do not cross the placenta. An exception is thyrotropin-releasing hormone. Several are potentially hydrolyzed by placental proteases and hydrolases. Similarly, indole and catecholamines are largely oxidized by placental enzymes. Maternal thyroid and steroid hormones are transferred in small amounts across the placenta, but their influence at physiologic concentrations is negligible. At pharmacologic dosage, hormones exhibit a variety of effects in fetuses, including teratogenicity. The indirect effect of changes in maternal endocrine activity is exemplified by the diabetic, where increased maternal glucose entering the fetal circulation will ultimately result in pancreatic beta-cell hypertrophy and increased insulin production.

(6) The fetal endocrine system has limited effects on the maternal organism. This is most clearly seen in the increasing amounts of estrogens in the maternal circulation with advancing pregnancy, and their metabolic effects in the mother. Some of the other fetal hormones, e.g., cortisol and thyroxine, may reach the maternal circulation in small amounts. The effects of fetal endocrine pathology as manifested indirectly through altered concentrations of fetal metabolites reaching the mother appear to be minimal.

GONADAL ENDOCRINE ACTIVITY, ITS HYPOTHALAMIC-PITUITARY CONTROL, AND SEX DIFFERENTIATION

The role of hormones in differentiation and development is dramatically exemplified by the phenotypic expression of male genetic sex through androgenic control. Reproductive tissues, anatomic structures of hormone-independent origin, become dependent upon testicular androgens for their stabilization, further differentiation, and proliferation. Patterns of

neurohypophyseal function are imprinted in a "male" direction by testicular activity. The synthesis and kinetics of enzymes in diverse organs become sex-related; i.e., their activities are determined by the presence or absence of testosterone during prenatal development. Target tissues respond either to testosterone, the secreted hormone, or to dihydrotestosterone, or 17β-estradiol, derivatives produced in the target tissue. Hormonal regulation proceeds by classic mechanisms, and effects are found at the enzymic and metabolic levels without necessarily recognized structural correlates. A period of presumably autonomous secretory activity is followed by gonadotropin, i.e., trophic hormone regulation, and temporal sequence of "critical periods" in target-tissue responsivity is observed. The existence of male pseudohermaphrodites as a consequence of enzyme deficiencies that result in insufficient testosterone synthesis and incomplete masculinization of the male fetus offers genetic evidence for the essential role of testicular testosterone in male phenotypic differentiation.

GONADAL DIFFERENTIATION

Prior to differentiation, the gonad is bipotential, being composed of medullary tissue (the future testes) and cortical tissue (the future ovary). During gonadal differentiation, one type of tissue proliferates while the other regresses, the tissue identity being dependent upon the genotype.

Primary differentiation of the indifferent embryonic gonads into testes and ovaries is poorly understood. Genes on both the sex chromosomes and on autosomes are involved. The Y chromosome is required for testes differentiation, but it is uncertain whether the genetic determinants act directly to induce differentiation or indirectly by activating genes on other chromosomes. Wachtel has assigned the initiation of testes differentiation to the H-Y antigen, a cell-surface component found in the tissues of all mammalian males. The quantity of H-Y antigen per cell surface appears to be related to the number of Y chromosomes; the antigen shows widespread phylogenetic conservation, and its presence offers an explanation for phenotypic XX males through possible Y-chromosome to autosome translocation. Whether the H-Y antigen is indeed a primary inducer or only an indicator of testicular differentiation still must be resolved.

The gonads of vertebrates other than mammals can be functionally reversed from their genetic sex, but the mammalian gonad has lost this plasticity, perhaps as a protection against the feminizing influence of maternal and placental estrogens. Irrespective of genetic sex, the persistence of medullary sex cords leads to androgen production, demonstrating that hormone production is controlled by the structure of the gonadal tissue and not its sex-chromosomal complement.

Germ cells do not influence the differentiation and proliferation of the fetal Leydig cells. To the extent that Leydig cells are the sole androgen-producing cells, the endocrine activity of the testes is independent of the presence of germ cells. This is quite different in the ovary. Here, the female germ cells induce the development of the follicle cells, and of the primordial and graafian follicles. These are the future endocrine apparatus of the ovary, and they probably develop the capacity for estrogen synthesis in utero. In the absence of germ cells, as in Turner's syndrome (XO constitution), the rudimentary gonad is devoid of hormonal activity.

DEVELOPMENT OF TESTICULAR ACTIVITY AND GENITAL-TRACT DIFFERENTIATION

The classic experiments of Jost in the fetal rabbit established conclusively the dependence of male phenotypic sex differentiation on fetal testicular hormones. Further, as shown by the impairment or absence of masculinization following decapitation during or prior to the critical period of sex differentiation in fetal rabbits, pituitary activity influences testicular activity. In contrast, differentiation into the female phenotype required no ovarian or steroidal stimulus.

In human beings, fetal testis differentiation occurs at 6 weeks of gestation. The beginning of Leydig-cell cytodifferentiation and the capacity of in vitro pregnenolone conversion to testosterone at 8 weeks is coincident with the onset of Wolffian duct and mesonephric tubule differentiation. Based on studies in the fetal rabbit by Wilson's group, Leydig cells differentiate functionally coincident with cytodifferentiation in steroidogenic capacity (through testosterone synthesis), in steroidogenic responsivity to LH (luteinizing hormone), and in development of smooth endoplasmic reticulum. Leydig cells increase greatly in number between the 10th and 18th weeks of gestation. This morphologic observation correlates well with testosterone concentrations in serum and testes (peak values at 12 to 15 weeks) and in vitro testicular capacity for testosterone synthesis (maximal at 17 to 21 weeks). The period of increasing testicular activity encompasses the passage of genital-duct, urogenital-sinus, and external-genitalia differentia-

tion. A more or less rapid decline to low levels by 24 weeks occurs then in all testicular parameters studied. In the rat, and perhaps in the human, 3β-hydroxysteroid dehydrogenase–$\triangle$-steroid isomerase activity is initially rate-limiting; this limitation in testosterone production is removed concurrently with the onset of genital-duct differentiation. The inference may be drawn that in the testicular feminization syndrome the defect must be manifest by the onset of testicular secretory activity, i.e., by 8 weeks of gestation.

Testicular testosterone has as a primary role the virilization of the male fetus. This is accomplished partially by secretion of the hormone into the fetal circulation and perhaps partially by secretion into the lumen of the epididymides and Wolffian ducts. Testosterone may also be required in larger amounts for completion of maturation of the spermatogenic tubules and for spermatogenesis itself.

The mechanism of testosterone action in genital-duct differentiation is characterized by increased uptake of testosterone by Wolffian or genital ducts, the presence of specific testosterone-binding proteins in ductal cytosol, and inhibition of testosterone uptake and virilization by the antiandrogen cyproterone acetate. 5α-Steroid reductase activity, which leads to dihydrotestosterone formation, appears in the Wolffian duct only after stabilization (about 12 weeks) and is not detectable in epididymides. In the urogenital sinus and external genitalia, 5α-steroid reductase activity precedes the period of differentiation. Thus, testosterone seems to be the active hormone inducing Wolffian-duct and epididymal differentiation and stabilization, while tissue conversion to dihydrotestosterone is necessary for later Wolffian-duct proliferation, and for the differentiation and growth of prostate, seminal vesicles, and external genitalia. Studies of androgen action and of the effects of mutations in humans and mice indicate that phenotypic male differentiation of the reproductive tract requires testosterone, 5α-steroid reductase, androgen-receptor proteins, androgen receptor-chromatin interaction, and mesenchyme-epithelium contact.

TESTICULAR MÜLLERIAN DUCT REGRESSION FACTOR

In addition to the production of testosterone, the fetal testis produces a factor of partially defined composition which causes Müllerian duct regression. The factor is a species of nonspecific glycoprotein of molecular weight between 150,000 and 300,000 daltons. It is produced by the seminiferous tubules, as shown in organ culture experiments with tubules separated from interstitial cells. In human fetuses, this factor can be demonstrated in the media of cultured testes from fetuses of all gestational ages studied (7 to 26 weeks). Careful time-sequence studies have shown that the regression factor is probably synthesized by the spermatogenic tubules shortly after their differentiation, which suggests that formation of this factor is the first endocrine function of the embryonic testes.

OVARIAN ENDOCRINE ACTIVITY

The germ cells enter meiotic prophase at the end of the first trimester; primordial and then graafian follicles appear in the second half of pregnancy. Some evidence, from in vitro incubation experiments, indicates that the synthesis of the steroidogenic enzymes required for ovarian estrogen formation coincides with the appearance of follicles. This would be expected in view of the known functions of follicular granulosa cells. Evidence exists for in utero ovarian secretory activity in only a few mammals (horse, giraffe). However, ovarian capacity for estrogen formation (aromatization) appears at the same developmental stage in the rabbit fetus as testicular capacity for testosterone synthesis. A functional role for aromatization remains to be uncovered. The acquisition of unique enzyme profiles at the same time in both gonads suggests regulation by common factors.

In the rat, the capacity of the uterus to bind estradiol increases from birth until about 10 days after birth. The production of these receptors seems to be independent of ovarian activity. Presumably, specific estradiol-binding proteins appear in the human prior to birth as seen in the occasional hypertrophied uteri and withdrawal bleeding in the premature and term human newborn. In rats, administration of clomiphene and administration of diethylstilbestrol in humans, to pregnant mothers gave rise to multiple abnormalities of the reproductive tract in the female offspring.

MAMMARY-GLAND DIFFERENTIATION

As first shown by Raynaud, mammary-gland differentiation is directed by fetal testes. In intact female or in castrated male fetuses, anhormonal differentiation of the mammary-gland primordia takes place. The primordial buds penetrate the underlying mesoderm, retaining their connections to the surface epidermal epithelium. In male or androgen-treated female rodents (not humans), the mammary-gland buds lose their connections with the epithelium and remain as isolated nodules in the mesenchyme. In human beings, breast development is retarded in girls with the adrenogenital syndrome and fairly pronounced in cases of testicular feminization. These differences are not due to adult sex hormones but are a result of androgen action during the critical period of mammary-gland differentiation. Neumann et al. consider this sex difference to be caused by a differential production of pituitary prolactin and, secondarily therefore, of mammary-gland development. He suggests that fetal androgens increase the threshold of inhibition of the hypothalamic prolactin inhibitory factor to estrogens. The equal frequency of transient milk secretion in the newborn human male and female indicates that a functional difference between the two sexes at birth does not exist.

SEXUAL DIFFERENTIATION OF THE BRAIN

Definitive studies in rodents (mice, rats, guinea pigs) have shown the postnatal androgenic suppression of the cyclic nature of pituitary-gonadotropin secretion in adult females. Conversely, male rats castrated within 5 days after birth exhibit a cyclic gonadotropin-release pattern as adults. Extensive work has established the locus of androgenic action to be in the hypothalamus. According to current concepts, the amygdala or ventromedial area of the hypothalamus secretes gonadotropin-releasing hormones tonically and is responsible for the arrhythmic and basal secretion of pituitary gonadotropins. The preoptic area of the hypothalamus, which integrates the various neural and hormonal stimuli, is activated by estradiol (with or without progesterone) to activate in turn the amygdala to release a surge of gonadotropin-releasing hormone. This is the positive-feedback mechanism of estradiol which, in females, ultimately leads to ovulation. Androgens cause changes in the preoptic region such that the later response to high estrogen levels is abolished. The active hormone appears to be 17β-estradiol or possibly 2-hydroxyestradiol. The hypothalamic or limbic system can convert testosterone to estradiol, and estradiol receptors are present during this critical period of hypothalamic sex differentiation. Hypothalamic estradiol arising intracellularly from testosterone within the limbic system might be biologically more effective since peripherally circulating estradiol is bound to plasma-binding proteins. In primates, including human beings, hypothalamic sex differentiation occurs during fetal life.

DEVELOPMENT OF GONADOTROPIN PRODUCTION AND ITS HYPOTHALAMIC CONTROL

Recent work from the laboratories of Grumbach and Kaplan and of Faiman and Winter and their collaborators has provided some clarification for the relationship of gonadotropin levels to testicular endocrine function in the human fetus. LH concentrations increase in fetal pituitary glands with peak values attained at 15 to 24 weeks in the female and 20 to 24 weeks in the male. In both sexes, LH appears in fetal serum and amniotic fluid at about 11 to 12 weeks; concentrations rise to maximum levels at 12 to 16 weeks (3 to 30 ng/mL), and then decline in the latter half of pregnancy. Serum HCG values decrease steadily from their highest concentrations at 11 to 15 weeks (up to 600 ng/mL) till term, but remain higher than those of LH. In sum, adenohypophyseal LH must contribute significantly to serum LHHCG concentrations toward and after midgestation.

Pituitary and serum FSH (follicle-stimulating hormone) concentrations are highest during the 15th to the 21st weeks of gestation. Serum FSH levels ranged largely between 15 and 50 ng/mL as compared with less than 1 ng/mL in newborns. These levels of FSH are of the same order of magnitude as found in oophorectomized or postmenopausal women.

The human fetal pituitary has the capacity to respond to hypothalamic LHRH (LH-releasing hormone) before midgestation, and immunoreactive LH-RH is detected in hypothalami of 8-week-old fetuses. A hundredfold increase in content occurs by midgestation. Since the hypothalamohypophyseal portal system may not be fully developed until 18 weeks, the extent of hypothalamic control of pituitary-tropin production prior to midgestation is unclear.

The pituitary concentrations of LH and FSH exhibit an interesting sex difference: both hormones, but particularly FSH, are found in higher concentrations in sera of midgestation female fetuses. The period of high FSH concentrations in fetal pituitaries and sera coincides with that of the rapid growth of seminiferous tubules in males, and of the intense transformation of oogonia into primordial follicles in the female. This sex difference may be a reflection of an inhibition by testicular androgens, acting perhaps directly on the pituitary since hypothalamic LHRH levels do not differ between the two sexes.

The temporal and quantitative relationships between testicular synthetic activity, testis and serum testosterone concentrations, pituitary and serum LH levels, and serum HCG concentrations permit a schema of the endocrine-somatic interrelationships during sexual differentiation. Normal differentiation and development of male internal sex structures, signaled and maintained by the onset and increase in testicular androgen production, are either independent of gonadotropin stimulation or dependent primarily on placental HCG. During the later stages of genital differentiation (12 to 16 weeks), pituitary LH secretion occurs and may influence Leydig-cell function. LH (and FSH) release at midgestation is either autonomous or stimulated by a large LHRH production. As fetal development advances, the negative-feedback system in the hypothalamic-pituitary-gonadal axis is established, leading to diminished-LHRH secretion and the decline in serum FSH and LH levels seen in both sexes after midgestation. This negative-feedback system is fully matured postnatally. The concomitant decline in testosterone secretion in male fetuses is a reflection of decreased gonadotropic stimulation, although additional influences such as prolactin or estradiol may directly inhibit Leydig-cell function.

Observations in anencephalic and apituitary fetuses further support an influence of fetal hypothalamic-pituitary-gonadotropic activity on later gonadal development. Pituitary FSH and LH content of anencephalics is extremely low, about 2 percent of that found in newborn infants. In such fetuses, testes are frequently hypoplastic and undescended with reduced numbers of Leydig cells. Underdevelopment of the penis and scrotum may be found. However, male ductal, tubular, and accessory glandular development and differentiation are normal. (An alternative hypothesis put forth originally by Solomon states that the rate-limiting step for testosterone synthesis by the younger fetal testes is the concentration of circulating placental C_{21} steroids with no direct effects exerted by HCG or LH.) In the female, small ovaries with hypoplastic primordial follicles are often encountered.

SEX STEROIDS OF NONGONADAL ORIGIN

These steroids may be divided into two categories: those of maternal and those of fetal origin.

Testosterone and particularly some of its active derivatives (e.g. methyltestosterone) cross the placenta. Hence, any such compound administered to the mother during critical stages of sex differentiation can produce varying degrees of masculinization or teratogenic effects.

Sex steroids of fetal origin consist of placental

androgens and estrogens, and of adrenocortical androgens. Both classes of steroids are rapidly sulfurylated and hydroxylated by fetal tissues, thereby preventing any pronounced sexual biologic activity. However, the withdrawal bleeding seen in many female newborns, and the mild breast stimulation in newborns of both sexes, indicate concentrations of circulating free estrogens sufficient to exert moderate physiologic effects. In the adrenogenital syndrome, the excess concentrations of circulating androgens result in clitoral hypertrophy and partial fusion of labia majora in female fetuses. In the rare cases of a generalized deficiency of 3β-hydroxysteroiddehydrogenase–$\triangle$-steroid isomerase, testosterone production is reduced or absent. Such newborns are generally male pseudohermaphrodites.

FETAL ADRENAL CORTEX AND ITS FUNCTIONS

The adrenal cortex of the human fetus (1) contains a histologically distinct zone, the fetal zone, which occupies most of the total gland and largely involutes during the first month after birth, and (2) is deficient in 3β-hydroxysteroid–$\triangle$-steroid isomerase activity, resulting in the production of large amounts of 3β-hydroxy-$\triangle^5$-steroids, particularly dehydroepiandrosterone. Fetal zones of various gestational duration have been described in other primates, edentates, and some Felidae; a reduction in adrenal weight before or after parturition is not uncommon among mammals in general. Adrenal C_{19}-steroid production is also found in sheep and guinea pig fetuses and perhaps also in other mammals with long periods of gestation.

The definitive cortex appears concurrently with or shortly after the fetal zone is recognized at 6 weeks of gestation. Throughout roughly the first half of pregnancy, the fetal zone is the principal steroid synthetic component of the adrenal cortex. The ultrastructural correlates of biosynthetic processes appear in the definitive cortex at about midgestaton. Subsequently, however, the extent of rough endoplasmic reticulum and mitochondria formation exceeds that seen in the fetal zone. An intense period of growth of the adrenal cortex takes place during the second half of gestation, proportionally greater in the definitive cortex which reaches 20 percent of the entire gland before parturition. This growth period reflects pituitary ACTH stimulation. The definitive cortex remains after parturition to develop into the adult adrenal cortex.

STEROID BIOSYNTHETIC CAPACITY AND FUNCTION

Extensive in vivo and in vitro studies have shown in fetal adrenal tissue the complete complement of enzymes required for de novo C_{19}-steroid and corticosteroid biosynthesis. C_{19}-steroid synthesis in vitro is found by the eighth week of gestation. The capacity for cortisol formation from progesterone appears in the adrenal cortex by 11 weeks. However, steroid biosynthesis in the fetal adrenal cortex differs from steroid biosynthesis in the adult gland in three important ways:

1. The activities of 3β-hydroxysteroid dehydrogenase and $\triangle$-steroid isomerase are inhibited, perhaps by the high titers of circulating estrogens. Estradiol competitively inhibits these two enzymes in vitro. This inhibition leads to the accumulation and secretion of $\triangle^5$-3β-hydroxysteroids, particularly of dehydroepiandrosterone.
2. Placental progesterone serves as a precursor for the synthesis of cortisol and other $\triangle^4$-3-ketosteroids.
3. In addition to synthesis from endogenous acetyl coenzyme and cholesterol, placental pregnenolone is a potential precursor of dehydroepiandrosterone.

There is increasing evidence that the proliferation of the definitive cortex during the third trimester is associated with the ability to synthesize cortisol and corticosterone de novo.

Postnatally, the involution of the fetal zone is correlated with decreased $\triangle^5$-3β-hydroxysteroid production. There is some evidence that the decline in functional capacity of the fetal zone begins during late pregnancy. The definitive cortex corresponds in its functional capacity to the adrenal cortex of the adult. The fetal zone appears as an incomplete, transient, steroid-producing gland; its function, if any, remains an enigma.

Cord serum cortisol values of about 7 ng/mL have been reported for the early second-trimester period. Following cesarean section near or at term, cortisol concentrations are about 20 to 30 ng/mL.

Labor increases these concentrations to 60 to 150 ng/mL. At 36 to 40 weeks of gestation, umbilical arterial concentrations of dehydroepiandrosterone (free and sulfate), 16α-hydroxydehydroepiandrosterone (free and sulfate), and pregnenolone sulfate are about 100 to 350 ng/mL each. Except for dehydroepiandrosterone sulfate, which is similar to the adult, the other two Δ^5-3β-hydroxysteroids exceed adult values from twenty- to fiftyfold. In anencephalic fetuses or after maternal cortisol administration, the serum Δ^5-3β-hydroxysteroid values are markedly depressed. Fetal serum exhibits approximately 20 percent less binding capacity for cortisol than does adult serum.

PLACENTAL TRANSFER OF CORTISOL

Maternal cortisol is transported across the placenta in minimal quantities. The relative concentrations of corticosteroid-binding proteins in maternal and fetal circulations, and the concentration of maternal cortisol required to effect transfer, make a maternal-to-fetal transfer of little physiologic significance. Such cortisol as is transferred is at least partially oxidized to cortisone by placenta, liver, and other tissues. The ratio of cortisol to cortisone is less than unity in the fetal circulation, as compared with greater than 10 in the maternal circulation. Fetal to maternal cortisol transport is favored by (1) higher concentrations of corticosteroid-binding proteins in maternal as compared with fetal plasma, (2) displacement of bound cortisol by progesterone which is higher in fetal plasma (2 μg/mL), and (3) increase in both maternal corticosteroid-binding proteins and placental progesterone with advancing gestation. Thus, there appears to exist a fetal-to-maternal cortisol gradient, which would favor fetal pituitary ACTH synthesis and release by diminishing fetal blood cortisol levels.

ACTH PRODUCTION AND REGULATION OF FETAL ADRENAL ACTIVITY

The question of pituitary regulation of fetal adrenal activity has not been completely answered. ACTH has been detected in pituitary glands of 8- to 10-week-old fetuses, and is present in term cord plasma (161 pg/mL) at concentrations three times as great as in maternal plasma (56 pg/mL). The fetal adrenal cortex develops normally in anencephalics up to 20 weeks of gestation, suggesting that development is either autonomous or dependent on extrapituitary factors. At about midgestation, the further development and growth of the adrenal becomes dependent upon pituitary factors, as seen clearly in the reduced weight and absent fetal zone in term anencephalics. One pituitary factor appears to be ACTH: (1) ACTH administration causes enlarged adrenals in surviving anencephalics with prominent "fetal zones"; (2) adrenal steroid production in vitro responds to ACTH stimulation; (3) maternal cortisol administration decreases umbilical arterial C_{19}-steroid sulfates and maternal

urinary estriol concentration; and (4) maternal metyrapone administration results in increased umbilical androgen and urinary estrogen levels, effects not seen in anencephaly. HCG has also been shown to cause changes in adrenal morphology and perhaps function. In rats and sheep, a functional hypothalamic pituitary-adrenal axis, including a negative-feedback loop, is unequivocally established during the fetal period.

Recently, α-melanocyte-stimulating hormone (α-MSH) and corticotropinlike intermediate lobe peptide (CLIP) have been implicated in fetal adrenal function. α-MSH has the amino acid sequence that is identical to the amino-terminal tridecapeptide of ACTH. CLIP is exactly the same as the carboxy-terminal residues, 18 to 39 region, of ACTH. Fetal pituitaries, which have a pars intermedia, contain large concentrations of α-MSH and CLIP. A marked decrease in these two peptides and a rise in ACTH content occur at parturition. CLIP or α-MSH have been advanced as the trophic hormone maintaining the fetal zone, the diminishing production of either hormone leading to the neonatal involution of the fetal zone.

FETOPLACENTAL STEROID UNIT

The concept of the fetoplacental unit, introduced by Diczfalusy, consists of viewing the placenta and fetus as one metabolic unit with respect to steroid metabolism. Neither placenta nor fetus alone synthesizes significant quantities of steroid hormones from acetate. The placenta has a very limited capacity to synthesize cholesterol from acetate, and the fetal adrenal (fetal zone only?) cannot convert Δ^5-3β-hydroxysteroids to Δ^4-3-ketosteroids. The placenta and fetus complement each other and thus elaborate most of the hormonally active steroids.

Plasma cholesterol is metabolized by the placenta to progesterone. Progesterone, and perhaps some pregnenolone, pass from the placenta into both maternal and fetal organisms for further metabolism. In the fetus, progesterone is a substrate for adrenal cortisol production, some testosterone formation, and peripheral metabolism to hydroxylated and largely sulfurylated products.

Pregnenolone, of endogenous and placental origin, is converted to dehydroepiandrosterone and its sulfate in the fetal adrenal. The source of fetal adrenal pregnenolone has not been settled; experimental support can be provided for a placental or a de novo adrenal origin. The secreted dehydroepiandrosterone sulfate, either per se or after hydroxylation at carbon 16 by the fetal liver, is carried by the fetal circulation to the placenta. Here, the sulfates are hydrolyzed to the free forms, oxidized to androst-4-ene-3,17-dione and its 16α-hydroxyderivative, and aromatized to estrone (in equilibrium with estradiol) and estriol. Some of the fetal C_{19}-steroids are converted to estrone in the fetal liver, thereby contributing a small amount to the total estrogen pool. Maternal C_{19}-steroids are of course also aromatized in the placenta; they account for more than 50 percent of estrone plus estradiol found but less than 10 percent of estriol. As the fetus grows, the maternal contribution to the placental substrate declines so that at term about 85 percent of the daily estrogen formation is of fetal origin. The estrogens are secreted into both the maternal and fetal circulation; those reaching fetal tissues undergo additional hydroxylation reactions and are sulfurylated.

This view of the fetoplacental unit applies to the midgestation fetus. Whether de novo fetal synthesis of steroid hormones plays a greater role at term, and whether this concept applies to fetal testicular function are unanswered questions.

The determination of maternal estrogens, particularly estriol, has been a valuable indicator of fetal viability. The combined activities of the placenta, the fetal adrenal, and the fetal liver are the theoretical basis for this clinical application.

ENZYME ACTIVATION AND INDUCTION BY CORTISOL

An integral aspect of development is the synthesis and activation of diverse enzymes required for the maintenance of homeostasis and function in the adult organism. The initiation of activity of such enzymes is induced, or "switched on," by hormones. This process of enzyme activation (or induction; in most instances, proof of an increase in enzyme content as distinct from activity is lacking) occurs throughout development until sexual maturation. The number of enzymes activated prior to birth depends upon the species examined. Greengard lists three periods for enzyme development in the rat liver: late fetal, neonatal, and late suckling. The activating hormone may not be identical with the adult regulating hormone; e.g., fetal liver tyrosine aminotransferase is induced by glucagon, but its adult activity is regulated by cortisol. Conversely, the enzymic response to a particular hormonal stimulus may change with age.

Glucocorticoids have been shown to activate or induce enzymes in a number of developing tissues and a variety of species. Examples which illustrate the wide diversity are glutamine synthetase in chick embryonic neural retina, phospholipidogenic enzymes of the brain, alkaline phosphatase and sucrase in chick, mouse, and human intestinal epithelium, argininosuccinate synthetase of the urea cycle in rat liver, lung lecithin or surfactant synthesis in several species, norepinephrine methylation by phenylethanolamine-N-methyltransferase in rat and rabbit adrenal medulla, and glycogenic enzymes of mammalian liver. Cortisol has also been implicated in regulating (1) fetal liver glycogen accumulation (see Hormonal Effects on Carbohydrate and Lipid Metabolism below); (2) the decay in intestinal capacity to absorb antibodies and other macromolecules during maturation; (3) the involution of the thymus; and (4) the onset of parturition.

HORMONAL CONTROL OF CARBOHYDRATE AND LIPID METABOLISM: INSULIN, GLUCAGON, CATECHOLAMINES

INSULIN

In the pancreas, the first islets make their appearance during the 10th week of pregnancy, with alpha and beta cells being recognized during the 12th to 15th weeks. A capillary circulation within the islets is established at 14 to 17 weeks. Insulin is detected radioimmunologically at the time that beta cells are recognized histologically, i.e., at 12 weeks. Insulin is present in fetal plasma by 12 weeks of gestation. There is a steady increase in insulin content of human fetal pancreases from 12 weeks to term. However, these increased tissue concentrations do not correlate with serum levels, which remain fairly stable throughout pregnancy (1 to 29 μU/mL).

In the premature and term human infant, as in fetal sheep, monkeys, and other species, the pancreatic response to glucose administration as reflected in plasma insulin levels is limited. Insulin levels rise slowly and remain elevated up to 2 hours, even after blood glucose has declined. The response to glucose is greatly potentiated with prior infusion of glucagon which, alone, is practically inactive. A continuous amino acid infusion to premature infants causes much greater elevation of plasma insulin concentrations than a continuous glucose infusion.

In summary, insulin is secreted during most of fetal life. The regulation of insulin synthesis and release remains inadequately understood. Pancreatic response to stimuli active in the adult is limited and sluggish, and the termination of the response appears variable. Both postnatal development of the pancreas and in utero inhibitory factors may be involved. However, as clearly seen in the newborn of poorly controlled diabetic mothers, and from the recognition that insulin is required for cell growth, physiologically significant amounts of insulin are secreted during in utero existence.

GLUCAGON

At term, 30 percent of the islet cells in human fetuses are alpha cells. The concentrations and regulation of plasma glucagon levels remain to be established. Glucagon does not cross the placenta. Hypoglycemia, norepinephrine, and arginine stimulate pancreatic glucagon secretion, but hyperglycemia does not depress plasma glucagon levels.

EPINEPHRINE AND NOREPINEPHRINE

Chromaffin cells invade the human adrenal cortex at 8 weeks' gestation, with subsequent organization of the medulla. At term, 1 to 2 percent of the entire adrenal gland consists of medullary tissue. Both epinephrine and norepinephrine are found in late first- and in second-trimester medullary tissue, with norepinephrine predominating. Ganglionic chromaffin cells become competent to synthesize epinephrine only after penetration into the adrenal cortex. This occurs quite early in human development, possibly explaining the presence of epinephrine in human fetal medullary tissue early in pregnancy. However, there is evidence that epinephrine is not secreted in significant quantities prior to midgestation. Pressor amines with norepinephrine predominating can be demonstrated in extraadrenal chromaffin bodies before they appear in the adrenal medulla.

In rat fetuses, adrenal epinephrine formation from norepinephrine is induced by glucocorticoids. A similar role for cortisol in the human fetus has not been described. Indirect evidence from experiments in sheep suggests that hypoglycemia and hypoxia stimulate catecholamine secretion by the adrenal medulla. Similarly, in the human newborn, hypoglycemia will result in as much as sevenfold increase in epinephrine excretion, while under normoglycemic conditions norepinephrine predominates.

HORMONAL EFFECTS ON CARBOHYDRATE AND LIPID METABOLISM

Glucose is the single major substrate for postimplantation embryonic and most of fetal energy metabo-

lism. Most pathways of glucose utilization are developed during early embryonic life. Storage, as glycogen, begins at the end of the first trimester, and lipogenesis during the last trimester. Hepatic glycogen accumulation continues through term to reach 8 to 18 percent of liver weight. Lipogenesis results in the rapid gross appearance of white and brown adipose tissue with fat-containing lobulated cells. The 11-week-old liver can convert pyruvate to glucose, but gluconeogenesis from lactate remains low until after birth. Several enzymes of glucose metabolism exhibit little activity until late in gestation or, depending on species, during the neonatal period.

Hormones do not play a recognized role in embryonic carbohydrate metabolism. At some period of development, carbohydrate and lipid metabolism come under hormonal regulation. During fetal life, two hormonal effects have been distinguished. One effect involves insulin, and perhaps somatomedin C, the other the hormones promoting glucose availability.

Insulin probably participates in the regulation of glucose uptake by fetal tissue. In experiments with mammalian fetuses, insulin administration promoted hypoglycemia, tissue glucose utilization, overall growth, and lipogenesis. The newborn of a poorly controlled diabetic mother is characterized by pancreatic hypertrophy, increased size, and fat deposits. Maternal hyperglycemia leads to elevated fetal blood glucose levels, with resultant increased insulin production, growth, and lipogenesis. Conversely, the newborn with defective pancreatic function shows signs of starvation, i.e., normal circulating glucose levels but reduced utilization. The rate of glucose utilization under conditions of adequate nutrition and the influence of insulin are limiting factors in regulating growth.

In several species, glucocorticoids are required for hepatic glycogen accumulation. A number of enzymes catalyzing glucose utilization or synthesis have been induced or activated by cortisol, glucagon, or epinephrine in mammalian fetuses, particularly in rats. Greengard postulates that glucagon may be the hormonal stimulus for the onset of certain enzymic activities, with glucocorticoids playing a permissive role. Growth hormone, somatomedins, and somatostatin, both through direct action on carbohydrate-lipid metabolism, and via their indirect effects on insulin and glucagon production, may well exert important, yet-to-be-defined controls on fetal energy metabolism.

In the human fetus, these mechanisms probably develop well before term. The fetus responds to maternal hypoglycemia or hypoxia with glucose secretion, i.e., increased blood concentrations, suggesting a prenatal capacity for glycogenolysis and, perhaps, limited gluconeogenesis. Catecholamine or glucagon release appears to be stimulated by such acute changes in the fetal environment.

Maternal blood glucose concentrations determine the glucose level in fetal blood. A positive maternal-fetal concentration gradient exists, and fetal levels follow changes in maternal blood glucose concentrations. Glucose is transferred across the placenta by facilitated diffusion. In late gestation, some fatty acids probably cross the placenta.

It is clear that the enzymic and hormonal potential for postnatal regulation of glucose and fat metabolism, and maintenance of glucose homeostasis, is developed prior to birth. The full realization of this potential is completed soon after birth, the rapidity and magnitude of pre- to postnatal activation varying with individual mammalian species. According to current concepts, the fetal separation from the mother results in decreased blood glucose concentrations. This acts as a signal for glucagon and catecholamine secretion, with the latter perhaps being dependent on a splanchnic nerve stimulation. The two hormones activate one or more enzymes, catalyzing glycogenolysis and leading to hepatic glucose secretion. A tendency toward normoglycemia is reestablished. The same hormones activate rate-controlling enzymes of gluconeogenesis and lipolysis, ultimately leading to lactate reutilization and increased plasma free fatty acids. The latter are then increasingly utilized as a metabolic fuel as hepatic glycogen stores are depleted. Glucose administration or elevated insulin levels will retard these adaptations to extrauterine existence. The newborn continues initially a fetal pattern of sluggish response to insulin stimulation in its glucose utilization; presumably, the transition to the adult response is dependent upon cell-membrane changes and the induction or stimulation of key glucose-utilizing enzymes.

NEUROENDOCRINE DEVELOPMENT, GROWTH HORMONE, PROLACTIN, AND NEUROHYPOPHYSEAL HORMONES

Profound changes in our understanding of neuroendocrine chemistry and physiology are occurring. The synthesis and secretion of pituitary hormones are controlled by hypothalamic and cortical releasing hormones or factors, some stimulatory and others inhibitory in nature. Some of these releasing hormones are found also in pancreas and intestines. Neuronal cells as synthesizers of a large spectrum of neurotransmitters, neurons as conduits for chemical messages, and the molecular mechanisms of neuroendocrine interaction are being recognized and clarified for their roles in neurophysiologic events. The endorphins were discovered, a class of opiate-like peptides of brain and pituitary origin which are potent releasers of immunoreactive growth hormone (HGH), prolactin, and vasopressin. The biosynthesis of diverse proteins including some hormonal peptides begins with the formation of a high-molecular-weight precursor, which is then posttranslationally proteolytically cleaved in one or more steps to yield the active molecule(s). Such high-molecular-weight precursors have been found in fetal pituitaries (e.g., "big" HGH and prolactin), as have subunits of glycoproteins (e.g., β subunit of LH). ACTH and β-endorphin may arise from one precursor molecule. Each of these recent findings, whether of biochemicals, or molecular events, or of ultrastructural correlates, represents a new potential locus of regulation, and for determination of fetal development or maldevelopment. This is a frontier of developmental endocrinology.

NEUROENDOCRINE DEVELOPMENT

Decapitation of fetal rabbits or rats, and hypophysectomy of sheep and monkey fetuses, arrests or reverses the morphologic and functional maturation of the thyroid, adrenals, and testes, with little effect on the pancreas, ovaries, growth, and skeletal maturation. The same findings are seen in human anencephalics. In the latter, the plasma concentrations of such pituitary hormones as have been studied (e.g., HGH, FSH, ACTH) are lower by one order of magnitude than those of normal newborns, and do not respond to physiologic stimuli.

The cells of the anterior pituitary are recognizable as the classic acidophil, basophil, and chromophobe cells during the 8th to 11th weeks of gestation. This is considerably later than the appearance of the primordia of both the anterior and posterior pituitary glands during the fifth week of gestation. A sequence of synthetic activity has been described: follicle-stimulating, luteinizing, adrenocorticotropic, and growth hormones detectable by the eighth to tenth week by radioimmunoassay methods, and prolactin, MSH, and thyrotropic hormone by the 12th to 14th week. Serum concentrations indicate secretion of HGH, FSH, LH, and TSH (thyroid-stimulating hormone) by the tenth week of gestation.

Hypothalamic-releasing-hormone synthesis occurs early in organogenesis. TRH (thyroid-releasing hormone) and LHRH have been detected in 4½-week-old fetuses, somatostatin in 9-week-old fetuses. The tissue concentration of somatostatin increases with age during the second quarter of gestation; such an increase is not seen with TRH or LHRH. The releasing factors, in addition to their presence in the hypothalamus, are also variably present in cerebrum and cerebellum.

The onset of hypothalamic-releasing hormone secretion is uncertain. Close anatomic apposition of primordial pituitary and hypothalamus and the existence of a neurohemal complex interdigitating this area would permit transmission of neurohumors in 8- and 9-week-old fetuses. There is concurrent development of the portal system and of hypothalamic nuclei and tracts during subsequent weeks. Monoamine fluorescence is found in the 10-week-old hypothalamus, and specimens from 11- to 15-week-old fetuses are rich in dopamine but low in norepinephrine and serotonin. Neurosecretory granules have been described in hypothalamic tracts at 16 weeks. The hypothalamic monoaminergic network, neurosecretory neurons and median eminence, and the hypophyseal portal system are established during the 16th to 20th week of gestation.

GROWTH HORMONE

Human growth hormone (HGH) is present in serum and pituitaries from the tenth week of gestation onward. There is an approximate 1000-fold increase in immunoreactive pituitary content by term to values at acromegalic levels. Biologically active HGH content also increases with advancing gestation. HGH concentrations reach a maximum in fetal serum at 15 to 29 weeks (approximately 50 to 250 ng/mL), followed by a significant decline toward term (33.5 ± 4.2 ng/mL). The concentration of HGH in serum does not correlate with that of the pituitary. Grumbach envisages that HGH synthesis and secretion begin in the fetal pituitary early in gestation. This secretion may be autonomous or under GHRF (growth hormone–releasing factor) control. By midgestation, the median eminence has sufficiently matured to effect a rather uncontrolled rate of GHRF secretion with concomitant intense stimulation of HGH secretion by pituitary acidophils. In the late-gestation fetus, neural inhibitory influences become operative, together with competence of the hypothalamic monoaminergic neuronal network resulting in diminished HGH synthesis and release. Decreased HGH secretion may be induced by diminished secretion of GHRF, by increased release of somatostatin, or by both mechanisms. During the first year, a fully functional mechanism is attained, as seen by the acquisition of sleep-mediated growth hormone release. The development of the neurotransmitter mechanisms effective in the adult, i.e., L-dopa stimulation, and alpha and beta adrenergic receptors, occurs during the perinatal period. In anencephaly, serum HGH is depressed (7 ng/mL), supporting the concept of hypothalamic control of HGH secretion near term. The maturation of pituitary HGH production and its neural regulation is another illustration of neuroendocrine development.

The feedback control of HGH production is incompletely understood. Glucose infusion increases HGH concentrations in fetal human and monkey blood. This response is the direct opposite of that found in the adult; an adequate explanation is lacking. Shortly after parturition, hyperglycemia produces the adult response of suppression of HGH output.

A need for HGH in the fetus has not been demonstrated. Growth and skeletal maturation in the decapitated animal (rats, rabbits, sheep, monkeys) or in the anencephalic or apituitary human fetus are essentially normal. However, in view of the known actions of HGH in the adult, a role in the hormonal control of energy, of anabolic metabolism, and of heteropolysaccharide synthesis is probable. Both HGH and somatostatin are regulatory factors for insulin and glucagon secretion. HGH may exert a physiologic role in fetal skeletal development through stimulating the production of somatomedins, a group of peptides with anabolic functions; e.g., it may promote proteoglycan sulfation and protein synthesis in cartilage, and stimulation of adipose cells. Fetal plasma contains somatomedins. A hereditary form of dwarfism has been described with normal HGH but reduced plasma somatomedin levels. Clearly growth depends on the integrated actions of many hormones and their effectors. The detailed understanding of the endocrine homeostasis involved in "growth" will make a fascinating future chapter.

PROLACTIN

Immunoreactive prolactin has been detected in 90-day human and 88-day-old sheep fetal pituitaries. This correlates reasonably well with the presence of lactotropes in the pituitary as identified by histochemical means. Prolactin content in human fetal pituitaries increases from the 13th to 30th weeks of gestation. A significant correlation between prolactin and HGH content exists, with HGH concentrations being 100- (early gestation) to 300-fold (late pregnancy) higher. Fetal serum prolactin levels are fairly constant until the third trimester, when a steady and rapid increase occurs. Near term, fetal, and maternal levels of serum prolactin are similar. The rapid rise in prolactin late in gestation can be correlated directly with the increase in circulating estrogens. A similar temporal estradiol-prolactin relationship is seen in sheep and rhesus monkeys. Hence, estradiol is an important modulator of prolactin production. Conversely, a specific hypothalamic factor seems not to be essential for prolactin synthesis and release during gestation since serum prolactin levels are comparable in normal and anencephalic fetuses.

VASOPRESSIN AND OXYTOCIN

Vasopressin—in the relatively few species studied—can be detected in pituitaries or plasma of fetuses by midgestation. Immunoreactive but not bioactive vasopressin concentrations in the fetal pituitary are greater than those of the adult. This may reflect the presence of arginine-vasotocin, which was recently discovered in pituitaries of human, sheep, guinea pig, and seal fetuses. Arginine-vasopressin and arginine-vasotocin are detectable by 12 weeks of gestation. The ratios of pituitary vasopressin to vasotocin concentrations rise from less than 1 before midgestation to well above 2 by term. Vasotocin production ceases in the perinatal period. Vasotocin in mammalian fetal pituitaries is an example of functional phylogenetic recapitulation during ontogeny; mammals had been thought not to synthesize vasotocin. Pineal tissue may also be a source of vasotocin.

In younger fetuses, the vasopressin/oxytocin ratios (28:1 in the human being) are much more than in the adult but decline toward adult values (less than 1) by birth. This may be explained by the observation that the supraoptic nucleus develops earlier than the paraventricular nucleus.

In the late-gestation fetal sheep, monkey, and human being, vasopressin metabolism is characterized by high pituitary and plasma concentrations, a high production rate, and a strong response in vasopressin release to changes in plasma osmolality or volume. High plasma vasopressin levels have been described at birth after normal vaginal delivery (23 μU/mL by bioassay; 80 μU by radioimmunoassay), and relatively low levels in neonates born by cesarean section (approximately 0.8 μU/mL or 20 μU). Cord blood from an anencephalic fetus did not contain detectable amounts of vasopression. This has been interpreted as a fetal response to the "stress" of vaginal delivery.

In the term fetus and newborn, the vasopressin control system appears to be functional. Neonates respond to isotonic dextran or hypertonic saline by changes in free water clearance without altered glomerular filtration rate, suggesting that both hypothalamic osmoreceptors and cardiac volume receptors are functional at birth. The renal tubule contains vasopressin and alpha- and beta-adrenergic receptor sites. Certain differences from the adult are noted: (1) High concentrations of vasopressin in fetal plasma at term as compared with maternal vasopressin levels, and (2) low maximal renal tubular excretory capacity with a low rate of glomerular filtration.

The exact function of vasopressin in the fetus is unknown. It has been postulated that these pressors play a role in amniotic fluid accumulation by passing into the fetal urine to the embryonic membranes, where they cause water uptake into the amniotic cavity. A constrictor effect on the umbilical circulation which secondarily effects placental separation from the uterus has also been suggested.

Immunoreactive and biologically active *oxytocin* is present in cord blood at term. Concentrations of both oxytocin and vasopressin in umbilical arterial blood exceed those in venous blood, indicating fetal pituitary origin. Maximal levels are observed at vaginal delivery, with lowest levels before the onset of labor (approximately 5 μU oxytocin activity per milliliter). An association between labor and fetal posterior pituitary secretory activity exists. A role for fetal oxytocin, which can readily pass the placenta to reach the myometrium, in promoting parturition has been suggested.

THYROID HORMONE METABOLISM
FUNCTIONAL DEVELOPMENT

Thyroid development is characterized by precolloid (6½ to 10½ weeks), early colloid (10½ to 11½ weeks), and follicular growth periods (after 11½ weeks). Colloid formation occurs abruptly and rapidly with 90 percent of follicles containing colloid by 11½ weeks. Although iodide uptake is seen during the precolloid stage, a dramatic increase accompanies early colloid deposition, to reach a maxmimum content in the gland between 20 and 24 weeks of gestation. Distinct from intrathyroidal concentration, the rate of iodide uptake increases throughout gestation until term.

Organic binding of radioiodine as iodotyrosines and iodothyronines is activated at about the same time as the iodide-trapping mechanism, i.e., around day 70 of gestation. The concentrations of intrathyroidal mono- and diiodotyrosine, thyroxine, and triiodothyronine increase during further gestation. Secretory activity appears concomitantly with synthesis. It is of interest that thyroglobulin is synthesized as early as day 29 of gestation.

Thyroxine is found in sera of 7-week-old fetuses and increases until term ($\pm$ 110 ng/mL). Serum thyroxine levels are about 20 ng/mL between the 11th and 20th weeks of gestation. The rise in fetal serum total thyroxine generally parallels the rise in concentration of serum thyroid-binding globulin (TBG). TBG is present also at 7 weeks; its binding capacity at term is tenfold greater (25 μg per 100 mL). Free serum thyroxine increases moderately, about $1\frac{1}{2}$ times, during the second and third trimesters of pregnancy, and constitutes about 0.025 percent of total thyroxine concentrations. In contrast to thyroxine, triiodothyronine (3,5,3'-triiodothyronine) is not present in detectable quantities in fetal serum until the third trimester (about 0.5 ng/mL cord blood). Instead, reverse triiodothyronine (3,3',5'-triiodothyronine) is found in larger concentrations (about 2 ng per milliliter of cord blood) and tends to parallel serum thyroxine levels during the third trimester. It seems that the monoiodination pathway of thyroxine to triiodothyronine begins to develop in utero and is stimulated to adult levels by exposure to the extrauterine environment (serum triiodothyronine/reverse triiodothyronine ratios are 0.3 at term, 4 at 1 month postpartum, and 3.2 for adults).

TSH PRODUCTION AND REGULATION OF THYROID FUNCTION

The fetal pituitary acquires its capacity for TSH synthesis early. Cell cultures from 4- to 18-week-old fetuses demonstrated TSH synthesis by 14 weeks. TSH can be detected in 12- to 8-week-old pituitaries and is present in sera of 9- to 10-week-old fetuses. TSH concentrations increase three- to fourfold in both pituitaries and sera at 18 to 22 weeks of gestation, with serum levels of about 10 μU per milliliter of serum. As a consequence of elevated TSH output, fetal thyroidal radioiodine uptake and thyroxine secretion increase

at this time. The raised TSH production probably reflects maturation of the hypothalamus and pituitary portal system since TRH is observed in the hypothalamic TRH, and pituitary TSH content tends to increase in unison with advancing gestation. At term, mean serum TSH levels have declined to about 10 μU/mL.

The sum of available data suggests that the early development of the thyroid gland and thyroglobulin synthesis are not TSH-dependent. Iodide trapping and organification, while presumably of autonomous establishment, are activated and their increased activity sustained by TSH. The temporal correlation of increased thyroidal activity, plasma thyroxine, and TSH concentrations, the development of the pituitary portal system about midgestation, and the changing serum thyroxine-triiodothyronine/TSH ratios point to the midportion of human pregnancy through the first postnatal month as the period of maturation of the hypothalamic-pituitary thyrotropin system. Peripheral monoiodination develops perinatally such that triiodothyronine/reverse triiodothyronine ratios increase rapidly. The lack of TSH transfer across the placenta, and the minimal transport of iodothyronines, make any significant contribution of the maternal system to the fetal thyroid hormone–TSH pool unlikely. The role of placental thyrotropin in fetal thyroid physiology is unknown. At term, there exists an apparent fetal-maternal gradient for thyroxine and TSH, but a reverse gradient for free triiodothyronine.

ROLE OF THYROID HORMONES IN DEVELOPMENT

Thyroid hormones are required for normal growth and general maturation, and are particularly important for the maturation of certain organ systems, notably the central nervous system, skeleton, and skin. Developing animals suffering from the effects of hypothyroidism show growth delay, neurologic and behavioral abnormalities, retardation in bone age, and deficiency in hair. Brain structure and weight, dendritic development, vascularization, and myelination are retarded or abnormal. RNA (ribonucleic acid), protein, and phosphalipid synthesis is diminished or characterized by altered patterns of synthesis. Centers of ossification in the femur, kneecap, and other bones make a delayed appearance.

Thyroid hormones have recently been shown by Oppenheimer's group to exert their primary effects on the control of gene expression and on mitochondrial activity. Triiodothyronine rapidly enters cells and binds directly to intramuscular chromatin, stimulating transcription and protein synthesis. Activity of numerous enzymes in different organs is stimulated following thyroid-hormone administration, presumably reflecting the profound effects of the hormone on protein synthesis in several tissues more than direct action on each enzyme. However, thyroxine does induce several enzymes, e.g., mitochondrial α-glycerophosphate dehydrogenase, liver urea-ornithine cycle enzymes, and liver enzymes involved in energy metabolism. It is in inducing specific enzymes as well as a more generalized protein synthesis resulting in cell proliferation and increased metabolic rates that the effects of thyroid hormone on promoting growth and development are to be found. This is most dramatically shown by tadpole metamorphosis, which can be induced by as little as 0.8 mg thyroxine per liter of medium.

The need for thyroxine appears to arise at a relatively late stage of mammalian development. This would explain why it is difficult to demonstrate any effect of thyroid deficiency in fetal life in species in which the young are born in a rather immature state. In human beings, congenital aplasia of the thyroid leads to delayed ossification of those bones which begin to ossify shortly before birth. Enamel formation and teeth mineralization are deficient in children with neonatal hypothyroidism. Since myelination of the human central nervous system occurs during the last weeks of gestation, an effect of prenatal thyroid deficiency on brain development would not be surprising. However, there is very little objective evidence which permits differentiating between effects of prenatal and early postnatal thyroid hormone lack (or excess). Most human cases, including frank cretinism, are not diagnosed within the first weeks after birth. This may soon change with recent advances in neurochemistry, the expanded analysis of material obtained by amniocentesis, and the further exploitation of the fetal sheep model.

An additional difficulty in assessing fetal needs for thyroid hormone is in the evaluation of maternal contributions to the total pool of circulating thyroid hormones in the fetus. Small amounts of triiodothyronine and perhaps thyroxine cross the human placenta. The quantities involved are insufficient to replace the secretory activities of the fetal thyroid; the quantitative needs for triiodothyronine in regulating fetal metabolic events and processes remain to be ascertained. The existence of inductive and regulatory activities which manifest themselves grossly only at the late stages of development remains to be shown.

PARATHYROID HORMONE, CALCITONIN, AND REGULATION OF CALCIUM AND PHOSPHATE METABOLISM

Calcium levels in fetal plasma are greater than maternal levels in all species studied (primates, herbivores, rodents). In sheep but not in the human being, part of this concentration differential is explained by higher fetal levels of plasma calcium-binding proteins. In rodents, fetal plasma calcium reaches lowest levels with the onset of skeletal ossification, then rises to maximum concentrations at the end of gestation. Fetal plasma phosphate levels exceed those of the mother in human beings and sheep, and it is noteworthy that virtually no phosphate is found in sheep and human fetal urine. It is clear that important differences exist between fetal and adult calcium and phosphate metabolism.

The placenta may exert a major regulating activity in determining fetal calcium metabolism. Calcium infusions or the maternal administration of parathyroid hormone (PTH) or calcitonin have little effect on fetal rat or guinea pig calcium levels. Calcium 45 exchanges slowly in all species studied. Placental permeability for PTH is minimal; changes in maternal circulating PTH concentrations exert negligible responses in fetal calcium or phosphorus concentrations. It seems that fetal calcium concentrations are relatively independent of change in maternal plasma calcium levels. Phosphate passes across the placenta by active transport.

Information on parathyroid activity and effects in the fetus is sparse. Parathyroid cell differentiation occurs about midgestation in the human fetus. Diverse observations with human and animal material, including PTH concentrations in human cord blood, suggest that fetal parathyroid glands are competent to secrete PTH. Calcitonin has been detected in human and pig fetal thyroids.

The need for and role of PTH and calcitonin in fetal calcium and phosphate metabolism remain to be established. Radioimmunoassays will clarify the production of PTH and calcitonin during earlier gestational periods. The value to fetal homeostasis of mobilization of fetal skeletal calcium or of renal response to PTH is not apparent. Calcium and phosphate metabolism in the adult is regulated by PTH acting at least in part through its regulation of $1\alpha,25$-dihydroxycholecalciferol levels. The synthesis, metabolism, and activity of the dihydroxycholecalciferols in the developing fetus remain to be elucidated.

OTHER HORMONES

Several hormonal substances, more or less well characterized in the adult, have not been investigated adequately in the human fetus. From observations in animal preparations, it seems likely that *erythropoietin* production is established in prenatal life. The *renin-angiotensin-aldosterone* system similarly is developed before birth. Both humoral systems depend on kidney maturation for their activities; kidney development is quite variable among mammals. The capacity for *aldosterone* production exists in the human fetal adrenal cortex. *Serotonin* increases in human fetal tissues with advancing pregnancy. A regulatory role for any of these hormonal substances in human fetal physiology has not been established.

IMMUNOLOGY OF PREGNANCY

ZEEV KOREN

The fetus, in all but highly inbred colonies of laboratory animals, is by virtue of its paternally inherited antigens an allograft within its mother's body, and should be immunologically rejected. Yet the birth of normal young is sufficient proof that this problem has been solved in mammalian evolution. This is particularly unusual because of the fine discriminating capacity of the mammalian immune system, which is capable of recognizing as foreign a protein which differs from isologous protein in respect to only a single amino acid. This coordinated biological mechanism permits the mammalian fetus to survive and flourish in utero when challenged. It is currently a subject of intensive study and controversy in reproductive biology.

Four classical hypotheses have been put forward:

1. The fetus is antigenically immature.
2. The uterus is an immunologically privileged site.
3. The mother is immunologically inert.
4. The fetus and mother are separated by a physical barrier.

Over the years, as experimental evidence has accumulated, these basic hypotheses have been modified, expanded, and refined in more sophisticated terms. To reflect this progress, the third hypothesis will be rephrased to suggest that there is a maternal immunologic state, rather than that the mother's immune system is inert. This discussion will hold to the basic format of reviewing interrelated facets of the four hypotheses.

ANTIGENICALLY IMMATURE FETUS

If, during its stay in the uterus, the fetus did not develop transplantation antigens, the problem of immunologic incompatibility would, of course, not arise. There is little doubt that the embryo possesses transplantation antigens; the only question is how early in life they develop. This question has been approached by transplanting embryonic tissues of different ages into hosts and subsequently looking for an immunologic response to the supposed fetal antigens. It is important to be certain that the embryonic graft will not mature and develop transplantation antigens in situ. To minimize or obviate this possibility, various techniques have been applied, among them (1) inactivation of transplanted tissue by irradiation; (2) determination of the ability of an embryonic cell preparation to absorb specific antibodies; and (3) direct visualization of the antigenic sites on the cells by fluorescent antibody procedure or some other method.

These techniques have all demonstrated the presence of transplantation antigens very early in embryonic development. In the human fetal cells transplantation antigens have been demonstrated at 6 weeks' gestation and are probably present immediately after conception. Fetal red cells containing ABO and Rh antigens exist early in pregnancy and can be found in the maternal bloodstream at 8 weeks of pregnancy. It should be stressed that multiparous women frequently show antibodies to HLA antigens displayed on cells of the fetus. There is the possibility that these antigens are present in a modified form—lesser quantities are displayed on the surface of embryonic cells than on adult tissue. In mice, skin homografts from infant donors transplanted to adult-compatible mice may long outlive grafts from adult donors. This suggests a qualitative as well as quantitative difference between antigens of embryonic and adult tissues that may account for differences in immunogenic behavior. More relevant to the question of allograft rejection of the fetus is the antigenic status of the extraembryonic tissue, particularly the placenta. In the placenta, maternal and fetal tissue come together, and hence one would suspect that this interface would be the primary focus of any immunologic reaction. However, in general, grafting experiments conducted with placental tissue or cell suspensions have been too crude to be very informative. Dancis et al. have presented findings indicative of potential immunologic competence and hemopoietic function of the placenta. However, much more investigation is needed for an understanding of the role that the placenta plays in immunologic and other defense mechanisms. About all that can be currently stated is that the fetus possesses transplantation antigens, is indeed immunogenic, and the differences in quantity and immunogenic quality cannot explain successful fetal survival.

THE IMMUNOLOGICALLY PRIVILEGED UTERUS

There are only a few known sites where heterologous or even homologous tissue can live for prolonged periods, protected from the usual rejection phenomena. These include the hamster cheek pouch, the anterior chamber of the eye, and the brain. The explanation for the privileged immunologic behavior of these sites is that they lack lymphatic drainage, which is the route graft antigens utilize to provoke host response.

However, the presence of vascular connections between the graft and host ensures that prior host immunity to the graft donor will lead to expression of allograft immunity and rejection. The uterus does not prevent fetoplacental cells from entering into the mother, and indeed has a good vascular supply and lymphatic drainage. Exfoliation of trophoblastic cells has been demonstrated in normal pregnancies. In addition, the uterus is not essential for the normal development of the fetus. This fact can be deduced from evidence of spontaneous and experimentally induced extrauterine pregnancies, some even proceeding to term with cesarean delivery of normal infants.

Experimental work involving transplantation of nonembryonic tissue provides evidence that transplantation immunity is expressed in the uterus and the mother can be sensitized to paternal antigens via the uterus. However, the possibility that at the implantation site the development of decidua involves some modification in immunologic reaction has been suggested (Beer, Billingham). This, however, cannot be considered a major factor in fetoplacental survival as deduced from placenta accreta (no decidual formation and deep penetration of villi into the myometrium).

MATERNAL IMMUNOLOGIC STATE

The existence of a state of generalized immunosuppression in the pregnant female is easy to dis-

prove. Various types of in vivo grafting or in vitro cytotoxic tests with maternal lymphoid cells demonstrate retention of a functional immune response. For example, pregnant women will easily reject skin grafts from unrelated males (i.e., not their husbands).

Moreover, maternal lymphocytes have been repeatedly shown to be reactive against foreign antigens. Indeed, some experiments show cytotoxicity of maternal lymphocytes to trophoblastic cells from the same gestation. Such response could indicate that the immune system of the mother is normal and the fetus is antigenic. If this is the case, then either the mother's response to the fetus is suppressed by other factors or a specific immunologic tolerance develops. This immune response of the mother protects rather than rejects the fetus. However, other experiments have shown a decreased maternal response against other foreign antigens. A reduction of T-cell activity was shown in pregnancy. The tuberculin reaction, which is a measure of cell-mediated immunity, is also depressed during pregnancy. The phytohemagglutinin-induced lymphocyte transformation rate is reduced in pregnancy. Depressed lymphocyte transformation could be due to fewer T cells being stimulated during pregnancy and a proportionate increase in B cells, which are primarily concerned with defense against foreign bacteria (Finn et al.).

It is possible that the mother develops sensitized T cells to destroy the fetus, but these cells are prevented from interacting with the fetoplacental unit by blocking antibody or excess antigen. Excess antigen can bind with the antigen receptors on the T cells and block their ability to bind to the target cells. Also, antibodies can cover antigenic sites of the fetoplacental unit cells, and in this way prevent attachment by the sensitized T cells. A possibility exists that a blocking antibody, or some other factor, might also coat the phytohemagglutinin receptor site on the lymphocytes to protect the fetus from the potentially destructive effects of the occasional sensitized lymphocyte that would penetrate the placental barrier.

Is there a role for the binding of noncytotoxic antibody to fetoplacental sites in the protection of the fetus from rejection? Hellstrom et al. suggest that a specific factor, possible blocking antibody, may be capable of giving the fetus protection against destruction by maternal sensitized lymphocytes that may have penetrated the placenta. It can be assumed that these blocking antibodies fail to destroy the trophoblastic cells in the presence of complement. In this way, the fetoplacental unit can be protected from immunologic damage. In mice it has been shown that antigenically foreign embryos not damaged in vivo by maternal lymphocytes can be destroyed in vitro, thus demonstrating that the sensitized T cells exist. This enhancement-mediated mechanism may also play a role in the development of tolerance. There is good evidence that although the pregnant female is not immunologically inert, she may occasionally react less vigorously to allografts. This effect has been attributed to corticosteroid hormones, particularly cortisone, which is secreted in increased amounts during pregnancy. Cortisone induces a transient fall in the number of circulating lymphocytes and causes lymphoid tissue involution. It has been suggested that high steroid hormone concentrations in the vicinity of the fetoplacental unit, due to the endocrine functions of these tissues, may play a role in protecting the fetus from immunologic destruction (Zipper et al.). Experimental work has involved administering superphysiologic doses of estrogen, progesterone, and HCG to skin of tumor-graft-bearing animals and watching for changes in immunologic reactions (Beer, Billingham). Results have been negative as often as positive, and peripheral test grafts may not be biologically analogous to the situation in utero.

Work with human patients has demonstrated the postpartum appearance of antitrophoblast antibodies (Hulka et al.). Thus it seems that during pregnancy, antibodies can *bind* freely but *without* a deleterious effect on the fetus. The significant change in immunologic maternal response produced by pregnancy seems to express itself in maternal T cells that can both suppress and help in the production of antibodies and cell-mediated immunity. According to Gershon, those exerting this inhibitory influence are called suppressor T cells. They can exert both antigenic specific and nonspecific suppression.

SEPARATION OF FETUS AND MOTHER BY A PHYSICAL BARRIER

As technology becomes more sophisticated, the nature of this so-called barrier becomes more and more complex. At the microscopic level, the most obvious feature is the so-called placental barrier which prevents mixing of fetal and maternal circulations. Thus, it would *seem* that the fetus is not a vascularized allograft and the efferent pathway from the mother's immune system would be blocked. However, fetal and placental cells have been found in the maternal circulation, and maternal antibodies have access to the fetal circulation.

Recently, a controversy has arisen over the permeability of the placenta to maternal cells. In a strain of mice *homozygous* for a chromosomal marker, it was reported that maternal cells were found in tissues of F_1-hybrid progeny, which should be *heterozygous* for the marker. It should be noted that although maternal cells were identified in the fetus, they could not be identified as immunocompetent cells. In order for maternal lymphocytes to pose a threat to the fetus, sufficient numbers would have to be transferred transplacentally at a time when the fetus was itself not immunocompetent to react against these cells. Thus, the fetus may be protected by (1) the placental separation of the maternal from the fetal circulation, which imposes severe limitations on the number of maternal cells transferred; and (2) breakdowns in this placental barrier which occur, at least in humans, *late* enough in gestation that the fetus is capable of destroying the maternal intruders immunologically. It should be noted that in other mammalian species, such as mice, immunocompetence does not develop until after birth, so this second mechanism does not apply.

At the *microscopic* level, the structure of the placental barrier has been extensively studied. The trophoblastic layer is believed to present an unbroken frontier to the maternal tissues, although some maintain that as pregnancy proceeds, there are focal areas of trophoblastic erosion. It has also been noted that exfoliation of trophoblastic cells does not seem to provoke a maternal immune response. Trophoblast has been shown to endure transplantation into a host preimmunized against the donor's antigens. Furthermore, pure trophoblastic grafts do not seem to be able to immunize a host to the foreign antigens of the donor. Thus, it has been concluded that either trophoblast does not possess histocompatibility antigens or these antigens are somehow *masked* so that they are not exposed to the maternal immune system (Simmons, Russell).

Two closely related major phenomena associated with trophoblast tissue involve the control of its invasiveness and the avoidance of immunologic rejection. At the time of implantation, primitive trophoblast is highly invasive and erodes the uterine mucosa to obtain nourishment for the developing embryo. Among the many factors that appear to control the invasive activity and differentiation of primitive cell trophoblast, the genetic dissimilarity between the trophoblast and the mother plays an important role. The possibility exists that not only is the invasive activity of trophoblast changed, but also that young trophoblast changes its surface structure, and thus the transplantation antigens are changed.

Evidence has been accumulated by using fluorescent-staining procedures and antisera techniques that trophoblast has organ-specific antigens (Koren et al.). Trophoblast does seem to express transplantation antigens, although it is refractory to rejection as a homograft. Assuming, then, that the trophoblast by itself is antigenic but incapable of expressing it, an intriguing theory has been presented of a "fibrinoid-like layer" which surrounds the trophoblastic cells and separates them from the maternal vascular system. The fibrinoid component is thought to mask, hide, and prevent the trophoblast from expressing its antigenicity. This fibrinoid layer is an acellular mucopolysaccharide rich in hyaluronic and sialic acids and is believed by some to envelop every trophoblastic cell. Others dispute the continuity of this layer and also point out that it is not present at all stages of implantation. In the mouse, it characteristically develops 2 days postimplantation and degenerates focally late in gestation (Kirby). Proponents of the fibrinoid barrier propose that it masks the expression of histocompatibility antigens and that the lack of an immune response to transplanted trophoblast can be reversed by pretreating the cells with neuraminidase to degrade the fibrinoid mucopolysaccharide and expose the antigens. It should be noted that the effect of neuraminidase on trophoblastic fibrinoid is another current controversy. Currie and Bagshawe suggest that fibrinoid acts as a barrier not only to the expression of antigens but to the cytotoxic effects of lymphocytes on trophoblastic cells. It was suggested that this latter type of barrier was an electrostatic one—that the high negative charge due to anionic mucopolysaccharide components repelled lymphocytes, which also have a negative surface charge. This attractive, but very speculative, theory was challenged as representing an oversimplification. Jones and Kemp cited a variety of cogent biochemical and biophysical objections to the modus operandi of sialomucin in the "self-isolation" of fetal trophoblast. In their theory, cells are probably held together by chemical bonds, and this accounts for the firm adhesion of trophoblast to genetically different endometrium. By the intercellular bridges that unite trophoblast and maternal cells, the trophoblast is recognizing its "genetic disaffinity" and responds by separating itself by a layer of sialomucin—a membrane that renders the surface of trophoblastic cells nonadhesive by marking the adhesive sites. This fact also prevents maternal lymphocytes from adhering or interacting immunologically with trophoblast. In con-

clusion, it appears that placental tissue can be antigenic. Maternal tolerance, obviously still an enigma, cannot be explained by a single factor but must be considered a complex mechanism influenced by several factors.

REFERENCES

Adam PAJ: Control of glucose metabolism in the human fetus and newborn infant. *Adv Metab Disord* 5:184–276, 1971.

Alexander DP et al.: Calcium, parathyroid hormone and calcitonin in the foetus, in *Foetal and Neonatal Physiology,* eds. KS Comline et al., Cambridge: 1973, pp. 421–429.

Assali NS (ed.): *Pathophysiology of Gestation,* New York: Academic, 1972.

Baird D: The Galton Lecture 1970: the obstetrician and society. *J Biosoc Sci* 3(suppl 3): 93–111, 1971.

Beer AE, Billingham RE: *The Immunobiology of Mammalian Reproduction,* Foundation of Immunology Series, Englewood Cliffs, N.J.: Prentice-Hall, 1976.

Bloch E: *In vitro* steroid synthesis by gonads and adrenals during mammalian fetal development. *Excerpta Medica Int Congress Ser* 132:675–679, 1967.

———: Fetal adrenal cortex: Function and steroidogenesis, in *Functions of the Adrenal Cortex,* vol. 2, ed. K McKerns, New York: Appleton-Century-Crofts, 1968, pp. 721–774.

Brown-Grant, K: Recent studies on the sexual differentiation of the brain, in *Foetal and Neonatal Physiology,* eds. KS Comline et al., Cambridge: 1973, pp. 527–545.

Caldeyro-Barcia R, Poseiro JJ: Oxytocin and contractility of the pregnant human uterus. *Ann NY Acad Sci* 75:813, 1959.

Cardiologic aspects of pregnancy. *Prog Cardiovasc Dis* 16:363, 1974.

Challis JRG, Torosis JD: Is α-MSH a trophic hormone to adrenal function in the foetus? *Nature* 269:27, 1977.

Chard T: The role of posterior pituitaries of mother and foetus in spontaneous parturition, in *Foetal and Neonatal Physiology,* ed. KS Comline et al., Cambridge: 1973, pp. 569–583.

Chesley LC, Duffus GM: Posture and apparent plasma volume in late pregnancy. *J Obst Gynaecol Br Commonw* 78:408, 1971.

Csapo A: The placenta and the initiation of labor. *Ned Tydschr Verlosk* 65:229, 1965.

———: The diagnostic significance of the intrauterine

pressure: I & II. *Obstet Gynecol Surv* 25:403, 515, 1970.

————: The regulatory interplay of progesterone and prostaglandin F$_{2\alpha}$ in the control of the pregnant uterus, in *Uterine Contraction—Side Effects of Steroidal Contraceptives,* ed. JB Josimovich, New York: Wiley, 1973.

————: Prostaglandins and the initiation of labor. *Prostaglandins* 12:149, 1976.

Currie GA, Bagshawe KD: The making of antigens on trophoblast and cancer cells. *Lancet* 1:708, 1967.

Dancis J et al.: Hematopoietic cells in mouse placentae. *Am J Obstet Gynecol* 100:1110, 1968.

Daniel EE, Renner SA: Effect of the placenta on the electrical activity of the cat uterus in vivo and in vitro. *Am J Obstet Gynecol* 80:229, 1960.

Davies IJ et al.: Specific binding of steroids by neuroendocrine tissues, in *Subcellular Mechanisms in Reproductive Neuroendocrinology,* eds. F. Naftolin et al., Amsterdam: Elsevier, 1976, pp. 263–275.

Davison JS et al.: Gastric emptying time in late pregnancy and labour. *J. Obstet Gynaecol Br Commonw* 77:37, 1970.

Dawber RP, Conner BZ: Pregnancy, hair loss and the pill. *Br Med J* 4:234, 1971.

Dawes GS: *Foetal and Neonatal Physiology,* Chicago: Year Book, 1968.

————, Shelly HJ: Physiological aspects of carbohydrate metabolism in the foetus and newborn, in *Carbohydrate Metabolism and Its Disorders,* vol. 2, ed. F Dickens et al., New York: Academic 1968, pp. 87–121.

Diczfalusy E: Steroid metabolism in the foeto-placental unit, in *The Foeto-Placental Unit,* eds. A Pecile, C Finzi, Amsterdam: Excerpta Med Found, 1969, pp. 65–109.

Duenholter JH, Pritchard JA: Human fetal respiration. *Obstet Gynecol* 42:746, 1973.

Dure-Smith P: Ureters in pregnancy. *N Engl J Med* 284:395, 1971.

Finn R et al.: Immunological responses in pregnancy and survival of fetal homograft. *Br Med J* 3:150, 1972.

Fisher DA et al.: Ontogenesis of hypothalamic-pituitary-thyroid function and metabolism in man, sheep and rat. *Recent Prog Horm Res* 33:59–116, 1977.

Freinkel N: Homeostatic factors in fetal carbohydrate metabolism, in *Fetal Homeostasis,* vol. 4, ed. RM Wynn, New York: Appleton-Century-Crofts, 1969, pp. 85–140.

Frenberg A, Fisher DA: Thyroid hormone metabolism in the foetus, in *Foetal and Neonatal Physiology,* ed. KS Comline et al., Cambridge, 1973, pp. 508–526.

Gershon RK: T cell control of antibody production, in *Contemporary Topics in Immunobiology,* eds. MC Cooper, ML Warner, New York: Plenum Press, 1974.

Gillman J: The development of the gonads in man, with a consideration of the role of fetal endocrines and the histogenesis of ovarian tumors. *Carnegie Contrib Embryol* 32:81–131, 1948.

Greengard O: The developmental formation of enzymes in rat liver, in *Biochemical Actions of Hormones,* vol. 1, ed. G Litwack, New York: Academic, 1970, pp. 53–88.

Gustavii B: Missed abortion and uterine contractility. *Am J Obstet Gynecol* 130:18, 1978.

Heany RP, Skillman TG: Calcium metabolism in human pregnancy. *J Clin Endocrinol Metab* 33:661, 1971.

Hellstrom KE et al.: Abrogation of cellular immunity to antigenically foreign mouse embryonic cells by a serum factor. *Nature* (London) 224:914, 1969.

Hill AV: The heat of shortening and the dynamics constants of muscle. *Proc Roy Soc, B* 126, pp. 136–195, 1938.

Heymann MA et al.: Closure of the ductus arteriosus in premature infants by inhibition of prostaglandin synthesis. *N Engl J Med* 295:530, 1976.

Holly RG: Dynamics of iron metabolism in pregnancy. *Am J Obstet Gynecol* 93:370, 1965.

Hulka JF et al.: Antibodies to trophoblasts during the postpartum period. *Nature* (London) 191:510, 1961.

Hytten FE, Leitch I: *The Physiology of Human Pregnancy,* 2d ed., Oxford: Blackwell, 1971.

Ibbertson HK: Thyroid function, in *Human Reproductive Physiology,* ed. RP Shearman, Oxford: Blackwell, 1972, pp. 478–524.

Jones BM, Kemp RB: Self-isolation of the fetal trophoblast. *Nature* (London) 221:829, 1969.

Jones KJ, Smith DW: Recognition of the fetal alcohol syndrome in early infancy. *Lancet* 2:999, 1973.

Josso N et al.: The anti-Müllerian hormone, in *Morphogenesis and Malformation of the Genital System,* eds. RJ Blandau, D Bergsma, New York: Alan R Liss, 1977, pp 59–84.

Jost A: Problems of fetal endocrinology: The gonadal and hypophyseal hormones. *Recent Prog Horm Res* 8:379–418, 1953.

———— et al.: Studies on sex differentiation in mammals. *Recent Prog Horm Res* 29:1–34, 1973.

Kaplan SL et al.: The ontogenesis of human fetal hormones: I. Growth hormone and insulin, *J Clin Invest* 51:3080–3093, 1972.

———— et al.: The ontogenesis of pituitary hormones and hypothalamic factors in the human fetus: Maturation of central nervous system regulation of anterior pituitary function. *Recent Prog Horm Res* 32:161–243, 1976.

Kirby DRS: Transplantation and pregnancy, in *Human Transplantation,* eds. FT Rapaport, J Daussel, New York: Grune & Stratton, 1968.

Koren Z et al.: *Am J Obstet Gynecol* 104:50, 1969.

Levina SE: Sexual differentiation in epiphyseal and hypothalamic regulation of the secretion of follicle-stimulating hormone and luteinizing hormone by fetal hypophyses cultured *in vitro,* in *Hormones in Development,* eds. M Hamburgh EJW Barrington, New York: Appleton-Century-Crofts, 1971, pp. 547–552.

Liggins GC: Endocrinology of the foeto-maternal unit, in *Human Reproductive Physiology,* ed. RP Shearman, Oxford: Blackwell, 1972a, pp. 138–197.

————: The fetus and birth, in *Reproduction in Mammals,* vol. 2, eds. CR Austin, RV Short, Cambridge, 1972b, pp. 72–109.

————: Foetal participation in the physiological controlling mechanisms of parturition, in *Foetal and Neonatal Physiology,* eds. KS Comline et al., Cambridge: 1973.

Lindheimer MD, Katz AL: Current concepts: The kidney in pregnancy, *N Engl J Med* 283:1095, 1970.

Lowry PJ et al.: Structuring and biosynthesis of peptides related to corticotropins and β-melanotropins. *Ann NY Acad Sci* 297:49–62, 1977.

McNaughton MC: Endocrinology of the foetus, in *Foetus and Placenta,* eds. A. Klopper, E. Diczfalusy, Oxford: Blackwell, 1969, pp. 557–602.

Maternal Nutrition and the Course of Pregnancy. Committee on Maternal Nutrition, Food and Nutrition Board Washington: National Research Council. National Academy of Sciences, 1970.

Mitchell FL: Steroid metabolism in the fetoplacental unit and in early childhood. *Vitam Horm* 25:191–270, 1967.

Mitchell MD et al.: Rapid increases in plasma prostaglandin concentration after vaginal examination and amniotomy. *Br Med J* 2:1183, 1977.

Murphy BEP: Steroid arteriovenous difference in umbilical cord plasma. Evidence of cortisol production by the human fetus in early gestation. *J Clin Endocrinol Metab* 36:1037–1038, 1973.

Murray JM, Weber A: The cooperative action of muscle proteins. *Sci Am* 230:59, 1974.

Myant NB: The thyroid and reproduction in mammals, in *The Thyroid Gland,* vol. 1, eds. R Pitt-Rivers, WR Trotter, Washington: Butterworth, 1964, pp. 283–302.

Naftolin F et al. (eds.): Androgen aromatization by neuroendocrine tissues, in *Subcellular Mechanisms in Reproductive Neuroendocrinology,* Amsterdam: Elsevier, 1976, pp. 347–355.

Neumann F et al.: Sexual differentiation. Morphology of development and maturation of endocrine organs, in *Endokrinologie der Entwicklung und Reifung,* ed. J Kracht, New York: Springer, 1970, pp. 58–82.

Niswanger JW, Langmade CF: Cardiovascular changes in vaginal deliveries and cesarean sections. *Am J Obstet Gynecol* 107:337, 1970.

Nora JJ, Nora AH: Can the pill cause birth defects? *N Eng J Med* 291:731, 1974.

Oakey RE: The progressive increase in estrogen production in human pregnancy: An appraisal of the factors responsible. *Vitam Horm* 28:1–36, 1970.

Oppenheimer JH: Thyroid hormone action at the cellular level. *Science* 203:971–979, 1979.

Parboosingh J, Doig A: Renal nyctohemeral excretory patterns of water and solutes in normal human pregnancy. *Am J Obstet Gynecol* 116:609, 1973.

Parry E et al.: Transit time in the small intestine in pregnancy. *J Obstet Gynaecol Br Commonw* 77:900, 1970.

Raynaud A: Effet des injections d'hormones, sexueles a la souris gravide, sur le developpement des ebauches de la glande mammaire des embryons. *Ann Endocrinol* (Paris), 8:248–253, 1947.

Rovinsky JJ: Blood volume and hemodynamics of pregnancy, in *Scientific Foundations of Obstetrics and Gynaecology,* ed. EE Philipp et al., London: Heinemann, 1970, pp. 332–342.

Rubi RA, Sala NI: Ureteral function in pregnant women. *Am J Obstet Gynecol* 113:335, 1972.

Ruthman LA et al.: Placental and fetal involvement by maternal malignancy. *Am J Obstet Gynecol* 116:1023, 1973.

Ryan KJ: Endocrine control of gestational length. *Am J Obstet Gynecol* 109:299, 1971.

Saldana I et al.: On the mechanism of mid-trimester abortions induced by the prostaglandin impact. *Prostaglandins* 3:847, 1973.

Schulman H, Romney SL: Variability of uterine contractions in normal human parturition. *Obstet Gynecol* 36:215, 1970.

Schwarz BE et al: Progesterone binding and metabolism in human fetal membranes. *Ann NY Acad Sci* 286:304, 1977.

Shepard TH: Development of the human fetal thyroid,

in *Hormones in Development,* eds M Hamburgh, EJW Barrington, New York: Appleton-Century-Crofts, 1971, pp. 767–780.

Short RV: Sex determination and differentiation, in *Reproduction in Mammals,* vol. 2, eds. CR Austin, RV Short, Cambridge: 1972, pp. 43–71.

Simmons R, Russell PS: The immunologic problem of pregnancy. *Am J Obstet Gynecol* 85:583, 1963.

Skowsky WR et al.: Vasopressin metabolism in the foetus and newborn, in *Foetal and Neonatal Physiology,* ed KS Comline et al., Cambridge: 1973, pp. 439–447.

Solomon S et al.: Formation and metabolism of steroids in the fetus and placenta. *Rec Prog Horm Res* 23:297–348, 1967.

Souma JA et al.: Comparison of thyroid function in each trimester of pregnancy. *Am J Obstet Gynecol* 116:905, 1973.

Spellacy WN: Diabetes and pregnancy. *Am J Obstet Gynecol* 113:855, 1972.

Ueland J et al.: Cardiorespiratory response to pregnancy and exercise in normal women and patients with heart disease. *Am J Obstet Gynecol* 115:4, 1973.

Vasicka A, Kretchmer HE: Uterine dynamics. *Clin Obstet Gynecol* 4:17, 1961.

Villee DB: Development of endocrine functions in the human placenta and fetus. *N Engl J Med* 281:473–484, 533–541, 1969.

Wachtel SS: H-Y antigen and the genetics of sex determination. *Science* 198:797–799, 1977.

Walker DG: Developmental aspects of carbohydrate metabolism, in *Carbohydrate Metabolism and Its Disorders,* vol. 1, ed. F Dickens et al., New York: Academic, 1968, pp. 465–496.

Wilson JD: Sexual differentiation. *Annu Rev Physiol* 40:279–306, 1978.

Winter JSD et al.: Sex steroid production by the human fetus: Its role in morphogenesis and control by gonadotropins, in *Morphogenesis and Malformation of the Genital System,* eds. RJ Blandau, D Bergsma, New York: Alan R Liss, 1977, pp. 41–58.

Zipper J et al.: Intrauterine grafting in rats of autologous and homologous rat skin. *Am J Obstet Gynecol* 94:1056, 1966.

10

Nutrition and Reproduction

RONALD A. CHEZ

NUTRITIONAL ASPECTS OF PRIMARY CARE
Nutritional standards
Assessment of nutritional status
Diet guidance and counseling
  Adolescence
  Cultural influences
  Faddism
  Lactose intolerance
  Economically deprived
  Obesity
  Hospital care

NUTRITIONAL RELATIONSHIPS IN THE NONPREGNANT WOMAN
Menstrual function and nutrition
  Menarche
  Amenorrhea
Oral contraception and metabolism and nutrition
  Metabolic changes
  Vitamins
  Minerals

NUTRITIONAL RELATIONSHIPS IN THE PREGNANT WOMAN
Hormonal changes and influence
General and individual requirements
  Weight gain
  Energy
  Minerals
  Sodium

Iron
Vitamins
Clinical management considerations
  Relevance
  Recommendation
  High-risk patients
Lactation
  Normal metabolism
  Abnormal metabolism

Nutrition is a term which encompasses the essential components of diet, the medical science related to the flux of substrate fuel for energy in the maintenance of health, and the art of feeding people. The interrelationships between nutrition, normal metabolism, and disease states increasingly stimulate questions relevant to the daily practice of medicine. Most of these questions are about dietary intake and do not lend themselves to resolution. The current list includes the relationship between:

1. Saturated fats and cholesterol content and coronary artery disease
2. Salt intake and the etiology and treatment of hypertension
3. Fiber content and intestinal carcinoma
4. Dietary phosphate/calcium ratio and osteoporosis

5. Iron-enriched flour and bread and prevention of iron-deficiency anemia
6. Animal and vegetable fats and carcinogenesis
7. Child-feeding practices and the incidence of subsequent adult cardiovascular disease, obesity, and diabetes mellitus
8. Fluoride, calcium, and glucose content and caries and periodontal disease
9. The general safety of food additives and their role in behavioral dysfunction
10. Pesticide residues on food and seafood pollutants and toxic levels of chemical intake.

The physician is asked by patients to explain these controversies, resolve discrepant information, and apply therapeutic measures. These are not easy tasks because the basic information is not always provided during formal medical education. Research in nutrition is hampered by difficulties in identifying and controlling the variables of food intake and nutrition definition. Every phase of research is affected, including the definition of the fed versus the fasted state, the evaluation of the antecedent health of the subject, the inability to recognize early deficient clinical states and the unavailability of appropriate laboratory assays, the degree of dietary restrictions resulting from cultural, social, and ethnic influences, the logistics of cross-sectional and longitudinal studies, the amount of physical activity, and the characteristics of the environment including the season of the year. The net result is a minimum of valid information.

In spite of these difficulties, the relationship of nutrition to the physiologic function of the woman in her reproductive years has enjoyed increasing scientific attention. There is sufficient information about the nonpregnant and the pregnant state to define basic requirements and standards, to assess clinical status, and to counsel and treat in the presence of deficiency and disease.

NUTRITIONAL ASPECTS OF PRIMARY CARE

NUTRITIONAL STANDARDS

The most frequently used system to define nutritional needs is the United States Recommended Daily Allowance (RDA). Its focus is on the amounts of vitamins, minerals, and energy sources needed to maintain good health. Previously, the concept had emphasized minimum intake necessary to prevent deficiencies. The RDA was established by the Food and Nutrition Board of the National Academy of Sciences–National Research Council. As new knowledge is developed, the data are updated. The data in Table 10–1 are statistical and derived from large populations. The recorded values are set at 2 standard deviations above the estimated *mean* requirement, or basically the highest daily nutrient need for the population. Therefore, the RDA is a guide to interpret the nutrient value of food normally eaten, not the required goal for all.

The table should be viewed flexibly for each individual. In addition to the variable of sex, age, weight, and height, one must add physical activity, abundance of food supply, variety of food supply, and the presence of pregnancy. Notice that 36 kcal per kilogram of body weight is recommended for the nonpregnant woman. This increases to 54 kcal per kilogram of body weight for the young teenager. The amount of protein recommended varies from 0.8 to 1.0 g per kilogram of body weight through this same age range and increases to 1.3 to 1.7 g/kg in pregnancy.

ASSESSMENT OF NUTRITIONAL STATUS

The adequacy of the patient's nutrition can be assessed by history, physical examination, and laboratory workup. A device for an immediate estimate of diet is to ask about the food intake in the previous 24 hours. This information can provide data about the manner in which the food is selected, the time of ingestion, and the amount of calories. It suffers from an assumption that this period is characteristic of the usual daily pattern. A more helpful history is one recorded by the patient over 1 week of time. Fill-in questionnaires which allow the amount of food consumed and recorded to be totaled and scored by composition are available. One such tool is published by the American College of Obstetricians and Gynecologists.

There are signs on physical examination that indicate malnutrition. The relationship of weight to height compared with standard tables is one (Table 10–2). Dry brittle hair of abnormal color suggests protein and calorie deficiency as does nondependent edema. Iron and folate deficiency result in signs of anemia and filiform papillary atrophy of the tongue. Gums that are red and swollen between the teeth are

TABLE 10-1   Recommended Dietary Allowances

	Nonpregnant females				Pregnancy	Lactation
	11–14 yr*	15–18 yr†	19–22 yr‡	23–50 yr§		
Energy, kcal	2400	2100	2100	2000	+300	+500
Protein, g	44	48	46	46	+30	+20
Vitamin A, IU	4000	4000	4000	4000	5000	6000
Vitamin D, IU	400	400	400		400	400
Vitamin E, IU	12	12	12	12	15	15
Ascorbic acid, mg	45	45	45	45	60	80
Folacin, μg	400	400	400	400	800	600
Niacin, mg	16	14	14	13	+2	+4
Riboflavin, mg	1.3	1.4	1.4	1.2	+0.3	+0.5
Thiamine, mg	1.2	1.1	1.1	1.0	+0.3	+0.3
Vitamin B_6, mg	1.6	2.0	2.0	2.0	2.5	2.5
Vitamin B_{12}, μg	3	3	3	3	4	4
Calcium, mg	1200	1200	800	800	1200	1200
Phosphorous, mg	1200	1200	800	800	1200	1200
Iodine, μg	115	115	100	100	125	150
Iron, mg	18	18	18	18	d	18
Magnesium, mg	300	300	300	300	450	450
Zinc, mg	15	15	15	15	20	25

*Weight, 44 kg (97 lb); height, 155 cm (62 in).
†Weight, 54 kg (119 lb); height, 162 cm (65 in).
‡Weight, 58 kg (128 lb); height, 162 cm (65 in).
§The increased requirements of pregnancy cannot usually be met by ordinary diets; therefore, the use of supplemental iron is recommended.
Source: Food & Nutrition Board: *Nutrition in Maternal Health Care.*

associated with vitamin C deficiency, and lack of riboflavin causes fissuring of the angles of the lips and inflammation of the tongue. The condition of the teeth as reflected in amount of decay and periodontal disease provides information about calcium, fluoride, and glucose levels as well as personal hygiene. A goiter suggests iodine deficiency. Enlarged wrists are a clue to vitamin deficiency, and follicular hyperkeratosis of the skin of the extremities is a clue to lack of vitamin A.

Both the availability of laboratory aids and the extent to which the physician wishes to confirm the working diagnosis vary between practice locales. A patient whose diet is deficient in meats, nuts, dairy products, and dry beans will probably be deficient in high-quality protein. Similarly, lack of meats, cereals, dry beans, and green leafy vegetables, all good sources of iron, result in iron deficiency and anemia. Assays to measure levels of serum iron, hemoglobin concentration, serum albumin, and percent of saturation of transferrin are readily obtainable in most laboratories. Such data will confirm an impression of a patient at nutritional risk. The subsequent section on vitamins and minerals in pregnancy details our current ability to assay these nutrients specifically.

DIET GUIDANCE AND COUNSELING

The primary therapy of undernourishment is counseling and the prescription of food. Food is intimately involved in the religious, ethnic, cultural, and social aspects of our lives. The purchase of food is a repetitive element of the monthly budget. Counseling about diet requires tolerance, sensitivity, and patience; it need not be solely the province of the physician and can often be done more effectively by another member of the health team particularly a nutritionist. There are special considerations in several identified groups of patients that require additional attention.

ADOLESCENCE

The perimenarchal girl is undergoing her last growth spurt. As her skeletal mass, tissue mass, blood volume, and physical activities increase, her demands for calories, protein, calcium, and iron increase. Her biochemical preparation for these changes is a result of her nutrition in childhood. Her ability to meet the current nutrient demands will affect the associated

TABLE 10–2 More than 85 Percent and Less than 120 Percent Standard Weight for 17- to 24-Year-Old Nonpregnant Females

| Height | | <85% | | >120% | |
cm	in	kg	lb	kg	lb
140	52.2	38.0	84	53.8	118
142	56.0	39.0	86	55.0	121
144	56.7	40.0	88	56.4	124
146	57.5	40.7	90	57.6	127
148	58.3	41.8	92	59.0	130
150	59.1	42.8	94	60.4	133
152	60.0	43.8	96	61.8	136
154	60.7	44.6	98	63.0	139
156	61.5	45.6	100	64.4	142
158	62.2	46.6	103	65.8	145
160	63.0	47.7	105	67.4	148
162	63.8	49.0	108	69.1	152
164	64.6	50.0	110	70.6	155
166	65.4	51.0	112	72.1	159
168	66.2	52.0	114	73.6	162
170	66.9	53.4	118	75.4	166
172	67.7	54.6	120	77.2	170
174	68.5	56.0	124	79.1	174
176	69.3	57.5	127	81.2	179
178	70.1	59.1	130	83.4	184
180	70.9	60.6	134	85.6	189
182	71.7	61.9	137	87.4	193
184	72.4	63.2	139	89.3	197
186	73.2	64.5	142	91.1	201
188	74.0	65.7	145	92.8	205
190	74.8	66.7	147	94.2	208
192	75.6	67.7	149	95.6	211
194	76.4	68.7	152	97.0	214
196	77.2	69.5	153	98.2	217
198	78.0	70.4	155	99.4	219
200	78.7	71.2	157	100.6	222
202	79.5	72.0	159	101.6	224

Source: *Assessment of Maternal Nutrition.*

growth pattern. Since this is by definition her preconceptional period, success in nutrition planning will best prepare her for childbearing.

The young teenager has limited knowledge about nutrition and not much enthusiasm for the deliberate planning of three balanced meals a day, is prone to food fads, and is joyfully tempted by junk foods. Junk food is a term applied to snack food with an excess calorie/protein ratio. Composed almost entirely of carbohydrates and fats to the exclusion of proteins, such foods' vitamin content is also inadequate. Junk food has become synonymous with fast-food-chain food and this may not be accurate. Specifically, a hamburger, french fries, and "milk" shake provide 1200 cal, 40 g of protein, and 40 g of fat. Substituting fried chicken for the hamburger results in the same calories with a 60 percent increase in protein and a 30 percent increase in fat. A 10-inch pizza has less fat and up to 70 g of protein with its 1200 cal. Therefore, many of the daily RDA requirements are met with such meals. However, all of these meals have an excess of fat, are deficient in water-soluble vitamins as well as vitamin D, and have excess salt content. In counseling the teenager, a physician can use this information positively to provide diets which are compatible with her eating habits and those of her peers. The physician should also consider active local lobbying to provide fruit- and milk-vending machines in those schools in which these machines presently dispense junk foods.

CULTURAL INFLUENCES

It is not surprising to learn that food, an intimate part of our everyday lives, is endowed with special values through folklore. What is surprising is how few of these folk beliefs are discerned by the medical provider. Unrecognized, they may dilute patient compliance with therapy and interfere with prophylactic measures. In the extreme, they have the potential of doing harm. Direct questioning is necessary to learn about relationships between cultural and religious backgrounds and dietary patterns. Asked in a frank and nonjudgmental manner, these questions allow the physician's therapy to more effectively consider such backgrounds when possible and to provide corrective information that can be used by the patient. Even so, there may be willful withholding of practices if the health provider is not viewed as sympathetic. Food preferences and taboos surround female reproductive function and all are not necessarily harmless.

The hot-cold theory of disease is prevalent in women in the South and of Latin-American origin. This concept extends to foods. For instance, cold foods are thought to impede menstrual flow. This belief extends to the 40 days postpartum, during which time they are to be avoided. Cold foods, also called acid or drying foods, include fruits and leafy vegetables. Therefore, their absence in the diet provides the potential for vitamin deficiency. The Chinese philosophy of Tao includes the concept of duality. Foods are classified into Yin and Yang. A number of foods with high vitamin C content as well as lamb and shellfish are considered taboo during pregnancy; again the potential for a deficiency exists if they are avoided.

FADDISM

Patients' beliefs about special foods, prestige foods, and body-image foods result in unusual dietary habits. There are patients who exaggerate their consumption of certain foods to the exclusion of a balanced diet with an end result of malnutrition. It is also important for the physician to recognize the food faddist, but the definition may be affected by the prejudices and food practices of the physician. There is ample room for misinterpretation in the semantics of current food regimens. Direct, candid questioning of the person for details of individual macrobiotic, lactovegetarian, nondairy, fruitarian, natural, raw or low-heat cooked, and yogurt diets is required. Reference sources should be frequently consulted to determine the actual daily caloric, mineral, and vitamin content of the related dietary regimens.

LACTOSE INTOLERANCE

Milk and milk products are valuable foods which are both cost effective and metabolically efficient. Lactose is the major disaccharide present in these foods. Lactase is required for its hydroxylation into glucose and galactose. There is some blurring of distinction between the pathology of lactase deficiency, lactose intolerance, and milk intolerance. A deficiency of the enzyme lactase is present in the majority of adult blacks and Orientals, resulting in lactose nondigestion or malabsorption. The deficiency can be associated with a clinical picture of cramping, bloating, diarrhea, and flatulence after ingesting milk. Awareness of this counterproductive phenomenon is important when counseling about the value of milk products in these races. Use of other high-protein and high-calcium foods, including those derived from milk, in which lactose has been consumed or metabolized in the manufacturing process is necessary.

ECONOMICALLY DEPRIVED

Awareness of food intolerances is particularly pertinent to those people who are impoverished and for whom food is a relatively large part of their costs. The Department of Agriculture (USDA) provides food supplements in the form of food stamps and a special program for women, infants, and children called WIC. Medical referral is necessary for patient participation. There are local and regional offices of the USDA throughout the country. Local health departments and the social service personnel at the hospi-

tals in the community are reliable sources of information. These programs need expanding to preconceptional women at risk, an appropriate focus for medical lobbying.

OBESITY

Obesity, defined as greater than 20 percent weight for height in standard tables (Table 10–2), or by the measurement of triceps skin-fold thickness with calipers, is a bona fide health hazard of epidemic proportions. Imagined obesity, defined by the patient's self-image or that of the commercials to which she is exposed, can result in unhealthy, self-prescribed eating practices. Both forms of obesity are ubiquitous in medical practice, and both require a chronic commitment of time and effort by the patient and her physician. The constant confrontation with popularly publicized weight-reduction schemes frequently serves to emphasize the lack of supportive or discriminatory data in the medical literature to validate stated claims. However, fuel homeostasis is a subject of increasing investigation, and publications are available for more intensive study.

Energy homeostasis is a function of fuel supply and fuel expenditure. The energy supply is obtained from food ingested, with endogenous stores making up any deficit. Excess calories from any carbohydrate-fat-protein composition result in the extra carbon atoms stored as fat. There is no apparent limit to the capacity for storage. When excess, it is recognized clinically as obesity. However, one poorly accessible factor in determining balance is the individual's endogenous metabolic rate and the efficiency of her basal fuel consumption. The concept of a "caloristat" is one attempt to clarify this. A second concept is that of an "aminostat," a specific metabolic orientation toward protein or lean body mass sparing.

The metabolic fuels of the body are muscle protein, adipose tissue, triglycerides, and liver glycogen. The actual energy substrates are glucose, glycerol, free fatty acids, ketones, and select amino acids including alanine, glutamine, and the branched chain group. The actual flux of these components is a function of the fed versus the fasted state. The primary hormone modifiers are insulin and glucagon. Their interactions with cell receptors determine net catabolic or anabolic states in the forms of glycogenolysis, gluconeogenesis, lipogenesis, lipolysis, and the degree of protein sparing via contrasting rates of synthesis and breakdown.

Weight-reduction regimens result in loss of water, glycogen, protein, and fat in various proportions. The caloric value or quality of the actual weight lost is not conveniently measured in the office. Because of the energy value of fat, 9 kcal/g, weight loss of 1 pound, or 0.45 kg of fat, equates to an energy deficit of 3500 kcal on the consumption-expenditure ledger. However, the energy value of 0.45 kg weight loss can range between 1900 and 3400 kcal. This is a function of such variables as amount of kcal consumed, the protein-fat-carbohydrate proportions of these calories including the ketogenic potential of the diet, the degree and type of voluntary activity, the number of days of calorie restriction and the extent of that restriction, and the degree of initial obesity. Therefore, the eventual goal, the mobilization of endogenous fat for fuel takes time as does a slow but steady weight loss.

Further, there is always water and protein loss with weight loss. In spite of commercial claims, the appropriate place for protein-supplemented fasting diets is not clear. There may be a protein sparing effect, but this takes place after at least some loss of lean body mass. At this time, an isocaloric mixture of proteins and carbohydrates is preferable.

The long-term treatment of obesity is fundamentally behavioral with the setting of realistic goals of both food consumption and physical activity that are compatible with home and work life. The prescription of diuretics and anorectic medicants should be sparing and short term if used at all. Obese patients frequently are malnourished. Dieting can enhance or create this condition. Supplements, particularly of water-soluble vitamins and minerals such as zinc and chromium, should be prescribed. In a society which is oriented toward immediate gratification and instant success, persistent motivation to maintain a weight-reduction program can exhaust the imagination and patience of the health provider.

HOSPITAL CARE

The concept of protein sparing is relevant to the nutritional status of postoperative hospitalized patients. Gynecologist-obstetricians occasionally confront situations of severe trauma or disease necessitating several days or more of intravenous therapy for nutrient and fluid requirements. The potential for malnourishment exists. Intravenous nutrition has advanced markedly with the current availability of isotonic crystalline amino acid mixtures and fat emulsions. Improved wound healing, resistance to infections, and preservation of lean body mass are all potential benefits derived from appropriate parenteral nutrition.

These benefits may be particularly pertinent to the chronic care of gynecologic oncology patients. Proper nutritional support can enhance tolerance to therapy, lessen surgical complications, and perhaps improve tumor response to treatment. However, the radiologic and chemotherapeutic management of the disease itself frequently is accompanied by anorexia, nausea, and diarrhea. Depression may lead to further lack of interest in food. A semistarved state can develop, and aggressive management is essential. The imagination and attention of the health team to enhancing food intake, perfecting the necessary delivery systems, and devising optimal formulations constitute an integral part of total patient care. A physician attempting to do this in the hospital situation may be dismayed at the lack of effectiveness of the nutrition service component in the hospital. The usual situation is one of inadequate or nonexistent interdisciplinary communication, understaffing, lack of valid assessment, and poorly defined responsibilities for patient education. Improvement as a team effort is necessary and required.

NUTRITIONAL RELATIONSHIPS IN THE NONPREGNANT WOMAN

MENSTRUAL FUNCTION AND NUTRITION

MENARCHE

One of the dominant hypotheses as to what triggers sexual maturation in girls relates to their nutritional status. Specifically, a critical weight of approximately 48 kg of which the proportion of body fat is approximately 17 percent has been suggested as the trigger for both the initiation of the weight spurt and menarche. Others believe that the height-for-weight ratio may be the important factor, of which the percentage of total body protein identified as lean body mass is essential. Undernutrition is associated with delayed menarche, delay in regular ovulation, delay in skeletal growth, and diminished adolescent growth spurt.

The basic concept of a critical metabolic signal for the body to initiate ovulatory-reproductive function makes biologic sense—that is, a delay of reproductive capacity until sufficient stores are available to provide fuel for the conception which nature anticipates. The absolute and relative increase in fat content of the young woman's body from menarche to late teens reinforces this biologic premise. However, the data that support these statements are derived primarily from retrospective data on weight and menarche rather than from directly observed measurements, and the actual metabolic criteria remain unknown.

AMENORRHEA

In the menstruating woman, among the etiologies that have been identified with secondary amenorrhea are chronic undernutrition and acute weight loss. Patients with weight loss-associated amenorrhea have both direct and indirect laboratory evidence of hypothalamic dysfunction, while pituitary and end-organ function remain normal. This evidence includes abnormal thermoregulation and water conservation as well as delayed increases in luteinizing hormone and thyrotropin levels after releasing hormone stimulation. Menses usually reappears with reacquisition of weight. Therefore, food is an essential therapy for this disease process. These facts also support the concept of minimum weight for height and presumably percent of fat stores for normal hypothalamic-pituitary-ovarian function.

An exaggeration of the effect of diet restriction on menstrual function occurs with anorexia nervosa. This serious disease of psychologic origin may be a more common cause of amenorrhea in the adolescent than is presently recognized. Self-imposed starvation with its associated weight loss should be specifically ruled out in the diagnostic workup of women with amenorrhea. Although the actual cause is not known, hypothalamic dysfunction can be readily documented in the laboratory. In addition to the tests mentioned above, other findings include decreases in the basal blood levels of luteinizing hormone, thyroid stimulating hormone, and triiodothyronine. Liver function may also become abnormal with chronic starvation. Therapy is primarily psychiatric and is directed toward the abnormal ideations about food and body image.

Obesity and menstrual dysfunction including anovulation are clinically associated. Since one theory for obesity is a defect in the hypothalamic noradrenergic nerve centers identified with sensations of satiety and hunger, this relationship may be primarily hypothalamic in origin. However, another theory invokes the fact that adipose tissue is a site where peripherally circulating androstenedione is aromatized to estrogens. As the fat deposits increase, the amount of estrogen produced from androgen conversion increases. Resultant high levels of estrogen provide a negative feedback to the hypothalamus with anovulation and oligomenorrhea occurring in the patient.

Therapies resulting in controlled weight loss are effective in restoring normal function.

ORAL CONTRACEPTION AND METABOLISM AND NUTRITION

The combination pill is the most effective single method of reversible contraception that is presently available. This is its primary benefit to the patient. There are risks, and they relate to the fact that because the pill is not a local or mechanical method, systemic changes occur in the nonreproductive organs. The combination pill is composed of two steroids. These steroids, one of two synthetic estrogens and one of five 19-nortestosterone progestins (Chap. 33), cause changes in carbohydrate, lipid, and protein metabolism, some of which are adverse. They also modify vitamin and mineral metabolism and are anabolic in some women. Therefore, the use of oral contraception has the potential of modifying total body nutrition.

As with other areas in this chapter, published studies on the changes in nutrition in women using oral contraception are not consistent in their findings. One of the main variables is that over 30 brands of pills are available with a number of different permutations in the amount, type, and potency of the two combined steroids, thus making data comparison difficult.

METABOLIC CHANGES

In general, the metabolic changes are in the same direction as those that occur in pregnancy, but the extent of the changes is modest. Circulating levels of triglycerides are increased secondary to both increased hepatic production and decreased rate of clearance, the latter probably in part a function of changes in circulating levels of insulin and glucagon. The increased hepatic synthesis of cholesterol results in increased circulating levels, and there are also increased levels of phospholipids and lecithin. On stopping the pill, a patient's return to base-line values requires about 3 months. The clinical implications of these lipid changes are pertinent to the pathology of the cardiovascular system, the question of enhanced atherogenesis, and the incidence of increased coronary artery disease.

These steroids stimulate hepatic endoplasmic reticulum to the point of hyperplasia. As a result, circulating levels of the carrier proteins, lipoproteins, and blood coagulation factors including plasminogen and fibrinogen are increased. Serum levels of albumin, haptoglobulin, and a number of amino acids are decreased. The latter may be secondary to the increased anabolic state that is induced by steroids. In some patients, the associated weight gain is undesirable enough to stop the drugs. These changes take about 8 weeks to revert to normal after stopping the pill. The clinical implications include the relationship of these changes to hypertension, thrombosis, and embolism.

The changes in carbohydrate metabolism include increases in concentrations of fasting blood sugar, insulin, and growth hormone, and a decrease in glucagon. According to the number of high risk or potentiating factors present in the woman and the rigor of the challenge, 10 to 50 percent of women will evidence abnormal glucose tolerance testing while on the pill. Eight weeks are required for reversal of these changes after stopping. The clinical implications include acceleration of both latent diabetes mellitus and atherogenesis.

The changes briefly sketched above do not occur to the same extent in all women. Also, neither the extent of each steroid's potency in humans nor the net interactions between the two steroids when combined can be effectively measured. An additional area of uncertainty is the importance of the antecedent and continuing state of nutrition of the patient. There are conflicting suggestions that the magnitude of these metabolic changes is less in a patient who is already malnourished; that the pill will intensify persisting states of undernourishment; and that enhanced nutrition will protect against adverse consequences of the laboratory-detected changes. Research data are lacking, but in the interim, it should be assumed that an appropriate balanced nutrition is preferable to other alternatives.

VITAMINS

There are changes in vitamin and mineral metabolism in women using the pill. Whether these changes are descriptive without clinical implications is uncertain. Further, whether a decrease in levels is synonymous with the term deficiency depends on such factors as changes in individual substrate turnover, changes in tissue levels compared to circulating levels, changes in gastrointestinal absorption, and changes in carrier binding. Also, antecedent nutrition, concurrent food intake, and duration of pill use have impact.

Serum vitamin A levels are increased. This is apparently secondary to an increase in lipoprotein and therefore an increased opportunity for binding. However, liver levels of vitamin A are decreased, suggesting a relative deficiency. The serum levels of thiamine and B_{12} are decreased. The tissue levels of these vitamins may not be changed and it is uncertain why serum levels decrease since absorption does not seem adversely affected. The erythrocyte levels of riboflavin are decreased.

The plasma, leukocyte, and platelet levels of vitamin C are decreased. This may be secondary to an increased rate of metabolism enhanced by ceruloplasmin, an oxidant of vitamin C. The level of ceruloplasmin is increased by hepatic synthesis. The erythrocyte, plasma, and tissue levels of folate are also decreased. This decrease is believed to be secondary to enhanced metabolism by intestinal enzymes. Folate is important in erythropoiesis as well as in the biosynthesis of the biogenic amine, norepinephrine. Clinical implications of deficiency include anemia and the possibility of changes in the relationship of norepinephrine to adrenergic function in general, hypothalamic function specifically.

Vitamin B_6 levels are also decreased and there is some evidence of functional pyridoxine deficiency on testing, caused by an increase in turnover of the vitamin as well as by estrogen interfering with its binding to cell receptor. Pyridoxal phosphate is important to a number of decarboxylase- and transaminase-dependent pathways. The tryptophan-serotonin metabolic pathway is pyridoxine dependent as is the tryptophan-nicotinamide pathway. In the former, there is a decrease in tryptamine excretion, a finding in patients with depression. In the latter, there is an increased excretion of the side products of the pathway including kynurenic acid and xanthurenic acid. The latter complexes with circulating insulin and decreases insulin's biologic activity. The clinical implications related to the associated lethargy and depression which interfere with successful compliance by pill takers on the one hand, as well as the increased incidence of abnormal glucose tolerance testing on the other, are both areas that require more research.

MINERALS

In mineral metabolism, circulating levels of transferrin are increased secondary to hepatic synthesis. Withdrawal bleeding with the pill tends to be less in volume than that occurring normally with menstruation. The patient with good nutrition therefore has an opportunity to enhance her iron stores, and serum levels of iron are increased in pill users. Copper levels are increased secondary to the increased production of its binding protein, ceruloplasmin. Zinc plasma levels are decreased but erythrocyte levels are increased. The significance of this shift and why it occurs is not clear.

The therapeutic issue that relates to nutrition and metabolism in the pill user is the appropriate role of supplementation during pill use. For those substrates where depletion of stores occurs, the deficiency will persist for 3 to 4 months while overall metabolism returns to the prepill base-line state. Most patients on reversible contraception are theoretically preconceptional and a number of patients do stop the pill in order to conceive. There is concern about a patient who enters pregnancy with depleted stores of minerals and vitamins. If a patient is marginally deficient when she starts using the pill, will the metabolic changes intensify this deficiency and amplify any adverse effects? There is a possibility that the patient already marginally deficient will be at less risk from metabolic changes and the extent to which they will occur.

It is tempting to supplement these patients, particularly with vitamin C, folate, zinc, and the B vitamins. With regard to vitamin B_6, there have been studies suggesting that supramaximal pharmacologic doses of pyridoxine will cause the abnormal glucose tolerance to revert to normal and will ameliorate any associated depression. However, caution has to be advised inasmuch as vitamin B_6 is a coenzyme of a number of enzyme pathways in gluconeogenesis and the Embden-Meyerhof cycle. One net result of an increase in metabolism is a lowering of circulating amino acids, an effect not to the advantage of the already malnourished patient. At present, the institution and preservation of good eating habits with appropriate balanced caloric intake is the most essential and appropriate therapy in patients on the pill. This therapy should suffice without the need for supplementation.

NUTRITIONAL RELATIONSHIPS IN THE PREGNANT WOMAN

HORMONAL CHANGES AND INFLUENCE

Pregnancy can be viewed in terms of new organ growth with its associated formation of new cells in the form of placenta and fetus, and the enlargement of already existing maternal cells. This tissue growth requires nutrients for energy and chemical components for structure. The hormonal changes associated with pregnancy modify maternal intermediary metabolism to provide these essentials. The effects from the hormonal secretions of the mother, fetus, and placenta are:

1. Increased specific protein synthesis in the reproductive tract and breast to provide sites of exchange for the conceptus during the antepartum and postpartum period
2. Sparing of carbohydrate, the primary fuel for the fetus, during the same period
3. Modified fat metabolism to ensure an available source of maternal energy during periods of decreased intake.

The increased synthesis of protein in estrogen-sensitive tissues is secondary to cytoplasmic and nuclear binding of estrogens. The synthesis of new proteins by the rough endoplasmic reticulum results in an anabolic state. There is a gradual rise in circulating red blood cell mass stimulated by the synergism between placental lactogen and erythropoietin. Human placental lactogen and pituitary prolactin initiate milk protein synthesis in the breast. The overall result is a net maternal positive nitrogen balance of as much as 250 g by the end of pregnancy.

Fasting blood glucose levels gradually decrease during pregnancy. There is increased conversion to lipids for maternal storage and constant and increasing utilization by the fetus. Orally ingested glucose results in a greater and more prolonged maintained increase in plasma glucose levels than occurs in the nonpregnant. Although basal insulin values are increased in most studies, there is both a peripheral and an hepatic resistance to insulin action. These changes are partly the result of the marked increase in estrogen concentration and the presence of placental lactogen with its growth-hormone-like anti-insulin activity.

In the first half of pregnancy, the main change in lipid metabolism is an increase in lipogenesis from the relative hyperinsulinism. This accumulation reaches a maximum before the third trimester. Later, these fatty acids become an important fuel for the mother as lipolytic activity in the maternal fat depots increases during the day and with overnight fasting, an effect mediated by placental lactogen. Recycling of unused free fatty acids occurs in the presence of excess supply. The enhanced availability and the utilization of fatty acids by the mother to spare glucose accentuate ketone body formation. A large statistical evaluation of data collected from a number of perinatal centers has implicated ketonuria as positively correlated with decreased infant neurologic development and intelligence quotients. These data have been used to support the opposition to purposeful weight-reducing regimens in pregnancy which by definition would require ketogenic dietary regimens. They also have been used to indict those who fail to encourage a maternal weight gain of more than 20 pounds. This issue will remain unresolved until we learn the frequency of ketonuria in normal pregnancy, the ability of the mother and fetus to use ketones as fuel, and whether the fetal nervous system is exclusively dependent on glucose.

Descriptive terms of "accelerated starvation" and "facilitated anabolism" have been used to dramatize the extent of interplay in intermediary metabolism during the pregnant woman's 24-hour day. The mother, eating 3 meals a day and "fasting" for 8 to 10 hours overnight, is accommodated or protected by hormone changes to ensure her fuel supply. The fetus, to a large extent protected through its placental transport mechanisms, is exposed to a relatively unchanging supply of glucose and amino acids with minimal diurnal variations. In optimal circumstances of maternal nutrition and freedom from disease, fetal growth and development progress well. There is a margin of reserve or safety in this growth when suboptimal conditions are extant. However, eventually, the mother is spared to the detriment of her fetus. The range of pathology varies from diminished fetal size at birth and diminished fetal brain development to premature labor with its associated perinatal morbidity and mortality. It is the combined responsibility of the obstetrician and the patient to ensure that proper nutrition prevent these phenomena from happening.

GENERAL INDIVIDUAL REQUIREMENTS

WEIGHT GAIN

Normal healthy women allowed to eat to satisfy their appetites consistently gain between 22 and 28 pounds during pregnancy. After minimal weight change in the first trimester, the subsequent rate of weekly increments is relatively constant at slightly less than 1 pound per week. The pattern is more important clinically than the total weight gain. Failure to gain weight and acute excessive increases in weight are both signs of potential pathology. The compo-

nents of this gain are fluid, fat, and cell protein. The distribution of gain is uneven. Maternal tissue and fluid accumulation occurs primarily in the second trimester and is manifest as an increase in blood volume and cells, fat storage, and uterine and breast growth. The weight gain in the third trimester is dominated by the fetus, placenta, and the amniotic fluid. These features are all illustrated in Fig. 10–1.

ENERGY

The accumulated total weights that have been assigned to each component in normal pregnancy are protein 1 kg, fat 3 kg, and water 6 kg. The energy cost of pregnancy must therefore relate to these additional requirements superimposed on the basal metabolic or basal maintenance rate of the woman. The isocaloric kcal per day requirement increases during pregnancy, and the manner in which it is expended changes according to the trimester. The average additional fuel requirement during gestation increases from approximately 100 kcal daily in the first half of pregnancy to about 300 kcal daily in the second half. This can be calculated as a 10 to 15 percent increase for the nonpregnant woman who is initially in isocaloric balance between 1800 and 2200 kcal per day. The total is estimated to be between 68,000 and 75,000 kcal. The variables include the extent of the woman's physical activity, her prepregnant weight, and the ambient temperature.

MINERALS

We are beginning to learn more about the normal pregnancy-associated physiologic changes in the metabolism of minerals as laboratory methodology improves. However, the concentration, measurements, and assays of biochemical function of these elements do not yet correlate with pathologic conditions of pregnancy nor even nutritional status. Therefore, the pertinence of apparent deficiencies in trace metals to the practice of obstetrics is uncertain.

Plasma zinc levels gradually decrease after the first trimester; whether this decrease reflects a change in body stores is unclear. The basis for the recommendation to increase zinc uptake in pregnancy is also unclear. Serum levels of copper gradually increase as does its glycoprotein, ceruloplasmin. Low serum copper levels can be caused by hypoproteinemia. There is preliminary data suggesting a correlation between low levels of copper with threatened abortion and severe placental insufficiency.

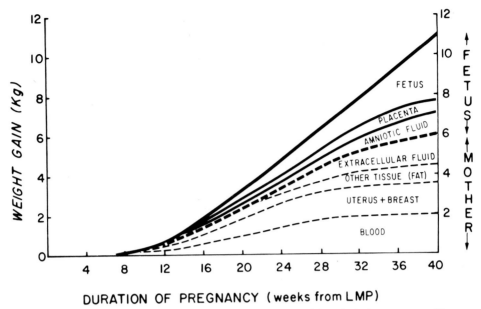

FIGURE 10–1 Pattern and components of average maternal weight gain during pregnancy. *(From Pitkin.)*

The biopotent fraction of plasma chromium is nicotinic acid complex, also called glucose tolerance factor. Plasma levels of this factor are governed by its release from stores, a function of glucose load and circulating plasma levels of insulin, and its peripheral utilization. The direction of these changes in pregnancy is unclear. Urinary levels of chromium may be accurate indices of nutritional status in the nonpregnant state; standards are not yet available in pregnancy.

Other trace metals which will be receiving more research attention in humans because of their associations in animal growth experiments are manganese, magnesium, tin, nickel, and selenium. The hope is that disease states can either be predicted or prevented by defined biologic associations secondary to deficiencies.

The importance of iodine in pregnancy is less subtle. The nutritional status of iodine can be assessed with 24-hour urinary excretion rate studies. The absolute excretion rate of iodine is the same in pregnancy and nonpregnancy. A level of less than 40 μg per 24 hours is diagnostic of inadequate iodine stores and intake. In pregnancy, iodine deficiency results in lower serum thyroxine values and elevated plasma thyroid stimulating hormone levels. Both the mother and the fetus develop goiter. Uncorrected hypothyroidism of the newborn is associated with mental retardation. Iodinized table salt is a readily available therapy in endemic goitrogenic areas and a prophylactic measure in other locales.

The fetus requires about 30 g of calcium, almost all of it in the last trimester. There is increased maternal calcium pool turnover and increased intestinal absorption of calcium during pregnancy. The fetus will acquire the calcium it needs by active transport across the placenta. To avoid depletion, the mother needs to ingest about 2 g of calcium a day. The patient's exposure to sunlight and the status of her vitamin D metabolism in general play supportive roles. The calcium requirement should be met by appropriate planning with an emphasis on dairy products. The use of oral calcium salt supplements is an adequate substitute for food.

SODIUM

Sodium is an essential element in pregnancy. The nonedematous pregnant woman accumulates about 6 L of water, close to 4 L of this divided between interstitial fluid and blood volume. Sodium is a major cation for osmotic equilibrium in interstitial fluid. Along with the fluid, 20 g of sodium must be retained; this retention is an integral part of the normal physiology of pregnancy. The retention is secondary to a marked increase in aldosterone secretion, probably a counter-response to the increased level of the natriuretic hormone, progesterone. A positive sodium balance of up to 1 g per week occurs near term. Any excess is excreted by the kidney.

As a general principle of good eating habits, excessive salting of foods should be discouraged in all patients because of its relationship to essential hypertension. This does not translate into an admonition that salt restriction during pregnancy should be encouraged. Lower extremity edema is a normal accompaniment of pregnancy in the majority of women and is explainable by physiologic changes. Further, it has not been shown that either the use of salt restriction or diuretics results in a change in the incidence of the toxemia. However, the relationship between salt metabolism and essential hypertension in the nonpregnant woman continues to make the original hypothesis attractive.

Dietary manipulation to avoid or treat toxemia of pregnancy has had a number of phases including excess red meat, no meat, high protein, water restriction, and excess as well as restricted salt. A present standard approach emphasizes a high protein caloric diet, allowing the woman to salt her food to taste. However, since toxemia of pregnancy remains a prevalent disease of unknown etiology a variety of dietary approaches are used in its management.

IRON

As much as 1 g of iron is needed for the tissue growth requirements of pregnancy. This is divided between the fetus and its blood volume (250 mg), the umbilical cord and placenta (50 mg), maternal red blood cell mass (500 mg), and daily maternal excretion (200 mg). Because iron is transported by the placenta to the fetus, maternal depletion will occur if there are inadequate maternal stores or ingestion. The sequence after bone marrow stores are depleted is an increase in iron absorption by the gut, a decrease in serum iron levels, an increase in serum binding capacity, a decrease in saturation of serum transferrin to below 16 percent, a decrease in the rate of erythropoiesis, and finally, a decrease in red blood cell size, hemoglobin content, and hemoglobin concentration. Therefore, the most sensitive indicator of iron nutritional status is the bone marrow iron stores. The last step, microcytic hypochromic iron-deficiency anemia, is the most overt clinical indicator of deficiency.

Absent or very low stores can be found in up to half of apparently healthy young nonpregnant women. The dominant cause is failure to replace the iron lost during menstrual blood flow, combined with inadequate iron ingestion either secondary to a deficient diet or through lack of an iron-containing medicine. Without supplementation in pregnancy serum iron

levels, erythrocyte count, hemoglobin concentration, hematocrit, and percent of transferrin saturation all decrease. Serum iron binding capacity increases as does gut iron absorption. Iron supplementation will modify these changes with serum iron remaining constant, total iron binding capacity increasing to a lesser extent, and the percent saturation of transferrin remaining in the normal range of greater than 20 percent. Also, hemoglobin concentration will not decrease. However, it is possible for the patient with initial severely depleted bone marrow stores not to have replenished them at term in spite of supplementation.

Iron supplementation is recommended for all pregnant women regardless of their initial hemoglobin values at the time of conception. Usual diets cannot provide enough iron for absorptive needs. Oral supplements resulting in 30 to 60 mg of elemental iron are required; ferrous sulfate is the least expensive preparation. Some patients develop gastric distress following oral iron and their compliance with the prescription decreases when this occurs. To increase absorption, the alternate use of injectable iron dextran preparations must be balanced with their associated risks of skin staining, pain, and hypersensitivity. The rate of incorporation of iron is not influenced by the route employed. As discussed elsewhere in this book, the finding of anemia requires a diagnostic workup to define etiology accurately.

VITAMINS

The prescribing of vitamins to the pregnant woman is so ingrained that the physician not doing so may jeopardize the patient's confidence in the care and ability of her doctor. The enhanced maternal metabolism and fetal growth-maintenance needs do place an extra demand on vitamin requirements. However, the exact effects of normal pregnancy on vitamin needs have been difficult to assess accurately by laboratory methodology.

Vitamin A levels have been reported to both increase and not change during pregnancy. If a low intake occurs over prolonged time, serum vitamin A levels will decline as will the levels in breast milk. Levels of vitamin D, or 25-hydroxycholecalciferol, its biologically active circulating metabolite, are not changed by pregnancy. However, changes do occur secondary to such variables as season of the year, sunlight exposure, and the vegetable-animal product content of the diet. Tocopherol serum levels, which reflect vitamin E, increase without a change in intake, suggesting a change in metabolism or transport.

Serum vitamin C levels decline by less than 15

percent during pregnancy. The most reliable index of thiamine nutrition is erythrocyte transketolase stimulation measurements, and preliminary data indicate no change from the nonpregnant state. Urinary thiamine levels decrease with gestation, and there is a direct correlation between these levels and dietary intake. Similarly, urine concentrations of riboflavin correlate with diet. Although the reason is unknown, urinary levels increase in midtrimester and decrease near term. The laboratory procedures to evaluate niacin and nicotinic acid deficiency are insufficient at present, and reliable statements about metabolism in pregnancy are not available.

Vitamin B_{12} and folic acid have particularly important roles in erythropoiesis. B_{12} deficiency from dietary practices is rare, but should be considered in patients on strict vegetarian diets. Serum levels of B_{12} decrease in pregnancy. Serum levels of folic acid correlate directly with ingestion, but erythrocyte levels are less variable and therefore provide a more accurate comment on actual tissue levels. Both serum and erythrocyte levels fall in pregnancy; this can be prevented with supplementation. The concentration of vitamin B_6 in whole blood erythrocytes, plasma, and urine all fall in pregnancy. As discussed under Oral Contraception, metabolites of tryptophan-xanthurenic acid, kynurenine, and hydroxykenurine all increase in the presence of pyridoxal phosphate deficiency. Xanthurenic acid binds insulin and thereby decreases the functional metabolic activity of circulating insulin. Recent clinical investigation has been directed at large doses of vitamin B_6 to reverse the relative glucose intolerant state. The pertinence of this to the incidence of gestational diabetes mellitus is unclear.

The translation of this information to the medical care of the pregnant woman is not clear. It is not certain if a change in circulating or urinary levels of a vitamin reflects increased requirements, a change in transport and binding, a change in turnover and metabolic clearance rate, or an actual change in tissue reserves. The latter factor is pertinent only to the fat-soluble vitamins which are stored and not the water-soluble vitamins which require daily replenishment. In addition to difficult methodology, other influential variables such as cigarette smoking, oral contraceptive or other medicine use prior to conception, age and parity, the extent of vitamin-supplemented food intake, and season of the year affect the interpretation of values.

Nevertheless, thoughtful scientists have provided RDA criteria as seen in Table 10–1. The general consensus is that vitamins are relatively cheap to purchase, deficiency is difficult to detect, laboratory assays are costly, and there is a safety margin between therapeutic dose and overdosage. However, excess intakes of the fat-soluble vitamins A and D are stored and can reach toxic levels. The physician should be thoughtful before prescribing more than 10,000 IU per dosage unit of A and more than 400 IU per dosage unit of D. Excess vitamin A can cause anorexia, dry cracking skin, alopecia, and bone pain. Anorexia, weight loss, polyuria, soft tissue and vascular calcification, and anemia are some of the findings with excess vitamin D.

A balanced 2200- to 2400-kcal daily diet will supply a sufficient quantity of vitamins and make supplementation unnecessary. Or from another view, vitamin pills cannot substitute for an inadequate diet and are a misdirected focus in that circumstance.

CLINICAL MANAGEMENT CONSIDERATIONS

RELEVANCE

A primary goal of prenatal care is term delivery of an appropriate for gestational age weight baby who is mature and fully developed. This is to be accomplished without insult to the mother, who will have been properly prepared for successful lactation. The probability of a good perinatal outcome is directly related to newborn birth weight. Perinatal morbidity and mortality increase as birth weight decreases. The incidences of developmental dysfunction and low intelligence quotient also increase as birth weight decreases; therefore, fetal nutrition also affects subsequent childhood and adolescence.

Both maternal weight gain and prepregnant weight affect birth weight. Specifically, birth weight increases as maternal weight gain increases. It also increases as prepregnant weight increases. These two factors act independently, but they are also additive. A high prepregnant weight (greater than 20 percent standard values for height) will counterbalance to some extent the negative effect on birth weight of inadequate weight gain during pregnancy. An underweight woman beginning pregnancy can minimize this negative influence on birth weight with purposeful caloric supplementation.

RECOMMENDATION

The guidelines for weight gain are a gain of at least 10 pounds by 20 weeks' gestation, and a gain of at least 20 pounds by term. The rate should be approximately 1 pound per week after the tenth week. It is helpful to plot these values sequentially on a grid. The caloric content of the daily diet should result in these standards. About 200 g of the diet should be carbohydrate to provide for maternal fat storage and to minimize maternal fat utilization near term. At least 1.0 g of protein per kilogram of body weight is recommended, with 1.3 preferable and up to 1.7 g/kg best for the young pregnant teenager. The argument over daily total calories opposed to amount of protein as more important to birth weight is not resolved; probably, both have equivalent importance. Daily iron, 30 to 60 mg elemental, and folic acid, 400 to 800 μg, supplementation should be prescribed. Weight-reduction diets, salt-restriction diets, and diuretics should be avoided.

HIGH-RISK PATIENTS

Nutrition counsel is an integral part of prenatal care and it requires attention at each visit. Inappropriate weight-gain patterns, iron-deficiency anemia, and clinical signs of vitamin deficiency are important diagnostic clues that require a conscientious search by the physician. There are factors in the initial examination that signal the woman at an increased risk. These factors include high parity, conceptions at a frequency of greater than 15-month intervals, low prepregnant weight of less than 15 percent of standard weight, obesity, addiction to tobacco, alcohol, and street drugs, low income with economic deprivation, adolescence, and food faddism including pica. During pregnancy, hyperemesis, inappropriate fetal growth patterns, and multiple pregnancy are high-risk factors.

Of more importance than actual chronologic age of the adolescent is her biologic age. This is calculated as her age in years minus her age at menarche. A result of less than 4 years places her and her fetus at particular risk.

Pica is the repeated excessive ingestion of matter without caloric value. The reason for this seemingly insatiable craving is uncertain; there may be a relationship to the patient's culture in some instances. Items eaten include laundry starch, clay, dirt, ice, raw rice, and cornstarch. Large quantities of these materials displace food nutrients from the diet and also cause satiety. The result is inadequate intake of substrates, resulting in deficiencies of essential nutrients and depletion of iron stores. Both malnutrition and anemia are the clinical consequences. For pica, as in the case of all of these special patients, therapy consists of increased active counseling and the use of

supplemental iron salts. Frequently, there is a need for financial assistance to help the patient purchase food.

LACTATION

NORMAL METABOLISM

An integral part of mammalian pregnancy is lactation and nursing. The metabolic changes that occur in human pregnancy anticipate that nursing will take place. Of the mother's 24-pound weight gain, 18 pounds is accounted for by the weight of the products of conception. The additional 6 pounds is in the form of fat deposits. They serve as a partial source of energy for the production of milk during the initial months of lactation.

Between 25 and 40 percent of women in the United States initially breast-feed; less than 20 percent continue past 3 months postpartum. These numbers are influenced by psychosocial perceptions, social class, availability and cost of commercial formulas, degree of physician interest and direction, infant's apparent well-being, and the extent of the woman's activities outside the home. Most women decide during their pregnancy that they wish to breast-feed and begin preparing with self-education materials and childbirth preparation courses. For some women, nipple-rolling exercises in the last trimester can be helpful.

In the first year of life, human milk production gradually decreases from 850 to 500 mL per day. The caloric density of human milk is about 0.7 kcal/mL. A high degree of metabolic efficiency, approximately 90 percent, results in a daily maternal cost for production of this milk of 660 down to 430 kcal. The additional daily maternal food ingestion to meet this need is directly related to the adequacy of the woman's antepartum fat stores. Approximately half of the caloric requirements will come from these stores because of the fat component of milk. Therefore, the lactating woman's diet should be increased by the amount necessary to maintain her weight. That is, maternal weight should be monitored as a clinical sign that the caloric intake is adequate. At least 20 g of protein should be included in the diet as should calcium-containing foods. In addition, supplements of water-soluble vitamins, vitamin D, and iron should be prescribed. There is no relationship between excess fluid intake and increased milk volume; fluids sufficient to satisfy thirst are sufficient.

ABNORMAL METABOLISM

There is a lack of consensus as to whether the quality or composition of the milk, the quantity of milk produced, and the duration of breast-feeding are related to maternal nutrition. Most authorities believe that there is no relationship between milk composition and whether a woman is adequately nourished or undernourished. The two exceptions are the intake of water-soluble vitamins and the percentage of polyunsaturated fatty acids in the diet. Maternal ingestion of both is directly related to their concentration in milk. If there is inadequate maternal caloric intake, maternal body fat will be mobilized. As body stores are used, the pattern of fatty acids in the milk will reflect the pattern of fat deposits as the body tissues are depleted. If the woman is severely malnourished and her fat stores are depleted, the fat content of the milk will decrease with no change in either the protein or lactose concentration. Because fat accounts for approximately one-half of the calories of human milk, any decrease in fat concentration will result in fewer calories being supplied to the infant. Since calories in the infant are required for basal maintenance as well as growth, the potential exists that growth may be adversely affected as a result of the infant's inappropriate use of milk proteins for caloric needs.

The quantity of milk is related to a number of factors which include physiologic ones such as the feeding schedule. Further, approaches that measure the volume of milk produced by weighing the baby and its excreta, or by mechanically emptying the breasts with pumps are not sensitive or consistently accurate. Therefore, valid information in this area has been difficult to obtain. A decrease in maternal intake of calories will decrease the volume of milk produced; this occurs without a change in composition. The volume of milk will then increase when the diet is increased. There is some recent evidence that an increase in the protein content of the diet, and not just calories, is more specific to increasing the volume of milk output. Therefore, the quantity of milk is probably sensitive to maternal nutrition.

The length of time a mother is able to breast-feed because she has sufficient milk also is influenced by a number of factors. Social and cultural ones play a dominant role. Again, valid data are lacking because of the difficulty in recognizing and controlling the multiple variables. However, it appears that maternal nutrition influences the duration of breast-feeding, with decline of milk production occurring earlier in those women who show poor weight gain during pregnancy, who have excess weight loss in the postpartum period, and who do not achieve body weights greater than their prepregnant weights during the time they are lactating.

The use of the combination pill is not recommended in the nursing woman. Most studies recorded a decrease in volume of milk produced, and a decrease in the amounts of fat, calcium, and protein. The disadvantages of decreased quantity and quality do not justify the apparent benefits of the pill for most patients.

Breast-feeding is enjoying a vogue of renewed interest and utilization. As with other areas of human reproduction, it lends itself to anecdotal information and prejudices. Breast-feeding has attracted research time and money because of its contraceptive potential inasmuch as lactating women are amenorrheic for longer periods of time than are nonnursing mothers. Surprisingly, there is relatively little research available about composition during changes in maternal homeostasis. It can be difficult to obtain valid controlled data in this area, but the lack of data may also be a subtle comment about the status and importance of breast-feeding in the scientific and medical world. It is probable that maternal nutrition is the dominant factor in the quality, quantity, and duration of breast-feeding. The impact of breast-feeding on populations throughout the world is immense. The need for more data is consistent with the potential seriousness of both maternal depletion and relative infant malnutrition as a consequence of inadequate breast-feeding.

REFERENCES

Assessment of Maternal Nutrition, Chicago: Amer Coll Obstetricians & Gynecologists, 1978.

Burke GS, et al.: Nutrition studies during pregnancy. *J Nutr* 38:453, 1949.

Camerini-Davalos RA, Cole HS (eds.): *Early Diabetes in Early Life,* New York: Academic, 1975.

Eastman NJ, Jackson E: Weight relationships in pregnancy. *Obstet Gynecol Surv* 23:1003, 1968.

Food and Nutrition Board: *Recommended Daily Allowances,* 8th ed., Washington: Nat Acad Sci, 1974.

Frisch RE, McArthur JW: Menstrual cycles: Fatness as a determination of minimum weight for height necessary for their maintenance or onset. *Science* 185:949, 1974.

Hytten FE, Leitch I : *The Physiology of Human Pregnancy,* Oxford: Blackwell, 1971.

Hytten FE, Lind T: *Diagnostic Indices in Pregnancy,* Basel: Ciba-Geigy, 1973.

Jacobson HN: Diet in pregnancy. *N Engl J Med* 297:1051, 1977.

Kane FJ Jr: Evaluation of emotional reactions to oral contraceptive use. *Am J Obstet Gynecol* 126:968, 1976.

Laboratory Indices of Nutritional Status in Pregnancy, Washington: Nat Acad Sci, 1978.

Law DH: Total parenteral nutrition. *N Engl J Med* 297:1104, 1977.

Lindheimer MD, Katz AL: Sodium and diuretics in pregnancy. *N Engl J Med* 288:891, 1973.

Luke B: Guide to better evaluation of antepartum nutrition. *JOGN Nurs* 5:37, 1976.

Maternal Nutrition and the Course of Pregnancy, Washington: Nat Acad Sci, 1970.

Moghissi KS, Evans TN (eds.): *Nutritional Impacts on Women,* Hagerstown, Md.: Harper & Row, 1977.

Nutrition in Maternal Health Care, Chicago: Amer Coll Obstetricians & Gynecologists, 1974.

Osofsky HJ: Relationships between nutrition during pregnancy and subsequent infant and child development. *Obstet Gynecol Surv* 30:227, 1975.

Pitkin RM: Nutritional support in obstetrics and gynecology. *Clin Obstet Gynecol* 19:489, 1976.

Podell RN, et al.: A profile of clinical nutrition knowledge among physicians and medical students. *J Med Educ* 50:888, 1975.

Snow LF, Johnson SM: Folklore, food, female reproductive cycle. *Ecol Food Nutr* 7:41, 1978.

Spellacy WN: Effects of oral contraceptives, estrogens, and progestogens on protein, carbohydrate, and lipid metabolism, in *Human Reproduction,* eds. ESE Hafez, RN Evans, Hagerstown, Md.: Harper & Row, 1973.

Standards for Ambulatory Obstetric Care, Chicago: Amer Coll Obstetricians & Gynecologists, 1977.

Van Itallie TB, Yang MU: Diet and weight loss. *N Engl J Med* 297:1158, 1977.

Vigersky RA, et al.: Hypothalamic dysfunction in secondary amenorrhea associated with single weight loss. *N Engl J Med* 297:1141, 1977.

Wray JD: Maternal nutrition, breast-feeding, and infant survival, in *Nutrition and Human Reproduction,* ed. WH Mosley, New York: Plenum, 1977.

11

Infection

WILLIAM J. LEDGER

The primary approach to the understanding of infectious disease involves identification of the responsible microbiologic pathogen. In the preantibiotic era, the most revered medical scientists were the investigators searching for the specific microbiologic agents in infectious processes. Microbiologic investigations first isolated and characterized pathogenic bacteria. Later advances in technology permitted the identification of viral and other nonbacterial agents, eliminating much of the confusion that existed in the understanding of many infectious diseases. For example, the recovery of a viral agent clarified the nature of the pathogen in influenza and eliminated further fruitless investigation for a bacterium that would fulfill Koch's postulates. This search for infectious agents was not a purely academic exercise, for the discovery of identifiable microbiologic cause in infection led to the development of useful treatment entities, including vaccines and antitoxins.

The discovery of antibiotics added a whole new dimension to the practice of medicine. Ehrlich's dream of a "silver bullet" against microorganisms had been realized. There was a striking reduction in the fatality rate for many of the bacterial pathogens. For the first time, patients afflicted with pneumococcal and beta-hemolytic streptococcal infections had a high survival rate. The striking results with antibiotics and the virtual elimination of fatal infectious disease led to widespread clinical usage of these antimicrobial agents in patients with confirmed or suspected bacterial infection.

This therapeutic enthusiasm for antimicrobial agents accelerated physician preoccupation with host-pathogen relationships that Weinstein and Dalton have characterized as the overemphasis on the bug and the drug. The standard care for the patient with an infectious disease was to determine the site of infection, the organism responsible, and then prescribe an appropriate antibiotic. These important considerations will be the major theme of this chapter. However, the reader should evaluate host-pathogen relationships in the light of the ever-increasing knowledge of the variations of host susceptibility to infection.

HOST FACTORS

Many studies document wide variations in host susceptibility to bacterial and viral agents. No gynecologist-obstetrician whose practice experience is limited to women of upper socioeconomic background should be so provincial as to attribute the paucity of infection in patients solely to his or her own medical and surgical skills. Patients of a lower socioeconomic class might have an unfavorable impact upon therapeutic results. For example, it seems clear that infectious morbidity is greater in the presence of malnutrition, particularly protein-calorie malnutrition. Exciting new developments in infectious disease are the research breakthroughs that offer a more complete explanation for these clinical observations. Specific studies by Selvaraj and Bhat have demonstrated de-

creased bactericidal and glycolytic activity of leukocytes as well as the lack of leukocytosis in malnourished patients with infection. Sirisinha et al. have demonstrated lower complement levels in malnourished infants. In addition, Tafari et al. have shown a failure of growth inhibition by amniotic fluid from the urban poor of Addis Ababa, Ethiopia. Because of its therapeutic implications to physicians, the most exciting discovery is the finding that some of these host defense inadequacies can be reversed by an improved diet, particularly increased protein intake. This finding should lead to future studies in nutritional aspects of preventive medical care. The new interest in improved nutrition in the pregnant female to both reduce the incidence of hypertensive disease of pregnancy and improve fetal survival may have an added value in the area of infectious morbidity.

This variation in host response to infectious agents is not limited to the malnourished. There are a number of systemic illnesses that can markedly influence the major mechanisms protecting the body from infection. For example, patients with acute or chronic leukemia may be more at risk for infection because of the depression of the humoral immune response (i.e., the circulating immunoglobulins), the cellular immune response, or specific leukocytic bactericidal function. Alteration of one or another of these functions may account for the clinically virulent disease processes seen in oncology patients on a gynecology service. This diminishment of host defense mechanisms is not limited to concurrent host disease, for the appearance of the immunosuppressed patient in the hospital setting, a result of advances in organ transplant technology, has been accompanied by the appearance of difficult-to-manage infectious problems with a new group of pathogenic microbiologic agents. Such examples should serve as a constant reminder of the multiplicity of factors in infectious disease. Consideration for the "bug and drug" is important to the clinician, but host factors play a significant role in infectious disease in gynecology and obstetrics.

MICROBIOLOGY OF THE GENITAL TRACT

Gynecologists and obstetricians have always had an interest in the microbiology of the genital tract, spurred by an awareness of pertinent clinical problems. Investigators in the preantibiotic era evaluated the normal flora of the lower tract to determine if the severe beta-hemolytic streptococcal infections of the postpartum period were the result of organisms endogenous to the patient, i.e., normal flora. The Lancefield grouping of streptococci represented a laboratory breakthrough in the identification and classification of bacteria, for it confirmed that the microorganisms responsible for puerperal sepsis were in many cases introduced from exogenous sources. This finding had great clinical significance and served as an important stimulus to the establishment of strict aseptic techniques by labor room personnel, designed to lower the risk of the introduction of these organisms into the genital tract. The resulting reduction of puerperal infectious morbidity and mortality was noted clinically before the availability of antibiotics for clinical practice. Another example of the stimulus of a clinical problem occurred with the reintroduction of intrauterine contraceptive devices into clinical practice in the early 1960s. This development was accompanied by a number of studies of the bacteriology of the genital tract. These evaluations attempted to determine the normal bacterial flora of the uterus and to evaluate the alterations, if any, associated with the insertion of an intrauterine foreign body. These studies did much to delineate both the location and the types of bacteria in the female genital tract. In each of these examples, the awareness of clinical problems (puerperal sepsis, and the possible relationship of intrauterine contraceptive devices to pelvic infection) led to basic research into the normal microbiology of the adult female genital tract. The results of these investigations extended beyond the narrow confines of the original clinical problems and have contributed to our understanding of the microbiology of the human genital tract.

There is ample evidence from many studies to demonstrate that the vagina has a normal flora; however, the nature of this flora is not clear. Preantibiotic era studies indicated that the vagina of the newborn infant was sterile, with bacteria being recovered at 12 to 14 hours of life. A number of studies have delineated change in bacterial flora associated with different life cycles. Prepubertal girls have a higher incidence of colonization with *Bacteroides,* particularly *B. fragilis* and *B. melaninogenicus,* which are infrequently found in mature and postmenopausal women. In all ages, anaerobes seem to be a significant component of the bacterial flora.

It is difficult to equate tissue changes in the glycogen content with alterations noted in the types of bacteria recovered from the vagina. Much of the scientific support for variations in glycogen content throughout a woman's life cycle was based upon qualitative histochemical studies of either tissue biopsies or exfoliated cells. Recently, an attempt was made by Gregoire et al. to quantitate the vaginal con-

TABLE 11-1 Mean Values of Glycogen ± SE Expressed as Micrograms of Glycogen per 100 mg of Tissue Wet Weight

Stage of cycle	Upper vagina (number of observations)	Lower vagina (number of observations)
Proliferative	1122 ± 292 (14)	1473 ± 214 (10)
Secretory	1321 ± 330 (16)	1667 ± 228 (13)
Postmenopause	1150 ± 208 (18)	1243 ± 242 (15)

tent of glycogen in women during the reproductive and the postmenopausal years by measuring the glycogen present in tissue biopsies. The same biochemical techniques in animals, with glycogen expressed in micrograms per 100 mg of tissue wet weight, revealed wide variations in glycogen content in different segments of the reproductive cycle. In this study, no statistical differences could be demonstrated in the glycogen content of the human vagina during different phases of the reproductive and life cycle (see Table 11–1). This finding is incompatible with attempts to designate cyclic vaginal glycogen as the major factor in the changing microbiologic flora of the vagina.

Another shortcoming of any theory which includes a "normal" microbiologic flora of the vagina, and a "pathogenic" flora associated with symptoms, is the failure to document the influences of social class and sexual activity upon the microbiologic findings. Walsh et al. demonstrated wide differences in the types of microorganisms recovered from the vaginas of pregnant women, depending upon their social class (see Table 11–2). Whether the differences are due solely to socioeconomic factors or the result of variations in sexual activity is not known. The re-

TABLE 11-2 Incidence of Microorganisms Recovered from the Lower Genital Tract of Pregnant Women

Isolate	Group I, %	Group II, %
Lactobacillus species	93.3	84.4
Streptococcus group D	32.6	22.9
Anaerobic streptococci	5.8	37.8
Escherichia coli	12.6	38.0
Proteus vulgaris	1.4	6.3
Micrococcus species	4.5	7.5
Bacteroides	0	8.0
Mycoplasma	0	8.0

covery of large numbers of "pathogenic" bacteria from asymptomatic nonpregnant women was noted in a study (Willson et al.) of endocervical cultures of women just prior to the insertion of an intrauterine device (see Table 11–3). It is possible that the gap between classic theory and investigative fact is related to heterosexual activity of the female population under study. This seems to be the situation with *Mycoplasma,* a group of genital tract organisms that have recently been intensively studied. These organisms, infrequently recovered from the vaginas of prepubertal girls or sexually mature virgins, are found in increasing numbers of women as the number of male sexual contacts increases. This finding in the evaluation of *Mycoplasma* is probably not unique. Leppäluoto has demonstrated marked changes in the bacterial forms seen in vaginal cytologic smears obtained shortly after intercourse. Such changes may account for the wide variety of microbiologic results obtained in surveys of different groups of women. In view of the microbiologic data presented in Tables 11–2 and 11–3, there seems to be little concrete evidence to suggest a "normal" vaginal flora and a "pathogenic" flora of enteric organisms that produce symptoms. Many of the organisms residing in the vagina are capable of causing serious infectious disease when host defense mechanisms are altered either locally or systemically.

There is still another shortcoming to the published surveys of the bacterial flora of the vagina. Microbiology is a demanding investigative discipline. The isolation and identification of microorganisms may depend upon the rapid transport of the sampled material to the laboratory, use of appropriate media, or both. This is quite different from clinical biochemistry, where a blood or urine specimen can be stored for long periods and yield reproducible results when many chemical parameters are analyzed. In microbiology, such storage would quickly result in the loss of the viability of organisms. With anaerobes, for example, the critical time lag between surface specimen collection and plating can be measured in minutes. Separate investigations of the vagina have revealed the recovery of aerobic and anaerobic bacteria, *Mycoplasma,* yeast, viruses, protozoa, and other microbiologic forms. To survey one patient for all viable microbiologic forms would require many swabs and a full bedside laboratory of appropriate media and tissue cultures, plus a main laboratory filled with many technicians skilled in the nuances of isolation and identification of these various microbiologic forms. Recently, the most informative studies of the lower genital tract have been limited in their microbiologic scope. A clearer future picture of the "normal" microbiologic vaginal flora may require a union of many separate studies, each investigating one facet of microbiology.

In addition to concerns about the microbiology of the vagina, the reintroduction of the intrauterine device into clinical practice stimulated research to uncover the dynamics of the microbiology of the upper genital tract. The classic teaching had been that the nonpregnant uterus is normally sterile, being contaminated by such events as a dilatation and curettage. There was concern in the early 1960s, that still persists, that there might be a relationship between the intrauterine device and pelvic infection. To clarify this picture, studies were instituted to determine the normal bacterial flora of the lower and upper genital tract. Although Bollinger recovered bacteria from the endometrial cavity of nonpregnant women using a transcervical approach, his results were not duplicated by Mishell et al. when the cervical approach was

TABLE 11–3 Lower Genital Tract Cultures from 200 Nonpregnant Clinic Patients

Isolate	Numbers	Incidence, %
Staphylococcus aureus	18	9
Coagulase-positive	5	2.5
Coagulase-negative	13	6.5
Staphylococcus albus	23	11.5
Coagulase-positive	1	0.5
Coagulase-negative	22	11.0
Diphtheroides	25	12.5
Bacteroides	35	17.5
Streptococci		
Nonhemolytic	27	13.5
Viridans	11	5.5
Anaerobic	14	7
Hemolytic,		
not Group A or D	17	8.5
Group A	1	0.5
Group D	1	0.5
Enterococci	4	2
Coliform bacteria		
Escherichia coli	16	8
Aerobacter aerogenes	11	5.5
Proteus vulgaris	5	2.5
Pseudomonas	1	0.5
Hemophilus vaginalis	1	0.5
Lactobacillus	6	3
Clostridium welchii	2	1
Neisseria gonorrhoeae	1	0.5

avoided in specimen collection. In fact, the dynamics of the clearance of bacteria from the uterus following the insertion of an intrauterine device suggest that the uterus has efficient mechanisms for ridding itself of any bacteria that manage to survive the antibacterial effects of cervical mucus and enter the cavity of the endometrium. These studies do not suggest a passive state of constant sterility of the upper genital tract but instead a dynamic system of local host defense mechanisms, including the cervical barrier, backed up by the efficient bacterial clearing action of the uterus if this cervical barrier has been breached. The discrepancy between the number of women exposed to the known pathogen *Neisseria gonorrhoeae* and the much smaller number that develop symptomatic salpingo-oophoritis suggests these mechanisms function and protect women against infection.

ACUTE LOCALIZED INFECTIONS

GONORRHEA

The gram-negative diplococcus *Neisseria gonorrhoeae* is the most important pathogen for the non-pregnant female. This designation is based upon two considerations: the numbers of women involved and the serious results of the infections. It is likely that only a minority of cases of this communicable disease are reported by physicians. In 1974, the Center for Disease Control estimated that 2.7 million cases actually occurred in the United States. Numerically, it is the most serious infectious disease problem in the country. *Neisseria* gonorrhea infections are usually not life-threatening, but upper genital tract invasion may result in salpingo-oophoritis, with resultant tubal occlusion and/or pelvic abscess formation. Tubal factor infertility may be the longterm residual effect of such attacks.

The female host response to *Neisseria* gonorrhea is variable and seems dependent upon poorly delineated factors. The vaginas of women of childbearing age are relatively resistant to invasion by this organism, while its introduction into the vaginas of females with lower systemic estrogen levels, when premenarchal or postmenopausal, can result in a symptomatic purulent vulvovaginitis. The widely accepted picture of the asymptomatic response of the nonpregnant woman to *Neisseria* gonorrhea in the lower genital tract may not be completely accurate. The concept of

the asymptomatic "carrier" does not correlate with the findings of Curran, who found culture-positive women, with no clinical evidence of salpingo-oophoritis, who were symptomatic with either urinary tract symptoms or abnormal uterine bleeding. It is possible that the defense mechanisms of the entire genital tract are called into play early in the protection against this organism. Whatever the mechanisms, it is clear that only a minority of women of childbearing age exposed to *Neisseria* gonorrhea will develop symptomatic salpingo-oophoritis.

VAGINITIS

One of the most common complaints of patients seen in a daily office practice is the itching and discomfort of symptomatic vaginitis. Although not life-threatening, these infections unquestionably diminish the quality of life for the patient involved. Because of this, women with this problem deserve the interest and attention of the physicians they consult.

There is an increasing physician awareness of the vaginitis due to the gram-negative aerobe, *Hemophilus vaginalis (Corynebacterium vaginale)*. The pioneering studies of Gardner and Dukes, in 1955, demonstrated the pathogenicity of this organism in the production of symptomatic vaginitis, and provided firm ground for the recognition of a distinctive vaginitis syndrome. There is not uniform acceptance of this organism as a pathogen for it can be recovered from women free of symptoms. Symptomatic patients frequently have a diffuse leukorrhea, usually gray, which can be associated with an offensive odor. Usually, these women did not have evidence of *Candida* or trichomonads on the wet-mount microscopic preparation of vaginal secretions and remained symptomatic despite the application of either local or systemic agents. Physician recognition that a specific bacterial offender might be responsible for symptoms in such patients led to an increased utilization of helpful diagnostic studies. Attempts to recover this organism in the microbiology laboratory with appropriate culture techniques have increased the frequency of diagnosis. These diagnostic advances have not been academic exercises alone, for a number of effective antibacterial agents can be employed in such patients, including the tetracyclines, ampicillin, and metronidazole. The latter agent was the most effective of all regimens evaluated in a recent report by Pheifer et al.

Vaginal infections due to the fungus *Candida albicans* are a frequent cause today of symptomatic vaginitis in the sexually active female. In this clinical situation, the host-pathogen relationship has not been clearly established. The confirmed microbiologic presence of these ubiquitous life forms is not synonymous with infection, for they can be recovered from the vaginas of asymptomatic women. However, when they have numerically become a more dominant form, severe symptoms may result. There seem to be specific life situations in which these *Candida* infections become problematic for women. The most dramatic example occurs when patients receive antibiotics for an infection elsewhere. Systemic antibacterial agents selectively reduce the competing bacterial population of the vagina and allow the overgrowth of *Candida albicans*. In addition to situations in which problems are created by the use of systemic medications, both pregnancy and uncontrolled diabetes have been shown to be associated with an increased frequency of *Candida* vaginitis. Although a number of factors may be involved, at least one may be the increased frequency of glycosuria in these patients. Hesseltine demonstrated many years ago that the placement of a carbohydrate solution into the vagina permitted *Candida* overgrowth and was associated with clinical symptoms. Most clinicians are convinced that oral contraceptive ingestion increases the incidence of *Candida* vaginitis. This has been attributed to the "pseudopregnancy" state caused by the pill or, alternatively, to increased heterosexual activity with more than one male partner. There is no uniformity of opinion about this relationship, for Spellacy et al. were unable to document this association. Fortunately for the clinician and patient, these infections can be suspected clinically by the gross appearance of a curd-like white discharge in a patient with vulvar pruritus and inflamed vulva. The presence of mycelia in a potassium hydroxide wet-mount preparation of vaginal secretions or the growth of *Candida* on Sabouraud's medium should confirm the clinical suspicion of a *Candida* vaginitis. A number of antifungal agents, particularly nystatin applied locally, are effective against these fungi and may be utilized for cure.

An irritating, uncomfortable vulvovaginitis may result from exposure to the protozoon *Trichomonas vaginalis*. Women with this infection will seek the physician's advice for an irritating vulvovaginitis and a malodorous discharge. The presence of trichomonads can be suspected by the finding of an inflamed vagina with punctate lesions and confirmed by the presence of motile trichomonads in the wet-mount preparation of vaginal secretions. A great therapeutic advance has been the introduction of metronidazole, a systemic agent with great clinical effectiveness

against these vaginal infections and a low frequency of serious immediate side effects. There continues to be concern about oncologic effects of these drugs in animals and mutagenic effects in bacteria. A new therapeutic concept has been the realization that male sexual partners may be asymptomatic carriers of these organisms. This has caused concurrent treatment of the male and female sexual partners to effect cure in patients who have previously been noted as treatment failures.

SOFT-TISSUE INFECTIONS OF THE LOWER GENITAL TRACT

Infection of the paraurethral (Skene's) and the vaginal (Bartholin's) accessory glands may cause acute symptoms. The surface epithelium of these glands becomes infected and inflamed secondary to the invasion of a pathogen such as *Neisseria gonorrhoeae*. Changes in the anatomy of these glands as a result of inflammation may cause the outflow of secretions to be retarded or to stop entirely. Following this, soft-tissue infection may develop, with inflammation and abscess formation. Accurate microbiologic studies of such patients frequently isolate a wide spectrum of organisms, particularly anaerobes, that are considered normal vaginal flora. When these infections occur, antibiotics may be very helpful in preventing the spread of soft-tissue inflammation, but the cornerstone of acute care is to establish operative drainage of the abscess and maintain an ostium so that future retention of secretions in these glands will not occur.

OTHER INFECTIONS OF THE LOWER GENITAL TRACT

There are a number of other microorganisms that can cause symptomatic infections of the lower genital tract. In most instances, both the laboratory recovery of these organisms and the patient's symptoms are related to sexual activity, i.e., the infectious agents are not considered normal vaginal flora. There is a wide range of these microbiologic agents.

Viruses are responsible for the formation of the herpes vesicles in the lower genital tract and the sometimes large cauliflower like masses of condyloma acuminatum. These lesions can cause symptoms when the vaginal vesicles of herpes simplex rupture and become secondarily infected or when the genital warts of condyloma acuminatum grow until there is vaginal outlet obstruction and infection with necrosis of the condyloma. Although widely used for the treatment of genital herpes, dye and phototherapy have not been established as effective therapy and may alter the virus in tissue.

More serious lower genital tract infection in the woman can result from sexual exposure to lymphogranuloma venereum, an organism more complex than a virus. If untreated, the infection can progress from a single papule or vesicle in the vagina to progressive disease, with the formation of draining fistulous sinuses, perirectal and ischiorectal abscesses, and eventually anorectal strictures and/or elephantiasis of the labia and clitoris. Such women in the past became perineal cripples with an unsatisfactory sexual prognosis, and colostomy was often necessary to provide uncomplicated bowel function. *Chlamydia,* the genus of the pathogenic organisms, is classified somewhere between bacteria and viruses. Unlike bacteria, these organisms will not grow on artificial media in the laboratory; and unlike viruses, they contain DNA, RNA, and enzymes. Fortunately for clinician and patient, these organisms are susceptible to antibiotics including tetracycline and clindamycin. Early treatment can result in cure and the prevention of disfiguring vulvar lesions.

Mycoplasmataceae are interesting organisms to the bench research worker in microbiology because of their variance from bacteria, with a lack of a cell wall, but their clinical significance is still unclear. The role of *Mycoplasma* in genital tract infection has not been delineated. It has been noted that *Mycoplasma* can frequently be recovered from the vaginas of asymptomatic, sexually active women. It may have a role in symptomatic vaginitis for women from whom both trichomonads and *Mycoplasma* have been isolated, and who showed no clinical improvement when the trichomonads were eliminated by oral metronidazole. Both T *Mycoplasma* and *Mycoplasma hominis* have been recovered from Bartholin abscesses. If prospective studies establish the role of these organisms in symptomatic disease, then systemic antibiotic therapy will be indicated. All *Mycoplasmataceae,* including the T *Mycoplasma* and *M. hominis,* are sensitive to tetracycline. Alternatively, lincomycin is effective against *M. hominis,* and erythromycin is effective against T *Mycoplasma.*

A serious, debilitating infection of the lower genital tract (chancroid, soft chancre) may result from

contact with the gram-negative aerobic bacillus, *Hemophilus ducreyi.* Frequently seen in tropical climates, these infections are fortunately rare in the temperate zone. This organism is a highly contagious agent with great virulence, and a genital infection rapidly progresses to painful vaginal lesions and infected inguinal nodes with suppuration and drainage. With this poor prognosis, it is fortunate that this organism is sensitive to both the sulfa drugs and tetracyclines, for clinical cures have been demonstrated with these agents.

Granuloma inguinale, another infection of the lower genital tract, results from infection due to the bacterium, *Donovania granulomatis.* This is a slowly progressive disease, with ulceration, profuse vascular granulation, and eventual extensive fibrosis formation. These organisms are sensitive to tetracyclines and if treatment can be initiated early in the course of the disease, cure can be achieved without the residual effects of fibrosis in the anogenital region. Host-pathogen relationships have not been clearly established in this infectious entity. The venereal transmission of the disease has not been apparent from evaluation of marital partners of patients with this infection; in fact, few have the disease.

Exposure to the spirochete *Treponema pallidum* will often result in a primary lesion (chancre), which usually presents as a painless ulcer on the labia or the cervix. If this lesion is undetected, the infection may progress to a secondary form in 6 to 8 weeks after the initial exposure, the condyloma latum, with the appearance of raised papules on the vulva. Neither the chancre nor the condyloma latum has any direct significance for the patient, for these are not progressive lesions leading to lower genital tract disfigurement. They have public health significance, since they may be the source of infection to susceptible sexual contacts, but more important, they represent a relatively asymptomatic stage of a treatable disease which can have serious systemic organ system sequelae in future years, if untreated.

URINARY TRACT INFECTIONS

Urinary tract infections are the most frequent infectious problem of women. The clinical significance of these infections is not limited to the numbers of women involved, for untreated or inadequately treated urinary tract infections may result in a protracted period of convalescence for the patient and, in some cases, permanent kidney damage.

There are a number of factors involved in the high frequency of female urinary tract infections. The data available on asymptomatic bacteriuria in women suggest that heterosexual activity may play a role. Indeed, the proximity of the relatively short female urethra to the sexual canal, the vagina, suggest that the introduction of microorganisms into the bladder can occur as a result of intercourse. The recently noted association by Curran of lower urinary tract symptoms and unsuspected lower genital tract gonorrhea must be borne in mind by physicians. The evaluation of such patients must include appropriate cultures for *Neisseria gonorrhoeae*. In addition to the alterations in the exposure of the urinary tract to microorganisms during coitus, there are probably other factors involved. Lapides has demonstrated a diminution in the bacterial clearing mechanisms of the bladder with overdistention, an event that occurs commonly because of the infrequent voiding patterns of many adult women. Lapides has advocated a program of compulsory frequent voiding in addition to initial chemotherapy for women with recurrent urinary tract infections. Stamey et al. have focused upon the appearance of pathogenic bacteria in the vagina near the urethra. Their data suggest that (1) the introitus of the normal premenopausal women is rarely colonized with *Enterobacteriaceae,* and (2) the first step in the subsequent development of bacteriuria is establishment of a pathogenic flora on the introitus. Kass and Schneiderman previously demonstrated the bladder invasion of introital bacteria with the presence of an indwelling urethral catheter, and Stamey believes that a similar invasion occurs after the establishment of an abundant pathologic flora in women without catheters. Undoubtedly, all these mechanisms play a role in the frequency of urinary tract infection in women. In patients with recurrent urinary infections, the diagnostic workup should include an evaluation for urinary tract abnormalities, either congenital or from the presence of stones which may be the source of the recurring problem. It is important to document these abnormalities, for they may be corrected by operative intervention.

There still is controversy about the microbiologic confirmation of urinary tract infections. The controversy revolves about the inherent dangers of catheterization as a diagnostic technique in women. Kass and Schneiderman have shown convincingly that carefully collected, clean-voided urine with more than 100,000 bacteria per milliliter has an 80 percent chance of representing bladder bacteriuria; two con-secutive clean-voided specimens with the same number of bacteria or more had 91 percent confidence limits, and three specimens with this number had a 95 percent confidence level. This confidence level approaches that of a single catheterization. This poses a diagnostic dilemma for many clinicians. Can they accept the technique of a clean-voided urine, with an error of 1 in 5 when positive, with the subsequent risks of unnecessary antibiotic therapy, or should they utilize the technique of catheterization and risk introduction of infection? An alternative system, suprapubic puncture, with an extremely low risk of infection, is probably infrequently done in clinical situations because of patient discomfort and inconvenience to the physician. At present, many services use a clean-voided specimen for the screening of asymptomatic women but will rely upon a catheter urine for the evaluation of the symptomatic febrile patient.

The burden of evidence suggests that the majority of organisms responsible for urinary tract infections are *Enterobacteriaceae*. In the patient having her first episode of a urinary tract infection, the predominant pathogen is *Escherichia coli*. Surveillance studies of an inpatient gynecologic service revealed that the *E. coli* strains recovered from the urinary tract of gynecologic patients were less resistant than those recovered from a renal unit during the same period (1969–1970). This undoubtedly reflects the comparative youth of the patients and the predominance of first episodes of urinary tract infections among this group. The only notable exception to this general trend was among oncology patients who were generally older, with a high proportion of resistant organisms.

A number of factors contribute to a favorable prognosis for cure among women with urinary tract infections. Most obstetric and gynecologic patients are young with normal urinary tracts, and the majority of the organisms recovered are relatively sensitive to available antibiotics. In addition, most systemic antibiotics are concentrated and excreted via the kidneys and urinary tract so that high levels of antibiotics are available at the site of infection. A general rule of care has been to follow treatment with appropriate cultures 2 days after therapy has been started and again a week after therapy is completed to be certain that the patient's infection has been eradicated. Further cultures at monthly intervals and then at 3- and 6-month intervals should be done to guard against reinfection. Normally, patients with symptoms limited to the lower urinary tract are treated for 10 to 14 days with oral agents, such as sulfa drugs or nitrofurantoins. In patients with clinical evidence of upper urinary tract involvement, a parenteral form of an antibiotic should be utilized, with similar limits to the length of therapy, depending upon clinical and laboratory evidence of cure.

SYSTEMIC INFECTIOUS DISEASE AFFECTING THE REPRODUCTIVE SYSTEM

Antibiotics have had a tremendous impact upon the frequency of infectious problems from a nonpelvic site with eventual pelvic manifestations. In the preantibiotic era, primary peritonitis with residual adhesion formation in the pelvis was not infrequently seen in girls under the age of 10 years. The offending organisms were usually the beta-hemolytic streptococcus or the pneumococcus. The pathologic physiology of such patients was not clearly established. For example, nearly half of the pneumococcal cases occurred in girls with nephrosis. One theory had been that this peritoneal infection was initiated by the upward entry of pneumococci through the vagina, uterus, and fallopian tubes. A more feasible explanation is that such infections are hematogenous, with the peritonitis and pelvic infection resulting from this bloodstream spread. This seems more reasonable, particularly in view of the usual antecedent history of an upper respiratory tract infection in patients with a streptococcal peritonitis. This disease entity has virtually been eliminated by the introduction of systemic antibiotics, particularly penicillin, with its initial and continuing dramatic bactericidal actions upon the beta-hemolytic streptococcus and the pneumococcus. Young girls are infrequently seen with such acute symptoms, and the residual effects of such infections are not an important factor in an infertility practice.

TUBERCULOSIS

The classic example of a pelvic infection with the primary infectious source elsewhere is tuberculosis. Most pelvic tuberculosis results from infection with *Mycobacterium tuberculosis*. The primary site of infection is the lung, with the pelvic infection secondary to hematogenous spread. The theory of infection, as presented in most gynecologic texts, has been that the fallopian tubes are the first pelvic site infected

and that they serve as a continued source of downward pelvic infection into the endometrial cavity which is frequently able to clear itself of infection following menstrual sloughing. This theory was based upon the microbiologic and morphologic evidence in women with pelvic tuberculosis that the fallopian tubes were more frequently involved than the uterus (see Table 11–4). Indeed, based upon a report of Solomons in 1935, preantibiotic literature advocated the removal of tuberculous fallopian tubes as treatment for tuberculous endometritis. In 1961 Sharman cast some doubt on this operative approach for cure when four patients treated with salpingectomy alone had persistent endometrial tuberculosis. It is possible that theories based upon histologic and microbiologic techniques may reflect the shortcomings of these techniques. For example, Vollum's experience with known infected material was that histologic evidence was positive in 51 percent, the culture was positive in 52 percent, and guinea pig inoculation in 58 percent. To add to the diagnostic difficulties is the finding that less than 50 percent of patients with genital tract tuberculosis have radiologic evidence of pulmonary tuberculosis. A tubercullin skin test in all patients with pelvic tuberculosis should be positive. Schaefer has advocated that patients should not be diagnosed as having genital tuberculosis unless the diagnosis is confirmed by histologic and/or bacteriologic examinations of uterine and tubal tissue or secretions. In light of the diagnostic study inadequacies and the unfavorable clinical experience with salpingectomy alone, it is possible that the varying rates of recovery of *Mycobacterium tuberculosis* from fallopian tubes and endometrium reflect microbiologic shortcomings and are not a true pathophysiologic picture of a descending infection. It is conceivable that endometrial and tubal involvement occur at similar times via hematogenous routes, but the monthly slough and regeneration of the endometrium make diagnostic attempts less than 100 percent effective. Another alternative explanation may be the variation in pelvic organ susceptibility. Witness the low incidence of ovarian in-

TABLE 11–4 Frequency of Tuberculosis in Genital Organs

Organ	Frequency, %
Fallopian tubes	90–100
Uterus	50–60
Ovaries	20–30
Cervix	5–15
Vagina	1

volvement (see Table 11–4). The infrequency of this disease in American medicine makes it unlikely that any prospective study will be large enough to yield the answers to these unsolved problems of the pathologic physiology of pelvic tuberculosis.

Tuberculosis is undoubtedly the most important communicable disease in the world. This designation is based upon numbers, for large segments of the world's population have this disease. Indeed, it has been estimated that one-half of India's population has tuberculosis. The recent worldwide upsurge in gonorrhea may threaten the numerical preeminence of tuberculosis, but there can be no question about the potential seriousness of tubercular infections. It is estimated that nearly 10,000 Americans and 500,000 inhabitants of India die annually from this infection. Few disease entities illustrate the importance of host factors in infection as well as tuberculosis. At the turn of the century, the mortality rate from this disease in the United States was 194.1 per 100,000 cases. Prior to the introduction of chemotherapeutic agents, there had been a steady decline in both the total number of people with infections and the mortality rate. This was thought to be due in part to the improvement in living standards of the general population. The tremendous socioeconomic dislocations of World War II temporarily reversed these trends, and in the immediate postwar period this was reflected in gynecologic practice by an upsurge in the number of infertile women with genital tuberculosis. Recent infertility statistics indirectly suggest that the percentages of infected women have markedly decreased, but in countries like India, with the problems of poverty and inadequate food supply, genital tuberculosis remains a frequently seen problem.

Although these host-pathogen relationships are important, few diseases have been as dramatically altered by systemic antibiotics as genital tuberculosis. In the preantibiotic era, the diagnosis of pelvic tuberculosis afforded a grim prognosis for the patient. She was irreversibly sterile, and cure would be accomplished only by operative removal of the infected pelvic organs with the attendant dangers of prolonged postoperative fistulous sinus drainage. The long-term use of systemic chemotherapeutic agents dramatically altered this picture. Cures without relapses were seen in the absence of operative intervention and even more striking were the reports of pregnancies following chemotherapeutic treatment of genital tract tuberculosis by such authorities as Stallworthy. Even Schaefer, a skeptical commentator on many poorly documented reports of pregnancy following treatment of alleged pelvic tuberculosis, now

believes pregnancy can follow adequate treatment of minimal genital disease. The reproductive prognosis in women with pelvic tuberculosis is still not good. Conception is infrequent; pregnancy loss, including abortion and ectopic pregnancy, is not uncommon.

GASTROINTESTINAL DISEASE

In addition to sequelae of the hematogenous spread of microorganisms, pelvic infection can result from disease of the gastrointestinal tract.

Appendicitis may have long-term implications for the health and functioning of the female genital tract. This is particularly true when there has been a delay in both the initial diagnosis and the operative intervention. A ruptured appendix with free spillage of infected material into the peritoneal cavity elicits a series of responses from the peritoneum in an attempt to localize and wall off the contaminating substances. The immediate result of such a mechanism is favorable and may be lifesaving for the patient. This ability to localize the infection is lessened during pregnancy because of the anatomic changes in the location of the appendix, reflecting changes in the peritoneal cavity relationship secondary to the growing pregnant uterus. This lessened ability of the peritoneum to wall off the infection when the appendix is no longer a pelvic organ is at least one factor in the high mortality rate in pregnant women with a ruptured appendix. The favorable short-term response of the peritoneum in nonpregnant women with appendicitis may have serious long-term implications for the fertility of such patients. One or both tubes may be nonfunctional because of involvement in the mass of tissue, including the dense adhesions, omentum, and bowel that wall off the infection. In less severe cases, peritubal adhesions may kink and distort the fallopian tubes, preventing the normal mechanisms of tubal pickup of ova and transportation of spermatozoa and ova so that union is impossible.

Diverticulitis of the colon may have secondary genital tract effects. It is a disease of aging, seldom seen in women under the age of 35. If abscess formation and rupture occur, there may be massive contamination of the peritoneum. Numerically, the most common microorganisms of the lower bowel are the anaerobes, outnumbering aerobes by nearly 1000 to 1, with different *Bacteroides* frequently isolated. This fact should be a consideration in the choice of systemic antibiotics for such patients. This massive contamination of the peritoneal cavity will be accompanied by the same immediate and long-term effects in the female genital organs as following the rupture of an appendix. In addition to these emergency situations, diverticulitis may secondarily involve genital tract organs. Ovarian abscess formation secondary to diverticulitis has been noted in postmenopausal women. Indeed, diverticulitis should be considered in the differential diagnosis of the postmenopausal woman with signs and symptoms of pelvic inflammatory disease.

The hazards of modern urban living, with increased incidence of penetrating abdominal trauma from such agents as knives or bullets, can have an impact upon the long-term health of the female genital tract. Bowel injury, with fecal spillage into the peritoneal cavity, results in the same massive bacterial contamination seen with a ruptured appendix or a ruptured abscess secondary to diverticulitis. The host defense mechanisms of the peritoneum may again result in pelvic adhesion formation. Thadepalli et al. have demonstrated the primary importance of anaerobes in patients with bowel injuries, and this should guide the selection of antibacterial agents while these patients are being prepared for primary operative care of the bowel injuries.

POSTOPERATIVE INFECTIONS

At present, nosocomial or hospital-acquired infections constitute the bulk of the inpatient infectious problems seen in a gynecology service. This may reflect a change in the number of women hospitalized for community-acquired infections. For example, although Mickal and Sellmann at the New Orleans Charity Hospital have reported no diminution in the numbers of women operated upon for ruptured tubo-ovarian abscess, there does seem to be a decrease in the absolute numbers of women admitted to the inpatient service of the Los Angeles County-University of Southern California (LAC-USC) Medical Center with the more serious sequelae of salpingo-oophoritis. Much more dramatic has been the abrupt drop in the caseload of women with infected abortions since the liberalization of the indications for hospital-performed pregnancy terminations. This relative increase in the number of women with nosocomial infections requires new attitudes on the part of the physician. There must be an awareness of our direct responsibility for these infections, for they reflect

the acquisition of disease in individuals previously free of infection. The benefits of hospitalization must outweigh this ever-present hazard. In addition to our individual responsibilities for patient care in the hospital, the gynecologist-obstetrician must recognize the expense and strain these infections impose upon our system of health care delivery. Altemeier estimated the cost of postoperative wound infections in the United States to be $9.83 billion in 1967 alone. In view of the importance and magnitude of this problem, it is necessary for all physicians to recognize both the scope and the details of the problem.

The starting point for the understanding of nosocomial infections is the formation and implementation of a system for the surveillance of infection on an inpatient service. This is necessary because of the inadequacy of the individual practitioner in the assessment of hospital-acquired infections. A number of available statistics suggest that there are attempts, conscious or otherwise, to minimize the extent of these problems. A survey by Ledger and Child of over 12,000 women undergoing hysterectomy in 1970 found a large discrepancy between the nearly 50 percent of women receiving systemic antibiotics during their hospitalization and the less than 10 percent with diagnosed sites of infection. This survey was performed before prophylactic antibiotics became a popular form of therapy, and the figures reflect therapy of suspected infection. These attempts to diminish hospital-acquired infections include dependence upon definitions of temperature morbidity as a delineation of actual morbidity and the frequent use of systemic antibiotics without prior culture. A most important observation by Ohm and Galask is the difficulty in establishing the primary site of infection when prior antibiotics have been used. These realities of daily practice necessitate a system of surveillance. The ingredients for a successful system include a clinical service willing to do indicated microbiologic studies before starting antimicrobial therapy, a clinical microbiology laboratory that is equipped for appropriate laboratory testing, particularly anaerobe methodology, and a hospital administration which will financially support these activities, particularly the important surveillance officer.

A surveillance system can provide a great deal of useful data for clinicians. Evidence indicates that most postoperative infections can be detected early in the postoperative course, prior to the patient's discharge from the hospital. In addition, this system can document both the number of women with infection and the number of patients who require systemic antibiotics. Such data may yield valuable information on

TABLE 11–5   Risk Factors of Various Operative Procedures

Operative procedure	Total number of patients	Patients receiving antibiotics	Percentage of total
Laparotomy and laparoscopy	510	40	7.8
Abdominal hysterectomy	150	43	28.7
Vaginal hysterectomy	76	33	43.4
Radical hysterectomy	16	13	81.3
Radical vulvectomy	13	12	92.3
Exenteration	10	10	100

the risk factors of different operative procedures (see Table 11–5). If the clinical microbiology laboratory performs standardized antibiotic sensitivity testing, the information can document both the relative frequency of organisms recovered from infectious sites and the range of antibiotic sensitivity of these bacteria. Such data can be a valuable aid to the clinician in antibiotic selection for the individual patient with a hospital-acquired infection. Finally, a surveillance system may provide the first hint of an epidemic infection due to one particular organism. The characterization of organisms from similar sites of infection gives needed information for a rational approach to an epidemiologic problem. For example, the appearance of many wound infections, due to a variety of organisms, with many operative teams involved, makes it unlikely that efforts to focus upon one hospital environmental factor (such as the face mask of the surgeon) will eliminate the problem.

A critical factor in the success of any surveillance system of hospital-acquired infections in a gynecology service is the ability to document all postoperative infections. Most gynecologist-obstetricians properly dislike hospital-acquired infections and minimize these problems. The wound drainage that precedes the defervescence of a patient's postoperative fever becomes a seroma. Alternatively, systemic antibiotics eliminate the fever of a patient with a suspected pelvic cellulitis that is never coded or acknowledged in the recorded postoperative course of the patient. Much of the confusion about morbidity stems from a definition based upon temperature elevation borrowed from the preantibiotic era of obstetrics. Because this definition might include patients with atelectasis, who do not require systemic antibiotics, many evaluations of gynecologic morbidity have contained their own modifications of the obstetric temperature definition so that only "real" morbidity is recorded. This is a self-serving mechanism of evaluation, for it grossly underestimates the extent of hospital-acquired infections. To accurately report

nosocomial infections, it is important to document all postoperative morbidity and to record, if possible, the use of systemic antibiotics in postoperative patients. This will provide a more accurate picture of gynecologic practice.

The evaluation of the postoperative temperature response can yield valuable information about patterns of practice and an indirect assessment of the extent of hospital-acquired infections. Ledger and Kriewall reported the technique of the fever index, a quantitative measure of the total quantity of fever that can be compiled using a Fortran computer program and the standard postoperative temperature records. The results, expressed in degree-hours, provide an indirect measure of morbidity and can be used to evaluate a number of events. For example, patients without a clinical diagnosis of postoperative infection can be compared to those with a diagnosis of infectious postoperative cellulitis who required systemic antibiotics. Despite some overlap, it is apparent that this measure indentifies two different patient populations (see Fig. 11–1). In addition, this measure can be used to evaluate two treatment regimens to indirectly determine the impact of a studied therapy (see Fig. 11–2). This measure provides a more exact evaluation of postoperative infections than is available from standard temperature definitions of morbidity or their modifications for gynecologic patients.

Another important ingredient in the understanding of hospital-acquired infections in gynecology is the recognition that the majority of pathogens are organisms endogenous to the patient. In the preantibiotic era, gram-positive cocci such as streptococci and pneumococci were causes of serious infection. Their relationship to infection was clear and the concept of a bacterial pathogen was unquestioned. The overwhelming effectiveness of antibiotics against these gram-positive pathogens has led to dramatic changes in the nature of pathogenic bacteria. Altemeier has documented the greater incidence of serious hospital-acquired infections due to gram-nega-

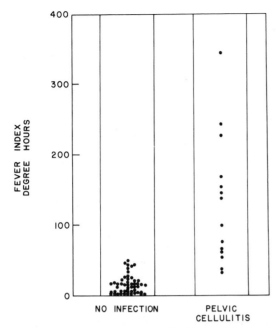

FIGURE 11–1 Postoperative fever index in two patient populations. In one, there was no clinical diagnosis of infection, and no antibiotics were utilized. In the other, a diagnosis of postoperative pelvic cellulitis was made, and the patients received systemic antibiotics before they were discharged. Although there is overlap, this technique of evaluation demonstrates two different patient populations.

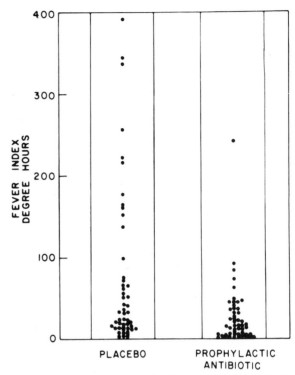

FIGURE 11–2 The postoperative fever index in 50 patients given prophylactic cephaloridine in vaginal hysterectomy is contrasted with that in 50 control subjects. The evaluated values of degree hours were seen more frequently in those patients receiving placebo.

tive organisms such as *E. coli,* and there is increasing awareness of *Bacteroides fragilis* as a cause of severe infection in gynecology and obstetrics. These bacteria, normal inhabitants of both the gastrointestinal and lower genital tracts can cause infection when host defense mechanisms have been compromised. Recognition of this endogenous source of bacterial infection is important in the understanding of postoperative gynecologic infections.

RESPIRATORY TRACT INFECTIONS

Compromises in host defense mechanisms during and after operation may result in postoperative respiratory tract infection. The most dramatic changes, because of their sudden onset and the extensiveness of lung involvement, are due to spillage of gastric contents in the respiratory tract while the patient is anesthetized. The tissue-necrotizing effects of the highly acidic gastric contents may permit overgrowth and infection due to organisms frequently found in the oral cavity that normally are easily cleared by the intact

respiratory tract. Less dramatic and serious in their manifestations, but much more frequent in numbers of patients involved, are the lung changes of atelectasis. These alterations, including collapsed, poorly perfused alveoli, can be suspected in the patient who has a temperature elevation early in the postoperative course and who may have a low arterial PO_2. Increasing patient efforts of deep inspiration as well as attempts to clear the upper respiratory tract of secretions seem to prevent progression of this problem. Usually, atelectatic areas will be cleared by the patient, but in some instances progression to a pneumonitis may occur, necessitating the use of systemic antibiotics. The most ominous development in postoperative pulmonary infections was the discovery that the aerosols of machines for respiratory assistance, such as the apparatus for intermittent positive-pressure breathing, may become heavily contaminated with microorganisms. When these organisms are delivered under pressure to the respiratory tract, a serious pneumonia with highly resistant bacteria such as *Serratia marcescens* may result. In some instances these infections have resulted in the death of the patient.

URINARY TRACT INFECTIONS

The normal physiology of the urinary tract may be adversely compromised following elective gynecologic operations. Inability to void following operative dissection and repair of the base of the bladder requires catheterization to ensure adequate drainage. Utilization of the urethral route for entrance and constant drainage of the bladder has been shown by Kass and Schneiderman to be associated with the upward migration of enteric organisms with pathogenic potential that may reside in the vagina. In addition, an open system of catheter drainage will allow organisms to ascend through the catheter. A number of measures have been employed to reduce the risk of this procedure. Systemic antibiotic prophylaxis has been attempted, and there is some suggestion that this has significant impact upon the actual bladder infection rates in short-term catheterization. However, there is the risk of a selection of more serious resistant organisms as pathogens. Alternatively, local antisepsis has been tried. The development of a closed collecting system for urinary tract drainage seems to decrease the incidence of bladder invasion by bacteria, and some services use the triple lumen catheter for constant irrigation of the bladder with an antibacterial solution. Another approach to the problem of adequate bladder drainage has been to utilize transabdominal needle puncture and suprapubic drainage of the bladder. Although Hofmeister et al. could not demonstrate any difference in the incidence of postoperative bladder infections, Mattingly et al. have shown a benefit with fewer bladder infections. It has been a personal impression that observation of the postoperative patient's ability to void is easier with the suprapubic drain than with the urethral catheter.

BLOODSTREAM INFECTIONS

Medical advances in intravenous parenteral nutrition capabilities have been accompanied by an increase in the number of hospital-acquired infections. Most studies demonstrate an incidence of infection at the site of entry to the vein and secondary bacteremia that is directly related to prolonged periods with indwelling intravenous needles. The entry seems related to the passage of skin bacteria along the needle tract, although contaminated intravenous fluids due to defective manufacturing standards and contaminated lipid solutions for intravenous nutrition have been implicated. The ability to maintain adequate nutrition with venous fluids alone has been lifesaving in the care of seriously debilitated patients with either severe intraabdominal infection or gynecologic malignancy. However, the potential ill effects of such efforts should always be apparent to the clinician. Physicians should never take a casual attitude toward the insertion of an intravenous cannula. This is an invasive operative procedure, requiring the same attention to surgical sterility as an abdominal incision. Additionally, attention should be directed toward the length of time these foreign objects are permitted to reside in a vein. This physician concern should be translated into a decrease in the incidence of upper extremity infection and thrombophlebitis. Evaluation of the elemental diet, utilizing the stomach and the first 3 feet of small bowel for absorption, may provide an alternative method for maintaining the nutritional status of these seriously ill patients.

A potentially lethal infectious complication may occur as the result of the utilization of blood products in postoperative gynecologic patients. This is not an infrequent event. A recent survey of over 12,000 women undergoing hysterectomy revealed that 16 percent of these patients received one or more blood transfusions during hospitalization. In a cooperative study of patients receiving transfusion, the number who acquired symptomatic hepatitis was 2.8 percent, with death occurring in 0.1 percent. The source of the blood donors is related to the number of recipients who develop hepatitis. Commercial blood is accompanied by a high rate of hepatitis, and many authorities believe this source should not be used. A recent diagnostic breakthrough has been the discovery of a number of antigens associated with serum hepatitis (SH) or hepatitis B. The presence of specific viral antigen in blood used for transfusion is associated with a high risk for the development of serum hepatitis. Exclusion of both commercial blood and blood which is positive for hepatitis antigen has resulted in a decrease, but not a total elimination, of hepatitis in recipients, for it provides no means for eliminating the patient with type A hepatitis or hepatitis, not A or B. A logical first step in the elimination of hepatitis in hospitalized patients would be to emphasize measures that would decrease the number of blood transfusions in hospitalized patients. The frequent association of abnormal genital tract bleeding and anemia with conditions requiring operative intervention makes it unlikely that all transfusions on a gynecology service can be eliminated, but the high frequency, 6 percent of the total, of 1-unit transfusion in the nationwide hysterectomy study suggests that the utilization of blood products by gynecologists can be reduced.

ABDOMINAL WOUND INFECTIONS

There are a number of well-delineated risk factors in the production of the postoperative abdominal wound infection. A wound infection reflects the end stage of the combination of bacterial inoculum, devitalized tissue, blood products, and foreign material in the wound. The sum of all these factors may overwhelm local host defense mechanisms and result in a clinical wound infection. Cruse and Foord have gone beyond theoretical considerations to delineate the clinical factors that increase the risk of abdominal wound infection for the postoperative patient undergoing aseptic operation. The risk factors include increasing age and obesity of the patient, length of time of the operation, significant intraoperative bleeding and shock, the use of cautery, shaving of the operative site, the use of abdominal adhesive drapes, and the use of drains. In addition, a surveillance study of gynecologic infections related postoperative wound infections to the extent of operative field contamination (see Table 11–6). Further evidence that implicates an endogenous source of organisms recovered from wound infections is the bacteria recovered from abdominal wounds following hysterectomy. The coagulase-positive staphylococcus is not a frequent isolate. The majority of the organisms recovered from infected wounds are considered normal inhabitants of the lower genital tract.

A number of efforts have been directed toward the elimination of postoperative wound infections due to endogenous organisms. These methods include attempts to more completely eliminate vaginal bacteria preoperatively as well as stressing the importance of meticulous operative technique. In the past decade, there has been renewed interest in the use of systemic antibiotics to prevent postoperative infections, including those of the abdominal wound in operations with a microbiologically contaminated field. Polk and Lopez-Mayor convincingly demonstrated a striking reduction in all postoperative infections following colon resection. In gynecology, Allen et al. showed a reduction in all postoperative morbidity when prophylactic antibiotics were given to patients undergoing elective abdominal hysterectomy. Decisions on the utilization of systemic antibiotics as prophylaxis on any gynecologic service will be dependent upon the evaluation of the risk of this widespread use of antibiotics and the potential benefit.

The clinical management of patients with a postoperative abdominal wound infection is usually straightforward. The wound should be opened to permit the drainage of purulent material and inspected to determine if the fascia is still intact. In most cases, this operative therapy will suffice and the wound will close by secondary intent. Aerobic and anaerobic microbiologic cultures of all wounds should be obtained, both for individual patient documentation and to be certain that exogenous organisms such as the group A beta-hemolytic streptococcus or the coagulase-positive *Staphylococcus aureus* are not involved. The presence of an inflamed wound edge, with progression of the inflammation, is a warning sign that streptococci are involved, and operative drainage alone may not suffice for cure. Frequently, these infections are mixed, with a coagulase-positive staphylococcus in addition to the streptococcus. Because of this, a choice of antibiotics prior to the definitive microbiologic culture report should include an agent which is effective against penicillinase-producing staphylococci. A frequently used antibiotic in this situation is one of the cephalosporin derivatives. Other more serious infectious wound complications may occur in which a spreading infection is accompanied by tissue or fascial necrosis. Rapid operative intervention is needed in these cases.

TABLE 11–6 Incidence of Wound Infections Related to Cleanliness of Operative Field

	Total cases	Wound infections	Percentage of total
Clean operative field			
Adnexal surgery	257	11	4.7
Herniorrhaphy	259	12	4.2
Contaminated operative field			
Total abdominal hysterectomy	337	35	10.4
Colectomy	98	32	32.7

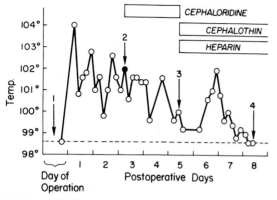

FIGURE 11–3 The early postoperative course of a patient with a group A beta-hemolytic streptococcus wound infection. A total abdominal hysterectomy and bilateral salpingo-oophorectomy were performed at 0.1; the red inflamed wound was opened at 0.2; heparin was started at 0.3 because of concern about pulmonary embolism; at 0.4 the patient became afebrile and remained so for the rest of her hospitalization.

The responsibility of the gynecologist does not end with individual patient care if exogenous organisms are involved. The recovery of bacteria such as the group A beta-hemolytic streptococcus or the coagulase-positive staphylococcus from a wound infection poses two additional problems to the clinician. Those patients shed large numbers of highly infectious organisms from their wound sites and may be a source of colonization of preoperative patients who will soon be undergoing elective operations. Because of this, these patients should be isolated until they have had the necessary treatment to eliminate these microorganisms. There may be clinical hints that the organism involved is the group A beta-hemolytic streptococcus. The sudden onset of fever in the postoperative period and the rapid discovery of a draining abdominal wound should alert the gynecologist to this possibility (see Fig. 11–3). The other responsibility is the possibility that these infections may be a result of an asymptomatic carrier among the hospital staff. A cluster of infections with a common organism demands epidemiologic investigation.

PELVIC INFECTIONS

Postoperative pelvic infections can be the most serious hospital-acquired infections on a gynecologic service. These infections range from a well-localized vaginal cuff collection to large pelvic abscess formation with rupture and intraperitoneal contamination. Because of the severe nature of these infections

and their potential lethality, it is important for the clinician to delineate risk factors in women who are candidates for elective gynecologic operations.

Youth does not protect women against postoperative pelvic infections. Instead, a number of studies have documented a greater risk of infection in younger women. For example, Taylor and Hansen found febrile morbidity and pelvic abscesses to be more common in women under the age of 35 than in those over 50. Their findings were not unique. Pratt and Galloway had higher postoperative morbidity rates in women less than 36 years of age, and Hall et al. discovered anaerobic postoperative pelvic infections to be more common in women under the age of 40. White et al. found postoperative febrile morbidity after hysterectomy to be much more common in women under the age of 35. Opinions about this age factor are not unanimous, for one study by Bolling and Plunkett of women undergoing vaginal hysterectomy could demonstrate no difference in the temperature-related morbidity of premenopausal and postmenopausal patients. However, this increased risk because of youth has been noted in recent evaluations of patients with infections serious enough to warrant operative intervention. Nearly all the women with hospital-acquired infections were premenopausal.

An additional factor related to age is the continued activity of the ovaries following pelvic surgery. The retention of adnexa in premenopausal women undergoing hysterectomy is not uncommon, particularly since many of the indications for operation are for pathologic processes limited to the uterus. The justification for adnexal retention is based upon the clinical sense that these ovaries function postoperatively, a feeling that has been confirmed by postoperative hormonal studies. The most striking relationship of this adnexal retention and postoperative infection has been in the patient with a postoperative adnexal abscess. Much of the emphasis in such situations has been placed upon mechanical factors (i.e., the capsule of the ovary is breached by ovulation) or operative trauma, permitting the entry of contaminating organisms, with the eventual development of an adnexal abscess. Other developments in infectious disease research suggest that alternative factors may play a role. Alexander and associates have demonstrated a cyclic variation in leukocytic bactericidal function and the relationship of this diminished leukocytic function to bacteremia in patients on a burn unit. If a cyclic variation in female host defense mechanisms can be demonstrated, it is possible that this variation will be related to cyclic ovarian function. This represents an exciting possibility for future study to diminish the incidence of hospital-acquired infections.

There is evidence that the social class of the patient population may influence the incidence of postoperative pelvic infection. A number of studies of hospital-acquired infections on a gynecology service suggest this is a factor. In their evaluation of the ovarian abscess, Willson and Black found this complication to follow 1 in 600 of vaginal hysterectomies on the private service as compared to 1 in 36 on the clinic service. Hall et al. found postoperative anaerobic pelvic infections to occur eight times more frequently in the clinic than on the private service. White et al. found an increased incidence of fever and vaginal cuff infections following vaginal hysterectomy and an increase in wound infections following abdominal hysterectomy on the clinic service. Not everyone is convinced that these variations are solely due to differences in the social classes of the population samples, for the clinic population is cared for by residents in training. To refute this concern about physician experience, Allen et al. could document no difference in postoperative morbidity based upon the level of experience of the resident performing the operation although there is the bias that the more difficult cases are done by the more senior house officers. A recent study by Ledger and Child demonstrated an increased number of black women with fever posthysterectomy who required antibiotics in both teaching and nonteaching hospitals. Although these differences may reflect social class, at least a portion of this variance may be due to sickle-cell trait and disease, for the problems with fever and antibiotic use occurred most frequently in patients with a positive sickle-cell preparation. Further study is needed to more clearly delineate all the elements of postoperative morbidity.

Another factor in postoperative morbidity seems to be the ability to secure adequate hemostasis at the time of operation. Pratt and Galloway and Taylor and Hansen all documented increased blood loss at the time of vaginal hysterectomy in young women. A number of factors may be involved in this apparent relationship of inadequate hemostasis and postoperative infection. Prolonged intraoperative hypotension will enhance the growth of anaerobic organisms in the vagina. Postoperatively, clotted blood is a good culture medium. In addition, breakdown products of blood, specifically hemoglobin and the ferric ion, can enhance the virulence of contaminating organisms. All these factors may weight the balance in favor of bacterial pathogens over local host defense mechanisms at the operative site.

A final factor in postoperative pelvic infections seems to be the vaginal approach to operation. All the aforementioned studies, linking age and morbidity, found vaginal hysterectomy to be associated with a higher incidence of pelvic infection. This danger of a serious infection is not limited to the patient undergoing hysterectomy, for Roe et al. reported postoperative abscess formation following a vaginal tubal ligation. The greater risk of bacterial contamination of the operative field has been theorized as a contributor to this morbidity.

A new development in the attempts to diminish postoperative pelvic infections is the utilization of preventive antibiotics in high-risk patient populations. This pattern of practice represents a break with medical tradition that decries this use of powerful systemic antimicrobial agents. The most heated opponents state the lack of justification because of low postoperative morbidity with good operative techniques. In addition, studies demonstrating poor results with the long-term use of antibiotics in hospitalized patients have been quoted in which more infections, not fewer, resulted from prophylactic antibiotics. Advocates can cite serious infectious morbidity following elective gynecologic operations, and a number of recent studies have demonstrated a decrease in postoperative infectious morbidity with the pre- and postoperative use of antibiotics. The employment of prophylactic antibiotics in operative procedures was based upon the original experimental work of Burke. He demonstrated in an animal model a critical time limit in the effectiveness of systemic antibiotics to prevent lesions caused by the local infection of bacteria (see Fig. 11–4). All the successful clinical regimens in gynecology have had in common the preoperative administration of antibiotics, so that an effective wound level of antibiotic can be achieved while an operation is performed in a field contaminated by bacteria. There is not complete agreement on the length of time antibiotics are needed for prophylaxis. The reported preventive regimens have varied from the day of operation (Ledger et al.) to 7 full days of therapy (Bolling, Plunkett). However, one comparative study showed no differences in postoperative morbidity when a course limited to the day of operation was evaluated against a prolonged treatment regimen. The mechanism of protection of this regimen against postoperative infection seems more dependent upon tissue antibiotic levels than upon complete elimination of surface bacteria from the vagina, for bacteria can be recovered from the vaginal cuff of a patient receiving prophylactic antibiotics at the end of the operation. A number of antibiotics have

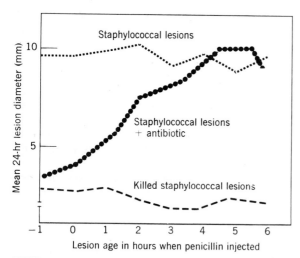

FIGURE 11–4 In guinea pigs, dermal lesion size increases with delay in administration of antibiotics and after interdermal inoculation with staphylococci.

been effective as prophylaxis in gynecologic operations including the cephalosporins, ampicillin, tetracycline, metronidazole, and a combination of penicillin and streptomycin. Two effective regimens of prophylaxis utilized either cephalosporins alone (antimicrobials which are ineffective in the laboratory against the gram-positive aerobe, the enterococcus, as well as the gram-negative anaerobe, *Bacteroides fragilis*) or cephalosporins in combination with metronidazole, whose antibacterial activity is limited almost completely to anaerobic organisms. The clinical results in each case were similar. This discrepancy between the clinical results and the microbiologic findings suggests that the pathogenicity of these organisms may be dependent upon the establishment of infection by a mixed flora of bacteria. The variety of effective antibiotics for prophylaxis in gynecology is a good omen, for it means that different antibiotic regimens can probably be effectively used on any gynecologic service.

The selection of alternative antibiotics may prevent the overuse of one or a combination of agents for prophylaxis, resulting in the selection of a resistant pathogen. One recent example of the selection of a resistant organism, *Klebsiella aerogenes,* was noted by Price and Sleigh in a neurosurgical service with an almost exclusive use of penicillin products. The indication for the use of preventive antibiotics depends upon the infectious problems of a specific gynecologic service. Good results with antibiotic prophylaxis have been reported in women undergoing vaginal hysterectomy, and one report demonstrated improved

results in women who have had an abdominal hysterectomy. However, Ohm and Galask have not found prophylactic antibiotics particularly helpful in abdominal hysterectomy. The critical clinical decision in this regard depends upon the degree of severity of the postoperative infectious problems. These have not been so frequent or extensive following abdominal hysterectomy to cause our gynecology service at the LAC-USC Medical Center to support this utilization at the present time. Prospective studies delineating the role of antibiotic prophylaxis in extensive gynecologic oncology operations have not been reported as yet.

An alternate preventive measure to systemic prophylaxis is the use of a closed suction drainage system at the vaginal cuff. This has resulted in a marked diminution postoperatively of infections involving the pelvis. Despite all preventive efforts, some postoperative pelvic infections will continue to be seen on a gynecologic service. The proper care of these problems will depend upon the knowledge and recognition of the extent of the infectious problems seen. Most postoperative pelvic infections follow hysterectomy and begin at the microbiologically contaminated vaginal operative site. The extent of infection is dependent upon both the pathogenicity of the contaminating organisms and the amount of foreign and necrotic material in the wound site. Infections may be limited to the vaginal cuff or may spread from this primary site into the pelvis with extensive infection, occasional pelvic abscess formation from an infected hematoma, or infection of the retained adnexa. The pathogenic organisms in these situations are usually endogenous to the vagina (see Table 11-2), although on occasion serious infections can be caused by an organism such as the group A beta-hemolytic streptococcus, which is frequently introduced from exogenous sources.

Also at high risk for postoperative pelvic infection are patients undergoing surgery for primary infection of the uterus or adnexa. This may be the result of a community or hospital-acquired infection. There can be massive bacterial contamination during the efforts at operative removal, and this permits seeding of any pelvic hematoma that may be a residual of the operation, with a resulting pelvic infection.

All the physician's therapeutic efforts in patients with postoperative pelvic infection should be based upon an assessment of the extent of infection, with subsequent efforts directed toward aiding host defense mechanisms. This need can be satisfied by a careful pelvic examination in the postoperative patient. The extent of the infection can be grossly delineated with appropriate vaginal drainage established. Generally, an infected collection of material at the vaginal apex can be treated adequately by operative drainage alone. In fact, Hall et al., in their evaluation of anaerobic pelvic infections, felt systemic antibiotics had little impact on the resolution of these infections. If there is evidence of extensive pelvic induration, particularly when purulent material is not discovered on examination, the diagnosis of pelvic cellulitis should be made and systemic antibiotics prescribed for the patient. If the patient has temperature elevations late in the postoperative period, repeated examinations should be performed to rule out the presence of a pelvic abscess. The introduction of ultrasonography into clinical practice has been a helpful addition to the care of these women. If an adnexal abscess is formed that is unresponsive to therapy, intraperitoneal rupture and death can result. Because of this potentially lethal result, laparotomy may be indicated in the patient who remains febrile beyond the first 5 to 7 postoperative days, despite the use of appropriate antibiotics with a mass high in the pelvis.

INFECTIONS OF THE PREGNANT WOMAN

Prior to the explosion of scientific information in the last century, a sense of mystery surrounded the phenomenon of pregnancy. As physicians observed gross changes in the pregnant woman's appearance and function, many theories were advanced about the effect of pregnancy upon specific disease entities. Many studies compared the response of the pregnant woman to that of the woman in the nonpregnant state. For the purposes of this chapter, the question is directed toward the influence, if any, of pregnancy upon systemic infectious disease. Answers can be found in the careful documentation of infection in pregnant and nonpregnant women.

There are many examples to indicate that systemic viral infections are associated with a poorer maternal prognosis during pregnancy. The recurrent pandemics of influenza, sparked by the appearance of immunologically different influenza strains, permit the recording of the impact of systemic viral disease on the pregnant woman in the preantibiotic and postantibiotic eras. In the worldwide influenza pandemic of 1918, Harris reported a maternal mortality rate of 27 percent, which increased to 50 percent when

pneumonia developed. Despite the availability of antibiotics, the Asian influenza pandemic of 1957 had a serious impact upon pregnant women. In New York City for example, Bass and Moloshok reported that the incidence of clinical infection was 50 percent higher in pregnant than nonpregnant women and that the mortality rate was greater. Nearly universal vaccination in Western countries over the decades has helped to eliminate smallpox as an entity in America. Prior to this control through immunization, there was evidence that the disease was associated with a higher mortality rate in pregnant women. Another accomplishment in preventive medicine has been the control of poliomyelitis with the widespread utilization of vaccines. Despite an occasional outbreak, polio has to all intents and purposes disappeared from the United States scene. There is good evidence from the prevaccine days that pregnant women were not only more susceptible to the disease but had a higher death rate. All these clinical observations suggest that systemic host defense mechanisms have been altered and modified in some manner by pregnancy.

The remarkable success of antibiotics in controlling bacterial disease makes it difficult to evaluate the influence of pregnancy upon such entities in these days of systemic chemotherapeutic agents. Studies in the preantibiotic era by Finland and Dublin indicated that serious bacterial infections, such as pneumonia, were less well tolerated by the pregnant woman. Antibiotics have been so effective that a finer measure than the death rate is needed to delineate the influence of pregnancy upon bacterial infections. In addition, close attention must be paid to organ system changes caused by pregnancy that could influence the host response to bacterial infections.

The immunologic competence of the host is dependent upon both humoral and cell-mediated responses. Techniques have been developed for the measurement of many host defense mechanisms and have been utilized for the study of pregnant women.

Much of the stimulus for these studies has come from the observed survival of a foreign protein graft, the fetus, in the host, the pregnant woman, for the entire gestation. Although the lack of rejection of the fetus by the maternal host is still incompletely understood, a number of suspected hypotheses have been eliminated after study. For example, the uterus is no longer held to be a privileged site for graft acceptance. In addition, the striking hormonal changes of pregnancy may modify graft acceptance, but they cannot explain the tolerance of the fetus by the mother for the entire length of the pregnancy. Continued detailed studies of this complex fetal-maternal relationship should provide some insight on the changes of the humoral and cellular responses of the pregnant woman when exposed to viruses, bacteria, and fungi. (See also Koren's contribution to Chap. 9.)

The clinical significance of changes in the response of pregnant women to bacterial agents is not known. A more fruitful examination of the pregnant woman's response to infection may be apparent in an organ system evaluation of the influence of physiologic changes upon the severity of bacterial infections seen during pregnancy.

ORGAN SYSTEM CHANGES

There is a remarkable variation in the susceptibility of pregnant and nonpregnant women to gonorrhea. In the nonpregnant state, approximately 20 to 40 percent of women exposed to the gonococcus will develop salpingo-oophoritis, while documented salpingo-oophoritis is rare in the pregnant woman. This infrequent phenomenon is not a result of a lack of invasiveness of the gonococcus during pregnancy, for disseminated gonococcal infection, particularly arthritis, is seen in pregnant women. It is likely that changes in local host defense mechanisms of the uterus during pregnancy, particularly the composition and secretion of endocervical mucus, account in part for the differences between the upper genital tract disease attack rates found in pregnant and nonpregnant women. The specific nature of the local tissue changes has not been elucidated as yet.

RESPIRATORY TRACT

The respiratory tract of the pregnant woman undergoes many changes from the nonpregnant state. There is an increase in tidal volume and in the respiratory rate. Although these variations would seem to be protective, there is good evidence (Finland, Dublin) that bacterial pneumonias are more severe in pregnant women. In addition to changes in defense mechanisms of the respiratory tract, the influence of pregnancy upon gastrointestinal physiology can have a dramatic effect upon either antepartum or postpartum lung function. A delayed gastric emptying time may contribute to the increased frequency of aspiration pneumonia in the anesthetized pregnant patient. This dreaded complication is usually recognized at the time of operation, but occasionally may not be ap-

parent to the personnel in charge of anesthesia in the operating room. The rapid postpartum onset of fever, tachypnea, and the appearance of diffuse changes on roentgen examination of the chest within a few hours of operation will yield the diagnosis. Antibiotics are indicated in such patients and at least some investigators believe that systemic adrenocortical steroids decrease the adverse effects of the highly acidic gastric contents upon the respiratory tract.

URINARY TRACT

The urinary tract of the pregnant woman undergoes vast changes in function which undoubtedly influence the ability to ward off infection. There is a marked dilatation of the collecting system—i.e., renal pelvis, ureter, and bladder—combined with a decrease in ureteral peristalsis and a slowing of the passage of urine from the kidney to the bladder. This results in an increased volume of residual urine within the renal collecting system at all times for the pregnant woman. Since urine is an excellent culture medium for enteric bacteria, this provides an excellent environment for the growth of bacteria and resulting symptomatic infection.

Infections of the urinary tract of antepartum patients occur frequently. In addition to pregnancy changes of the urinary tract, heterosexual activity and the short female urethra may combine to provide for the introduction of a nidus of bacteria into the bladder that will initiate the process of asymptomatic bacteriuria, progressing to symptomatic lower urinary tract infection, and finally to symptomatic upper urinary tract infection. The magnitude of the clinical problem is reflected in the observation that pyelonephritis is the most common infectious entity requiring admission on an antepartum service.

PYELONEPHRITIS

There are suggestions that preventive measures can be taken to decrease the incidence of pyelonephritis in pregnant women. Kass and Schneiderman have demonstrated that between 5 and 10 percent of pregnant women will have significant bacteriuria. These asymptomatic bacteriuric pregnant women have a much highe. incidence of pyelonephritis later in pregnancy than pregnant women without bacteriuria. A trial of systemic chemotherapeutic treatment of women with asymptomatic bacteriuria led to a reduction in the number of patients subsequently developing pyelonephritis. In view of these results, it seems logical that antepartum care should include screening for bacteriuria followed by appropriate chemotherapy. Because of the error inherent in a single screening culture of voided urine (an accuracy of approximately 80 percent) and the risk of infection from the use of the catheter to obtain urine for culture, some compromise may be needed. Since many good commercial systems are available for the culture of voided urine, two consecutively positive cultures (i.e., colony count above 100,000) from a carefully collected urine could be obtained before the patient is subjected to systemic chemotherapy. A portion of the second urine sample should be refrigerated and submitted for culture and identification if the second screening urine is positive and systemic chemotherapy is given. This same microbiologic concern about the identification of the organism should be followed in the posttreatment period through delivery and the postpartum period.

Despite these efforts to identify and treat a high-risk population, some pregnant patients with pyelonephritis will still be seen. In addition to a justifiable concern about the proper choice of antimicrobial agents, physicians should be aware of possible derangements of renal physiology in these women. Kass and Schneiderman have demonstrated a decrease in the concentrating abilities of the kidneys of women with bacteriuria. It is a frequent clinical observation that patients with pyelonephritis are dehydrated with an increased insensible fluid loss due in part to the high fevers preceding hospitalization that have been compounded by bouts of nausea and vomiting. Whalley et al. demonstrated a markedly diminished renal function in some patients with pyelonephritis. Serum electrolytes should be evaluated to help guide the selection of intravenous fluids, since copious amounts may be necessary to replace prior fluid losses and ensure sufficient urine output. Most studies indicate that *Escherichia coli* is the most common microorganism recovered from these women. Unless these patients have had frequent urinary tract infections in the recent past requiring systemic antimicrobial therapy, these organisms are not highly resistant and are usually responsive to treatment with such single agents as ampicillin or a cephalosporin. Evaluation of initial bacterial isolates and their susceptibilities, plus the finding of a sterile urine culture after 48 hours of therapy, is a good indication of an appropriate antibiotic choice. The necessary length of antimicrobial chemotherapy has not been established as yet. A 10-to 14-day therapeutic course of antibiotics with microbiologic evidence of cure seems effective. Recently, Hilliard and Harris demonstrated benefit in long-term systemic antibiotic prophylaxis in patients with pyelonephritis.

OTHER URINARY TRACT INFECTIONS

The most frequent site of infection in the postpartum patient is the urinary tract. A number of labor and delivery phenomena influence this occurrence. During labor, the patient's bladder is elevated out of the pelvis, and there is direct trauma to the bladder base by the presenting part of the fetus. Delivery is frequently accompanied by events that can lead to a postpartum urinary tract infection. There can be delivery trauma to the base of the bladder and the urethra. Anesthesia, particularly continuous regional anesthesia, may remove the sensation of bladder filling and prevent the use of voluntary muscles for voiding in the immediate postpartum period. Unfortunately, this diminished maternal neurologic competence coincides with the mobilization of extracellular fluid and the diuresis seen immediately postpartum. A final complicating factor is the uncomfortable episiotomy incision, which can further inhibit voluntary efforts at voiding. All these events may have varying degrees of impact on the voiding mechanisms of a postpartum patient. In some patients, the result will be an overdistended bladder, requiring subsequent catheterization, and the eventual development of a postpartum urinary tract infection.

An approach to the control of this problem requires measures of prevention. Steps should be employed to eliminate the problem of the patient with an overdistended bladder during labor and in the immediate postpartum period. The major components of such a preventive program are an awareness by the attending physician and nursing staff. Bladder overdistention should be guarded against, and patients should be encouraged to void during labor. The nationwide trend toward natural childbirth with a decreasing emphasis upon regional anesthesia during labor may be a favorable development toward postpartum urinary tract health, for these patients should be able to resume normal voiding activity sooner than the previously anesthetized patient. Perhaps a portion of the present-day problems has been related to an overemphasis on the dangers of the urethral catheter. There unquestionably is a demonstrable risk of urinary tract infection with each catheter insertion, but is this risk any greater than the problems of the overdistended bladder in the postpartum period when the catheter has not been used in a patient unable to void? This question needs to be answered by prospective study in patients during labor, delivery, and the immediate postpartum period. Despite all these preventive efforts by the physician and nursing staff, there will remain the occasional patient who develops postpartum urinary tract infection.

The cornerstone to the care of such patients is precise diagnosis and treatment. The diagnosis of a urinary tract infection in a febrile postpartum patient is too often made on the basis of the cellular findings, i.e., white blood cells on microscopic examination of a voided urine. These findings are followed by the use of powerful systemic antibiotics. The immediate result of such a policy is both obvious and favorable, for the patient becomes afebrile and is a clinical cure. The dangers of such a therapeutic philosophy are subtle and may not be immediately evident. The use of powerful systemic antibiotics in a patient with an uncomplicated urinary tract infection is probably not necessary for cure, and frequent use of these agents increases the risks for the development of a population of resistant organisms in the ward or hospital.

Evaluations of normal postpartum patients without microbiologic evidence of infection include cystoscopy and microscopic examination of urine. To diagnose infection in the postpartum patient, the significant microscopic finding is the presence of bacteria in an uncentrifuged urine sample, not white blood cells in a properly collected urine specimen. The most definitive diagnostic technique is the significant bacterial colony count, particularly in the patient with symptoms of a lower urinary tract infection. In such a woman, treatment is based upon adequate antimicrobial therapy, with agents such as sulfa drugs or nitrofurantoins whose antibacterial activity outside the urinary tract is limited. Most postpartum urinary tract infections occur in women without a chronic history of such difficulties, and the organisms recovered are usually not resistant. The most important single item in the history that dictates an alternative initial therapeutic approach is recent antibiotic therapy during pregnancy. These patients may have less susceptible bacteria, and more powerful bactericidal agents may be necessary to eliminate these organisms. A restrictive policy on the use of antibiotics for all other patients should only be employed if microbiology laboratory facilities are available to screen these patients after treatment to be sure that the bacteriuria has been eliminated.

UTERUS

During pregnancy the uterus undergoes many changes that can influence its response to infecting microorganisms. The tremendous growth rate, with a marked increase in vascularity, provides a vast range of potential problems. If improper instrumentation is used to terminate the pregnancy, a vessel laceration followed by hematoma formation in the uterine wall or the abdominal cavity may provide a fertile ground for the multiplication of bacteria. The introduction of foreign substances into the genital tract to terminate a pregnancy may result in widespread tissue necrosis, with the subsequent creation of an environment favorable for the growth of anaerobic organisms. In addition to these uterine wall changes there is the production of amniotic fluid, which forms a protective buffer around the fetus. The volume of this new body secretion ranges from approximately 100 mL at 14 weeks to 1000 mL at term. Separate studies of the amniotic fluid indicate it is inhibitory to bacterial growth. Kitzmiller et al. believed this was due to a lack of sufficient nutrient, but Larsen et al. have shown a loss of this inhibitory property with simple dilution of amniotic fluid alone. This antibacterial factor seems to be a zinc-protein complex with a molecular weight of less than 10,000. Of interest is the observation that this complex seems to be inhibited by the presence of phosphate. In addition to these changes in the normal state, there is evidence that the presence of meconium enhances bacterial growth. It seems unlikely that amniotic fluid immunoglobins play a major role in this protective mechanism, for only small amounts are found in normal amniotic fluid. Spore et al. have shown that the uterus has a remarkable ability to clear itself of bacteria postpartum. These physiologic changes influence the uterine response to infectious agents during pregnancy and the postpartum period and should be recognized in any evaluation of infections of the pregnant uterus.

ABORTION

Abortion, the termination of pregnancy when the fetus is in a nonviable state, may be associated with significant infectious morbidity. The scope of the problem of the infected abortion has undergone vast changes in the past few years with the introduction of both more acceptable contraceptive techniques and more liberal indications for the hospital termination of an unwanted pregnancy. The overall result in most urban centers has been a steady decline in the total number of women with an infected abortion as well as a decrease in the maternal mortality from sepsis. Parallel to this development has been the realization that physician termination of pregnancy may be accompanied by significant infections and even death.

The severity of infection following a community-acquired infected abortion is dependent upon the extent of tissue damage and the virulence of infecting organisms. Large amounts of poorly perfused tissue or a large extrauterine hematoma resulting from the abortion attempt set the stage for a serious infectious problem. This development is frequently seen in women whose pregnancies have progressed beyond the 12th week or who have been exposed to such tissue-necrotizing abortefacients as an intrauterine soap douche. Concomitantly, the introduction of one of many normal bacterial inhabitants of the vaginas of sexually active women into traumatized tissue of the upper genital tract may result in a serious pelvic infection.

Despite the extensive number of articles on the community-acquired infected abortion, there is evidence that knowledge on this subject is incomplete. It is likely that the significance of anaerobic organisms other than *Clostridium perfringens* has been grossly underestimated by the microbiologic techniques relied upon in most clinical studies. The emphasis of most reports on the infected abortion has been upon gram-negative aerobes such as *Escherichia coli* and the potential dire results from such infection. A carefully done anaerobic microbiologic study of patients with infected abortions by Rotheram and Schick indicated that anaerobic cocci and *Bacteroides* can frequently be recovered from the endocervix and bloodstream. The implications for antibiotic coverage because of this observation should be borne in mind in the care of the patient who fails to respond to standard therapeutic measures.

The care of the patient with an infected abortion is based upon a careful evaluation of the extent of the infection. Attempts to delineate this aspect of diagnosis are dependent upon pelvic examination and the use of roentgen examination of the abdomen. The physical examination will provide a measure of the size of the uterus and the possibility of extrauterine involvement. It also permits the physician to obtain aerobic cultures of the uterine contents and provides the chance to examine a Gram stain of infected exudate from the uterus. For anaerobic organisms, material may be obtained by needle culdocentesis. The roentgen examination in many cases will provide a great deal of information. Free gas, suggesting a uterine perforation, may be present, or the film may reveal

the presence of gas in the uterine wall suggesting a clostridial myometritis. Both of these discoveries have serious prognostic impact and usually are a factor in the decision for more extensive operative intervention.

The therapeutic approach to the patient with an infected abortion is aggressive, both in the medical and operative aspects. This is based upon the consideration that in a few instances, the patient with an infected abortion may develop evidence of septic shock that progresses to disseminated intravascular coagulation (DIC) and death. The general trend in the care of these patients has been to utilize large doses of potent antibiotics. Concern has been voiced about the theoretic considerations when bactericidal antibiotics are used in patients with infections, because of the possible massive release of endotoxin. Despite this, most services use bactericidal drugs without difficulty. This therapeutic aggressiveness has been carried over into the operative care of such patients. Although Neuwirth and Friedman cautioned against early curettage in patients with an infected abortion, most recent evaluations indicate that this is not only acceptable but preferable therapy. One of the most feared microorganisms in women with an infected abortion is *Clostridium perfringens*. Infections with this pathogen may be associated with the systemic release of toxin, intravascular hemolysis, renal failure, and death. In the 1960s, a significant emphasis in the literature was on the early clinical recognition of this infection followed by operative extirpation of the pelvic organs. The results of this regimen as measured by patient survival have been excellent. However, questions about the necessity of this aggressive operative approach have been raised by O'Neill and Schwarz, by Pritchard and Whalley, and in a recent report from England. The report from Philadelphia (O'Neill, Schwarz) suggests that the isolation of *Clostridium perfringens* from the infectious site is not always associated with illness requiring more therapy than curettage and antibiotics. The report from Dallas (Pritchard, Whalley) agrees with this and further suggests that when clostridial infection is associated with renal failure, hysterectomy will not add to survival. These conclusions seem pessimistic, for we have seen survival in such an event; in most instances, curettage and antibiotics will suffice, even when a *C. perfringens* bacteremia is noted. Good results were reported in the English study in which surgical extirpation was not utilized in infected abortion patients with serious pelvic infection.

A major concern of all physicians caring for women with an infected abortion is the development of endotoxic shock. Since the initial description by Studdiford and Douglas, there has been increasing awareness of this entity. A number of varied pharmacologic approaches have been used in patients with septic shock, including vasoconstrictors, vasodilators, and adrenal steroids. There is evidence in animal experiments and in one human trial that steroids are beneficial. The cornerstone of therapy in patients with septic shock remains the adequate and complete removal of the nidus of infection. This is usually accomplished by curettage alone, but in the patient who remains critically ill despite adequate antibiotic coverage, extirpation of the pelvic organs may be necessary for cure.

Pregnancy termination in the hospital has been accompanied by infectious morbidity. The extensive statistical base of the New York City experience as well as the surveillance system established by the Center for Disease Control suggest that factors related to infectious morbidity include physician inexperience, increasing length of gestation when the termination is performed, and the abortion technique utilized. Suction curettage within the first 12 weeks of pregnancy carries far less maternal risk than the intraamniotic injection of various substances, hysterotomy, or hysterectomy in pregnancies beyond 12 weeks. The infectious complications following abortion seem to fit into a number of distinct clinical categories.

Serious infections can result from the introduction of potent exogenous microorganisms into the genital tract at the time of the performance of the pregnancy termination. For example, a serious pelvic infection due to the group A beta-hemolytic streptococcus in a patient who had a laminaria tent[1] inserted prior to suction curettage has been reported. In addition, deaths from a coagulase-positive staphylococcus sepsis following the intraamniotic injection of hypertonic glucose have been noted. If these grampositive organisms are recovered from the site of infection in a cluster of patients with sepsis following therapeutic abortions, the personnel involved in the performance of the pregnancy terminations should be screened for the presence of the organisms so that appropriate preventive steps can be taken to avoid an epidemic of these serious infections.

Another group of serious infections is found in patients whose pregnancy termination attempts have been accompanied by significant soft-tissue dam-

age. Uterine perforation, often associated with curettage performed after 12 weeks of gestation, may be followed by a serious pelvic infection. The seeding of the upper genital tract with microorganisms at the time of the procedure, combined with a significant amount of poorly perfused tissue or blood clot formation, may result in an extensive pelvic abscess. Many patients with these posttraumatic infections may be successfully treated with systemic antibiotics alone, but frequently drainage of a pelvic abscess or the removal of extensively infected pelvic organs may be required for cure. An infrequent but feared complication of suction curettage is unrecognized uterine perforation, with bowel injury from the subsequent intraperitoneal manipulation with the suction tip. Neither the small nor the large bowel is sterile, and the colon in particular contains far greater numbers of contaminating organisms than the vagina. The result may be an extensive pelvic abscess. In the large bowel, anaerobes are numerically the most common microorganisms with *Bacteroides fragilis* present in large numbers. This fact should be a part of the antibiotic planning for such patients. The key to successful therapy in these women is the early recognition of the perforation with immediate laparotomy so that persistent contamination of the peritoneal cavity from the injured bowel does not continue. Without this operative care, systemic antibiotics alone in these patients will not suffice for cure.

Serious infections have followed the intraamniotic injection of hypertonic solutions. The early experience with pregnancy termination was followed by a report by MacDonald and O'Driscoll of death due to *C. perfringens* sepsis in a patient who had received the intraamniotic injection of a hypertonic dextrose solution. Concern about bacterial growth enhancement in amniotic fluid by this carbohydrate solution led to its abandonment. The instillation of hypertonic saline into the amniotic cavity has not been free of infectious problems. Steinberg et al. demonstrated the frequent occurrence of bacteremia associated with maternal fevers following this intraamniotic injection of salt. Other studies clearly show the potential infectious dangers of this technique. Wentz and King have demonstrated myometrial necrosis with the inadvertent injection of hypertonic salt into the uterine musculature rather than the amniotic cavity. This necrosis creates a favorable environment for significant anaerobic infection. In addition to local pelvic changes, investigators have demonstrated alterations in maternal clotting mechanisms following the intraamniotic injection of concentrated salt solution. These clotting changes are of more than theoretical

---

[1]This is a dried seaweed which swells with absorption of water and is used to dilate the cervix. It can sometimes be contaminated and is hard to sterilize except by gas techniques.

concern, for maternal deaths with DIC have been reported, and there has been a similar case at the LAC–USC Medical Center.

One clinical development has been the use of hysterectomy, by either the vaginal or abdominal route, as a means of pregnancy termination. Any major operative procedure is accompanied by the possibility of postoperative infectious morbidity, but enthusiastic proponents of vaginal hysterectomy for pregnancy termination cite a low incidence of infectious problems. Such reports are of particular interest, because of the established difficulties with postoperative pelvic infection in nonpregnant premenopausal women undergoing this procedure. If significant differences in the posthysterectomy infection rate of pregnant and nonpregnant women can be established, an attempt should be made to determine the impact of pregnancy changes upon the host response to contaminating organisms at the time of operation.

PREMATURE RUPTURE OF MEMBRANES

For the pregnancy that progresses beyond the 20th week of gestation, the greatest risk for maternal infection is the premature rupture of the membranes. When the membranes are intact, the amniotic fluid has a significant degree of antibacterial activity. This has been noted in laboratory studies, and it seems obvious to clinicians in view of the low incidence of problems following the invasive diagnostic procedure transabdominal amniocentesis. However, when the integrity of the amniotic sac has been lost, it is possible for the normal microbiologic flora of the vagina to ascend into the amniotic cavity and infect this fluid as well as the membranes. In the past, the dominant microbiologic pathogens were thought to be the gram-negative aerobe *E. coli* and gram-positive aerobic cocci. There was special concern about the potentially lethal but fortunately rare infections due to such virulent pathogens as the *Staphylococcus aureus*. The lethal potential of the combination of stillbirth and a *C. perfringens* intraamniotic infection has also been reported. In addition to the concerns about these infrequent pathogens, there has been a new awareness in obstetrics of the importance of anaerobic organisms in uterine infections, particularly the gram-negative rod, *Bacteroides fragilis*. Currently, the most serious infections on an obstetric service in terms of prolonged hospitalization and the necessity for operative removal of pelvic organs are associated with *B. fragilis* infections.

An approach to the proper management of patients with premature rupture of membranes requires knowledge of the factors influencing infectious morbidity and mortality of both mother and fetus. In many instances, physician decision making is unnecessary, for when the membranes rupture near term, 80 percent of the patients are in labor within 24 hours. This figure drops to 50 percent when the patient is not at term. In those patients without spontaneous labor, the physician must make therapeutic choices that will result in a healthy mother and fetus. For the premature fetus the physician decision must weigh the hazards of existence outside the uterus against the potential for the development of amnionitis and intrauterine fetal infection, when further fetal maturity is sought in utero. Although the dominant concern of most studies has been the duration of membrane rupture, one evaluation of premature rupture of membranes by Sacks and Baker showed that fetal survival correlated better with the length of gestation when membrane rupture occurred than with the more traditional evaluation of the time interval between membrane rupture and delivery. In addition, the cooperative study indicated that fetal infection in this population had an impact upon only a small percentage of the total number. There is an urgent need to delineate these high-risk patients by diagnostic studies. The primary maternal concern is also infection. The physician deciding to terminate the pregnancy must be aware of the increasing risk of infection following repeated examinations of an unfavorable cervix during induction attempts, particularly when there is either failure of uterine activity or evidence of fetal jeopardy that necessitates cesarean section. These concerns must be weighed against the intrapartum development of an intraamniotic infection in women with premature rupture of membranes when intervention has been avoided. Again, the evidence seems overwhelming that only a small number of the women are at risk to develop an infection. In addition to these elements in decision making, there is evidence of a different maternal and fetal prognosis when a clinic and private population are evaluated, with a poorer prognosis in the clinic population. All these factors must be considered before a therapeutic choice can be made in the treatment of premature rupture of membranes.

A new aspect of this decision making has resulted from a number of rapidly developing areas of expertise in obstetrics. These are improvements in the assessment of fetal lung maturity and evidence of increasing fetal-survival rate in the nursery with the atraumatic delivery of prematures coupled with improved nursery survival of smaller and smaller babies. These developments have had an impact upon the management of the patient with premature rupture of membranes and will undoubtedly result in further modifications in the future. Many centers have adopted a policy of the use of steroids to enhance lung maturity in concert with elective delivery of a premature infant. They report a lessened incidence of respiratory distress in the infants so treated. We have attempted to be selective in the patients of less than 32 weeks' gestation by employing transabdominal amniocentesis after real-time B scan confirms the presence of fluid. If bacteria and white blood cells (WBC) are indicative of bacterial contamination, the pregnancy is terminated. If the fluid is clear, then we await the onset of labor. This approach has yielded a prolonged intrauterine existence in many instances with the eventual delivery of a mature, uninfected baby. When labor ensues in the patient with premature rupture of the membranes, we do not use prophylactic antibiotics, but treat the symptomatic patient. In the woman with amnionitis, we set no time limit for delivery unless there is evidence of maternal or fetal deterioration.

POSTPARTUM UTERINE INFECTIONS

In the postpartum patient, a common and important site of infection is the uterus. Because of this frequency, it is important to delineate risk factors in the production of endometritis.

There are a number of influences upon the incidence of a postpartum uterine infection. Prolonged rupture of the membranes, with a prolonged labor, particularly when accompanied by frequent vaginal examinations, increases maternal risk. There seems to be a difference in the severity of postpartum uterine infection in clinic patients, especially when delivery is accomplished by cesarean section. The increasing utilization of invasive techniques during labor, i.e., the indwelling intrauterine catheter to measure intraamniotic fluid pressures, and a fetal scalp electrode, may have an impact upon infectious morbidity. It is difficult to isolate the role of the intrauterine catheter in infection. The monitored obstetric patient invariably is in a high-risk category with such problems as premature rupture of the membranes or prolonged labor and more frequently requires cesarean section. Although one study by Gassner and Ledger showed an increase in maternal infection rate in monitored patients, this same study could not demonstrate any increase in the infection rate with monitoring when the influence of the length of time of membrane rupture was negated. In addition to concern for the mother, there are fetal concerns. A recent study by Chan et al.

demonstrated no variation in fetal morbidity following intrapartum monitoring. Another report by Cordrero and Hon showed a low incidence of fetal scalp infection following monitoring. Two recent evaluations from Houston and Los Angeles indicate a higher incidence of scalp infection than previously noted. Obviously, continued surveillance of this potential problem is necessary.

The goal of the obstetrician should be to lessen the impact of factors that increase maternal postpartum morbidity. This can be achieved by obstetric management that stresses infrequent examination and avoids prolonged labor with a long interval of membrane rupture. Despite these efforts, patients will still be seen with postpartum endomyometritis.

The care of a woman with a postpartum endomyometritis is dependent upon both accurate diagnosis and appropriate care. Diagnosis is based upon a careful clinical examination with the collection of uterine and blood samples for microbiologic study. A keystone of care is the removal of any retained products of conception and the establishment of adequate uterine drainage, for the postpartum uterus has demonstrably efficient mechanisms for the clearance of bacteria.

In addition to these concerns about adequate operative drainage, antibiotics are indicated for the treatment of women with a postpartum endomyometritis. In most instances, the decision to use antibiotics is based upon clinical findings before microbiologic studies are available. The initial choice of antibiotic agent or agents by the physician is usually empirical and is based upon past experience in similar clinical situations. Most obstetric textbooks cite the anaerobic streptococcus as the most frequently recovered organism from such patients, based upon preantibiotic era studies of Schwarz and Dieckmann. However, a recent survey of postpartum infections by Sweet and Ledger indicates that *E. coli* is the most common organism recovered, coagulase-negative staphylococci, enterococci, anaerobic cocci, and *Bacteroides* being frequently isolated. There is a considerable difference in the severity of infection following delivery that is dependent upon the route. Figure 11–5 shows the marked difference in the fever indices of these two populations. Because of this, we have adopted a philosophy of care that attempts to diminish the use of potent antibiotic agents. In patients delivering vaginally who develop a postpartum uterine infection, we usually employ either ampicillin or a cephalosporin as the sole agent. In patients developing an endomyometritis following cesarean section, we have utilized a combination of penicillin and

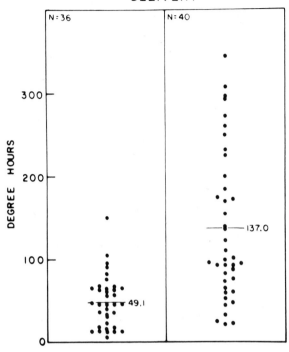

BACTEREMIA BY ROUTE OF DELIVERY

N=36　　　N=40

DEGREE HOURS

300

200

100

0

137.0

49.1

VAGINAL DELIVERIES　CESAREAN SECTIONS

FIGURE 11–5 The temperature response of a patient with a right ovarian vein thrombophlebitis treated with both heparin and antibiotics. At 0.1 the administration of ampicillin and heparin was begun. At 0.2 exploratory laparotomy was performed and tetracycline was added to the regimen. At 0.3 heparin therapy was reinstituted. The patient became afebrile on the seventh day of hospitalization and remained so for the remainder of her hospital course.

an aminoglycoside, but a recent study of this population at the LAC-USC Medical Center showed better results with clindamycin and an aminoglycoside as initial therapy. The frequent serious infections following cesarean section have sparked interest in prophylactic antibiotics. Although febrile morbidity is reduced, there is evidence that serious infections are not prevented. Because of this, we have no enthusiasm for this use of antibiotics.

SYSTEMIC MATERNAL INFECTIONS AFFECTING THE FETUS

Systemic maternal infections may have a profound influence upon the well-being of the fetus. The immediate adverse effects of such infections on the fetus may be directly related to the transplacental passage of organisms or associated indirectly when maternal infection results in either abortion or premature labor with the delivery of a premature infant, depending upon the length of gestation when the infection is acquired. In addition to these short-term results, the transplacental passage of microorganisms may cause long-term disability for the surviving infant.

BACTERIAL INFECTIONS

Systemic maternal bacterial infections can yield poor fetal results without evidence of direct bacterial infection of the fetus. The septic pregnant patient with pyelonephritis has an increased incidence of premature labor and delivery, affecting the fetus adversely. Proposed theories for this premature labor include the reflex release of oxytocin either due to maternal fever or blood volume changes, and the effect of endotoxin release upon uterine activity, but the exact mechanisms have not been established as yet. Prevention through routine screening for bacteriuria and aggressive treatment of maternal pyelonephritis should have a great impact upon the numbers of women with this problem. Although Kass and Schneiderman have suggested that asymptomatic bacteriuria without pyelonephritis is associated with low-birth-weight infants, a prospective study by Elder et al. utilizing either tetracycline or placebo in bacteriuric pregnant women demonstrated no fetal benefit from maternal tetracycline therapy.

There is evidence in some clinical conditions of transplacental passage of bacteria, with a resulting fetal infection. Most obstetrician concern in the past has been directed toward the spirochete *Treponema pallidum* and the resulting intrauterine fetal syphilis. One study from the 1940s indicated that transplacental infection does not take place before the 18th week of pregnancy, but recent evaluations indicate that the spirochete may infect the fetus before this stage of gestation. The previous gonorrhea epidemic in the United States preceded by a number of years a rise in the incidence of syphilis acquired in utero and recent reports indicate that this is the current reality. Because of this, it has been suggested that the serologic status of the mother be evaluated at the time of the first prenatal visit, in the third trimester, and during labor, providing the opportunity for the detection and treatment of syphilis acquired during pregnancy. Other bacterial pathogens may be accompanied by transplacental passage and fetal infection. One of these organisms, *Salmonella typhosa,* may require more obstetrician attention in future years. It has been reported that maternal infections may result in fetal infection with intrauterine fetal death. Recently, an epidemic of *S. typhosa* infections has been reported in Mexico, and an increasing number of patients have been seen in urban areas close to Mexico, such as Los Angeles. In a recent 1-year survey of bacteremia on an obstetric-gynecologic service at the LAC-USC Medical Center, there were three pregnant women with a *S. typhosa* bacteremia. A major concern in the care of these patients expressed by Overturf et al. is the frequent resistance of *S. typhosa* to chloramphenicol, the former drug of choice in such situations. Presently, intravenous ampicillin remains effective, but continued microbiologic surveillance will be necessary. Other bacterial pathogens may cause pregnancy problems. An infrequent event, the transmission of tuberculosis to the fetus, may result in neonatal death. Maternal *Listeria monocytogenes* and *Vibrio fetus* infections may result in fetal infections or death. The role of *L. monocytogenes* in pregnancy wastage may extend beyond this, for it has been implicated in women with habitual abortion. Physician awareness of these transplacental bacterial infections is necessary for appropriate diagnostic testing and antibiotic selection.

In the 1970s, the group B beta-hemolytic streptococcus has been implicated in maternal-fetal transmission of disease. Baker et al. reported severe neonatal infections with rapid fetal demise despite appropriate antibiotics. The exact mechanisms of this maternal-fetal transmission have not been established. It is assumed that contamination of the fetus occurs during passage through the vagina with labor and delivery, followed by asymptomatic newborn incubation in the nursery, and terminated by clinical signs of fetal sepsis and rapid death despite appropriate antibiotics. The absence of maternal antibodies to these organisms and heavy vaginal colonization in mothers whose infants have this infection suggest vertical transmission between mother and fetus. However, epidemiologic studies have posed questions about the universality of this sequence of events. For example, the group B beta-hemolytic streptococcus has not been recovered from the vagina of every mother whose newborn infant has died of this disease. In addition, there obviously is a marked difference in either infant susceptibility or the virulence of the group B beta-hemolytic streptococcus, for it is presently estimated that neonatal death from this infection occurs in 1 in 1000 deliveries and this organism can be recovered from the vaginas of 5 percent or more of pregnant women. The lethality of these newborn infections has led some pediatricians to recommend third-trimester vaginal cultures of all pregnant women with penicillin treatment for both mother-to-be and the male sexual partner, but the effectiveness in eliminating maternal colonization has not been demonstrated in a prospective study.

VIRAL INFECTIONS

Maternal viremia can have direct and immediate adverse effects upon fetal survival. In the first trimester, a maternal infection with a number of viral agents including rubella, mumps, poliomyelitis, and smallpox can be followed by fetal infection and death. In addition to these agents, a documented increase in stillbirths with maternal acquisition of hepatitis in the third trimester has been observed. To date, the only effective therapy has been preventive immunization, and this should only be utilized for nonpregnant women. The use of attenuated live virus, such as cowpox, during pregnancy is not recommended, for it has been accompanied by stillbirth, abortion, and congenital infection.

Maternal viral infections with transplacental fetal infection can have adverse effects upon the newborn. Intrauterine exposure to rubella, cytomegalovirus, or Coxsackie B virus may first manifest itself clinically in the nursery, with death resulting from pneumonia or hepatitis. In addition to this transplacental transmission of virus, there is evidence that fetal exposure to active maternal herpes simplex lesions of the lower genital tract during delivery may be followed by newborn viremia and death. Cesarean section for such women in labor whose membranes have been ruptured less than 6 hours has been demonstrated by Amstey and Monif to be of benefit.

Maternal viremia during pregnancy can be accompanied by adverse effects upon the newborn without causing mortality. The classic example is first-trimester maternal rubella, which may be associated with microcephaly, congenital heart disease, deafness, and mental retardation. Cytomegalovirus acquired during pregnancy may result in microcephaly, hydranencephaly, and microphthalmia. The availability of a rubella vaccine stimulated hopes that a significant segment of pregnancy malformations could be prevented, but the ability of the vaccine to establish and maintain an effective antibody titer to prevent maternal viremia has not been documented by long-term clinical studies. However, since the introduction of this vaccine, there have been no rubella epidemics in the United States comparable to that of 1964.

MYCOPLASMAL INFECTIONS

A definitive role of maternal *Mycoplasma* infestation in fetal loss has not yet been established. However, two recent studies suggest that these organisms can have a role in pregnancy wastage. Braun et al. found an increased incidence of low-birth-weight infants among mothers who were culture-positive for lower genital tract *Mycoplasma* during pregnancy when compared to culture-negative women. A much more indirect, but still intriguing possibility of an association of genital tract *Mycoplasma* recovery with pregnancy wastage was engendered by a study by Elder et al. In an attempt to determine the role of bacteriuria in pregnancy wastage, tetracycline or placebo was given to a group of pregnant women both with and without significant bacteriuria. To everyone's surprise, the incidence of low-birth-weight infants was far lower in the pregnant women without bacteriuria who received tetracycline. There are a number of explanations for these results. Tetracycline is effective against both *Mycoplasma hominis* and T *Mycoplasma,* and its use in pregnant women could have eliminated these organisms with a resulting beneficial fetal effect. Alternatively, this broad-spectrum antibiotic could have an effect upon *Chlamydia.* Another possibility is that this observation occurred by chance and will not be duplicated in future studies. Prospective studies of the treatment of *Mycoplasma*-positive pregnant women are now being carried out and should better delineate the relationship between maternal genital tract infection and adverse fetal effects.

PROTOZOAL INFECTIONS

Maternal protozoal infection may have an unfavorable impact upon the fetus. Maternal malaria may result in embryonic death, abortion, or premature delivery, without transplacental passage of the *Plasmodia.* These poor pregnancy results are thought to be secondary to the high fevers and circulating toxins in these women. Maternal *Toxoplasma gondii* can have profound effects upon the fetus. Toxoplasmosis is able to cross the placenta and infect the fetus in utero, resulting in neonatal death or a newborn with central-nervous-system (CNS) damage. In the United States, exposure of susceptible women to this protozoan seems related to the ingestion of poorly cooked meat or close household contact with a cat. At least one evaluation of this infectious problem by Kimball et al.

has advocated that these exposures be avoided by pregnant women.

ANTIBIOTIC THERAPY AND CHEMOTHERAPY

An awareness of the biologic nature of different bacteria should improve our understanding of the bacterial-antibiotic relationships. The introduction of antibiotics into clinical practice was accompanied by a dramatic reduction in the number of serious, life-threatening infectious diseases due to gram-positive organisms. Traditional concerns about such gram-positive pathogens as the streptococcus and pneumococcus were replaced by an awareness of the rise in hospital-acquired infections due to gram-negative organisms, such as *E. coli.* Lorian has suggested that the widespread use of antibiotics with major activity against the bacterial cell wall may have influenced this emergence of pathogens, because of basic differences in bacterial structure and physiology. The gram-positive coccus has a thick cell wall with a rigid layer of mucopeptides and an intracellular osmotic pressure of 20 atm, while the gram-negative bacillus has a much thinner cell wall and an intracellular pressure of only 5 atm. These variations between gram-positive and gram-negative bacteria should be borne in mind in the evaluation of different groups of antibiotics.

SITES OF ACTIVITY

Antibiotics can be categorized on the basis of their major site of activity against bacteria, but this is an oversimplification, since there are many examples of antibacterial agents with more than one mode of action. Antibiotics with activity against the cell wall of bacteria have been effective in the treatment of infection. This clinical effectiveness is reflected by their widespread usage in hospitalized gynecologic-obstetric patients. The most frequently used agents with this site of activity are the penicillins and cephalosporins. The cell-wall activity of these antibiotics results in bacterial destruction only in the presence of actively dividing cells. When these antibacterial agents are exposed to metabolically active bacteria, cell-wall synthesis is selectively stopped, while protein synthesis and increase of cell volume continues. The final result is the bursting of the cell. The relative ineffectiveness of penicillin against gram-negative organisms is based in part upon the minimal amount of the susceptible mucopeptide component in the cell wall of gram-negative organisms and the low intracellular osmotic pressure of these bacteria. The greater effectiveness against gram-negative organisms of such penicillin derivatives as ampicillin and carbenicillin or the cephalosporins is probably related to the ability of these antibiotics to penetrate the lipopolysaccharide layer of gram-negative bacteria and then attack alternate sites within the bacterial cell.

Another group of antibiotics serves as detergents acting on the barrier function of the cell membrane. Agents with this action include polymyxin, colistin, and the polyene antifungal agents amphotericin and nystatin. The antibiotics polymyxin and colistin, infrequently used by gynecologists and obstetricians, probably have similar antibacterial actions. These surface agents destroy the effectiveness of the osmotic barrier of the cell membrane. The effectiveness of these agents against sensitive microorganisms seems to be dependent upon the phospholipid fraction of the cell which determines the cell binding of the antibiotic. The antifungal agents similarly bind to the cell membrane, causing leakage of essential intracellular material and fungal death.

A large and varied number of antibiotics act on bacterial ribosomes, and modify the molecular mechanisms of replication, information transfer, and protein synthesis. Within this large group of antibiotics with impact upon bacterial protein synthesis, individual antibiotics act on a number of different intracellular mechanisms. In the "normal" bacterial cell, messenger RNA conveys the coding for the manufacture of protein from nuclear DNA to cytoplasmic ribosomes where proteins are manufactured. Chloramphenicol interferes with messenger RNA attachment to the ribosome complex. Another step in protein synthesis involves transfer RNA conveying and linking amino acids to the messenger ribosome complex in the proper sequence for the manufacture of proteins. The tetracyclines, erythromycin, lincomycin, and clindamycin interfere with this attachment of amino acid-transfer RNA complex to the ribosome. This inhibition of synthesis of protein could be antagonistic to the action of antibiotics such as penicillin whose major impact is on the cell wall, but who depend upon continued intracellular production of protein to result in cell bursting. This theoretical concern about antibiotic antagonism is seldom a clinical problem, for in

higher concentrations, penicillin interferes with intracellular protein synthesis as well as the cell wall. The aminoglycosides, streptomycin, kanamycin, neomycin, and gentamicin, cause bacteria to misread the genetic code. These antibiotics bind to the ribosome and result in the production of faulty proteins. This and additional mechanisms result in the death of sensitive bacteria, and probably account for successful clinical results when these agents are used in combination with bactericidal antibiotics such as penicillin.

SELECTION OF AGENTS

Selection of antibiotics for a patient with an infection requires a long-term view of possible consequences. In addition to the immediate concern about cure for the individual patient, there are considerations about the impact of the repeated use of a similar antibiotic or combination of antibiotics on a gynecologic-obstetric service. This broad view of the choice of antibiotics can be difficult for the individual practitioner, for as physicians we have been trained to evaluate therapy on the basis of individual patient response. A drug used for treatment is justifiably considered successful if the patient is cured. With this background, it may be difficult for a doctor to comprehend criticism of antibiotic choices that have resulted in cure. The long-term considerations focus upon the question of the development of bacterial resistance with its serious future implications for an inpatient service. There is ample evidence that the excessive use of an antibacterial agent on a surgical service can result in the emergence of organisms resistant to that antibiotic. A survey by Gardner and Smith of a surgical service with an observed use of kanamycin in 72 percent of hospitalized patients recorded a significant increase in the number of *Klebsiella* isolates resistant to kanamycin. Another report by Price and Sleigh noted a rise in *Klebsiella aerogenes* isolates on a neurosurgical service using semisynthetic penicillin and ampicillin in most patients undergoing operation.

Despite the unwarranted optimism of physicians that the drug industry will continually develop new and more effective antibiotics, physician concern should be directed toward preventing the development of resistant bacterial strains to present effective antibiotics. The basis for minimizing the appearance of resistant strains is a restrictive use of antibiotics. This can be implemented by making two major therapeutic commitments. First, antibiotics should not be employed in clinical circumstances in which host defense mechanisms alone will suffice. In gynecology and obstetrics there are many situations in which systemic antibiotics will not significantly alter the patient's convalescence. For example, a clinical entity exists in the postpartum obstetric patient, the lochial block, in which there will be prompt defervescence of fever with the establishment of uterine drainage alone. In gynecology, the fever of atelectasis will resolve with efforts to improve the patient's pulmonary clearance mechanisms, while most postoperative abdominal wound infections or vaginal cuff collections can be resolved by operative drainage of the site of infection alone. In these circumstances, treatment with systemic antibiotics is not required.

Another important commitment is the restriction of the choice of antibiotics for the patient needing systemic therapy. For example, many hospital-acquired lower urinary tract infections can be effectively treated with agents with limited activity outside the urinary tract without resorting to more powerful systemic antibacterial drugs. In addition, some classes of antibiotics should be reserved for specific clinical situations. The semisynthetic penicillins should only be employed in the patient with the high likelihood of having a coagulase-positive staphylococcus infection. Clindamycin and chloramphenicol should be reserved for use in the patient in whom there is a high suspicion of a *Bacteroides fragilis* infection. Gentamicin should be restricted to patients with suspected gram-negative sepsis, particularly on the oncology service where resistant gram-negative aerobes are frequently recovered. These guidelines of therapy should have a favorable impact upon antibiotic usage on a clinical service.

ADMINISTRATION OF AGENTS

The major elements in rational antibiotic usage in gynecology and obstetrics are an exact diagnosis of the site of infection and an awareness of the range of organisms involved in the infectious process. This requires careful clinical examination of all patients as well as the use of appropriate laboratory tests in the evaluation. Appropriate microbiologic cultures are important for the proper care of individual patients and in addition yield a sense of the range of antibiotic sensitivities of organisms recovered from specific infectious sites. This knowledge of potential pathogens is valuable in the selection of antibiotics for seriously ill patients. A helpful guide to the selection of anti-

biotics for commonly recovered pathogens in gynecologic and obstetric infections has been suggested by Mead and Louria.

There are a number of situations in which clinical findings should dictate a proper initial choice of antibiotics before the microbiologic identification of organisms can be completed. Although mastitis in the postpartum patient is most commonly diagnosed long after the patient's discharge from the hospital, the offending microorganism is usually a hospital-acquired, penicillin-resistant *Staphylococcus aureus*. These microbiologic data call for the use of a penicillinase-resistant antibiotic such as cloxacillin, but studies have demonstrated similar clinical effectiveness when agents such as ampicillin were employed. Patients with a postoperative abdominal wound cellulitis often have more than one organism involved, including a penicillinase-producing, coagulase-positive staphylococcus as well as a streptococcus. In this clinical setting an antibiotic such as one of the cephalosporins should be used. In postoperative and postpartum pelvic infections, the presence of a foul, fecal odor and clinical or roentgen evidence of gas formation should suggest the presence of anaerobes in the infection site. Gram's stain of the smear of the purulent exudate is a helpful guide in the initial selection of antibiotics, for penicillin and penicillinlike antibiotics are effective against most gram-positive anaerobes, while antibiotics such as chloramphenicol or clindamycin will be indicated when gram-negative rods, suggestive of *B. fragilis,* are seen.

In addition to these clinical hints in individual patients, there is evidence that knowledge of the range of potential bacterial pathogens can help in the choice of antibiotics. For example, two recent surveys of both an obstetric and gynecologic service demonstrated that the majority of *E. coli* recovered from patients with hospital-acquired lower urinary tract infections were not highly resistant. The therapeutic decision to use such agents as sulfa drugs or the nitrofurantoins in such situations is more defensible with this information available. In an evaluation of obstetric infections, the most commonly recovered microorganisms were *E. coli,* viridans streptococci, the enterococcus, peptostreptococcus, coagulase-negative staphylococcus, and *Bacteroides*. Knowledge of this range of pathogens should be an important aid in the initial choice of antibiotics. It is important to increase physician awareness of the significance of enterococci. Most recent infectious disease literature has been obsessed with an emphasis upon anaerobic infections, particularly those due to *B. fragilis*. Our philosophy has been to utilize a penicillin-aminoglycoside combination as initial therapy in most non-pregnant patients with hospital-acquired infections. The use of antibiotics effective against *Bacteroides* has been reserved for initial therapy in patients with clinical evidence of sepsis or for seriously ill patients with suspected pelvic abscess formation. This policy diminished the overall use of such agents on a gynecologic-obstetric service, and perhaps will delay the appearance of resistant organisms.

The dictum, primum non nocere, is especially applicable to physician selection of antibiotics. These agents, which have been so effective in the treatment of infectious disease can cause life-threatening reactions in susceptible women.

ADVERSE REACTIONS

Penicillin administration may result in a wide variety of patient reactions ranging from an uncomfortable skin rash to anaphylaxis and death. All physicians should have some concept of the frequency of these adverse results. A study by Rudolph and Price of reactions to nearly 100,000 administrations of penicillin demonstrated that penicillin allergy was accompanied by a significant number of reactions; a history of previous exposure to penicillin did not confer reduced reaction rate, and death from anaphylaxis occurred in 1 patient among 94,655 administrations of the drug. The greater effectiveness of ampicillin against some gram-negative organisms led to widespread clinical usage. This has created a therapeutic dilemma because of the increased number of skin rashes in patients receiving this drug when compared to ordinary penicillin. This creates concern about the future selection of penicillin for such patients, for it is difficult on clinical grounds to sort out this ampicillin allergy from a true penicillin reaction. Although the cephalosporins have been touted as a substitute for use in the patient allergic to penicillin, there is a similar chemical configuration, and cross-reactivity and sensitivity occur frequently enough to cause most infectious disease experts to look for alternative antibiotics.

In addition to allergic reactions, serious toxicity can result from the administration of either the penicillins or cephalosporins. The report by Weinstein et al. of favorable results against gram-negative aerobes with massive doses of penicillin G stimulated interest in this therapy in obstetric and gynecologic patients. In older patients, particularly those over 50, impaired renal clearance may result in high serum and CNS levels and seizures. This has been a rare phe-

nomenon in a young patient population with good renal function. The cephalosporins, particularly cephaloridine, can be nephrotoxic, especially when high serum levels are maintained in the presence of unsuspected renal impairment.

The aminoglycosides can result in serious eighth nerve and renal toxicity. This is often related to elevated serum levels of the antibiotics and occurs most freqently in clinical situations in which standard doses have been given to a patient with unrecognized impaired renal function. In an attempt to avoid this toxicity, determination of the peak and trough levels of antibiotic should be obtained in women under treatment. This provides a more scientific basis for the calculation of dosage.

There is special concern about maternal toxicity associated with the use of high doses of tetracycline during pregnancy. Prospective studies utilizing intravenous tetracycline before any adverse dose-related toxicity had been reported noted liver toxicity and death. This has led to a marked loss of enthusiasm for the use of tetracyclines in pregnant women.

The toxic effects of chloramphenicol upon the bone marrow have resulted in a diminished use of this antibiotic in patients with serious infections. There probably is some bone marrow suppression of blood-forming elements in every patient receiving this agent, but the life-threatening bone marrow aplasia occurs infrequently, about once in 20,000 to 100,000 administrations of the drug. A major clinical concern about these reactions is that they are frequently irreversible and may result in death, despite appropriate therapy. For this reason, use of chloramphenicol is restricted to patients with infections for which it is clearly the drug of choice.

Clindamycin, an alternative drug for use in *Bacteroides fragilis* infection, has been noted to have selective sites of toxicity. There may be biochemical evidence of liver toxicity, and a severe enterocolitis has been seen in patients receiving this medication orally. Recent studies suggest that the enterocolitis is caused by an enterotoxin produced by *Clostridium difficile,* which is resistant to clindamycin. This knowledge of the etiology of the disease should enable us to determine the best approaches for prevention and treatment.

EFFECTS ON THE FETUS

The use of antibiotics in the pregnant patient carries a special set of concerns for the practicing physician. Since there is no selective placental barrier against the maternal-fetal transfer of antibiotics, at least a portion of maternal serum levels of antibiotics will be delivered to the fetus. If maternal labor and delivery follow closely the administration of antibiotics, the newborn will be required to detoxify and excrete these exogenous chemicals with a liver that is not mature. Sulfa drugs are conjugated in the liver by the same enzyme system that conjugates bilirubin. This competition for a limited number of the same liver enzyme sites may result in hyperbilirubinuria of the newborn. The long-term administration of tetracycline to the pregnant woman may result in diminished long bone growth for the fetus as well as a deposition of the medication in the developing teeth of the fetus; this deposition will be visible in the newborn. In addition to these concerns about direct toxic effects upon the fetus, there is the problem of the impact of maternal antibiotic administration during labor upon newborn reactions in the nursery. Invasive maternal monitoring techniques and a greater willingness for cesarean section for fetal indications have been accompanied by a greater incidence of more serious postpartum maternal infections. There is increasing interest in the preventive use of antibiotics in such patients, but preoperative administration carries with it the problem of serum antibiotic levels in the newborn. This may complicate an already difficult diagnostic problem of neonatal sepsis which depends upon a positive blood culture. This is a matter that requires prospective study to delineate the proper therapeutic approach to such problems.

REFERENCES

Alexander JW et al.: Periodic variation in the antibacterial function of human neutrophils and its relationship to sepsis. *Ann Surg* 173:206, 1971.

Allen JL et al.: Use of a prophylactic antibiotic in elective major gynecologic operations. *Obstet Gynecol* 39:218, 1972.

Altemeier WA: Current infection problems in surgery. *Proceedings Int Conf on Nosocomial Infections,* Center for Disease Control, Baltimore: Waverly Press, 1971, p. 82.

_____ et al.: Gram negative septicemia: A growing threat. *Ann Surg* 166:530, 1967.

Amstey MS, Monif GRG: Genital herpes virus infection in pregnancy. *Obstet Gynecol* 44:394, 1974.

Baker CJ et al.: Suppurative meningitis due to streptococci of Lancefield group B: A study of 33 infants. *J Pediatr* 82:724, 1973.

Bass MH, Moloshok RE: In *Medical, Surgical and Gynecological Complications of Pregnancy,* eds. AF Guttmacher and JJ Rovinsky, Baltimore: Williams & Wilkins, 1960, p. 526.

Bolling DR Jr, Plunkett GD: Prophylactic antibiotics for vaginal hysterectomies. *Obstet Gynecol* 41:689, 1973.

Bollinger CC: Bacterial flora of the non-pregnant uterus: A new culture technique. *Obstet Gynecol* 23:251, 1964.

Braun P et al.: Birth weight and genital mycoplasmas in pregnancy. *N Engl J Med* 284:167, 1971.

Burke JF: The effective period of preventive antibiotic action in experimental incision and dermal lesions. *Surgery* 50:161, 1961.

Chan WH et al.: Intrapartum fetal monitoring. Maternal and fetal morbidity and perinatal mortality. *Obstet Gynecol* 41:7, 1973.

Cordrero L, Hon EH: Scalp abscess: A rare complication of fetal monitoring. *J Pediatr* 78:533, 1971.

Cruse PJE, Foord R: A five year prospective study of 23,649 surgical wounds. *Arch Surg* 107:206, 1973.

Curran J: Personal communication.

Elder HH, et al.: The natural history of asymptomatic bacteriuria during pregnancy: The effect of tetracycline on the clinical course and the outcome of pregnancy. *Am J Obstet Gynecol* 111:441, 1971.

Finland M, Dublin TD: Pneumococcic pneumonias complicating pregnancy and the puerperium. *JAMA* 112:1027, 1939.

Gardner HL, Dukes CD: Hemophilus vaginalis vaginitis. *Am J Obstet Gynecol* 69:962, 1955.

Gardner P, Smith AH: Studies on the epidemiology of resistance (R) factors. *Ann Intern Med* 71:1, 1969.

Gassner CB, Ledger WJ: The relationship of hospital acquired maternal infections to invasive intrapartum monitoring techniques. *Am J Obstet Gynecol* 126:33, 1976.

Gibbs RS et al.: Antibiotic therapy of endometritis following cesarean section: Treatment successes and failures. *Obstet Gynecol* 52:31, 1973.

Gregoire AT et al.: The glycogen content of human vaginal epithelial tissue. *Fertil Steril* 22:64, 1971.

Hall WL et al.: Anaerobic postoperative pelvic infections. *Obstet Gynecol* 90:1, 1967.

Hammerschlag MR et al.: Anaerobic microflora of the vagina in children. *Am J Obstet Gynecol* 131:853, 1978.

Harris JW: Influenza occurring in pregnant women. *JAMA* 72:978, 1919.

Harter CA, Benirschke K: Fetal syphilis in the first trimester. *Am J Obstet Gynecol* 124:705, 1976.

Hawkins DF et al.: Management of septic chemical abortion with renal failure. *N Engl J Med* 292:722, 1975.

Hesseltine HC: Biologic and clinical importance of

vulvovaginal mycoses. *Am J Obstet Gynecol* 34:855, 1937.

Hilliard GD, Harris RE: Utilization of antibiotics for prevention of symptomatic postpartum infection. *Obstet Gynecol* 50:205, 1977.

Hofmeister FJ et al.: Foley catheter or suprapubic tube. *Am J Obstet Gynecol* 107:767, 1970.

Kaspar DL, Baker CJ: Correlation of maternal antibody deficiency with susceptibility to neonatal group B streptococcal infection. *N Engl J Med* 294:753, 1976.

Kass EH, Schneiderman LJ: Entry of bacteria into the urinary tracts of patients with inlying catheter. *N Engl J Med* 256:556, 1957.

Kimball AC, et al.: Congenital toxoplasmosis: A prospective study of 4,048 obstetric patients. *Am J Obstet Gynecol* 111:211, 1971.

Kitzmiller JL et al.: Retarded growth of *E. coli* in amniotic fluid. *Obstet Gynecol* 41:38, 1973.

Lapides J: Pathophysiology of urinary tract infections. *Univ Mich Med Cent J* 39:103, 1973.

Larsen B et al.: Bacterial growth inhibition by amniotic fluid. *Am J Obstet Gynecol* 119:492, 1974.

Ledger WJ, Child M: The hospital care of patients undergoing hysterectomy. An analysis of 12,026 patients from the professional activity study. *Am J Obstet Gynecol* 117:423, 1973.

———, Headington JT: Group A beta-hemolytic streptococcus. *Obstet Gynecol* 39:474, 1972.

———, Kriewall TJ: The fever index—A quantitative indirect measure of hospital acquired infections in obstetrics and gynecology. *Am J Obstet Gynecol* 115:514, 1973.

———, Peterson EP: The use of heparin in the management of pelvic thrombophlebitis. *Surg Gynecol Obstet* 131:1115, 1970.

———, et al.: The fever index. A technique for evaluating the clinical response to bacteremia. *Obstet Gynecol* 45:603, 1975.

———, et al.: Guidelines for antibiotic prophylaxis in gynecology. *Am J Obstet Gynecol* 121:1038, 1975.

———, et al.: The prophylactic use of cephaloridine in the prevention of pelvic infections in premenopausal women undergoing vaginal hysterectomy. *Am J Obstet Gynecol* 115:766, 1973.

———, et al.: The surveillance of infection of an inpatient gynecology service. *Am J Obstet Gynecol* 113:662, 1972.

———, et al.: A system for infectious disease surveillance on an obstetric service. *Obstet Gynecol* 37:769, 1971.

Leppäluoto P: The coitus-induced dynamics of vaginal bacteriology. *J Reprod Med* 7:169, 1971.

Lorian V: The mode of action of antibiotics on gram-negative bacilli. *Arch Intern Med* 128:623, 1971.

Lusk RH et al.: Clindamycin-induced enterocolitis in hamsters. *J Infect Dis* 137:464, 1978.

MacDonald D, O'Driscoll MK: Intra-amniotic dextrose—a maternal death. *J Obstet Gynaecol Br Commonw* 72:452, 1965.

Mattingly RF et al.: Bacteriologic study of suprapubic drainage. *Am J Obstet Gynecol* 114:732, 1972.

McCracken GH: Group B streptococci: The new challenge in neonatal infections. *J Pediatr* 82:703, 1973.

Mead PB, Louria DB: Antibiotics in pelvic infection. *Clin Obstet Gynecol* 12:219, 1969.

Mickal A, Sellmann AH: Management of tubo-ovarian abscess. *Clin Obstet Gynecol* 12:252, 1969.

Mishell DR Jr et al.: Intrauterine device: A bacteriologic study of the endometrial cavity. *Am J Obstet Gynecol* 96:119, 1966.

Neuwirth RS, Friedman EA: Septic abortion. *Am J Obstet Gynecol* 85:24, 1963.

Norden CW et al.: Predictive effect of urinary concentrating ability and hemagglutinating antibody titer upon response to antimicrobial therapy in bacteriuria of pregnancy. *J Infect Dis* 121:588, 1970.

Ohm MJ, Galask RP: The effect of antibiotic prophylaxis on patients undergoing total abdominal hysterectomy. I. Effect on morbidity. *Am J Obstet Gynecol* 125:442, 1976.

Okada DM et al.: Neonatal scalp abscess and fetal monitoring. *Am J Obstet Gynecol* 129: 185, 1977.

O'Neill RJ, Schwarz RH: Clostridial organisms in septic abortion. *Obstet Gynecol* 35:458, 1970.

Overturf G et al.: Antibiotic resistance in typhoid fever. *N Engl J Med* 289:463, 1973.

Pheifer TA et al.: Nonspecific vaginitis. *N Engl J Med* 298:1429, 1978.

Polk HC, Lopez-Mayor TF: Postoperative wound infection: A prospective study of determinant factors and prevention. *Surgery* 66:97, 1969.

Pratt JH, Galloway JR: Vaginal hysterectomy in patients less than 36 or more than 60 years of age. *Am J Obstet Gynecol* 93:812, 1965.

Price DJE, Sleigh TD: Control of infection due to *Klebsiella aerogenes* in neurosurgical unit by withdrawal of all antibiotics. *Lancet* 2:1213, 1970.

Pritchard JA, Whalley PJ: Abortion complicated by *Clostridium perfringens* infection. *Am J Obstet Gynecol* 111:484, 1971.

Roe RE et al.: Female sterilization. I. The vaginal approach. *Am J Obstet Gynecol* 112:1031, 1972.

Rotheram EA, Schick SF: Nonclostridial anaerobic bacteria in septic abortion. *Am J Med* 46:80, 1969.

Rudolph AH, Price EV: Penicillin reactions among

patients in venereal disease clinics. *JAMA* 223:499, 1973.

Sacks M, Baker JH: Spontaneous premature rupture of the membranes. *Am J Obstet Gynecol* 97:888, 1967.

Savage WE et al.: Demographic and prognostic characteristics of bacteriuria in pregnancy. *Medicine* 46:387, 1967.

Schaefer G: Tuberculosis of the female genital tract. *Clin Obstet Gynecol* 13:965, 1970.

Schumer W: Steroids in the treatment of clinical septic shock. *Ann Surg* 184:333, 1976.

Schwarz OH, Dieckmann WJ: Puerperal infection due to anaerobic streptococci. *Am J Obstet Gynecol* 13:467, 1927.

Selvaraj RJ, Bhat KS: Metabolic and bacterial activities of leukocytes in protein-calorie malnutrition. *Am J Clin Pathol* 25:166, 1974.

Sharman A: Latent or subclinical genital tuberculosis in female infertility. *Proc R Soc Med* 54:301, 1961.

Sirisinha S et al.: Complement and C-3-proactivator levels in children with protein-calorie malnutrition and effect of dietary treatment. *Lancet* 2:1016, 1973.

Solomons B: Sterility, with special reference to surgical possibilities. *Surg Gynecol Obstet* 60:352, 1935.

Spellacy WN et al.: Vaginal yeast growth and contraceptive practices. *Obstet Gynecol* 38:343, 1971.

Spore WW et al.: The bacteriology of the postpartum oviducts and endometrium. *Am J Obstet Gynecol* 107:572, 1970.

Stallworthy J: Fertility and genital tuberculosis. *Fertil Steril* 14:284, 1963.

Stamey TA et al.: Recurrent urinary infections in adult women. *Calif Med* 115:1, 1971.

Steinberg CR et al.: Fever and bacteremia associated with hypertonic saline abortion. *Obstet Gynecol* 39:673, 1972.

Studdiford WE, Douglas GW: Placental bacteremia; a significant finding in septic abortion accompanied by vascular collapse. *Am J Obstet Gynecol* 71:842, 1956.

Study group: Metronidazole in the prevention and treatment of *Bacteroides* infections in gynaecological patients. *Lancet* 2:1540, 1974.

Swartz WH, Tanaree P: T-tube suction drainage and/or prophylactic antibiotics: A randomized study of 451 hysterectomies. *Obstet Gynecol* 47:665, 1976.

Sweet RL, Ledger WJ: Puerperal infectious morbidity. *Am J Obstet Gynecol* 117:1093, 1973.

Tafari N et al.: Failure of bacterial growth inhibition by amniotic fluid. *Am J Obstet Gynecol* 128:187, 1977.

Taylor ES, Hansen RR: Morbidity following vaginal hysterectomy and colpoplasty. *Obstet Gynecol* 17:346, 1961.

Thadepalli H et al.: Abdominal trauma, anaerobes, and antibiotics. *Surg Gynecol Obstet* 137:270, 1973.

Vollum RL: Bacteriological diagnosis of tuberculous endometritis. *J Clin Pathol* 7:226, 1954.

Walsh H et al.: Further observation on the microbiologic flora of the cervix and vagina during pregnancy. *Am J Obstet Gynecol* 96:1129, 1966.

Weinstein L, Dalton AC: Host determinants of response to antimicrobial agents. *N Engl J Med* 279:467, 1968.

_____, et al.: Clinical and bacteriologic studies of the effect of "massive" doses of penicillin G on infections caused by gram-negative bacilli. *N Engl J Med* 271:525, 1964.

Wentz AC, King TM: Myometrial necrosis after therapeutic abortion. *Obstet Gynecol* 40:315, 1972.

Whalley PJ et al.: Transient renal dysfunction associated with acute pyelonephritis of pregnancy. *Obstet Gynecol* 46:174, 1975.

White SC et al.: Comparison of abdominal and vaginal hysterectomies. *Obstet Gynecol* 37:530, 1971.

Willson JR, Black JR: Ovarian abscess. *Am J Obstet Gynecol* 90:34, 1964.

_____ et al.: The effect of an intrauterine contraceptive device on the bacterial flora of the endometrial cavity. *Am J Obstet Gynecol* 90:726, 1964.

12

Neoplastic Growth

SEYMOUR L. ROMNEY   SHELDON C. SOMMERS

This chapter is intended to provide an overview of cancer in the human female with a particular focus upon the genital tract. Conceptually, the objective has been to present the pathophysiology of female malignant neoplastic disease in terms of basic mechanisms, cellular changes, disturbed function, and diagnostic signs and symptoms. Unfortunately, this is not, as yet, totally possible. To achieve such a reality, the specific etiology—including carcinogens, mutagens, hormonal milieu, host immune responses, and other as yet unknown variables—would have to be known, and the interrelated metabolic responses fully elucidated. Such considerations remain to be clarified and are challenges for the future. The emphasis is upon gynecologic malignant diseases in general. Where specific organ site cancer is mentioned, the expectation is that the reader will find material to supplement or reinforce the discussions in other parts of the text. The general aspects of carcinoma and sarcoma of specific organ sites are presented in Chaps. 40 (Vulva and Vagina), 41 (Cervix), 42 (Uterus), 43 (Trophoblast), 44 (Fallopian tube), 45 (Ovary), and 46 (Breast). In each of those chapters, the discussion involves a review of the current status of malignant disease in various organs. In addition, in Chap. 47 (Principles of Cancer Therapy), the rationale and general considerations of treating cancer in women are presented. Consistent with the design of the text, a more comprehensive discussion of any particular neoplasm is assured if the reader will use the index and cross-references to various parts of the book.

Cancer is a disease of multifactorial origin, characterized by the insidious development of precursor, proliferative lesions, which unpredictably and irreversibly undergo malignant transformation during the course of stem cell renewal. The transformation is a biologic function in contrast to the abnormal morphologic changes which are subjectively identified as representing potentially lethal lesions by light and electron microscopy.

A considerable effort has been focused upon precursor lesions in order to understand the sequential events and cellular alterations that constitute the natural history of each neoplasm. The criteria for distinguishing degrees of cellular dysplasia, the presence of in situ malignant lesions, or for establishing the presence of microinvasion are not sharp nor totally objective. This may result in controversy, which can only be eliminated when there are more objective criteria to characterize the malignant state.

Malignant disease represents a potential hazard for the female from birth through the advanced years. An ever-present problem for the physician is recognizing the reality that an abnormality in function or detectable morphology may reflect the presence of a neoplasm, either benign or malignant. Benign tumors lack biologic aggressiveness and produce symptoms or signs related to their local, in situ manifestations. Malignant tumors—in part depending upon host genetics, degrees of differentiation, tumor volume, ability to permeate lymphatic or vascular channels, as well as immunologic response—are capable of irreversibly destroying the economy of the body and causing death.

Sarcoma botryoides, a rare tumor, can be encountered in the neonate, but in general, malignancies are seen more frequently with advancing years. One of the consequences of reducing mortality from infectious diseases and improving the management of metabolic degenerative disorders has been a prolongation of the average life-span. With this has come an increased incidence of malignant disease.

CANCER EPIDEMIOLOGY

Cancer has been the second leading cause of death in the United States in the past three decades. It is the primary cause of approximately one-sixth of all deaths, and the leading cause of mortality among females in the age group 30 to 54 years. In this age group, cancer death rates have been recently declining, but in the ages over 55, there has been an increase. Currently the incidence of malignant disease is increasing more rapidly than reported cure rates. In the age group 30 to 49, mortality rates for women, in general, exceed those for men, largely due to the numerous deaths from cancer of the breast and of the genitourinary organs. Respiratory cancer mortality is currently being reported more frequently among women. In the past decade, a doubling of the death rates from lung cancer among white women in the general population has been noted, rising from 6.2 to 12.4 per 100,000. Mortality from cancer of the breast remains unchanged and is still the leading primary malignancy among women, with an annual death rate of approximately 23 per 100,000.

Different organ sites and different age groups have shown variable responses to efforts at cancer detection, diagnosis, and therapy. However, in the major sites, namely rectum, lungs, stomach, pancreas, female breast, uterus, prostate, ovary, and blood (leukemia), mortality rates increase progressively with age and are highest in the oldest age group. In the United States and Canada, cancer death rates have about doubled with each 10-year advance in age. In Table 12-1, the probability of eventually developing and dying of cancer by site, race, and sex has been determined.

INCIDENCE AND SURVIVAL TRENDS

Accuracy of reported incidences (and death rates) depends to a significant degree upon the record-keeping practices in hospitals, the ability of tumor registries to obtain the essential follow-up data from the responsible clinics and physicians, and the transfer of such information to responsible agencies such as state health departments, the Division of Vital Statistics, U.S. Department of Health, Education, and Welfare, the American Cancer Society, *World Health Statistics Report,* etc. A comparison of incidence rates for common sites by race and sex and of rates

TABLE 12–1 Probability at Birth of Eventually Developing and Dying of Cancer of Major Sites, by Race and Sex, United States, 1973

Site of cancer	White males, %	Black males, %*	White females, %	Black females, %*
Eventually developing				
All sites	29.4	26.6	30.8	23.8
Esophagus	0.4	1.1	0.2	0.3
Stomach	1.2	1.5	0.9	0.9
Colon-rectum	4.4	2.9	5.2	3.6
Pancreas	1.1	1.1	1.0	1.0
Lung	6.1	6.0	1.6	1.3
Breast	—	—	8.1	5.2
Cervix uteri	—	—	1.5	3.0
Corpus uteri	—	—	2.2	1.1
Other uterus	—	—	0.3	0.3
Ovary	—	—	1.5	0.9
Prostate	5.1	6.4	—	—
Bladder	2.4	0.8	0.8	0.5
Kidney	0.8	0.5	0.5	0.4
Eventually dying				
All sites	17.6	16.4	16.2	14.1
Esophagus	0.4	0.9	0.2	0.3
Stomach	0.8	1.1	0.6	0.8
Colon-rectum	2.2	1.5	2.8	2.0
Pancreas	1.0	0.9	0.9	0.8
Lung	5.4	4.7	1.5	1.2
Breast	—	—	3.1	2.3
Uterus	—	—	1.0	1.9
Ovary	—	—	1.0	0.6
Prostate	1.8	2.4	—	—
Bladder	0.7	0.4	0.3	0.3
Kidney	0.4	0.2	0.3	0.2

*Life Tables employed and data on eventually dying of cancer are for nonwhite males and females.
Sources: U.S. National Center for Health Statistics: Vital Statistics of the United States, 1973, Washington, D.C.: U.S. Govt. Printing Office, 1975. Cutler SJ, Young JL, Jr, eds.: *Third National Cancer Survey: Incidence Data.* National Cancer Institute Monograph no. 41, U.S. Department of Health, Education, and Welfare Publication no. 75–787, Washington, D.C.: U.S. Govt. Printing Office, 1975.

of change over several decades is seen in Table 12–2.

A cooperative study, designed to examine the broad experience of more than 100 hospitals of various types and sizes in different parts of the country, conducted by the biometry branch of the National Cancer Institute (Myers, Axtell), has provided important information concerning trends in survival related to age, sex, stage of disease, and therapy for 48 forms of cancer. Specific data are available for cancers of the genital organs (Asire, Shambaugh). The value of the report is related to the fact that the participating tumor registries used a carefully designed common protocol that included acceptable criteria for report-

ing data. It contains the follow-up results and calculated 10-year survival rates obtained from 219,493 cancers (excluding nonmelanotic skin cancers and carcinomas in situ) which were diagnosed and treated in the various participating hospitals in the 10-year period from 1955 to 1964. More than two-thirds of all the cancers were diagnosed in persons 55 years of age or older. In the older age group, the proportion of cancers in males exceeded that in females. Of the males 50 percent with newly diagnosed cancers were 65 years of age or older, compared with 41 percent of females. In the age group 15 to 34, the survival rate decreased with age even after adjusting for normal mortality expectations. The relative 5-year survival

Table 12–2 Comparison of Incidence Rates* for Common Areas in the NCI Surveys of 1947 and 1969 for Selected Sites of Cancer, by Race and Sex

Site	Race	Males				Females			
		Rate in 1947	Rate in 1969	Change in rate	Change in rate, %	Rate in 1947	Rate in 1969	Change in rate	Change in rate %
All sites	White	282.0	300.8	18.8	6.7	294.0	255.5	−38.5	−13.1
	Black	248.0	337.2	89.2	36.0	287.0	242.9	−44.1	− 15.4
Esophagus	White	6.1	4.4	−1.7	−27.9	1.7	1.4	−0.3	−17.6
	Black	7.5	15.1	7.6	101.3	1.8	3.4	1.6	88.9
Stomach	White	31.4	12.9	−18.5	−58.9	17.3	5.8	−11.5	66.5
	Black	34.4	17.8	−16.6	−48.3	18.0	7.9	−10.1	−56.1
Colon-rectum	White	43.2	45.1	1.9	4.4	38.5	34.4	−4.1	−10.6
	Black	25.8	38.6	12.8	49.6	23.2	35.5	12.3	53.0
Pancreas	White	8.8	10.7	1.9	21.6	5.6	6.8	1.2	21.4
	Black	10.8	14.0	3.2	29.6	3.4	7.7	4.3	126.5
Lung	White	28.7	67.0	38.3	133.4	6.5	13.5	7.0	107.7
	Black	22.3	74.4	52.1	233.6	3.8	11.9	8.1	213.2
Female breast	White	—	—	—	—	70.0	72.5	2.5	3.6
	Black	—	—	—	—	47.8	60.1	12.3	25.7
Cervix uteri	White	—	—	—	—	38.4	15.3	−23.1	−60.2
	Black	—	—	—	—	74.6	34.2	−40.4	−54.2
Corpus uteri	White	—	—	—	—	22.4	21.5	−0.9	−4.0
	Black	—	—	—	—	15.6	11.3	−4.3	−27.5
Ovary	White	—	—	—	—	14.7	13.3	−1.4	−9.5
	Black	—	—	—	—	9.0	10.4	1.4	15.6
Prostate	White	36.4	44.7	8.3	22.8	—	—	—	—
	Black	50.7	78.8	28.1	55.4	—	—	—	—
Kidney†	White	5.6	7.8	2.2	39.3	3.1	3.7	0.6	19.4
	Black	4.3	7.1	2.8	65.1	3.0	3.6	0.6	20.0
Bladder	White	16.3	19.7	3.4	20.9	7.0	5.2	−1.8	−25.7
	Black	4.4	9.6	5.2	118.2	5.6	3.2	2.4	−42.9

*Per 100,000 population standardized for age on 1950 U.S. Census population.
†Estimated by the authors of this article.
Sources: Cutler SJ, Davesa SS: Trends in Cancer Incidence and Mortality in the U.S.A., in *Host Environment Interactions in the Etiology of Cancer in Man*, eds. R Doll, I Vodopija, Lyon: International Agency for Research on Cancer, 1970. Cramer DW, Cutler SJ: Incidence and histopathology of malignancies of the female genital organs in the United States. *Am J Obstet Gynec* 118:443–460, 1974.

rate[1] decreased from 58 to 33 percent. In patients under 15 years of age, the survival rate was low, as low as for patients 65 years of age or older.

[1]Relative survival rate is the survival rate observed in a group of patients; it reflects mortality from all causes.

Adjustment for "normal" mortality expectation does not alter the high case-fatality rate seen in the first 2 years after diagnosing cancer. Female cancer patients have an overall better prognosis than males. The 5-year survival rate for males (31 percent) is lower than the 10-year rate for females (42 percent). This applies to all patients regardless of whether they have localized or "all stages combined" disease. The distinct survival advantage of female patients with cancer is due largely to the nature of the primary sites involved. For the male, the four leading cancer sites (lung, prostate, colon, and bladder) have 5-year survival rates of 8, 51, 43, and 56 percent respectively. The four leading female sites (breast, uterine cervix, colon, and uterine corpus) have survival rates of 62, 60, 48, and 75 percent respectively. Comparative aspects of incidence and mortality by site and sex are seen in Fig. 12-1.

AGE AND SEX DIFFERENTIALS IN MORTALITY

Regardless of the specific cause, mortality among males is greater than among females at every stage of life except in the advanced years. Women outlive men in general, and with longevity cancer becomes a greater threat. Acute leukemia is responsible for a significant mortality in the childhood years. This form of cancer is also seen significantly in all the older age groups. Although the sex differential in mortality is relatively small in the preschool years, it rises to a

peak in the 15 to 24 age group and then declines. In the advancing years, once past childbearing, the sex mortality differential reveals a female bias. Women appear to have advantages in resistance to most common diseases. Men are confronted with environmental hazards resulting from occupation, life-style, and general behavior. As a result, sex differentials in mortality show considerable variability as to the principal cause of death.

With changing occupational behavioral patterns and life-styles, the sex differential may be narrowed in terms of cancer incidence and mortality. The cancer mortality by site, sex, and age for the major neoplasms which are encountered clinically is seen in Table 12-3. Among females, the increased mortality with age in all cancer sites is not as striking as it is in males. In the United States and Canada, lung cancer is responsible for the highest death rates among males. Approximately seven times more lung cancer has been reported among men than women. Cancer of the stomach involves twice as many men as women, and the female mortality rate is approximately half that observed in males. The death rates for cancer of the small bowel and colon, including the rectum, are only moderately lower in women. This sex differential is even greater in many other countries.

FIGURE 12-1 Comparative cancer incidence and mortality rates in females and males *(American Cancer Society)*.

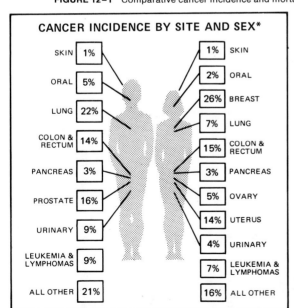

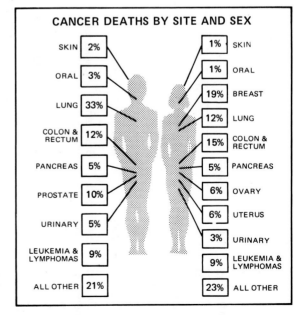

*Excluding nonmelanoma skin cancer and carcinoma in situ of uterine cervix.

TABLE 12–3 Mortality for the Five Leading Cancer Sites in Major Age Groups by Sex, United States, 1975

	Under 15		15 to 34		35 to 54		55 to 74		Over 75	
	Male	Female	Male	Female	Male	Female	Male	Female	Male	Female
Site	Leukemia	Leukemia	Leukemia	Breast	Lung	Breast	Lung	Breast	Lung	Colon and rectum
Number	648	505	746	540	10,070	8344	40,924	15,867	12,226	11,174
Site	Brain and nervous system	Brain and nervous system	Brain and nervous system	Leukemia	Colon and rectum	Lung	Colon and rectum	Colon and rectum	Prostate	Breast
Number	420	333	426	522	2496	4102	12,700	11,830	10,835	7404
Site	Lympho- and reticulo-sarcoma	Bone	Testis	Brain and nervous system	Pancreas	Colon and rectum	Prostate	Lung	Colon and rectum	Lung
Number	64	73	402	324	1326	2430	8299	10,851	8426	3582
Site	Bone	Kidney	Hodgkin's disease	Uterus	Brain and nervous system	Uterus	Pancreas	Uterus	Stomach	Pancreas
Number	54	48	391	303	1254	2397	6216	5515	3037	3367
Site	Kidney	Connective tissue	Skin	Hodgkin's disease	Stomach	Ovary	Stomach	Ovary	Pancreas	Uterus
Number	44	35	252	230	1057	2371	4799	5690	3031	2935

Source: Vital Statistics of the United States, 1975.

BLACK AND WHITE DIFFERENTIALS IN INCIDENCE AND MORTALITY

There is a significant disparity in both cancer incidence and cancer death rates between whites and blacks in the United States. An inference seems justified that variations are due to environmental influences and not biologic differences. Life-style, socioeconomic circumstances, occupational pursuits, and the accessibility and utilization of health care are important associated epidemiologic variables.

Among white women, aged 25 to 44, malignancies are the leading cause of death, accounting for approximately three-tenths of all deaths. Among white males in this age group, malignancies account for approximately one-eighth of the total deaths. The male death rate is one-fifth lower than that seen in the females. The excess cancer mortality in this relatively young age group of both white and black is largely related to malignancies of the reproductive organs and the breast.

In the 45- to 64-year-old age group, white men have a mortality rate twice that of women. Heart disease, cancer, and accidents account for this difference. Heart disease, cancer, and accidents are also encountered more frequently in black men in these years. Cancer of the prostate is a particular problem for black males. Both the incidence and the mortality rate in blacks are higher than in whites, and when the disease is diagnosed, it is generally at an advanced stage.

Cancer of the breast has a greater incidence in higher socioeconomic groups, and this is reflected by an increased incidence of breast cancer in white women. However, recent data suggest that more breast cancer is currently being seen in black women. Cancer of the cervix is notably a disease of lower socioeconomic groups, associated with early onset of sexual activity, multiple partners, and early age of first pregnancy. While the availability of Pap screening and the initiation of mass screening programs have resulted in the earlier diagnoses of invasive disease, poor women in general have frequently not availed themselves of the benefits. Overall survival is poorer in blacks than whites.

Endometrial carcinoma is more frequently seen among affluent women. Because the role of exogenous estrogens continues to be controversial, caution is indicated when prescribing hormonal preparations over extended periods of time. More white than black women have corpus cancer. A greater incidence of ovarian cancer is recorded in higher socioeconomic groups, and white women have a higher incidence. A comparative picture of cancer diagnosed early for selected sites with 5-year survival rates is given in Table 12–4.

ESTIMATED CANCER DEATHS

It is estimated that in 1979 approximately 400,000 deaths resulted from cancer. The cancer incidence by sex and site is seen in Fig. 12–1. A comparison of the death trends by site in the United States in females and males is presented in Fig. 12–2.

PATHOPHYSIOLOGY

Malignant neoplasms are characterized by autonomous aggressive growth capable of widespread infiltration and tissue destruction. Uncontrolled, undiagnosed, and untreated, their tendency is to propagate via lymphatics or bloodstream. Metastatic foci are produced, representing secondary tumors which are histologically identical to the primary tumor. Invasive tumors are composed of two specific elements, the uncontrolled proliferating cells and a benign vascular stromal element.

An inflammatory stromal response characteristically is noted in the region of tumor invasion (Fig. 12–3). This reaction, provoked by tumor cells, becomes more extensive as the tumor grows and surrounds the entire peripheral zone of the tumor, impinging upon the neighboring tissues. The inflammatory response is organized on the invasive side of the tumor, where it revascularizes the neoplastic elements so as to sustain oncogenesis. Thus, strictly speaking, neoplastic invasion does not destroy the vascular connective tissue but transforms it to its advantage (Folkman). In contrast, nonconnective tissue elements, epithelium, fat, muscle, or nerves, are irreversibly destroyed when invasion occurs. Tissue compression, atrophy, and necrosis occur. Characteristically, invasive neoplasms simultaneously have features of new growths and inflammations. Unfortunately, however, an immunologically ineffective inflammatory response is provoked by the malignant cells, which remain autonomous in the interaction. Thus, cancers are simultaneously neoplastic and inflammatory, but the inflammation, protective elsewhere, is turned to the advantage of the cancer cells.

TABLE 12-4 Percent of Cancer Cases Diagnosed in a Localized Stage and 5-Year Survival Rates† by Race and Sex for all Stages and Localized Stage for Selected Sites, End Results Group, 1955–1964

Site of cancer	Race	Males			Females		
		Percent diagnosed in localized stage	5-year survival rate		Percent diagnosed in localized stage	5-year survival rate	
			All stages	Localized stage		All stages	Localized stage
All sites	White	38	31	59	42	47	74
	Black	29	21	49	32	37	69
All sites adjusted‡	White	38	31	59	42	47	74
	Black	29	22	51	32	36	68
Esophagus	White	34	3	5	37	7	12
	Black	25	1	3	30	4	7*
Stomach	White	17	9	38	20	12	41
	Black	10	7	36*	11	11	53*
Colon-rectum	White	43	41	67	42	46	72
	Black	34	31	59	31	36	67
Pancreas	White	14	1	4	15	2	5
	Black	11	1	3*	14	3	8*
Lung	White	18	8	20	19	11	34
	Black	17	6	16	13	6	10*
Female breast	White	—	—	—	45	62	84
	Black	—	—	—	31	47	77
Cervix uteri	White	—	—	—	52	60	79
	Black	—	—	—	40	51	78
Corpus uteri	White	—	—	—	74	72	83
	Black	—	—	—	51	40	63
Ovary	White	—	—	—	28	32	72
	Black	—	—	—	25	28	74*
Prostate	White	57	51	64	—	—	—
	Black	48	41	58	—	—	—
Bladder	White	76	56	68	72	56	71
	Black	53	29	46	47	27	48*
Kidney	White	43	35	63	48	38	60
	Black	43	39	67*	47	42	71*

*Rates have standard error between 5 and 10 percent.
†Adjusted for normal life expectancy.
‡White and black male figures are adjusted to the site distribution of the total male cancer cases. White and black female figures are adjusted to the site distribution of the total female cancer cases.
Source: Axtell LM, et al.: *Treatment and Survival Patterns for Black and White Cancer Patients Diagnosed 1955 Through 1964.* Publication no. 75–712 U.S. Department of Health, Education, and Welfare, Washington: U.S. Govt. Printing Office, 1975.

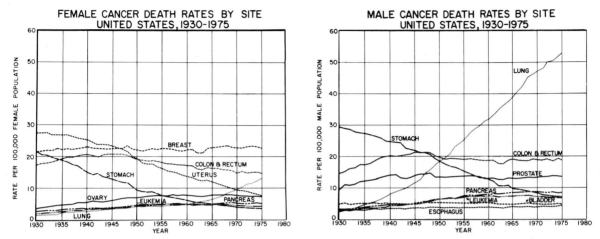

FEMALE CANCER DEATH RATES BY SITE
UNITED STATES, 1930-1975

MALE CANCER DEATH RATES BY SITE
UNITED STATES, 1930-1975

FIGURE 12-2 Female and male cancer death rates by site, United States, 1930–1975. Rates for the population standardized for age on the 1940 U.S. population. National Vital Statistics Division and Bureau of the Census, United States.

FIGURE 12-3 A benign keratomatous skin tumor has abundant lymphocytic infiltration along one margin. ×150, H&E.

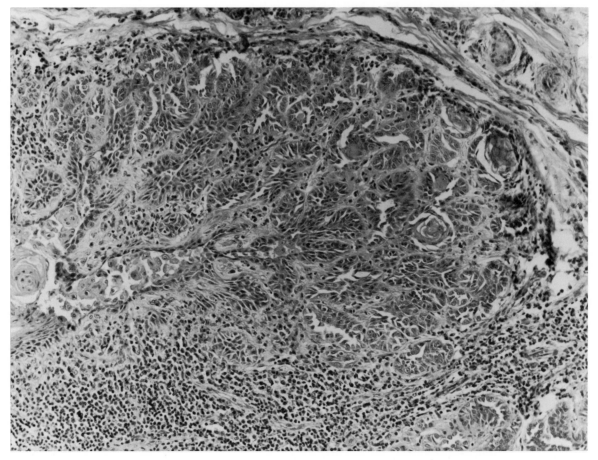

CANCER BIOLOGY

Cancer biology is one of the great scientific adventures of this century and will occupy the lifetime of many scientists. All vertebrates have malignant neoplasms and their development usually involves both host and environmental factors interacting in multistage processes.

Cancer is not uniform throughout the human population. Epidemiologic genetic studies indicate that malignant neoplasms afflict about 20 percent of the adults investigated. Heredity is most important in cancers that develop with little or no environmental contribution and least significant when strong environmental agents are involved, such as x-radiation or ultraviolet light. Inheritance of unstable nuclear deoxyribonucleic acid (DNA), or a tendency for individual chromosomes to break and exchange portions, or to be present in abnormal numbers (such as XO, XXY, trisomy 21, etc.) increases the likelihood of cancer development. Sometimes, as in xeroderma pigmentosum, an inherited inability to repair DNA correctly and completely after damage by physical, chemical, or infectious agents initiates the carcinogenic process.

"Cancer families" have been described with specific site susceptibilities. For example, endometrial carcinoma and gastrointestinal carcinoma, the latter in both sexes, are inherited as a genetic dominant. Such cancer families make up 10 to 15 percent of all cases of endometrial carcinoma. In general, individuals from cancer families develop malignancies at a younger age than in the general population and tend also to have multiple primary cancers. Such individuals may also possess certain physical peculiarities such as benign tumors, connective-tissue overgrowths, or malformations. Apparently, specific chromosomal defects, certain limited tissue susceptibilities, and particular types of multiple primary cancers are involved. The medical implications of careful family histories, family studies, and certain laboratory tests for improved cancer screening and case finding are important (Lynch).

In inbred rodents cancer viruses, or oncogenes, are inherited. Cat leukemia is horizontally transmitted. C-type viruses cause lymphomas, leukemias, and sarcomas under appropriate experimental conditions. Viral vaccines administered to mothers protect their offspring from otherwise high incidences of the heritable cancers. In rabbits there are GS antigens, which are considered footprints of similar viruses, but the actual presence of virus is as yet unproved. In human cancer, oncogenes and cancer viruses transmitted by inheritance have not been demonstrated (Meier, Huebner).

Cells of tissues that manifest mitotic activity are at a greater risk of cancer development. Neurons and myocardial cells do not divide mitotically after birth and scarcely ever undergo recognizable neoplastic transformation. The thyroid epithelium is active mitotically until an individual reaches the age of about 20 years. X-radiation damage before that time is followed by a significant number of thyroid carcinomas, while radiation exposure thereafter induces fewer thyroid carcinomas (Sommers).

CARCINOGENS

To designate any substance a carcinogen requires recognition of the particular animal or other species at risk, the route of administration, the dose given, the duration of observation, the development of unequivocal malignant neoplasia acceptable both morphologically and biologically, and the exclusion of other possible causative agents such as viruses. Comparable numbers of untreated controls must be studied with equal care. Extrapolation of results from rats to man without knowledge of the particular experimental or physiologic conditions and the biologic differences involved is dangerous.

CARCINOGENESIS

The sequence of events in carcinogenesis is described as (1) initiation or neoplastic transformation and (2) growth promotion. *Transformation* refers to an irreversible heritable alteration in DNA, often considered to be a mutation. Most mutations are lethal, but a minority permit or encourage active cell replication. *Initiation* is a carcinogenic property of irradiation (cosmic rays, x-rays, ultraviolet light, infrared, laser, and heat waves), physical agents (asbestos, plastic film), chemical agents (polycyclic hydrocarbons like benzpyrene, nitrosamines, aniline dyes, arsenic, nickel and a host of other substances), and infectious agents (parasites like schistosomes, tuberculosis bacilli, and certain viruses like the Epstein-Barr herpes type). Some of these also have promoter activity.

Some carcinogens are notably organ specific, such as asbestos for lung and pleura and aniline dyes for urinary bladder. Others like x-radiation may cause cancer of many tissues such as skin, bone, gonads, breast, colon, etc. True carcinogens are cell transformers which means that the nuclear DNA is irreversibly altered and cell proliferation continues to replicate the abnormality.

Promoters are substances that encourage and accelerate the proliferation of transformed cells. Promoters are sometimes loosely called *cocarcinogens,* but the latter term is properly restricted to substances that in the presence of a carcinogen stimulate the outgrowth of visible, recognizable cancers. Cocarcinogens are recognized under controlled experimental situations in which cancer does not occur except in their presence (Boutwell). Compared with carcinogens, of which perhaps 800 to 1000 are known, promoters are legion. Many are growth stimulants, such as insulin, other hormones, vitamins, proteins, polypeptides, and amino acids. A number of promoters such as those in fetal calf serum have not been isolated or characterized. Without spontaneous mutations or induced cell transformations, promoters do not produce cancers; hence, they do not cause cancer.

Spontaneous mutations also may initiate carcinogenesis. In tissue culture experiments, repeatedly subcultured normal cell lines are often eventually transformed. Experimentally, animal cell lines infected with an oncogenic virus and also exposed in tissue culture to a chemical carcinogen transform and grow more rapidly than when exposed to either agent alone. XXY human cells with unstable DNA exposed in vitro to SV40 virus were transformed, but human cells with stable DNA were not. There are multiple possible interactions between stable or unstable chromosomal DNA and one or more carcinogenetic initiators or cell-transforming agents. Neoplastic transformation alone does not lead to the development of a recognizable cancer. The altered cells must grow, and some proliferating clones must have a competitive metabolic advantage or no neoplasm will result.

As worked out in multiple stages for skin, the carcinogenetic sequence of initiation, cell structural transformation, promotion of growth, and the emergence of a recognizable neoplastic tumor involve six or seven steps (Burch; also see Fig. 12–4). Mathematical analysis of the age incidences of certain human carcinomas, such as those of cervix and breast, also indicates a five- or six-stage process. Endometrial carcinoma in rabbits and women requires about one-seventh of the life-span from initiation to clinical recognition, or 10 years in humans (Fig. 12–5) (Sommers, 1973a). Carcinoma of the cervix seems to develop over a 7- to 14-year period to the in situ stage; then, in approximately an additional 10 years, it becomes invasive and clinically overt. The slow preclinical progression of precancerous and early cancerous growths offers great opportunities for prevention, diagnosis in early stages, and better cancer control.

CANCER AND HORMONES

Cancer and its relation to hormones has been studied for nearly 100 years. In respect to mouse breast carcinoma, the model demonstrates three chief complementary pathogenetic mechanisms: (1) heredity, (2) a milk factor virus, and (3) hormones. To provide fully developed normal mouse mammary tissue, five types of hormone are necessary: thyroid, adrenal corticosteroids, pituitary somatomammotropin, progesterone, and estrogens. Castrated female mice of strains inbred for high incidence of breast cancer developed few breast tumors, while usually unaffected male mice injected with estrogen developed breast cancers.

ESTROGEN: HORMONE OR CARCINOGEN?

Estrogens have had considerable attention focused on them. In terms of their widespread clinical usage in steroid contraception, in postmenopausal replacement therapy, in osteoporosis, and in cancer therapy, these potent compounds may be among the most frequently used pharmacologic agents. Never before have so many women been prescribed a hormonal compound of this nature for daily consumption. Hormones, including estrogens, have not been found to be cell transformers. There are no hard data proving that they initiate carcinogenesis; consequently, they do not represent carcinogens. Currently, in the highly charged emotional atmosphere of concern with drugs, food additives, and environmental influences which may have pathogenic effects, any substance that has epidemiologic, statistical, incompletely proved, or questionable relation to any cancer is likely to be stigmatized as a carcinogen. Controlled, documented data are essential in this area.

Estrogens are growth promoters in common with many other substances. A reliable opinion that links estrogens more closely to cancer is that of Furth, who considers that greater mitotic activity in a tissue increases the chance of spontaneous mutations. This would seem more likely to be true, if at all, of individuals with chromosomal or DNA instability, as mentioned previously. An alternative theory, for which, aside from lymphoreticular cancers, evidence is lacking, is that, in proliferative or repair states as they age, all humans develop neoplastic cells, but these

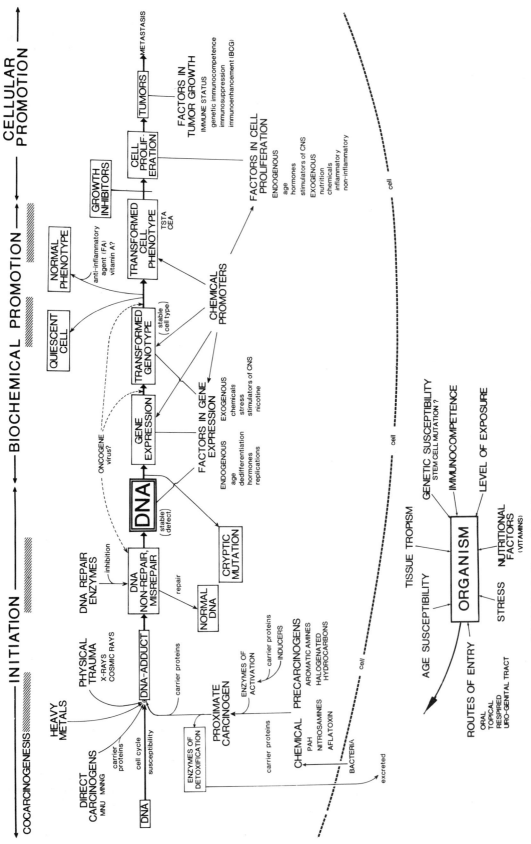

FIGURE 12–4 The multiple influences and stages of carcinogenesis, particularly of epithelial cells, are schematized. (Courtesy of Drs. Carol Henry and John H. Kreisher, Microbiological Associates, Bethesda. Md.)

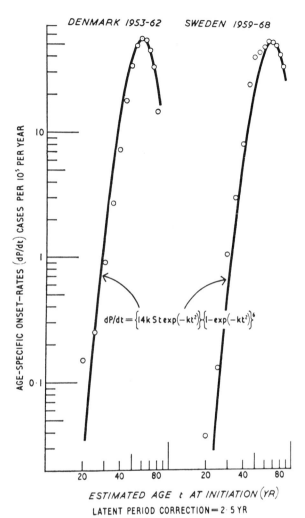

FIGURE 12-5 The graphic demonstration of the age of onset of endometrial carcinoma in Denmark and Sweden has been estimated to indicate seven steps in the initiation of this cancer. *(From Burch, p. 198, reprinted with permission.)*

do not survive to become cancerous if the immunologic surveillance mechanisms are functioning normally.

UNOPPOSED HYPERESTROGENISM

Unopposed estrogen refers to an experimental or clinical condition in which premenarchal or postmenopausal endogenous or exogenous estrogen activity is present without counterbalancing progesterone. In women of childbearing age or in sexually mature animals, unopposed estrogen is often associated with a failure of ovulation and successive anovulatory or anestrous cycles. Estrogen-secreting tumors

at any age provide unopposed excessive estrogen. In the normal menstrual cycle, the last 14 days are a time of progesterone predominance, and in pregnancy there is a 9-month interval of progesterone predominance. At these times, breast duct and endometrial gland proliferation are restrained.

This may be one reason why successful childbirth before age 20 is an epidemiologic protective factor against breast carcinoma and why endometrial carcinoma is more common in the never pregnant and those with infrequent ovulation. Women with higher estriol levels appear to have less risk. Endogenous estrogens are vital in the development and health maintenance of all females.

EXOGENOUS ESTROGENS

In the past 20 years, many physicians have philosophically supported the view that all women should always have as much exogenous estrogen as they need. Recent reports have served to bring a new understanding concerning the therapeutic use of exogenous estrogens and have pointed to issues that make this question much more complicated. The publicity surrounding conjugated estrogens administered to perimenopausal women and the claims of an increased risk of endometrial carcinoma constitute a serious scientific controversy (Antunes et al.; Hutchison, Rothman; Jick et al.; Ziel, Finkle). The epidemiologic statistical retrospective case-control studies were not of high quality. The reports included nonrandom cancer patients, biased controls, a failure to correct for hysterectomized women, and in one series a review that provided only a 74 percent consensus on the cancer diagnosis. Horwitz and Feinstein reported for curetted women who had or had not presented with vaginal bleeding that the risk of endometrial carcinoma was the same in the women who took or did not take estrogens. The major evidence that the reported trend might be more widespread than suspected came from studies reviewing the incidence of endometrial carcinoma in regional tumor registries. Tumor registries have the advantage of recording results annually concerning patients from a restricted isolated region so that data come in more quickly. A review of the incidence of endometrial cancer in six tumor registries, ranging from Connecticut to Hawaii, indicated that all were showing a marked increase in incidence. The fact that the risk of developing endometrial cancer parallels the increasing use of exogenous estrogens (Fig. 12–6) lends further confirmation to this association. Gusberg and Hertz have both postulated a relationship with unopposed estrogen for

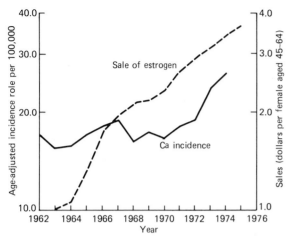

FIGURE 12-6 Comparison of trends in age-adjusted incidence rate of endometrial cancer (upstate New York, 1962–1974) to estrogen sales in wholesale dollars per female aged 45 to 64 in the United States, 1962 to 1975. *(From P. Greenwald.)*

many years and have offered evidence based on an association of atypical endometrial hyperplasia or adenocarcinoma of the endometrium with such conditions as granulosa theca-cell tumors of the ovary, the Stein-Leventhal polycystic ovarian syndrome, and clinical syndromes associated with anovulation including obesity, diabetes mellitus, and infertility.

The pathologic changes that may develop with unopposed and excessive estrogen stimulation are in particular endometrial cystic and adenomatous hyperplasia, and perhaps dysplasia. Endometrial hyperplasia is the common precursor stage of endometrial carcinoma. However, about 85 percent of women with endometrial hyperplasia do not develop carcinoma. Both in rabbits and women, further changes not dependent on estrogen are necessary for carcinoma to evolve (Sommers, 1978). Thus estrogen per se does not cause endometrial carcinoma, but is a permissive factor as part of the endocrine environment in which this cancer ordinarily develops.

Excess estrogen, unopposed by progesterone, also stimulates the breast to develop fibrocystic disease. This hyperplasia has a statistical relation to breast carcinoma, but, as already mentioned, heredity, host resistance, and other factors seem more closely related to mammary carcinogenesis in humans and rodents.

ESTROGEN HYPOTHESES

Of the three major estrogens, estriol is the least growth stimulating and in fact inhibits the effects of estradiol and estrone. The contention of Lemon and coworkers has been that, in animals and women, higher circulating estriol levels are associated with less breast carcinoma. The ratio of blood estriol to total estrogens is found to be lower in women with breast carcinoma. This theory has considerable vitality. It seems more persuasive than that of Bulbrook and his group, who believe that a low ratio of urinary androsterone to etiocholanolone is an indicator of breast carcinoma susceptibility. McDonald, Siiteri and colleagues have advanced the estrone hypothesis. They suggest that unopposed estrone cytoplasmic receptor, binding with transfer of the complex, is the active influence that affects targeted endometrial nuclei. In developing their concept of the hormonal milieu of endometrial carcinoma, they emphasize that significant estrone production, resulting from increased aromatization of plasma androstenedione, derives from extraglandular sites. They associate such findings with the epidemiologic stigmata of endometrial carcinoma, i.e., ovarian abnormalities, anovulation, and obesity (McDonald, Siiteri; Siiteri, Schwarz, McDonald). None of these theories is proved or disproved and endocrine investigations continue. The difficulty may be what was already hinted, namely that hormones are only a second-order or third-order correlate in endometrial or breast carcinoma development. Local target-cell overresponsiveness, chromosomal DNA instability, and their consequences are probably more cogent. Prospective studies are needed. Meanwhile, administration of lower dosages of estrogen and cyclic progesterone is suggested.

DIETARY FACTORS IN HORMONE-DEPENDENT CANCERS

Most of the experimental work relating diet to hormone-dependent cancers has been concerned with mammary cancer. Studies with animals have shown that increasing the level of fat in the diet stimulates mammary tumor development. The effect of caloric restriction in reducing cancer incidence is a general one, influencing most kinds of tumors, but the stimulation by dietary fat is more selective for certain types of tumors. The effect of dietary fat appears to be largely independent of caloric intake. The high fat diet is most effective when given after animals have been exposed to a carcinogen. This suggests that dietary fat acts as a promoting agent, producing a more favorable environment for the development of latent tumor cells. Unsaturated fats seem to be more effective than saturated fats in promoting mammary tumorigenesis.

Epidemiologic data in diverse female populations show a positive correlation between dietary fat intake and age-adjusted mortality from breast cancer in different countries. Similar but less significant correlations have been observed between fat intake and ovarian and prostate carcinoma. Breast-cancer mortality has a positive correlation with total caloric intake, and with intakes of animal protein and simple sugars. Such epidemiologic data provide clues to the possible influence of different dietary components on carcinogenesis.

TUMOR ANTIGENS AND TUMOR MARKERS

Tumor antigens have been sought for over 50 years, and each scientific generation has claimed success, only to be disappointed. Cancers produce and secrete a variety of polypeptides, proteins, enzymes, hormones, and other substances. Ectopic hormones, placental trophoblastic hormones, or their subunits and isoenzymes, among other materials identified by blood bioassays or radioimmunoassays, have been proposed as tumor markers.

Membrane-bound cancer cell antigens offer more promise. In various C-type, oncogene-related animal cancers, immunofluorescent histologic techniques identify specific tumor antigens localized in cell membranes. Human ovarian and lung carcinomas possess cellular antigens that appear tumor specific. They are responsible for a localized immune reaction around the tumor cells. The connective tissue stroma contains lymphocytes, macrophages, and plasma cells that are the histopathologic indicators of host immunologic resistance reactions (Ioachim). Localized immune reactions appear more important in certain human cancers than any generalized immune process that might exist throughout the body.

Efforts to identify and isolate antigens which are specific for ovarian cancer have been made since Witebsky's studies in the 1930s. Most patients with ovarian cancer are first diagnosed in advanced stages, and the importance of trying to identify antigens of value in early detection of these tumors has stimulated active investigations. To be useful for immunodiagnosis, the cancer antigen must either circulate in the bloodstream prior to the spread of intact viable cells or must, while still localized in the ovary, elicit an immune response involving the formation of specific antibodies that can be identified. The results to date have not been clinically useful (Penn).

A tumor marker is a substance present in a tumor which circulates and can be quantitated in the serum or urine with the expectation that the amount of the substance will correlate with viable cancer. It is not essential that the substance be specific for a single cancer only. The best example of a useful tumor marker is human chorionic gonadotropin (HCG). The HCG produced by choriocarcinoma has not been identified as being any different from that produced by normal placenta. Moreover, as measured in all bioassays and most radioimmunoassays, it cannot be differentiated from pituitary LH (luteinizing hormone). In spite of this, the accurate and sensitive measurement of HCG in the blood or urine of a patient with gestational trophoblastic neoplasm is essential for the accurate diagnosis, management, and follow-up of these patients. Sequential HCG beta subunit titers are accurate indices of the presence of trophoblastic neoplasms and of the effectiveness and success of chemotherapy protocols. They represent the only widely applicable blood test for a specific type of cancer. As a trophoblastic polypeptide, HCG is not a tumor antigen.

The goal is to identify a tumor marker which is specific for each cancer. In spite of lack of specificity, there are circulating substances that have been found useful in following the clinical course of patients with specific diseases and occasionally useful in differentiating cell types. Among these are plasma α-fetoprotein, carcinoembryonic antigen (CEA), and as noted, the beta subunit of HCG, which are all important in differentiating germ-cell tumors of the ovary and testis. A reasonable prediction of what can be expected in the near future from tumor markers comes from the experience with CEA (Neville, Laurence). This antigen was first used in conjunction with colon cancer but was shown subsequently to be present not only in other malignancies, but also in normal tissues. However, its practical usefulness has been relegated mostly to sequential follow-up tests to investigate recurrences after colon and other cancer surgery. Successful treatment can apparently be correlated by observations which include disappearance of circulating CEA, and by subsequent monitoring of CEA levels. The CEA levels often give evidence of recurrence prior to any clinical manifestation.

CANCER AND VIRUSES

VIRAL GENOMES

Viral genomes involve distinctly different types of viruses that are hidden from ordinary test evaluation. Sometimes viral antigens (GS, for example) found in tumors are suggestive evidence of viruses that eventually can be grown out in tissue culture. At other times tumors possess an enzyme, reverse transcriptase or revertase, that is considered an activity of a hidden viral genome. It is reported that human breast carcinomas contain a GS antigen that links this type of neoplasm to the mouse mammary tumor virus (Mesa-Tejeda et al.).

In human cancers, proof of a viral genome has been long forecast. However, its documentation is still awaited. The evidence that viruses produce human malignancies is, for the most part, limited to observations in the laboratory. Immunologic methods, including complement-fixation tests and neutralizing antibody and cytolytic techniques, are useful in detecting a virus and identifying its proteins and antiviral antibodies. Purified antigens and specific immune serums are essential for tumor identification and clinical screening, but these are difficult to produce. Specific enzyme assays (such as for RNA-directed and DNA polymerase) and methods to identify the nucleic acids of adenoviruses in human tumors are techniques also being investigated. The epidemiologic and etiologic association of viruses and some cancers is impressive but still inconclusive. Oncogenic DNA viruses (papovaviruses), adenoviruses, poxviruses, and other herpesviruses have received attention.

The papovaviruses are small DNA viruses including papilloma, polyoma, and simian vacuolating virus. The papilloma virus produces the common wart and laryngeal papilloma in man. The other viruses have particular properties that are valuable in oncogenetic studies. The adenoviruses are human viruses capable of causing acute respiratory and ocular disease in man, but not cancer. They have been shown to be carcinogenic in other mammals.

In addition to the herpes simplex virus (HSV), the Epstein-Barr herpesvirus (EBV) has stimulated major interest. EBV is a small virus, discovered by electron microscopy in cultured Burkitt's lymphoma cells. However, it has demonstrated little biologic activity, except in cell culture, where it can convert peripheral lymphocytes to lymphoblastoid cells. In humans, the only cancers presently believed to have viral etiology involving Epstein-Barr herpesvirus are Burkitt's lymphoma and anaplastic nasopharyngeal carcinoma. The former is chiefly an African and the latter a Chinese and Southeast Asian type of cancer. EBV is related to herpes simplex virus. Poxviruses are the largest animal viruses, and they have a predilection for epidermal cells. Whether a lytic, proliferative, or oncogenic response results depends on the type of poxvirus. Vaccinia causes proliferation initially and then cell lysis. The poxviruses multiply in the cytoplasm independent of cell nucleic acid synthesis. This location in the cytoplasm permits analysis of replication by electron microscopy and autoradiography. Cells infected with poxvirus may display altered morphology and loss of mitotic and contact inhibition.

HERPES INFECTION IN CARCINOMA OF THE CERVIX

Considerable epidemiologic evidence suggests that cervical cancer can be considered a venereal disease. Carcinoma of the cervix has long been known to be increased in women with venereal diseases such as syphilis and with increased vaginal trichomoniasis, while the incidence is low in nuns and Jewish women. A substance or viral agent transferred to the cervix during sexual intercourse may cause the disease, and this hypothesis has resulted in an intensive search for such a factor (Kessler). Among viruses, HSV has been implicated. Two similar but antigenically distinct types of this virus have been identified, HSV-1 and HSV-2. Type 1 causes most oral and cutaneous herpetic infections. Type 2 causes most genital infections. Both types have been implicated in carcinoma of the cervix.

A strong association between antibodies to HSV-2 and cancer of the cervix has been reported (Rawls et al.; Nahmias et al.). Also, immunofluorescent HSV-2 antigen is found in cervical carcinoma cells but not in noncancer controls. However, a conclusive causal relationship remains difficult to establish. Among women with the disease 80 percent or more have such antibodies, but in control groups the prevalence rate has usually been about 30 percent. Women in low socioeconomic groups have a high incidence of carcinoma of the cervix. Most reports provide little information about the patients studied and even less on selection of controls. Early sexual activity, pelvic inflammatory disease, multiple sexual partners, and multiparity have all been implicated.

There is a need for prospective studies with proper controls to examine all the variables associated with sexual activity including age, race, and socioeconomic status. In two studies, the prevalence rates of HSV-2 antibodies in patients with the disease were 80 to 100 percent, while controls were 30 and 62 percent respectively (Royston, Aurelian). Requiring further explanation is the fact that lower prevalence rates have been found among women with carcinoma in situ, suggesting that the virus infection may be a secondary complication. Most recently, it has been reported that New Zealand women with either carcinoma in situ or invasive disease have HSV-2 antibody prevalence rates of only about 30 percent. In this study, controls have a rate of 23 percent. Although the discrepancy may be attributable to differences in methodology, these findings, even if substantiated, would not exclude HSV-2 as a cause of cervical carcinoma but rather would suggest that the virus acts independently and directly and may be one of several causes of the disease (Aurelian). The case for an etiologic role of HSV-2 at present is incomplete, circumstantial, and unproved. HSV-2 may turn out to be a passenger virus, a promoter, or an epiphenomenon. Further evidence is awaited.

TUMOR CELL KINETICS

Once the initiation and promotion of neoplastic growth have resulted in cancer development, the tumor grows. Cancer cells grow and divide in the same manner as normal cells. The unique abnormality of the malignant cell is a loss in cell regulation, which varies from one type of tumor to another. Cell replication cycles and tumor volume doubling times have been utilized to measure cancer growth. Cell kinetic studies involve a special terminology and sophisticated mathematics. Some general conclusions developed from the investigations of animal and human cancers are:

1. Various human cancer cell reproductive times are not uniformly faster than those of normal human cells, and at times are slower. Cancer is not a disease of abnormally rapid cell reproductive cycles.
2. Within primary cancers, only a portion of the cells have unlimited reproductive capacity and are said to be clonogenic. A majority of the cancer cells are often partly differentiated and replicate less actively; within the tumor, they may be located adjacent to a proportion of resting cancer cells that may divide slowly or never.
3. Cancers may have high rates of cell death. Tumor volume doubling times have been measured, utilizing sequential x-rays or skin calipers. Among the major findings are these:
   a. Human cancer transplants into conditioned animals grow more rapidly than metastases, which in turn grow faster than primary cancers.
   b. Some primary cancers expand in lag, log, and plateau phases that obey the general laws of population growth.
   c. Tumor volume increases at least 15 times more slowly than is predicted from the cancer cell cycle

times. This notable discrepancy is believed to be caused by a reduced fraction of replicating tumor cells, the death of from 50 to 99 percent of new cancer cells produced, or the exfoliation or migration of cancer cells out of tumors.

Mathematical models developed for breast, endometrial, and other human cancers correlate well with the measurements of tumor volume doubling times (Terz et al.). Breast carcinomas exist in fast- and slow-growing types. Studies demonstrate that individual human cancers of various tissue and histopathologic types possess a wide spectrum of growth, as well as different degrees of aggressiveness from slight to extreme (Burch; Sommers, 1973b).

Defective replication causes dividing tumor cells to fail to develop or maintain a fully mature state. When unregulated proliferations of cells achieve a critical cell mass, they lose their intrinsic contact inhibition, the ability to repress cell migration which is normally present. To a greater or lesser degree, loss of contact inhibition results in malignant cells invading normal tissues. The more-differentiated cells grow more slowly. Conversely, the greater the deficiency in cell regulation, the more undifferentiated are the cells and the more rapidly they proliferate (Prehn, Prehn).

PRECURSOR LESIONS

In the vulva and vagina, precursor conditions of squamous-cell carcinoma most commonly appear grossly as keratoses, ulcerations, or leukoplakia. Microscopically the analogous alterations are an irregular and laggardly epithelial keratinization with a surface scale of hyperkeratotic and nucleated parakeratotic material. At ulcer margins and in leukoplakia, an additional epithelial thickening by the downgrowth of pegs composed of basal and precornified epithelium is found (Fig. 12–7). The severity of epithelial dysplasia is estimated by noting (1) the degree of loss of cell stratification and polarity; (2) the extent of nuclear enlargement and hyperchromatic polyploidy; and (3) the number and location of mitoses. If these are multinucleated syncytial epithelial cells of Bowen's type, the condition may be recognized as Bowen's disease type of carcinoma in situ. Ordinarily there is an infiltration of lymphocytes and plasma cells just beneath the dysplastic epithelium.

In the uterine cervix, precursors of squamous-cell carcinoma appear grossly and microscopically similar to the changes just described. What is distinctive is

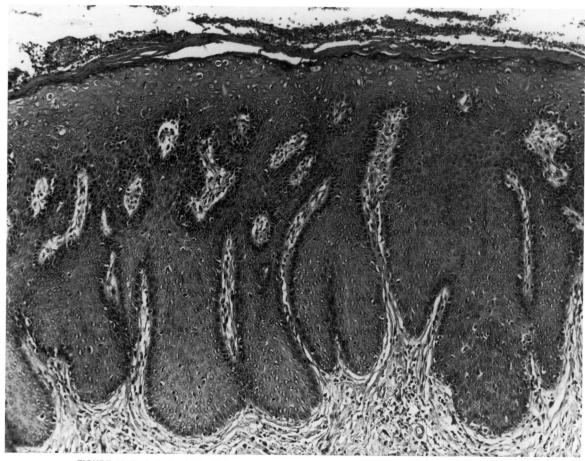

FIGURE 12–7 In leukoplakia of the uterine cervix, vulva, and elsewhere there is thickening of the epithelium, surface hyperkeratosis, and irregular or laggardly squamous-cell maturation. ×150, H&E.

the tendency to form a mosaic of foci of different microscopic lesions at the portioendocervical junction. These comprise thickened layers of basal-cell hyperplasia, laggardly dysplastic keratinization, epithelial thickening, hyperkeratosis, and parakeratosis in adjacent areas. Failure of nuclear maturation and the usual pyknotic nuclear shrinkage, plus irregular cell arrangement, sizes, and staining occur to various degrees. So long as keratin is formed in the most superficial one- or two-cell layers, the conservative interpretation is dysplasia, not carcinoma in situ, and all the above changes are regarded as reversible (Fig. 12–8). Erythroplasia of Queyrat is a red velvety area that microscopically has a monotonous thin epithelial covering that appears to be entirely composed of basal cells. Probably it is a dysplasia. Note that squamous metaplasia and epidermidalization of endocer-

vix have not been mentioned, since they do not appear to be cancer precursors in humans.

Endocervical carcinoma-precursor conditions are not often recognized or well characterized. Some microglandular proliferations after oral contraceptives appear ominous but, evidently, are not precancerous. Most other endocervical atypias are also not precancerous, and the pathologist should avoid overinterpreting cytologic peculiarities as significant.

The endometrium has been studied in detail for 80 years and a great deal has been written about its carcinoma precursors. Most gynecologic pathologists agree that the acidophilic clear-cut glands with abnormally pale nuclei are a cancer precursor. The condition is called carcinoma in situ by Hertig and coworkers, Vellios, Johannessen, and Sommers. Something very similar is termed atypical adenoma-

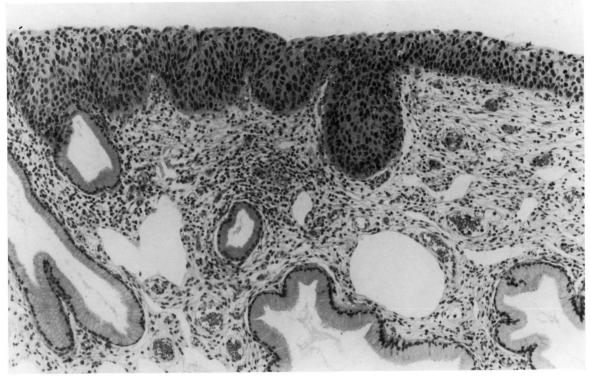

FIGURE 12–8 Cervical dysplasia is recognized by the failure of cell maturation except at the very surface where the cells are flat and thus squamous. Nuclear variations also are notable.×150, H&E.

tous hyperplasia by Gusberg and Kaplan. Lesser precursor conditions include outpouched glands with linings of irregularly enlarged epithelium possessing prominent nuclei. In endometrium, chronic inflammation is attended by a false atypicality of epithelium. Squamous metaplasia of the endometrium is not a precancerous lesion.

In the fallopian tube, as in the endocervix, carcinoma precursors are poorly defined. In tuberculous salpingitis, for example, epitheliel atypism is so characteristic that it suggests a search be made for tubercles, but it is not precancerous.

Ovarian epithelial precursors of carcinoma are occasionally seen by chance. They include (1) germinal inclusion cysts whose epithelium is stratified or papillary, with enlarged and abnormally hyperchromatic nuclei, and sometimes psammoma bodies; (2) endometriosis with focal atypical changes as described for uterine endometrium; (3) papillarity and cytologic atypia of parts of mucinous cyst linings; and (4) sheets of proliferated granulosa cells too small to constitute a tumor.

Borderline lesions are conditions that micro-

scopically are not clearly classified as either cancer or noncancer. One example is verrucous carcinoma of vulva, vagina, or cervix. From the bulky, partly necrotic, and dirty appearance of the lesions, the clinical impression is clearly a cancer. But microscopically, owing to the mild degree of squamous-cell proliferation and to lack of invasion, biopsies are diagnosed as epithelial hyperplasia pathologically (Fig. 12–9). Not until the gynecologist and pathologist exchange information that these lesions show a gross carcinoma and a microscopic hyperplasia can they be identified as borderline verrucous carcinoma. Clearly, borderline lesions are histopathologically controversial because microscopic interpretation will vary with every change from basal-cell hyperplasia to carcinoma in situ in the effort to distinguish each morphologic subentity. In the best interest of the patient, a specific diagnosis is obviously desirable and the "borderline" designation should not be used since it results in confusion from pathologist to gynecologist. Confronted with this dilemma when receiving biopsy material, it is reasonable for the pathologist to request a rebiopsy for additional tissue. If the borderline

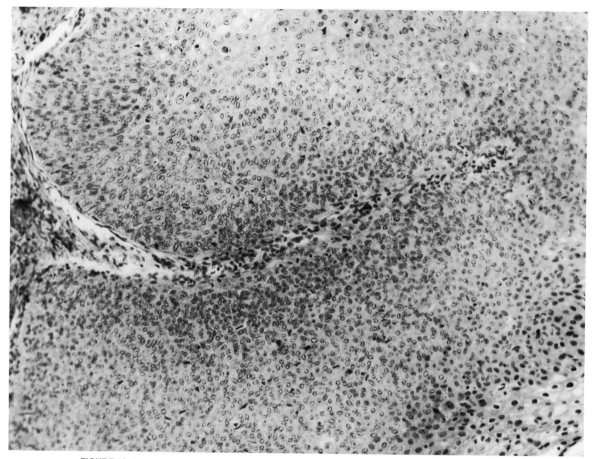

FIGURE 12–9 In verrucous carcinoma of cervix, no invasion of the stroma is seen, at the left margin. Cytologically also, the epithelium is hard to recognize as carcinomatous. × 150, H&E.

impression emerges from study of the histologic material of surgical specimens, it is desirable that the slides be reviewed in consultation and if necessary a consensus diagnosis and prognosis be assigned.

VAGINAL CYTOLOGY

Studies of animal and human cells have many research applications, including the measurement of cell reproductive cycles, DNA injury and repair, virus culture testing substances for mitogenic activity, analyzing enzyme deficiencies, and investigating chromosomes. In pregnancy, aspirated amniotic cells can be used to search for karyotypic abnormalities such as trisomy 21 (Down's syndrome). In gynecology, diagnostic cytology predominantly involves the Papanicolaou method of examining smears of vaginal cells (Papanicolaou, 1949). Material aspirated from the va-

gina, sometimes scrapings from the cervix, or endocervical mucus is smeared on glass slides, air-dried, or dropped into an alcohol-ether fixative. The Pap smears are then stained either with hematoxylin and eosin or Papanicolaou's stain, cover slipped, and scanned microscopically for atypical or neoplastic cells.

Vaginal cytology is an art that requires about 6 months of initial training; the diagnostic ability increases thereafter with constant application. It is distinct from tissue histopathology, and competence in one field does not necessarily reflect skill in the other. Most professional cytologists are not physicians but highly trained technologists. Pathologists check their findings.

Cervical smears are the greatest public health cancer case finding method of the twentieth century. Their use communitywide in the United States, Canada, and other countries has greatly reduced the incidence of invasive cervical carcinoma, which once was the most common cancer of women (Dickinson).

In practice the stained cervical smears are scanned microscopically so that the entire slide is examined. From a predominance of the superficial, large, polygonal vaginal epithelial cells, the presence of ample estrogen effect is inferred. If smaller, rounded parabasal cells predominate, the presence of an inactive or atrophic vaginal mucosa is recognized. Abundant neutrophilic leukocytes or purulent exudate indicate vaginal or cervical inflammation. Should nothing else be found, this is a "negative" cervical smear or Papanicolaou class I.

A relative abundance of parabasal, basal, and other partly matured epithelial cells results in the report of an "abnormal, not atypical" vaginal smear, or Pananicolaou class II. When some parabasal or other immature vaginal epithelial cells have relatively enlarged nuclei, perhaps hyperchromatic or containing nucleoli, the smear is designated as "atypical cells, probably benign," or Papanicolaou class III. Some laboratories divide the atypicality into (a) slight, (b) moderate, and (c) severe. So much individual variation in interpretation exists among cytologists and institutions that these subcategories lack reproducible criteria, and sometimes this leads to clinical misinterpretation or overreaction. When a number of the epithelial cells are notably atypical, with variable sizes and shapes of the nuclei, heavy nuclear staining, and some with nucleoli, the smear is reported as "atypical cells, possibly malignant," or Papanicolaou class IV. The changes are considered not clearly neoplastic, and repeat smears, or cervical biopsies, or both are required to make a more definite diagnosis (Papanicolaou, 1954).

Extreme cytologic atypism in vaginal smears, with recognizable neoplastic cells singly or in clusters, is diagnosed as a vaginal smear "positive for tumor cells" or Papanicolaou class V. Often there is considerable necrosis, blood, and purulent exudate as well. Expert cytologists may designate positive smears as having squamous-cell carcinoma or adenocarcinoma cells present. The exfoliated cells are not themselves invasive, and the presence of other similar cells left behind to invade the cervix or vagina is inferred (Fig. 12–10). The Papanicolaou test is best regarded as a screening method, with treatment based on confirmatory biopsies (Task Force Report).

Cervical carcinoma in situ can be recognized in vaginal smears (Gray). The epithelial cells have notably enlarged and variable nuclei, which tend to be pale rather than heavily stained. The distinction from invasive carcinoma cells is difficult and requires ex-

perience. The report would read "tumor cells present; carcinoma in situ" or Papanicolaou class V (carcinoma in situ).

As noted, vaginal or endocervical adenocarcinoma cells may be accurately recognized in Pap smears. Endometrial adenocarcinoma also can be diagnosed in vaginal smears with accuracy varying in different laboratories from 60 to 85 percent. Less often, since the distance from the vagina is greater, tubal adenocarcinoma and ovarian cancer cells of various types can also be diagnosed by Pap smears. Sometimes metastatic carcinoma cells to the ovary, uterus, or vagina are recognized (Ng; Shingleton et al.).

Skilled cytologists can also diagnose several nonneoplastic conditions from vaginal smears, including trichomoniasis, candidiasis, the presence of intrauterine devices or foreign bodies, pregnancy, and abortion. To some extent changes of various phases of the menstrual cycle are recognizable (Valicenti, Priesterm).

STAGING TUMORS

Because of the need to individualize, select, and evaluate specific therapeutic modalities, the anatomic extent and the cellular morphology of each tumor must be determined. This has resulted in the development of internationally accepted "staging criteria," designed to standardize clinically the anatomy of a cancer and to establish whether it is noninvasive (in situ) or, if invasive, to characterize the magnitude of spread. Localized extension, relationships to adjacent viscera, as well as possible regional or distant lymphatic or hematogenous metastatic spread are estimated. The classification and staging recommendations approved in 1971 by the International Federation of Gynecology and Obstetrics (Cancer Committee, FIGO) are now widely used. The stagings for the various gynecologic malignancies are identified in the various chapters with specific neoplasms. An equally important consideration is the need to determine the degree of tumor differentiation histologically and cytologically. The latter provides an estimate of the biologic aggressiveness of the neoplasm. Both of these factors influence decisions regarding choices of therapy.

While the scheme potentially serves the valuable purpose of identifying extent of tumor involvement, there are circumstances in individual patients where the tumor bulk volume is not accurately defined by any of the current staging criteria. Moreover, it is ap-

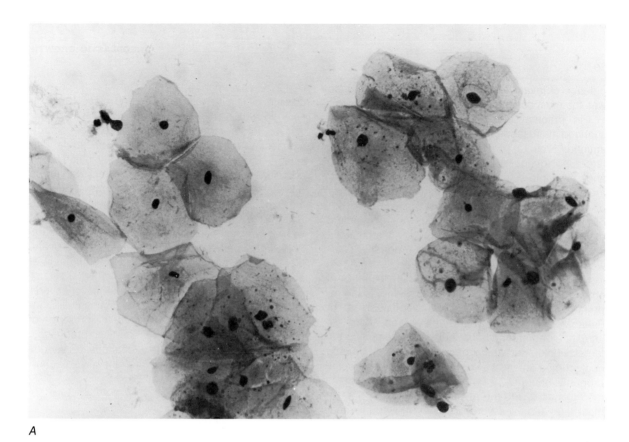

A

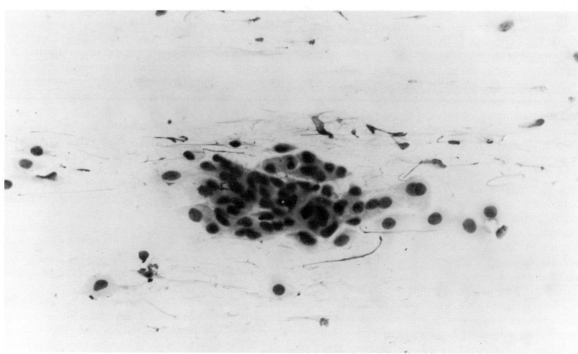

B

FIGURE 12–10 *A.* A normally estrogenized vaginal smear is composed of large polygonal cells with small dark nuclei. ×400, Papanicolaou stain. *B.* In the absence of estrogen, the vaginal smear has an atrophic appearance. ×400, Papanicolaou stain.

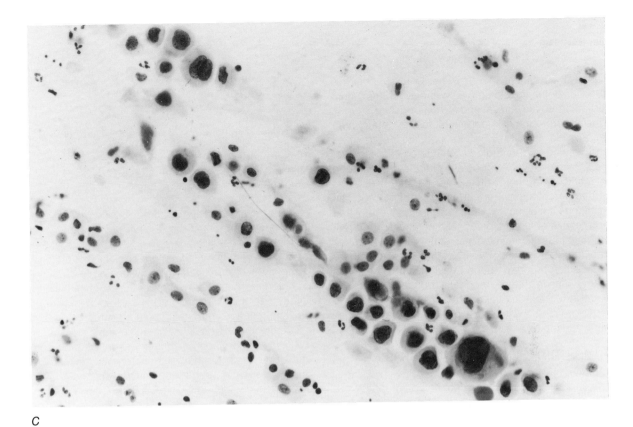

C

D

FIGURE 12–10 *C.* Vaginal smear shows clear-cut atypical cells recognizable as carcinoma in situ of cervix. ×400, Papanicolaou stain. *D.* Very atypical vaginal smear includes cells with irregular and giant nuclei, one engulfing another cell. This is diagnostic of invasive carcinoma of cervix. ×400, Papanicolaou stain.

parent that tumor aggressiveness, tumor-host response, optimum biologic conditions for maximum
radiotherapeutic effectiveness (tumor-tissue oxygen
tension) are equally important factors in determining
therapeutic outcome. Thus, a specific tumor mass
and volume and its biologic characteristics may not
be accurately evaluated by any of the current criteria
for clinical staging or histological grading, degrees
of dedifferentiation. The net effect is that in specific
instances it may not be valid to compare therapy and
end results of tumors, given the limitations of current
staging classifications. This reality should also be
considered in any comparative analysis of therapeutic results reported among institutions. For these
many reasons, the important concept that has
emerged is that the therapy of all tumors should be
individualized, based on a careful evaluation of as
many factors as possible.

TUMOR DIFFERENTIATION AND GRADING

The clinical importance of tumor cell differentiation is
that the more mature specialized cells that differentiate have a reduced growth activity and invasiveness. This is expressed by saying a tumor is named
from the best-differentiated portion and graded from
the least-differentiated part.

Cells of both benign and malignant neoplasms
differentiate to varying extents within tumors. For example, a familiar benign skin proliferation called seborrheic keratosis is composed largely of basal cells
of the epidermis. Sometimes there are also many
partly or completely keratinized cells. A similar condition, solar keratosis, has few basal cells and many
differentiated keratinized cells and surface keratin.
Comparable variations in differentiation occur in skin
basal-cell carcinomas, which may have foci of keratin
differentiation or intermingled keratinized squamous-
carcinoma cells.

Tumor grading is a numerical summary of the relative degree of cancer differentiation and growth activity. Broders, who originated a popular method,
used over a dozen cytologic criteria, and had four
grades of carcinoma, grade I the best- and grade IV
the least-differentiated. The Broders method is cumbersome, and survival with grade III and IV cancers
is sometimes nearly identical. Hence the method of
Ewing, who employed only three grades, is easier to
apply. To illustrate how a tumor is graded, the criteria
for squamous-cell carcinoma, of the cervix, skin,
esophagus, or elsewhere, are given below.

Since some tumors may have both keratin pearls
and tumor giant cells, one may have to compromise
in such cases on grade II (Fig. 12–11).

	Grade I	Grade II	Grade III
Keratin pearls	Present	Absent	Absent
Individual keratinized cells	Many	Few	Rare
Tumor giant cells	Absent	Absent	Present
Mitoses per high power field of tumor	<4	2–4	>4

The most objective grading criterion is the mitotic count, since it is reproducible among observers
and laboratories. However, among institutions, there
is so much variation in tumor grading, that the method
is mainly useful between one gynecologist and one
pathologist. The subtlety of grading is such that if one
is told that for carcinoma grade I the treatment should
be such, but for grade II it should be something else,
this reasoning is to be viewed with skepticism.

The combination of clinical cancer staging and
pathologic tumor grading is a more powerful method
of prognosticating cancer case survivals and choosing among competing therapies. It represents a great
advance in the clinicopathologic analysis and management of a variety of cancers.

LYMPHATIC AND VASCULAR INVASION

In carcinomas of the cervix and endometrium, both in
biopsies and resected specimens, it is important to
search microscopically for tumor invasion of lymphatics and blood vessels. As Barber and coworkers have
shown for both sites, the presence of vascular invasion in tissue specimens reduces the 5-year survivals
after surgery alone by about half (Fig. 12–12). Hence,
lymphatic or blood vessel invasion or both are now
considered indications for prophylactic chemotherapy, or radiation therapy, or both.

Pathologically, the tumor cell nests must lie in
endothelium-lined spaces. Lymphatics generally do
not contain red blood cells, while veins and venules
occur in pairs close to an artery or arteriole. Vascular
invasion is not restricted to advanced stages of carcinoma, since it is significant prognostically, for example, in apparently confined cervical squamous-
cell carcinoma, stage IB.

More widespread vascular invasion is common
in autopsied cases of carcinoma of the cervix, endometrium, and fallopian tube. Characteristically, gynecologic sarcomas invade blood vessels and metastasize to lungs. Generalizations concerning ovarian
cancers are not possible, but many do not show vascular spread.

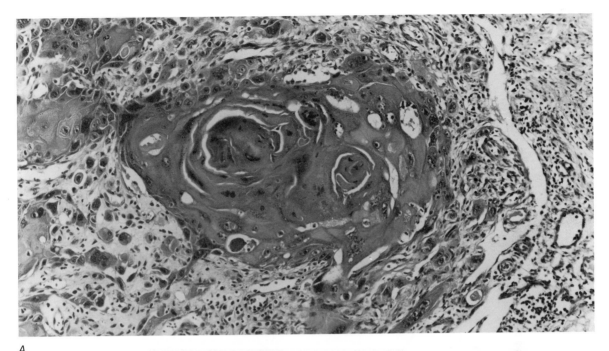

A

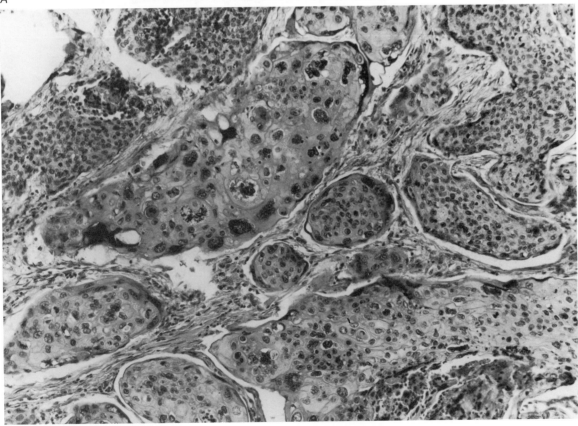

B

FIGURE 12–11 *A.* Well-differentiated squamous-cell carcinoma of cervix has abundant keratin in the tumor cells, which locally form a concentric pearl. *B.* In poorly differentiated squamous-cell carcinoma of cervix there is less keratin, more cytologic variation, mitoses, and tumor giant cells. ×150, H&E.

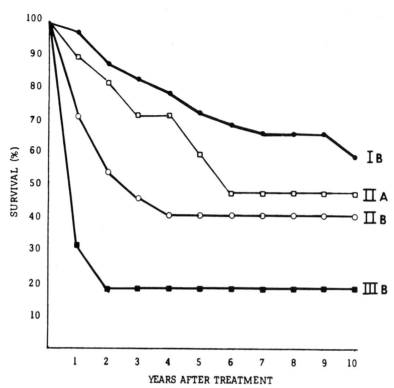

FIGURE 12–12 In favorable stage IB carcinoma of cervix, the 10-year survival is about 60 percent. However, if the tumor invades vessels, only two-thirds as many survive as when vessels are not invaded. *(From Barber et al., reprinted with permission.)*

Probably various cancers desquamate showers of malignant cells that enter the vascular system, but most or all of these tumor emboli fail to lodge and grow as metastases. The success of radical hysterectomy and pelvic lymph-node resection rests on the tendency of cervical carcinomas to reach regional lymph nodes but to spread no further for some time. Giant histological sections of such cases show tumor foci in intermediate lymphatics removed by the radical surgery, and sometimes immobilized by radiation therapy.

CANCER IMMUNITY

There is increasing evidence that immunological mechanisms are is capable of inhibiting aspects of oncogenesis or neoplastic growth (Penn).

A consequence of the use of immunosuppressive drugs in successful renal transplantation has been the development of primary malignant tumors in some recipients. The overall global incidence of malignancies in this group of patients is about 1 percent. The impression exists that because the recipient's immune response is deficient, tumors are seen in rela-

tively younger individuals. Carcinomas of the skin, lip, and cervix have been reported. Lymphomatous tumors have also been encountered, including histiocytic or reticulum-cell sarcomas of the brain. Whenever immunosuppressive drugs are administered for a year or longer, the possibility that the patient may develop a malignant tumor should be recognized. The finding of a high incidence of lymphoreticular neoplasms in infants having immunodeficiency syndromes also constitutes evidence of an immune defense role in malignancies. Despite therapy which can support infant survival for a number of years, many of these children succumb to a neoplasm. Long-term remissions, possibly due to immune resistance, have been reported in patients with hypernephroma, neuroblastoma, malignant melanoma, choriocarcinoma, and Burkitt's lymphoma.

Current concepts of the immunologic response focuses upon the T- and B-cell systems. In the T-cell system, stem cells are transformed in the thymus to *T lymphocytes,* which contain antibody-type receptors. These cells are involved with cell-mediated immunity. The T-cell system is responsible for delayed hypersensitivity reactions and the rejection of organ and skin grafts. It is also thought to be involved in autoimmune diseases. These cells are responsible for the development of immunity to most virus diseases and to chronic fungus or mycobacterial lesions. Lymphocytes of thymic derivation include cytotoxic and killer lymphocytes, some directed against cancer cells (Hellstrom et al.). In human breast cancer patients with resectable tumors, the proportion of blood T cells is reduced, suggesting lowered host-cellular immunity. In Japanese women, who have fewer and less aggressive breast carcinomas than American women, aside from increased blood estriol there is indirect evidence of increased cellular immunity including more effective T cells.

The B-cell system involves B lymphocytes derived from bone marrow. B lymphocytes are transformed into plasma cells in response to a specific antigen, and are capable of producing large amounts of antibody. Part of the local tumor immune reaction involves local antibody secretion. Macrophages are the third cellular arm of the local cancer immune reaction. While mechanisms of macrophage function are more difficult to measure and hence uncertain, evidence indicates that histiocytes participate in human breast carcinoma immune reactions both in the tumor and in the regional axillary lymph nodes.

In summary, certain human cancer antigens, mostly membrane-bound and noncirculating, have been identified. The host reaction to these antigens is local, involving T lymphocytes, plasma cells, and macrophages. In different patients, cancer aggression may be sluggish, moderate, or great. Host resistance also may be great, moderate, slight, or absent. The major biologic considerations in cancer prognosis are determined by (1) the interplay between individual tumor aggressiveness and different degrees of host immune resistance; (2) the extent of cancer spread and invasion; (3) the site and histopathologic type of cancer; (4) the histologic and nuclear grades of the tumor; and (5) the presence or absence of lymphatic and blood vessel invasion. Were it possible to assess accurately each of these variables, then estimating survival in the individual case would be more accurate than probability statistics (see Chap. 47).

RADIATION AND CYTOTOXIC EFFECTS ON CANCERS

Ionizing radiation in its various forms (grenz rays, x-radiation, α and β radiation, isotopes, atomic, pi-meson, etc.) has profound damaging effects on susceptible cells. Besides surgery, it is the best means known for controlling cancer. The mechanism of ra-

diation damage is via the production of chromosome breaks, ionization products of cell water, with swelling and rupture of cell nuclei and cell walls. The cells most damaged are those with relatively more nuclear chromatin and less cytoplasm (lymphocytes, basal cells, granulosa cells), immature cells (marrow blasts, germ cells) and those undergoing frequent mitoses. Because cancers have more of these cell categories, they are damaged more than the adjacent normal tissues.

Cells vary in their radiosensitivity or radioresistance. Nerve cells, myocardium, and cartilage are notably resistant. Lymphocytes and gonadal cells are notably sensitive. Many other cell types have an intermediate radiosensitivity. It is not possible or desirable to generalize about radiation responsiveness of individual tumor types, since this must be learned empirically. In general, undifferentiated and rapidly growing cancers with many mitoses respond best to radiation therapy. Escape of cancers from radiation therapeutic control involves the recurrence of a much less differentiated and more anaplastic neoplasm in some cases.

Cytotoxic tumor effects of cancer chemotherapy often are radiomimetic (see Chap. 47). This means that chemical interference with nuclear metabolism produces cytologic and histopathologic changes resembling those of ionizing radiation (Fig. 12–13). The stromal effects of radiation such as dense scars with large fibroblastic cells, vascular dilatation or telangiectasia, and the loss of specialized cells or histologic features are usually absent after radiomimetic drugs. Not all chemotherapeutic agents are radiomimetic; some simply cause the death and dissolution of cells. It is interesting that a few chemotherapeutic agents also produce nuclear gigantism and atypia of uninvolved tissue cells, such as the pulmonary alveolar and renal tubular epithelium.

Current cancer therapeutic modalities and regimens which can produce progressive cytotoxicity can frequently be associated with iatrogenic malnutrition, independent of any metabolic effect of the tumor, per se. Anorexia and weight loss in association with malnutrition can occur as a part of the morbidity of an aggressive course of radiotherapy and/or chemotherapy.

Active intervention of iatrogenic nutritional problems is essential for general systemic support and may increase the patient's tolerance to anticancer therapy. Several approaches have been suggested utilizing elemental dietary support and total parenteral nutrition, including hyperalimentation, in the care of patients undergoing radiotherapy and chemotherapy.

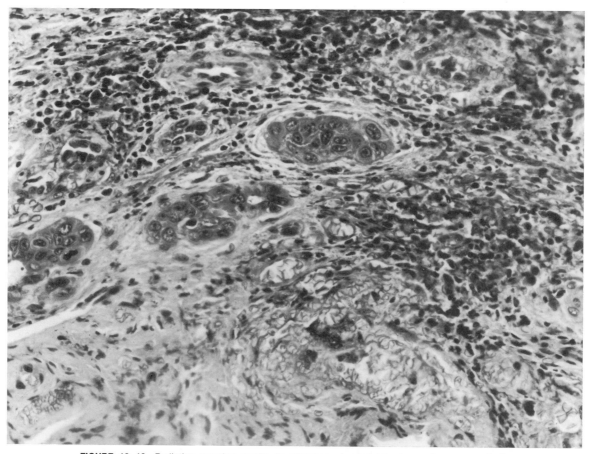

FIGURE 12–13 Radiation reaction results in dilatation of small blood vessels, seen centrally, dense fibrosis with hyaline change, and degenerative changes in some of the squamous-carcinoma cells present in oval nests. ×150, H&E.

CLINICOPATHOLOGIC CORRELATIONS OF GYNECOLOGIC TUMOR SYMPTOMS

Most women with gynecologic problems related to precursor or neoplastic lesions have one or more of three major symptoms: pain, vaginal flow, or a mass. *Pain* in young, female adults, truly originating in the genital tract, most often arises from smooth muscle spasm. Myometrial cramping contractions occur when menstrual blood and necrotic endometrium are being ejected through a narrow endocervical canal. This may be functional dysmenorrhea. However, structural dysmenorrhea involves pain from myometrial spasms associated with the presence of a foreign body, polyp, or tumor. The tumor may originate in the endometrial cavity or the endocervix.

Torsion of an ovarian cyst results in acute abdominal pain as the blood supply to the cyst and adjacent parametrial structures is reduced and anoxia stimulates sensory nerves. A similar tourniquet-type of pain follows the infarction of an ovarian tumor or a myometrial leiomyoma. The latter event is most common in a rapidly growing fibroid tumor during pregnancy or postpartum, and the leiomyoma typically undergoes so-called red degeneration.

Chronic pelvic pain accompanies the distention of the fallopian tubes and obstruction of their lumens by tumor, pus, or adhesions. Part of the pain is from interference with tubal peristalsis; part is from traction or peritoneal adhesions between tubes, ovaries, omentum, uterus, and sometimes bowel. As fibrous adhesions contract and pull on the involved organs, pain results from stimulation of the nerves and interference with the blood supply locally.

Pain originating in endometriosis may confuse the diagnostic problem of a tumor mass. Foci of hemorrhage into small nests of endometrium scattered beneath the peritoneum, in bowel serosa, or in vaginal stroma stretch the connective tissue or rupture into the free space nearby and cause pain from the irritant effect of blood locally. In older women, dull pain is often related to the stretching and distorting effect of large, multiple uterine leiomyomas which may obscure the presence of an ovarian carcinoma. They may also be perceived as a pelvic mass accompanied by irregular vaginal bleeding of uncertain etiology.

Unfortunately, the ovary is virtually never the cause of pain unless twisted on its pedicle. Thus, ovarian cancer is often symptomless in its early stages and not discovered when the disease could be curable.

Abnormal vaginal flow may be bloody, mucoid, or watery. Any type of vaginal bleeding in a woman between 12 and 60 years old is likely to be considered menstrual by the patient and physician. In perimenopausal or older women, this can be a dangerous assumption. Ordinarily menstruation should last not less than 2 or more than 7 days. Other causes of vaginal bleeding, either intermittent or constant, represent the whole spectrum of gynecologic diseases from congenital anomalies, mechanical problems, infections, degenerations, and endocrine problems to benign and malignant neoplasms. Interference with the endometrial blood supply of a hyperplastic or carcinomatous endometrium, polyps, and submucous tumors leads to capillary and venous rupture and hemorrhage that subsequently appears in the vagina.

Vaginal mucus or mucopurulent secretion usually reflects infection and inflammation of the vagina, cervix, or both, and may arise secondary to the presence of a tumor. These are catarrhal reactions comparable to the excess mucus discharge in nasopharyngeal inflammations. The neoplasm or bacterial, viral, parasitic, or mechanical agents irritate the mucous glands of vagina and endocervix to hypersecretion.

Watery discharge in older women may be indicative of tubal carcinoma; the retained secretions in the tumor rupture into the uterus. The finding is rare even when tubal carcinoma is present.

A pelvic *mass* is the least common presenting complaint among the three major gynecologic symptoms affecting women. Few women palpate their own abdomens. Every physician in practice needs to be mindful that the most common abdominal tumor in a woman of childbearing age is a pregnancy. Statistically, uterine leiomyomas or fibroid tumors are clinically the most likely pelvic tumors found by vaginal examination among women in the childbearing years.

This neoplasm, whether palpable or not, affects practically half of all women. Cysts of the ovary may fluctuate in size as the watery fluid in follicular or serous cysts, or the blood contained in luteal or endometriotic cysts, is temporarily resorbed or discharged. Dermoid ovarian cysts (benign teratomas) are full of sebaceous material that is fluid at body temperature. They are usually so distended as to imitate a solid tumor. Pedunculated subserous uterine fibroids or tubal cysts may appear to change in position. Sometimes solid tumors lose their original pedicle and are vascularized from adjacent structures, as in the so-called wandering fibroid.

Everyone involved in the health care of women must remember that in a woman of any age, particularly after 40, a palpably enlarged ovary or ovarian mass had best be considered cancer first, until it is ruled out. This approach is at present the best hope for ovarian cancer control. The physician must find this sign, because the patient will not volunteer the information.

CANCER CACHEXIA

Cachexia occurs in one-third to two-thirds of cancer patients and is characterized by anorexia, increased metabolism, negative protein balance, and an increased energy expenditure despite a reduced caloric intake. Marked asthenia, significant loss of body fat and lean body mass, anemia, and accompanying water and electrolyte abnormalities are common. Anorexia and a sense of fullness cause oligophagy with resultant reduction in caloric intake, which contributes to the tissue wasting. Weight loss can only be temporarily treated and reversed by hyperalimentation. Complications of the disease and its treatment may contribute to further malnutrition and increased energy and/or nitrogen loss. However, it is the autonomous neoplasm that profoundly influences a systemic derangement of the patient's metabolism, and it continues to grow in the presence of progressive cachexia and malnutrition.

It has been proposed that the pathogenesis of cancer cachexia involves the production of peptides and other small molecules by the cancer cells. Through allosteric transitions and resulting activations and inactivations of normal cell enzymes, the metabolism of the host is deranged. Energy-consuming biochemical reactions occur in the normal cell and result in the release of intermediary metabolites (amino acids, peptides, etc.) into a metabolic pool used by the cancer cell for its growth. It has been further hypothesized that the cancer cell is less vulnerable to allosteric effects and that host metabolites entering the cancer cell are totally consumed.

REFERENCES

Antunes CM et al.: Endometrial cancer and estrogen use. *N Engl J Med* 300:9, 1979.

Asire AJ, Shambaugh EM: Cancer of the female genital organs. *Cancer Patient Survival,* U.S. Department of Health, Education and Welfare Publication, report no. 5, pp. 77–992, 1976.

Aurelian L: Virions and antigens of herpes virus type 2 in cervical carcinoma. *Cancer Res* 33:1539–1947, 1973.

Barber HR et al.: Cancer of the endometrium. *Tex Med* 70:41–56, 1974.

——: Vascular invasion as a prognostic factor in stage 1B cancer of the cervix. *Obstet Gynecol* 52:343-348, 1978.

Boutwell RK: The function and mechanism of promoters of carcinogenesis. *CRC Crit Rev Toxicol* 2:419, 1974.

Broders AC: The microscopic grading of cancer, in *Treatment of Cancer and Allied Diseases,* vol. 1, ed. GE Pack, New York: Hoeber, 1940, p. 55.

Bulbrook RD, Hayward JL: Abnormal urinary steroid excretion and subsequent breast cancer. *Lancet* 1:519, 1967.

Burch PRJ: *The Biology of Cancer.* Baltimore: Univ Park Press, 1976, p. 189.

Dickinson LE: Control of cancer of the uterine cervix by cytologic screening. *Gynecol Oncol* 3:1, 1975.

Ferenczy A: Diagnostic electron microscopy in gynecologic pathology. *Pathol Annu* 14:353–381, 1979.

Folkman, J: Tumor angiogenesis: therapeutic implications. *N Engl J Med* 285:182–186, 1971.

Furth J: Personal communication, 1976.

Gray LA (ed.): *Dysplasia, Carcinoma in Situ and Micro-Invasive Carcinoma of the Cervix Uteri.* Springfield, Ill.: Charles C Thomas, 1964.

Greenwald P: Endometrial cancer after menopausal use of estrogens. *Obstet Gynecol* 50:239, 1977.

Gusberg SB, Kaplan AL: Precursors of corpus cancers IV. Adenomatous hyperplasia as stage O of the endometrium *Am J Obstet Gynecol* 1963.

Hellstrom I et al.: Demonstration of cell mediated immunity to human neoplasms of various histological types. *Int J Cancer* 7:1, 1971.

Hertig AT, Sommers SC: Genesis of endometrial carcinoma: I. Study of prior biopsies. *Cancer* 2:946–956, 1949.

—— et al.: Genesis of endometrial carcinoma III. Carcinoma in situ. *Cancer* 2:946–971, 1949.

Hertz R: Pharmacology of the endometrium. *Gynecol Oncol* 2:264–271, 1974.

Horwitz RI, Feinstein AR: Alternative analytic methods for case-control studies of estrogens and endometrial cancer. *N Engl J Med* 229:1089, 1978.

Hutchison GB, Rothman KJ: Correcting a bias. *N Engl J Med* 29:1129, 1978.

Ioachim HL: The stromal reaction of tumors: An expression of immune surveillance. *J Natl Cancer Inst* 57:465, 1976.

Jick H et al.: Replacement estrogens and endometrial cancer. *N Engl J Med* 300:218, 1979.

Johannessen JV: Urogenital system and breast, in *Electron Microscopy in Human Medicine,* vol. 9, New York: McGraw-Hill, 1980.

Kessler II: Perspectives on the epidemiology of cervical cancer with special reference to the herpesvirus hypothesis. *Cancer Res* 34:1091, 1974.

Lemon HM et al.: Reduced estriol excretion in patients with breast cancer prior to endocrine therapy. *JAMA* 196:1128, 1966.

Lynch HT (ed.): *Cancer Genetics,* Springfield, Ill.: Charles C Thomas, 1976.

McDonald PC, Siiteri PK: The relationship between extraglandular production of estrone and the occurrence of endometrial neoplasia. *Gynecol Oncol* 2:259–263, 1974.

Meier H., Huebner RJ: Host-gene control of C-type tumor virus—expression and tumorigenesis: Relevance of studies in inbred mice to cancer in man and other species. *Proc Natl Acad Sci USA* 68:2664, 1971.

Mesa-Tejeda R et al.: Detection in human breast carcinoma of an antigen immunologically related to a group-specific antigen of mouse mammary tumor virus. *Proc Natl Acad Sci USA* 75:1529, 1978.

Myers MH, Axtell LM: *Cancer Patient Survival,* U.S. Department of Health, Education, and Welfare Publication, Report no. 5, 77:992, 1976.

Nahmias AJ et al.: Antibodies to herpes virus hominis type 1 and 2 in humans. Women with cervical cancer. *Am J Epidemiol* 91:547–552, 1970.

Neville AM, Laurence DRJ: Carcinoembryonic antigen. *Int J Cancer* 14:1, 1974.

Ng ABP: The cellular detection of endometrial carcinoma and its precursors. *Gynecol Oncol* 2:162, 1974.

Papanicolaou GN: Cytologic diagnosis of uterine cancer by examination of vaginal and uterine secretions. *Am J Clin Pathol* 19:301, 1949.

————: *Atlas of Exfoliative Cytology,* Cambridge, Mass.: Harvard Univ Press, 1954.

Parsons L, Sommers SC: *Gynecology,* Philadelphia: Saunders, 1978, p. 998.

Penn I: Occurrence of cancer in immune deficiencies. *Cancer* 34:858, 1974.

Prehn RT, Prehn LM: Pathobiology of neoplasia. *Am J Pathol* 80:529, 1975.

Rawls WE et al.: Herpes type 2 antibodies and carcinoma of the cervix. *Lancet* 2:1142-1143, 1970.

Royston I, Aurelian L: The association of genital herpes with cervical atypia and carcinoma in situ. *Am J Epidemiol* 91:531–538, 1970.

Shingleton HM et al.: The contribution of endocervical smears to cervical cancer detection. *Acta Cytol* 19:261, 1975.

Siiteri PK et al.: Estrogen receptors and the estrone hypothesis in relation to endometrial and breast cancer. *Gynecol Oncol* 2:228-238, 1974.

Sommers SC: Effects of ionizing radiation upon endocrine glands, in *Pathology of Irradiation,* ed. CC Berdjis, Baltimore: Williams & Wilkins, 1971, p. 408.

————: Carcinoma of endometrium, in *The Uterus,* eds. HJ Norris et al., Baltimore: Williams & Wilkins, 1973a, p. 276.

————: Growth rates, cell kinetics, and mathematical models of human cancers. *Pathobiol Annu* 3:309, 1973b.

————: Postmenopausal estrogens and endometrial cancer, in *Estrogens and Cancer,* ed. SG Silverberg, New York: Wiley, 1978.

Task Force Report: Cervical cancer screening programs. *Can Med Assoc J* 114:1003, 1976.

Terz JJ et al.: Analysis of the cycling and noncycling cell population of human solid tumors. *Cancer* 40:1462, 1977.

Valicenti JF, Jr, Priesterm SK: Psammoma bodies of benign endometrial origin in cervicovaginal cytology. *Acta Cytol* 21:550, 1977.

Vellios F.: Endometrial hyperplasias, precurors of endometrial carcinoma. *Pathol Annu* 7:201–229, 1972.

Witebsky E: Disponibilität und Spezifität alkoholloslicher Strukturen v. Organgen u. bosärtige Geschwülsten. *Z Immunol* 62:35–73, 1929.

Ziel HK, Finkle WD: Increased risk of endometrial carcinoma among users of conjugated estrogens. *N Engl J Med* 293:1167, 1975.

13

Psychosomatic Mechanisms

JAMES L. MATHIS

DEVELOPMENT OF CONCEPTS

PRESCIENTIFIC ERA

The builders of the Egyptian pyramids knew that the mind, an organ which they erroneously believed to be located in the anatomic heart, was the center of thought and feeling, and they correctly observed that the brain (properly located) controlled the muscles and their actions. This early concept of the anatomic and physiologic separation of thinking and feeling (heart) from somatic function (brain) set a pattern of thought which still exists. Today we know that thoughts and feelings come from the cortical and limbic areas of the brain, but the ghost of ancient belief survives when we refer to romance as residing in the heart and speak of strong emotions as "heartfelt."

The ancient Egyptians did not allow their misconceptions to impede treatment when they established a Pir-Ankh (House of Life) at Dendera where both inpatients and outpatients were treated and where the close relationship of emotional and physical aspects of disease was recognized. The Greeks borrowed heavily from their Egyptian predecessors and continued to practice a medicine which recognized the intermarriage of the psyche and the soma. Their attempts at explanations were based upon an imperfect knowledge of anatomy and physiology, demonstrated by the concept of the wandering uterus in the etiology of hysteria. The Romans copied the Grecian practices, but their theoretical concepts of mind-body unity remained part mystical, part spiritual, and usually were explained in mysterious ways.

In 1818, Johann Christian Heinroth was the first to use the term "psychosomatic." His understanding of the term unfortunately was consistent with the prevailing philosophy of his age in that he considered the body to be the somatic abode of the soul. Sin, he believed, caused disease, which affected the soul and, in turn, the body. This connection of sin-soul and disease-body, based on man's unending attempts to explain observable, but mysterious, phenomena, has not been dissipated completely by modern science. Its legacy remains to haunt us when we are faced with symptomatology and/or somatic changes which we cannot explain precisely in cause-and-effect terminology.

SCIENTIFIC ERA

Lipowski has written that the history of psychosomatic medicine can be divided into three phases. Before 1920, psychosomatic medicine was a branch of philosophy. In the second phase, from 1920 to 1955, clinical anecdotes and imaginative speculations led to systematic study in two directions, the psychodynamic and the psychophysiologic. Psychodynamic concepts evolved largely from anecdotal material and uncontrolled studies, but the psychophysiologic aspects were developing from more scientifically rigorous methods of research. The third phase of psychosomatic medicine (since 1955) has been characterized by an emphasis on the study of psychophysiologic responses to environmental stimuli and holistic focus which includes the sociologic, the psychologic, and the biologic.

The concept of "psychosomatic disease" as a diagnostic entity now is considered obsolete by most authorities. The preferred concept is that the onset and the course of all illnesses are influenced by psychosocial factors and that the illness becomes an additional factor of stress in a reverberating system. Psychosomatic medicine then becomes a scientific discipline concerned with the study of the relationships of the biologic, psychologic, and sociologic determinants of health and disease. Lipowski further describes it as a set of postulates and guidelines embodying a holistic approach to the practice of medicine. In the specialty of gynecology and obstetrics, almost every condition and symptom can be highly charged emotionally and/or be of social significance to the patient and her family.

ETIOLOGIC FACTORS

The preface to a further discussion of psychosomatic mechanisms must include this statement: Most students of psychosomatic medicine do not believe that emotions cause physical illness. Such an oversimplified concept of direct causality has not stood the test of controlled studies. This is not to negate the important etiologic role played by the emotions, but rather to place them in the proper perspective as contributory factors in the complicated reverberating system of the human organism. Present thinking is based upon three basic concepts: psychosocial stress, psychophysiologic response specificity, and individual susceptibility. Let us look at each of these concepts in more detail.

PSYCHOSOCIAL STRESS

Psychosocial stress may be defined as a reaction to a situation in which external and/or internal stimuli (including unconscious forces) activate emotions and elicit physiologic changes which threaten health and survival. The concept implies that social stimuli and psychologic states (internal conflicts and frustrations) can upset homeostasis and force the individual to make adaptive adjustments. This set of circumstances may be, but is not necessarily, traumatic; it is only necessary that the end result be an attempt at some form of adaptation. The effect on the individual's health depends upon the capacity to cope, the environmental supports, and upon the highly private meaning of the stressful events to that individual. It is this individualized meaning of the stressful event or situation which determines the activation of emotions. For example, an event which infuriates one person may produce fear or depression in another.

EVOKED EMOTIONS

At least five major categories of subjective meanings have been identified. They are threat, gain or relief, loss, challenge, and insignificance. The emotions evoked may include fear, anger, grief, anxiety, depression, guilt, and shame, alone or in combination. Both the subjective meaning and the evoked emotions will be determined by the sociocultural setting, past experiences and learning, and the basic personality attributes of the individual. For example, a spontaneous abortion may be perceived as a gain or relief by one woman, but as a great loss by another.

The woman experiencing the loss may react by anger, grief, or depression depending upon her personality and her background experiences.

DEFENSIVE BEHAVIORAL PATTERNS

The emotions play the leading role in the mediation of dysfunctional effects on the body and on illness behavior by their tendency to produce preparation for one of three defensive behavior patterns: flight, fight, or inactivity (immobility). The emotions elicited by the psychosocial stress are accompanied by physiologic reactions which may have one or more of the following effects:

1. Once perceived, they may augment, reduce, or change the quality of the emotion.
2. They may precipitate, make manifest, exacerbate, or ameliorate a pathologic bodily process.
3. They may motivate overt behavior, healthy or unhealthy.
4. They may set in motion ego mechanisms of defense and coping strategies aimed at relief of the distress, such as denial, suppression, intellectualization, or isolation.
5. They may be communicated as somatic symptoms that foster adoption of the sick role.

Thus in simplified form we have this possible chain of events: Psychosocial stress may have symbolic meaning to an individual and may lead to one or more of the dysphoric emotions mentioned above. The emotions activate preparation for fight, flight or inactivity. Simultaneously, the emotions have physiologic concomitants involving cardiovascular, respiratory, glandular, and/or musculoskeletal systems which may produce one of the states listed above. The symptoms (physiologic responses) may join the vicious circle as added stress factors.

We will return to the mediation of these states after a look at the concepts of specificity and susceptibility.

PSYCHOLOGIC SPECIFICITY

This concept refers to the tendency of an individual to respond to a given stimulus situation with a reasonably predictable set of psychologic and physiologic reactions. The tendency is based on the following variables:

1. Stimulus response specificity—a stimulus evokes similar responses in many individuals.

2. Individual response specificity—the relatively fixed psychologic and physiologic response characteristics of a given individual. These characteristics depend upon genetics, developmental history, past exposure to traumatic events and illnesses, unconscious conflicts, attitudes, behavioral patterns, available social supports, and all that vast multitude of variables which make up an individual's personality or life-style.
3. Current psychophysiologic state of the individual—the presence of such factors as fatigue, emotional state, level of autonomic arousal, other problems, and/or physical illnesses. The response of a pregnant woman to a given situation might be quite different in her nongravid state.

INDIVIDUAL SUSCEPTIBILITY TO DISEASE

Epidemiologic studies show a positive correlation between life changes and susceptibility to illness or injury. But in a group of individuals subjected to similar stresses and changes, not all will become ill. There is clearly a marked individual variation in resistance to pathology of all types. The hypothesis of individual susceptibility proposes not only a variation from one person to another in resistance to illness, but a variation in a given individual from one time to another.

It may be that certain personality patterns increase susceptibility to certain types of illness, and it may be equally true that a wide range of life events which are interpreted as stressful may increase the probability of an illness in any individual. For example, there is good evidence to support the hypothesis that increased susceptibility to coronary artery disease and an increased mortality from that condition are associated with type A behavior patterns. Individuals who are highly competitive and time-pressured, who react with hostility to frustrations, and who are achievement- and goal-oriented as well as deadline-oriented are called type A. However, even if this concept is accepted, it does not exclude the possibility of a variation in susceptibility that is unrelated to personality characteristics.

MEDIATING MECHANISMS

Acceptance of the basic hypothesis that psychosocial factors have a complex but definite influence on the physiologic balance of the human organism raises another question: By what means? The near-mystical explanations of pioneers such as Groddeck no longer suffice for practitioners trained to rely on statistical analyses and controlled studies. Current psychophysiologic research efforts attempt to answer the question by focusing primarily on neurophysiologic, neuroendocrine, and immune-mediating mechanisms. New answers are producing more questions and further complicating the field, but one fact appears evident: Psychosocial stimuli produce immediate effects on the autonomic nervous system and profound alterations in the hormone balance of the organism, thus secondarily affecting *all* metabolic processes. Figure 13–1 is an oversimplified but workable summary of the mediation from stimulus to end organ.

CLINICAL EXAMPLES

AMENORRHEA

Let us relate the diagram to a common gynecologic condition, amenorrhea without demonstrable organic cause.

A 31-year-old single female with a very responsible teaching position in a major university spent an unplanned night with an old boyfriend. "Unplanned" means that she was not taking contraceptive pills and that no other preventive measures were conveniently available. The effects of wine, roses, and old memories overcame her usual pedantic approach to life, and the next day she became frightened when she realized that she had exposed herself to a situation which could be embarrassing and possibly threatening to her career. The stimulus for this patient had been external, the unprotected sexual intercourse, and she perceived it cortically as an overt threat to her future well-being. The conscious knowledge that the intercourse had occurred near her expected time of ovulation translated in her limbic system into anger and fear, with fear far outweighing the anger she felt at herself for her uncharacteristic, thoughtless behavior. Her first impulse was to fight, that is, to call a physician and get something done at once to prevent pregnancy. However, another emotion generated in her limbic system, shame, promoted inaction; so she did nothing. Centers in her hypothalamus stimulated her autonomic nervous system so that she developed a rapid heartbeat, sweaty palms, shaky hands, expe-

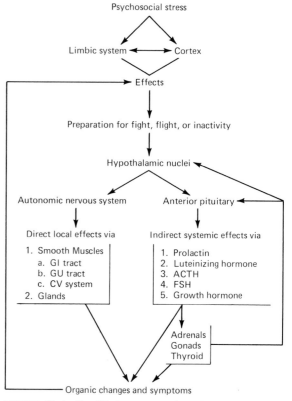

FIGURE 13–1 Simplified summary of psychosomatic mechanisms.

rienced difficulty in going to sleep, and felt as if she were facing impending disaster; she had the physiologic signs and symptoms of overt anxiety or fear. She noted no great change in her appetite, but began to eat voraciously even when not physically hungry.

The hypothalamic message to the pituitary gland probably produced a decrease in luteinizing hormone and/or a reduction in follicular stimulating hormone. (There are conflicting reports in the literature as to which occurs most frequently.) Other glands may have been affected, but this central-nervous-system signal to the ovaries resulted in a cessation of endometrial growth so that the next expected menstrual period did not occur.

The lack of a menstrual period on its expected date (the symptom) now became an added stress, reinforcing the chain of events set in motion by the primary stimulus. The original stimulus had resulted in autonomic-nervous-system hyperactivity with all its concomitants, including overeating and a gain of approximately 4 pounds in 2 weeks. The symptoms of acute anxiety changed with the missed menstrual period, and she became very despondent and lethargic;

her previous overeating turned into a positive aversion toward food.

A negative pregnancy test and a few brief sessions with a knowledgeable and understanding physician interrupted the pathophysiologic chain and allowed the return of homeostasis. This young lady was a relatively stable and mature individual so that no further complications occurred.

PSEUDOCYESIS

Let us look at another situation which is more complex. One theory about pseudocyesis is that it occurs most often in a woman who consciously wishes to be pregnant, but at the same time harbors some strong conflicting negative attitude, frequently unconscious, related to pregnancy, and childbearing. The history of Mrs. Jack may illustrate the probable mechanisms by which the symptoms are produced.

Mrs. Jack was a 32-year-old female who had been married for 13 years without a pregnancy despite a total lack of use of contraceptive measures. Both she and her husband had completed infertility workups, but no abnormalities had been detected in either of them. Although her husband had resigned himself to the idea of no children, Mrs. Jack had not completely despaired. She interpreted Mr. Jack's lack of hope to mean that he had lost interest in her and that he would find himself another woman who could bear him children. This occurred to her consciously and produced overt fright. Mrs. Jack had both an external and an internal stimulus. The external one was the thought that she might lose her husband, and the internal one was an unconscious feeling of being an imperfect woman because of her infertility. She was a barren woman in a family where fecundity was the rule. (Each of her seven siblings had at least three children.) On a conscious level she saw her marriage in jeopardy; on an unconscious level, her self-esteem was threatened.

Mrs. Jack was a devout member of a fundamental religious sect. She attended a religious meeting at which she addressed the congregation and asked for their prayers that she might bear a child. The minister assured her that her prayers, strengthened by those of the congregation, would be answered without fail, if she but had sufficient faith. Now a third threat was added to Mrs. Jack's psychosocial stress. The previous threats of the loss of her husband and the loss of her self-esteem became complicated by the knowledge that a failure to become pregnant would be a certain sign of her lack of faith.

Mrs. Jack's limbic system had more than sufficient reasons for generating fear, but once Mrs. Jack left the religious gathering, her discomfort evaporated and she was at peace with the world. All doubts disappeared from consciousness (denial and suppression), and she immediately began to prepare for motherhood, in spite of warnings from her husband that she might be disappointed again. Her faith apparently was rewarded in approximately 2 weeks when her expected menstrual period did not occur. She was overjoyed.

Mrs. Jack did not see a physician for 5 months, despite urging from family and friends. She gained 25 pounds; her breasts enlarged and became more sensitive; she walked with a noted degree of lordosis; and her abdomen looked as if she were about 4 months pregnant. The belated pelvic examination by her family physician revealed a normal-sized uterus. The pregnancy test was negative. Mrs. Jack stalked out of the office when this was communicated to her and did not see another physician for over 2 months. She then saw four different doctors in 2 weeks, adamantly refusing to accept the idea that she was not pregnant.

It is probable that Mrs. Jack's hypothalamic centers had signaled the pituitary gland to reduce its output of luteinizing hormone and perhaps to increase its output of prolactin. We are certain that at least three pituitary hormones, prolactin, adrenocorticotropic hormone (ACTH), and growth hormone are highly sensitive to stressful situations, and there is much reason to include luteinizing hormone in this group. (Two other target-gland hormones, testosterone and cortisol, also have proved to be highly sensitive to stress.) It seems logical to assume in Mrs. Jack's case that luteinizing hormone and prolactin played major roles in her symptom production, but it is a fact rather than an assumption that a true pseudopregnancy had developed.

There is little reason in this case to theorize that there was any notable amount of direct autonomic-nervous-system stimulation from the hypothalamus. The overt anxiety which we saw in the young professor with the missed menstrual period following unprotected intercourse did not exist in Mrs. Jack. The physiologic changes were sufficient to allow Mrs. Jack's denial system to produce the reality she consciously wanted.

Other clinical examples of specific conditions seen in a gynecology-obstetrics practice would add little to an understanding of the mechanisms involved in psychosomatic conditions. There is even the danger of implying that psychosomatic mechanisms refer only to certain diagnostic entities. That message would be the exact opposite of the one we wish to convey. Perhaps this can be emphasized by a very common, often frustrating clinical situation not specific to females.

PAIN OF MUSCLE TENSION

All physicians are familiar with the complaints of pain in the low back, the posterior part of the neck, and the occipital region of the head. Finding an organic lesion which can be given full credit for the discomfort is the exception rather than the rule. The examining physician commonly finds only spastic muscles, sometimes with definite spots of acute sensitivity (trigger points?). Few physicians need to be told that prolonged muscle spasm produces rather intense pain; most of them know this from a personal experience at one time or another. The pain is real.

It has been known for many years that sustained skeletal muscle tension leads to pain without pathologic involvement of either the blood vessels or the muscles. Experiments have shown that prolonged muscular contractions mechanically obstruct blood flow in small vessels and produce relative ischemia of the muscles. This ischemia appears to be associated with shifts of electrolytes across the cell membranes and to an accumulation within the muscle of metabolic products usually dissipated in the presence of adequate blood flow and oxygen. It is postulated that these metabolic products play a significant role in the production of the pain.

One study showed that the backache syndrome most commonly appeared in settings characterized by threatening life situations evolving from difficulties in personal and social adjustments. Positive measures could not be taken to resolve the difficulties under the assumption that such action would produce insecurity and/or frustrations. There was a fear of retaliation or punishment for the angry feelings. Thus there were contrasting forces at play. There was the normal impulse to move or to act as a result of the intense feelings, but simultaneously there was a restraining need to prevent the action. Spasticity of the muscles resulted from the opposing impulses to move and to resist the movement.

There is no specific personality type involved in muscle tension pain, but it appears more likely to occur in individuals who depend on activity involving the musculature for their basic satisfactions. For instance, the women in one series of low-backache studies all related memories of having been "tom-

boys" usually interested in vigorous competitive play and sports. They were doers rather than watchers.

The lack of a specific personality type does not preclude a relatively specific response to the stressful stimulus. The "spastic muscle people" showed a remarkable consistency of response in that all of them wanted to perform actions involving the musculature, such as running or fighting, but because of the nature of their situation, they were unable to do so. Result: a contracted musculature.

SOMATOPSYCHIC MECHANISM

If we are dealing with a reverberating system, then it follows that the term "psychosomatic" must have its counterpart in "somatopsychic." Just as psychosocial factors play a role in the susceptibility to and the etiology of organic conditions, so do organic conditions produce their own psychosocial components. These components may lead to or be a part of secondary conditions which are not directly related on the surface to the original situation. For example, the strikingly beautiful young wife of a physician did not consult an obstetrician until the seventh month of her pregnancy. Her original beauty was well masked by a gain of almost 60 pounds by this time. The weight gain was not the result of fluid retention; it was due to gluttonous overeating which began the moment she suspected that she was pregnant.

The pregnancy had been "accidental." She had agreed with her husband prior to marriage that there would be no children. She had no specific career aspirations, and had normally wished to have a family, but the husband was almost pathologic in his demand that they remain childless. She had made the bargain with him in the courting days with the lack of rational thinking so commonly seen when youthful hormones overwhelm the cortex. His attitude did not change; in fact, it appeared to grow stronger after 4 years of marriage, just as her desire for a baby appeared to increase. Pregnancy resulted when she "forgot" to take her contraceptive pill.

She did not tell her husband that she was pregnant until it was far too late to have an abortion. Her rapid weight gain successfully camouflaged the pregnancy from an inattentive husband for 7 months. The overeating had not been a conscious move on her part, but her fear of what her husband would do when he discovered that she was pregnant was quite real and conscious. Gorging herself with food was her hypothalamic response to the mixed effects of fear, apprehension, and joy which occurred when she knew that she was pregnant.

CONCLUSION

One practical aspect of this concept of psychosomatic medicine is that it is pertinent to every patient. It is doubly significant to the patients of the gynecologist-obstetrician who so frequently deals in the emotion-laden areas of sexuality and reproduction. The physician who gives primary care to females must be alert constantly to the interplay among the biologic, the psychologic, and the sociologic factors. The theory of somatic versus psychic medicine is no longer tenable. Each factor must be considered from all aspects of cause and effect. The relative significance of these factors will vary from patient to patient and from time to time in a given patient. The science of psychosomatic medicine is to recognize and assay the relative weight of the factors. The art is to understand them and to empathize with the patient who has them. Only then is the physician capable of constructive intervention.

REFERENCES

Dorpat TL, Holmes TH: Backaches of muscle tension origin, in *Psychosomatic Obstetrics, Gynecology and Endocrinology,* ed., WS Kroger, Springfield, Ill.: Charles C Thomas, 1962, p. 425.

Lader M: Psychophysiological research and psychosomatic medicine, in *Physiology, Emotions and Psychosomatic Illness,* Ciba Foundation Symposium 8, Amsterdam: Assoc. Sci. Publ. 1972.

Lipowski ZJ: Psychosomatic medicine in the 70's: An overview. *Am J Psychiatry* 134:233, 1977.

_____ et al. (eds.): *Psychosomatic Medicine: Current Trends and Clinical Applications,* New York: Oxford Univ. Press, 1972.

Mathis JL: Psychiatry and the obstetrician-gynecologist. *Med Clin North Am* 51:1375,1967.

Rahe RH: Epidemiological studies of life change and illness. *Int J Psychiat Med* 6:133,1975.

Sachar EJ: Hormonal changes in stress and mental illness. *Hosp Pract* :49, 1975.

Sheehan D, Hackett T: Psychosomatic disorders, in *The Harvard Guide To Modern Psychiatry,* ed., A Nicholi, Cambridge, Mass.: Belknap Press, 1978, p. 319.

Silverman S: *Psychological Aspects of Physical Symptoms,* New York: Appleton-Century-Crofts, 1968, pp. 3–30.

PART THREE

Approach to the Patient

14

Patient Evaluation

JOHN VAN S. MAECK

Today's woman is demanding a greater role in her own health care. It is no longer acceptable for the gynecologist to examine, diagnose, and treat the patient without reference to her interest in understanding her body and its problems (see Chaps. 9, 30, and 31).

When the patient seeks the gynecologist-obstetrician for a periodic health exam, rather than for an acute problem, the physician has an ideal opportunity to establish a relationship of reciprocal respect which can assure the woman's creative participation in her own health care and her return to the physician at appropriate intervals throughout her life.

How the physician perceives his or her function in the total health care system will to a large extent determine the character of the medical care provided. This chapter attempts to define the particular role and responsibilities of the obstetrician-gynecologist as a provider of regular, periodic, preventive care within an ideal system of comprehensive care meant to insure that *no current or potential* patient problem is overlooked.

If the patient is to be at the center of her own health care, and if all her problems are to be listed and followed systematically, a careful record must be kept which is understandable to the patient and to other physicians. In our society many women receive most or all of their medical care from the gynecologist-obstetrician. He or she may be the only doctor a woman sees at regular intervals for preventive health care, so maintenance of the health records will fall to the gynecologist, who is thus perceived as the primary physician. This does not mean *comprehensive care* is provided—no specialist can do that. But one must be prepared to identify for the patient all significant health problems, which one cannot afford to miss, including those of medical, social, and psychological origin. The physician will manage those within his or her capabilities and will refer other problems to other members of the health care system. The patient will be treated as a complete human being whose gynecologic and/or obstetric problems may be related to conditions or illnesses outside the reproductive system, and whose environment and psyche have direct bearing on her health.

The gynecologist-obstetrician must see patients as needing continuing, not episodic care, and therefore manage current problems such as pregnancy and identify potential problems which may be eliminated before becoming clinically significant (for example, identification and treatment of cervical dysplasia before it becomes invasive cancer). To offer this kind of service, the physician must not only develop a comprehensive screening procedure which is applicable and appropriate to the patient at the time of periodic examination, but must educate patients in the value of periodic examination.

THE OFFICE PRACTICE

In planning for the ambulatory care of the patient, the gynecologist-obstetrician must, of course, hire and train a capable staff, acquire equipment, and develop a business system; but above all must develop a system of medical record keeping far more precise than random note taking. Records are the vital part of the physician's practice, and significantly affect the quality of service. Properly used, the medical record can assure the complete gathering of relevant data, formulation of a list of all problems, plans for treatment, and thorough follow-up which will better define problems and sometimes alter treatments. The record thus provides clear, concise communication with other members of the health team: organized to show all relevant facts and the logic in dealing with them, the doctor's medical record stands at the core of the practice.

THE PROBLEM-ORIENTED RECORD

The problem-oriented medical record (Weed), in philosophy and format, is ideal for this kind of record keeping. It systematizes the approach to patient care and is designed to assure that none of the factors involved in patient care is overlooked. It is structured so that all data are organized around the patient's problems, rather than around the source of the information, so that the problem list forms an excellent key, or index, to the rest of the record.

The problem-oriented medical record is logically based upon the four phases of medical practice (Weed): (1) the data base, which includes the chief complaint, patient profile (how she spends her day and related social data), the present illness(es), past history and systems review based on a series of explicit and related questions, the defined physical examination, and base-line laboratory tests; (2) the development of a numbered problem list derived from the data base; (3) the formulation of initial plans, all numbered to match the problems to which they apply; and (4) a follow-up of each problem with appropriate progress notes (also numbered and titled to match problems) at each subsequent visit.

COMPREHENSIVE PATIENT CARE

Assuming that the gynecologist-obstetrician is concerned with continuing comprehensive care of patients, even though this is not the primary function of the doctor, it is necessary to assure that *all* appropriate information about each patient is obtained and appropriately recorded. The collection of such data may best be accomplished by means of a questionnaire, either self-administered or completed with the help of the office nurse or other members of the office staff (Bjorn).

Whether the patient comes to the physician for acute illness, contraceptive advice, premarital counseling, or periodic health examination, certain information will always be collected and should be standard. The precise character of the questionnaire will vary with the physician's breadth of interest in comprehensive care of patients, the methods of practice, or with the particular health characteristics peculiar to a certain patient population of a particular geographic area. The broader and more comprehensive the questionnaire when combined with the appropriate laboratory tests and physical examination, the greater the assurance (when properly used) that all significant problems will be identified. Its construction should reflect all that has happened to the patient's health, past and present, and should include questions which may identify potential problems.

STANDARD DATA BASE EXAMPLE

The content for a possible standard data base for the gynecologist-obstetrician is listed in outline form below, and includes certain minimum initial laboratory tests and procedures, all of which are designed to identify problems of the past and present as well as potential problems of the future.

Identification. Name (last, first, maiden), address, age, phone number, religion, occupation, referring physician, primary physician.

Social history. Married, separated, single, widowed, living with a partner.

Operations. Date, place, doctor, type of operation, result.

Hospitalization. Date, illness, result, follow-up.

Pregnancies. Dates, number of pregnancies, period of gestation, number of abortions, number of children living, their weight at birth, sex, maternal/fetal complications.

Drug Reactions, Allergies, Immunizations. Polio, rubella, tetanus, smallpox, etc.

Patient profile.

Living Situation. Alone, with parents, spouse, friend, other. Change in marital status; children: problems—drugs, school, behavior, sexual; recurrent illness; present medications.

Present Means of Support. Self, spouse, part-time work, pension, savings, welfare, other.

Level of Education, Level of Satisfaction. Occupation, family, health care system.

Collection of the following information concerning the patient's past medical history in relationship to current, past, and potential illness would seem to have particular value.

Gynecologic (Genital System).

Current. Menstrual abnormalities, dysmenorrhea, discharge-itching, sexual activity and orientation, dyspareunia, pelvic pain, protrusion. Breasts: discharge, lumps, pain.

Past. Menses: onset, interval, duration, LMP (last menses), LRMP (last regular menses), contraception, venereal disease, abnormal cytology. Breasts: lactation.

Potential. Family history of cancer. Early and varied sexual activity.

Urinary.

Current. Dysuria, urgency, incontinence, hematuria.

Past. Renal disease, recurrent urinary-tract infection, hematuria.

Potential. Family history of polycystic disease.

Endocrine.

Current. Changes in weight, abnormal hair growth, change in sexual function.

Past. Thyroid disorder, diabetes mellitus, menstrual disorders.

Potential. Exposure to radioactive material. Family history of diabetes mellitus, hirsutism.

Gastrointestinal.

Current. Abdominal pain, melena, nausea, vomiting, diarrhea, changes in bowel habits.

Past. Ulcer, gallbladder disease, jaundice, other liver diseases, diverticulosis, colitis.

Potential. Family history of cancer, rectal polyps.

Hematopoietic.

Current. Ecchymosis, abnormal bleeding, enlarged lymph nodes, vitamin B^{12}, "liver injection."

Past. Bleeding problems.

Potential. Family history of pernicious anemia, sickle-cell disease, hemophilia.

Cardiovascular.

Current. Chest pain, dyspnea, edema (feet and ankles), varicose veins, leg ulcer.

Past. Rheumatic fever, other heart disease, hypertension, phlebitis, embolic disease.

Potential. Family history of hypertension, heart attack. Limited physical activity, cigarette smoking, mental tension, high blood cholesterol.

Mouth-Throat-Larynx.

Current. Hoarseness, sore mouth or tongue, lump in neck.

Past. Recurrent pharyngitis.

Potential. Heavy smoker.

Respiratory.

Current. Chronic cough, hemoptysis, dyspnea.

Past. Tuberculosis, heavy smoker, asthma.

Potential. Smoking. Family history of cystic fibrosis.

Neurology.

Current. Headache, dizzy spells, drugs for seizures.

Past. Seizures, paralysis, nervousness.

Potential. Family history of Huntington's chorea.

Psychiatric.

Current. Anxiety, depression, difficulty sleeping, weeping, suicidal thoughts, overuse of alcohol, other drugs.

Past. Nervous breakdown, attempted suicide, psychiatric treatment.

Potential. Drug abuse. Family history of alcohol problem, suicide, mental problems before age 60.

Musculoskeletal.

Current. Joint pain or swelling, stiff neck, backache.

Past. Gout, other diseases or injuries.

Potential. Arthritis.

Family History. Number of siblings, blood relatives deceased under age 60 and/or with hereditary disease.

Initial Physical Examination. General appearance, height, weight, blood pressure, thyroid, lymph nodes, heart, lungs, breasts, abdomen, vulva, urethra, perineum, vagina (lesions, support, discharge), cervix (position, erosion, ulcer, laceration), uterus (size, shape, position, mobility), adnexa (position mass, tenderness), parametria, cul-de-sac, anorectal, extremities.

Initial Laboratory Tests. Cervicovaginal cytology, urinalysis (protein, glucose), hematocrit, or hemoglobin, and serological test for syphilis.

PREGNANCY, STANDARD DEFINED DATA BASE

The data base for the obstetric patient requires information in addition to that which has been listed above, and includes the following: The expected date of confinement, onset of fetal motion, history of nausea, vomiting, indigestion, constipation, headache, bleeding (specify), vaginal discharge, edema, abdominal pain, urinary symptoms, history of "German measles", herpes, or other virus infections, history of radiation (specify), history of accidents, particularly accidents or trauma to the abdomen or pelvis.

Lab tests: Rubella titer, blood and Rh type, cultures for *Neisseria*.

THE PATIENT INTERVIEW

Use of the questionnaire, answered by the patient prior to a visit, saves time for both doctor and patient, and allows their initial interview to begin at a deeper level than mere history taking. The doctor who carefully reviews the questionnaire before the patient arrives will be able to identify problems and potential problems about which more probing questions can be asked.

For whatever reason the patient has sought care, the physician should presume her to have "pain," physical or psychological, She may have anxiety concerning her state of health induced by the propaganda from one of the health institutions which promote periodic health checkups; she may be worried about "how can I sleep with my lover and not become pregnant?" or the "pain" may have been produced inadvertently by another physician who has identified an abnormal Pap smear and referred the patient to the gynecologist for evaluation and management.

The interview may be initiated with a question such as "Do you have a problem?" or "What is your problem?" thus promptly identifying the reason for the consultation.

Through skilled guidance and attentive listening the physician will determine the present illness by identification of the onset and duration of the chief complaint, associated symptoms, made worse or relieved by what, and whether or not the illness was modified, if at all, with treatment.

By creating a warm, but professional atmosphere, and by avoiding a condescending manner, the doctor should be able to inspire the patient with a sense of confidence which will allow her to begin to confide "secrets" which may have significant bearing on her illness. A series of logically arranged, explicit and related questions can follow which will give a complete systems review. Throughout the questioning she should be encouraged and allowed to express anxieties regarding her role as a woman, her sexuality, her family and children, and her perception of herself in society. How she spends her day and her perception of its value should be learned. For example, does she feel she is limited to mundane chores and depressed about it; how does she feel about the younger (older) generation?

THE PHYSICAL EXAMINATION

The Role of the Nurse

Upon completion of the interview the nurse guides the patient to the area where she may undress and put on an examining gown. She is asked to empty her bladder to facilitate pelvic examination, and the obtained specimen is examined for protein and sugar and bacteria. The nurse should obtain the patient's height, weight and blood pressure, and a specimen of blood for hematocrit and other tests included in the standard data base.

The nurse then conducts the patient to the examining room and may describe to the patient the procedures involved in the examination. Depending upon her role and training, she may discuss with the patient the value and technique of self-breast examination. Oftimes the nurse finds these few moments alone with the patient an opportunity to identify certain anxieties or problems not previously communicated to the physician or entered on the questionnaire. The patient should not be left alone any longer than necessary awaiting the arrival of the physician and the examination.

The Breast Examination

With the patient in the sitting position, the doctor can assess the character of the skin, and the hair and its distribution. The head and neck including the thyroid and lymph nodes are examined. The heart and lungs are examined and careful inspection of the breasts is made. The latter are observed for asymmetry, dimpling, or retraction of the breast surface, nipple, or areola. This portion of the examination is facilitated by having the patient lean forward, placing both hands on her hips to cause retraction of the pectoralis major muscles. She should then sit erect with the heels of her hand together, pressing firmly toward the midline. The presence and assistance of a nurse throughout the examination is helpful, particularly for the reticent, embarrassed patient. Explanation by the physician of what is being done and demonstration to the patient of how she may examine her own breasts may convert embarrassment to self-education.

Palpation of the breast, a most important part of the examination, must be performed with the patient supine, so positioned that the breasts form an even layer on the chest wall. The patient's arms are initially at her sides and later elevated to a position perpendicular to her thorax and then eventually above her head. Each breast is then carefully palpated—all quadrants of the breasts, areola, and nipple, gently and precisely. If the hands are cold, they should be warmed. Palpation is best performed with the fingers extended, using the sensitive palmar surface of the terminal digit for the evaluation of breast tissue and the identification of size, shape, consistency, demarcation, and mobility of abnormal masses.

After many examinations the physician will come to distinguish normal thickening of supporting breast tissue in the inferior aspects of the pendulous breasts as distinguished from pathology. The most experienced clinician, on the other hand, will not infrequently have difficulty differentiating localized physiologic enlargement from true neoplasm. A breast mass which is not clearly within physiologic bounds should be further evaluated by mammography, thermography, aspiration, or surgical biopsy. Upon completion of the palpation of both breasts, the axillae and the supraclavicular areas should be explored thoroughly, reaching the apex of the axilla beside the chest wall and behind the pectoralis major muscle. Elevation and lowering of the arm will assist in this exploration. At the finish of the breast examination the patient should be told of the findings. Any concern on the part of the physician will be detected by the patient. If significant abnormality is not found, she should be reassured. If an abnormality is detected, the patient should be advised of its character and the recommendation for management.

Examination of the Abdomen

The abdomen is then palpated in all four quadrants in search of mass or tenderness. Notation is made of previous surgical scars and the presence or absence of hernia. The abdominal palpation is conducted with the flat of the hands and fingers and every effort made to avoid "poking."

The Pelvic Examination

The trepidation with which some women approach the pelvic examination can be allayed by the physician and the supporting nurse. If the physician can communicate that the pelvic examination is an examination which happens to take place in the genital area, the gynecologist will have done much to alleviate anxiety. It is helpful for the doctor to explain what is going to be done, but it is usually advisable not to demonstrate the instruments used in the examination unless requested by the patient. Terms of endearment and other forms of condescension should be avoided. If a step in the examination will be painful, the patient should be told so; false assurances should never be given.

With the help of the nurse, the patient's feet are placed in stirrups in preparation for the pelvic examination. This part of the examination should be conducted in a sensitive but matter-of-fact way, without embarrassment to patient or physician. The nurse should behave as matter of factly as for the preceding portion of the examination and avoid creating an atmosphere suggesting that the patient's survival will depend upon the nurse's hand-holding assistance. It is especially important that the woman undergoing her first pelvic examination not be hurt or frightened.

Inspection of External Genitalia. Having inspected both groins during the examination, the external genitals are inspected with good light. It is preferable that the gynecologist place an arm or elbow on the patient's leg or thigh prior to touching the pudenda to avoid startling the patient, who will respond with involuntary muscular contraction. The labia are separated, the introitus inspected along with the urethra and clitoris. Notation is made of the perineal body, whether or not scarred, and the presence or absence of hymenal remnants.

Insertion of Speculum. A warmed, nonlubricated bivalve vaginal speculum is then inserted into the vaginal introitus as the fingers of the opposite hand gently spread the labia. The speculum size will vary depending upon whether the woman is virginal, parous, or the vagina atrophic. The posterior blade of the speculum is inserted into the introitus with pressure against the perineal body and canted at approximately a 45° angle (see Fig. 14–1). Ordinarily the natural lubrication at the introitus will assist this insertion. Any discomfort on the part of the patient should be quickly noted and corrected by the examiner.

Inspection of the Cervix. The speculum may now be inserted to its hilt as it is gradually rotated so that its handle points directly posterior. Opening the speculum should then expose the cervix with minimum difficulty or discomfort. Occasionally slight suprapubic pressure will assist in pushing the fundus and its cervix lower into the pelvis to aid in exposing the cervix. With slight rotation of the speculum and manipulation, the cervix can be seen throughout its circumference, as can the vaginal fornices.

Taking the Pap Smear. At this point a specimen for vaginal cytology is obtained. The patient should have been instructed to refrain from douching or using vaginal creams or medications at least 48 hours prior to examination, for otherwise the cytologic examination will be compromised. The endocervix is swabbed with a cotton-tipped applicator which is then smeared on a slide and immediately fixed. Commercial aerosol hair sprays are effective and inexpensive fixatives. The portio vaginalis is then firmly scraped circumferentially with the tip of a tongue blade or Ayre's spatula. These scrapings are smeared and fixed. Finally a swab of the posterior fornix or "vaginal pool" is taken and similarly smeared and fixed. Three separate glass slides may be used or all three specimens may be smeared on one or two slides, but fixation must be rapidly accomplished to prevent drying. The smears are then accurately labeled. A specimen obtained by scraping the lateral vaginal walls gives a somewhat more accurate cytologic interpretation of the endocrine status.

The cervix is further examined for lacerations, cysts, erosions, polyps, or other abnormalities. The speculum is then gradually withdrawn, allowing the inspection of the fornices about the cervix and the lateral wall in search of laceration, cysts, or ulcerations of the vagina.

Digital examination is performed by inserting the middle finger into the vaginal introitus, followed by the index finger unless the vagina is virginal or otherwise too small. The cervix is reached, its consistency, configuration, and position noted. The cervix may be moved from side to side to identify the pres-

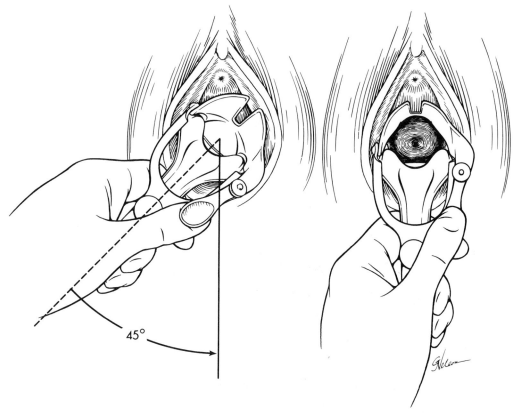

FIGURE 14-1 Insertion of the speculum; inspection of the cervix. To avoid discomfort the speculum is inserted at an angle which will decrease its transverse diameter at the introitus, beyond which it can easily be rotated to the midline. The cervix is exposed by opening the blades with thumb pressure. The cervix is inspected and specimens obtained for cytologic examination (see text).

ence of tenderness. The fornices are explored for mass, tenderness, or distortion.

Pelvic Support. Attention is paid at this point to the character of the pelvic support, especially in parous women or those with complaints of pelvic pressure. Pressure on the perineal body may give a view of the anterior wall. Relaxation can be made more apparent by having the patient bear down, increasing the intrapelvic pressure. The pubococcygeus muscles are palpated to evaluate their function in pelvic support. Notation is made of vaginal lacerations, scars, or other distortion.

Palpation of Uterus and Ovaries. With the opposite hand placed gently on the abdomen, the gently palpating extended fingers are swept toward the symphysis, while at the same time the vaginal hand elevates cervix and uterus. It is through this maneuver that the anterior fornix, and in the not-too-obese pa-

tient, the uterine fundus, can be palpated between the two hands (see Fig. 14-2). Its absence suggests a retroverted uterus which may be verified through palpation of the posterior fornix and by rectovaginal examination (see Fig. 14-3). Having "grasped" the fundus between his vaginal fingers and abdominal hand, the examiner outlines the configuration of the corpus and estimates the size, mobility, and the presence or absence of tenderness. Each lateral pelvis is then examined in an attempt to identify adnexa. With the vaginal fingers exploring the right fornix, the abdominal hand sweeps the contents of the right pelvis toward the vaginal hand (see Fig. 14-4). The ovary when identifiable can be palpated between the two hands and its compression usually gives a twinge of discomfort. If one side is known to be tender, it should be examined last. The normal fallopian tube can rarely be palpated.

Similar exam of the left pelvis may be facilitated by reversing hands.

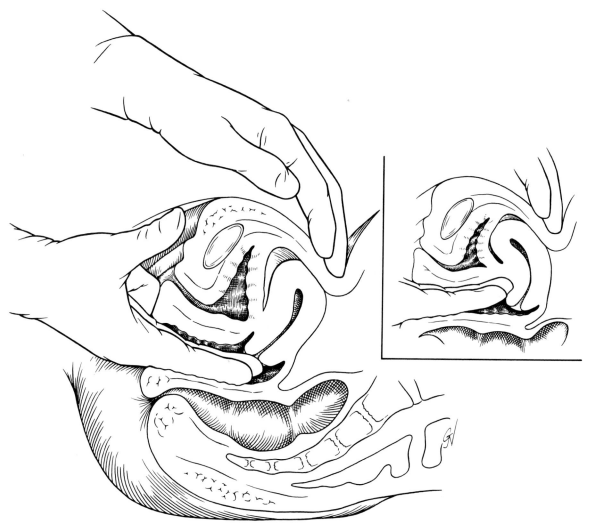

FIGURE 14–2 Bimanual examination. Palpation of cervix to determine size, shape, consistency, and its relation to axis of vagina. Inset. Palpation of uterus for size, shape, consistency, mobility, tenderness. Its anterior position is best determined when the corpus can be ''grasped'' between the fingers of the two hands.

The Rectal Examination. Upon completion of the bimanual examination, the middle finger, after adequate lubrication, may be inserted gently and slowly into the anal canal. Note is made of mass in the anal canal or lower rectum; reaching farther into the rectal canal, the posterior cul-de-sac can be palpated as can the cervix. The corpus of the retroverted uterus can often be identified by this maneuver as can mass, induration, or tenderness. The combined rectovaginal examination facilitates the evaluation of parametria, as well as outlining adnexal masses. The uterosacral ligaments are palpated near their insertion and inspected for nodularity and tenderness.

As the fingers are withdrawn, the rectal finger is inspected for the presence of blood and mucus and the presence or absence of hemorrhoids is noted.

The physician removes excess lubrication from the anogenital area and the patient may sit up. The lower extremities can be then inspected for the presence of varicose veins, ulceration, or other abnormalities.

Throughout the examination, the physician pays particular attention to the patient's response to the examination. Abnormal pelvic tenderness is oftimes identified by change of expression on the patient's face during the bimanual examination. It is frequently

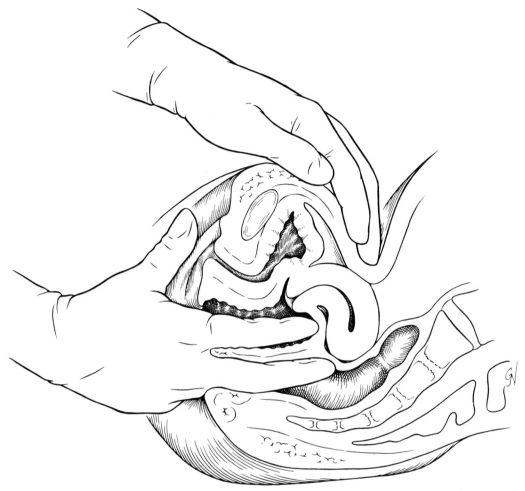

FIGURE 14–3 Bimanual rectovaginal examination. The retroverted or retroflexed corpus uteri can best be identified as shown. The finger in the rectum can identify the corpus in the cul-de-sac of Douglas when the abdominal fingers fail to locate a "mass," the corpus, anteriorly.

difficult for a patient to relax her abdominal or perineal muscles during the pelvic examination. The patient should be encouraged not to hold her breath and at times a deep expiration will be helpful. The greatest assistance in obtaining such relaxation is in gaining the patient's confidence that she will not be inadvertently or carelessly hurt.

THE ASSESSMENT

Development of Problem List

Upon finishing the examination, the doctor will have completed the data base collection, except for initial laboratory tests. In certain acute or emergency situations, portions of the data base may be incomplete, to be filled in at a later visit. The physician will review the positive findings of the questionnaire, the notes which have been made during the interview, and the positive findings of the examination and from this, develop a problem list. This will include any *abnormal symptom, physical finding,* or *laboratory test;* it will include any *psychosocial problem;* but it will only include a diagnosis when the physician has enough data to be certain of one. Each problem is listed only at the level proved by the facts, and is not upgraded to a diagnosis until ample evidence is gathered for its substantiation. Obviously, an incorrect diagnosis in the problem list can lead to mismanagement. When such a list of problems is numbered and dated with

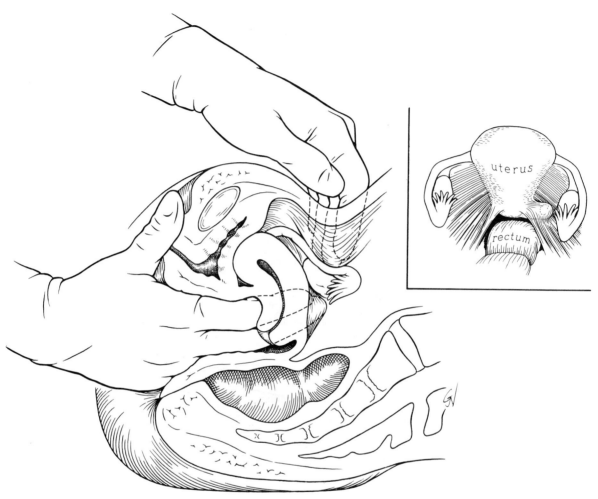

FIGURE 14-4 Bimanual examination. Examination of adnexa, parametria and lateral pelvic wall. The vaginal fingers explore "through" the right vaginal fornix as the abdominal fingers "sweep" the adnexa toward the vagina. The parametria (cardinal ligaments) and uterosacral ligaments are examined for mobility, tenderness, nodularity; the pelvic wall for configuration, mass, or tenderness.

an indication as to whether each is active or resolved, it will accurately reflect the doctor's knowledge of the patient's health at that moment because it includes all the significant previous illnesses, operations, or abnormal symptoms and findings. At subsequent visits there may be additions to the active problem list and previous problems may have been resolved. Those not resolved remain as active problems to be dealt with either by the gynecologist-obstetrician or the appropriate consultant by referral. An accurate problem list which reflects the patient's health status at any particular time becomes the essential ingredient of patient care and patient education.

PREVENTIVE MEDICAL CARE

The obstetrician, in fulfilling the role of primary physician to women, has assumed an increasing role in preventive medical care. The impetus for this responsibility relates in part to the significance of early cancer detection by means of a simple, effective breast and pelvic examination and the cytologic smear. National publicity and educational programs over years have created an unusual awareness on the part of many women who, quite naturally, seek the help of their gynecologist-obstetrician. Examinations have been extended now to include certain aspects of preventive medicine in general, and some of these have proved of real merit in either the prevention or early detection and treatment of disease.

In deciding whether or how often to screen for a particular problem at the periodic examination, the physician must weigh, for any given population of patients, the statistical incidence of the disease, its susceptibility to treatment once identified, the accuracy with which it can be diagnosed, the human risk involved, and the resources spent in its identification.

Failure of a particular screening procedure to identify a disease when it is present can lead to unjustified reassurance, delaying both diagnosis and treatment. Erroneous identification of disease may result in unnecessary treatment which is costly, unpleasant, or even harmful. For example, death from hemorrhage or anesthesia could occur as the result of a cone biopsy performed for a Pap test incorrectly labeled as abnormal. Many screening tests have very low yields and are expensive in terms of manpower and dollars.

The patient should be made aware of limitations of the examination, and surely should know its results and implications—whatever they may be. The tendency of the patient who has been told of a "normal" examination to ignore future signs or symptoms may be a real hazard of the periodic health examination.

THE PLACE OF GYNECOLOGIC CANCER DETECTION IN THE PERIODIC HEALTH EXAMINATION
(See also Chap. 12)

The accuracy of the cytologic examination and the detection of both the invasive and preinvasive lesions of cervical cancer have been the most important reason for periodic health examination. The techniques and management of the cytologic examination are discussed in detail in Chap. 41. Its effectiveness in identifying early cancer of the endometrium, the ovary, and the fallopian tube diminishes in approximately that order. It must not be assumed, therefore, that a negative Pap smear means no cancer is present. Accuracy probably does not exceed 95 percent, even in the presence of invasive cervical lesions—which further emphasizes the importance of careful history taking and careful physical examina-

tion. A patient should be made aware that self-examination kits or Pap tests done by other than trained professionals can overlook serious disease.

Endometrial cancer (Chap. 42) usually presents itself through symptoms of abnormal bleeding. Patient education in recognizing the symptoms can do much toward early detection. Physician delay continues to be a most important factor in diagnosis and, accordingly, in treatment delay. Careful identification of historical factors which relate to family history, menstrual aberrations, infertility, and certain physical characteristics, including obesity, assist in identifying the patients of higher risk.

Ovarian and tubal carcinoma are much more silent in their genesis and too often are discovered only after their masses preclude optimum cure and survival (see Chap. 44). Careful pelvic examination and attention to early symptoms often will afford clues leading to earlier diagnosis. Unfortunately, the accurate diagnosis of ovarian or tubal carcinoma depends almost exclusively upon laparotomy and histologic examination. Nonetheless, the gynecologist ought not and must not defer this procedure in the presence of persistent findings.

CARCINOMA OF THE BREAST
(See also Chap. 46)

Because the breast examination is so much a part of obstetric and gynecologic examination, and because of awareness that endocrine changes associated with reproduction may subtly manifest themselves in breast tissue, the specialist has frequent and unique opportunities to find and differentiate early malignant disease. It seems unfortunate that more gynecologists and obstetricians have not been trained and do not assume the responsibility for management of breast diseases.

Involvement of the patient herself in the identification of breast cancer is important since approximately 90 percent of malignant breast lesions are discovered by the patient. Unfortunately, these self-identified lesions are too often far advanced.

The need for better patient education and participation in early detection is obvious and is perhaps of equal, if not greater, importance than current procedures such as radiologic mammography and xerography. Careful, conscientious, regular examination by the patient and the physician is still the most valuable means of detection of breast cancer.

THE PLACE OF OTHER PROCEDURES IN THE PERIODIC HEALTH EXAMINATION

Preconceptional Care. Plans and programs for the identification of potential problems can include a preconceptional survey examination for certain diseases which may preclude safe pregnancy for either mother or fetus. The identification of maternal diabetes, prior to conception, for example, would seem to give an advantage to both patients.

Education and medical assistance in the spacing and planning of pregnancy is demonstrably advantageous not only to the woman, but to her offspring. The prevention of pregnancy or its abortion can be a significant preventive health measure where there are diseases of the cardiovascular, pulmonary, or renal systems which in themselves threaten her well-being.

Blood pressure. Periodic recording of blood pressure and the confirmation of abnormal elevation in women of whatever age is a simple, inexpensive health care measure. There is increasing evidence that the progression of hypertensive cardiovascular disease can be ameliorated or controlled with appropriate health and pharmacologic measures.

Anemias. Detected and characterized with minimal effort and expense, most, if not all, anemias can be appropriately treated and controlled.

Glaucoma. Glaucoma can be detected and arrested prior to irreversible progression to blindness. Tonometry testing for this disease can be performed by appropriately trained technicians at the time of the periodic health exam, but the examination itself is not without some hazard.

Several other screening mechanisms have been proposed in the interest of preventive health care (Wolf). Their value in cost-effectiveness is subject to careful scrutiny. For example, it may be important to have an ECG by age 25, for comparison at a later date. Spirometry (FEV_1) at 5-year intervals after age 25 in heavy smokers can be of real prognostic value. PA and lateral x-ray examination of the chest should be obtained by age 25. Value thereafter in patients without symptoms and no significant history is open to question. PPD testing annually when negative is of greater value in the detection of pulmonary tuberculosis infection than routine chest x-rays. The overall survival from pulmonary carcinoma is not greatly influenced by routine chest x-rays (Boucat). Of much greater value would be the effect of changing the behavior of the chronic smoker.

Triglyceride and cholesterol blood levels obtained at 5-year intervals after age 25, especially for patients who have a family history of cardiovascular disease, would seem to have real diagnostic merit.

Multiphasic laboratory screening tests have great appeal to those concerned with preventive health care. However, the long-term benefits in terms of morbidity and mortality are not readily demonstrable. Furthermore, the unexpected abnormal screening result in itself presents a significant problem and if followed up by the physician, infrequently leads to a positive diagnosis (Schneiderman).

In consideration of any or all screening procedures, the value of each becomes much more apparent in those patients who have positive past or family history of related disease—thus the emphasis on careful history collection and evaluation. Probably the most valuable contribution to the screening periodic health examination is that of the experienced physician who, however briefly, is willing to "look and listen."

PATIENT EDUCATION: THE GYNECOLOGIST-OBSTETRICIAN AND THE PATIENT

Probably the most effective preventive health care measure for women is education in how to take care of themselves. It seems true that physicians have been so busy caring for the crises that relatively little time has been given to the task of patient education. Also unfortunate has been the classic contract between the doctor and the patient in which the patient puts herself in the doctor's hands to be taken care of. The relationship has often been described as that of child to parent. The patient trusted and obeyed the doctor without question; the physician soothed and reassured without explaining. As a result the patient could make no contribution to her own *preventive* health care, and in the case of an acute problem, often did not understand what was required of her, and may thus have hindered treatment.

In the past few years both patients and doctors have begun to realize the value of time spent educating the woman about her own body. A patient with a basic understanding of how her reproductive system works will be better able to understand problems that arise, to follow the physician's explanations and instructions, and to take part in any decision making that may be necessary. The woman who has received careful instruction in self-examination of the breast is better able to actively participate in her health care.

Not all instruction will come from the doctor, of course. The physician who is committed to providing the best possible preventive health care will find the Problem-Oriented Medical Record System a valuable tool for the patient's education and her problem management. Her own copy of her problem list should give her considerable insight into her own state of health.

REFERENCES

Barber HRK, Graber EA: The PMPO syndrome. *Obstet Gynecol* 38:921, 1971.

Bjorn JC, Corss HD: *The Problem Oriented Private Practice of Medicine,* Chicago: Modern Hospital Press, 1970.

Boucat KR, Weiss W: Is curable lung cancer detected by semiannual screening? *JAMA* 10:224, 1973.

Cutler SJ et al.: Increasing incidence and decreasing mortality rates for breast cancer. *Cancer* 28:1376, 1971.

Gershon-Cohen J: Imperative changes in detection methods for breast cancer. *South Med J* 64:387, 1971.

Gilbertsen VA, Kjilsberg J: Detection of breast cancer by periodic utilization of methods of physical diagnosis. *Cancer* 28:1552, 1971.

Graham RM:Diagnosis of ovarian carcinoma by cul-de-sac aspiration, in *Ovarian Cancer,* eds. F Gentil, AC Junqueira, New York: Springer-Verlag, 1968, p. 122.

Haagensen CO: *Carcinoma of the breast: A monograph for physicians.* Am Cancer Soc 1958, p. 7.

Martin PL: How preventable is invasive cervical cancer? *Am J Obstet Gynecol* 113:541, 1972.

Schneider J, Twiggs LB: The costs of carcinoma of the cervix. *Obstet Gynecol* 40:851, 1972.

Schneiderman LJ et al: The abnormal screening laboratory results. *Arch Intern Med* 129:88, 1972.

Weed LL: *Medical Records, Medical Education and Patient Care,* Cleveland: Case Western Reserve, 1969.

Wolf, GA Jr: A look at multiphasic screening. *Hosp Med Staff* 13, 1972.

_____: Why do multiphasic screening? *Hospitals* 46:65, 1972.

15

The Fetus and Newborn

E. J. QUILLIGAN M. A. SIMMONS

NORMAL GROWTH AND DEVELOPMENT

FERTILIZATION AND IMPLANTATION

Ovulation occurs roughly at midcycle during a normal 28-day cycle. Just prior to ovulation the ovum has undergone the first maturation division (meiotic), which is a reduction division (22+ X chromosomes) (Fig. 15–1). At ovulation, the ovum, surrounded by the zona pellucida and cumulus oophorus, is shed, technically into the abdominal cavity, but in actual fact it is picked up almost immediately by the fimbriated end of the fallopian tube. The ovum and its surrounding layers are then transported by tubal ciliary and tubal muscular action to the ampullary portion of the fallopian tube, where they are met by spermatozoa that have undergone both maturation divisions and capacitation. The sperm penetrates the zona pellucida by releasing enzymes (hyaluronidase) from its acrosome (Fig. 15–2). The sperm then attaches to the membrane of the ovum and penetrates into the cytoplasm of the ovum. With this, the ovum undergoes a second maturation division (meiotic), and the ovum nucleus is now called the female pronucleus. The penetrated sperm head forms the male pronucleus (Fig. 15–3). With penetration of the first sperm, the ovum reacts to inhibit further sperm penetration. The male and the female pronuclei meet in the center of the ovum, lose their membranes, and the chromosomes intermingle. The fertilized ovum now has 44+ XX or XY chromosomes. Several mitotic divisions take place so that about 3 days after ovulation a solid ball of about 16 cells is present (morula).

During cell division the zygote has been propelled through the fallopian tube to the uterus by tubal muscular and ciliary action. The fourth day following fertilization fluid from the uterus enters the morula, creating a cystic space. The zygote is now called a blastocyst. The blastocyst has an outer cell mass of trophoblastic tissue and an inner cell mass destined to become the embryo.

During the latter half of the menstrual cycle the endometrium has undergone the changes described in Chap. 42 and is ready for the blastocyst to implant.

On the fifth day the zona pellucida disappears, and on the sixth day the blastocyst attaches to the endometrium (Fig. 15–4). The blastocyst usually attaches with the inner cell mass next to the endometrium. The reason for the location of the adhesion be-

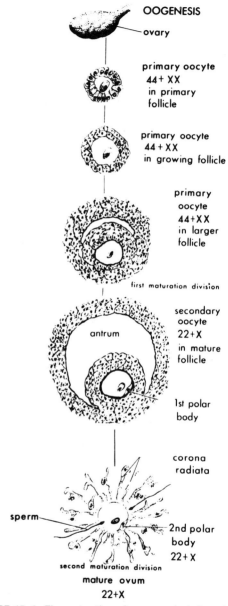

FIGURE 15–1 The maturation of an ovum including chromosomal complement at each stage. *(From The Developing Human: Clinically Oriented Embryology, KL Moore, Philadelphia: Saunders, 1973.)*

tween blastocyst and uterus is poorly understood. The adhesion itself seems to be due to a sticky substance on the blastocyst wall remaining after the zona pellucida disappears.

Following adhesion, the trophoblastic tissue of the blastocyst penetrates the superficial uterine epithelium. The mechanism for the trophoblastic inva-

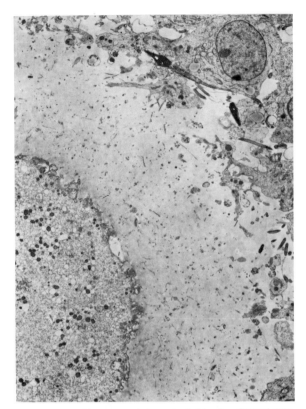

FIGURE 15–2 Human oocyte inseminated in vitro. Several spermatozoa are identifiable in the cumulus oophorus and at the outer aspect of the zona pellucida. ×3600. *(Courtesy of L. Zamboni.)*

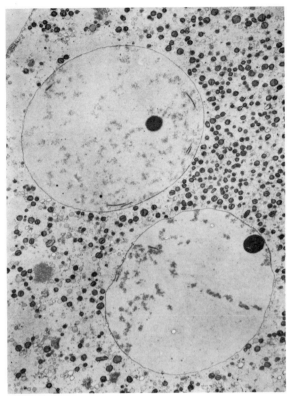

FIGURE 15–3 Fertilized human egg in binuclear stage. The two binuclei are next to one another in the peripheral portion of the egg cytoplasm. ×4800. *(Courtesy of L. Zamboni.)*

sion appears to be an excretion by the trophoblastic tissue of a substance which will destroy endometrial cells. There is also apparently a reaction in the endometrium facilitating the process. When the embryo has invaded the endometrium, a fibrin coagulum covers it, and finally the endometrial lining grows over the invasion site.

PLACENTATION

After implantation, trophoblastic proliferation continues. With this continued cell division, small fluid-filled spaces appear within the syncytiotrophoblasts (lacunae) (Fig. 15–5). The tropholastic tissue gradually surrounds or invades small maternal vessels (venulae or capillaries) with bleeding into the lacunae. Further trophoblastic growth causes erosion of progressively larger maternal vessels until veins and spiral arteries are reached. Thus a very sluggish circulation is established on the maternal side of the placenta at about 11½ days. By 22 days spiral arteri-

FIGURE 15–4 Attachment of blastocyst to the endometrial wall. Note inner cell mass is immediately adjacent to the endometrium. *(From The Developing Human: Clinically Oriented Embryology, KL Moore, Philadelphia: Saunders, 1973.)*

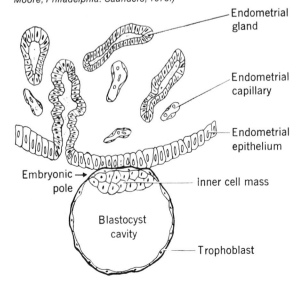

Endometrial gland

Endometrial capillary

Endometrial epithelium

Embryonic pole

Inner cell mass

Blastocyst cavity

Trophoblast

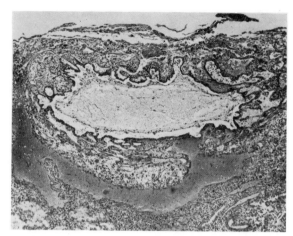

FIGURE 15-5 Section of an early embryonic implantation with lacunae formation.

oles have been tapped but still open into clefts in the cytotrophoblastic shell. The trophoblastic shell becomes thinner, and by 6 weeks the spiral arteries open directly into the intervillous space (Fig. 15-6).

With implantation certain changes occur in the endometrium. The glands become more tortuous and tightly packed, and the stromal cells become swollen and polyhedral. This is known as the decidual reaction of the endometrium. The decidua is divided by its relationship to the embryo; the decidua basalis lies directly beneath the invading trophoblastic tissue (placenta), the decidua capsularis lies over the remainder of the trophoblasts, and the decidua parietalis occupies the rest of the endometrium.

On the seventh or eighth day the trophoblastic tissue differentiates into cytotrophoblastic and syncytiotrophoblastic layers. The syncytiotrophoblastic layer is a continuous one, having cells which are non-dividing, and lacking membranes between cells. The cytotrophoblasts are the actively dividing cells which lie beneath the syncytiotrophoblastic layer, replenishing it. These two layers bud outward and form the primary villi. They lie within the lacunae, and as they continue to bud and add mesenchyme, secondary and tertiary villi are formed. During the third week capillaries develop within the mesenchymal core of the villi, and a fetal circulation is established shortly thereafter (Fig. 15-6). With both a maternal circulation through the interconnected lacunae and a fetal circulation, a mechanism is available for maternal-fetal exchange of nutrients and wastes.

Some of the villi traverse the entire width of the intervillous space and reach the deep surface of the endometrium, cytotrophoblasts penetrate the syncy-

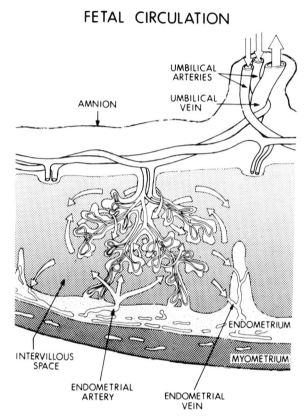

FETAL CIRCULATION

MATERNAL CIRCULATION

FIGURE 15-6 Fetal and maternal placenta circulation. *(By permission of Ortho Foundation.)*

tiotrophoblastic layer, and there attach tightly to the maternal endometrium (decidua). They become anchoring villi and serve to keep the conceptus firmly attached to the uterus.

The placenta thus developed is called a hemochorial placenta. It interposes three layers between maternal and fetal blood: trophoblast, mesenchyme, and fetal capillary epithelium.

FETAL DEVELOPMENT

By the seventh day cells at one pole of the blastocyst form a mass distinct from the trophoblastic tissue. This is called the inner cell mass and is destined to form the embryo, amnion, and yolk sac, while the trophoblastic tissue forms the chorion and placenta. At this same time, 7½ days, a small space is seen at the upper pole of the inner cell mass; this is the amniotic space. On the inner surface a layer of flattened cells develop, the endoderm. The remaining cells of the inner cell mass are ectoderm; later they also give origin to mesoderm. The ectodermal cells are involved in the formation of the amnion while the endodermal cells form the yolk sac. In man extraembryonic mesoderm forms from trophoblastic tissue and fills the old blastocyst space. The yolk sac is involved in fetal nourishment until a fetal circulation is established. The fetal vessels and blood elements develop from the yolk sac and extraembryonic mesoderm.

The ectoderm eventually forms the central nervous system and skin. Endoderm lines all the hollow viscera and forms liver and lungs, while mesoderm forms muscle and connective tissue.

Table 15–1 lists the various organs and their period of development. It is apparent that organ formation is almost complete by 12 weeks. It is important to recognize the various developmental stages, because teratogens present at certain times during pregnancy may result in aberrant development of the organ developing at that time. During the first 2 weeks, noxious influences usually result in fetal death. From 3 to 8 weeks major morphologic abnormalities will occur, and from 8 weeks till term minor defects may occur.

Some agents have demonstrated their teratogenic potential in the human; many others may be teratogenic in the human, but the principal studies have been performed in other species. To be safest the pregnant woman should avoid any drugs not absolutely essential, particularly during the first 60 days of her pregnancy.

The influence of irradiation is dependent on the doses given and the period of gestation when the fetus is irradiated. In Hiroshima those children who were calculated to have received 10 to 19 rads in early pregnancy had significantly smaller head sizes, and when the dose rose above 200 rads there was 50 times the expected incidence of mental retardation. Even diagnostic radiation may be hazardous to the fetus. Diamond et al. reported that when the mother had received diagnostic radiation during her pregnancy the child had twice the chance of dying and three times the incidence of leukemia of an unirradiated child.

The antibiotics which can potentially cause difficulty in the fetus are tetracycline, the sulfas, and clindamycin. Tetracycline causes a staining of the deciduous teeth, hypoplasia of the enamel, and possibly shortening of the long bones (Winthrop et al.). The sulfas and clindamycin will displace bilirubin from albumin. This raises the free bilirubin in the newborn and could lead to kernicterus at a lower total blood-

TABLE 15–1 Sensitivity of Fetal Organs to Teratogens

Organ	Period of development, in weeks	
	Most sensitive to teratogens	Less sensitive to teratogens
CNS	2–5	5–38
Eye	4–8	8–38
Ears	6–12	12–20
Palate	7–12	12–16
Heart	3–6	6–12
Arms	4–8	8–12
Legs	4–8	8–12
Teeth	7–12	12–20
External genitalia	7–16	16–38

bilirubin level. Since these antibiotics cross the placenta, it is not prudent to give them to the mother, particularly if premature labor, a septic infant, or a sensitized erythroblastotic infant is anticipated.

The androgenic agents will cause masculinization of the female fetus (clitoral hypertrophy and tubal fusion). They are seldom used at present but were formerly given to prevent abortion.

The antitumor agents have been used as abortifacients, and in general they do cause abortion; however, if they do not, a congenital anomaly almost always occurs. The anomaly is usually a skeletal or central-nervous-system (CNS) defect (Thersch). Some other agents and their effects or possible effects on the fetus are listed in Table 15–2.

GROWTH OF FETUS AND PLACENTA

The size the fetus reaches at term is a function of several factors, both genetic and environmental. In clinical medicine there has been considerable interest in attempting to relate fetal growth to characteristics within the placenta; however, it is perhaps more useful to look first at certain general characteristics of placentation and fetal growth.

Organ development involves several distinct phases which are arbitrarily separated out of a continuum of development. These phases include differentiation, growth, maturation, and aging. In each of these phases there are varying contributions from cell division or hyperplasia, from cell growth or hypertrophy, and from cell differentiation. Three phases of placentation can be clearly defined: the period of im-

TABLE 15–2 Effects of Agents on Fetal Development

Agent	Effect on fetus	Reference
Cigarette smoking	Decreased fetal weight	Abernathy Jr.: *Am J Public Health* 56:626, 1966.
Narcotic addiction	Withdrawal symptoms	Cobrinik, RW et al.: *Pediatr* 24:288, 1959.
Lysergic acid diethylamide (LSD)	Increased chromosome breaks?	Tjio et al.: *JAMA* 210:849, 1969.
Diphenylhydantoin	Cleft lip?	Mirkin BL: *J Pediatr* 78:329, 1971.
Adrenal corticosteroids	Cleft lip? Adrenal insufficiency	Bongiovanni et al.: *Fertil Steril* 11:181, 1960.
Stilbestrol	Vaginal adenosis	Herbst AL et al.: *N Engl J Med* 284:878, 1971.
Coumadin	Fetal bleeding	Gordon RR et al.: *Brit Med J* 2:719, 1955.
Thiazines	Bone marrow depression	Rodriguez SU et al.: *Brit Med J* 2:719, 1955.
Alcohol	Mental retardation	Jones KL et al.: *Lancet* Nov 3, 1973, p. 999.
Oral contraceptives	Limb reduction	Albanil M: et al.: *Fertil Steril* 28:791, 1977.
Lithium	Cardiovascular abnormalities	Weinstein MR et al.: *Am J Psych* 132:529, 1975.

plantation (or differentiation); a second phase of rapid placental growth; and a third stage of maturation, in late gestation, characterized by a marked growth in function of the organ without much change in the size. How do these various stages of placental development affect subsequent growth of the organ and affect the growth and development of the fetus?

First one may consider the stage of implantation. Some clues as to how implantation may affect subsequent growth of the fetus and placenta have come from the studies in sheep where the unique anatomy permits some quantitation of the relationship between implantation and final size of the placenta. The non-pregnant uterus of the sheep has approximately 100 potential implantation sites which are grossly visible and distributed equally in both uterine horns. Even among singlet gestations there is great variability in the number of potential sites actually used for the formation of the miniature placentas or cotyledons, the sum of which makes up the total placental mass. Several studies have shown that the final size of the placenta at the end of gestation is at least in part a function of the number of implantation sites used initially; that is, there is a linear relationship between the number of cotyledons developed and the total size of the placenta. If, in a single pregnancy, 20 cotyledons are formed, the total weight of that placenta is considerably less than in a pregnancy in which 60 or 80 cotyledons are used. Alexander has shown that factors such as the age of the mother and the sex of the fetus influence the total number of placental cotyledons developed in a pregnancy. Her studies and our own have shown that when there are fewer implantation sites used, there is compensatory growth within each

FIGURE 15–7 Relationship of the fetal weight/placental weight ratio to the weight of the placenta in the last week of gestation. *(From Kulhanek.)*

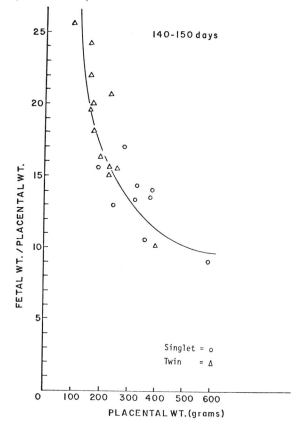

cotyledon; that is, the DNA (deoxyribonucleic acid) per cotyledon and the average cotyledonary weight are inversely related to the cotyledonary number. Despite this compensatory growth, the total weight of the organ and the total DNA are reduced in placentas utilizing fewer implantation sites. This same compensatory growth of individual cotyledons is seen in twin placentas. The placenta of each twin is smaller than the placenta of a singlet fetus, although the total amount of placental tissue, combining both twin placentas, is greater than the singlet placenta. It has been well documented that the individual cotyledons are larger, both in weight and DNA content, in twin placentas than in singlet placentas. Similarly, in experiments which restrict by surgical reduction the number of implantation sites in a sheep, the result is a small placenta at term and a small fetus. Thus in this species, which has been most intensively studied, it can be clearly demonstrated that there is a cause-and-effect relationship between placental weight reduction and fetal weight reduction. It is of interest that it is a restricted number of sites of implantation which lead to small placentas and thus to small fetuses, rather than the poor growth of individual cotyledons, a phenomenon which has not been observed in any studies.

In man, monkey, and sheep species a clear relationship can be shown between fetal weight and placental weight at a constant gestational age, particularly near term. The fetal weight/placental weight ratio is much higher when the placenta is small, and this relationship holds true regardless of whether one is comparing small placentas in singleton pregnancies or small placentas in twin pregnancies. Figure 15–7 presents data on the fetal-placental weight ratio as placental weight decreases. The relationship is not different for singletons and twins. Thus, a fetus attached to a small placenta tends to be growth-retarded when compared to a population of normal fetuses, although it is able to achieve a larger size than predicted by the weight of its placenta alone. The data in Fig. 15–7 show the impact of placental maturation (the attainment of maximal organ function) upon fetal growth.

It has already been stressed that in all species the placenta decreases or stops its rate of growth completely in late gestation, at a time when fetal growth continues at a rapid rate. However, in Fig. 15–8 data are presented on the measurement of the diffusing capacity of the placenta to urea in the sheep, showing that, unlike placental weight and placental DNA, the diffusing capacity to urea increases markedly in late gestation. Figure 15–9, taken from the work by Aherne and Dunnill, shows similar measurements of total trophoblastic surface area of the human placenta against gestational age. There is a

FIGURE 15–8 Relationship of fetal weight to the urea-diffusing capacity of the placenta (milligrams of urea crossing the placenta in 1 minute for a given transplacental concentration difference of urea). *(From Meschia et al.)*

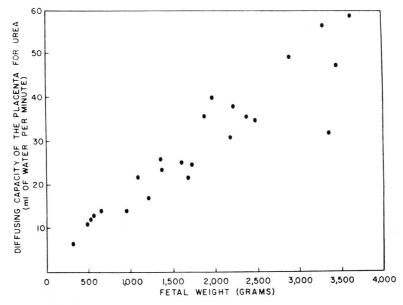

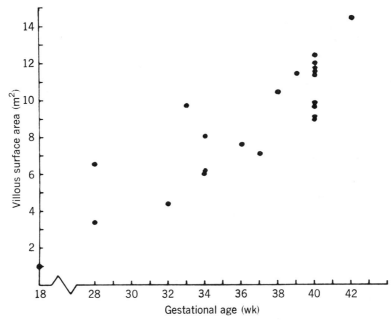

FIGURE 15-9 Relationship of total villous surface area of the placenta to gestational age. *(From Aherne et al.)*

marked increase in total surface area in late gestation, in contrast to the minimal changes in total placental weight or total DNA. The increase in the diffusing capacity of the placenta in late gestation is a function of both increased folding of trophoblasts and an increased surface area, coupled with a reduction in the diffusing distance from the fetal capillaries to the maternal blood. It should be emphasized that at a given fetal age placental permeability per kilogram of fetal weight is less than normal when the placenta is small, emphasizing the cause-and-effect relationship between small placentas and small babies (Fig. 15-10).

Several different levels of architecture contribute to the marked increase in surface area during late gestation. These include the gross folding of the trophoblast into villi and the microvillous formation on each trophoblastic cell. Figures 15-11 and 15-12 depict these different levels of architecture.

Fetal growth is characterized by a continuous increase in the proportion of total body weight represented by cells. For this reason, as gestation progresses, and continuing in postnatal life, there is an increase in the ratio of intracellular to extracellular water volumes, decreasing the percentage of body weight represented by extracellular fluid volume. Figure 15-13 presents these changes in body composition as a percentage of body weight. The changes in

FIGURE 15-10 Among fetuses of approximately the same age there is a positive correlation between urea permeability per kilogram of fetal weight and total placental DNA (first order regression analysis). *(From Kulhanek et al.)*

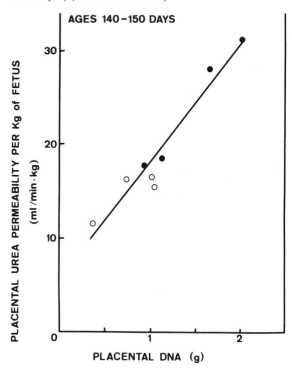

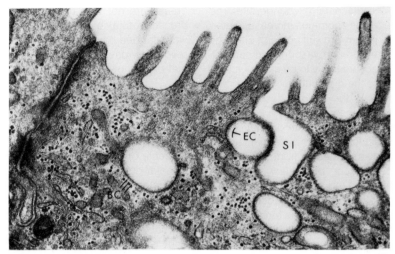

FIGURE 15–11 Scanning electron micrograph of the villous portion of the 40-day yolk sac. The individual folds are readily discernible; the fold on the right is branched. Outlines of the endoderm cells covering the folds are evident since the apical portion of each cell protrudes in a domelike fashion. ×500. *(From King et al.)*

cell number and cell size in the various organs of the fetus during gestation have not been adequately studied in man.

PLACENTAL PHYSIOLOGY

A basic characteristic of mammalian development is the formation of the placenta, across which nutrients for growth and waste products of metabolism are ex-

FIGURE 15–12 Apical region of the endoderm cells at high magnification. A delicate layer of filamentous material is present on the microvilli. Several stages of invagination of the apical cell membrane are shown. Because of their proximity to the cell surface, most of the saccules shown here are probably still open to the uterine lumen out of the plane of section. A junctional complex is present where the two epithelial cells are apposed. 41 days of gestation. ×44,000. *(From King et al.)*

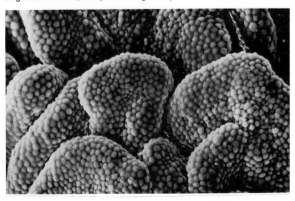

changed. Transplacental exchanges are accomplished as a function of both perfusion and permeability. Placental perfusion is a composite of uterine blood flow and umbilical blood flow. Permeability is a characteristic of the placental membrane.

PLACENTAL PERFUSION

The magnitude of the changes required in maternal circulation during pregnancy can be appreciated best in the reproductive tissues. Uterine blood flow in sheep increases from approximately 20 mL per minute in the nonpregnant state to approximately 1000 mL per minute at term, a fiftyfold change which is di-

FIGURE 15–13 Composition of fetus at various ages with values expressed as percent of body weight. *(From Weil et al.)*

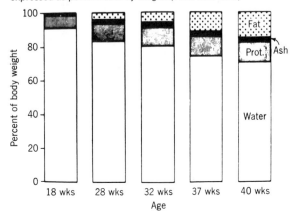

rected primarily to the placental exchange site. The factors which produce this enormous increase in uterine blood flow in pregnancy are still unclear, although growth of the vascular bed and vasodilation secondary to an estrogen effect are likely to be major factors. Figure 15–14 presents the distribution of uterine and umbilical blood flows to the various tissues of the ovine uterus in late pregnancy. The effect of estrogens upon uterine blood flow is quite dramatic (Fig. 15–15). Since the vascular bed of the pregnant uterus is almost maximally vasodilated, it is not surprising that hypotension can reduce blood flow markedly. Similarly, norepinephrine and epinephrine cause a marked decrease in blood flow by vasoconstriction. However, acute changes in arterial gas tensions have very little effect upon the uterine vascular bed. The marked vasoconstriction of the uterine vascular bed in response to catecholamines illustrates the fact that adaptive measures in the maternal circulation are geared to her survival, not necessarily to the short-term advantage of the fetus.

UMBILICAL BLOOD FLOW

Umbilical blood flow increases markedly during gestation, and most of this blood is distributed to the placental exchange site. At term, greater than 90 percent of the umbilical flow is distributed to the placenta (see Fig 15–14). The factors responsible for this in-

crease are not well documented, but a gradual increase in fetal blood pressure and a growth of the vascular bed have both been implicated. Changes in respiratory gas tensions have little effect upon umbilical blood flow.

PLACENTAL PERMEABILITY

In the previous section on fetal and placental growth, the increase in area and decrease in thickness of the placenta during gestation were stressed. Just as the alveolar surface area of the lung increases in early postnatal life proportional to body size, so the total surface area of the trophoblast increases in proportion to the increase in fetal body weight. However, the trophoblast has a much larger surface area per unit body weight than the alveoli and is much thicker, reflecting the enormous variety of metabolic functions within the trophoblast. It should be emphasized that measurements of the urea-diffusing capacity have shown an increase which is proportional to body weight. Thus both physiologic measurements and morphometric measurements in man and other mammals have confirmed a close relationship between placental development and fetal growth.

Placental permeability has been studied in a number of ways. In man, there are obvious restrictions on experimental design which impose certain difficulties in evaluating the rate at which drugs or other compounds cross the placenta. We will come back to the special features of human placental permeability but first let us look in more detail at placental transfer in other mammals. Measurements of the clearance of compounds across various organs of the body (placenta, kidney, and lung) have proven useful in describing some of the unique characteristics of these organs.

Placental clearance (C) is defined as the quantity of a substance crossing the placenta (q) per unit concentration difference between umbilical arteries and maternal arteries ($a - A$). Thus, the clearance of a substance will be a function of both permeability of the placenta to that substance and perfusion of the placenta, represented by umbilical and uterine blood flows. If the placental permeability is very low, then permeability will become the major determinant of clearance and the substance will be considered membrane- or diffusion-limited. In this case the clearance will be virtually independent of changes in umbilical or uterine blood flow. The greater the permeability, the greater the placental clearance, until a maximal clearance is reached. This maximum clearance represents a flow-limited clearance, since it will

FIGURE 15–14 Distribution of uterine and umbilical blood flows in a pregnant sheep at term with a fetus weighing 3000 g. Percents are of either total umbilical or total uterine blood flows distributed to the structure. *(From Makowski et al.)*

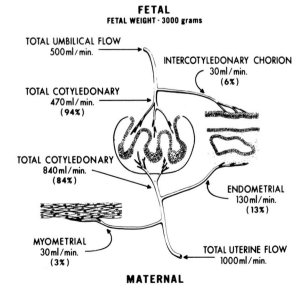

FETAL
FETAL WEIGHT · 3000 grams

TOTAL UMBILICAL FLOW
500 ml/min.

INTERCOTYLEDONARY CHORION
30 ml/min.
(6%)

TOTAL COTYLEDONARY
470 ml/min.
(94%)

TOTAL COTYLEDONARY
840 ml/min.
(84%)

ENDOMETRIAL
130 ml/min.
(13%)

MYOMETRIAL
30 ml/min.
(3%)

TOTAL UTERINE FLOW
1000 ml/min.

MATERNAL

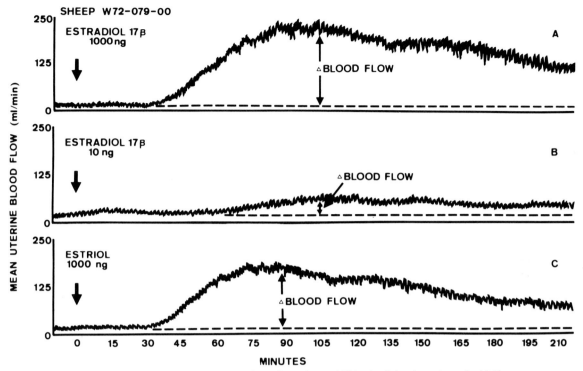

FIGURE 15-15 Effect on uterine blood flow of two doses of 17β-estradiol and one dose of estriol injected into the lumen of one uterine artery. Injection period 1 minute. *A* Response elicited by 1000 mg *B* The effect of 10 mg injected the following day. *C* Response elicited by 1000 mg of estriol. The response was quantitated by measuring the peak delta blood flow elicited by each dose. *(From Resnik et al.)*

be determined only by the magnitude and pattern of uterine and umbilical blood flows. Clearly, since a flow-limited clearance represents a maximum value for a given placenta, all compounds that are flow-limited by virtue of a high placental permeability would have identical placental clearances. This has been shown to be the case for the clearance of antipyrine and tritiated water across both the sheep and primate placentas, whereas urea, sodium, and chloride are all markedly membrane-limited. The relationship between the two venous concentrations (umbilical vein and uterine vein) are of special importance. Even in the case of antipyrine and tritiated water, where placental clearance is flow-limited, the two venous streams tend toward, but do not achieve, equilibration. Thus the placenta simulates a somewhat inefficient concurrent-flow system. The fact that the two venous streams do not equilibrate completely is due in large part to "shunts" within the two circulations; that is, umbilical and uterine blood flows are distributed to tissues other than the placenta, and the outflow from these tissues is mixed in the uterine and umbili-

cal veins with the outflow from the placenta. Since the magnitude of these "shunts" in the uterine circulation is quite large, it should be emphasized that the best reference point for interpreting changes in umbilical venous concentrations is not the maternal arterial blood, but the uterine or ovarian venous blood.

FETAL METABOLISM

As a starting point for discussion of fetal metabolism, let us consider first the data on fetal metabolic rate and the more general topic of fetal respiration. The oxygen consumption per kilogram of body weight during fetal life is approximately the same as that of newborn infants during the first few days of postnatal life, i.e., 6 to 8 mL at standard temperature and pressure (STP) of oxygen per minute per kilogram of fetal body weight. To meet these needs the fetus is completely dependent on the continuous delivery of oxygen across the placenta. Under normal conditions with a well-oxygenated mother, oxygen transport across the placenta is primarily flow-limited, but with maternal hypoxia produced by disease or by exposure to high altitude, oxygen transport across the placenta becomes primarily membrane-limited. The total oxygen uptake by the umbilical circulation increases as gestation progresses and the fetus grows. For the sheep fetus in late gestation, fetal oxygen consumption increases approximately 0.7 mL of oxygen at STP per minute per day. This can be altered by maternal starvation. Just as in adult man or in newborn animals, the fetal oxygen consumption falls with exposure to maternal starvation. Thus, a reduction in metabolic rate represents a general adaptation of mammals to starvation.

The fetus must maintain an adequate oxygen uptake in the presence of very low oxygen tensions in the umbilical circulation. Even the most arterialized blood of the fetus has a low P_{O_2} because, as described earlier, the placenta simulates a somewhat inefficient concurrent-flow system. Thus, the umbilical venous outflow tends to equilibrate with the uterine venous blood. This is illustrated in Fig. 15–16, which shows that as uterine venous P_{O_2} is varied by altering the oxygen concentration in the inspired air and/or by altering the oxygen affinity of maternal blood, the umbilical venous P_{O_2} is always lower than the uterine venous P_{O_2}. Figure 15–16 also illustrates the fact, confirmed by other data, that the uterine venous/umbilical venous P_{O_2} difference is not reduced at low uterine venous oxygen tensions, supporting the fact that there is a residual diffusion limitation to oxygen transfer at low oxygen tensions. The fact that umbilical venous P_{O_2} tends to equilibrate with uterine venous blood explains why acute inhalation of oxygen by the mother cannot increase umbilical venous P_{O_2} to levels approaching maternal-arterial blood. Thus, oxygen inhalation by the mother does not carry the danger of increasing fetal oxygen tensions to levels that would produce vasoconstriction of fetal vessels. In fact, it has been shown that maternal oxygen inhalation can improve fetal oxygen consumption, and this procedure remains one of the mainstays of therapy for fetal distress.

FETAL CARBON DIOXIDE PRODUCTION AND ACID-BASE BALANCE

In health, the fetus is characterized by an oxygen consumption which cannot be increased by increasing the oxygen concentration in the inspired air of the

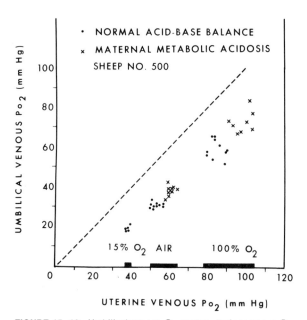

FIGURE 15–16 Umbilical venous P_{O_2} versus uterine venous P_{O_2} in a sheep with (1) normal acid-base balance (mean uterine venous pH, 7.42; range, 7.46 to 7.36), and (2) maternal metabolic acidosis (mean uterine venous pH, 7.15; range, 7.22 to 7.02). Mean umbilical venous pH was 7.39 (range, 7.43 to 7.34) in the normal state and 7.40 (range, 7.42 to 7.37) during maternal acidosis. *(From Rankin et al.)*

mother. Thus, normally the fetus is not hypoxic in the sense that its metabolic requirements for oxygen are adequately met. The fetus excretes CO_2, a waste product of metabolism, by means of a P_{CO_2} gradient across the placenta. The umbilical venous P_{CO_2} again tends to equilibrate with uterine venous P_{CO_2}, although remaining slightly higher. Thus, when one compares the arterialized blood of the fetus (umbilical venous blood) with arterial blood of the mother, the P_{CO_2} is higher in the fetal circulation. Since the standard bicarbonate concentration of fetal blood is within the normal adult range, the fetal pH is slightly lower than in the adult, reflecting the small but significant difference in P_{CO_2}. It should be stressed that the normal fetus has no evidence of a metabolic acidosis. Fetal blood thus has the characteristics of a mild, uncompensated respiratory acidosis. The placenta is relatively impermeable to ions such as sodium, chloride, and bicarbonate. Put more precisely, their placental clearances are much less than that of antipyrine or tritiated water, which are flow-limited. P_{CO_2} in fetal blood changes rapidly in response to changes in maternal blood P_{CO_2} levels. Since bicarbonate concentration in fetal blood cannot change as rapidly, the pH differences in fetal blood may be in the same or opposite direction from changes in maternal blood pH, depending upon whether the changes in maternal blood are principally respiratory or metabolic. Maternal respiratory acidosis or alkalosis will lower or raise fetal pH respectively. Maternal metabolic acidosis or alkalosis with appropriate compensatory changes in maternal P_{CO_2} will move the fetal pH.

FETAL NUTRITION

The determination of metabolic quotients is being used in many nutritional studies in both man and other mammals. Essentially, a metabolic quotient is a ratio of two whole-blood arterial-venous differences, one difference for the test substance expressed in terms of the oxygen required for its aerobic metabolism and the other the arterial-venous difference of oxygen. Thus, the fetal glucose/oxygen quotient is given as

$$\frac{6 \times \Delta \text{ glucose}}{\Delta \text{ oxygen}}$$

where Δ glucose equals the umbilical arterial-venous difference of glucose (mM/mL blood) and Δ oxygen equals the umbilical arterial-venous difference of oxygen (mM/mL blood). In recent years, studies on metabolic quotients across the umbilical circulation have radically altered our ideas of fetal metabolism. It had been assumed from very indirect evidence that glucose was the sole metabolic fuel of the mammalian fetus. However, recent studies in sheep have shown that the umbilical glucose/oxygen quotient is equal to 0.46; that is, only 46 percent of the fetal oxygen consumption could be accounted for by glucose uptake. With maternal starvation and its accompanying maternal hypoglycemia, the glucose/oxygen quotient falls to less than 0.2. As one might expect from these data, the respiratory quotient of the fetus is less than 1, supporting the fact that carbohydrate is not the predominant fuel in fetal life. A cautionary note should be added, though, concerning the interpretation of respiratory quotients. In a rapidly growing fetus one cannot make the required assumption that the accumulation of carbon for growth is negligible when compared to the amount of carbon excreted by the fetus. Thus, even if the respiratory quotient were 1, it would not imply the metabolism solely of carbohydrate.

Another major source of fuel to the fetus is the catabolism of amino acid. Amino acids are used in fetal life both for growth and, through catabolism, as a source of energy. Again, this represents a departure from traditional concepts of perinatal biology. In the past, a number of studies have shown that newborn infants during early postnatal life had a very low urea-excretion rate. This had been interpreted as reflecting the fact that the newborn, growing rapidly, was using nitrogen for growth. Since placental clearance equals

$$\frac{\dot{q}}{a - A}$$

the urea-production rate of a fetus can be determined ($\dot{q}$ urea) by independent measurements of placental clearance and the concentration difference for urea between the two arterial circulations. Estimates of the urea-production rate in humans have been made from the combination of urea clearance measurements in primates and $a - A$ measurements in humans (Jones). Figure 15–17 summarizes the data in humans, showing that in fetal life there is a higher urea-production rate than in either newborn infants or adults. These observations in the fetus are new and contrary to the common belief that glucose is the major metabolic fuel of the fetus. In fact, amino acid catabolism could account for 10 to 25 percent of the oxygen consumption in the primate fetus.

In species other than the rabbit or guinea pig, transplacental fatty acid transport is limited. Thus, fatty acids do not provide a significant portion of fetal substrate needs. Essential fatty acids are supplied in satisfactory quantities.

More recently, lactate has been demonstrated to provide up to 25 percent of carbon substrate for fetal metabolism (Burd et al.). The source of this lactate is the placenta which converts nearly one-third of its glucose uptake (from the uterine circulation) to lactate. Acetate may also provide up to 10 percent of fetal substrate requirements (Chav, Creasy).

FIGURE 15–17 The urea-excretion rates in newborn infants (NB) and adults represent only urinary excretion; the rate in the fetus represents an estimate of transplacental urea excretion. *(The data for the figure were obtained from the following studies: for the fetus from Gresham et al: J. Pediatr 79:809–811, 1971, and for the adult and newborn from McCance and Widdowson, Cold Spring Harbor Symp Quant Biol 19:161, 1954.)*

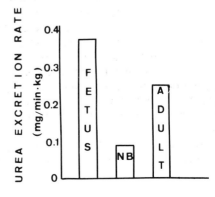

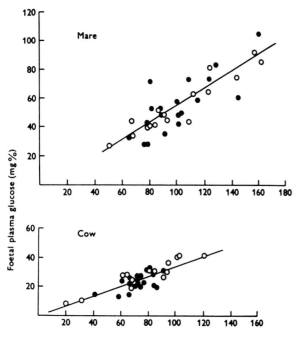

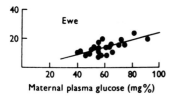

FIGURE 15–18 The relation between maternal and fetal plasma glucose levels in mare, cow, and ewe. ● = values from chronic preparations; ○ = values from acute preparations (chloralose anesthesia) with fetus undisturbed in utero. Two to three values are included per experiment. Regression lines were fitted by the method of least squares. *(From Silver et al.)*

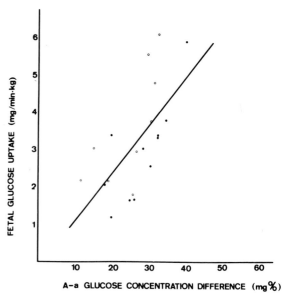

FIGURE 15–19 Relationship of fetal glucose uptake to the concentration of glucose between maternal-arterial and fetal-arterial blood, in milligrams per 100 mL of blood. ● = twin; ○ = single. *(From Battaglia et al.)*

For most substances which contribute to growth in fetal life, little is known about constants which regulate their rates of placental transfer. However, a fair amount of information has been collected for glucose transfer across the placenta. Figure 15–18 compares the relationship between umbilical-arterial and maternal-arterial glucose concentrations in three different animals (Silver et al.). While there are differences among the three species, two points of similarity should be emphasized. First of all, in all three groups there is a linear relationship between the fetal and maternal glucose concentrations; the greater the maternal glucose concentration, the greater the fetal glucose concentration. Secondly, in all three animals the slopes of the lines are much less than identity lines; that is, as maternal glucose concentration increases, fetal glucose increases,

but not proportionately. Thus, a larger concentration difference develops between the two circulations as the maternal concentration rises. The significance of this point is brought out in Fig. 15–19, where fetal glucose uptake is plotted against this driving force, the $A - a$ concentration difference (Battaglia). As the concentration difference increases, the glucose uptake by the fetus increases. Thus, we have the first example of how something done to the mother (an alteration in maternal glucose concentration) can change fetal metabolism in a predictable fashion.

DISEASES OF THE FETUS

ERYTHROBLASTOSIS FETALIS

The majority of fetuses and newborns who develop serious erythroblastosis fetalis are the product of an Rh-negative mother and Rh-positive father. If the fetus is also Rh-positive, fetal cells entering the maternal circulation may elicit an antibody response to the Rh blood factor. This transplacental passage of fetal cells is usually greatest at delivery, but may occur during pregnancy prior to the onset of labor. The antibodies (gamma G globulin, IgG) cross the placenta into the fetus, where they destroy fetal red cells. Other incompatibilities can exist between fetal and maternal blood such as ABO, Kell, Duffy, and other antigens. ABO incompatibility does not cause hydrops fetalis; however, it may be associated with significant jaundice in the newborn. The Kell and Duffy antigens are infrequent but may occasionally be associated with severe disease so they should not be ignored. However, since the occurrence is less frequent or the fetal difficulty less marked, Rh erythroblastosis will form the basis for the following discussion.

The incidence of Rh-negative women in the general population varies from 1 to 34 percent, depending on the ethnic origin. Only about 6 percent of those pregnancies are sensitized. It is unusual for the first pregnancy to be affected unless the mother has received prior Rh-positive blood; however, an occasional first pregnancy will be affected without a history of the mother receiving blood. The problem may appear in any subsequent pregnancy. However, more than one-half of the women who subsequently become sensitized will demonstrate this during the second pregnancy (Freda). In addition, about one-third of the infants who die do so in the first sensitized pregnancy. Thus, it is very important to recognize the

pregnancy at risk for significant erythroblastosis fetalis.

A logical approach to the detection of the fetus in jeopardy begins by recognizing the sensitized mother. This is accomplished by obtaining an Rh type (she will be negative) and Rh antibody titer at the first prenatal visit. A significant titer is any titer if the woman has had a previous erythroblastotic fetus, or a titer of 1:8 or greater during the pregnancy, with titers repeated every 2 weeks. If the mother has a significant titer, the fetus may be affected, and the physician should begin to follow it by obtaining amniotic fluid specimens for their bile chromogen content. The timing of the first amniocentesis should be between 20 and 24 weeks. About 5 mL of fluid is removed by transabdominal amniocentesis, placed in a darkened tube, and sent to the laboratory for spectrophotometric bile chromogen analysis. This is done by observing the increase in optical density above an expected baseline at 450 nm (ΔOD_{450}), on a semilogarithmic graph (Fig. 15–20) (Liley, 1961). One plots this ΔOD_{450} opposite the proper weeks of gestation on a Liley nomogram (Fig. 15–21). Repeat amniocenteses are performed every 2 weeks in zone I, weekly in zone II, and every 3 to 7 days in zone III to confirm the ΔOD_{450} and the trend with advancing gestational age. Fetuses in zone I are in no difficulty, can be

FIGURE 15–20 Optical density measurement of amniotic fluid from a sensitized Rh-negative patient. *(Courtesy of B. Weiss.)*

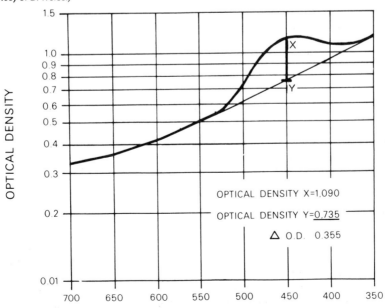

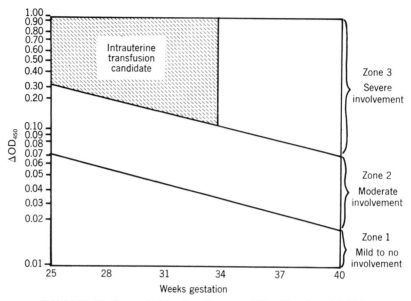

FIGURE 15–21 Zones of ΔOD_{450} from the work of Liley. *(Courtesy of B. Weiss.)*

delivered when spontaneous labor starts, and will seldom need an exchange transfusion after birth. The fetuses in zone II can also be delivered in term. However, they have more likelihood of needing an exchange transfusion and may require an immediate exchange. Therefore, it is prudent to terminate these pregnancies under optimal conditions at between 37 and 39 weeks' gestation with a mature lecithin/sphingomyelin (L/S) ratio and a favorable cervix and presenting part. If a fetus lies in upper zone II and goes into zone III or is in zone III initially, this usually signifies the fetus is very anemic [8 g Hb (hemoglobin) or less]. With profound anemia the fetus may develop edema of the subcutaneous tissues, hepatosplenomegaly, and may expire. In order to prevent this, Liley (1963) suggested giving a blood transfusion to the fetus. This is done by placing O-negative cells into the peritoneal cavity of the fetus; from there they reach the circulation, probably through lymphatic channels. The transfusions start about the 24th to the 32d week of gestation and continue every 10 to 14 days until the fetus is mature enough to survive in a nursery (33 to 35 weeks). Using the intrauterine transfusion, 35 to 40 percent of those fetuses who previously might have succumbed to severe erythroblastosis are delivered with a good blood count and without edema. When profound edema of the fetus has occurred (fetal hydrops), intrauterine transfusion is rarely of benefit. The care of the newborn is discussed later in this chapter under hyperbilirubinemia.

In the future, there should be few infants affected with erythroblastosis caused by Rh antibodies. This is due to the use of gamma globulin with a high titer of anti-Rh. Pollack et al. found that giving this (300 μg gamma G) to nonsensitized Rh-negative mothers within 72 hours of delivering Rh-positive infants prevented sensitization in a subsequent pregnancy in almost every case. As stated previously, the major fetal maternal exchange of erythrocytes seems to occur at delivery. The anti-D globulin prevents antibody formation in the mother, perhaps by coating these cells or by blocking antibody production sites. An excess of anti-D globulin can be detected by the presence of a positive indirect Coombs' test after giving hyperimmune gamma globulin. This will frequently assist the physician in ascertaining that there has not been an overwhelming fetal-maternal bleed. The major reason that hyperimmune gamma globulin occasionally is not effective is thought to be a large fetal-maternal bleed. This is more likely to occur if the placenta is manually removed or the placental end of the severed umbilical cord is not allowed to drain freely. Occasionally, a significant maternal bleed, which may result in Rh sensitization, occurs prior to delivery, in which case the newborn may show anemia. If any of the above circumstances are present (manual placental removal or fetal anemia), maternal blood should be drawn and stained (Kleihauer-Betke stain) for the percent of fetal cells. If the calculated fetal cells in the maternal circulation exceed 30 mL, the mother should receive an added 300 μg of gamma G for every additional 30 mL of fetal blood or fraction thereof in the maternal circulation.

ABNORMAL FETAL GROWTH

EVALUATION OF INTRAUTERINE GROWTH RATE

Within obstetrics there has been a long-standing interest in the evaluation of the progress of a pregnancy in terms of both the size of the baby and the duration of the pregnancy. The conventional approach included an estimation of gestational age from a careful menstrual history and an evaluation of the size of the infant by abdominal palpation. However, by 1960 clinical studies had stimulated obstetricians and neonatologists to move to a much more careful evaluation of the size and gestational age of an infant. This impetus came from a number of quite different studies appearing in the clinical literature within a few years of each other.

As data on the birthweight/gestational age distribution of infants appeared, it became clear that a large number of infants were born with low birthweights, not from premature onset of labor and a preterm delivery, but rather from a slow rate of intrauterine growth. Furthermore, the problems of the relatively large birthweight infant born prematurely came to light from such studies. Neonatal hypoglycemia was first ascribed to an association with the maternal disease of toxemia, but it was soon recognized as one of several metabolic problems related to small-for-gestational-age (SGA) infants regardless of the associated maternal disease.

Given the impetus from the birthweight/gestational age studies and from the observation of hypoglycemia as a problem associated with SGA infants, obstetrics in the 1960s sharpened its tools for the antenatal recognition of marked deviations in intrauterine growth rate. First came ultrasound in 1963, which became more and more firmly established for the measurement of fetal size. Figure 15–22, from the report of Campbell and Dewhurst, shows how repeated determinations of fetal biparietal diameter by ultrasound can provide the obstetrician with two separate pieces of information: first, the size of the infant, and second, an estimate of gestational age obtained from the growth curve of the biparietal diameter. This same study has shown that the antenatal recognition of retarded fetal growth by the use of ultrasound enables the obstetrician to identify a group of patients with ap-

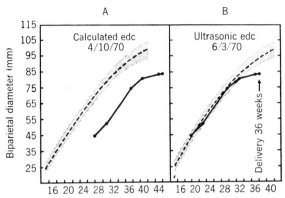

Figure 15–22 Growth of the biparietal diameter *(A)* according to the original calculated EDC; *(B)* according to the revised ultrasonic EDC. *(From Campbell et al.)*

proximately ten times the perinatal mortality rate among all patients studied by ultrasound examinations. Similarly, after transabdominal amniocentesis became firmly established in the management of Rh-sensitized pregnancies, it began to be used to evaluate the maturity of the infant, supplementing the estimate obtained from the menstrual history. The amniotic fluid concentrations of many different substances have been investigated as possible indicators of gestational age. The most widely used test today is the L/S ratio of the amniotic fluid. It usually reaches a ratio of 2:1 at about 35 weeks and indicates fetal pulmonary maturity. Recently Hallman and coworkers have further refined the test with the measurement of phosphatidyl inositol and phosphatidylglycerol. When the latter is detectable in amniotic fluid, fetal lung maturity is almost invariably present. This test is particularly helpful in the offspring of the diabetic because in this situation respiratory distress may develop when the L/S ratio is greater than 2:1 but does not develop when phosphatidylglycerol is present.

There is considerable current interest in clinical obstetrics and pediatrics for the evaluation of the velocity of growth rather than linear growth. For a more complete discussion of this, the reader is referred to Falkner's work. He has shown the increased sensitivity obtained for detecting abnormal rates of growth by charting the velocity of growth for various anthropomorphic measurements, rather than charting linear growth. Figure 15–23 presents data on the velocity of growth of fetal body weight during gestation. It brings out very clearly the rapid rate of growth in midpregnancy and the slower rate of fetal growth in the latter part of pregnancy. As was stressed in a previous section, this lower rate of fetal growth should not be inter-

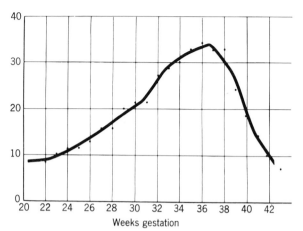

FIGURE 15–23 Mean daily fetal growth (in grams) during previous week of gestation. *(From Hendricks.)*

preted as indicating placental insufficiency in normal pregnancy. It is likely that such studies, aimed at evaluating the velocity of growth for various anthropomorphic measurements of infants in utero, will enable obstetricians in the next few years to determine when a fetus begins the rapid phase of growth in utero. One will be able to ask whether there are differences in clinical outcome among infants who begin the rapid phase of intrauterine growth earlier or later in gestation. This would be similar to the questions that have been asked in postnatal life concerning the onset of puberty in children and the occurrence of the puberty growth spurt at different postnatal ages.

SMALL-FOR-GESTATIONAL-AGE INFANTS

Let us turn next to a consideration of the specific problems of infants whose growth rates are at variance with the general population. We recognize that infants whose birth weights are small for gestational age (SGA infants) consist of a very heterogeneous group from the point of view of clinical problems. Many terms have come to be used to describe such babies: intrauterine growth retardation, small-for-dates, small-for-gestational-age, fetal malnutrition, dysmaturity, and placental-insufficiency syndrome. General descriptive titles which do not imply etiology are preferred, considering our limited knowledge of intrauterine factors which lead to SGA infants. SGA infants vary widely in body proportions. Some have head circumferences and body lengths proportionately reduced when compared to body weight. Others have reduction in birth weight without comparable reduction in skeletal proportions. At this time we cannot

ascribe specific management problems to one or another group of such infants. A few of the factors which lead to the delivery of SGA infants have begun to be described. It has already been stated that the slower rate of fetal growth in late gestation should not be interpreted as evidence of placental insufficiency. "Bigger" does not equal "better" when applied to the interpretation of growth rates in man. A maximal rate of growth may not be equated with an optimal rate of growth. In postnatal life, we recognize the fact that children have different and specific rates of growth at various stages of development. We are not tempted to equate bigger size or faster maturation with optimal development.

Some of the obstetric factors which clearly affect infant size include maternal size and maternal parity. It is known, for example, that infant birth weight increases from the first to the fourth pregnancies. In addition, mortality and morbidity change from the first to the fourth pregnancies, with the lowest rate of prenatal pathology occurring with the second pregnancy. Lobl et al. have shown the striking effect of maternal age on infant birth weight in primiparous pregnancy. Thus, when the median maternal age reaches 38 years there is a marked increase in SGA infants. In contrast, teenage pregnancies are complicated by an increased incidence of premature onset of labor and the delivery of preterm infants of normal size with no associated intrauterine growth retardation. Multiple pregnancy is another obvious cause of SGA infants. Figure 15–24 shows the effect of multiple pregnancy

FIGURE 15–24 Mean birthweight of single and multiple fetuses related to duration of gestation (cubic curves fitted by method of least squares). *(From McKeown et al.)*

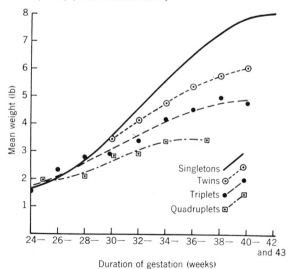

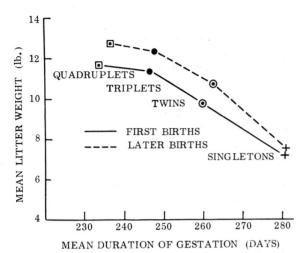

FIGURE 15-25 Mean litter weight and mean duration of gestation of first and later births. *(From McKeown et al.)*

on infant birth weight. Figure 15-25 presents comparable data on the time in gestation for the onset of labor with increasing numbers of fetuses. Taken together, these data emphasize the need for an obstetric and pediatric team in the management of multiple pregnancies, since the outcome can then be anticipated and will include the dual problems of prematurity and SGA infants. A team of physicians will be required, not only because several infants may require resuscitation, but also for the management of specific problems of prematurity and intrauterine growth retardation. There may be additional complications such as twin-twin transfusion syndrome, etc. Toxemia is associated with SGA infants, particularly when the onset of symptoms and signs occurs early in pregnancy. The older, multiparous patient with chronic hypertensive vascular disease is most at risk. Other causes of SGA infants include congenital infections and chromosomal abnormalities. When the birth weights of infants infected with rubella virus are compared with the birth weights of previous siblings, the incidence of intrauterine growth retardation associated with rubella infection rises from 30 to 60 percent (Turner).

A large number of congenital infections may lead to intrauterine growth retardation, especially when associated with severe signs and symptoms in the infant. Similarly, there is an increased incidence of SGA infants in association with all the chromosomal trisomies and with many of the syndromes associated with congenital anomalies and short stature in later life. Severe placental pathology is a relatively uncommon cause of intrauterine growth retardation, but occasionally its effect can be striking. This is particularly true with large chorioangiomas of the placenta or with placentas associated with multiple small infarcts.

The obstetric management of pregnancies in which intrauterine growth retardation is suspected includes, first and foremost, attempts to confirm both the size of the infant and the gestational age. A useful test in this regard is repeated ultrasonic examinations with estimation of biparietal diameter, since this can be used both as an estimation of the size of the infant (from the velocity of growth of the biparietal diameter) and an estimation of gestational age. Transabdominal amniocentesis is used for additional evidence of the maturity of the infant by the measurement of the L/S ratio. The clinical significance of changes in various endocrinologic tests with intrauterine growth retardation is still unclear. However, such pregnancies should be monitored for intrapartum fetal distress by continuous fetal heart rate and intraamniotic pressure measurements. The incidence of fetal distress and birth asphyxia occurring during labor and delivery is quite high, presumably as a reflection of the various obstetric complications often present. Physicians involved in the delivery should anticipate the potential problem of meconium-aspiration pneumonitis (see Resuscitation, later in this chapter).

The neonatal management problems presented by SGA infants occur in the following general order: first, there is the problem of managing birth asphyxia and CNS depression secondary to birth asphyxia in the delivery room. The resuscitation of the infant may be further complicated by meconium-aspiration pneumonitis, since these relatively mature babies may pass meconium into a small amniotic fluid volume during labor and in response to asphyxia make strong gasping efforts, filling the tracheobronchial tree (see Resuscitation). Another problem is hypoglycemia. It is a reasonable practice to begin all SGA infants on an infusion of 10% glucose at 100 mL/kg per day for the first 12 to 24 hours of life. As the infant recovers from birth and shows good sucking and swallowing movements and sustained, vigorous hunger cries, he should be weaned to milk feedings and the intravenous infusions of glucose gradually tapered. Occasionally, despite an infusion of 10% glucose, an infant will develop hypoglycemia; thus all SGA infants should be followed with frequent measurements of blood glucose concentration. Ideally, blood glucose concentration should be maintained over 40 mg per 100 mL at all times. Some SGA infants, particularly male infants, will develop signs and symptoms associated with marked polycythemia and hyperviscosity. When capillary hematocrits greater than 75 or central hematocrits greater than 65 are noted, the polycythemia should be treated by a small exchange transfusion with plasma calculated to lower the central hematocrit to 50. Follow-up studies have suggested a poor outcome after neonatal polycythemia regardless of whether exchange transfusion was employed. Since the nutritional requirements of SGA infants are still ill-defined, we would prefer to have these babies on demand feedings whenever possible.

LARGE-FOR-GESTATIONAL-AGE INFANTS

The excessive-sized or large-for-gestational-age (LGA) infant is a much more difficult clinical group to define, in part because there is great variability in the 90th percentile in studies of gestational age-birth-weight distribution for different populations of infants. Also, the problems of LGA infants have received much less attention. In general, large infants show an increase in all body proportions, including body length and head circumference as well as birth weight. The infant born to a diabetic mother is an exception to this, since these infants have an increase in total body fat leading to an increased weight-length ratio. Follow-up studies on such infants in later childhood suggest that this alteration in body proportion persists throughout childhood. In contrast to SGA infants, who may be born with placentas varying markedly in weight, all LGA infants are born with large placentas, presumably reflecting the fact that total mass of placental tissue provides an absolute restriction on the maximum attainable size of the infant. LGA infants have a significantly higher mortality rate than infants appropriately grown. Much of the increased mortality may be attributed to mechanical problems arising at the time of delivery. Long labors associated with cephalopelvic disproportion may lead to severe fetal asphyxia and/or birth trauma in the infant, generally in the area of the head and neck. Head trauma may range all the way from a massive intracranial hemorrhage to a cephalohematoma whose only complication may be hyperbilirubinemia. The increased mortality rate of large infants includes the increased mortality rate of infants weighing approximately 3 kg and born prematurely. Such infants rarely receive the attention they deserve, since from size alone they appear to be appropriately grown term infants. However, such preterm LGA infants should be observed in intensive-care nurseries. Other obstetric trauma associated with the head or neck area includes peripheral nerve injuries of the cervical or brachial plexus (Erb's

palsy). One of the more serious complications of such injuries involves unilateral or bilateral phrenic-nerve paralysis, for which respirator care may be required. Peripheral nerve injuries should be followed carefully until full recovery of function in a limb is documented. During the recovery phase, attention should be paid to introducing passive exercises to avoid functional loss from immobilization.

Physicians can be forewarned of the likelihood of an LGA infant if there is an obstetric history of large-birth-weight babies. Since it is known that infant birth weight increases with increasing parity, a woman who has had an LGA infant in a first pregnancy can be suspected of having another excessive-sized infant in a subsequent pregnancy. When an LGA infant is suspected from abdominal examination or from a MacDonald's measurement (the distance along the curvature of the abdomen from the symphysis pubis to the top of the fundus), the diagnosis should be confirmed when possible by ultrasonic examination and estimation of biparietal diameter. If an LGA infant is recognized during the pregnancy, it is essential that the progress of labor be followed carefully and charted appropriately. Cesarean section is frequently necessary to avoid birth trauma.

Thus far three problems have been clearly associated with LGA infants: transposition of the aorta, Beckwith's syndrome, and maternal diabetes. Transposition of the aorta, a congenital cardiovascular anomaly, was shown in 1961 to be associated with LGA infants; the reason for this is unknown. Beckwith's syndrome, first described in 1963, is characterized by infants who are large in body weight and length and have associated anomalies including umbilical abnormalities, macroglossia, renal enlargement, and severe hypoglycemia in the neonatal period. Microcephaly and facial flame nevus are additional anomalies often present in Beckwith's syndrome. The unusual anomalies help to distinguish these infants from infants of diabetic mothers, who also are of large size and who often have hypoglycemia. Hypoglycemia in infants of diabetic mothers can be managed similarly to hypoglycemia occurring in SGA infants. Another common problem in infants of diabetic mothers is hypocalcemia; Tsang et al. reported an incidence of 60 percent in class B to D diabetics. A calcium concentration below 3 meq/L represents fairly severe hypocalcemia needing treatment. In practice, we would treat all infants with signs of jitteriness or tetany and calcium concentrations under 4 meq/L. Another problem is hypercoagulability, with or without associated polycythemia. For reasons which are still unknown, the infant of the diabetic mother is much more prone to complications related to clot formation and embolization. Vascular accidents, such as renal vein thrombosis, occur almost exclusively in infants of diabetic mothers. Only when hypercoagulability is coupled with an increased hematocrit and hyperviscosity has it been our practice to lower the capillary hematocrit by an appropriate small-volume exchange transfusion with plasma. It should be emphasized that many of the problems of LGA infants can be minimized or prevented by better management of labor and delivery and by prompt recognition of problems in the nursery area. Unfortunately, we still tend to equate "big" babies with "well" babies and thus still provide less observation to LGA infants than their mortality and morbidity rates would warrant.

ASPHYXIA

The fetus in utero has what appears to be a deficiency of oxygen. The arterial oxygen tension is about 25 mmHg in contrast to the maternal arterial P_{O_2} which is between 90 to 100 mmHg. Yet the fetal-tissue oxygen tension is normal and the fetus has a pH quite close to that of the mother (about 7.35). The fetus compensates for its lower P_{O_2} by an increased flow rate. This is accomplished by an increased cardiac output through widely dilated fetal vascular beds (particularly in the placenta and central nervous system). When the fetal oxygen tension drops, the fetus has peripheral vasoconstriction and CNS and coronary vasodilation, thus tending to protect the central nervous system and heart. The peripheral vasoconstriction further limits the oxygen supply to peripheral tissues (muscle, skin, gastrointestinal system, and renal system) forcing them to use anaerobic metabolism with the conversion of glucose to lactic acid. This lactic acidemia lowers the pH (metabolic acidosis). Continued lack of oxygen will cause reduced fetal cardiac efficiency with less oxygen pickup at the placenta, more anaerobic metabolism, increasing acidosis, and a continued downward spiral to CNS damage, and finally death of the fetus.

As pointed out earlier in this chapter, fetal O_2 supply is dependent on maternal intervillous space (IVS) blood flow, maternal-fetal oxygen pressure difference, placental surface area and distance between fetal and maternal blood. Since the prime factor in fetal oxygenation is maternal IVS blood flow, anything which interrupts maternal flow will cause some fetal hypoxia. The phenomenon most commonly responsible for an acute change in uterine blood flow is a uter-

ine contraction; blood flow is reduced by the increased myometrial pressure on the maternal arteries and arterioles. Thus, with each uterine contraction the fetus becomes relatively hypoxic. The fetal tolerance or response to hypoxia is based on the level and duration of oxygen lack and the available substrate for anaerobic metabolism, glucose. Since in a normal fetus the depth and duration of oxygen deficiency are small and the glucose reserves in the form of cardiac and hepatic glycogen are good, there is usually no response in the fetus and no difficulty associated with normal labor. If the contractions of labor are too frequent or last too long, then the fetus has a more significant drop in oxygen tension. This is usually associated with a deceleration of the fetal heart rate occurring late in the uterine contraction cycle (Chap. 28) and fetal acidosis.

Maternal uterine blood flow will also decrease when the patient becomes hypotensive, i.e., supine hypotension or following conduction anesthesia. In this situation it is important to restore circulating blood volume. This can be done by getting the uterus off the inferior vena cava (lateral position), thus allowing adequate venous return from the lower extremities, and giving crystalloids (5% dextrose in water or normal saline) intravenously.

In maternal vascular disease (hypertensive) there may be a chronic reduction of uterine blood flow leading not only to a chronically lower arterial P_{O_2} in the fetus but also to reduced glycogen stores. In this situation the fetus may not be acidotic when the uterus is quiescent; however, with uterine activity asphyxia is more profound and the fetal ability to tolerate it (with anaerobic metabolism) is reduced. Thus late decelerations and acidosis in the fetus are apparent sooner, and so is the likelihood of fetal brain damage. A situation similar to the above exists in the fetus with an abnormally small placenta or a placenta which has large infarcted areas. In essence, then, fetuses with chronic reduction in oxygen tolerate stress very poorly. This has led to the stress test (oxytocin-induced uterine contractions, maternal exercise, or maternal inhalation of 15 percent oxygen) for the elucidation of the compromised fetus. In this test one observes fetal heart rate and uterine activity during the antepartum period. If contractions are not spontaneously present they are induced with oxytocin to a frequency of 3 every 10 minutes. If the fetus has no late decelerations in response to these contractions, the test is considered a negative contraction stress test; it correlates very well with a fetus which will not die in utero within the next week (false-negative rate 6 to 10 per 1000). If the fetus shows late decelerations with the contractions, the fetus may or may not be compromised (there is a 50 percent false-positive rate). Recently, nonstress monitoring has become important in antepartum monitoring. In the non-stress test one observes the fetal heart rate response to fetal activity. A fetus that is well will move twice or more in a 20-minute period and the fetal heart rate will accelerate 15 beats per minute or more. A reactive fetus has a 0.2 to 1 percent chance of dying within 1 week of the test. As with a positive stress test, a non-reactive fetus does not necessarily indicate a sick fetus; in fact, it usually is not.

The therapy of fetal asphyxia depends on the etiology of the oxygen lack. In some instances simple maneuvers such as reducing the oxytocin infusion or turning the patient on her side will suffice. Increasing the maternal-arterial P_{O_2} by giving the mother pure oxygen to breathe through a mask may be beneficial through the elevation in the gradient between mother and fetus. If the fetus does not respond to conservative measures and continues to have late decelerations or shows acidosis, it should be delivered.

FETAL INFECTIONS

There are a variety of fetal infections which can cause problems in the newborn. Some are acquired trans-placentally, others after rupture of the membranes, and still others during the passage through the birth canal. A few of these will be discussed in more detail.

VIRAL INFECTIONS

Rubella

The virus of German measles is the most significant teratogen of all the viruses studied to date. The fetus becomes infected following maternal viremia through a placental and then fetal infestation with the virus. Since the fetus has an incompetent immunologic system, the virus persists for long periods, even up to an infant age of 19 to 20 months (Cooper et al.).

The percentage of fetuses affected depends on the date in gestation that the virus is acquired. Sever et al. found that if the maternal rubella was 0 to 28 days before conception, three of seven fetuses were normal. There was one congenital rubella syndrome, one abortion, and one stillbirth, and one infant had multiple infections for the first year of life. If the maternal infection was in the first trimester, about one-half either had congenital rubella or were aborted. If the infection was during the second trimester, about 20 percent had the stigmata. During the third trimester all fetuses that were followed were normal.

The fetal problems encountered also depend on the age of viral acquisition. During the first trimester congenital heart disease, cataracts, hearing loss, microcephaly, and mental retardation have all been reported. During the second trimester (early, 15 to 16 weeks) the above may be present but after 16 weeks hearing loss (nerve deafness) becomes the major problem.

Since a large proportion of those mothers infected with rubella during the first trimester may have an abnormal child and since it is now possible to legally abort patients, it is very important to establish with certainty whether rubella really is present. There are other viruses such as Coxsackie which will closely mimic the rubella virus without producing congenital anomalies. The diagnosis of rubella may be made by culturing the nasopharyngeal secretions. The nasopharynx and stool are positive for virus from 8 days before the rash to about 6 to 8 days after the rash disappears. The serum is positive for virus from 3 days prior to the rash to the onset of rash; thus it is not as useful as the nasopharynx to prove the disease (Heggie and Robbins). Another method of diagnosing in retrospect the presence of rubella is by following maternal antibody titers. The titer of antibodies will begin to rise within a week following the viremia and rises progressively for several weeks following the infection. Thus, if maternal antibody titers have increased fourfold within 2 weeks after a suspicious rash, a presumptive diagnosis of rubella may be made. The presence of a single antibody titer means only that the individual has had rubella at some time in the past, and conversely the presence of a negative titer indicates an individual susceptible to the disease. It is recommended that an antibody titer be drawn during the first prenatal visit. Subsequent sero-conversion then indicates a recent viremia.

The immunization of young girls with negative titers of rubella antibody is possible using attenuated strains of the virus. It is now recommended that this be done particularly for women in their reproductive years with a negative rubella titer. It is very important that pregnancy be prevented for 6 months after immunization because the fetus may become infected transplacentally with the virus. Fortunately, to date, none of the stigmata associated with the virus have been reported.

Cytomegalovirus

Cytomegalovirus infection is very common in pregnant women: cervical, 12 percent; urine, 6 percent; breast, 6 percent; and pharyngeal, 2 percent. The virus does cross the placenta and causes intrauterine infection with an incidence of 0.5 to 1.5 percent; however, a more common route of infection is acquisition of the virus during the birth process, 5 to 7 percent. The vast majority of infants infected with cytomegalovirus are thought to have few if any sequelae; however, recent studies by Reynolds with long-term follow-up of a small number of children (18) show a significant number may have hearing impairments or reduced intelligence levels. Overwhelming infection in the newborn can cause death, severe brain damage, or perceptual organ damage.

The presence of disease may be diagnosed by observing the virus in the tissues at autopsy where it appears as intranuclear or intracytoplasmic inclusion bodies in large swollen cells. The intranuclear bodies have a halo sign while the intracytoplasmic bodies are granular and basophilic staining. They may be found in almost any organ of the body but are particularly frequently seen in the brains of infants dying of the disease. The virus can be isolated and grown in culture and rising antibody titers may indicate infection.

Herpes Simplex

The herpes simplex type 2 virus is found in the reproductive tract (vagina and vulva) of many females, both pregnant and nonpregnant. There may be vesicular or ulcerative lesions that yield virus which may be cultured. Inclusion bodies may be seen on vaginal smear and the patient may have an antibody titer to the herpesvirus.

If active infection is present in the birth canal, the fetus may become infected during labor and delivery. The incidence of fetal infection in the presence of active disease is unknown. Fetal infection frequently results in death or brain damage and thus should be avoided. If active vaginal infection is present, the infant should be delivered by cesarean section rather than subjected to the possibility of acquiring the disease during passage through the birth canal. It is important that this be done before the membranes rupture or at least within 4 hours after their rupture. If the membranes have been ruptured longer than 4 hours or if there is evidence of virus in the amniotic fluid, vaginal delivery is recommended.

PROTOZOAL INFECTIONS

Toxoplasmosis

Toxoplasma gondii is a protozoal infection that is present in meats (pork and mutton particularly) and cat feces. The mode of maternal infestation is by eating partially cooked infected meats or through feline contact. The protozoa may infect the placenta and then the fetus if the mother has an acute infection (Feldman). If the fetus is infected (incidence 0.2 to 18 per 1000 live births) chorioretinitis, hydrocephalus, and cerebral calcifications may be the result. There may also be growth retardation, hepatosplenomegaly, and anemia. The death rate is 10 to 15 percent. Ten percent of the infants recover normally and the remaining 75 to 80 percent have some degree of central-nervous-system damage. This high degree of neurologic damage has led some to suggest all pregnant women be examined serologically for evidence of previous infection. If antibodies are present there is no danger; if absent the mother should avoid partially cooked meat and contact with cats. The current therapy with pyrimethamine and sulfadiazine has not been fully evaluated for efficacy and safety in pregnancy. In the newborn it may or may not prevent the disastrous sequelae of this disease.

SPIROCHETAL INFECTION

Syphilis

The incidence of syphilis has risen in recent years in the adult population, and thus it is very important that every pregnant mother have a blood test for antibodies both early in her pregnancy and also at 32 weeks. The screening test usually performed is a flocculation test (VDRL or Kline). If this is positive, a complement-fixation test (Kolmer) or *Treponema pallidum* immobilization test is usually done to confirm the diagnosis. If one of these is positive the mother should receive penicillin therapy or, if she is allergic to penicillin, erythromycin.

The spirochete does cross the placenta and infect the fetus. If the mother is actively treated the fetus has no difficulty; however, if the mother remains untreated the fetus may die in utero from overwhelming infection, may have symptoms of the disease at birth, or may develop symptoms within the first few weeks or months of life. The lesions most frequently involve skin, mucous membranes, hematologic systems, bone, and viscera. The frequently described rhinorrhea is due to infection in the nasal mucous membrane. Further progession destroys nasal cartilage and thus leads to the development of the saddle nose. The cutaneous lesions may be macular, nodular, circinate, or annular, and usually involve the palms of the hands, soles of the feet, face, or diaper area. Spirochetes can be recovered from these skin lesions. There may be hepato- or splenomegaly. X-ray of the long bones shows typical periostitis.

The diagnosis of infection will usually be suspect from the findings in the infant; however, a positive diagnosis may be made by spirochete identification, the presence of a specific gumma in the fetus, a higher serologic titer in the fetus than in the mother, or a rising titer in the newborn. Treatment is with penicillin and should not be delayed since therapy in the first few months of life may prevent serious problems later in infancy, such as pneumonia alba, saddle nose, etc.

ADAPTATION OF THE INFANT TO EXTRAUTERINE LIFE: "BIRTH SHOCK"

Many of the adaptations of the infant to extrauterine life represent acute and drastic changes in physiology; others are more subtle. The first expansion of the fluid-filled lung with air and the flooding of the lung with blood through the pulmonary circulation are adjustments which must occur within moments of delivery. Similarly, changes must occur in the general circulation: from a heart in which the right and left ventricles work in parallel and cardiac output is represented by the combined output of both ventricles to one in which the ventricles function in series and cardiac output is represented by the output of either ventricle. These are changes which are also fairly acute and occur as a result of closure of the foramen ovale and ductus arteriosus. The changes in the circulation occur more gradually than expansion of the lungs, generally being completed over some hours during the first day of life.

However, many other organs besides the circulation and the lungs are affected at this time. For example, cerebral function is affected by a number of different changes; the input to the brain from tactile, visual, and auditory stimuli is tremendously increased; cerebral blood flow, which is high in fetal life compared to that of the adult, falls at birth as arterial P_{O_2} rises and arterial P_{CO_2} falls. The concentration of glucose in the blood falls, thus the supply of glucose to the brain, which is represented by the product of cerebral blood flow times concentration, decreases. In addition, CNS function may be affected by varying degrees of intrauterine asphyxia or by various drugs which were used to medicate the mother during labor and delivery.

Gastrointestinal tract and liver functions are also altered with delivery. Prior to delivery, umbilical venous blood represented the blood containing the nutrients for growth (carbohydrates, fats, and amino acids) which perfused the fetal liver. Due to a series of organ buffers, this blood had a very constant concentration of nutrients, in the absence of maternal disease. For example, the maternal liver acts on the widely fluctuating concentrations in maternal-portal venous blood and tends to stabilize maternal-arterial concentrations; the placenta in turn is perfused by this arterial blood. The fetal liver then acts as a final buffer in adjusting fetal-arterial concentrations of carbohydrates, fats, and amino acids reaching the rapidly growing tissues in fetal life. By contrast, after birth the infant feeds intermittently; milk enters the GI (gastrointestinal) tract, is digested and absorbed into portal venous blood. Thus, the newborn liver is presented with nutrient concentrations which fluctuate widely from hour to hour. This requires that some essential endocrine adjustments be made in order to once again stabilize arterial concentrations in this new environment.

One can look to similar changes in other organ systems which are provoked by the transition from intra- to extrauterine life. It is not surprising that even the normal term baby delivered after an uncomplicated labor and delivery shows a period of recovery lasting some hours after birth. Some of these adjustments include changes in CNS reactivity, respiratory rate and pattern, presence or absence of bowel sounds, etc. For this reason the nurses can obtain a great deal of information about a baby if the infant is kept in an isolette for the first 4 or 5 hours after delivery, and not swaddled in blankets. This permits observations to be made on the infant's respirations, abdominal distention, color, activity, etc. Then, if the baby develops no problems and behaves normally, routine basinet care can begin. The "low risk" nursery can be more properly regarded as an observation nursery, with the observations being more intense during the first few hours after birth.

There are two problems in babies where the subsequent course can be altered markedly by proper observation and supportive care during this recovery period. The first problem is the relatively frequent one of birth asphyxia. When an infant has suffered some degree of asphyxia, during passage through the birth canal or during resuscitation, proper support, including the adjustment of oxygen concentrations, environmental temperature, and maintenance of glucose intake and hydration can make a marked difference in the severity of the signs the baby will continue to show over the next few days. If hypoglycemia, cooling, and hypoxia are prevented during the first 6 to 8 hours after birth, the infant will recover far more quickly from the combined stress of asphyxia and birth.

Pharmacologic problems are another general area requiring close observation during this time. We are just beginning to appreciate the multitude of ways in which an infant can be poisoned, either chronically in addicted mothers with the subsequent development of withdrawal signs, or acutely as in the case of local anesthetics or magnesium sulfate given to the mother. In the case of the withdrawal syndromes, sedation and supportive care are all that are required. With the acute intoxications, exchange transfusion of the infant may be necessary. Again, close observation during these first 4 to 6 hours immediately after birth by personnel that are trained to recognize changes in CNS "state" is all-important in alerting the physician to consider a variety of possible etiologies.

RESUSCITATION

It cannot be emphasized too strongly that whenever a high-risk pregnant patient is to be delivered, a physician whose *sole* concern will be the care of the infant should be present at the delivery. The effort is directed at five areas. In order of urgency these are (1) ventilation, (2) circulation, (3) temperature, (4) glucose regulation, and (5) hydration. In the presence of meconium staining of the amniotic fluid, resuscitation of the newborn should begin prior to completion of the delivery. After delivery of the infant's head but before the shoulders and chest leave the birth canal, nasopharyngeal and oral suction with a rubber catheter and De Lee trap should be undertaken. Using this approach, the incidence of meconium aspiration pneumonitis can be reduced (Carson et al). Each of these five areas will require more attention by the physician and nursing personnel as the severity of neonatal depression increases. Most of the infants who make weak respiratory efforts initially, but whose heart rates are over 100 per minute, will not require more than pharyngeal suctioning and supplemental oxygen. Their body temperature should be supported as in those with more severe CNS depression from intrapartum asphyxia. Temperature support consists first of drying the skin thoroughly with a towel, since the evaporative heat losses of the skin wet with amniotic fluid are enormous. It has been our practice to supplement the more traditional warmer with a radiant heater from above the infant in the belief that reliance upon two sources of heat support may increase the

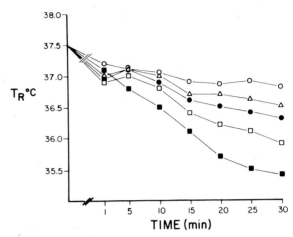

FIGURE 15–26 Mean deep body temperatures (T_R) of each group during the first 30 min of life. T_R is on the ordinate and time postdelivery on the abscissa. ■ = wet infants in room air; □ = dry infants in room air; ● = wet infants under the radiant heater; △ = dry infants wrapped in a blanket; ○ = dry infants under the radiant heater. *(From Dahm et al.)*

safety factor somewhat. The effectiveness of various forms of temperature support in the delivery room is demonstrated in Fig. 15–26 (Dahm and James). A cool environment may stress the infant in a number of ways: by increasing his metabolic rate and heat production, and by provoking a redistribution of blood flow from skin (and possibly from the splanchnic bed) to core tissues, thus increasing the potential for metabolic acidosis. A warm environment can and should be provided to all newborn infants, but it is especially important for the infant with varying degrees of birth asphyxia.

VENTILATION

Infants who do not begin spontaneous and adequate ventilation after brief suctioning of the oral and nasal pharynx particularly when there is meconium present will require intubation, cleansing the lower airway, and positive pressure ventilation. Someone *other than* the physician breathing for the baby should listen to the chest and confirm that air is being delivered in adequate amounts to both lung fields. In the initial resuscitation of severely depressed infants, 100 percent oxygen should be used until the physician is certain he has been able to correct the hypoxia. It is important to emphasize that during a resuscitation the physician controls the inspiratory phase; that is, he pushes air into the lungs, but the expiratory phase is out of his control, and this phase is very slow in fluid-filled lungs. For this reason it is important to breathe for the infant at a rate slow enough to allow expiration, a rate of 30 to 40 breaths per minute. If this is exceeded, one ends up with a barrel-chested infant, hyperexpanded, with little or no air moving in or out.

CIRCULATION

The infant with a high risk of mortality or morbidity because of size, gestational age, severe asphyxia, or erythroblastosis, etc., cannot be managed properly without access to the arterial circulation. This is required for respiratory gas measurements and secondarily is often used for blood pressure measurements and for infusions. Umbilical arterial catheterization remains the method of choice. It is simple and if proper technique is observed carries quite a low risk of complications. Table 15-3 presents a checklist of the precautions one should observe in arterial catheterization. Infants with birth asphyxia are often hypotensive. This should be treated by a rapid infusion of plasminate until whole blood is typed and available. It is extremely rare for sodium bicarbonate or epinephrine to be required during resuscitation. If the lungs have been properly ventilated and the hypotension of severe asphyxia corrected with volume expansion, the infant will rapidly metabolize lactate which is a perfectly suitable substrate for aerobic metabolism.

HYDRATION AND GLUCOSE REGULATION

After the baby with birth asphyxia has been resuscitated, it is wise to ensure adequate glucose intake

TABLE 15-3 Precautions with Umbilical Artery Catheters

1. Number 3½ French polyvinyl catheter, end hole, saline-filled.
2. Sterile preparation of umbilical stump and surrounding 6 cm of skin with organic iodide or tincture of iodine.
3. Radiologic confirmation of position in abdominal aorta.
4. On-line 0.2-μm filter between infusate and catheter.
5. Infusion by a constant-infusion pump with rapid start time.

and hydration by an infusion of 10% glucose at approximately 80 mL/kg per day. The larger and more mature babies will often move to nipple feeding far more quickly, and then the intraarterial or peripheral venous infusion can be discontinued. However, babies who have had severe birth asphyxia will have a prolongation of the normal GI adjustments occurring after birth. They should not be fed until bowel sounds are normal and other aspects of the physical exam satisfactory. It is much easier to prevent than to treat problems of hypoglycemia and dehydration. Thus, the goal is to establish an adequate glucose and water intake by intravenous or intraarterial infusions. This enables the physician to evaluate the possibility of oral feedings more objectively and without the additional pressure of impending hypoglycemia or dehydration.

METABOLIC DISORDERS IN THE NEWBORN

Disorders in metabolic adjustments of the newborn infant are the most common problems encountered in a modern nursery. The necessary adjustments from intrauterine to extrauterine life are extensive, and often the conditions of extrauterine life impose stresses upon an infant with which he cannot cope. In addition, abnormalities of the prepartum period (e.g., maternal diabetes) and intrapartum period (e.g., asphyxia) may add further stresses which become apparent only in the neonatal period.

WATER AND ELECTROLYTE HOMEOSTASIS

HYPONATREMIA

Water crosses the placenta readily, while ions such as Na^+, Cl^-, and K^+ cross very slowly. Therefore, rapid administration of hypotonic fluids to a patient in labor or during delivery can be associated with hypotonicity and hyponatremia in the neonate. There is no net deficit in the infant's sodium pool, but rather a dilutional hyponatremia. Administration of hypotonic fluids (5 or 10% dextrose in water) to a patient in labor should be done with caution and at a rate that does not exceed the ability of the maternal kidney to excrete water. When rapid fluid administration is required during labor, isotonic fluids (Ringer's lactate, normal saline, etc.) are more appropriate.

Hyponatremia in the fetus or newborn infant is a reflection of maternal hyponatremia, not of changes in maternal total body sodium. Occasionally, routine maternal diuretic therapy and a salt-restricted diet may be associated with neonatal hyponatremia. Sporadic therapy with potent diuretics likewise is unlikely to result in neonatal hyponatremia, but an aggressive diuretic regimen, which is occasionally used in preeclampsia, can lead to significant neonatal hyponatremia. Frequently, a combination of these risk factors occurs in a given patient, and thus the cumulative risk of neonatal hyponatremia is high.

Neonatal hyponatremia is nearly always a result of water overload rather than sodium deficit. It occurs frequently in an intensive-care nursery and generally is iatrogenic, from excessive water administration either in the intrapartum period or in the nursery. CNS insults, such as asphyxia, intracranial hemorrhage, meningitis, or birth trauma, may also be associated with hyponatremia, presumably as a result of inappropriate antidiuretic hormone (ADH). A low-salt syndrome with associated hyponatremia can occur in infants who require aggressive diuretic therapy. Abnormal sodium losses can also occur in infants with surgical diseases requiring constant gastric or high-intestinal drainage, if not corrected by appropriate fluid replacement.

In most cases hyponatremia is a benign disorder and is not associated with significant management problems, morbidity, or mortality. Diuretic-induced low-salt syndrome is an exception; an infant who requires such therapy (congestive heart failure, biliary atresia, etc.) and develops hyponatremia is a most difficult management problem. Continued diuresis is difficult in such a situation, and any attempt to correct the sodium deficit only aggravates the expanded extracellular volume. Symptomatology from neonatal hyponatremia is rare. We have not seen seizures occur in association with it. Efforts to correct the sodium concentration should be directed at water restriction and slow return of the sodium to normal levels. Such efforts should be tempered, however, by the knowledge that most hyponatremia is entirely benign, and any restriction of fluid should not be done at the risk of causing other problems, e.g., hypoglycemia, which carry significant risks. The routine administration of isotonic or hypertonic fluids in an effort to repair sodium deficits is generally contraindicated in the newborn period. Prevention of hyponatremia by appropriate fluid administration is the most sensible approach.

HYPERNATREMIA

Hypernatremia is always of iatrogenic origin and carries a significant mortality risk. Because maternal hypernatremia is exceedingly rare, hypernatremia rarely occurs in the immediate newborn period. It is usually a result of sodium bicarbonate administration to the infant for correction of neonatal acidosis.

The incidence of hypernatremia is dependent upon the indications used for sodium bicarbonate administration. By tempering our use of bicarbonate in the management of acidosis, we have reduced our incidence of hypernatremia from 8.8 percent to 0.6 percent. During the years when aggressive bicarbonate therapy was practiced at our hospital, the mortality rate associated with hypernatremia was 80 percent, with a 100 percent mortality in infants with sodium concentrations over 160 meq/L. The dangers of hypertonicity in the face of dehydration are clear, but only anecdotal evidence exists about the risks of hypertonicity in the presence of normovolemia. The experimental evidence implicating hypertonicity in the etiology of intracranial hemorrhage is fairly well established. In association with the decline in incidence of hypernatremia on our neonatal intensive-care unit, the incidence of intracranial hemorrhage fell from 13.6 percent to 2.6 percent. Since the occurrence of hypernatremia is directly related to the use of sodium bicarbonate, the risks of neonatal acidosis have to be balanced against the risks of hypernatremia and hypertonicity. We limit sodium bicarbonate administration to patients with a *metabolic* acidosis and prefer not to exceed 5 meq/kg per day.

The treatment of hypernatremia is a difficult problem. The risks of rapid correction with the administration of hypotonic fluids are greatly feared but not well documented. Similar reservations exist for the rapid correction by exchange transfusion. A prudent approach is to lower the sodium concentration to normal over a 24-hour period by administration of fluids of appropriate tonicity.

FLUID AND ELECTROLYTE REQUIREMENTS

Regimens for fluid administration in the neonate reflect the recognition of the large insensible water losses which occur even in the infant who is relatively unstressed, and the inability of the immature kidney to concentrate efficiently. It is important in the face of immature renal function to provide fluid intake that meets insensible water losses and allows the kidney to excrete a moderately hypotonic urine (~150 mosm/L).

Traditionally it has been felt that in the first 2 days of life only small amounts of fluid need to be supplied exogenously. The fasting and thirsting regimen of the 1950s has now fallen into disfavor, but in general fluid administration volumes are reduced during the first 2 days of life. There has also been a tendency to withhold electrolyte administration for the first 2 days, but this seems unwise, given the volumes of water now recommended over the first 2 days.

In general, volumes of 75 mL/kg per day, increasing to 100 mL/kg per day over the first 2 days, meet a neonate's requirements without threatening the concentrating or diluting capacity of the immature kidney. A similar empiric system would provide between 100 and 120 mL per day per 100 calories metabolized. Sodium can be supplied at the rate of 3 meq per 100 mL fluid administered and potassium at the rate of 1 to 2 meq per 100 mL of fluid. Approximately half of the anion supplied should be metabolizable (HCO_3^-,) rather than in the form of Cl^-.

All empiric maintenance fluid regimens assume insensible water losses of 40 to 50 mL/kg per day and thus do not apply to infants who are under stress. Neonates allowed to remain outside a neutral thermal zone can easily double their heat production and thus their insensible water losses. Insensible water losses as high as 200 mL/kg per day have been described in very small infants. Recent nursery practices, such as the use of phototherapy or of open radiant heaters and the trend toward low-humidity incubators, have introduced additional factors increasing insensible water losses.

It is clear that empiric regimens are only a guide. Not only do unusual losses modify the initial empiric approach, but infants may vary quite markedly in their maintenance fluid requirements. Changes in serum protein concentration (or total serum solids), serum osmolality, and serum electrolytes must be followed in evaluating an infant's water and electrolyte balance.

Careful recording of urine output and urine specific gravity is the easiest and most reliable parameter in following hydration. Urine-flow rates of less than 2 mL/kg per hour or greater than 5 mL/kg per hour are regarded as abnormal, and appropriate corrective steps are taken. Urine-specific gravities outside the range 1.005 to 1.011 (reflecting a urine osmolality of approximately 150 mosm/L) are similarly abnormal and are followed closely and treated appropriately. Normal newborns may lose up to 10 to 12 percent of their body weight in the first 5 days of life because of alterations in water spaces. Such changes should also be expected, perhaps in exaggerated form, in

preterm infants. Therefore, close monitoring of body weight in an effort to allow appropriate weight loss (1 to 3 percent of body weight per day) is a reasonable objective.

ACID-BASE HOMEOSTASIS

The relationship between maternal and fetal blood pH, [HCO_3^-], and P_{CO_2} has been discussed in previous sections. Clearly, maternal acid-base status must be evaluated for a proper interpretation of fetal scalp pH measurements. Usually acidosis in the fetus or newborn infant is a result of poor oxygenation, with a shift to anaerobic metabolism and the resulting production of lactic acid, etc. Cord blood P_{CO_2} is not a reliable predictor of intrapartum acid-base status, as transient cord compression can lead to elevations in P_{CO_2} in the infant which are of little physiologic significance. A low pH and a negative base excess are better measures of significant intrauterine acidosis.

Disorders of acid-base balance occur in many neonatal diseases. The respiratory distress syndrome is characterized by hypercapnia ($\uparrow P_{CO_2}$), and a coincident metabolic acidosis often exists. When such a metabolic acidosis is identified, the probability of underperfusion of tissues from inadequate cardiac output or a maldistribution of cardiac output should be considered. Treatment requires support of intravascular volume and serial measurements useful in evaluating circulatory status (blood pressure, central venous pressure, urine output, and urine-specific gravity). The adminstration of alkali should be restricted to the correction solely of a *metabolic* acidosis and limited in total osmolar load. Hypercapnia alone affects the in vivo standard bicarbonate concentration (or calculated base excess), and thus the negative base excess measured in an infant must be corrected for the level of hypercapnia before evaluating the degree and type of acidosis with regard to a choice of therapy. Unfortunately, there are no reliable data on the risks of acidosis itself. Since acidosis often occurs simultaneously with hypoxia and poor perfusion, it is difficult to distinguish independent hazards from acidosis. In a child who is adequately oxygenated and perfused, there is no rationale for the rapid or aggressive treatment of acidosis per se. It should be obvious that acidosis resulting from CO_2 retention (respiratory acidosis) can be effectively treated, if indicated, only by intervention with ventilatory techniques designed to lower the P_{CO_2}.

Other causes of acidosis can occur in the neonatal period. Late metabolic acidosis of prematurity remains an incompletely understood entity. This is an acidosis characterized by a depletion in the total bicarbonate pool, which occurs infrequently in premature infants who are otherwise well, in the second or third week of life. It is apparently secondary to retention of anionic products of protein catabolism (SO_4^{2-}, PO_4^{3-}). Protein intakes of over 5 g/kg are most commonly associated with this syndrome. The pH in such infants is usually around 7.25, with a serum bicarbonate of 12 to 15 meq/L. The acidosis may be associated with poor weight gain. It can be corrected rapidly either by eliminating protein intake for 24 hours or by the addition of 1 to 3 meq/kg per day of oral $NaHCO_3$ to the diet.

Persistent metabolic acidosis in a newborn should prompt an immediate search for an inborn error of metabolism. Disorders in amino acid catabolism (tyrosinemia, phenylalanemia, maple syrup urine disease, etc.), urea cycle enzymes (ornithine transcarbamylase deficiency, argininosuccinicaciduria), and shortchain organic acid catabolism (methylmalonic aciduria, propionic aciduria) can all cause acidosis in the newborn period. Any child with a persistent metabolic acidosis should have such causes ruled out.

GLUCOSE HOMEOSTASIS

The glucose required by the fetus is met by transplacental glucose uptake, so an abrupt change necessarily occurs at the time of birth, coincident with the loss of the placenta. A normal newborn has hepatic glycogen stores of approximately 2 to 3 g/kg which, in the absence of additional glucose supply or exogenous glucose administration, would meet the newborn's glucose requirements for only 12 to 24 hours. Recent work has demonstrated that active gluconeogenesis is present in the normal newborn infant.

Hypoglycemia is a common, serious, and *preventable* occurrence on an intensive-care nursery service. The exact incidence of hypoglycemia depends upon the definition one prefers, and there continues to be controversy about how low a "normal" glucose can be. Problems in the timing and method of collection, specimen handling, and laboratory methodology further compromise efforts at defining normal glucose levels. In the past, values above 20 mg per 100 mL in low-birth-weight and above 30 mg per 100 mL in term infants have been regarded as normal. Recently many have challenged the concept of 2 standard deviations below the mean as a normal glucose concentration. Such a definition is of little bi-

ologic significance and may significantly underestimate abnormal glucose levels. When considering the glucose levels present during fetal life, it is difficult to regard concentrations of glucose as low as 20 mg per 100 mL as physiologic. Furthermore, one should not expect a simple relationship between glucose concentration and clinical symptoms. Glucose supply to the brain will be a function of both concentration and cerebral blood flow. In the newborn period both blood flow and concentration are changing. Clinically we are able to measure only concentration. Thus, we have regarded blood glucose levels of < 30 mg per 100 mL as an absolute indication for therapy and aim to maintain glucose concentrations above 40 mg per 100 mL.

Using a definition for hypoglycemia of 30 mg per 100 mL (see Fig. 15-27), Lubchenco et al. have confirmed that SGA infants of all gestational ages have a high incidence of hypoglycemia. In addition, LGA infants who are preterm are also at high risk for hypoglycemia. There was no greater incidence of hypoglycemia in other LGA age groups and only a minimally increased incidence in the preterm, appropriate-for-gestational-age group.

FIGURE 15-27 Incidence of hypoglycemia in newborn infants, classified by birth weight and gestational age. Glucose levels < 30 mg per 100 mL prior to first feeding. *(From Lubchenco et al.)*

INCIDENCE OF HYPOGLYCEMIA PRIOR TO FIRST FEED
(Glucose < 30 mgm%)

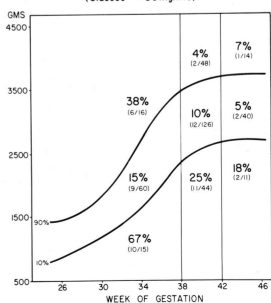

The etiology of hypoglycemia in the SGA infant is thought to be deficient glycogen stores. Although increased glucose demand could play some role, most studies do not confirm a hypermetabolic state in SGA infants, and thus increased glucose utilization is probably not of significance in the production of hypoglycemia. It seems unlikely that deficient glycogen stores alone account for the high incidence of hypoglycemia in SGA infants. With relatively limited glycogen stores in all preterm newborn infants, it is probable that other deficits exist in carbohydrate homeostasis. Recent evidence suggests that such infants may have a defect in gluconeogenesis and cannot respond to a falling blood glucose concentration with increased utilization of gluconeogenic substrate (alanine, glycine, glutamine, lactate).

Infants of appropriate size for gestational age who have had significant intrapartum stress are also at higher risk for the development of hypoglycemia. This phenomenon may be due to glycogen depletion or to exhaustion of hormonal regulation mechanisms. Hypoxia and hypothermia can also be associated with hypoglycemia. Similar mechanisms have been implicated in the production of hypoglycemia in infants with erythroblastosis fetalis, although these infants are known to have islet-cell hyperplasia and may be hyperinsulinemic. By the criteria of the usual clinical neurologic examination, neonatal hypoglycemia is often "asymptomatic"; therefore all infants at risk of hypoglycemia require routine glucose determinations. Such general clinical signs as cyanosis, jitteriness, lethargy, abnormal cry, apnea or abnormal respiratory pattern, and poor feeding may be seen in symptomatic infants. Initial screening with Dextrostix is adequate for identification of those infants with a glucose concentration less than 40 mg per 100 mL, and infants so identified must then have a laboratory glucose determination performed.

Treatment for hypoglycemia relies on the administration of exogenous glucose. Usually the infusion of a 10% dextrose solution, initially at rates of 100 to 150 mL/kg per day, is adequate to raise the glucose concentration to acceptable levels. The administration of higher glucose concentrations is rarely necessary, but if a bolus of concentrated glucose seems indicated, it should be diluted to 20% dextrose and infused slowly over a 5- to 10-minute period. After a stable and satisfactory blood glucose level has been established, a 10% dextrose infusion at a rate of 100 mL/kg per day is continued and then gradually tapered. Frequent blood sugar determinations should be made, and if hypoglycemia again supervenes, the infusate concentration of dextrose should be increased gradually.

The use of glucagon for the treatment of hypoglycemia is ill-advised. Since many newborns with hypoglycemia have deficient glycogen stores, glucagon will not be effective in raising the blood glucose concentration. Even in infants with adequate stores, the amount of glucose mobilizable by glucagon is small in comparison to the amounts that can be administered exogenously. Similar arguments can be made against the use of epinephrine, and such therapy is not indicated. In the patient with refractory hypoglycemia, the intravenous administration of hydrocortisone in a dosage of 2 to 5 mg/kg per day in four divided doses is sometimes successful.

In the infant of the diabetic mother, hypoglycemia results from quite different pathophysiologic mechanisms. Persistent elevated glucose levels in the mother cause a constant stimulation of the fetus' islet cells and consequent hyperinsulinemia. As long as the transplacental glucose supply is adequate, the only apparent hazard from the hyperinsulinemia is the excessive glycogen and adipose tissue which is deposited, leading to excessively large infants. However, the removal of the constant glucose supply at birth leaves the infant hyperinsulinemic in the absence of adequate substrate, and hypoglycemia frequently results.

After delivery there is a more profound fall in blood glucose in infants of insulin-dependent diabetics than of gestational diabetics, but both groups have significantly lower glucose concentrations than normal neonates by 2 hours of age. The majority of such infants raise their glucose levels spontaneously by 4 hours of age without exogenous glucose administration.

The approach to therapy in the hypoglycemia of infants of diabetic mothers varies considerably. Close monitoring of blood glucose and early oral feeding seem entirely acceptable in asymptomatic infants. However, in those infants with glucose levels below 30 mg per 100 mL it has been our policy to administer intravenous 10% dextrose. The use of intravenous glucose runs the risk of rebound hyperinsulinemia and a protracted course in the weaning of the infant from parenteral glucose therapy.

The morbidity rate in infants of diabetic mothers is increased, but this seems more related to the other complications in such patients (congenital anomalies, prematurity, respiratory distress syndrome, hyperbilirubinemia, clotting disorders, hypocalcemia) than to the disorder in carbohydrate metabolism.

Although neonatal hypoglycemia may contribute to neurologic handicaps, it is likely that some of the coexistent problems in SGA infants (congenital anomalies, intrauterine infection, etc.) and stressed infants (hypoxia, shock, etc.) may be more responsible than hypoglycemia per se for the poor outlook. Nonetheless, hypoglycemia remains an easily preventable and treatable entity, and no infant should be allowed to develop hypoglycemia in the present-day nursery.

Other disorders of carbohydrate metabolism can occur in neonates. Beckwith's syndrome is associated with hypoglycemia, and leucine-sensitive hypoglycemia can also occur in the newborn. Several infants with refractory hypoglycemia have proved to have islet-cell tumors, occasionally in extrapancreatic sites. Rarely, such an infant has no identifiable tumor but responds to subtotal pancreatectomy.

The occurrence of transient diabetes in the newborn is well described. Most often these infants are SGA, recover spontaneously, and require no prolonged insulin therapy. On rare occasions permanent diabetes mellitus, with life-long insulin dependence, begins in the newborn period. Ketosis in the newborn period is rare in infants with either transient or permanent diabetes.

CALCIUM HOMEOSTASIS

The fetus has calcium concentrations (total calcium, ionized calcium and ultrafilterable calcium) proportional to but slightly higher than those in the mother, presumably as a result of active calcium transport across the placenta. Any abnormality in maternal calcium balance may be reflected in the fetus. In normal infants, the calcium concentrations fall after birth to below normal adult levels, presumably as a result of parathyroid suppression. Calcium concentrations in the newborn remain low for the first 2 to 3 days of life and then gradually rise to normal levels.

Even in the absence of maternal parathyroid disease, "early" hypocalcemia (within the first 48 hours of postnatal life) is a common finding in premature infants, SGA infants, infants of diabetic mothers, and infants with neonatal asphyxia. The etiology of hypocalcemia in these infants had been presumed to be due to parathormone resistance. However, recent studies suggest that these infants do respond to parathormone and suggest that the primary defect is in parathormone output by the neonatal parathyroid gland. Since newborns, particularly infants with asphyxia or other perinatal stresses, may have elevated serum phosphate concentrations, serum calcium concentrations are depressed when an immature parathyroid cannot induce phosphate excretion by increasing parathormone output. In addition, premature infants (particularly those under 32 weeks of gesta-

tional age) have much lower total body calcium stores, and their dietary calcium intakes are also quite low.

A rare cause of early-onset hypocalcemia is maternal hyperparathyroidism. A high maternal calcium level may cause a high fetal calcium concentration which stimulates fetal parathyroid function. After birth, a significant fall in the newborn's calcium concentration occurs. Hypocalcemia in the first day of life without obvious cause (prematurity, intrauterine growth retardation, asphyxia) should prompt a search for maternal hyperparathyroidism. The occurrence of "early" hypocalcemia may be the first clue to the diagnosis of an otherwise symptom-free maternal disease. A diagnosis can be made in the mother by serum Ca, P, and alkaline phosphatase levels.

In contrast to the obvious symptoms in late-onset hypocalcemia, infants with early-onset disease may be symptom-free. Routine determination of calcium levels in low-birth-weight and premature infants have identified a great number of infants who were not obviously symptomatic. Up to 35 percent of low-birth-weight infants have serum calcium concentrations less that 7 mg per 100 mL. When these infants do have symptoms, they are generally those of increased irritability, high-pitched cry, and jitteriness. Hypocalcemia has been shown to be associated with a higher incidence of apnea in such infants (Fig. 15–28).

The existence of late-onset hypocalcemia has been well recognized for many years and is due to

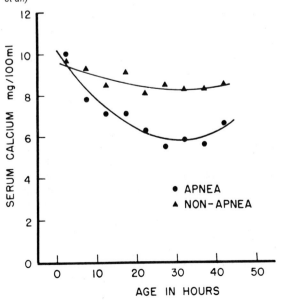

FIGURE 15–28 Relationship of serum calcium concentration to age in hours for infants with and without apnea. *(From Gershanik et al.)*

the excessive phosphate loads in cow's milk formulas. Not only are absolute phosphorus concentrations higher in cow's milk than in human milk (500 mg/L vs. 150 mg/L), but the calcium/phosphorus ratio is also much lower (1.3 vs. 2.3). The added phosphate load exceeds the neonatal kidney's ability to excrete phosphate, leading to hyperphosphatemia and hypocalcemia. Late-onset hypocalcemia occurs between 1 and 2 weeks of age in otherwise healthy infants. These infants develop irritability, jitteriness, a high-pitched cry, poor feeding, frank clonus, and finally seizures. They are hyperreflexic on physical examination and may have a demonstrable Chvostek's sign.

The definition of hypocalcemia varies considerably among different newborn centers. Normal calcium concentrations are approximately 5 meq/L or 10 mg per 100 mL. However, it is the ionized, non-protein-bound fraction of this total serum calcium that is of physiologic importance. Since approximately 40 percent of serum calcium is protein-bound, total serum calcium is highly dependent on total serum protein concentration. There are often instances when low serum protein concentrations are associated with apparent hypocalcemia, but ionized calcium concentration remains normal and the patient is free of symptoms. The McLean-Hastings nomogram can be used to assess the impact of hypoproteinemia on total and ionized serum calcium concentrations. Since newborns are frequently hypoproteinemic, it is important to consider the degree of hypoproteinemia before diagnosing hypocalcemia. When they become available for clinical use, calcium electrodes will simplify diagnosis by measuring calcium activity directly.

The decision to treat hypocalcemia is empiric. In the presence of seizures, immediate intravenous administration of calcium is indicated. Infants with other signs (jitteriness, irritability, etc.) should also be treated. There is no evidence that asymptomatic hypocalcemia carries any risk if it is not treated. However, we have elected to treat any infant with a calcium concentration below 7.5 mg per 100 mL, assuming a total protein content of at least 4 g per 100 mL. Calcium gluconate (*not* calcium chloride, the use of which should be discouraged in the newborn) is given intravenously in a dose of 100 to 150 mg/kg every 6 to 8 hours until the infant's calcium concentration has stabilized in the normal range. Oral administration of calcium may be added in such infants.

Other causes of neonatal hypocalcemia are quite rare. Familial hypoparathyroidism is not usually evident in the nursery. However, one form of hypoparathyroidism is being recognized more frequently in the nursery. Di George's syndrome is a disorder of the development of the third and fourth pharyngeal arches which leads to partial or complete absence of the thymus and parathyroid glands, often in association with anomalies of the aortic arch. These infants, who have characteristic features of a subtle midline nasal cleft and a short upper lip with a fish-mouth appearance, may have severe cardiac problems. They develop hypocalcemia in the nursery and, because of impaired cellular immunity, often have severe infections.

MAGNESIUM HOMEOSTASIS

Neonatal hypomagnesemia is being recognized with increasing frequency. The pathophysiology of magnesium regulation is similar to calcium regulation. Hypomagnesemia generally coexists with hypocalcemia; in our nursery, hypomagnesemia has never been found in the absence of hypocalcemia, although this has been described at other centers.

Normal serum magnesium concentrations must be defined in each laboratory. The approach to therapy is similar to the rationale used in the treatment of hypocalcemia; that is, treatment is restricted to symptomatic infants. Magnesium sulfate can be given in a dose of 100 mg/kg intravenously and repeated every 6 to 8 hours as required.

As parenteral hyperalimentation becomes more routine, the occurrence of hypomagnesemia could become more common. Hyperalimentation solutions should have adequate magnesium supplements, and hypomagnesemia should be ruled out in any child who exhibits neurologic signs while receiving hyperalimentation.

Although hypercalcemia is rarely encountered in the newborn age group, the occurrence of hypermagnesemia can be a problem in the infant. Babies delivered from toxemic or eclamptic pregnancies in which magnesium sulfate has been used can have hypermagnesemia. Generally the elevation in serum magnesium concentration is modest and of no clinical significance. Levels over 8 meq/L can be associated with serious problems. Careful monitoring of maternal serum magnesium concentrations should be encouraged. Hypermagnesemia in infants can cause hypotonia, hyporeflexia, primary apnea, and, in concert with its mild diuretic effect, urinary retention. Treatment is entirely supportive, with careful attention to serum calcium levels. Usually the neuromuscular depression improves spontaneously over the first 6 to 12 hours of life. Severe hypermagnesemia can be treated successfully by exchange transfusion.

PYRIDOXINE DEFICIENCY AND DEPENDENCY

Investigation of the disorders in pyridoxine (vitamin B_6) metabolism provides an excellent example of the complex interrelationships of fetal and maternal metabolism. Pyridoxine deficiency as a cause of seizures in infants was well described in the mid-1950s; the large group of infants with such seizures were all on a diet markedly deficient in pyridoxine. Their seizures and abnormal EEGs responded promptly to replacement therapy with pyridoxine. Primary pyridoxine deficiency in the neonatal period became rare as infant formulas were routinely supplemented with pyridoxine and then prepared in a manner that did not destroy the vitamin.

Although it is uncommon, pyridoxine deficiency in a mother can lead to diminished stores in the fetus and result in a neonate at risk of seizures soon after birth. It is now clear that long-term therapy with isoniazid can lead to pyridoxine deficiency, and therefore any mother on isoniazid therapy should have routine pyridoxine replacement. Infants born to mothers receiving isoniazid should be considered at risk of pyridoxine deficiency.

During the same period of time, several infants with neonatal seizures which responded to pharmacological doses of pyridoxine were identified. It may be that some of these infants were pyridoxine-dependent because they had adjusted to high concentrations of pyridoxine during intrauterine life, secondary to an excessive maternal intake of the vitamin. This would then be an example of a substance provided in excess during pregnancy that can lead to significant symptomatology in the newborn period when high concentrations are withdrawn.

It is now clear that most infants with such "pyridoxine dependency" have a deficit in the apoenzyme which binds the cofactor to pyridoxine and that their dependency is not related to maternal pyridoxine intake or serum concentration. "Pyridoxine dependency" is one example of an increasingly common group of vitamin-resistant syndromes, all of which are characterized by at least partial correction with pharmacological doses of the respective vitamin (vitamin B_{12} in the responsive form of methylmalonic aciduria, vitamin D in vitamin D–resistant rickets). When such dependency exists in the newborn, seizures are invariable and respond promptly to pyridoxine administration.

Seizures in the newborn can be of diverse etiology, but those seizure states due to hypoglycemia, hypocalcemia, and pyridoxine deficiency or dependency can be reversed rapidly. In any infant with seizures, blood specimens for glucose, calcium, and magnesium should be obtained and then, preferably with EEG monitoring, glucose, calcium, and pyridoxine should be administered serially. If a specific injection results in clinical improvement accompanied by disappearance of seizure activity on the EEG, a presumptive diagnosis can be made. In infants with pyridoxine dependency, continued high-dose supplementation is necessary.

HYPERBILIRUBINEMIA

Bilirubin is the final product in the catabolism of heme, with 1 g of hemoglobin yielding 34 mg of bilirubin. Damaged, abnormal, antibody-sensitized, or senescent erythrocytes are removed from the circulation into the reticuloendothelial system, where hemoglobin is catabolized to bilirubin. In adults, up to 90 percent of bilirubin production results from such destruction of circulating erythrocytes. In the newborn, as much as 30 percent of bilirubin production comes from sources other than the circulating red-cell mass. Bilirubin is transported from the reticuloendothelial system to the liver by albumin, where it is cleared by the parenchymal cells of the liver. Here bilirubin is rapidly conjugated to glucuronate and excreted into the bile in the conjugated or polar form. Minimal excretion of unconjugated bilirubin occurs via any pathway.

Exact estimates of intrauterine fetal bilirubin production are not available, but it is assumed that there is a significant production of bilirubin under normal conditions even though fetal bilirubin levels are not elevated. Unconjugated lipid-soluble bilirubin crosses the placenta more readily than the conjugated water-soluble form. Thus the "immaturity" of the conjugation mechanism in the fetus is an adaptive mechanism for transplacental excretion of this waste product. Bilirubin appears in the amniotic fluid early in gestation and is detectable until just before term. The exact pathway for bilirubin appearance in amniotic fluid is unknown, but its presence has been of great clinical benefit in monitoring Rh-isoimmunized pregnancies.

The rapid increase in bilirubin concentration immediately after birth in hemolytic disease demonstrates the quantitative importance of intrauterine transplacental bilirubin excretion. The normal adult pathways for bilirubin excretion (hepatic conjugation and subsequent excretion into the biliary tree) are less active in the newborn, and unconjugated hyperbilirubinemia (greater than 2 mg per 100 mL) occurs universally in the neonate. The immaturity of glucuronyl transferase in the newborn has been regarded as the primary cause of "physiologic jaundice." The hyperbilirubinemia usually peaks on the third or fourth day of life and then falls rapidly as the conjugation mechanism matures. Recently, other causes of physiologic hyperbilirubinemia have been suggested. There is clearly an increased load of bilirubin in the newborn period resulting from the shortened red-cell survival and the increased red-cell volume of the newborn. Diminished gastrointestinal function may lead to a significantly increased enterohepatic circulation of bilirubin and thus elevated bilirubin concentrations. It has been shown that the abrupt changes in the circulatory supply to the liver which occur at birth may lead to impaired liver function; i.e., if the ductus venosus remains patent, portal blood bypasses the liver, resulting in diminished bilirubin clearance.

Hyperbilirubinemia occurs occasionally in breast-fed infants. Most of the time this is a reflection of the decreased caloric intake and decreased stools until breast-feeding is well established. No specific therapy is required unless the bilirubinemia is extreme. Rarely the elevated bilirubin occurs because the breast milk contains concentrations of Δ^5, pregnanediol, which inhibits glucuronyl transferase. Rare cases of a maternally derived plasma factor which also inhibits conjugation have been described.

The differential diagnosis of hyperbilirubinemia continues to be a difficult problem in neonatal medicine. The occurrence of jaundice is such a common finding in newborn infants that potential pathologic causes must be ruled out in a great number of infants. Table 15–4 lists various etiologies associated with hyperbilirubinemia in the newborn. Because of the variety of causes of jaundice in the newborn, no infant can be regarded as having physiologic jaundice without careful thought and investigation. Often jaundice is the first clue to serious illness in an infant, such as sepsis, galactosemia, or hypothyroidism.

The attention paid to bilirubin by pediatricians reflects the seriousness of the potential sequelae to hyperbilirubinemia. Unlike the adult, who seems to be relatively resistant to toxic effects of bilirubin, the newborn infant is usually sensitive to central-nervous-system damage from high serum bilirubin concentrations. Kernicterus is technically a pathological diagnosis (staining of basal ganglia), but it has certain clinical correlates which are nearly pathognomic, including athetotic cerebral palsy and deafness.

TABLE 15–4 Etiology of Hyperbilirubinemia

I. Increased bilirubin production
  A. Hemolytic processes
    1. Isoimmunization (Rh, AO, BO; minor group)
    2. Red-cell enzyme defects (GGPD, pyruvate-kinase)
    3. Hereditary red-cell deformities (spherocytosis, elliptocytosis
    4. Oxidant-induced hemolysis (vitamin K_3, etc.)
    5. Hemolysis associated with infection
  B. Sequestered hemoglobin sources (cephalohematoma, concealed hemorrhage)
  C. Polycythemia syndromes
  D. Fetal transfusion syndromes (maternal-fetus, placental-fetus, twin-twin)
  E. Increased enterohepatic circulation
    1. "Physiologic jaundice"
    2. Intestinal obstruction (atresia, meconium plug syndrome, meconium ileus)
    3. Delayed feeding with fasting
II. Decreased bilirubin excretion
  A. Abnormalities of bilirubin conjugation
    1. "Physiologic jaundice" (delayed maturation of glucuronyl-one-transferase)
    2. Breast-milk jaundice
    3. Crigler-Najjar syndrome
  B. Liver circulatory changes (persistent patency of ductus venosus)
  C. Infection (congenital or acquired viral and bacterial)
  D. Inborn errors of metabolism
    1. Galactosemia
    2. Tyrosinosis
    3. Hypermethioninemia
  E. Hypothroidism
  F. Neonatal hepatitis (including α_1-antitrypsin deficiency)
  G. Biliary atresia and choledochus cyst
  H. Cystic fibrosis

There are undoubtedly far more subtle neurologic sequelae to the occurrence of hyperbilirubinemia, but these are difficult to establish.

Because of the tight binding between unconjugated bilirubin and albumin, it is rare for bilirubin to be deposited in the extravascular space in adults, even in the face of significant elevations in indirect (unconjugated) bilirubin. The newborn is at high risk for such extravascular, and in particular CNS, deposits because of the low serum albumin levels common in neonates, particularly prematures. The combination of unusually high unconjugated bilirubin concentrations plus low serum protein concentrations increases the risk of significant CNS deposition of bilirubin. Other substances, particularly organic anions, also compete with bilirubin for albumin-binding sites, so that the presence of high levels of free fatty acids, certain drugs (sulfa, aspirin, benzoate), and other hemolytic products (hemopexin) may act to displace bilirubin from albumin to extravascular sites.

Therapy for hyperbilirubinemia depends primarily on accurate diagnosis of etiology. Obviously, if bacterial sepsis is the etiology, care must first be directed to treatment of infection and then, if appropriate, to the lowering of bilirubin concentration. This becomes increasingly important in present-day nurseries, where effective therapy for lowering bilirubin concentration is sometimes routinely used and can obscure signs of potentially serious illness. In the past, clinical studies clearly demonstrated an increased risk of kernicterus at bilirubin concentrations greater than 20 mg per 100 mL. This value was used as a limit beyond which bilirubin concentration should not be allowed to rise. However, small prematures with low serum protein concentrations may be at high risk of bilirubin encephalopathy at concentrations significantly less than 20 mg per 100 mL. Recent investigators have tried to develop methods of predicting the quantity of bilirubin potentially available for diffusion out of the intravascular space. These include column chromatography on Sephadex for measurement of "free" bilirubin concentration, and the various binding capacities (PSP, HBABA) and saturation index measures. Odell has emphasized that in the *absence of hemolytic disease,* a ratio between indirect bilirubin and total serum proteins of less than 3.7 is associated with salicylate binding indices within the safe range in most cases. This ratio can be determined simply in any hospital, and we have used it as yet another parameter in reaching a decision about definitive therapy for bilirubin concentrations less than 20 mg per 100 mL. In the presence of asphyxia, hypotension, acidosis, hypothermia, or marked prematurity, one's indication for definitive therapy must be less restrictive, as all these factors increase the risk of bilirubin encephalopathy.

With hemolytic disease (in particular, Rh isoimmunization) exchange transfusions serve two purposes: first, the removal of sensitized red cells with a markedly shortened life-span which, in essence, represent "potential" unconjugated bilirubin; and second, the removal of already formed unconjugated bilirubin from tissues. When intrauterine transfusions have been done several times, it may not be necessary to carry out an exchange transfusion after birth to satisfy the first purpose, since some of these infants have almost nothing but donor Rh-negative cells in their peripheral blood. In these babies, the first exchange and all subsequent exchange transfusions can be done for the removal of bilirubin. When intrauterine transfusions have not been done, or when the infant at birth still has over 50 percent of his cells represented by sensitized cells, a first exchange should be carried out shortly after birth, provided the infant has been shown to be severely sensitized by amniotic fluid bilirubin analyses. The older criteria of anemia, cord bilirubin concentration, etc., are less useful since the advent of intrauterine transfusions and amniotic fluid bilirubin concentration measurements. While intrauterine transfusions and amniotic fluid analyses have altered the approach to the first "early" exchange transfusion, the indications for the subsequent "late" exchange transfusions are unaltered, since these procedures are carried out to remove already formed bilirubin. Definitive therapy for hyperbilirubinemia in hemolytic disease means exchange transfusion, which is universally effective in lowering serum bilirubin concentrations. Disadvantages of exchange transfusion include the various stresses it places on the infant from the necessary manipulation, potential catheter accidents (bleeding, perforation of abdominal structures, long-term thrombotic or fibrotic damage) and metabolic effects of stored blood (ACD, CPD, or heparinized). Exchange transfusions with donor blood volumes equal to twice the infant's estimated blood volume are carried out via the umbilical vein. Pretreatment with albumin infusion or addition of albumin to the unit of blood (1 g of albumin per kilogram body weight) will improve the efficiency of bilirubin removal.

Recently, phototherapy has been widely and effectively used for the treatment of hyperbilirubinemia. In infants where bilirubin concentrations justify therapeutic intervention, phototherapy is now the modality of choice. In the presence of hemolytic disease, "prophylactic" phototherapy has been shown to reduce the number of exchange transfusions required. The bilirubin concentration which will require phototherapy will vary with the individual infant. Potential complications, both short-term and long-term (such as impaired fluid and temperature regulation, obscuration of diagnostic signs, effects on biologic rhythms, etc.), must be weighed before instituting this effective and easy-to-overuse form of therapy.

RESPIRATORY DISORDERS OF THE NEWBORN

The transition from intrauterine life acts as a biologic test which may lead to the recognition of metabolic problems in the infant. Similarly, neonatal respiratory disorders are a reflection of the abrupt adjustments to air breathing required immediately after delivery. Respiratory diseases continue to be the leading causes of death in the newborn, particularly in the premature infant. Much of the clinical research in neonatology has been directed as the management of idiopathic respiratory distress syndrome (hyaline membrane disease), since it accounts for about two-thirds of the total cases of neonatal respiratory diseases. As is clear from Table 15–5, the causes of respiratory symptoms are myriad, and any infant with such symptoms requires complete differential diagnosis before settling on a diagnosis of idiopathic respiratory distress syndrome (IRDS). Indeed, many causes of respiratory distress are not even of pulmonary origin. Tachypnea, cyanosis, and labored breathing are commonly associated with metabolic problems, and their severity can be as impressive in these conditions as in pulmonary disease. With hypothermia, hyperthermia, hypoglycemia, acidosis, and asphyxia, the respiratory symptomatology is often of short duration if appropriate therapy is carried out. The contrast in subsequent course with IRDS is particularly important in weighing a decision to transfer an infant with early respiratory problems. Frequently the prompt diagnosis and correction of problems in temperature regulation, acid-base status, or glucose concentration can reverse respiratory symptoms and thus avoid needless transport of an infant to a secondary or tertiary medical center.

RESPIRATORY ADJUSTMENTS AT BIRTH

During intrauterine life the lungs are not only fluid-filled and devoid of air, but pulmonary blood flow is very low; most of the blood supply to the lung arises from the bronchial circulation. Because of the high pulmonary vascular resistance relative to placental vascular resistance, blood is shunted from the pulmonary artery through the ductus arteriosus to the aorta. Thus, at delivery, adjustments must include not only rapid expansion of previously fluid-filled alveoli, but also a fall in pulmonary vascular resistance to al-

TABLE 15–5 Respiratory Distress in Newborns

I. Pulmonary causes
   A. Hyaline membrane disease
   B. Transient tachypnea of newborn ("wet lung" syndrome)
   C. Pneumonia, congenital or acquired
   D. Aspiration syndromes (meconium, amniotic fluid)
   E. Spontaneous pneumothorax
   F. Transient persistence of fetal circulation
   G. Phrenic nerve paralysis
   H. Upper airway obstruction
      1. Choanal atresia
      2. Lingual thyroid
      3. Cord paralysis
      4. Laryngeal web
      5. Tracheal web
      6. Vascular rings
   I. Lung cysts
   J. Diaphragmatic hernia
   K. Mediastinal masses
      1. Teratoma
      2. Bronchogenic cysts
      3. Esophageal duplication
   L. Congenital lobar emphysema
   M. Hypoplasia and agenesis
II. Nonpulmonary causes
   A. Asphyxia, either fetal or neonatal
   B. Hypo- or hyperthermia
   C. Hypoglycemia
   D. Acidosis
   E. Congenital heart disease
   F. Central-nervous-system lesions
   G. Pharmacological (withdrawal syndromes, intoxications)
   H. Acute intrapartum hemorrhage

low perfusion of the pulmonary arterial tree. Respiratory movements are made during intrauterine life, and a large number of studies are underway to evaluate the pattern of fetal respirations and their relationship to fetal maturity and fetal distress. At this time the relationship of these respiratory movements to the initiation of breathing is not known. The relative importance of various stimuli for the first breath remains unclear. Chemical (P_{O_2}, P_{CO_2}, and pH), tactile, and thermal stimuli may all be important in the initiation of breathing. Compared to normal restful breathing, the intrathoracic pressures required for the first breath are large. Distending pressures of -70 cmH$_2$O have been documented during the first breath, and subsequent breaths are associated with pressures much above the -10 cmH$_2$O common during restful breathing. The requirement for such large initial expansion pressures reflects the importance of stable, noncollapsing, air-filled alveoli in decreasing the distending pressures needed during each inspiration. The stability of the alveoli, and the resistance to complete collapse during expiration, is a property of the lung due to the presence of surfactant, a phospholipid which lowers surface tension.

IDIOPATHIC RESPIRATORY DISTRESS SYNDROME

IRDS, or clinical hyaline membrane disease, remains the major single cause of neonatal mortality in preterm infants, despite two decades of research. The incidence of IRDS depends in large part on the definition used in various centers. IRDS is more common in infants under 1500 g and 36 weeks of gestational age. Most studies show an incidence of approximately 20 percent in infants under 1500 g, 5 to 10 percent in infants 1500 to 2000 g, and less than 1 percent in infants 2000 to 2500 g. Mortality rates improved during the 1960s from rates of approximately 60 percent to rates of 30 to 35 percent, and recent studies have reported mortality rates of 10 percent or less, reflecting newer methods of ventilatory support.

Although there has been considerable controversy over the etiology of hyaline membrane disease, the primary importance of deficient surfactant has become well established. Pulmonary hypoperfusion can be an additional factor in the pathophysiology of IRDS, probably secondary to the diffuse alveolar collapse (atelectasis) resulting from surfactant deficiency. Increasing concentrations of lecithin in the developing lung are associated with pulmonary maturity. Lecithin/sphingomyelin ratios in amniotic fluid, the lipids presumably originating from the lung, have been used clinically to assess pulmonary maturity in the human fetus.

The infant with IRDS has respiratory difficulty beginning immediately after birth, with tachypnea, retractions, alar flaring, expiratory grunting, and cyanosis. Coexistent hypotension, hypothermia, and hypoglycemia are common. The characteristic radiologic features include diffuse atelectasis with a characteristic reticular-granular or ground-glass appearance, and hypoexpansion. Progressive disease may result in complete opacification of the lung fields. Laboratory findings document the severity of the intrapulmonary right-left shunt ($\downarrow P_{O_2}$ in spite of increased inspired oxygen concentration), existence of hypoventilation ($\uparrow P_{CO_2}$), and inadequate systemic tissue perfusion ($\downarrow$ pH and $\downarrow$ base deficit).

In the past, IRDS worsened over the first 36 hours, then stabilized, and if the infant were alive at the end of 72 hours, recovery could be expected. Recent therapeutic advances have altered this pattern of evolution of the disease; infants with IRDS may be severely ill for over a week and still recover. The treatment for IRDS includes meticulous attention to supportive care: temperature support, glucose regulation, hydration, support of intravascular volume with colloid and blood administration, and supplemental oxygen administration. Infants who develop persistent hypoxemia despite these efforts will require ventilatory support, usually with some form of continuous positive airway pressure (CPAP), delivered by endotracheal tube, face mask, nasal prongs, or head box, or continuous negative pressure (CNP) to the chest wall. If hypoxemia continues despite such CPAP or CNP support, assisted ventilation with positive end expiratory pressure (PEEP) is required.

The correction of acidosis is commonly regarded as an essential aspect of therapy in IRDS, reflecting a concern over possible [H+] effects on increasing pulmonary vascular resistance, further reducing pulmonary perfusion. Respiratory acidosis is the usual accompaniment of IRDS and can be treated only by an improvement in effective ventilation. Sodium bicarbonate should be administered in amounts calculated to correct only a metabolic acidosis (see Fig. 15–25), and total sodium administration should be restricted to less than 8 meq/kg per day. Some centers use antibiotics routinely because of the frequent occurrence of infection in infants with IRDS (perhaps associated with necessary manipulations, such as umbilical artery catheterization, endotracheal intubation, and frequent suctioning) and the difficulty in excluding the existence of pneumonia. We have not treated routinely with antibiotics but do carry out frequent blood cultures and granulocyte counts because of the high risk of infection.

Although maternal administration of corticosteroid has recently been suggested for prevention of IRDS, there is no effect of steroid treatment on the course of prognosis in infants with IRDS, and such therapy is not indicated.

Many complications are associated with IRDS, including hemorrhagic disorders resulting in disseminated intravascular coagulation, intracranial hemorrhage, and pulmonary hemorrhage. While spontaneous pneumothorax does occur, the incidence of pneumothorax, pneumomediastinum, pneumopericardium, and even pneumoperitoneum increases when ventilatory intervention is required. Retrolental fibroplasia is a direct result of oxygen toxicity in premature infants. It occurs when arterial P_{O_2} levels are not monitored frequently and kept above 100 mmHg. Recently, another complication of oxygen therapy has become common which is unrelated to arterial P_{O_2} levels. Bronchopulmonary dysplasia is secondary to a direct effect of inspired oxygen on the bronchial tree and results in a pulmonary fibrotic process that can cause long-lasting pulmonary sequelae.

TRANSIENT TACHYPNEA

Transient tachypnea of the newborn can present a clinical picture nearly indistinguishable from IRDS. Infants with transient tachypnea are also premature and frequently have been delivered by cesarean section. They demonstrate tachypnea, retraction, flaring, grunting, and cyanosis. On x-ray, their lungs appear hazy, normal, or hyperexpanded. There are prominent hilar bronchovascular markings. Although such infants may be hypoxic in room air, it is rare for significant shunting to be demonstrated by persistent hypoxia in 100 percent inspired oxygen concentrations. P_{CO_2} values may be slightly increased. Treatment consists of general supportive care, with supplemental oxygen administration. The disease is self-limited and carries an excellent prognosis.

PNEUMONIA

Pneumonia is by far the most common serious infection in the newborn and may be either congenital or acquired. Although occasionally reported in infants delivered with apparently intact membranes, most cases of congenital pneumonia follow prolonged rupture of the membranes. The infecting organisms reflect the vaginal flora; group B streptococci, staphylococci, and *E. coli* predominate. Occasionally congenital pneumonia may be caused by *Listeria*, syphilis, and tuberculosis.

Acquired bacterial pneumonias can occur unassociated with premature rupture of membranes and in infants of any gestational age. Bacterial pneumonias can be superimposed on other varieties of respiratory distress and occur more frequently when ventilatory assistance with a respirator or CPAP apparatus is used. Gram-negative organisms predominate, with *E. coli*, *Aerobacter-Klebsiella*, and *Pseudomonas* frequent pathogens.

The documentation of viral pneumonias in the newborn has become more common. Although pneumonia with congenital herpesvirus and cytomegalovirus infections has been known for a number of years, acquired viral pneumonias have been recognized only recently. The viruses implicated in such infections follow the epidemiology of viral infections prominent in the community at the time. Respiratory syncytial virus has been a particularly troublesome agent and can occur in epidemic form in the nursery. Pneumonias secondary to adenovirus and parainfluenza virus infections have also been well documented. The usual radiologic findings of pneumonia are present. Bronchopneumonia with patchy infiltrates in both lung fields is most common. Pleural effusions can occur secondary to bacterial pneumonias, and such effusions commonly have the appearance of transudates rather than empyema. The white-cell counts in neonatal empyema fluid may be misleadingly low. Pleural effusions are uncommon in the newborn from causes other than infection and should be regarded as infectious until proved otherwise. Treatment requires the appropriate choice of antibiotics based on culture evidence, as well as general supportive care.

ASPIRATION SYNDROMES

Meconium aspiration is a severe problem in the newborn infant. Often babies born after the passage of meconium are asphyxiated, causing CNS depression. They may have a poor cough and gag reflex, thus further predisposing them to respiratory complications from any aspirated material. Meconium-aspiration pneumonia is often a devastating, progressive disease with signs of marked tachypnea, retractions, cyanosis, and increased A-P diameter. The chest x-ray shows bilateral hyperexpansion, coarse and streaky infiltrates, and patchy areas of hyperlucency alternating with atelectasis (honeycombing). The appearance of air trapping and emphysema may become progressively worse.

Clinically, the emphasis should be on prophylaxis. When meconium staining is recognized, a physician should be present at delivery whose sole concern is care of the infant. It is important to empty the oral cavity and pharynx of secretions. If meconium is found, laryngoscopy and tracheal suctioning should be carried out. This should be done prior to the use of positive pressure resuscitation.

Once meconium-aspiration pneumonia is diagnosed, therapy is entirely supportive. In general, a disease characterized by air trapping and hyperexpansion contraindicates the use of CPAP or PEEP. Sometimes ventilator therapy with high inspired oxygen concentrations is required.

Aspiration of milk feedings continues to be a recurrent problem in small preterm infants. Careful nursing care with expert feeding technique and a slow progression to nipple feeding can reduce its incidence markedly. When an infant aspirates repeatedly, one should suspect persistent pharyngeal incoordination from a CNS problem or an H-type tracheoesophageal fistula.

TRANSIENT PERSISTENCE OF THE FETAL CIRCULATION (PFC SYNDROME)

Although many pulmonary disease processes in the neonate are associated with right-left shunting at the ductal and foramen levels because of increased pulmonary vascular resistance, recently a group of infants have been identified who seem to have this physiologic derangement as a primary disease process. These infants are often near term, born after complicated pregnancies or intrapartum periods. They demonstrate respiratory distress beginning at birth and worsening over the first 24 hours of life. They most often have little problem with ventilation (normal or low P_{CO_2}) but have such profound hypoxemia that they may be diagnosed as having cyanotic congenital heart disease.

The radiograph classically shows oligemia of the lungs, but occasionally an alveolar pattern of pulmonary edema may be present. The heart size may also be slightly enlarged.

Therapy should be directed at the correction of hypoxemia with proper ventilatory support. In severe cases, the use of a pulmonary vasodilator may be required.

INFECTION IN THE NEWBORN

Localized suppurative infection (meningitis, omphalitis, pneumonia, otitis) has been recognized as a common occurrence in the newborn for over a century, but the existence of generalized septicemia in the neonate, with definite clinical signs, was not appreciated until the classical studies by Dunham were published in 1933. The ability to recognize septi-

cemia diagnosed by appropriate cultures and eventually to treat sepsis effectively with antibiotics followed the early descriptions by Dunham. In present-day nurseries there is a high index of suspicion of infection in any infant who appears ill.

Infection continues to carry a high mortality, even with earlier recognition and aggressive treatment. The occurrence of significant infection in the newborn is estimated to be approximately 1 in 500 live births, but if preterm births alone are considered, the incidence rises to about 1 in 200 live births. In the preantibiotic era, mortality approached 100 percent. Even after the introduction of antibiotics, mortality rates of over 60 percent were associated with septicemia, meningitis, and pneumonia. Recent reports have suggested a significant improvement in outcome, although mortality rates of 50 percent in isolated epidemics are still reported.

The neonate demonstrates a unique susceptibility to infection, but the causes of this susceptibility are still under study. There has been documentation of impaired immunoglobulin production, low complement levels, poor opsonization, diminished phagocytic ingestion and killing, and inadequate inflammatory response. An intact epidermis and respiratory mucosal lining is the first line of defense against invading pathogens. Thus, with the common use of intubation, suction catheters, feeding tubes, arterial and central venous catheters, and venipuncture, it is not surprising that these barriers are often violated, predisposing to invasions by bacteria. Even without such manipulation, the infant is uniquely susceptible to invasion through the unprotected umbilical stump, which may often be the site of superficial suppuration and potential source of septicemia.

Obstetric factors also predispose to subsequent neonatal infection. After 24 hours of ruptured membranes the incidence of amniotic fluid infection and neonatal infection increase. The risk of such infection, both to the mother and the infant, has to be balanced against the risk of early delivery in terms of fetal size and maturity. Maternal bleeding, prolonged labor, and difficult operative deliveries have also been implicated in increasing the risk of neonatal infection. Recently, cases of scalp infection have occurred following intrauterine fetal ECG monitoring with scalp electrodes.

Ascending infection or infection acquired in passage through the birth canal are the most common sources of perinatal infection, with a striking association between maternal vaginal flora and organisms subsequently identified in infant infection. This association holds for both viral and bacterial infections, and for "congenital" infections, as well as for infection not immediately apparent at birth. Occasionally, infants become infected with organisms responsible for an intercurrent maternal infection. *E. coli* subtypes responsible for maternal urinary-tract infection have been found in association with neonatal septicemia. Rarely, perinatal bacterial infection can be of transplacental origin; with tuberculosis, *Listeria*, syphilis, and *Vibrio fetus* infections being clearly established. In contrast, viral infections are usually of transplacental origin, with cytomegalovirus and rubella the most common. Congenital toxoplasmosis and malaria are of transplacental etiology. Certain fungal infections have also been associated with placental invasion. Herpesvirus infection is usually acquired during passage through the birth canal, but rare cases of presumed transplacental origin have been reported.

The organisms responsible for bacterial infection in the neonate have undergone an intriguing evolution. In early reports the pyogenic cocci (beta-hemolytic streptococcus and *Staphylococcus aureus*) were the most common pathogens. Beginning in the early 1950s, gram-negative organisms (particularly *E. coli*) began to be more common. In the 1960s *E. coli* and *Aerobacter-Klebsiella* were most prominent, with *Pseudomonas* a frequent complication of respiratory therapy or of long-term debilitation. Recently, the group B beta-hemolytic streptococcus has been increasingly diagnosed in septic infants with some recent reports showing it to be the most common cause of neonatal infection. In addition, *Hemophilus influenzae* infections, previously quite rare, have been appearing.

Although the congenital viral syndromes associated with rubella and cytomegalovirus have been recognized for a number of years, recent attention has been focused on acquired viral infection in the nursery. Infection with enteroviruses (Coxsackie, echo), adenoviruses, parainfluenzae, respiratory syncytial virus, and herpesvirus have all been shown to be responsible for various neonatal illnesses. The occurrence of viral infections in the nursery reflects the existing epidemiology of viral illness in the community. Often epidemics of viral illness in the community will rapidly become apparent in the nursery.

In parallel to the change in the organisms responsible for neonatal sepsis, there has been the emergence of resistance patterns to different antibiotics. The appearance of penicillin resistance among staphylococci is the best-known example, but the gram-negative organisms responsible for neonatal infections have also been altered in terms of antibiotic sensitivity. The universal susceptibility of gram-neg-

ative organisms to kanamycin has slowly changed, and some centers now report more than 30 percent of *E. coli* resistant to kanamycin. Similar changes have occurred with ampicillin sensitivity; nearly all *Klebsiella* are now resistant. It is essential to monitor both the organisms responsible for infection in the nursery and their change in antibiotic resistance patterns.

The signs of septicemia or of isolated infections in the newborn are often nonspecific. Lethargy, irritability, weak or shrill cry, poor feeding, regurgitation or vomiting, respiratory distress, apnea, cyanosis or mottling, abdominal distention, diarrhea, petechiae, jaundice, and temperature instability (hypothermia or fever) are all frequent accompaniments of septicemia. It is uncommon to have signs or physical findings specifically referable to the site of infection. Thus, meningismus is not seen in the presence of meningitis; abdominal tenderness is not always associated with peritonitis; polyuria or frequency is not a specific sign of urinary-tract infection; ear pulling is not seen with otitis media. On physical exam, there may be signs of poor perfusion of skin and other organs such as hypotension; tachycardia; pale, cyanotic, and clammy skin. With meningitis, the fontanel may be full or tense; in pneumonia rales can occasionally be heard.

Diagnosis depends on a high index of suspicion. Often infants with such nonspecific findings are treated, only to have negative cultures subsequently associated with a benign course. Definitive diagnosis of the etiology of the infection requires confirmation by appropriate culture. Various ancillary aids may prove helpful. After 24 hours of age, absolute granulocyte counts (neutrophils and bands) greater than 12,000 or less than 2000 should make one highly suspicious. A pronounced shift to immature granulocytes, even if the total granulocyte count is within the normal range, should be regarded with suspicion. Similarly, there may be thrombocytopenia, jaundice (often with an elevated conjugated fraction of bilirubin), and anemia (with evidence of hemolysis). In the presence of prolonged rupture of membranes, some centers have found polymorphonuclear leukocyte counts, as well as gram stains on gastric aspirates valuable as a guide to possible infection. Others have recommended frozen section of the cord as a reliable guide to significant intrauterine amnionitis or screening by poly counts from external ear swabs.

Cultures of blood (preferably from two sites), pharynx, spinal fluid, and urine, as well as culture of any specific suppurative site are adequate for diagnosis. With the recent emergence of anaerobic organisms as pathogens in obstetrics, it is important to use appropriate anaerobic techniques in addition to routine culture methods when dealing with potential perinatal infection. In screening for infection after premature rupture of membranes, we culture the surface of the placenta, include a cord blood culture drawn with a needle and syringe, and an additional surface skin culture of the infant.

Viral cultures are as important as routine bacterial cultures in the search for etiology in a "septic" infant. As is apparent in Fig. 15-29, it is impossible to distinguish clinically between viral and bacterial sepsis. Identical signs occur in septic infants, whether of bacterial or viral etiology. The return from viral cultures at our hospital has been as rewarding as routine bacterial cultures in confirming the etiology of an illness. The identification of an infant with sepsis is important not only because of the advent of antiviral chemotherapy, but also as a precaution for strict isolation procedures, particularly for women who may be pregnant.

Treatment of infants with sepsis depends on proper choice of antibiotics and general principles of supportive care. The choice of antibiotics to administer until specific etiology is documented depends on the epidemiology and antibiotic resistance patterns in the nursery. The most common approach at present is the use of ampicillin and kanamycin. Some centers have seen the emergence of such significant resistance to these antibiotics that they use gentamicin as the initial choice. In the presence of meningitis it has often been necessary to administer intrathecal antibiotics.

Supportive care includes careful temperature support; colloid and blood administration; attention to parameters of perfusion status (blood pressure, central venous pressure, urine output); monitoring of coagulation status (to detect disseminated intravascular coagulation); ventilation support as indicated; maintenance of glucose requirements; and gastrointestinal suction when abdominal distention is present.

FIGURE 15-29 Manifestations of disseminated herpes simplex and Coxsackie B infections in the neonatal period. *(From Overall et al.)*

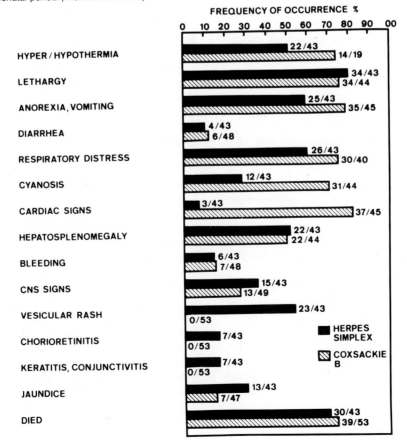

REFERENCES

Aherne W, Dunnill MS: Quantitative aspects of placental structure. *J Path Bact* 91:123–39, 1966.

Alexander G: Studies on the placenta of the sheep (Ovis aries L.) Placental size. *J Reprod Fertil,* 7:289, 1964.

Battaglia FC, Meschia G: Foetal metabolism and substrate utilization, *Foetal and Neonatal Physiology, Proceedings of the Sir Joseph Barcroft Centenary Symposium,* Cambridge, 1973, pp. 382–397.

Burd LI et al.: Placental production and foetal utilisation of lactate and pyruvate. *Nature,* 254(5502):710, 1975.

Campbell S, Dewhurst CJ: Diagnosis of the small-for-dates fetus by serial ultrasonic cephalometry. *Lancet* 2:1002–1006, 1971.

Carson BS et al.: Combined obstetric and pediatric approach to prevent meconium aspiration syndrome. *Am J Obstet Gynecol,* 126:712, 1976.

Cooper LZ et al.: Rubella. Clinical manifestations and management. *Am J Dis Child* 118:18–29, 1969a.

——.: Transient arthritis after rubella vaccination. *Am J Dis Child* 118:218–225, 1969b.

Dahm LS, James LS: Newborn temperature and calculated heat loss in the delivery room. *Pediatrics* 49:504–513, 1972.

Diamond EL et al.: The relationship of intra-uterine radiation to subsequent mortality and development of leukemia in children. A prospective study. *Am J Epidemiol* 97:283–313, 1973.

Falkner F: Velocity growth. *Pediatrics,* 51:746, 1973.

Feldman HA: Toxoplasmosis. *Pediatrics* 22:559–574, 1958.

Freda VJ: The Rh problem in obstetrics and a new concept of its management using amniocentesis and spectrophotometric scanning of amniotic fluid. *Am J Obstet Gynecol,* 92(3):341, 1965.

Gershanik JJ et al.: The association of hypocalcemia and recurrent apnea in premature infants. *Am J Obstet Gynecol* 113:646–652, 1972.

Hallman M et al.: Phosphatidyl-inositol and phosphatidylglycerol in amniotic fluid: Indices of lung maturity. *Am J Obstet Gynecol,* 125(5):613, 1976.

Heggie AD, Robbins FC: Natural rubella acquired after birth. Clinical features and complications. *Am J Dis Child* 118:12–17, 1969.

Hendricks CH: Patterns of fetal and placental growth: The second half of normal pregnancy. *Obstet Gynecol* 24:357–365, 1964.

Jones MD Jr et al.: Urinary flow rates and urea excretion rates in newborn infants. *Biol Neonate* 21:321–329, 1972.

King BF, Enders AC: The fine structure of the guinea pig visceral yolk sac placenta. *Amer J Anat* 127:394–414, 1970.

Kulhanek JF: Gestational changes in DNA content and urea permeability of the sheep placenta and their relationship to fetal growth. PhD thesis, University of Colorado, Boulder, 1972.

—— et al.: Changes in DNA content and urea permeability of the sheep placenta. *Am J Physiol* 226:1257–1263, 1974.

Liley AW: Liquor amnii analysis in the management of the pregnancy complicated by rhesus sensitization. *Am J Obstet Gynecol,* 82:1359–1370, 1961.

——: Errors in the assessment of hemolytic disease from amniotic fluid. *Am J Obstet Gynecol,* 86:485–494, 1963.

Lobl M et al.: Maternal age and intellectual functioning of offspring. *Johns Hopkins Med J,* 128:347, 1971.

Lubchenco LO, Bard H: Incidence of hypoglycemia in newborn infants classified by birth weight and gestational age. *Pediatrics,* 47:831, 1971.

Makowski EL et al.: Measurement of umbilical arterial blood flow to the sheep placenta and fetus in utero. Distribution to cotyledons and the intercotyledonary chorion. *Circ Res* 23:623–631, 1968.

McKeown T, Record RG: Observations on foetal growth in multiple pregnancy in man. *J Endocrinol* 8:386–401, 1952.

Meschia G, et al.: The diffusibility of urea across the sheep placenta in the last two months of gestation. *Q J Exp Physiol* 50:23–41, 1965.

Odell GB: Influence of binding on the toxicity of bilirubin. *Ann NY Acad Sci,* 226:225, 1973.

Overall JC Jr, Glasgow LA: Virus infections of the fetus and newborn infant. *J Pediatr* 77:315–333, 1970.

Pollack W et al.: Results of clinical trials of RhoGAM in women. *Transfusion* 8:151–153, 1968.

Rankin JH et al.: Relationship between uterine and umbilical venous PO2 in sheep. *Am J Physiol* 220:1688–1692, 1971.

Resnik R et al.: The stimulation of uterine blood flow by various estrogens. *Endocrinology* 25:1192–1196, 1974.

Reynolds DW et al.: Subclinical congenital cytomegalovirus (C-CMV) infection: A microbiologic and clinical long term study. *Pediatr Res* 7(4):372, 1973.

Sever JL et al.: Rubella in the collaborative perinatal research study: II. Clinical and laboratory findings in children through three years of age. *Am J Dis Child* 118:123–132, 1969.

Silver M et al.: Placental exchange and morphology in ruminants and the mare, in *Foetal and Neonatal Physiology, Proceedings of the Sir Joseph Barcroft Centenary Symposium,* Cambridge, 1973, pp. 245–271.

Thiersch JB: Therapeutic abortions with a folic acid antagonist, 4-aminopteroyl-glutamic acid (4-amino P.G.A.) administered by the oral route. *Am J Obstet Gynecol* 63:1298–1304, 1952.

Tsang RC et al.: Hypocalcemia in infants of diabetic mothers. *J Pediatr,* 80(3):384, 1972.

Turner G: Recognition of intrauterine growth retardation by considering comparative birth-weights. *Lancet* 2:1123, 1971.

Weil WB Jr, Helmrath TA: *Pediatrics,* 15th ed., eds HL Barnett, AH Einhorn, New York: Appleton-Century-Crofts, 1972, pp. 28–34.

Witkop CJ et al.: The frequency of discolored teeth showing yellow fluorescence under ultra-violet light. *J Oral Ther Pharmacol* 2:81–87, 1965.

16

Infancy and Childhood

PAUL F. BRENNER

Gynecologic problems occur infrequently in the infant and young child but are often serious, requiring careful evaluation by special techniques. The reproductive tract of the newborn female remains under the hormonal influence of the mother for the first 2 to 3 weeks of life, making examination easier then than later. Any abnormality of genital development must be detected and evaluated at this time so that the infant can be raised in the proper sex.

Physicians and parents alike tend to avoid subjecting the young girl to a vaginal examination even when symptoms are present. A special blend of gentleness, painstaking explanation, and the ability to relate to children is required to prevent physical or emotional trauma, but examination is usually possible without anesthesia.

The special problems of sexual development, infections, injuries, tumors, and precocious puberty will be considered, with particular emphasis on diagnoses which have prognostic or therapeutic significance.

ETIOLOGY OF ABNORMAL SEXUAL DEVELOPMENT

The sex of an individual is determined by a series of factors which include genetic sex, gonadal sex, morphology of the internal genitalia, morphology of the external genitalia, endocrine sex, sex of rearing, and gender role. In the normal individual all these factors are in agreement. In the individual with an intersex disorder there is disagreement among the first four factors. An abnormality of endocrine sex (i.e., androgen-producing ovarian tumors) does not necessarily result in an intersex disorder. The first five determinants are classified as organic and the last two as psychological. An individual with concordant organic determinants may assume a gender role opposite to that of the genetic sex, gonadal sex, and the morphology of the internal and external genitalia solely as the result of a psychological disorder.

Sexual development occurs in three stages: (1) gonadal development, (2) development of the internal genitalia, and (3) development of the external genitalia. The genetic sex, set at the time of fertilization, normally determines the sex of the gonad. Germ cells, originating in the entoderm of the yolk sac, migrate to the undifferentiated gonad. The undifferentiated gonad is bipotential and may become either an ovary or a testis. Location of the germ cells in the medullary portion of the undifferentiated gonad and the regression of the cortex lead to the development of a testis. Location of the germ cells in the cortex portion of the undifferentiated gonad and the regression of the medulla lead to the development of an ovary. The differentiation of the bipotential gonad to either an ovary or a testis occurs during the first 12 weeks of pregnancy, with the development of the testis (6 to 7 weeks) preceding that of the ovary (11 to 12 weeks).

The development of the internal genitalia is determined by the presence or absence of secretions of the testis. All embryos possess dual primordia, the Wolffian and the Müllerian ducts. Androgen secretion from the testis results in the development of male internal genitalia derived from the Wolffian ducts. The vas deferens, seminal vesicles, and the epididymis are derived from the Wolffian primordia. Müllerian-inhibiting factor (MIF) secreted by the testis results in the regression of the Müllerian duct system. The fallopian tubes, uterus, and a portion of the upper vagina are derived from the Müllerian primordia. Normally the presence of the testis results in Wolffian duct development and Müllerian duct regression, and the absence of the testis results in Müllerian duct development and Wolffian duct regression. The differentiation of the internal genitalia occurs between 8 and 16 weeks of pregnancy (Figs. 16–1 to 16–4).

The development of the external genitalia is determined by the presence or absence of androgen. The external genital anlagen are common to both sexes. In the presence of androgen, the glans penis

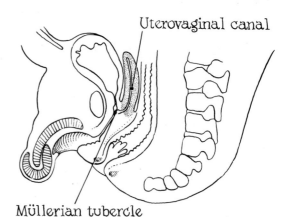

FIGURE 16–1 Müllerian tubercle, 50 mm, 10½ weeks. Point at which Müllerian ducts abut against urogenital sinus marks opening of future vagina. Urogenital sinus is lengthy, connects with urethral groove on underside of phallus. *(Courtesy of CM Dougherty.)*

develops from the genital tubercle, the shaft of the penis from the genital folds, and the scrotum from the genital swellings. In the absence of androgen, the clitoris develops from the genital tubercle, the labia minora from the genital folds, and the labia majora from the genital swellings. Development of external genitalia occurs early in the second trimester of pregnancy.

When the genetic and gonadal sex do not agree with the morphology of the internal and external genitalia, the Klebs classification is applied. Patients with an intersex disorder in which the gonads are testes, are classified as male pseudohermaphrodites. When the gonads are ovaries and the external genita-

FIGURE 16–2 Beginning of vagina, 70 mm, 12 weeks. A solid cord of cells produced by sinus epithelium pushes cranially displacing Müllerian epithelium. Length of sinus to its junction with urethral groove is appreciably shortened. *(Courtesy of CM Dougherty.)*

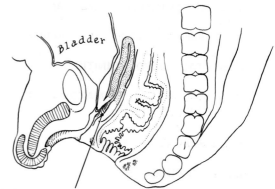

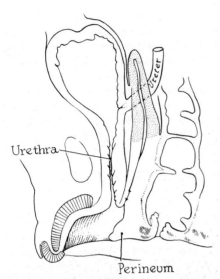

FIGURE 16–3 Formation of vaginal vestibule, 106 mm, 16 weeks. Displacement of Müllerian epithelium in urethrovaginal canal is near completion. The lengthened vagina has brought the junctional region closer to urethral groove. Phallus is relatively smaller while the urethral groove is larger in its ventral-caudal dimension. *(Courtesy CM Dougherty.)*

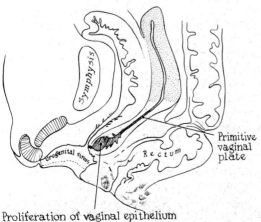

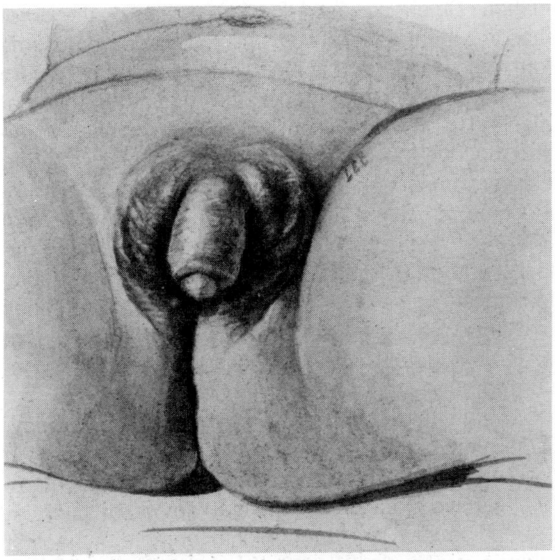

FIGURE 16–5 Masculinized female external genitalia. Clitoris is enlarged; labioscrotal folds are enlarged; skin is wrinkled and pigmented. *(From CM Dougherty and R Spencer: Female Sex Anomalies, Hagerstown, Md.: Harper & Row, 1972.)*

lia are male, the individual is designated a female pseudohermaphrodite (Fig. 16–5). When the histology of the gonads reveals both testicular and ovarian tissue, the individual is classified as a true hermaphrodite.

Abnormal sexual development results from either disorders of gonadal development or disorders of fetal endocrinology. The former are the result of major

FIGURE 16–4 Canalization of the vagina, 131 mm, 16 weeks. The solid cord of sinus epithelium is canalized by central desquamation starting at caudal end. The large vagina causes pressures on sinus wall at point where it will eventually open. *(Courtesy CM Dougherty.).*

chromosomal abnormalities which occur at random and are not hereditary. The latter are the result of genetic defects and are frequently hereditary. Disorders of fetal endocrinology are associated with a normal karyotype.

DISORDERS OF GONADAL DEVELOPMENT

Chromosomal errors may occur during meiosis or mitosis (see also Chap. 6). Meiosis is the division of germ cells that produces gametes with a haploid chromosome complement. A gamete may lack a sex chromosome as the result of failure of two sex chromosomes to separate, called nondisjunction, or as the result of failure of a sex chromosome to be incorporated into the new cell when the cell membranes are formed during anaphase, called anaphase lag. Following nondisjunction of sex chromosomes, a gamete either lacks a sex chromosome or contains an extra sex chromosome. Structural abnormalities as well as abnormal numbers of human chromosomes lead to disorders of gonadal development. Structural modification of sex chromosomes includes deletion of either the short or long arm, isochromosome formation of either the short or long arm, and ring formation. Deletions result from a portion of the chromosome being broken off and lost. Isochromosome formation is the result of the division of the centromere in a transverse rather than in the normal longitudinal plane. The isochromosome is then composed of either the long arms alone or only the short arms. A ring chromosome is formed when the free ends of a chromosome remaining after partial deletion fuse to form a circle. When chromosomal errors occur during mitosis, both of the cells are retained in the organism. Mosaicism is the occurrence of two or more cell lines of different karyotypes in one individual derived from a single zygote. Nondisjunction or anaphase lag occurring during mitosis leads to mosaicism.

Spermatogenesis starts at the time of puberty. Each germ cell divides to form four male gametes. In the female, meiosis starts during the fourth month of fetal life and stops during the first meiotic division. At puberty, a few ova each month complete the first meiotic division and begin the second meiotic division. The second meiotic division is not completed unless the egg is fertilized. Each germ cell during oogenesis forms one egg and three polar bodies.

Disorders of gonadal development include Klinefelter's syndrome, gonadal dysgenesis, true hermaphroditism, and male pseudohermaphroditism. Male pseudohermaphroditism may result from a Y-chromosome defect (mixed gonadal dysgenesis) or from a primary gonadal defect. Klinefelter's syndrome and gonadal dysgenesis do not cause ambiguous external genitalia in the newborn, but true hermaphroditism and male pseudohermaphroditism do cause intersex disorders.

KLINEFELTER'S SYNDROME

Klinefelter's syndrome occurs in 1 out of every 400 newborn male infants. Individuals with Klinefelter's syndrome appear normal at birth and the morphology of the internal and external genitalia is normal male. At puberty they develop gynecomastia, small testes and aspermia. The scrotum is normal size but the testes are small, usually less than 1.5 cm in the greatest diameter. Histologic examination of the testis reveals hypoplastic, hyalinized tubules and usually Leydig cell hyperplasia. The phallus is normal size, and erection and ejaculation, lacking sperm, are possible, although libido is frequently diminished. They ultimately achieve normal height and pubic hair development but the amount of body hair is decreased. The characteristic chromosome abnormality associated with Klinefelter's syndrome is the presence of an extra X chromosome. All patients with this disorder have at least two X chromosomes and a Y chromosome present in at least some of their cells. Most Klinefelter patients have the karyotype 47 XXY. The levels of gonadotropins are increased and the concentration of testosterone in the circulation of patients with Klinefelter's syndrome is below the normal male range. The risk for gonadal tumors is not increased in Klinefelter's syndrome.

GONADAL DYSGENESIS

Gonadal dysgenesis occurs in 1 out of every 5000 newborn infants. Individuals with gonadal dysgenesis are born with normal female internal and external genitalia. The gonads are represented as bilateral streaks. A normal number of germ cells migrate to the undifferentiated gonad, but they atrophy at a much faster rate than usual. The absence of ovarian follicles results in hypoestrinism, sexual infantilism, and primary amenorrhea. There is a great diversity in the clinical spectrum and karyotype findings of individuals with gonadal dysgenesis. Gonadal dysgenesis may be further classified as Turner's syndrome with the karyotype 45X, gonadal dysgenesis due to structural chromosome abnormalities or mosaicism, pure gonadal dysgenesis with the karyotype 46XX, and gonadal dysgenesis with the karyotype 46XY.

Turner's syndrome is characterized by streak gonads, sexual infantilism, short stature, and multiple congenital anomalies which may include a shield chest, webbed neck, lymphedema of the hands and feet, a short fourth and/or fifth metacarpal, hypoplastic nails, pigmented nevi, congenital heart disease, cubitus valgus, low posterior hairline, inner epicanthal folds, a palate with a high, narrow arch, small chin, low-set ears, and ptosis (Fig. 16–6). Patients with Turner's syndrome have an increased incidence of diabetes and Hashimoto's thyroiditis. The features of this syndrome can present in a combination of clinical symptoms or alone. Findings at birth suggesting Turner's syndrome include cardiac malformations, the most common of which is coarctation of the aorta, webbing of the neck, and lymphedema of the hands and feet. Increase in height does not keep pace with the chronological age, and the final height usually does not exceed 58 inches. At puberty the effects of estrogen lack become apparent: absence of secondary sex characteristics, primary amenorrhea, infantile external genitalia, and thin vaginal mucosa.

The most common karyotype of patients with gonadal dysgenesis is 45X associated with Turner's syn-

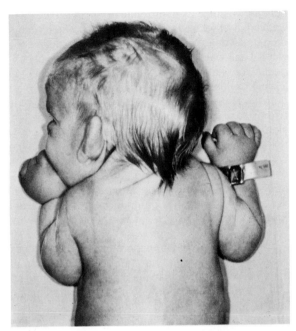

FIGURE 16–6 Newborn infant with gonadal dysgenesis. Loose skin, low hairline, low-set ears, and puffiness of hands are typical stigmata. *(Courtesy of Rowena Spencer.)*

drome. As the result of mosaicism and variation in the extent of structural defects, a wide spectrum exists in the clinical presentations of gonadal dysgenesis. Occasional individuals with gonadal dysgenesis may have a normal female karyotype 46XX (pure gonadal dysgenesis) or a normal male karyotype 46XY. Individuals with gonadal dysgenesis and a normal karyotype have, in common with those with a chromosomal defect, streak gonads, sexual infantilism, elevated levels of gonadotropins, and very low concentrations of estrogen in the peripheral circulation. They have normal stature, however, and lack the anomalies commonly associated with Turner's syndrome.

TRUE HERMAPHRODITISM

By definition the gonads of the true hermaphrodite contain both ovarian and testicular tissue. An ovary and a testis or an ovotestis may be present. The karyotype is usually 46XX. The development of the internal genitalia corresponds closely to the histology of the ipsilateral gonad. A uterus is nearly always present. The development of the external genitalia is generally more male than female, but the findings of hypospadias, cryptorchidism, incomplete labioscrotal

fusion, and inguinal hernia indicate an intersex disorder. If gonadal tissue is not removed prior to puberty, approximately three-fourths of patients with true hermaphroditism have breast development, one-half menstruate, and one-fourth ovulate. Spermatogenesis is very infrequent.

MALE PSEUDOHERMAPHRODITISM, GONADAL TYPE

Two types of male pseudohermaphroditism are due to a disorder of gonadal development. The first is mixed gonadal dysgenesis which is the result of a Y-chromosome defect. The gonads of these individuals are comprised of a testis on one side and streak gonad on the other. The internal genitalia are usually normal female with oviducts, uterus, and the upper portion of the vagina present. The external genitalia are ambiguous and usually more closely resemble female structures. The second type of male pseudohermaphroditism resulting from a disorder of gonadal development is a primary gonadal defect. These individuals have a normal male karyotype, 46XY, absent gonads, and no Müllerian duct derivatives. The external genitalia are ambiguous and usually more closely resemble male structures.

DISORDERS OF FETAL ENDOCRINOLOGY

Inappropriate androgen can cause problems of intersex. Androgen excess in the gonadal female fetus causes varying degrees of virilization, Androgen deficiency in the gonadal male fetus results in a spectrum of aberrations departing from complete virilization. Disorders of fetal endocrinology produce female pseudohermaphroditism with partial virilization and male pseudohermaphroditism with partial failure of virilization.

FEMALE PSEUDOHERMAPHRODITISM

The female pseudohermaphrodite is a genetic female, karyotype 46XX, and a gonadal female with normal ovarian differentiation. The internal genitalia are normal female with oviducts and a uterus present and with complete Wolffian duct regression. The appearance of the external genitalia is incongruous with the genetic and gonadal sex to a varying extent. The spectrum of morphologic changes of the external genitalia range from clitoromegaly in the mildest form through incomplete fusion of the labioscrotal folds, but with maintenance of separate vaginal and urethral orifices; progressive fusion of the labioscrotal folds with the creation of a urogenital sinus into which the urethra and cervix both exit; pseudoscrotal formation with perineal hypospadias; and finally formation of a penile urethra in the most advanced forms of virilization of the genetic and gonadal female fetus (see also Chap. 9).

The female pseudohermaphrodite must have been exposed to an excessive quantity of androgen while in utero. The most common source of the excess androgen is production by the fetus itself. Congenital adrenal hyperplasia is the most common cause of female pseudohermaphroditism and the most frequent etiology of ambiguous external genitalia in the newborn (Fig. 16–5). It is the only intersex disorder that can be life-threatening, and therefore it is mandatory to establish diagnosis as soon after birth as possible. Patients with congenital adrenal hyperplasia have normal female internal genitalia, and the virilized external genitalia can be corrected surgically. Female pseudohermaphroditisms due to congenital adrenal hyperplasia or nonadrenal causes are the only intersex disorders that carry the possibility of completely normal sexual function, including coitus and conception. Left untreated, patients with congenital adrenal hyperplasia have accelerated growth in their early years and are much taller than their peers. The distal epiphyses close prematurely, and these patients are ultimately considerably shorter than average. A male neonate with congenital adrenal hyperplasia does not usually have ambiguous external genitalia and frequently is not diagnosed at birth unless there is a family history of this disease.

Congenital adrenal hyperplasia is an autosomal recessive disorder which is the result of an enzyme deficiency in the synthesis of cortisol. The pathways of adrenal steroid biosynthesis are outlined in Fig. 16-7. The enzyme deficiency results in a decrease in cortisol synthesis, which reduces the negative feedback on the pituitary. Increased ACTH (adrenocorticotropic hormone), stimulating the zona reticularis of the adrenal gland, increases androgen production, which virilizes the external genitalia. Enzyme deficiencies in cortisol synthesis which result in ambiguous external genitalia include 21-hydroxylase deficiency with-

out salt wasting, 21-hydroxylase deficiency with salt wasting, 11-hydroxylase deficiency, and 3β-ol-dehydrogenase deficiency. The 21-hydroxylase deficiency without salt wasting is the most common form of congenital adrenal hyperplasia. Deficiencies of either the 21-hydroxylase enzyme with salt wasting or the 3β-ol-dehydrogenase enzyme are life-threatening. The 11-hydroxylase deficiency is associated with hypertension. Congenital adrenal hyperplasia is diagnosed by demonstrating an increase in steroid precursor in the cortisol pathway preceding the locus of action of the deficient enzyme and an increase in adrenal androgen. The 17α-hydroxyprogesterone in the serum and its urinary metabolite pregnanetriol are elevated when there is a 21-hydroxylase or 11-hydroxylase deficiency.

In female pseudohermaphroditism, if the excess androgen is not of fetal adrenal origin, it may be of maternal origin either from the ingestion of androgens or the production of androgen from an ovarian tumor. Very rarely the underlying etiology of female pseudohermaphroditism with partial virilization is never determined, and may be idiopathic.

DIAGNOSIS

Recognition of ambiguous external genitalia in the newborn may be overlooked in the delivery room. Size of the phallus, position of the urethral orifice, the degree of hypospadias, the extent of labial scrotal fusion, the presence of testes in the scrotum bilaterally, the presence of a uterus, and the presence of an inguinal hernia should be part of the initial examination of the neonate. A penis has a midline ventral frenulum and the clitoris has two lateral folds which extend to the labia minora. Fusion of the labial scrotal folds always forms from a posterior to anterior direction. Cryptorchidism is considered a minor anatomic abnormality when it is unilateral, a uterus is absent, and the genital development is otherwise normal. Cryptorchidism should be considered an early indication of an intersex disorder if it is bilateral, or if it is unilateral and a uterus is present. Hypospadias is a minor anatomic abnormality when both testes have descended into the scrotum, a uterus is absent, and the development of the external genitalia is otherwise normal. Hypospadias should be considered an early indication of an intersex disorder if it is associated with cryptorchidism, a palpable uterus, or a defect in scrotal fusion.

It is very uncommon for an ovary to be situated outside the abdominal cavity. In the first weeks of life, if a uterus is present, it is slightly enlarged due to stimulation of the high circulating levels of maternal estrogen. The uterus may be palpated by gentle rectal examination using the little finger. Intersex disorders in which a uterus is present include true hermaphroditism, mixed gonadal dysgenesis, and female pseudohermaphroditism. Intersex disorders in which a uterus is absent include male pseudohermaphroditism resulting from a primary gonadal defect, a defect in testosterone action, or a defect in testosterone biosynthesis. Abnormalities in the synthesis or action of MIF do not result in ambiguous external genitalia.

Evaluation of the neonate with ambiguous external genitalia must be conducted in order to determine as early as possible the existence of a life-threatening disorder and the sex for rearing. Congenital adrenal hyperplasia may be a serious threat to the life of the neonate, and therefore it is mandatory to confirm or exclude this diagnosis as soon after birth of an infant with ambiguous external genitalia as possible. Measurement of elevated serum levels of 17α-hydroxyprogesterone or increased excretion of its urinary metabolite pregnanetriol, increased excretion of 17-ketosteroids, and elevated serum levels of testosterone have been used to diagnose congenital adrenal hyperplasia. The concentration of 17α-hydroxyprogesterone in the peripheral circulation is the preferred test to establish this diagnosis, but this assay is not always available.

Serum progesterone determinations can be used in place of 17α-hydroxyprogesterone. For the proper interpretation of the results, the normal value of these laboratory parameters at various time intervals after birth must be available (Table 16–1). In a neonate with a karyotype 46XX, serum concentrations of 17α-hydroxyprogesterone which exceed 7 ng/mL, concentrations of testosterone which exceed 50 ng per 100 mL, urinary excretion of 17-ketosteroids greater than 4 mg per day, and excretion of pregnanetriol greater than 0.5 mg per day are diagnostic of congenital adrenal hyperplasia. The normal daily urinary excretion of 17-ketosteroids is presented in Table 16-1. The salt-losing form of congenital adrenal hyperplasia

TABLE 16–1 Urinary 17-Ketosteriod Excretion

Age	Normal excretion, mg/day
<1 month	< 4.0
1–12 months	< 0.5
1–5 years	< 1.0
6–9 years	< 2.0
10–15 years	<10.0
>15 years	<15.0

is not usually apparent until the end of the first week of life. The infant with an enzyme deficiency in the cortisol pathway fails to thrive and does not regain its birth weight in the first 7 to 10 days of life.

The genetic sex of a newborn suspected of having an intersex disorder must be determined. Nuclear chromatin counts are not reliable in the first 2 days of life as normal female counts are characteristically low at this time. The karyotype is the preferred method of determining the genetic sex. Intersex disorders which have a normal female karyotype, 46XX, include true hermaphroditism and female pseudohermaphroditism. Male pseudohermaphrodites have a male karyotype, 46XY. Urethroscopy and a vaginogram are indicated to determine if the urethra and the vagina are separate. Finally, it may be necessary to recommend exploratory laparotomy to distinguish between true hermaphroditism and nonadrenal female pseudohermaphroditism, or between true hermaphroditism with a male karyotype and various forms of male pseudohermaphroditism.

TREATMENT PRINCIPLES

The psychological determinants of sex, sex of rearing, and gender role are usually related to the appearance of the external genitalia. Therefore, once a neonate is identified as having an intersex disorder, it is of the greatest importance to assign the sex of rearing of an individual as soon after birth as possible in order to prevent psychological trauma. The assignment of the sex of the infant should be made while the newborn is still in the hospital in order to obviate a change in gender role later in life which can produce serious psychological sequelae. All female pseudohermaphrodites have the potential of normal sexual function and fertility and should be raised as females. For infants with all other intersex disorders, the sex assigned to the infant should be decided primarily on the potential of the external genitalia for normal coitus, as these patients are usually infertile. It is easier for the surgeon to create functional female external genitalia than functional male external genitalia. Therefore, most patients with an intersex disorder other than congenital adrenal hyperplasia and with more than a mild form of ambiguous external genitalia should be raised as female. The amputation of the phallus of these infants should be performed soon after birth in order to avoid psychological trauma to the infant and the parents.

Hermaphrodites with a Y sex chromosome are at increased risk for gonadal tumors, either dysgerminoma or gonadoblastoma. The risk of tumor formation in individuals with intersex disorders with a Y chromosome increases at the time of puberty except for testicular feminization. Individuals with mixed gonadal dysgenesis and male pseudohermaphroditism should have their gonads removed prior to puberty. Gonadal tumors rarely occur in individuals with testicular feminization before the age of 25, and gonadal steroids produced by these individuals promote breast development. Therefore, the removal of these gonads can be safely delayed until after the age of 20. Patients with ambiguous external genitalia who do not have a Y chromosome are not at increased risk for gonadal tumor formation and do not need their gonads extirpated.

MALE PSEUDOHERMAPHRODITISM, ENDOCRINE TYPE

The male pseudohermaphrodite is a genetic male, karyotype 46XY, and a gonadal male with normal testicular differentiation. To a varying extent, the appearance of the external genitalia is incongruous with the genetic and gonadal sex. The spectrum of morphologic changes of the external genitalia includes hypospadias in the mildest form; posterior migration of the urethral orifice and failure in the fusion of the labioscrotal folds; urogenital sinus formation and clitoromegaly; and, in the greatest change from the normal male phenotype, completely feminized external genitalia.

Male psuedohermaphroditism with partial failure of virilization may be the result of abnormalities in the synthesis or action of MIF, defects of testosterone action, or defects in testosterone biosynthesis (see also Chap. 9). Alterations in the synthesis or action of MIF do not cause ambiguous external genitalia. The morphology of the Wolffian duct derivatives and the morphology of the external genitalia are normal male. Regression of Müllerian duct derivatives fails to occur, and oviducts and a uterus frequently are present in an inguinal hernia.

A defect in testosterone action is the most common cause of male pseudohermaphroditism. The alteration of normal testosterone action can result from a complete androgen-binding protein defect (complete testicular feminization), and partial androgen-binding protein defect (incomplete testicular feminization), or a 5α-reductase enzyme deficiency which mediates the conversion of testosterone to dihydrotestosterone. Individuals with complete testicular feminization are genetic males, karyotype 46XY, and gonadal males with bilateral testes. There is com-

TABLE 16-2 Classification of Intersexuality

I. Disorders of gonadal development
  A. Klinefelter's syndrome
  B. Gonadal dysgenesis
    1. Turner's syndrome
    2. Mosaicism
    3. Pure gonadal dysgenesis
  C. True hermaphroditism
  D. Male pseudohermaphroditism
    1. Primary gonadal defect
    2. Y chromosomal defect
II. Disorders of fetal endocrinology
  A. Female pseudohermaphroditism with partial virilization
    1. Congenital adrenal hyperplasia
      a. 21-Hydroxylase deficiency without salt wasting
      b. 21-Hydroxylase deficiency with salt wasting
      c. 11-Hydroxylase deficiency (hypertensive)
      d. 3β-ol-Dehydrogenase deficiency
    2. Nonadrenal female pseudohermaphroditism
      a. Maternal androgenization
        (1) Exogenous androgen
        (2) Virilizing tumors
      b. Idiopathic
  B. Male pseudohermaphroditism with partial failure of virilization
    1. Abnormalities of Müllerian inhibitory factor synthesis or action
    2. Defects of testosterone action
      a. Complete androgen-binding protein defect (complete testicular feminization)
      b. Partial androgen-binding protein defect (incomplete testicular feminization)
      c. 5α-Reductase deficiency
    3. Testosterone biosynthesis defect
      a. Pregnenolone synthesis defect (lipoid adrenal hyperplasia)
      b. 3β-Hydroxysteroid dehydrogenase deficiency
      c. 17α-Hydroxylase deficiency
      d. 17–20 Desmolase deficiency
      e. 17β-Hydroxysteroid dehydrogenase

plete regression of the Müllerian duct derivatives, and the internal male genitalia are also absent. The vaginal vault is usually reduced in depth and the appearance of the external genitalia is normal female. An inguinal hernia may be present at birth. Growth and breast development are normal but axillary, pubic, and body hair are sparse. Failure to menstruate usually leads these phenotypic females to seek medical consultation.

The partial androgen-binding protein defect has been designated male incomplete pseudohermaphroditism, type I. This partial defect in the cell receptor leads to varying degrees of ambiguous external genitalia as well as to varying degrees in the development of the male internal genitalia. There is complete suppression of Müllerian duct derivatives. All of these individuals experience breast development at puberty. The deficiency of the 5α-reductase enzyme has been designated male incomplete pseudohermaphroditism, type II. This enzyme deficiency is an autosomal recessive disorder found in certain families. All the individuals are born with normal male internal genitalia, ambiguous external genitalia, bilateral undescended testes, and lack of a phallus. At puberty there is marked virilization, absence of breast devel-

opment, phallic growth, and descent of the testes into the scrotum. In general these individuals with male incomplete pseudohermaphroditism, type II, are capable of adequate male sexual function and in some cultures are raised as males.

Defects in the biosynthesis of testosterone are due to an enzyme deficiency. The location of these enzyme alterations in the pathways of testosterone synthesis are demonstrated in Fig. 16–7. The individuals with these rare disorders of fetal endocrinology have male gonads, complete regression of the Müllerian duct derivatives, ambiguous external genitalia, and may develop breasts at puberty. Defects in the biosynthesis of testosterone are autosomal recessive disorders. A classification of intersex disorders is presented in Table 16–2.

FIGURE 16–7 Pathways of adrenal steroid biosynthesis.

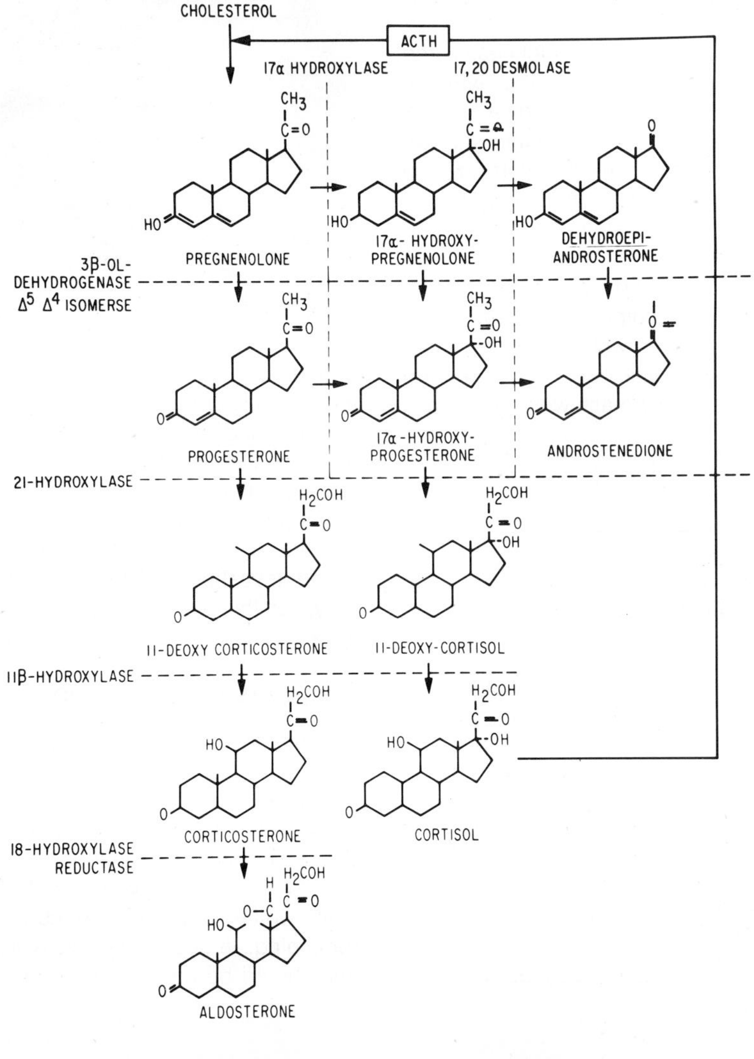

CONGENITAL ANOMALIES OF THE FEMALE GENITAL ORGANS

Congenital anomalies of the female reproductive organs which do not result in ambiguous external genitalia are infrequently diagnosed prior to puberty. These anomalies are not associated with major chromosomal errors but may be associated with abnormal development of the urinary system. Primary amenorrhea, pain, or pregnancy wastage usually lead the patient to seek medical evaluation. These developmental abnormalities may be classified as (1) failure of normal canalization; (2) failure of the development of Müllerian duct derivatives; and (3) failure of fusion of Müllerian duct derivatives (Table 16–3).

FAILURE OF NORMAL CANALIZATION

Anomalies of the Hymen

The appearance of the orifice and the thickness of the hymenal membrane vary considerably. The hymenal aperture may be single, may be divided by a septum (septate), may contain multiple small openings (cribriform), or may be imperforate. The cribriform hymen is thick and rigid, and has multiple minute openings. The egress of menses may be painful or blocked and coitus may not be feasible. An imperforate hymen prevents the escape of vaginal desquamate, cervical mucus, and blood. A mucocolpos may form in the neonate and a hematocolpos will form when menstruation occurs. As the vagina becomes distended with blood, it creates a pelvic mass which becomes

TABLE 16–3 Congenital Anomalies of the Female Genital Organs (Normal External Genitalia)

I. Failure of canalization
  A. Imperforate hymen
  B. Transverse vaginal septum
  C. Absence of the vagina
  D. Cervical atresia
II. Failure of the development of Müllerian duct derivatives
  A. Bilateral
    1. Absence of oviducts, uterus, vagina
    2. Absence of the uterus
  B. Unilateral—Unicornuate uterus
III. Failure of fusion of Müllerian duct derivatives
  A. Arcuate uterus
  B. Septuate uterus
  C. Bicornuate uterus
  D. Uterus didelphys

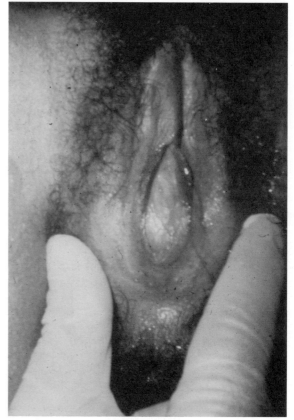

FIGURE 16–8 Imperforate hymen.

palpable abdominally. Girls with an imperforate hymen usually complain of primary amenorrhea, cyclic cramps, and eventually pelvic pain or even urinary retention. Examination of the external genitalia reveals a bulging, tense hymen without any visible aperture (Fig. 16–8). The treatment of an imperforate hymen is surgical incision and release of the menstrual blood. Investigation of the urinary tract is not necessary, for this abnormality is not associated with an increased incidence of urinary tract anomalies.

Transverse Vaginal Septum

Transverse septa of the vagina are usually incomplete. The septa may cause dyspareunia or hemorrhage as the result of vaginal lacerations at the time of delivery, and they may be an incidental finding during a pelvic examination. When discovered, they should be excised. Even when the septa are removed some women may have extensive vaginal scar tissue remaining. In such cases delivery by cesarean section should be considered if they become pregnant.

Congenital Absence of the Vagina

Failure of the vagina to develop is usually associated with the absence of the uterus and oviducts, but in some patients vaginal agenesis may be present with a hormonally responsive uterus. The recommended treatment has been the surgical formation of a neovagina and the connection of the cervix to the neovagina. Whenever a neovagina is created, it will quickly constrict if the patient cannot keep the vagina dilated either by regular coitus or by the use of vaginal dilators or vaginal stent. Maintenance of the patency of the cervical os into the neovagina may be difficult in patients with a uterus. Some surgeons have found that in the presence of complete vaginal agenesis, attempts to preserve fertility are associated with considerable morbidity and mortality, and at the time the neovagina is created they recommend extirpation of the uterus and tubes. Such patients are frequently found to have endometriosis at the time of laparotomy.

Congenital Cervical Atresia

This rare lesion if associated with functional endometrium, results in a hematometra, pain, reflux of the endometrium through the oviducts, and possibly endometriosis. There is no communication between the uterine cavity and the vaginal vault to allow the normal flow of menstrual blood. Surgical attempts to create a communication between the uterus and vagina almost never result in the patient's ability to conceive and are often associated with considerable morbidity or with additional surgical intervention. Hysterectomy with the preservation of ovarian function may be necessary.

FAILURE OF THE DEVELOPMENT OF MÜLLERIAN DUCT DERIVATIVES

Absence of the Oviducts, Uterus and Vagina

Complete absence of the oviducts, uterus, and vagina causes primary amenorrhea and sterility, and leads to problems with coitus. The cyclic hypothalamic-pituitary-ovarian function, appearance of the external genitalia, growth pattern, and development of secondary sex characteristics are normal in these patients. Absence of the uterus and/or vagina does not cause symptoms prior to puberty. The first clinical signs may be the inability to have intercourse and/or the absence of spontaneous menstruation. While an artificial vagina may be created surgically, the failure of the uterus to develop renders these women sterile. If the vagina is congenitally absent, the patient should be evaluated for associated anomalies of the urinary tract and skeletal system. Women with vaginal agenesis have a 50 percent incidence of upper urinary tract abnormalities; 15 percent have an absent kidney, and 10 percent have a vertebral defect. Treatment of congenital absence of the uterus and vagina requires the creation of a neovagina. This is usually accomplished surgically, but nonsurgical methods using vaginal cylinders of gradually increasing diameter have been successful. No matter how the artificial vagina is created, the patient must be motivated to keep it dilated or the cavity will be quickly obliterated. Therefore, surgery is often delayed until a time when the woman has a reasonable expectation of maintaining the neovagina's patency by regular coitus.

Absence of the Uterus

Congenital absence of the uterus must be distinguished from testicular feminization. Both conditions are associated with a normal female phenotype and an absent uterus. The distinction can be made by a karyotype determination or the measurement of blood testosterone. Women with congenital absence of the uterus have a female karyotype, XX, and female levels of testosterone. Patients with testicular feminization have a male karyotype, XY, and male levels of testosterone. Women with congenital absence of the uterus are sterile.

Unicornous Uterus

The unicornous uterus may be accompanied by a rudimentary horn or by a Müllerian duct remnant in the lateral wall of the vagina lined by endometrium. The rudimentary horn may or may not communicate with the uterus, and its endometrial lining may or may not be responsive to cyclic hormonal stimulation. A blind rudimentary horn responsive to cyclic hormone levels can cause severe dysmenorrhea because there is no passage for menstrual blood. Treatment consists of surgical excision of the rudimentary horn. A cyst in the lateral wall of the vagina lined by endometrium can fill with blood, enlarge, and occupy most of the vaginal vault. The cystic remnant of the Müllerian duct has to be excised or opened. While even minor anomalies of the genital organs may be associated with urinary tract maldevelopment, the asymmetric malformations of the uterus are the ones most likely to be associated with urinary tract anomalies.

FAILURE OF MÜLLERIAN DUCT DERIVATIVES TO FUSE

Anomalies resulting from the failure of normal fusion of the genital organs derived from the Müllerian ducts occur during the second to fourth month of fetal development. The degree of separation may range from slight (arcuate uterus), partial (septate uterus and bicornuate uterus), to total (uterus didelphys). The septate uterus is the partial lack of fusion which is expressed inside the uterus only. The bicornuate uterus is the partial lack of fusion which is expressed externally and internally and is associated with a single cervix. Uterus didelphys is the complete duplication of the uterus and cervix and may be accompanied by duplication of the vagina. Abnormalities due to failure of fusion of Müllerian duct derivatives usually do not have clinical significance until the patient desires children. All degrees of failure to achieve normal fusion increase the incidence of obstetric complications, particularly abnormal presentations and premature labor. The septate uterus is frequently associated with pregnancy wastage characterized by both first- and second-trimester abortions. Surgical excision of the septum is the treatment for women with a septate uterus and a history of recurrent abortion. Patients may attempt to become pregnant 6 months following metroplasty with a 60 to 80 percent expectancy of a full-term gestation. Delivery should be by cesarean section. Surgical therapy is ill-advised, however, for women with a septate uterus who have a history of infertility. The bicornuate uterus is associated with an increase in second-trimester losses. Anomalies resulting from the failure of fusion of Müllerian duct derivatives rarely cause infertility (Table 16–4).

PREPUBERTAL VULVOVAGINITIS

The most common complaint of premenarchal patients seen in the pediatric gynecology clinic is vulvovaginitis. At least three factors place young girls at high risk for vaginal infections: the relatively unprotected introitus, the thin unestrogenized vaginal mucosa, and, most important of all, the failure of children to be properly instructed in proper perineal hygiene. For instance following defecation, bacteria are carried toward the vagina if children wipe from rectum to vagina.

As a result of these factors vulvovaginal infections in children are most frequently caused by nonspecific mixed bacteria normally found in the rectum. There are also a wide variety of specific causes of vulvovaginitis in children. If they have had a recent streptococcal or staphylococcal infection elsewhere in the body, particularly in the upper respiratory tract, these organisms can also be found in the vagina. Monilial vaginitis is rare in the prepubertal child, and when it occurs it should be considered an indication to screen the child for carbohydrate intolerance, diabetes mellitus. *Trichomonas* vaginitis is also an infrequent cause of leukorrhea in young girls. There is still debate as to whether gonococcal vaginitis in the prepubertal girl is more often due to contact from contaminated inanimate objects, bed linen, or sexual contact. A family history of parasites and additional complaints or findings of perianal pruritus or irritation suggest pinworms (*Enterobius vermicularis*) as the etiologic agent of the vulvovaginitis, and a "Scotch tape test"[1] is indicated to identify the pinworm eggs.

Congenital anomalies which result in a communication between the vagina and rectum or the blad-

[1] A Scotch tape test is one in which adhesive tape is attached, sticky side out, to an applicator. The applicator is then applied to the perianal area and pinworm eggs adhere to the sticky tape for identification.

TABLE 6–4 Obstetrical Problems Caused by Failure of Müllerian Duct Derivatives to Fuse

Anomaly	Abnormal obstetric presentation	Second-trimester abortion	First-trimester abortion	Infertility
Separate uterus	Inc.*	Inc.	Inc.	—
Bicornuate uterus	Inc.	Inc.	—	—
Uterus didelphys	Inc.	—	—	—

*Inc. = Increased.

der can cause a vaginal discharge. A foreign body, whether tissue paper or a solid object like a button, can produce a discharge which is characteristically purulent and bloody. A bloody, purulent discharge may rarely be the result of a tumor. Finally, a vaginal discharge in the premenarchal child is not always pathological, but may be physiological. The vaginal mucosa and cervix are quite sensitive to estrogen. The amount of vaginal desquamate is increased in the first few weeks of life from exogenous estrogen of maternal origin, and in the months immediately preceding puberty as the result of increased endogenous levels of estrogen producing a physiological leukorrhea.

All children with leukorrhea require a careful history as to the character of the discharge, the presence of blood, the method of perineal hygiene, recent streptococcal or staphylococcal infections, venereal disease in the members of the immediate family, parasites among the family, perineal pruritus, and the possibility of a foreign body in the vagina. The external genitalia and perineum are inspected and a gentle rectal exam performed. If a discharge is present at the introitus, a wet mount using saline and a wet mount using potassium hydroxide are prepared and examined for yeast and *Trichomonas.* A gonorrhea culture on chocolate agar, a culture of Stewart's medium, and a Gram stain are collected. A history and perineal findings suggesting pinworms are followed with the Scotch tape test. With a cooperative child a soft plastic eyedropper can be placed in the vagina to collect the discharge. Glass instruments should not be placed in the vagina of a young girl. The further management of prepubertal vulvovaginitis depends on the character of the discharge and whether any foreign body has been placed in the vagina. Any time either the child or her parent indicates the patient may have placed a foreign body in the vagina or whenever there is blood with the discharge, the vagina must be inspected. Vaginoscopy with the child awake is frequently successful using a variety of instruments, including specially designed vaginoscopes, Killian's nasal speculum, or the author's preference, the veterinary otoscope (Fig. 16-9). Should vaginoscopy prove unsuccessful with the child awake, she must be scheduled for vaginoscopy under anesthesia. The Kelly air urethroscope is an excellent instrument for examination of the vagina of the young anesthetized patient. If the discharge is not mixed with blood and there is no history of a foreign body, vaginoscopy is not included as a mandatory part of the initial exam.

Children with nonspecific vulvovaginitis need to

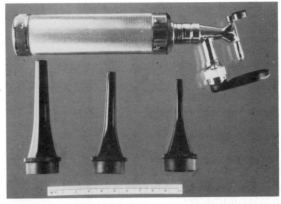

FIGURE 16-9 Veterinary otoscope. Attachments are 4, 7, and 9 mm in outer diameter and 75 mm in length.

be carefully instructed on proper perineal hygiene. The importance of wiping the perineum from front to back, away from the vagina, following defecation must be stressed. Underpants made of cotton, which absorbs discharge, are better than the synthetic fibers such as nylon which hold the discharge against the vulvar tissue. The underpants should be changed as frequently as necessary during the day. Both the underpants and the toilet tissue should be white and should not contain dyes which may prove irritating to the vulva. The child's clothing should be loose-fitting, and skirts are preferred over skin-tight slacks. Sitz baths two to four times a day in warm water bring temporary relief of symptoms, but soaps should be avoided. If vulvitis is present, the application of 1% hydrocortisone cream or Mycolog cream after each sitz bath is recommended. Systemic antibiotics are advocated for the treatment of the bacterial vaginitis. Oral liquid preparations may be administered in divided doses, the total dose depending on the weight of the patient (ampicillin 50 mg/kg per day for 10 days). Even if the vaginitis fails to respond completely, the vulvitis is generally improved, enhancing the possibility of a satisfactory vaginoscopy without anesthesia if necessary.

In addition to the history of a foreign body and the presence of blood in the discharge, persistent leukorrhea which fails to respond to therapy is an indication for vaginoscopy. If a specific etiology is not found by vaginoscopy, the persistent vulvovaginitis is treated with estrogen applied locally for 14 consecutive nights. The estrogen may be administered as a conjugated estrogen (Premarin) cream or as half of a Furacin-E urethral suppository, which is inserted into the vagina. Specific treatment is available for pinworms (pyrvinium pamoate), monilial vaginitis (nystatin), *Trichomonas* vaginitis (metronidazole), and streptococcal, staphylococcal, and gonococcal vaginitis (penicillin). Foreign bodies require removal. Gonococcal vaginitis proved by culture is an indication to search for gonorrhea in other members of the immediate family. Gonococcal vaginitis may be the result of sexual assault.

VULVAR LACERATIONS, HEMATOMAS AND LABIAL ADHESIONS

When a child who has sustained a recent vulvar laceration is seen in the emergency room, the attending physician is tempted to secure hemostasis and repair the laceration under local anesthesia. It is rare for a child to cooperate in a repair under these conditions. Even when a single pumping vessel is identified as the source of the bleeding in a small laceration, the doctor is best advised to repair the laceration under general anesthesia. If there is any question as to the possible injury to the vagina, urethra, or bladder, these structures must be examined while the patient is anesthetized.

Most vulvar hematomas in children are the result of "straddle" injuries. The extent of the hematoma must be clearly defined, which includes inspection of the perineum and a rectal examination. If in 3 to 4 hours the hematoma has not expanded and the child is able to void clear urine spontaneously, a nonsurgical approach employing ice packs is sufficient. An enlarging hematoma is an indication for operative intervention in order to evacuate the hematoma and identify and ligate the sites of active bleeding.

In young girls before the age of 8, the labia can become adherent as the result of adhesions. Labial fusion may partially or completely occlude the vaginal orifice. As long as the child can void spontaneously without discomfort, there is no need for treatment. Most cases will resolve without treatment when the endogenous estrogen levels increase in early puberty. Attempts at manual separation of the labia are condemned, for not only do they traumatize the patient physically and emotionally but they almost always fail: more scarring occurs, and the labia fuse once again. If labial adhesions lead to problems of

voiding, then estrogen cream should be administered topically for 14 consecutive nights.

ALLEGED SEXUAL ASSAULT

The physical, psychological, and social sequelae of sexual assault require a multidisciplinary medical approach to the patient. Care of the victim of a sexual assault should include immediate medical attention, privacy, confidentiality, and adequate follow-up. In a medical center, a team composed of a physician, nurse, social worker, and security officer is optimal to meet these goals. This team faces many responsibilities in the care of alleged victims of sexual assault, but it is not their responsibility to prove or disprove that rape occurred. This is a matter for the judicial system, not for the medical profession.

The sexual assault of a child is even more devastating than that of an adult. The child may never completely recover from the physical and emotional traumas sustained during the attack. For any victim of an alleged sexual assault, the physician's first responsibility is to identify and treat any life-threatening problems. If the patient does not face a threat to her life the physician's task is the careful documentation of the extent of the injuries and the collection of evidence. When the child has not sustained pelvic bleeding and there is no evidence of vaginal penetration, vaginoscopy for the collection of evidence, including cultures for gonorrhea, with the child awake, can be attempted. If the first attempt is unsuccessful, no further efforts at vaginoscopy are advised. When the child has sustained pelvic bleeding or there is evidence of vaginal penetration, the patient should be anesthetized for the collection of evidence and the repair of the traumatized tissue. The collection of evidence includes a smear to be examined for sperm, a dry swab for the chemical determination of acid phosphatase (a component of semen), a saline swab for ABO typing, and a culture for gonorrhea. The young girl who has been vaginally traumatized must be examined for penetration of the peritoneal cavity and for possible total avulsion of the upper vaginal vault. If the peritoneal cavity has been entered, there will be evidence of crepitus and intraperitoneal gas. Avulsion of the upper vaginal vault causes the child marked discomfort in walking or talking, and she will develop an ileus.

PRECOCIOUS PUBERTY

Precocious puberty is the development of secondary sex characteristics at an earlier age than that found in 99.5 percent of the population. The precise definition can be determined by subtracting 3 standard deviations from the mean age at which a specific pubertal event occurs. For example, if in a given population the mean age at which breast budding is first noticed is 11.2 years ± 1.1 years (standard deviation), then a girl in this population would be considered to have precocious puberty if her breast development began prior to 8 years. Differences in the mean age at which the events of puberty occur are found in the literature, and this acounts for the discrepancies in the definition of precocious puberty. Precocious puberty will here be defined as the appearance in girls of breast budding prior to the age of 8, or menarche before the age of 9.

Precocious puberty is either isosexual, in which the secondary sex characteristics are in agreement with the genetic sex, or heterosexual, in which the secondary sex characteristics are in disagreement with the genetic sex. Girls with clinical evidence of hirsutism or masculinization have heterosexual precocious puberty. Clinical evidence of heterosexual precocious puberty requires the patient to be evaluated for the etiology of the androgen excess. Therapy is selected to remove or suppress the source of the androgen.

Incomplete precocious puberty is the appearance of a single pubertal event, either breast development (premature thelarche), axillary hair growth (premature adrenarche), or pubic hair growth (premature pubarche). There is no evidence of an estrogen effect on the advancement of bone age or the maturity of the cells in the vaginal desquamate. Premature thelarche and premature adrenarche are benign conditions which do not require treatment. Although the mechanism is unclear, approximately half of the patients with premature pubarche have organic brain disease.

Isosexual precocious puberty may be due to causes within the central nervous system, referred to as true or cerebral isosexual precocious puberty, or to causes outside the central nervous system, referred to as pseudoisosexual precocious puberty. Sexual maturation progressing to menstruation occurs in both true and pseudoisosexual precocious puberty. Except in hypothyroidism there is an initial rapid in-

crease in height. Early in the disease the patients are taller than their peers, but under the influence of estrogen the distal epiphyses fuse prematurely and the patients ultimately are short in stature. In true precocious puberty there is cyclic function of the reproductive axis, and ovulation and fertility are feasible. In the pseudo form the reproductive axis is suppressed and follicular maturation and ovulation do not occur. Causes of pseudoisosexual precocious puberty include estrogen-secreting ovarian tumors, estrogen-secreting adrenal tumors, iatrogenic causes, hypothyroidism, McCune-Albright syndrome, and the hemihypertrophy syndrome of Wilkins. Causes of true isosexual precocious puberty include organic brain disease, but many cases are constitutional.

Ten percent of girls with isosexual precocious puberty have the pseudo form. The most common cause of pseudoisosexual precocious puberty is an ovarian tumor which secretes estrogen. Granulosa-theca cell tumors of the ovary produce estrogen and in prepubertal girls are palpable by rectal-abdominal examination. Choriocarcinoma of ovarian or extragonadal origin produces human chorionic gonadotropin (HCG) which stimulates the ovary to secrete estrogen. These tumors may be diagnosed by measurement of the increased amounts of HCG in the urine or serum. Some investigators accept estrogen-producing adrenal tumor as a cause of isosexual precocious puberty. If this lesion does occur, it is extremely infrequent. Estrogens are frequently a component of cleansing creams, cosmetics, and preparations for diaper rash. Pharmaceutical products may contain estrogen primarily or may be contaminated with estrogen. Any of these sources may cause isosexual precocious puberty and only by a meticulous history can they be identified.

A marked reduction of thyroid hormone secretion occurs in hypothyroidism. Removal of the negative-feedback effect of thyroid hormone on the hypothalamus and pituitary gland leads to an increase in thyroid-releasing hormone (TRH) and thyroid-stimulating hormone (TSH), and accompanying this pituitary stimulation there may be an increase of gonadotropins and/or prolactin. Thus ovarian cysts due to gonadotropin stimulation may be associated with hypothyroidism. Once the patient becomes euthyroid, the cysts regress spontaneously. Hypothyroidism as the etiology of precocious puberty is almost always found in girls. The bone age is retarded.

Albright's syndrome is the combination of areas of fibrous or cystic dysplasia of bone, café-au-lait spots in the skin, and sexual precocity. This rare syndrome occurs more commonly in girls and is characterized by facial asymmetry, skeletal deformities, and brown spots on the face, neck, shoulders, and back. The hemihypertrophy syndrome of Wilkins is the rare combination of unilateral sexual precocity and vascular anomalies.

Of girls with isosexual precocious puberty, 90 percent have the true form, and of these, 90 percent have a diagnosis of constitutional precocious puberty. The underlying etiology is unknown. The onset of symptoms may occur at any age but is rare in the first 12 months of life. The course of the disease may be rapid or slow; very rarely, spontaneous remissions have occurred. The disease is not detrimental to the general health of the patient but is a source of emotional trauma for both the patient and her family. Approximately half these girls have abnormal EEG (electroencephalogram) tracings. The diagnosis is one of exclusion as there is no pathognomonic laboratory test. The remaining 10 percent of patients with true isosexual precocious puberty have organic brain disease which may be tumor, congenital defect, obstructive lesion, or a postinfection lesion. They almost always have neurologic evidence of the disease prior to the sexual precocity. A neurologic exam usually denotes the cause.

The specific diagnosis of a patient with isosexual precocious puberty requires a careful history, physical examination, and a few properly chosen laboratory tests. Incomplete forms of sexual precocity can be diagnosed by examinations several months apart which indicate that only one pubertal change is present, accompanied by evidence of a lack of a peripheral estrogen effect. The bone age is in agreement with the patient's chronologic age, indicating an absence of an estrogen effect on bone maturity. A retarded bone age indicates girls with isosexual precocious puberty due to hypothyroidism. Advancement of bone age beyond the 95th percentile for the patient's chronological age indicates a periph-

eral estrogen effect. A serum follicle-stimulating hormone (FSH) measurement can separate true from pseudo causes of isosexual precocious puberty. In true forms the sensitivity of the hypothalamus to the negative feedback of endogenous estrogen decreases; as a result, gonadotropin-releasing hormone and gonadotropins increase. In the pseudo forms the exquisite sensitivity of the hypothalamus to circulating estrogen persists and gonadotropins remain very low. Specific causes of pseudoisosexual precocious puberty can be identified, based on unique findings in the history and physical examination. An abnormal neurologic exam suggests the presence of organic brain disease. Finally, the diagnosis of constitutional precocious puberty is one in which all other causes are excluded. Diagnostic tests used in the evaluation of patients with precocious puberty are outlined in Table 16–5.

The treatment of isosexual precocious puberty depends upon the etiology. Incomplete forms are usually self-limiting, may regress spontaneously, and do not require treament. Ovarian and adrenal estrogen-producing tumors are surgically removed. Once an iatrogenic source is identified, it is eliminated. Hypothyroid patients, including those with ovarian cysts, are managed medically with thyroid hormone replacement therapy. Unfortunately most central-nervous-system (CNS) lesions resulting in sexual precocity are untreatable.

By far the most common cause of precocious puberty in girls is constitutional. Ideally, treatment would result in the inhibition of ovulation, the cessation of menses, the regression of secondary sex characteristics, and the prevention of estrogen effect on bone. Estrogen at first produces a growth spurt, but with premature epiphyseal closure the patients are ultimately of short stature. The earlier the disease is manifested, the shorter will be the patient's final height. Medroxyprogesterone acetate, danazol, and cyproterone acetate have been used in the treatment

TABLE 16–5 Isosexual Precocious Puberty

Bone age retarded	Bone age normal (Incomplete form)	Bone age advanced	
		FSH low (pseudo form)	FSH normal (true form)
Hypothyroidism	Precocious thelarche Precocious adrenarche Precocious pubarche	Ovarian Adrenal Iatrogenic Fibrous dysplasia Hemihypertrophy	CNS disease Constitutional

of constitutional precocious puberty. Danazol is not recommended as it causes virilization. Cyproterone acetate is not always reliable in suppressing menstruation and is not yet available in the United States. Medroxyprogesterone acetate, 100 to 200 mg injected intramuscularly every 2 to 4 weeks, causes the inhibition of ovulation and the cessation of menstruation but does not always produce regression of secondary sex characteristics and does not retard premature fusion of the distal epiphyses. Use of medroxyprogesterone acetate may be associated with suppression of adrenal cortical function and a prolonged delay in the recovery of the reproductive axis after the medication is discontinued. Advantages and disadvantages must be considered on an individual basis.

TUMORS OF THE GENITAL TRACT

Tumors of the genital tract rarely occur in the premenarchal child. Some tumors are benign, asymptomatic, and regress spontaneously, and others may be life-threatening requiring radical treatment if there is to be any chance for survival. Practically every type of tumor of the genital tract reported to occur in the adult female has been found during the first two decades of life. Selected tumors of particular significance to children and adolescents are presented here.

Congenital cysts of the external genitalia may be present in as many as 0.6 percent of newborn female infants. These are hymenal cysts, paraurethral cysts, or very rarely clitoral cysts. Congenital cysts are usually single, less than 2 cm in diameter, and white or pale yellow in color with blood vessels visible on their surface. They almost always are asymptomatic, and if left alone they regress spontaneously shortly after birth. Occasionally paraurethral cysts enlarge and cause urethral obstruction. Urinary retention and the persistence of the cysts for longer than 2 months indicates need for a urologic investigation and surgical intervention.

Sarcoma botryoides is a rare but highly malignant tumor, most commonly found in young girls. The tumors originate from multiple sites in the upper portion of the vagina and cervix and the lesions cause symptoms of vaginal bleeding and/or discharge. The reluctance to perform vaginoscopy on a young girl many times has led to delays up to several years in establishing the correct diagnosis. Initial inspection

of these tumors reveals a cluster of polyps which belie the rapidity with which they can grow and metastasize. The tumor may expand to occupy the entire vagina, and it may spread to the parametrial, pelvic, femoral and paraaortic lymph nodes as well as to organs located outside the pelvis. The only hope for survival of more than a few years for patients with this tumor is radical surgery, usually exenteration. Reluctance to commit a young child with sarcoma botryoides to extensive surgery is understandable but will usually result in her death.

More than two decades ago, diethylstilbestrol (DES) was administered to pregnant women for the management of threatened abortion. In 1971 Herbst et al. reported that young girls in their first three decades of life who were products of these DES-treated pregnancies were at increased risk for vaginal adenosis and clear-cell adenocarcinoma of the vagina. In these in utero DES-exposed offspring, the incidence of vaginal adenosis may be as high as 90 percent, but the incidence of vaginal carcinoma is less than 0.1 percent, much less than the original reports indicated. Any patient whose mother received DES or any other nonsteroidal estrogen in the first half of the pregnancy which resulted in the birth of the patient should begin semiannual pelvic examinations at age 14 years or at the time of menarche, whichever comes first. The pelvic examination should include inspection, palpation, Papanicolaou smear, and Schiller stain of the vagina. Colposcopy is the most reliable method of diagnosis of vaginal adenosis. Vaginal biopsies are obtained as indicated by Schiller stain and colposcopy. Vaginal adenosis does not require specific treatment but does demand consistent follow-up.

The most common genital neoplasm in childhood is the ovarian tumor. One-third of the ovarian tumors in children are physiologic cysts and two-thirds are true neoplasms. As in the adult, ovarian neoplasms may be derived from epithelium, germ cells, and gonadal stroma. Prior to puberty, most ovarian neoplasms are of germ-cell origin, half of which are malignant. The benign germ-cell neoplasms are mature cystic teratomas (dermoids). Ovarian tumors of epithelium and gonadal stromal origin are infrequent in children. Ovarian neoplasms of stromal origin may be overrepresented in most series because they are associated with sex-hormone production and the striking clinical sequelae thereof and are therefore likely to be reported. The treatment of benign ovarian neoplasms is to remove the tumor while conserving as much normal ovarian tissue as possible. Extirpation or irradiation of the pelvic organs when the tumor is malignant is a difficult decision when the patient is a child. Radical treatment for ovarian cancer should not be delayed for a young girl, however, if it offers a reasonable opportunity for cure.

REFERENCES

Congenital Anomalies of the Female Genital Organs

Gerbie AB: Congenital anomalies of the female genital tract. *Pediatric Ann* 3:20, 1974.

Jones HW Jr, Jones GES: Double uterus as an etiological factor of repeated abortion; indication for surgical repair. *Am J Obstet Gynecol* 65:325, 1953.

Jones WS: Obstetric significance of female genital anomalies. *Obstet Gynecol* 10:113, 1957.

Maciulla GH et al.: Functional endometrial tissue with vaginal agenesis. *J Reprod Med* 21:373, 1978.

McRae MA, Kim MH: Dysmenorrhea in uterus unicornis with rudimentary uterine cavity. *Obstet Gynecol* 53:134, 1979.

Rock JA, Jones HW Jr: The clinical management of the double uterus. *Fertil Steril* 28:798, 1977.

Woolf RB, Allen WM: Concomitant malformations: The frequent simultaneous occurrence of congenital malformations of the reproductive and urinary tracts. *Obstet Gynecol* 2:236, 1953.

Ylikorkala O, Viinikka L: Pituitary and ovarian function in women with congenitally absent uterus. *Obstet Gynecol* 53:137, 1979.

Ambiguous External Genitalia

Donahoe PK, Hendren WM: Evaluation of the newborn with ambiguous genitalia. *Pediatr Clin North Am* 23:361, 1976.

Federman DD: *Abnormal Sexual Development: A Genetic and Endocrine Approach to Differential Diagnosis,* Philadelphia: Saunders, 1967.

Imperato-McGinley J, Peterson RE: Male pseudohermaphroditism: The complexities of male phenotype development. *Am J Med* 61:251, 1976.

Jaffe RB: Disorders of sexual development in *Reproductive Endocrinology: Physiology, Pathophysiology and Clinical Management,* eds. SSC Yen and RB Jaffe, Philadelphia: Saunders, 1978.

Manuel M et al.: The age of occurrence of gonadal tumors in intersex patients with a Y chromosome. *Am J Obstet Gynecol* 124:293, 1976.

Park IJ, et al.: An etiologic and pathogenic classification of male hermaphroditism. *Am J Obstet Gynecol* 123:505, 1975.

Walsh PC et al.: Familial incomplete male pseudohermaphroditism, Type 2. Decreased dihydrotestosterone formation in pseudovaginal perineoscrotal hypospadias. *N Engl J Med* 291:944, 1974.

Wilson JD et al.: Familial incomplete male pseudohermaphroditism, Type I: Evidence for androgen resistance and variable clinical manifestations in a family with the Reifenstein syndrome. *N Engl J Med* 290:1097, 1974.

Prepubertal Vulvovaginitis

Altchek A: Pediatric vulvovaginitis. *Pediatr Clin North Am* 19:559, 1972.

Capraro VJ: Vulvovaginitis and other local lesions of the vulva. *Clin Obstet Gynecol* 1:533, 1974.

———, Capraro EJ: Vaginal aspirate studies in children. *Obstet Gynecol* 37:462, 1971.

———, Gallego MB: Vulvovaginitis in children. *Pediatr Ann* 3:74, 1974.

Davis TC: Chronic vulvovaginitis in children due to Shigella flexneri. *Pediatrics* 56:41, 1975.

Felman YM et al.: Gonococcal infections in children 14 years and younger. *Clin Pediatr* 17:252, 1978.

Sexual Assault

Breen JL et al.: The molested young female: Evaluation and therapy of alleged rape. *Pediatr Clin North Am* 19:717, 1972.

Burgess A, Holmstrom L: Rape trauma syndrome. *Am J Psychiatry* 131:981, 1974.

Capraro VJ: Sexual assault of female children. *Ann NY Acad Sci* 142:817, 1967.

Hogan WL: The raped child. *Med Aspects Human Sexual* 8:129, 1974.

Robinson HA et al.: Review of child molestation and alleged rape cases. *Am J Obstet Gynecol* 110:405, 1971.

Soules MR et al.: The forensic laboratory evaluation of evidence in alleged rape. *Am J Obstet Gynecol* 130:142, 1978.

Woodling BA et al.: Sexual assault: Rape and molestation. *Clin Obstet Gynecol* 20:509, 1977.

Precocious Puberty

Bidlingmaier F et al.: Plasma gonadotropins and estrogens in girls with idiopathic precocious puberty. *Pediatr Res* 11:91, 1977.

Hayles AB: Precocious sexual maturation in juvenile hypothyroidism. *Fertil Steril* 27:1220, 1976.

Madden JD, MacDonald PC: Origin of estrogen in isosexual precocious pseudopuberty due to a granulosa thecacell tumor. *Obstet Gynecol* 51:210, 1978.

Pintor C et al.: Adrenal and gonadal steroids and puberty response to LHRH in girls: II. Precocious puberty. *J Endocrinol Invest* 2:143, 1978.

Richman RA et al.: Adverse effects of large doses of medroxyprogesterone (MPA) in idiopathic isosexual precocity. *J Pediatr* 79:963, 1971.

Werder EA et al.: Treatment of precocious puberty with cyproterone acetate. *Pediatr Res* 8:248, 1974.

Tumors of the Genital Tract

Breen JL, Maxson WS: Ovarian tumors in children and adolescents. *Clin Obstet Gynecol* 20:607, 1977.

Dewhurst CJ: Tumors of the genital tract in childhood and adolescence. *Clin Obstet Gynecol* 20:595, 1977.

DiSaia PJ et al.: *Synopsis of Gynecologic Oncology,* New York: Wiley, 1975.

Herbst AL et al.: Adenocarcinoma of the vagina: Association of maternal stilbestrol therapy with tumor appearance in young women. *N Engl J Med* 284:878, 1971.

Merlob P et al.: Cysts of the female external genitalia in the newborn infant. *Am J Obstet Gynecol* 132:607, 1978.

17
Adolescence

DIANE S. FORDNEY

BIOLOGIC ADOLESCENCE (PUBERTY)

ADOLESCENT GYNECOLOGIC PROBLEMS
Precocious or premature puberty
Delayed sexual development
Delayed menarche
Primary amenorrhea
  Chromosomal abnormalities
  Congenital anomalies of the reproductive tract
  Vaginal anomalies, hematometra, congenital
  cervical hypoplasia, uterine anomalies
  Vaginal agenesis
  Neuroendocrine mechanisms—anorexia
  nervosa
  Primary amenorrhea with virilization
Secondary amenorrhea; chronic oligo-ovulation
Menorrhagia
Dysmenorrhea
Abdominal or pelvic pain
Infections
  Cystitis
  Vulvitis
  Vaginitis
  Other infections
Sex-related problems of adolescence
  Sexual activity of teenagers
  Contraception
  Pregnancy
  Abortion
  Sexually transmitted diseases

Adolescence is a loosely defined life stage representing, to most minds, the teenage years. Depending on how it is separated into its defining components, the age range can be earlier or later and can be much more or much less than a decade. Adolescence is a concept derived from sociology, biology, and psychology. Sociologically, adolescence begins in dependency and ends in independence with respect to economics, the development of social relationships, the culmination of educational efforts, and in the achievement of life experience. Biologically, however, it starts from the first sign of sexual maturation and ends when complete somatic growth is attained. The biologic epoch can be very much shorter than one defined by social criteria. Finally, psychological implications of adolescence include the basic emotional transition from childhood to adulthood and the behavioral impact of Western society's prolonged economic and social dependency for an individual who is biologically mature. The importance of these considerations in meeting the gynecologic needs of adolescents is manifested by parental inquiries about preparation for their child's impending puberty, and in the way physicians view the adolescent. The conflict between traditional roles of child versus parent affects the provision of care in ways not applicable to older women. The anguish of parents, the patient, and social institutions over the problems related to sexual activity in the child/woman adolescent complicates the provision of health services.

Fifty percent of the population of this country is under the age of 30, and 25 percent falls in the age group between 12 and 20 (U.S. Bureau of the Census). Within this age group most young women seeking medical care will see a gynecologist. Their contact with other medical professionals is minimal because young people are usually healthy, and their medical or physical concerns center on the changes attendant to achieving sexual maturity. Between 25 and 40 percent of all obstetric and gynecologic patients are in this adolescent category (Hollingsworth, Kreutner). Most of these are involved in the management of sex-related problems such as contraception, pregnancy, abortion, and venereal disease. The older the adolescent, the more likely she is to appear for care of a preventive nature such as contraception and routine examinations. The younger adolescents are seen for specific concerns, such as fear of pregnancy or actual pregnancy, body normalcy, menstrual disorders, and vaginitis. For all of these patients, there are implications beyond those seen in the older woman. For many, their first contact with an adult medical setting includes the emotionally loaded pelvic examination. How this is accomplished may have profound implications on their willingness to participate in the preventive aspects of medicine later. The first encounter with a menstrual disorder or a vaginal problem is always more stressful than later problems when women are more experienced in bodily function and dysfunction. Good medical management requires correct information, the certainty that the adolescent understands, and appropriate treatment. It can only be accomplished by an approach that is perceptive of the young woman's concerns and fears, and that is marked by compassion, nonjudgmental education, and tolerance.

BIOLOGIC ADOLESCENCE (PUBERTY)

Major changes occur in adolescents as a result of both sexual maturation and physical somatic growth. All children between the ages of 9 and 15 have rapid height and weight growth. Superimposed on that is the "adolescent growth spurt" which occurs usually between the ages of 12 and 13 years in girls. While there are great variations among individuals, rapid growth rarely begins before the age of 8 or after the age of 13. Typically, a girl will begin to show accelerated growth shortly after the age of 9 to 10, achieve

peak velocity by age 12, show the superimposed growth spurt from 12 to 13, and then continue a decelerated growth after age 14 (U.S. Public Health Service). When the sex steroid–induced adolescent growth spurt ends, the non-steroid-related rapid height growth phase begins to decelerate as well. This is due to gradual closure of long bone epiphyses which is induced by sex steroids (Frisch). Children whose accelerated growth begins early or late can, at the same chronologic age, have very different physical appearances. At one extreme, a 14-year-old girl can look like a child; another at the same age may seem to be fully adult. Since both extremes are prevalent, the concerns of the physician who sees young people may vary greatly. There is an interesting disparity between early and late developers in terms of overall height and weight. Early developers have their height spurt early, but it is more rapid over a shorter period of time. Late developers achieve a higher initial somatic height by virtue of a more prolonged somatic rapid growth phase prior to their growth spurt. Eventually, they will be as tall or slightly taller than the earlier developers, but with a less acute spurt. Since the fastest weight gain occurs for the late developer at the same mean weight but at an older age than for the early developer, the late developer experiences a shorter duration of weight accumulation before the end of the growth stage. Thus they weigh less at age 16 than the early developers. Weight accumulation proceeds much more steadily during the rapid growth phase of adolescence and does not participate in the height growth spurt related to sex steroids (Frisch). Most body systems show a steady overall rapid growth between the ages of 9 and 15 with some notable exceptions. The brain and skull as well as the lymphatic tissues of the body reach their peaks early. The brain and skull have achieved 90 percent of adult size by the age of 8 and show a very slow continuing growth pattern from that time on. The lymphoid system shows a marked spurt between the ages of 7 and 11 but then declines to age 18 when it resumes its earlier level of development. During the time when other structures in the body are growing rapidly, the lymphatic tissue is atrophying. A third exception is the reproductive system structures which grow disproportionately faster than all other organ systems (Tanner).

Hormonal changes in puberty account for the reproductive system's growth acceleration. The childhood pituitary is capable of producing follicle-stimulating hormone (FSH) and luteinizing hormone (LH), although the amounts produced are half those of adults (Yen, Visic; Reiter, Kulin). About 2 years before the onset of any pubertal change, there is a steady increase in the production of FSH and LH, initially as nighttime surges. This increase is caused by the release of FSH- and LH-releasing factors from the hypothalamus, a process which is undeveloped or suppressed in childhood (Ross, Van de Wiele). Small amounts of estrogen tried experimentally in childhood markedly suppress the hypothalamus because of an increased sensitivity of hypothalamic receptors for steroids. Studies have shown that one-twentieth to one-eighth of the dosage of estrogen required to suppress FSH secretion in adults will accomplish that same diminution in children (Kelch; Reiter, Kulin). While the child's ovary is capable of responding to FSH and LH, it responds poorly as compared with the adult's (Gaul; Emans, Goldstein). Thus gonadotropin production, as well as ovarian production of estrogen in response to gonadotropins, requires a change in hypothalamic and ovarian sensitivity at the onset of sexual maturation. The one event is a decrease in hypothalamic sensitivity to circulating steroids; the other is an increased sensitivity of the ovary to gonadotropins. Soon after the FSH levels rise, a concomitant increase in plasma estradiol level occurs. When the ovary is producing sufficient levels of estradiol, it suppresses hypothalamic FSH- and LH-releasing factors, thus decreasing the gonadotropin levels. This in turn results in a rapid increase in LH-releasing factor and an eventual surge or cyclic LH increase that results in ovulation (Jenner). While this LH surge is necessary for ovulation and eventual menarche, it is the much earlier production of estrogen that is responsible for the development of secondary sexual characteristics and reproductive organ growth. Another major hormonal event which occurs during puberty is an increase in adrenal androgens, responsible for the appearance of pubic and axillary hair.

The stages of sexual maturation were best described by Marshall and Tanner in 1969 following detailed observations of 192 English schoolgirls. The Tanner stages for female sexual maturation are as follows:

Stage B1—preadolescent with elevation of nipple papilla only
Stage B2—breast budding, the elevation of the breast and nipple into a small mound with enlargement of the areolar diameter
Stage B3—further enlargement of the breast with no separation of the contours of the mound and areola, the "conical" breast
Stage B4—further enlargement with projection of

the areola to form a secondary mound above the level of the breast
Stage B5—mature stage in which there is projection of the nipple only, resulting from recession of the areola to the general contour of the breast

The breast developmental stages describe *thelarche*. The mean age for breast budding is 10 to 11 years, with age 8 marking the lower limit and age 14 the upper limit of normal variation in development of breast buds (stage B2). A child who shows breast development before the age of 8 may have precocious puberty; one with no breast budding by age 14 may have delayed puberty.

Adrenarche, the development of pubic and axillary hair, is characterized by Tanner as follows:

Stage PH1—none
Stage PH2—sparse growth of long, straight or only slightly curled hair along the labia majora
Stage PH3—thicker, coarser, and curled hair extending over the junction of the pubis
Stage PH4—adult-type hair spreading over the mons pubis but not onto the medial aspect of the thighs
Stage PH5—hair has spread to medial surface of thighs

Breast development typically appears before pubic hair growth. This is quite variable however. Breast budding may appear as much as 2 years before pubic hair appears, or both may occur simultaneously, or breast budding may happen even 2 years after the appearance of pubic hair. In the most typical case, pubic hair appears 1 year after breast budding. Axillary hair may appear just before or just after menarche.

On an average, *menarche* (the onset of menstruation) occurs 2 years after breast budding although menarche *always* followed the age of peak height growth in all girls studied (Fig. 17–1). It must be remembered that the relationship of thelarche, adrenarche, and menarche is quite variable between individuals. Although one usually predicts that more young women will undergo menarche at stage B3 breast and pubic hair development, only 35 percent did so in Tanner's series. There are strong data to suggest that the critical variable for menarche is body weight, rather than stage of breast and pubic hair development. Girls who have early and late sexual development have the same mean weight of about 103 pounds at the time of menarche.

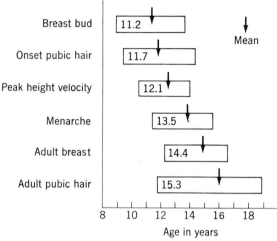

FIGURE 17–1 Sexual maturation in the female. *(From EO Reiter, HA Kulin: Sexual maturation in the female. Normal development and precocious puberty. Pediatr Clin North Am 19:583, 1972.)*

The mean age of menarche in this country appears to be decreasing by 0.4 year with each decade. Currently, the mean age of menarche is 12.7 years (Reiter, Kulin). The expected range for the onset of menarche in this country is 8 to 17 years, but for the vast majority, onset occurs in the 11 to 14 age range. Older reports state that menstruation may be anovulatory for the first year or two, but more recent evidence indicates that about half of the menstrual cycles in the first year following menarche are ovulatory. This does not mean, however, that the interval between menstrual periods is regular. In fact, infrequent or irregular menstruation is the rule during at least the first year or two following menarche. While the cause of this is most likely lack of maturation of the ovarian-pituitary-hypothalamic axis, it is also true that adolescents seem more susceptible to stress or environmental interference with ovulation. Such things as travel, fatigue, weight change, or stressful life situations may lead to adolescent hypothalamic oligomenorrhea. Mean body weight seems to be highly correlated with the onset of menarche, but other factors have also been implicated. Poor diet, which is not strictly related to weight, can result in delayed menstruation. It has been theorized that an adequate diet is the major factor responsible for decreased age at menarche in most of the Western world.

The age at menarche of the girl's mother and other female relatives is highly correlated with the age of onset of menarche, presumably on a genetic basis. Other factors, such as urban versus rural living, temperate versus extreme climate, daylight cycles, and blindness have all been provocatively reported as having influences on menarche. Factors associated with social class seem to affect physical growth and menarche. Certainly good nutrition, regular meals, sufficient sleep, and exercise, which are most often found in more affluent households, may be the major factors accounting for class differences. One association with earlier onset of menarche is an earlier achievement of full somatic growth as well as greater adult size than in previous generations (Zaccharias).

Due to high levels of estrogen in the soon-to-be-menarchal woman, the remainder of the internal and external genitalia undergo significant changes. In childhood the fatty pads of the labia majora completely cover the labia minora on visual observation. The clitoris, however, is relatively obvious. With significant levels of estradiol, the labia minora grow selectively larger than do the labia majora with protusion of the minor lips through the major and an apparent, but not real, decrease in clitoral prominence. The vaginal barrel of the child is covered by thin squamous epithelium and has no rugae. Estrogen produces cornification and thickening of vaginal epithelium which results in the formation of rugae and the onset of a physiologic clear, translucent vaginal discharge. Accompanying this is a decrease in vaginal pH from a level of about 7 to one of 4.0 to 5.0. The cornification and acidification of the vaginal epithelium is largely protective to the vagina and the susceptibility to pathogens is greatly reduced.

The squamocolumnar junction of the endocervix undergoes profound changes during adolescence. From the onset of puberty into the early twenties, the junction may migrate as much as a centimeter up and down the endocervical canal. Basically, the squamous-cell epithelium of the exocervix migrates into the endocervical canal so that the squamocolumnar junction becomes an endocervical structure. However, there is great variation from woman to woman and from month to month in the same woman in the location of this junction. In childhood the uterine cervix is two to three times as long and is the same diameter as the uterine fundus. Following the influence of estrogen, the uterine fundus eventually becomes two to three times as long, and two to three times as wide as the cervix. Additionally, the endometrium changes from the atrophic basal epithelial cells of childhood to the proliferative type of the estrogenized adult. Fallopian tubes increase dramatically in length and diameter as an effect of estrogen. Only the ovary itself appears to continue to grow at a rate commensurate with overall somatic growth and is not directly stimulated by estrogen. The major growth of these organs occurs prior to the onset of menarche before progesterone production. Thus, progesterone apparently has very little effect on the differential and rapid growth rate of reproductive organs (Tanner).

ADOLESCENT GYNECOLOGIC PROBLEMS

This section will deal with those gynecologic problems which are specific to adolescents. There is a fairly well-circumscribed group of problems which are presented to the clinician and which separate adolescents from older patients. No attempt will be made to describe problems adolescents share with older women unless those conditions are commonly found in adolescents.

PRECOCIOUS OR PREMATURE PUBERTY

Although gynecologists are not likely to be primarily involved in cases of precocious puberty, they will be involved in consultation. Significant sexual development culminating in menarche before the age of 8 is defined as precocious. There are two categories of precocious puberty. The first is isosexual precocity where the patient has normal pubertal development including menses; the second is heterosexual precocity in which the girl has evidence of virilization with or without changes characteristic of female normal puberty. Heterosexual precocity may include premature thelarche or premature adrenarche. Premature menarche should never be diagnosed unless there is pubic hair or breast development. Vaginal bleeding in children with no sexual development requires meticulous evaluation for vaginal, cervical, and uterine disease.

Isosexual precocity is usually caused by premature development of the hypothalamic-pituitary-ovarian axis. The normal pubertal process occurs, but too early. Eighty percent of precocious puberty is due to such premature activation of the reproductive axis for unknown reasons. Most of these patients have abnormal electroencephalograms, and some have a defined central-nervous-system disorder such as tumor or hamartoma (Lin). Although the idiopathic state exists most often, it is imperative that thorough exami-

nation be made to exclude organic disorders. For example, cerebral disorders including brain tumors, postinfectious encephalitis, hydrocephalus, polyfibrous dysplasia, and neonatal asphyxia occur in roughly 5 to 10 percent of cases.

A second group of isosexual precocity cases does not involve premature maturation of the hypothalamic-pituitary-ovarian axis. In these children there is unopposed estrogen or androgen stimulation, and the child is not potentially fertile. Common causes include adrenal or ovarian tumors such as granulosa-cell tumors, arrhenoblastomas, and cysts. Gonadotropin-producing tumors have been reported rarely, and choriocarcinoma is usually rapidly fatal. On occasion, other medical conditions, such as hypothyroidism, are found. Iatrogenic precocious puberty can be induced by ingestion of estrogen- or androgen-containing substances (Cloutier, Hayles; Ross, Van de Wiele).

Appropriate treatment of hypothyroidism, idiopathic estrogen administration, and steroid-producing tumors and cysts will often cause regression of puberty, but sexual development to the point of treatment may remain. Brain tumors are only rarely treated successfully. In cases of idiopathic precocious puberty, it is generally felt that the administration of medroxyprogesterone acetate will cause cessation of menses and regression of breast development. It may also reduce premature epiphyseal closure although reports are conflicting (Cloutier, Hayles). Side effects to progestational agents are considerable, however, and their use is questionable, at least in the older, 6- to 8-year-old child with precocious puberty (Richman).

Heterosexual precocity is due to androgen production from either an adrenal or ovarian source which causes some features of puberty to develop. These features include acne, hirsutism, or clitoromegaly, as well as the development of pubic and axillary hair. The condition can be caused by congenital adrenocortical hyperplasia, adrenal tumors, and ovarian tumors such as arrhenoblastoma, or Sertoli cell tumors. Again, ingestion of exogenous steroids must be ruled out. Congenital adrenocortical hyperplasia (CAH) is the most common cause. Typically, an elevated 17-ketosteroid level is identified which can be suppressed by dexamethasone. In addition, elevated urinary pregnanetriol and increased serum 17-hydroxyprogesterone are often found. If there is an adrenal or ovarian tumor, the 17-ketosteroid level cannot be suppressed. Plasma testosterone elevation may help to distinguish between ovarian and adrenal sources of androgen. Treatment of these conditions would include excision of ovarian or adrenal tumors, elimination of exogenous androgens, or glucocorticoid replacement by hydrocortisone in cases of congenital adrenal hyperplasia. Further premature sexual development will not continue once adequate therapy is instituted (Jenner; Emans, Goldstein).

Premature thelarche and premature adrenarche may sometimes be seen in young children and confused with precocious puberty. Usually premature thelarche is seen in a very young girl, between the ages of 1½ and 4 years of age, and the breast development may be either symmetrical or asymmetrical. There is no other evidence of puberty or estrogen effect in these children. Although the etiology is not clear, the condition is thought to be due to increased sensitivity to low levels of endogenous estrogen. Small luteinized ovarian follicles may be responsible in some instances, as well as small amounts of exogenous estrogen ingestion by the child. The breasts do not continue to develop nor do other signs of sexual maturation occur; follow-up is the only course indicated. In premature adrenarche, there may be the appearance of pubic or axillary hair without any other sign of either estrogenization or virilization. Most children with this condition have a slight increase in urinary 17-ketosteroid production and increased plasma dehydroepiandrosterone and dehydroepiandrosterone sulfate. Thus, premature adrenarche has indeed occurred, but it is not followed or accompanied by precocious puberty since the accelerated bone age, breast growth, and other evidences of estrogenization are missing. Appropriate management consists of reassurance and follow-up. Pubertal development at adolescence can be expected to be normal (Sigurjonsdottir, Hayles; Rosenfeld; Capraro).

DELAYED SEXUAL DEVELOPMENT

Although sexual maturation and menarche may be delayed until ages 17 to 19 where there is either a strong familial history of late development, chronic medical illness, malnutrition, or preexistent known neuroendocrine disease such as brain tumor, cases of delayed puberty should be investigated at an earlier age. If there is no evidence of breast budding or pubic hair by the age of 15, a careful evaluation is required (Hollingsworth, Kreutner). This condition is labeled as delayed sexual development. If menarche is delayed beyond the age of 17, it is diagnosed as primary amenorrhea and requires evaluation, even though there may be signs of secondary sexual development. At whatever age a young girl appears

concerned about delayed sexual maturation or delayed menarche, the minimal evaluation should include a thorough history and examination of the genital structures, including rectovaginal bimanual examination, to eliminate the possibility of undiagnosed medical or other illness, or of congenital anatomic defects involving the reproductive system. With the ever-increasing earlier onset of sexual activity, young girls who have not had at least this brief evaluation and who are otherwise normal may well endure both physical and mental trauma by age 16 or 17 if they have unsuspected congenital anomalies. In the 15-year-old girl with delayed sexual development, there are five major groups of causes. The first of these consists of chromosomal abnormalities such as Turner's syndrome. The second is ovarian failure. The third group is comprised of abnormalities of neuroendocrine maturation. The fourth group is comprised of chronic medical conditions and malnutrition, and the fifth is influenced by genetic or familial factors.

Chromosomal abnormalities, with gonadal dysgenesis or streak ovaries, are found in roughly 25 percent of young women with the diagnosis of delayed sexual development (Chaps. 6 and 32). About half of these will have Turner's syndrome with XO karyotyping. Turner's syndrome has other accompanying classic physical findings including short stature, webbed neck, low hairline, short fourth and fifth metacarpals, low-set ears, narrow and high-arched palate, cardiac anomalies, renal anomalies, and an increased incidence of medical conditions such as hypertension, achlorhydria, Hashimoto's struma, and diabetes mellitus. Such an individual may undergo adrenarche by the age of 15 or 16 but will show no significant estrogenization. The other 40 to 50 percent of patients with gonadal dysgenesis have either a mosaic karyotype or other sex-related chromosome anomalies such as XXX or XXY or a mosaic combination of these (Engel, Forbes). Typically, the young woman with X-chromosome anomalies will have a normal cervix, uterus, and vagina capable of responding to estrogens. However, that is not always the case and there may be associated vaginal or uterine agenesis. Such an individual is appropriately treated with replacement estrogens. Once secondary sexual characteristics have developed, the addition of a progestational agent during the last 5 days of each 30-day period will give cyclic withdrawal bleeding. The usual dosage might be Premarin, 0.3 mg a day, 25 days out of a 30-day month, with medroxyprogesterone added on days 20 to 25 of the cycle. It should be noted that increasing Premarin dosage to 1.25 mg per day may be necessary to improve breast development and to allow sufficient estrogen stimulation of the endometrium to induce withdrawal bleeding (Federman; Rothchild, Owens). Although an increased risk of endometrial carcinoma has been reported in postmenopausal women taking conjugated estrogen, there has been no evidence to indicate that cyclic administration of estrogens in low doses, combined with a progestational agent at the end of each estrogen period, is associated with endometrial carcinoma in younger women. It is possible to induce secondary sexual characteristic development and menstruation through such a regimen, but this woman is unable to conceive since she has no functional gonad. The young woman who has an associated vaginal anomaly, agenesis, or hypoplasia will also be denied normal sexual functioning until such a situation is corrected. These young women need ample opportunity to discuss the psychological problems involved with issues of infertility and vaginoplasty at length, either with the gynecologist or with a counselor knowledgeable about the psychological problems associated with anatomic abnormalities.

Ovarian failure is recognized as a cause of sexual development retardation in a significant number of cases. Histories of prior abdominal radiation, total body irradiation, or chemotherapy suggest the diagnosis of ovarian failure. There are more cases of ovarian failure of unknown etiology than there are cases associated with ovarian ablation or damage from iatrogenic factors. These may represent intra- or extra-uterine vascular accidents to the gonad, or they may be cases of gonadal dysgenesis with chromosomal abnormalities that cannot be substantiated. FSH and LH levels are typically elevated in the absence of a functional ovary, and treatment and management considerations are identical with those for gonadal dysgenesis. Although most cases of ovarian failure have abnormal or absent ovaries, there are two situations in which the ovary appears to be fairly normal. The first of these is an extremely rare condition caused by a 17α-hydroxylase deficiency associated with adrenal insufficiency, hypertension, and elevated plasma progesterone levels. Investigation of another syndrome reveals apparently normal ovaries which do not respond to FSH and LH, the "resistant ovary" syndrome. Possible explanations for this include an absence of receptors for gonadotropins in the ovary, or biochemical alteration of gonadotropin structure (Grumbach, Van Wyck; Wilkins, Fleischmann).

Neuroendocrine abnormalities which can cause delayed sexual maturation include organic brain disease, absence of gonadotropin-releasing factors, gonadotropin deficiencies, panhypopituitarism, and chronic medical or psychological disease which alters hypothalamic maturation. Brain tumors are rare causes of delayed sexual maturation, and evaluation with visual fields, skull and sella turcica radiography, or sophisticated CAT (computerized axial tomography) scans are used to determine their presence or absence. A tumor may not be evident at the time of first contact with the patient, and evaluation for brain tumor should be repeated at appropriate intervals.

The group of neuroendocrine disorders identifying specific deficiencies in gonadotropins or gonatropin-releasing factors is referred to as *hypogonadotropic hypogonadism* (Emans, Goldstein). These are diagnosed when there is no evidence of an underlying lesion. Because of the expense and side effects of agents causing ovulation, such as clomiphene citrate or human menopausal gonadotropin, and the practical unavailability of gonadotropin-releasing factors, young women diagnosed as having hypogonadotropic hypogonadism are best treated from the age of 15 with substitution estrogen-progesterone therapy. If the condition persists into adulthood, ovulation can be produced by using agents specifically designed to induce ovulation for the purpose of conception.

Chronic medical illness, malnutrition and psychologic stress usually cause delayed sexual maturation because the child has failed to attain the critical weight necessary for the onset of sexual maturation. Correction of the medical or psychological problem will result in increased somatic development and sexual maturation. The gynecologist's role is primarily as diagnostician with a high index of suspicion that such conditions may be the underlying problem.

Finally, *familial causes* of delayed sexual maturation considered to have a genetic basis is a diagnosis to be made after excluding other factors. A family history of late onset of sexual development must be present, and thorough evaluation must confirm that the patient is normal.

The major components of medical evaluation for delayed sexual maturation include the medical history, physical examination, psychologic screening, karyotyping, laboratory assessments for medical illness suspected from history and physical examination, serum FSH and LH, sellar tomograms, visual fields, and diagnostic laparoscopy. If all of these are normal, the diagnosis of familial delayed sexual maturation is appropriately made. The girl and her parents may be reassured, provided appropriate 6-month follow-up is maintained.

In summary, in a young woman with no signs of secondary sexual development by the age of 15, it is imperative to begin evaluation. Fully 75 percent of such individuals will be found to have a specific etiology. If not appropriately evaluated at this time, the child may not seek help until age 16 to 18 when she is likely to present with primary amenorrhea, or perhaps not until adulthood when fertility is sought. In many of these conditions, there is a significant possibility of severe physical harm, or death, and in all of them there is significant psychologic stress produced by passing through adolescence without signs of normal sexual development. These psychological consequences of delay can produce an even greater problem in management.

DELAYED MENARCHE

Delayed menarche is the term used in the evaluation of a young woman who has not begun to menstruate by the age of 17 but who has some pubertal development. Because the time interval from the onset of secondary sexual characteristic development and menarche is 2 to 3 years, a young woman presenting at age 17 who began breast development at age 14 and who has a normal history and physical examination, including a full pelvic examination, can be reassured that she will begin to menstruate soon. Similarly, if her breast development did not begin until she reached age 16, she may be within the group of individuals who will not begin to menstruate until 18 or 19. It is important, however, to obtain her medical history with reference to familial onset of menarche, stress, under- or overeating, and drugs, and to ascertain that her sexual development has been steady and progressive. A young woman who began breast development at the age of 11 or 12 and is not menstruating by age 16 would not normally be in that group of individuals who have delayed menarche from familial factors. Because she has some signs of sexual development, the differential diagnosis is unlike that of the woman who has no sexual development. Most young women seen at the age of 16 without menses but with sexual development belong to the group with late but normal menarche. However, anomalies of the reproductive tract are common findings in these individuals; therefore, a thorough pelvic examination to eliminate uterine or vaginal agenesis is necessary. If this examination is normal and reveals good vaginal estrogenization, if there is normal hair distribution, and if there is no evidence of other disease, obesity, psy-

chological problems, or an underlying organic basis for delayed menarche, further evaluation can be delayed until the age of 17 to 18. Education of the parent and the young woman in the expected sequence of maturation, reassurance that she appears to be following her own normal curve of development, and regular follow-up are appropriate.

PRIMARY AMENORRHEA

Primary amenorrhea is defined here as the failure to achieve menarche by the age of 17. Classically, amenorrhea has been described as menarche delayed beyond the age of 18, but the more recent literature uses the younger age because 70 percent of young women evaluated at age 17 will be shown to have an abnormal factor responsible for the amenorrhea (Hollingsworth, Kreutner). By 17, both the young woman and her parents are usually greatly concerned and embarrassed by the absence of menses and want evaluation, treatment, and the onset of menses as soon as possible. Thus, there are good medical, psychologic, and social reasons to evaluate the patient by age 17. There are five major causes for primary amenorrhea: chromosomal genetic abnormalities, congenital reproductive tract anomalies, neuroendocrine factors, virilizing conditions, and pregnancy. Pregnancy is included because Behrman found at least 1 out of 30 young women with primary amenorrhea to be amenorrheic because of pregnancy. Pregnancy must always be considered in the evaluation of amenorrhea in an adolescent. Chronic medical disease, malnutrition, and drugs are not included because most patients without disease in childhood or in their earlier teens have achieved sufficient somatic growth and weight to have begun menses, although they may present with secondary amenorrhea or oligomenorrhea by age 18. Many young women who have delayed sexual maturation or no sexual maturation may not present until the ages of 17 or 18, at which time evaluation of conditions such as gonadal dysgenesis and ovarian failure, which should have been diagnosed earlier, must be included.

CHROMOSOMAL ABNORMALITIES

In addition to chromosomal conditions producing primary amenorrhea without sexual development, there are chromosomal conditions which produce individuals who may have normal secondary characteristic development, slight secondary sexual development in which estrogen effect has occurred but not at adequate levels, or virilizing effects superimposed on a phenotypic female. Various authors have found a 25 percent incidence of these disorders in young women with primary amenorrhea (Behrman; Jacobs; Phillip).

Sex Chromosome Abnormalities

Individuals who have mosaic cell lines of Turner's syndrome (XO/XX, XO/XXX/XX, etc.) may sometimes develop a few hypoplastic secondary sexual features from estrogenization. The gonads in these individuals are seen to be either a combination of a streak and a hypoplastic gonad or two hypoplastic gonads which on biopsy appear to be atretic. Apparently, in this instance, the gonad allowed some estrogen production during puberty but then became atrophic, resulting in actual or impending ovarian failure. Should such an individual's ovaries continue to produce adequate levels of estrogen, they are potentially fertile. The occurrence of XO mosaic genotypic individuals with hypoplastic gonads capable of minimal secondary sexual development and then deestrogenization, or with hypoplastic gonads capable of ovulation is rare (Wilkins, Fleischmann).

The most classic example of an individual with primary amenorrhea and normal sexual development is that of the androgen-insensitivity syndrome or "testicular feminization." Although some of these individuals may have been diagnosed at birth because of genital ambiguity, or in childhood because of labial or groin masses, there are a significant number of these young women who present with primary amenorrhea. Breast development is entirely normal, but pubic hair may be somewhat diminished. There is no uterus, and the vagina may vary from complete absence to blind pouches of varying sizes without a cervix and uterus at the apex. In these individuals the gonad, which may be located in the labia, the groin, or the abdomen, is a normal testis which produces normal amounts of androgens. The congenital defect is a somatic one in which body cells are unresponsive to the androgen and thus will not virilize. Instead, the testosterone is degraded into estrogens, which cause feminization of the individual. The defect was operant during intrauterine life because production of testosterone by the fetal gonad usually results in a male phallus and accessory organs. However, the other intrauterine function of fetal testes, production of Müllerian duct-inhibiting substance, is intact. Female reproductive organs did not develop. The external genitalia may be phenotypically ambiguous at birth but are usually of normal female appearance because of maternal estrogen effect. Once the diagnosis is established, management consists of counseling in regard to infertility and vaginoplasty, and performance of gonadectomy. Gonadectomy is essential because up to 25 percent of gonads in Y-bearing individuals that remain intraabdominal or in the groin develop malignant germ-cell tumors. Because such tumors are highly malignant and it is difficult to evaluate these gonads for malignant change, most authorities feel that maintenance of the gonads is dangerous. Once the gonadectomy is performed, the individual must have replacement therapy with an estrogen preparation (Federman).

A final chromosomal cause of primary amenorrhea consists of true hermaphroditism. In these individuals, the gonads have both ovarian and testicular elements. The majority of such individuals are reared as males although there is often external genital ambiguity. Individuals presenting with primary amenorrhea are those who are phenotypically normal females in whom the Y chromosome or the testicular tissues has been either totally or relatively inactivated. They appear to be normal females in secondary sexual development or present a mixed picture with mild to moderate virilization. Although karyotyping in the past has indicated that most of these individuals were chromosomally XX, more recent studies using improved techniques find a much higher percentage of XX/XY mosaicism. The gonad in a true hermaphrodite may be either an ovary on one side and a testis on the other, an ovotestis on one side with the corresponding gonad being either an ovary or a testis, or they may be bilateral ovotestes. These young women usually have a normal uterus, but it may be absent or hypoplastic. Similarly, the vagina may be normal, it may be only a sinus duct, or it may be absent, depending on the extent of the intrauterine influence of the Y chromosome. Testicular tissue must be removed because of the risk of malignancy. It is theoretically possible, if one gonad is known to be an ovary by biopsy, to allow that to remain, and once the testis or ovotestis is removed, for the young woman to assume an ovulatory menstrual cycle (Jones).

Patients with a Y chromosome are best told that that is part of their problem. Their gender identity is usually unswervingly female, and they accept the Y chromosome as the cause of the problem without shaking that identity. If their identity is ambiguous because their sex of rearing was confused by genital ambiguity, they are usually relieved to have a biologic explanation for their ambiguity. Counseling for gonadectomy, infertility, and for other procedures that are necessary is almost impossible if physicians try to avoid discussion of the Y chromosome. All patients sooner or later want to understand and read about their condition and to know how to label it. Similarly, most are too intelligent not to figure out what "a piece of one of your X chromosomes is missing" really means. Trust is essential in patient management and can be fragile.

CONGENITAL ANOMALIES OF THE REPRODUCTIVE TRACT

Clinicians in a lifetime of practice will probably see two or three of the major congenital reproductive tract anomalies and five to ten of the minor ones. In the group of adolescents presenting with primary amenorrhea, the incidence of genital tract anomalies is significant. When added to those individuals who are diagnosed as having intersex problems with associated maldevelopment of portions of the female reproductive tract, the incidence may approach 40 percent of primary amenorrhea. To put it another way, if one estimates the current adolescent population at 30 million and the conservative incidence of major reproductive tract anomalies such as failure of uterine and vaginal development to be 1 in 5000 individuals, there would be approximately 6000 adolescent cases in the United States. If one adds the more common problems such as imperforate hymen, and vaginal and uterine septi, the population is probably closer to 20,000 young women with such problems. Any portion of the genital tract may develop in an abnormal fashion during embryogenesis in an otherwise totally normal individual. When sex chromosome-related abnormalities are present, the incidence of reproductive tract developmental problems increases. Management problems include not only the appropriate medical or surgical management of the anomaly and any reconstruction that is required, but also the issues of possible infertility and the profound damage to self-esteem and expectations of a young woman who is not diagnosed until the late teens. An advantage to the early diagnosis of these conditions is the opportunity for parental counseling to ensure sensitive and honest preparation of the individual in order to help her adjust to the loss of her expectation of menstruation, normal sexual functioning, and pregnancy. Because there is an association of reproductive tract abnormalities with urinary tract abnormalities, the young woman discovered to have either should be evaluated for the presence of the other.

VAGINAL ANOMALIES, HEMATOMETRA, CONGENITAL CERVICAL HYPOPLASIA, UTERINE ANOMALIES

Imperforate hymen is one of the relatively common anatomic anomalies resulting in primary amenorrhea. In these individuals there are normal secondary sexual characteristics and development, but menses do not occur in 2 to 3 years. They have monthly episodes of severe abdominal pain and distention. If the problem is not recognized early, the young woman with an imperforate hymen and primary amenorrhea may present with a large abdominal mass representing hematometra with hematocolpos. The treatment is to make a cruciate incision in the hymen so that the flaps thus created will pull away from each other and not readhere. This procedure should be performed in an operating room under general anesthesia to minimize physical and psychologic distress to the young woman. The procedure will also facilitate the removal of old blood which may require suction evacuation of the uterus. If there has been significant hematometra with associated oviductal dilation, there is a risk of postoperative infection. Because of this risk of infection, it is important that the initial surgical approach to the hymen be the definitive one and that full evacuation of old menstrual blood be accomplished. If the initial incision is inadequate to allow complete drainage, bacteria may enter and cause a devastating upper tract infection (Underwood, Kreutner; McKusick). There is also a risk of endometrial, peritubular, and intratubular adhesions which may result in infertility; however, most patients will be fertile. Such young women should be checked for symptoms of persistent abdominal pain and counseled appropriately.

When *vaginal septa* occur, they are either vertical or transverse. Only transverse septa are a cause of primary amenorrhea (Jones, Heller). A transverse septum can be confused with a blind vaginal pouch rather than an imperforate vaginal septum with a uterus above it. Cervical atresia is rare. It may consist of absence of the cervix, even though the uterine fundus has developed, or there may be a transverse septa or ablation of the endocervical canal in a hypoplastic cervix (Asplund). Such patients invariably develop hematometra and its attendant episodic abdominal pain. Treatment is problematic, and the prognosis is poor.

In the individual who does not have a vagina but does have a uterus, it is preferable to use transabdominal drainage of hematometra because perineal drainage complicates eventual vaginoplasty. The attendant scarring tends to obliterate the plane used for development of a new vagina. Even though the possibility of attaching the neovagina to the uterus exists in these young women, infertility is almost universal. Hysterectomy is not usually advised as a first procedure, but, because of complications, pain, and frustration, it is common at a later date. Drainage offers the conservative initial approach both from the psychological standpoint of acceptance of the anomaly and in the hope that sterility will not occur.

Primary amenorrhea may be due to several abnormalities of the uterine fundus. The first of these is *uterine agenesis,* which usually coexists with cervical and vaginal agenesis as well. Sterility is final, and there are no alternatives. However, counseling is essential and vaginoplasty in those individuals with a hypoplastic or absent vagina is indicated. There may be absence or hypoplasia of the oviducts. Although uterine hypoplasia and agenesis usually occur in an otherwise normal individual, as many as one-third of cases coexist with sex-chromosome abnormalities. It is important to establish the karyotype of the individual.

Uterine hypoplasia is a cause of primary amenorrhea, presumably because of insufficient endometrium to respond to endogenous estrogen. If the individual has fully developed secondary sexual characteristics and adequate circulating estrogen, and in addition has a patent cervix, an attempt can be made with estrogen, to stimulate endometrial growth, although results are inconsistent and poor. The response to this regimen is less than 25 percent and the risks of the estrogen should be explained to the individual. The hypoplastic uterus which does not respond to endogenous or exogenous hormone is associated with infertility as well as amenorrhea (Jeffcoate, Lerer). Because there is a small minority of women whose menstruation is so minimal as not to be recognized, occurring as a slightly brown discharge for a few hours, or who give no evidence of menstruation at all and yet are fertile, biopsies of the endometrium of an individual with a hypoplastic uterus can often yield useful information. Absence of endometrial cells can be determined. Biopsies at 2-week intervals may show a change from estrogenic proliferation to secretory progestational change. Such women may well be able to conceive without further medical attention.

In the case of a bicornuate uterus or *uterine septi* associated with primary amenorrhea, both uterine horns are usually hypoplastic and thus do not undergo a sufficient endometrial response for menstruation. There may be a uterine horn which undergoes endometrial stimulation but which does not have access to the endocervical canal. Or, if a uterine septum is responsible for primary amenorrhea, there may be obstruction of the menstrual flow through the cervix by the septum. When there is a septum preventing egress of menstrual flow through the cervix, surgical removal of the septum by hysterotomy effectively resolves the problem and is not associated with increased infertility (Jones).

VAGINAL AGENESIS

An important reproductive tract anomaly associated with primary amenorrhea is vaginal agenesis. The agenesis may be total so that there is no vaginal dimple or pouch, or it may be partial with a small dimple seen at the introitus, or there may be development of the lower third of the vagina. Usually with total vaginal agenesis, there is also uterine fundal and cervical agenesis. Similarly, while most cases of vaginal and uterine agenesis are unrelated to chromosomal abnormalities, between 20 and 30 percent of individuals with a vaginal abnormality do, in fact, have chromosomal abnormalities. In the absence of sex-related chromosomal abnormalities, the ovaries are almost always normal.

For women with vaginal agenesis or hypoplasia, the timing of vaginoplasty is of great importance. Older literature and textbooks often suggest the procedure be deferred until the young woman is ready to marry. With the age of first sexual contact diminishing and the incidence of premarital intercourse increasing, it is probably harmful to give such advice to a young woman today. Similarly, if the young woman is born without a functional vagina, she should be informed of this at the time the diagnosis is made. It is necessary, whether vaginoplasty is planned in the near future or not, to allow time for integration and adjustment to this profoundly distressing information. Beyond that, in a series of 27 young women with vaginal agenesis or hypoplasia, Fordney reports that 70 percent of the young women had not been told that they had no vagina at the time of initial diagnosis. Of the young women over the age of 16, 75 percent had attempted intercourse before knowing they had no vagina, 50 percent of them three times or more. It would seem that the ideal time for vaginoplasty is when full somatic growth has been attained, full sexual maturation has been accomplished, and before the onset of sexual contact. The most suitable age, therefore, would probably be 15 or 16. An assumption that a young woman who has had to undergo vaginoplasty will be more likely to have premarital intercourse than if she had been born with a vagina is naive. It is almost as naive as assuming that a young woman will be able to go through late adolescence and early adulthood, casual dating, courtship, development of a relationship, and commitment to marriage without being in any way inhibited or concerned about the fact that she has neither a vagina nor sexual experience. A young woman faced with knowledge that she is not sexually functional and usually also with the knowledge that she will be infertile not only needs time and counsel to adjust to these conditions, she also needs to know how she will deal with the issue of no vagina in a social or sexual relationship with a potential partner. She needs to be rehearsed in how she will function sexually after the vaginoplasty, how she will deliver whatever information she decides to relay to her partner, and how she will talk with him about her infertility when contemplating marriage. Thus, deferral of definitive medical management until impending marriage is also a mistake, because it defers the coping skill needed to approach these critical life issues. In addition, the knowledge that the lack of a vagina *can* be corrected, and then that it *is* corrected, is of tremendous therapeutic value in the young woman's life adjustment. These things are more appropriately dealt with in the mid-teens rather than in the late teens. As will be discussed later, teenagers make their decisions about premarital sexual intercourse in a context totally unrelated to medical advice and often despite conditioning toward premarital virginity. If the patient's decision is to wait, or if her decision is to have vaginoplasty but to maintain virginity until marriage, both decisions are reasonable and can be respected whether or not she undergoes vaginoplasty at an earlier age.

There are currently two approaches to *vaginoplasty,* surgical and nonsurgical. The surgical approach is most generally in use in this country. It is usually accomplished by a dissection from the perineum to a depth of 12 to 14 cm between the bladder and the rectum. The cavity thus formed is then lined with a split thickness graft from the thigh. The graft is applied on a mold made of balsa or styrofoam and allowed to remain in situ for 6 weeks, at which time the stint is removed. The new vagina at the end of this period is lined with epithelium under estrogen influence and appears to be normally cornified vaginal squamous epithelium with a rugated appearance. It is capable of serum transudation for vaginal lubrication during sexual stimulation.

Following the removal of the stint, the young woman is advised to reinsert it at bedtime to prevent stenosis of the vagina as long as she is not having frequent intercourse (McIndoe). A reason for the common decision to defer vaginoplasty until the onset of regular sexual activity is to avoid a prolonged period of the use of a bedtime vaginal stint to prevent stenosis. The complications of surgical vaginoplasty are numerous and occur in about 25 percent of cases. These include complete stenosis of the vagina if stint dilatation is not continuously used postoperatively. This is a tragic complication since a second surgical attempt is usually unsuccessful or only partially successful. Other complications include infection, sloughing of portions of the graft, thus necessitating regrafting, damage to the bladder or to the rectum, and dyspareunia from scarring even if there is no significant stenosis.

The alternative approach was first described by Frank in 1930 and uses progressive self-dilation of the perineal area to create a vagina. The procedure was developed because of Frank's astute observation that there were young women in his practice who had no vagina, later married, and through repetitive efforts to have intercourse developed adequate vaginal pouches. The patient is instructed to press a dilator against the perineum at the area of either the vaginal pouch, dimple, or where the vaginal introitus would be, up to 20 or 30 times during three to four intervals during the day. She is instructed to apply pressure for a few seconds until she feels discomfort, then to follow the pressure with dorsoventral and lateral movement of the dilator for 30 seconds to a minute. Dilators range from a size compatible with the pouch or equivalent to the size of the index finger in diameter and progress to dilators larger in both diameter and length. Although there are reports in the literature stating that this method is not always successful, the problems with its utility seem to center around two things. The more important of these is the need for constant demonstration and verification of correct use of the dilators, combined with counseling not only about the dilatation procedure but about other issues surrounding the patient's problem. Where 45-minute appointments are given once a week, 5 to 10 minutes are spent on checking progress and 35 to 40 minutes in discussing reactions and concerns. It is necessary to establish trust and rapport to have the method work. It is also necessary to use a dilator which is as atraumatic as possible. For example, glass dilators have a distinct disadvantage not only because they can break, but because the young woman is always fearful that they will. She is likely to use the glass dilator inefficiently or not at all. Because she also fears that by pressing in the vaginal area she may hurt herself, it is important to establish that the dilator is totally under her control at all times, even during the demonstration, and that when it hurts enough so that she is uncomfortable, she can stop. The patient will not in the course of self-dilation injure herself. Rarely, a patient applies the dilator so zealously that she develops small mucosal abrasions at the end of the forming pouch, accompanied by spotting. She should be cautioned about this and reassured that it is a minor problem, as well as be instructed in how to avoid it. Most young women are able to accomplish this self-dilation in 12 to 15 weeks, although it may take 2 weeks to a month to progress from just touching the genital area to being able to insert the index finger to the depth of 2 cm and then to use the equivalent-sized plastic dilator. Once progress is being made, the patient moves rapidly, changing the dilator diameter and length approximately every week or 2 weeks. The diameter of a forming vaginal pouch increases more easily and more rapidly than does its length once the 4 cm depth level is reached. This is a second problem which sometimes arises in the use of this technique. The vaginal pouch length seems to be limited from 6 to 8 cm. The normal vagina in a supine patient begins at a 45° angle from the introitus to the sacral promontory, then changes direction to become more parallel to the abdominal wall. The young woman attempting to accomplish her entire dilatation with a thrust of 45° toward the sacral promontory will find that she makes very little progress beyond the 6 cm level. She must be instructed to insert to 4 to 5 cm and then to press down on the portion of the dilator outside the vaginal pouch, reorienting the internal end of the dilator before continuing to press up to find and develop the plane between the bladder and the rectum. In this way, a vaginal depth of between 10 to 14 cm can be achieved, which is generally adequate for sexual function. In my own series, the ultimate depth achieved was adequate for all but one woman who required a partial surgical vaginoplasty for increased depth. Fibrous bands in the area of the pelvic diaphragm in two androgen-insensitivity syndrome patients halted progress until surgical release of these bands, followed by continuing dilatation, was accomplished.

Several authors feel that the nonsurgical vaginoplasty is greatly preferable to the surgical in that there are no significant complications reported, and the provision of adequate counseling is guaranteed (Wabrek et al.; Fordney). After development of the new vagina, there appears to be no problem with scarring or stenosis and the young women do not need to maintain continuous dilatation or intercourse; finally, even if the resultant pouch is not totally adequate for sexual function, partial surgical vaginoplasty is still available, but it will occur above the area of the levator sling which is the area associated with most complications of surgery. Additionally, the nonsurgical approach is more economical. For those physicians hesitant to counsel about psychological adjustment and rehearsal needs, the incorporation of a health educator or an individual trained in counseling skills is an excellent addition to the treatment program. Even though the psychological reactions to the condition may appear to be bizarre, ranging from grief to depression to anxiety and hostility, the reactions are totally appropriate for the impact of this congenital anomaly on a patient's life. Psychiatric referral is not necessary unless there are no other counseling services available, or unless other serious psychologic conditions exist.

NEUROENDROCRINE MECHANISMS— ANOREXIA NERVOSA (See also Chap. 7)

Primary amenorrhea may be caused by the same neuroendrocrine abnormalities discussed under delayed sexual maturation. However, in some cases, low levels of gonadotropins may induce estrogen changes, such as minimal breast development and slight maturation of vaginal mucosa. These levels may have appeared normal at the onset of puberty; then menarche fails to occur due to diminished estrogen secondary to reasons such as organic central-nervous-system tumor, idiopathic hypopituitarism, systemic disease, psychological problems, or excessive weight loss or gain. Such individuals fail to have withdrawal bleeding after an injection of progesterone and have low levels of gonadotropins. Treatment should be directed to the underlying cause of hypogonadotropism.

The syndrome of weight loss of at least 25 percent of body weight and amenorrhea in an otherwise healthy woman under the age of 25 is termed *anorexia nervosa*. Treatment should be directed to the underlying cause of hypogonadotropism. Diagnosis and treatment of suspected conditions other than the psychological factors have been previously discussed. Anorexia nervosa is a significant behavioral cause of amenorrhea in the adolescent. Such young women have high energy and freely admit a neurotic aversion to obesity. They tend to be excellent students and to be compulsively neat, but they develop a feeling that they are worthless and unattractive; they seem to fix on obesity as a problem even when they weigh well below a normal weight. Such young women often admit to self-induced vomiting, and psychosomatic examination may reveal severe intrafamily stress or psychosexual problems. Because they are not eating, they have severe weight loss which leads to cachexia, hypotension, bradycardia, and resultant genital atrophy and amenorrhea. Neuroendocrine studies document impaired hypothalamic function not only in FSH and LH but also in TSH (thyroid-stimulating hormone) following stimulation by releasing factors. This is an abnormal response in individuals who have normal to low-normal gonadotropic and thyroid hormone values. Adrenal function may also be abnormal with increased levels of plasma cortisol. Although forced feeding by intragastric tubes may be necessary to avoid death by starvation when 40 percent or more of the body weight is lost, this measure is not indicated in earlier stages of the condition. The most encouraging psychotherapeutic approach has been with behavior modification in which systematic exercises geared at changing specific forms of behavior are utilized. Vigersky has written a recent monograph on anorexia nervosa. Depression is also associated with diminished levels of gonadotropins and while treatment with psychotherapy is not encouraging, there are reports of improvement following antidepressant medication used on a short-term basis to reverse the depression, followed by psychotherapy. Menses return after cessation of the antidepressants, which can themselves cause amenorrhea.

PRIMARY AMENORRHEA WITH VIRILIZATION
(See also Chap. 7)

Signs of virilization in a young woman with primary amenorrhea are seen with three conditions. These are androgen production by the ovary, usually from an androgen-producing tumor; increased androgen production by the adrenal, either by tumor or by a symptomatically late form of congenital adrenal hyperplasia; and much more rarely virilization accompanying mixed gonadal dysgenesis or some form of XX/XY mosaicism. Occasionally, polycystic sclerotic ovary syndrome (PCO) may be a cause of primary amenorrhea. The differentiation of PCO from congenital adrenal hypoplasia, adrenal tumor, or ovarian tumor is made by the assessment of 17-ketosteroids which are usually normal or only slightly elevated in PCO syndrome. In addition, in PCO, 17-ketosteroids suppress

partially or not at all when dexamethasone is given, but will be suppressed if congenital adrenal hyperplasia exists. Plasma testosterone levels are often elevated but not as high as would be seen with virilizing ovarian or adrenal tumors. The extent of virilization is less than would be found with a masculinizing tumor. A rare form of virilization associated with primary amenorrhea is seen with an incomplete form of testicular feminization or Reifenstein's syndrome, this condition being the result of a partial defect at the cytoplasmic receptor level in 17-ketosteroid reductase or 5α-reductase. These individuals usually have breast development and varying degrees of masculinization (Wilson; Saez). There are rare instances of male pseudohermaphroditic individuals with ambiguous genitalia and XY karyotype who have breast development at puberty along with clitoral enlargement and virilism. In these individuals there is a 17β-hydroxylase steroid defect with impaired conversion of androstene-dihydrotestosterone (Knorr et al.).

SECONDARY AMENORRHEA; CHRONIC OLIGO-OVULATION
(See also Chap. 7)

Secondary amenorrhea is defined as amenorrhea of at least 4 months' duration occurring after menarche. This group of disorders is marked by chronic anovulation. It is much more common than primary amenorrhea and is more amenable to treatment. The most frequent cause of secondary amenorrhea in adolescence, other than pregnancy, is hypothalamic amenorrhea or chronic anovulation. While infrequent menses are not unusual during the first several years after menarche, if the condition persists for longer than 2 years, evaluation is indicated. The adolescent hypothalamus is more sensitive to environmental stimuli than is that of the more mature woman in whom the hypothalamic-pituitary-ovarian axis has been well established.

Post-birth control pill amenorrhea in adolescents results from suppression of ovulation and interference with a not fully mature endocrine axis. Once regular periods have been established and secondary amenorrhea occurs, the most common etiologies are pregnancy and stress. It is therefore essential to evaluate not only the sexual history of the adolescent in whatever language is appropriate to her, but familial, school, and social pressures that may be affecting ovulation. Beyond this, the etiologies of secondary amenorrhea are the same as those causing primary amenorrhea with the exceptions of sex-chromosome abnormalities and vaginal and congenital anatomic anomalies.

MENORRHAGIA (See also Chap. 20)

Oligo-ovulation can lead to extremely heavy and prolonged bleeding. These bleeding episodes are not truly menstrual since the bleeding pattern is a dysfunctional one concordant with unopposed estrogen stimulation for a long period of time. On rare occasions, when the adolescent is anemic, bleeding heavily, and hypotensive, dilatation and curettage (D&C) is the fastest and most effective method for stopping the bleeding. Such an individual has both acute and chronic blood loss and vascular instability. Some authors advocate the oral administration of 2.5 mg estrogen combined with progesterone every 4 hours until bleeding stops, or the intravenous administration of estradiol. The response, however, is variable, and there may be concern about the side effects of the agent as well as the risk of allowing heavy bleeding to continue for another 24 hours. Dilatation and curettage is effective because it removes the irregularly shedding endometrium and possibly also induces uterine contraction by a mechanical stimulus. For less severe bleeding episodes, a regimen utilizing 0.3 to 0.6 mg of Premarin daily for 10 days with the addition of 10 mg of medroxyprogesterone daily for the last 5 days will usually result in a cessation of bleeding, followed by a normal amount of menstrual-like bleeding associated with the steroid withdrawal. Such individuals may then be cycled at 4- to 6-week intervals with 5 to 10 days of a progestational agent. This allows maturation of the hypothalamus without interference with ovulation. Alternatively, these women may be allowed to react to their own hormones with the understanding that amenorrhea for 6 weeks to 2 months should be treated by progesterone to induce withdrawal bleeding. It may be necessary to first administer estrogen to "repair" the endometrium by stimulating it into a normal proliferative state and then to "mature" it with the progesterone so that normal bleeding will follow withdrawal of the steroids. When combined estrogen and progesterone administration does not stop bleeding, D&C is indicated.

Another approach to the hormonal management of polymenorrhea is the administration of a combined estrogen-progestational preparation until bleeding stops (Jones; Speroff). The disadvantage of this method is that it usually takes longer to control bleeding, and side effects such as nausea and vomiting may become a problem. Progesterone alone, although it will eventually cause the endometrium to develop an atrophic change, may not be appropriate therapy for two reasons. A patient will often continue bleeding for as long as a month, even though the bleeding may diminish, and high levels of progesterone may induce atrophy of the endometrium along with a depression of gonadotropins so that normal cycling may not resume for several months.

In secondary amenorrhea in adolescence due to chronic anovulation, the management problem is not anovulation but rather the dysfunctional bleeding that follows it. Rarely blood dyscrasias will present with heavy menstrual bleeding in adolescents.

DYSMENORRHEA (See Chap. 35)

Dysmenorrhea, or painful menstruation, may be either primary or secondary. Primary dysmenorrhea refers to painful menstruation that develops near menarche and which is not associated with organic pathology. The typical history given by such young women indicates that for the first year or two after menarche, they did not have dysmenorrhea. That period coincided with anovulatory menstrual cycles; primary dysmenorrhea became a problem once the woman was menstruating regularly and cyclically. Bickers first found that hypercontractility of the uterus and dysmenorrhea were present only when there was a corpus luteum. Later it was found that suppression of ovulation by estrogens, androgens, or the oral contraceptives produced relief from the symptom in most cases. Most adolescents have some cycles with such severe dysmenorrhea that school attendance is difficult or impossible. Typically, just prior to or with the onset of menstrual bleeding, continuous heavy lower abdominal midline pain is superimposed upon periodic severe cramping pain. The symptoms persist for a few hours to 2 to 3 days. Associated symptoms in severe cases are nausea, vomiting, diarrhea, and often the vagal symptoms of pallor, weakness, and sweating. While young women with primary dysmenorrhea describe a physiologic premenstrual syndrome of bloating, intestinal irritability, and aching in the lower back, buttocks, or lower pelvis radiating down into the medial aspect of the thighs, it is unusual for disabling pain to occur prior to the onset of menses.

Etiology of Dysmenorrhea

Possible proposed etiologies include cervical stenosis, and for this reason dilation of the cervix has been recommended. Studies have failed to establish presence of an obstruction, and the treatment of dysmenorrhea by cervical dilation has been unrewarding. Uterine hypoplasia was also considered a cause of dysmenorrhea. However, the period when the uterus is most likely to be small, the first year or two following menarche, is the time when dysmenorrhea is absent. Jeffcoate and Lerer found hypoplasia of the uterus in only 3 percent of almost a thousand patients with primary dysmenorrhea. Perhaps the two most widely held theories about primary dysmenorrhea have been that it is of psychologic origin or is the result of estrogen-progesterone imbalance. Despite large studies which have tried to evaluate psychologic factors or psychoneurosis in primary dysmenorrhea, it has never been demonstrated that psychoneurotic features are associated. What has been demonstrated is that the induction of relaxation, overcoming muscular and psychologic anxiety and tension, diminishes the severity of pain. The estrogen-progesterone hormonal imbalance theory could not explain why pain occurred with the onset of menses rather than the week before when these hormones were in a changing state. The observations that young women whose mothers had severe dysmenorrhea were most likely to have severe dysmenorrhea, the fact that primary dysmenorrhea tends to disappear in the vast majority of women in their twenties and thirties or after childbirth, and that young women who engaged in athletics had a lower incidence of primary dysmenorrhea were used as arguments for a psychogenic origin.

The cause of dysmenorrhea has been clarified recently. A significant increase in endometrial prostaglandin (PG) and prostaglandin $F_{2\alpha}$ ($PGF_{2\alpha}$) was found in the luteal phase with an even greater increase during the first phase of menstruation. Prostaglandin $F_{2\alpha}$ is known to stimulate profound uterine contractions and is believed to cause pain by the production of uterine muscle ischemia.

Jones and Wentz infused $PGF_{2\alpha}$ into normal women and caused the symptoms of lower abdominal and leg cramps, nausea, vomiting, and diarrhea which make up the primary dysmenorrhea syndrome. Administration of PG inhibitors such as indomethacin, ibuprofen, and flufenamic acid in clinical trials have been highly successful in eliminating the syndrome (Halbert et al.).

Treatment of Dysmenorrhea

Antiprostaglandins have recently been used for the treatment of dysmenorrhea. The medication is begun with the onset of menstrual bleeding or the onset of discomfort but before disabling dysmenorrhea; it is continued until discomfort is gone. For the average patient whose dysmenorrhea exists for 1 day, a 1- or 2-day course of therapy appears to be adequate.

There are young women who experience considerable pain with menstruation but who are not disabled by that pain. For them, mild analgesic and anti-inflammatory agents like aspirin, 10 to 15 mg every 4 to 6 hours, combined with a muscular relaxation technique such as a hot bath for 20 minutes, controls symptoms. The relaxation breaks up a characteristic pain, anxiety, and muscle tension reaction secondary to release of sympathetic nervous system factors which appear to aggravate the uterine discomfort associated with primary dysmenorrhea. Anxiety and muscle tension also worsen the symptoms of primary dysmenorrhea by producing uterine anoxia. Strong analgesic agents are usually contraindicated since they do not attack the pathophysiology and may produce dependency. The use of oral contraceptive agents, unless also necessary for contraception, is probably not indicated except in the most resistant cases. Some adolescents complaining of "cramps" may in fact seek oral contraceptives for treatment for dysmenorrhea as a socially acceptable way of obtaining oral contraceptives.

Secondary dysmenorrhea accounts for 5 percent or fewer of dysmenorrhea symptoms. As in older women, it is usually seen in association with observable pelvic pathology. Endometriosis is uncommon in the adolescent.

ABDOMINAL OR PELVIC PAIN
(See Chap. 1)

In the adolescent, pelvic or abdominal pain is more frequently associated with nongynecologic disorders than it is with gynecologic problems unless the adolescent is sexually active. If she is sexually active, all the pregnancy-related disorders as well as sex-related disorders must be included in the differential. The association of pelvic or abdominal pain with a solid pelvic mass in the non-sexually active menstruating teenager is most frequently seen in association with germ-cell tumors of the ovary, 25 percent of which are malignant, or with functional cysts. Uterine sarcoma and vaginal adenocarcinoma are rare but occur disproportionately in this age group. As is true of all pelvic masses, the differentiation between functional ovarian cysts and pathologic cysts is made by a combination of size, fixation, symptoms, and course. Young women with a pelvic mass who are having severe abdominal pain and who do not respond in a few hours of observation should undergo laparoscopy to rule out the possibility of hemorrhage into a cyst, torsion of a cyst, leaking of a cyst, pregnancy-related problems such as ectopic gestation, or a sex-related condition such as tuboovarian abscess. A frequent cause of pelvic pain in teenagers is mittelschmerz, or ovulatory pain. In these cases, the pain is described as aching to sharp with a sudden onset that lasts from a few minutes to 6 to 8 hours. On occasion the pain may persist for a day or two. The pain is believed to be due to peritoneal irritation from spillage of follicular fluid or bleeding from the follicle as it ruptures with ovulation. Usually the diagnosis is easily made because of the recurrent nature of the discomfort at midcycle. If the patient is being evaluated for the first episode of pain or for a very severe episode, other causes of pelvic and abdominal pain must be considered. For the young woman with recurrent mittelschmerz, a recommendation of pelvic heat by heating pad in combination with mild analgesics will afford symptomatic relief.

INFECTIONS (See Chap. 11)

CYSTITIS (See Chap. 38)

Unless it has been a problem in childhood due to abnormalities in the urinary system, cystitis in adolescents is a hallmark of the onset of sexual activity. The urethra is vulnerable to bacterial contamination and irritation, and the initiation of intercourse is commonly associated with urethritis and cystitis. It is necessary to obtain a culture and to begin treatment with an agent such as a sulfa compound or a broad-spectrum antibiotic such as ampicillin or tetracycline. Often, addition of the urinary antiseptic dye, Pyridium, will provide quick relief from urgency and pain. So-called honeymoon cystitis tends to be more of a problem in the first few years of sexual activity, although many women find that without some care they may have recurrent episodes of cystitis or urethritis throughout their childbearing years. Perhaps the most important advice to give to young women who develop coitally related cystitis is to void immediately after intercourse. The urethral flushing by urination has been shown to decrease the incidence of cystitis significantly. Repetitive episodes of cystitis require evaluation of the urinary tract by intravenous pyelogram and cystoscopy (Kreutner).

VULVITIS

Vulvitis is inflammation of the vulva and is seen in young women complaining of itching, burning, redness, and swelling of the vulva. The term is reserved for those cases in which there is no underlying vaginitis to cause chemical irritation of the vulva by the discharge. The most common cause in adolescents relates to dressing habits. Teenagers today spend much of their time in tight-fitting blue jeans which can mechanically abrade the vulva from pressure. In the presence of normal physiologic discharge, abrasion often leads to irritation. Another form of vulvar irritation comes from use of pantyhose without cotton crotches, or nylon and rayon underpants which are nonabsorbent and which, when wet, act as minute abrasives causing vulvar irritation. Finally, summertime vulvitis is seen in association with hours spent in tight, wet bathing suits which cause a mechanical irritation of the vulva in the presence of moisture. There may be a superimposed infection from *Candida albicans* in the pubic and vulvar area, or a secondary infection with bacterial organisms. If such infections occur, topical application of the appropriate fungicide or antibiotic cream is indicated, but the prime therapy should be geared to changing dress patterns. Useful instructions for the young women include wearing underwear with absorbent cotton crotches, avoiding tight-fitting clothing, and avoiding spending long periods of time in wet swimming suits. Symptomatic relief can be obtained with warm water sitz baths. Local application of a cortisone preparation such as 1% hydrocortisone in a hydrophilic base will alleviate the inflammation. Vulvitis or vulvodermatitis may also result from allergic or chemical reactions to agents such as bubble bath, scented toilet paper, soaps, feminine hygiene deodorants, and medicated tampons. The adolescent is likely to appear with a complaint related to these agents when she is beginning to experiment with many of these products. Their use should be discouraged.

VAGINITIS (See Chaps. 11 and 40)

Although in prepubertal girls the most common causes of vaginal infection are bacteria, primarily enteric but also including *N. gonorrhoeae,* the common vaginal infections for the teenager become those of adult women. Chief among these is *Candida albicans,* resulting in a characteristic curdy, white, heavy, somewhat malodorous discharge with itching and burning. The most common source of infection is the gastrointestinal tract, as *Candida* is a ubiquitous organism with a marked preference for moist areas. The vagina is a natural target, and in association with antibiotic treatment, stress, trauma, or mechanical irritation to the vagina and vulva, it frequently will become infected. The occurrence of *Candida* vaginitis with antibiotic treatment is so common as to suggest to the practitioner that prophylactic administration of a fungicidal agent be considered when it is necessary to place a young woman on broad-spectrum antibiotics.

Non-coitally related bacterial vaginitis can include *Hemophilus vaginalis,* which is common in the adolescent and is characterized by grayish, malodorous discharge with abundant gram-negative bacteria and positive culture. Clue cells comprised of epithelial cells with multiple adherent bacteria on them also support this diagnosis. The treatment of choice is ampicillin or local triple sulfa cream. *Mixed bacterial* infections are rare unless there is a foreign body present. In the teenager the foreign body most often seen is a lost tampon.

While *Trichomonas vaginalis* is usually considered to be a venereal disease, non-sexually active women may develop the infection by communal living or shared linens as the protozoon survives fairly well outside the body. Appropriate treatment is metronidazole, 250 mg three times a day for 10 days, and if the teenager is sexually active, her sexual partner should be treated as well.

The presence of gram-negative diplococci in the vagina or *Neisseria gonorrhoeae* on culture implies sexual activity, and a teenager, unlike a child, is at risk for uterine and tubal infection. Appropriate therapy would be full treatment for gonorrhea, along with counseling in how to avoid reinfection through the use of the condom with sexual contact.

Teenagers are subject to all the viral genital infections. A viral organism may be the cause of vaginitis which is symptomatic but culture negative. *Herpesvirus hominis* 2 (HVH2) is the most common venereal disease of adolescent girls. It is diagnosed by the severe pain attending the primary vesicular and ulcerated lesions of the vulva, introitus, anus, vagina, or on the cervix. There is no specific cure for genital herpes although there are promising trials with ultrasound, zinc paste, and immune serums. Multiple other therapies have been proposed in the

last 10 years, all of which have proved to be ineffective. Recurrence rates are high because of the survival of the virus in the dorsal horn of the spinal cord and in the perineal nerve roots. Suggestions for symptomatic treatment include analgesics, sitz baths, and many other agents. Teenagers must be cautioned that they are carrying an infectious disease when they have lesions and should avoid all sexual contact during those periods.

Cytomegalovirus (CMV) infections can cause urethritis, cervicitis, and endometritis and occur in 6 to 8 percent of sexually active women. Like HVH2, CMV is responsible for a number of serious fetal infections and may cause congenital anomalies in infants. It, too, poses a serious management problem since there is no curative treatment. Unlike herpesvirus, the problems are primarily those of potential risk to a child should the teenager conceive, rather than to the infected teenager. Because of concern about increasing numbers of infected young men and women and the resultant harm to potential infants, it is advisable that a viral culture confirm the presence of CMV or HVH2 in a young woman and that she use the condom to minimize spread of the agent (Stern, Mackenzie).

OTHER INFECTIONS

Condylomata acuminata, or venereal warts, are caused by a papilloma virus and are transmitted by sexual contact. The lesions usually begin as small plaques on the vulva and around the anus; at times they involve the vagina and cervix. They frequently coexist with other organisms causing vaginitis, such as *Trichomonas,* and they can be painful or bleed. Treatment in a nonpregnant adolescent consists of local application of a 20 to 25% solution of podophyllin in tincture of benzoin; this is left in place from 1 to 4 hours and removed by bathing. If the lesions are very large, it is unwise to attempt podophyllin removal of the entire lesion at one time since the resulting inflammation and cellulitis can be disabling. Staged application of podophyllin to small areas is advised, or surgical excision or cryosurgery should be considered.

A second viral agent causing lesions in teenagers is *molluscum contagiosum,* which appears as small seedy tumors. Transmission is either sexual or by close physical contact. The lesions are small, white, translucent, and have a central umbilication. They usually appear on the abdominal wall or genitalia and often occur with lymphadenitis. Lesions can be removed by curettage or can be painted with 0.7% solution of cantharidin.

Adolescents are more likely to develop *pediculosis pubis* than are adults. The reason may be a lack of knowledge about general hygiene, specifically of sexual hygiene. The patient develops severe itching in the pubic and vulvar area primarily in the haired regions, and adult lice and eggs can be identified on the hair shafts. Treatment with 1% gamma benzene hexachloride as a shampoo, cream, or a lotion is extremely effective. All linens, bedclothing, and underclothing must be decontaminated at the same time. Pediculosis pubis is sometimes confused with the mite *Sarcoptes scabiei,* or scabies, which is spread in the same fashion as pubic lice and is common with poor hygiene. Observation of cutaneous mite burrows confirms the diagnosis. It, too, is adequately treated with 25% benzyl benzoate or 1% gamma benzene hexachloride (Hollingsworth, Kreutner).

SEX-RELATED PROBLEMS OF ADOLESCENCE

During adolescence, multiple personality and social changes occur. These factors intersect with medical care delivery systems in problems associated with sexual experimentation and mental health. The adolescent age group has the highest incidence of death and injury by automobile or other physical trauma. Adolescents also have the highest incidence of suicide. Suicide is often unanticipated because community expectation for young people does not include suicide, and the warning signs are often interpreted as temporary unpleasant stages of development. Adolescent usage of culturally forbidden agents, or agents restricted to "adults," such as alcohol and drugs, are major problems. For most teenagers, experimentation with alcohol and drugs follows a pattern of exposure and retreat, characterized by poor impulse control and overindulgence, and, later, by declining use. For some individuals, however, the use of harmful agents when identity, personality, and attendant control structures have not yet fully developed can lead to abuse or to the tragic waste of lives (Grinder).

Those areas in psychological and social development of the adolescent that relate to sexual experimentation and to associated problems include body image, cognition, sex role development, role models, and peers. Major development of cognitive abilities occurs in adolescence. The teenager is beginning to

sort information gained from the world around her and to apply it to her own place in that world. She is learning how to process data, but until late adolescence, that process is frequently faulty when overridden by other concerns. The adolescent is developing an appropriate sex role identity and sex role behavior. Much of this is learned from the family, but much stereotypic learning comes from media and other female role models in the American society (Naffziger, Naffziger). Unfortunately, the development of female sex role identity in American culture includes a high value on physical desirability, motherhood, interaction with the opposite sex on a sexual level, and deferral of decision making to males. Adolescent self-image is often marked by conflicts between values and perceived social adulthood. Most parents try to caution their daughters to be careful in the extent of allowed intimacies and warn of the problems of sex. However, there is frequently a second message of "be popular," "date," and the teenager sees the model of the father's family role as more important than that of the mother. For some, the quality of the relationship with parents and significant adults makes it easy for the adolescent to internalize and absorb parental and adult standards. For others, the deficiencies or hypocrisies of adult role models cause them to reject the entire fabric of intergenerational morality, or to accept it only partially. All humans learn to some degree by trying out certain forms of behavior to see how they fit. New situations, particularly situations with ambivalent social messages, tempt adolescents to experimentation. What happens to them as a result may determine whether or not the experiment is maintained or stopped. A classic example of this would be the young woman who has been warned that if she is sexually active before marriage, her parents will know or she will have immediate problems. Most parents are unaware of their children's sexual behavior for some time after it has begun, and only rarely is first intercourse followed by pregnancy or venereal disease. What does occur is a mounting anxiety and alienation. The behavior is repeated for reasons that have nothing to do with fear or absence of punishment, but the emotional response to the behavior may be strongly flavored by guilt and fear. During adolescence, the peer group becomes more important than it has been earlier or will ever be again in terms of goals, attitudes, and behavior of the individual. The marked physical and social changes that occur in adolescence, combined with a recognition of imperfection in parents, increases bonding among peers and increases distance with younger children or adults. Intimacy with parental figures is thus decreased when the peer group replaces it. A problem for teenagers is that they, as individuals, have difficulty in assimilating, responding to, and formulating a plan of action for their myriad new decisions and experiences, and their peer advisers have the same difficulties. These changes and problems have a major influence in a teenager's decision to become or not to become sexually active (Grinder).

For 50 percent of females, some form of sexual activity up to and including intercourse has begun by the age of 17 (Sorenson). There have always been very strong social pressures on the teenager to engage in sexual games and overtures, and a young woman finds herself between these pressures and the very strong social message that, as a teenager, she is not ready for sex. Traditionally, education about sexual activity has been, "Thou shalt not because it's bad," or "Thou shalt not because terrible things will happen to you." Neither of these dictums effectively influences sexual behavior. The prohibitive direct messages are seen by teenagers to be false and do not address the basic issues of what it means to be sexually active.

Responsibility for one's actions is a critical developmental difference between adult and adolescent sexual behavior. Not all adults are responsible, and not all adolescents are irresponsible, but with sex-related problems like pregnancy, adults more readily accept the responsibility of contraception or the responsibility of having and rearing the child. For adolescents to make responsible decisions about sexual involvement, they need more accurate information. Being told, on the one hand, that sex is bad and dangerous and, on the other hand, that it's what everybody wants and that it's something so special that it is forbidden until certain conditions are met probably gives it an increased interest value. More interest is aroused in this way than would be achieved by a discussion of the physical pleasures, by detailed sex information, or by speaking of the pleasurable psychological aspects involved in communicating with another individual at a level of intimacy that also includes intercourse. Introduction to the fact that there are major decisions to be made about whether or not children are desired as a result of sexual intercourse, along with information about whether or not the teenager can integrate being a parent with her other goals, is necessary in order for that individual to make a decision about sexual activity, or to protect herself from pregnancy as a consequence.

Venereal disease, while presented as a danger, is rarely discussed in terms of effective ways of prevention because such a discussion would imply approval of teenage sexual activity. The social importance of sexual responsibility must be presented repetitively, universally, and must be integrated with other developmental concerns. It is incredible that in a society where 1 out of 5 teenagers is pregnant prior to marriage, where 25 percent of teens have venereal disease, and where 25 percent of all abortions performed are on teenagers, responsible adults still believe that if they say "don't" loud enough, teenagers will not engage in sexual activity. Vital information that adolescents need to make responsible decisions about sexual behavior is either not given at all, or is given too late (Zelnick, Kantner). It is necessary to provide honest and open discussions, probably before menarche, to allow the teenager time to integrate the material before wrestling with the pressures of immediacy. Clinicians need to support, if not to institute, community education.

SEXUAL ACTIVITY OF TEENAGERS

The sexual activities of adolescents, especially as related to pregnancy or venereal disease, have long been subject to study. Behavior patterns are changing rapidly, with marked differences occurring in periods of time as short as 4 to 5 years. Generally, the trend is for earlier and more sexual activity among adolescents. Many adolescents who become sexually active, whether with nonintercourse activity such as nude petting, oral or digital sexual stimulation, or intercourse, find themselves in conflict with their basic values. This conflict, however, while causing them pain, guilt, and anxiety, does not significantly deter them from experimentation. There is evidence that genital petting of any kind is followed in not more than 2 years, and usually in 1 year or less, by intercourse. Data for the year 1974–1975 showed that 10 percent of 13-year-old females, 17 percent of 14-year-olds, 24 percent of 15-year-olds, and 51 percent of 19-year-olds were intercourse active (Vener, Stewart; Dreyfoos). These rates of sexual activity occur across all social and economic classes. The vast majority of adolescent women become sexually active before they seek contraceptive information from medical health systems, usually for periods as long as a year earlier. The precipitating event for seeking contraception is fear of pregnancy or venereal disease. Unfortunately, all too many young women *are* either pregnant or victims of venereal disease at the time they appear for medical help. Almost all physicians will provide contraceptive information and techniques to teens who are sexually active and request it. However, it is equally important that teenagers who are seen for any reason prior to the onset of sexual activity be informed not only of methods but of the fact that these will be available to them when needed. This allows the young person easier access to contraception.

CONTRACEPTION

The two factors that determine whether or not an adolescent will become pregnant are the number of years that she has been sexually active and whether or not she uses contraception. Of the 50 percent of teenagers who are coitally active by the age of 19, about half stated that they had not used a contraceptive the last time they had intercourse (Vener, Stewart; Kantner et al., Lincoln et al.). Four out of five of these adolescents said that they had had sexual relations without using contraception at some time in the past. Among the minority who stated they had always used some form of contraceptive, the methods used in order of descending frequency were withdrawal, douche, and rhythm, with only rare consistent use of other methods. Among younger teenagers appearing for contraception for the first time at a variety of teen clinics, approximately 70 percent had never used contraception and had been sexually active at a frequency of four times a month for a year before coming in for contraception (Fordney-Settlage).

The reasons that these young women do not use contraception has been a subject of much controversy and inquiry. A commonly held psychodynamic theory is that because there is ambivalence about the desirability of becoming pregnant, they are inefficient users of contraception. However, in studies in which teenagers were asked the reason, 40 percent indicated that they became pregnant because they thought they could not become pregnant because of their age, infrequent coital contact, or because of the time of month in which they had intercourse. The basics of reproduction were misunderstood by the majority of this sample. Out of 10 teenagers, 3 said that access to contraceptives was a major problem, indicating that they were either unaware of how to get contraceptives or felt too exposed to get them from drugstores or professionals (Kantner et al.). Indeed, one survey has shown that significant numbers of contraceptives used, as well as information about more effective contraceptive methods, are obtained through other teenagers (pill sharing) (Zelnick, Kantner). Another 23 percent of teens stated they did not use contraception because they felt it interfered with their own or their partner's pleasure. Only 12 percent

of teenagers admitted a moral or medical objection to the use of contraception. Only 10 percent or 1 in 11 of pregnant teenagers didn't mind getting pregnant, and 6 percent or 1 in 15 nonpregnant teenagers said they did not use contraception because they were trying to have a baby (Kantner et al.). Thus failure to use contraception in teens has very little to do with a decision to have a child. Offering contraceptive availability, when contraception and sexual activity are not yet an issue, could be important to young teenagers seeking medical attention for other reasons.

Parents are frequently concerned but unable to discuss sex and contraception realistically with their children. Only one-fifth of the states which require health education mandate sex education. Only one state prohibits sex education instruction in public schools, and only two which mandate sex education forbid teaching about birth control. Of the 29 states and the District of Columbia which require teaching health education in school, only 6 mandate the teaching of some form of family life or sex education. Other states specify that sex education is a local option. Often state and local policy is so hedged with restrictions as to make sex education a nonreality (Lincoln et al.; Pomeroy, Landman). Therefore, hundreds of localities fail to provide sex education and/or birth control education altogether, or they restrict it severely. It is left to private physicians, clinics, and community groups which are alert to the problems of teenage sexuality and pregnancy to provide sex information to the teenagers they see. Their access is limited to a small portion of the teenagers who require such counseling. A survey of high school teachers who participated in health education courses revealed that only 30 percent mentioned birth control methods or abortion; only 6 in 10 sex education programs discussed birth control. A wide variety of topics such as human reproduction, adolescent changes, venereal disease, anatomy and physiology of reproduction, dating, necking, and petting, were discussed. Eight out of ten parents said they support the teaching of sex education in schools including birth control, and an equal number of these parents said they support the provision of contraceptives to unmarried teenagers (Lincoln et al.).

In those areas where there are comprehensive multiservice programs for pregnant teenagers, three-fourths did not offer contraceptive services or abortion counseling. Seven in ten did offer instructions about family planning, but the service was not provided. In the mid-1970s, only one-third of teenagers using contraceptives had ever obtained a birth control method from a clinic or a physician. A married teenager often obtains birth control aids from a private physician, but only 15 percent of the unmarried do so (Kantner et al.; Zelnick, Kantner). Their own perception of "wrongness" about their sexual activity may well be a major bar to obtaining services from physicians. Although reports vary, most obstetricians and gynecologists will provide contraception to unmarried teenagers but of physicians in other specialties, at least a third will not.

The methods of contraception available to teenagers are the same as those for older women. However, their usefulness has to be tempered with knowledge of risks and problems that are more prevalent among teenagers than among older women. Concern about parental permission, which implies parental knowledge, where to keep either pills or diaphragm and jelly, how to make sure contraceptive material is available where intercourse is taking place, inhibition about the use of coitally related methods, and failure to include male adolescents in contraceptive planning are major difficulties adolescent females encounter in contraception. There are parents who will help their adolescents secure contraceptive methods, but the vast majority of teens find themselves unable to speak to their parents about their need even in the face of pregnancy, and they are left on their own to get a method.

There has been a marked trend away from condom usage among male adolescents. Prior to the advent of the birth control pill in the early 1960s, most males having coital contact with adolescent women used the condom if contraception was used. It is no longer common for the young man to carry condoms in case his sexual partner has no birth control method. Sorenson's report on teenage sexual activity would indicate that fewer than 10 percent of males consider this a realistic responsibility. Thus, at least on initial contact, the burden of contraception falls to the young women. Sexual activity is beginning earlier and may involve more partners, but there has been a shift in the double standard to serial monogamy in which the vast majority of sexually active young people are involved in monogamous relationships for a period of 1 to 2 years before a different sexual relationship evolves. In the context of sex-with-feeling, or a higher level of commitment in sexually involved adolescents, there is the possibility that the young man may be included in contraceptive planning and that methods which involve shared responsibility can be used effectively. Little information exists on the effect of the inclusion of the male partner in contraceptive decisions or contraceptive use-effectiveness, but those who have involved the male find much less discontinuation of use of contraceptives than the 60 percent discontinuation rates reported in female-only programs (Lane et al.).

Specific Contraception Methods (See Chap. 33)

The majority of adolescents attending family-planning clinics request and receive *oral contraception*. This is also the method most frequently prescribed by private physicians. The advantages of oral contraceptives include the highest effectiveness, use that is non-coitally related, and convenience. The disadvantages in the teen population include the fact that their lives are not as orderly as those of adult women, and the possibility of missing a pill or pills during the month is greatly increased. Most teenagers need to hide pills from their parents, often resulting in the pills being unavailable when the teenager needs to take them. In addition, many teenagers are not sufficiently mature or motivated enough to use the method properly. It is also a poor choice for individuals having infrequent intercourse because they are the most likely to discontinue the method. Undesirable side effects for teens are the same as for adults, with the addition that in a young woman who has not had regular menstrual cycles for 1 or 2 years prior to starting the pill, there is high incidence of anovulation following cessation of oral contraceptive use. The 1 in 10,000 incidence of anovulation following the use of the pill is usually related to women with a prior history of oligo-ovulation. The effect of oral contraceptives in suppressing ovulation will continue or prolong oligo-ovulation in adolescents due to immature development of cyclic activity of the hypothalamic-pituitary-ovarian axis. For teenagers who, having been informed of various kinds of contraceptive methods, prefer to take the pill, all side effects need to be explained. It is wise to initiate the oral contraception with one of the lower dose, estrogen-containing pills, with less than 50 μg of estrogen. If breakthrough bleeding becomes a problem, then the 50-μg estrogen pill or a higher level is necessary (Nelson).

Many adolescents select *IUDs* because they, too, are not coitally related, and there is a very high effectiveness rate, with motivation required only for insertion. The copper-7 device is the sole device small enough to avoid expulsion in the adolescent who has never been pregnant. If other devices are used, they should be restricted to adolescents who have been pregnant. The nulligravida has a higher incidence of pain, bleeding, and expulsion, irrespective of the type of device used, and appears to have a greater risk of developing pelvic inflammatory disease (Williamson). The sexual adventurer, the woman who is having intercourse with multiple partners, is at higher risk for becoming infected with *Neisseria gonorrhoeae,* and there is indication that with the IUD there is a higher incidence of salpingitis than with other contraceptive methods (Eschenbach). The risk of infection is of major concern because of the infertility that accompanies even well-treated salpingitis. Studies contrasting salpingitis in patients with and without an IUD show a two- to fivefold increase in those women wearing an IUD. This disadvantage may be partially offset if the teenager is instructed to use contraceptive jelly or foam with the IUD when having intercourse with a new partner, or with one who is not engaged in a monogamous sexual relationship. Contraceptive jellies and foams have a protective effect against gonorrhea.

Barrier methods available to teenagers include condom, condom and foam or vaginal jelly, and diaphragm and vaginal jelly. *Diaphragms and jellies* are being selected more frequently in the older adolescents, the 17 to 19 age group, because of increased awareness of the risks of oral contraceptives and IUDs, and an ever-increasing desire to avoid agents which may have a long-term effect on the body. Occasionally, young women using the diaphragm and jelly will experience an increased incidence of urinary tract problems, and some become allergic to the contraceptive agent in the cream or jelly. If the young woman can be instructed to use the diaphragm and jelly whether or not coitus is anticipated in order to avoid the coitally related disadvantage of this method, this method can be highly effective in the adolescent population (Lane et al.). The foams or jellies alone are associated with slightly higher failure rates but still provide a good degree of pregnancy prevention, and they offer the advantage of protection against venereal disease. *Foaming suppositories* have been highly touted, but there are now reports that they, too, have an unacceptably high failure rate, a disturbing incidence of irritation and odor, and probably should not be recommended to young women who will be choosing vaginal foam as a contraceptive method.

The *condom* alone is less effective in pregnancy prevention than the other mechanical methods but does afford great protection against the contraction of venereal disease. The use of *condom and foam* and *condom and jelly* affords contraceptive effectiveness approaching that of the IUD. However, young people rarely plan to use the condom for birth control. Complaints of lack of naturalness and lack of sensitivity

with the condom are more prevalent than are information about its contraceptive and venereal disease effectiveness. In addition, since the male adolescent rarely comes in for birth control information, if the condom is used as a birth control method, it must be at the insistence of the female. While theoretically the use of the condom and foam in adolescent population is desirable because of the ready availability of the agents, ease of transporting them, and effective contraception and venereal disease protection, it is sadly true that most female adolescents are not able to persuade their sexual partners to use condoms. Whether this is due to male rejection of the condom or the inability of teenage girls to ask them to use the method is unclear.

In the process of selection of contraception by the teenager, all variable methods should be offered and discussed at some length. Questions and fears, usually relating to a friend's use of a particular method, need to be discussed frankly and openly. Much greater access to the physician must be given when starting a teenager on a contraceptive method. She may need to be seen at monthly and bimonthly intervals as she selects and rejects one or two methods. Here, as elsewhere in adolescent gynecology, the availability of educators and counselors working with physicians and with the adolescent in groups or individually can vastly improve the medical service and reduce the physicians' work load.

Postcoital Contraception

Postcoital contraceptive requests occur more frequently with teenagers than with other populations. The request usually follows the initial coital encounter, coital encounters spaced at great intervals, or rape. Rape occurs more frequently in the 12- to 19-year age group than it does for any other age group, and is less related to sexual desirability than it is to the increased vulnerability of the teenage girl. Rape is a condition of aggression rather than of sexual desire, and the teenage girl is much less able to anticipate and protect herself from situations in which aggression will be successful than is a more mature woman.

The postcoital contraceptive methods are three, high dose estrogen administration or "morning after" pill, postcoital IUD insertion, and menstrual extraction. While the administration of high-dose estrogen is the most commonly used, there are reservations about the desirability of this treatment. Estrogen must be given, preferably within 24 hours and not later than 72 hours, after unprotected intercourse. It must be continued for 5 days, and the doses are either diethylstilbestrol, 25 mg twice a day, or conjugated estrogens, 25 mg twice a day. This dosage may be associated with nausea and vomiting, fluid retention, headaches, dizziness, breast tenderness, and menstrual irregularity. The failure rate is about 0.3 percent when all doses are taken; however, the patient discontinuation rate is much higher. In addition, the patient is subjected to all the possible long-term effects of estrogen administration because of the very high dosage required. A consideration of menstrual extraction is an alternative to the morning-after pill because of very low complications and few side effect problems. The insertion of a copper-7 IUD has been suggested as an alternative in postcoital contraception, but experience with this has been limited and the failure rate seems to be higher than with the morning-after pill or menstrual extraction (Emans, Goldstein).

PREGNANCY

Each year more than one million 15- to 19-year-old women become pregnant, 10 percent of all women in this age group. Two-thirds of those pregnancies are conceived out of wedlock. In addition, 30,000 girls younger than 15 get pregnant. These pregnancies are resolved in ways very different from the way pregnancies were resolved 20 years ago, or even 10 years ago. In the past, up to 75 percent of such pregnancies were resolved by "shotgun" marriages, and concomitantly 75 percent of those marriages ended in marital dissolution. In 1974–1975, 28 percent of teenage pregnancies resulted in births with conception following marriage, and 10 percent resulted in marital births conceived before marriage; 20 percent delivered out of wedlock, and of these 8 percent of the babies were given up for adoption. Finally, 27 percent of teenage pregnancies were terminated by induced, and 14 percent by spontaneous abortion. While teenage births rates have declined since the beginning of the 1960s following a general U.S. fertility trend, the decline has been limited to the older adolescents, those 18 to 19 years old. Among girls of 14 to 17, fertility has remained constant, and among girls younger than 14 birthrates have risen slightly, although barely above the 1 per 1000 mark. A very substantial part of adolescent childbearing now occurs out of wedlock in the 14- to 19-year-old age group. Only 10 percent of the pregnancies in unmarried 15- to 19-year-old women were intended, and it is assumed that the percentage of intended births to girls 14 and younger must be very small.

Overall, nearly 4 million sexually active 15- to 19-year-old women are at risk of an unintended pregnancy each year, and half a million 13- and 14-year-old girls have that same risk. Stated another way, 1 in 6 of those at risk actually do get pregnant in each year. The number of adolescents at risk for pregnancy is greater than ever before, the number of those who will bear the child out of wedlock is greater than ever before, and the number of those who wanted the child and who planned the pregnancy is very small. The medical disadvantages of pregnancy in teenagers such as low birth weight, toxemia, anemia, poor diet, inadequate prenatal care, and prematurity contribute to a 60 percent higher maternal mortality rate and a two- to threefold increase in infant death rate. Social and economic disadvantages of teen pregnancy include lack of job skills, a doubled incidence of school dropouts, unemployment, welfare dependency, a lasting lower socioeconomic status, and larger family size (Lincoln et al.).

The clinician who cares for the pregnant teenager must take the time to discuss with her the various options available, considering all the needed information and facilities.

ABORTION (See Chap. 33)

Abortion is an option for the pregnant teenager, with roughly 25 percent choosing pregnancy termination. In the United States, at least 30 percent of all abortions each year are obtained by teenagers (Tietze). Legalization of abortion has enabled more young women to avoid the adverse consequences of early pregnancy and of recourse to illegal abortions. Legal abortion is still not equally available in all parts of the country, and economic considerations coupled with social constraints have mitigated against the young and the poor. It is estimated that almost 25 percent of teenagers were unable to get abortion services in 1975 (Center for Disease Control). Most of these delivered unwanted, out-of-wedlock infants. Some resorted to self-induced or illegal abortions with the attendant morbidity and mortality risks.

Adolescents seek abortions at later stages of pregnancy than do older women. While there are no significant differences reported in abortion complications of teenagers by stage of gestation at the time of termination of abortion, over 40 percent of young women under the age of 20 are more than 13 weeks pregnant when aborted; in older age groups, only 20 percent are at such an advanced stage. When abortions are done in the second trimester, medical complications are three to four times greater than complications in the first trimester (Tietze). Late abortions may be increased because of fear of family or health professionals' reaction to the pregnancy, and because of ignorance about how to obtain an abortion. For some, there seems to be denial of the pregnancy until denial is no longer possible, an inability to justify an abortion on moral grounds, and ambivalence centering around a need to establish female identity, with pregnancy as a means of doing this. There is sometimes pressure from peers, family members and even boyfriends not to have an abortion.

Postabortion anxiety and depression are fairly universal among women 24 to 48 hours after the abortion. This reaction is greatest in women who have abortions in the second trimester, and it denotes a need for counseling and professional support at 48 hours after the abortion. Long-term depressive reactions have been seen in adolescents following abortion. These reactions may occur anytime from 3 months to 1 year. They may appear at the due date of the aborted fetus. It is important that support services include long-term telephone and letter contact, with interviewing at a later date (Sarrel).

SEXUALLY TRANSMITTED DISEASES
(See Chap. 36)

Gonorrhea

In the late 1960s and 1970s, there have been increasing rates of gonorrhea, the 15 to 19 and 20 to 25 age groups having the largest rates. The total teenage group of 10- to 19-year-olds shows a disproportionate rise in the frequency of gonorrhea. Sexual activity at a younger age and with more partners is implicated. However, probably more significant is the departure from barrier methods of contraception such as diaphragm and jelly, condom, or foam to birth control pills and IUDs. These are the most popular forms of birth control, and the pill particularly is the method most commonly used among the adolescent population. It gives little or no protection from gonococcal infection. Although some infected young women experience urethritis, vaginitis, or lower pelvic peritoneal abdominal pain, roughly 80 percent are asymptomatic or have only a mild vaginal discharge. The endocervix is the most frequent site of primary gonorrhea, but the urethra, vagina, rectum, introital glands, eye, and oropharynx are also reported sites. Routine screening with Thayer-Martin media and immediate incubation at 5 to 10% CO_2 is recommended to culture for *Neisseria gonorrhoeae* as the organism

is fragile. Use of transport media and nonincubated samples may miss as many as 20 percent of positive cases.

The treatment for uncomplicated gonorrhea is penicillin G, 4.8 million units IM, 20 to 30 minutes after a dosage of 1 g of probenicid orally. If the patient is allergic to penicillin, she may be given spectinomycin 2 g IM, cephaloridine 4 g IM for 2 days, or kanamycin 2 g IM. An oral single-dose regimen using ampicillin, 3.5 g, with probenicid, 1 g administered simultaneously, is also effective. Fortunately, only about 10 percent of infected girls have severe complications of gonorrhea, such as endometritis, salpingitis, and peritonitis. Disseminated gonococcal infection occurs in 1 to 3 percent of patients and is the commonest cause of arthritis in adolescents and young adults. The onset of arthritis during menses or pregnancy should call attention to this possibility. During pregnancy the fetus is also at risk and can suffer fatal consequences if the infection is untreated. Therapy for disseminated or complicated gonorrhea is a minimum of 10 million units of aqueous penicillin every 24 hours intravenously for at least 3 days. When clinical improvement occurs, the patient can be placed on oral ampicillin, 500 mg every 6 hours for at least 10 days. Patients with acute salpingitis may require antibiotics intravenously for a longer period of time. A repeat culture 7 to 10 days after therapy is essential since treatment failures occur in 1 to 5 percent of patients, and penicillin-resistant strains of organism have been isolated in some individuals (Stern, Mackenzie).

Syphilis

Syphilis has been on the decline steadily since about 1945 (Center for Disease Control). The 10- to 90-day incubation period, which allows contact with health professionals for treatment of gonorrhea prior to the development of the primary chancre, along with the likelihood of contracting syphilis and gonorrhea at the same time, has had a great deal to do with the steady decline in clinical syphilis. Penicillin therapy of gonorrhea aborts syphilis. Physicians have stopped using the VDRL (Venereal Disease Research Laboratory) test at the first clinic visit in most programs, except for pregnancy care. If the patient has gonorrhea, it is very important to obtain the VDRL 6 weeks later. The VDRL is easy to perform, inexpensive, well controlled, and is an excellent screening test. Treatment of primary stage syphilis is the same as for secondary and early stages of late disease, benzathine penicillin G, 2.4 million units IM. Aqueous penicillin

G, a total of 4.8 million units, given as 600,000 units daily for 8 days is also effective. Patients allergic to penicillin can be given tetracycline or erythromycin, 500 mg four times a day for 15 days. Although treatment for acute gonorrhea eradicates syphilis in the incubation stage, it must be remembered that it does not eliminate established syphilis (Stern, Mackenzie).

The other sexually transmitted diseases now more common than syphilis and gonorrhea are discussed earlier in this chapter and also in Chap. 36.

REFERENCES

Asplund J: The uterine cervix and isthmus under normal and pathologic conditions. *Acta Radiol Suppl* 91:8, 1952.

Behrman SJ: Adolescent amenorrhea. *Trans NY Acad Sci* 142:807, 1967.

Bickers W: Primary dysmenorrhea. *Va Med Mon* 69:423, 1942.

Capraro V: Premature thelarche. *Obstet Gynecol Surv* 26:2, 1971.

Center for Disease Control: *Abortion Surveillance.* Atlanta, 1976.

————: Morbidity and Mortality. Atlanta, 1974.

Cloutier MD, Hayles AB: Precocious puberty. *Adv Pediatr* 17:125, 1970.

Dreyfoos JG: Women who need and receive family planning services: Estimates at mid-decade. *Fam Plann Perspect* 7:172, 1975.

Emans SJH, Goldstein DP: *Pediatric and Adolescent Gynecology.* Boston: Little, Brown, 1977.

Engel E, Forbes A: Cytogenetic and clinical findings in 48 patients with congenitally defective or absent ovaries. *Medicine* 44:135, 1965.

Eschenbach DA: Acute pelvic inflammatory disease: Etiologies, risk factors and pathogenesis. *Clin Obstet Gynecol* 19:147, 1976.

Federman D: *Abnormal Sexual Development.* Philadelphia: Saunders, 1968.

Fordney DS: Vaginoplasty by self-dilation. Treatment results of 27 women with vaginal agenesis, in preparation.

Fordney-Settlage DS et al.: Sexual experience of younger teenaged girls seeking contraceptive assistance for the first time. *Fam Plann Perspect* 5:223, 1973.

Frank RT: The formation of an artificial vagina without operation. *Am J Obstet Gynecol* 35:1053, 1938.

Frisch RE: Critical weight at menarche, initiation of the adolescent growth spurt and control of puberty, in *Control of the Onset of Puberty,* ed. MM Grumbach, New York: John Wiley, 1974.

Gaul C: Clinical experience with the use of hypothalamic releasing hormones. *Recent Prog Horm Res* 28:173, 1972.

Grinder RE: *Adolescence.* New York: John Wiley, 1978.

Grumbach MM, Van Wyck JJ: Disorders of sex differentiation, in *Textbook of Endocrinology,* ed. R Williams, Philadelphia: Saunders, 1974.

Halbert DR et al.: Dysmenorrhea and prostaglandins. *Obstet Gynecol Surv* 31:77, 1976.

Hollingsworth DR, Kreutner AKK: Gynecologic problems of adolescent girls. *Curr Probl Pediatr* 8(12):7,1978.

Jacobs PA: Primary amenorrhea, a study of 101 cases. *Fertil Steril* 16:795, 1965.

Jeffcoate T, Lerer S: Hypoplasia of the uterus with special reference to spasmodic dysmenorrhea. *J Obstet Gynaecol Br Empire* 52:97, 1945.

Jenner MR: Plasma estradiol in prepurbertal children, pubertal females, and in precocious puberty. *J Clin Endocrinol* 34:521, 1972.

Jones H, Heller R: *Pediatric and Adolescent Gynecology.* Baltimore: Williams & Wilkins, 1968.

Jones GS: Endocrine problems of the adolescent. *Md State Med J* 16:45, 1967.

————, **Wentz AC:** The effect of PGF$_{2a}$ on corpus luteum function. *Am J Obstet Gynecol* 114:393, 1972.

Kantner JF et al.: Unprotected intercourse among unwed teenagers. *Fam Plann Perspect* 7:32, 1975.

Kelch RP et al.: Studies on the mechanisms of puberty in man, in *Gonadotropins,* ed. BB, Saxena, New York: John Wiley, 1972.

Knorr D et al.: Reifenstein's syndrome, a 17-beta hydroxysteroid-oxyreductase deficiency? *Acta Endocrinol (Suppl)* 173:37, 1973.

Kreutner AK: Examination of the adolescent, in *Adolescent Obstetrics and Gynecology,* eds., DR Hollingsworth, AK Kreutner, Chicago: Year Book, 1978.

Lane ME et al.: Successful use of the diaphragm and jelly by a young population: Report of a clinical study. *Fam Plann Perspect* 8:81, 1976.

Lin N: Prevalence of EEG abnormality in idiopathic precocious puberty and premature pubarche. *J Clin Endocrinol Metab* 25:1296, 1965.

Lincoln R et al.: *11 Million Teenagers.* New York: Alan Guttmacher Institute, Planned Parenthood Federation of America, 1976.

Marshall WA, Tanner JM: Variations in pattern of pubertal change in girls. *Arch Dis Child* 44:291, 1969.

McIndoe A: Treatment of congenital absence and obliterative conditions of the vagina. *Br J Plast Surg* 2:254, 1950.

McKusick VA: Hydrometrocolpos as a simply inherited malformation. *JAMA* 189:813, 1964.

Naffziger CC, Naffziger K: Development of sex role stereotypes. *Fam Coord* 23:251, 1974.

Nelson JH: Selecting the optimum oral contraceptive. *J Reprod Med* 11:135, 1973.

Phillip J: Primary amenorrhea, a study of 101 cases. *Fertil Steril* 16:795, 1965.

Pomeroy R, Landman RC: Public opinion trends: elective abortion and birth control services to teen-agers. *Fam Plann Perspect* 4:24, 1972.

Reiter E, Kulin H: Gonadotropins during adolescence: A review. *Pediatrics* 51:260, 1973.

Richman R: Adverse effects of MPA in idiopathic isosexual precocity. *J Pediatr* 79:963, 1971.

Rosenfield R: Plasma 17-ketosteroids and 17-beta-hydroxysteroids in girls with premature development of sexual hair. *J Pediatr* 79:260, 1971.

Ross G, Van de Wiele R: The ovaries, in *Textbook of Endocrinology*, ed. R Williams, Philadelphia: Saunders, 1974.

Rothchild E, Owens R: Adolescent girls who lack functioning ovaries. *J Am Acad Child Psychiatry* 11:88, 1972.

Saez JM: Familial male pseudohermaphroditism with gynecomastia due to testicular 17-ketosteroid reductase defect I. Studies in vivo. *J Clin Endocrinol Metab* 2:604, 1971.

Sarrel P: Adolescence, in *Gynecology and Obstetrics, The Health Care of Women*, eds. SL Romney et al., New York: McGraw-Hill, 1975.

Sigurjonsdottir TJ, Hayles AB: Premature pubarche. *Clin Pediatr* 7:29, 1968.

Sorenson RC: *Adolescent Sexuality in Contemporary America*. New York: World, 1973.

Speroff L: Dysfunctional uterine bleeding, in *Clinical Gynecologic Endocrinology and Infertility*, eds. L Speroff et al., Baltimore: Williams & Wilkins, 1973.

Stern MS, Mackenzie RG: Venereal disease in adolescents. *Med Clin North Am* 59:1395, 1975.

Tanner JM: *Growth at Adolescence*. Oxford: Blackwell, 1962.

Tietze C, Lewit S: Early medical complication of legal abortion: Highlights of the joint program for the study, in *Abortion and the Law*, ed., JD Butler, Cleveland: Case Western Reserve Law Review, 1973.

———, Murstein MC: Induced abortion. 1975 factbook. *Rep Popul Fam Plann* 14, 1975.

Underwood P, Kreutner A: Neoplasms and tumorous conditions of the lower genital tract and uterus, in *Adolescent Obstetrics and Gynecology*, eds. A Kreutner, A Hollingsworth, Chicago: Year Book, 1978.

U.S. Bureau of the Census: *Population Estimates*, ser. P-25, no. 614, 1975.

U.S. Public Health Service: *Vital and Health Statistics: Height and Weight of Youths 12–16 Years*, U.S. Department of Health, Education, and Welfare Publication no. HSM 73-1606, 1973.

———: *Vital and Health Statistics*, ser. 11, no. 147, 1975.

Vener AM, Stewart CS: Adolescent sexual behavior in middle America revisited: 1970–1973. *J Marr Fam* 36:728, 1974.

Vigersky RA (ed.): *Anorexia Nervosa, A Monograph of the National Institute of Child Health and Human Development*. New York: Raven Press, 1977.

Wabrek AJ et al.: Creation of a neovagina by the Frank non-operative method. *Obstet Gynecol* 37:408, 1971.

Wilkins L, Fleischmann W: Ovarian agenesis: Pathology, associated clinical symptoms and the bearing on the theories of sex differentiation. *J Clin Endocrinol Metab* 4:357, 1947.

Williamson HO: Contraception, in *Current Therapy*, ed. HF Conn, Philadelphia: Saunders, 1976.

Wilson JD: Familial incomplete male pseudohermaphroditism type I. Evidence of androgen resistance and variable clinical manifestations in a family with the Reifenstein syndrome. *N Engl J Med* 290:1097, 1974.

Yen SSC, Visic WT: Serum FSH levels in puberty. *Am J. Obstet Gynecol* 106:134, 1970.

Zaccharias L: Age at menarche. *N. Engl J Med* 28:868, 1969.

Zelnick M, Kantner JF: The probability of premarital intercourse. *Soc Sci Res* 1:335, 1972.

18

The Reproductive Years

MARY JANE GRAY

THE SETTING: THE OFFICE VISIT

PROBLEMS RELATIVE TO SEX
Sexual counseling
Rape
Contraception and sterilization

GYNECOLOGIC INFECTIONS
Vulvovaginitis
Pelvic infections

PROBLEMS RELATING TO PREGNANCY
Unplanned pregnancy
Spontaneous abortion
Ectopic pregnancy
Antepartum care
Postpartum care
Infertility

PROBLEMS OF MENSTRUATION
Dysmenorrhea
Primary dysmenorrhea
Secondary dysmenorrhea
Premenstrual tension
Variations in bleeding
Amenorrhea, primary and secondary

NEOPLASIA
Tumors of the uterus
Ovarian tumors
Disorders of the breast

PSYCHOLOGICAL ISSUES
Relationship of crises to menses
Depression

MEDICAL PROBLEMS OF THE REPRODUCTIVE YEARS
Common causes of death
Risk factors
The problem list

Once a woman becomes sexually active, the need for contraceptive advice, sexual counseling, and pregnancy detection followed by abortion or antepartum care makes her a captive patient. For most women between menarche and menopause the doctor who takes care of these needs is the primary physician. Just how important a woman's gynecologic and obstetric medical needs are during the reproductive years is shown in Fig. 18–1. Menstrual dysfunction and tumors are potential hazards for all women. Increasingly the modern woman expects to be counseled and educated and to receive emotional support as well as traditional medical care. As women struggle to integrate their goals of personal fulfillment and independence with the age-old roles of wife and mother, many resent the range of problems associated with menstruation and childbearing which encumber the route.

Physicians have often been content to practice routine gynecology, taking Pap smears because they are easy to obtain and explain but ignoring the fact

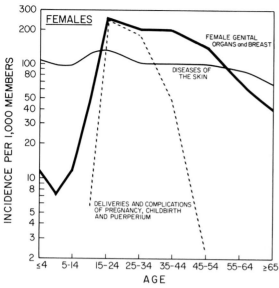

FIGURE 18–1 Incidence of attended illness or preventive care by diagnostic category, showing age and sex. *(From HH Avnet, Phys Serv Pattn & Illn Rates, Group Health Insurance, Inc., 1967)*

that the woman's greatest health problems may relate to drugs and alcohol, to unwanted pregnancies, to poor diet, or to lack of exercise, as well as the fact that the leading causes of death in this age group are accidents and suicide. Women have too often found physicians condescending, judgmental, and unsympathetic in their lack of comprehension of women's problems (Chap. 2).

The problems of the young- and middle-adult years fall under several headings which are considered here in broad scope and in detail elsewhere in the text.

THE SETTING: THE OFFICE VISIT

Although the desirability of the annual checkup is widely acknowledged, many women postpone a visit until a problem arises. Just under the surface lurks fear of cancer, of pregnancy, of venereal disease, or of not being "normal." A generation of "DES (diethylstilbestrol) daughters," frightened and not quite understanding the risks, is seeking evaluation of problems. All this anxiety is compounded by the more general fear of not being understood by an unsympathetic physician. The gynecologic history requires that the woman reveal her actions and feelings, past and present, as they relate to sex. Because of the

wide variation in ethical and religious customs and a legal code reflecting the sexual mores of an earlier era, a woman faces an unknown doctor with apprehension about how she will be received, and she may be reluctant to be honest with the doctor or other office personnel.

Obtaining a History. Uncovering the real reason the patient chose to see a physician at a particular time is necessary if the visit is not to be wasted. It is also essential to obtain a detailed data base for long-range care. A checklist or self-administered questionnaire may serve as a screening history, but it should be used as a springboard from which to talk with the patient. Consideration of the gynecologic history is to be found in Chap. 14.

Physical Examination. Gynecologic emergencies (pain, bleeding, itch) may be treated on an interim basis after a limited examination. If the physician is to assume primary care for the woman, however, a complete examination including, as a minimum, weight, blood pressure, general appearance, thyroid, breasts, lymph nodes, heart, lungs, abdomen, pelvis, rectum, and extremities should be recorded. A Pap smear should be taken at least annually. All women during the menstrual years need frequent hemoglobin determinations because of the recurring blood loss. Urinalysis should be routine. The recent increased incidence of gonorrhea suggests the need for frequent gonococcus (GC) cultures in all patient populations.

Patient Teaching. Many young women are eager to learn more about themselves and their reproductive tracts. The pelvic examination can be an educational exercise if it incorporates the use of a mirror to demonstrate pelvic anatomy, and is followed by the doctor's discussion of physiology, sexual activity, and contraception. This technique encourages questions from the patient and helps reveal sexual attitudes. An excellent movie by Sarrel demonstrates the use of the pelvic examination as a teaching exercise.

Summarizing the Data. After the data have been collected, the physician should go over the findings with the patient, reassuring her when results are normal, suggesting possible solutions to her problems, and giving her the information she needs to participate in the decisions concerning her care. A *problem list* should be compiled and appended to the front of the chart. A complete and up-to-date problem list containing, as it does, an instant summary of all positive findings, saves time and makes safer both the physician's response to telephone inquiries and coverage by an alternate physician.

PROBLEMS RELATIVE TO SEX

SEXUAL COUNSELING

Traditionally the young woman who became engaged sought a gynecologist for a premarital examination. In addition to a legally required test for syphilis, this consisted of a history, physical examination, including pelvic examination, contraceptive and sexual advice, as well as a lesson in basic anatomy and physiology. Now the physician must be prepared to extend sexual and relationship counseling to a much wider group, including those involved in nonmarital and homosexual relationships.

Not only do women seek help for the problems encountered in relationships and in understanding their complexities, but at a time when a high proportion of marriages end in divorce and other relationships terminate with almost equal pain, the physician must be prepared to listen and counsel women about these problems also. Often the woman needs to hear that a failure in marriage need not mean the end of her world; rather that if she remarries, she has an excellent chance that the second marriage, undertaken in maturity, will be happier than the first. Or that perhaps she will find an independent existence as satisfying. The knowledge that children may be less harmed by divorce than by overt or hidden fighting by parents may also be helpful. Nonetheless, the period of dissolution of any long-standing relationship is likely to be a time of distress which the physician can help ameliorate.

Couples with family histories of hereditary diseases will seek help in understanding the genetic risks they may encounter if they plan to have children. Many of these problems are best referred to special clinics or genetic counselors. Genetic problems are considered in more detail in Chaps. 6 and 32.

Sex is instinctive; sex is easy. Almost any two human beings who are physically and psychologically normal and who care about each other can work out a good sexual relationship. However, many psychosocial factors may inhibit the sexual response and make sex difficult. Problems often start in the area of communication and in the context of the interpersonal relationship.

Evaluating Sexual Problems. Sexual difficulties are usually brought first to the physician. If one listens attentively and sorts out the problems of ignorance ("How often should we have intercourse?" "Is he perverted because he wants oral sex?") from the major relationship stresses ("I don't reach an orgasm—I hate him" or "Sex isn't as good as it used to be—he comes to bed drunk every night"), the physician can treat those areas in which he feels competent and refer the others to a marriage counselor or psychiatrist. The message to be conveyed is that sex is a proper area for concern and that dysfunction in this area requires the thoughtful attention of patient and physician. The doctor will often want to discuss these problems with the partner and may want to see the couple together. Problems of marital and sexual counseling are taken up in Chap. 34. Vincent's book *Sexual and Marital Health* will be helpful to the novice at sexual counseling and Kaplan's *The New Sex Therapy* will be valuable for a more theoretical approach to sexual therapy.

Female Sexual Dysfunction

Lack of Penetration. Inability to penetrate the vagina may, rarely, be caused by an anatomic problem—a rigid or anomalous hymen or an absent vagina. More often the cause is *vaginismus,* or spasm of the muscles at the vaginal introitus. Pain on initial attempts at intercourse causes muscle tightening which in turn causes increased pain when attempts at intercourse continue. Thus a cycle is set up in which the muscle spasm makes intercourse impossible and the attempts painful. The diagnosis can usually be made by the spastic response to the examiner's finger. Although the patient may have multiple problems, systematic desensitization techniques (Jones, Park) have been very successful in treating this condition.

Frigidity or Low Libido. *Frigidity* may be defined in various ways, but the term is most often used to indicate a complete lack of libido or interest in sex and should be differentiated from *orgasmic dysfunction,* failure to reach orgasm. The former condition in a mature woman often indicates psychiatric problems. Kaplan has defined low libido as an arousal dysfunction which may signal nonspecific withdrawal from sex. It may reflect poor information about sex, be situational, or may reflect a general inhibition of all pleasurable activity. Treatment is difficult and a psychiatrist may be needed.

Orgasmic Dysfunction. Women have become increasingly aware of the female potential for orgasmic sexual response and find that *orgasmic dysfunction* poses a threat to their self-image. Masters and Johnson's studies on the female sexual response are classics in this field. Therapy is not easy. It involves making the woman comfortable with her sexuality and with sexual pleasure, as well as strengthening her relationship with her partner. Group therapy for "preorgasmic women" has also proved effective (Heiman; Barbach).

Dyspareunia. *Dyspareunia* means painful intercourse. Treatment depends upon clarification of the cause by history and by examination. Pain on penetration is often caused by insufficient lubrication because of the woman's inhibited sexual response, to inadequate foreplay, or to diminished estrogen levels at the menopause. Minor degrees of vaginismus may permit penetration with pain. Any vulvar or vaginal infection such as monilia or trichomonas (Chap. 40) may irritate the mucous membranes and produce pain. Scars from episiotomies, tears, or other surgery may be tender. Frequently repeated intercourse may also produce local irritation, contributing to pain.

Pain on deep penetration may be the result of cervical or uterine pathology, endometriosis, ovarian neoplasms, or pelvic congestion with a tender retroverted uterus. Aching pain after coitus may result from pelvic congestion when sexual arousal occurs without orgasm and resolution.

Honeymoon Cystitis. "Honeymoon cystitis" refers to the cystitis which sometimes develops following initial coitus. The short female urethra is easily traumatized during intercourse so that bacteria are introduced into the bladder. If such infections are recurrent, a complete investigation of the urinary tract should be undertaken after the anatomic relationship between the urethra and the hymen is checked. Sometimes such infections can be stopped by instructing the woman to void immediately after intercourse, thus preventing ascending urinary-tract infections. Treatment is the same as for other cystitis.

RAPE

The number of women seeking medical care following rape has increased markedly. This reflects both an increase in crimes of violence and a greater willingness on the part of rape victims to admit that the act has taken place and to seek help. Nonetheless, it is agreed that only 10 to 20 percent of rapes are reported.

The *legal* definition of rape requires (1) penetration of the penis into the female genitalia, (2) lack of consent, and (3) compulsion, either through force or threats (Woodling).

The rape victim needs medical help to treat injuries and to prevent venereal disease and pregnancy. Medicolegal evaluation of her situation for documentation is also necessary if the crime is to be prosecuted. In addition, counseling services or the support of a concerned physician are most important in helping the woman deal with feelings of anger, disgust, and loss of self-esteem over the event. Follow-up care is essential.

Initial medical evaluation starts with a sympathetic but objective history and complete physical evaluation, including a pelvic examination. The latter must describe evidence of trauma, the condition of the external genitalia and vagina, and must include the collection of specimens for examination to establish coitus and/or ejaculation. A detailed protocol for such an examination is given in Hilberman's *The Rape Victim*. Local law-enforcement agents can provide information regarding local medicolegal procedures. The physician should be aware, however, that recent documentation by Groth of the high incidence of sexual dysfunction during rape make the results of such tests suspect.

Penicillin therapy (or an alternative for those allergic to penicillin, Chap. 36) should be given to prevent venereal disease. Note should be made of the time in the menstrual cycle, with an assessment of the likelihood of conception. The "morning-after pill" (Chap. 33) should be considered if there is a high risk of conception.

In many cities rape counseling centers are available to help give immediate support to the victim and assist with emotional follow-up. Where these centers do not exist, other support systems must be found to help the woman deal with the practical problems and the feelings engendered.

CONTRACEPTION AND STERILIZATION (See Chap. 33)

At a given period in her life, a woman usually either wants *to be* or wants *not to be* pregnant. Many, however, are ambivalent about pregnancy and their roles as women. These women may fail to use adequate contraception for varied reasons.

The physician who is reluctant to prescribe contraceptives for single women should consider the consequences of a pregnancy for the woman. The worse the relationship in which coitus is taking place, the more disastrous a resulting pregnancy.

The Teenager

Among the young who are unmarried, guilt about being sexually active, apprehension about the pelvic examination, and fear of being refused or of receiving a "parental" lecture by the physician may be factors discouraging the request for and use of contraceptives. There is little evidence that the availability of contraceptives is a major factor in initiating intercourse. Almost always, sex comes first and a concern for the consequences follows. Contraception is a fundamental right of the woman concerned, and the decision to use it a step toward responsibility. Some young women do not want to think of themselves as being prepared for intercourse and do not want their friends or partners to so view them. The question, "What would you do if you found yourself pregnant?" may help the woman who is having unprotected intercourse face her problem.

Family Planning

Marriages are more likely to survive if pregnancy can be avoided for the first 2 years. Couples may continue to practice contraception in order to complete education, start careers, or buy houses. Women in their late twenties sometimes need to be reminded that infertility increases from about 5 percent at age 20 to a figure of 30 percent at age 35, and that fetal and maternal risks increase with age. They may still wish to defer pregnancy but should understand the risks as well as the advantages in doing so. Women with progressive medical conditions such as diabetes and heart disease should be advised to have their families as early as is compatible with their life situation, if indeed childbearing and rearing seem personally desirable and medically acceptable.

Choice of Method

Finding the best method of contraception for a couple involves consideration of many factors. For those women for whom pregnancy would be very distressing, the oral contraceptive pill remains the most dependable method of contraception. On the other hand, the IUD (intrauterine device) may be the choice if a woman has had problems with the pill, is of borderline intelligence, poorly motivated, or likely to be unreliable because of psychiatric problems, alcohol, or drugs. Details concerning technology and methods are to be found in Chap. 33.

Oral contraceptives decrease lactation in some women and occasionally a hyperinvoluted postpartum uterus may be perforated with an IUD. Contraception for the woman who is spacing pregnancies rather than preventing them need not always be totally effective. There is a place here for the diaphragm or foam and condom

Sterilization

Once the couple is sure that they want no more children, sterilization for the woman or her husband is preferable to contraception. In recent years, approximately 15 percent of men and 15 percent of women in the United States have been sterilized. Tubal ligation is easy during the puerperium when the uterine fundus lies just under the abdominal wall. Laparoscopy makes it no more difficult as an interim procedure. Although vasectomy involves a more minor operation, the woman is the one who becomes pregnant and therefore has the greater stake in avoiding conception.

Some couples are presently marrying with the firm decision that they do not want children. If they have thought through the consequences of this decision, the physician should be willing to help them achieve this goal without feeling responsible for their life-style.

GYNECOLOGIC INFECTIONS

VULVOVAGINITIS (See Chap. 40)

The acute itching, irritation, pain on urination, and dyspareunia associated with vaginal infections make these conditions gynecologic emergencies; every effort should be made to see the patient and treat her within 24 hours. Only acute cystitis is comparable in the amount of constant discomfort which it causes. The two most common of the vaginitides are *Trichomonas vaginalis vaginitis* and *monilial vaginitis*.

Trichomonas Vaginitis. Trichomonas vaginitis is caused by the protozoan flagellate *Trichomonas vaginalis,* which differs from other strains of trichomonas in that the organism is capable of living only in the female vagina and the male urethra and is generally transmitted by intercourse. In the female, the discharge is typically thin, bubbly, and green but can vary in appearance. It is usually accompanied by marked irritation of the mucous membranes. Pruritis, dyspareunia, and urinary difficulties are usual. The diagnosis is made by identifying the motile organism in a wet drop preparation. The organism has a characteristic appearance on a Pap smear and its presence is generally reported when found there.

Monilial Vaginitis. Although the fungus responsible for vaginal thrush is properly named *Candida albicans,* the commonly used terms "monilia" for the infectious agent and "moniliasis" for the disease originated with the previous terminology, *Monilia albicans.* The term "yeast" is also used, but is incorrect. The organism is ubiquitous, being found in cultures from skin, gastrointestinal tract, dust, pets, food, and water. It can be cultured from the vaginas of 16 percent of women who have no clinical infection. The occurrence of occasional mycotic infections of the glans penis suggests that intercourse may sometimes be a source of infection.

The organism requires glucose or glycogen for growth; it tends to recur during the secretory part of the menstrual cycle. Pregnant women harbor the organism twice as frequently as the nonpregnant; women on the contraceptive pill show an increased susceptibility; diabetics are particularly susceptible. Broad-spectrum antibiotics, which reduce the normal vaginal flora, decrease the competition for glycogen and favor the fungus; as a result, many infections follow systemic antibiotic therapy. Reports suggest that up to 75 percent of women treated with antibiotics experience symptoms.

The clinical recognition of monilial vaginitis in symptomatic women is usually easy. The discharge is white, thick, and curdlike; the mucous membranes are red and endematous. The typical mycelia may be identified in wet smears to which 10% KOH or NaOH is added, or the organism can be grown on Sabouraud's or Nickerson's media. A number of vaginal creams are moderately effective. The infection is easy to control but difficult to eradicate. Repeated recurrences should cause the physician to suspect diabetes in women not on oral contraceptives and may necessitate another method of contraception in the women who are.

Hemophilus vaginalis. A pleomorphic gram-negative bacillus, *Hemophilus vaginalis* is generally considered to be pathogenic in the vagina, producing a vaginitis with a grey discharge and a disagreeable odor. The diagnosis is made by finding granular epithelial cells identified by Gardner as "clue cells." The infection responds to systemic or local antibiotic therapy.

Gonorrhea. Gonorrhea, the commonest of the classic venereal diseases, may cause a purulent vaginal infection, but symptoms are often absent. The incidence is increasing, with an estimated 2 million new cases annually. *Neisseria gonorrhoeae* is identified by intracellular gram-negative diplocci on smears taken from the cervix and urethra or, more accurately, by culture on Thayer's or Transgrow medium. Transmission is by sexual intercourse and the sexual partner must be treated. Antibiotic therapy consists of

penicillin after pretreatment with probenecid (Chap. 36).

Venereal Warts. Venereal warts *(condylomata acuminata)* are caused by a virus transmitted by intercourse. The incubation period is 30 days or more. Similar in appearance to warts on other parts of the body, these can cause pain on intercourse and occasionally cause misleading interpretations of Pap smears. Treatment consists of topical application of podophyllin.

Genital Herpes. The type 2 herpes virus infects primarily the genitalia of both male and female, being transmitted by intercourse. After an incubation period of 2 to 7 days, multiple small vesicles appear which break to leave painful ulcers with sharp edges. The infection may be confirmed by virus cultures and antibody titers, but the lesions are usually so typical that the diagnosis can be made clinically. The infection tends to recur, often precipitated by physical or emotional trauma. Oral-genital contact makes possible genital infections with the type 1 virus and vice versa.

There are two long-range sequelae to genital herpes in the female. If a baby is delivered through a herpes-infected vagina, the infant has a high probability of becoming infected and dying. Cesarean section can protect the infant.

Many studies have found an increased incidence of cancer of the cervix in women who have antibodies indicating previous herpes type 2 infections. Therefore, women with these infections must be urged to have frequent Pap smears for life.

Unfortunately, there is no safe, effective treatment for genital herpes infections. The severe pain and edema must be treated symptomatically.

Other Vulvovaginitis. In some women with vaginal irritation, discharge, and itching, the search for the etiologic agent remains unsuccessful. Sometimes allergic reactions to detergents, contraceptive jellies, vaginal douches, or deodorant sprays can occur. In some women psychogenic factors seem to be important. Women with a tendency to have recurrent vaginal infections should be advised to wear cotton underclothes and avoid pantyhose, tight-fitting pants, and wet bathing suits, all of which increase genital moisture.

PELVIC INFECTIONS

Gonorrhea

The most common cause of acute and chronic salpingitis remains the gonococcus. This organism travels up the female genital tract during the menses, infecting the endometrium and spreading into the fallopian tubes. If antibiotic treatment is not instituted promptly, the infection spreads to the peritoneal surfaces of the pelvis causing abscess formation involving tubes, ovaries, and other pelvic organs. The differential diagnosis of *pelvic inflammatory disease* (PID) from other kinds of pelvic peritonitis is difficult. Ectopic pregnancy, ruptured follicle cyst, acute appendicitis, and diverticulitis need to be considered. Since specific treatment of some of these is surgical, a correct diagnosis must be established by whatever tests are indicated (Chap. 11). Antibiotic therapy must be instituted promptly to salvage tubal function since gonorrheal salpingitis remains a leading cause of infertility.

Postabortal and Postpartum Infections

Another common cause of pelvic peritonitis is puerperal infection following abortion or delivery. Such infections may be caused by a number of different organisms, including streptococci, coliform organism, staphylococci, and clostridia. Women who get such infections become acutely ill and must be hospitalized and treated appropriately (Chap. 11).

IUD Infections

The possibility of the intrauterine device serving as a nidus for infection has been of concern since IUDs were first used many years ago. It has now been shown that the incidence of pelvic infection is indeed increased fivefold in women with IUDs in place, that these are often unilateral, and that the incidence increases with the length of IUD use. Therapy consists of IUD removal after appropriate antibiotic therapy has been started. *At least* 6 months should elapse before another intrauterine device is inserted.

PROBLEMS RELATING TO PREGNANCY

UNPLANNED PREGNANCY

The woman who finds herself with an unexpected pregnancy may feel guilt, shame, or despair; she may face rejection, loss of education, loss of job, breakup with her partner. An additional child may increase her work at home for 20 years and cause postponement of plans for her personal growth. It may be an inconvenience or a major disaster. Some women quickly readjust their views and accept the pregnancy without major regret, but others cannot.

Abortion Counseling

Now that abortion is a widely available option, early documentation of pregnancy is important. The woman needs time to consider her best course, yet must know that abortion *after* 12 weeks carries a four- to fivefold risk of complications and death compared with an early suction dilatation and curettage (D and C). Thus, the questions to consider are as follows. (1) Is she pregnant or is her period delayed for some other reason? (2) Does she want the pregnancy to continue? An immunologic pregnancy test together with a pelvic examination will answer the first question; a sympathetic physician or counselor can enable her to look at her attitudes toward the pregnancy. Psychological studies on women who have had abortions show that psychiatric complications occur chiefly in those women with problems antedating the pregnancy, and that women feel guilty afterward only if they consider the action wrong in their particular circumstances. Statistics showing that maternal mortality from early abortion is significantly lower than that after term delivery are reassuring to those who elect termination (Chap. 33).

Out-of-wedlock pregnancies include not only the single woman, but the widowed and divorced. Despite the stereotype of illegitimacy occurring in the teenager, the rate is higher in the older age group where the percentage of women having intercourse is higher. Some will elect to continue the pregnancy and raise the child; others will opt for adoption or abortion. If a woman thoroughly understands the alternatives, she can usually be helped to find a course with which she can live comfortably.

SPONTANEOUS ABORTION (See also Chap. 15)

At least 1 in 5 early pregnancies ends in spontaneous abortion. The incidence is higher if those instances in which a slightly delayed period followed by heavier-than-usual bleeding are included. It has been demonstrated that a high percentage of aborted fetuses have chromosomal abnormalities, and many have developmental abnormalities.

Spontaneous abortions usually occur in the first trimester, the patient having developed cramps and bleeding. If bleeding is heavy or the cervix is dilated, suction curettage can be rapidly carried out. The value of exogenous hormonal therapy for threatened abortion has never been demonstrated. The woman who has had one abortion can be assured that her chance of repeating is not greater than that of the population at large. After three consecutive abortions, however, the woman is considered to be a *habitual aborter* and a detailed investigation of her problem should be carried out (Chap. 27).

ECTOPIC PREGNANCY

Ectopic pregnancy, meaning literally a misplaced pregnancy, is the term which includes tubal pregnancy, ovarian pregnancy, abdominal pregnancy, and cervical pregnancy, according to the site of implantation. The commonest of these is tubal pregnancy, occurring approximately once in 200 gestations, the incidence varying in part with the regional incidence of salpingitis. Any interference with tubal mobility may predispose to ectopic pregnancy. As the gestational sac grows, the tube can expand only limitedly before it ruptures, accompanied by tearing into its blood supply; the result is intraabdominal hemorrhage. Bleeding may be profuse, making ectopic pregnancy a major cause of maternal death.

The therapeutic goal is diagnosis before rupture followed by prompt surgical removal of the involved tube. Whenever signs and symptoms compatible with an early gestation are present, together with abdominal pain, the diagnosis of ectopic pregnancy must be considered and appropriate tests carried out (Chaps. 23, 44). An IUD prevents uterine pregnancies but not tubal pregnancies, making ectopic pregnancy relatively if not actually more common in women in whom IUDs have been inserted. If abdominal signs and symptoms appear before a period has been missed, or if vaginal bleeding mimics a normal period, the differentiation from an acute appendix or salpingitis may be difficult. Abdominal pregnancy is thought to follow tubal abortion with reimplantation of the gestation on the peritoneal surface of the pelvic viscera.

ANTEPARTUM CARE

Once the diagnosis of pregnancy has been established and the decision to continue the pregnancy made, the physician contracts to care for the woman during her antepartum course, for delivery and for 6 weeks postpartum (Chaps. 28 and 29). Since many of the complications of pregnancy occur as emergencies, the pregnant woman needs to understand how she can reach a doctor 24 hours a day.

Pregnancy Fears

Although pregnancy and delivery now involve a 1 in 5000 chance of dying, we are only three generations removed from the era in which women commonly died in childbirth and during puerperium. This accounts for the prevalence of folklore—much of it frightening—with which women are bombarded. The social isolation in which childbirth occurred during the recent past has added a fear of the unknown to the old wives' tales. For some women, feminine identity relates to success in childbearing and they approach labor and delivery not only with the fear of pain and death, but also with the concern that they will not "measure up." Epinephrine inhibits uterine contractions, so fear itself compounds problems for the anxious.

Most women, even if they want to be pregnant, find themselves ambivalent about the pregnancy and the expected baby. The nausea and fatigue of early pregnancy may be difficult. The decision as to how long to work may be pressing. Later, distortion in body size may upset the woman and sometimes her husband. The thought of the continuing responsibility of a child is frightening to both. Much of this anxiety can be alleviated by discussion with an empathetic physician.

High-risk Pregnancy

Another important function of antepartum care is to screen for medical and obstetric problems. Hypertension, diabetes, and systemic disease pose increased risks for mother and infant (Chap. 30) and require special handling. The young primigravida, the woman over 40, and the multigravida who has more than four previous deliveries encounter higher risks. Increased medical and obstetric monitoring of mother and fetus in these groups will improve results.

As pediatricians improve the survival rates of premature infants, and as ultrasonic and amniotic fluid assays become more reliable methods of assessing fetal maturity, the indications for rescuing a baby from a hostile intrauterine environment by early delivery increase. Such decisions require cooperation between obstetrician and pediatrician as well as the informed participation of the patient and her husband (Chaps. 15, 28).

Education for Childbirth

The education of the pregnant woman is an important part of antepartum care. Recent studies correlating fetal growth and outcome with diet and weight gain during pregnancy may explain part of the high fetal wastage among the poor. Some patients relate more easily to midwives and nurses than to a hurried physician; thus teaching is often better done by the paramedic.

At a time when monitoring and intervention are improving fetal salvage, a reaction against the scientific impersonality of hospitals and doctors has been manifested by training programs for "natural" or "prepared" childbirth, using husbands as coaches and a minimum of medication and procedures. In some, the reaction extends to a desire for a home delivery among friends, despite increased risks to mother and child. Classes which help parents prepare for labor and delivery can offer knowledge and emotional support, and may help restore childbirth to the place of a physiologic body function in which a physician is ready to intervene whenever complications arise. If the medical profession can integrate the best from both approaches, patients and their offspring will profit and some of the joy can be restored to childbirth.

POSTPARTUM CARE

General Instructions

When the recently delivered woman is discharged from the hospital, she should have full instructions regarding her activities and what to expect in the normal course of events (Chap. 29). Excessive bleeding, thrombophlebitis, and fever are the major late puerperal problems. In addition, breast pain and tenderness in the woman who is breast-feeding may indicate a mastitis or abscess.

Resumption of Intercourse

Tradition has forbidden coitus for 6 weeks postpartum. Realistic appraisal of sexual behavior shows that this dictum is rarely followed. It is safe for a patient to start intercourse after her bleeding stops and her perineum is no longer tender. Contraception started in the hospital or a change in the postpartum visit from 6 weeks to 1 month after delivery may better serve the patient's needs. Family planning must always be discussed so that the medical as well as social reasons for spacing children are understood (Chap. 33).

Postpartum Depression

Depression varying from "third-day blues" to true psychosis may occur after delivery and may require hospitalization. The rapid drop in estrogen and progesterone postpartum suggests a mechanism parallel to that causing premenstrual depression. The stress in coping with a new baby, however, is often a major factor in these reactions. Women sometimes need to be reminded that husbands feel neglected postpartum, and that maternal involvement with the infant to the exclusion of the husband may start a pattern of misunderstanding ending in divorce. At the same time, the husband must assume responsibility for part of the care of the baby and for emotional support of his wife.

Special Counseling

If the pregnancy has ended in a stillbirth or an abnormal or retarded child, the physician must help the couple resolve their doubts and guilt over this. Frequently genetic counseling (see Chap. 32) is necessary to aid the couple in assessing their problems and understanding the risks of future pregnancies. Sometimes a couple are drawn together by such a tragedy, but more often the parents need help in discussing the many threatening issues involved. A parent may try to help a handicapped child to the exclusion of the rest of the family and needs to understand that such a relationship damages all, including the involved child.

INFERTILITY (See also Chaps. 8 and 27)

Eighty percent of normal women having regular unprotected intercourse will be pregnant within 1 year. The remainder are said to be *infertile*. Approximately half will eventually conceive and are therefore only *relatively infertile*. If an absolute barrier to pregnancy exists, the woman is said to be *sterile*. Great care should be taken, however, in telling any woman who has a uterus, a tube, and an ovary that she cannot become pregnant. Many a woman has been surprised to find herself pregnant after such a misguided statement. A detailed workup of the young infertile couple may be deferred until they have lived together for 2 years, but an older couple with fewer potentially fertile years should be investigated promptly.

The Male Factor

The husband is asked to bring in an ejaculated semen specimen to be analyzed for sperm count, motility, and morphology. These tests are traditionally performed by a urologist and should always precede the more elaborate tests of the female reproductive tract, since male factors account for 30 to 40 percent of barren marriages. Some men are so threatened, however, by the notion that they may be sterile that they refuse to cooperate. The relativity of infertility is demonstrated when some infertile couples divorce and remarry and each proves fertile with a new spouse.

Study of the Woman

A workup of the woman starts with a screening history and physical examination followed by a careful gynecologic evaluation. The sex history may turn up factors contributing to infertility, such as infrequent intercourse, avoidance of the fertile portion of the cycle because of mittelschmerz, postcoital douching, the use of contraceptive jellies, or the somewhat less spermicidal lubricating jellies. A history of previous pelvic infections should be carefully noted. Ovulation is established by basal body temperature charts and endometrial biopsy; tubal patency is checked by insufflation of gas or by a radiopaque medium injected under fluoroscopy. Various other studies such as laparoscopy are often indicated. These procedures require special timing in the menstrual cycle and several months for completion.

Psychogenic Infertility

Many psychogenic causes of infertility have been postulated, and certainly infertile women are frequently anxious and upset. It is often difficult to know which comes first, the infertility or the feeling of inadequacy. Tubal spasm and hypothalamic inhibition of ovulation have been suggested as possible mechanisms for psychogenic infertility. The theory that adoption is frequently followed by pregnancy is unsupported by most statistical analyses.

Artificial Insemination

Sometimes the cause of infertility is clearly attributable to the husband and the question of artificial insemination arises. There are legal, moral, and psychological implications associated with this procedure; it should be performed only by those who can help the couple recognize and work through their feelings toward the insemination and the resulting infant.

Adoption

Adoption is an alternative to childlessness sought by many couples. They should be encouraged to start proceedings as early as possible after carefully considering their motives in seeking children.

PROBLEMS OF MENSTRUATION
(See also Chap. 35)

DYSMENORRHEA

Dysmenorrhea, painful menstruation, is one of the most common conditions the physician is called upon to treat. Up to 80 percent of women have some discomfort associated with menses, and perhaps 10 percent of women are incapacitated enough to lose time from school or work.

PRIMARY DYSMENORRHEA

Primary or *essential dysmenorrhea* has its onset shortly after the menarche, the very first periods frequently being anovulatory and painless. The peak incidence occurs during the late teens with some spontaneous improvement afterward. The relief following the birth of a baby may be dramatic (Chap. 35).

The most frequent symptom of dysmenorrhea is uterine cramps, low in the midline. Although estrogen and progesterone assays are normal, recent studies have demonstrated the association of incoordinate uterine contractions with dysmenorrhea. Prostaglandin $F_{2\alpha}$, present in endometrium and menstrual fluid, is capable of inducing contractions in the nonpregnant uterus, and this compound has been found in increased amounts in many women with dysmenorrhea. Although dysmenorrhea is usually associated with ovulatory periods, pain may also occur in anovulatory patients with the passage of clots. Many women complain of pelvic aching and backache, possibly related to the increased blood supply in the pelvis. If pain is severe, other symptoms such as nausea, vomiting, and headache occur. Urinary frequency and diarrhea are sometimes noted. Some of these symptoms are mediated by the autonomic nervous system. All are intensified if the patient is tense. The pain threshold of the woman involved is an important variable. In addition, ignorance of reproductive physiology and anatomy, the attitudes with which she has been indoctrinated, and her overall stability are factors modifying her perception of this basic physiologic phenomenon.

Management. The goal of therapy in the treatment of dysmenorrhea is to enable the woman to maintain her usual activity. After a complete evaluation, it is reassuring to these women to learn that dysmenorrhea is usually associated not with pathology but with normal ovulatory periods. They must be assured that their symptoms can be relieved.

Aspirin is the mainstay of the treatment of mild to moderate dysmenorrhea. In addition to its analgesic action, it is possible that specific antiprostaglandin action accounts for its effectiveness. For the sexually active woman, oral contraceptives relieve dysmenorrhea as a "good" side effect of the pill. Suggestions for therapy may be found in Chap. 35.

Women have been victimized by old wives' tales and need to be assured that it is safe to bathe and wash hair during menstruation, to swim, to exercise, to have intercourse, and, in short, to behave like healthy human beings.

SECONDARY DYSMENORRHEA

Secondary dysmenorrhea refers to painful periods beginning some years after menarche, usually as the result of pathology in the reproductive organs—polyps, benign smooth muscle tumors, pelvic inflammatory disease, adenomyosis, or endometriosis. The latter disease has been thought to produce pain 2 to 3 days before the period begins as the result of cyclic changes in the displaced endometrial tissue (Chap. 38). In women with secondary dysmenorrhea, the exact diagnosis is made by methods which include D&C examination under anesthesia, and laparoscopy. Therapy will depend on the lesion found and the age and desire for childbearing. If the uterus must be preserved despite severe dysmenorrhea, interruption of the pain-mediating nerves of the pelvis by presacral neurectomy may be considered.

Pain from IUDs. A common cause of secondary dysmenorrhea in the nulliparous woman is the presence of an intrauterine contraceptive device. Normally, cramping diminishes with each successive cycle after insertion, but if it continues, it may force removal of the IUD. If cramps have not been a problem and the patient begins to complain of uterine pain months or years after the device was inserted, the presumptive diagnosis of endometritis should be made. If the uterus is tender, antibiotics should be employed and the device removed.

PREMENSTRUAL TENSION

Premenstrual tension consists of a constellation of symptoms which reach their peak before the onset of bleeding and may include headache, backache, irri-

tability, insomnia, depression, and fluid retention (Dalton). Up to 90 percent of women report symptoms during the premenstrual phase of their cycle. The incidence increases somewhat with increasing age. Women with personality and psychiatric problems are more incapacitated than others. Depending on the predominant symptoms, these women may be helped by diuretics, tranquilizers, or hormonal manipulation. Counseling with attention to personal problems is frequently helpful (Chaps. 13 and 26).

VARIATIONS IN BLEEDING

The years from 20 to 40 are associated wth more regular and normal periods than either adolescence or premenopause. Nevertheless, deviation from a woman's own normal cycle is a problem frequently presented to the gynecologist.

Menstrual Terminology. The usual menstrual blood loss ranges from 20 to 80 mL; amounts significantly greater than this are considered pathologic. *Menorrhagia* or *hypermenorrhea* refers to heavy bleeding at regular cyclic intervals. Scant periods are termed *hypomenorrhea*. *Polymenorrhea* refers to periods occurring more frequently than an 18-day cycle. If cycles are more than 40 days in length, they are designated as *oligomenorrhea*. Iron-deficiency anemia is a frequent accompaniment of heavy periods and must always be considered and treated. The term *metrorrhagia* applies to bleeding between periods. Cycles can be designated as ovulatory or anovulatory, depending on whether ovulation with lutealization of the follicle takes place. Anovulatory periods tend to be heavier and less regular, but endometrial biopsy, basal body temperature, or other tests for progesterone effects are necessary to make the differentiation (Chap. 35).

Dysfunctional Uterine Bleeding. Dysfunctional uterine bleeding is the term applied to abnormal bleeding for which no organic pathology of the genital tract can be found. It is frequently anovulatory, although occasionally secretory or mixed-type endometria can be found on biopsy or curettage. The diagnosis is made after eliminating systemic disease and pelvic pathology by careful examination and D&C. The curettage is curative in about 60 percent of women; hormonal therapy is required in the rest. In the young woman with a negative Pap test, hormonal therapy may be safely tried before D&C.

Metrorrhagia. Premenstrual spotting may be a symptom of luteal insufficiency. In some women, the midcycle hormonal dip may cause midcycle spotting or bleeding. Irregular bleeding, especially if accompanied by cramps, can be caused by endometrial polyps. Cancer of the endometrium (Chaps. 12 and 42) usually involves irregular bleeding but occurs infrequently before the age of 40. Increasing menorrhagia is commonly associated with leiomyomata and adenomyosis (see below). D&C is necessary for diagnosis in these conditions.

Postcoital Bleeding. Bleeding after intercourse characteristically denotes cervical disease—polyps, erosion, dysplasia, or cancer. Pap smear and biopsy are followed by cautery or cryosurgery for benign disease; more radical therapy is required for malignant disease.

AMENORRHEA, PRIMARY AND SECONDARY

Amenorrhea (lack of menses) can be primary or secondary. *Primary amenorrhea* describes failure to initiate periods; it is usually investigated during adolescence and may reflect genetic and developmental problems. The most common cause of *secondary amenorrhea* in the previously regular woman is pregnancy, and this diagnosis must always be considered regardless of history since the disapproval with which pregnancy out of wedlock is viewed may tempt the woman to deny sexual activity.

Psychogenic Amenorrhea

Amenorrhea with a psychogenic basis may occur in women under stress, probably mediated through the hypothalamus with a reduction in gonadotropin levels, and possibly through an increase in prolactin secretion. Special forms of psychogenic amenorrhea include *pseudocyesis* or false pregnancy, occasionally seen in women with an overwhelming desire to be pregnant, and *anorexia nervosa,* most often found in the late adolescent, coupling lack of appetite and resulting cachexia with amenorrhea.

Polycystic Ovaries

Polycystic or *Stein-Leventhal ovaries* (Chap. 7) are an infrequent cause of oligomenorrhea or secondary amenorrhea, associated with infertility and occasionally with obesity and hirsutism. The ovaries are characteristically smooth, round, and white. Urinary 17-ketosteroid levels may be slightly elevated. Some polycystic ovaries secrete slightly increased amounts of androgens, accounting for the hirsutism. Definitive diagnosis is made on laparoscopy. Clomiphene and gonadotropin are used for treatment with a high incidence of success.

Menopause

Secondary amenorrhea in all women at the *menopause* is a sign of ovarian failure. Such failure usually occurs between ages 45 and 52, but may occur prematurely in ovaries which contain an inadequate number of germ cells on a genetic basis. High gonadotropin levels are diagnostic of this condition. It is obvious that the infertility in this condition cannot be treated, but hormonal substitution therapy may be necessary to prevent atrophy of estrogen-dependent organs, to relieve hot flashes, and to defer osteoporosis. The discovery of an apparent association of an increased incidence of endometrial cancer with the use of estrogen therapy at the menopause has complicated the management of this period for both the woman and her physician. The patient needs to be helped to make an informed choice (Chap. 35).

Other Endocrine Amenorrheas (See also Chap. 7)

Most *endocrimopathies,* in severe form, may cause secondary amenorrhea. The gynecologist sees endocrine problems primarily as they affect the female genital tract. Those genetically determined such as Turner's syndrome (Chap. 6) and the *adrenal genital syndrome* will usually be diagnosed before adolescence; others may occur at any time.

Hyperadrenalcorticism. Cushing's syndrome, or *hyperadrenalcorticism,* may be the result of adrenal hyperplasia, adrenal tumor, or a pituitary basophilic adenoma which affects the adrenal via the production of ACTH (adrenocorticotropic hormone). Classically, the syndrome consists of obesity of the trunk, striae, hypertension, decreased glucose tolerance, and secondary amenorrhea, although not all of these need to be present in the same patient. Diagnostic tests are first directed toward identifying the type and location of pathology by attempting to suppress the adrenal cortex with steroids. Menses usually return after treatment and these women may conceive and carry a pregnancy normally.

Sheehan's Syndrome. Sheehan's syndrome is a type of panhypopituitarism secondary to pituitary necrosis in women who have been in hemorrhagic shock postpartum. The diagnosis is made on the basis of the obstetric history, together with the presence of hypothyroidism, hypoadrenalism, and amenorrhea. Women with this syndrome fail to lactate, show marked weakness and weight loss, and lose axillary and pubic hair. The diminished endocrine function can be documented and replacement therapy instituted.

Pituitary Tumors. Recent sensitive assays for prolactin together with techniques for obtaining tomograms of the sella turcica have made possible the detection of microadenomas of the pituitary. These lesions are found in 2 percent of autopsies of individuals without symptoms of pituitary dysfunction. The incidence has been reported to be 40 percent in women with amenorrhea and galactorrhea (Davaja). Patients with larger lesions may have headaches and visual field defects requiring surgery. The hyperprolactinemia and amenorrhea associated with the microlesions can be reversed by the ergot alkaloid Bromocriptine. Criteria for treatment have not been worked out, but prolactin levels should be obtained in all women with prolonged secondary amenorrhea.

Thyroid Abnormalities. Both hypo- and hyperthyroidism can interfere with menstrual function and fertility. Systemic symptoms will suggest these problems, but thyroid function studies should be included in the evaluation of menstrual dysfunction to determine which women have sufficiently abnormal thyroid function to warrant treatment.

NEOPLASIA

Women today live with the knowledge that a woman has a 1 in 4 lifetime chance of developing cancer and a 1 to 10 risk that it will be in the female sex organs including the breast. Nonetheless, neoplasia in the premenopausal woman is more often benign than malignant. Furthermore, one of the biological advantages of the female is the fact that she develops her malignancies in organs such as the breast, the cervix, and the uterus, which are readily accessible to diagnostic procedures and treatment. (For a more comprehensive discussion of malignant diseases, see Chap. 12.)

TUMORS OF THE UTERUS

Polyps

The occasional cervical polyp can be easily removed in the physician's office. It should always be sent for pathologic examination, although it will usually be benign.

Dysplasia

Since the introduction of the Pap smear, neoplastic change in the cervix can be followed at the cellular level. The cytologic smears document the progression of the premalignant lesions of mild dysplasia to severe dysplasia to carcinoma in situ, over a period of approximately 10 years. Mild dysplasias are seen in the late teens or twenties. Initial studies with oral contraceptives suggested that their use might be associated with an increased incidence of carcinoma of the cervix. Further evaluation of the problem has shown that the correlation is with early sexual activity and multiple partners rather than with the contraceptive pill itself. Abnormal smears in the young woman require evaluation by biopsy directed by colposcopy, or by a cone biopsy which includes the entire squamocolumnar junction. After evaluation, the premalignant lesion can be treated by cautery, cryosurgery, or cone biopsy.

Carcinoma in situ

Hysterectomy is the preferred treatment for carcinoma in situ in the woman who has completed childbearing, since the untreated lesion usually progresses to invasive cancer. The uterus has no known function other than its role in pregnancy, although the menstrual period has a psychological impact on most women. Once it is explained that the hormonal function of the ovary is totally separate from the childbearing capacity of the uterus, most women are ready to exchange loss of menstruation for freedom from cancer.

Invasive Carcinoma of the Cervix

Invasive cervical cancer is most often found in parous women starting in the mid-twenties and occurring in increasing incidence with increasing age. Radical surgery or radiation is required for treatment. The earlier the stage at which these lesions are diagnosed, the less the posttherapy disability and the greater the survival rate (Chaps. 41 and 47). Invasive cancer of the cervix can be cured in 90 percent of stage I tumors, with an overall cure rate of 50 percent. A major factor in treatment delay has been the reluctance of some physicians to examine women who are bleeding. This attitude cannot be tolerated.

Leiomyomata Uteri (See also Chap. 42)

Routine pelvic examination may reveal a pelvic mass. Attempting to differentiate those masses originating in the uterus from those in the ovary and determining which require surgery may be difficult. The ultrasonic scan is a tool which may help.

Uterine enlargement in the young woman who is not pregnant is usually caused by *leiomyomata uteri,* benign smooth muscle tumors. These tumors tend to grow slowly until the menopause, after which they usually regress. They reach a size sufficient to be detected or to cause symptoms most commonly in the fourth and fifth decades. Myomata may grow more rapidly during pregnancy or under the hormonal stimulation of the contraceptive pill. Asymptomatic leiomyomata generally do not require therapy, but the woman's case should be followed regularly and the size and location of the tumors noted carefully in her record for future comparison.

The most common symptom related to leiomyomata is menorrhagia. Although bleeding is sometimes prolonged and irregular, the pattern is usually that of a gradually increasing flow frequently associated with iron-deficiency anemia. Treatment usually consists of hysterectomy, although myomectomy may be considered in the childless woman.

Cancer of Endometrium

Apparently increasing in incidence as cancer of the cervix has decreased, cancer of the endometrium is usually a malignancy of the menopausal and postmenopausal years. Those conditions which lead to continuous, unopposed estrogen stimulation of the endometrium may produce uterine cancer even in younger women. Therefore, all unexplained uterine bleeding requires the physician to perform dilatation and curettage or, similar procedure to rule out this diagnosis (Chap. 42).

OVARIAN TUMORS

Ovarian Enlargement

Ovarian enlargement may indicate a wide range of conditions from a follicle cyst through a variety of benign, questionably malignant, or very malignant tumors, reflecting the varied embryologic potential of ovarian tissue. In the young woman, the cyclic growth and resolution of the normal follicle with its occasional persistence form the basis of most ovarian enlargement found on routine examination. Since these cysts resolve spontaneously, surgery is not indicated unless they are symptomatic as the result of hemorrhage into the cyst, torsion, or rupture with bleeding into the peritoneal cavity. If the ovary is 7 cm or more in diameter, if a cyst persists, or if the tumor is solid,

it warrants laparoscopy, sometimes followed by laparotomy because of the possibility of malignancy (Chap. 45).

DISORDERS OF THE BREAST

In our society, the milk-producing function of the human breast has been largely displaced by its sexual function. Cancer of the breast is the fifth most common cause of death in women, falling just behind cancer of the gastrointestinal tract. The symbolic nature of the breast and the sense of mutilation associated with mastectomy make this malignancy more feared than an intestinal neoplasm (Chap. 46).

Self-examination

Women now expect routine breast palpation as an important part of the physical examination and wish to be taught self-examination. They should perform such an examination monthly following menstruation since most breasts are tender and lumpy premenstrually. Women need to know that they are looking for a change from their own normal state, usually in the form of a distinctive lump or mass. Pain is not an important symptom of cancer of the breast. The relationship of early diagnosis to cure must be stressed because some women are so paralyzed by fear of cancer that they procrastinate even after they have found a mass.

Cystic Disease of the Breast

Cystic disease of the breast is the cause of most nodules and is considered in detail in Chap. 46 and in Haagensen's *Diseases of the Breast.* Studies by Franz have shown that 19 percent of women with clinically normal breasts show gross evidence of cysts at autopsy, and an additional 34 percent show microcysts or intraductal metaplasia or proliferation. Clinically palpable cysts are infrequent before the age of 25 and reach peak incidence in the years from 35 to 50, reflecting the need for estrogen stimulation for growth. They are most prominent in the premenstrual phase of the cycle, and may or may not be tender. The cysts are usually multiple and bilateral and may range up to 7 or 8 cm in diameter.

The treatment in persistent or painful cystic disease is aspiration. If the fluid is clear and the cyst disappears, the diagnosis may be considered confirmed. If the tumor is solid, excisional biopsy is required. Haagensen states that the incidence of carcinoma of the breast is four times as high in women with cystic disease as in those without, although others disagree. He believes that both conditions result from an abnormal response to hormonal stimulation rather than from cancer developing within the walls of the cysts. Certainly cystic disease makes the diagnosis of cancer more difficult for both patient and physician.

Other benign diseases of the breast requiring biopsy for diagnosis include adenosis, fibrous disease, fibroadenomas, intraductal papillomas, and fat necrosis.

Cancer of the Breast

Cancer of the breast is almost unknown below the age of 20 and steadily increases thereafter, reaching a slight plateau about the menopause and then rising sharply. Repeated pregnancy seems to protect against it, as does lactation. The increased incidence associated with late age of menopause suggests that the number of menstrual periods experienced by a woman during her lifetime, with the accompanying cyclic hormonal fluctuation, may be a factor in etiology. A genetic factor is well documented. Although the estrogen stimulation of oral contraceptives produces breast tenderness in some women, recent studies suggest that the incidence of carcinoma of the breast is no higher in women who have been on the pill than on controls.

When a nodule is suspected of being malignant, the patient must have immediate biopsy. Mammography and thermography may help in clinical diagnosis. Women are generally aware that the traditional radical mastectomy is being challenged, but they should understand the risks involved and should not be left to decide therapy on an irrational basis. The physician in turn must understand the woman's concern with her sexual image as related to her breasts and must be prepared to help her adjust to a damaged body image.

Problems with Breast Size

Many women express concern over their breast size. To some it is reassuring to learn that there is little correlation between size and function and that most women who want to breast-feed will be able to do so. Others feel pressure from husbands and peers to augment their breast size. Hormonal stimulation beyond that normally occurring in the regularly menstruating woman will upset menses without increasing breast contours. Plastic surgical procedures carry some risk, may interfere with breast-feeding, and rarely seem indicated. An exception is the reduction mammoplasty in the woman with heavy pendulous breasts which cause discomfort, limit physical activity, and make clothes impossible to fit (see Chap. 46).

PSYCHOLOGICAL ISSUES

Many thoughtful individuals are reassessing woman's place in our society and wondering to what extent her special problems relate to the hormonal changes to which she is constantly subjected, and to what extent rigidly defined "feminine" behavior, as taught in our various institutions, leads her into uncomfortable roles. Women worked on assembly lines during World War II, retreated in family "togetherness" during the 1950s, reassessed their condition in the 1960s and are searching for new ways of life for the 1970s.

RELATIONSHIP OF CRISES TO MENSES

Dalton has studied crises in women's lives and has found a doubling in the incidence of crimes, industrial accidents, surgical and medical emergencies, suicide attempts, and all psychiatric hospitalizations during the premenstrual and menstrual periods. Whether or not she is correct in concluding that low progesterone levels are etiologic, such a clustering of events in this portion of the cycle does suggest a hormonal component. An interesting parallel exists with postpartum psychosis and menopausal symptoms. Wide mood swings can be leveled with the combination-type contraceptive pills, but may cause an increase in depression. Hormonal effects on EEGs have been demonstrated, but the precise mode of action remains to be worked out. The effect of estrogen in reducing monoamine oxidase activity may be important.

DEPRESSION

Depression is the most common psychiatric problem in women at any age, with suicide a leading cause of death in the age group under consideration. More women attempt suicide and are hospitalized for depression than men. Perhaps the theory that repressed rage leads to depression is correct, or perhaps some of these women find so little reward in traditional feminine roles and routine jobs that depression becomes a way of life. Bart has found a marked correlation between depression in housewives and maternal role loss, with the greatest incidence in those who have overprotective relationships with their children. Chesler has studied the relationship between women's roles and their psychiatric hospital admissions.

The physician must be aware of the signs of depression and be sensitive to the woman, allowing her to discuss her problems and referring her for further help as needed. Often the depressed woman tries to hide her distress. Fatigue, disturbances of sleep, and lack of libido, together with fluctuations in weight, are likely to be the symptoms complained of to the doctor. Suicidal thoughts, if elicited, must be taken seriously.

The psychological state obviously influences function in other areas such as motivation to prevent pregnancy, the acceptance of pregnancy itself, sexual satisfaction, menstrual dysfunction, and reaction to menopause. These topics will be discussed elsewhere (Chaps. 13, 26, 34.)

MEDICAL PROBLEMS OF THE REPRODUCTIVE YEARS

Since many women of the reproductive years obtain all their medical care from gynecologists, it is important for these physicians to be familiar with the relative frequency of significant disease during these years. Table 18–1 is an adaptation of a table from Robbins and Hall's *How to Practice Prospective Medicine* and lists the chief causes of death in women 40 to 44 years of age, together with the factors increasing and decreasing these risks.

COMMON CAUSES OF DEATH

Of the 14 most common causes of death, accounting for 60% of all deaths of women, cancer of the breast, cervix, and endometrium are traditionally diagnosed by the gynecologist. Cardiovascular disease has come into increasing focus since risks have appeared to be increased by the use of contraceptive pills, especially in women over 30 who smoke.

RISK FACTORS

It is of great importance to the physician and the patient to be able to identify risk factors associated with

these common causes of death. Those factors in Table 18–1 marked by an asterisk are the ones which are subject to modification. Some, such as the use of seat belts, not smoking, and temperance in the use of alcohol, are part of general health education which needs to be constantly reinforced by the physician. Others such as depression and alcoholism can be detected by the sensitive doctor and referred for counseling. Hypertension, diabetes, and rheumatic heart disease may be better managed by an internist. Transient hypertension associated with the use of the oral contraceptive pill can be reversed, however, by discontinuing the pill.

Obesity. Frustrating to both patient and physician, exogenous obesity often relates to poor eating habits and sedentary life patterns with a strong psychological overlay of compulsive eating. Screening for hypothyroidism or other endocrine problems should be done only if some question of etiology remains after the history and physical examination. The plan should be directed toward reeducation in eating habits. Crash diets for rapid weight loss and anorectic agents can be harmful; they have little place in treatment. Often groups which use behavioral techniques are more effective than the physician in motivating women to lose weight.

Anemia. Anemia is one of the most common problems of the middle years. In the female, iron deficiency secondary to gynecologic or obstetric bleeding, acute or chronic, is the most common type. Failure to respond to iron therapy within 6 weeks after initial studies indicates the need for further workup.

Recurrent Urinary-tract Problems. Any woman with a history of urinary-tract infection in the past should be screened with a urine culture when seen for a general evaluation, despite the absence of symptoms. The frequency of asymptomatic urinary-tract infection is high and symptoms should always be sought. An acute urinary-tract infection includes dysuria, frequency of urination with or without fever, and back pain. The presence of pyuria and bacteria with or without albuminuria is sufficient evidence of infection to start the patient on therapy for 10 days. The patient must understand the reasons for completing the full course of prescribed medication since frequently she will stop taking medicine as soon as symptoms subside. A culture should be obtained 2 weeks after completion of therapy to assure that asymptomatic infection is not continuing. If the culture is positive and the colony count over 100,000, sensitivities should be determined and the appropriate antibacterial agent

Table 18–1 Deaths per 100,000 40- to 44-Year-Old Women, 10-Year Period

Rank	Cause of death	Rate	%	Increased risk	Decreased risk
1	Cancer of breast	351	11.6	Mothers or sisters with disease	*Self-examination
2	Arteriosclerotic heart disease	297	9.8	*Elevated blood pressure *Elevated cholesterol *Sedentary *Diabetic *Smoker *Overweight	Low cholesterol Exercise Nonsmoker Underweight
3	CNS (central nervous system) vascular disease	200	6.6	*Elevated blood pressure *Elevated cholesterol *Diabetic *Smoker	
4	Cancer of cervix	136	4.5	Low social and economic status *Teenage intercourse	Jewish Annual Pap smear
5	Rheumatic heart disease	133	4.4	Murmur Rheumatic fever	
6	Cirrhosis of liver	133	4.4	*Alcoholic	Nondrinker
7	Cancer of gut	109	3.6	History of polyps Rectal bleeding	*Annual sigmoidoscopy
8	Auto accidents	103	3.4	*Heavy alcohol *Nonuse of seat belts	Nondrinker Seat belts
9	Suicide	91	3.0	*Often depressed Family history of suicide	
10	Cancer of lungs	60	2.0	*Smoker	Nonsmoker
11	Pneumonia	60	2.0	*Alcoholic Emphysema	
12	Hypertensive heart disease	49	1.6	*Smoker *Elevated blood pressure *Overweight	
13	Cancer of endometrium	45	1.5	*Irregular vaginal bleeding	
14	Lymphosarcoma and Hodgkin's disease	42	1.4		
15	Other causes	1211	40.1		
	Total causes	3020	100.		

*Indicates area for physician's intervention.
Source: Adapted from Robbins and Hall.

used. Recurrence of a second urinary-tract infection within a period of several months is an indication that additional culture and sensitivities should be obtained and consideration given to obtaining an intravenous pyelogram.

Diabetes Mellitus. Because of the importance of diabetes, problems in carbohydrate intolerance should be included among the more common problems in this age group. As part of the routine screening data base, a blood sugar should be obtained on all patients 1 hour following the oral administration of 50 g of dextrose. In this screening, it is not infrequent to find borderline elevations of blood sugar. Women showing this symptom frequently have a family history which is positive for diabetes. They are often overweight or actually obese. The usual plan with minor elevations of blood sugar is to repeat the blood sugar evaluation 2 hours after a prescribed test meal containing at least 100 g of carbohydrate. If this result is normal, the patient is started on a weight-reducing plan and the blood sugar is rechecked in 6 months. The effect of birth control pills in producing carbohydrate intolerance in a prediabetic individual is similar to that noted in pregnancy. If the blood sugar remains elevated following the test meal, a 3-hour oral glucose-tolerance test should be done to confirm the diagnosis and to establish the renal threshold.

THE PROBLEM LIST

The need for a solid data base from which to construct a problem list is obvious. The list should incorporate both established diagnoses and prevalent risk factors to keep the physician abreast of the woman's medical and emotional needs and to allow the doctor to help her make plans to achieve and maintain optimal health.

REFERENCES

Barbach LG: *For Yourself: The Fulfillment of Female Sexuality,* New York: Anchor Press, Doubleday, 1976.

Bart P: Depression in middle-aged women, in *Woman in Sexist Society: Studies in Power and Powerlessness,* eds. V Gornick, BK Moran, New York: Basic Books, 1971

Chesler P: *Women and Madness,* New York: Doubleday, 1972.

Dalton K: *The Premenstrual Syndrome and Progesterone Therapy,* Chicago: Yearbook Med Publ, 1977.

Davaja V et al.: Significance of galactorrhea in patients with normal menses, oligomenorrhea, and secondary amenorrhea. *Amer J Obstet Gynecol* 20:509, 1977.

Haagensen CD: *Diseases of the Breast,* Philadelphia: Saunders, 1971.

Heiman J et al.: *Becoming Orgasmic: A Sexual Growth Program for Women,* Englewood Cliffs, New Jersey: Prentice-Hall, 1976.

Hilberman E: *The Rape Victim, 1976.* Washington, D.C.: Amer. Psychiatric Assoc.

Jones WW Jr, Park PM: Treatment of single partner sexual dysfunction by systematic desensitization. *Obstet Gynec* 39:411, 1972.

Kaplan HS: *The New Sex Therapy: Active Treatment of Sexual Dysfunctions,* New York: Brunner/Mazel, 1974.

_____: Hypoactive sexual desire. *J Sex Mar Ther* 3:3, 1977.

Masters W, Johnson V: *Human Sexual Inadequacy,* Boston: Little Brown, 1970.

Vincent C: *Sexual and Marital Health,* New York: McGraw-Hill, 1973.

Woodling BA et al.: Sexual assault: Rape and molestation. *Clin Obstet Gynecol* 20:509, 1977.

19

The Later Years

RAYMOND H. KAUFMAN   PAUL C. WEINBERG

Since the turn of the century, life expectancy has increased from 47 to 71 years, multiplying the numbers of the aged in the population. According to National Council on Aging (NCOA) data, 12 million of those over 65 are women. Since the gynecologist-obstetrician is more and more frequently the primary care physician, it is essential that these specialists now become even more knowledgeable in all aspects of the aging process, especially the psychosocial milieu in which older women find themselves.

The organic aspects of aging are best considered by the gynecologist in the categories of general systemic diseases and local genital diseases. Health and function can be adversely affected by chronic debilitating diseases such as arthritis, atherosclerosis, stroke, chronic pulmonary disease, and the organic brain syndrome. Fortunately, in patients so affected, there are better modalities of medical management and rehabilitation than in the past. These patients require careful assessment and counseling so that their chronic disease does not impose greater loss of function than is unavoidable. They frequently feel that remaining active, especially sexually, can be dangerous because of their chronic disease. The risks are far less than they believe. Highly individualized evaluation is needed to determine the real risks in this patient population. (See also Chap. 35.)

PHYSICAL CHANGES OF AGING

As a woman goes through and passes the menopause, a series of changes take place in her body, some of which are related to a hypoestrogenic state and others to the general degenerative alterations in the cardiovascular and musculoskeletal systems. There tends to be a gradual redistribution of fat from the upper body, arms, neck, and breast to the midsection, the abdomen, thighs, and buttocks. The collagenous and elastic tissues of the body also undergo alterations resulting in loss of tissue elasticity and tone. The skin becomes lax and wrinkled. Intolerance to cold increases as age advances.

Changes occur in the musculoskeletal system of the aging woman. There is a progressive decrease in the number of individual striated muscle fibers. The gradual weakening of muscles, including the back muscles, leads to postural changes of the spine. There is loss of bone mineral and mass. Most cross-sectional studies of osteoporosis have concluded that there is a linear relationship between bone loss and aging. Meema et al. are of the opinion that the loss of ovarian function rather than age, per se, is the more important factor in the development of involutional osteoporosis in women. It would appear that the rate of bone loss, initially, may be greater after an artificial menopause. As in the male, aging is associated with degenerative changes in the cardiovascular system which lead to atherosclerosis and its systemic complications.

In terms of the genitalia, atrophy of the Müllerian structures and the external genitalia occurs as a result of a hypoestrogenic state. The introitus and vagina narrow and lose their elasticity. The vaginal mucosa thins significantly and is not well lubricated. Such sequelae cause frequent episodes of vaginitis with associated leukorrhea. Many of the complications related to the hypoestrogenic state can be prevented or delayed by the use of exogenous estrogens.

ESTROGENS IN THE POSTMENOPAUSAL WOMAN

In 1970, there were 28 million women over the age of 50. These women have an average life expectancy of 28 years beyond the menopause. Thus, the potential use of estrogens by the postmenopausal woman is enormous (see also Chap. 35). The controversy that

has arisen during the past few years as to the possible relationship of exogenous estrogens and the development of endometrial carcinoma, however, has caused concern in the minds of many individuals. Not all postmenopausal women require estrogen. Studies indicate that 50 to 60 percent of women 5 years after their last menstrual period are still producing adequate endogenous estrogens; 40 percent of women 10 years after their last menstrual period are also producing adequate endogenous estrogens. These estrogens are being generated by the peripheral conversion of androstenediol to estrogen within the fat. In the 40 to 50 percent of women whose endogenous estrogen production is deficient, symptoms of inadequate estrogen may become manifest. Such symptoms include hot flashes, irritability, night sweats, and insomnia. In the symptomatic female, consideration should be given to the use of exogenous estrogens, remembering the caveat of their possible relationship to the development of endometrial carcinoma.

RELATIONSHIP TO ENDOMETRIAL CANCER

Voluminous evidence has accumulated relating the use of exogenous estrogens to the development of endometrial adenocarcinoma (see also Chaps. 12 and 42). Between 1940 and 1970, the incidence of endometrial carcinoma was stable. In the years 1969 to 1973, there was a 50 percent increase in the occurrence of invasive endometrial carcinoma and a 100 percent increase in the occurrence of in situ endometrial adenocarcinoma. The studies of Mack et al., Ziel and Finkle, Smith et al., and Antunes et al. have indicated that the estrogen-user has five times the risk (or more) of developing endometrial adenocarcinoma than the nonuser. This risk appears to increase in direct proportion to the length of time the estrogen has been taken and to the dose of estrogen given. There are many controversial aspects of these studies that make some investigators feel that the relationship of the use of exogenous estrogen to endometrial carcinoma is not valid. Prior to the prescription of exogenous estrogen for any postmenopausal woman, however, this point of concern should be fully discussed with the patient.

ESTROGEN ADMINISTRATION

Despite the theoretical risk of the association between the use of estrogens and endometrial carcinoma, their judicious use in the symptomatic patient appears justified to us. Ideally, the smallest dose that will relieve the patient's symptoms should be used for the shortest period of time possible. A wise precautionary measure is to sample the endometrium by office biopsy prior to instituting estrogen, repeating this on an annual basis to be sure that the endometrium is not being unduly stimulated by the hormone. Some investigators prefer to use a progestational agent cyclically to cause bleeding on a periodic basis. As yet, there is not sufficient evidence to suggest that this will be of benefit in the prevention of endometrial adenocarcinoma.

If abnormal bleeding occurs in the patient receiving exogenous estrogens, it should be immediately investigated with a thorough pelvic examination, cervicovaginal smear, and endometrial biopsy, and at times with fractional uterine curettage, rather than ascribing the bleeding to the effect of estrogen.

In addition to their value in alleviating the previously mentioned symptoms associated with menopause, exogenous estrogens are of immense help in improving the integrity of the vulvovaginal tissues. Furthermore, the studies of Lindsay et al., and Meema et al. suggest that exogenous estrogens are of considerable value in preventing the development of osteoporosis.

VULVOVAGINAL DISEASE

As already indicated, failing ovarian function, leading to a decrease in the production of estrogen and progesterone, results in atrophic changes of the vulva and vagina (see also Chap. 40). There is atrophy of the labia majora and thinning of hair over these as well as the mons pubis. Frequently, the atrophy is progressive with almost complete disappearance of the labia minora. The clitoris also atrophies. The vaginal mucosa gradually thins, losing the normal rugal patterns seen in younger women. Associated with thinning of the vaginal mucosa, secondary bacterial infection may occur in the vagina leading to the development of atrophic vaginitis with its coexisting mucopurulent discharge. Simultaneous with the atrophy of the vulvar tissues, the skin and mucosal surfaces become highly sensitive to external irritants resulting in pruritus and scratching. These changes, especially those occurring within the vagina, can be reversed by topically applying estrogen cream. Just one-half an applicator of an estrogenic cream, used on a weekly

basis, will lead to thickening of the mucosal tissues of the vagina and vulva.

VAGINAL ATROPHY

Frequently, the atrophic changes result in marked narrowing of the introitus and vagina; this is especially true in the woman who has abstained from intercourse for a long period of time. Severe dyspareunia often results when coitus is attempted. This problem is sometimes resolved by the use of graduated dilators or finger dilatation to stretch the introitus. In addition, a water-soluble lubricant should be used with coitus. Furthermore, as mentioned above, the use of an intravaginal estrogen cream may be of help.

PELVIC RELAXATION

One of the problems in the aging woman is related to relaxation of the supporting tissues of the pelvic floor. These changes tend to occur concomitantly with decrease in estrogen production and the associated atrophy of the supporting structures, resulting in loss of their connective tissue elasticity and tone (see also Chaps. 38 and 39). The onset of symptoms may be slow and insidious, but not infrequently, the elderly woman will suddenly notice a protrusion coming from her vagina. In others, the process is a totally gradual one, slowly becoming more pronounced over a long period of time. The patient may be completely asymptomatic, or she may complain of symptoms related to pelvic relaxation such as pelvic heaviness, backache, urinary stress incontinence, and difficulty in defecation.

TREATMENT OF PELVIC RELAXATION

When pelvic relaxation is symptomatic, consideration should be given to surgical correction of the defect. This is usually best accomplished by vaginal hysterectomy, anterior colporrhaphy, and colpoperineorrhaphy. In performing these surgical procedures, the physician's consideration should be directed toward repairing the defects while still allowing continuation of coital activity. On occasion, in treating the elderly

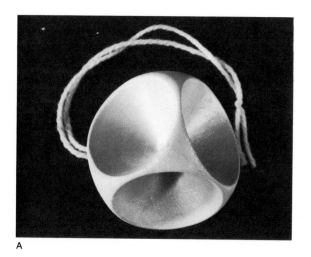

A

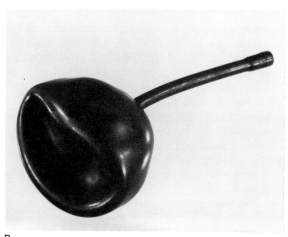

B

FIGURE 19-1 Several pessaries used for conservative management of "genital prolapse": *A* Cube or Bee-Cell pessary. *B* Inflatable balloon pessary. *C* Ring pessary.

female with total genital prolapse who no longer desires continued sexual activity, consideration can be given to the LeFort operation (partial colpocleisis). In the individual with symptomatic pelvic relaxation who is a poor medical risk because of severe illness, the use of intravaginal pessaries is another alternative (Fig. 19–1). At times, these pessaries help hold prolapsed genital tissues in a more anatomic position. They do act as foreign bodies within the vagina, resulting in irritation and trauma to the tissues, and for this reason they must be frequently removed, the vagina and pessary cleansed, and the pessary replaced.

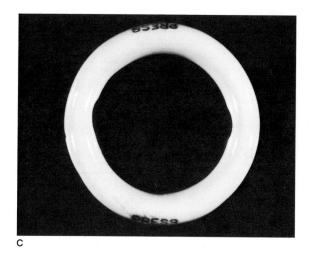

C

POSTMENOPAUSAL BLEEDING

Postmenopausal bleeding should be a warning of possible genital malignancy (see also Chaps. 20, 41, and 42). Generally, one-third of the patients will have a malignancy of the genital tract; one-third will have a benign neoplasm, such as endometrial hyperplasia or polyp; and one-third will reveal no pathologic cause as the source of bleeding.

Because of this association of genital malignancy with postmenopausal bleeding, a careful workup of the patient is mandatory. This should in-

clude a thorough pelvic examination, cervicovaginal cytology (an endocervical aspirate is most valuable), an office endometrial biopsy, and/or biopsy of any grossly suspicious lesion seen on the vulva, vagina, or cervix. Should the office endometrial biopsy prove negative, a thorough fractional uterine curettage should be performed. One of the very common errors committed by the physician is to ascribe postmenopausal bleeding to the use of exogenous estrogen with consequent delay in diagnosis of a genital malignancy. As previously cited, even in the patient receiving estrogens, a thorough evaluation should be performed.

OVARIAN CARCINOMA

One of the most insidious genital malignancies is ovarian carcinoma (see also Chap. 45). Early ovarian carcinomas are usually fortuitously found. By the time a significant-sized adnexal mass can be palpated or the patient complains of abdominal distention, pain, or vaginal bleeding, the disease is already far-advanced. For this reason, the clinician must look with suspicion on any palpable ovary in the postmenopausal female. The ovary decreases markedly in size after the menopause, reaching a diameter less than 2 cm by 1 cm, usually not palpable. When an enlarged ovary is felt, this is cause to suspect an ovarian neoplasm, and surgical exploration should be performed.

PSYCHOSOCIAL CONSIDERATIONS

Psychosocial considerations are all important in this aging population of women (see also Chaps. 26 and 34). Of this group, 95 percent still live in the community and are not institutionalized; over 80 percent are still self-mobile.

Butler has considered the psychodynamics of public attitude toward aging. Generally, the aging are stereotyped as attitudinally rigid, useless, and nonproductive. When the young themselves age, these attitudes become internalized, and at the worst, self-hatred or at the least, a markedly diminished self-image evolves.

Harris, in a poll sponsored by NCOA, found that most of the public considers the principal features of aging to be illness, slowing down, wrinkles, and gray hair.

SEX AND THE ELDERLY

Although 60 percent of the population over 65 are still sexually active, only 5 percent of Harris's sample perceived this fact. Thus, the myth that the aged are neuter is reinforced.

Of the 12 million women over 65, 6 million live alone and 1.5 million are single or divorced. Since there are more than 150 women to every 100 men in this age group, finding a marital partner can be difficult. The difficulty is compounded by the culturally sexist attitudes of our society that condone men's marrying younger women, but do not allow women this same freedom with younger men. The disadvantage is further emphasized by the fact that in this age group 78 percent of males are married as opposed to 39 percent of females. The myths, stereotypes, and sexism applied to the aging population have been appropriately called "ageism." Its most extreme aspect is the attitude toward and ignorance of sexual function in the later years.

Physiologically, both male and female are capable of coital function into the very late years. Of those still with partners, over 60 percent do continue coital activity. In the male, erection may take longer and ejaculation be less frequent, but orgasm may be as pleasurable as previously. In the female, there are longer arousal times to lubrication and less vasocongestion, but if these changes are explained and understood, they need not lead to performance anxieties. Continued sexual activity at this age represents a very meaningful self-assertion, a real outlet for passion, caring, and relating to another human. These are the very kinds of relationships of which the aging are largely deprived.

OTHER PROBLEMS

The small group (5 percent) that are necessarily institutionalized face even more obstacles. Nursing-home personnel in general insist upon segregation, furnish little privacy, discourage conjugal visits, and are appalled at masturbation as a sexual outlet. These attitudes are representative of the bias and stereotyping of the aged as "sexless."

Prescribing drugs to the aging requires assiduous care. With the controversy regarding estrogen's role in increasing the incidence of uterine cancer, cardiovascular disease, and hypertension, one must balance risks against benefits. Confronted with the anxieties and the depressive states of the older ages, tranquilizers and other psychotropic agents must be cautiously and judiciously prescribed, frequently in low dosage.

The physician who assumes a role in caring for this group of aging citizens needs to be as learned as possible in the psychobiology of aging and to help see that patients have as fulfilling a life as their mental and physical status will allow.

REFERENCES

Antunes CMF et al.: Endometrial cancer and estrogen use. *N Engl J. Med* 300:9, 1979.

Butler RN: in *The Aging Reproductive System,* ed. EL Schneider, New York: Raven Press, 1978, pp. 1–8.

Harris L: *The Myth and Reality of Aging in America.* Washington, National Council on Aging, 1975.

Horwitz RI, Feinstein AR: Alternative analytic methods for case-control studies of estrogens and endometrial cancer. *N Engl J Med* 299:1089, 1978.

Lindsay R et al.: Long-term prevention of postmenopausal osteoporosis by oestrogens. *Lancet* 1:1038, 1976.

Mack TM et al.: Estrogens and endometrial carcinoma in a retirement community. *N Engl J Med* 294: 1262, 1976.

Meema S et al.: Preventive effect of estrogen on postmenopausal bone loss. *Arch Intern Med* 135: 1436, 1975.

Rosenberg L et al.: Myocardial infarction and estrogen therapy in postmenopausal women. *N Engl J Med* 294: 1256, 1976.

Siiteri PK, MacDonald PC: Role of extra glandular estrogens in human endocrinology, in *Handbook of Physiology,* Sec. 7, eds. RO Greep, EB Astwood, Baltimore: American Physiology Society, 1973, pp. 615–629.

Smith DC et al.: Association of exogenous estrogens and endometrial carcinoma. *N Engl J Med* 293: 1164, 1975.

Ziel HK, Finkle WD: Increased risk of endometrial carcinoma among users of conjugated estrogens. *N Engl J Med* 293: 1167, 1975.

PART FOUR

Manifestations of Disease

20

Bleeding and Amenorrhea

PAUL G. McDONOUGH

BLEEDING

Genital bleeding patterns which depart from established or preconceived norms are one of the most common health care problems of women. Evaluation requires some knowledge of physiologic bleeding patterns, pathologic aberrations, and the spectrum of causes contributing to menstrual disturbances in different age groups.

PHYSIOLOGIC BLEEDING PATTERNS

Menarche or first menses usually occurs at 13.5 years of age. The mean for the normal ovulatory menstrual interval is 29 ± 2 days. The menstrual interval may range from 21 to 44 days and still be consistent with cyclic ovulation (Ross et al.). The average duration of flow is 5 ± 2 days and is relatively constant for a given individual. Average blood loss at menses is 30 to 100 mL. The average age for cessation of menses is 49 with ranges from 35 to 55 years (Fluhmann).

PATHOLOGIC ABERRATIONS

Departure from these norms for onset, rhythm, quantity, and cessation of menses should be recognized and investigated.

PREMENARCHAL BLEEDING

The appearance of genital bleeding prior to the normal age of onset for menarche is called premenarchal bleeding. One should distinguish between occurrences of bleeding with and without development in this pediatric age group. Sexual development in childhood denotes the premature release of ovarian estrogens, secondary to increases in pituitary gonadotropins and, rarely, to an autonomous estrogen-producing ovarian tumor (McDonough). Premenarchal vaginal bleeding in the absence of sexual development usually has local causes.

Nonspecific vulvovaginitis is caused by a foreign body or pinworm *(Enterobius vermicularis)* and may produce a blood-tinged discharge. Organisms, such as beta-hemolytic streptococcus, *Staphylococcus aureus,* or *E. coli,* may be transferred to the vagina from an upper-respiratory infection, skin lesion, or fecal contamination.

Specific vulvovaginitis caused by *Neisseria gonorrhoeae, Candida albicans, Trichomonas vaginalis,* or herpesvirus type 2 is less frequent, but each may produce a blood discharge, especially herpesvirus type 2 infections.

Prolapsed urethra tends to occur in the 2 through 6 age group. Bright red blood is noticed on the diaper or underpants of the child. The large, protuberant urethra may fill the introitus and resemble a prolapsed cervix.

Sarcoma botryoides (rhabdomyosarcoma) is a rare vaginal malignancy usually occurring under the age of 5 years.

PATHOLOGIC BLEEDING DURING ADOLESCENCE AND REPRODUCTIVE YEARS

Disturbance in Quantity of Menses: Hypermenorrhea and Hypomenorrhea

Etiology of Hypermenorrhea. *Submucous Uterine Myoma.* Menses may appear normal for the first 3 to 5 days of the flow. Just as the menstrual flow seems to be diminishing, it suddenly starts anew with increased quantity.

Blood Dyscrasia. Some patients with primary or secondary thrombocytopenia may be unable to control menstrual "shedding" and they develop hypermenorrhea. Less frequently, sex-linked factor IX deficiency and von Willebrand's disease (vascular hemophilia) also result in hypermenorrhea (Horowitz, O'Leary). Curettement of the uterus should be avoided in blood dyscrasia since there is a high risk of intrauterine infection. Especially with secondary thrombocytopenia, bleeding is better controlled by hormonal therapy.

Endometrial Polyp. Bleeding tends to occur at the conclusion of menses and consists of "trail off spotting." Hysterography or hysteroscopy is sometimes required for proper diagnosis.

Adenomyosis. Whether infiltration of the myometrium with endometrial glands predisposes to hypermenorrhea is still uncertain. A premenopausal female with the clinical triad of hypermenorrhea, dysmenorrhea, and a tender enlarged uterus is common. Hormonal therapy may aggravate pain, although this is not consistent. The pathology specimen reveals increased uterine weight and abundant endometrial glands in the uterine myometrium. Correlation of the clinical and pathologic findings on a physiologic basis is unclear.

IUD. The presence of an intrauterine device will produce cyclic hypermenorrhea in approximately 10 percent of patients.

Corpus Luteum Dysfunction. In some instances hypermenorrhea may result from erratic and prolonged production of progesterone during the luteal phase of the cycle. The true incidence of cyclic hypermenorrhea from this cause is difficult to estimate since diagnosis requires evidence of biphasic BBT (basal body temperature) with persistent temperature elevation during menses, persistent secretory changes in the endometrium 5 days after onset of menses, and fluctuating luteal-progesterone levels which remain elevated during menses. The phenomenon is called "irregular shedding," or perhaps more accurately, erratic progesterone-withdrawal bleeding.

Estrogen-Withdrawal Bleeding. Cyclic ovulatory hypermenorrhea can be closely mimicked by estrogen-withdrawal bleeding. Complete failure of ovulatory LH (luteinizing hormone) will result in estrogen-withdrawal bleeding, which rarely has a rhythmic pattern. Estrogen-withdrawal bleeding is usually painless and associated with a monophasic BBT.

Etiology of Hypomenorrhea. Ovulatory hypomenorrhea is not common; it tends to be associated with oral contraceptives and endometrial sclerosis.

Oral Contraceptives. The combined oral contraceptive produces glandular regression in the endometrium with a decrease in menstrual flow.

Endometrial Sclerosis. The only symptom of endometrial scarring (Asherman's syndrome) following postpartum or postabortal curettage may be cyclic hypomenorrhea. Endometrial sclerosis usually is evidenced by frank amenorrhea, but degrees of scarification of the endometrium may result in cyclic spotting.

Endocrinopathy (Cushing's syndrome). Endocrine disturbances most often produce oligomenorrhea or complete cessation of menses. In certain instances of hypercortisolism, hypomenorrhea may be the only menstrual aberration. Cortisol overproduction, if unaccompanied by adrenal androgen excess, seems to have the least effect on menstrual rhythm.

Disturbance in Rhythm of Menses: Oligomenorrhea and Polymenorrhea

Oligomenorrhea is a decrease in the number of menses per unit of time. The same causes as those for amenorrhea are operative, and the diagnostic workup discussed under amenorrhea is applicable.

Polymenorrhea is an apparent increase in the number of menses per unit of time. Discerning the cause of polymenorrhea is not easy. The use of a basal body temperature chart is an invaluable diagnostic adjunct.

Biphasic Basal Body Temperature (Pseudopolymenorrhea). A biphasic graph enables one to discern menses at each end of the graph. Intermenstrual bleeding is strong evidence of a local lesion within the genital tract. The normal midcycle estrogen drop may occasionally produce physiologic spotting, but it is most important that a careful search of the genital tract be made in all patients for the presence of a chronic inflammatory or neoplastic lesion. Cervical endometriosis may produce intermenstrual bleeding, but such spotting is likely to be postcoital and to occur during the luteal phase of the cycle. Endometrial neoplasia in the form of benign polyps, submucous myomas, or malignancy may be the explanation for erratic bleeding superimposed on an ovulatory cycle. The problem of ovulatory polymenorrhea needs to be approached systematically and may include colposcopy, hysterography, hysteroscopy, and fractional curettage. Endocervical polyps are a relatively frequent cause of polymenorrhea; they can be exposed by inserting a small pediatric Foley catheter into the uterus and partially insufflating the balloon. As the catheter is gradually withdrawn the symmetrical friction of the balloon against the endocervical canal causes covert endocervical polyps to prolapse sufficiently for diagnosis and excision.

Rarely, polymenorrhea with a biphasic temperature graph may be the result of a shortened proliferative phase or premature degeneration of the corpus luteum. No treatment is necessary unless the short menstrual interval is troublesome. Estrogen can be given from cycle days 3 to 10 to prolong the proliferative phase, or progesterone can be given after ovulation to prolong the luteal phase. Oral contraceptives will block ovulation and artificially restore the interval to normal. Clomiphene citrate (Clomid) may be used in this situation.

Monophasic Basal Body Temperature with Polymenorrhea. Frequent bleeding with a monophasic temperature graph usually signifies organic pathology or continuous estrogen production with erratic estrogen-breakthrough bleeding. Pregnancy complications and neoplasia should be a first consideration in menstrual disturbances with indecipherable polymenorrhea. After diagnosis has excluded pregnancy, endometrial biopsy or curettage, depending upon the age group, is usually the best approach to monophasic polymenorrhea. Periodic progestin therapy for 5 to 10 days at 30- to 40-day intervals can be effective, but usually progestin-estrogen combinations are necessary to control estrogen-breakthrough polymenorrhea if curettage is unsuccessful.

PERIMENOPAUSAL BLEEDING

Infrequent or absent ovulation is common in the perimenopausal years. Occasionally there is also some shortening of the cycle interval caused by a shortening of the follicular phase. Consequently, in the transition from ovulatory menses to irregular cycles of the perimenopausal period and finally to amenorrhea, one may see hypermenorrhea, shortened interval, and finally more prolonged intervals with oligomenorrhea and anovulation (Sherman et al.).

POSTMENOPAUSAL BLEEDING

Bleeding in any woman over 45 years of age who has been amenorrheic for one year or longer should be considered postmenopausal. The principal concern in the postmenopausal patient is the possible presence of malignancy. Premalignant and malignant lesions associated with postmenopausal bleeding are adenomatous endometrial hyperplasia, with or without atypia, endometrial carcinoma, and malignancies of the tube, ovary, cervix, vagina, and vulva.

Benign lesions such as cervicitis, cervical and endometrial polyps and submucous myomas may produce bleeding in the postmenopausal female. Atrophic vaginitis is a frequent finding with advanced age and may produce bleeding, especially if associated with trauma. Cytologic studies, cystoscopy, proctoscopy, and fractional curettage should be negative before the bleeding is ascribed to atrophic changes in the vagina.

Exogenous estrogen therapy with breakthrough bleeding is a frequent cause of dysrhythmic postmenopausal bleeding. Patients should receive diagnostic evaluation as outlined below.

APPROACH TO DIAGNOSIS (MANAGEMENT)

Unanticipated genital bleeding creates considerable patient apprehension. The physician with a clear concept of normal menstrual rhythms must decide which bleeding patterns require investigation. The different etiologies of atypical uterine bleeding tend to vary in frequency depending upon the age of the patient. For pedagogic purposes, the causes of abnormal bleeding can be placed under four broad generic headings.

Complications of Pregnancy. Recognition of the possibility that trophoblastic tissue may be present in any site or any form in every patient with atypical bleeding is vital. Cause may be an intrauterine pregnancy, ectopic or molar gestation. Some form of testing for HCG (human chorionic gonadotropin) is a primary consideration.

Benign or Malignant Neoplasia. All processes involving tissue growth, including chronic infections of the cervix, are categorized under this heading.

Blood Dyscrasia. Though rare, this group is designated as a special category and should not be overlooked in diagnosis.

Dysfunctional Uterine Bleeding. Accounting for all other arrhythmic uterine bleeding, dysfunctional bleeding is the result of anovulation or of disturbances in corpus luteum function. It is the most prevalent cause of bleeding abnormalities. This is not surprising when one realizes that the mechanism for cyclic ovulation is so delicately timed that even mild disturbances may interfere with the cycling mechanism. Failure of release of pituitary follicle-stimulating hormone (FSH) and of LH results in sporadic or chronic anovulation. As a consequence of ovulation failure, progesterone is produced, resulting in irregular and unopposed stimulation of the endometrium by estrogen. Erratic estrogen-withdrawal or estrogen-breakthrough bleeding is the result. Anovulatory bleeding episodes tend to be painless; however when estrogen-withdrawal bleeding follows a protracted period of amenorrhea, it can be quite heavy and associated with pain. The sequelae of chronic anovulation are varying degrees of endometrial hyperplasia, infertility, and occasionally anemia.

The relative frequency of the three broad organic causes of bleeding and dysfunctional bleeding vary in different age groups. Consequently, patient care must be individualized along the following guidelines.

BLEEDING DURING CHILDHOOD

In the age group where bleeding occurs but sexual development is absent, visual examination of the vagina and cervix is mandatory. This can be facilitated by use of the Huffman vaginoscope. Material should be collected for bacteriologic and cytologic studies. In difficult cases where local bleeding is a problem, general anesthesia and the use of a direct vision endoscope with recirculating water to distend the vagina provide for maximal visualization (McDonough).

Bleeding accompanied by premature sexual development requires skull x-rays, thyroid studies, and determination of gonadotropin levels in blood or pooled urine. Pelvoabdominal examination is necessary to rule out a rare estrogen-producing ovarian tumor (McDonough).

BLEEDING DURING ADOLESCENCE

Organic disease in adolescence is infrequent, and anovulation is the rule rather than the exception. Today, complications of pregnancy and vaginal adenosis are more frequent in this group than in past years.

Menstrual abnormalities during adolescence usually fall into the categories below.

Mild Abnormalities of Interval and Duration

Slight shortening or lengthening of the menstrual interval is a frequent occurrence, either as the result of anovulation or an ovulation disturbance with a short luteal phase.

Management. In addition to compiling history, physical examination, and cytologic studies for these patients, the physician will do the following:

1. Establish the level of blood loss with a hemoglobin determination.
2. Prepare a menstrual calendar to record the bleeding days. (This is a most useful adjunct, as it helps clarify discrepancies in the menstrual history provided by the adolescent and that provided by her mother.)
3. Review the menstrual calendar every 3 months offering reassurance if needed.
4. In selected instances, with well-motivated patients, a basal body temperature may be taken for one cycle to ascertain the ovulatory or anovulatory nature of the bleeding. Most patients with mild alterations in their menstrual pattern respond to reassurance and the problem resolves with time.

Oligomenorrhea during Adolescence

It is not unusual for the adolescent to experience 3 or 4 months of amenorrhea followed by a normal menstrual flow. Anovulation is frequent in this age group and often is associated with polycystic ovaries. If there is extended amenorrhea or heavy estrogen-withdrawal bleeding, medroxyprogesterone acetate (Provera) or norethindrone acetate (Norlutate), 10 mg, may be prescribed daily for the first 5 days of alternate months. This therapy provides physiologic progesterone withdrawal, then allows a month free of any therapy so these spontaneous menses can occur, marking a return of the normal cyclic mechanism. It is important to stress to these patients that if withdrawal bleeding fails to occur after a progesterone challenge, endogenous estrogen levels may have decreased to the point where evaluation for hypoestrogenism is necessary. A concise evaluation of a failure to bleed following progesterone consists of skull x-ray, thyroid function study, and measurement of serum FSH. Enthusiasm for investigating the failure of progesterone to provoke a withdrawal period should

not cause the physician to overlook the possibility of pregnancy.

Polymenorrhea and Hypermenorrhea during Adolescence

Occasionally, bleeding during adolescence may be of a quantity sufficient to cause anemia. Anovulation is the most frequent cause, but others should not be overlooked, including complications of pregnancy, blood dyscrasia, hypothyroidism, trauma to the genital tract, polycystic ovarian disease, or a uterine intracavitary defect (submucous myoma or endometrial polyp).

Investigation. A complete history and pelvic examination to establish that the bleeding is coming from the uterus will be followed by pregnancy test, triiodothyronine (T_3) and tetraiodothyronine (T_4) tests, and hematologic evaluation to corroborate anemia and rule out blood dyscrasia. The most common blood dyscrasia in adolescents is primary or secondary thrombocytopenia.

Management. Anovulatory bleeding of serious magnitude, associated with a drop in hemoglobin, must be arrested promptly. Progestins are given in large doses initially to accomplish hemostasis, then cyclically for 6 months to produce regular withdrawal bleeding (McDonough). (See Chaps. 7, 42.)

Dilatation and curettage (D&C) is rarely needed in this age group unless the diagnosis is obscure or the bleeding intractable to the point of shock. Hormonal therapy usually brings about complete arrest of bleeding within 24 to 48 hours. Only if the physician feels that he does not have time to allow for this latent period is D&C justified.

BLEEDING DURING REPRODUCTIVE YEARS (AGE 20 TO 35)

The physician's approach to this age group is modified by (1) increased concern that atypical bleeding may be the result of some complication of pregnancy; and (2) concern that with protracted anovulation, varying degrees of endometrial hyperplasia and, rarely, endometrial carcinoma may develop. The latter concern applies principally to the hirsute patient in the fourth decade of life who has a long history of anovulatory bleeding. For these reasons, endometrial biopsy should be used frequently for this age group, especially if the patient does not respond promptly to hormonal therapy. Bleeding during the reproductive years may be approached categorically as that which is responsive to hormonal therapy and that which is intractable and unresponsive to such therapy.

Bleeding Responsive to Hormonal Therapy

The initial approach to the problem of bleeding in the 20 to 35 age group should include the patient's history and a pelvic examination with appropriate cytologic studies. In addition, most patients should have these tests:

1. A vaginal smear taken from the lateral vaginal wall to be evaluated for hormonal effect.
2. Pregnancy testing.
3. T_4, T_3 tests.
4. Endometrial biopsy, especially for anovulatory polymenorrhea, for oligomenorrhea if the vaginal smear is remarkably estrogenic (>40 percent superficial cells), or if there is a suspicion of an incomplete abortion. Patients with biphasic ovulatory polymenorrhea should have a complete fractional curettage, preceded by cytologic studies, colposcopy, and hysteroscopy.
5. Measurement of 17-ketosteroids and serum testosterone if the menstrual abnormality is associated with hirsutism.

Management. Anovulatory bleeding in this age group can usually be controlled by 5-day courses of Provera, 10 mg, or Norlutate, 10 mg daily in alternate months. While the patient is on therapy, it is helpful to follow the pattern of bleeding with a menstrual calendar. If bleeding is not occurring at predictable times after the 5-day courses of progestin, then an estrogen-progestin combination should be given on days 5 through 25.

Bleeding unresponsive to cyclic estrogen-progestin should be treated with Ortho-Novum 10 mg. A proper course of therapy with a gradual step-down of dosage usually extends over a period of 6 to 9 months. If pregnancy is desired in this age group, then inducing ovulation with clomiphene citrate (Clomid) is the treatment of choice if spontaneous ovulation fails to occur.

Bleeding Intractable and Unresponsive to Hormonal Therapy

Occasionally, patients during the reproductive years have protracted polymenorrhea or hypermenorrhea and are unresponsive to estrogen-progestin combinations. These patients require a complete systematic evaluation and inspection of the genital tract so as to rule out any abnormal, surreptitious cause of bleeding. Evaluation consists of (1) hematologic studies to rule out blood dyscrasia; (2) 2-hour postprandial blood sugar and blood urea nitrogen (BUN) to rule out systemic disease; (3) T_4, T_3, TSH (thyroid-stimulating hormone) tests to rule out hypothyroidism; (4) HCG testing to rule out persistent or residual trophoblastic tissue (pregnancy); and (5) admission to the hospital for genital-tract study.

Intractable bleeders with anemia unresponsive to hormonal therapy are studied in the operating room in a four-step sequence consisting of (1) hysteroscopy for careful evaluation of the lower genital tract; (2) a combined pelvic pneumoperitoneum and hysterogram to outline simultaneously the internal-external uterine contour and to rule out unsuspected intracavitary defects and Müllerian abnormalities; (3) laparoscopy to identify any unrecognized pelvic pathology—endometriosis, pelvic inflammatory disease, polycystic ovarian disease, or unrecognized fibroids; and (4) careful fractional D&C with prior iodine staining of the lower genital tract and biopsy of any suspicious areas. Selective biopsy may also be done on the basis of prior colposcopic examination.

Management. Usually this complete surveillance of the genital tract will identify a specific abnormality or provide a basis on which to modify the endocrine therapy. If scant amounts of endometrial tissue exhibiting stroma necrosis, decidual response, and inflammatory cells are obtained, then reepithelialization of the endometrium is indicated. This is accomplished by giving a gradually increasing dose of estrogen over a period of 25 days, followed by a 5-day course of a progestin for three or four cycles of therapy. Clomid therapy may follow the last course of sequential estrogen if resumption of ovulation is desired.

Abundant endometrial tissue at the time of curettement and histologic evidence of hyperplasia are the indications for endometrial neutralization, which can be accomplished with the Ortho-Novum regime. If this is unsuccessful, Depo-Provera intramuscularly, 100 to 200 mg every 2 weeks for 6 months, can be used in selected instances to control intractable bleeding. Megestrol acetate (Megace), 20 mg daily, is an equally effective oral agent for endometrial neutralization. Hysterectomy is a final choice for these patients.

BLEEDING DURING THE PERI- AND POSTMENOPAUSE (AGE 35 OR OLDER)

A careful fractional curettage or judicious endometrial biopsy is mandatory in all patients in this age group.

Bleeding at this time in life may be a cyclic hypermenorrhea or a rhythmic disturbance. It is important to distinguish cyclic hypermenorrhea from anovulatory uterine bleeding. Cyclic hypermenorrhea is associated with normal cycle length and ovulation. The basal body temperature chart is biphasic, and progesterone values remain elevated during the bleeding phase. Curettage is not effective, and these patients are best treated with observation or Norlutate, 10 mg, for cycle days 15 through 25. Cyclic hypermenorrhea unresponsive to D&C and hormonal therapy may require hysterectomy because some of these patients have covert submucous myoma, endometrial polyps, or severe adenomyosis.

Prolongation of the menstrual interval and diminution of the flow are a relatively constant phenomenon in this age group. Attempting to separate physiologic anovulatory perimenopausal bleeding patterns from disorders caused by organic pathology is difficult. Any deviation from an oligorhythmic bleeding sequence requires a careful fractional D&C or judicious endometrial biopsy to rule out malignancy and evaluate undue endometrial proliferation. If endometrial histology is negative for cancer or adenomatous hyperplasia but reveals mild forms of endometrial hyperplasia, the patient can be placed on cyclic therapy with a progestin. After 1 year of therapy, another sampling should be taken to assess the status of the endometrium. If good neutralization is found the endometrium should be observed for 1 year off therapy and be rebiopsied at the end of that year, or if bleeding recurs. Continued hyperplasia should be reassessed by a second fractional D&C with appropriate therapy, usually hysterectomy, instituted on the basis of the findings. There is no reason to procrastinate with bleeding abnormalities in this age group.

AMENORRHEA

A delay in the initiation of menses at the time of puberty or the interruption of an established menstrual pattern constitutes amenorrhea. Failure to initiate menses, interruption of a normal cyclic pattern of menses, or premature cessation of menses all constitute unphysiologic amenorrhea. Arbitrarily dividing menarchal failure and the interruption of a normal cyclic menstrual pattern into primary and secondary amenorrhea is largely semantic since the same etiologic factors may be operative in either instance.

An arbitrary rule stating what constitutes significant pathologic amenorrhea is difficult to establish and has very little use clinically. An interruption of the recycling mechanism due to pregnancy should be diagnosed as soon as possible. A delay of 3 to 6 months in the diagnosis of other causes of amenorrhea does not create any harm or undue anxiety for the patient if the presence of pregnancy has been eliminated. If normal or abnormal trophoblast is suspected in spite of a negative routine pregnancy test, then the more sensitive β subunit HCG determination should be performed.

ETIOLOGY

Amenorrhea which precludes the onset of the first menstrual period tends to have its etiology in genetic causes or anatomical maldevelopments of the genital tract. In contrast, the interruption of an established cyclic pattern of menses is usually psychogenic in origin. The spectrum of pathology seen in association with amenorrhea is varied, but certain well-defined categories are recognizable. These categories can be broadly grouped into eugonadotropic amenorrhea, hypergonadotropic amenorrhea, hypogonadotropic amenorrhea, and amenorrhea occurring in association with androgen excess. The first two groups are more often associated with menarchal delay, the hypogonadotropic group with secondary amenorrhea. Androgen-excess diseases may produce primary or secondary amenorrhea but are more frequent in the latter category.

EUGONADOTROPIC AMENORRHEA

Nonfunctional Uterus

Congenital—Rokitansky Syndrome. The most frequent anatomical cause of primary amenorrhea is the Rokitansky-Kuster-Hauser syndrome (McDonough). Rokitansky syndrome is characterized by hypoplasia and failure of fusion of the two Müllerian anlagen. The bilateral hypoplastic discrete uteri in these individuals are associated with total vaginal agenesis. Ovarian endocrine and exocrine functions are normal. Developmental abnormalities of the kidneys occur frequently, with the most common renal malformation being a solitary ectopic kidney located in the pelvis. The etiology of the Rokitansky syndrome remains obscure. The high frequency of sporadic cases tends to incriminate an autosomal-recessive gene or an environmental factor that affects early development of the mesonephric and paramesonephric system. Rokitansky-syndrome individuals are usually asymptomatic except for menarchal delay and have normal somatic and sexual development. Total absence of the vagina is usually the only physical finding. Cytogenetic studies confirm a normal 46XX karyotype, and a basal body temperature graph is biphasic. The diagnosis of Rokitansky syndrome can usually be made clinically; laparoscopic visualization of the pelvic structures is not a necessity. Extirpation of the rudimentary uterine nubbins is not indicated since these uteri are rarely the site of malignancy, uterine fibroids, covert hematometra, or symptomatic herniation into the inguinal canal. A vagina can be created for these patients by mechanical dilatation or surgery.

Acquired Nonfunctional Uterus. Endometrial sclerosis in the acquired nonfunctional uterus is caused by intrauterine adhesions that partially or completely obliterate the uterine cavity. These adhesions are usually caused by overzealous postpartum curettage or induced abortions complicated by endometritis. Bleeding does not occur after estrogen-progesterone treatment, and the diagnosis is confirmed by hysterography or hysteroscopy. The exact incidence of endometrial sclerosis, or Asherman's syndrome, is not known, but it probably constitutes a small percentage of patients with amenorrhea (Asherman). Tuberculosis may occasionally cause sufficient endometrial scarification to produce target-organ or anatomical amenorrhea. In some instances the destruction of the endometrium produces sclerotic changes without significant distortion of the intracavitary portion of the uterus on hysterosalpingography. Hysteroscopy, in experienced hands, may be necessary for the proper diagnosis. Rarely, nonviable hyalinized or calcific villi may remain in the uterus after a missed abortion and produce anatomical amenorrhea. Pregnancy testing is negative in these patients and endometrial biopsy or curettage is necessary to reveal the abnormality.

Endometrial refractoriness caused by temporary involution of endometrial glands may follow discontinuation of oral contraceptives or after the use of injectable synthetic steroids such as Depo-Provera. This form of amenorrhea is the result of target-organ unresponsiveness and must be distinguished from the hypothalamic pituitary-oversuppression syndrome also produced by oral contraceptives.

Functional Uterus with Obstruction

Among patients with amenorrhea secondary to an obstructed genital tract, those having an imperforate hymen, or a transverse vaginal septum constitute the largest patient category. The vast majority of patients with obstructed genital tract have primary amenorrhea; however, acquired genital-tract obstruction with secondary amenorrhea may occur following a cervical conization or as the result of malignancy.

Patients with imperforate hymen may have normal sexual development, pelvic pain, urinary frequency, and a physician may find a bulging mass on the perineum with Valsalva maneuver.

Transverse vaginal septum, a failure of canalization of the distal third of the vagina with a proximal hematocolpos and hematometra, is not always precisely recognized. Visual inspection of the introitus in transverse vaginal septum reveals no apparent vagina and no change in perineal contour or distension of the introitus with Valsalva maneuver. The Valsalva maneuver is important in distinguishing transverse vaginal septum from imperforate hymen. Transverse vaginal septum is rigid and presents a solid core of uncanalized tissue extending over the last 3 to 5 cm of the lower vagina. The proximal vagina, distended with trapped menstrual blood, is felt high on rectal examination. The treatment of transverse vaginal septum involves surgical dissection of the uncanalized distal vagina, identification of the patent upper vagina, and sufficient mobilization of tissue to bring the upper vagina down to the level of the introitus. The frequent occurrence of transverse vaginal septum in blood relatives suggests a genetic etiology, probably autosomal-recessive inheritance. Renal malformations may accompany transverse vaginal septum but not with the same frequency as in Rokitansky syndrome.

Diagnostic needling of any obstructed genital tract should be performed only prior to definitive surgical correction. Preliminary needling without definitive plans for surgery may convert a proximal hematocolpos into a proximal pyocolpos. Delays in diagnosing amenorrhea caused by genital-tract obstruction will result in continued menstrual reflux. An aseptic inflammation with accompanying endometriosis may impair future fertility.

Patients with eugonadotropic amenorrhea clearly demonstrate the necessity for visual inspection of the introitus and palpation of the cervix in all patients with primary amenorrhea. To rule out endometrial sclerosis or Asherman's syndrome, all eugonadotropic patients with biphasic temperature charts and secondary amenorrhea should have sounding of the uterus and hysterosalpingography or hysteroscopy performed. If hysterography is normal, an endometrial biopsy should accompany these studies in order to rule out instances of protracted missed abortion with residual nonactive trophoblastic tissue. Endometrial tuberculosis is a rare disease, but histologic and fluorescent studies help identify the bacterium.

HYPERGONADOTROPIC AMENORRHEA (PRIMARY OVARIAN FAILURE)

In the past, the majority of patients with ovarian failure were considered to be Turner or quasi-Turner phenotypes with demonstrable sex-chromosome abnormalities. Radioimmunoassay techniques for serum gonadotropins have expanded our vistas and identified increasing numbers of phenotypically and cytogenetically normal 46XX females with amenorrhea and primary ovarian failure (McDonough et al.). Patients with amenorrhea resulting from ovarian failure can be divided on the basis of the cytogenetic findings.

Ovarian Failure with Abnormal Chromosomes

Short stature is the principal clinical finding in individuals with primary ovarian failure and structural deletions of their sex chromosomes. Other somatic anomalies such as webbed neck, shield chest, etc., may or may not accompany the diminished stature. Sex-chromosome karyotypes ranging from 45X to 45X/46XX and 45X/46XY have been described in these individuals. Sex-chromosome mosaicism is the most frequent overall chromosomal abnormality, but 45X remains the principal single-cell line abnormality (McDonough et al.). Privations or deletions of sex-chromosome material tend to be causally related to ovarian failure and short stature. A careful search for a Y-cell line should be made in all Turner or quasi-Turner phenotypes with ovarian failure regardless of the presence or absence of masculinization. Identification of a Y chromosome or XY-cell line in a phenotypic female dictates prophylactic extirpation of the "rudimentary ovaries" or streaks. Perhaps future techniques to identify Y genetic material, such as the immunologic determination of H-Y antigen, may assist in the identification of patients who are at risk for dysgenetic gonadal tumors (Saenger et al.). Because of the scope and limitations of present techniques to identify nonfluorescent, genetically active Y material, physicians must continue to follow all chromosomally abnormal amenorrheic patients closely. Pelvic examination and periodic x-rays of the pelvis will help detect early dysgenetic ridge tumors in patients with an unrecognized Y-cell line. The periodic x-rays in such individuals may also facilitate early detection of calcification, suggesting the presence of a gonadoblastoma (McDonough et al.).

It is not possible among the chromosomally incompetent ovarian-failure patients with menses to draw any correlates between those individuals with primary and secondary amenorrhea with respect to their sex-chromosome morphology. This broad spectrum of ovarian function probably includes degrees of interference with germ-cell migration, mitotic activity in the genital ridge, abnormal meiotic pairing, and overutilization of primary oocytes. The degree of interference with each of these events cannot be specifically measured in its relation to the deletion of sex-chromosome material.

In addition to recognizing hypergonadotropic amenorrhea, the principal responsibilities of the physician to the chromosomally abnormal, short-statured group are to identify associated cardiovascular and renal malformations, to extirpate rudimentary streaks in Y-cell-line patients, and to provide continued surveillance for ridge tumors in all patients by careful periodic examination and roentgen studies of the pelvis.

Ovarian Failure with Normal Chromosomes

Individuals who are phenotypically and cytogenetically normal and have ovarian failure are said to have chromosomally competent ovarian failure. It is conceivable that this group may be a large heterogeneous group, larger than is apparent from the literature with different causes producing the ovarian failure. Patients with normal chromosomal complements, 46XX or 46XY, tend to be tall since epiphyses stay open in the absence of ovarian steroids and the presence of a normal genetic complement. The normal chromosomal karyotype ensures normal stature, which is further augmented by delayed epiphyseal fusion resulting from primary ovarian failure. In order to establish the diagnosis of chromosomally competent ovarian failure, one must measure serum FSH in every hypoestrogenic female having either primary or secondary amenorrhea. An elevated serum FSH on two consecutive determinations is diagnostic of primary ovarian failure. A buccal smear should be performed as a minimum to distinguish the cytogenetically normal 46XX and the less-frequent 46XY forms of gonadal failure.

46XY Forms. *Swyer's Syndrome (XY Gonadal Dysgenesis).* Gonadal failure with XY karyotypes is infrequent but important to mention because of the high risk of dysgenetic ridge tumor and the diagnostic confusion with forms of androgen-insensitivity syndromes. XY ovarian failure seems to be inherited as a sex-linked gene. Individuals with XY forms of gonadal dysgenesis should have prophylactic extirpation of the rudimentary streaks because of the high frequency of tumor formation. The palpation of a cervix or Müllerian system, sexual infantilism, and low-normal serum testosterone levels differentiate XY gonadal dysgenesis (Swyer's syndrome) from testicular feminizing syndrome (Espiner et al.).

Congenital Androgen-insensitivity Syndrome. Patients with congenital androgen-insensitivity syndrome (testicular feminizing syndrome) have only slight elevations in serum LH and are gonadal males. Testicular tissue in these individuals is active in suppressing Müllerian development. In spite of adequate androgen production, cytosol receptors for testosterone are defective and a hairless phenotype is present. Both XY gonadal dysgenesis and XY androgen-insensitivity syndrome probably represent a spectrum of male pseudohermaphroditism. They both require removal of the gonads.

46XX Forms. The etiology of ovarian failure in phenotypically normal 46XX individuals may be diverse. Familial instances do occur, but a heterogeneous group of causes is probably present in the sporadic cases (McDonough).

Multiple affected siblings, the frequency of consanguinity, associated neuroauditory abnormalities, and XX cells in gonadal culture indicate that some XX forms of ovarian failure are distinct genetic entities and are probably related to a single autosomal-recessive gene (ibid.). The report of identical twins discordant for ovarian failure suggests that environmental factors may be operative in some instances (McDonough et al.). These environmental factors could occur in utero or could represent an environmental insult occurring later in neonatal life or early infancy. Environmental factors could prevent migration, interfere with early mitotic activity in the gonadal ridge, disrupt meiotic pairing, or destroy the follicular apparatus of the fully developed ovary. The precise contribution of environmental factors, such as infection or teratogens, will only be ascertained after careful historical scrutiny of all sporadic cases of ovarian failure. In a few instances, autosomal chromosomal aberrations have been identified in individuals with ovarian failure. Most of these aberrations have been normal variants of chromosomal morphology that are not related to the gonadal problem. The modifying role of autosomal variants or abnormalities in females having normal sex chromosomes and ovarian failure is still speculative. Rarely, systemic diseases such as β thalassemia and mucopolysaccharidosis may provide enough infiltration to the

ovary to produce ovarian failure. Autoimmune ovarian failure is difficult to document but should be a consideration when ovarian failure occurs in association with a multiple endocrinopathy. A small number of patients with functional ovarian failure will exhibit large numbers of primordial follicles on ovarian biopsy. This group of patients, thought to have an ovarian cell-membrane receptor defect, have been described literally in the expression "ovarian insensitivity syndrome" or "Savage syndrome" after the original case study (Koninchx, Brosens). The receptor defect, if present, does not seem to be an all-or-none phenomenon to judge from the amount of breast development described in some patients with Savage syndrome. Further studies may help to elucidate the nature of the abnormality and to establish whether the gonadotropin-resistant ovary is a unique form of ovarian failure.

A rare cause of hypergonadotropism is a deficiency in 17-hydroxylation, which prohibits the production of androgens, estrogens, and some adrenal steroids. Patients with this deficiency have increased levels of desoxycorticosterone and progesterone as a consequence of the enzymatic block in steroidogenesis. The absence of estrogens in the periphery results in hypergonadotropism.

Amenorrhea caused by ovarian failure in individuals with normal sex chromosomes is basically a functional or biochemical diagnosis. Serum gonadotropin measurements should always precede ovarian visualization and biopsy. One should not place undue reliance on ovarian morphology and histology. The morphology of ovarian hypodevelopment is varied; even to the experienced eye, the ovaries may resemble those seen in hypogonadotropic hypogonadism. A functional diagnosis of hypergonadotropism is a better index to the disturbance level than are subjective interpretations of ovarian morphology and histology.

HYPOGONADOTROPIC AMENORRHEA

The third category of patients with amenorrhea includes patients with low or undetectable base-line gonadotropins. Low levels of pituitary gonadotropins are seen in the prepubertal child, but once hypothalamic maturity has occurred, low or absent gonadotropins are unphysiologic. In some patients, hypothalamic pituitary maturity is never achieved and an irreversible form of hypogonadotropism persists. Other patients with hypogonadotropism are initially normal but develop acquired hypogonadotropism as a result of diverse etiologies. Included in the latter category are patients with low base-line FSH and LH and some patients with hypothalamic pituitary dysfunction who have low serum FSH and tonically elevated serum LH.

Congenital Hypogonadotropism (Kallmann's Syndrome)

Irreversible or monotropic failure of gonadotropins is referred to as Kallmann's syndrome or isolated gonadotropin deficiency (IGD). These patients are unable to effectively synthesize gonadotropins, presumably because of a defect in the hypothalamus. They may have associated olfactory-sensory defects. The nature and extent of the olfactory defects are determined to a considerable degree by the working definition of anosmia, since the spectrum of normal odor detection varies considerably from one expert to another. It is more important for diagnostic purposes to focus on the persistently low gonadotropin levels. Single-dose gonadotropin releasing factor (GnRF) challenge in such patients usually results in no gonadotropin release. In some patients with Kallmann's syndrome, repeated challenges or constant infusions of GnRF may result in a blunted gonadotropin response (Boyer et al.). The abbreviated response to GnRF stimulation, noted especially in pooled urinary gonadotropins, is sufficient to continue the argument over whether the defect is hypothalamic or pituitary in origin (Kulin, Santner). Perhaps further studies of dynamic hypothalamic pituitary function will delineate the anatomical area of dysfunction. Other genetic syndromes, such as Prader-Willi and Laurence-Moon-Biedl, are associated with irreversible hypogonadotropism but are exceedingly rare, and other aspects of each syndrome, principally mental retardation, supersede the hypogonadotropism in importance.

Acquired Hypogonadotropism

Pituitary Tumors and Pituitary Necrosis. Central nervous system lesions associated with acquired hypogonadotropism are most frequently pituitary and/or parapituitary tumors. Galactorrhea may be seen in association with amenorrhea in some of these patients. Pituitary tumors are important to recognize because they pose a threat to the life of the patient, and prognosis is directly related to the time of diagnosis. The most common pituitary tumor which produces amenorrhea in the younger age group is the craniopharyngioma which may grow rapidly into the suprasellar area. Fortunately, most craniopharyngiomas calcify and are usually apparent on routine x-rays of the sella turcica. The rapid growth of this tumor makes periodic

skull x-rays imperative in all patients with menarchal delay or brief menstrual histories. Other pituitary tumors, such as chromophobe adenomas and prolactin-producing adenomas, tend to grow slowly over a longer period of time. Amenorrhea or amenorrhea with galactorrhea may antedate the neurological symptoms by many years. Radiologic views of the sella turcica and serum prolactin are important diagnostic adjuncts in the follow-up of all patients with persistent hypogonadotropism. Hypogonadotropism accompanied by hyperprolactinemia is an indication that further studies of the central nervous system, including polytomography of the sella turcica, visual fields, and computerized axial tomography are required.

Persistent hypogonadotropic hyperprolactinemia may also occur in association with growth-hormone- and ACTH-producing pituitary tumors. Careful physical examination is necessary in all amenorrheic patients to detect signs of growth-hormone or cortisol excess. Growth-hormone levels can be measured in the morning, before and after 30 minutes of exercise. High basal levels of growth hormone and paradoxical responses to stimulation and suppression studies should prompt further radiologic evaluation of the central nervous system. ACTH-dependent adrenal hyperplasia can be screened utilizing morning plasma-cortisol levels before and after evening suppression with 1 mg of dexamethasone. High morning levels or poor suppression with dexamethasone indicates the need for getting further daytime blood levels and free urinary cortisol levels. Hyperpituitarism caused by growth hormone and ACTH production is rare, but early recognition is important. Morning sampling for growth-hormone and cortisol levels is beset with limitations but serves as an important screening technique in the evaluation of persistent hypogonadotropic amenorrhea.

Radiologic enlargement of the sella turcica in association with hypogonadotropism may also occur in patients with empty sella syndrome, carotid artery aneurysms, and primary hypothyroidism. Secondary enlargement of the pituitary may develop in primary hypothyroidism, presumably as a compensatory mechanism. The measurement of TSH is important in differentiating sellar enlargement due to primary hypothyroidism from a true intrasellar tumor since the former responds readily to thyroid-replacement therapy (Keye et al.).

Postpartum ischemic infarction and necrosis of the pituitary can occur in association with obstetric shock syndromes. This hypogonadotropic amenorrhea usually has varying degrees of insufficiency of other pituitary tropic hormones, manifested clinically by lactation failure, genital atrophy, hair loss, hypotension, hypoglycemia, and anemia. Undetectable serum gonadotropins, low T_4, TSH, and low plasma-cortisol levels corroborate the clinical diagnosis of hypopituitarism caused by Sheehan's syndrome.

Drug-Induced Amenorrhea. Various drugs can induce amenorrhea by virtue of their effect on the hypothalamus, or by weight loss through anorexia. Phenothiazine derivatives, reserpine, and ganglionic blocking agents affect the hypothalamus and produce amenorrhea, sometimes with galactorrhea. These effects are usually reversible once the drug is discontinued. Other drugs, such as alcohol, digitalis preparations, cytotoxic drugs, and certain antibiotics, may produce amenorrhea through their anorectic effect.

The second large category of drug-related amenorrhea encompasses oversuppression syndromes following the use of oral or parenteral synthetic steroids. Fewer than 1 percent of women taking oral contraceptives develop amenorrhea during or after taking the pill, regardless of the length of time it was taken. In this 1 percent, the hypothalamic pituitary axis is suppressed by the exogenous steroids and remains so after the medication is discontinued. This condition of oversuppression may persist for prolonged periods of time. It is important to distinguish postpill amenorrhea from that caused by endometrial involution. In the latter, endogenous estrogen levels are normal but the endometrium is unresponsive because of the glandular regression induced by the synthetic steroid. Postpill target-organ amenorrhea usually has a good prognosis with spontaneous cure. In postpill amenorrhea resulting from hypothalamic pituitary oversuppression, most patients have spontaneous recovery of menstrual function within several months. In others, ovulation or pregnancy can be induced by ovulation-inducing drugs.

Psychogenic Amenorrhea. It is universally accepted that stress factors may produce amenorrhea. Nevertheless, the precise biochemical intermediaries involved in mood changes and gonadotropin production are unknown. The anatomic areas within the limbic system and hypothalamus that affect emotional expression are the same areas that contain steroid receptors and some enzymes involved in steroid metabolism.

Psychogenic amenorrhea may occur in association with acute or chronic emotional stress. It may also have a strong nutritional component related either to weight loss or weight gain. Neuroendocrine aberrations resulting from stress may produce temporary or prolonged disturbances in gonadotropin and prolactin production. Disturbances producing psychogenic amenorrhea tend to fall into four basic patterns.

Stress-Induced Tonic LH (Short Term). Temporary interruption of the recycling mechanism may occur as a result of sudden psychic stress. Cyclic LH is replaced by stress-induced continuous LH production. In most instances, failure of the recycling mechanism is brief in duration and there is prompt recovery after 1 or 2 months.

Stress-Induced Tonic LH (Long Term). If stress factors persist, long-term tonic LH stimulation will produce a clinical picture not unlike polycystic ovarian disease. Amenorrhea will persist and the patient may note mild facial hirsutism with acne. Continued pulsatile LH production will increase ovarian production of Δ^4-androstenedione, testosterone, and estrogen. Vaginal hormonal cytology will reveal many superficial cells; bleeding will still occur after use of progestation agents. Hyperprolactinemia in some patients with persistent LH elevations suggests a pseudocyesis-type syndrome.

Stress-Induced Hypogonadotropism. Eventually psychic stress may induce loss of both cyclic LH and tonic LH release from the pituitary, resulting in low base-line levels of FSH and LH. Acquired hypogonadotropism of this type also may occur as the result of nutritional factors, especially weight loss with or without significant psychopathology.

Anorexia may be a symptom of any systemic disease or may be the result of drugs and medications. The weight loss which occurs secondary to the anorexia may produce low-gonadotropin amenorrhea. Anorexia in the absence of illness or drug therapy is usually psychogenic in origin, and is usually seen before a patient is 25 years of age. Anorectic individuals have lost at least 25 percent of their original body weight and exhibit a distorted attitude toward eating and weight gain that overrides all hunger. They take pleasure in refusing food and losing weight, are hyperkinetic with overactivity, and have an inappropriate perception of body image. Physical examination may reveal light lanugo hair growth, especially over the back and malar eminences. Bradycardia and low body temperature are present.

Gonadotropin profiles in severe weight-loss amenorrhea reveal low LH values and low or normal FSH in serum. There is a failure of pulsatile LH output especially during sleep, and a delayed LH response to gonadotropin-releasing hormone stimulation. The ACTH adrenal axis is altered similarly by decreased pulsatile ACTH and some loss of diurnal variation in plasma-cortisol levels. The metabolic clearance rate for cortisol is reduced, apparently in some attempt at internal homeostasis. Elevated serum levels of growth hormone are seen in some of the patients with this anorexia or "Twiggy syndrome." Other findings which have been described are hypercholesterolemia, carotenemia, hypoglycemia, low serum T_3 levels, and increased catechol estrogens (Warren, Vande Wiele; Fisherman). The increased formation of catechol estrogens in these patients is important since they may compete for estrogen-binding sites centrally and inhibit the biological inactivation of catecholamines. Prolongation of catecholamine activity could provide for continued stimulation of dopamine receptors and explain some of the aspects of the anorexia syndrome.

Even in apparent postpill amenorrhea, the roles of weight loss and psychological factors should receive serious consideration. Women of low body weight may be at particular risk for developing postpill amenorrhea.

Stress-Induced Hypogonadotropic Hyperprolactinemia. Some individuals with stress-acquired hypogonadotropism have elevated levels of serum prolactin. The hyperprolactinemia may precede or follow the hypogonadotropism. Pituitary tumors should be the first suspect in hyperprolactinemic patients, although stress-related neuroendocrine dysfunction may produce a comparable pituitary profile (Zacur et al.). Time and further study should help delineate the true frequency of stress-induced hyperprolactinemia with amenorrhea.

Psychogenic amenorrhea may be associated with elevated LH levels and low FSH; with low LH and normal or slightly elevated FSH; and with low-gonadotropin–high-prolactin profiles. These patterns are usually seen in different patients, but a single individual may pass sequentially through any two or three of the patterns.

Systemic Illness—Endocrine (Thyroid or Adrenal Hyper- or Hypofunction). Amenorrhea may occur as a result of a systemic endocrinopathy involving some extragonadal endocrine gland. Abnormalities in thyroid function, either hyper- or hypothyroidism, may produce amenorrhea. Adrenal cortisol overproduction and underproduction may interfere with normal cyclic gonadotropin production and produce amenorrhea. Thyroid evaluation is an essential part of the diagnostic workup of amenorrhea, but plasma-

cortisol values are indicated when the clinical picture, including blood pressure and blood sugar, suggest cortisol overproduction.

Systemic Illness—Nonendocrine. The precise role of systemic illness in the etiology of amenorrhea is not always easy to decipher. Generalized systemic illnesses involving poor nutrition, malabsorption syndromes, cardiac disease, renal disease, severe infection, or neoplasia may produce amenorrhea. It is difficult to determine whether the amenorrhea is directly related to the illness or is caused by psychogenic factors, weight loss, or drug therapy. In most systemic disease there is anorexia which may be largely responsible for the hypogonadotropism. The endocrine abnormalities seen in anorexia nervosa usually cannot be distinguished from those in starvation due to other causes. Amenorrhea should not be attributed to any systemic illness until other causes have been eliminated.

Amenorrhea and Galactorrhea. Amenorrhea and galactorrhea are cardinal symptoms in several syndromes—Chiari-Frommel, Ahumada-DelCastillo, and Forbes-Albright syndromes. Although these eponyms have been in common usage, they serve very little purpose now, and most of them can be collectively categorized as amenorrhea-galactorrhea syndromes. The development of a sensitive, specific radioimmunoassay for serum prolactin has aided in the identification of patients with amenorrhea-galactorrhea syndromes who may have prolactin-producing pituitary tumors. All patients with elevations in serum prolactin, regardless of the presence or absence of galactorrhea, should be identified and evaluated for pituitary tumors.

ANDROGEN EXCESS

The last category of patients with amenorrhea is the group with androgen overproduction, adrenal or ovarian in origin. Adrenal androgen overproduction may result from a virilizing adrenal tumor or congenital adrenal hyperplasia. Virilizing ovarian tumors are rare. The principal cause of ovarian androgen overproduction is the androgenic ovary syndrome. Patients with polycystic ovaries are an etiologically complex and clinically heterogeneous group. Patients with polycystic ovary syndrome usually have normal thelarche. Pubarche is excessive and is followed by sequential growth of hair on the upper lip, chin, intermammary area, and extremities. Serum LH levels are tonically elevated with normal or slight elevations of serum testosterone and urinary 17-

ketosteroids. The vaginal smears are remarkably estrogenic with 25 to 40 percent superficial cells. Presumably, this group of hirsute patients with amenorrhea has a constant tonic "leak" of LH which stimulates ovarian production of the weak androgen Δ^4-androstenedione and produces morphologic polycystic ovaries. Increased blood production rates for testosterone and estrone follow as a result of the increasing formation of the prehormone Δ^4-androstenedione. Increased testosterone production results in hirsutism, and the increased rates of blood production for estrone provide for a well-estrogenized genital tract. Evaluation of patients who have androgen overproduction involves principally the measurement of 17-ketosteroids in urine, serum testosterone, and serum LH (Yen, Vela). In a small number of patients with elevated 17-ketosteroids, urinary pregnanetriol values are indicated to rule out "late onset" or "late diagnosed" congenital adrenal hyperplasia (McDonough).

APPROACH TO DIAGNOSIS (MANAGEMENT)

GENERAL

History

Historical factors are of paramount concern in evaluating the patient with amenorrhea. Drugs the patient has taken, including oral contraceptives, as well as evidence of psychic stress, must receive primary consideration. Marked changes in body weight should receive careful attention. Psychosocial history should focus on the months preceding the development of amenorrhea.

Physical Examination

Most patients with amenorrhea have a normal physical appearance. Any signs of (1) androgen overproduction, (2) cortisol overproduction, (3) galactorrhea, (4) hypothyroidism, (5) acromegaly, (6) weight loss and/or weight gain, (7) short stature (with or without associated somatic anomalies), and (8) sexual infantilism should be carefully investigated.

Evaluation of Endogenous Estrogen

Pivotal in the diagnosis of all amenorrheas is the evaluation of the patient's endogenous estrogen. The vaginal smear, cervical mucus, or endometrium can be used in a bioassay of the patient's estrogen. Of these bioassays, the vaginal smear is probably the most

sensitive index since it exhibits a relatively linear response to increases in endogenous estrogen. Measuring estrogen quantity by endometrial histology is difficult and endocervical mucus may be limited because of the frequent occurrence of endocervicitis. A progesterone-challenge test is the most frequently used clinical bioassay of endogenous estrogen, but it is important to understand the scope and limitations of this test. The progesterone challenge must be performed with a "pure or C21" progestin such as progesterone in oil or Provera. The 19-norsteroid compounds are not reagent-pure and may have some intrinsic estrogenic contamination, either in their preparation or metabolism. The response to 10 mg of Provera daily for 5 days or 100 mg of progesterone in oil is a suitable test, but this must be carefully scrutinized to make certain that the withdrawal menses is of sufficient quantity and time span to suggest adequate endogenous estrogen levels. Patients with relatively poor endogenous estrogen may occasionally manifest a positive but limited response to a progesterone challenge. Conclusions about endogenous estrogen on the basis of progesterone withdrawal must be guarded in limited-response situations. Target-organ failures are best evaluated by prolonged high-dose estrogen challenges. Endometrial sclerosis must ultimately be diagnosed by hysterography or hysteroscopy. Failure to bleed following estrogen priming does not always indicate the presence of target-organ disease. Long-term hypoestrogenic patients may have a refractory endometrium requiring considerable estrogen priming before displaying a positive response. This is especially true in the weight loss–hypoestrogenic amenorrheas. Overproduction of catechol estrogens in these patients may have an antiuterotropic effect.

The measurement of peripheral estrogenic steroids has very little practical role in ascertaining quantity of endogenous estrogen. The intermediary metabolism of estrogens is extremely complex. Interpreting a single blood level of a specific estrogen is difficult and of limited value in patient management. Normal or low estrogen values are difficult to interpret, but unusually high serum values for total estrogen or estradiol may be helpful in detecting an estrogen-producing ovarian tumor. A peripheral bioassay such as the vaginal smear or progesterone-challenge test will better serve the clinician. In certain situations, indirect quantitation of peripheral estrogen can be obtained by measuring the appropriate feedback hormones, serum FSH in particular. In a few patients the target-organ effects of estrogen may be normal but serum FSH levels markedly elevated with hypergonadotropism. These patients are categorized as having euestrogenic forms of ovarian failure (Falk). Their cases emphasize the differential sensitivity of target tissues, including the hypothalamus, to estrogen. Differences in target-organ sensitivity and the limitations of chemical estrogen assays show the need to measure serum FSH where hypoestrogenism is suspected.

SPECIFIC

Once pregnancy has been excluded, amenorrheic patients can be divided prognostically into normal and low estrogen groups. The prognosis for spontaneous cure is good in the normal group and guarded in the hypoestrogenic category. The sequential workup of each group is designed to uncover the most frequent and serious etiologies associated with normal or low estrogen production. Etiologic overlap occurs frequently since temporary euestrogenism is a transitional stage for severe forms of hyper- and hypogonadotropism.

Low Estrogen Group

Patients with low endogenous estrogen must be evaluated for central nervous system disease or hypergonadotropic forms of ovarian failure. Initial evaluation includes skull x-rays, T_4, T_3, and serum gonadotropins. Plasma-cortisol levels are obtained if the clinical phenotype suggests cortisol overproduction or if blood pressure or blood sugar is elevated. If serum gonadotropins indicate hypergonadotropism, then cytogenetic studies should be performed on all patients, especially individuals below 63 inches in height (McDonough; McDonough et al.). If serum gonadotropins are low, the physician should pause temporarily in the diagnostic workup and intensify the psychosocial and nutritional history. The frequency of psychogenic amenorrhea warrants this expense of time before further sophisticated endocrine and central nervous system evaluation are undertaken. The majority of patients with acquired monotropic failure of gonadotropins will be found to have psychogenic or weight-loss amenorrhea. If hypogonadotropism persists, then serum prolactin levels must be obtained to identify the "silent hyperprolactinemic" individuals who are at risk for prolactin-producing pituitary tumors. The measurement of 17-ketosteroids in urine may be indicated in rare patients with hypogonadotropism in order to identify androgen overproduction in the absence of hirsutism. The latter may occasionally be important in the diagnosis of rare

adrenal tumors when clinical evidence of androgen overproduction is limited. If hypogonadotropic hyperprolactinemia persists, levels of growth hormone at rest and after 30 minutes of exercise should be obtained. Further endocrine evaluation should be combined with visual field studies and polytomography of the sella turcica. The combination of tomographic findings, persistent low gonadotropins, elevated serum prolactin, and blunted growth hormone–ACTH responses to hypoglycemic testing suggest a central nervous system lesion. Decisions concerning further invasive studies of the central nervous system will be based on this information for each patient, as well as on the clinical course of the patient's illness.

Normal Estrogen Group

The majority of patients with normal endogenous estrogen experience temporary interruptions of the recycling mechanism with tonic elevated LH. In some instances the tonic LH elevation may be protected with androgen overproduction on the part of the ovary. Although endogenous estrogen levels in this group are normal, some screening of the central nervous system with sellar x-rays should be performed in order to eliminate patients who may have early pituitary tumors. Evaluation for hypothyroidism is still necessary since hypothyroid patients may be euestrogenic. Plasma-cortisol levels are performed if clinical evidence of hypercortisolism is present. Interference with ovarian estrogen production may be a late finding in some cortisol-excess diseases. If skull x-rays and thyroid evaluation are normal, a pause in the evaluation is justified while a pure progestin or C21-compound is administered on a cyclic basis. A synthetic progestin such as Provera can be administered, 10 mg daily, for the first 5 days of every other month over a 6-month time span. Withdrawal menses following the administration of alternate-month Provera serves to relieve anxiety, confirms that endogenous estrogen is adequate, and indicates a patent responsive genital tract. Alternate months during which no Provera is given allow spontaneous menses to occur. The majority of patients with temporary interruption of the recycling mechanism experience spontaneous menses during or following the alternating 6-month trial of a pure progestin.

If there is clinical evidence of androgen overproduction, then tests for serum LH, serum testosterone, and 17-ketosteroids should be requested. In some patients with androgen overproduction, the vaginal smear is unusually good, exhibiting more than 40 percent superficial cells. Endometrial biopsy should be performed to rule out undue degrees of endometrial hyperplasia. Endometrial biopsy and uterine sounding are also indicated in those patients who have a good vaginal smear but do not bleed after a progesterone challenge. These are the patients who may have acquired forms of endometrial sclerosis (Asherman's syndrome) or a missed abortion with residual hyalinized villi.

Interruption of the normal menstrual rhythm with resulting arrhythmic bleeding or amenorrhea is a ubiquitous problem. Clearly definable causes are not apparent in all patients. The diagnostic approach should involve a constant vigilance for pregnancy and its complications, for malignant neoplasia, pituitary tumors, and obstructed genital tract pathology. The search for serious pathology should be tempered by an awareness of the role of psychosocial and nutritional factors in temporary or protracted interruptions of the recycling mechanism. Continued studies in the area of neuroendocrinology may help clarify the physiopathology of dysfunctional bleeding and psychogenic amenorrhea.

REFERENCES

Asherman JD: Amenorrhea traumatica (atretica). *J Obstet Gynec Br Commons* 55:23, 1948.

Boyar RM et al.: Clinical and laboratory heterogeneity in idiopathic hypogonadotropic hypogonadism.

Espiner EA et al.: Familial syndrome of streak gonads and normal male karyotypes in five phenotypic females.

Falk RJ: Euestrogenic ovarian failure. *Fertil Steril* 28:502, 1977.

Fishman J et al.: Influence of body weight on estradiol metabolism in young women. *J Clin Endocrinol Metab* 41:989, 1975.

Fluhmann CF (ed): *The Management of Menstrual Disorders,* Philadelphia: Saunders, 1956.

Horowitz HE, O'Leary D: Von Willebrand's disease. A critical evaluation of diagnostic criteria. *NY State Med* 65:2236, 1965.

Keye, WR et al.: Amenorrhea, hyperprolactinemia and pituitary enlargement secondary to primary hypothyroidism. *Obstet Gynec* 48:697, 1976.

Koninchx R, Brosens IA: The "gonadotropin resistant ovary" syndrome as a cause of secondary amenorrhea and infertility. *Fertil Steril* 28:926, 1977.

Kulin HE, Santner SJ: Timed urinary gonadotropin measurements in normal infants, children and in patients with disorders of sexual maturation. *J Pediatr* 90:760, 1977.

Marshall WA, Turner JM: Variations in pattern of pubertal changes in girls. *Arch Dis Child* 44:291, 1969.

McDonough PG: Dysfunctional uterine bleeding, in *Current Therapy,* ed HF Conn, Philadelphia: Saunders, 1977, p. 851.

_____: Menarchal delay, in *Current Problems in Obstetrics and Gynecology,* vol, no 1, ed. RW Kistner, Chicago: Year Book, 1977.

_____: Primary ovarian failure, in *Endocrine Causes of Menstrual Disorders,* ed. J Givens, Chicago: Year Book (in press).

_____: Sexual precocity. *Clin Obstet Gynec* 14:1037, 1971.

_____ et al.: Gonadoblastoma (gonocytoma III): Report of a case. *Obstet Gynec* 29:43, 1967.

_____ et al.: Phenotypic and cytogenetic findings in 82 patients with primary ovarian failure—changing trends. *Fertil Steril* 28:638, 1977.

_____ et al.: Twins discordant for 46,XX gonadal dysgenesis. *Fertil Steril* 28:251, 1977.

Ross GT et al.: Pituitary and gonadal hormones in women during spontaneous and induced ovulatory cycles. *Rec Prog Horm Res* 26:1, 1970.

Saenger P et al.: Presence of H-Y antigen and testis in 46,XX true hermaphroditism, evidence for Y chromosomal function. *J Clin Endocrinol Metab* 43:1234, 1976.

Sherman BM et al.: The menopausal transition: Analysis of LH, FSH, estradiol, and progesterone concentrations during menstrual cycles of older women. *J Clin Endocrinol Metab* 42:639, 1976.

Warren MP, Vande Wiele RL: Clinical and metabolic features of anorexia nervosa. *Am J Obstet Gynec* 117:435, 1973.

Yen SCC, Vela P: Inappropriate secretion of FSH and LH in polycystic ovarian disease. *J Clin Endocrinol Metab* 30:435, 1970.

Zacur H et al.: Galactorrhea-amenorrhea: Psychological interaction with neuroendocrine function. *Am J Obstet Gynec* 125:850, 1976.

21

Shock

DENIS CAVANAGH   MANUEL R. COMAS

Every gynecologist-obstetrician must be familiar with the early signs and the correct management of shock. Because of failures in the recognition and treatment of this condition, many women die every year. In addition to the toll in avoidable maternal deaths in obstetrics, shock accounts for a large number of deaths among gynecologic patients. It is also worthy of note that some of the most serious complications of pregnancy such as Sheehan's syndrome, bilateral renal cortical necrosis, and acute tubular necrosis are associated with this process. The early diagnosis and the proper management of the patient in shock requires an understanding of the basic concepts of the syndrome. We will attempt to cover these aspects of shock in this chapter.

GENERAL CONSIDERATIONS

DEFINITION

Shock is a condition in which there is a disparity between the circulating blood volume and the capacity of the vascular bed. This results in hypotension and, more important, in reduced tissue perfusion of vital organs with cellular hypoxia. If uncorrected, this condition will lead to a progressive failure of cellular metabolism and eventually to vital organ damage and death. In this definition it will be noted that the emphasis is placed on the failure of tissue perfusion, rather than on the rise in heart rate and the fall in blood pressure which usually accompany it.

INCIDENCE

The exact incidence of shock in gynecologic and obstetric patients is unknown. It has a variable though not infrequent occurrence. In some complications, such as rupture of the uterus, shock is almost always present, whereas it complicates only 2.5 to 6.4 percent of cases of septic abortion (Douglas and Bechman).

The presence of shock will complicate any underlying disease process, causing physiologic disturbances and increasing the threat to the life of the patient. In the pregnant woman the living fetus is additionally at risk, for maintenance of adequate placental perfusion is essential to fetal health.

ETIOLOGY AND CLASSIFICATION

Shock may arise from any one of multiple causes. Hypovolemia secondary to hemorrhage or dehydration is the most common cause. Shock may also be due to infection, cardiac failure, hypersensitivity (anaphylactic or allergic), neurogenic disturbances, or blood flow impedance.

There are many classifications of shock. The classification in Table 21–1 has advantages for the physician providing for the health care of women. It is based on the initiating hemodynamic event and includes complications seen in gynecologic and obstetric patients. While the classification is convenient as a general guide, some overlap occurs. Note that the conditions given in the table may operate independently or in combination.

TABLE 21–1 Classification of Shock States in Obstetrics and Gynecology*

I Hypovolemic shock
   A Hemorrhagic shock: associated with postpartum or postabortal hemorrhage, ectopic pregnancy, placenta previa, abruptio placentae, rupture of the uterus, dysfunctional uterine bleeding, benign and malignant uterine neoplasms, rupture of ovarian neoplasms, and obstetric and gynecologic surgery
   B Fluid loss shock: excessive vomiting, diarrhea, diuresis, or too-rapid removal of ascitic fluid
   C Supine hypotensive syndrome: compression of inferior vena cava by pregnant uterus
   D Shock associated with disseminated intravascular coagulation: intrauterine dead fetus syndrome and amniotic fluid infusion
II Septic shock (endotoxic shock): associated typically with infected abortion, chorioamnionitis, pyelonephritis, and postpartum endometritis; may be hypovolemic; has cardiogenic component
III Cardiogenic shock
   A Failure of left ventricular ejection
      1 Cardiac arrest (asystole or ventricular fibrillation)
      2 Myocardial infarction
   B Failure of left ventricular filling
      1 Cardiac tamponade: associated with coagulation defects
      2 Pulmonary embolism: associated with infusion of air or fat, or with thrombophlebitis associated with pregnancy, use of hormones, extensive pelvic surgery, or sickle-cell disease
IV Neurogenic shock
   A Chemical injury: associated with aspiration of gastrointestinal contents
   B Drug-induced: associated with spinal anesthesia
   C Inversion of uterus with vasomotor collapse
   D Electrolyte imbalance: associated with hyponatremia from any cause

*When a pregnant woman is in shock, the fetus is also in shock.

HEMODYNAMIC CHANGES IN NORMAL PREGNANCY

Pregnancy causes profound alterations in the circulatory system. Some of these changes seem to promote the development of shock, while others have definite protective implications.

Most hemodynamic changes of pregnancy appear to be due to the presence of a modified arteriovenous shunt at the placental site and obstruction to venous return by the gravid uterus. In normal pregnancy the systolic blood pressure is generally reduced, and the diastolic pressure is invariably lower. The pulse rate is elevated by 12 to 20 beats per minute. Blood volume is maximal from 32 to 36 weeks of gestation, and cardiac output is greatest from 25 to 27 weeks. The total workload on the heart is increased in spite of the reduction of peripheral resistance. Peripheral blood flow is increased, and in addition, the capillaries and precapillary arterioles show increased vasomotor activity. Increased capillary fragility probably occurs during the third trimester and certainly during labor. As will be seen later, certain changes in the coagulation mechanism may predispose to the development of disseminated intravascular coagulation.

PATHOGENESIS OF SHOCK

As stated previously, shock is caused by a critical reduction in the perfusion of tissues by blood. It is therefore important to review first how the microcirculation normally perfuses the tissues and then how this process is affected by shock.

A microcirculatory unit consists of blood vessels arranged in serial and parallel fashion and includes arterioles, metarterioles, precapillary sphincters, capillaries, arteriovenous anastomoses, venules, and collecting venules. Figure 21–1 shows a diagram of a microcirculatory unit.

Functionally, the components of the microcirculation may be classified as resistance vessels, exchange vessels, shunt vessels, and capacitance vessels. The *precapillary resistance* elements include small arteries, arterioles, and precapillary sphincters. The first two elements determine the extent of total tissue blood flow, while the sphincters, by adjusting the number of capillaries open, determine the distribution of capillary blood flow, extent of capillary flow velocity, capillary surface area available, and mean extravascular diffusion distance. *Postcapillary resistance* vessels include the muscular venules and small veins. Their strategic position, immediately postcapillary, enables them to markedly influence capillary pressure. The ratio of precapillary to postcapillary resistance determines the capillary hydrostatic filtration pressure. The *exchange vessels* are

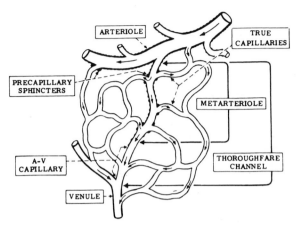

FIGURE 21–1 Diagram of a microcirculatory unit. *(From E. Selkurt: Physiology, 3d ed., Boston: Little, Brown, 1971; after R Chambers and BW Zweifach.)*

the capillaries and venules. The exchange between the vascular and extravascular compartments is carried out through their walls in a variable manner. In any given tissue the venous end of the exchange vasculature is more permeable to water and solutes than is the arterial end. The *shunt vessels* include arteriovenous anastomoses, preferential channels, and even capillaries when they receive blood flow greatly in excess of their exchange capacity. Flow through these vessels bypasses the effective exchange circulation of tissue and therefore is considered nonnutritional. Because of their great distensibility, the veins are the major capacitance or storage elements of the circulation. The venous component of the microcirculatory system is estimated to contain about 70 percent of the total body blood volume.

MICROCIRCULATORY CHANGES IN HEMORRHAGIC SHOCK

In general, the economy of the body is maintained by a process of "negative feedback"; that is, the response to a noxious stimulus tends to cancel or correct the abnormal state. After severe hemorrhage the patient enters a state of primary, or *reversible,* shock. The resulting hypotension stimulates stretch receptors monitoring blood pressure in the carotid sinus and aortic arch. These receptors supply information to the vasomotor center in the medulla via the ninth and tenth cranial nerves. The vasomotor center provides a response designed to restore the blood pressure to its former value. The efferent limb of this reflex is mediated through the sympathetic nervous system, resulting in an increase in the rate and force of cardiac contraction which improves the effective cardiac output. This sympathetic discharge also constricts the peripheral arterioles and increases the tone of the venules and small veins. Blood flow through nonvital organs is diminished, and the large venous reservoir is emptied into the central circulation. This also causes a fall in the hydrostatic pressure across the tissue capillaries, and fluid will then move from the extravascular compartment into the circulation.

Control of blood flow through the brain and the heart is mediated almost entirely by local factors; therefore, these organs do not participate in the "sympathetic squeeze." The three defense mechanisms brought into play are (1) selective organ ischemia, (2) immediate autotransfusion from increased venomotor tone, and (3) delayed autotransfusion from transcapillary refilling. These mechanisms tend to correct hypovolemia, improve cardiac output, and sustain blood pressure and therefore the perfusion of vital organs. At this stage transfusion and control of hemorrhage are usually effective in restoring the normal circulatory balance.

Other responses help stabilize the plasma volume. Increased release of antidiuretic hormone (ADH) by the pituitary and aldosterone by the adrenal cortex results in the conservation of sodium and water by the kidneys. It can be seen that all the above-mentioned responses are examples of negative feedback mechanisms functioning to correct the departure from the normal state.

If early and adequate measures are not taken to correct the disparity between the circulating blood volume and the capacity of the vascular bed, secondary, or *irreversible,* shock will develop. When the initial compensatory mechanisms fail, "positive feedback" cycles are established in which the initiating stimulus is increased by the response. The sequence of events is as follows: The available blood volume continues to fall. Excretion of metabolites is deficient from areas undergoing severe vasoconstriction. The accumulation of these metabolites eventually constitutes a powerful stimulus for metabolic vasodilation of the metarteriole and the precapillary sphincter in spite of the persistence of increased sympathetic tone. Postcapillary resistance elements, however, apparently continue in a state of constriction long after the precapillary sphincters have begun to dilate, thereby causing the blood to be pooled in the capillary bed. This will increase the capillary hydrostatic pressure and decrease or even reverse the fluid shift from the extravascular to the vascular space. Venous return to the heart is further decreased, with a conse-

quent drop in cardiac output and blood pressure. As the diastolic pressure falls, coronary artery blood flow is reduced, producing myocardial anoxia and eventually cardiac decompensation. This cardiac injury can be overwhelming and self-perpetuating.

In the final stage of irreversible hemorrhagic shock, the postcapillary venules become unresponsive to sympathetic stimulation, and the microcirculation is then subjected to the unopposed effect of endogenous vasodilator substances. The capillary and venule spaces expand, resulting in progressive pooling of blood and stagnant hypoxia. At this time no amount of blood replacement, ventilation, drugs, or surgical manipulation will reverse the course, and the patient will soon die of cardiorespiratory failure.

MICROCIRCULATORY CHANGES IN SEPTIC SHOCK

The previously described effects of hemorrhagic hypovolemic shock on the microcirculation are a classical example of the low-output shock syndrome. It is possible to have shock without hypovolemia and even with a hyperdynamic circulatory state. This can be seen in certain patients with septic (endotoxin) shock. As a response to gram-negative sepsis, cardiac output may be temporarily increased. The blood flow to the area of sepsis may be doubled or even tripled. When the patient goes into shock the blood volume may be relatively normal, and the velocity of blood through certain areas may be increased.

Septic shock is caused by endotoxin, a lipopolysaccharide-protein complex derived from the disintegration of the cell wall of gram-negative bacteria. It has been shown to have many effects in the experimental animal, but some of these effects are species-specific with the lower animals and are not particularly applicable to man.

In an effort to clarify the pathophysiology of septic shock in the primate, Cavanagh et al. (1970) have studied the subhuman primate. They have shown that bolus doses of endotoxin given intravenously to the baboon cause profound hypotension, diminish myocardial contractility, increase the release of [³H]norepinephrine (a tracer for endogenous catecholamines), increase the peripheral and renal resistance to blood flow, initiate intravascular coagulation, and cause deposition of fibrin in the glomeruli of the kidney. Thomas had previously shown in lower animals that endotoxin produces a local and generalized Shwartzman reaction. Lillehei and McLean suggested severe vasospasm in small vessels as the basic mechanism of action of endotoxin, citing the known sympathomimetic effects of the substance. Other important aspects of the pathogenesis of septic shock will be considered later in this chapter.

DISSEMINATED INTRAVASCULAR COAGULATION

Disseminated intravascular coagulation (DIC) is more accurately called intravascular coagulation fibrinolysis syndrome (ICF), but DIC is the term most widely used in gynecology and obstetrics. DIC accompanies practically every clinical and experimental situation in which shock is seen. DIC is an apparently paradoxic situation in which thrombotic and thrombolytic mechanisms are initiated simultaneously so that intravascular coagulation and a hemorrhagic diathesis are present at the same time.

This is often a difficult concept to grasp. There are two great paradoxes in DIC. First, that the stimulation of the clotting mechanism results in a bleeding defect. Second, that the treatment of this bleeding defect with an anticoagulant may be appropriate in some cases. It should be remembered that the hemostatic process functions in a remarkably interdependent manner. The presence of activated coagulation factors serves to initiate the "clot-dissolving," or fibrinolytic mechanism, probably to ensure control of the clotting mechanism. When the thrombotic and thrombolytic mechanisms are in balance, hemostasis is assured. Normally both processes are limited to a local area of injury. Through the action of a variety of stimuli, however, these two processes can be triggered within the vascular bed. In pregnant patients intravascular coagulation is almost always primary, with fibrinolysis being a secondary response. The bleeding diathesis results from the consumption of coagulation factors, the pathologic activity of the fibrinolytic system, and the anticoagulant effects of some of the by-products generated by this process.

Many synonyms for "DIC-like syndromes" are still commonly used. Such terms as hypofibrinogenemia, afibrinogenemia, or even defibrination syndrome simply describe the consumption of factor I, or fibrinogen. On the other hand, the term fibrination syndrome places more weight on the thrombotic implications of DIC than on the bleeding defect.

In 1965 McKay introduced the concept of multiple causality resulting in a common end point, when he described DIC as an "intermediary mechanism of disease which is not necessarily bound to a single disease entity, but may be responsible for much of the pathology, morbidity and mortality attributed to the antecedent disease." This is a very attractive concept. DIC can be a rapidly progressive entity with the potential to cause great injury to vital organs. On the other hand, we cannot ignore the underlying disease process that stimulated the development of the consumption coagulopathy. In gynecologic and obstetric patients, aggressive treatment of the primary disease usually saves the patient's life and brings DIC under adequate control.

Triggering Stimuli

What are the stimuli which can initiate DIC? The list has continued to lengthen since the mid-1950s, when research interest in this process began to grow. These stimuli are classified today in the general categories of infusion of tissue extracts, endothelial damage, anoxia, bacterial endotoxins, chemical and physical agents, hemolytic processes, immune reactions, and thrombocytopenia.

Figure 21–5 lists conditions in gynecology and obstetrics that are commonly associated with DIC. Some of these conditions, such as endotoxin shock, hemorrhagic shock, intrauterine dead fetus syndrome, and amniotic fluid infusion are discussed in this chapter. Other conditions associated with DIC, such as abruptio placentae, saline-induced abortion, and eclamptogenic toxemia, are described elsewhere (see Chaps. 30 and 33). It should be mentioned that a very small number of cases have been reported in which DIC has been associated with hydatidiform mole, degenerating myomas, and advanced gynecologic malignancies. Consumption coagulopathy has also been reported in neonates whose mothers suffered from toxemia, abruptio placentae, and Rh isoimmunization.

Incidence

The exact incidence of DIC in gynecologic and obstetric patients is not known. It may be invariably associated with abruptio placentae and cases of amniotic fluid infusion in which the patient survives the embolic episode. It is seen with less frequency in the other diseases.

Pathophysiology

To understand the pathophysiology of DIC it is important to review briefly the normal mechanism of hemostasis. Hemostasis is the general term applied to the lifesaving process which stops the flow of blood from injured vessels. To be effective, hemostasis requires

Table 21-2 Coagulation Factors Present in Plasma and Serum*

Factors present in plasma	Normal values, mg/100 mL	In normal serum
I Fibrinogen	200–400	Absent
II Prothrombin	75–125	< 5%
V Labile factor, proaccelerin	75–125	Absent
VII Stable factor, proconvertin	75–125	Present
VIII Antihemophilic globulin (AHG)	50–200	Absent
IX Plasma thromboplastin component (PTC) Christmas factor	50–200	Present
X Stuart-Prower factor	75–125	Present
XI Plasma thromboplastin antecedent	70–130	Present
XII Hageman factor	70–130	Present
XIII Fibrin-stabilizing factor, fibrinase	50–200	Absent
Platelets	150,000–400,000/mL	Absent

*Roman numerals indicate standard or international nomenclature for coagulation factors. Missing are III, thromboplastin, a tissue factor not normally present in circulating plasma or serum in significant amounts; IV, calcium ion, present in all tissues and fluids; and VI, not included in current nomenclature.

(1) normal blood vessels and normal extravascular tissues, (2) platelets which are normal in quality and quantity, and (3) adequate levels of coagulation factors. Table 21–2 shows the coagulation factors present in plasma and serum with their normal range of concentration.

The Thrombotic Process. For descriptive purposes the coagulation process can be divided into *three* phases: the vascular phase, the platelet phase, and the coagulation phase.

In *the vascular phase,* when an injury occurs to a small vessel and results in the extravasation of blood, three responses follow which help limit the injury. Vasoconstriction markedly reduces blood flow through the area. Next the escape of blood into the relatively rigid extravascular supporting tissue increases the pressure within these structures and helps collapse capillaries and venules. Last, various substances such as tissue thromboplastin (factor III) and adenosine diphosphate (ADP) are released from the injured tissue and help to initiate the final coagulation phase.

In *the platelet phase,* platelets adhere to the surface of the injured vessel and aggregate to one another almost instantaneously after an injury. This results in the formation of a platelet plug which may provide temporary or complete hemostasis, depending on the extent of the injury. Factors encouraging platelet adhesion and aggregation are ADP (derived from injured tissues) and the anti-VW factor, which is lacking in von Willebrand's disease.

Platelets have other functions in normal coagulation. They release adenosine triphosphate (ATP) as well as ADP and various phospholipids, collectively known as platelet factor 3. They also release thrombasthenin, a contractile protein which is responsible for clot retraction.

The coagulation phase is necessary for the formation of a firm thrombus which will later be the structural basis for the reconstructive process.

The mechanisms involved in the interactions of the coagulation factors are not entirely known. However, when activated, each factor sequentially activates the factor next in line in a "waterfall sequence." This is the so-called "cascade theory" of coagulation. Two pathways, extrinsic and intrinsic, are involved in this sequence.

Figure 21–2 shows how this is accomplished. *The extrinsic pathway* involves a rapid process in which the procoagulant material comes from the tissues and is not ordinarily present in the bloodstream. *The intrinsic pathway* is a slower process in which the coagulation proteins, which normally circulate in inactive form, are sequentially activated. The end result of both pathways is the deposition of fibrin.

The coagulation phase begins with the phenomenon of surface activation of factor XII (Hageman factor). This involves a molecular rearrangement of this factor, causing factor XI to be converted to its activated form factor XIa, sometimes called plasma thromboplastin antecedent. In vivo, factor XII is activated by contact with skin or any collagenous struc-

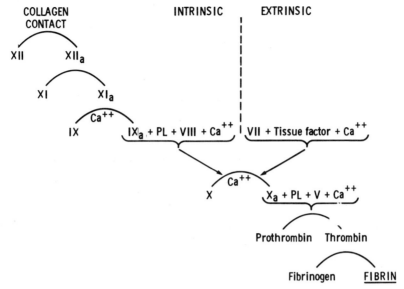

FIGURE 21-2 Scheme of intrinsic and extrinsic blood coagulation. PL, platelet factor 3, or phospholipid.

ture. In vitro, it occurs when it is exposed to electronegative surfaces, such as glass.

The activation of factor XI initiates the activation of factors IX (plasma thromboplastin component) and VIII (antihemophilic globulin). Together with calcium and platelet factor 3, factors IX and VIII are involved in the conversion of factor X into its enzymatic form. Factor Xa of Stuart and Prower forms a particulate complex (prothrombinase), with factor V (accelerator globulin), calcium, and platelet phospholipid. Prothrombinase then initiates the conversion of prothrombin into thrombin.

A functionally identical prothrombinase can be produced in a matter of seconds by activation of the extrinsic pathway. This pathway bypasses the activation of factors XII, XI, IX, and VIII. Tissue thrombo-

plastins released after injury interact with calcium and factor VII (serum prothrombin conversion accelerator), and the resulting complex causes activation of factors X and V and platelet phospholipid into prothrombinase.

Figure 21-3 shows the final sequence of the coagulation process. Under the effects of the prothrombinase complex, factor II (prothrombin) is activated to thrombin. This then reacts with factor I (fibrinogen) in the following manner: four peptides are split from fibrinogen, leaving only fibrin monomers. These monomers and peptides form a visible but unstable fibrin polymer (soluble fibrin). Finally, factor XIIIa (fibrin-stabilizing factor) brings about the formation of a stable fibrin polymer (insoluble fibrin). This insoluble fibrin gives rise to the permanent hemostatic plug.

FIGURE 21-3 Final sequence of the coagulation process.

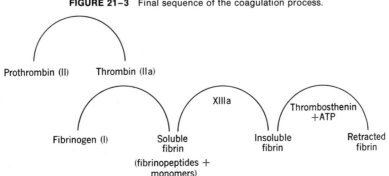

The last stage in the coagulation process is that of clot retraction, which may help bring together the margins of the injury. This takes place under the influence of a contractile protein (thrombasthenin) and ATP supplied by the platelets.

The Thrombolytic Process. Normally, the formation of fibrin is not a continuous process. The coagulation process is limited so that the clot does not propagate beyond the site of the wound. There are proteolytic enzymes in tissue and leukocytes which act as antithrombins, antithromboplastins, and inhibitors of prothrombinase. The reticuloendothelial system and liver macrophages help remove some activated coagulation factors from the circulation.

The fibrinolytic system is considered the major physiologic means of disposing of fibrin after hemostasis has been secured (Fig. 21–4). Fibrinolysis can be carried out by leukocytes, but most of it is carried out by the activation of a potent plasma protease called plasmin (Alkjaersig et al.; Holemans, Silver). This exists in normal plasma in the form of an inactive precursor, plasminogen, which can be activated by hypoxia, tissue extracts, bacterial enzymes (streptokinase and urokinase), activated factor XII, thrombin, and hypoglycemia.

Plasminogen is deposited within the clot during the clotting process. When activating substances from plasma, blood vessels, or tissue penetrate the clot, plasminogen is converted into its active form, *bound plasmin,* and localized secondary fibrinolysis occurs.

Normally, antiplasmins in plasma rapidly destroy free plasmin but are ineffective against bound plasmin, which is thus free to perform its physiologic function.

The lysis of fibrin clots by plasmin results in the formation of partially digested fragments of fibrin, which are known as fibrin degradation products (FDP), or fibrin split products (FSP). These products can also be formed by the lytic action of plasmin on fibrinogen. Normally, only minimal amounts of FDP are found in the circulation. When present in large quantities they act as powerful anticoagulants. They impair the aggregation of platelets and their release of phospholipids, ATP, and ADP. Fibrin degradation products also interfere with plasma thromboplastin formation, the thrombin-fibrinogen reaction, and the polymerization of fibrin. They form inactive complexes with fibrin monomers which are known as soluble fibrin monomer complexes (SFMC).

In pregnancy, the majority of cases of DIC are initiated by the entrance into the circulation of tissue extracts or fluids rich in thromboplastin content. This occurs in abruptio placentae, the intrauterine dead fetus syndrome, septic abortion, and amniotic fluid infusion. A similar mechanism is also probably operative in eclamptogenic toxemia, molar pregnancy, ruptured uterus, and saline-induced abortions. The entrance of thromboplastic substances into the circulation causes activation of the extrinsic pathway. In amniotic fluid infusion, the fluid has a high content of collagenous cellular debris and other particulate matter, which may cause platelet aggregation and the activation of factor XII and the intrinsic pathway. In hemorrhagic and septic shock there is endothelial damage and platelet aggregation, which initiate DIC by activation of the intrinsic pathway.

Once DIC is established, coagulation will proceed in vivo much as it does in vitro. Initially a state of hypercoagulability exists during which platelets, fibrinogen, and factors V, VIII, and XIII are eventually consumed, sometimes almost to the point of total depletion.

As intravascular coagulation develops, there is a greater chance of thromboembolism. Thus, the activation of the fibrinolytic system is a protective mechanism. We have noted that plasminogen can be activated by the initiating tissue extracts factor XIIa, and thrombin. In DIC, plasmin is produced in quantities which exceed the capacity of the antiplasmins. Circulating plasmin causes proteolysis of hemostatically important fibrin plugs, as well as circulating fibrinogen in the presence of factors V and VIII, and results in the release of FDP into the circulation.

The end result of this process is a bleeding dia-

FIGURE 21–4 Activation mechanism of the thrombolytic system.

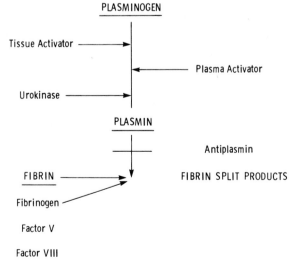

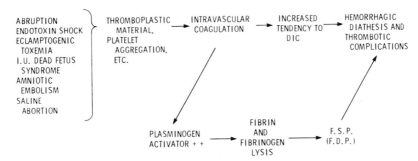

FIGURE 21-5 Pathogenesis of disseminated intravascular coagulation.

thesis which complicates the primary illness, particularly in the presence of an open wound. Several important clotting parameters are affected. The platelet phase is impeded by the thrombocytopenia. Circulating plasmin lyses whatever fibrin may have been deposited at the wound's margin. The generation of new fibrin is imperfect because of the depletion of the consumable factors and the presence of circulating anticoagulants (FDP). Figure 21-5 summarizes the pathophysiologic features of DIC.

Diagnosis of DIC

The cardinal manifestation of DIC is abnormal bleeding. This is usually demonstrated by a marked increase in vaginal bleeding. During surgery the patient will exhibit bleeding from the incisional margins, other operative areas, and venapuncture sites. Hematuria, bleeding from the gums, and ecchymoses are not uncommon. Shock is frequently seen. Mental confusion reflects cerebral anoxia, and convulsions may occur. In chronically ill patients, particularly those with disseminated malignancies, there may be seen a premonitory stage of hypercoagulability manifested by thromboembolic phenomena.

Confirmation by laboratory tests is essential, not only to establish the presence and severity of the disease but also to follow and evaluate its course. No single laboratory test is diagnostic for DIC. In the full-blown syndrome the diagnosis of DIC is easy, since almost all tests will be abnormal. However, specific identification of which process poses the greater threat to the patient, intravascular coagulation or fibrinolysis, may be very different.

Table 21-3 lists laboratory tests which are helpful in the diagnosis and management of DIC. Some are simple to perform, and should be immediately available to the physician. Others require experienced laboratory personnel and may take over 24 hours to perform.

When suspicion of DIC is strong or when clinical evidence of coagulopathy is present, the following tests can be helpful: (1) quantitative determination of fibrinogen, (2) clotting time, (3) clot lysis time, (4) peripheral smear for platelets and red blood cell morphology, (5) quick prothrombin time determination, (6) partial thromboplastin time determination, and (7) thrombin time.

In the absence of adequate laboratory facilities, the clot observation of a peripheral smear can be used effectively. A 5-mL sample of blood is placed in a 15-mL test tube which is then inverted four or five times. The clotting mechanism is abnormal if there is no clot within 6 minutes, or if the clot which forms is not solid and lyses within 1 hour. The clot size is abnormal if it occupies less than 45 percent of the total volume of the blood. The clot stability is abnormal if, after standing for half an hour, it will not withstand inverting the test tube several times.

Table 21-3 Laboratory Tests for DIC

Test	Result
Clotting time	Normal (5–15 minutes)
Clot retraction	Poor (disintegrates in 15–60 minutes)
Fibrinogen	Usually decreased
Thrombin time	Usually prolonged
Prothrombin time	Usually prolonged
Partial thromboplastin time	Usually prolonged
Factor consumption	Factors V, VIII, and XIII reduced
Platelets	Usually decreased
Red blood cell morphology	Often abnormal
FDP (ESP)	Present
Euglobulin clot lysis	Usually shortened
Plasminogen	Usually decreased

The clotting time, as determined in the clot observation test, provides evidence of fibrinogen levels. If the clotting time is less than 6 minutes, the fibrinogen level is probably more than 150 mg per 100 mL. If the clotting time is more than 6 minutes and the clot is poor, the fibrinogen level is probably 100 to 150 mg per 100 mL. If there is no clot in 30 minutes, the fibrinogen level is probably less than 100 mg per 100 mL. In this respect, however, it must be kept in mind that the quality of the patient's fibrinogen is very important. The influence of fibrinogen on the clotting process is much greater than that of its first derivative, even though there is little difference in molecular weight. Therefore, it is important to remember that even though a patient demonstrates a fibrinogen level of 200 mg per 100 mL, a significant degree of DIC may still exist.

In a normal blood smear with Wright's stain, four to ten platelets should be seen per high-power field. Fewer than four platelets per high-power field implies thrombocytopenia. This can easily be confirmed by a regular platelet count. Thrombocytopenia is characteristic of intravascular coagulation but is not found in a pure fibrinolytic syndrome. Platelets are slow to return to normal when the process is controlled. In DIC the passage of the red blood cells through fibrin "meshes" changes their shape. Peripheral blood smears may show "helmet-shaped," "tear-shaped," and fragmented red blood cells (schistocytes). When microspherocytes are seen in septic patients, *Clostridium welchii* infection should be strongly suspected, particularly in the presence of hemoglobinemia and hemoglobinuria. In pure pathologic fibrinolysis, the red blood cell morphology is normal.

One of the most consistent findings in DIC is the appearance of FDP. These can be detected in serum by using the "Fi test," and their reaction with antifibrinogen serum in the presence of latex particles produces agglutination. Semiquantitation may be achieved by using serial dilutions of serum. Prolongation of TT (thrombin time), in the absence of heparin treatment, and with normal fibrinogen levels, usually reflects significant circulating concentrations of FDP.

The *ethanol gelation test* and *protamine sulfate test* are also available for the detection of FDP. They detect the formation of complexes between soluble fibrin monomers and FDP.

Fibrin monomers are normally formed by the action of thrombin and are the precursors of polymerized fibrin. For these monomers to remain soluble, inhibitors of polymerization such as FDP must be present. The finding of these complexes specifically indicates DIC.

HEMORRHAGIC SHOCK

PATHOPHYSIOLOGY

The central event in hemorrhagic shock is loss of blood from the vascular space with diminution of circulating blood volume. In its compensated phase, hemorrhagic shock includes elevation of circulating catecholamines with widespread arteriolar vasoconstriction (Bauer et al.). Liberation of renal pressor substances helps sustain this vasoconstriction (Simeone), and cerebral vessels are spared by this process. There is also an influx of extravascular fluid into the vascular compartment, the net effect being the accommodation of the vascular space to available circulating volume. Venous return and cardiac output are thereby maintained. Tachycardia also helps maintain cardiac output. In this phase of shock, administration of intravenous fluids and electrolytes achieves homeostasis readily, provided that hemorrhage is controlled.

With continued blood loss, hemorrhagic shock enters the primary stage of *early decompensation*. Peripheral vasoconstriction, influx of extravascular fluid into the vascular space, and tachycardia no longer preserve adequate circulating volume because of the continued fall in the circulating blood volume. With tissue hypoxia, increased capillary dilatation occurs, possibly as a result of the local histamine liberation. This further increases the disparity between the available blood volume and the capacity of the vascular bed so that venous return and cardiac output are further reduced. The process is intensified by sequestration of fluid through capillary walls damaged by hypoxia.

If allowed to continue, the process enters the secondary stage of *late decompensation*, in which arteriolar and capillary tone is lost, with vast expansion of the capillary bed and therefore of the vascular compartment in general. Marked tissue acidosis occurs, at times associated with DIC and stimulation of the fibrinolytic system. The transition from this phase into the stage of irreversible shock is not clearly defined, and can only be gauged by the success or failure of adequate therapeutic measures. Irreversible hemorrhagic shock is signaled by evidence of organ death in the form of hepatic, renal, cardiopulmonary, or central nervous system failure.

CLINICAL PICTURE

In its early phases, hemorrhagic shock is featured by a relatively normal blood pressure, with tachycardia and diaphoresis. The patient appears restless and anxious. This "compensated" shock is easily managed by volume replacement. If untreated, it is followed by the hypotensive, decompensated phase. In its early stages, the decompensated phase readily responds to adequate volume replacement. Later in the evolution of this process, however, a less satisfactory response is elicited, even though treatment is intensified, and the patient may enter the secondary, or irreversible, stage. Hemorrhagic shock is characteristically reversible until very late in its evolution. For this reason, vigorous therapy should always be initiated as soon as this diagnosis is made, even in an apparently exsanguinated patient.

MANAGEMENT

The essentials of management are to stop bleeding and replace blood. After the diagnosis of hemorrhagic shock has been made, hemostasis is essential. However, this may not be attainable without major surgery. It may be necessary to defer surgical intervention until measures for control of shock have been initiated unless definite evidence of intraabdominal bleeding is present. When indicated, such measures as oxytocin administration for uterine atony, or repair of a cervical laceration, should be undertaken without delay.

Replacement of intravascular fluid volume is essential and ideally blood loss should be replaced with compatible blood. This should always be done through a large bore needle (18 gauge) or indwelling polyethylene catheter (16 gauge) to allow prompt adequate replacement. Early in the development of hemorrhagic shock, this may be accomplished by the administration of intravenous fluids and electrolytes. Five percent glucose in normal saline solution is of value, with sodium bicarbonate added as needed to combat acidosis. Ringer's lactate solution is less suitable, since anaerobic metabolism in the shock state produces large amounts of lactate. The conversion to

bicarbonate which occurs during normal aerobic metabolism is inefficient in this situation.

With more severe degrees of hemorrhagic shock adequate blood replacement becomes essential. Properly typed and cross-matched blood should be used. In the face of severe hemorrhage this should be as fresh as possible. Sufficient blood should be given to replace the estimated blood loss, or until all clinical evidence of shock has subsided. When blood is not available, serum albumin, dextran, or 3% saline may be used.

In the obstetric patient, because of her ability to compensate for blood loss, the arterial blood pressure is a poor guide to the management of hemorrhage. This is particularly true in the patient with abruptio placentae, in whom central venous pressure monitoring is a much more accurate guide to replacement. Early and adequate replacement is especially difficult in these patients because of the tendency to underestimate blood loss.

Other therapeutic measures should include oxygen administration by nasal catheter at a flow of 4 to 5 liters per minute and positioning the patient in the modified Trendelenburg position (feet elevated, head down). Vasopressors are not indicated since peripheral vasoconstriction already exists. Therapy should be monitored with repeated readings of central venous pressure, checked initially every hour and less frequently as the patient improves. Hourly urinary output should be recorded as well as frequent measurements of pulse, respirations, and blood pressure. Blood volume estimations are useful in early shock but are quite inaccurate in late shock. Hemoglobin and hematocrit determinations are of little value in determining the magnitude of acute blood loss, but a base-line determination followed by daily measurements provides some guidance as to the adequacy of therapy. The best immediate guide to therapy is the clinical appearance of the patient. Tachycardia and diaphoresis are especially useful signs. Blood pressure alterations frequently appear only when the process is more advanced.

When therapeutic measures to combat shock have been initiated, surgical efforts should be undertaken to attain hemostasis, with the magnitude of the surgical procedure depending upon the underlying condition. Indeed, it is sometimes impractical to await response to medical measures, as in severe hemorrhage associated with rupture of the gravid uterus. In such cases control of hemorrhage must be achieved at exploratory celiotomy. On entering a blood-filled abdomen, manual compression of the aorta against the vertebral column will often allow better visualization of the bleeding site after the removal of clots.

After examination of the involved area, the decision can be made regarding corrective measures. Identifiable bleeding points can be controlled with proper suturing. If the gravid uterus has ruptured, total abdominal hysterectomy is usually indicated. In rare cases, when the defect is small, repair may be attempted. However, there is always the hazard of repeated rupture during a subsequent pregnancy.

Hypogastric artery ligation is successful in certain situations in which hysterectomy is impossible or undesirable. This is achieved by isolating the bifurcation of the iliac arteries. The internal iliac artery is identified, and its anterior division is ligated close to its origin. Few adverse effects are to be expected from this procedure. The incision into the peritoneum should be made over the external iliac artery and carried proximally lateral to the ovarian vessels. The ovarian vessels are ligated bilaterally prior to bilateral ligation of the hypogastric arteries. The ureters should always be identified prior to bilateral hypogastric ligation; they are usually easily located where they cross the common iliac artery.

FLUID LOSS SHOCK

Fluid loss shock may be seen in association with excessive vomiting, diarrhea, diuresis, or too-rapid removal of ascitic fluid. The diagnosis is obvious, and management consists of adequate fluid replacement.

SUPINE HYPOTENSIVE SYNDROME

Although not associated with hemorrhage or infection, this condition may cause alarm in the antepartum period. This temporary hypotensive state is due to reduced venous return to the right auricle from the pressure of the gravid uterus on the inferior vena cava. Typically the patient is lying on her back in bed or on an examining table and while her blood pressure is being taken, an acute hypotensive episode occurs. The situation is quite alarming to attendants unfamiliar with the supine hypotensive syndrome, but the blood pressure returns promptly to the normal range when the patient is turned to her side. A woman

should be discouraged from lying on her back in late pregnancy, because this position may cause hypotension in the mother and distress to the fetus.

THE INTRAUTERINE FETAL DEATH SYNDROME

Most fetuses deliver spontaneously soon after intrauterine demise. Tricomi and Kohl have shown that 75 percent of patients will go into spontaneous labor by the end of the second week after fetal death, and 93 percent will do so by the end of the third week.

If the dead fetus is retained in utero longer than 5 weeks the mother may develop DIC. This results from the passage into the maternal circulation of small but repeated infusions of thromboplastic material from the degenerating placenta and dead fetus. This usually is a slow process, and the coagulopathy develops over a period of days to weeks. When the fetus is retained longer than 5 weeks Pritchard has found that the likelihood of significant DIC occurring is about 1 in 4.

Until recently, the management of these patients has been conservative. The obstetrician usually awaits the onset of spontaneous labor, doing serial fibrinogen determinations after the fourth week. Thereafter, most have chosen a policy of delivery if labor has not ensued by this time. This prevents the development of DIC and certainly relieves the emotional stress upon the mother. Our usual method is the intravenous administration of an oxytocin solution in increasing concentrations until labor is safely established. We do not recommend the use of intraamniotic hypertonic saline injection to induce labor. Stander, et al. have conclusively shown that significant DIC can develop when this technique has been used in elective second-trimester abortions. Experience with intraamniotic prostaglandin $F_2\alpha$ indicates that it may be effective in initiating labor and free of harmful effects on the maternal coagulation mechanism.

If the patient develops a coagulation defect, the treatment described by Jimenez and Pritchard may be helpful. Heparin is administered intravenously for 2 to 3 days to block the action of the initiating procoagulant substances. This usually restores fibrinogen and other coagulation factors to normal levels. When this occurs labor can be stimulated and delivery safely accomplished. Fibrinogen replacement therapy is rarely indicated and can usually be limited to the patient who is admitted in labor and whose condition is complicated by a bleeding defect, or to the patient who bleeds excessively after delivery because of the presence of a consumption coagulopathy. The danger of hepatitis following the use of human dried fibrinogen must always be kept in mind, and cryoprecipitate should be used.

AMNIOTIC FLUID INFUSION

In 1926, Meyer first reported a case of amniotic fluid embolism producing sudden death in a 21-year-old multipara. Lushbaugh and Steiner established this diagnosis firmly in 1941 with a series of eight well-documented cases.

The mortality rate for this syndrome is very high; 50 percent of patients may die at the time of embolization, while more than half of the survivors die subsequently. Amniotic fluid infusion accounts for approximately 10 percent of all deaths associated with pregnancy.

Fortunately amniotic fluid infusion (embolism) is rare. Predisposing factors include multiparity, hypertonic uterine contractions, oxytocin induction or stimulation of labor, traumatic delivery, meconium staining of the amniotic fluid, large babies, and intrauterine death.

The diagnosis is difficult, and the situation is complicated by the tendency of many physicians to attribute unexplained maternal death or unexplained obstetric shock to amniotic fluid infusion. The usual clinical picture includes marked dyspnea and cyanosis and a relative absence of chest pain. There may be convulsions and profuse hemorrhage. The blood usually does not clot.

There is hardly any time for confirmatory tests. As stated before, the infusion is usually massive and over half of the patients die at the time of the original incident. Most cases are confirmed at autopsy with the finding of fetal squames and other debris plugging the pulmonary capillaries. A high index of suspicion is essential if one is to save the patient surviving the initial embolization. Previously normal obstetric patients who suddenly go into profound shock, particularly immediately after delivery, and exhibit evidence of a coagulation defect should be presumed to have amniotic fluid embolism.

In the survivors of the initial episode, a radiograph of the chest may show perihilar infiltrates, but this is infrequent and may also be seen in pulmonary edema. In 1947, Gross and Benz reported that aspiration of

blood from the right ventricle may confirm amniotic fluid embolization. The blood usually separates into three layers with amniotic debris floating over the buffy coat of white blood cells. Most physicians are understandably reluctant to perform this procedure in a severely ill patient, but it may promptly confirm the diagnosis. In 1966, Altchek and Litwak suggested the use of pulmonary scanning with macroaggregated ^{131}I albumin to demonstrate perfusion defects, and help establish the diagnosis in surviving patients. However, it was not until 1973, when Gregory and Clayton again reported on the use of this technique, that the method became more widely accepted. Coagulation studies performed in these patients usually confirm the presence of DIC. Coagulation factors are rapidly depleted with fibrinogen, platelets, and factors V, VIII, and XIII being particularly affected. The activation of the fibrinolytic system is instantaneous, and patients may continue to bleed from circulating fibrinolysins after intravascular coagulation has been controlled by heparin administration and replacement with fresh blood, fresh frozen plasma, and possibly fibrinogen.

The treatment of these patients should have two objectives: to support the cardiovascular system and to control the coagulopathy. The support of the cardiovascular system in shock patients is discussed elsewhere in this chapter. Obviously, if the patient is bleeding profusely, administration of fresh whole blood in sufficient quantities to maintain an effective circulating blood volume is essential. If fresh whole blood is not available, then replacement with stored bank blood, platelet packs, and fresh frozen plasma should be carried out when there is evidence of a severe coagulopathy.

Gregory and Clayton recommend the administration of heparin immediately upon clinical suspicion of amniotic fluid embolism. They follow the initial recommendation of Reid et al., who recommended administering 50 to 75 mg heparin intravenously to help neutralize the clotting effects of the amniotic fluid entering the circulation. It is unlikely that this dosage will produce any alterations in the thrombin component of the clotting mechanism. This should be given within 10 minutes after evidence of respiratory distress in a patient suspected of amniotic fluid embolism. If the blood fails to clot after heparinization, fibrinogen should be given. The use of antifibrinolytic agents should be reserved for patients who show laboratory evidence of circulating fibrinolysins in spite of adequate control of DIC. In pregnant patients, primary fibrinolysis is rare, and secondary fibrinolysis is part of a defense mechanism.

ENDOTOXIC SHOCK
(SEPTIC SHOCK)

Endotoxic shock is a syndrome resulting from sepsis due to gram-negative bacteria. The most common organisms involved are *E. coli, Aerobacter aerogenes, Proteus mirabilis* or *P. vulgaris,* and *Pseudomonas aeruginosa* (Koch). Endotoxic shock in the young patient is relatively rare. When it does occur it is usually in association with pregnancy. The most common cause is septic abortion, but it is also seen with chorioamnionitis and pyelonephritis. In 1956, Studdiford and Douglas first drew attention to "acute circulatory collapse" in association with septic abortion.

Shock associated with infection is called septic shock. By usage, this term is now applied to the characteristic clinical picture associated with gram-negative infection and is frequently called gram-negative shock, or endotoxic shock.

The seriousness of septic shock is well recognized, with mortality rates in reported series ranging from 11 to 82 percent (Coleman; Shubin and Weil). The variations in mortality rates are attributable to differences in patients, the underlying disease process, the promptness of diagnosis, and the method of management.

The relatively young gynecologic or obstetric patient with septic shock may be expected to respond more readily to therapy than an older, debilitated patient, and this has been the general experience. However, even in relatively healthy young people the mortality rate is considerable, and recovery is achieved only by prompt diagnosis and aggressive management.

PATHOPHYSIOLOGY

Wise et al. were among the first to report shock, without blood loss, in gram-negative sepsis. The correlation of vascular collapse in septic abortion with gram-negative sepsis was made by Studdiford and Douglas. Their association of the two conditions was based on the work of Good and Thomas who had produced shock in conjunction with renal cortical necrosis by repeated injection of sublethal doses of endotoxin.

For the past decade, two main mechanisms have been presented to explain the findings in endotoxic shock: selective vasospasm and DIC. Selective vasospasm in small arteries and veins was proposed by Lillehei and MacLean to explain the hemorrhagic necrosis observed in the intestines of dogs dying from the effects of endotoxin. Their observations led to their suggestion that vasopressors should not be used in endotoxic shock but that glucocorticoids should be beneficial because of their vasodilating effects (Lillehei et al.). Studies of peripheral resistance in patients with endotoxic shock, however, have yielded conflicting data, with depression (Wilson et al.), elevation (Udhoji and Weil), and marked variation (Hopkins et al.) having been reported.

Disseminated intravascular coagulation was proposed by McKay et al. because of the correlation between autopsy findings in patients dying of endotoxic shock and the changes of the generalized Shwartzman reaction in experimental animals, as studied by Thomas and coworkers (Good and Thomas, 1952 and 1953; Thomas; Thomas and Good).

Since conclusive data applicable to the clinical situation are lacking, attempts have been made to clarify the mechanism of endotoxic shock through studies in the baboons (Cavanagh et al., 1970). This animal is ideally suited to such studies, inasmuch as the coagulation profile closely resembles that of the human being, and the animal is large enough so that hemodynamic and biochemical changes can be measured with accuracy and relative ease. In these studies a single lethal dose of potent coliform endotoxin was given intravenously. From these studies it has become apparent that selective vasospasm, DIC, and reduced myocardial response to sympathetic stimuli all play an important part in the pathogenesis of endotoxin shock in the primate (Evensen et al.; Gilbert; Hampton and Matthews; Hinshaw et al.; Ts'ao and Kline). Studies by Bachmann and by Cavanagh et al. (1970) show that in the primate the kidney is a primary target organ in endotoxic shock; thus, acute tubular necrosis is more commonly associated with endotoxic shock rather than shock associated with postpartum hemorrhage.

In therapeutic studies, the value of methylprednisolone with and without low-molecular-weight dextran has been demonstrated (Rao et al.; Rao and Cavanagh). Studies by Rao et al. support the idea that aspirin in clinical dosage appears to protect against coliform endotoxin, and there is no doubt that complement plays an important part in the pathogenesis of septic shock. For a more complete account of the pathophysiology of septic shock, see the monograph by Cavanagh et al. (1977).

CLINICAL ASPECTS

Prevention

Since the mortality rate in endotoxic shock is so high, it is important to prevent the condition wherever possible. Patients with a diagnosis of infected abortion should be treated vigorously with antibiotics, and the septic focus should be removed early. Large doses of aqueous penicillin G, 30 to 60 million units per day in intravenous fluids (or ampicillin, 1 to 2 g every 4 to 6 hours) and gentamicin 60 to 80 mg every 8 hours intravenously, usually provide adequate antibiotic therapy. Curettage should be performed early, preferably within 6 hours after initiation of antibiotic therapy. Oxytocin may also be used to aid in expelling products of conception using 20 units in each liter of intravenous fluids. An elevation of temperature over 102°F should prompt close observation and monitoring for the development of endotoxic shock. The potential for endotoxic shock in the patient with an infected abortion should always be kept in mind, and aspiration curettage should be followed by careful sharp curettage because it is effective in removing infected residual products.

Chorioamnionitis can frequently be prevented by induction of labor following spontaneous premature rupture of the membranes. Induction should be performed, even in the afebrile patient, if there is no contraindication and the estimated fetal maturity is over 36 weeks. Induction may also be indicated when the estimated fetal maturity is 32 to 36 weeks, since the intrauterine hazard of infection may be greater than the extrauterine problem of prematurity. These cases must be considered individually, however, and it should be remembered that the incidence of chorioamnionitis is higher among patients in lower socioeconomic groups (see Chap. 30).

Pyelonephritis in pregnancy is partially the result of urinary stasis due to mechanical pressure on the ureters by the uterus. Renal intracalyceal pressure can be reduced, therefore, by having the patient lie on her side. Although the disease is bilateral, the right side is usually more involved, and the patient is more comfortable lying on her left side. Adequate antibiotic therapy is essential in this situation, but the choice of antibiotics is difficult during pregnancy since certain agents (tetracycline, sulfisoxazole, etc.) have been reported to produce adverse effects on the fetus. Patients with this complication should be admitted to the hospital and may be given 1 g ampicillin intravenously every 4 to 6 hours unless the urine culture reveals an ampicillin-resistant organism (see Chap. 31).

History

Patients who have undergone illegal abortions, and even a few who have had legal abortions, will frequently present with a vague or even contradictory clinical history. The menstrual history may be falsified. Patients with chorioamnionitis should be asked about time of rupture of membranes and onset of symptoms. In pyelonephritis the onset of flank pain, dysuria, and chills as well as the estimated date of confinement are important historic facts. Postpartum endometritis is often associated with manual exploration of the uterus and even more commonly with intrapartum chorioamnionitis.

Physical examination

The patient is usually febrile with a temperature above 102°F. Normal or subnormal temperature in association with shock is a grave prognostic sign and warrants early aggressive management. Local findings depend upon the site of infection. In *infected abortion* there is suprapubic tenderness, and local or generalized abdominal rebound tenderness is frequently encountered. On speculum examination the cervix is bluish and soft; tenaculum marks may be visible. The external os may exude a foul-smelling discharge. Products of conception may be found in the cervical canal or vagina. Bleeding may be minimal if the products of conception have been expelled or removed. Foreign bodies such as gauze and catheters may be found. Bimanual examination reveals marked tenderness. The internal os may admit one finger. The uterus is enlarged and soft, and manipulation of the cervix or corpus uteri elicits excruciating pain. Broad ligament tenderness is evidence of parametritis and pelvic cellulitis. Rarely, thrombosed veins are palpable.

In *chorioamnionitis* the findings are similar, with evidence of local or generalized peritonitis and a markedly tender uterus. Fetal heart tones are sometimes absent.

Postpartum endometritis is usually associated with a subinvoluted, tender uterus and signs of peritonitis.

In *pyelonephritis,* loin tenderness will usually be elicited.

Clinical Classification of Septic Shock

With the onset of shock, the patient's appearance is a useful guide to the type of treatment required. From a clinical viewpoint septic shock may be classified as primary or secondary. Primary (reversible) shock is subdivided into the early (warm-hypotensive) phase and the late (cold-hypotensive) phase. Secondary shock is also known as irreversible shock.

Primary Shock: Early or Warm-Hypotensive Phase. In the early (warm-hypotensive) phase, the patient is hypotensive, alert, and apprehensive. Her face is flushed and her skin is warm. Temperature is usually in the range of 101 to 105°F (38.4 to 40.6°C). Profuse sweating is not uncommon. A "shaking chill" coinciding with the temperature peak may be seen. There is a moderate tachycardia, usually 100 to 110 beats per minute (about 20 percent of these patients have a pulse rate under 72 beats per minute). The pulse pressure remains satisfactory, and the urinary output is adequate at this stage.

Primary Shock: Late or Cold-Hypotensive Phase. In this late phase of primary shock, the clinical picture is one of cold hypotension. The patient is hypotensive, pale, and clammy. The temperature is often subnormal. She gradually becomes less alert and less apprehensive. As the blood pressure drops, oliguria may supervene. The triad of hypotension, tachycardia, and oliguria is typically present in this phase.

Secondary (Irreversible) Shock. Prolonged cellular hypoxia and anaerobic metabolism associated with endotoxic shock are manifested by metabolic acidosis and excess blood lactate levels. Irreversible shock should be strongly suspected in all patients who have elevated arterial blood lactate levels. Anuria, cardiac or respiratory distress, and coma are grave prognostic signs.

Careful monitoring of the patient in endotoxin shock is essential. The clinical measurements most useful in our experience are listed in Table 21–4.

Laboratory Studies

On admission a complete blood count should be done. Urine is taken for urinalysis, culture, and sen-

Table 21–4 Clinical Measurement for Monitoring Endotoxic Shock

Clinical measurement	Frequency
Pulse rate	Every 15 minutes
Blood pressure and pulse pressure	Every 15 minutes
Central venous pressure	Every 30 to 60 minutes
Blood volume	Early in course
Urinary output	Every hour

sitivities at the time of insertion of an indwelling catheter. Smear of cervical discharge is obtained, along with culture and antibiotic sensitivities, and blood cultures are obtained at times of rigors or temperature peaks. Base-line chemistry studies include serum electrolytes, blood urea nitrogren, and uric acid. An electrocardiogram and chest x-ray should be obtained. When septic abortion is suspected, a plain film of the abdomen in the upright position is indicated to rule out the presence of gas under the diaphragm suggestive of uterine perforation or the possibility of a foreign body, such as a rubber catheter, in the peritoneal cavity. Other studies should be obtained according to requirement and availability. Ideally, a blood coagulation profile, arterial blood lactate levels, blood gas analyses, and blood volume measurements should be obtained in severely hypotensive patients and should be repeated as often as necessary. It should be remembered that blood volume measurements are unreliable in the later stages of endotoxic shock because of circulatory stagnation and sequestration of fluid.

MEDICAL MANAGEMENT

The success of treatment will depend largely upon the promptness of diagnosis. Thus, every effort should be made to observe the infected patient closely for the early signs of shock. Treatment is directed to the needs of the particular patients. *If a removable septic focus is present, surgery is the keystone of treatment.* In such situations as pyelonephritis, when the septic nidus cannot be removed, therapy is medical by necessity.

The essential steps in management are as follows:

1. Ensure that the patient has an adequate airway. If necessary, an endotracheal tube should be passed or a tracheostomy performed.
2. Adequate fluid and blood replacement should be carried out using the central venous pressure, the urinary output, and the blood volume estimation as guides. Blood, plasma, or 5% dextrose in saline should be given as indicated. Low-molecular-weight dextran provides volume replacement and reduces sludging in the microcirculation. Metabolic acidosis is common and becomes progressive if not corrected; in this case 0.45% saline, with one or two ampules of sodium bicarbonate added, is useful. Sodium bicarbonate acts rapidly and provides good buffering action. Lactate should not be used for correction of acidosis in

these patients, but tromethamine (THAM) is sometimes of value.

3. Antibiotics should be selected according to the organisms found on the Gram-stained smear, and on the basis of the previously known antibiotic sensitivities from similar organisms in the hospital in which the patient is being treated. The intravenous route and massive dosage must be employed. Penicillin (or ampicillin) and chloramphenicol have been found to be the most generally useful drugs. Penicillin should be given as crystalline penicillin G in a dosage of 10 million units every 4 hours in intravenous fluids. Chloramphenicol is given as an intravenous bolus, 1 g in 100 mL saline every 6 to 8 hours. As an alternative to penicillin, 2 g ampicillin may be given every 6 hours intravenously. Nephrotoxic drugs should be avoided in the presence of oliguria.

It should be remembered that most crystalline penicillin is supplied in the form of the potassium salt. If this is being used, remember that 60 million units of potassium penicillin G contains 90 meq potassium, which may create a hazard in the presence of renal failure. Therefore, the sodium salt should be used whenever possible.

It has been suggested that bactericidal drugs should not be employed in septic shock, since massive destruction of organisms could lead to massive liberation of endotoxin. This hypothesis, however, has not been borne out by experience in clinical practice.

4. Glucocorticoids should be given in pharmacologic doses. There is some evidence that the synthetic corticosteroids are more effective than hydrocortisone. Methylprednisolone sodium succinate (Solu-Medrol), 15 to 30 mg per kilogram of body weight per day, or dexamethasone (Decadron), 3 to 6 mg per kilogram of body weight per day should be given by continuous intravenous infusion after an initial intravenous loading dose of 125 mg methylprednisolone sodium succinate or 20 mg dexamethasone. These drugs probably exert a beneficial effect in at least three ways: (a) by a specific antiendotoxin effect at the cellular level, (b) by their inotropic action on the heart, and (c) by improving renal perfusion. Abrupt discontinuance after up to 72 hours has produced no ill effects in our experience; therefore, there seems to be no need to follow a regimen of gradual withdrawal.

5. Vasomotor drugs should be given as indicated by the clinical state of the patient. In septic shock the primary aim of therapy is improvement of tissue perfusion rather than the restoration of "normal" blood pressure. The choice of drug will depend on the patient's appearance and will involve either a vasopressor or vasodilator agent. It would appear that in the warm-hypotensive phase, a vasopressor rather than a vasodilator is indicated. Metaraminol (Aramine) is a useful vasopressor in the management of this condition. It is given only in sufficient quantities to maintain systolic blood pressure at the lower limit that ensures an adequate urinary output.

When a patient is seen in the cold-hypotensive phase, however, generalized vasoconstriction is present, and there is usually an element of hypovolemia. Volume replacement together with vasodilator drugs in small doses is the treatment of choice at this stage. Chlorpromazine (Thorazine) in a dose of 5 to 10 mg intravenously every half hour, as needed, is the best vasodilator in our experience. When the central venous pressure is elevated and the pulse rate is in the normal range, isoproterenol (Isuprel) may be used for its inotropic and vasodilator (beta receptor) effects. Because it may produce cardiac arrhythmia, it should not be used if the pulse rate exceeds 120 beats per minute. Also helpful sometimes is L-dopamine, but this must be used with care in the form of an intravenous infusion.

6. Digitalization should be carried out when the central venous pressure is above 15 cm of water and tachycardia is present.

7. Heparin should be considered if clotting studies indicate the presence of a consumption coagulopathy, i.e., thrombocytopenia, hypofibrinogenemia, a fall in the fibrinogen factors (V, VIII, and XIII), and the presence of fibrin split products. If a full coagulation profile is not available, and the patient is not responding to the standard treatment outlined above, then heparin should be tried. Heparin should not be given routinely. There is no evidence that hypothermia or hyperbaric oxygen are of value in endotoxic shock.

SURGICAL TREATMENT

When septic shock is associated with a surgically removable nidus of infection, the focus must be excised. In cases of septic abortion the nidus should be removed, in the presence of adequate supportive measures, within 6 hours of diagnosis. Usually, dilatation of the cervix and evacuation of the uterus with ring forceps followed by digital and sharp curettage are adequate to extirpate the septic focus. Suction curettage is also effective. However, when the disease has advanced to the stage of micro-abscess formation in the myometrium, hysterectomy is the only effective surgical treatment.

Hysterectomy should be considered if (1) the patient continues in shock following curettage and adequate supportive measures, (2) the uterus is over 16 weeks' gestation size, (3) the uterus is perforated, (4) the patient is oliguric, (5) intrauterine *Clostridium welchii* infection is diagnosed, or (6) a corrosive or toxic douche has been used. The technique of hysterectomy should be appropriate for the particular problem. For example, in the presence of clostridial infection, pedicle size should be kept small so that a minimum of devitalized tissue is left behind.

Septic pelvic thrombophlebitis with involvement of both ovarian and hypogastric vessels is not uncommon in patients with long-standing septic abortions, postpartum endometritis, or chorioamnionitis. Septic pulmonary embolization may occur, and coalescing lung abscesses may be the ultimate cause of death. Ligation of the inferior vena cava and ovarian veins is suggested, heparinization being used postoperatively at 1000 units per hour via an infusion pump. Good results have been reported in septic pelvic thrombophlebitis with heparinization alone, but in these causes the diagnosis was generally presumptive. However, when there is evidence of septic pelvic thrombophlebitis, a trial of heparin for 24 hours is a reasonable course to follow.

In the presence of chorioamnionitis, if vaginal delivery is not accomplished within 12 hours, abdominal delivery should be seriously considered. It is best accomplished by low transverse cesarean section. In the presence of severe infection or endotoxic shock, cesarean hysterectomy should be performed. Ligation of the inferior vena cava and ovarian veins should be carried out if indicated.

In an occasional patient with persistent anuria, dialysis may be required. In this case, consultation with a nephrologist is indicated.

CARDIOGENIC SHOCK

CARDIAC ARREST

Sudden failure of the pumping action of the heart will lead to an immediate reduction in available blood volume. Heart failure may be due to myocardial infarction, cardiac tamponade, or massive pulmonary embolism, but when it occurs in a previously healthy person, it is usually referred to as cardiac arrest.

The general incidence of cardiac arrest during anesthesia is now about 1 in 1500. Cardiac arrest occurs between 5000 and 10,000 times annually in the United States. The total number of obstetric patients affected is unknown, but because most of these patients are healthy young women, the condition is probably less common than among surgical patients. When it occurs in obstetric patients, however, more than half of the mothers and even more of the babies will probably be lost.

Cardiac arrest lasting over 4 minutes at normal body temperature is rarely compatible with complete recovery. Prolonged cerebral hypoxia results in death or survival in a decerebrate state.

Predisposing Factors

1. Hypoxia frequently exists during the induction stage of anesthesia, and this is the most common time for cardiac arrest to appear in the obstetric patient.
2. Hypercapnia may develop during surgery and is sometimes evidenced by ventricular extrasystoles or bradycardia. In patients given large amounts of stored blood during anesthesia, a raised serum potassium level may contribute to cardiac arrest.
3. Certain anesthetics, particularly intravenous Pentothal Sodium, cyclopropane, chloroform, or Trilene, may cause cardiac arrest when heart disease is already present. The likelihood is increased further with these anesthetics if vasoconstrictive agents, such as epinephrine or vasopressin, are also used to effect hemostasis in the operative area.
4. Sympathomimetic agents such as epinephrine may contribute to cardiac arrest.
5. Cardiac arrest occurs about five times more commonly in women with heart disease.
6. Rapid blood loss may produce cardiac arrest.
7. Vagal stimulation, especially in the presence of hypoxia or hypercapnia, during such procedures as gynecography or laparoscopy, can also lead to cardiac arrest.

Prevention

1. Atropine, 0.65 mg, should be given preoperatively to all patients receiving a general anesthetic. Unless the patient is pregnant and the baby is premature, an anxious patient may be given up to 50 mg Demerol without causing significant fetal

depression. Special care must be taken with the cardiac patient.

2. When hypercapnia and hyperkalemia are present, the patient should be given 20% glucose and 3% sodium chloride solution intravenously. This, in addition to piperoxan hydrochloride (1 mg per kilogram of body weight), will help prevent a posthypercapneic rise of the serum potassium level at room air.

3. The stomach should be empty before the general anesthetic is administered because aspiration of vomitus may lead to asphyxia and cardiac arrest.

Diagnosis

The most important single factor in improving the survival rate in association with cardiac arrest is early diagnosis. Vascular instability as evidenced by hypotension and abnormal cardiac rate or rhythm, respiratory difficulty, and muscular twitching commonly precede arrest. The alert anesthetist will recognize these danger signs, and prompt action will avert catastrophe. The anesthetist must observe the vital signs in all patients carefully throughout anesthesia. In obstetric cases it is particularly important the mother not be unattended while the baby is being resuscitated. It is essential that the anesthetist be especially alert during the induction stage of anesthesia, and immediately report the absence of a carotid pulse or recordable blood pressure. If these do not reappear within 1 minute, then the presence of cardiac arrest should be considered established. The diagnosis may also be made from the absence of heart sounds on auscultation and the absence of bleeding from the operative site.

When the abdomen is open and neither aortic pulsations nor heart impulses can be palpated, external cardiac massage is begun.

The establishment and maintenance of adequate respiration is the responsibility of the anesthetist. The establishment and maintenance of adequate circulation is the responsibility of the gynecologist-obstetrician. For success in treatment, teamwork is essential, and all members must be familiar with the steps to be taken. There is no time for discussion.

A *cardiac resuscitation set* should be available in every operating room and every delivery room.

Management of Established Cardiac Arrest

1. The administration of any drug which may have precipitated cardiac arrest is immediately stopped. If associated with pneumoperitoneum, the abdominal gas should be allowed to escape through a large cannula.

2. Full oxygen is given, and the lungs are artificially ventilated at a rate of 20 times per minute. If the patient is not already intubated, an endotracheal tube is inserted as soon as the color of the mucosa improves. If no mask or oxygen supply is available, mouth-to-mouth resuscitation should be instituted in an effort to inflate the lungs.

3. The head of the table is lowered slightly and the legs are raised to aid venous return.

4. With the patient in a shallow Trendelenburg position, external cardiac massage is begun.

The heel of the right hand, with the left hand on top of it, is placed on the sternum just above the xiphoid. Vertical pressure is exerted, using body weight, to push the sternum inward for a distance of about 1½ inches. This action forces blood out of the heart and into the lungs and the general circulation. When the pressure is released, the heart fills. Chest compression should be performed about 60 times per minute. If no help is available, the patient is pressure-ventilitated about four times between each minute of massage.

If an ECG tracing shows ventricular fibrillation and not arrest in asystole, a defibrillator should be called for and defibrillation carried out.

It is essential that every gynecologist-obstetrician be familiar with the management of cardiac arrest and that a cardiac resuscitation set and an electrical defibrillator be available for every minor operating room and delivery room. In summary, the plan of action is as follows:

1. Stop drug, e.g., Pentothal Sodium.
2. Put patient in Trendelenburg position and elevate the legs to 90° for 10 seconds or longer if an assistant is available.
3. Give oxygen by mask (or endotracheal tube if in place).
4. Carry out pressure ventilation at about 20 per minute. If necessary, an endotracheal tube should be passed and assisted ventilation continued.
5. Massage the heart at 60 to 80 times per minute by external compression.
6. Defibrillate with electric defibrillator (direct current 200 to 400 watt-seconds).
7. Provide supportive measures, e.g., compression of the aorta, blood, intravenous fluids, inotropic drugs. Sodium bicarbonate should be used for the treatment of metabolic acidosis.

8. *Results:* If adequate oxygenation and circulation are established within 4 minutes, about 50 percent of the patients will recover.

MYOCARDIAL INFARCTION

The diagnosis is established from the patient's history and electrocardiographic evidence of myocardial ischemia. An x-ray of the chest may show evidence of cardiac enlargement with pulmonary edema. Elevated levels of transaminase, in the absence of liver, pulmonary, or muscular damage, are also helpful in establishing the diagnosis. The patient is usually cold and clammy with a low blood pressure. If there is concomitant right-sided heart failure, the central venous pressure remains high.

CARDIAC TAMPONADE

This type of cardiogenic shock is due to an effusion into the pericardial sac. A discussion of the management of cardiac tamponade can be found in most medical textbooks and therefore will not be included in this section.

PULMONARY THROMBOEMBOLISM

Pulmonary infarction secondary to thromboembolism is one of the most serious and sinister complications found in gynecologic and obstetric patients. It affects women of all ages and is an important cause of death. With the present widespread use of oral contraceptives, pulmonary embolization is now being reported in teenagers. It is an important cause of maternal death, and after major gynecologic surgery 5 to 10 percent of patients develop clinically detectable venous thrombosis.

Pulmonary thromboembolism can occur without any obvious clinical evidence of thrombosis in the veins of the pelvis or the lower extremity. If the thrombosis results in partial vein occlusion, few local symptoms may occur. Current studies of postoperative patients with ^{125}I-labeled fibrinogen scanning have identified silent venous thrombosis of the lower extremities in approximately 35 percent of cases studied (Flanc et al.; Mattingly, Wilkinson). This is understandably frustrating, since thromboembolism can be a preventable disease if the susceptible patient and the onset of the initial venous thrombosis can be identified clearly. Although pulmonary infarc-

tion may occur during pregnancy, labor, or the post-partum period, it most frequently develops in the first 10 days of the puerperium.

Pathogenesis

In 1854, Virchow pointed to a triad of factors contributing to the formation of venous thrombosis. These factors still are true today: (1) alteration in the coagulation factors of the blood, (2) trauma to the vessel wall, and (3) venous stasis.

Numerous changes in blood-clotting factors due to oral combined-hormone contraceptive therapy have been reported and are summarized in Table 21–5. The changes in coagulation factors during pregnancy are discussed earlier in this chapter. Changes in blood coagulation in the postoperative state include an increase in some of the intrinsic coagulation factors, especially factors VIII, IX, and X. Fibrinogen, circulating fibrinolysin inhibitors, and platelet adhesiveness and aggregation are also increased within 72 to 92 hours following surgery. Tissue necrosis secondary to the surgical procedure may result in the release of thromboplastinlike substances.

Gynecologic surgery, whether for benign or malignant disease, frequently results in trauma to the walls of the pelvic veins. There are extensive venous

Table 21–5 Clotting Factor Changes with Combined Estrogen-Progesterone Tablets

Increased clotting factors

Fibrinogen (I)
Prothrombin (II)
Proconvertin (VII)
Antihemophilic globulin (VIII)
Plasma thromboplastin component (IX)
Stuart-Prower factor (X)

Related substances which are increased

Fibrinolysin
Antifibrinolysin
Plasminogen
Platelet aggregation and sensitivity
Venous disability

Decreased factors

Antithrombin III
Heparin tolerance
Clotting time
Venous flow rate

Source: MacDonald.

collateral vessels in the female reproductive organs, and postoperative pelvic infection which frequently develops, contributes to venous thrombosis. Major trauma to the pelvic and groin veins occurs during the lymphadenectomy which accompanies radical surgical treatment of cervical and vulvar cancer. Pelvic thrombophlebitis may be seen as a complication of sepsis during pregnancy, especially with chorioamnionitis and infected abortion.

Venous stasis plays an extremely important role in the production of venous thrombosis. It results in platelet aggregation with adhesion to the vein wall, and the release of procoagulant substances which form an initial platelet, fibrin, and erythrocyte network. This process eventually leads to thrombus formation.

It is obvious that the increasing uterine mass in pregnancy results in diminished venous return from the lower extremities and the pelvic veins. Patients with large ovarian and uterine neoplasms also suffer from this pressure effect. Immobilization during the preoperative, operative, and postoperative periods is directly related to the frequency of thromboembolic complications. Breneman does not recommend that the patient be admitted to the hospital for prolonged preoperative investigations as his study showed an increase of venous thrombosis in these patients. Diagnostic evaluations should be carried out on an outpatient basis. If the patient has been hospitalized, ideally she should be operated upon after a period of at least 3 weeks of normal activity outside the hospital.

Venous return from the lower extremities falls to approximately one-half its normal rate during pelvic surgery. This is due to the positioning of the patient and to the loss of muscle tone secondary to deep anesthesia and the use of muscle relaxants. Tight packing of the intestines in the upper abdomen may put pressure on the inferior vena cava, leading to stasis in the veins of the pelvis and lower extremities. The surgeon or his assistants may lean on the patient's thighs or hips during surgery, still further diminishing return from the lower extremities. It should be obvious that the longer the operative period, the greater the risk to the patient.

The degree of postoperative immobilization is directly related to the incidence of thromboembolism. Radical vulvectomy patients have a particularly high incidence of pulmonary embolization. These patients are frequently immobilized for as long as 3 weeks because of infection and necrosis in the groin areas.

Once venous thrombosis is established, the size of the clot is increased by platelet aggregation, which results in an extremely large friable clot. Pulmonary embolization arises from fragmentation of this clot or detachment of the entire clot from the vessel wall. If the embolus is small, the patient may suffer few symptoms and survive. If a large portion of the clot becomes detached, a major branch of the pulmonary artery may be occluded. This will cause reflex spasm of other branches of the pulmonary artery and frequently death, probably in association with cardiac arrest.

Diagnosis

Pulmonary infarction always presents a problem in diagnosis. This is unfortunate, since many patients will die from a recurrent episode while the physician debates the possibility of pulmonary embolization.

A very high index of suspicion is necessary. It is important to define the high-risk patient who is likely to develop thromboembolic disease. The following factors have been shown to increase the incidence of pulmonary embolization: age over 45 years, obesity, immobility or paralysis, pulmonary disease, cardiac disease, diabetes mellitus, malignancy, ascites, polycythemia, varicose veins, a history of thrombophlebitis, prolonged air travel, hormone therapy, and pregnancy. As mentioned previously the type and length of operation and type of anesthesia used also correlate well with the incidence of pulmonary embolization. If these high-risk factors are kept in mind, then the diagnosis of pulmonary embolization will be easier to establish in the patient who suddenly experiences chest pain or dyspnea. It should be obvious that prophylactic measures should be taken to prevent the initial thrombosis in these patients.

Clinically, small emboli may be asymptomatic. When symptoms arise, tachypnea or dyspnea is the earliest and most common feature. If the embolus is large, there may be an increase in pulmonary artery pressure which eventually will cause right ventricular strain or failure. Return to the left ventricle is impaired, the left ventricular output will fall. The patient then exhibits the usual signs and symptoms of shock: tachycardia, hypotension, coldness of the skin, and diaphoresis. Cyanosis may frequently accompany pulmonary thromboembolism. Impairment of coronary blood flow may result in angina. Diminished cerebral circulation causes confusion syncope, frequently with a feeling of impending doom. Hemoptysis and pleuritic chest pain occur after the segment supplied by the blocked artery is infarcted.

Examination of the chest may be negative or may reveal the presence of a faint friction rub with rales. With time there may be tenderness of the intercostal muscles overlying the area of pleural reaction. Neck veins are frequently distended and the central venous pressure may be elevated as a result of right ventricular failure. Pleural effusions are uncommon at an early stage but eventually may become quite massive. Abdominal examination may reveal marked muscle guarding simulating the rigidity seen in acute abdominal conditions. Examination of the legs may reveal edema of the foot or calf, tenderness along the femoral vein, or calf pain on dorsiflexion of the foot (Homan's sign). Pain in the calf may be elicited in venous thrombosis by placing a sphygmomanometer around the thigh and pumping it to a pressure of 160 mmHg (Lowenberg's sign). Excessive pressure on the calf and repeated attempts to elicit Homan's sign may cause embolization and therefore are to be discouraged. Pelvic examination may reveal the presence of uterine and parametrial tenderness consistent with pelvic infection, and the possibility of septic pelvic thrombophlebitis must be considered.

Roentgenographic examination of the chest may be useful in confirming the suspicion of pulmonary infarction. It must be emphasized that emboli frequently may not produce roentgenographic changes for days. On the other hand, frank consolidation, pleural effusion, and elevation of the diaphragm may be observed. Serial chest x-rays are required for demonstration of progressive pulmonary parenchymal changes, as well as dilatation of the main pulmonary artery and right ventricle. However, all these changes are nonspecific and may be seen in congestive failure, atelectasis, and pneumonitis.

An electrocardiogram may be of help in the differential diagnosis between pulmonary and myocardial infarction. In pulmonary embolism it may be normal or merely show a sinus tachycardia. In massive pulmonary embolization it may show right-axis deviation and right-axis strain with peaked P waves and occasionally ST segment changes indicative of right ventricular strain or ischemia. Acute cor pulmonale is almost always due to pulmonary embolization, provided a recent previous ECG tracing is known to be normal.

With pulmonary embolism the serum lactic dehydrogenase (LDH) and serum bilirubin levels may be elevated, while the serum glutamic oxaloacetic transaminase (SGOT) level is usually normal. A normal SGOT value 24 to 48 hours after the onset of chest pain almost always excludes myocardial infarction. Szucks et al. have shown that this trio of laboratory tests is only diagnostic in about 12 percent of known cases of pulmonary embolization. The LDH

level is usually elevated, but this is too nonspecific to be of diagnostic value. Arterial blood gas estimations showing low P_{O_2} and P_{CO_2} are nearly constant in acute embolism.

Scanning of the lungs with [131]I- or technetium-labeled macroaggregates of albumin has increased the diagnostic accuracy in recent years. The technique demonstrates abnormalities in the distribution of blood flow and areas of pulmonary artery obstruction, but the evidence is only presumptive, since this technique cannot differentiate between pulmonary embolization and other disease processes producing segmental decreased arterial flow, i.e., pneumonia, atelectasis, pneumothorax, carcinoma, or granulomatous diseases. However, it has greater sensitivity than the chest x-ray and will provide better screening for pulmonary abnormalities if the patient's condition permits its use.

Recently, pulmonary arteriography has been used to provide positive angiographic evidence of the extent and anatomic location of the pulmonary embolus in patients having equivocal findings suggestive of pulmonary embolization and in those with massive pulmonary embolism who may require immediate embolectomy. Many feel that pulmonary arteriography is the most definitive diagnostic study and should be employed whenever there is a serious question as to diagnosis. The pulmonary artery pressure can also be measured using this technique. McIntyre and Sasahara have reviewed this subject. However, most authorities feel that in acute embolism the combination of a positive lung scan and a low P_{O_2} and P_{CO_2} in arterial blood is the best guide to rapid and accurate diagnosis.

Treatment and Prevention

Prevention consists of the identification of the patient who is at high risk and/or the early recognition and treatment of thrombophlebitis. Mattingly and Wilkinson suggest that if thromboembolism is to be prevented, then once the high-risk patient is identified, prophylactic measures must be directed toward the most significant causative factors, namely, venous stasis in the lower extremities.

In the surgical patient, the most practical method for improving venous return from the legs is to elevate the legs 15° above the horizontal or to place the patient in the Trendelenburg position with the legs straight rather than bent at the knee. Cushioning of the heel with a pillow on the operating table will prevent compression of the deep leg veins in the calf.

Several techniques such as galvanic calf stimulation, encasing the legs in a plastic envelope with rhythmic alterations of pressure, or passive flexion and extension of the foot have been shown to improve circulation in the lower extremities during surgery.

Various drugs have been utilized in an effort to prevent surgical thrombophlebitis in the high-risk patient. Some of these drugs are heparin, sodium warfarin, dextran, and salicylates (Bonnear, Walsh; Gordon-Smith et al.; O'Brien; Sevitt, Gallagher).

In our experience the use of low-dose heparin at 3000 USP units given 2 hours before surgery, and every 8 hours thereafter for the subsequent 5 postoperative days, is an effective method of preventing postoperative venous thrombophlebitis. We agree with Gordon-Smith et al. that the incidence of venous thrombosis in the operative patient can be lowered sixfold with preoperative heparinization. Bleeding is not a problem since this dosage has a negligible effect on the clotting time.

A patient with a deep venous thrombosis should receive anticoagulant therapy if it is not contraindicated by one of the following factors: (1) blood dyscrasias (2) ulcerative lesions of the gastrointestinal tract (3) subacute bacterial endocarditis (4) severe hypertension with a history of encephalopathy, and (5) severe hepatic or renal disease. An acceptable method of anticoagulation in the patient with deep-vein thrombosis is as follows: 5000 to 10,000 units of heparin given intravenously every 4 to 6 hours. The dose is adjusted depending either on the clotting time or on partial thromboplastin time (PTT) performed 30 minutes prior to the administration of heparin. The goal of therapy is to maintain a clotting time or PTT two or three times that of normal. Alternatively, a patient may be given 10,000 units intravenously and then approximately 1000 units of heparin per hour depending upon the 6-hour clotting time or PTT. On the fifth day the patient is started on an oral anticoagulant, usually sodium warfarin, and combined therapy is maintained for about 5 days. At this time, the heparin is gradually discontinued, and the patient is maintained on the oral anticoagulant until symptoms of thrombophlebitis have subsided for 6 weeks. During this period, the prothrombin time should be determined twice weekly to adjust the dose and to keep the prothrombin time 2 to 2½ times normal. The patient is also kept on bed rest with the leg elevated until all symptoms have subsided.

In cases of iliofemoral thrombosis, immediate surgical therapy may be necessary to prevent propagation of the clot into the vena cava with pulmonary embolization. However, anticoagulant therapy should be tried first. Then thrombectomy may still be performed to remove the obstructing thrombus, and the previous anticoagulation will reduce the chances of postthrombectomy embolism or the disabling postphlebitic syndrome.

Treatment of Acute Pulmonary Thromboembolism. If acute pulmonary embolism occurs, the initial and immediate treatment is 10,000 to 15,000 USP units of intravenous heparin. This immediately improves lung perfusion while the alveolar oxygen concentration is enhanced by the use of nasal oxygen or a respirator. A decrease in the respiratory rate and an increase in the arterial PO_2 within 30 minutes indicate improvement and a more favorable prognosis. If the patient's condition deteriorates, pulmonary embolectomy may be required as an immediate lifesaving procedure. Other therapeutic adjuvants are as follows: 10 mg morphine sulfate is given and repeated in 1 hour if necessary to allay pain and anxiety. Rapid intravenous digitalization should be carried out using Cedilanid (lanatoside C). An initial dose of 0.8 mg is given intravenously, followed by 0.4 mg at 4-hour intervals to a total of 1.6 mg. If the patient survives the initial shock, she is started the next day on 0.25 mg digoxin daily. For hypotension, Aramine (metaraminol) 100 mg in 5% glucose is ideal because of its inotropic effect which improves coronary arterial perfusion and myocardial function. Aminophylline, 250 to 500 mg intravenously, may be used to alleviate dyspnea.

If the patient survives, anticoagulation with heparin is continued as before. An oral anticoagulant (sodium warfarin) is started after 1 week of heparin therapy, which is tapered off over the next 72 hours. The patient is then maintained on sodium warfarin for a period of 6 months to 1 year at a dosage level which decreases the prothrombin time to approximately 25 percent of normal.

When it is believed the embolus has arisen from the legs, the patient is confined to bed, with the legs elevated, for about 5 days.

Ligation or plication of the inferior vena cava is preferable to unilateral or even bilateral femoral ligation, even when the thrombosis is present in the deep veins of the lower leg. Indications for ligation of the vena cava are (1) thrombosis above the level of the superficial femoral vein if not responsive to thrombectomy, (2) septic thrombophlebitis of the pelvic veins, (3) embolism occurring from the lower extremities despite the use of prophylactic anticoagulant therapy. In cases of recurrent embolization, venography, pulmonary arteriography, and cardiac catheterization should be performed to rule out sites of thrombus formation proximal to the proposed site of ligation.

Although there are numerous methods for interruption of the vena cava, the serrated vena cava clip has gained some preference. It is effective in arresting large and potentially lethal emboli, and rarely gives rise to late sequelae such as disabling leg edema and ulceration (Bowers, Leb; Miles, Elsea). The transjugular insertion of a heparinized silastic umbrella into the inferior vena cava has been recommended by Mobin-Uddin et al. This procedure avoids celiotomy and is particularly indicated for persons with severe cardiac disease who have suffered a pulmonary embolism.

AIR EMBOLISM

Fortunately, this condition is rare. It may occur following delivery if air enters the venous sinuses from the placental site after manual removal of the placenta or as a result of pumping blood to a patient being treated for hemorrhagic shock. Air embolism has also been reported in pregnant women following blowing into the vagina during sexual activities, and following uterotubal insufflation in infertility patients.

Although a small amount of air may be introduced into the circulation with relative impunity, a large accumulation of air in the right side of the heart interferes with cardiac valvular function. In addition, the presence of air in the pulmonary artery obstructs the flow of blood to the lungs.

Management

1. The patient's head should be lowered to minimize the possibility of cerebral air embolism.
2. The patient should be placed in the left lateral position in an effort to release the air lock in the pulmonary outflow tract.
3. A large-bore needle (18 gauge) may be inserted into the right ventricle to achieve release of the trapped air. This can also be done by running a central venous pressure catheter into the right ventricle.
4. An emergency thoracotomy should be performed if improvement is not seen within 2 minutes. This will permit direct aspiration of air from the right side of the heart.
5. A good airway should be obtained by using a pharyngeal endotracheal tube. Adequate oxygen administration is essential.

NEUROGENIC SHOCK

ASPIRATION OF VOMITUS

Aspiration of vomitus is the most common cause of death associated with general anesthesia. It can also occur in the presence of high spinal anesthesia.

Cause

1. General anesthesia with a full stomach. During the course of labor the stomach may take 12 hours or even up to 48 hours to empty.
2. With high spinal anesthesia, the patient may be unable to expel vomitus refluxing into the pharynx from the stomach. Thus, it should be kept in mind that spinal anesthesia does not necessarily protect the patient from the dangers of aspiration.

Prevention

1. All solid foods should be eliminated and oral fluids limited during labor.
2. Unless contraindicated, regional anesthesia should be given to patients who have eaten within 12 hours.
3. If general anesthesia is essential for delivery of a particular patient, and she has eaten within 12 hours, a large-caliber stomach tube should be passed. The patient will then empty her stomach spontaneously or the contents can be aspirated. In addition, a cuffed endotracheal tube should be used during anesthesia. The inflated balloon prevents aspiration should reflux of the stomach contents occur despite the foregoing precautions.
4. Combat hypotension following spinal or epidural anesthesia which can result in loss of consciousness with accompanying loss of protective upper respiratory tract reflexes.
5. Give 30 mL magnesium trisilicate orally about 30 minutes before induction. This will raise the pH of stomach contents. If the pH of the stomach contents is less that 2.0 and the patient aspirates a chemical substance, pneumonitis will develop.
6. Use pressure on the cricoid cartilage so that it is pushed cephalad and posteriorly in order to occlude the esophagus. This pressure should be applied from the time the patient is asleep until intubation has been completed and the cuff inflated.
7. The endotracheal tube should not be removed until the patient has regained consciousness.

8. Make sure that in addition to an ample supply of oxygen, a suction apparatus is available before inducing general anesthesia.

Management

1. The mask must be removed and the patient's head turned to one side. At the same time the table should be converted to a steep Trendelenburg position.
2. Using a jaw retractor, the fingers of the right hand are inserted behind the patient's last molar tooth to force the jaw open.
3. Solid material should be scooped out with gauze around the fingers of the anesthetist.
4. The pharynx should be suctioned rapidly with a large-caliber suction tip.
5. Oxygen should be given under pressure in an effort to break the associated laryngospasm. If a satisfactory response is obtained by this time, the patient is turned over to the semiprone position and postural coughing encouraged.
6. If respiratory distress develops, an endotracheal tube must be passed immediately and the tracheal contents aspirated.
7. If the pulse weakens or slows and cyanosis persists, a tracheostomy should be carried out. The trachea is quickly aspirated and oxgyen supplied through a soft rubber catheter. If difficulty persists, it is suggested that, if solid material is still present in the bronchi, bronchoscopy should be carried out without delay. Even if cardiac arrest occurs, closed chest cardiac massage should be performed as described previously.

Postoperative Care

1. An x-ray of the chest must be obtained immediately postoperatively.
2. Postural coughing must be encouraged.
3. The patient must be observed for clinical or radiographic evidence of lung collapse or pneumonitis, and these conditions should be treated.
4. If the pH of the material aspirated from the trachea is less than 2.0, or if wheezing and bronchospasm are present, one should assume that acid aspiration has occurred.

If acid aspiration has occurred, it must be appreciated that a serious problem exists, even though there is no solid material in the patient's stomach. Hydrocortisone, 200 mg, should be given intravenously immediately, followed by an additional 100 mg intravenously every 4 hours. This dosage should be continued until the chest x-ray reverts to normal or at least for 24 hours if the chest x-ray shows no significant changes. If bronchospasm occurs, the patient should be given a continuous intravenous infusion of aminophyllin, 500 mg in 500 mL 5% dextrose. In addition, positive-pressure ventilation should provide sufficient oxygen to maintain arterial oxygen tension at 90 to 100 mmHg.

Antibiotic coverage should be given to these patients on the basis of a Gram-stained smear and culture of the aspirate taken from the trachea. Ampicillin, 1 g every 6 hours, should be given intravenously unless contraindicated.

A chest x-ray is obtained every 12 to 24 hours. The right lung is more often affected than the left. Acid aspiration is indicated by soft, irregular mottling, and solid aspiration shows uniform densities with some degree of mediastinal shift.

The patient should be kept in the intensive care unit for continuous monitoring and treatment and is given oxygen, with a mechanical respirator being used as necessary. Blood gas determinations are made frequently, and a tracheostomy set is kept by the patient's bedside.

SPINAL HYPOTENSION

High spinal anesthesia resulting in respiratory paralysis and cardiogenic shock is second only to aspiration of vomitus as a cause of maternal anesthetic death. Spinal hypotension can occur with improperly given caudal or epidural anesthesia. The basic problem is that the capacity of the vascular bed is suddenly increased with the production of relative hypovolemia.

Prevention

1. All spinal anesthetics must be given slowly. With all types of drugs, the minimum dose for the effect desired should be used. It must be appreciated that the dose for spinal anesthesia in the pregnant woman is approximately half the dose needed for the same patient in the nonpregnant state.
2. The blood pressure must be taken every 30 seconds for at least 5 minutes after a spinal anesthetic has been given.
3. Spinal anesthesia should be avoided in women with essential hypertension in pregnancy, recent hemorrhage, or anemia.

Management

Following spinal anesthesia, the patient may suddenly become stuporous, cold, and hypotensive. Occasionally convulsions may occur. In such cases the following steps should be taken:

1. The patient's legs should be elevated 90 degrees. With this simple procedure about 700 mL of blood becomes immediately available to the rest of the circulation. The table should *not* be adjusted for the Trendelenburg position, and two pillows must be kept under the patient's head and shoulders.
2. Oxygen is given by mask.
3. The rate of intravenous infusion of 5% dextrose in water is increased.
4. Ephedrine, 12.5 mg, is given intravenously, and the same dose is repeated in 3 minutes if no blood pressure response is shown.
5. If hypotension persists, the patient is placed on her side in the left lateral position so that hypotension is not aggravated by compression of the inferior vena cava by the gravid uterus.
6. If cardiovascular collapse occurs, it should be treated as previously outlined.

INVERSION OF THE UTERUS

This condition is probably more common than is reported. Most cases are associated with mismanagement of the third stage of labor by placing excessive fundal pressure or excessive traction on the cord in an attempt to deliver the placenta.

REFERENCES

Alkajaersig N et al.: The mechanism of clot dissolution by plasmin. *J Clin Invest* 38:1086, 1959.

Altchek A, Litwak RS: Amniotic fluid pulmonary embolism. *Obstet Gynecol* 27:885, 1966.

Bachmann F: Aterogen, thrombogen, and pyridinolcarb treatment. *Proceedings of the First International Symposium, Tokyo 1969, Amsterdam.* Excerpta Medica, 1969, p. 87.

Bauer WE et al.: The role of catecholamines in energy metabolism during prolonged hemorrhagic shock. *Surg Forum* 20:9, 1969.

Bonnar J, Walsh J: Prevention of thrombosis after pelvic surgery by British Dextran 70. *Lancet* 1:614, 1972.

Bowers, RF, Leb SM: Late results of vena cava ligation. *Surgery* 37:622, 1955.

Breneman JC: Postoperative thromboembolic disease: Computer analysis leading to statistical prediction. *JAMA* 193:576, 1965.

Cavanagh D et al.: Rupture of the gravid uterus: An appraisal *Obstet Gynecol* 26:157, 1965.

_____, Rao PS: Septic shock (endotoxic shock). *Clin Obstet Gynecol* vol. 16: no. 2.

_____ et al.: Pathophysiology of endotoxin shock in the primate. *Am J Obstet Gynecol* 108:705, 1970.

_____ et al.: Septic abortion with endotoxic shock. *Aust NZ J Obstet Gynecol* 10:160, 1970a.

_____ et al.: *Septic Shock in Obstetrics and Gynecology,* Philadelphia: Saunders, 1977.

_____ et al.: *Obstetric Emergencies,* Hagerstown, Md.: Harper and Row, 1978.

Coleman BD: Septic shock in pregnancy. *Obstet Gynecol* 24:895, 1964.

Collins CG: Suppurative thrombophlebitis of the pelvis. *Am J Obstet Gynecol* 108:681, 1970.

DeCenzo JA et al.: Endotoxin shock. *Obstet Gynecol* 22:8, 1963.

Douglas GW, Bechman EM: Clinical management of septic abortion complicated by hypotension. *Am J Obstet Gynecol* 96:633, 1966.

Evensen, SA et al.: The effect of endotoxin on factor VII in rats: In vivo and in vitro observations. *Scand J Clin Lab Invest* 18:509, 1966.

Flanc C et al.: The detection of venous thrombosis of the legs using 125-I labeled fibrinogen. *Br J Surg* 55:742, 1968.

Gilbert RP: Endotoxin shock in the primate. *Proc Soc Exp Biol Med* 3:328, 1962.

Good RA, Thomas L: Studies on the generalized Shwartzman reaction II. The production of bilateral cortical necrosis of the kidneys by a single injection of bacterial toxin in rabbits previously treated with Thorotrast or Trypan blue. *J Exp Med* 96:625, 1952.

_____: Studies on the generalized Shwartzman reaction. IV. Prevention of the local and generalized Shwartzman reactions with heparin. *J Exp Med* 97:871, 1953.

Gordon-Smith JC et al.: Controlled trial of two regimens of subcutaneous heparin in the prevention of postoperative deep-vein thrombosis. *Lancet* 1:1133, 1972.

Gregory MG, Clayton EM: Amniotic fluid embolism. *Obstet Gynecol* 42:236, 1973.

Gross P, Benz EJ: Pulmonary embolism by amniotic fluid: Report of 3 cases with new diagnostic procedure. *Surg Gynecol Obstet* 85:315, 1947.

Gunter CA et al.: Cardiorespiratory and metabolic response to live *E. coli* and endotoxin in the monkey. *J Appl Physiol* 26:780, 1970.

Hampton JW, Matthews C: Similarities between baboon and human blood clotting. *J Appl Physiol* 21:1713, 1966.

Hinshaw LB et al.: Cardiovascular responses of the primate in endotoxin shock. *Am J Physiol* 210:335, 1966.

Holemans R, Silver, MJ: in *Dynamics of Thrombus Formation and Dissolution,* eds. SA Johnson, MM Guest, Philadelphia: Lippincott, 1969, p. 307.

Hopkins RW et al.: Hemodynamic aspects of hemorrhagic and septic shock. *JAMA* 191:731, 1965.

Jimenez JM, Pritchard JA: Pathogenesis and treatment of the coagulation defects resulting from fetal death. *Obstet Gynecol* 32:449, 1968.

Koch ML: Bacteremia due to bacterial species of genera *Aerobacter, Escherichia, Paracolobactrum, Proteus* and *Pseudomonas. Antibiotic Med* 2:113, 1956.

Lillehei RC et al.: Physiology and therapy of bacteremic shock. *Am J Cardiol* 12:599, 1963.

_____, McLean LD: The intestinal factor in irreversible endotoxin shock. *Ann Surg* 148:513, 1958.

Lushbaugh CC, Steiner PE: Additional observations on maternal pulmonary embolism by amniotic fluid. *Am J Obstet Gynecol* 48:833, 1942.

MacDonald R: *Scientific Basis of Obstetrics and Gynaecology,* Baltimore: Williams & Wilkins, 1971, chap. 13.

Mattingly RF, Wilkinson EJ: Thromboembolism in pelvic surgery. *Clin Obstet Gynecol* 16:162, 1973.

McIntyre KM, Sasahara AA: The hemodynamic response to pulmonary embolism in patients without previous cardiopulmonary disease. *Am J Cardiol* 28:288, 1971.

McKay DG: *Disseminated Intravascular Coagulation: An Intermediary Mechanism of Disease,* New York: Hoeber-Harper, 1965.

_____ et al.: Endotoxin shock and the generalized Schwartzman reaction in pregnancy. *Am J Obstet Gynecol* 78:546, 1959.

Miles RM, Elsea PW: Clinical evaluation of the serrated vena cava clip. *Surg Gynecol Obstet* 132:581, 1971.

Mobin-Uddin K et al.: Transcaval interruption with umbrella filter. *N Engl J Med* 286:55, 1972.

O'Brien JR: A trial of aspirin in postoperative venous thrombosis (abstr.). *Third Congress of the International Society on Thrombosis and Haemostasis,* August 22, 1972, p. 42.

O'Driscoll K, McCarthy JR: Abruptio placentae and central venous pressures *J Obstet Gynecol Br Commonw* 73:923, 1966.

Owen CA, Bowie EJW: The intravascular coagulation—fibrinolysis syndromes in obstetrics and gynecology. *Current Concepts,* Kalamazoo: Upjohn Company, 1976.

Phillips LL, Quigley HJ: Coagulation disorders in pregnancy, in *Advances in Obstetrics and Gynecology,* vol. 1, eds. CC Marcus, SL Marcus, Baltimore: Williams and Wilkins, 1967.

Pritchard JA: Fetal death in utero. *Obstet Gynecol* 14:573, 1959.

Rao PS, Cavanagh D: Endotoxin shock in the subhuman primate. II. Some effects of methyl prednisolone administration. *Arch Surg* 102:486, 1971.

_____ et al.: unpublished data.

Reid DE et al.: Intravascular clotting and afibrinogenemia, the presumptive lethal factors in the syndrome of amniotic fluid embolism. *Am J Obstet Gynecol* 66:465, 1953.

Sevitt S, Gallagher NG: Prevention of venous thrombosis and pulmonary embolism in injured patients: A trial of anticoagulant prophylaxis with phenidione in middle-aged and elderly patients with fractured necks of the femur. *Lancet* 2:981.

Shubin, H, Weil MH: Bacterial shocks: A serious complication in urological practice. *JAMA* 185:850, 1963.

Simeone FA: Hemorrhagic shock. *Amer J Cardiol* 12:589, 1963.

Stander RW et al.: Changes in maternal coagulation factors after intraamniotic injection of hypertonic saline. *Obstet Gynecol* 37:660, 1971.

Studdiford WE, Douglas GW: Placental bacteremia: A significant finding in septic abortion accompanied by vascular collapse. *Am J Obstet Gynecol* 71:842, 1956.

Szucks MM et al.: Diagnostic sensitivity of laboratory findings in acute pulmonary embolism. *Ann Intern Med* 74:161, 1971.

Thomas L: The physiological disturbances produced by endotoxins. *Ann Rev Physiol* 16:467, 1954.

_____, Good RA: Studies on the generalized Shwartzman phenomenon. I. General observations concerning the phenomenon. *J Exp Med* 96:605, 1952.

Tricomi V, Kohl SG: Fetal death in utero. *Am J Obstet Gynecol* 74:1092, 1957.

Ts'ao CH, Kline DL: Plasminogen activator formed by reaction of streptokinase with human plasminogen. *J Appl Physiol* 26:634, 1969.

Udhoji VN, Weil MH: Hemodynamic and metabolic

studies on shock associated with bacteremia. Observations on 16 patients. *Ann Intern Med* 62:966, 1965.

Virchow R.: *Handbuch der Speziallen Pathologie und Therapie,* V. II, Stuttgart: Enke, 1854.

Wilson RF et al.: Hemodynamic measurements in septic shock. *Arch Surg* 91:121, 1965.

Wise RI et al.: The syndrome of vascular collapse due to gram negative bacteria. Its management with L-norepinephrine and antibiotics. *J Lab Clin Med* 40:961, 1952.

22

Pain

RICHARD W. STANDER

BREAST

Breast pain is one of the most common complaints
heard by those responsible for the health care of

women. Although breast pain is seldom the initial harbinger of mammary cancer, it is fear of cancer that often prompts patients to report the symptom of pain upon its earliest appearance. Evaluation of the pain and appropriate diagnostic measures will usually reveal the cause to be other than cancer. Thus informed, the patient may be relieved of significant anxiety.

NONLACTATING BREAST

CYCLIC PAIN

Cyclic discomfort in the nonlactating breast is the most common type of breast pain encountered. It may occur at any time during the reproductive years but is more common in the fourth and fifth decades than in earlier years. This discomfort tends to be bilateral and related to menses in that pain appears during the progestational phase of the cycle, increases as the menstrual period approaches, and is alleviated or obviated with the onset of menstruation. The pain is clearly related to ovarian endocrine activity. A similar discomfort may be induced in postmenopausal patients treated with estrogen and may also be observed during the initial days of birth control pill ingestion. This type of pain is often self-limited and is not incapacitating.

More severe forms of cyclic pain may accompany chronic cystic mastitis (see Chap. 46). These lesions may appear late in the third decade and increase in frequency until the menopause. A variety of physical findings may be present in patients with breast pain accompanying chronic cystic disease.

NONCYCLIC PAIN

Persistent breast pain is usually unilateral and is often related to solitary breast lesions, most of which are benign. When pain is accompanied by erythema at the periphery of the areola and temperature elevation, one should suspect periductal mastitis. This is the most common inflammatory condition of the nonlactating breast.

Persistent breast pain may be found after trauma or surgery and results from fat necrosis. Concomitant induration and varying degrees of skin adherence are usually noted. Fat necrosis with resulting discomfort

may also occur spontaneously, particularly in women with large, pendulous breasts.

Pain accompanying breast cancer usually indicates advanced disease and is seldom noted with early lesions.

LACTATING BREAST

Generalized breast pain is common during the period between delivery and the onset of lactation. Known as the period of engorgement, it produces extreme discomfort requiring the use of ice packs and/or analgesics.

Caking of the breast may occur during the initial days of lactation, resulting in unilateral or bilateral discomfort. Irregular firm areas will be noted throughout the breasts, although there will be no local or systemic signs of inflammation.

Mastitis during lactation is accompanied initially by diffuse pain throughout the affected breast, induration, erythema, and temperature elevation. As the process becomes localized, and if abscess formation ensues, diffuse pain gives way to pain of a more circumscribed nature (see Chap. 30).

HEADACHE

Excluding headache secondary to obvious maladies such as meningitis or cerebral tumor, the symptom of headache resulting from vascular causes or tension is commonly reported to the gynecologist.

MIGRAINE HEADACHE

Migraine headache is a type of vascular headache which is episodic and of relatively brief duration. Between episodes there are intervals of complete freedom from symptoms. In many patients, there are associated transient neurologic or gastrointestinal symptoms. Migraine headache is rare before the age of 10 and afflicts females more often than males. The maximum incidence tends to be in the third and fourth decades, with attacks declining in frequency thereafter. Frequency of migraine headaches also tends to decrease during pregnancy. These headaches often occur in those with obsessive-compulsive characteristics. Although an allergy is rarely the cause, there is a high incidence of allergy in the family and medical history of migraine sufferers. It is well known that sodium and water retention may trigger attacks in those who are prone. As a consequence, in ovulating females, migraine headaches are seen more frequently in the immediate premenstrual portion of the menstrual cycle. It has also been noted that administration of steroids as used in contraceptive pills may be associated with migraine headaches.

Prior to onset of headache, neurologic symptoms of the "classical" migraine may be present. These may include blurring of vision in one or both eyes, bright colors, central scotomas, tunnel vision, homonymous hemianopia, or even complete blindness. A variety of other symptoms, including parasthesias have been described. Quite often, however, premonitory neurologic symptoms are minor or entirely lacking.

The headache is often unilateral but may be bilateral. It may be occipital or frontal in location and may involve the upper part of the neck. It has a throbbing quality that is aggravated by lying down or physical effort. It may last for a period of a few hours to 1 or 2 days. Photophobia may accompany the pain. Nausea is often present at some time during the attack and may lead to vomiting of a protracted nature. Although severe abdominal pain is rare, it may appear early in migraine headache and be mistaken for an abdominal emergency.

In rare instances when migraine headaches are seen in the prepubertal female, attacks tend to disappear with the onset of menstruation. At the other end of the reproductive spectrum, onset of migraine headaches may be noted in the perimenopausal period. Under these circumstances, recurrent attacks are seldom present for more than a year or two and may be secondary to vascular instability accompanying the irregular production of ovarian steroids.

TENSION HEADACHE

These headaches are usually of a persistent or continuous nature rather than throbbing or intermittent. Patients may liken them to a sensation of weight or pressure on the head or describe them as a tight band around the head. They are often accompanied by a sense of mental or physical fatigue and may be aggravated by mental effort, stuffy atmospheres, or emotional stresses. In certain individuals the symptoms of tension headache may be subconsciously perverted

or exaggerated, resulting in a description of pain that may seem bizarre, e.g., the sensation of "a nail being driven into my skull."

HEADACHE SECONDARY TO ARTERIAL HYPERTENSION

In the nonpregnant female, significant headache secondary to hypertension is often found in the malignant phase of the disease. It is characteristically occipital in location, throbbing in nature, and is most frequently present upon awakening. It may last only a short while and tends to improve as the day progresses. Onset of headaches of this type in late pregnancy may represent an exacerbation of essential hypertension, but in patients who have been previously normotensive throughout pregnancy, such headaches may represent the first symptom of a rapidly developing toxemia of pregnancy (see Chap. 30).

ABDOMINAL AND PELVIC PAIN

ACUTE ABDOMINAL PAIN

Evaluation of acute abdominal pain and an early correct diagnosis are of utmost importance. Acute cholecystitis, appendicitis, perforation of bowel, twisted ovarian cyst, or ectopic pregnancy may be readily dealt with if diagnosis is promptly made and appropriate treatment is carried out. Significant delay in diagnosis will increase the chances of morbidity and mortality. Vital to a correct diagnosis is an accurate history with special attention paid to the following.

Onset of Pain. Sudden onset of pain is most frequently caused by perforation of a hollow viscus or by ischemia such as might occur from mesenteric thrombosis. In disorders involving obstruction of a hollow viscus or inflammation of its walls, the onset of pain may be more insidious, requiring several hours to reach its peak. This pattern may be seen in intestinal obstruction, acute cholecystitis, appendicitis, and salpingitis.

Character of Pain. Colic is the most commonly seen type of abdominal pain and is caused by muscular contraction of an obstructed hollow viscus such as intestine, ureter, gallbladder, or appendix.

Location of Pain. Pain involving the entire abdomen from the onset or shortly thereafter suggests a generalized reaction to an irritating fluid flooding the peritoneal cavity, as with rupture of a tuboovarian abscess. If pain initially located in the epigastrium then shifts to the right lower quadrant, local inflammation of the parietal peritoneum is indicated; depending upon the location, this type of pain may represent a localized inflammatory process such as cholecystitis, peritonitis, or appendicitis.

Referred abdominal pain provides some insight into the location of the primary disease process. Midepigastric pain is associated with structures innervated by T_6 through T_8, such as stomach, duodenum, pancreas, liver, and biliary tree. Periumbilical pain may stem from disorders in structures innervated by T_9 and T_{10}, such as colon, bladder, uterus, and lower ureters.

Vomiting. Vomiting may accompany any kind of severe abdominal pain. It tends to occur early in appendicitis and cholecystitis. With obstructive lesions, vomiting is more likely to appear later, and it increases in frequency as obstruction increases.

Gynecologic History. Acute abdominal pain following a delay in menses suggests ectopic pregnancy. Abdominal pain with onset during or shortly after menstruation may indicate acute salpingitis.

ACUTE ABDOMINAL PAIN RELATED TO THE GASTROINTESTINAL TRACT

APPENDICITIS

Epigastric discomfort without evidence of right lower quadrant tenderness may be the first symptom of appendicitis. This is usually followed by anorexia, then nausea and vomiting. In a matter of hours, pain generally shifts to the right lower quadrant and tenderness will be elicited upon deep palpation over McBurney's point. A low-grade fever and leukocytosis are generally present. The appearance of generalized abdominal tenderness at this time suggests perforation with peritonitis, while palpation of a right lower quadrant mass may indicate abscess formation with the inflammatory process localized in a specific portion of the abdomen. Only 40 percent of patients follow this "classical" pattern of developing abdominal symptoms. Atypical abdominal pain may occur when the appendix is not in its usual position. In pregnancy, the gravid uterus carries the mobile cecum and ap-

pendix upward so that characteristic right lower quadrant pain may not occur. A retrocecal appendix can mimic disease of the gallbladder or duodenum, while inflammation of a pelvic appendix can imitate diverticulitis or disease of the fallopian tube or ovary or may produce symptoms involving the bladder. In such atypical cases, the diagnosis may be evident by doing *serial* abdominal, pelvic, and rectal examinations supported by appropriate laboratory studies.

ACUTE DIVERTICULITIS

Acute diverticulitis most often involves the sigmoid colon, and pain is referred to the left lower quadrant. Although it may appear with no preceding symptoms, in many individuals it follows a long history of symptoms of irritable colon and occurs with increasing frequency with advancing years. Fever and leukocytosis are common. Constipation and nausea frequently are observed, but vomiting is uncommon. Diverticulitis is less likely to lead to perforation and peritonitis than is appendicitis. It normally subsides after a few days, but the patient is subject to recurrent attacks.

ACUTE CHOLECYSTITIS

Acute cholecystitis is usually accompanied by pain in the right upper quadrant and in the epigastrium. In 90 percent of cases it is associated with a gallstone impacted in the cystic duct. The pain is steady in nature, but obstruction of the cystic duct by infection or stone will superimpose pain of a colicky nature. Nausea, vomiting, and mild temperature elevation are often seen in severe attacks. Leukocytosis is common, and bilirubinemia and bilirubinuria are usually detected several hours after the attack.

ACUTE PANCREATITIS

The presenting picture of acute pancreatitis is extremely variable, ranging from rapid onset of severe epigastric pain, followed by shock and cyanosis, to repeated episodes of deep epigastric pain accompanied by vomiting. Pain is often referred to the interscapular area. This picture is often attributed to alcoholic gastritis, since acute pancreatitis is frequently seen in alcoholics. In addition to alcoholism, acute pancreatitis is frequently encountered with peptic ulcer and cholelithiasis and as a postoperative complication, particularly following surgical procedures on the stomach or the biliary tree. Fever and leukocytosis generally accompany an acute attack. Marked elevation of serum amylase is frequently encountered but generally returns to normal in 48 to 72 hours.

PERFORATION OF PEPTIC ULCER

Perforation of peptic ulcer occurs less frequently in females than in males. Ninety percent of patients with perforation give a history of dyspeptic symptoms compatible with ulcer and preceding perforation by months or years. In an occasional patient, however, perforation may be the first sign of ulcer.

As gastric contents escape, severe pain first appears in the epigastrium and then spreads rapidly to involve the entire abdomen. The patient appears to be severely ill with shallow respirations and a rigid abdomen. Fluid may be detectable in the flanks on physical examination, and liver dullness may not be percussible if a large amount of air has escaped into the peritoneal cavity. In most cases, intraabdominal air can be detected with upright or lateral decubitus x-rays.

PAIN ASSOCIATED WITH INTESTINAL OBSTRUCTION

Intestinal obstruction is heralded by the onset of colicky abdominal pain followed by abdominal distention, vomiting, and constipation. Regardless of the cause of obstruction, several widely accepted generalizations have been made concerning intestinal obstruction.

1. The higher the obstruction and the more acute the obstruction is, the earlier vomiting will appear.
2. The lower the obstruction and the greater the abdominal distention, the more likely it is to be associated with constipation.
3. Vomiting with intestinal obstruction first consists of gastric contents, followed by bile, and then material with a fecal odor.
4. At the onset of mechanical intestinal obstruction, bowel sounds are high pitched and are maximal when the patient is suffering an identifiable attack of colicky pain.

ACUTE PAIN ASSOCIATED WITH THE URINARY TRACT—URETERAL COLIC

Severe pain may be caused by a sudden increase in intraluminal ureteral pressure, most often as a result of a ureteral calculus, but also from inflammation, trauma, or pressure from a source external to the ureter. Typically, there is sudden onset of pain in the back at the costovertebral angle. Pain may remain localized there if obstruction occurs where the ureter crosses the pelvic brim. Obstruction at a lower site may result in ipsilateral abdominal pain. Obstruction at the ureterovesical junction may cause additional pain to be referred to the labium majus on the affected side.

ACUTE PAIN ASSOCIATED WITH THE REPRODUCTIVE TRACT DURING PREGNANCY

ECTOPIC PREGNANCY (See Chap. 30)

Implantation of the ovum in a site other than the uterine cavity may produce pain. With tubal implantation, the most common type of ectopic pregnancy, the initial pain is caused by peritoneal distention as the fallopian tube is unable to accommodate the enlarging products of conception. Invasion of the wall of the fallopian tube by trophoblastic elements also contributes to lower abdominal and pelvic pain which may be dull and aching at first but will progress to a sharp and localized pain as pregnancy advances. At this point tubal rupture is imminent. When rupture occurs, the localized abdominal pain tends to be temporarily relieved and is replaced by generalized lower abdominal and pelvic pain as hemoperitoneum progresses following rupture. Most often, pain is preceded by a period of amenorrhea, and pregnancy is suspected. This is followed by spotting or irregular bleeding and the onset of pain. The pain may be intermittent for a period of several days or progress rapidly and become severe within a few hours. If blood or the mass is in the cul-de-sac, abdominal and pelvic pain may be accompanied by an urge to defecate. On abdominal examination, there is usually tenderness or guarding in one or both lower quadrants, but seldom is an abdominal mass present. Pelvic examination generally reveals marked pelvic tenderness on motion of the cervix. Adnexal tenderness is present and is generally more pronounced on one side, although a specific mass can be palpated in only about one-half of the cases. Nausea and vomiting are rare.

Abdominal pregnancy may also be associated with abdominal pain which has a more insidious onset and appears later in pregnancy. Partial or complete bowel obstruction may result with classic symptoms of intermittent colicky pain or colicky pain progressing to the ileus with associated vomiting.

In both forms of ectopic pregnancy, leukocytosis and low-grade fever with progressive anemia may indicate internal bleeding (see Chap. 30).

ABRUPTIO PLACENTAE

Acute abdominal pain in late pregnancy may result from premature separation of the placenta with formation of retroplacental hematoma and infiltration of the myometrium by blood. It may also occur prior to or during any stage of labor. Seldom associated with abdominal trauma, it occurs more frequently in patients with hypertensive disorders complicating pregnancy, i.e., essential hypertension or toxemia of pregnancy. The degree of abdominal pain correlates with the degree of premature separation. Pain is mild or absent with minimal separation and is usually severe when associated with total premature separation of placenta. The pain is unremitting and may be referred to any area of the abdominal wall over the gravid uterus and occasionally is referred to the back. Abdominal findings vary from mild tenderness elicited upon abdominal palpation of the uterus to severe pain with boardlike rigidity of the uterus. In total abruption, fetal heart tones will be absent. Aberrations of fetal heart tones may be present if premature separation is incomplete. Vaginal bleeding usually accompanies the onset of pain, but on occasion it may not be noted until several hours after the pain began. Shock and a falling hemoglobin or hematocrit may reflect the degree of intrauterine blood loss more accurately than an estimation of the rate of vaginal blood loss (see Chap. 30).

UTERINE RUPTURE

Acute abdominal pain in pregnancy may result from uterine rupture. This catastrophic event may precede the onset of labor when there is a history of previous uterine incision such as cesarean section. The uterus may rupture during labor at the site of a defective uterine scar or as a result of obstructed labor or the injudicious use of oxytocics. The pain of uterine rupture is often described as an acute tearing sensation that is extremely brief. If the fetus is extruded into the abdominal cavity as a result of uterine rupture, fetal heart tones will disappear following the acute pain (see Chap. 30).

OTHER CAUSES

Acute abdominal pain originating in the reproductive tract during pregnancy can also occur from degeneration of a leiomyoma or torsion of an ovarian cyst.

Although many of the causes of acute abdominal pain stemming from the gastrointestinal tract can be observed during pregnancy, an additional cause of pain may be listed for pregnancy. Although rare, it should be mentioned that sudden onset of pain in the right upper quadrant of a patient with toxemia of pregnancy may herald impending convulsion. This pain is thought to be secondary to stretching of the liver capsule by an abnormal intracapsular accumulation of fluid (see Chap. 30).

ACUTE PAIN ASSOCIATED WITH THE REPRODUCTIVE TRACT IN THE NONPREGNANT WOMAN

ACUTE SALPINGITIS

Acute salpingitis most often results from gonococcal infection. Infection may be confined to the cervix until the time of menstruation at which time it may ascend to the fallopian tubes via the endometrial cavity. Acute salpingitis produces severe lower abdominal pain which gradually increases over several hours. Abdominal findings include severe lower abdominal tenderness and guarding. Vomiting is infrequent in the early stages of the disease, and bowel sounds are usually normal. Pelvic examination will usually reveal a copious purulent discharge emanating from the external os of the cervix; and motion of the cervix will elicit exquisite pelvic tenderness. Evaluation of the pelvis is difficult because of acute pain, but lack of a discrete mass helps differentiate acute salpingitis from a twisted ovarian cyst. Fever and leukocytosis generally accompany acute salpingitis (see Chaps. 11 and 44).

DEGENERATING FIBROID

Uterine fibroids are the most common pelvic neoplasms in the female. Growth is slow, although the aggregate uterine mass may reach a very large size. Pelvic discomfort from uterine fibroids most often occurs because of encroachment upon adjacent bladder or rectum. On occasion, however, acute abdominal and/or pelvic pain results from necrosis secondary to loss of blood supply. In such instances, pain may be constant and severe, and bimanual palpation of the uterus may elicit extreme tenderness. Low-grade fever and leukocytosis may be observed (see Chap. 42).

TORSION OF OVARIAN CYST

Acute lower abdominal and pelvic pain with a rapid onset may occur when an ovarian cyst is deprived of its blood supply through torsion of its pedicle. Pain may be severe and constant if infarction occurs or it may be mild and intermittent if torsion is incomplete. Although torsion with acute pain is often the first symptom of an ovarian tumor, the patient may give a long-standing history of vague abdominal or pelvic discomfort prior to the onset of acute pain. A tender adnexal mass is usually palpated upon pelvic examination, and mild temperature elevation and leukocytosis usually accompany infarction (see Chap. 45).

CHRONIC OR RECURRENT ABDOMINAL PAIN

PAIN RELATED TO GASTROINTESTINAL TRACT (See also Chap. 31)

A variety of symptoms may arise from ingestion of food, ranging from expression of organic disorders of the gastrointestinal tract to functional abnormalities related to stress. An accurate history, with respect to type and location of pain, temporal relationship to food ingestion, and type of food that produces discomfort, will often allow the physician to narrow the field of diagnostic possibilities and order appropriate specific laboratory tests.

PEPTIC ULCER

The pain of duodenal ulcer is cyclic and tends to recur several times daily throughout cycles that last several weeks. Between cycles, the patient may be free of pain for several months.

The pain of uncomplicated peptic ulcer is referred to the epigastrium. If pain is referred to the back, perforation is suggested. The epigastric pain is not colicky unless obstruction is present and is variously described as "hunger pains" or as being "burning" or "boring" in nature. Characteristically, the onset of pain is initially quite mild and often is first noticed before the evening meal. As symptoms progress, discomfort will be noted 1 to 4 hours after meals and is relieved by antacids or vomiting.

CHOLELITHIASIS AND CHOLECYSTITIS

A wide variety of symptoms may be encountered with chronic disease of the gallbladder. Cyclic episodes of pain in the right upper quadrant, fever, and mild jaundice may be noted. On the other hand, symptoms may be very mild, with cyclic episodes of discomfort which are indistinguishable from other disorders. Typical biliary colic arises in the epigastrium and radiates to the right upper quadrant and the right subscapular region. Discomfort is often produced as a result of ingestion of fatty foods. However, it should be remembered that abdominal discomfort after the ingestion of foods with a high fat content is more often a result of functional disease of the gastrointestinal tract than of chronic gallbladder inflammation or cholelithiasis.

CHRONIC OR INTERMITTENT INTESTINAL OBSTRUCTION

Intermittent episodes of colicky abdominal pain may signify partial or incomplete obstruction of bowel. During the episodes of colicky pain, increased peristalsis will be detected by hyperactive bowel sounds upon abdominal auscultation. In the very thin patient, visible evidence of hyperperistalsis may be noted upon close examination of the abdominal wall. Although postoperative adhesions are cited as the most common cause of intermittent partial obstruction, inflammatory diseases such as regional ileitis, neoplasm, recurrent incomplete volvulus, and vascular disorders (thrombosis without infarction) are among possible underlying causes.

CHRONIC PANCREATITIS

Symptoms may exhibit as clearly defined bouts of acute pancreatitis frequently associated with acute alcoholic bouts. Conversely, the milder form may produce cyclic episodes of epigastric pain with vomiting which may be mistaken for gastritis. Although an elevated serum amylase may be found early in an attack, pancreatic function decreases with each succeeding episode, and the chances of detecting amylase elevation progressively diminish. In long-standing cases of recurrent pain secondary to chronic pancreatitis, diminution in pancreatic function may be signaled by the onset of diabetes mellitus and steatorrhea.

IRRITABLE COLON

Also known as spastic colon and functional bowel disorder, this is the most common cause of chronic, recurring abdominal pain. The pain is often colicky in nature, although it is not directly related to food ingestion. It generally involves the left lower quadrant but may appear anywhere in the hypogastrium. On occasion, the pain may be referred to the right or left upper quadrant if the hepatic or splenic flexure of the colon is involved. The pain is secondary to incoordinate function of large bowel and may be associated with bloating, constipation, or diarrhea alternating with constipation.

CHRONIC PAIN ASSOCIATED WITH THE REPRODUCTIVE TRACT DURING PREGNANCY

Cramping abdominal or pelvic pain at any time during pregnancy may result from uterine contractions. Cramping pain early in pregnancy may represent the earliest symptom of impending abortion, especially if accompanied by uterine bleeding. If the process of abortion progresses, this pain will increase in intensity. Back pain in conjunction with cramping abdominal pain suggests that the process of cervical dilatation has begun.

Cramping abdominal pain later in pregnancy may represent only an exaggeration of physiologic events, since the uterus contracts continuously in both the nonpregnant and pregnant state. However, cramping pain which is progressive in frequency and intensity may signal the onset of premature labor or, at term, the spontaneous onset of normal labor.

Chronic or recurrent pelvic pain may stem from physiologic alterations of the pelvic girdle during pregnancy. This may appear as hip pain, back pain, or pain referred to the symphysis pubis. Although most often described as dull and aching, such pain can occasionally be sharp and lancinating, resulting in significant disability to the patient and consternation on the part of the family.

CHRONIC PAIN ASSOCIATED WITH THE REPRODUCTIVE TRACT IN THE NONPREGNANT WOMAN

PELVIC TUMORS

Unless infarction or torsion of a pedunculated subserous fibroid produces acute abdominal pain, discomfort from uterine fibroids is likely to be described as an "aching" or "heaviness in the pelvis." Progressive constipation may be noticed if there is significant encroachment upon the rectum or sigmoid colon by enlarging fibroids. Anterior enlargement may encroach upon the bladder and cause increased urinary frequency or in extreme cases incontinence. In the same context, ovarian tumors seldom cause severe abdominal pain unless torsion and loss of blood supply, hemorrhage into a cyst, or rupture and intraperitoneal spillage have occurred. Large tumors may cause rather indefinite discomfort in the lower abdomen and pelvis, but most benign ovarian tumors are asymptomatic and are discovered during routine pelvic examination. Malignant ovarian tumors are unlikely to cause pain until metastases involve other structures.

PAIN SECONDARY TO CHRONIC INFLAMMATION

Chronic pelvic inflammatory disease can produce intermittent pain and disability. Pain may be related to formation of pelvic adhesions which may involve bowel as well as reproductive structures. Such pain will frequently be found in a patient who gives a history of acute pelvic inflammatory disease with repeated episodes of abdominal pain and fever. The pain of chronic inflammatory disease may also be caused by chronic distention of the fallopian tubes with pus or sterile fluid. Exacerbation of pelvic pain due to chronic inflammatory disease may accompany menstruation or result from intercourse.

PELVIC CONGESTION

Pelvic discomfort may appear in a cyclic fashion in relation to menses, but this is not true dysmenorrhea, since symptoms tend to abate with onset of flow. The discomfort is more common in women in the fourth and fifth decades and is characterized by onset of generalized pelvic discomfort beginning 7 to 10 days prior to the onset of menstruation. Backache and discomfort in the upper portion of the lower extremities may also be associated with pelvic pain. Symptoms often become worse during periods of stress and anxiety. Although many regard this cyclic discomfort as psychosomatic in origin, there seems to be an association between pelvic discomfort and salt and water retention that commonly occurs during the days immediately preceding menstruation. An additional factor that might be important in the production of pain is alteration of pelvic blood flow by autonomic changes influenced by ovarian steroids. The pelvic and back discomfort caused by pelvic congestion are often relieved by lying down and may be exacerbated by intercourse. Although pelvic pain may be the sole premenstrual symptom, it is more often a part of the constellation of "premenstrual tension" in which irritability, depression, weight gain, and breast tenderness complete the picture (see Chap. 18).

DYSMENORRHEA

Pain associated with menstruation may be functional in nature or associated with various lesions of the reproductive tract.

Functional (primary) dysmenorrhea is a common cause of disability in women, causing significant loss of time from school in younger women and loss of important productivity in others. Primary dysmenorrhea tends to appear during adolescence but is usually not present at the menarche. This type of discomfort is associated with ovulatory menses, and menses are often anovulatory for several months after the onset of menstrual periods.

The pain of functional dysmenorrhea is of a cramping nature, primarily centered over the low abdomen but often radiating to the back and thighs. Onset of pain is gradual, and discomfort may be noted prior to the onset of uterine bleeding. Pain usually reaches its maximum during the first 24 hours of flow and in most cases has subsided by the second day of menstruation. In some individuals associated symptoms of nausea and vomiting are present and are as distressing as the pain itself. Pain of functional dysmenorrhea is probably a result of periodic uterine hypoxia resulting from intense uterine contractions generated late in the secretory phase of the menstrual cycle and continuing well after the onset of menstruation. These contractions are of greater intensity and regularity than those occurring during the proliferative phase of the cycle (see Chap. 17).

Pain associated with menstruation may result from a variety of pelvic abnormalities. Among these abnormalities are endometrial polyp, uterine fibroids (particularly of the pedunculated submucous variety), cervical stenosis, endometriosis, adenomyosis, and chronic pelvic inflammatory disease. Although special diagnostic aids may be necessary for a definitive diagnosis, a careful history and physical examination will help pinpoint the cause of painful menstruation.

Dysmenorrhea associated with endometrial polyp and submucous fibroid is generally seen in late reproductive years and often in women who have not suffered from dysmenorrhea previously. Those who have borne children may liken the cramping discomfort to pain associated with the uterine contractions of labor (see Chap. 42).

Menstrual pain associated with obstruction to menstrual flow secondary to stenosis of the cervix may occur in women who have undergone cautery or conization for diagnosis or treatment of cervical abnormalities. Symptoms generally do not appear for several months after the surgical procedure (see Chap. 41).

Dysmenorrhea associated with endometriosis usually does not precede the onset of flow and tends to increase in intensity throughout the menstrual period. Rather than being cramping, as pain associated with uterine contractions, it tends to be steady, and location of pain and radiation will depend upon the location of endometrial lesions (see Chap. 37).

PAIN ASSOCIATED WITH OVULATION (MITTELSCHMERZ)

Many women experience cyclic lower abdominal discomfort associated with ovulation. The pain is generally dull and affects the right lower quadrant more often than the left, although it may alternate in successive cycles in some individuals. It is rarely lancinating or incapacitating and generally lasts only a few hours. The exact relationship of the pain to the mechanisms of ovulation is unknown. It may result from increased intrafollicular pressure prior to follicle rupture or may be due to release of a small amount of follicular fluid into the peritoneal cavity. Scant uterine bleeding may precede, accompany, or follow the abdominal discomfort.

DYSPAREUNIA

Pain with intercourse may be due to organic lesions of the vagina and pelvis, but is most often a functional problem. In general, three types of dyspareunia are recognized.

Pain which is present upon attempts at vaginal penetration may be so severe as to prevent intromission. In functional dyspareunia, this may be caused by involuntary contraction of the levators and other pelvic muscles as a result of inhibiting psychic influences (see Chap. 26). Organic lesions that produce pain on initial vaginal penetration include an unusually thick or unyielding hymen and inflammatory conditions of the vagina such as those associated with *Trichomonas vaginalis* or *Monilia* infections. Congenital abnormalities such as vaginal septum may cause pain upon intromission. Scarring from episiotomy or perineorrhaphy may also cause dyspareunia. Painful intercourse may be associated with atrophic vaginal changes which may be found in the postmenopausal woman (see Chap. 40).

Discomfort may be felt only with deep penetration of the penis into the vagina. This may occur during periods of pelvic congestion prior to menstruation, as a result of endometriosis involving the uterosacral ligaments or pelvic peritoneal cul-de-sac, prolapse of the ovaries into the cul-de-sac, severe retroversion of the uterus, or chronic pelvic inflammatory disease (see Chaps. 37, 39, and 44).

A third type of pain may result from intercourse in which orgasm has not occurred. Vasocongestive changes in pelvic structures from sexual stimuli are generally relieved by the contracture of voluntary musculature associated with orgasm. Lack of orgasm and persistence of congestion may produce pelvic pain.

BACKACHE

PAIN ASSOCIATED WITH PREGNANCY

Low back pain may be associated with an otherwise normal pregnancy. It may be accompanied by discomfort in the pelvic girdle or may exist as an isolated symptom. Discomfort is generally low grade, nonradiating, and often described as a "dull ache" confined to the lumbar area. It occurs as a result of postural changes effected to compensate for the weight and location of the gravid uterus, bringing unusual strain to muscles and ligaments of the lumbar spine.

In others, low back pain may not appear until the postpartum period. Again, it tends to be localized, relieved in the supine position, and aggravated by physical activity. It is thought to be due to a weakness of the abdominal muscles and failure of their role in normal postural tone. Relief is gained as tone improves in the abdominal musculature.

PAIN UNASSOCIATED WITH PREGNANCY

Backache is among the most common complaints among both men and women. In the female, as in the male, it most often results from osseous and musculoligamentous disorders rather than intraabdominal or intrapelvic disease.

Among the more common causes of backache are trauma with resulting contusion of the lumbar muscles, back sprain in which a sudden thrust or fall stretches or tears the spinous ligaments, and back strain resulting from a long steady pull on the back muscles and ligaments from remaining in a bent or twisted position for long periods of time. Compression fractures of the spine may occur with minimal trauma when osteoporosis is present and vertebral bodies have become demineralized (see Chap. 19). Herniated nucleus pulposus may be a cause for acute back pain with a radicular component as an expression of nerve-root compression. Location of radiating pain depends on the level of the lesion. Osteoarthritis, a disease appearing in the fifth decade or later, may also cause backache.

Poor posture, improper shoes, awkward occupational attitudes, improper mattresses, and unnatural seating can all exert abnormal strain on muscles, ligaments, and joints leading to back pain of a chronic nature. As more women enter occupations requiring greater physical effort, one might anticipate an increasing number of job-related back complaints in the future health care of women.

Also important are certain static abnormalities in the production of backache. These include a short leg, functional scoliosis due to unequal size of the pelvic bones, foot strain, short hamstrings, contracted calf muscles, and contracted fasciae latae and iliotibial bands. Static abnormalities exert unusual tension on the low-lumbar and sacroiliac ligaments, especially when there is an increase of the normal lordosis or a functional scoliosis due to inequality of the pelvic level or a short leg. Only rarely do gynecologic disorders cause backache as a primary complaint. Backache may accompany functional dysmenorrhea or large intrapelvic tumors. Chronic pelvic inflammatory disease may be associated with back discomfort. Backache may also be among the complaints of those with uterine prolapse. In patients with known carcinoma of the cervix, back pain may result from invasion of lumbar lymph nodes. Osteoporosis in the postmenopausal patient may be associated with shortening or collapse of vertebral bodies, causing back pain.

REFERENCES

Haagensen CD: *Diseases of the Breast,* rev 2nd ed., Philadelphia: Saunders, 1974.

Menaker GJ: The physiology and mechanism of acute abdominal pain. *Surg Clin North Am* 42:241, 1962.

Wolf HG: *Headache and Other Head Pain,* 3d ed., New York: Oxford University Press, 1972.

23

Mass

LESTER SILBERMAN

Spleen
   Inflammatory
   Obstructive
   Neoplastic
   Miscellaneous
   Other Masses
Ascites

SPECIAL INVESTIGATIVE TECHNIQUES
Ultrasound
Laparoscopy
Culdoscopy
Pelvic pneumography

**DIFFERENTIAL DIAGNOSIS OF
ABDOMINOPELVIC MASSES**
Adnexa and cul-de-sac
   Palpation characteristics
   History
   Symptoms
   Investigative studies
Midline suprapubic area
   Papation characteristics
   History
   Symptoms
   Investigation
Midabdominal area
Epigastrium
Right upper quadrant
Left upper quadrant

CONCLUSION

INTRODUCTION

The term *mass* as applied to medicine may be defined in various ways. Medical dictionaries unsatisfactorily define it as "a lump or aggregation of coherent material" (Gould) or as "an aggregation of particles of matter characterized by inertia" (Stedman). To the patient, a mass, a lump, or a bunch is likely to be a source of concern which brings her to seek medical advice. To the physician, the identity or cause of the mass may be readily discernible. In many cases, however, the position of the mass beneath the skin covering, within the peritoneal cavity, or in other equally inaccessible areas makes the diagnosis a more difficult matter.

During the course of this discussion, masses which are of interest to the examining gynecologist will be discussed in brief detail. In addition, the techniques and special diagnostic studies available for the evaluation of the palpable mass will be considered.

TYPES OF MASS

Functional. The functional mass has no pathologic significance. It appears during the course of normal physiologic functioning and is usually temporary in nature. The main difficulty associated with the presence of a functional mass is that it may be confused with a mass of clinical significance. Typical examples of functional masses include the dilated cecum, follicular cysts of the ovary, and the gravid uterus.

Inflammatory. Infection of an organ or structure, especially with accumulation of pus and abscess formation, may cause enlargement of that structure to an abnormal and clinically observable degree. The inflammatory mass thus formed may also involve adjacent structures. For example, the salpingitis responsible for the formation of a palpable pyosalpinx may be accompanied by adhesions to adjacent intestine, omentum, and ovary, producing a mass much larger than the original pyosalpinx. An abscess formed as a result of a ruptured appendix may, in a similar manner, involve cecum, omentum, fallopian tube, or ovary.

Obstructive. Obstruction of the outflow tract of an organ may produce secondary swelling of that organ as material accumulates within it. Obstruction of Bartholin's duct with subsequent accumulation of fluid produces a Bartholin cyst. Obstruction of the cervical canal by scarring secondary to cautery or by a malignant process may result in a hematometria or, if infection supervenes, a pyometria.

Neoplastic. Tumor development or formation of a cyst within an organ, whether benign or malignant, may be perceived by the patient and physician as a newly developing mass. Often, efforts to diagnose any mass are directed toward exclusion of the presence of a malignancy.

Miscellaneous. Under this heading are included a number of different masses which do not fall under the previous four categories. This category would include organized blood clots in the cul-de-sac secondary to intraperitoneal bleeding, displaced organs (e.g., pelvic kidney) perceived as an abnormal mass, and hepatic cirrhosis.

PROBLEMS IN DIAGNOSIS

The identity of a mass may be obscured by the involvement of a number of varied structures within the confines of what one perceives as the palpable mass. Hence, a mass formed by a simple ovarian cyst adherent to a diverticular abscess may defy accurate diagnosis unless an exploratory laparotomy is performed. Many intraabdominal and intrapelvic masses may only be accessible through laparotomy, and there is often no way to distinguish which organ system is involved when the mass presents in a particular area of the abdomen.

The student and physician must learn to accept a certain degree of ambiguity. The diagnostic guess based solely upon intuition and luck is readily remembered when correct and quickly forgotten when incorrect. Unfortunately, such guesses are far too often incorrect. Students must discipline themselves to explore all the diagnostic possibilities and not let "intuition" so color the workup that other equally possible diagnoses are left unexplored. The words "I'm not sure" should not be considered an admission of defeat but an honest assessment of the situation.

CHARACTERIZATION OF THE MASS

A mass should be described, whenever possible, with reference to the following characteristics:

1. Size (measured in centimeters in all palpable dimensions)
2. Shape
3. Consistency (cystic, solid, nodular, etc.)
4. Location
5. Delimitation (the sharpness of the borders of the mass)
6. Mobility
7. Attachment to adjacent structures (skin fixation)
8. Tenderness

Additional characteristics obtained from the history are equally important. These will vary with the location of the mass, but some general comments concerning the patient's awareness of the presence of a mass can always be elicited. Is the mass painful or tender? Is the patient aware of enlargement or pressure? Are there other local or systemic manifestations related to the mass? These points will be discussed in more detail as masses connected with various organ systems are described.

SUMMARY

Determining the cause and pathogenesis of a palpable mass may often present a challenging problem, and a clear-cut diagnosis may not be possible without complicated diagnostic procedures or exploratory surgery. For purposes of evaluation and therapy, it is important to expend full effort toward discovering the correct diagnosis. In some cases the mass must be evaluated and removed simply to rule in or out the presence of malignancy, and in others the mass may simply be a reflection of a disease process which requires management other than surgery. In the following discussion certain systems of the body will be discussed in terms of different varieties of masses arising from each. Attention will be paid to the characteristic findings on palpation and associated symptoms and findings as well as on diagnostic studies used to define the origin of the mass.

Finally, we will consider each region of the abdomen in terms of the differential diagnosis of masses which may be found in that area.

EXTRAABDOMINAL MASSES

THYROID GLAND

Palpation of the thyroid gland should be included in the physical examination of a patient. It should be remembered that thyroid enlargement may be a normal physiologic concomitant of adolescence and pregnancy.

DIFFUSE THYROID ENLARGEMENT

Diffuse enlargement of the thyroid gland may be associated with the euthyroid, hyperthyroid, or hypothyroid state.

NODULAR ENLARGEMENT

The presence of a single nodule in the thyroid gland or of a multinodular goiter may also be associated with varying degrees of thyroid dysfunction. The differential diagnosis includes nodular goiter, benign adenoma, acute nonsuppurative thyroiditis, lymphocytic thyroiditis, and thyroid cancer. The nodules of a nodular goiter may be nonfunctioning or hyperfunctioning. Lymphocytic thyroiditis, or Hashimoto's disease, is believed to be an autoimmune disease with a preponderant occurrence in the female population. The thyroid is usually firm and lobulated. Either hypofunction or hyperfunction may be found. It is important to differentiate thyroid carcinoma from other benign conditions producing a nodular thyroid. Rapid progressive growth of a nodule, evidence of recurrent laryngeal nerve paralysis, and the presence of involved lymph nodes in the neck or supraclavicular area are all highly suggestive of the presence of thyroid carcinoma.

BREAST

INFLAMMATORY

Mastitis with Abscess

In mastitis a localized area of induration and erythema is found which is tender to palpation and generally associated with the onset of fever, chills, and generalized malaise. Without proper therapy, this infection may evolve into a breast abscess with palpable fluctuance and painful axillary lymphadenopathy. Tuberculosis involving the breast may also present as an indurated tumor, poorly delimited with overlying skin retraction, or as a central abscess.

NEOPLASTIC

Cysts

Of the multiple causes of mammary cysts, cystic breast disease is the most frequent. Cysts secondary to gross cystic disease of the breast are usually round and mobile with sharply defined borders. Tenderness is often a feature, especially during the premenstrual phase of the cycle. A reduction in size often follows menstruation. Galactoceles, which are cysts with a thick, creamy secretion, may be formed at the time of weaning; they are rounded structures with sharply defined borders and good mobility within the breast tissue. Fat necrosis results from breast trauma, producing a small, firm tumor in the more superficial breast tissue. Fixation with poor mobility may be found, but in contrast to carcinoma, the lesion tends to have sharp borders. Cyst formation can occur with calcification in the cyst wall. Biopsy is often necessary to distinguish fat necrosis from carcinoma. Dilatation of the mammary ducts in the area of the nipple and areola sometimes results in the formation of cystic tumors 1 to 3 cm in diameter. These tumors may be associated with a bloody discharge from the nipple as well as nipple retraction. Again, surgical exploration with excision and histologic examination is necessary to rule out carcinoma. Growth of a papilloma within a mammary duct can also cause dilatation of that duct and distention with serum or blood. Cysts as large as 10 or 12 cm in diameter have been reported but are rare. The characteristic symptoms of intraductal papillomas are nipple discharge with painful nipple retraction.

Solid Tumors

It is of utmost importance to differentiate solid benign tumors from malignant growths, since the success of therapy in breast carcinoma often depends on the stage of the disease at the time of surgery. Biopsy of a suspicious lesion should be freely performed. There are various characteristics, however, which strongly suggest the presence of malignancy. The degree of sharpness at the edges of the tumor is distinct in adenofibromas and cysts and indistinct in carcinoma, fibrous disease, and adenosis. The latter three conditions are also characterized by decreased mobility of the lesion within the breast tissue and fixation to surrounding tissue and skin. Retraction of the skin over the palpable lesion, evidence of inflammation over the lesion, and edema are all suspicious signs. A marked increase in the size and firmness of one breast is also characteristic of malignancy. Careful examination for changes in the nipple, discharge, and axillary and supraclavicular lymph-node enlargement should be performed.

LYMPHATIC SYSTEM

In the following discussion, attention will be focused on two areas in which the lymph nodes are likely to be of concern in the diagnosis of gynecologic disease. For the rest, it is sufficient to say that the presence of persistent, abnormally enlarged nodes may well necessitate a search for an inflammatory or neoplastic cause. In the latter category, both primary lymphatic tumors and metastatic tumors must be considered.

GROIN LYMPHATICS

The lymph nodes found in the groin area consist of two groups of glands: the superficial inguinal nodes, which lie along the inner two-thirds of the inguinal ligament, and the superficial femoral nodes, which are clustered around the entrance of the saphenous vein into the femoral vein. Efferent lymphatics pass through the fascia covering the femoral artery and vein to communicate with the external iliac nodes in the pelvis. The superficial femoral nodes drain the skin of the lower limb as well as, to some extent, the perineum and gluteal region. The superficial inguinal nodes drain the vulva, clitoris, perineum, and the lower third and a portion of the middle third of the vagina.

Infection

It is apparent that infected lesions of the lower limb and perineum are likely to result in groin lymphadenitis. Chancroid, primary syphilitic chancre, and granuloma inguinale are important vulvar lesions usually associated with nonsuppurative lymph-node enlargement. Lymphogranuloma venereum, on the other hand, is notable for the presence of suppurative lymphadenitis.

Neoplasm

Malignancies of the vulva, perineum, and the lower two-thirds of the vagina may involve the superficial inguinal nodes.

Supraclavicular Nodes

First described by Virchow in 1948, the supraclavicular fossa lymphaticus is recognized as a possible site of metastatic spread of malignancy. The left supraclavicular mode lies in close proximity to the thoracic duct near its point of drainage into the venous system. The thoracic duct drains lymphatics from the left supradiaphragmatic portion of the chest as well as from abdomen and pelvis. Involvement of the left supraclavicular node is believed to be secondary to retrograde drainage from the thoracic duct (see Fig. 23–1).

The right supraclavicular lymph nodes lie adjacent to the great lymphatic vein and drain the right supradiaphragmatic areas of the chest. Malignancies of the head, neck, breast, and thorax may metastasize to either right or left supraclavicular lymph nodes. Findings of adenopathy should evoke a systematic search for infection, lymphatic carcinoma, or metastatic disease.

PERINEAL MASSES

VULVA (see Chap. 40)

INFLAMMATORY

Condyloma Acuminata

These verrucous lesions, probably of viral origin, are commonly found on the vulva and in the perianal region. They consist of warty papillomatous skin lesions varying in size from 0.5 to 2 cm and occurring either singly, in small clusters, or when confluent, in large clusters. They become even larger during pregnancy, sometimes forming huge cauliflower masses which may pose a problem at the time of delivery. They tend to be associated with vaginal discharge, especially when caused by *Trichomonas* or *Monilia*. Such lesions are usually asymptomatic, although patients may report some associated pruritus.

OBSTRUCTIVE

Bartholin Cyst and Abscess

Occlusion of Bartholin's duct, usually secondary to chronic infection, may result in the formation of a Bartholin cyst. Accumulation of secretion within the gland and duct may produce a cyst over 5 cm in diameter, although most are smaller. These cysts are nontender and are located within the vulvar tissue, somewhat posteriorly. Unless the cyst is large enough to mechanically inhibit coitus, it is usually asymptomatic. Secondary infection, however, may lead to a Bartholin abscess with surrounding tenderness, induration, and erythema. Bartholin's gland may also be primarily infected, usually by the gonococcus, with abscess formation creating a picture similar to secondary infection of a Bartholin cyst.

Sebaceous Cyst

Obstruction of the duct of a sebaceous gland may result in a small, firm, cystic lesion which is found to

FIGURE 23–1 Location of left supraclavicular node.

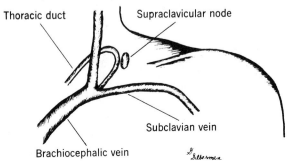

Thoracic duct

Supraclavicular node

Subclavian vein

Brachiocephalic vein

Silberman

contain a cheesy sebaceous material. These cysts usually appear on the inner surfaces of the labia majora and minora. They are generally asymptomatic and are less than 1 to 2 cm wide. Secondary infection may lead to abscess formation, sometimes necessitating surgical excision or drainage.

NEOPLASTIC

Benign Cystic Tumors

Wolffian-duct cysts are found on the vulva as well as in the vagina. They are usually small, thin-walled, and translucent, although some are larger. They may be located in the area of the hymen or near the clitoris or urethra, are usually asymptomatic, and require no treatment. Epidermal inclusion cysts result from entrapment of stratified squamous epithelium beneath the surface of the skin, often secondary to episiotomy repair or trauma. These small nodules are nontender and asymptomatic unless secondarily infected. A cyst of the canal of Nuck is a fluid-filled cyst in the inguinal canal or the labia majora and is formed when the round ligament carries with it a projection of peritoneum into the inguinal canal and labia. The projection becomes isolated and filled with fluid. Endometriosis involving the vulva may present as a nodular lesion which becomes particularly painful and tender at the time of menses.

Benign Solid Tumors

Benign solid tumors of the vulva are uncommon. Of these tumors, the fibroma is the most frequent. It may present as a small nodular lesion, but as it enlarges, it is likely to become pedunculated and undergo surface ulceration and necrosis with bleeding and discharge. The lesion is otherwise asymptomatic. A lipoma is a soft, slowly growing lesion which may appear anywhere on the vulva, and which also may develop a pedicle as it enlarges. Hydradenoma is a benign sweat-gland tumor with a slightly raised, brownish surface and a small, pointed center.

Malignant Tumors

Epidermoid carcinoma is the most common vulvar malignancy. Its gross appearance is varied, and in the early stages it can present as an elevated papule or small ulceration. With progression of the disease, a firm, indurated ulceration will develop. Biopsy is usually sufficient to make the diagnosis. Sarcoma of the vulva is rare but may arise from any of the lymphoid or connective-tissue elements of the vulva or

within a fibroma. Carcinoma within Bartholin's gland is also rare but differentiation from infection in the gland is extremely important.

ANORECTUM

INFLAMMATORY

Abscess

The pathogenesis of an abscess in the anorectal area usually begins with inflammation of an anal gland in the area between external and internal sphincters. Pus collection in this area may be difficult to palpate. However, spread of infection downward to the anal margin will result in the formation of a perianal abscess. This will be recognized as a protuberance which is tender, erythematous, and indurated and is sometimes mistaken for a thrombosed external hemorrhoid. Spread of infection from the intersphincteric area across the external sphincter may result in an ischiorectal abscess. The loose areolar tissue of this fossa allows a rather large collection, extending from the top of the fossa down to the perineal skin. Symptoms may develop even before the abscess can be visualized. With progression of the disease, erythema of the skin over the ischiorectal fossa is noted, terminating in a palpable fluctuant abscess. Upward infection from the intersphincteric area may produce a rectal wall abscess with symptoms of vague pain, painful defecation, and fever and malaise. The abscess is palpable on rectal or pelvic examination as a tender, fluctuant swelling in the lateral rectal wall (see Fig. 23–2).

FIGURE 23–2 Pathways of anorectal infection originating in intersphincteric area.

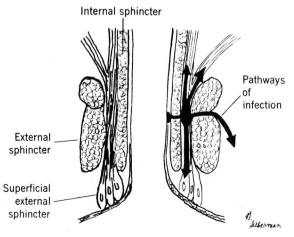

Internal sphincter

Pathways of infection

External sphincter

Superficial external sphincter

NEOPLASTIC

Carcinoma

Carcinoma of the anal region arises from squamous epithelium of the anal mucous membrane, in the glands or ducts, or from the transitional glands separating rectal and anal mucous membranes. These tumors, though quite small, are likely to cause symptoms of painful defecation or bleeding. Inappropriate therapy for thrombosed hemorrhoids or anal fistula is often carried out until the diagnosis of malignancy is ascertained by biopsy.

ABDOMINAL AND PELVIC MASSES

OVARY (see also Chap. 45)

FUNCTIONAL

Functional cysts, follicle or luteal, are usually asymptomatic although those of sufficient size may produce pelvic discomfort. Cysts may rupture producing pelvic pain which generally subsides within 24 to 48 hours. Bleeding associated with this rupture can produce hemoperitoneum and evidence of acute blood loss necessitating surgical exploration. A functional cyst may become torsed upon its vascular pedicle with resultant ischemic necrosis and signs of peritoneal irritation, again necessitating surgery. Hemorrhage into the cyst will produce acute enlargement and increased pain.

Most functional cysts undergo spontaneous resorption. Therefore, in the younger patient and in the absence of significant symptoms, cysts may be followed for 6 to 12 weeks without detriment to the patient. Resolution of the cyst is to be expected. In the middle-aged group, a shorter period of observation is desirable because of the increased risk of cancer. Postmenopausal women with adnexal cysts should be explored promptly.

INFLAMMATORY

Ovarian Abscess

Gonococcal, puerperal, or postsurgical pelvic infection with bacterial invasion of the ruptured follicle can result in ovarian abscess formation, palpable as an exquisitely tender nonmobile, poorly defined mass in either of the adnexal regions or the cul-de-sac. The inflammatory process of the ovary usually merges with a similar process in the fallopian tube with the formation of a tuboovarian abscess. The involvement is most often bilateral.

A history of recent exposure to gonorrhea or recent pelvic surgery or childbirth, associated with spiking fever, elevated white blood cell count, abdominal pain with rebound tenderness and guarding, and the characteristic findings on pelvic examination are sufficient for diagnosis.

NEOPLASTIC

Benign Cystic Tumors

This group of ovarian tumors is comprised of cystadenomas, both serious and mucinous, and cystic teratomas. The usual benign neoplastic cyst is 6 to 12 cm in diameter, generally nontender, and round to ovoid in shape. Its mobility tends to be limited by its size, the larger cysts being the less mobile. It has been suggested that cystic teratomas tend to occupy a more anterior position in the adnexal areas than do cystadenomas. All cysts, however, may be found in the adnexal regions or in the cul-de-sac.

These benign cysts vary in the symptoms they produce. When large enough, the cyst can cause vague feelings of pelvic discomfort or heaviness. Disturbances of menstrual function are not uncommon but are variable in nature. Torsion may occur as described with functional cysts. Secondary infection of the cyst, usually after torsion of the pedicle but occasionally through lymphatic or hematogenous routes, is less frequent. The infected cyst is palpable as an exquisitely tender pelvic mass and is associated with systemic signs of sepsis. Differentiation between this condition and pelvic inflammatory disease with tuboovarian abscess may be difficult, but one should remember that pelvic inflammation is usually bilateral.

Benign Solid Tumors

Ovarian fibromas and Brenner tumors are two benign solid tumors of the ovary. The size of these tumors varies from small nodules on the ovary noticed incidentally at exploratory surgery to huge growths, filling most of the pelvis and abdomen. They are firm, solid, nontender, and depending on their size, mobile. The larger tumors may produce pelvic discomfort and feelings of pelvic heaviness. Torsion may occur. An interesting, but as yet unexplained, association of fibroma of the ovary with hydrothorax (Meigs's syndrome) is seen infrequently. Although described originally in association with an ovarian fibroma, other tumors of the ovary may have a similar association.

Malignant Cystic Tumors

Serous and mucinous cystadenocarcinomas are the two most frequently encountered cystic malignant tumors of the ovary.

These tumors vary from 5 to 25 cm. The findings on pelvic examination will obviously vary, depending upon the extent of tumor involvement when the patient is seen. Early lesions with no capsule invasion will be indistinguishable from benign lesions on pelvic examination. The advanced lesion may present with tumor invading the parametria and cul-de-sac, giving the impression that the pelvis is a solid frozen mass. There are all gradations of findings between these two extremes.

Unfortunately, there are no characteristic symptoms associated with the development of ovarian carcinoma. Pelvic discomfort, abdominal swelling, vaginal bleeding, and loss of weight are usually hallmarks of more advanced disease. Ascites and pleural effusion, indicative of metastatic disease, are poor prognostic signs, although both may occur in the presence of benign lesions. Hepatomegaly, palpation of other intraabdominal masses, and x-ray evidence of metastatic spread appear late in the course of the illness.

The generally poor survival rate for treated ovarian malignancies makes it imperative that adnexal masses be diagnosed promptly, especially in that age group most at risk for ovarian malignancies. Exploratory laparotomy with gross and histologic examination is the best method for making this diagnosis.

Malignant Solid Tumors

In the ovary, adenocarcinoma as well as the more undifferentiated carcinomas are somewhat less frequent than cystic malignancies. Abdominal and pelvic findings, as well as symptoms associated with the malignancy, are similar to those of malignant cystic tumors.

Functioning Tumors of the Ovary

The association of evidence of abnormal androgen or estrogen secretion with a palpable adnexal tumor is one of the most fascinating occurrences in the field of gynecology. The elaboration of estrogen from a granulosa theca cell can result in precocious puberty in the child and uterine bleeding and hypertrophic breast changes in the postmenopausal woman. Arrhenoblastomas producing androgen result in defeminization and subsequent masculinization. Other ovarian tumors associated with androgen production and masculinization will be considered in Chap. 45.

MISCELLANEOUS

Endometrioma

Pelvic endometriosis with ovarian involvement is often associated with the formation on the ovary of a cystic mass filled with old blood, giving a chocolate-colored appearance to the contents of the cyst. These are palpable as adnexal or cul-de-sac masses, usually not more than 10 cm in greatest diameter, sometimes occurring bilaterally. Tenderness is not a distinctive feature, and mobility of the mass depends on the extent of the endometriosis-induced scarring in the pelvis.

PAROVARIAN CYST

Parovarian cysts are formed from the embryologic remnants of the mesonephric tubules and ducts embedded in the mesovarium and mesosalpinx. Cysts are found between the layers of the broad ligament. They may be palpable on pelvic examination as cystic structures which are nontender, mobile, and around 5 to 8 cm wide, although in rare instances they attain greater size. Torsion can occur, as with ovarian cysts. It is difficult to differentiate parovarian from ovarian cysts, and exploratory laparotomy may be necessary. Simple excision of the cyst is adequate therapy.

FALLOPIAN TUBE (See also Chap. 44)

INFLAMMATORY

Pyosalpinx and Hydrosalpinx

One of the unfortunate sequelae of acute pelvic inflammatory disease secondary to gonorrhea is the development of pyosalpinx or hydrosalpinx. Although the inflammatory process may involve the adnexa unilaterally, bilateral involvement is most common. Adnexal areas and the cul-de-sac may be filled with tender, cystic-feeling, retort-shaped masses extending toward the lateral pelvic walls. If the inflammation has been present for a relatively short time, the entire pelvis is likely to be tender, and movement of the uterus in any plane by the examining fingers will evoke varying degrees of discomfort. The uterosacral ligaments may be indurated and tender as well. When the process is of long duration and a hydrosalpinx is present, tenderness is likely to be a less prominent sign. In this case, retort-shaped masses may be easily palpated. The size of the palpable mass varies. The mass is likely to have little mobility.

A clear-cut history of acute pelvic inflammatory disease, followed by persistent pelvic pain or discomfort associated with the characteristic pelvic findings, suggests the diagnosis. Such a history, however, is not often available. Visualization of pelvic structures through a laparoscope may reveal the diagnosis in patients with suspiciously thickened or enlarged adnexa. Unilateral hydrosalpinx may be difficult to distinguish from an ovarian neoplasm, and exploratory laparotomy may become necessary in order to clearly define the problem. It is not uncommon for patients with bilateral hydrosalpinx to present with infertility secondary to tubal obstruction.

NEOPLASTIC

Benign Tumors

Benign neoplasms of the fallopian tube are relatively infrequent. Leiomyomas are the most common. Fibromas, lipomas, and cysts of various kinds have also been reported, but are rare. When large enough to be palpable, these tumors present as adnexal masses which are generally nontender and moderately mobile. They produce few or no symptoms but because of their location and the difficulty in distinguishing them from ovarian lesions, laparotomy is usually required for definitive diagnosis.

Malignant Tumors

Carcinoma of the fallopian tube is another relatively uncommon malignancy. The fallopian tube may be markedly enlarged, resembling a huge pyosalpinx on palpation. The mass is usually nontender and, because of a lack of surface tumor and adhesions, is moderately mobile. Symptoms related to carcinoma of the fallopian tube are often vague and noted in the more advanced lesions. A clear or blood-tinged watery discharge has been described as the classical symptom of fallopian tube malignancy. Abnormal vaginal bleeding is also a frequent symptom. Backache and sacral pain herald the occurrence of more advanced disease.

MISCELLANEOUS

Ectopic Pregnancy

Implantation of a fertilized egg in the fallopian tube sets the stage for an acute surgical emergency. Hemorrhage secondary to erosion by the trophoblast can spread into the lumen of the tube, the wall of the tube, or the peritoneal cavity. The acute distention of the fallopian tube caused by hemorrhage into it is probably responsible for the pain characteristic of the condition. Rupture of the fallopian tube or bleeding through the fimbriated end will result in a hemoperitoneum. Pelvic examination often will not reveal tubal enlargement because the adnexal structures on the affected side may be so tender that adequate palpation is not possible. Examination under anesthesia will reveal a small mass not usually larger than 5 or 6 cm, with the adjacent ovary also palpable. Clotted blood in the cul-de-sac may be palpable as an irregular, vaguely defined mass.

The combination of a recent period of amenorrhea followed by some abnormal uterine bleeding, lower abdominal pain, weakness, and shoulder pain make the diagnosis of ectopic pregnancy a likely possibility. Signs of acute blood loss, lower abdominal tenderness with guarding and rebound, and a cul-de-sac tap positive for nonclottable blood necessitate exploratory laparotomy. When the diagnosis is in doubt, laparoscopy may resolve the question without the need for further surgery.

UTERUS (See also Chap. 42)

FUNCTIONAL

Pregnancy

The most common midline mass found in a woman during the reproductive years of life is the pregnant uterus. Up until the eleventh to twelfth week of gestation, the uterus remains a pelvic organ; beyond that time it can be palpated above the pubic symphysis. Uterine enlargement is difficult to evaluate prior to 6 weeks after the last menstrual period. Isthmic softening and cyanosis of the cervix and vagina may hint at the presence of an intrauterine pregnancy, but enlargement at this early stage may not be appreciable. After 6 weeks, definite uterine enlargement is determined on repeated examinations, with softening of the fundus and normal mobility.

OBSTRUCTIVE

Obstruction of any part of the lower reproductive tract is designated as gynatresia. The obstruction may be congenital (imperforate hymen, transverse vaginal septum) or acquired (malignancy, senile contraction, or stricture post-radiotherapy, cautery, or surgery). Blockage will result in the accumulation of menstrual fluid with the formation of a hematocolpos or hematometra depending on the site of obstruction. Absence or cessation of menses, lower abdominal pain, and an enlarging mass in the presence of one of the above factors suggests the diagnosis. Secondary infection of the accumulated material can occur producing increased pain and systemic signs of sepsis.

NEOPLASTIC

Benign Tumors

Leiomyomas are smooth muscle tumors and are the most common benign neoplasms (see Chap. 42). Myomas are frequently multiple and range in size from less than a centimeter in diameter to those producing a uterine enlargement of 28 weeks' gestational size or more. When small and intramural or subserosal in location, these tumors are apt to cause minimal uterine enlargement, asymmetry, and irregularity of menses. Larger tumors will present as lower abdominopelvic masses with varying degrees of asymmetry and irregularity. Pedunculated myomas occupy positions in the adnexa or in the cul-de-sac, making them difficult to distinguish from ovarian tumors. Myomas are characteristically firm and rubbery in consistency with clear demarcation of their borders. With the exception of certain cases of degeneration, they are likely to be nontender.

Symptoms vary depending on the position of the tumors and include abnormal bleeding, feelings of pelvic pressure, urinary frequency, stress incontinence, and tenesmus.

Diagnosis is usually made by pelvic examination. Submucosal myomas may be suggested by the irregularity of the endometrial cavity at the time of curettage or by filling defect noted on a hysterosalpingogram done for infertility or habitual-abortion investigation.

Malignant Tumors

There are a number of malignant processes which involve the uterus, adenocarcinoma of the endometrium being the most common. Less common are trophoblastic disease and sarcoma, and other primary and metastatic malignancies are even more infrequent (see Chap. 42).

The most common symptom that is associated with malignancies of the uterus is abnormal uterine bleeding.

CERVIX (See also Chap. 41)

NEOPLASTIC

Polyps

Cervical polyps are benign, pedunculated lesions generally arising from the endocervical mucosa and are seen protruding through the external os. Polyps are generally small, measuring less than a centimeter in greatest dimension but occasionally growing to several centimeters in size. They may be single or multiple. The pedicle may be of varying lengths, occasionally long enough to allow the polyp to present at the vaginal introitus. Polyps have a bright, cherry-red color and are soft and fragile in consistency. They are apt to produce metrorrhagia especially after coitus or straining.

Although it is unusual to find malignancy in a cervical polyp, polyps should be removed and examined histologically.

Malignant Tumors

The gross appearance of the cervical carcinoma is quite variable. In early stages there may be no mass. As the disease advances, the area becomes firm, slightly elevated, granular, and somewhat friable to the touch. With increasing growth, the lesion may become erosive or exophytic and may spread to involve the entire cervix as well as adjacent vaginal mucosa. Bimanual examination at this time reveals the presence of a firm, irregular mass extending from the cervix and vaginal fornices to involve the parametria on one or both sides; this involvement spreads to the lateral pelvic walls as the disease progresses. Growth of tumor through the cul-de-sac to involve the rectum and anteriorly to involve the bladder may also be suspected on bimanual examination. An excavating lesion causes destruction of the cervix and upper vagina, giving the appearance of a shaggy, moth-eaten necrotic cavity. The exophytic lesion protrudes from the cervix in a typical cauliflower-shaped mass. An endophytic lesion shows little surface growth on the cervix but infiltrates the cervical stroma, producing a hard, sometimes stony induration. The earlier lesions may be easily defined as to size and shape, but more extensive involvement makes this difficult. The cervix in advanced cases may be immobile, whereas early lesions do not affect mobility.

The diagnosis of cervical cancer rests upon careful inspection of the cervix and vagina, exfoliative cytologic examination, and biopsy of suspicious cervical lesions.

VAGINA (See also Chap. 40)

FUNCTIONAL

Although not actually palpable masses, the results of pelvic relaxation—cystocele, rectocele, enterocele, and uterine prolapse—may appear at first glance to be abnormal masses. Palpation, however, will reveal that these outpouchings of vaginal wall are in fact produced by poor support of bladder, rectum, and small bowel, and by the cervix which has prolapsed down to or through the vaginal introitus, with no palpable evidence of mass. These conditions will be further considered in Chap. 39.

INFLAMMATORY

Condylomata Acuminata

These verrucous lesions are often found scattered throughout the vagina in association with similar lesions on the vulva. Histologically, they may be classified as papillomatous growths and are believed viral in origin. They have a warty appearance, and individual lesions are about 1 cm or less in diameter. Confluence of lesions, however, may produce large cauliflowerlike masses. The larger masses tend to occur in association with pregnancy and have on rare occasions produced problems at time of delivery.

OBSTRUCTIVE

Gynatresia

Occlusion of the genital canal has been discussed in the section on masses of the uterus secondary to obstruction. A mass in the area of the vagina, palpable on rectal examination as a fluctuant cystic structure filling the pelvis, is formed as a result of an imperforate hymen. At the time of menarche, symptoms of menses may appear in the absence of actual bleeding. The blood which accumulates behind the intact hymen distends the vagina, forming a hematocolpos. Each successive episode of bleeding further distends the vagina. The diagnosis depends upon the observation of a bulging hymen, behind which the bluish purple blood is visible. Treatment by an incision through the hymen confirms the diagnosis.

NEOPLASTIC

Benign Tumors

Inclusion cysts of the vagina are usually formed secondary to the retention of mucosal remnants beneath the surface of the epithelium during the repair of an episiotomy or laceration. These remnants become encysted and secrete a cheesy material which distends the cyst. They are small, not exceeding a few centimeters in diameter, and are generally nontender and asymptomatic.

Gartner's cysts arise from remnants of the lower Wolffian-duct system and are found along the anterolateral vaginal wall. They are nontender and vary from 1 to 5 cm in diameter. On infrequent occasions, these cysts become large enough to protrude through the introitus. The cyst contains a thin serous fluid.

Fibromas, myomas, and adenomyomas are infrequent solid tumors found within the vagina. They present as firm, nontender nodules of varying size. Diagnosis is generally made on the basis of excisional biopsy.

Malignant Tumors

Primary vaginal cancer is an uncommon tumor. The appearance of the carcinoma and its characteristics on palpation are varied; diagnosis is dependent upon biopsy and histologic examination.

GASTROINTESTINAL TRACT

FUNCTIONAL

Fecal Material in Large Bowel

Examination of the lower abdomen and pelvis may reveal an irregular mass due to the presence of fecal material in the descending and sigmoid colon. It is sometimes difficult to differentiate this from a pathologic lesion in either the large intestine or reproductive organs. The mass will most often be cylindric in shape, having a diameter of approximately 4 cm and lying obliquely in the left lower quadrant. On abdominal examination the mass is firm, but on pelvic examination it may be perceived as softer and more malleable. The mass is invariably nontender and is somewhat mobile. The redundancy of the sigmoid may allow it to be palpated in the adnexal region, in the cul-de-sac, or anterior to the uterus (see Fig. 23–3).

If doubt exists as to the nature of the mass, the diagnosis can most likely be ascertained upon examining the patient after several days. It will be helpful to administer an enema to the patient prior to examination.

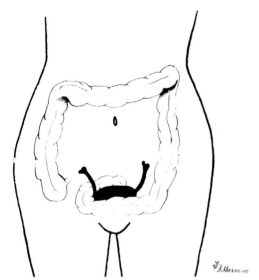

FIGURE 23–3 Redundant sigmoid colon palpable on pelvic examination anterior and posterior to uterus.

Gaseous Distention

Distention of the cecum with gas and fecal contents may produce a right lower quadrant and right adnexal mass. On palpation the mass may be round to cylindric in shape with a diameter of 6 to 8 cm or more. The consistency is soft and cystic, and peristalsis is sometimes palpable. The mass is not mobile and is generally nontender. There are no symptoms associated with gaseous distention. Reexamination of the patient after several hours or days will usually reveal the evanescent nature of the mass.

INFLAMMATORY

Diverticulitis

Diverticulosis is a common disease, with an incidence which increases with age. The sigmoid colon is the usual site for diverticulosis, and the descending colon, transverse colon, and cecum are involved in decreasing order. Inflammation of these diverticula by obstruction of the neck results in erosion and ulceration of the mucosa followed by infection and possible rupture and abscess formation.

The usual site for a mass secondary to diverticulitis is in the left lower quadrant and left adnexal region. The shape of the mass is likely to be irregular, and the size depends upon the size of the abscess and the involvement of adjacent bowel and pelvic organs in the inflammatory reaction. The consistency varies from soft and fluctuant to firm, and the mass is often poorly defined. The mass is nonmobile, adherent to the pelvic wall, and frequently tender.

Symptoms associated with diverticulitis may vary markedly. Patients with a diverticular abscess have presented with minimal gastrointestinal complaints; but the disease can produce more severe gastrointestinal symptoms, including bloody diarrhea, signs of generalized peritonitis, and obstruction.

A barium enema is the most valuable diagnostic tool in this disease and should be considered in all patients with left lower quadrant and left adnexal masses. X-rays, however, may not always reveal the true pathologic situation, and exploratory laparotomy may be required to confirm the diagnosis and treat the condition.

Appendiceal Abscess

The location of the mass secondary to an appendiceal abscess depends upon the position of the appendix. It may be felt high in the right pelvis, right lower quadrant, right adnexal area, or cul-de-sac. The appendiceal abscess frequently involves the adjacent bowel, omentum, and perhaps fallopian tube and ovary in the inflammatory process. The mass tends to be poorly delineated, and the size depends on the size of the abscess and involvement of adjacent organs. The configuration of the mass may alter significantly as the process progresses or resolves under medical therapy. The mass is usually somewhat firm as a result of the induration of surrounding structures. It is nonmobile and tender.

Diagnosis of an appendiceal abscess rests on a history consistent with acute appendicitis followed by right lower quadrant localization. On physical examination temperature may be normal or elevated. Abdominal examination will reveal signs of peritoneal irritation—tenderness, rebound tenderness, and decreased bowel sounds. Laboratory data will include an elevated white blood cell count with a shift to the left. Flat plate of the abdomen may reveal the abscess cavity. Definitive diagnosis usually rests on demonstration of the appendiceal abscess at the time of surgery.

NEOPLASTIC

Small Intestine

Neoplasms of the small bowel constitute only a small percentage of all tumors. These neoplasms, if malignant, are usually not palpable until late in the course of disease.

The location of the mass depends upon the size

of the lesion. A mass may be palpable anywhere within the abdomen or in the cul-de-sac. The size of the mass will vary.

Large Intestine

The formation of a palpable abdominal mass is most often a late manifestation in colonic neoplasms. By the time a mass is palpable, other symptoms have usually caused the patient to seek medical aid. The most common site of large intestinal masses is the rectum. The sigmoid colon and cecum are involved to a lesser extent, and the ascending, descending, and transverse colons are infrequently involved. The size and shape of the mass vary, depending on the size of the lesion, the presence of perforation, and the involvement of adjacent structures. The mass tends to be firm, with poor delimitation and mobility.

With rectal examination and sigmoidoscopy in the age group at risk, 75 percent of large bowel lesions are within reach. Colonoscopy and barium enema are useful for lesions in the more proximal large bowel.

LIVER

Enlargement of the liver is an important consideration in the diagnosis of the mass found in the right upper quadrant. Liver enlargement may be diffuse (typically found in hepatitis and biliary and vascular obstruction) or nodular (seen in carcinoma and postnecrotic regeneration with the formation of hyperplastic liver nodules). Liver function tests will be helpful in diagnosing disease causing liver enlargement. Radioisotope scanning and ultrasound have been used to delineate suspected lesions within the liver parenchyma, and liver biopsy has been an important tool in the diagnosis of obscure liver disease as well as malignancies within the hepatic parenchyma.

GALLBLADDER

INFLAMMATORY

Acute Cholecystitis

Ninety percent of cases of acute cholecystitis are associated with gallstones. A mass may be found in the right upper quadrant subcostal area in one-fourth of cases. This mass is tender, usually poorly defined, and nonmobile. The size of the mass depends upon the size of the gallbladder and the involvement of ad-

herent omentum. An x-ray of the abdomen may demonstrate calculi in the region of the gallbladder and an intravenous cholangiogram will show nonvisualization of the gallbladder.

NEOPLASTIC

Gallbladder Carcinoma

Eighty to ninety percent of cases of gallbladder carcinoma are associated with cholelithiasis. In approximately one-half the cases, a right upper quadrant subcostal mass is palpable.

PANCREAS

INFLAMMATORY

Pseudocysts of the pancreas are formed when rupture of a pancreatic duct secondary to trauma or infection releases fluid into the surrounding tissues. On palpation a vaguely defined cystic mass is felt in the midepigastrium. Tenderness is a variable feature, and the mass is poorly delimited. A history of pancreatitis or trauma with evidence of chronic pancreatitis can usually be obtained.

URINARY TRACT

FUNCTIONAL AND OBSTRUCTIVE

Distended Bladder

A filled or overdistended bladder may masquerade as a cystic mass, filling the anterior pelvis and displacing the uterus, fallopian tubes, and ovaries posteriorly and cephalad. It is essential to ask patients to void prior to pelvic examination unless the examination is designed to investigate the presence of stress incontinence. If the patient has voided and there is still a suspicion that the bladder is the cause of the anterior cystic structure, a catheter may be inserted under sterile conditions so that the urine in the bladder can be drained and measured.

NEOPLASTIC

Renal Cell Carcinoma

Carcinoma involving the kidney may be manifested as a palpable, firm, nodular flank mass. Adhesions and tumor may fix the mass so that no descent is noted on inspiration. Flank pain and hematuria are associated findings. Intravenous pyelograms may reveal the presence of the mass or the nonfunctioning of the involved kidney. Tomograms and arteriography give more information regarding the neoplasm, but definitive diagnosis rests on exploratory surgery with biopsy.

Bladder Carcinoma

Induration of the bladder palpable on pelvic examination may be caused by carcinoma within the bladder. Hematuria is the major complaint in the majority of cases. Definitive diagnosis is made by endoscopic visualization of the bladder with biopsy.

MISCELLANEOUS

Polycystic Kidney

Congenital polycystic renal disease is characterized by multiple cysts in the renal parenchyma, producing compression atrophy of renal tissue. The disease is bilateral in 90 percent of cases. Although far easier to palpate in the infant and child, the bilateral, irregular, flank masses may also be palpable in the adult. The history and characteristic physical findings plus x-ray evidence from intravenous or retrograde pyelography are usually sufficient for the diagnosis.

VASCULAR SYSTEM

Aortic Abdominal Aneurysm

Most abdominal aortic aneurysms arise below the level of the renal artery and hence, if large enough, are palpable abdominally. Aneurysms of this size may measure up to 20 cm or more. They are sometimes tender and are felt on palpation as an expansile, pulsatile mass. An aortic abdominal aneurysm must be distinguished from a mass which overlies the aorta and transmits aortic pulsation through it.

SPLEEN

INFLAMMATORY

Splenic enlargements secondary to infection have a variety of causes. Acute systemic infections such as typhoid and infectious mononucleosis, chronic infections such as tuberculosis and histoplasmosis, subacute bacterial endocarditis, and a variety of para-

sitic infections may all produce splenomegaly. The spleen is usually no more than 4 to 6 cm below the inferior costal margin. The clinical picture associated with splenomegaly often includes temperature elevation, the pattern of which may be characteristic of the particular disease present, and general malaise. More specific signs and symptoms, such as the periodic episodes of fever and chills associated with malaria or the evidence of septic emboli characteristic of subacute bacterial endocarditis, will all be more prominent in the picture than the splenomegaly. Diagnosis generally rests upon the clinical picture, chest x-ray, blood cultures, the variety of serologic and skin tests available, and other measures appropriate for investigating the specific disease.

OBSTRUCTIVE

Primary liver disease with portal hypertension may cause prominent splenic enlargement secondary to congestion of the spleen, with fibrosis and reticuloendothelial hyperplasia.

NEOPLASTIC

Cysts

Cysts of the spleen are rare. They are categorized as true cysts which are thought to be embryonic in origin, false cysts believed secondary to intrasplenic hemorrhage, and cysts which are secondary to parasites, notably *Echinococcus*.

Lymphomatous Tumors

Splenic enlargement may be but one feature of lymphatic carcinoma, notably Hodgkin's disease, lymphosarcoma, reticulum-cell sarcoma, or giant follicular lymphoma. The diagnosis in lymphatic neoplasm rests upon the histologic appearance of a suspicious lymph node.

Leukemia

Splenomegaly is most commonly found in chronic lymphocytic leukemia, but other forms of leukemia may show some degree of splenic enlargement as well. Examination of a peripheral blood smear and bone-marrow aspirate are important features of the workup for this group of diseases.

MISCELLANEOUS

Splenomegaly may be found in a variety of hematologic disorders such as chronic hemolytic states, polycythemia, thrombocytopenia, and a variety of chronic anemias. In addition, there is a group of rare storage diseases, such as Gaucher's disease, Niemann-Pick disease, amyloidosis, and certain collagen diseases, in which the excessive storage of metabolic products within the spleen is probably responsible for the enlargement.

It should be remembered that enlargement of the spleen often accompanies other systemic problems and is seldom the most prominent feature.

OTHER MASSES

Blood Clots

Hemoperitoneum can result from a variety of sources. In gynecology the most common causes are ectopic pregnancy and excessive bleeding from a corpus luteum. Trauma with injury to the spleen or other viscus and perforation of bowel, e.g., peptic ulcer disease, may also give rise to severe bleeding. Collection of blood and blood clots in the cul-de-sac may be palpable as an irregular, soft, doughy mass, poorly delimited and of variable size, which is by itself not particularly tender. If surgery is not performed, repeated examinations over a period of time will reveal a change in the size, extent, and consistency of the mass. Culdocentesis, in the presence of intraperitoneal bleeding, may often yield nonclotting blood. Laparotomy, often performed for both diagnosis and therapy of the intraabdominal bleeding, will reveal the true nature of the cul-de-sac mass.

Retroperitoneal Abscess and Neoplasm

A variety of tumors may be seen in the retroperitoneal region of the pelvis, including benign tumors such as fibromas, lipomas, and cystic teratomas and malignancies such as malignant teratomas, metastatic carcinoma, and bone and nerve tumors. In addition, abscesses may result from osteomyelitis or spinal tuberculosis. These retroperitoneal masses can be palpated on vaginal and rectovaginal examination. They are of varying size, depending on the type of tumor, and appear fixed to the sacral or parasacral areas posteriorly. Tumors resulting from inflammation are likely to be tender and are often associated with other systemic findings of infection. Radiologic investigation may reveal the presence of bony changes secondary to malignancy or infection. A barium enema will usually show the presence of a space-occupying lesion between the rectum and sacrum. The palpation of normal uterine and adnexal struc-

tures is often possible, suggesting that the origin of the tumor is not within the reproductive organs.

Urachal Cyst

The urachus is the remnant of the allantois, the lower end of which expands to form the bladder in the embryo. Incomplete obliteration of the urachus may result in cystic dilatation large enough to be felt as a lower abdominal mass. It is sometimes difficult to distinguish a mass in the anterior abdominal wall from one within the pelvis itself. Palpation of the pelvic organs should suggest the extraabdominal nature of the cyst.

Abdominal Wall Hematoma or Abscess

A hematoma in the rectal muscle may result from trauma or strain, which may be no more than an episode of coughing. Such an insult may not even be remembered by the patient. In addition, the hematoma may become infected, causing the formation of an abdominal wall abscess.

Foreign Body

The presence of a sponge, pad, or surgical instrument forgotten at the time of previous pelvic or abdominal surgery is an unfortunate and preventable surgical complication. Palpation of an irregular mass in the cul-de-sac or adnexal area in a patient who has previously undergone a surgical procedure should suggest a foreign body as a possibility. The patient may be asymptomatic or may have vague feelings of abdominal discomfort, evidence of persistent infection, or even signs or symptoms of intestinal obstruction. Since most materials used within the abdomen are radiopaque, or have radiopaque threads sewn into them, an x-ray of the abdomen will determine the diagnosis.

Omentum and Peritoneum

Primary malignancies within the abdomen commonly metastasize to the omentum and peritoneal lining. Metastatic involvement sufficient to produce a palpable abdominal mass is a sign of advanced disease and carries a grave prognosis. The tumor nodules are usually firm, irregular, and if superficial, well delimited.

ASCITES

There are numerous causes for accumulation of fluid in the peritoneal cavity, and the type of fluid accumulation varies with the situation. A transudate is common in venous obstruction, an exudate is often secondary to peritonitis, and chylous fluid is secondary to lymphatic obstruction.

Inflammatory Causes. Bacterial peritonitis may develop from primary inflammation in the gastrointestinal tract (appendicitis, diverticulitis) or may be associated with a ruptured viscus. Spontaneous bacterial peritonitis has also been noted. Chemical peritonitis may be secondary to pancreatitis or rupture of the biliary tree with escape of bile into the peritoneal cavity. Although now an infrequent illness, tuberculous peritonitis is another cause of ascites.

Obstructive Causes. Lymphatic obstruction secondary to thoracic duct trauma, mediastinal tumors, and parasitic infiltration may lead to the accumulation of chyle in the peritoneal cavity. The same picture has been found in cases of volvulus in which lymphatics of the bowel are obstructed. Vascular obstruction is a more common cause of ascites in which the character of the fluid is that of a transudate. Other causes of decreased venous return to the heart, such as congestive heart failure, tricuspid insufficiency, and constrictive pericarditis, may also result in ascitic-fluid accumulation. Cirrhosis accompanied by portal hypertension can cause ascites, but this is usually in association with decreased levels of circulating albumin secondary to decreased liver production of protein.

Neoplastic Causes. Peritoneal tumors, usually metastatic, and liver cancer, whether primary or metastatic, are frequently found in association with ascites. Multiple causes probably operate in these cases, including peritoneal irritation, lymphatic obstruction, vascular obstruction, and hypoalbuminemia.

Miscellaneous Causes. Hypothyroidism has been found to be related to the accumulation of peritoneal fluid. The presence of a solid ovarian tumor, classically a fibroma, for reasons not yet discovered, has also been associated with accumulation of fluid in pleural and peritoneal cavities.

Conditions Mimicking Ascites

Abdominal distention by intraabdominal neoplasms or intestinal obstruction may mimic some of the findings of ascites, but careful physical examination and specialized studies will rule out ascites in these cases.

Intrauterine pregnancy during its later stages can be distinguished by careful palpation of the abdomen for fetal parts and auscultation for the fetal heartbeat. Polyhydramnios may make these findings difficult, but ultrasound examination or an x-ray of the abdomen should easily differentiate the two conditions.

A large ovarian cyst which fills the abdomen may be difficult to distinguish from ascites. Certain clues, however, are present on physical examination. Ascites produces bulging at the flank, shifting dullness and some protrusion of the umbilicus, whereas the fluid within the ovarian cyst does not. X-ray of the abdomen will show a ground-glass appearance, with bowel floating in the ascitic fluid. Ultrasound may also succeed in differentiating free from encysted fluid. Occasionally the diagnosis can be made only on the basis of exploratory surgery.

Pancreatic pseudocysts may also be large enough to fill the abdomen and simulate ascites. Cysts formed in the mesentery are usually not palpable but occasionally may reach sufficient size to produce generalized enlargement and mimic ascites. Investigation, including x-rays and ultrasound, may also serve to make ascites a more or less probable diagnosis.

Abdominal distention secondary to intestinal obstruction should be easily distinguishable from ascites. The clinical picture of nausea and vomiting, absence of bowel movements, characteristic findings on palpation and auscultation of the abdomen, and radiologic examination should make the diagnosis obvious.

SPECIAL INVESTIGATIVE TECHNIQUES

In addition to routine radiologic studies, such as intravenous and retrograde pyelography, barium enema, and upper gastrointestinal series, there are several techniques which are more specifically aimed at providing information regarding the pelvic structures. Of these, ultrasound and laparoscopy are currently increasing in popularity among gynecologists. Culdoscopy and pelvic pneumography, despite less frequent usage, still have their proponents and remain important diagnostic devices in some clinical conditions.

ULTRASOUND (Donald)

History

In 1880, Pierre and Jacques Curie discovered that the application of a force or mechanical pressure to certain crystals produced an electric current. One year later it was noted that the passage of an electric current across the surface of such a crystal produced a high-frequency vibration wave. World War I saw the development of an ultrasound device designed to detect submarines. This, however, was not put into practical application until World War II, when the device known as sonar became more widely used. The medical use of ultrasound began in the 1960s, with several investigators independently developing equipment to obtain one-dimensional pictures detecting interfaces within the body and the distances from these to other interfaces and body surfaces. This is the so-called A-scan. Later a B-scan was devised which was capable of producing two-dimensional pictures, and more recent sophistication of ultrasound technology has resulted in marked improvement of the images obtained.

Principle

A focused high-frequency sound ranging from 1 million to 15 million vibrations per second is pulsed into the body. At interfaces within the body, sound striking the interface at 90° is reflected back to the source, where it is then recorded on an oscilloscope screen. The use of an appropriate storage device allows the reflected sound to record a picture of the areas struck by the ultrasonic beam as the scanner is moved across the abdomen.

Indications

Ultrasound examination is now used for a wide variety of obstetric problems. Partial characterization of cystic and solid tumors is possible from their ultrasound appearance. It is also possible to distinguish between the free fluid (ascites) and encysted fluid, as found in large ovarian neoplasms. Since malignancy, tuboovarian abscess, and endometriosis may all have similar characteristics on ultrasound, it is always necessary to correlate the ultrasound picture with the clinical findings.

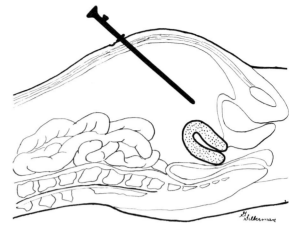

FIGURE 23–4   Laparoscopic examination.

LAPAROSCOPY (Horwitz)

History

The first attempt at endoscopic visualization of abdominal organs was made in 1901 by Kelling, who inserted a cystoscope into the abdomen of a dog and was able to view the abdominal contents. Nine years later he published a monograph dealing with similar experiences on human subjects, and in the same year Jacobaeus independently reported from Stockholm on his series of laparoscopy and thoroscopy. Numerous other authors have since reported their experience with the procedure as well as new developments in equipment and technique.

Equipment and Technique

Visualization of the pelvic and abdominal contents depends upon pneumoperitoneum for distention of the abdominal cavity. Carbon dioxide is usually used and is introduced through a small trocar inserted either just beneath the umbilicus or into one of the lower quadrants. Following pneumoperitoneum, the laparoscope is introduced via an incision in the subumbilical area. Fiberoptic light sources have improved visualization through the endoscope. The patient is placed in the Trendelenburg or head-down position so that the intestines slide away from the pelvis, permitting better visualization of the reproductive organs (see Fig. 23–4).

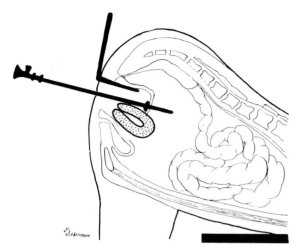

FIGURE 23-5 Culdoscopic examination.

Indications

Laparoscopy has been used to visualize normal organs, diagnose the presence of ectopic pregnancies, visualize suspected pelvic masses or malignancies, examine bowel and omentum, and diagnose the presence of pelvic inflammatory disease and endometriosis with their complications. With the development of specialized instruments, biopsies of suspected lesions, tubal sterilizations, and foreign-body removal have been accomplished. Morbidity of the procedure is low, and its value in avoiding more extensive surgery is estimated at 50 to 70 percent.

Contraindications

The presence of peritonitis or conditions in which adhesions between abdominal viscera and peritoneum might be suspected, such as surgical wounds in the area of laparoscope insertion, are contraindications to the technique.

CULDOSCOPY (Decker)

History

Successful endoscopic visualization of the pelvis via the cul-de-sac was first performed in the early 1940s. Drawing on the earlier experiences with both laparoscopy and colpotomy reported by various investigators, Decker succeeded in examining the pelvic organs through a lighted telescope-like device inserted through a cannula placed into the cul-de-sac by a

puncture wound in the posterior vaginal fornix. Further experience with the technique along with improved instrumentation and light sources resulted in increased sophistication and improved results.

Technique

The procedure may be carried out under spinal or local anesthesia. The patient is placed in the knee-chest position on the examining table with the head of the table tilted down, displacing the bowel from the pelvis. The cervix is grasped with a tenaculum, the posterior vaginal fornix is visualized, and a trocar is inserted between the uterosacral ligaments into the cul-de-sac. After successful puncture, the trocar is removed from its sleeve and replaced by the culdoscope, and the pelvic organs are examined (see Fig. 23-5.)

Indications

Culdoscopy has been used for the same indications as laparoscopy. Laparoscopy has replaced culdoscopy in most situations.

Contraindications

Inability of the patient to assume the knee-chest position is an obvious contraindication to culdoscopy, as is the presence of acute vulvar or vaginal infection or acute peritonitis. The presence of a palpable mass in the cul-de-sac or the absence of the typical stretching of the vaginal fornix on examination, suggesting the presence of adhesions, are indications that culdoscopy cannot be safely performed.

PELVIC PNEUMOGRAPHY (Decker; Levin)

History and Technique

The combination of an induced pneumoperitoneum and abdominal x-rays was introduced in 1919 by Orndoff and Stewart and Stein. It is a procedure infrequently utilized today but remains a valuable aid in the diagnosis of various pelvic abnormalities. The pneumoperitoneum can be induced by transabdominal puncture or through the uterus via a cervical cannula. Carbon dioxide is most frequently used because of its high solubility and rapid absorption from the peritoneal cavity. The needle is withdrawn, and the patient is placed in a prone position. The table is then tilted so that the patient's head is down, and several x-rays are taken. The head-down position causes the gas to rise and accumulate in the pelvis, serving to outline the pelvic structures.

Indications

Pelvic pneumography or gynecography is most helpful in the evaluation of suspected pelvic abnormalities in children and in virgin or obese adults in whom pelvic examination is difficult. It has also been used with success in the diagnosis of polycystic ovarian disease and ectopic pregnancy.

Contraindications

Transabdominal pneumoperitoneum is contraindicated in cases in which intrauterine pregnancy is suspected or shock or peritonitis is present. The transuterine route cannot be used in the presence of pregnancy, pelvic inflammatory disease, or acute vaginal or cervical infections.

DIFFERENTIAL DIAGNOSIS OF ABDOMINOPELVIC MASSES

In many cases the location and palpation characteristics of a palpable mass plus the symptoms caused by it give sufficient information so that it can be correctly identified. The presence of a number of structures in any area of the abdomen or pelvis and the absence of clear-cut symptoms may, however, make the diagnosis difficult without special investigative procedures such as x-rays, isotope scans, ultrasound, and exploratory surgery.

Extremely large masses may also defy diagnosis. Large ovarian cysts, pancreatic pseudocysts, hepatic hemangiomas, and other lesions can, despite their varied origins, attain such great size and so fill the abdomen that diagnosis without surgery is not possible. Fortunately, this situation is not a frequent occurrence.

There are a number of radiologic and other specialized studies which may aid the diagnosis of a palpable mass. The use of these studies should be weighed against the information they provide and the effect of this information on the management of the patient. The question of how the results of a study will alter the therapy should always be confronted. If, for example, a patient is to undergo laparotomy for a 10 cm, mobile cystic mass in the right adnexal area, will

the findings of an intravenous pyelogram, barium enema, or ultrasound scan alter the decision to operate or provide useful information for the surgeon? If the answer to this question is no, then the scheduling of the test should be reconsidered. Obtaining studies for purely educational purposes is not invalid, but these findings must be weighed against the financial burden placed on the patient.

ADNEXA AND CUL-DE-SAC

PALPATION CHARACTERISTICS

Certain characteristics of a cul-de-sac or adnexal mass are often similar. It is appropriate, therefore, to discuss the approach to investigation of a mass in either of these areas under one heading. Tables 23–1 and 23–2 list the possibilities which should be considered.

Identification of a mass as either cystic or solid will help to narrow the diagnostic possibilities. A cystic mass which is mobile is most likely to be ovarian or parovarian in origin. A cystic lesion which is nonmobile and adherent to other pelvic structures or to the lateral pelvic walls may represent an ovarian neoplasm, an inflammatory mass such as a tuboovarian abscess, or an endometrioma. A mass which is both solid and mobile can be a solid ovarian tumor, a pedunculated myoma, a benign bowel neoplasm, or even an unruptured ectopic pregnancy. A solid, nonmobile mass might suggest the presence of a bowel neoplasm, an inflammatory mass, a retroperitoneal neoplasm, or a solid, possibly malignant, ovarian tumor.

Tenderness is another important parameter. Distinct and often exquisite tenderness will be encountered upon palpation of a twisted ovarian or parovarian cyst, an ectopic pregnancy, and inflammatory lesions, whether reproductive or gastrointestinal in origin.

It is also important to distinguish and characterize the other organs palpable on pelvic examination. Palpation of a mass in addition to normal uterus and ovaries bilaterally indicates that the mass is extraovarian in nature. If the uterus is found to be irregular and asymmetric, it is likely that the solid mass adjacent and perhaps fixed to it is a pedunculated myoma. A mass which is adherent to the uterus may also be the result of inflammatory disease, malignancy, or endometriosis. Masses which are bilateral are often secondary to pelvic inflammatory disease, and bilateral retort-shaped cystic masses are partic-

TABLE 23–1 Conditions to Be Considered in the Diagnosis of a Palpable Adnexal Mass

	Cystic	Solid

Ovary	Functional cyst
	Neoplastic cyst
	  Benign
	  Malignant
	Endometrioma
	Ovarian abscess
		Neoplasm
		  Benign
		  Malignant
		Endocrine

Fallopian tube	Pyosalpinx/hydrosalpinx
	Tuboovarian abscess
		Inflammatory mass due to PID*
		Ectopic pregnancy
		Neoplasm
		  Benign
		  Malignant

Mesosalpinx	Parovarian cyst	
Uterus		Pedunculated myoma

Bowel	Sigmoid, cecal gas
	  or feces
	Diverticular abscess
	Appendiceal abscess
		Neoplasm
		  Benign
		  Malignant
		Diverticulitis
		Appendicitis

Miscellaneous	Abdominal wall abscess	Foreign body Abdominal wall hematoma

*Pelvic inflammatory disease

ularly characteristic of tuboovarian abscesses. Bilateral ovarian cysts are not uncommon. The adnexal mass or cul-de-sac mass noted in association with a fixed retroflexed uterus and palpable nodularity along the uterosacral ligaments in a patient whose history is suggestive of endometriosis is quite likely to represent a "chocolate cyst" of the ovary.

HISTORY

A careful history should be taken, noting signs and symptoms indicative of pelvic inflammation or endometriosis. A history of infertility may suggest endometriosis, pelvic inflammatory disease, leiomyomas, or even long-standing ovarian cysts. Previous pelvic surgery should raise the possibility of infection, or perhaps, a foreign body. Malignant disease elsewhere in the body, especially in the breast or gastrointestinal tract, might lead the examiner to suspect the presence of pelvic metastases.

SYMPTOMS

The patient's symptoms provide important clues to the identity of a mass. Fever, chills, and malaise suggest pelvic inflammatory disease or gastrointestinal disease such as diverticulitis or appendicitis. Torsion of an adnexal cyst may produce some temperature elevation, but in general it is lower than with inflammatory lesions. Most other causes of adnexal or cul-de-sac masses are not associated with temperature elevation. A history of weight loss and general debilitation is strongly suggestive of advanced malignancy.

Menstrual abnormalities include delay of normal menses associated with an ectopic gestation, a persistent corpus luteum, or a corpus luteum of pregnancy. A large cul-de-sac mass which is soft and tender, urinary retention, and a 10- to 12-week history of amenorrhea might well indicate the presence of an incarcerated pregnant uterus (see Chap. 30). Irregular vaginal bleeding, on the other hand, is often associated with ovarian neoplasms, uterine myoma, pelvic inflammation, and endometriosis.

The clinical picture of an acute abdomen with direct and rebound tenderness, guarding, and hypoactive bowel sounds may be found in association with pelvic inflammatory disease, torsion of an adnexal neoplasm, ectopic pregnancy, and diverticulitis or appendicitis with or without abscess formation.

The symptoms of diarrhea, nausea, vomiting, anorexia, or the passage of blood or mucus by rectum

TABLE 23–2 Conditions to Be Considered in the Diagnosis of a Palpable Cul-de-sac Mass

Ovary	Cyst
	Functional
	Neoplastic (benign, malignant)
	Endometrioma
	Solid
	Benign
	Malignant
	Endocrine
Fallopian tube	Ectopic pregnancy
	Pyosalpinx/hydrosalpinx
	Tuboovarian abscess
	Pelvic abscess
Uterus	Retroflexed uterus
	Subserosal or pedunculated myoma
Mesosalpinx	Parovarian cyst
Bowel	Fecal material in bowel
	Neoplastic (benign, malignant)
	Diverticulitis with pelvic abscess
	Appendicitis with pelvic abscess
Kidney	Ectopic kidney
Miscellaneous	Retroperitoneal abscess
	Retroperitoneal neoplasm

should suggest a gastrointestinal mass. Patients with diverticulitis, even with abscess formation, are sometimes remarkable for the minor degree of symptoms with which they present. Careful questioning in order to detect subtle changes is often rewarding. Malignancy is suggested by the presence of blood in the stool, anemia, and alterations in bowel habits. Pain with sciatic radiation may well indicate the presence of retroperitoneal neoplasm with bone and nerve-root involvement.

Endocrine abnormalities including hirsutism, clitoral hypertrophy, and deepening of the voice may point to one of the more unusual endocrine tumors of the ovary. Abnormal uterine bleeding, especially in the postmenopausal woman, noted in conjunction with an adnexal tumor, may suggest the presence of a granulosa-theca cell tumor.

The subjective feeling of shoulder pain in association with abdominal pain and a pelvic mass is characteristic of intraabdominal bleeding, usually secondary to an ectopic pregnancy or a bleeding corpus luteum.

INVESTIGATIVE STUDIES

Acute blood loss, whether intraperitoneal or external, is not reflected by the level of hemoglobin or hematocrit until a number of hours after the onset of bleeding. Therefore, the blood loss of patients with ectopic pregnancy or corpus luteum bleeding will not, in the acute state, be mirrored by the patient's hematocrit. This test, however, is certainly important as a baseline for subsequent assessment, before and after therapy, of the amount of blood the patient has actually lost.

The presence of infection originating in either the reproductive organs or gastrointestinal tract will usually result in the elevation of the white blood cell count and appearance in the peripheral blood smear of more immature forms of leukocytes. Unfortunately, leukocytosis is not always a reliable finding, and cases of pelvic infection with bilateral tuboovarian abscesses as well as diverticular or appendiceal abscesses are occasionally found with normal white blood cell counts and no shift to the left.

Culdocentesis involves tapping the peritoneal cavity through the cul-de-sac with a needle and syringe. The finding of nonclotting blood in the cul-de-sac confirms the presence of intraabdominal bleeding; when associated with a palpable mass, an ectopic pregnancy or a bleeding corpus luteum is strongly suggested. Pus in the cul-de-sac reflects pelvic or other intraabdominal infection. It should be stressed that the absence of fluid does not constitute a negative tap; in such cases the culdocentesis should be termed noncontributory. The absence of peritoneal fluid may mean either that no fluid is present or that the examining needle has not been accurately placed.

Radiologic studies may constitute an important part of the workup of an adnexal mass, especially if surgery is contemplated. The finding of pleural fluid on a chest x-ray suggests Meigs's syndrome or an effusion secondary to metastatic disease. Abdominal x-rays often reveal calcifications characteristic of an ovarian cystic teratoma or a uterine myoma. The full extent of the pelvic mass may be delineated, and air-fluid levels in an abscess cavity can also be seen. A barium enema should be considered in all cases of questionable left lower quadrant masses. It is not uncommon for a patient whose diverticulitis has advanced to abscess formation to present with minimal gastrointestinal signs and a mass which is fixed to the left pelvic wall. Proper diagnosis prior to laparotomy would allow for surgical consultation and appropriate bowel preparation. An intravenous pyelogram is an important study, especially when pelvic malignancy is a consideration. The presence of ureteral obstruction might well alter the type and extent of surgery performed and would certainly alert the surgeon to possible difficulties encountered during the dissection. On infrequent occasions the presence of an ectopic kidney in the pelvis will be seen on intravenous pyelogram and will resolve the evaluation of the cul-de-sac mass and avert surgery.

Ultrasound scanning of the abdomen and pelvis may give important clues to the identity of the palpable mass. The presence of an extrauterine gestational sac is presumptive evidence of an ectopic pregnancy. This examination can also help to sort out conditions in which uterine and ovarian abnormalities coexist.

Examination under anesthesia is an important diagnostic tool when thickness of the anterior abdominal wall and poor patient cooperation preclude adequate pelvic evaluation. With relaxation of the lower abdominal musculature and where deep palpation is not painful, the physician's ability to palpate pelvic structures is enhanced. If necessary, surgical exploration can then be accomplished under the same anesthesia.

Endoscopic visualization of pelvic structures through the laparoscope or culdoscope is of limited value when a significant mass is already clinically palpable. It can be useful to distinguish between a pedunculated myoma and a solid ovarian tumor or to detect a suspected mass that cannot be outlined clearly on bimanual examination.

The presence of a distinct persistent adnexal or cul-de-sac mass of significant size will usually necessitate surgical exploration, both for definitive gross and histologic evaluation and for therapy. The presence of solid adnexal tumors in which ovarian malignancy cannot be ruled out by other means also necessitates surgery.

MIDLINE SUPRAPUBIC AREA

Table 23-3 lists the possible causes of a midline suprapubic mass. Of these, intrauterine pregnancy, ovarian cysts, hematometria or pyometria, leiomyoma, and trophoblastic disease can enlarge to the size of 20 weeks' gestation or more. The remainder are usually much smaller and are palpable only on pelvic examination.

PALPATION CHARACTERISTICS

Findings on pelvic and abdominal examination will often suggest the diagnosis without the need for further specialized investigation. A mass which is contiguous with the cervix is likely to be of uterine origin, although occasionally, adherent ovarian tumors may be difficult to separate from the uterus. Irregularity and asymmetry of the mass make the diagnosis of uterine leiomyomas likely. The cystic soft anterior mass which displaces the uterus and adnexa may well be a distended bladder. Requesting that the patient void or, if that is not successful in reducing the size of the mass, emptying the bladder with a catheter will quickly settle this diagnosis. The characteristic feel of fecal material in a redundant sigmoid colon presenting as a series of somewhat doughy nodular masses stretched across the anterior cul-de-sac can be deceiving to the inexperienced examiner. The ability to feel the uterus and ovaries indicates that the mass is extragenital. Bowel or bladder masses and lesions of the lower anterior abdominal wall remain possibilities if this is the case. The cervix should be inspected for occlusion secondary to scarring or malignancy. Finally, it is always important with a mass which is the size of 20 weeks' gestation or greater to listen for fetal heart tones and palpate for fetal parts, always remembering that the most common supra-

TABLE 23-3 Conditions to Be Considered in the Diagnosis of a Palpable Midline Pelvic or Suprapubic Mass

Uterus	Pregnancy
	Hematometria, pyometria
	Neoplasm
	Benign (leiomyoma)
	Malignant
	Trophoblastic
Bladder	Distended bladder
	Neoplasm
	Cystitis (severe)
Ovary	Neoplasm
	Benign
	Malignant
Bowel	Fecal material in bowel
	Malignant neoplasm
Miscellaneous	Urachal cyst
	Abdominal wall hematoma or
	abscess
	Foreign body

pubic midline mass is the pregnant uterus. Sounding of the enlarged uterus when pregnancy has been ruled out may reveal the flow of blood or pus characteristic of a hematometrium or pyometrium.

HISTORY

A previous history of known pelvic abnormalities such as myomas or ovarian cysts will often suggest the diagnosis. The patient should be questioned regarding previous pelvic surgery with a view toward discovering the presence of a foreign body or a reason for cervical occlusion. A history of abdominal trauma may suggest the presence of an abdominal wall hematoma or abscess.

SYMPTOMS

Of all the conditions listed in Table 23–3, only pyometria is likely to be associated with temperature elevation. Enlarging abdominal girth is suggestive of pregnancy, ovarian cysts, or ascites. Questioning and examination for signs of pregnancy should always be performed in patients during their reproductive years. A period of amenorrhea with associated nausea, vomiting, and breast enlargement is clearly suggestive. Abnormal uterine bleeding may be indicative of the presence of myoma, pregnancy, or ovarian cyst. Pressure by a myoma on surrounding pelvic structures may produce stress incontinence, decreased bladder capacity, or feelings of tenesmus. When urinary retention is a possibility, the patient should be questioned concerning her pattern of urination during the several days prior to her examination. Frequent urination in small amounts with dribbling is characteristic of the overflow incontinence associated with an overdistended bladder. The small tumor palpable anteriorly unconnected with the cervix or uterus is certainly suggestive of a bladder tumor or the induration secondary to a severe cystitis. Alterations in bowel habits and bloody stools with a decreased caliber are indicative of a malignant gastrointestinal neoplasm.

INVESTIGATION

When pregnancy is suspected, it should always be remembered that the common immunologic test for pregnancy may be negative prior to 8 weeks and after 20 weeks of gestation. A more sensitive radioimmune assay can detect chorionic gonadotropin as early as 7 days after fertilization and can prove valuable in diagnosing an early pregnancy or differentiating an ectopic gestation from pain or a mass not associated with pregnancy. The presence of an early pregnancy will be typified by progressive uterine growth over several weeks after the initial finding of an enlarged uterus, and pregnancy tests will eventually become positive. Beyond 20 weeks abdominal palpation and auscultation over the mass will usually make the diagnosis of pregnancy obvious.

A flat film of the abdomen may reveal the presence of calcifications characteristic of cystic teratomas, calcified myoma, or fetal parts. It may also reveal the extent of the mass or the presence of a foreign body. A barium enema is extremely important in cases in which there is any suspicion of bowel lesion. An intravenous pyelogram may serve to outline the mass and examine the deviation and involvement of the ureters by it. The use of ultrasound in the diagnosis of early pregnancy, trophoblastic disease, in the determination of whether fluid is free or encysted, and in the discovery and partial characterization of ovarian neoplasms is becoming increasingly important.

If bladder disease is a possibility, endoscopic visualization of the bladder mucosa is a valuable part of the diagnostic process. Severe inflammation and bladder tumors are visible, and biopsies may be taken through the cystoscope.

When abnormal uterine bleeding is part of the clinical picture and pregnancy has been ruled out, dilatation and curettage should be performed to investigate the bleeding and assess the size and configuration of the endometrial cavity. Myometrial irregularities secondary to submucosal myomas can be appreciated by the examiner as the curette passes over them; sounding of the uterus will disclose enlargement and distortion of the cavity; and histologic examination of the scrapings is an indispensable method of discovering uterine malignancy.

The nature of most suprapubic midline masses is discernible by means of the above modalities of investigation. Sometimes, however, exploratory laparotomy is necessary to both confirm the diagnosis and treat the disease.

MIDABDOMINAL AREA

Table 23–4 lists the possibilities to be considered in the differential diagnosis of a mass palpable in the

TABLE 23-4 Conditions to Be Considered in the Diagnosis of a Midabdominal Mass

Bowel	Neoplasm (malignant)
Vascular	Aortic aneurysm
Miscellaneous	Omental malignancy (metastatic)
	Anterior wall hematoma or abscess
	Peritoneal malignancy (metastatic)

TABLE 23–5 Conditions to Be Considered in the Diagnosis of a Palpable Epigastric Mass

Bowel	Malignant neoplasm (gastric usually)
Pancreas	Pseudocyst
Vascular	Aortic aneurysm
Liver	Diffuse hepatomegaly
	Hepatic abscess
	Neoplasm
	Cyst
	Benign
	Malignant
Miscellaneous	Peritoneal malignancy (metastatic)

midabdominal or periumbilical area. For purposes of discussion, masses in this location are differentiated from those which arise in the pelvis and extend to or beyond the midabdomen. The latter masses have been previously discussed under the heading of midline suprapubic masses. Intestinal and omental neoplasms probably form the largest portion of masses in the abdomen. It is likely that by the time a neoplasm in either the bowel or omentum becomes large enough to be palpable, the malignancy is already far advanced and symptoms referrable to the malignancy are already present. The mass secondary to a malignant tumor is likely to be nodular, firm, and nontender. The pulsatile mass of an aortic aneurysm is usually easily palpable. In the thin patient with a prominent lordosis, the pulsating aorta over the lumbar vertebrae may be palpable on abdominal examination, simulating the presence of an aneurysm. The diagnosis, therefore, should not be made unless the expansile nature of the mass can be appreciated.

If omental tumor is a possibility, a careful search should be made on physical examination for the primary source of the metastatic lesion. Pelvic examination with special attention to the adnexal areas is quite important, the omentum being a common site for metastatic ovarian carcinoma. Questions regarding the presence of gastrointestinal symptoms, change in bowel habits, evidence of gastrointestinal bleeding, and signs or symptoms of intestinal obstruction may point toward a diagnosis of gastrointestinal neoplasm.

Radiologic investigation should include routine abdominal x-rays, a barium enema, and if obstruction is not present, an upper GI (gastrointestinal) series. This may serve to reveal either the presence of an extrinsic lesion or a tumor originating in the bowel.

When the nature of the mass remains unclear, exploratory laparotomy is necessary for diagnosis as well as therapy.

EPIGASTRIUM

The possibilities to be considered in the diagnosis of a mass in the epigastrium are listed in Table 23–5. Of these, masses originating in the liver and other causes of hepatomegaly will be considered in the next section. Gastrointestinal neoplasms, by the time they are palpable, are likely to be far advanced. A strong indication that a lesion is gastric in origin is the presence of hematemesis or black tarry stools. The patient will usually appear for medical aid long before the gastric tumor is palpable. Neoplasms of the transverse colon are likely to be responsible for lower GI hemorrhage, anemia, and signs and symptoms of intestinal obstruction. The presence of a vaguely defined cystic mass in the epigastrium in a patient with a history of pancreatitis or pancreatic trauma or in a patient with evidence of chronic pancreatitis should strongly suggest the presence of a pancreatic pseudocyst. Investigation of an undiagnosed epigastric mass should include tests for occult blood in the stool and x-rays of the upper and lower gastrointestinal tract, both for purposes of revealing intrinsic lesions and for outlining lesions extrinsic to the bowel.

RIGHT UPPER QUADRANT

Right upper quadrant masses most likely originate in the liver or gallbladder (Table 23–6). Palpable enlargement of a kidney secondary to carcinoma or polycystic disease is usually felt on deep palpation of the right lumbar region. A renal mass will usually descend with deep inspiration. It should be remembered that more than 90 percent of patients with polycystic renal disease will have bilateral involvement. Tumor involving the colon may be difficult to distinguish from the renal mass, as it may also occupy a

TABLE 23-6 Conditions to Be Considered in the Diagnosis of a Palpable Right Upper Quadrant Mass

Liver	Diffuse hepatomegaly
	Postnecrotic nodular regeneration
	Hepatic abscess
	Neoplasm
	Cyst
	Benign
	Malignant
Gallbladder	Cholecystitis
	Malignant neoplasm
Bowel	Malignant neoplasm
Urinary	Renal carcinoma
	Polycystic disease

TABLE 23-7 Conditions to Be Considered in the Diagnosis of a Palpable Left Upper Quadrant Mass

Spleen	Splenomegaly
	Neoplasm (rare)
Urinary	Renal carcinoma
	Polycystic disease
Bowel	Malignant neoplasm

position in the right lumbar region. Hepatomegaly or neoplasms of the liver occupy a more superficial position. Nodularity of the liver is often a sign of neoplasm, cyst, abscess, or regenerating hepatic nodules. Tenderness over the enlarged liver suggests acute enlargement secondary to vascular obstruction, congestive failure, or inflammatory conditions. Palpable liver pulsation is classically secondary to tricuspid regurgitation. Auscultation over the liver may reveal a bruit in the presence of arteriovenous fistulas or vascular tumors or secondary to the pressure of an enlarged liver on the aorta, and neoplastic infiltration of the liver capsule and peritoneum may result in the presence of a friction rub.

Signs and symptoms referrable to the liver or biliary tree will usually indicate the probable source of the palpable mass. Jaundice, signs of hepatocellular dysfunction, or bilary obstruction will frequently be obvious. A characteristic history of fatty food intolerance, previous episodes of sharp right upper quadrant discomfort, and perhaps transient episodes of jaundice are suggestive of gallbladder disease. Investigational studies include tests of liver function and special radiologic studies to visualize the gallbladder and demonstrate the presence of cholelithiasis. The barium enema is indispensable for the discovery of gastrointestinal malignancies. If the mass is most likely renal, an intravenous pyelogram or retrograde pyelography is an important part of the diagnostic workup.

LEFT UPPER QUADRANT

The most usual cause of a mass palpable in the left upper quadrant is splenic enlargement (Table 23-7). However, the origin of the mass may be renal or gastrointestinal. A thorough history and physical examination, as well as a peripheral smear, often point to

splenomegaly. Evidence of acute or chronic bacterial or parasitic inflammation, lymphatic neoplasm, leukemia, or liver disease may be apparent. Hematologic changes secondary to hypersplenism may be suggested by the examination of the blood and confirmed by more specialized studies as well as bone-marrow aspiration.

CONCLUSION

This discussion has attempted to summarize most causes of palpable masses that a physician comes in contact with. Palpable masses originating in the skin have not been dealt with, and the student is referred to the many excellent texts on dermatology which discuss these lesions. For obvious reasons, emphasis has been placed on masses in the abdomen and pelvis, for these are most likely to be a problem for the gynecologic practitioner. Common and uncommon lesions have been discussed. An unusual condition cannot be diagnosed unless it is included in the differential diagnosis.

It is important to stress again the value of keeping an open mind. To focus on a diagnosis without adequate information is to do both the patient and yourself a disservice. Intuition, based on knowledge and past experience, is an important tool in the practice of any branch of medicine, but intuition should never replace a logical and systematic approach to a problem in which all possibilities are carefully considered.

REFERENCES

Anderson WAD, Kissane JH (eds.):_Pathology,_ 7th ed., St. Louis: Mosby, 1977.

Beeson PB, McDermott W (eds.): _Textbook of Medicine,_ 14th ed., Philadelphia: Saunders, 1975.

Decker A: _Culdoscopy,_ Philadelphia: FA Davis, 1967.

Donald I: Diagnostic sonar in obstetrics and gynecology, in _Obstetrics and Gynecology Annual,_ ed. RW Wynn, New York: Appleton-Century-Crofts, 1972.

Gould Medical Dictionary, 3d ed., New York: McGraw-Hill, 1972.

Gusberg SB, Frick HC: *Corscaden's Gynecologic Cancer,* 4th ed., Baltimore: Williams & Wilkins, 1970.

Haagensen CD: *Diseases of the Breast,* 2d ed., Philadelphia: Saunders, 1971.

Horwitz ST: Laparoscopy in gynecology. *Obstet Gynecol Surv* 27:1, 1972.

Levin B: Roentgenologic aspects of gynecologic endocrinology, in *Textbook of Gynecologic Endocrinology,* 2d ed., ed. JJ Gold, New York: Harper & Row, 1977.

Maddrey W: Principal manifestations of liver disease, in *The Principles and Practice of Medicine,* 19th ed., eds. AM Harvey et al., New York: Appleton-Century-Crofts, 1976.

Novak ER et al. (eds.): *Novak's Textbook of Gynecology,* 9th ed., Baltimore: Williams & Wilkins, 1975.

Sabiston DC (ed.): *Textbook of Surgery,* 11th ed., Philadelphia: Saunders, 1977.

Stedman TL: *Medical Dictionary,* 22d ed., Baltimore: Williams & Wilkins, 1971.

Viacava ET, Pack GT: Significance of supraclavicular single node in patients with abdominal and thoracic cancer. *Arch Surg* 48:109, 1944.

Way S: The lymphatics of the pelvis, in *Scientific Foundations of Obstetrics and Gynecology,* eds. EE Philipp et al., Philadelphia: FA Davis, 1970.

Werner SC, Ingber SH (eds.): *The Thyroid,* 3d ed., New York: Harper & Row, 1971.

24

Genital Discharge and Pruritus

JAMES A. MERRILL

Discharge from the vagina and itching of the vulva or vagina are common reasons women see a gynecologist, although they are not always primary complaints. These two symptoms often appear together but may occur independently. There are both local and systemic causes for discharge and pruritus, and the symptoms are perceived by different women differently. In addition to disease states, physiologic variations, emotions, and the internal and external environments are influential in producing these symptoms. However, these are only *symptoms,* and treatment should be reserved until the cause has been established.

The patient's willingness or reluctance to seek medical advice because of genital discharge or pruritus is influenced by social and moral attitudes. Anxiety may arise from the misconception that discharge or itching represents venereal disease or cancer. In some circumstances, the patient may actually present with a complaint of vaginal or perineal malodor. This may or may not be associated with excessive or abnormal secretions and often is perceived only by the patient and not by those around her. In our present society, there are many who perceive any body odor as something offensive or "unclean."

DISCHARGE

In clinical practice, discharge refers to excessive or abnormal vulvovaginal secretions. *Leukorrhea* and *discharge* have been used synonymously. However, leukorrhea literally means "a flow of white substance" and should be used only when referring to an excessive amount of normal secretions. The more fastidious and compulsive the woman, the more likely she is to complain of a discharge, while other women appear oblivious of profuse discharge.

NORMAL DISCHARGE

Women with adequate endogenous or exogenous estrogen have vaginal secretions. There is a small amount of secretion from Bartholin's, sebaceous, sweat, and apocrine glands of the vulva; the vaginal epithelium; the cervix; and rarely the uterus and oviduct. Secretions of Bartholin's, sebaceous, sweat, and apocrine glands of the vulva vary with ovarian function and sexual stimulation. Vaginal secretions generally are white or greyish with a semisolid consistency due to clumps of superficial epithelial cells. The cervix secretes an alkaline glairy mucoid substance, influenced by ovarian steroid hormones and characteristically more abundant and less viscous at the time of ovulation. This secretion may be exaggerated in women receiving estrogen-dominant oral contraceptive tablets. The alkaline watery secretion from the uterus during the secretory phase of the menstrual cycle and the watery fluid from the oviduct contribute little to vaginal secretions.

The normal secretions from the vagina are acid with a pH range from 3.8 to 4.2. Physiologic vaginal secretions usually are not malodorous, although some women may claim an offensive odor. Microscopic examination of the discharge reveals clumps of desquamated squamous epithelial cells and a predominant *Lactobacillus* flora. Leukocytes are not seen characteristically. The amount of vaginal secretion increases at the time of ovulation, several days before menstruation, during pregnancy, and during sexual excitement.

An explanation of the nature of the discharge and the reassurance that no pathologic condition exists often relieves the symptoms of discharge and/or malodor.

ABNORMAL DISCHARGE

Table 24–1 lists causes of genital discharge (see Chap. 40). The three common types of vaginitis (trichomoniasis, candidiasis, bacterial vaginitis) ac-

count for the majority of complaints of discharge. Chronic cervicitis accounts for most mucoid discharge commonly not associated with itching, pain, or sensitivity. In recent years oral contraceptives, intrauterine devices, and genital herpes have emerged as causes of discharge.

PHYSIOLOGIC (HORMONAL) CAUSES

Newborn babies may have a mucoid vaginal discharge for 1 to 10 days after birth. This is the result of in utero stimulation of the infant's uterus and vagina by the high levels of maternal estrogen. Similarly, a mucoid discharge is not uncommon in girls a few years before and after the menarche. This is apparently due to increased estrogen production by the maturing ovary. It is a self-limiting phenomenon and requires only explanation and reassurance. Pregnancy and the use of oral contraceptive pills may substantially increase the cervical mucus production and secretion, resulting in a profuse watery or mucoid discharge. In some cases it may be necessary to withdraw the contraceptive pills or substitute a preparation with a relatively low estrogen content.

VAGINAL CAUSES

Vaginitis

The most common significant vaginal infection is candidiasis (produced by *Candida albicans*), now constituting approximately half of all cases of vaginitis. Pruritus is a more common symptom than discharge. It is generally thought that increased use of antibiotics and oral contraceptives accounts for the increased incidence of this infection by altering the normal bacterial flora or the pH of the vagina. However, Lapan reported no increase in incidence of candidiasis among patients receiving contraceptive pills. The discharge is commonly white and curdy with adherent plaques on the surface of the vagina. The diagnosis is confirmed by finding the typical spores and hyphae in a potassium hydroxide–wet smear preparation.

Trichomoniasis is less common as a cause of vaginitis than it once was. The *Trichomonas* parasite is found in the vagina far more commonly than it produces clinical vaginitis. Furthermore, it is clear that psychosomatic factors influence the development and recurrence of *Trichomonas* vaginitis. Since the disease may be transmitted by the male, the sexual partner must also be treated if recurrence of the infection is to be prevented. A typical discharge is frothy

TABLE 24–1   Causes of Genital Discharge

Physiologic
  Neonatal mucorrhea
  Premenarchal leukorrhea
  Premenstrual
  Pregnancy
  Oral contraceptive pills
  Puerperium
	Uterine
	  Pyometra
	  Carcinoma
	  Submucous myomas
	  Endometrial polyps
	  Intrauterine devices

Vaginal
  Candidiasis
  Trichomoniasis
  Hemophilus vaginalis
  Bacterial vaginitis
  Atrophic vaginitis
    Postmenopausal
    Postirradiation
    Pediatric
  Herpes
  Foreign body vaginitis
    Pediatric
    Adult
  Allergic and primary
    irritant reactions
  Vaginal adenosis
	Tubal
	  Hydrosalpinx (hydrops
	    tubae profluens)
	  Carcinoma
	
	Vulvar
	  Herpes
	  Pyodermas
	  Suburethral diverticulum
	  Urethritis
	  Bartholinitis
	  Condylomata acuminata
	  Syphilis
	  Granuloma inguinale
	  Lymphogranuloma
	    venereum
	  Chancroid
	  Carcinoma

Cervical
  Gonorrhea
  Chronic cervicitis
  Cervical polyps
  Carcinoma
	Fistulas
	  Urinary
	  Rectal

and greenish grey with punctate red foci on the surface of the vagina and cervix. The diagnosis is confirmed by identifying the motile *Trichomonas* parasites in a saline wet smear preparation.

A grey, homogeneous, malodorous discharge may result from *bacterial vaginitis.* Some authors have indicated that the common agent causing this is *Hemophilus vaginalis.* The diagnosis is suspected when numerous leukocytes are found in a saline preparation of discharge. Culture is often disappointing. Some authors believe that the presence of *Hemophilus vaginalis* is confirmed by findings of few, or no leukocytes and stippled or granulated epithelial cells in the wet saline smear. These have been called "clue cells."

Atrophic Vaginitis

Atrophic vaginitis is the superficial irritation and sometimes bacterial infection of a thin, poorly vascularized vaginal epithelium usually seen in postmenopausal or castrate women. The causative bacterial

agents are numerous and are rarely identified specifically. The discharge is usually watery but may be mucopurulent, and the patient complains of burning and itching in the vagina and vulva. The diagnosis is indicated by examination which reveals typical estrogen-deficient epithelium with telangiectasia and atrophy. The diagnosis is supported by examination of a saline-slide suspension of discharge which reveals numerous leukocytes, bacteria, and predominant *parabasal epithelial* cells.

Vaginitis in children resembles atrophic vaginitis in postmenopausal women. It is difficult to determine the specific cause for discharge and vaginitis in children, but the lack of estrogen stimulation of the vagina is a common underlying factor. *Trichomonas, Candida,* and mixed bacteria may cause vaginitis in the child, but represent a minor role. Gonorrhea should be considered and excluded but is an infrequent cause of discharge in children. The combination of a discharge, malodor, and sometimes scant bleeding should suggest the possibility of a foreign body in the vagina. This can usually be determined by rectal examination, direct inspection with a vaginoscope, or use of appropriate pediatric speculum and vaginal probing. Intestinal parasites, particularly pinworms, may cause vaginitis and discharge in children. The investigation of discharge in a child should include the microscopic examination of a Scotch-tape preparation to exclude pinworms, a microscopic examination of a saline suspension of the discharge, culture, and careful examination. Whatever the cause of the vaginitis in the child, local application of estrogen cream is often helpful in therapy.

Malodorous mucopurulent discharge may result from vaginitis secondary to a foreign body in the vagina of the adult. Such foreign bodies might include vaginal tampons which are forgotten, diaphragms, vaginal pessaries, and an assortment of unusual objects. The diagnosis is readily established by vaginal examination.

Reaction to vaginal douche solutions or other female hygienic medication may produce inflammation with resultant discharge. This reaction may be due to an allergy or the direct irritant effect of the substance. Certain contraceptive creams and foams cause an inflammatory response in some women. Too frequent douching, even with nonirritating substances, may also produce discharge from the vagina.

CERVICAL CAUSES (see Chap. 41)

Gonorrhea involving the endocervix produces a mucopurulent discharge, often without evidence of irritation of the vagina or vulva. Appropriate cultures are indicated. The most common cervical cause of discharge is *chronic cervicitis* which often represents the secretion from exposed endocervical epithelium. Although exposed endocervical epithelium (erosion) exists in adolescents more often than is generally appreciated, the disorder is most common among parous women. The amount of discharge is, to some extent, hormonally related and may be exaggerated by the use of oral contraceptive pills with a relatively high content of estrogen. The diagnosis is established by careful inspection of the cervix.

A characteristic symptom of *malignant neoplasm* of the lower genital tract is discharge. Any growth in this location may produce a continuous serous, mucoid, sanguineous, or purulent discharge. If the neoplasm becomes infected and necrotic, the discharge is characteristically purulent, malodorous, and offensive. This may represent a serious management problem in patients with far-advanced malignancy of the cervix, vagina, or vulva. On rare occasions, benign neoplasms, such as cervical polyps or sloughing submucous myomas, produce discharge.

UTERINE CAUSES

Intrauterine devices are rare causes of discharge, as is the accumulation and release of exudate (pyometra) or bloody fluid (hematometra) secondary to uterine malignancy or radiation therapy.

TUBAL CAUSES

An interesting, but exceedingly rare, type of discharge occurs with hydrosalpinx or carcinoma of the oviduct. The discharge is described as intermittent release of fluid, usually clear or blood-tinged. It is the result of periodic emptying through the uterus of the fluid contained in the diseased oviduct and is referred to as *hydrops tubae profluens*.

VULVAR CAUSES

Any of the various inflammatory diseases of the vulva may produce discharge as a result of draining sinuses or weeping lesions. However, in these circumstances, the primary complaint is usually pain, tenderness, or itching. The incidence of genital herpes is increasing. The primary vesicles of this infection may occur on the vulva, vagina, or cervix. The vesicles ulcerate, and the erythematous ulcerative lesions subsequently coalesce. The patient may complain of genital discharge, but vulvar pain, "tingling," and dysuria are the usual presenting symptoms. The diagnosis may be made by cytologic studies, culture, or serum antibody determination.

FISTULAS

Urinary or rectal fistulas may produce a discharge which is ordinarily recognized by its color and odor and is confirmed by careful inspection of the vagina and the bladder or rectum.

CLINICAL INVESTIGATION

Evaluation of a patient complaining of discharge is facilitated by examination of the patient when the discharge is most prominent and when there has been no prior medication or douching. The age of the patient will suggest certain causes, as indicated above.

The amount of discharge reported by the patient will be variable and is not necessarily related to the actual volume of secretion. Profuse discharge is common in acute trichomoniasis, urinary fistulas, and infected necrotic neoplasms. Itching or pruritus with discharge is most frequently due to candidiasis and is less often seen in atrophic vaginitis in postmenopausal patients and in acute trichomoniasis. Sudden onset of discharge suggests infection. Typically, the discharge of trichomoniasis commences or becomes worse during and after menstruation. Bloody discharge should alert the physician to the possibility of a neoplasm or foreign body.

The key to identifying the cause of discharge is a careful pelvic examination and gross and microscopic examination of the discharge. The physician should look for ulceration, edema, and excoriation of the vulva. The vagina and cervix should be carefully inspected for lesions as well as evidence of inflammation or foreign bodies. Curdy secretions suggest either normal vaginal secretion or candidiasis. White plaques, which are readily scraped from the epithelium, are pathognomonic of candidiasis but are seen in only about 20 percent of patients with this infection.

An opaque homogeneous discharge suggests trichomoniasis or bacterial vaginitis. Malodor with little discharge is a characteristic of *Hemophilus* vaginitis. The discharge of atrophic vaginitis is serous or watery, and discharge arising from endocervical glands is usually mucoid.

Wet mount preparations of vaginal secretions are essential. They should be prepared with physiologic saline and also with dilute (10 to 20%) potassium hydroxide (KOH). Both suspensions can be prepared on the same glass slide. A drop of discharge is placed on each end of the slide with a nonabsorbent applicator. Any curds or plaques in the secretion should be included. If the discharge is frothy, that area should be selected for sampling. The discharge is thoroughly mixed with saline at one end of the slide and with KOH at the other end of the slide. A cover slip is placed on both suspensions. The slide is then examined microscopically. Motile trichomonads, leukocytes, epithelial cells, bacteria, and granulated epithelial cells ("clue" cells) are best identified in the saline suspension (Fig. 24–1). The spores and hyphae of *Candida* are best identified in the KOH suspension (Fig. 24–2).

FIGURE 24–1 The microscopic appearance of *Trichomonas* in a saline suspension.

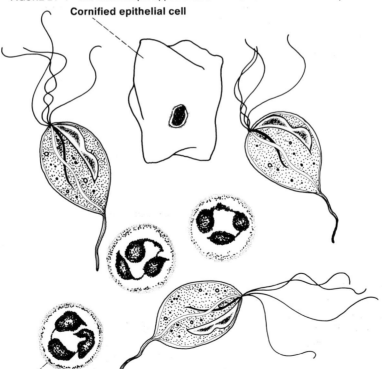

Cornified epithelial cell

Leukocyte

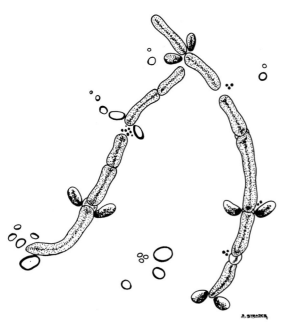

FIGURE 24–2 The spores and hyphae of *Candida albicans* as seen microscopically with KOH suspension.

Stained smears of vaginal secretions are rarely helpful in the diagnosis of genital discharge. Although trichomonads and *Candida* may be identified in the standard cytologic preparations (Pap smears) obtained for cancer diagnosis, this method is not reliable. However, cellular changes pathognomonic of genital herpes may be identified in similar preparations and do serve as a convenient and reliable method of diagnosing this disease.

Furthermore, cultures are rarely required in the differential diagnosis of genital discharge. Culture of the discharge may be revealing in the patient with persistent discharge for which a specific cause is not apparent by the methods of examination described. *Specific cultures* in reduced oxygen atmosphere to identify *Neisseria gonorrhoeae* are essential, of course.

Nickerson's medium has proved accurate and practical for identifying *Candida* species. Simple, single-vial culture tubes may be streaked with discharge, and a positive culture is identified by a color change following incubation at room temperature. Unfortunately, not all *Candida* is *Candida albicans*, which is the cause of vaginitis. This culture is seldom more reliable than careful examination of a KOH suspension.

Gardner and Dukes recommend Casman's blood agar with 5% defibrinated rabbit blood as the best medium for culturing *H. vaginalis*. Incubation must be in a reduced oxygen atmosphere. The success of culturing this organism is extremely variable.

Biopsy will be necessary if a suspected neoplasm is found.

PRURITUS

Genital pruritus is not uncommon. *Pruritus vulvae* is often considered a specific entity despite the fact that it is actually a manifestation of disease. At times, the pruritus is so severe as to produce an uncontrollable urge to scratch the affected area. In many patients, the itching becomes particularly intense at night in bed. Severe scratching during sleep is not uncommon. Pruritus of the vulva can be agonizing to the patient and frustrating to the gynecologist. Thoroughness and sympathetic persistence are required in the evaluation of this symptom. Too often, the physician is unable to find the specific cause or to satisfactorily treat it. Genital pruritus has many possible causes, and unless they are identified, the treatment is usually unsatisfactory. It is also important to distinguish generalized itching of the body or other areas of the body from localized pruritus of the vulva because the causes and treatment are different. Itching may be psychologic as well as physiologic. Patients with long-standing pruritus of the vulva appear to have a definite scratching habit.

Pruritus is defined as "itching, an uncomfortable sensation due to irritation of a peripheral sensory nerve." Pruritus should not be used to describe pain, burning, or tenderness. Pruritus exists if the patient indicates that the unpleasant sensation arouses a *desire to scratch*. The sensation of pruritus may be carried by the same nerve fibers which transmit the sensation of pain, but there is controversy over this possibility. Clinically, however, causes of pruritus of the vulva differ from those of pain. Itching leads to scratching, which in turn intensifies the itching, often creating a vicious circle. Vigorous scratching may produce pain.

CAUSES

Most pruritus is produced by the causes of vaginitis and vaginal discharge. The remaining cases (15 to 20 percent) provide perplexing problems in diagnosis

TABLE 24–2   Causes of Genital Pruritus

Pruritus associated with vaginal discharge
  Candidiasis
  Trichomoniasis
  Diabetes

Systemic

Psychosomatic

Skin diseases not specific to the vulva
  Psoriasis
  Lichen planus
  Seborrheic dermatitis
  Apocrine miliaria (Fox-Fordyce disease)

Chronic vulvar dystrophy
  Red
  White
  Red and white

Cancer of the vulva

Unusual infestations or infections
  Pediculosis pubis
  Scabies
  Insect bites

Allergy and local sensitivity
  Chemical
  Physical

Rectal or urinary disease
  Hemorrhoids and fissures
  Fecal incontinence
  Pinworms
  Urinary infection

and management (Table 24–2). Some causes are clearly defined but others remain uncertain or controversial.

Unfortunately, the vast array of commercial preparations women are encouraged to use on the vulva and vagina probably contributes to the development or aggravation of pruritus.

PRURITUS ASSOCIATED WITH VAGINAL DISCHARGE

Pruritus often accompanies vaginal discharge, but not always. Discharge from cervicitis, foreign bodies, neoplasms, and physiologic changes rarely produces itching. Itching associated with vaginal discharge is most frequently seen with vaginitis (discussed earlier in this chapter), which may account for up to 80 percent of all cases of genital pruritus. Actually the itch tends to occur inside the introitus and less often also on the vulva. Candidiasis involving the vagina or vulva is the most common infection which produces pruritus. In addition to the vagina, the infection may involve the labia majora, genitocrural folds, mons pubis, perianal region, and inner thighs. The lesions are usually beefy red and weeping with sharply demarcated edges. Besides pruritus, there may be burning, sensitivity, and pain.

Candidiasis of the vulva and vagina often develops in patients with diabetes mellitus and may produce the symptoms which lead to initial diagnosis of the diabetes. However, Gardner and Kaufman believe that diabetic vulvitis may also be a distinct entity persisting after the fungus infection has been eradicated. The cycle of infection-pruritus-scratching-pruritus may result in gross and microscopic changes in the vulvar skin similar to those seen in neurodermatitis.

SYSTEMIC

Diseases such as diabetes mellitus, severe anemia, avitaminoses A and B, Hodgkin's disease, leukemia, and jaundice are infrequently associated with varying degrees of pruritus of the vulva. Rarely a primary symptom, pruritus more often becomes manifest either after the initial diagnosis has been established or other systemic manifestations of the diseases are apparent.

Drug reactions occasionally include pruritus of the vulva but usually only in association with other more obvious manifestations of drug idiosyncrasy.

PSYCHOSOMATIC

Pruritus of the vulva may be a manifestation of unrecognized emotional conflicts or problems. Many emotional illnesses have a sexual basis or component, and pruritus of the vulva may occur with loneliness, sexual frustration, guilt over sexual practices, fear of venereal disease, or fear of cancer. Patients with vulvar pruritus of undetermined cause often fit a stereotype. They are perimenopausal or postmenopausal and live alone or with an unattentive family. They are compulsive, fastidious, and self-regimented, preferring "everything in its place and a place for everything." Their interests are few, and their activities limited. Probably more commonly, a psychologic overlay develops in the woman with intractable itching, contributing to anxiety and tension and further aggravating the symptom. A psychosomatic basis for vulvar pruritus *should always be considered,* but the diagnosis should not be decided until the more common possibilities have been excluded.

SKIN DISEASES NOT SPECIFIC TO THE VULVA

Skin diseases not specific to the vulva which may produce pruritus include such generalized dermatoses as *psoriasis, lichen planus,* and *seborrheic dermatitis.* Two to three percent of the population suffer from psoriasis. The scalp, ears, and extensor surfaces of the extremities are much more frequently involved than the genital area. When the vulva is involved, examination of other skin surfaces will reveal the characteristic lesions. Seborrheic dermatitis, although common elsewhere on the body, rarely involves the vulva. The rare lesions of lichen planus appear as slightly elevated, discrete white papules. Involvement of other areas of the body usually suggest the correct diagnosis.

Apocrine miliaria (Fox-Fordyce disease) is seen almost exclusively in women. It is rare, persistent, and intensely pruritic. The lesions are small, discrete dry papules located on the skin of the mons pubis and labia majora. The main symptom is pruritus which appears to be precipitated by emotional stimuli such as anger, fear, or sexual excitement. The disease develops during the reproductive years and usually involutes spontaneously. The cause is unknown, but the primary pathologic alterations appear to be obstruction or altered function of terminal sweat ducts. The differential diagnosis includes neurodermatitis and lichen planus.

CHRONIC VULVAR DYSTROPHIES

Some of the most intense and persistent cases of pruritus of the vulva are found in patients with chronic epithelial dystrophies of the vulva. These lesions are variously identified as *leukoplakia, leukoplakic vulvitis, kraurosis vulvae, lichen sclerosus et atrophicus, primary atrophy,* and *atrophic* and *hyperplastic vulvitis.* In the past, these lesions were considered to have significant potential for malignancy, but at present, this potential appears to be quite minimal. Of greater significance is the chronic discomfort and disability caused by the itching. It is convenient to group all these lesions under the term "chronic epithelial dystrophy of the vulva," as suggested by Jeffcoate. The lesions may be designated further as *red, white,* or *red and white.* The advantage of this nomenclature is that it is easily understood. For an additional classification of the vulvar dystrophies, see Chapter 40.

The appearance of the vulva is variable and may change from time to time, depending particularly upon how much the patient rubs or scratches (Fig. 24–3). Although the lesions are usually limited to the vulva, they may extend to the inner thighs and rarely may involve the perianal region. The usual appearance of the vulva results from hyperkeratosis and chronic inflammation in the dermis. Much of the change in the vulva is due to frequent scratching and secondary infection as well as the atrophic changes which characteristically accompany estrogen deficiency in the postmenopausal woman. The skin and mucosal surfaces tend to become thin and almost translucent. Tissues are easily traumatized, excoriated, and fissured. The vulvar epithelium may appear thick, scaly, and crinkled or smooth, atrophic, shrunken, and rigid. Adhesions may develop about the clitoris, and the vaginal introitus may become stenotic. The vulva may be *red* with fissuring and excoriation secondary to frequent scratching. Edema may be present, particularly in the clitoral area. In other cases, the vulva may exhibit thickened *white* areas which may be diffuse or localized. The white areas are often slightly elevated. In still other cases, there may be combinations of the previously described changes, resulting in both *red* and *white* areas.

The causes of chronic vulvar dystrophies are obscure. They may include yeast infection, diabetes, estrogen deficiency, vitamin or other nutritional deficiencies, local allergic reactions, radiation, vaginal discharge, emotional problems, and even the scratch habit. Since several of these factors may exist simultaneously, all possible causes should be considered in a thorough evaluation of the patient. Many of the

FIGURE 24–3   The gross appearance of chronic vulvar dystrophy.

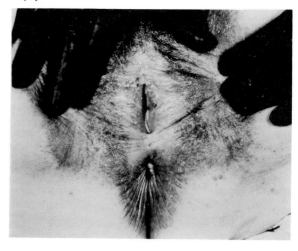

skin changes are secondary to chronic scratching. In Great Britain achlorhydria is reported to be a common factor in the production of chronic vulvar dystrophy, as are the anemias. Such an association has not been observed generally in this country.

CANCER OF THE VULVA

Pruritus may be the presenting complaint in a substantial number of patients with carcinoma of the vulva. Invasive cancer usually presents as an obvious ulcerative or exophytic lesion. Carcinoma in situ may resemble chronic vulvar dystrophy but more often presents as a slightly raised, red velvety lesion. In each circumstance, diagnosis is confirmed by biopsy.

UNUSUAL INFESTATIONS OR INFECTIONS

Pediculosis pubis is an infestation of the hair-bearing pubic area by the crab louse. A skin lesion may not be present, but the typical lesion consists of a maculopapular inflammation which may crust over. The scratching may produce secondary skin changes. The diagnosis is established by finding nits and parasites at the bases of hairs.

Scabies of the vulva is caused by mites which produce minute papules or vesicles.

Other *insect bites* from mosquitoes, chiggers, fleas, and bedbugs may also produce localized areas of pruritus in the genital areas.

Tinea cruris is a fungal infection involving the genitocrural areas, producing erythematous patches with vesiculation, crusting, and scales. The slightly pigmented or red lesions spread peripherally and coalesce, often healing in the center as they enlarge. They are well circumscribed with slightly elevated margins.

ALLERGY AND LOCAL SENSITIVITY

Local skin sensitivity to various materials such as douche solutions, hygienic sprays, soaps, antiperspirants, deodorants, detergents, therapeutic medications (gentian violet, podophylin), cosmetics, local anesthetics, lubricants, and contraceptive creams and foams may produce a contact dermatitis in the vulva or vagina and resultant pruritus. Rubber and synthetic fabrics may do likewise. Pruritic reactions to condoms and contraceptive diaphragms have been reported. Wearing pantyhose, especially if tight, accounts for some persistent complaints of genital pruritus. When allergic dermatitis follows contact with

poison oak or poison ivy, the vulvar reaction is similar to that seen elsewhere on the body.

RECTAL OR URINARY DISEASE

Hemorrhoids, anal fissures, and fecal incontinence may produce itching which is usually centered around the anus. Pinworms may produce itching in the child, as previously discussed. Urinary infection and urinary incontinence may produce irritation, maceration, and pain but rarely itching.

CLINICAL INVESTIGATION

Every effort should be made to identify the cause of genital pruritus before initiating treatment. Consideration of all possibilities leads to the special aspects of history taking and clinical examination. The history should include specific questions directed toward possible systemic diseases, evidence of nutritional deficiencies, emotional or marital-sexual problems, or contact with chemical or physical agents. In addition to careful inspection of the genitalia, examination of wet suspensions of vaginal discharge, skin scrapings, urinalysis for glucose, vaginal cytology for estrogen status, and inspection of pubic hairs for pediculi may yield diagnostic information. Biopsy of the vulva should be done whenever chronic epithelial changes are present. Therapy for vulvar dystrophy should not be initiated without prior biopsy. Only in this way is it possible to correctly diagnose and treat early cases of vulvar carcinoma. Vulvar biopsy is a simple procedure which can be accomplished readily in the office. The British recommend testing for gastric acidity. Routine hemogram should be taken, and other specific blood studies should be performed as indicated.

REFERENCES

Gardner HL, Kaufman RH: *Benign Diseases of the Vulva and Vagina,* St. Louis: Mosby, 1969.

_____, Dukes CD: *Haemophilus vaginalis* vaginitis. *Am J Obstet Gynecol* 69:962, 1955.

Janovski NA Douglas CP: *Diseases of the Vulva.* Hagerstown, MD,: Harper & Row, 1972.

Jeffcoate TNA: Chronic vulva dystrophies. *Am J Obstet Gynecol* 95:51, 1966.

Lapan, B: Is the "pill" a cause of candidiasis? *NY State J Med* 70:949, 1970.

25

Hirsutism, Alopecia, and Acne

A. BRIAN LITTLE

Hirsutism is the growth of hair in unusual places in unusual amounts; alopecia is the loss of hair. Both states may be associated with severe psychologic disturbance. The "normal," or desirable, amount of hair is generally determined culturally, but its quantity and distribution depend on genetic, racial, and hormonal factors. Hair on the face, breasts, or abdomen is considered undesirable in our culture. Hair on the head, legs, and pubis is accepted as normal; in fact hair of the scalp is carefully coiffured and displayed, and wigs are presently in vogue to augment the variations of hair style. Legs are shaved without qualm. Commonly, the gynecologist sees women with only mild to moderate degrees of hirsutism or temporal hair loss, and frequently any tests performed are normal. Confident reassurance of the patient is sufficient to relieve her anxiety and usually results in an acceptance of any mild variation from "normal."

HIRSUTISM

PHYSIOLOGY

All areas except the palms of the hands and soles of the feet grow hair of two types: vellus (lanugo) and terminal hairs. Terminal hairs are longer and coarser than vellus hairs but have a wide range of caliber and length (Van Scott). Hair on the head may grow 100 cm, whereas on the back it usually remains less than 3 cm. Vellus hair is always shorter. The roots for each type extend in depth corresponding to the overall length (i.e., 0.5 to 3.5 mm below the skin surface). In the female, terminal hairs have the appearance of lanugo in certain areas, such as the face.

The number of hair follicles on individuals does not change. Most hair follicles in women support lanugo only, rather than the coarser terminal hair. The appearance of terminal hair on the upper lip, cheeks, chin, chest, and abdomen is the most common evidence of hirsutism. This expression comes about by change in size (length and caliber) rather than through effects on the other parameters of hair growth, namely cycle and rate of growth.

The cycle of hair growth in man is characterized by a mosaic pattern of growth. It begins at birth in the growing (anagen) phase, and after a few days it enters the resting (telogen) phase. Then growth becomes mixed, and individual hairs develop their own pattern rather than the same pattern, as in animals who moult periodically. About 90 percent of the scalp is in the anagen phase and 10 percent is in the telogen phase at one time. The scalp anagen phase lasts about 3 years (0.3 mm per day), and the telogen phase lasts 3 months. Therefore, there is a specific loss of hair daily, as hairs involute (the catagen phase).

Changes in hair cycle lead to larger proportions of hair entering the telogen cycle and, in extremes, all anagen hairs may do so at one time. Such conditions occur in pregnancy (Lynfield), in severe illness, and after a high fever. About 3 months later there is often a large loss of hair. Regrowth, however, does occur in these situations. Some drugs, such as heparin, also lead to the conversion of anagen to telogen hairs (Tedhope et al.). Radiation also leads to hair loss, partly because of suppression of mitotic activity in the hair follicle and partly because of anagen conversion to telogen phase (Van Scott, Reinerton). [Total depilation occurs at about 300 R (roentgens) of irradia-

FIGURE 25–1 See text for discussion.

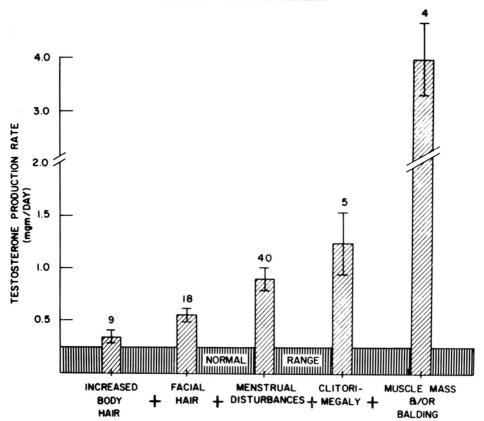

tion.] Chemotherapeutic drugs, antimetabolites, and alkylating agents reduce the rate of hair growth by their effects on the mitotic activity of matrix cells (Van Scott et al.). For example, methotrexate used in the treatment of choriocarcinoma can cause reduced hair growth.

Effects on the rate of hair growth must take into consideration that all scalp hairs, regardless of size, reproduce matrices (the epidermic root of the hair follicle) by mitosis once in 24 hours and, therefore, the rate of growth is the same, although a large hair will produce more length than a small hair each day. Starvation and extremely cold climates will reduce rate of hair growth. Hair-root metabolism in vitro has actually been used as a measurement of nutritional state.

The size of hair is also important. At puberty the length and coarseness of terminal hairs increase in the axilla and over the pubis, and in males the beard develops. Insofar as the size and length of the hair is proportional to the size of the general matrix population of cells, it can be understood that not all lengthening and coarsening are the result of androgenic stimulus, but as in the case of hirsutism following diphenylhydantoin (Dilantin) administration, the hyperplasia of the submucosal connective tissue is responsible (as it is for the gingival hyperplasia following Dilantin).

CAUSES

A useful classification of hirsutism and virilism in the female has been proposed by Israel (Table 25–1). As can be seen, except for familial and racial or genetic causes, hirsutism and virilism are caused by endocrinopathies or from the extremes of endocrine physiologic states (eg., pregnancy, puberty, menopause) or from the administration of drugs which imitate endocrine disease (with the exception of diphenylhydantoin). In most instances the final common pathway appears to be some form of androgenic stimulus. The gynecologist most commonly encounters adrenal hyperplasia, polycystic ovarian disease, exogenous hormone administration, and familial causes of hirsutism.

Androgenic stimulus to hair growth occurs as a result of increased total androgen production (e.g., congenital adrenal hyperplasia), an unusual sensitivity of the target organ (i.e., hair follicle) to normal circulating androgen (e.g., familial or racial cause) or a decreased estrogen secretion (e.g., in the menopause) resulting in a preponderance of androgen effect (Segré).

About one-third of all women have some excess hair growth which they disguise with beauty aids. Of

TABLE 25–1 Classification of Hirsutism and Virilism in the Female*

Type	Etiology	Clinical manifestations
Familial and racial	Genetic	Mild or moderate hirsutism
Physiologic	Puberty, pregnancy, menopause	Mild hirsutism
Adrenal	Hyperplasia	Mild hirsutism
		Achard-Thiers syndrome ("diabetes of bearded women")
		Female "pseudohermaphroditism"
	Hyperplasia and/or tumor	Cushing's syndrome and adrenogenital syndrome
Ovary	Polycystic ovary (Stein-Leventhal syndrome)	Mild hirsutism, amenorrhea, infertility, obesity
	Hyperluteinization	Hirsutism and/or virilization
	Hilar-cell hyperplasia	
	Tumor (arrhenoblastoma, adrenal rest, lutein cell)	
	Ovotestis (genetic)	Hermaphroditism
	Gonadal dysgenesis (genetic)	Virilism
Thyroid	Juvenile hypothyroidism	Mild hirsutism
Pituitary	Tumor	Acromegaly, hirsutism, Cushing's syndrome
Iatrogenic (drug)	Androgens, corticosteroids, diphenylhydantoin	Mild hirsutism

*Source: Israel.

this group, about 10 percent seek help and require evaluation. Most of the organic causes of hirsutism can be identified with a complete history, physical examination, and appropriate endocrine tests. There are a few who must be labeled idiopathic, since the causes cannot be characterized. Persons in this category were usually considered to have congenitally hypersensitive hair follicles. Recently, some patients have been found to have some identifiable pathophysiologic disturbance of androgen metabolism. The newer, more sensitive methods for the definition of androgen excess include the measurement of the metabolic clearance rates, the circulating concentrations, the production rates, and the interconversions of testosterone, androstenedione, and dehydroepiandrosterone (Kirschner and Bardin), plus the presence or absence of androgen receptors in cytoplasm and nucleus of target organs (see Chap. 27).

Some generalities of endocrine effect include the fact that growth hormone appears to be responsible for increased size of the individual hair. Luteinizing hormone (LH) is necessary for the change from prepubertal to adult hair. Thyroxine appears to increase growth rate, and adrenalectomy increases the number of hairs growing. Oophorectomy leads to the shedding of hairs. These generalities have been worked out mainly in animals, and in human beings they do not always follow such rules; in fact, in some cases no cause can be elucidated for either hair excess or loss on an endocrine basis (Lloyd).

Even with the removal of the cause, the hirsutism does not always diminish; when it does (as seen above in the physiologic cycle of hair growth), it takes a long time. For moderate degrees of hirsutism repeated application of a bleaching solution (hydrogen peroxide—ammonia), wax depilation, and rarely electrolysis is employed (Israel).

Hirsutism of pregnancy disappears rapidly postpartum. Although hirsutism that appears at the menopause persists, it usually is only slight. In contrast, women who are "somewhat hairy" become less "hairy" at the menopause.

RACIAL AND GENETIC PREDISPOSITION TO HIRSUTISM

The amount of hair that any woman will comfortably endure is determined racially and culturally. Even as Caucasians have much more beard growth than Mongol populations, so are there differences among families in each group (Lorenzo), and transplants of skin show inherent genetic traits of hairiness (Hamilton et al.). The actual growth of beard or axillary hair in each racial group shows considerable disparity. The disappearance of axillary and pubic hair with advancing age is more marked in Japanese women, for example, in comparison with Caucasians. This difference in hair growth is associated with a lower 17-ketosteroid excretion in Japanese women in comparison with American women, although circulating plasma testosterone appears to be the same (Lloyd). It should be remembered that production rates of testosterone may be increased in the presence of an elevated metabolic clearance rate with a constant circulating testosterone level (see Chap. 7).

MANAGEMENT

Although endocrine evaluation of androgen disorders will be considered in more detail in Chap. 7, certain tests may be carried out to determine ovarian and adrenal function in hirsute women. After a history including detailed menstrual cycle evaluation and careful physical examination observing those areas of increased hair, a pelvic examination should be done to palpate for enlarged ovaries. Laboratory tests are initially urinary 17-ketosteroid and 17-hydroxycorticosteroid excretion with subsequent plasma free and bound testosterone and additional sophisticated tests (e.g., dexamethasone suppression) as indicated.

Differential diagnosis should include androgen-producing tumors and end-organ hypersensitivity (idiopathic hirsutism, mixed adrenal and ovarian contribution to androgen production). A 24-hour collection of urine for 17-ketosteroids and 17-hydroxycorticosteroids should be evaluated. If the 17-ketosteroids are less than 20 mg per 24 hours, it is unlikely that adrenal disease is present; excess androgen production by the ovary is most likely. In rare instances, the adrenal may be involved in the presence of normal 17-ketosteroids, but in such cases the 17-hydroxycorticosteroids would be elevated (normal range: 4 to 12 mg per day). If the 17-hydroxycorticosteroids are elevated, Cushing's syndrome should be suspected. A rapid screening test is a plasma cortisol drawn at 8 A.M. following a single 1.0-mg dose of dexamethasone, given orally at 11 P.M. the night before; if circulating cortisol is less that 6 μg per 100 mL, it is diagnostic of adrenal hyperfunction. If the urinary 17-ketosteroids are greater than 20 mg per 24 hours and the patient does not have signs or symptomatic evidence of Cushing's syndrome, adrenal suppression with dexamethasone will confirm the adrenal contribution to androgen production. This may be done by the administration of 2.0 mg of dexamethasone qid (four times a day) for 5 days. The urinary 17-ketosteroid determination is repeated on the fifth day of suppression. If there is no suppression of 17-ketosteroids, a functioning adrenal tumor should be suspected and further evaluation proposed. If the urinary 17-ketosteroids suppress to 3 to 4 mg per 24 hours, adrenal hyperplasia is diagnosed and treatment of 5.0 mg prednisone daily should be given. Warnings relating to increased dosage requirement for infections, stress, and disease should be given to those patients on comparable adrenal steroid therapy. Following suppression, values of urinary 17-ketosteroids of 5 to 11 mg per 24 hours confirm abnormal ovarian production of androgens and testosterone precursors.

Plasma testosterones (0.2 to 0.8 ng/mL) may be elevated in patients with anovulation and hirsutism, but in at least 30 percent of such patients, testosterone may not be elevated and the variation is great. The additional measurement of free and bound testosterone provides further diagnostic evidence. In such abnormal cases where normal values of total testosterone are observed, the free moiety is greater than normal in hirsute women (increasing from 1.6 percent to 2.6 percent free). The MCR (metabolic clearance rate, see Chap. 7) and testosterone production rate will also be increased (see Table 25–2).

In idiopathic hirsutism in women, catheterization studies have been carried out on the ovarian and adrenal venous effluents and then compared with peripheral values of testosterone, androstenedione, dehydroepiandrosterone, Δ^5-androstenediol, and cortisol. The results indicate a major contribution of

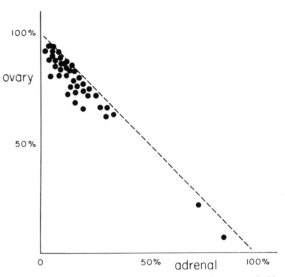

FIGURE 25–2 Origin of testosterone and its prehormones in idiopathic hirsutism.

ovarian, androgen, and other testosterone precursors including dehydroepiandrosterone.

The origin of testosterone and its prehormones are largely from the ovary in idiopathic hirsutism (see Fig. 25–2).

CENTRAL-NERVOUS-SYSTEM FACTORS

Increased hair growth is associated with areas of increased blood flow to the skin; whether this is mediated by androgen is not known, but certain types of brain damage and sympathectomy are known to

TABLE 25–2 Testosterone Parameters in Normal and Hirsute Women and Normal Men

	Normal women	Hirsute women	Normal men
Testosterone production rate, μg per day	250 (100–300)	600 (280–7000)	7000
Urinary testosterone glucuronide, μg per day	5	10–40	70
Plasma testosterone, ng per 100 mL	30 (15–60)	120 (30–400)	600 (400–1000)
Percent free testosterone (unbound to testosterone-binding globulin)	1.61	2.61	2.85
Metabolic clearance rate testosterone, L per day	600	800 (500–1200)	1100

cause increased hair growth even without altered blood flow.

Increases in hair growth are associated not only with some central-nervous-system diseases but also with severe psychologic reactions, and severe stress may be associated with hair loss. Patients with anorexia nervosa, a complex psychiatric disease that imitates hypopituitarism, may have hair growth on the shoulders, upper arms, back, and occasionally on the face. In this case complex factors apparently overcome what might be expected to be the loss of hair as a result of the associated inanition.

ALOPECIA

Alopecia is the loss of hair and is as upsetting to a woman as the excess growth of hair. It may result from physiologic or endocrine disorders, systemic diseases, local cutaneous disease or infection, and physical or chemical trauma.

PSYCHOLOGIC AND ENDOCRINE DISORDERS

Postpartum hair loss is common and results from a marked conversion from anagen phase (stimulated by pregnancy) to telogen phase at delivery. The resulting hair loss may be noticeable or even excessive. This is generally followed by complete regrowth of hair over the next 3 to 6 months.

Similar causes are probably responsible for the loss of hair in some newborn infants born with luxuriant hair who lose it completely, causing great concern to their mothers. This hair also regrows spontaneously.

Hypopituitary dwarfs have little hair, and patients who develop Sheehan's disease (postpartum hypopituitarism) (see Chap. 7) similarly lose axillary and pubic hair. On the other hand, patients with acromegaly often have increased coarser hair.

In extremes of androgen stimulation in women, in addition to hair appearing in unusual areas, baldness (as in the male) may also ensue. Alopecia areata has also been seen in women taking oral contraceptives, but this is probably coincidence.

In men, baldness is inherited as a sex-linked autosomal dominant trait, but in women it is a recessive trait, and baldness will occur in androgenic syn-

dromes if the genotype is appropriate. In fact, in middle-aged women hair loss may be a manifestation of this genetic inheritance, and although it rarely leads to baldness, it can be very upsetting.

OTHER CAUSES

Systemic lupus erythematosus, dermatomyositis, severe wasting, and lymphomas are associated with hair loss. Secondary syphilis will also cause alopecia areata. Porphyria cutanea tarda may be associated with hair growth.

Burns, x-rays, or the constant traction produced by certain hair styles may lead to hair loss. Chemotherapy, thallium, heparin, and excessive vitamin A intake may also cause temporary loss.

Local infection and skin diseases occasionally produce alopecia.

ACNE

Acne, the common lesion of adolescence, appears to be the result of androgenic stimulation of the sebaceous glands which begins during puberty. Almost 75 percent of all young women and men have some acneiform changes in the skin, usually of the face, at puberty. The usual onset is by the appearance of "blackheads," or comedones, on the skin. Pustules, inflammatory papules, and cysts may last throughout adolescence into the early twenties. In some men and women, the scarring of the face is disfiguring.

The usual sequence of events is that of marked increase in secretion and size of the sebaceous glands in response to the increased androgen production at puberty. These glands become blocked with their own secretion and dilate with keratin, lipids, and large numbers of *Corynebacterium* and *Staphylococcus albus*. The dilated glands or cysts break into the surrounding tissues of the dermis, spreading the inflammation. The enlargement of follicles, their rupture into and derangement of the epidermis, and the continued chemical and bacterial inflammation with the formation of cysts and tissue healing and replacement leads to a vicious circle which may persist for many years. Recurrent infection of the apocrine glands in the axilla and around the anus is most difficult to manage.

Since estrogen will usually diminish the sebaceous glands' sensitivity to androgens, it can then be given in combination as a contraceptive pill or alone to reduce the amount of acne on an adolescent's face. This may be added to the usual management of local therapy, drainage of pustules, and combating infection with antibiotics in difficult problem cases.

REFERENCES

Hamilton JB, Terada H: Interdependence of genetic aging and endocrine factors in hirsutism, in *The Hirsute Woman,* ed. RB Greenblatt, Springfield, Ill.: Thomas, 1963, pp. 20–47.

Israel SL: *Diagnosis and Treatment of Menstrual Disorders and Sterility,* 5th ed., New York: Hoeber-Harper, 1967, pp. 311–317.

Kirschner, MA, Bardin CW: Androgen production and metabolism in normal and virilized women. *Metabolism* 21:667, 1972.

Lloyd CW: Central nervous system factors in hirsutism. *Clin Obstet Gynecol* 7:1085, 1964.

Lorenzo EM: Familial study of hirsutism. *J Clin Endocrinol Metab* 31:556, 1970.

Lynfield YL: Effect of pregnancy on the human hair cycle. *J Invest Dermatol* 35:323, 1960.

Segré EJ: *Androgens, Virilization and the Hirsute Female,* Springfield, Ill.: Thomas, 1967.

Tedhope GR et al.: Alopecia following treatment with dextran sulfate and other anticoagulant drugs. *Br Med J* 1:1034, 1958.

Van Scott EJ: Physiology of hair growth. *Clin Obstet Gynecol* 7:1062, 1964.

_____, Reinerton RP: Detection of radiation effects on the hair roots of the human scalp. *J Invest Dermatol* 29:205, 1957.

_____, et al.: The growing hair roots of the human scalp and morphologic changes therein following Amethopterin therapy. *J Invest Dermatol* 29:197, 1957.

26

Psychosexual Symptoms

LAWRENCE S. JACKMAN

INADEQUACY OF MIND-BODY DICHOTOMY

Traditional medical approaches to emotionally related, psychophysiologic, and psychosexual symptoms have emphasized the need to differentiate such problems from organic disease in order to facilitate diagnosis and therapy. This extension of the mind-body dichotomy creates a compartmented, simplistic, and cumbersome classification of problems that has only limited usefulness in actual patient management.

When symptoms involving the female reproductive tract, fertility management, and sexually related problems are considered, a diametrically opposite view offers a better working model with which to evaluate and assist the patient. In this view, virtually all reproductive tract complaints and problems are likely to have strong and important psychological and emotional connections. These cause, maintain, or complicate the problem, add special significance for the patient, and may possibly have long-term effects on her self-image, attitude, behavior, and adaptability in gender-specific and sexually related areas of life.

Recent research in the field of biofeedback, although inconclusive so far in regard to therapeutic applications, nevertheless has clearly demonstrated in the laboratory what most workers have intuitively believed: the mind has power over somatic processes and events, and this power blurs the distinction between voluntary and involuntary responses. That such power can be controlled by training implies that it already exists in the untrained individual. Thus the mind can indeed directly affect vascular flow and glandular secretion, to name but two areas, although the precise mechanisms and pathways involved remain to be worked out.

Symptoms that originate in psychosocial stress and that, in a behavioral model, can be viewed as responses to stimuli are themselves stimuli for a subsequent level of response. Thus they function in the reverberating interaction of psychosomatic mechanisms described by Mathis (Chap. 13). This model leads to the concept of self-reinforcing negative feedback loops, or vicious cycles, which serve to maintain and prolong the problem. The model offers a useful explanation of the common clinical observation that the problem often persists long after the "cause" is eliminated. For example, a microorganism may flourish in the vagina and produce an inflammatory response. This leads to vaginal discharge and dyspareunia and causes the patient to seek medical attention. The examination is also painful. An appropriate medication is prescribed and the organism is eliminated. The patient remains fearful of pain with coitus, however, and her anxiety inhibits the vaginal lubrication which accompanies the excitement phase of sexual response. This inhibition of physiologic response produces further mucosal irritation with coitus. The dyspareunia persists and the patient returns. Reexamination now shows no definable organic cause. Various inappropriate treatment strategies at this juncture are represented by such advice as, "There is nothing wrong now so stop worrying," "You must be imagining the symptom," "Take more medicine because it is not completely healed," and "Perhaps referral to an expert in this field might help."

Psychologic mechanism may thus produce, reinforce, and/or maintain symptoms which may have, or may once have had, an organic etiology as well.

TREATMENT BY DECONDITIONING

Primary vaginismus (vaginismus without antecedent physical disease) is perhaps the paradigm of a psychophysiologic symptom affecting the reproductive system and is an illuminating example of the interaction of mind and body.

Vaginismus can be defined as a spasm of the muscle groups investing the vagina, primarily the pubococcygeal portions of the levator sling muscles. Typically, the patient with severe symptoms states that she is unable to engage in sexual intercourse because of the pain she experiences at attempted intromission. Severe vaginismus is the female condition most often seen as a cause of failure to consummate a marriage.

Vaginismus is best understood in the classic behavioral terms of conditioned response. The stimulus is the anticipation by the woman that there will be vaginal penetration. Her learning (or mislearning) associates penetration with anxiety and fear. The circumstances, events, details, and consciousness of this association are variable and may or may not be clear to the patient or the physician. Regardless, the bodily response is a protective reflex spasm of the perivaginal muscle groups, closing the introitus and making penetration difficult or impossible. The spasm can and should be directly observed with the patient in the lithotomy position, and it is this observation which confirms the diagnosis.

This sequence in which anticipated penetration produces muscle spasm has the characteristic automaticity of a reflex arc; it would seem to be quite refractory to the patient's willful attempts to control or diminish it. There is nothing imaginary or unreal about it, as many sufferers and their frustrated sexual partners fear; it is an observable muscular phenomenon triggered by psychic associations.

Therapeutic approaches which focus on insight have been generally unsuccessful, but those which attempt to decondition the response, usually by self-administered progressive vaginal dilatation, often bring rapid and complete reversal. Facilitating the patient's own observation of the phenomenon with the aid of a mirror can be the first step in the process.

After the patient has demonstrated the muscular spasm for herself, she may need to be taught pertinent pelvic anatomy and physiology. She can be assured that a brief treatment program has good promise of success if she is willing to undertake it. She is then shown how to insert and retain a small (usually about 1 cm in diameter) vaginal dilator. Nightly practice with the dilator at home is prescribed, and the patient is seen at intervals to discuss her progress and exchange the dilator for the next larger one, until she can use a size equal to that of her partner's phallus. The situations which occurred at the time of the original mislearning may or may not come to light during the therapy, which is often successful in reversing the vaginismus in only a few weeks.

THE PRESENTATION GIVES CLUES

Psychologic mechanisms appear adequate to account for virtually any symptoms usually associated with organic reproductive tract abnormalities and disease processes. Thus the recurrent question for the dispenser of health care is not what symptoms suggest important connections to psychological and emotional processes, but rather which kinds of patient presentations suggest the usefulness of probing these areas in search of important connections. It should be noted that identification of such associations in no way rules out the concomitant presence of an organic disease factor. It simply clarifies the meaning of the problem for the patient and directs attention to areas which may require some consideration, discussion, and perhaps specific suggestions to the patient in order to complete the problem's resolution.

The patient's "presentation" includes all of the manifestations of the problem. Specifically, it includes her way of talking about the problem, her choice of terms and idioms, her feelings in relation to it, her thoughts concerning it, the way she modifies her behavior to accommodate the problem, her facial expressions and posture when the problem is discussed, the bodily tensions she reveals when the problem is examined, and the associations to the problem from her past and her family's past.

An examination of the presentation of the patient with vaginitis might reveal that she *describes* her symptoms in vague general.terms ("I have pain down there"), *feels* embarrassed and ashamed of her condition, *thinks* that she is being punished for a real or imagined sexual transgression, *withdraws* from social interactions with sexual overtones, *looks* anxious and *exhibits* a closed body posture when discussing the problem, *reveals* muscle tension in her abdomen, pelvis, and thighs when the examination is about to begin or in progress, and *remembers* other shame and anxiety-evoking situations, whether real or imagined, from the past.

The critical next step is to pay attention to the various aspects of this presentation and to the context in which the patient views the problem. This can lead to an appreciation of the emotions and psychophysiologic and social forces behind the problem. Such a contextual framework can function to the person's benefit or detriment, but it must be clarified if it is to be either supported or modified in treating the patient.

The skillful clinician will observe and attempt to elucidate the various aspects of the patient's presentation. The question then becomes not whether but to what extent management of these aspects is indicated for each patient.

INAPPROPRIATE PRESENTATIONS

The single most useful observation about presentations is unfortunately linked to an entirely subjective and culturally determined judgment: appropriateness. When one or more aspects of the patient's presentation is not appropriate, the importance of nonorganic factors is usually increased. Probing in these areas is then likely to be fruitful.

The designation of appropriateness depends entirely on one's frame of reference. Thus, a further caution must be given: one cannot conclude that a behavior is inappropriate except in the context of the social milieu in which the patient exists. Appropriateness is very much a learned and conditioned response and is not strictly a function of circumstances. For example, in the Amish country of Pennsylvania, there is often a striking silence in the hospital labor suite. For Amish women, it is appropriate to experience labor silently and without complaint. However, in the labor rooms of hospitals serving the Hispanic women of New York, the wailing and screaming can shatter the composure of the uninitiated. These women have been conditioned to express vocally and loudly their experience of the birthing process. Appropriateness in this situation is not a function of sensory input of uterine contractions but rather of the expectation which the women bring to the experience.

The health professional, also the product of an upbringing and subculture, brings his or her own expectations and values to the situation. When these personal biases about appropriateness are left unexamined, they distort and render worthless the observation of the patient's presentation.

Presentation involves both voluntary and involuntary components. Of the two, involuntary ones are by far the more useful to observe for clues clarifying the connections between the symptoms and the mental and emotional experiences, especially if the patient is attempting to disguise the connections because of embarrassment or shame. The portions of the presentation which are least conscious, such as body posture, are much less well disguised than, for example, facial expression.

Although each individual has a unique presentation, recurrent patterns can serve as a guide for the clinician. More reaction than one might anticipate in a certain situation, or less, are equally inappropriate and are therefore valuable observations. Too many questions and too few may both point the way to an otherwise unexplored problem area. Laughter at sad news, an apparent lack of concern about a serious matter, a dramatic emotional outpouring in response to a minimal physical problem should all alert the professional to important psychophysiologic relationships for this individual in these circumstances. Giving a diagnostic label is of almost no practical use in such cases. Such labels lump patients with supposedly similar problems together. In the process, the individual patterns that require understanding in order to achieve a satisfactory resolution of the problem are neglected. Nevertheless, certain recurrent and striking patterns offer useful examples of the phenomenon of inappropriate presentation.

THE ANXIOUS PATIENT

The patient who exhibits anxiety or fear out of all proportion may simply reflect her own lack of understanding of the proceedings and their significance, or she may be providing an important clue to psychological and emotional connections. The best way to differentiate these two states is to observe her response when the necessary information has been provided and any misunderstandings or misinterpretations have been resolved. When the inappropriate anxiety persists despite these educational measures, the likelihood of some anxiety-reinforcing thinking or emotional patterns is increased.

For example, an overwrought patient called her physician and stated almost hysterically that she had discovered a "lump" and begged for an immediate examination. This was conducted later the same day and revealed an infected sweat gland on the labia majora. The patient was assured of the relatively trivial nature of the lesion, and hot wet compresses and a topical antibiotic ointment were prescribed. She failed to show the anticipated relief from her anxiety, and called the physician's office daily to discuss the progress of the treatments and to press for further verbal assurances that "the disease is not serious." This inappropriate anxiety about a pimple prompted an invitation for a further interview during which she was able to discuss her fear that the condition was a deserved punishment for a sexual transgression. She visibly relaxed as soon as the story was out, began to

laugh at herself for her irrational fear, and had an uneventful recovery.

THE ANGRY PATIENT

The patient who brings anger to the medical interview and examination also brings a valuable clue to the emotional charge she has invested in some part of the process, whether to the condition or illness, the biologic system involved, or the need for medical attention. Some women, among them ardent feminists, have, for example, seen the need for a gynecologic examination by a physician as a defeat for their preferred system of self-examination and care. In addition, they may have experienced truly insensitive treatment by physicians in the past, and they now transfer their earlier feelings to the present encounter.

This anger will be felt by the health professional whether it is openly or covertly expressed, and it is likely to engender a correspondingly hostile attitude.

At this point, the professional who is consciously aware of his or her own reactions need only notice that the process is occurring in order to suspect that emotional connections play an important part in this situation for this patient. Sharing the awareness of the process ("I notice you seem very angry about being here") may help her discuss and make clear those past and present connections which can obstruct a successful outcome.

An often useful strategy in dealing with an angry patient is simply to accept the anger without judgment. This is generally more helpful than explaining to a patient why her anger is unnecessary or inappropriate or misplaced, all of which often produce even more anger. In other words, resistance often reinforces the anger and causes it to persist, while acceptance without judgment may move the interaction beyond this barrier.

For example, a new patient who presented herself for routine periodic examinations and contraceptive technology was instructed to disrobe in a changing room and then await the doctor's examination. She angrily stated that this was a degrading and sexist practice and that she wished to disrobe in the presence of the male physician and female attendant. Further, she wanted to be examined in the nude and without the use of a gown or drape sheet.

Acknowledging the patient's reaction without being judgmental, the doctor said, "I can see you are angry and that this is important to you. Let's do it your way." The patient's anger immediately appeared to diminish and the examination proceeded. Later, in the consultation room, she talked about how her anger, stemming from an unpleasant interaction some years before, had kept her from listening to and remembering most of what doctors said to her about herself and even influenced her, like a small child having a tantrum, to refuse to take prescribed medications. Her unique preexamination behavior was never repeated.

THE SEDUCTIVE PATIENT

When a patient presents herself in a sexually seductive manner and the presentation is not consciously or unconsciously supported by the physician, she offers evidence of her style of dealing with situations and individuals. For her, sexuality is an important aspect of situations that for others are very different, for example, a visit to a doctor. Such an individual is likely to sexualize pelvic sensations and symptoms, and, conversely, she may expect and look for such symptoms in response to sexually stressful situations. The mental connections and forces that support her presentation of herself as a sexually interested and possibly available individual in the situation remain to be identified, but the possibility that psychosexual factors support her problem should be seriously entertained. Her actual sexual behavior may have nothing to do with her symptoms, but it is likely that she believes or suspects such a connection.

The usefulness of seductiveness as a diagnostic clue to the patient's psychosexual world is invalidated if the health professional overtly or covertly encourages it. Participation makes the behavior appropriate, thus robbing it of any useful diagnostic value.

Seductiveness is not infrequently a clue to strong psychological drives to control and be in charge of one's life. This is especially true in situations in which control must be given up. Hospitalized patients give up control of aspects of even basic biologic behaviors such as eating and elimination. They are given specified treatments at defined intervals, and are almost always made dependent on the medical staff.

One strategy, not necessarily conscious, of regaining control is, by seductiveness, to control the one who controls. Although this may have an overtly sexual character, it may also take a somewhat different form. For example, a patient told her physician that she trusted him totally, although she had never been able to trust a doctor before, that she was sure he knew what was best for her, and that she was prepared to do whatever he suggested by way of treatment. This presentation is the equivalent of a small child's asking her father to take care of her. It is as sure a control as is any sexual advance.

THE PATIENT AS "EXPERT"

Not infrequently, inappropriateness is shown by the patient's assuming the role of self-proclaimed expert. In this role, she may attempt to restrict what diagnoses and therapies will be acceptable. "Don't tell me it is emotional. I am sure there is an infection there somewhere, and I want you to find it." Although one should never forget that there may be organic pathology which has, in fact, not been identified in such a patient, it is also likely that the patient is giving a clue as to what diagnosis or treatment would be most threatening to her. Why it is threatening and what makes it so becomes the crucial psychologic connection for understanding where the problem lies.

A woman who refused to accept a diagnosis of "tension" for her strange pelvic sensations insisted on a series of laboratory tests and consultations. Then she revealed that her husband had suffered severe incapacity as the result of a meningeal tumor which had been erroneously diagnosed as "tension headaches" for a period of some months. Her mother had undergone a hysterectomy for "tumors." These experiences supported her determination to discover an organic cause for her symptoms.

In another example, a patient in shock with a boardlike abdomen, was seen in an emergency department. Immediate surgery was performed and a ruptured and bleeding ovarian cyst was resected. Postoperatively the patient at first made an uneventful recovery. However, she showed little animation and appeared lifeless and withdrawn during the physician's daily rounds despite careful attention to her dress and appearance. On the day before discharge, she developed two distinct but vague complaints for which no simple explanation could be found. Now suspecting somatization of an emotional malaise, the physician opened a discussion of her life situation. After an initial denial, she revealed her reluctance to return home to the burden of her chronically unhappy marital relationship, a situation she had so far not admitted directly to anyone. She was thankful for the patience and understanding of the physician, despite there having been no advice or solution offered, and she was discharged the following day without somatic complaints.

BEHAVIOR OF THE PATIENT BETWEEN VISITS

Sometimes the importance of psychologic factors is revealed by inappropriateness of the patient's behavior between rather than during her visits for health care. Discrepancies between her knowledge, understanding, stated desires and goals, and her actual performance should lead to the suspicion that an unexplored and unresolved psychosexual factor plays an important part in the maintenance of the problem. The literature on provision of abortion services is replete with discussions of the problem of "repeaters," women who seek termination of unwanted pregnancies again and again despite intensive family-planning education and provision of effective contraceptive technology. Obviously, some unaddressed and unresolved psychological and emotional connection impels these women into contraceptive failure. If the problem is left unresolved, the medical effort in behalf of such women is incomplete and unsatisfactory.

THE DEPRESSED PATIENT

The reverse of emotional excess is the flatness of affect which frequently accompanies depression. Although probably more common than displays of emotional excess, it is less flamboyant and may require a greater professional alertness in order to be a useful sign.

ACHIEVING PERSPECTIVE

So far we have examined inappropriate presentations as a clinical sign of psychosexually connected problems. At the same time, the presentation itself often becomes a new problem. This develops when the inappropriateness is permitted to control the interaction, which then becomes about the presentation instead of about the patient's symptoms. This shift of focus can be prevented or reversed by the professional at any time by the conscious awareness that it has occurred. The act of observation of the phenomenon shifts the observer to a secondary or *meta* level of communication; from this perspective, attention automatically is refocused on the patient's problems.

Any of the common inappropriate presentations may be present in barely discernible forms which require careful observation on the part of the professional, or they may be so obvious and dominant that they obscure other aspects of the patient. When "professionally inappropriate" reactions occur among the caregivers in response to their patients, the interaction is altered and the care is likely to be modified. These responses occur in a mechanical fashion, and can control behavior unless they are recognized. The author recalls colluding unconsciously with fellow residents to avoid visiting on daily rounds a certain terminally ill young woman who stirred feelings of helplessness in all of us. Instead, we managed her condition by reliance on secondhand data, nursing reports, and laboratory results, and we never confronted the care of the patient herself.

In another instance, a pregnant woman was seen for routine prenatal care. At each visit she was angry and complained about various real and imagined injustices. The office hours were inconvenient, the receptionist not courteous, the nurse forgetful, the room too warm, and so forth. She had for a long time been in psychotherapy to help her deal with her hostility and considered herself "much better than before." Quickly the professional staff developed a dislike for her attitude, which then supplanted her physical condition as the focus of her visits. When this shift came to conscious awareness at a staff conference, the necessary perspective was gained to include the hostility within the framework of this woman's presentation of herself. When it was accepted for what it was, it ceased to be an obstruction to her obstetric care. When she was hospitalized for a period of time because of bleeding in the third trimester, she was encouraged to keep a written list of complaints and grievances but found it too much trouble and gave up the project, much to her own amusement.

It seems paradoxical that, as in the above example, acceptance of the troublesome element in a presentation will often serve to eliminate it, and there is an increasing recognition of the usefulness of this approach. It is certainly the common clinical experience that the opposite strategy, telling the patient to be different, meets with limited success. In fact, it seems to be inherent in the very nature of the phenomenon that emotionally charged material is usually illogical yet persists tenaciously against logical interventions. Accepting the presentation as it is exerts a kind of formal control over the relationship, allows the possibility of guided change toward a more appropriate presentation, and facilitates an effective therapeutic interaction.

RECOGNIZING PRESENTATIONS

That human beings first develop the ability to communicate with others at the nonverbal level is self-evident. Infants and small children recognize patterns of openness, rejection, anger, affection, etc. long before they understand the meaning of language. These nonverbal pattern-recognition skills become secondary to language and often recede to an unconscious awareness but are never lost as growth and maturity occur. They are easily recultivated into a most useful tool of clinical observation by anyone who is willing to pay attention to a personal experience with a patient, and who can also recognize major personal biases which may influence that experience. Since the ability is already present, it is not essential that the professional first become knowledgeable in the literature of nonverbal communication. Stated more simply, when the professional has the experience of liking the patient, the patient is presenting herself as likable; when the professional repeatedly feels confused, the patient is likely to be presenting herself in a confusing way. When the patient characteristically fails to carry out prescribed treatment, she is presenting herself as a person who seeks advice but does not take it. And if the patient looks or acts or sounds like another person in the professional's past or present life, care must be taken not to misinterpret this presentation because of that likeness.

Health professionals, particularly those without intensive training in psychologic or psychiatric techniques, often fear that opening discussions in these areas may create problems where they did not already exist, or may precipitate new and unexpected problems better left undiscovered. Actually, when the patient's presentation suggests the importance of nonorganic factors in her problem, she is probably also asking for guidance or clarification of these aspects, whether the inappropriateness be conscious or covert. Should the probing activate a significant response, one can be certain that the difficulty already existed. Should it prove fruitless, it can be acknowledged honestly as an educated but erroneous guess and dismissed.

"Primum non nocere" is the time-honored maxim of clinical practice. The exploration of psychosexual factors in gynecologic symptoms falls well within the intent of the maxim; it is an essential aspect of effective care.

REFERENCES

Haley, Jay: *Strategies of Psychotherapy,* New York: Grune & Stratton, 1963.

————: *Uncommon Therapy,* New York: Norton, 1973.

Watylawick P et al.: *Principles of Problem Formation and Problem Formation and Problem Resolution,* New York: Norton, 1974.

PART FIVE

Specific Problems

27

Reproductive Failure

JAMES C. WARREN

Reproductive failure occurs when a given couple cannot produce viable offspring. It manifests itself in two general categories: failure to become pregnant and failure to carry the pregnancy to viability.

It is estimated that approximately 15 to 20 percent of all couples in the United States seek medical assistance because of reproductive failure. Thus, we have a problem of considerable magnitude. No one dies of infertility and (possibly for this reason) there is a tendency among physicians to approach such problems in a more casual manner than disease states which produce physical morbidity and mortality. Nevertheless, failure to reproduce thwarts a basic human instinct and is a source of anguish, guilt, and broken marriage. Therefore, it deserves a rigorous approach and careful consideration.

INABILITY TO BECOME PREGNANT

Couples who are unable to establish a pregnancy may be infertile or sterile. Infertility is an involuntary reduction in reproductive ability. Sterility is *total* inability to reproduce. Note that infertility is a relative term while sterility is absolute. In either case, the situation may be reversible or not reversible.

The possibility of infertility or sterility is generally entertained only after the couple in question have tested their capacity to establish a pregnancy by trying for an appropriate period of time. It must be remembered that there are four general factors which influence the anticipated physiologic performance of couples in terms of fertility: age of the wife, age of the husband, frequency of intercourse, and duration of coital exposure.

Fertility is low in the young woman (possibly because of anovulation), increases to a peak at 24 years of age, and then declines with a rapid fall after age 30 (Table 27–1). The same maximum is seen in the male at age 25 with a similar type of decline (Table 27–2). Also, note that the best conception rates occur when intercourse occurs four or more times weekly (Table 27–3). Of course it is possible that some of the effects of aging are related to frequency of intercourse. Given a group of couples 25 years of age having intercourse three times a week (without contraception), approximately 50 percent should be

TABLE 27–1 Fecundability (Fertility) Rate and Mean Delay in Conception

Age at marriage	Fecundability rates per 1000 women	Mean conception delay, months
12-15	90	13.4
16	93	11.7
17	128	10.4
18	121	9.2
19	151	8.7
20	180	7.2
21	209	6.4
22	226	6.4
23	203	6.0
24	276	5.3
25	214	6.4
26	180	8.9

Source: SJ Behrman, RW Kistner.

TABLE 27–2 Percent of Conceptions Occurring in Less Than 6 Months at Various Age Levels

Age of husband	Number of cases	Conception in less than 6 months, %
Under 25	126	74.6
25-29	132	47.7
30-34	76	38.2
35-39	55	25.5
40 and over	44	22.7
All cases	433	48.5

Source: J MacLeod, RZ Gold: The male factor in fertility and infertility VI. Semen quality and certain other factors in relation to the ease of conception. *Fertil Steril* 4:10, 1953.

pregnant within 6 months. To advance in age or have less frequent intercourse will decrease the chances of success. The performance of a couple who seek consultation should be evaluated in light of these factors. If it is significantly below projected expectations (this means a couple trying seriously for 12 to 18 months without success), a diagnosis of infertility should be entertained and an evaluation conducted.

REQUIREMENTS FOR PREGNANCY

Certain requirements must be met to establish pregnancy. It is useful to keep them in mind.

1. The male must produce and mature satisfactory numbers of normal, motile spermatozoa.

TABLE 27–3 Percent of Conceptions in Less Than 6 Months for Various Rates of Intercourse

Average frequency of intercourse	Number of cases	Conceptions in under 6 months, %
Less than once a week	24	16.7
Once but less than twice	109	32.1
Twice but less than 3 times	123	46.3
Three times but less than 4 times	100	51.0
Four times and over	72	83.3
All cases	428	48.40

Source: J MacLeod, RZ Gold: *Fertil Steril* 4:10,1953.

2. He must have patent conduits and enough potency to ejaculate spermatozoa from the urethra into the vagina
3. The spermatozoa must reach the cervix, pass through the cervical mucus, and ascend through the uterus and oviduct at a time appropriate to meet the ovum.
4. The spermatozoa must be capable of penetrating and fertilizing the ovum.
5. The female must ovulate an ovum which has access to a patent oviduct.
6. The fertilized ovum must move into the uterus, find an endometrium prepared for implantation, implant, develop normally, and produce a glycoprotein gonadotropin in its trophoblastic portion capable of rescuing the corpus luteum.

This is a complex series of events requiring integrity of several structures. A moderate or sporadic defect in any one can cause infertility; a severe, consistent defect can result in sterility.

EVALUATION OF THE INFERTILE COUPLE

An investigation done by a physician knowledgeable in the fields of infertility and reproductive biology serves three important purposes for couples who have not achieved a pregnancy:

1. It may explain the cause of the infertility.
2. It may suggest the appropriate therapy.
3. It may allow an estimate for the probability of success.

The only way to evaluate the infertile couple is with a thorough, rational, orderly examination of *both* partners. Physicians who are not willing to take this responsibility seriously should refer these patients to those who do. Incomplete examinations usually involving a remunerative D&C (dilatation and curettage) and a few x-rays rarely explain the cause of infertility. The physician is responsible for proceeding in an orderly fashion and trying to minimize cost. The couple is responsible for careful cooperation in the testing. Under these circumstances comes the best chance for success. During the evaluation which proceeds from history to physical examination to a series of specific tests, it is valuable to keep in mind causes for failure and evaluate each of them as completely as possible at each step. These causes and their approximate incidence are given in Table 27–4.

TABLE 27–4 Causes of Infertility and Their Approximate Incidence

I. Male factors 40 percent
   A. Decreased production of spermatozoa
      1. Varicocele
      2. Testicular failure
      3. Endocrine disorders
      4. Cryptorchidism
      5. Stress, smoking, heat, systemic infections
   B. Ductal obstruction
      1. Epididymis, postinfection
      2. Congenital absence of vas deferens
      3. Postvasectomy
      4. Ejaculatory duct, postinfection
   C. Failure to deliver into vagina
      1. Ejaculatory disturbances
      2. Hypospadias
      3. Sexual problems (i.e., impotence)
   D. Abnormal semen
      1. Volume problems
      2. Necrospermia and agglutination
      3. High viscosity
II. Ovulation factors, 20 percent
   A. Anovulation
   B. Inadequate corpus luteum
   C. Amenorrhea with low estrogen production
III. Tubal obstruction or dysfunction, 20 percent
   A. Pelvic inflammatory disease, tuberculosis, puerperal infection
   B. Congenital
   C. Endometriosis
   D. Peritonitis (ruptured appendix or viscus, surgery)
IV. Cervical and uterine factors, 10 percent
   A. Myomata, polyps, developmental abnormality of endometrial cavity, synechiae
   B. Abnormalities of cervix
      1. Obstruction (surgical, new growths)
      2. Destroyed endocervical glands (surgical, infections)
V. Vaginal factors, < 5 percent
   A. Congenital absence of vagina
   B. Imperforate hymen
   C. Vaginismus
   D. Vaginitis
VI. Immunologic incompatibility, 5 percent
   A. Spermatozoa-immobilizing antibodies
   B. Spermatozoa-agglutinating antibodies
   C. ABO incompatibility
VII. Nutritional and metabolic factors, < 5 percent
   A. Thyroid
   B. Diabetes
   C. Severe nutritional disorders

These are the factors that must be evaluated. More than one cause may be responsible in a given couple, and the effect of any cause or combination of causes may be moderate or severe and correctable or noncorrectable. In any evaluation of the infertile couple, the entire list should be investigated.

HISTORY AND PHYSICAL OF THE FEMALE PARTNER

It is usually the woman who first presents herself for assistance, and thus one usually starts with her. The history should ascertain duration, frequency, and success of coital exposure. Ask about use of lubricants (possibly spermatocidal), postcoital activities (douching, especially with spermatocidal solutions), fertility and diabetes in other members of the family, general health, and reasons for desiring pregnancy. On physical examination evaluate general health status, habitus and contours, thyroid size, hirsutism, and abdominal scars. Test for glucose in the urine. During the physical, evaluate factors by examination and questioning.

Vagina. Evaluate the hymen, look for vaginismus, a vaginal septum, vaginitis. Ask about pain on intercourse.

Cervix and Uterus. Ask about frequency and amount of menstrual bleeding, previous vaginal surgery, and dysmenorrhea and dyspareunia. Light menstrual periods or spotting with a history of onset after a D&C or interuterine infection suggests the presence of intrauterine synechiae. History of previous cervical surgery (conization, cautery, D&C) raises the possibility of destruction of cervical glands with obstruction or decreased mucus production. Extremely heavy menstrual periods may be due to a submucous fibroid or polyp, or anovulation. Severe dysmenorrhea suggests cervical stenosis or endometriosis. Severe dyspareunia suggests endometriosis, intrapelvic disease, and vaginismus. The cervix should be open with no evidence of scarring or infection and with mucus appropriate for day of the cycle (see below). Evaluate the fundus as to size, shape, position, and fixation. Look for a plastic string indicating unknown or forgotten IUD. Feel carefully on rectovaginal examination for tender uterosacral nodules because they, especially with a fixed posterior fundus, strongly suggest endometriosis.

Tubal. History of tubal infection, tuberculosis, ruptured appendix, other abdominal infection, or finding an abdominal scar suggests possibility of tubal obstruction. Palpate for tubal enlargement and tenderness.

Ovulation. Presence of menstrual periods rules out congenital absence of vagina and imperforate hymen as well as ovarian and pituitary failure. Regular menstrual periods; mittelschmerz; watery vaginal discharge at midcycle; prodromal signs such as breast tenderness, backache, ankle edema, moodiness; being able to predict onset of the period and cramping with the period are reasonably reliable subjective signs of ovulation. On examination, note if ovaries are normal size and mobile. If one ovary is larger than the other, consider the possibility of the presence of corpus luteum or endometriosis.

SCREEN OF THE INFERTILE COUPLE

It is preferred to have both members of the couple at the first visit, but often it is the wife who comes alone. She is started on the screening program and her husband is requested to return for seminal analysis. On the first visit, after history and physical, the factors that must be evaluated are explained, and the screening procedure (that generally takes two or three cycles) is started. Methodology for the components of the screen is given in the supplement at the end of this chapter.

If the wife is having menstrual periods at reasonable intervals, she is instructed to start taking rectal basal body temperatures (BBT) on the fifth day of her next cycle. (It is explained that the metabolic thermometer is shaken down the night before, the temperature taken for 4 minutes immediately on awakening, and that day 1 of a cycle is always the day menstrual bleeding starts.) She is asked to record temperatures carefully and return with her husband (after 2 days of abstinence from intercourse and douching) 1 to 2 days before the projected ovulation day (i.e., day 13 if the cycle, by history, is 28 days). At that visit a seminal sample is taken from the husband, and the wife is evaluated in terms of opening of the cervix, amount and consistency of mucus, ferning response, and spinnbarkheit. If pelvic examination of the wife is normal and she has no history of peritoneal or pelvic infection, the Rubin test is done at that visit. Afterward, the endometrial cavity is gently explored with sound to seek synechiae or other distorting lesions. If she has a history of peritonitis, previous surgery, or pelvic masses, one may defer the Rubin test and use laparoscopy, culdoscopy, or (if physical

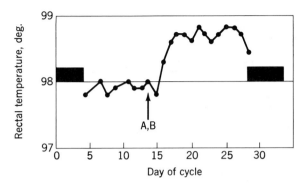

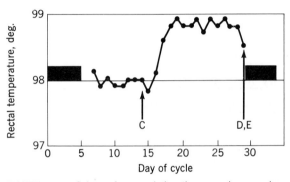

FIGURE 27–1 Scheme for completing the screening examination in two menstrual cycles. Shown is a plot of the patient's basal body temperature for two consecutive cycles. *A* Cervical score of 10, Rubin ⊗, endometrial cavity normal. *B* Seminal analysis: 4.0 mL volume, 45×10^6 spermatozoa per mL 70% motility, 65% normal morphology. *C* Huhner test reveals 12 motile spermatozoa per hpf. *D* Biopsy reveals 28-day endometrium. *E* Seminal analysis adequate, agglutinating and immobilizing antibodies negative.

findings are minimal and sedimentation rate normal) possibly hysterosalpingogram for the screen of tubal patency. Tubal manipulation may cause a flare-up of quiescent pelvic inflammatory disease.

During the second cycle the patient repeats the BBT, and once again returns without douching 1 or 2 days before ovulation for a postcoital (Simms-Huhner) test. Mucus is taken from a point as high up in the cervical canal as possible and examined for the presence of motile spermatozoa.

The patient continues her BBT and returns the day before the onset of the next menstrual period for endometrial biopsy. Many patients can pick this day without difficulty. If not, one must select the day from the BBT curve, or the woman must come within 2 hours of the onset of the menstrual period for the biopsy. If the menstrual period comes at an inopportune time, the physician must try again at the end of the third cycle. Finally, agglutinating and immobilizing

spermatozoa antibody testing is done at the same time a second seminal analysis is carried out (see below). An evaluation where everything was successfully done during the first two cycles is shown in Fig. 27–1.

If the patient has amenorrhea with patent vagina and palpable uterus, one must decide whether the amenorrhea is due to ovulation failure, destruction of the endometrial cavity, or cessation of estrogen production. For this purpose one may (in the absence of vaginitis) do a maturation index, scraping cells from the upper third of the vagina for grading (as to superficial, intermediate, and parabasal) and administering 100 mg of progesterone in oil. The patient returns in 3 weeks. A normal menstrual period (usually occurring within 3 to 8 days of the progesterone injection) and an estrogenic maturation index indicate ovulation failure. Little or no bleeding and an estrogenic maturation index suggest Asherman's syndrome and signal a gentle probing of the endometrial cavity to evaluate patency. Little or no bleeding and a maturation index displaying low estrogen production (superficial cells less than 15 percent) indicate cessation of estrogen production. If the patient has ceased producing estrogen, determination of gonadotropin levels, preferably blood FSH (follicle-stimulating hormone) (Goldenberg) which best differentiates between ovarian and pituitary failure, is indicated. Then evaluations of tubal patency, seminal quality, and antibodies are carried out as above.

REVIEW OF DATA OBTAINED ON THE SCREEN

At this point, the screen which has evaluated ovulation, tubal, uterine, cervical, vaginal, antibody, nutritional, and male factors is reviewed. A decision is made as to whether each factor is adequate, inadequate, or borderline. One form used for this review is shown in Fig. 27-2. It gives the results of the scan of the couple shown in Fig. 27-1.

If both seminal analyses are above acceptable levels (volume greater than 2.0 mL, liquefaction within 45 minutes, concentration above 20 million per mL, 60 percent motility with 40 percent showing good forward progression, 60 percent showing normal morphology), male factors are declared adequate. This decision is further substantiated if the postcoital test reveals five or more progressive motile spermatozoa per high-power field and the antibody testing is negative. If the seminal requirements above are not

<u>INFERTILITY EVALUATION</u>
Department of Obstetrics-Gynecology
Washington University School of Medicine

Name _____ Suzie Brown _____ Age of wife 26 husband 28 ___

A.I.U.

A.   Hx: Duration _____ Married 4 yrs, trying for 2 yrs

        Coital Pattern _____ 2-3 times/wk, orgasm (+)   A

    Previous Data _____ No previous workup

    _____ General and pelvic exam negative (9-17-73)

B. 1. Ovulation Hx _____ M.P. every 27-30 days   Subjective signs (+)   A

                      Find _____ BBT x 2 look ovulatory (Oct, Nov '73)

                      _____ EB on day 29 (11-26-73) = 28 day endometrium

    2. Tubal   Hx _____ No surgery, PID, or peritonitis   A

                      Find _____ Rubin (+) 10-14-73

    3. Cervix   Hx _____ No surgery, abortion   A

                      Find _____ Cervical score=10 (10-14-73, 1 day preovulation)

                      Post-Coital 12 motile, 3 nonmotile/hpf (11-11-73, 1 day preovulation)

    4. Uterus   Hx _____ Normal size M.P.   A

                      Find _____ Normal sounding of cavity (10-14-73)

    5. Vagina   Hx & Find _____ Patent, no vaginitis or vaginismus (9-17-73)   A

    6. Male   Hx _____ Negative   A

                      Find _____ #1 (10-14-73) 40×10^6/ml, 70% motile, 65% normal

                      _____ #2 (11-26-73) 50×10^6/ml, 65% motile, 60% normal

    7. Immuno   Hx _____ Neg   A

                      Find: Sperm _____ Isojima, Kibrick, FD neg (11-26-73)

    8. Metabolic Hx _____ Neg   A

                      Find _____ Glucose in urine = neg   PBI = 6 µg%

C. Further Investigation ____ <u>All factors of screen are adequate. Will do</u>

_____ <u>laparoscopy in January 1974</u>

_____

_____

_____

_____

D. Final Conclusion _____ <u>1-2-74: NOTE: M.P. due Dec 23, 1973 has not come.</u>

_____ <u>BBT up and remains up.</u>

_____ <u>Pregnancy test this a.m. = ⊕</u>

_____

_____

_____

E. Plan _____ <u>Return to referring OB-GYN</u>

_____

_____

_____

FIGURE 27–2 Summary form used for evaluation of each factor in the screening examination.

clearly adequate, we turn to further investigation and possible therapy of the male.

If BBTs are both clearly biphasic and the elevation persists for 12 days, cervical score at the time of ovulation is 9 to 12, and endometrial biopsy shows a full-blown secretory endometrium with good predecidual change in stromal cells and secretory exhaustion in the glands, one concludes that normal follicular development and ovulation are occurring. If the cervix (examined just before ovulation) is pouting, cervical mucus is copious with good spinnbarkheit and 4+ fern reaction, and postcoital test is satisfactory, one concludes that cervical factors are adequate. If the Rubin test reveals free flow of gas at less than 100 mmHg, the patient complains of shoulder pain on sitting up, and probe of the endometrial cavity with a uterine sound reveals no abnormalities, one concludes that tubal and uterine factors are adequate. Lastly, if there is no vaginitis or vaginismus and antibody tests are negative, one concludes that these factors are adequate. If any of the female requirements above are clearly inadequate, turn to further investigation and possibly therapy of the specific factor. If any factor seems borderline on the screening examination, testing pertinent to it is repeated in an attempt to assign to it the status of adequate or inadequate.

If all the factors of the screen, both male and female, seem adequate and yet the couple has clearly demonstrated their incapacity to reproduce, carry out extensions of the screening examination as follows:

1. Thyroid evaluation of both partners [T_4 (tetraiodothyronine) by column or by competitive binding protein].
2. Glucose tolerance test in the female.
3. Mycoplasma culture.
4. Laparoscopy on the female. On day 6 or 7 of the cycle, with the patient in the semilithotomy position, one performs a hysterogram or does hysteroscopy to reevaluate the endometrial cavity. Then with the laparoscope, careful evaluation of the pelvis is made and tubal patency tested by inserting methylene blue in the cervix and noting whether it spills out from both tubes. This procedure reveals intrauterine abnormalities, unexpected tubal obstruction, peritu-

bal adhesions which limit approach of the fimbriae to the ovary, and silent endometriosis.

On occasion there is a couple that seems to be completely adequate even at this stage of the investigation. It is a mistake to assure them that all is well, especially if they have been unsuccessful for 2 to 3 years in obtaining a pregnancy. The poor (50 to 60 percent) subsequent pregnancy rate in such couples (Jones, 1962) indicates that there really is something wrong—we just do not know what it is.

If specific factors are inadequate, one now investigates and treats these problems. Every factor that is not clearly adequate must be considered.

FURTHER INVESTIGATION AND THERAPY OF THE MALE

The screening evaluation usually allows us to place the male into one of the following groups:

1. All seminal factors are adequate.
2. There are relative or borderline seminal defects: spermatozoa count 10 to 19 million per milliliter, motility 35 percent, abnormal forms 50 percent.
3. There are severe seminal defects: azoospermia, aspermia, severe oligospermia (1 to 2 million per milliliter), no motility.

Examination of men in category 1 should center on review of potency, frequency of intercourse, presence of hypospadias, and postcoital test. In those with borderline defects one should first reexamine the scrotum and penis carefully and repeat seminal analysis twice at 4-week intervals (after 48 hours of abstinence) to be sure that the patient really belongs in this category. A careful search is made for stress, excessive smoking, alcohol intake, heat to scrotum, or a recent viral or infectious illness. As oligospermia caused by these factors may be reversible, it is wise to relieve them (i.e., a 4-week vacation) and then reevaluate. It is important in this reevaluation to remember that the lag period between spermatogenesis and delivery in the ejaculate is 10 to 12 weeks. If these simple measures do not result in a seminal sample that clearly comes up to the requirements of adequacy, the male is termed infertile and the workup is begun.

The initial step of this workup is a careful examination (with the man standing) to detect varicocele (use the Valsalva manuever), congenital absence of the vas deferens, postinflammatory changes, and testis size. If the physical is normal and testes at least 50 percent of normal size, evaluate serum FSH, testosterone, T_4, and prolactin. If history suggests congenital adrenal hyperplasia, evaluate 24-hour urinary ketosteroids and pregnanetriol. If testes are small, Barr chromatin or chromosomes should be evaluated and donor insemination discussed.

CAUSES OF MALE INFERTILITY

A sensible and usable evaluation of etiologic factors in male infertility in a large series of patients has been reported by Dubin and Amelar (1971). The cause and incidence are given in Table 27-5. Remarks to follow refer to that table.

Varicocele. Note that in Amelar's experience varicocele was by far the most common cause of male infertility. In this disorder oligospermia, decreased motility, and tapered head forms (MacLeod, 1965) are found. Surgical correction results in improved spermatozoa quality in 80 percent with a pregnancy rate approximating 50 percent. The size of the varicocele appears to have no influence on the outcome of therapy (Dubin, Amelar, 1970).

Volume and Viscosity Problems. When semen volume is low (<1.0 mL) with otherwise normal characteristics, homologous intracervical insemination and capping may lead to pregnancy. If there is no success, one can turn to donor insemination (see below). Most volume problems present as high volume (>5.0

TABLE 27–5 Causes of Male Subfertility 1965–1970, 1294 Cases

Causes	No. of cases	%
Varicocele	512	39
Semen volume problems	157	11.8
Endocrine abnormality	111	8.6
Sexual problems	64	5.1
Ductal obstruction	96	7.4
Testicular failure	176	14.0
Ejaculatory disturbance	24	2.0
Cryptorchidism	56	4.4
Spermatozoa agglutination	10	0.8
Necrospermia	15	1.3
High spermatozoa density	2	0.2
High seminal viscosity	1	0.1
Unknown	70	5.4

Source: L Dubin, RD Amelar 1971.

mL) with impaired quality. Because the first portion of this ejaculate is usually (90 percent of the time) the best, a split ejaculate (see below) is taken. If the first, or for that matter either, portion consistently yields 2 to 3 mL that meet adequate requirements, a trial of homologous insemination with this fraction is in order. High viscosity of the seminal fluid is rare, but Amelar (1962) has reported pregnancy in one case after Alevaire (mucolytic respiratory mist) douche.

Endocrine Problems. Endocrine disorders comprise hypopituitary states, adrenogenital syndrome, and hypothyroidism. The majority of Amelar's patients in the endocrine category displayed low gonadotropin levels. He reports that treatment of the *hypogonadotropic* patient is successful 30 percent of the time. With the current availability of both human menopausal gonadotropin and chorionic gonadotropin, it is reasonable to surmise that future results with combined therapy will yield a higher degree of success in men in this category. Patients with adrenogenital syndrome may or may not have the "congenital" variety but should display significantly elevated ketosteroids and pregnanetriol. The spermatozoa pattern resembles that of varicocele. Treatment with glucocorticoids appears to be effective (Amelar, 1966). Hypothyroidism is actually a very rare cause of infertility. While hypothyroid males should be treated and treatment is effective, giving Cytomel to euthyroid males is a *waste of time.*

Sexual Problems. The moderately high incidence of sexual problems emphasizes the necessity of a careful history of actual success at coitus that should be taken independently from both partners. While some of these problems are best treated by the psychiatrist, it is well to remember that diabetes mellitus, perineal surgery, diseases of the nervous system, and certain drugs may be responsible.

Obstruction. Ductal obstruction is suggested by a history of infection or surgery and confirmed by physical examination. An enlarged obstructed epididymis usually results from gonococcal or tuberculous infection. The resultant azoospermia can sometimes be corrected by epididymovasostomy, if testis biopsy reveals spermatogenesis. Absence of the vas deferens usually results in a low semen volume as the associated absence of the seminal vesicle leaves only prostatic fluid in the ejaculate. No successful treatment of this disorder is available. Vasectomy repair (in terms of appearance of spermatozoa in the ejaculate) is successful from 40 to 80 percent of the time, but pregnancy rates approximate a lower figure (see Male

Sterilization in Chap. 33). Possible implications of an autoimmune mechanism in this finding are discussed below.

Testicular Failure. The causes of testicular failure as indicated in the series of Dubin and Amelar are shown in Table 27-6. When other causes for decreased production of spermatozoa (Table 27-4), ductal obstruction, failure to deliver into the vagina, and seminal volume and viscosity problems have been ruled out as a cause for the infertility of an azoospermic male, a testis biopsy is indicated unless the couple declines, prefers donor insemination, or the Barr chromatin pattern and chromosome analysis reveal Klinefelter's syndrome.

Patients with Klinefelter's syndrome demonstrate a positive Barr chromatin pattern, are XXY or some variant thereof on chromosome analysis, and have small testes, gynecomastia, and generally elevated FSH levels. No treatment is available except donor insemination.

Germinal aplasia is probably the most common cause of testicular failure. The physical examination is normal, the semen azoospermic, and FSH may be elevated. Diagnosis of this disorder and maturation arrest (arrest at a specific stage of spermatogenesis) can be made only on testis biopsy.

Ejaculatory Disturbance. Complete aspermia (no ejaculate) results from the more common retrograde ejaculation, a lesion in the nervous system (paraplegia, syringomyelia), or ejaculatory duct obstruction. Aspermic men (especially with a history of prostatic surgery) should be checked for retrograde ejaculation by having them empty the bladder after ejaculation. The urine is centrifuged and a spermatozoa count done on the resuspended sediment. Infertility due to retrograde ejaculation has been treated by la-

TABLE 27–6 Testicular Failure

Type	No. of cases	% of entire series
Germinal cell aplasia	44	3.4
Klinefelter's syndrome	32	2.7
Infantile testis (chromatin negative	20	1.5
Mumps orchitis	32	2.5
Maturation arrest	24	1.8
Testis tumor	8	0.7
Surgical injury	16	1.4

Source: L Dubin, RD Amelar 1971.

vage of the bladder with sodium bicarbonate, effecting ejaculation, recovering spermatozoa by lavage, and carrying out artificial insemination (Bourne). While ejaculatory duct obstruction is rare, a rectal examination in those with this disorder may disclose distended seminal vesicles, and stripping may open the obstruction.

Cryptorchidism. A testis which remains cryptorchid after puberty will be sterile. Because early diagnosis and treatment will prevent sterility, aggressive approach with gonadotropins followed by surgery if not effective is indicated by age 6.

THERAPY OF TESTICULAR FAILURE

Attempts at treatment consist of stimulation and suppression of testis function. Stimulation may be effected with human menopausal gonadotropins (Glass), luteinizing hormone–releasing hormone (Zárate) and clomiphene citrate (Palti, Wieland). Suppression involves the use of testosterone enanthate.

The physician should always consider stimulation first because suppression may produce permanent azoospermia. If FSH is not elevated (i.e., not above 20 mIU/mL), gonads are at least 50 percent of normal size, and absence of germinal cell aplasia is shown (by observation of some sperm in the ejaculate or testis biopsy), clomiphene is probably the best first choice of treatment. Regimen may be one tablet every other day or one tablet daily, 25 days of each month. Medication is continued for 3 to 4 months, at which time seminal analysis and serum FSH are again evaluated. If seminal analysis is unchanged and FSH is elevated, clomiphene (or for that matter, LRF and gonadotropins) will not be effective. On this regimen, improvement in seminal analysis is reported to be 75 percent and the incidence of subsequent pregnancy to be 42 percent, if wives are normal (Paulsen). If chomiphene therapy, as defined above, does not elevate either sperm concentration or FSH, it is logical to turn to LRF (but not possible at this time because the compound is not available) or to gonadotropins.

When the FSH is initially clearly elevated, if the sperm count fails to improve with clomiphene (under conditions where FSH and serum testosterone become elevated) or if there is failure with human menopausal gonadotropins, the physician should think about suppression. Probably the best regimen is one that follows the guidelines of Heller (Rowley) as modified by Paulsen (personal communication). It involves intramuscular administration of testosterone enanthate, 200 mg per week for 16 to 20 weeks. Seminal analysis is done every 4 to 6 weeks. Counts are suppressed during therapy and "rebound" occurs after 3 to 36 months.

Using this overall spectrum of therapies one can still not be overly optimistic about pregnancy. The overall success rate is only about 40 percent (in 1 to 2 years) as compared with 80 percent (in 6 months) when artificial insemination with donor sperm is used (Strickler).

FURTHER INVESTIGATION AND THERAPY OF THE FEMALE

Factors which play a role in the infertile female are evaluated reasonably well by the complete screening procedure, if it is carried out as described above. Should any of the results be equivocal, it is best to carefully repeat them. If any factors are deemed inadequate, further investigation and possibly therapy for these are indicated. Such investigations and therapy are developed by category below.

OVULATION FACTORS

These are manifested in three general categories:

1. Ovulation failure (normal estrogen production)
2. Hypoestrogenic amenorrhea
   a. Low gonadotropins
   b. High gonadotropins
3. Inadequate corpus luteum

Patients in any of these categories should have an evaluation of serum prolactin.

If pregnancy is desired, treatment of ovulation failure and low-gonadotropin hypoestrogenic amenorrhea is induction of ovulation using specific drugs (glucocorticoids or thyroid), clomiphene, LRF, or human gonadotropin. In the low-gonadotropin hypoestrogenic group, or in any patient who shows lactation, or elevated serum prolactin, skull x-rays and polytomograms should be obtained to rule out tumor of the pituitary or hypothalamus before therapy. The patient with hypoestrogenic amenorrhea who has elevated gonadotropins (two plasma FSH determinations above 40 mIU/mL—see Fig. 27-3) almost certainly has ovaries that are bereft of follicles and is not a candidate for further therapy. The patient with an inadequate corpus luteum requires support of the corpus luteum with human chorionic gonadotropin (HCG) or of the endometrium with progesterone.

Ovulation failure is marked by a history of erratic bleeding episodes (which may extend to oligomenor-

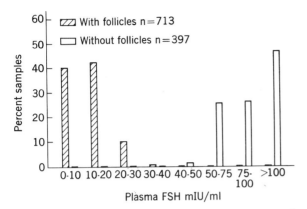

FIGURE 27–3 Distribution of plasma FSH (radioimmunoassay) in samples from women with secondary amenorrhea with and without follicles (*n*, number of samples). *(From Goldenberg et al.)*

rhea or hypermenorrhea), a BBT curve which is not biphasic, and the finding of a proliferative endometrium on biopsy done just before or within 2 hours after the onset of a spontaneous bleeding episode. Withdrawal bleeding occurs 3 to 8 days after administration of progesterone. In a variant of ovulation failure sometimes referred to as *follicular luteinization,* the BBT may be elevated for 4 to 6 days, then fall with onset of bleeding and a biopsy that shows early secretory endometrium. It is of interest that a similar syndrome can be caused in the laboratory animal by administration of doses of LH (luteinizing hormone) smaller than those clearly required for ovulation (Ying). Sections of the ovaries of animals so treated demonstrate many retained ova. For this reason, follicular luteinization is included here as a variant of ovulation failure, although there is no absolute evidence as to whether ovulation does or does not occur in the woman who demonstrates this disorder.

Hypoestrogenic low-gonadotropin amenorrhea is marked by a history of no bleeding, with little or no response to progesterone, a flat BBT curve, a maturation index indicating little or no estrogen production, and a low-grade proliferative or atrophic endometrium on biopsy.

The inadequate corpus luteum is characterized by an endometrial biopsy which shows the endometrium to be 3 or more days retarded at onset of menses (i.e., absence of predecidual stroma) when dated by appropriate criteria (Noyes, 1950, 1956).

Treatment of Ovulation Failure

One first searches for a specific cause. Hypothyroidism is such a case but is seen rarely. Treatment of hypothyroidism with thyroid preparations brings

about a dramatic response; similar treatment of euthyroid patients is a waste of time. Obesity and hyperandrogenic states must also be considered. History may correlate deterioration of the menstrual periods with weight gain. Weight loss is sometimes associated with a return of normal menses.

Women with excessive androgen production often have hirsutism, acne, defeminization, and even virilization. Laboratory evaluation includes urinary 17-ketosteroids, 17-hydroxycorticoids, and determination of serum-free and total testosterone (Paulson). If values are elevated, one can carry out sequential suppression tests with glucocorticoids (adrenal source) and Enovid-E (ovarian source). Ovarian size should be carefully reevaluated. Catheterization of adrenal and ovarian vein to determine the site of androgen production in hirsute women has indicated that the major source is ovarian the overwhelming majority of the time, while, rarely, androgens originate from the adrenal (Kirschner). Further, dexamethasone significantly suppresses blood free testosterone even in one-third of those whose androgens are of ovarian origin. In those cases where clear suppression of blood testosterone (and ketosteroids, if elevated) to normal levels by dexamethasone occurs, it is reasonable to provide a clinical trial of suppression using 0.5 mg at bedtime. If the patient returns after 2 to 3 months with regular ovulatory periods, treatment is carried out for a total of 8 months. If therapy induces regular menses, the urinary steroids often stay normal (and sometimes hirsutism improves) for months or years thereafter. This situation and congenital adrenal hyperplasia are the only indications for such medication.

In the great majority of anovulatory women, no distinct etiology is defined. Anxiety and other psychogenic problems may be responsible for many of the idiopathic cases.

Hypoestrogenic low-gonadotropin amenorrhea results from failure of gonadotropin synthesis or release by the pituitary. It may result from damage to the pituitary or hypothalamus by tumor, infection, vascular occlusion, or trauma. It may also result from extreme hyperandrogenic states (adrenal or ovarian tumor and congenital adrenal hyperplasia) in which cases distinct virilization is present. A syndrome with associated lactation has also been reported in primary hypothyroidism. The mechanism is explained by the observation that thyrotropin-releasing factor (TRF) (which is elevated in primary hypothyroidism) promotes pituitary release of prolactin as well as thyroid-stimulating hormone (TSH). Another cause is the "postoral contraceptive therapy amenorrhea syndrome." This syndrome of amenorrhea which lasts in excess of 1 year after contraceptive therapy appears to occur with an incidence approximating 1 percent. In an intensive study of 69 such patients, Shearman (1971) found that 11 had copious galactorrhea but x-ray of the sella was normal in all cases. Most patients in this category had low gonadotropins and low estrogen production but the majority responded normally (estrogen production) to a standardized gonadotropin stimulation test while a few gave the excessive response usually associated with the Stein-Leventhal syndrome. One patient had a spontaneous cure after 72 months. An occasional patient in this category has high gonadotropins; such patients represent premature menopause which just happens circumstantially at this time.

Ovulation failure and hypoestrogenic amenorrhea are discussed together because the basic therapies have certain factors in common. Except those who respond adequately to thyroid, weight loss, or dexamethasone, the armamentarium consists of clomiphene citrate, human gonadotropins, and the decapeptide LRF which is now under investigation.

Use of Clomiphene. This drug is currently the mainstay for treatment of ovulatory failure. It is a weak estrogen and therefore a competitive antiestrogen. While the exact mechanism of action is not established, the ultimate effect is via the hypothalamus or pituitary to cause the gonadotropin surge (both LH and FSH) required to induce ovulation. Induced ovulation, as indicated by the temperature nadir, generally occurs 5 to 10 days after withdrawal of the drug when it is given in 5-day cycles (Insler).

The best results are achieved in anovulatory patients whose vaginal smears show estrogen production and who demonstrate withdrawal bleeding on progesterone, especially those with Stein-Leventhal syndrome. If serum prolactin values are normal, clomiphene should also be the initial drug used with low-gonadotropin amenorrheas and postcontraceptive syndromes, after x-ray of sella to rule out pituitary neoplasm.

The basic strategy is to start with 50 mg of clomiphene daily for 5 days. The drug is given on the fifth day of a menstrual cycle induced by 100 mg of progesterone intramuscularly or a suitable oral progestation agent. Progress is followed by the basal body temperature. If no ovulation occurs, the regimen is repeated. If again there is no ovulation, dosage is subsequently increased to 100 mg daily, 150 mg daily, and 200 mg daily, testing each dosage for one or two cycles. When the basal body temperature in-

dicates that ovulation has occurred, the same dose is repeated so that cervical mucus can be examined and a postcoital test done just prior to ovulation. An endometrial biopsy is taken at the approach of the menses. The *lowest* dosage that gives a sharp biphasic BBT curve and a well-developed secretory endometrium on biopsy should be designated as the maintenance dose. It is continued for 6 to 8 months with intercourse every 2 days during the fertile week, monitoring of BBT, and an occasional premenstrual biopsy. Too often clomiphene is given for a month or two and put aside if no pregnancy occurs. Lamb has shown the value of continuing the therapy by comparing cumulative conception rates on clomiphene with those seen after removal of an IUD and those of young married women (see Fig. 27-4).

Nevertheless, in a given patient, none of the dosages above may effect the normal ovulatory response. Three ovulatory and three anovulatory responses to clomiphene can occur. They have been nicely reviewed by Murray and Osmond-Clarke:

O_1 Normal ovulatory response.

O_2 Ovulation with poor estrogenic response—low estrogenic vaginal smear; scanty, cellular cervical mucus at ovulation.

O_3 Short luteal phase—luteal phase persists only 7 to 10 days after normal estrogenic response (similar to the naturally occurring inadequate corpus luteum discussed below).

A_1 Luteinized follicle—normal estrogenic response followed by a poor luteal phase which persists only 4 to 6 days before bleeding.

A_2 Follicular response—rise in estrogenic index but no luteal phase and no bleeding.

A_3 No response.

It should be noted that unless one does frequent vaginal smears or evaluates cervical mucus, one would interpret both A_2 and A_3 as just "no response." Naturally the best conception rate (70+ percent) is seen in patients with the O_1 response. In the O_2 group pregnancy rates are 10 to 15 percent, and in all other groups pregnancy is rare or does not occur without additional therapies.

Approximately 15 percent of women who receive clomiphene develop faulty cervical mucus secretion and poor spermatozoa penetration corresponding to the O_2 group above (Graff). The great majority of these women develop this problem only after clomiphene therapy, and results of their Huhner tests deteriorate significantly after therapy. This response can proba-

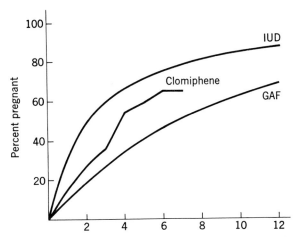

FIGURE 27-4 Cumulative conception rate calculated by the life table method for anovulatory women treated with clomiphene, fertile women after removal of an intrauterine device (IUD), and a representative sample of young married women not using contraception (GAF). *(From Lamb et al.)*

bly be attributed to the antiestrogenic effects of clomiphene which are even more profound on the vaginal smear and even seen in the endometrium (Lamb). Kistner (1968) has suggested treating those with the O_2 response with small doses of estrogen (0.1 to 0.2 mg of diethylstilbestrol daily). We have done this, but results have not been spectacular. Insler et al. treated patients who failed to conceive on five cycles of clomiphene (and whose cervical mucus was suppressed) with large doses of ethinyl estradiol. He used 75 to 150 μg per day starting on the fourth day of a 5-day clomiphene schedule and continuing until the BBT first showed a rise. With this regimen ovulation occurred, cervical scores and Huhner tests improved significantly, slope of the thermal shift and length of the luteal phase were unchanged, and 24 percent of the patients became pregnant within three cycles. This problem is approached by using clomiphene on days 5 to 9, then following it with conjugated estrogens (Premarin) on days 10 to 14, using 1.25, 2.5, or even 5.0 mg per day. With this regimen, ovulation is not interfered with and mucus is often improved. Before starting any treatment with estrogens, it is wise to recall that the antiestrogenic effect of clomiphene is responsible for the suppression of cervical mucus. The incidence will be intensified by excessive dosage.

Reasonable success (50 percent) can be obtained in the O_3 group by giving HCG after ovulation as in the case of the inadequate corpus luteum. Groups A_1 to A_3 are best approached by increasing clomiphene dosage or adding HCG. It is well to remember that ovulation requires an intact positive estrogen feedback mechanism (that is, the estrogen surge from the developing follicles must induce an LH surge). In patients who lack this mechanism, substitution of 10,000 IU of HCG 8 days after the last clomiphene dose may be effective. Thus, patients who fall into group A_3 require more clomiphene; those in groups A_1 and A_2 may profit by the addition of HCG.

In patients with low estrogen production who do not bleed after progesterone, results with clomiphene are less impressive, but before going to gonadotropins, an all-out effort should be made using 100 mg of clomiphene for 9 days and 10,000 IU of HCG approximately 8 days after the last pill (Kistner, 1965).

Complications of clomiphene citrate include hyperstimulation with enlarged ovaries and occasional ascites, hot flashes, flushes, multiple pregnancy, blurring of vision, and scotomata. Hyperstimulation and multiple pregnancy are not nearly as common as seen with use of gonadotropins and are minimized by judicious and progressive regulation of dosage with frequent examination of the patient.

Use of Gonadotropins. If clomiphene alone or with estrogen or HCG in various permutations does not produce the normal ovulatory response and the desired pregnancy, one may try human gonadotropins. There are two exceptions to this statement. The first is the hypoestrogenic patient with elevated serum FSH levels. Such patients have ovarian failure and will, of course, not respond. The second exception is the polycystic ovary syndrome (Stein-Leventhal syndrome). Fortunately, the response to clomiphene is usually good in this syndrome, and if no pregnancy occurs in 12 months, wedge resection of the ovaries is indicated. Gonadotropins should be avoided because of hypersensitivity of these patients to exogenous gonadotropins and problems that follow treatment (Keettel; Gemzell; Taymor; Jones, et al., 1969).

Human gonadotropins are available as Pergonal which contains 75 IU of FSH and 75 IU of LH per ampule. Treatment is expensive and should be carried out only by those interested and experienced in its use. The ideal patient is one who has low levels of endogenous gonadotropins. The amount required varies from 1000 to 3000 IU of FSH generally given over a 10- to 12-day period. Urinary estrogen is usually monitored, particularly later in the course of therapy as increasing amounts are used. Total urinary estrogen values between 50 and 100 μg per 24 hours signal that the follicle is ripe for ovulation. At this time, after a day of rest, 10,000 IU of HCG is given. Pregnancy rates in four to six cycles approximate 35 percent. The major complications of therapy are hyperstimulation syndrome and multiple pregnancy.

Use of LRF. After the decapeptide LRF was purified from sheep hypothalami, the amino acid sequence was determined, synthetic material was made, and clinical trials were carried out. The drug can be used to test pituitary reserve and responsiveness. It has been shown to induce ovulation, and pregnancy has been reported following its use. It would appear to be especially valuable in the hypogonadotropic woman who does not respond to clomiphene but whose pituitary is capable of responding to LRF by releasing LH and FSH. It has the advantage over gonadotropins that it can be synthesized in vitro. Further, sublingual administration may be possible. At present it is not available for clinical use in the United States.

The Inadequate Corpus Luteum. The inadequate corpus luteum syndrome has been described by Jones (1962) and later shown to be associated with a poor pregnancy rate. In this disorder, which may occur with or without clomiphene stimulation, the luteal phase is shortened by at least 3 days as revealed by endometrial biopsy and BBT. Two possible etiologies have been put forward: first, inadequate FSH production during ovular ripening (Strott) and second, an inadequate LH surge at ovulation time (Friedman). The diagnosis is made by careful observation of BBT and taking the trouble to do the endometrial biopsy just before onset of the menstrual period. This abnormality appears to occur in some patients on an infrequent basis and under this condition may be of no consequence. On the other hand, when it occurs regularly, it appears to be a cause of both infertility and loss of pregnancy (discussed below). Two major therapeutic methods have been suggested. Jones has favored use of 25 mg progesterone vaginal suppositories twice daily through the luteal phase and reported an 80 percent pregnancy rate in the naturally occurring syndrome. One must agree that such a course is preferred to synthetic progestins, some of which may actually be luteolytic. HCG may also be used—10,000 IU immediately after ovulation or 5000 IU starting after ovulation and continuing every 2 to 3 days until just before the expected menses (to avoid a pseudopregnancy). When this situation arose in response to clomiphene therapy (the O_3 group above), no pregnancies were seen in 52 patients. When HCG was given in the immediate postovular phase, almost 50 percent of the patients conceived.

TUBAL FACTORS

There are four basic types of tubal obstruction; obstruction at the cornu, obstruction in the isthmus, fimbrial obstruction, and peritubal adhesions. Site of the obstruction is usually delineated by hysterosalpingogram (cornual and isthmal), laparoscopy, or culdoscopy (fimbrial obstruction and peritubal adhesions). There are various surgical techniques for each with permutations involving use of splints, prostheses, and postoperative hydrotubation. Success rates (pregnancy) vary from 5 to 40 percent (Clyman).

There are a few points to be made. First, the incidence of pelvic adhesions following surgery, especially that done for minimal or questionable reasons, suggests that one should be hesitant to perform laparotomy on the young woman who has not yet had her family unless the indications are quite clear. Resections of functional ovarian cysts, uterine suspensions, removal of small subserous fibroids, wedge resection of the ovaries before trial with clomiphene, and unnecessary appendectomies all take a toll on reproductive capacity. Second, aggressive therapy of gonorrhea early in its course is always in order. If reparative tubal surgery is done, avoidance of powder and foreign bodies, meticulous care in handling of tissues, fine instruments, and complete hemostasis are mandatory. While it is impossible at this time to make an unequivocal statement, occasional use of prostheses seems reasonable if raw surfaces must be left, as does postoperative hydrotubation with hydrocortisone and antibiotic mixtures.

ENDOMETRIOSIS

Endometriosis appears to be associated with infertility in that it is seen more frequently in the infertile patient and does cause tubal adhesions and distortions. In the infertile patient who is otherwise normal, this possibility should be considered and laparoscopy or culdoscopy carried out. It is found in about one-third of patients in this category.

There are two choices for therapy, hormonal and surgical. In patients with minimal or asymptomatic endometriosis, pregnancy rates are very good (85 percent) after conservative surgery (Ranney). They are also very good following medical therapy (Moghissi). With more extensive disease, there is some debate as to the most effective form of therapy. It is a good idea to gauge the extent of the disease with laparoscopy, and reasonable to try medical therapy first in those instances where little or no tubal or ovarian involvement is seen. It may even be considered when ovarian endometriomas do not exceed 1 to 2 cm in size. Medical therapy can be carried out with oral medroxyprogesterone acetate (Provera), 10 mg three times a day or Danazol, 400 mg twice daily for 6 months. The patient then, in the absence of recurrence of severe pain and pelvic findings, tries to achieve pregnancy for a 1-year period. If pregnancy is not achieved, conservative surgery should be performed. If ovarian endometriomas are larger than 1 to 2 cm or if significant tubal distortion and adhesions are present, conservative surgery probably offers the best outcome. This surgery should effect complete resection of all endometriosis present, and protect from adhesions by uterine suspension and elevation of the ovary by a suture placed in the ovarian ligament attaching it to the posterior surfaces of the uterus. Danazol has worked well in causing the regression of endometriomas. A recent paper (Dmowski) suggests that Danazol is better than Provera for patients who can afford it. Indeed, the pregnancy rate of patients with larger ovarian endometriomas after Danazol therapy may be comparable to that after surgery, unless there are extensive adhesions.

CERVICAL FACTORS

Infertility may result from obstruction of the cervical canal as well as production of an abnormal or hostile mucus. Obstruction may be due to endocervical polyps, endometriosis, or tuberculosis (rare), or it may follow surgical procedures (conization, aggressive cauterization, D&C) presenting as stenosis or synechiae. The latter are often associated with intrauterine synechiae. Abnormal mucus may result from infection, surgical destruction of endocervical mucus glands, or preovulatory estrogen deficiency. Obstruction is usually detected when one attempts the sounding and Rubin test procedures. Abnormal mucus is detected by examination of cervical mucus and postcoital test just prior to ovulation. With endocervicitis, numerous leukocytes are present in the cervical mucus.

Obstruction may be treated by gentle cervical dilatation, and polyps may be removed by gentle endocervical curettage. If cervical synechiae are present, evaluation of the endometrial cavity by hysterogram or hysteroscopy is indicated. Figure 27-5 shows Asherman's syndrome following a D&C. Note the IUD in the peritoneal cavity. Because of the obliterated cavity it had no room to coil and penetrated the fundus like a

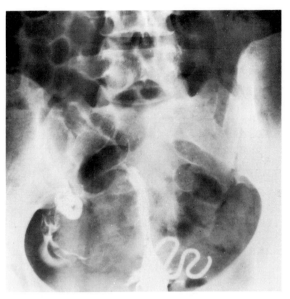

FIGURE 27–5 Asherman's syndrome as indicated by hysterogram which also shows free IUD in the peritoneal cavity.

spear on insertion. Treatment consists of dilatation of the cervix and endometrial cavity, breaking up of synechiae, and insertion of a Foley catheter or intrauterine contraceptive device (Louros; Comninos) with administration of generous doses of estrogen.

Cervical erosions and lacerations associated with preovulatory mucus of good quality do not require treatment. Similar lesions with thick, leukocyte-laden preovulatory mucus should be treated. Primary attempt is made with locally applied agents. If this is unsuccessful, broad-spectrum systemic antibiotics may be tried. If these fail, electrocauterization or cryosurgery is indicated, but great care should be taken to avoid deep penetration of the endocervical canal which only results in further destruction of endocervical glands or stenosis. After the infection is cleared, it may be both useful and informative to cycle the patient with generous dosage of estrogen for one or two cycles (2.5 to 5.0 mg of conjugated estrogens daily for 24 days with 50 mg of Provera on the last day) and note the response. Production of a copious mucus of good quality indicates that the glands are capable of responding.

If the endocervix is not infected, preovulatory mucus of poor quality indicates an inadequate preovulatory estrogen surge or destruction of endocervical glands. Here, the estrogen regimen above may be informative. An immediate response indicates the former, its absence favors the latter. With damaged endocervical glands, several high-dosage estrogen cycles *may* improve the quality. Inadequate preovulatory estrogen surge is an endogenous problem similar to the suppression of cervical mucus sometimes seen with clomiphene. One may try to improve quality by administration of 0.1 to 0.2 mg of diethylstilbestrol from day 5 to 15 of the cycle. The BBT must be followed carefully, however, as even these low doses may delay or inhibit ovulation. In those instances where response to generous estrogen dosage shows that the glands are intact and the diethylstilbestrol inhibits ovulation with little or no improvement of mucus, it is reasonable to try clomiphene, 50 mg daily, days 5 to 9 and Premarin 1.25 to 5.0 mg daily, days 10 to 14. If the primary structures of the cervical and hypothalamic estrogen receptors turn out to be dissimilar, it is conceivable that we may someday come up with a real "cervical estrogen" for use in this situation.

There is one important point to be made. One should start treatment programs such as those above only after being convinced that preovulatory cervical mucus is of poor quality. This can be done only by repeatedly observing the cervix late in the follicular phase. If a single observation or observations at the wrong time of the cycle (when the mucus frequently looks poor even in the normal, fertile woman) are allowed to serve as the basis for this type of therapy, the result may be a long and fruitless therapeutic misadventure.

UTERINE FACTORS

Lesions that severely distort or obliterate the endometrial cavity may cause infertility. They may be detected on sounding the cavity at the time of the Rubin test and confirmed by hysterogram. Polyps and pedunculated submucous myomas can be removed with ovum forceps at D&C. Synechiae are treated as described above. Nonpedunculated submucous myomas and congenital abnormalities may be corrected abdominally. Needless to say, such a step should be taken only after a complete evaluation reveals no other cause for the infertility (see also Repeated Abortion below).

Uterine retroversion, in the absence of fixation by adhesions, pelvic inflammatory disease, or endometriosis, is rarely a cause of infertility. Nevertheless, there are a few patients with retroverted nonfixed uteri who insist that even without contraception they become pregnant (and do so with great ease) only with the pessary. Therefore, manual correction and placement of a Smith-Hodge pessary for 6 months is reasonable in the patient with a retroverted uterus, particularly if the fundus is in a position where it causes

dyspareunia and possibly lessens the frequency of intercourse, or if postcoital tests are poor. If pregnancy does not occur despite the fact that the pessary maintains the uterus in an anterior position, there is nothing to be gained by a surgical uterine suspension. The fixed, retroverted uterus is an indication for laparoscopy.

Tuberculous endometritis is now very rare in the United States but is found in incidences from 5 to 8 percent in sterile women in some parts of the world. It is almost always secondary to a pulmonary infection. It may be diagnosed by both histologic and bacteriologic methods. If one has reason to suspect the disease, dilatation and curettage should be conducted in the luteal phase of the cycle with some tissue submitted to histologic study employing regular staining procedures and those specific for acid-fast bacilli. The remainder is submitted for bacteriologic studies. Chronic (nongranulomatous) endometritis is usually attributable to a specific etiologic factor such as pelvic inflammatory disease, IUD, or postpartum and postabortal states (Cadena). It is appropriate to insist on plasma cell infiltration to make the diagnosis. Its role as a serious cause of infertility in the absence of pelvic inflammatory disease remains to be proved.

VAGINAL FACTORS

In congenital absence of the vagina, rectal examination usually reveals absence of significant uterine rudiments, and indeed the urethra can be palpated almost directly in front of the rectum. Approximately 90 percent of these patients have no functional endometrial tissue. Because the ovaries are normal, they demonstrate normal development of other secondary sexual characteristics, and no masses are palpated on rectal examination. The hallmark of this variety of the disorder is the complete absence of abdominal and pelvic pain. In patients without endometrial tissue, a vagina can be constructed (after intravenous pyelogram to rule out pelvic kidney). While such an artificial vagina allows coitus, there is obviously no chance of pregnancy. A small percentage of patients with congenital absence of the vagina do have rudimentary uterine and endometrial tissue. The characteristics of this variety are recurrent abdominal pain and palpable pelvic masses. Presence of functional endometrial tissue is an indication for laparotomy. In a few cases, reconstructions have been carried out, but for the most part, extirpation of the uterine rudiments is indicated, and sterility persists.

When examination of the perineum reveals absence of a satisfactory vagina but rectal examination reveals not the easily accessible urethra but rather a bulging mass below the level of the cervix, one immediately considers imperforate hymen and partial agenesis of the vagina. In the former case, incision of the hymen will be accompanied by a gush of dark blood from the hematocolpos. To treat the latter disorder, the procedure described by TeLinde and Mattingly is recommended.

While nonsurgical approaches to the construction of the artificial vagina are difficult and require extreme cooperation on the part of the patient, one encounters more success with the small but patent hymen and the testicular feminization syndrome where a small vaginal pouch (1- to 3-cm depth or so) already exists. When the hymenal orifice is small but clearly patent, progressive dilatation can be effected by the use of liberally lubricated Young's dilators. Ideally, such disorders should be picked up on premarital examination.

Vaginismus is diagnosed by history or its presence at the time of pelvic examination. It is treated initially by generous stretching of the vagina using Young's dilators or by desensitization techniques. If coital problems persist after stretching to the point where the vagina admits two examining fingers, psychiatric evaluation is indicated. Vaginitis is categorized by gross appearance, smears, and cultures, and appropriate treatment given.

ANTIBODY PROBLEMS

While activity in the area of immunoreproduction has intensified in recent years with an abundant literature, there is much controversy as to testing methods, results, significance, controls, and mechanisms involved. One of the problems is that at least 12 antigenic substances have been isolated from human ejaculate (Li). Some are intrinsic and some are seminal plasma antigens which only coat the spermatozoa. A second arises from the variable methodology used by various investigators. Nevertheless, there is emerging evidence that antibodies against spermatozoa may be responsible for infertility in human beings (Behrman, 1973).

ANTIBODY TESTING

Studies in human beings have generally evaluated circulating antibodies which show immobilizing or agglutinating activities against the spermatozoa. Attempts to show that such activities are pertinent to infertility have compared incidence in fertile couples,

infertile couples with and without other demonstrable causes, women with no coital exposure, prostitutes, and men after vasectomy. The basic premise is that an activity which shows low incidence in fertile couples and young girls and high incidence in couples who are infertile, prostitutes, and men with previous vasectomy may be pertinent as a cause of infertility.

Immobilizing Antibody. This type of antibody appears to correlate best in terms of its pertinence to infertility. The recommended technique for exploration of human infertility problems is that of Isojima et al. (1968). Motility values after incubation of the patient's inactivated serum, spermatozoa, and complement for 60 minutes at 37°C are determined and compared with an incubation in which inactivated normal human serum replaces that of the patient. A control for detection of nonspecific activity is run by leaving out complement. In this case, there should be no immobilization. The spermatozoa immobilizing factor, as demonstrated by this test, is present in IgG (gamma-G globulin) and IgM (gamma-M globulin) fractions (Isojima, 1972).

Agglutinating Activity. There is a definite tendency for washed spermatozoa from several mammalian species to agglutinate in a head-to-head fashion, especially if suspended in normal serum (Bedford) in the absence of any antibodies whatsoever. Separation of this natural phenomenon from one induced by agglutinating antibodies requires extremely careful adjustment of test conditions and even then may be fraught with problems and ambiguities.

The recommended test is that of Kibrick, Belding, and Merrill which utilizes suspension of spermatozoa in a gelatin solution to minimize disruption of weak unions. Spermatozoa, fresh gelatin, and serum at various dilutions are mixed, incubated, and observed for macroscopic agglutination. This test, which must be carefully controlled, has been widely used in human studies. The agglutinin it detects is present in the IgG fraction (Boettcher).

A microscopic method to evaluate spermatozoa agglutination was introduced by Franklin and Dukes who initially reported that almost 80 percent of women with unexplained sterility displayed this factor in their serum. In their later work (Dukes and Franklin) the incidence was 67 percent in women with unexplained infertility as compared with approximately 20 percent where another cause for the infertility could be shown. Others have found differences of lesser magnitude (Schwimmer; Isojima, 1969), or no significance (Hanafiah). There is debate about specificity and significance of this test, possibly because of differences in methodology. The factor apparently responsible for this effect occurs in the beta globulin fraction (Boettcher).

EFFECTS IN THE MALE

Autoantibodies in the male may be responsible for (1) interference with normal spermatogenesis or (2) direct effects on the spermatozoa which prevent pregnancy.

Autoimmune Aspermatogenesis. Using the guinea pig model with adjuvant, Freund demonstrated that the adult testis of the same or a different animal of the same species, on being homogenized and injected, caused immune aspermatogenesis with degenerative changes in the seminiferous tubules. Interstitial tissue was unaffected. The animals displayed circulating antibodies and cutaneous hypersensitivity reactions. Immature testis homogenate does not elicit autoimmune spermatogenesis, suggesting that the antigen is present only at or after the secondary spermatocyte stage (Katsch, 1960). Antispermatogenic antigen of guinea pig testis has been purified to homogeneity by Katsch and coworkers (1972). It is a glycopeptide with a molecular weight of approximately 12,600. With Freund's adjuvant, microgram amounts produce autoimmune aspermatogenesis. Similar bilateral testicular lesions have been induced in other species by unilateral injection of Freund's adjuvant (Eyquem, Kreig; Menge, Christian). Finally, in men, similar systemic immunization produced antibody formation and in some cases aspermatogenesis (Mancini).

Thus, it is possible that trauma, infection, or occlusion of the ductus or vas might induce autoimmune azoospermia. Increases in circulating spermatozoa antibody (both immobilizing and agglutinating) have been reported in such conditions. Further, although reanastomosis after vasectomy is reversible (in terms of motile spermatozoa in the ejaculate) in 70 percent of cases, spermatozoa concentration and pregnancy rates are low (see Chap. 34).

Effects on the Spermatozoa. Whether presence of spermatozoa antibodies in the serum of men with otherwise normal spermatozoa parameters is a lesser form of the antoimmune disorder discussed above remains to be seen. Finally, antigens of the ABO blood group system have been found on spermatozoa. There is debate as to whether they are inherent components of the spermatozoa cells which would allow segregation of the cells into distinct populations or merely absorbed from seminal plasma. Their possi-

ble role in infertility is yet to be established, although hemagglutinins have been reported in cervical mucus (Solish).

Therapy of the Male. In a recent series (Ansbacher), follow-up of some 200 infertile couples revealed that 13 husbands demonstrated antibodies. Four of eight with agglutinating antibody (Kibrick) subsequently fathered a child, while none of five with immobilizing antibodies (Isojima) did. The only potential therapy for men with autoimmune antibodies in serum and seminal fluid has been reported by Schoysman. Seventeen men were given testosterone injections which caused azoospermia and eliminated the source of the antigen. Titers went down, and after therapy normal semen quality returned in nine, with five attaining a pregnancy.

EFFECTS IN THE FEMALE

Studies on agglutination and immobilization of spermatozoa cells by sera of the female partner of fertile and infertile couples as well as virgins and prostitutes have been made by several investigators trying to effect a correlation with infertility. Table 27-7 indicates correlation of immobilization and agglutination (Kibrick) tests with infertility. The immobilization test correlates well. There are also suggestions that presence of immobilizing antibodies may be associated with reduced penetration of cervical mucus (Kremer test). With the Kibrick method, the high positive incidence in groups which are negative by immobilization parameters suggests nonspecificity. Nevertheless, the two methods probably detect different immunologic responses, and both tests should be used in the infertile couple.

There is a good deal of controversy over microscopic agglutination (Franklin-Dukes) as to its specificity, significance, correlation with infertility, and as to whether it is even affected by an antibody. The findings of some investigators mentioned above and those shown in Table 27-7 suggest that it is worthless. Nevertheless, Dukes and Franklin (1968) continue to find higher activity in couples with unexplained infertility (67 percent) than in couples who are fertile (9 percent) or have an organic cause for infertility (16 percent). Further, they continue to see 60 to 70 percent pregnancy rates if titers fall on condom therapy (Franklin, personal communication). Possibly the controversy arises from differences in methodology.

Origin of Antibodies in the Female. The general supposition is that vaginal spermatozoa inoculation gives

TABLE 27–7   Percentage of Positive Results by Sperm Immobilization Tests, Complement Fixation, and Franklin-Duke's and Kibrick's Agglutination Tests

Type of patient	SIT*	Franklin-Dukes' agglutination test	Kibrick's agglutination test
Sterile			
Unexplained sterility	7/36 (19.4%)	9/34 (26.5%)	6/10 (60%)
Patients with a cause of sterility	1/65 (1.5%)	13/58 (22.4%)	4/11 (36.4%)
Patients whose clinical tests were not completed	0/23 (—)	4/23 (17.4%)	9/16 (56.3%)
Control			
Pregnant women	0/19 (—)	5/19 (26.3%)	7/13 (53.8%)
Unmarried girls	0/16 (—)	1/16 (6.3%)	2/18 (11.1%)

*SIT, sperm immobilization test.
Source: Isojima, 1969.

rise to serum antibodies which also exist in the reproductive tract. Indeed, immunization via the vagina with production of systemic antibody response has been shown in the guinea pig by Behrman and Otani and in the mouse by Bell. Whether these antibodies are produced locally remains to be seen. While immunoglobulins have been found in cervical mucus by Lippes and coworkers (Tourville), they have not been identified as antibodies to semen components.

Therapy. The only therapy of the isoantibody state in the female employed so far is condom therapy, popularized by Franklin and Dukes. After 6 to 12 months of condom use, 50 to 75 percent of women demonstrate lower or negative titers, and then the condom is not used during the fertile week (days 11 to 18 of a 28-day cycle). If titers fall with the condom, 75 percent of women with agglutinating antibody achieve a pregnancy, while only 30 percent of those with immobilizing antibodies do so.

Many authors report that experiences with sperm antibody testing have not been very satisfactory. We have used the methods of Isojima, Kilbrick, and Franklin and Dukes faithfully. On original testing we find one of these tests positive in about 20 percent of our patients. Unfortunately, 80 percent of these positive tests are not abnormal on repeat testing. Therefore, we only employ condom therapy after two positive tests. We currently hold that there really are cases of infertility attributable to immunologic cause, but the tests we use are not always satisfactory in detecting them.

ARTIFICIAL INSEMINATION

Artificial insemination may be conducted with spermatozoa from the husband or from a donor.

ARTIFICIAL INSEMINATION WITH HUSBAND'S SPERMATOZOA (AIH)

This approach may be utilized when impotence, severe hypospadias, or poor coital techniques cause failure of deposition of appropriate numbers of spermatozoa in the vagina. Presence of one of these conditions is suspected when seminal analysis is normal but the postcoital test consistently reveals absence of spermatozoa in cervical mucus of good quality (2 hours after coitus).

Another indication for AIH is retrograde ejaculation. The patient empties his bladder and ejaculates. The bladder is then lavaged with a small amount of saline containing sodium bicarbonate to render the solution alkaline. Spermatozoa are concentrated, resuspended, and deposited in the vagina. A few pregnancies have been reported with this technique.

The technique can also be carried out using a "split ejaculate sample" of the male. If the ejaculate can be collected in two "halves," the first half will generally be richer in spermatozoa and acid phosphatase (from the prostate), while the second will be richer in fructose (from the seminal vesicle). In some 90 percent of men, the first half of the ejaculate has a higher spermatozoa concentration, motility is better, and the percentage of abnormal forms lower. Some 5 percent of men have ejaculates that are approximately equal, and in 5 percent the second sample is better. In men with high-volume ejaculates where analysis of the total ejaculate is somewhat below accepted levels and in the absence of any demonstrable etiology in the wife, one may submit split ejaculates to analysis. If the first portion on two occasions displays spermatozoa concentrations two or three times the second portion with better motility and morphology (falling well above the minimal acceptable limits), it is reasonable to try split ejaculate insemination. Alternatively, the husband may use a withdrawal coital technique in which he attempts to deliver approximately the first half of his ejaculate before withdrawal of the penis. There are several papers reporting successes with its use (as an example, see Amelar, 1965). Unfortunately, none of these studies has divided such couples into two groups and compared incidence of pregnancy in randomly selected couples in which whole ejaculate was used

with that of randomly selected couples in which split ejaculate was used. Nevertheless, in the male who cannot otherwise be improved, this technique is worth a trial before turning to the use of donor spermatozoa.

ARTIFICIAL INSEMINATION WITH DONOR SPERMATOZOA (AID)

The ideal couple for AID is one in whom male factors appear to be entirely responsible for the infertility. The male is clearly subfertile, azoospermic, or aspermic, and his condition cannot be improved, while no abnormalities are found in the wife. It may also be tried after prolonged infertility in the face of persistent agglutinating or immobilizing antibodies with no other demonstrable cause. If the wife's serum contains antibodies to the husband's spermatozoa, antibody testing should be done with spermatozoa samples from proposed donors; those without reaction are used. The third situation for its employment is the Rh-negative woman (whose husband is Rh-positive and

TABLE 27–8 Definition of Cervical Scoring System*

Parameter	0	1	2	3
Amount of mucus	None	Scant; a small amount of mucus can be drawn from the cervical canal	Dribble; a glistening drop of mucus seen in the external os; mucus easily drawn	Cascade; abundant mucus pouring out of the external os
Spinnbarkheit	None	Slight; uninterrupted mucus thread may be drawn approx. ¼ of the distance between the external os and vulva	Moderate; uninterrupted mucus thread may be drawn approx. ½ of the distance between the external os and vulva	Pronounced; uninterrupted mucus thread may be drawn for the whole distance between the external os and vulva
Ferning	None; amorphous mucus	Linear; fine linear ferning seen in a few spots; no side branching	Partial; good ferning with side branches in parts of the slide, linear ferning or amorphous mucus in other parts	Complete; full ferning of the whole preparation
Cervix	Closed; mucosa pale pink, the external os hardly admits a thin applicator		Partially open; mucosa pink, the cervical canal easily penetrable by an applicator	Gaping; mucosa hyperemic, the external os patulous

*A score of 10 to 12 just prior to ovulation is considered adequate.
Source: V Insler et al.: The cervical score: A simple, semiquantitative method for the monitoring of the menstrual cycle. *Int J Gynaecol Obstet* 10:223, 1972.

probably homozygous) who has either a high-titer or anti-D antibody or who has lost a previous pregnancy with erythroblastosis. Here one must be very careful to use an Rh-negative donor.

Before initiating AID, testing of the woman should be carried out to document ovulation and eliminate uterine, cervical, tubal, and vaginal factors as contributing etiologies for the infertility. Knowing the ovulation day is very important in both AID and AIH. It can be determined by analysis of sequential basal body temperature curves which allow one, in most instances, to project the day of ovulation (the day of the temperature nadir). Artificial insemination is carried out two or three times each cycle at daily or 2-day intervals around the ovulation day.

Donors should be healthy young males who physically resemble the husband in terms of hair color, eye color, and general body build. They should be free of disease and instructed never to donate spermatozoa if there is exposure to venereal disease. The Rh type of the wife should be determined in advance. If she is Rh-negative, it is preferable to use an Rh-negative donor and imperative to do so if she demonstrates anti-D antibody. Donors should abstain from sexual relations for 2 to 3 days in advance of giving spermatozoa. Insemination is conducted with a cervical cap or by deposition of spermatozoa in the cervix using a syringe and polyethylene tubing. Any materials used must be well washed, rinsed, and air dried. Cervical caps are commercially available. The freshly collected sample is placed in the cap and the cap placed over the cervix. The string is left protruding from the vagina so that it can be used to remove the cap 12 hours after insemination. Inseminations should be carried out monthly for 6 to 8 months to yield success rates which approximate 75 percent. If pregnancy does not occur in 8 months, there is a good chance that some undetected female factor for failure has been missed in the preliminary tests. In these cases it is wise to complete the evaluation of the female including hysterogram and laparoscopy. Remember that with randomly selected 25-year-old couples, the mean delay in conception time approximates 5 months.

Frozen Spermatozoa. The use of frozen spermatozoa samples offers several potential advantages. The major advantage is constant availability of spermatozoa for insemination without programming and the expense that is incurred with a fresh sample when the programming is incorrect. At the present time, the use of frozen spermatozoa appears to be only 50 to 60 percent as effective in accomplishing pregnancy per unit of time as does the use of fresh spermatozoa. The

motility of the thawed spermatozoa is reduced and declines more rapidly than that of fresh spermatozoa so that insemination should be conducted daily. Recent advances in methodology include the use of various protective agents such as glycerol and egg proteins as stabilizers and development of complicated programs for the freezing and thawing of spermatozoa. The few reported series of pregnancies resulting from use of frozen spermatozoa indicate no greater incidence of fetal abnormality than when fresh spermatozoa are utilized. Freeze-program techniques have been widely used in the insemination of farm animals. Advances in cell biology will almost certainly provide us with a safe, efficient way to freeze and store spermatozoa over the next decade.

Legal Aspects. In many states the legal status of artificial insemination is in some question. The physician planning to enter into artificial insemination should do so in good faith after he has been assured by the couple that they sincerely want it. It is our policy to provide at least a 4-week waiting period for further discussion as to whether they wish to proceed. Written consent of the wife and husband is secured. A satisfactory format for this consent is that of Behrman (1968). Donors should be kept anonymous, and AID should not be performed in the inharmonious marriage. Psychologic consequences of this procedure are at present undefined, but a report of several years ago indicates that divorce rates among couples who obtain children via artificial insemination with donor spermatozoa were lower than in the population at large. Our own experience with a query to patients who achieved pregnancy with donor insemination also indicated that the majority felt it had strengthened their marriages (Strickler).

GENERAL STRATEGY OF MANAGEMENT

The screening procedure described above should be carried out on every infertile couple. Every factor must be listed as (1) adequate, (2) inadequate, or (3) unresolved. Factors in the last category should also be reevaluated as adequate or inadequate. Then a necessary review of all inadequate factors should be carried out to establish etiology if possible and allow classification of each inadequacy as to (1) mild or severe, and (2) correctable or uncorrectable. Severe correctable inadequacies are corrected, and a 6- to 12-month trial for pregnancy is made. If mild correctable inadequacies coexist, attempts to correct them may or may not be indicated before this trial. This decision depends upon the difficulty and possible complications of the attempt.

As an example, consider a situation where the wife is anovulatory and appears to have been so for the entire 3 years since marriage (severe, probably correctable). She also has a 3-cm leiomyoma which distorts the endometrial cavity (mild, probably correctable) and cervicitis with mucus that is heavily laden with leukocytes during the preovulatory period (mild, probably correctable). The husband's seminal analysis is repeatedly 10 percent below acceptable levels for count and morphology, and postcoital tests are adequate (mild, possibly correctable). The strategy involves attempts at induction of ovulation, therapy for the cervicitis, and a try for pregnancy. This decision is based on the fact that any month a woman does not ovulate she does not become pregnant and that treatment of the cervicitis is easy and has no expected complications. To remove the sessile myoma abdominally may lead to peritubal adhesions that make matters *worse*. Attempts to improve the husband (other than easily instituted general health measures or medication if he has one of the rare hypothyroid or adrenal hyperplasia problems) are difficult and time-consuming. If one obtains a good ovulatory response to therapy and clears up the cervicitis with no pregnancy after 8 to 12 months, one would then think about trying to correct the mild inadequacies.

There are no clear statistics to aid one in handling a couple with four inadequacies as described above. Therefore, therapy becomes a matter of logic, and the minimum requirement is to find every inadequacy, decide whether it is mild or severe, and determine its etiology, if possible, to predict correctability.

Couples with severe uncorrectable inadequacies present in the wife (i.e., hypoestrogenic amenorrhea with high gonadotropins, congenital absence of the vagina, failed attempt at tuboplasty) should be invited to consider adoption. Severe uncorrectable inadequacies in the husband (i.e., azoospermia with no germinal elements present on testis biopsy, congenital absence of the vas, immobilizing autoantibodies with no response to testosterone therapy) are best approached by adoption or AID, depending upon the couple's desires.

Even when defects are severe and uncorrectable, it is wise to project low probability of success rather than zero probability unless one is sure that the latter is warranted. With no uterus, premature menopause, germinal aplasia, and absence of the vas, the zero is warranted. With apparent tuboplasty failure or immobilizing antibodies, however, pregnancy is unlikely but may occur. If a man is told he cannot possibly make his wife pregnant and then she does become pregnant, he may have some concern as to who is really responsible. Thus one avoids the zero prognosis unless one is absolutely sure.

UNANSWERED QUESTIONS

As indicated above, the role of certain inadequacies in a given infertile couple must be assigned as mild or severe. Sometimes this can be done using clinical follow-up information on reported series of cases. Information exists on series of patients with complete tubal obstruction, Klinefelter's syndrome, germinal aplasia, and intrauterine synechiae which obliterate the endometrial cavity. With numerous other situations the role cannot be so well defined because of inconsistencies in analysis, unavailability of large, well-controlled series, and disagreements between studies. All this is complicated by the fact that some infertile couples have failed to become pregnant only by chance and when they finally do so the therapy gets credit.

UNKNOWN FACTORS CAUSING INFERTILITY

Even after a thorough workup no definite cause for infertility may be found in up to 20 percent of cases. While a majority of these couples will achieve a pregnancy without therapy, the 30 to 40 percent who have tried unsuccessfully for over 2 years continue childless year after year. Failure to delineate the cause is not surprising as many of our present testing methods are crude and empirical. A great number of questions pertaining to reproductive failure are presently unanswerable and untestable.

TUBAL TRANSPORT

Factors controlling tubal transport of both spermatozoa and ova and other facets of tubal physiology are incompletely understood in the mammal, and practically nothing is known in the human being. The work of Greenwald has shown that in numerous mammalian species, administration of estradiol in small dosages changes the rate at which eggs are transported through the tube and into the uterus. In the rabbit, 25 μg of estradiol cyclopentylpropionate clearly accelerates the rate at which the ovum is transported through the tube. In 80 to 100 percent of all animals, 50 μg of the same steroid is effective in preventing pregnancy, and 100 μg is capable of blocking the ova so that they remain in the tube at the junction of the ampulla and isthmus. While variations of estrogen production in the normal human cycle may or may not be of this degree, it is possible that minor alterations in the hormonal environment shortly after ovulation, particularly if persistent in a given female, may serve as a subtle cause of infertility.

PHEROMONES

A *pheromone* is a hormonal substance secreted by one individual which stimulates a physiologic or behavioral response in another individual of the same species. As compared with endocrinology, the study of pheromones is sometimes designated as exocrinology. Pheromones have been shown to affect pregnancy rates as follows. A group of female rats in estrous are mated and then subdivided into two subgroups. One is put into contact with strange male rats (each female caged near a male other than the male with whom she had coitus). If this maneuver is carried out before implantation, presence of the strange male will have a marked effect in reducing pregnancy rates and litter sizes. This is mediated via the olfactory system of the female in response to a substance in the urine of the male rat. Rendering the female anosmic nullifies the response. The ultimate molecular mechanism by which it is effected remains to be seen, but its pertinence to pregnancy is clear.

Pheromones, in the form of sex attractants, have been demonstrated in the primate. If a male monkey is placed in a cage adjacent to a female in estrous, he will perform various types of repetitive work in order to gain access to her cage. Michael demonstrated that the stimulus was present in the washings of the vagina of the estrous monkey but absent in the washings of the vagina of the castrate monkey. He identified these compounds as short-chain fatty acids. His subsequent studies revealed that the generation of these short-chain fatty acids was due to bacteria in the vagina of the monkey. On application of vaginal antibiotics (which killed the bacteria), the stimulus to the male disappeared. There have been some attempts to carry out similar studies in the human being, but so far the role of pheromones in human infertility remains undecided.

IMPLANTATION

Molecular aspects of implantation in the mammal are incompletely understood. If a female rat is castrated after mating, progesterone and a small amount of estrogen are required to effect implantation of fertilized ova. Ferrando froze the uteri of rats by a quick-freeze technique. After the freezing, implantation was no longer facilitated by estradiol but was by the administration of histamine. This suggests that estradiol works through a histamine mechanism to facilitate implantation. It further suggests that a given woman might lack some necessary factor involved in this mechanism. While we would be completely unable to evaluate or distinguish such a situation, it could, if persistent, prove to be a severe inadequacy responsible for infertility.

METABOLIC DEFICIENCIES IN SPERMATOZOA

We are able at present to count spermatozoa and to evaluate motility and morphology. In order to achieve pregnancy, the spermatozoa must penetrate the egg to fertilize it. Recent studies, particularly by Williams and coworkers, have indicated that the capacity of the spermatozoa to gain access to the cytoplasm of the egg depends upon the availability of certain hydrolases in the spermatozoa acrosome. These enzymes allow the spermatozoa to penetrate the corona cells which surround the egg as well as the zona pellucida. One of the hydrolases, known as *acrosin,* is a trypsin-like proteolytic enzyme. Various body fluids contain acrosin inhibitors. It is entirely possible that a male could have spermatozoa which appear normal in terms of numbers, motility, and morphology and yet lack this proteolytic enzyme necessary for fertilization. We have no way to routinely test for such a possibility at present. Our workup would lead us to conclude that male factors are normal when in fact this is not true.

Causes akin to these are probably responsible for those cases of infertility which we cannot explain. There is reason to surmise that the percentage of patients in whom the cause of infertility is unknown will diminish over the coming decade.

INABILITY TO CARRY PREGNANCY TO VIABILITY

It is sometimes difficult to separate, with certainty, patients who fail to conceive and implant (establish a pregnancy) from those who lose it in the first few days (abort). While the history of a slightly delayed menstrual period in which the onset of bleeding that is heavier than normal with passage of "tissue" is suggestive, it is neither absolute nor always obtained. A pregnancy may be lost late in the period of gestation, but other chapters in this book deal with such events. Here we are concerned about wastage in the early part of pregnancy, which is referred to as *abortion*.

SPONTANEOUS ABORTION

Spontaneous abortion is termination of pregnancy before the 20th week without voluntary action on the part of the pregnant woman or some other person to effect its interruption. The fetus resulting from such an event will have a weight not exceeding 500 g and a crown-to-rump length of 16.5 cm or less. While spontaneous abortion is only one expression of pregnancy wastage, it is a major one.

INCIDENCE AND TIME OF OCCURRENCE

It is difficult to state an absolute occurrence rate for spontaneous abortion for two reasons. First, abortions occurring in the first few weeks of conception may not be recognized as such but interpreted as merely a heavy period. Second, the possibility of intervention is difficult to eliminate. Within these limitations, the distribution of fetal loss in the United States in 1964 as given by Stickle is presented in Fig. 27-6. It indicates a total abortion rate of 27 percent, with most occurring in the first few weeks of gestation and a marked decrease after the 12th week. The embryo may have died several days before the actual event of abortion. This is particularly true in the case of "missed abortion."

FIGURE 27-6 Cumulative outcome of pregnancy by number of weeks elapsed since conception. *(From Stickle.)*

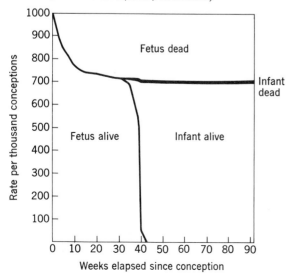

CAUSES OF SPONTANEOUS ABORTION

Basically abortion results from either defective germ cells or faulty maternal environment. While an etiology cannot be assigned in all cases, recent progress, especially in cytogenetics, has tremendously improved our ability to do so.

Chromosomal Abnormalities

During the first trimester of pregnancy, the proportion of abortuses reported to display chromosomal anomalies ranges from 20 to 65 percent (Boué 1970; Carr). The largest percentage (about half) are trisomic for a chromosome, usually in chromosome groups A, B, and C, groups in which trisomes are not seen in living offspring. A considerable number are monosomic for X (45XO), but some of these monosomics do reach term to be born with Turner's syndrome. A considerable number demonstrate polyploidy (usually triploid). A few possess mosaic patterns, autosomal monosomy, and translocations. It is in the last case that one occasionally finds specific translocations in the parents.

Women who have a spontaneous abortion with an abnormal karyotype appear to be subsequently no less fertile than those who have an abortion with a normal karyotype (Boué 1973), nor do they have a greater tendency to abort again. When consecutive abortions in given women are karyotyped, the general normal or abnormal chromosomal nature is usually repeated (8 of 11 normal twice, 14 of 17 abnormal twice), but if two consecutive anomalies are found, they are almost always different except when one of the parents is a translocation carrier.

These observations have led to some acceptance of first-trimester abortion as an early protective mechanism to eliminate abnormal individuals from the species. Obviously no therapy will allow the pregnancy to be carried to term with successful outcome, nor is such an event desirable.

Uterine Fundal Abnormalities

While not a common cause of abortion, developmental abnormalities of the uterus (bicornuate uterus) and intrauterine defects (myomas, polyps, synechiae) which distort the endometrial cavity may result in abortion. While uterine hypoplasia and retroversion have been mentioned as causes of abortion, no proof for their implication exists. The exception is fixed retroversion which may lead to incarceration. The presence of an intrauterine contraceptive device increases the probability of abortion, especially if it is not removed when pregnancy is diagnosed.

Cervical Abnormalities

Amputation of the cervix (fortunately now rarely done in childbearing years) is associated with early abortion. Weakness of the cervical connective tissues resulting from laceration at delivery, vigorous dilatation at D&C or possibly congenital reasons may cause the syndrome of "the incompetent cervix." Here, abortion occurs after the 14th to 16th weeks of pregnancy in the absence of vigorous contractions.

Infection

A dozen viruses have been implicated as causes of early abortion (Sever), the most notable of which are rubella, cytomegalovirus, and herpes. Syphilis is recognized as a cause of abortion after the fourth month. While mycoplasmas, listeriosis, and epidemics of "flu" and other febrile disorders have been suggested as causes, they remain to be proved.

The Inadequate Corpus Luteum

Mentioned above as a cause of infertility, this syndrome has also been associated with repeated abortions in the first trimester (Moszkowski). If biopsy taken near the onset of the menstrual period consistently reveals an endometrium that is 3 days or more retarded, therapy with vaginal progesterone or HCG is indicated.

Hormonal and Nutritional Factors

There is evidence that maternal diet and fetal development are related, as severe starvation in animals increases fetal resorption rates. Thus, it is feasible that *severe* malnutrition predisposes to abortion. The roles of specific deficiencies or folic acid, ascorbic acid, and tocopherol in abortion are uncertain.

Many years ago in a study of women who were hypothyroid by basal metabolic rate, but not myxedematous, Litzenberg and Carey indicated that one-third of those who conceived aborted, some repeatedly. More recent studies by Jones and Man confirm the fact that hypothyroid women have a higher incidence of abortion, prematurity, and stillbirth.

Numerous studies have probed the possibility that analysis of hormone levels in early pregnancy can be used to predict abortion. Further, there have been suggestions that specific deficiencies of these hormones (progesterone, estradiol, HCG) may cause abortion and their administration may prevent abor-

tion. These arguments remain to be proved. Klopper demonstrated that long-term prognostication of the outcome of pregnancy by determination of estriol and pregnanediol in the first few weeks of pregnancy was not possible.

On the other hand, once abortion threatens, assay of plasma HCG in early pregnancy gives a good short-term prediction (lower values in cases which will subsequently abort), while plasma estradiol and progesterone allow only uncertain predictions. These lower values probably result from, rather than cause, deterioration of the products of conception.

Removal of the corpus luteum before the 55th day of gestation in the human female (Csapo) results in excessive myometrial contractility and abortion. It is possible that a specific deficiency of progesterone with otherwise normal products of conception could occur and result in an abortion that would be preventable if massive progesterone therapy was given. While such successes have been reported (particularly in habitual abortion), these apparent successes seem to be due to absence of the appropriate controls. In the sixties it was believed that the abortion that can be prevented by progesterone is rare, if it exists at all (Goldzieher; Shearman, 1963). A recent study does, however, clearly indicate that in a population of patients including women who had suffered earlier abortion and premature delivery, a synthetic progestin, Delalutin, when given in dosages of 250 mg per week starting after the 14th week of pregnancy, did improve fetal birth weight and survival. This prospective double blind shows that therapy significantly improves fetal outcome (Johnson).

Psychiatric Causes

Tupper and Wiel found that women with repeated abortions regularly fell into two groups: the basically immature woman who cannot accept the responsibility of motherhood, and the independent, frustrated woman who yearns for the rewards of the male world and feels that maternity is unsatisfying. The tendency of such women to abort was increased if they were ignored by husband, friends, or doctor. Tupper and Wiel's observations indicate that attention and supportive therapy are effective in preventing pregnancy loss.

REPEATED ABORTION

There are patients who have repeated and even consecutive spontaneous abortions. The term *habitual abortion* became attached to the situation where three or more spontaneous abortions had taken place. Unfortunately, this led to projected mathematical models constructed by Malpas and by Eastman which predicted that the percentage of patients who will abort after 0, 1, 2, and 3 previous abortions is approximately 10, 15, 40, and 80, respectively. This gloomy outlook is based on the concept that this is a clinical syndrome where chance plays little role. Further, the assumed projections of Malpas and Eastman were used to establish control values for numerous studies of various methods of treatment for this disorder. Because the projections were too high, the literature abounds with invalid "cures" ranging from folic acid to synthetic progestins. Warburton and Fraser, making a more precise analysis, provided percentages of women who will abort as 12, 24, 26, and 26, after 0, 1, 2, and 3 previous abortions, respectively. While even these data may represent only approximations, they give a more realistic appraisal of expected success rates.

It seems that women who suffer repeated abortion actually fall into two groups, a large group occurring by chance and a small group where some consistent factor is responsible.

EVALUATION

A single spontaneous abortion, especially if the embryo displays chromosomal anomalies, is usually ascribed to chance, and after a few months, pregnancy is again tried. After a second or third abortion, the patient will be anxious for an evaluation. Perusal of the causes above suggests the following special studies necessary in the clinical evaluation of such patients:

1. Chromosome evaluation of both parents seeking a translocation carrier, preferably using Giemsa banding and quinicrine techniques.
2. Hysterogram to look for abnormalities of the endometrial cavity.
3. Evaluation of the cervix for incompetency. A history of repeated losses of pregnancy, usually after the 14th week, in which the pregnancy appears to "fall out" accompanied by ballooning of the membranes and a report of few or no contractions is strongly suggestive of the disorder. In the nonpregnant state, the cervix may admit a large Hegar dilator (9 or better) with ease and appear gaping on inspection.
4. BBT and endometrial biopsy 1 day before the expected menstrual period to detect the inadequate corpus luteum.

5. Serologic test for syphilis.
6. Thyroid function tests.
7. Blood type of husband and wife.
8. Hemoglobin and glucose tolerance test.

THERAPY

If the husband is found to be a translocation carrier, AID may be tried. If other causes are eliminated and double uterus or myoma appears to be the etiologic factor, unification operation or myomectomy should be performed. The incompetent cervix should have a cerclage placed with a Shirodkar- or McDonald-type operation just after the 14th week of pregnancy when there is a lesser chance of causing retention of a genetically abnormal conceptus. The inadequate corpus luteum is treated with vaginal progesterone (see above). Syphilis and thyroid dysfunction are treated. In the case of ABO incompatibility with several previous abortions, one may try donor insemination with a compatible donor.

Finally, when the patient becomes pregnant, efforts should be made to give her a maximal feeling of security. She should be seen frequently and advised to avoid mental and physical strain as well as coitus (the latter prescription should be time-limited). She should rest 1 to 2 hours both morning and afternoon. The value of some of these steps may be moot, but they are not inappropriate. Fortunately, the outcome of the next pregnancy is considerably better than the formulas Eastman and Malpas suggest. With elimination of distinct causes and careful supportive care of the patient, one can anticipate viable infants in 65 to 75 percent of cases.

METHODS FOR THE INFERTILITY WORKUP

I. General instructions to the patient
   A. It is important to follow instructions carefully.
   B. Day 1 of a cycle is the first day of menstrual bleeding.
   C. The patient should never douche within 2 days of an appointment unless specifically instructed to do so.
   D. The patient should always bring BBT records to an appointment.
II. The basal body temperature
   A. The patient should obtain a metabolic thermometer and learn how to read it.
   B. The thermometer should be shaken down the

night before and kept on the bedside table.
C. Temperature is to be taken rectally for 4 minutes immediately on awakening from day 5 of the cycle until the onset of the following menstrual period.
D. Menstrual periods, sleepless nights, illness, coitus, spotting, bleeding, watery vaginal discharge, and low unilateral abdominal pain (mittelschmerz) should be indicated on the record.
E. Interpretation
   1. Examples of ovulatory and anovulatory cycles are shown in Fig. 27–7. The clear biphasic nature in the ovulatory cycle is due to the thermogenic effect of progesterone.
   2. The day of ovulation is taken as the temperature nadir.
   3. The slope of the thermal shift is usually such that 1 to 4 days elapse between the nadir and the sustained high phase.
   4. Sustained high temperature should last at least 10 days.

If the above requirements are met, one concludes that ovulation with a normal corpus luteum has probably occurred.

III. Rubin test and cervical evaluation
   A. The patient, keeping an accurate BBT, comes in just before ovulation (0 to 2 days before temperature nadir).
   B. Place a dry speculum into the vagina.
      1. Color and degree of opening of cervix evaluated.
      2. Amount of cervical mucus determined.
      3. Spinnbarkheit evaluated (see Table 27–8).
      4. Ferning evaluated by smearing mucus from cervical canal (as high as one can go) on slide for drying and subsequent microscopic examination.
      5. The cervical score is calculated in accordance with Table 27–8 and recorded.
      6. It is important to evaluate the BBT later to be sure that evaluation was really carried out within 0 to 2 days before ovulation.

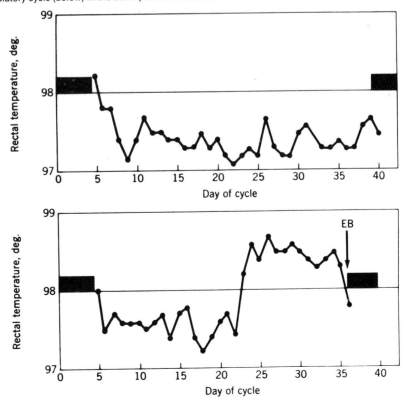

FIGURE 27–7 Basal body temperature indicating a 40-day anovulatory cycle (above) and a 36-day ovulatory cycle (below) in the same patient in successive months.

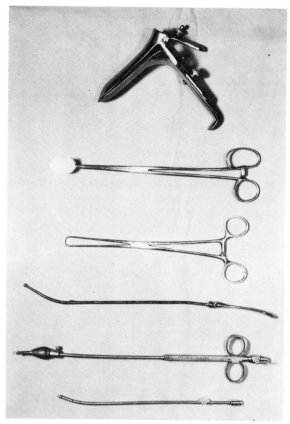

FIGURE 27–8 Instruments for Rubin test and endometrial biopsy. From top to bottom: speculum, dressing forceps, tenaculum, uterine sound, cannula, Novak curette.

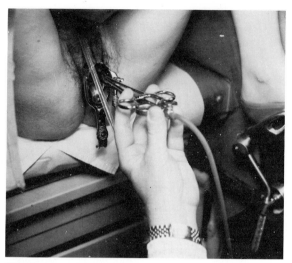

FIGURE 27–9 Patient with cannula in place for Rubin test.

C. The Rubin test (equipment shown in Fig. 27–8)
 1. Gentle pelvic examination is done to ascertain position of fundus.
 2. The anterior lip of cervix is seized with single-tooth tenaculum.
 3. The uterine sound is inserted, and contours of the endometrial cavity carefully evaluated.
 4. The insufflator is inserted into cervical canal, fixed by fingers against tenaculum, and valves opened (Fig. 27–9).
 5. Both sides of lower abdomen are auscultated briefly to ascertain normal bowel sounds (stethoscope with long tubing held by assistant).
 6. The valve on the insufflation apparatus is opened slowly allowing CO to run into uterus. (*Never use air!*) Allow pressure to rise to 100 mmHg over 1 to 2 minutes.

  a. If gas can be heard escaping from fimbrial ends of tubes, continue insufflation at low pressure until 200 mL of gas is instilled.
  b. If gas cannot be heard and no flow is apparent, continue application and allow the pressure to slowly go to (but not above) 200 mmHg. Wait 2 minutes: gas flow may be heard and fall in pressure noted if obstruction is spastic and relieved. Similar finding may be seen with hydrosalpinx, but patient will generally complain of persistent pelvic pain in this case.
D. Interpretation
 1. Free flow of gas below 100 mmHg with escape noises heard bilaterally and shoulder pain almost immediately on sitting up are acceptable as an indication of tubal patency.
 2. Sudden escape of gas at pressures below 150 mmHg with escape noises heard bilaterally and shoulder pain almost immediately on sitting up are acceptable as tubal spasticity that is spontaneously released and interpreted as tubal patency.

If one of these situations is not obtained, the test may be repeated one or two times on days 6 to 9 of the subsequent cycle. If subsequent tests are negative or if severe or lingering pelvic pain accompanies the test referred to in D2 above, the patient is scheduled for hysterosalpingography or laparoscopy.

The Rubin test is only a screening procedure. If there is any doubt, further workup is indicated. A history of peritonitis, appendicitis, or abdominal surgery suggests the possibility of peritubal adhesions which may be extremely difficult to detect. History or palpable findings suggesting pelvic inflammatory disease are a special signal to bypass the Rubin test.

IV. Endometrial biopsy

    A. Biopsy is done when the patient anticipates onset of menstrual period within 24 hours or within 2 hours of onset of a period if it starts without warning.

    B. A carefully kept BBT record should be biphasic.

    C. The speculum and tenaculum are placed as for Rubin test after position of fundus is ascertained. Cervix washed with Betadine.

    D. Uterine cavity gently sounded for depth and patency.

    E. The curette is inserted until it touches fundus, gentle pressure is exerted to bring it into contact with endometrium, and it is removed with a single stroke. Strive for tissue from the upper fundus.

    F. Tissue is teased from curette with an obliquely broken applicator stick. Forcing it out with a syringe and fixative only serves to hopelessly fragment it.

    G. If there is a history to suggest previous endometritis or tuberculosis, a four-quadrant biopsy is done, removing tissue after each stroke.

    H. Endometrium should be dated by the criteria of Noyes et al. Surface must be present.

    I. Look at the slides yourself. If biopsy is taken at the onset of menstruation, the presence of secretory exhaustion in glands and a good deciduoid reaction in stroma indicate ovulation and rule out the inadequate corpus luteum syndrome. The presence of subnuclear vacuoles with minimal intraglandular secretion suggest a luteinized follicle or the response to an injection of progesterone in an otherwise anovulatory woman.

    J. Review timing with the patient and BBT record later to be sure that onset of menstrual period really came within 24 hours of the biopsy. The point is that even though the morphology of the endometrium is compatible with the fifth postovulatory day, if the menstrual period comes 8 to 9 days later, the patient may have actually had a good ovulatory cycle. The biopsy was done too soon and should be repeated with the onset of menses of the following cycle.

V. Seminal analysis

    A. The sample is collected by masturbation, after 3 days of abstinence, in a washed, well-rinsed, dried glass container. No other collection device or method is acceptable.

    B. Liquefaction should occur within 30 to 45 minutes.

    C. Volume should be determined in a calibrated glass cylinder.

    D. Concentration is determined by counting in a hemocytometer chamber using a standard white cell pipette which dilutes the sample 1:20. Dilution is effected with a solution of 4% sodium bicarbonate and 1% phenol in distilled water. Counting is done in the red cell field of the Neubauer chamber, recording all the spermatozoa cells with 5 blocks (each of 16 small squares). Six zeros are placed behind the number counted giving concentration in millions per milliliter.

    E. Motility is evaluated by placing a drop of semen on a clean slide and using a cover slip. Under high dry objective, the percent motility in several fields is estimated.

    F. Morphology: Smears are air dried, fixed in 10% Formalin (1 minute), rinsed in distilled water, stained in Meyer's hematoxylin for 2 minutes, and rinsed again in distilled water. Two hundred cells are counted, and normal morphology recorded as percent of total.

    G. Interpretation: MacLeod has been responsible for modification of acceptability levels in seminal analysis to lower and more realistic terms. He has recently written an authoritative review of the subject (1971). At the present time reasonable or acceptable quality depends on attainment of the following:

        1. A volume of 2.5 to 5.0 mL.

        2. Spermatozoa concentration of 20 million per milliliter.

        3. Spermatozoa motility seems to be a most important parameter in semen quality. Minimal acceptable standards at present are 60 percent motility with at least 40 percent of the spermatozoa in a specimen showing good forward progression.

        4. Normal morphology should be observed in 60 percent of spermatozoa in a sample.

There is a strong relationship between head-shape morphology and motile activity in spermatozoa. It has been pointed out that systemic disturbances (liver disease, infections, allergies, stress) may induce changes of germinal epithelium function and head structure of spermatozoa (MacLeod, 1966). These effects are often temporary, coming on within 2 to 3 weeks and disappearing in several weeks or months. Thus, if defects are found on examination, recent illness or infections of any kind should be eliminated as possible causes, and the analysis repeated.

VI. Postcoital test
   A. Performed 0 to 2 days before ovulation as projected from previous BBT records.
   B. The couple (having abstained for 3 days) has intercourse 2 hours in advance.
   C. Mucus sample taken from cervical canal *as near the internal os as possible* with gentle aspiration (Davajan).
   D. Mucus put on slide, covered with cover slip.
   E. Warm to 37°C for 5 to 10 minutes.
   F. Examine 10 high-power fields noting number of progressively motile and immotile spermatozoa per high-power field.
   G. Similarly examine few drops of the vaginal pool.
   H. Interpretation of postcoital test: If five or more motile spermatozoa are present per high-power field, the result is satisfactory. If no motile spermatozoa are seen in cervical mucus and none in vagina, suspect faulty coital technique.

REFERENCES

Amelar RD: Coagulation, liquefaction and viscosity of human semen. *J Urol* 87:187, 1962.

_____: Further evaluation: The adrenal cortex, in *Infertility in Men,* Philadelphia: Davis, 1966, p. 80.

_____, Hotchkiss RS: The split ejaculate. *Fertil Steril* 16:46, 1965.

Ansbacher R et al.: Clinical significance of sperm antibodies in infertile couples. *Fertil Steril* 24:305, 1973.

Bedford JM: Nonspecific tail–tail agglutination of mammalian spermatozoa. *Exp Cell Res* 38:654, 1965.

Behrman SJ: Techniques of artificial insemination, in *Progress in Infertility,* eds. SJ Behrman, RW Kistner, Boston: Little, Brown, 1968, p. 273.

_____, Menge AC: Immunologic aspects of infertility, in *Human Reproduction,* eds. ESE Hafez, TN Evans, Hagerstown, Md.: Harper & Row, 1973, p. 237.

_____, Otani Y: Transvaginal immunization of the guinea pig with homologous testis and epididymal sperm. *Int J Fertil* 8:829, 1963.

Bell EB: Immunological control of fertility in the mouse: A comparison of systemic and intravaginal immunization. *J Reprod Fertil* 18:183, 1969.

Boettcher B et al.: Human sera containing immunoglobulin and nonimmunoglobulin sperm-agglutinins. *Biol Reprod* 5:236, 1971.

Boué JG, Boué A: Chromosome abnormalities in spontaneous human abortions. *Presse Med* 78:635, 1970 (French).

_____ et al.: Outcome of pregnancies following a spontaneous abortion with chromosomal anomalies. *Am J Obstet Gynecol* 116:806, 1973.

Bourne RB et al.: Successful artificial insemination in a diabetic with retrograde ejaculation. *Fertil Steril* 22:275, 1971.

Cadena D et al.: Chronic endometritis. *Obstet Gynecol* 41:733, 1973.

Carr DH: Chromosome abnormalities and spontaneous abortions, in *Human Population Cytogenetics,* eds. PA Jacobs et al., Baltimore: Williams & Wilkins, 1970, pp. 104–118.

Clyman MJ: Tubal reconstructive surgery for infertility, in *Pathways to Conception,* ed. AI Sherman, Springfield, Ill.: Charles C Thomas, 1971, p. 110.

Comninos AC, Zourlas PA: Treatment of uterine adhesions (Asherman's syndrome). *Am J Obstet Gynecol* 105:862, 1969.

Csapo AI et al.: The significance of the human corpus luteum in pregnancy maintenance: I. Preliminary studies. *Am J Obstet Gynecol* 112:1061, 1972.

Davajan V, Kunitake GM: Fractional in-vivo and in-vitro examination of postcoital cervical mucus in the human. *Fertil Steril* 20:197, 1969.

Dmowski WP and Cohen MR: Antigonadotropin (Danazol) in the treatment of endometriosis. *Am J Obstet Gynecol* 130:41, 1978.

Dubin L, Amelar RD: Varicocele size and results of varicocelectomy in selected subfertile men with varicocele. *Fertil Steril* 21:606, 1970.

_____, _____: Etiologic factors in 1294 consecutive cases of male infertility. *Fertil Steril* 22:469, 1971.

Dukes CD: Antispermatozoal antibody, in *Progress in Infertility,* eds. SJ Behrman, RW Kistner, Boston: Little, Brown, 1968, p. 701.

_____, Franklin RR: Sperm agglutinins and human infertility: Female. *Fertil Steril* 19:263, 1968.

Eastman NJ: Habitual abortion, in *Progress in Gyne-*

cology, eds. JV Meigs, SH Sturgis, New York: Grune & Stratton, 1946, vol. 1, p. 262.

Eyquem A, Krieg H: Experimental autosensitization of the testis. *Ann NY Acad Sci* 124:270, 1965.

Ferrando G, Nalbandov AV: Relative importance of histamine and estrogen on implantation in rats. *Endocrinology* 83:933, 1968.

Franklin RR, Dukes CD: Antispermatozoal antibody and unexplained infertility. *Am J Obstet Gynecol* 89:6, 1964.

Freund J et al.: Aspermatogenesis in the guinea pig induced by testicular tissue and adjuvants. *J Exp Med* 97:711, 1953.

Friedman S, Lopez-Manzanara R: *Hormonal studies and treatment of the short luteal phase (SLP).* Presented at the Fifty-fifth Annual Meeting of the Endocrine Society, Chicago, June 20–22, 1973.

Gemzell C.: Induction of ovulation using human pituitary or urinary FSH. *Clin Obstet Gynecol* 10:401, 1967.

Glass SJ, Holland HM: Treatment of oligospermia with large doses of human chorionic gonadotropin. *Fertil Steril* 14:500, 1963.

Goldenberg RL et al.: Gonadotropins in women with amenorrhea. *Am J Obstet Gynecol* 116:1003, 1973.

Goldzieher JW: Double-blind trial of a progestin in habitual abortion. *JAMA* 188:651, 1964.

Graff G: Suppression of cervical mucus during clomiphene therapy. *Fertil Steril* 22:209, 1971.

Greenwald GS: Species differences in egg transport in response to exogenous estrogen. *Anat Rec* 157:163, 1967.

Hanafiah MJ et al.: Sperm-agglutinating antibodies in 236 infertile couples. *Fertil Steril* 23:493, 1972.

Insler V et al.: Cycle pattern and pregnancy rate following combined clomiphene-estrogen therapy. *Obstet Gynecol* 41:602, 1973.

Isojima S: Relationship between antibodies to spermatozoa and sterility in females, in *Immunology and Reproduction,* ed. RG Edwards, London: International Planned Parenthood Federation, 1969, p. 267.

_____ et al.: Immunologic analysis of spermimmobolizing factor found in sera of women with unexplained sterility. *Am J Obstet Gynecol* 101:677, 1968.

_____.: Further studies on sperm-immobolizing antibody found in sera of unexplained cases of sterility in women. *Am J Obstet Gynecol* 112:199, 1972.

Johnson JWC et al.: Efficacy of 17α-hydroxyprogesterone caproate in the prevention of premature labor. *N Engl J Med* 293:675, 1975.

Jones GS, Pourmand K: An evaluation of etiologic factors and therapy in 555 private patients with primary infertility. *Fertil Steril* 13:398, 1962.

_____ et al.: Elucidation of normal ovarian physiology by exogenous gonadotropin stimulation following steroid pituitary suppression. *Fertil Steril* 20:14, 1969.

Jones WS, Man EB: Thyroid function in human pregnancy. *Am J Obstet Gynecol* 104:909, 1969.

Katsch S: Localization and identification of antispermatogenic factor in guinea pig testicles. *Int Arch Allergy Appl Immunol* 16:241, 1960.

_____ et al.: Purification and partial characterization of aspermatogenic antigen. *Fertil Steril* 23:644, 1972.

Keettel WC et al.: Observations on the polycystic ovary syndrome. *Am J Obstet Gynecol* 73:954, 1957.

Kibrick S et al.: Methods for the detection of antibodies against mammalian spermatozoa. *Fertil Steril* 3:419, 1952.

Kirschner MA, Jacobs JB: Combined ovarian and adrenal vein catheterization to determine the site(s) of androgen overproduction in hirsute women. *J Clin Endocrinol Metab* 33:199, 1971.

Kistner RW: Further observations on the effects of clomiphene citrate in anovulatory females. *Am J Obstet Gynecol* 92:380, 1965.

_____; Induction of ovulation with clomiphene citrate, in *Progress in Infertility,* 2d ed., eds. SJ Behrman, RW Kistner, Boston: Little, Brown, 1968, p. 407.

Klopper A, MacNaughton M: Hormones in recurrent abortion. *J Obstet Gynaecol Br Commonw* 72:1022, 1965.

Kremer J: A simple sperm penetration test. *Int J Fertil* 10:209, 1965.

Lamb et al.: Endometrial histology and conception rates after clomiphene citrate. *Obstet Gynecol* 39:389, 1972.

Li TS, Behrman SJ: The sperm- and seminal plasmaspecific antigens of human semen. *Fertil Steril* 21:565, 1970.

Litzenberg JC, Carey JB: The relation of basal metabolism to gestation. *Am J Obstet Gynecol* 17:550, 1929.

Louros NC et al.: Use of intrauterine devices in the treatment of intrauterine adhesions. *Fertil Steril* 19:509, 1968.

MacLeod J: The clinical implications of deviations in human spermatogenesis as evidenced in seminal cytology and the experimental production of these deviations, in *Excerpta Medica International Congress Series* n. 133, *Proceedings of the Fifth World*

Congress on Fertility and Sterility, Stokholm, June 16–22, 1966, p. 563.

———: Seminal cytology in the presence of varicocele. *Fertil Steril* 16:735, 1965.

———: Human male infertility. *Obstet Gynecol Surv* 26:335, 1971.

Malpas P: A study of abortion sequences. *J Obstet Gynaecol Br Commonw* 45:932, 1938.

Mancini RE et al.: Immunological and testicular response in man sensitized with human testicular homogenate. *J Clin Endocrinol Metab* 25:859, 1965.

Menge AC, Christian JJ: Effects of auto- and iso-immunization of bulls with semen and testis. *Int J Fertil* 16:130, 1971.

Michael RP et al.: Pheromones: Isolation of male sex attractants from a female primate. *Science* 172:964, 1971.

Moghissi KS, Boyce CR: Management of endometriosis with oral medroxyprogesterone acetate. *Obstet Gynecol* 47:265, 1976.

Moszkowski E et al.: The inadequate luteal phase. *Am J Obstet Gynecol* 83:363, 1962.

Murray M, Osmond-Clarke F: Pregnancy results following treatment with clomiphene citrate. *J Obstet Gynaecol Br Commonw* 78:1108, 1971.

Noyes RW: Uniformity of secretory endometrium. *Obstet Gynecol* 7:221, 1956.

——— et al.: Dating the endometrial biopsy. *Fertil Steril* 1:3, 1950.

Palti Z: Clomiphene therapy in defective spermatogenesis. *Fertil Steril* 21:838, 1970.

Paulsen DF: Clomiphene citrate in the management of male infertility: Predictors for treatment selection. *Fertil Steril* 28:1226, 1977.

Paulson JD et al.: Free testosterone concentration in serum: Elevation is the hallmark of hirsutism. *Am J Obstet* 128:851, 1977.

Ranney B: Endometriosis 1. Conservative operations. *Am J Obstet Gynecol* 107:743, 1970.

Rowley MJ, Heller CG: The testosterone rebound phenomenon in the treatment of male infertility. *Fertil Steril* 23:498, 1972.

Schoysman R: Treatment of male infertility due to auto-agglutination of spermatozoa, in *Proceeding of the Sixth World Congress on Fertility and Sterility,* ed. I Halbrecht, Tel Aviv: Israel Academic Press, 1970, p. 112.

Schwimmer WB et al.: An evaluation of immunologic factors of infertility. *Fertil Steril* 18:167, 1967.

Sever JL: Viruses and the fetus. *Int J Gynaec Obstet* 8:763, 1970.

Shearman RP: Prolonged secondary amenorrhea after oral contraceptive therapy. *Lancet* 2:64, 1971.

———, Garrett WJ: Double-blind study of effect of 17-hydroxyprogesterone caproate on abortion rate. *Br Med J* 1:292, 1963.

Solish GI: Distribution of ABO isohaemagglutinins among fertile and infertile women. *J. Reprod Fertil* 18:459, 1969.

Stickle G: Defective development and reproductive wastage in the United States. *Am J Obstet Gynecol* 100:442, 1968.

Strickler RC et al.: Artificial insemination with fresh donor semen. *N Engl J Med* 293:848, 1975.

Strott CA et al.: The short luteal phase. *J Clin Endocrinol Metab* 30:246, 1970.

Taymor ML: Gonadotropin therapy. Possible causes and prevention of ovarian overstimulation. *JAMA* 203:362, 1968.

TeLinde RW, Mattingly RF: Congenital absence of the vagina, in *Operative Gynecology,* 4th ed., Philadelphia: Lippincott, 1970, p. 466.

Tourville DR et al.: The human female reproductive tract: Immunohistological localization of γA, γG, γM, secretory "piece," and lactoferrin. *Am J Obstet Gynecol* 108:1102, 1970.

Tupper C, Wiel RJ: The problem of spontaneous abortions. IX. The treatment of habitual aborters by psychotherapy. *Am J Obstet Gynecol* 83:421, 1962.

Warburton D, Fraser FC: Spontaneous abortion risks in man: Data from reproductive histories collected in a medical genetics unit. *Am J Hum Genet* 16:1, 1964.

Wieland RG et al.: Idiopathic oligospermia: Control observations and response to cis-clomiphene. *Fertil Steril* 23:471, 1972.

Williams WL.: Biochemistry of capacitation of spermatozoa, in *Biology of Mammalian Fertilization and Implantation,* eds. KS Moghissi, ESE Hafez, Springfield, Ill.: Charles C Thomas, 1972, pp. 19–53.

Ying SY, Meyer RK: Effect of steroids on neuropharmacologic blockade of ovulation in pregnant mare's serum (PMS)-primed immature rats. *Endocrinology* 84: 1466, 1969.

Zárate A et al.: Therapeutic effect of synthetic luteinizing hormone-releasing hormone (LH-RH) in male infertility due to idiopathic azoospermia and oligospermia. *Fertil Steril* 24:485, 1973.

28

Prenatal Care

E. J. QUILLIGAN

IDENTIFYING THE HIGH-RISK PATIENT
Patient history
Physical examination
   Diagnosis of pregnancy
   Estimation of the pelvic capacity
Patient counseling
   Physical activity
   Coital activity
   Bathing
   Douching
   Smoking
   Employment
   Alcohol
   Clothing
   Dental Care
   Breast care
   Drugs
   Diet

SYMPTOMS IN EARLY PREGNANCY AND THEIR THERAPY
   Nausea and vomiting
   Headache
   Urinary frequency
   Constipation
   Skin changes
   Laboratory work
   Subsequent visits

TESTS OF FETAL STATUS
   Plasma estriol

Oxytocin challenge test
Tests of fetal maturity
Tests for placental localization

LABOR

The broad objective of prenatal care is to ensure for the mother and fetus a normal period of gestation and a healthy conclusion of that gestation, providing the community with a new member who is capable of reaching his or her full genetic potential. During this period the health care team has the opportunity to provide both the physical and psychologic support necessary to reach the above objective.

Whether the amount of prenatal care significantly influences achieving this objective is difficult to measure precisely. In the study of 140,000 pregnancies in New York City there was a positive correlation between the amount of prenatal care and perinatal mortality regardless of social class. On the other hand, in the collaborative perinatal study there was essentially no difference in either perinatal mortality or neurologic damage at 1 year regardless of the time of registration in pregnancy for prenatal care. Two factors may be operational to make these statistics difficult to interpret: (1) patients with disease tend to register earlier in pregnancy for care than the normal, thus loading the statistics against early care, and (2) the vast majority of pregnant patients are normal, tending to obfuscate small differences.

The broad objective of prenatal care might be subdivided into rather specific goals:

1. To recognize and treat any disease present in the mother or fetus.
2. To provide education about the pregnancy to the family.
3. To provide necessary psychologic support for the patient.

The realization of these specific goals frequently requires the efforts of a group of physicians and/or paramedical personnel because the obstetrician and gynecologist may not have the time or in-depth knowledge necessary to render ideal care. The other physicians who may form a part of the health care team include the internist, pediatrician, and anesthesiologist. The paramedical personnel involved may include nurse-midwives, nurses, dietitians, and social workers. The group should be organized by the obstetrician around the individual patient and her problem; frequent communication between group members is mandatory for optimal care.

During the prenatal period the obstetric care group has the opportunity to establish a relationship with the patient which will enhance the joy of pregnancy and enable a smoother medical course. This can be accomplished only if the obstetric group makes an effort to educate the patient and her husband about her pregnancy, thus ensuring an actively participating couple in all modes of medical management. A classic example of the benefits of a team approach with dedicated individuals was seen in the Yale experience with teenage pregnancies (Sarrel). Through use of physicians, social workers, dietitians, and teachers a perinatal loss of 8 per 1000 was reported. This contrasts with the 38 to 59 per 1000 perinatal mortality reported in other series of teenage pregnancies. In addition, these girls had a low incidence of prematurity (10.88 percent) and toxemia (5.0 percent), again in contrast with other series. They also had in general short, uncomplicated labors (mean time in labor 8.7 hours).

IDENTIFYING THE HIGH-RISK PATIENT

From a medical standpoint, recognition of the patient who will present a problem during her pregnancy is very important so that she can receive special medi-

TABLE 28-1 Risk Factors

Past history—general

1. Diabetes
2. Hypertension
3. Age
   a. > 35 years
   b. < 16 years
4. Renal disease
5. Malnutrition
6. Other maternal medical problems such as collagen diseases, etc.
7. Low socioeconomic group

Past history—pregnancies

1. Previous abortion
2. Previous premature delivery
3. Previous abruptio placentae
4. Greater than gravida 4
5. Previous cesarean section
6. Previous erythroblastosis

Present pregnancy

1. Anemia
2. Diabetes
3. Hypertension
4. Other maternal diseases
5. Bleeding
   a. Early—threatened abortion
   b. Late—placenta previa or abruptio placentae
6. Malpresentation
7. Erythroblastosis
8. Deficient prenatal care

Intrapartum factors

Maternal factors
1. Moderate to severe toxemia
2. Hydramnios or oligohydramnios
3. Amnionitis
4. Uterine rupture
5. Mild toxemia
6. Premature rupture of membranes > 12 hours
7. Primary dysfunctional labor
8. Secondary arrest of dilatation
9. Meperidine (Demerol) > 300 mg
10. Magnesium sulfate ($MgSO_4$)
11. Labor > 20 hours
12. Second stage > 2½ hours
13. Clinical small pelvis
14. Medical induction
15. Precipitous labor > 3 hours
16. Primary cesarean section
17. Repeat cesarean section
18. Elective induction
19. Prolonged latent phase

TABLE 28–1 Risk Factors *(Continued)*

20. Uterine tetany
21. Pitocin augmentation

Placental factors
  1. Placenta previa
  2. Abruptio placentae
  3. Postterm > 42 weeks
  4. Meconium-stained amniotic fluid (dark)
  5. Meconium-stained amniotic fluid (light)
  6. Marginal separation

Fetal factors
  1. Abnormal presentation
  2. Multiple pregnancy
  3. Fetal bradycardia > 30 minutes
  4. Breech delivery total extraction
  5. Prolapsed cord
  6. Fetal weight < 2500 g
  7. Fetal acidosis pH ≤ 7.25 (stage I)
  8. Fetal tachycardia > 30 minutes
  9. Operative forceps or vacuum extraction
 10. Breech delivery spontaneous or assisted
 11. General anesthesia
 12. Outlet forceps
 13. Shoulder dystocia

TABLE 28–2 Tabulation of Scores for Perinatal Deaths and Surviving Infants

	Survivors	Survivors	Deaths	
Score	Apgar 4+	Apgar <4	Fetal	Neonatal
0	222	2	0	0
1	258	4	1	3
2	159	2	3	4
3	78	1	6	2
4	38	5	8	5
5	12	4	9	12
6	4	3	17	7
7	0	0	11	7
8	0	0	9	10
9	0	0	9	11
10	0	0	4	6

Source: Goodwin et al.

cal care and the special tests which will benefit her pregnancy. Between one-third and one-half of the patients who subsequently will develop problems during their pregnancy can be recognized during their first prenatal visit. Several authors (Nesbitt and Aubry; Goodwin et al.; Hoebel et al., 1973) have developed risk indices. An example of the type of information necessary for such a risk index is seen in Table 28-1.

In Nesbitt's series of 1001 patients, 30 percent fell into a high-risk category on the first visit. Those 300 patients had 50 percent of the maternal complications, 42 percent of the complications of labor, 50 percent of the perinatal deaths, and 46 percent of the morbid infants. To look at the opposite side of the coin, these statistics also show that 50 percent of maternal complications occurred in patients classified as low risk during the first prenatal visit. Goodwin's risk index includes the present pregnancy in his scoring system, thus providing a continually updated risk index. In the lowest-risk pregnancy there was no perinatal mortality, and in the highest-risk there was 100 percent perinatal mortality (Table 28-2). There was also good correlation between risk index and Apgar score at birth (Table 28-3).

Hoebel and his colleagues continue to place the fetus in a high-risk category if any difficulty develops during labor. They demonstrated the importance of this continual assessment by showing a perinatal mortality of 35 per 1000 live births when the pregnancy was low risk antenatally but became high risk during labor, compared with a perinatal mortality of 22 per 1000 live births when the pregnancy was high risk antepartum and low risk intrapartum, a significant reduction.

PATIENT HISTORY

The knowledge required to develop this risk index must be gained from a careful history and physical examination. The history should contain as essential data the patient's name, age, and date of her last normal menstrual period. It is important that one obtain a careful menstrual history from the patient. This should include the time of onset of first menstruation, the du-

TABLE 28–3 Mean Scores for Perinatal Deaths and Surviving Infants*

All perinatal deaths (144)	6.2
Neonatal deaths (67)	6.5
Fetal deaths (77)	5.9
Perinatal deaths, major congenital anomalies (18)	3.6
Perinatal deaths <2500 g (55)	7.2
Surviving infants <2500 g (26)	3.9
Surviving infants >4000 g (24)	1.9
Surviving infants, Apgar score >4 (771)	1.2
Surviving infants, Apgar score <4 (21)	3.0

*Figures in parentheses indicate number of pregnancies studied.

ration of the menstrual cycle, whether the cycle is regular or irregular, the length of menstrual flow, a rough approximation as to the amount of menstrual flow, and whether the patient was using some form of contraceptive device prior to the onset of this gestation. If the menstrual periods have been regular and if the cycle is approximately 28 to 30 days, calculation of the estimated date of confinement (EDC) is possible by counting forward 280 days from the first day of the last normal menstrual period. From a practical standpoint, this can be done more easily by subtracting 3 months and adding 7 days to the first day of the last normal menstrual period. It is important to realize that ovulation usually occurs 14 days before the next menstrual period; thus if a woman has a 35-day cycle, she would ovulate on day 21 rather than day 14. Since all calculations of date of confinement are based on an average 27-day cycle, for the individual with a long or short cycle the number of days that her cycle is longer or shorter than 28 days must be added to or subtracted from her EDC. Next in the history it is important to obtain a very careful account of the course of any previous pregnancies.

Previous Pregnancies

The history should include answers to the following questions.

1. When did the previous pregnancies occur (year)?
2. What was the duration of pregnancy (weeks)?
3. Did any significant problems develop such as bleeding, hypertension, diabetes, or premature labor?
4. Were the labors spontaneous or induced? Reason for induction.
5. How long did the labor last?
6. Were there any complications during previous labors such as bleeding or slow labor?
7. Were the infants delivered vaginally or by cesarean section? Reason for cesarean section.
8. What type of anesthetic was used for delivery?
9. What was the condition of the infant(s) at birth?
10. Were there any postpartum problems in the mother such as infection in uterus, bladder, or breasts? Was there bleeding? If so, what was the amount and the time postpartum? Thrombophlebitis? Episiotomy pain?
11. Did the infant have problems in the nursery? Infection? Jaundice? Respiratory distress?
12. Was the child breast fed? Any problems?
13. Current health of the children? Emotional and intellectual development?

Present Pregnancy

The following points should be covered.

1. Symptoms of pregnancy: Nausea and vomiting, breast enlargement or fullness, constipation, urinary frequency.
2. How does patient feel about the pregnancy? Planned or unplanned? Contraceptive failure?
3. Bleeding during the present pregnancy? Amount, character, and time after last normal menstrual period.

This part of the history should be followed by a complete review of systems as in any history and a complete review of the past history of the patient with regard to any significant diseases or operations and a review of the social history of the patient (see Chap. 14).

PHYSICAL EXAMINATION

Following the history, a complete physical examination should be done (see Chap. 14). The pelvic examination should direct itself toward (1) the diagnosis of pregnancy, (2) an estimation of the capacity of the pelvis, and (3) any general abnormalities that might be present.

DIAGNOSIS OF PREGNANCY

Several signs are said to be characteristic of pregnancy on pelvic examination. These are cyanosis of the cervix, softening of the lower uterine segment (Hegar's sign), and enlargement of the uterus. Cyanosis of the cervix can occur with a variety of conditions and thus is not necessarily pathognomonic of pregnancy. Softening of the lower uterine segment, on the other hand, is frequently one of the first definitive signs of pregnancy. The isthmus of the uterus between the corpus and the cervix becomes quite soft early in pregnancy (about 6 weeks). This softening is in contrast to the remainder of the uterus which has its normal consistency. Uterine enlargement, of course, is the most important sign of pregnancy; however, this is a sign that is best judged over time, i.e., progressive uterine enlargement, which usually does not begin until about 6 to 8 weeks after the last normal menstrual period. The uterus then increases progressively so that by 3 months it is above the symphysis pubis, soft and globular, by 4 months halfway to the umbilicus, and at 5 months it is at the umbilicus.

During pregnancy fundal growth usually follows the MacDonald rule which states that the height of the fundus in centimeters above the top of the symphysis is in a ratio of 8 to 7 of the duration of the pregnancy in weeks. This rule is most accurate between 16 and 36 weeks of pregnancy. Fetal growth in terms of weight increases progressively with uterine enlargement.

ESTIMATION OF THE PELVIC CAPACITY

First, an approximate measurement of the distance from the underside of the symphysis pubis to the promontory of the sacrum is taken. In the majority of instances this is a distance greater than 12 to 12.5 cm and gives one an indication as to whether the anterior-posterior diameter of the pelvic inlet is adequate (Fig. 28–1). Next, it is wise to palpate the bony sidewalls of the pelvis to determine whether they are divergent, convergent, or straight as one progresses from the pelvic inlet to the pelvic outlet (Fig. 28–2). It is also important to palpate the ischial spines and to make some estimate of the distance that exists between the ischial spines. The ischial spines are the narrowest point of the midpelvic diameter and may be the point of maximum constriction in the birth passage. The curve of the sacrum should be determined because it is a sacrum which is hollow rather than flat which gives an adequate anterior-posterior diameter to the midpelvis. Finally, one can measure the distance between the ischial tuberosities as an approximation of the transverse diameter of the pelvic outlet (Fig. 28–2B). While checking on the pelvic outlet, it is also wise to determine roughly the angle of the pubic rami. This gives the physician an estimate of the anterior triangle of the pelvic outlet. Though clinical pelvimetry is important and should always be performed,

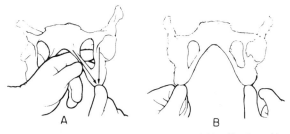

FIGURE 28–2 The intertuberous diameter. *A* Identification of ischial tuberosity at the point of convergence of pubic rami and pelvic side walls. *B* Measurement of intertuberous diameter. *(From CM Steer, Moloy's evaluation of the pelvis, in Obstetrics, 2d ed., Philadelphia: Saunders, 1959.)*

it is important to remember that true evaluation of the pelvis always awaits labor. It is the proportion between fetal size and pelvic capacity plus the power of the uterine contractions which determine whether a given fetus will traverse the birth canal. Finally, it is important that a *routine pelvic examination* be performed as has been described in Chap. 14 to note any pathology that might be present. It is particularly important that a Papanicolaou smear be done since cervical neoplasia can occur in the pregnant as well as the nonpregnant individual.

To recapitulate, the diagnosis of pregnancy should always be uppermost in the physician's mind when the patient has missed a menstrual period. There will frequently be additional symptoms such as nausea, vomiting, breast tenderness, urinary frequency or constipation, and general lethargy. Positive physical findings may be softening of the lower uterine segment and/or enlargement of the uterus. In some instances, particularly in early pregnancy, the diagnosis of pregnancy can only be suspected by history and physical examination.

Confirmation of the gravid state is then obtained by measuring the output of human chorionic gonadotropin (HCG) in the urine (a hormone excreted only by trophoblastic tissue). This is usually done by an immunologic assay. Several types are available including latex inhibition, latex agglutination, hemagglutination inhibition, beta subunit, and radioreceptor assay. The radioreceptor and beta subunit assays are the most sensitive and accurate currently available. The radioreceptor assay measures levels to 100 mIU HCG per milliliter and the beta subunit assay is positive with values of less than 10 mIU HCG per milliliter of serum. The more rapid latex tests are less sensitive, 2000 to 3000 IU HCG per liter of urine, but are less time-consuming and expensive. They are in general adequate for pregnancy screening because of a low false-positive rate. The hemagglutination inhibi-

FIGURE 28–1 The diagonal conjugate diameter of the inlet. *A* When the examining finger definitely reaches the promontory, the true conjugate diameter may be estimated by subtracting 1 to 1.5 cm from the measured length of the diagonal conjugate diameter. *B* If the examining finger fails to reach the promontory, the measured length of the finger to base-of-thumb span may give the length of the anterior-posterior diameter of the inlet. *(From CM Steer, Moloy's evaluation of the pelvis, in Obstetrics, 2d ed., Philadelphia: Saunders, 1959.)*

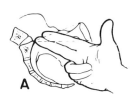 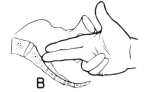

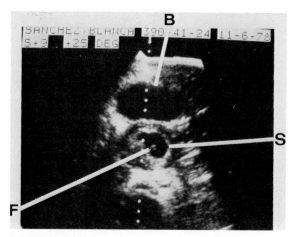

FIGURE 28-3 Ultrasound gestational sac (S) with fetus (F) present in center; B, maternal bladder.

tion test is positive with 500 to 1000 IU HCG per liter of urine.

Later in gestation, fetal presence can be diagnosed by fetal movement (14 to 22 weeks), the presence of the fetal heart (12 to 14 weeks by ultrasonics and 18 to 24 weeks by stethoscope), and the presence of a gestational sac on ultrasonic B scan (6 to 8 weeks, Fig. 28–3).

PATIENT COUNSELING

Following an adequate history and physical examination, the physician should counsel the patient on what to expect during the pregnancy. Many patients have ideas totally out of context with the facts as to what they can and cannot do during the pregnancy. Unfortunately, old wives' tales frequently dominate the thinking of the patient at this time, and she may, for example, believe that should she raise her hands above her head during the pregnancy she will strangle the baby. It is well in this initial conversation to try to discover as many of the misconceptions that the patients have about pregnancy as possible and then give them a set of specific instructions as to what they should expect during the pregnancy. Instructions should be given in regard to physical activity, sexual activity, travel, diet, and what changes the patient might expect to occur as a natural result of the pregnancy.

PHYSICAL ACTIVITY

The patient may engage in that physical activity during her pregnancy which she engaged in prior to her pregnancy, recognizing of course that she may tire more easily and should not permit herself to become overly fatigued. Swimming, golf, tennis, and walking are all excellent exercises for the pregnant woman, and in fact she should be encouraged to have some degree of exercise every day. This will keep muscle tone at an optimum and many feel assists in the labor and delivery process. It is unwise to initiate new sports requiring a great deal of coordination and balance during a pregnancy, such as skiing, because balance will be disturbed in many individuals by the enlarging conceptus and significant falls could prove harmful to the patient.

COITAL ACTIVITY

Coital activity can be maintained throughout pregnancy unless the patient is bleeding, threatening premature labor, has ruptured membranes, or finds it too uncomfortable for her. There is no evidence at the present time, given the above exceptions, that coital activity has any adverse effect, either for the mother or the fetus.

BATHING

The patient may be permitted to bathe throughout her pregnancy, using either showers or tub baths. Tub bathing will not cause infection in the vagina or uterus as the bath water does not enter the vagina of the patient.

DOUCHING

Douching should be avoided during pregnancy unless there is very specific vaginal tract infection requiring it. In that instance specific instructions should be given regarding the douche so that the pressure of water in the vagina is extremely low. This can be accomplished by keeping the douche bag no more than 6 inches above the level of the vagina while douching.

SMOKING

Smoking during pregnancy should be avoided not only because of the deleterious cardiovascular and pulmonary problems possible in anyone who smokes, but because there is evidence that infants of smoking mothers are smaller than of nonsmoking mothers (Simpson). Some studies have reported a higher perinatal mortality in smoking mothers; however, it is difficult to sort out the multiple factors in a smoking mother which may also influence perinatal mortality such as social class, maternal age, etc. Yerushalmy recently reported that mothers who subsequently started smoking gave birth to smaller infants than control nonsmoking mothers.

EMPLOYMENT

Heavy physical labor should be avoided during pregnancy; however, the positions most women occupy can be continued until the individual becomes too fatigued or uncomfortable. This usually is late in the third trimester. If employment is maintained, frequent periods of rest should be available. One hour of rest at midday in the lateral recumbent position may significantly reduce the incidence of toxemia of pregnancy.

ALCOHOL

Alcohol in moderation does not harm either mother or fetus; however, chronic alcoholism may be associated with an increase in congenital malformations.

CLOTHING

Clothing should be comfortable and not constricting. Stockings which constrict just above the knee should not be worn as they will aggravate the venous stasis already present in the lower extremities. A well-fitting brassiere should be worn throughout the pregnancy. Significant enlargement of the breasts occurs, which without support will result in the breakdown of elastic tissue and in sagging breasts following the pregnancy. Low-heeled, comfortable shoes should be worn. A natural lumbar lordosis occurs during pregnancy, and high-heeled shoes will accentuate this, frequently causing low-back pain.

DENTAL CARE

Routine dental care may be given during pregnancy. It is not recommended that the patient receive any sleep anesthetics in the dentist's office (Pentothal sodium or nitrous oxide) as they may lead to maternal hypoxia and thus fetal damage.

BREAST CARE

In addition to a well-supporting brassiere, the mother who wishes to nurse her child should toughen her nipples. This should be started at about the sixth to seventh months and can be accomplished by vigorous massage of the nipple and areola for 3 to 5 minutes daily.

DRUGS

Unless absolutely essential, drugs of all types should be avoided during pregnancy. In general, all drugs cross the placental barrier; only the amount varies. Many drugs will have immediate effects on the fetus or newborn, and some may have long-term effects (Table 28–4). There has recently been shown a striking increase in vaginal adenosis and adenocarcinoma of young women whose mothers received diethylstilbestrol during their pregnancy.

DIET

For many years some physicians have made a fetish of having the patient gain only 15 to 20 pounds above her ideal weight during pregnancy. The 15 to 20 figure was arrived at by adding together the average weight of a term fetus (7½ pounds), the weight of amniotic fluid (2 pounds), and increased maternal weight (breasts and uterus) and fluid (1 to 6 pounds). Thus, a woman who was 30 pounds overweight would be required to lose 10 pounds during her pregnancy. There is no evidence that nonfluid retention weight gain is harmful to the fetus. On the contrary, there is

TABLE 28–4

Drug	Fetal or neonatal effect
Aminopterin	Abortion, congenital defects
Methotrexate	Malformation: skull, face, extremity
Mercaptopurine	Abortion
Azathioprine	Abortion
Cyclophosphamide	Abortion
Barbiturate	Respiratory depression
Opiate	Respiratory depression
Methadone	Withdrawal symptoms
Heroin	Withdrawal symptoms
Diphenylhydantoin	Cleft lip, microcephaly
Streptomycin	Deafness
Tetracycline	Stained teeth
High doses of ascorbic acid	Withdrawal scurvy
Synthetic vitamin K	Kernicterus
19-Nortestosterone	Female clitoral hypertrophy
Diazepam	Fetal muscular weakness
Magnesium sulfate	Fetal muscular weakness
Lithium	Cardiovascular abnormalities
Oral contraceptives	Limb reduction defects.

evidence that undernutrition may be harmful to the conceptus. The studies of Niswander et al. indicate that the fetal birth weight has a significant relationship with the maternal prepregnancy weight, thus perhaps implicating diet since childhood. Other studies, such as those done around the starvation that occurred in Holland during World War II (Smith) and the siege of Leningrad (Antonov), definitely lead to the conclusion that the fetus born during significant nutritional privation is lighter in weight for his or her gestational age. However, recent studies by Stein and Susser have failed to show any neurologic or intellectual deficit in the Dutch. Studies done in Guatemala by Lechtig and coworkers point toward total caloric intake as one of the major factors in weight of the newborn rather than any specific component such as protein. In addition to these human observations, recent work by Winick in rats indicates that protein deprivation in the mother when pregnant or lactating will be associated with a decrease in brain cell numbers shown by a reduced DNA content. This is also true of children who die of malnutrition. Patients in the lower socioeconomic group as well as teenage pregnant patients are the most likely to have a deficient diet, thus may be the prime candidates for dietary counseling during their gestation. The earlier this counseling can be performed, the more advantageous to the patient and her fetus. The Food and Nutrition Board of the National Research Council has made certain recommendations for diet during pregnancy. Diet can be based somewhat on the age and activity of the individual. Those recommendations are given in Chap. 10 (Table 10-1).

Protein

Adequate protein intake during pregnancy may be essential for optimum fetal health. As stated above, Winick noted a decrease in brain DNA in the fetus of those rats made protein-deficient during gestation and/or lactation. The effects seemed much worse if both prenatal and neonatal deprivation occurred. The DNA reduction is present in both gray and white matter of the brain as well as heart, liver, kidney, and placenta. Winick noted a reduction in placental cell numbers in a malnourished population in Chile. Between 60 and 65 g of protein are recommended daily during pregnancy. This should be in the form of meat, milk, eggs, fish, and cheese for optimal amino acid composition. A correctly balanced diet should include the following: 1 quart of milk (whole or skim), two servings of meat (fish once a week), and one egg per day.

Iron and Folic Acid

The increased erythropoiesis in the patient as well as the movement of iron into the fetus for its erythropoiesis necessitates that the patient absorb approximately 6 mg of iron per day. Since only about 10 to 20 percent of the iron from food is absorbed and most diets contain no more than 15 to 18 mg of iron per day, supplementation is necessary. It has been recommended by the National Research Council that 30 to 60 mg of elemental iron be given as a supplement. This can be taken in the form of ferrous sulfate, 300 mg three times a day. In addition, a daily supplement of 200 to 400 μg of folic acid is suggested by many to prevent folic acid deficiency during pregnancy (see Chap. 10).

Assuming again that the patient eats an adequate diet, it is not necessary to further supplement with other vitamins or calcium. In discussing diet with the patient, she must be given specific dietary instructions. Many types of sample diets are available. Table 28-5 shows the type of dietary instructions a patient needs to receive.

SYMPTOMS IN EARLY PREGNANCY AND THEIR THERAPY

NAUSEA AND VOMITING

One of the most common symptoms of early pregnancy is some light nausea and vomiting during the first trimester. The etiology has been thought at various times to be (1) the high levels of circulating steroids in pregnancy (estrogen), (2) the high level of gonadotropin present during the first trimester of pregnancy (HCG), and (3) emotional. The latter is probably operative only when the nausea and vomiting of pregnancy become excessive (hyperemesis), that is, to the point where the patient needs to be admitted to the hospital (ketonemia and ketonuria). Ketonuria has been shown by Churchill and Berendes to be associated with a reduced intelligence quotient when comparing them with offspring of nonketonuric mothers. The majority of people who experience nausea and vomiting find it present early in the morning or during the day when the stomach is empty; thus one of the precepts is to keep some food in the stomach most of the time. It is frequently beneficial to the patient if she will eat six small meals per day instead

TABLE 28–5 Eat This Way Every Day

Eat these foods	Eat these amounts
Milk group	
Milk	
Expectant mother over 18 years	1 qt (4 cups)
Expectant mother under 18 years	1¼ qt (5 cups)
Whole milk, nonfat milk, evaporated milk, nonfat dry milk	
Cheddar and Monterey Jack cheeses (1 slice = 1 cup milk)	
Meat group	
Meat, fish, fowl, cheese, beans, peanut butter	2 servings
A serving is:	
2 to 3 oz of cooked meat, fish, or fowl	
½ cup cottage cheese	
1 cup cooked dry beans or peas	
4 tbsp peanut butter	
2 to 3 oz liver	
Egg or another small serving of meat	
Vegetable-fruit group	
Dark green and deep yellow vegetables and fruits	½ cup
Broccoli, greens, spinach, sweet potato, yams, yellow squash, pumpkin,	
carrots, cantaloupe,* dried apricots*	
Citrus fruits or other high vitamin C foods	½ cup
Orange or juice, grapefruit or juice, greens, broccoli, green	
peppers,*chili peppers,* strawberries,* cantaloupe*	
Other fruits and vegetables	2 servings
White potato, cabbage, tomato, corn, green beans, green peas,	(1 cup)
apple, banana, prunes, raisins	
(and other vegetables, fruits, or juices)	
Bread-cereal group	
Whole grain or enriched bread and cereals	5 servings
A serving is:	
1 slice bread ½ cup macaroni or spaghetti	
1 tortilla ¾ cup ready-to-eat cereal	
½ cup cooked cereal ½ cup rice, enriched or converted	
½ cup grits	
Other foods to complete your meals	
Coffee or tea	As you wish
Margarine, butter, salad dressing, dessert, additional servings of bread,	As you wish, if not gaining
fruit, meat, milk, and other foods.	too much weight

*Where the price is low.

of three large meals as she is accustomed to doing. It is also important for her to have some dry food in her stomach almost as soon as she awakens in the morning; therefore, it has been suggested that the patient keep either dry toast or soda crackers at her bedside, which she can eat immediately upon awakening. It is also helpful in many of these patients to separate their liquid and solid intake by as much as one-half hour. If these minor measures do not control the nausea and vomiting, there are mild antiemetics available which are beneficial. Some antiemetics (meclizine, cyclizine, and chlorocyclizine) have been shown to be teratogenic in animals and should be avoided. However, others such as doxylamine succinate plus pyridoxine hydrochloride (Bendectin) and chlorpromazine (Thorazine) may be very helpful in prevention of ketonemia. Prompt admission of the patient to the hospital and intravenous alimentation should also be utilized to avoid ketonemia.

HEADACHE

Headache is a common symptom of early pregnancy. Usually it is frontal in nature, is quite mild, and is controlled easily with aspirin. Persistent or severe headaches may indicate more serious trouble and should be investigated.

URINARY FREQUENCY

Urinary frequency is also a very common complaint early in pregnancy. It does not necessarily indicate that the patient has inflammation in the urinary tract; however, this should always be checked as it has been demonstrated by Kass and others that roughly 6 percent of pregnant women will have asymptomatic bacteriuria. This incidence is high enough and the consequences of acute pyelonephritis serious enough that each pregnancy should have a clean-catch urine examination on the first or second visit (see below). Should it be determined that the patient has bacteria in her urine, she should be adequately treated with antibiotics for a period of 10 to 14 days and the urine rechecked at frequent intervals during pregnancy to assure the management team that the patient has remained free from urinary-tract infection.

CONSTIPATION

Constipation is another very frequent complaint during pregnancy. It is due mainly to the decreased transit time of food through the large intestine and thus the absorption of large amounts of water. It can easily be counterbalanced by having the patient increase her water intake, and it has been suggested that the patient drink from five to seven glasses of water or liquids per day. If this mild measure does not help, then frequently the bulk foods, such as bran flakes, or a mild laxative, such as milk of magnesia, will be efficacious.

SKIN CHANGES

The patient may notice a pigmentation in a butterfly distribution around the face, particularly over the bridge of the nose and around the eyes, or a darkening of the skin in the midline of her abdomen, or a darkening of the nipples on her breast. These are all perfectly normal signs of pregnancy, and the patient should be reassured that they are not indicative of pathology. The face mask is called chloasma.

LABORATORY WORK

The following laboratory work should be performed on the first visit: hemoglobin or hematocrit, clean-catch urinalysis, as previously mentioned, including determination for sugar and albumin as well as an examination for bacteria and white and red blood cells in the urine, serology, blood type and Rh, Papanicolaou smear of the cervix, and, in high-risk populations, culture of the cervical mucus for *Neisseria gonorrhoeae*. On this visit it has also been suggested that unless a patient is known to have had rubella, a rubella titer be done. If the titer is positive, the physician can assume (1) the patient has had rubella in the past or (2) the patient recently had rubella. Another similar titer in 2 to 4 weeks will confirm the former. If no titer is present and the patient develops symptoms plus a titer, active infection can be assumed, and the patient may wish to have an abortion since the chance of congenital malformation is high. On each subsequent visit the urine should be examined for sugar and albumin. At 32 weeks a repeat hematocrit should be done.

SUBSEQUENT VISITS

If it is determined at this visit that the patient is low risk and all her laboratory work as well as physical examination appear to be normal, the patient may be seen at monthly intervals until she is approximately 6 to 7 months pregnant; then she should be seen twice monthly until the ninth month, during which time she should be seen every week. At each of the succeeding prenatal visits it should be ascertained whether the uterus is increasing in size. This can best be done by measuring the height of the fundus above the symphysis, stretching a tape measure from the top of the symphysis to the top of the fundus. Assuming the same physician makes the measurements each time, there should be a progressive increment of growth in the uterine fundus throughout pregnancy until the 36th to 38th weeks. From about the 24th to the 32nd to 33rd weeks the height of the uterine fundus in centimeters will approximate the weeks of gestation of the pregnancy, assuming that there is a single fetus present and there is not an excess amount of amniotic fluid (hydramnios).

During an examination for the height of the uterus, it is well to attempt to determine the position of the fetus in the uterus using the maneuvers of Leopold (Fig. 28–4). In this situation the obstetrician determines what fetal part is in the lower uterine segment, usually the vertex, what part is in the fundus of the uterus, usually the breech of the fetus, which side the back of the fetus is on, and, conversely, which side the small parts are on, plus the location of the cephalic prominence of the fetus. During this maneuver one will palpate as much as possible the size of the fetus, and it is well with each prenatal visit to attempt to estimate the size of the fetus in grams. The patient's blood pressure should be taken in the upper arm with the patient in the lateral recumbent position. Normally the pressures remain essentially unchanged throughout pregnancy with perhaps a slight decrease in both systolic and diastolic pressures in the second trimester. Any elevation of diastolic greater than 15 mmHg above the baseline or systolic elevation greater than 30 mmHg above the baseline signals pregnancy-induced hypertension and should be evaluated or treated as described in Chap. 30. A pressure greater than 140 systolic or 90 diastolic should receive similar attention. Gant and coworkers have suggested that an elevation in diastolic pressure greater than 20 mmHg which occurs when the patient turns from the lateral recumbent to the dorsal position is associated with a significant rise in the incidence of pregnancy toxemia.

A clean-voided, first specimen of urine should be obtained and checked for albumin and sugar at each visit. Presence of albumin may also signal the onset of developing toxemia of pregnancy, and the presence of sugar in the first voided specimen in the urine is an indication to do a glucose tolerance test.

One should check with the patient to determine whether the fetus is active; usually it becomes active sometime around the 16th to 20th week. This may also assist in determining the gestational age of the fetus. As well as asking whether the fetus is active, it is well to listen for the fetal heart rate. This is usually heard sometime around the 20th to 24th week of gestation if a conventional stethoscope is used, and at approximately the 12th week of gestation if an ultrasonic stethoscope is used.

The patient should be questioned to determine whether any problems have developed since the previous visit. She should particularly be questioned concerning the presence of any vaginal bleeding, headache, abdominal pain, and/or urinary-tract pain. Some problems which arise during pregnancy that bother the patient, such as mild ankle edema, may be perfectly normal and call for no therapy, while other problems, such as bleeding, may be quite significant and necessitate investigation as well as therapy.

At some point during the process of prenatal care, the physician and the patient should discuss the types of anesthesia available during labor and delivery so that together the patient and the physician may make a rational choice of anesthesia for delivery (see Chap. 29). The physician and the patient should discuss the events that will happen to the patient when she is admitted to the hospital for her delivery, since particularly with the first child this can be a very traumatic experience. In many hospitals a tour of the facilities is given, which can be very helpful in educating the patient concerning her hospital experience. An educated individual is usually less apprehensive and more cooperative. This state of mind can be very important in the smooth conduct of a labor and delivery.

If at any time during the prenatal care the patient develops any problem, she must be placed in a high-risk category and given appropriate care for that particular condition. Those patients who fit into the high-risk category from the beginning of their prenatal care are usually managed by a group, depending upon the complication of the pregnancy. For instance, the diabetic patient is usually managed by a group consisting of internist, obstetrician, dietitian, nurse, and perhaps social worker. These high-risk pregnancies should be managed by obstetricians as well as other members of the medical group who are thoroughly familiar with the latest advances in maternal management during pregnancy and who also possess the ability to assess the fetus as the pregnancy progresses. In the past few years the advent of amniotic fluid sampling, fetal heart rate monitoring, and estriol monitoring during pregnancy has permitted the obstetric care team to have some assessment of the intrauterine fetus and to manage the pregnancy from the standpoint of both the mother and the fetus on a much more rational basis.

TESTS OF FETAL STATUS

PLASMA ESTRIOL

Estriol is an estrogen formed in large quantities by the fetoplacental unit during pregnancy. The fetal adrenal gland produces a precursor, dehydroepiandroste-

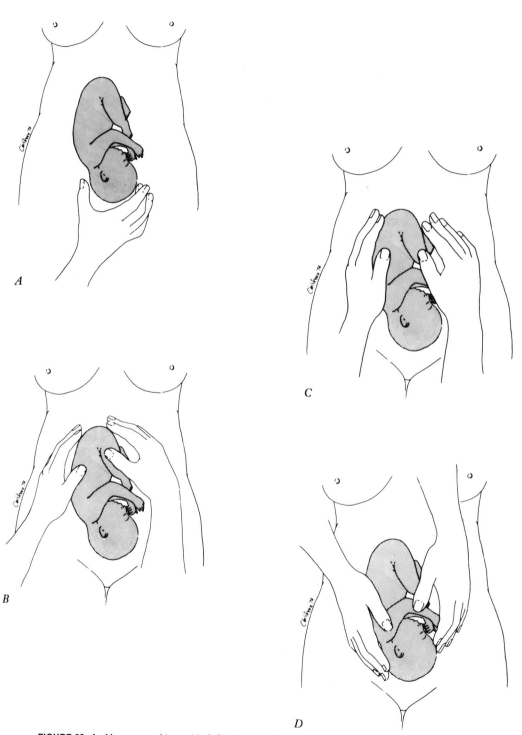

FIGURE 28–4 Maneuvers of Leopold. *A* Determination of the part occupying the lower uterine segment, in this case the vertex. *B* Determination of the fetal part occupying the uterine fundus. *C* Palpation of the fetal back and small parts. *D* Determination of the cephalic prominence, that is, the part of the fetal head palpated first as the hands are directed posterior. If the fetal back and cephalic prominence are on the same side, the fetal position is occipital anterior.

rone, which is hydroxylated in the 16 position by the fetal liver and aromatized to estriol in the placenta.

The amount of estriol in the maternal urine and plasma usually rises progressively throughout pregnancy (Fig. 28-5). The value of the test has been questioned by some authors; however, we find the test helpful if done frequently enough and by a reliable laboratory. We are currently determining plasma-unconjugated estriol using a radioimmunoassay. The test must be done on a daily basis when managing the diabetic and at least twice weekly in hypertensive states and in postdate pregnancies.

In our laboratory, a significant decrease is a value that is greater than 40 percent below the previous 3 days' mean in diabetics and a 50 percent drop in postdate pregnancy. The percentage has been determined by selecting a value greater than 2 standard deviations from normal in a group of normal patients. We have also found that a value below 11 ng/mL is associated with fetal jeopardy.

OXYTOCIN CHALLENGE TEST

This test is based on the supposition that late decelerations of the fetal heart rate with uterine contrac-

FIGURE 28-5 Unconjugated plasma estriol values during pregnancy.

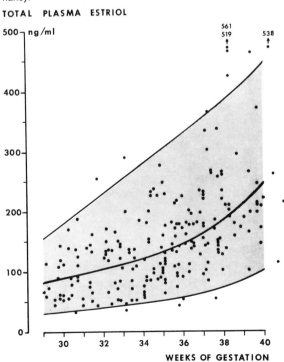

TOTAL PLASMA ESTRIOL

tions (see Chap. 29) indicate fetal hypoxia. The test is performed weekly. The patient is placed supine in bed and the blood pressure checked every 5 minutes for 15 to 20 minutes to rule out supine hypotension. An external fetal monitor (ultrasound or microphone) is placed on the abdomen to continuously monitor fetal heart rate, and an external tocodynamometer (TKD) is placed on the abdomen to monitor uterine activity (see Chap. 29). A base-line fetal heart and uterine activity pattern is established for 15 to 20 minutes. Intravenous oxytocin is then given by an infusion pump starting at the rate of 0.5 mU per minute. The rate of oxytocin infusion is doubled every 20 minutes until the patient is having three contractions per 10-minute period. If there are no late decelerations for 30 minutes, it is considered a negative test. If late decelerations of the fetal heart occur (see Chap. 29), the test is read positive (Ray et al.). Using the test in the above manner, the false-negative rate is about 7 to 10 per 1000, i.e., there will be 7 to 10 unexpected fetal deaths within 1 week of a negative test. The false-positive rate is 50 to 70 percent in contrast to the low false-negative rate. Paul and coworkers found only five fetuses out of 21 had fetal distress when delivered within 1 week of a positive test. Thus, a positive test does not necessarily call for immediate intervention. Our own tendency is to intervene when the infant is premature only when both the estriol is falling and the oxytocin challenge test is positive. If the infant is mature, pregnancy is interrupted when either test is abnormal.

More recently a nonstress method of fetal evaluation has been developed. This test is based on the premise that a well fetus will have a cardiac acceleration associated with fetal activity. The test is done by observing fetal activity on the TKD channel (see Fig. 28–6) and an associated fetal cardiac acceleration of 15 beats per minute or greater. The definition of fetal normality we are currently using is two accelerations of 15 beats per minute or greater associated with fetal activity in a 20-minute period. The test is easier to perform than the contraction stress test and seems to have an equally low false-negative rate. The false-positive rate is quite high since the state of activity and medication will significantly alter fetal activity.

TESTS OF FETAL MATURITY

Several tests of fetal maturity have been proposed and utilized: the first date the fetal heart rate is heard, quickening, appearance of fetal epiphysis by x-ray, biparietal diameter of the fetal head by A scan and real-time ultrasound, amniotic fluid phospholipids,

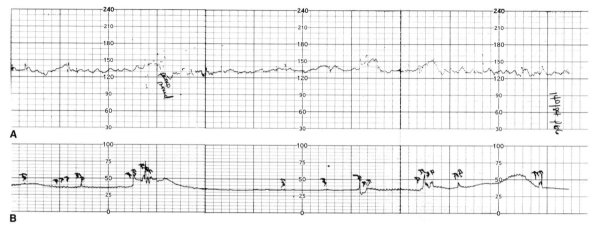

FIGURE 28-6 Fetal activity with associated fetal cardiac acceleration: *A* Fetal heart rate. *B* Uterine activity. Note fetal movement (FM) on uterine activity channel.

amniotic fluid creatinine, and percentage of fetal fat-containing cells in the amniotic fluid. This is not a complete list by any means. Table 28-6 lists the values for these tests.

The preferred is the amniotic fluid lecithin/sphingomyelin ratio (L/S ratio) which indicates the maturity of the fetal lung. Lecithin is the surface-active material of the lungs. Without it the alveoli tend to collapse and respiratory distress follows. The amount of lecithin in amniotic fluid seems to reflect the amount present in the fetal alveoli. In Donald's series, if the L/S ratio was greater than 2, they found a 0.3 percent incidence of hyaline membrane disease at autopsy and a 3.7 percent incidence of respiratory

distress syndrome. This test requires a chromatographic procedure; it thus must be performed in a laboratory and requires hours for the result. A recent modification, the shake test, can be done immediately, at the bedside, and the results seem promising. The test consists in mixing 1 ml of amniotic fluid and 1 ml of absolute ethyl alcohol, shaking, and observing after 15 minutes. If small bubbles are present, the test is positive, and the incidence of respiratory distress syndrome very low. Recently Gluck and associates have demonstrated the value of phosphatidylinositol and phosphatidylglycerol in determining fetal pulmonary maturity.

TESTS FOR PLACENTAL LOCALIZATION

In the patient who develops vaginal bleeding during the last trimester of her pregnancy, the obstetrician needs to know the placenta location. The test currently used is real time ultrasonic scanning. The test is based on the fact that pulses of ultrasound will be reflected back when they strike surfaces of differing densities. These returning pulses can be detected and stored on a storage oscilloscope. A picture can thus be formed by moving the pulsing crystal over the mother's abdomen. Gottesfeld tested this technique for placental detection and found it very accurate (> 95 percent). The technique has also been used to detect fetal central-nervous-system anomalies such as anencephaly and hydrocephaly and anomalies of pregnancy such as hydatidiform moles. Since to date little if any effect on the fetus has been demonstrated from use of the instrument over short time periods at

Table 28–6   Tests of Fetal Maturity

Observation	Significance
Fetal heart	Heard at 20 weeks by stethoscope
Quickening	Begins 14 to 16 weeks
Fetal distal femoral epiphysis	Seen at 36 weeks by x-ray
Fetal proximal tibial epiphysis	Seen at 38 weeks by x-ray
Fetal biparietal diameter	Reaches 8.5 cm at 36 weeks by ultrasound
Amniotic fluid lecithin/sphingomyelin ratio	2.0 or more when lungs mature
Amniotic fluid creatinine	2.0 mg per 100 mL or greater after 36 weeks
Amniotic fluid fat cells	18% after 38 weeks

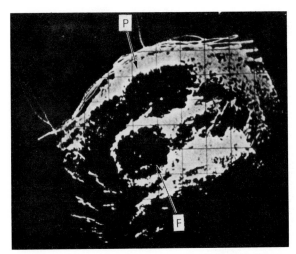

FIGURE 28-7 Ultrasonic B scan at 38 weeks' gestation. Note anterior placenta (P) and fetus (F) in vertex presentation.

present energy levels, and the accuracy is high, this is the preferred technique for placental localization (Fig. 28–7).

LABOR

At some time during the last trimester the patient should be told of the premonitory signs of labor. She may notice the onset of uterine activity which is rhythmic, and indeed approximately 80 percent of labors start with the onset of rhythmic uterine activity. This is felt as lower abdominal or low-back tightening or pain. The patient may notice the onset of a bloody show, which is the passage of a small amount of blood in mucus. This usually precedes the onset of labor by as much as 72 hours. If a bloody show follows pelvic examination, it may have little or no significance; however, it should always be reported to the physician. The patient may have a spontaneous rupture of her membranes, in which case there will be a sudden loss of a large amount of relatively clear fluid which the patient cannot control. If the patient is not in labor and reports that her membranes have ruptured, she should be seen immediately and only a sterile speculum examination should be done to confirm rupture of the bag of waters. One may see fluid coming from the cervical os or take a small amount of fluid from the vaginal pool to check for ferning (a fern

pattern seen through the microscope of fluid dried on a glass slide). The pH of fluid can also be checked, and it should be alkaline if it is amniotic fluid. Further vaginal examinations should not be done until the patient is in active labor since repeated examinations enhance the development of chorioamnionitis. In most instances at term the patient will be in spontaneous labor within 24 hours of rupture of her membranes; however, if she is not, labor should be induced using a well-controlled intravenous oxytocin infusion. If the patient is prior to 36 weeks and rupture of the membranes is confirmed, some physicians prefer to deliver the patient, while others observe the patient. If observation is chosen, the patient must be monitored closely for infection and instructed not to put anything into her vagina.

To sum up, good prenatal care should (1) assist the physician to recognize quickly the complications of pregnancy and to treat those complications, (2) assist the patient to understand what is happening to her during the pregnancy, and (3) maximize the patient's participation in the events happening during this pregnancy through a thorough understanding of the processes involved.

REFERENCES

Antonov AN: *J Pediatr* 30:250, 1947.
Churchill JA, Berendes JW: Intelligence of children whose mothers had acetonuria during pregnancy, in *Perinatal Factors Affecting Human Development,* Scientific Pub. No. 185, Washington: Pan American Health Organization, 1969.
Donald IR et al.: *Am J Obstet Gynecol* 115:547, 1973.
Gant NF et al.: *Am J Obstet Gynecol* 120:1, 1974.
Gauthier R, Evertson L, and Paul R: *Am J Obstet Gynecol* 133:34, 1979.
Goodwin JW et al.: *Can Med Assoc J* 101:57, 1969.
Gottesfeld KR et al.: *Am J Obstet Gynecol* 96:538, 1966.
Hallman M et al.: *Am J Obstet Gynecol* 125:613, 1976.
Herbst AL et al.: *N Engl J Med* 284:878, 1971.
Hoebel CJ et al.: *Am J Obstet Gynecol* 73:808, 1957.
_____ et al.: *Am J Obstet Gynecol* 117:1, 1973.
Infant Death: An Analysis by Maternal Risk and Health Care, Washington: National Academy of Sciences, 1973.
Kass EH: *Arch Intern Med* 105:194, 1960.
Larson SM, Help WB: *Am J Obstet Gynecol* 93:950, 1965.

Lechtig A et al.: *Am J Obstet Gynecol* 125:25, 1976.

Maternal Nutrition and the Course of Pregnancy, Washington: National Academy of Sciences, 1970.

Nesbitt REL, Aubry RH: *Am J Obstet Gynecol* 103:972, 1969.

Niswander KR: *Obstet Gynecol* 33:482, 1969.

Ray MR et al: *Am J Obstet Gynecol* 114:1, 1972.

Sarrel PM: *Am J Obstet Gynecol* 105:575, 1969.

Simpson WJ: *Am J Obstet Gynecol* 73:808, 1957.

Smith CA: *Am J Obstet Gynecol* 53:599, 1947.

Smith RW: *Obstet Gynec* 35:537, 1970.

Stein A, Susser M: *Pediatr Res* 9:70, 1975.

Winick M: *Nutrition and Development,* New York: Wiley Interscience, 1972.

Yerushalmy J: *Am J Obstet Gynecol* 112: 277, 1972.

29

Perinatal Care

TOM P. BARDEN

NORMAL LABOR

DEFINITION

Labor is the physiologic process by which the uterus expels, or attempts to expel, its contents, the products of conception after 20 weeks' gestation, through the cervical opening and vagina to the outside world. Normal labor is characterized by periodic, involuntary uterine contractions which produce gradual cervical effacement and dilatation, as well as descent of the fetal presenting part; however, any one of or all these changes may occur to some degree prior to the onset of labor. The most consistent symptom of labor is discomfort associated with contractions, but there are occasional patients who experience minimal pain with labor contractions. Uterine contractions during labor usually occur at intervals of less than 10 minutes and become more frequent in more advanced labor. Contraction intensity and patient discomfort also tend to increase during normal labor. The cervix is usually not dilated more than 1 to 2 cm prior to the onset of labor, but in occasional patients, dilatation may be advanced prior to the onset of clinical labor. Labor is arbitrarily divided into three stages: (1) from onset of labor to complete dilatation of the cervix, (2) from complete dilatation to birth of the fetus, and (3) from birth of the fetus to delivery of the placenta.

PHYSIOLOGY

For an extensive discussion of the mechanism of onset, see Chap. 9.

Uterine Contractility

The uterus is an actively contractile organ not only in labor but throughout pregnancy and also during the nongravid menstrual cycle. The studies of Reynolds (1949), Alvarez and Caldeyro-Barcia, Csapo and Sauvage, and Hendricks (1966) have provided the current knowledge of uterine contractility. They used either external or internal methods of recording either the average intrauterine pressure or the pressure changes of specific areas of the myometrium. (See Fig. 29–1.) During early pregnancy there are very mild, painless contractions occurring at a rate of about one per minute, with occasionally somewhat more intense contractions which are also painless. The latter are commonly referred to as *Braxton Hicks*

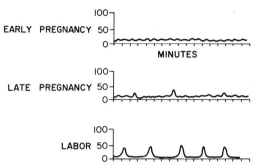

FIGURE 29–1 Evolution of uterine activity during pregnancy.

contractions, and as pregnancy progresses, they gradually become more frequent. During the last few weeks of pregnancy, the Braxton Hicks contractions become more frequent and may occur at relatively regular intervals, simulating labor and producing false labor. The Braxton Hicks contractions are thought to be responsible for most of the cervical changes that usually precede the onset of labor. They are more common in multiparous patients, and although they tend to be painless, on occasion they are quite uncomfortable. The intensity of Braxton Hicks contractions, measured from the intrauterine cavity, are 10 to 15 mmHg. As labor gradually evolves from prelabor uterine activity, contractions become more intense and more frequent, as they do until delivery.

The term *tonus* refers to intrauterine pressure between contractions which average 8 to 12 mmHg (see Fig. 29–2). The intensity of a contraction is the maximal rise of intrauterine pressure above tonus which in labor usually is 25 to 50 mmHg. Contractions occur in labor at intervals of 2 to 10 minutes, or at a rate of one to five per 10 minutes. The tonus, intensity, and frequency of contractions are usually higher in primigravidas than in multiparas. When a patient lies on her side, contractions are less frequent and more intense than when she is supine.

The site of origin and propagation of uterine contractions has been described by Reynolds (1949) using a series of external tocotransducers and by Cal-

FIGURE 29–2 Terminology of intrauterine pressure recordings.

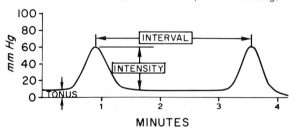

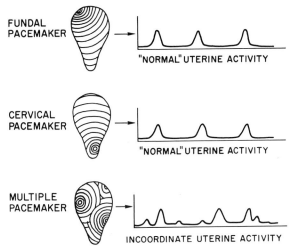

FIGURE 29-3 Relationships of uterine contractility to intrauterine pressure recordings.

deyro-Barcia and coworkers (1952, 1955) recording pressure, from microballoons inserted into the myometrium, of various uterine locations (see Fig. 29–3). A normal contractile wave originates in one cornual region and spreads downward through the entire myometrium in 10 to 15 seconds. This normal pattern of uterine contractility has been described as *descending gradient* or *fundal dominance* and is responsible for normal labor progress. If contractions develop from a pacemaker in the lower part of the uterus, normal cervical changes of labor do not occur despite the normal appearance of the intrauterine pressure recording. If multiple pacemakers are serially producing contractile waves, labor may not progress normally, and a typical "incoordinate" pattern may be recorded. It is generally not possible to discern the pacemaker location by palpation, and complex recording systems are generally not available. Normal progress of labor is the best evidence of normal uterine contractility.

ONSET OF LABOR

The most consistent symptom of early labor is an increasing awareness of contractions with increasing rhythmicity and frequency. Contractions generally occur at intervals of 10 minutes or less following the onset of labor. Contractions of active labor usually produce lower abdominal and low-back discomfort, in contrast to prelabor contractions which are usually painless. Vaginal passage of mucus, a small amount of blood, or amniotic fluid may be found around the time of the onset of labor. The cervix is usually not more than partially effaced and 2 cm dilated prior to the onset of labor, but occasional patients are further dilated prior to the development of regular contractions. The most consistent sign of active labor is evidence of progressive effacement and dilatation of the cervix, which is detected only by serial vaginal examinations.

PROCESS OF LABOR

Fetal Head

Dimensions of the fetal head are the largest of the fetus and are, therefore, most critical in its passage through the birth canal. The prominent upper portion of the skull, or cranium, is composed of pairs of frontal, parietal, and temporal bones, plus the upper portion of the occipital bone and the wings of the sphenoid bones. These bones are loosely joined by membranous sutures referred to as *sagittal* between the parietal bones, *frontal* between the frontal bones, *coronal* between the frontal and parietal bones, and *lambdoid* between the parietal bones and the occipital bone. The anterior fontanel is a diamond-shaped membranous space formed at the junction of the two frontal and two parietal bones. The smaller posterior fontanel is formed by the junction of the parietal bones and the upper portion of the occipital bone. The sutures and fontanels of the fetal skull are palpable at vaginal examination, and their orientation permits diagnosis of the fetal position in relation to the maternal pelvis. Areas of the fetal skull are referred to as the *occiput* over the occipital bone, the *vertex* in the midline between the posterior and anterior fontanels, the *sinciput* or *bregma* immediately anterior to the anterior fontanel, and the *mentum* or fetal chin (see Fig. 29–4). The term *attitude* refers to the relationship of the fetal head to the long axis of the body, ranging from complete flexion to various degrees of extension. The attitude of the fetal head determines the diameters which present to the pelvis in labor. In a term fetus of about 3250 g, the well-flexed fetal head measures about 9.5 by 9.5 cm in its transverse and anteroposterior dimensions. When the posterior vertex presents, its perpendicular diameter is the suboccipitobregmatic which extends from the anterior fontanel to the undersurface of the occipital bone, measuring 9.5 cm. When the anterior vertex or anterior fontanel presents, its perpendicular diameter is the occipitofrontal which measures 12.0 cm and extends from the nose to the posterior fontanel. With a

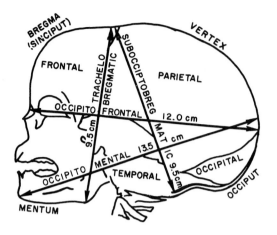

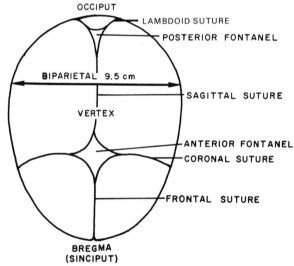

FIGURE 29–4 Topography of the fetal skull.

bregma presentation, the corresponding anteroposterior diameter is the occipitomental, extending from the chin to the region of the posterior fontanel, which measures 13.5 cm. In a face presentation, the perpendicular diameter is the trachelobregmatic, measuring 9.5 cm, which extends from the lower jaw to the anterior fontanel. The largest transverse diameter of the fetal skull is the biparietal which measures 9.5 cm and extends between the parietal bosses.

Maternal Pelvis

In addition to the size and presentation of the fetus, the mechanism of labor is strongly influenced by the shape and capacity of the birth canal. The curved passage is formed by the sacrum, coccyx, and two innominate bones with their associated ligaments and muscles. The linea terminalis is a bony ridge extending from the sacral promontory, along the arcuate line of the ilium to the crest of the pubis, which forms the division between the expansive false pelvis and the obstetrically significant true pelvis. The true pelvis is bounded posteriorly by the anterior surface of the sacrum, laterally by the inner surface of the ischial bones, and anteriorly by the pubic rami. The contour of the pelvic passage varies at different levels which are arbitrarily designated as planes of the inlet, midpelvis, and outlet (Fig. 29–5). The plane of the inlet, or superior strait, is bounded by the sacral promontory, linea terminalis, and upper border of the pubis.

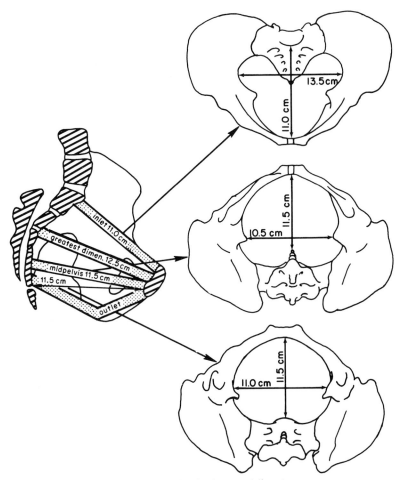

FIGURE 29–5 Pelvic planes and diameters.

It is approximately 13.5 cm wide and 11.0 cm in the anteroposterior diameter, forming a slightly heart-shaped ellipse. Inferior to the inlet, the pelvic capacity expands to the plane of greatest dimensions which extends from the posterior surface of the symphysis pubis to the sacrum at its level of greatest concavity. This plane measures approximately 12.5 by 12.5 cm. The birth canal then narrows to the midplane which extends from the posterior surface of the symphysis pubis, through the ischial spines, to the sacrum. The interspinous diameter of 10.0 to 10.5 cm represents the smallest dimension of the true pelvis and is the most critical plane through which the fetus must negotiate in its passage through the birth canal. The pelvic outlet consists of two triangular-shaped planes with a common base extending between the ischial tuberosities. The posterior triangle extends to the tip of the sacrum, and the anterior triangle is bounded by

the pubic arch. The average dimensions of the outlet are 11.0 cm between the ischial tuberosities and 11.5 cm from the pubis to the tip of the sacrum, which is designated the posterior sagittal diameter of the outlet.

Mechanisms of Labor

The relative dimensions of the fetus and maternal birth canal necessitate a complex series of overlapping movements of the fetal presenting part during its passage through the pelvis which are referred to as the *mechanisms of labor*. In 95 percent of patients, the fetal vertex presents, and it is most often in a transverse position at the onset of labor (Fig. 29–6). As labor progresses, descent and flexion are accompanied by internal rotation of the occiput anteriorly. With further descent and internal rotation, the head

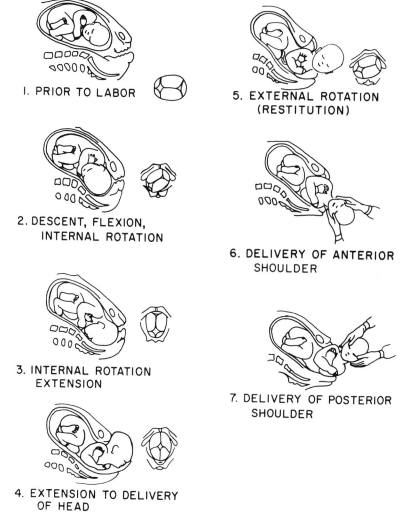

1. PRIOR TO LABOR

2. DESCENT, FLEXION, INTERNAL ROTATION

3. INTERNAL ROTATION EXTENSION

4. EXTENSION TO DELIVERY OF HEAD

5. EXTERNAL ROTATION (RESTITUTION)

6. DELIVERY OF ANTERIOR SHOULDER

7. DELIVERY OF POSTERIOR SHOULDER

FIGURE 29–6 Mechanism of labor for cephalic presentation.

begins to extend until it is born by extension in the occipitoanterior position. The fetal head then undergoes restitution to its original position, and thus becomes oriented with the fetal shoulders. As the fetal shoulders reach the muscular pelvic floor, they turn into the anteroposterior plane, and the fetal head turns by external rotation to the transverse position if this was not accomplished by restitution. Next, the anterior shoulder delivers under the symphysis pubis, followed by delivery of the posterior shoulder across the perineum. Expulsion of the remainder of the fetal body then occurs with ease. Occasionally the posterior shoulder may deliver first.

CLINICAL EVALUATION OF THE LABOR PATIENT

General Evaluation

Immediately after arriving at the hospital, the patient in labor should be screened for evidence of labor complications and status of labor. Ideally, a copy of her prenatal medical record should be on file in the labor suite. Historical items of immediate interest include the patient's age, parity, gestation, general health status, known allergies, complications of the pregnancy, the onset of labor, condition of membranes, character of vaginal bleeding or discharge, and time of her last meal. Initial physical evaluation should include observation of her general demeanor, blood pressure, temperature, uterine size and consistency, fetal presentation, fetal heart activity, nature of vaginal discharge or bleeding, extent of edema, and reactivity of deep tendon reflexes.

Pelvic Examination

Vaginal speculum examination should precede digital examination if the patient has not had an adequate pelvic examination earlier in the pregnancy, or if there is history of ruptured membranes. If cervical cytology smears have not been obtained earlier in pregnancy, they may be taken at this time; however, the major objective of this examination is to grossly identify and prevent delivery through a carcinoma of the cervix. Frequently blood or amniotic fluid will prevent satisfactory cytologic smears, and they must be repeated at the first postpartum examination.

The diagnosis of ruptured membranes is confirmed by observation of typical amniotic fluid pouring out of the cervical os with gentle pressure on the uterine fundus, or if the fetal presenting part is directly visualized through the partially dilated cervix. Ruptured membranes are strongly suggested if vaginal fluid, allowed to dry on a glass slide, produces a microscopic fern pattern due to amniotic fluid content of sodium chloride. The presence of blood may interfere with ferning. Amniotic fluid is slightly alkaline in contrast to vaginal secretions which are normally mildly acidic; thus Nitrazine Paper will turn from orange to blue when moistened by amniotic fluid. The presence of blood in this case will produce a false-positive test, as it is also alkaline.

Digital pelvic examination should be performed at the time of initial evaluation of a patient in labor unless it is contraindicated by clinical evidence suggestive of placenta previa. The examination is performed by inserting two fingers of the lubricated sterile gloved hand into the vaginal introitus while spreading the labia with the other hand. Widespread use of vaginal rather than rectal examinations for many years has confirmed that they are more comfortable, more informative, and not associated with a higher incidence of infection. The occasional patient who resists vaginal examination will usually permit rectal examination. The examination permits evaluation of pelvic dimensions, cervix, and fetal presenting part. Even though the pelvic dimensions were recorded earlier in pregnancy, it is prudent to review the findings at this time (see Fig. 29–7). Estimation of

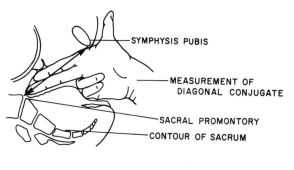

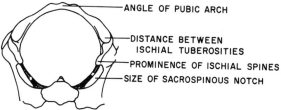

FIGURE 29–7 Evaluation of pelvic capacity.

the diagonal conjugate may be prevented by low station of the fetal presenting part, but when it is possible to measure this dimension, the anteroposterior dimension of the inlet may be presumed to be approximately 1.5 cm less. The sacrum is normally concave, but if it is found to be flat, the anteroposterior dimension of the midpelvis is usually shorter than normal. The ischial spines are palpated for an impression of their relative prominence and to determine the station of the presenting part. The term *station* refers to the relative level of the most dependent bony fetal structure to the ischial spines; it is described as zero station at the level of the spines or plus or minus the number of centimeters below or above the spines, respectively (see Fig. 29–8). An impression of the capacity of the posterior portion of the midpelvis is gained by judging the distance from the ischial spines to the sacrum, the sacrospinous notch, which is normally about 3 cm. Capacity of the anterior portion of the pelvis is estimated by palpating the angle of the pubic arch which is normally obtuse. The transverse dimension of the pelvic outlet is readily measured between the ischial tuberosities.

The cervix is examined for its location, consistency, relationship to fetal presenting part, effacement, and dilatation. The term *effacement* refers to the degree of thinning or "taking up" of the cervix during labor (see Fig. 29–9). The uterus is anatomically and functionally divided into a thick, active, upper segment and a thin, passive, lower segment. As labor

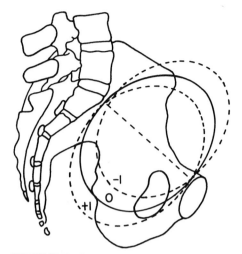

FIGURE 29–8   Station of fetal head.

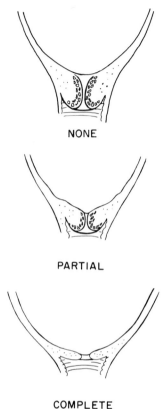

FIGURE 29–9   Effacement of cervix.

progresses, the cervix, starting with the internal os and progressing to the external os, is gradually incorporated into the lower uterine segment. The myometrial fibers of the lower segment become stretched, while those of the upper segment gradually become shorter. The cervix shortens from about 2 cm prior to labor to almost paper thinness in the primigravida, but with less thinning in a multiparous patient. The degree of effacement is commonly referred to as a *percentage,* but this is rather arbitrary, with interpretation varying among examiners. Considerable effacement of the cervix may occur from prelabor contractions, so that the extent of effacement does not necessarily indicate the stage of labor.

In normal labor the cervix dilates to accommodate passage of the fetus. Generally dilatation of 10 cm, referred to as full or complete dilatation, is adequate. *Cervical dilatation* is determined by sweeping the examining fingers across the cervical os to judge its average diameter. The cervix may be dilated several centimeters prior to the clinical onset of labor, but usually progresses from about 1 to 10 cm during the course of labor. The estimation of dilatation is fairly consistent from one examiner to another.

Vaginal examination also permits diagnosis of fetal presenting part, position, and attitude. The fetal presenting part is the portion of the fetus palpable through the cervical os. It determines the *presentation* which is described as cephalic, breech, oblique, or transverse. The term *lie* refers to the relationship of the long axis of the fetus to that of the mother, with longitudinal lie including cephalic and breech presentations. *Position* describes the relation of the fetal presenting part to the maternal pelvis by indicating

the location within the pelvis of an arbitrary point on the presenting part. (See Fig. 29–10.) The fetal landmarks are occiput in vertex presentations, brow or bregma in brow presentations, chin or mentum in face presentations, sacrum in breech presentations, and acromion in shoulder presentations. The maternal pelvis is divided into eight segments, namely, anterior, left anterior oblique, left transverse, left posterior oblique, posterior, right posterior oblique, right transverse, and right anterior oblique. The fetal position is generally abbreviated by indicating the fetal landmark, the side of the pelvis, and the segment of the pelvis occupied by the landmark [i.e., occiput left anterior (LOA) or sacrum right transverse (RST)]. In cephalic presentations the orientation of the fetal head is diagnosed by palpation of the various sutures and fontanels of the skull. The normal attitude of the fetal head is complete flexion so that the posterior vertex presents and the sagittal suture is palpable through the cervix. By moving the examining fingers along the sagittal suture, the posterior fontanel is located a short distance from the center of the cervical opening.

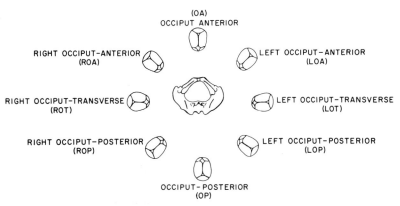

FIGURE 29–10 Position of fetal head.

The identity of the posterior fontanel is confirmed by extending the examining fingers beyond the membranous fontanel to palpate the two lambdoid sutures, not by palpating the midline frontal suture that is located beyond the anterior fontanel (Fig. 29–4). The size and shape of the fontanels are not reliable indications of their identity because of the frequent development of molding. *Molding* is an overlapping of fetal skull bones which occurs most commonly in primigravidas, especially when there is relative disproportion between the fetal head and maternal pelvis (see Fig. 29–11). Usually the anterior parietal bone overlaps the posterior, and the occipital and frontal bones are pushed beneath the parietal bones. The fetal head may also become distorted during labor by formation of a *caput succedaneum* in which the fetal scalp over the cervical os becomes edematous. Caput formation often makes it difficult to palpate the underlying sutures and fontanels of the fetal skull. After delivery, caput succedaneum may be confused with *cephalhematoma,* a rare complication in which hemorrhage occurs beneath the periosteum and is limited by periosteal midline attachment. In contrast, caput succedaneum usually extends across the midline over the portion of the scalp that presented against the cervical os.

Further Evaluation of the Labor Patient

Following the initial evaluation, a complete history and physical examination should be accomplished whenever time is not limited by advanced labor. If available, the history recorded earlier in pregnancy will suffice, but a physical examination should be done which includes visualization of optic fundi and thorough examination of the heart, lungs, breasts, and abdomen. If blood type is not known, it should be de-

termined at this time. In addition, the patient's hematocrit should be obtained as its level may influence the choice of analgesia and anesthesia. Urinary protein should be tested routinely.

General care during labor should provide optimal patient comfort plus optimal fetal and maternal safety. When a patient is admitted in early labor, a cleansing enema will minimize the likelihood of fecal expulsion on the fetus or episiotomy wound at delivery. The enema is omitted if labor is further advanced. The patient's vulva should be thoroughly cleansed

FIGURE 29–11 Molding, caput succedaneum, and cephalhematoma.

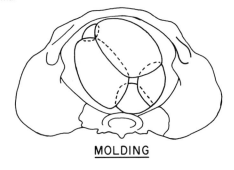

MOLDING

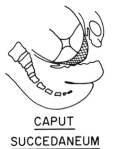

CAPUT
SUCCEDANEUM

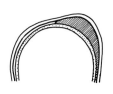

CEPHALHEMATOMA

with surgical soap. Although the shaving of pubic hair was common practice in the past, most obstetricians now agree that this procedure is neither necessary nor desirable. Thus, the patient is saved the discomfort of hair regrowth during the puerperium. The patient should be encouraged to void every 3 to 4 hours during labor. An occasional patient may require catheterization if unable to void in 6 to 8 hours and with obvious distention of the urinary bladder. In early labor, a patient may be given freedom of ambulation within the labor suite if a suitable exercise area exists. As labor becomes more active, and in every patient following use of analgesics, she should be confined to a labor bed with protective side rails. At this time, a slow intravenous infusion of Ringer's lactate solution or 5% dextrose in water should be started in a forearm vein to provide a readily accessible route for possible administration of medications, blood, or blood substitutes. Nutrition during labor should be limited to oral fluids in prodromal labor and to intravenous fluids only during active labor.

Pulmonary aspiration of gastric contents is the leading cause of anesthetic maternal mortality because of the frequency of vomiting during inhalation anesthesia. Vomiting is also common when hypotension develops with conduction anesthesia, in the supine position, and during second stage labor. Although aspiration of particulate material will produce an immediate state of pulmonary obstruction, the aspiration of gastric fluid with pH of 2.5 or less will produce the often fatal syndrome of acid aspiration, first described by Mendelson. The routine use of oral antacids during labor has proved very effective protection against the serious risk of pulmonary aspiration. An appropriate protocol consists of administration of an aluminum hydroxide–magnesium hydroxide liquid preparation, 30 mL orally on admission, and 15 mL every 2 hours until delivery.

Vaginal examinations should be repeated as infrequently as possible. In primigravidas the length of labor is generally more predictable than in multiparas, and therefore they require very few examinations, despite their longer labor. Assuming the patient presents in early labor, she need not be reexamined until her contractions become more uncomfortable, when she is likely progressing from the latent to active dilatation phase of labor. If that examination reveals advanced effacement and some progress of dilatation, she need not be reexamined more often than every 2 hours unless there is evidence of abnormally slow or rapid progress. When cervical dilatation is complete and the primigravida enters second-stage

labor, she will sense rectal pressure and begin pushing efforts with abdominal muscles. As the fetus descends to the perineal floor, the fetal presenting part gradually becomes visible. If labor progress has been normal, the patient does not need to be prepared for delivery until the fetal presenting part is definitely on the perineal floor. In a multiparous patient, the progress of labor is much more unpredictable. Vaginal examinations should be repeated at about hourly intervals until one is able to determine the efficiency of her labor. At the earliest symptom of rectal pressure with contractions, she should be reexamined to determine her progress. The multipara should be prepared for delivery when the cervix is dilated 6 to 8 cm, depending on the rapidity of labor. A vaginal examination should always be performed immediately after rupture of membranes to rule out evidence of cord prolapse.

The results of vaginal examinations, as well as notes on uterine activity, maternal and fetal vital signs, medications, and complications, should be recorded in either tabular or graph form. Maternal blood pressure, heart rate, and temperature should be recorded every 60 minutes. Fetal heart rate and uterine activity are most conveniently and accurately recorded by a labor-monitoring instrument, discussed in the next section; however, if monitoring equipment is not available, fetal heart rate should be recorded as the average rate during auscultation for 15 or 30 seconds at intervals of 15 to 30 minutes in first-stage labor and every 5 minutes during second-stage labor. Fetal heart rate should be sampled during, immediately after, and more remotely after uterine contractions in order to detect late decelerations due to fetal hypoxia.

Labor Monitoring

Electronic monitoring of fetal heart rate and uterine activity has been widely accepted as the most informative method of fetal surveillance during labor. The display of fetal heart rate calculated from consecutive beat-to-beat intervals provides detail not possible to perceive by intermittent, or even continuous, auscultation. Most of the available instruments provide a choice of external or internal sensors. In the external application, transducers are placed on the maternal abdominal wall. External monitoring is convenient and applicable under any obstetric circumstances, even when vaginal examinations are contraindicated. It is not possible to calibrate the external uterine pressure transducer, and the apparent intensity of con-

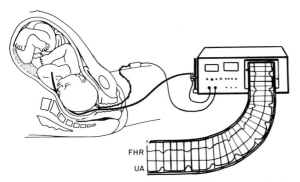

FIGURE 29-12 Labor monitoring, utilizing intrauterine catheter and fetal electrode.

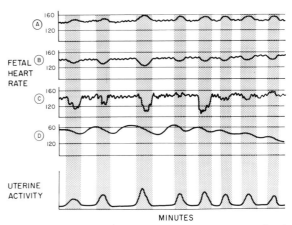

FIGURE 29-13 Patterns of fetal heart rate change associated with uterine contractions: *A* Acceleration. *B* Early deceleration. *C* Variable deceleration. *D* Later deceleration.

tractions depends on the location and firmness of its application. Fetal heart signals are detected by an ultrasonic transducer, which is less accurate than direct internal monitoring. Internal monitoring necessitates rupture of membranes and some cervical dilatation for application of an electrode to the fetal presenting part and vaginal insertion of a water-filled plastic catheter into amniotic fluid above the presenting part. The most convenient type of fetal electrode in current use has a sharp metal spiral tip which is rotated into the superficial layer of skin overlying the fetal presenting part (see Fig. 29-12). It is applied by palpation at vaginal examination. The electrode wires are attached to a leg plate and junction box which connects to the monitor. The intrauterine catheter attaches to a pressure transducer mounted on the side of the monitor. The pressure recording may be equilibrated to atmospheric pressure and accurately reflects changes in intrauterine pressure. The catheter and fetal electrode are easily removed at the time of delivery.

The permanent record displays fetal heart rate in beats per minute and uterine activity in millimeters of mercury for internal monitoring or an arbitrary scale for external monitoring. The terminology related to labor monitoring in common use at the present time is as follows:

Base-line fetal heart rate: the average rate between uterine contractions

Tachycardia: base-line fetal heart rate over 160 beats per minute

Bradycardia: base-line fetal heart rate under 120 beats per minute

Base-line variability: the heart rate variation from beat to beat (short term) and above and below the average rate on a time basis extending up to 1 minute (long term)

Periodic rate changes: fetal heart rate changes which are associated with uterine contractions (see Fig. 29-13)

Accelerations: periodic rate changes in which fetal heart rate increases during uterine contractions

Early decelerations: periodic rate changes in which fetal heart rate slowing during uterine contractions reflects the shape and intensity of the associated contractions

Late decelerations: periodic rate changes in which fetal heart rate slowing reflects the shape and intensity of the associated contractions starting in the midportion of the contraction cycle and persisting into the interval after contractions

Variable decelerations: periodic rate changes which do not reflect the shape or intensity of associated contractions, have variable time of onset, but return to base line by the end of contractions

Normal fetal heart rate responses in first-stage labor consist of normal base-line rate and base-line variability with the possibility of accelerations, early decelerations, or mild variable decelerations. During second-stage labor there is a normal increase of base-line variability and frequent occurrence of variable decelerations. Labor monitoring permits the early recognition and prompt treatment of abnormal fetal heart rate patterns which will be discussed in a later portion of this chapter.

ANALGESIA AND ANESTHESIA

Pain relief in labor and delivery is easily the most dynamic and heterogeneous subject in modern obstetrics. There are obvious extremes from "natural" labor without use of any medications to generous use of narcotic and amnesic drugs with inhalation anesthesia, and a variety of intermediate techniques, all frequently employed within the same obstetric unit. Some techniques have historically fallen into disrepute only to later emerge and gain acceptance, while methods that are popular in one area of the world may be rarely employed elsewhere.

The discomfort of labor and the requirements for analgesia vary considerably among patients. Such variations in response are undoubtedly influenced by a variety of psychic and physical factors such as the patient's basic personality, level of anxiety, physical state, confidence in attendants, degree of uterine activity, and labor complications. This variation in patient responses to labor justifies the use of various techniques which, when properly applied, will offer optimal relief of pain and safety for mother and fetus. The safety of the fetus must remain a constant concern, for virtually every drug administered to the mother during labor will have some effects on the fetus. A balance must be sought between humane relief of pain and optimal maternal and fetal safety. The agents or techniques to be used must be selected on a basis of individual requirements imposed by general health or disease states, the time from the patient's last meal to the onset of labor, known allergies, pregnancy gestation, stage and apparent progress in labor, and past experience with anesthesia. Analgesia in labor is rarely indicated prior to the active dilatation phase of labor. During the hours of latent-phase labor, when the cervix is primarily effacing because of relatively mild contractions, use of analgesics may significantly slow and prolong labor. Generally analgesic medication should not be given until the patient is 3 to 4 cm dilated and strong contractions are producing moderate discomfort. After medications have been given, the patient should remain in the labor bed with protective side rails in place. She should be encouraged to remain in the left or right lateral recumbent position, specifically avoiding the supine position in which uteroplacental blood

flow is compromised by uterine compression of the aorta and vena cava.

PSYCHIC TECHNIQUES

Hypnosis is an ideal method of pain relief in labor, with no adverse effects on mother, fetus, or the process of labor. However, hypnosis has proved to be impractical for general use in obstetrics due to the lack of good candidates, estimated at 15 to 20 percent of obstetric patients, and the impractical demand on time of professional personnel to properly prepare the patient.

The term "natural childbirth" is used in reference to many forms of self-control acquired by learned relaxation techniques. The concept was popularized by the book entitled *Childbirth Without Fear* by Grantly Dick-Read, published in 1940. This method suggests that childbirth pain is derived from learned fear and tension which may be controlled by appropriate preparation. More recently, the "psychoprophylactic method," popularized by Lamaze, is based upon developing a distraction mechanism against what is called the conditioned reflex of pain during labor. There are many interpretations of the methods of natural childbirth, from those advocating no medication for pain relief during labor and with minimal assistance at delivery to those which consider conduction analgesia-anesthesia and even forceps delivery permissible. There is a general consensus that patient awareness of labor physiology reduces anxiety, which in turn reduces appreciation of discomfort. Unfortunately, some patients who are unable to successfully apply a method of childbirth pain relief are forced to accept analgesia with a sense of failure.

SYSTEMIC DRUGS

A wide variety of systemic drugs have been used during labor for analgesia, sedation, ataraxia, amnesia, and inhibition of secretions. Maternal side effects of drug therapy may include respiratory depression, alteration of blood gas and acid-base status, effects on uterine motility, allergic manifestations, and interference with voluntary muscle control. Virtually all drugs pass freely to the fetal circulation, but they generally produce few apparent side effects until after delivery. Certain drugs produce predictable changes in fetal heart rate responses during labor and may confuse the diagnosis of fetal distress. Neonatal effects of the drugs administered to the mother during labor are influenced by their dosage and route of administration, the time interval from their use and delivery, maternal weight, neonatal weight, gestational age, labor and delivery complications, type of anesthesia used for delivery, and mode of delivery.

Barbiturates. These drugs are useful for their sedative or hypnotic actions when used in early labor to help differentiate prolonged latent-phase labor from false labor. Short-acting barbiturates, such as secobarbital (Seconal) and pentobarbital (Nembutal), 100 to 200 mg orally, will produce sedation to promote sleep for several hours. Patients in false labor will usually stop contracting, while those in latent-phase labor will progress to active-phase. If there is significant pain in early labor, a narcotic analgesic is more effective than the sedative action of a barbiturate. Barbiturates readily pass the placenta to attain fetal blood levels of about 70 percent of the maternal level. Repeated exposure to barbiturates may stimulate fetal liver enzymes concerned with formation of glucuronides which lead to increased conjugation of bilirubin. The accumulation of conjugated bilirubin, which does not cross the placenta, may produce neonatal jaundice. But this form of neonatal jaundice does not produce kernicterus and mental retardation as does excessive unconjugated bilirubin. The most significant danger of barbiturates in late pregnancy and labor is their long-lasting sedative effects in the neonate. Brazelton observed decreased sucking efforts for as long as 7 days in newborns exposed to barbiturates prior to delivery.

Morphine. This drug is occasionally useful in labor for its potent analgesic action. In patients having painful contractions but not progressing normally in labor, a period of comfortable rest afforded by administration of morphine, 10 to 15 mg intramuscularly, may promote a return to progressive labor. Morphine readily passes the placenta to attain maximum fetal and maternal blood levels by approximately 30 minutes after maternal intramuscular injection. The fetus is unable to conjugate morphine efficiently, and the level of the drug in the fetal brain is consistently higher than in the maternal brain. The use of morphine in late labor will produce neonatal respiratory depression unless the newborn is treated immediately by a narcotic antagonist. Naloxone hydrochloride (Narcan) is an effective narcotic antagonist without respiratory depressant effects of its own. The newborn dosage of naloxone is 0.01 to 0.02 mg/kg, intramuscularly or intravenously. The use of morphine to produce "twilight sleep" as described early in this century (Gauss) is no longer considered a safe or useful technique of analgesia. The approach, which utilized frequent repeated doses of morphine and

scopolamine throughout labor, usually resulted in severe neonatal depression.

Meperidine (Demerol). This drug is currently the most popular analgesic agent used during labor in the United States. Like morphine, it is a phenanthrene alkaloid of opium which produces central-nervous-system depression, particularly of the respiratory center. Meperidine readily crosses the placenta, but it tends to be less depressant to the neonate than morphine. When administered in dosage of 50 to 100 mg intramuscularly, repeated every 2 to 3 hours, it produces moderate analgesia without an appreciable effect on uterine contractility. It may also be administered intravenously to achieve more rapid onset of action. Its analgesic action is potentiated by simultaneous administration of an ataractic drug such as promethazine (Phenergan) or hydroxyzine (Vistaril). Neonatal depression due to meperidine is effectively reversed by administration of naloxone (see above).

Other analgesic drugs such as codeine, anileridine (Leritine), oxymorphone (Numorphan), and alphaprodine (Nisentil) are less popular, but are acceptable for use during labor. However, Nisentil produces more respiratory depression in the newborn than meperidine when given in equivalent analgesic doses.

ATARACTIC DRUGS

This group of drugs, useful in labor for their tranquilizing, antiemetic, and narcotic potentiating effects, includes phenothiazine derivatives such as promethazine, hydroxyzine, and triflupromazine (Vesprin), as well as the benzodiazepin derivative, diazepam (Valium). The usual intramuscular dosage of the compounds is promethazine 25 to 50 mg, hydroxyzine 50 to 100 mg, triflupromazine 50 to 100 mg, and diazepam 10 to 15 mg. These drugs are known to pass the placenta readily and all have been shown to affect newborn neurobehavioral states. The use of diazepam during late pregnancy and labor is associated with reduction of fetal heart rate base-line variability and neonatal hypotonia. There is no evidence that any of these drugs influence the quality of clinical labor. Their use during labor may reduce the dosage requirements for narcotic analgesics and the concomitant neonatal respiratory depression.

Scopolamine. A belladonna derivative, this drug is used for its amnesic and secretion-inhibiting actions. It is usually given by intramuscular injection of 0.4 mg in combination with meperidine and an ataractic drug. Scopolamine frequently produces restlessness, excitement, and even hallucinations, which may lead to self-inflicted injury if the patient is not carefully attended.

Atropine. A parasympatholytic agent, atropine is similar to scopolamine and is used in similar dosage for its secretion-drying action in preparation for inhalation anethesia. Both atropine and scopolamine readily cross the placenta to produce fetal heart rate tachycardia and loss of base-line variability, which are not inherently harmful to the fetus, but simulate signs of fetal distress which may prompt inappropriate intervention.

INHALATION ANESTHESIA

The use of this technique for normal delivery has become less common as regional anesthetic methods have become more popular. However, inhalation anesthesia remains very useful when there is a need for rapid administration or uterine relaxation. The use of any general anesthetic technique produces the hazard of aspiration of gastric content, leading to maternal death. This risk is greatly reduced by routine administration of antacids during labor (see section on labor management). All gaseous agents readily pass the placenta, and in some cases reach equilibrium more quickly in the fetus than in the mother. Such differences relate in part to factors such as protein-binding sites, lipid content, and solubility coefficients of maternal versus fetal blood. The effective anesthetic concentration of various inhalation agents is approximately 25 percent less in pregnant than in nonpregnant patients.

Nitrous Oxide. A nonflammable, pleasant-smelling, and safe agent, nitrous oxide will produce analgesia when administered in concentrations of 30 to 40 percent with oxygen. It is not effective for surgical anesthesia. Intermittent analgesia for pain with contractions is obtained when the patient takes several deep breaths of a nitrous oxide–oxygen mixture during the early portion of each contraction, then breathes room air between contractions. Nitrous oxide has no effect on uterine activity.

Halothane (Fluothane). This potent agent is useful in producing the uterine relaxation necessary for certain obstetric manipulations. However, at deep surgical levels there is reduced uterine response to oxytocics. Its use for delivery may be complicated by uterine atony and postpartum hemorrhage. In contrast to ethyl ether, halothane is several times more potent, induc-

tion is more rapid, and excessive secretions are not a problem. Halothane readily crosses the placenta and will produce neonatal depression related to time and dose.

Methoxyflurane (Penthrane). A potent, nonflammable, pleasant-smelling agent, methoxyflurane is capable of producing surgical anesthesia and uterine relaxation. It may be employed for analgesia during labor by use of a patient-held inhaler. It is not safe when used for long periods of time due to potential accumulation of inorganic fluorides and nephrotoxicity.

Other Inhalation Agents. Trichloroethylene (Trilene) is a nonflammable agent formerly used for analgesia during labor by administration through a patient-held inhaler. This agent is no longer recommended for use in obstetric patients because frequent neonatal depression follows its use during labor.

Ethyl ether is a flammable agent with a wide margin of safety, but it has several disadvantages when compared with other agents. It is very irritating to the respiratory tract and frequently triggers vomiting with the accompanying risk of aspiration. It is capable of producing excellent uterine relaxation, but induction time is very slow. Neonatal depression is common following ether anesthesia.

Cyclopropane is a flammable agent with a very narrow margin of safety, but the ability to support blood pressure. Its use is associated with cardiac arrhythmias and laryngospasm. Cyclopropane is no longer recommended for use in obstetrics.

INTRAVENOUS HYPNOTIC AGENTS

This group of agents is commonly used for rapid induction of anesthesia in conjunction with inhalation agents. The drugs include thiopental (Pentothal), thiamylal (Surital), and methohexital (Brevital), ultrashort- and short-acting barbiturates. Intravenous injection of these drugs permits rapid induction without stimulation of secretions or vomiting, but they also are respiratory and cardiovascular depressants. They do not produce the uterine relaxation necessary for obstetric manipulations. They may be used in combination with skeletal muscle relaxants, such as succinylcholine (Anectine), in order to produce a very light balanced anesthetic characterized by analgesia, amnesia, and some muscular relaxation.

Ketamine is a nonbarbiturate, rapid-acting hypnotic which does not inhibit laryngeal and pharyngeal reflexes. Side effects include an increase of blood pressure, heart and respiratory rates, salivation, nausea, and vivid but usually pleasant dreams (Little et al.).

REGIONAL TECHNIQUES

By far the most popular form of anesthesia for vaginal delivery, regional anesthetic techniques are also commonly employed for labor analgesia and operative delivery. Nerve block techniques permit the patient to be comfortable while fully conscious. The mother and fetus are generally not as subject to adverse effects of the agents used for regional anesthesia as with systemic drugs or inhalation anesthetic agents. Toxic responses to regional anesthetic agents are most commonly due to direct drug toxicity with high blood levels from rapid absorption or direct intravenous injection. Very rarely, patients develop anaphylactic reactions to these agents. Adequate personnel and equipment for resuscitation should be available before the use of any nerve block technique. The necessary equipment includes a source of oxygen, bag and mask, oral airway, laryngoscope, endotracheal tube, suction apparatus, cardiac defibrillator, and a complete selection of drugs. The proper use of local, pudendal, and paracervical block techniques are easily mastered by the obstetrician, but the proper use of lumbar and caudal epidural blocks requires more specialized training than is usually available except in anesthesiology training programs. The technique of lumbar subarachnoid block is less formidable to perform than epidural techniques, but it should not be used without full cognizance of the potential complications and their proper management.

The objective of regional anesthesia is to block sensory pathways involved with perception of pain during a particular portion of labor. Pain of first-stage labor is mediated predominantly through sympathetic nerves passing through uterine, cervical, and pelvic plexuses, hypogastric nerves and plexus, to the lumbar and lower thoracic sympathetic chain, entering the cord at the 11th and 12th thoracic nerves. To a lesser extent, pain of uterine contractions is mediated over parasympathetics of the pelvic nerve derived from the second, third, and fourth sacral nerves. Thus in first-stage labor, nerve blocks may be effected at the level of the cervical nerves by a paracervical block, or more effectively at the level of the cord by an epidural block. During second-stage labor and delivery, most pain sensation is transmitted by the pudendal nerve from the vagina and vulva through the

ischiorectal fossa and greater sciatic foramen to the second, third, and fourth sacral nerves. A bilateral pudendal nerve block generally provides adequate anesthesia for normal delivery, but a greater degree of comfort during delivery is provided by a block at the level of the spinal cord.

Among the wide variety of local anesthetic agents currently available, there are marked differences in potency, duration of action, and potential toxicity. Agents commonly used for regional anesthesia are lidocaine (Xylocaine), bupivacaine (Marcaine), and 2-chloroprocaine (Nesacaine).

Lumbar Epidural Block. This type of block has gained widespread popularity for obstetric analgesia-anesthesia due to its versatility throughout labor. By use of an indwelling epidural space catheter and intermittent administration of agents with high protein binding or rapid breakdown properties (bupivacaine and 2-chloroprocaine), one may produce a segmental block specific for first- or second-stage labor. The result of epidural analgesia, when properly administered, is excellent relief of discomfort without interference with uterine activity. In preparation for delivery, injection of a larger dose of the agent provides adequate anesthesia for vaginal or transabdominal delivery. From widespread obstetric experience, the use of epidural block anesthesia has been associated with longer second-stage labor and more frequent use of forceps for delivery.

Caudal Epidural Block. This technique may also be used for pain relief during labor, as well as for delivery. The block is administered through the caudal canal where there is some risk of inadvertent injection of the local anesthetic agent into the fetus. Therefore, most anesthesiologists prefer to use the lumbar technique.

Lumbar Subarachnoid Block. This technique involves a single injection of local anesthetic agent shortly before delivery. The resulting anesthetic is appropriate for vaginal or transabdominal delivery; however, if desired, the agent may be directed to a specific level by patient positioning following the injection. Although rarely attained, a block of only the vulva, perineum, and buttocks area is referred to as a "saddle block." Generally the level of anesthesia achieved is up to the tenth thoracic dermatome, or the level of the umbilicus, which produces adequate anesthesia for forceps manipulations and episiotomy repair. The level should extend to the sixth to fourth thoracic dermatome for cesarean section.

The most common complication of epidural and

subarachnoid blocks is the development of maternal hypotension due to the sympathetic block. This problem is minimized by rapid infusion of intravenous fluid prior to the procedure, along with lateral displacement of the uterus to prevent aortocaval compression following the block. Occasional patients develop an unrelenting headache following subarachnoid block as cerebral spinal fluid leaks through the needle wound of the meninges. The use of very small gauge needles for the procedure has nearly eliminated this problem.

Paracervical Block. This technique, also referred to as a "uterosacral block," is useful in first-stage labor during cervix dilatation-related discomfort. It serves to block sensory pathways in the vicinity of the cervix as local anesthetic agent is injected into each lateral vaginal fornix (see Fig. 29–14), using a needle guide that limits the depth of injection to less than 1 cm beneath the vaginal mucosa. An appropriate dose of lidocaine is 5 mL of a 1% solution on each side. The analgesia effect persists for approximately 1 hour. The block may be repeated, but excessive cumulative dosage of the agent must be avoided. Attempts to develop self-retaining catheters in the paracervical area for serial injections have generally failed due to their dislodgment as the cervix dilates and the fetal presenting part descends. The paracervical block technique is easily mastered by the obstetrician, but as with any regional anesthetic technique, there is a possibility of toxicity of the drugs. Paracervical block may be followed by a transient episode of fetal bradycardia (Rogers; Nyirjesy et al.; Shnider, Gildea). The exact mechanism of this fetal response to paracervical block is not known; however, the fetal bradycardia may be due to rapid absorption of the agent in the highly vascular paracervical area, uterine artery vasoconstriction, decreased uterine blood flow, and fetal hypoxia. Freeman and associates have suggested that the agent crosses the placenta to produce

FIGURE 29–14 Technique for paracervical block.

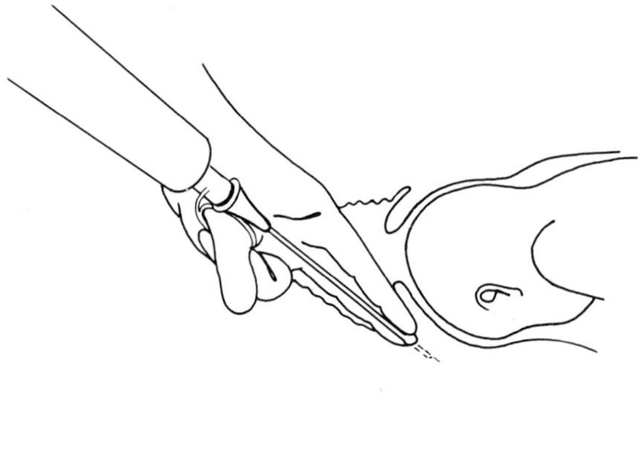

suppression of the fetal sinoatrial node, resulting in a temporary slowing of fetal heart rate. The fetal response usually subsides spontaneously within 10 to 15 minutes.

Pudendal Nerve Block. This is a convenient, simple, and relatively safe technique providing relatively adequate anesthesia for normal vaginal delivery, including most forceps manipulations. It is a technique to be applied by the obstetrician at the time of delivery or somewhat earlier in second-stage labor. One using the technique should be prepared to manage an occasional toxic reaction to the anesthetic agent. Any of the local anesthetic agents are appropriate for this block (see Fig. 29–15). It is readily performed by transvaginal injection of the agent, using a needle guide, to a bilateral site immediately posterior to the tip of each ischial spine. Prior to injection, aspiration which is free of blood assures extravascular injection. When episiotomy is anticipated, pudendal block may be complemented by local perineal infiltration to block branches of the inferior hemorrhoidal nerve.

Local Infiltration. When delivery is imminent and other techniques are impractical, local infiltration of the episiotomy site is useful. The infiltration requires injection of the local anesthetic agent throughout the

FIGURE 29–15 Technique for pudendal nerve block.

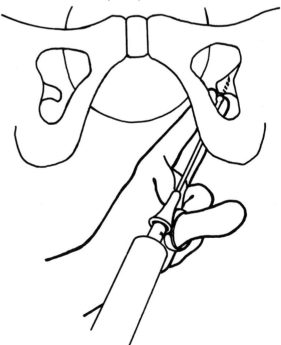

midline or mediolateral episiotomy area through a single skin injection site.

For an excellent review of the fetal and neonatal effects of regional anesthesia in obstetrics, the reader is referred to the article by Ralston and Shnider.

INDUCTION OF LABOR

Induction of labor is the deliberate initiation of labor prior to its spontaneous onset. It may be accomplished by medical administration of an oxytocic drug or by surgical amniotomy, and it is commonly referred to as *elective* or *indicated*. In contrast, the use of an oxytocic drug or amniotomy during labor is referred to as *stimulation of labor.*

Elective induction of labor refers to its initiation by any means when strictly for convenience of the patient and/or physician, and without a medical indication. Advocates of elective induction of labor have suggested it serves to provide optimal use of hospital facilities and personnel and to prevent uncontrolled deliveries. However, any complication of an elective procedure must be considered unacceptable unless there is evidence to indicate the likelihood of a more serious problem without the intervention. In review of 6860 elective inductions, Keettel and associates concluded that 39 of 92 perinatal deaths were primarily due to elective induction. In general, unexpected premature delivery has been the most frequent factor contributing to neonatal deaths following elective induction of labor and elective cesarean section delivery. The application of modern techniques of pregnancy dating would eliminate most of these neonatal deaths. In 1978, the Food and Drug Administration required a change in the labeling for injectable oxytocin which specifically excluded its use for elective induction of labor.

There is a consensus that induction of labor is contraindicated when there is obvious cephalopelvic disproportion, invasive carcinoma of the cervix, uterine scar of cesarean section or other hysterotomy, transverse presentation, or total placenta previa. Relative contraindications include fetal distress, unfavorable conditions of the cervix in a primigravida, high parity, poor application of the presenting part to the cervix, and suspected fetopelvic disproportion. If conditions favor an easy induction of labor, it may be indicated in management of fetal distress, but if cervical conditions are unfavorable, or fetal distress is more severe, optimal results may be obtained by operative delivery. Grand multiparity is generally considered to be a contraindication to induction of labor

due to the risk of uterine rupture; however, in some patients a delay of induction or operative delivery may represent a greater risk.

Indications for induction of labor are strongly influenced by other clinical circumstances. Premature rupture of membranes is generally the most common indication for induction of labor but is strongly influenced by gestation, estimated fetal weight, presence or likelihood of infection, condition of the cervix, and past obstetric history. Fetal jeopardy associated with erythroblastosis fetalis or placental insufficiency states, such as diabetes mellitus or toxemia of pregnancy, must be carefully weighed against the risk of potential prematurity imposed by induction of labor and delivery. Intrauterine fetal death may represent an indication for induction of labor if there is deterioration of the patient's psychologic state or increasing risk of a coagulopathy. Induction of labor for postterm pregnancy is recommended only when the gestation is firmly established and conditions are favorable for induction (see below), or if there is evidence of fetal or placental deterioration (i.e., abnormal fetal heart rate response or falling estriol levels).

The scoring system suggested by Bishop has proved a valid means of evaluating a patient prior to the induction of labor (see Fig. 29–16). A score of zero to 13, based on dilatation, effacement, consistency, and position of the cervix, and on station of the fetal presenting part, indicates increasing ease of inducibility. Friedman and associates subsequently concluded that the prime determinant of the score should be cervical dilatation with little or no influence by position of the cervix. Another method of evaluating patients for ease of induction of labor was suggested by Smyth and was based on the elapsed time until a uterine response occurred during a series of intravenous injections of oxytocin.

Induction of labor may occur following artificial rupture of the membranes, administration of an oxytocic substance, or a combination of the two methods. On occasions, labor will commence after simple manipulation of the membranes by "stripping," when membranes are separated from the small circumferential area within the cervical os by a vaginal examining finger. The mechanism of labor onset after stripping or rupture of membranes has been unclear until recently; however, evidence now suggests that fetal membranes and the adjacent decidua have the capacity for the synthesis of prostaglandins, which in turn are the primary oxytocic substances in control of human parturition. Methods using cathartics, repeated enemas, or drugs like quinine with stimulant effects on muscle other than uterine have been gen-

	Score			
Factor	0	1	2	3
Dilatation, cm	Closed	1–2	3–4	5 or more
Effacement, %	0–30	40–50	60–70	80 or more
Station	−3	−2	−1.0	+1, +2
Consistency	Firm	Medium	Soft	
Position	Posterior	Mid	Anterior	

FIGURE 29–16 Bishop scoring of inducibility of labor.

erally discarded because of their lack of effectiveness and undesirable side effects. Oxytocic drugs in common use at present include synthetic oxytocin, ergonovine (ergometrine), methylergonovine, and prostaglandins $F_{2\alpha}$ and E_2, with many restrictions on their use discussed later in this section.

Amniotomy is an effective method for induction of labor in patients at term with a high inducibility score. In a study by Booth and Kurdyak, 88 percent of patients at term were in active labor within 6 hours of amniotomy. Most would agree that this degree of success is achieved only when patients are close to spontaneous onset of labor. The technique involves perforation of membranes overlying the presenting part and palpable through the cervical os at vaginal examination. It may be accomplished by using a sterile metal or plastic amniotome or a long surgical clamp. Umbilical cord prolapse constitutes a major complication of amniotomy, but there is no convincing evidence that it is related to the timing of amniotomy with or between contractions. Some suggest that amniotomy between contractions is less apt to produce a gush of fluid, sweeping the cord down, while others reason that the fetal presenting part fills the pelvic inlet to prevent cord prolapse during contractions. Following amniotomy, a thorough vaginal examination should seek evidence of cord prolapse, and fetal heart rate should be carefully monitored for evidence of fetal distress. Other complications of amniotomy include subsequent ascending infection of the uterus and fetus, disruption of the placenta, fetal injury, fetal hemorrhage from a vasa previa, and inadvertent preterm induction of labor.

Synthetic Oxytocin

This octapeptide, first synthesized in 1953 by DuVigneaud, Ressler, and Trippett, is the most widely used oxytocic drug for induction of labor. In clinical use of oxytocin, it is important to recognize that patient sensitivity to its oxytocic action varies quite unpredictably. Dose-response studies reported by Cal-

deyro-Barcia and Sereno conclude that the human uterus is more responsive to oxytocin throughout pregnancy than in the nonpregnant state, and the response increases as pregnancy advances to maximum values between 32 and 36 weeks' gestation. The dosage of oxytocin required to successfully induce labor at term is generally in the range of 0.5 to 10 milliunits per minute, intravenously. Overdosage of oxytocin, which may occur at very low infusion rate, produces uterine hypertonus and abnormally frequent contractions. The term *tachysystole* is commonly used to refer to more than five contractions in a 10-minute period. Complications of excessive uterine stimulation include fetal distress, premature separation of the placenta, and uterine rupture.

Studies of Gonzalez-Ponizza and coworkers revealed that when oxytocin is infused intravenously, levels of it in the blood rise during the first 20 minutes and then stabilize. The same authors reported that when the infusion was stopped, the half-life of oxytocin was less than 4 minutes. Thus in use of oxytocin intravenously, it is recommended that the infusion be started at 0.5 milliunit per minute, and be increased by 1-milliunit increments every 20 minutes until labor-like uterine activity is reached. If overstimulation occurs, it generally subsides within a few minutes of stopping the infusion. Control of the intravenous dosage of oxytocin is best achieved by use of an infusion pump. If a pump is not available, dosage of oxytocin may be regulated by controlling the number of drops per minute. If 2.5 units of oxytocin are added to 1000 mL of 5% dextrose in water, each milliliter of solution contains 2.5 milliunits of oxytocin. If the infusion apparatus delivers 1 mL every 15 drops, an infusion rate of 3 drops per minute will deliver 0.5 milliunit of oxytocin per minute. A patient should be constantly observed for evidence of overstimulation during an infusion of oxytocin. Labor monitoring greatly facilitates adequate observation of the patient. As labor progresses, contraction frequency and intensity increase, and the dosage of oxytocin often must be reduced to prevent overstimulation.

Oxytocin may also be given by intramuscular injection, or by absorption through nasal or oral mucosa (Hendricks, 1960; Newman, Hon). When swallowed, it is deactivated in the alimentary canal. Despite their relative convenience over intravenous infusion, these other methods of administration of oxytocin are relatively less safe because of the unpredictable response and lack of control in the event of overstimulation.

Prostaglandins

The prostaglandins are a group of unsaturated hydroxy fatty acids which are present in almost all human tissues and may serve as hormones. It is of considerable interest that they appear in amniotic fluid at the onset of labor (Karim). In human beings and several other mammals, the largest quantity of prostaglandins is found in seminal fluid. It is known that prostaglandins E_1, E_2, $F_{1\alpha}$, and $F_{2\alpha}$ are oxytocic throughout human pregnancy. At present there is no evidence that prostaglandins have any advantage over intravenous oxytocin for induction of labor at term. However, intraamniotic prostaglandin $F_{2\alpha}$ and intravaginal prostaglandin E_2 have proved clinically useful for evacuation of the uterus in early pregnancy (Rutland, Ballard; Anderson, Steege).

ABNORMAL LABOR

DYSFUNCTIONAL LABOR

The terms *dystocia* and *dysfunctional labor* refer to difficult or abnormal labor which may be due to ineffective uterine activity, abnormal presentation or excessive size of the fetus, inadequate pelvic capacity, or a combination of these factors. These etiologic factors of dystocia are easily remembered as the three Ps or "powers, passenger, and passage." The interrelationships of these factors are complex and not fully understood. For example, when relative fetopelvic disproportion exists, the progress of cervical dilatation is often abnormal, despite apparently normal uterine activity as detected by palpation or by intrauterine pressure recording. It is important to recognize that none of the factors is absolute. A patient with a relatively small pelvis may have no difficulty in labor and delivery of a small fetus. Fetopelvic disproportion cannot be finally diagnosed until labor is in progress.

By simultaneously recording myometrial activity at various parts of the uterus, studies of Reynolds (1949, 1954) and Caldeyro-Barcia et al. have permitted our current understanding of uterine physiology and dysfunction. In a normal uterine contraction there is a gradient of diminishing activity from the fundus to the lower uterine segment (see Uterine Contractility above). Uterine dysfunction occurs when contractions are initiated from multiple pacemaker areas producing incoordinate activity, or by contractions originating in the lower uterine segment and sweeping upward to produce a reverse gradient of activity. The effectiveness of labor is also dependent on the frequency and intensity of contractions as well as the degree of uterine relaxation between contractions. Abnormal uterine activity is conveniently described as hypotonic, hypertonic, or incoordinate.

In hypotonic dysfunction, weak and infrequent contractions fail to produce normal labor progress. It may occur at various times in labor, but most often develops in advanced labor, associated with maternal exhaustion. This variety of dysfunction has been referred to as *secondary inertia* of labor. In early labor, hypotonic uterine dysfunction is essentially the same as false labor; however, in occasional patients, prolonged latent-phase labor may be due to hypotonic activity. Generally, hypotonic uterine activity responds well to uterine stimulation by oxytocic drugs.

Hypertonic uterine activity is associated with two varieties of uterine dysfunction. Excessive uterine activity may produce abnormally rapid labor, referred to as precipitate labor. This occurs most often in multiparous patients and is associated with increased fetal morbidity and mortality. There is no specific treatment of this condition. More often, hypertonic uterine activity occurs in early labor, producing unusually painful contractions and poor progress in labor. Studies indicate that these contractions originate in the lower uterine segment and have a reverse gradient of activity. This type of dysfunction has been referred to as *primary uterine inertia*. It responds best to sedation and is often accentuated by oxytocic drugs.

Incoordinate uterine activity is typical of early labor and often persists in mild degree throughout labor. Severe incoordination clinically resembles hypertonic dysfunction with painful contractions but failure of progress. There may be associated uterine hypertonus between the frequent and irregular contractions of this disorder, leading to fetal hypoxia and clinical fetal distress. Incoordinate uterine activity often responds to sedation, analgesia by drugs or regional block techniques, or even by a change in maternal position. Some advocate use of oxytocin stimulation, but most studies indicate that the abnormal pattern is accentuated by this form of treatment.

The most comprehensive study of the clinical features of normal or abnormal labor has been accomplished by Friedman (1967) who has studied labor on a basis of the rate of cervical dilatation. When cervical dilatation is plotted versus time, typical labor progress produces a sigmoid-shaped curve (see Fig. 29–17). The labor graph, as well as clinical labor, can be divided into several well-defined phases. The latent phase extends from the onset of labor to the beginning of the active phase, when the rate of dilatation accelerates from the linear rate of progress during the latent phase. During the latent phase uterine activity gradually becomes more coordinated, there is minimal discomfort, and the cervix effaces with minimal progress of dilatation. The latent phase is generally the most time-consuming portion of labor, lasting approximately 8½ hours in nulliparas and 5 hours in multiparas. The active phase is subdivided into an initial acceleration phase, a linear phase of maximum slope, and the deceleration phase occurring just before second-stage labor. The active phase lasts approximately 5 hours in nulliparas and 2 hours in multiparas. After complete dilatation, second-stage labor lasts approximately 60 minutes in nulliparas and 15 minutes in multiparas.

Dysfunctional labor occurs in various clinical forms which include prolonged latent phase, protracted active phase, secondary arrest of dilatation, and precipitate labor. From Friedman's analysis of labor graphs, *prolonged latent phase* may be defined as longer than 20 hours in nulliparas and longer than 13½ hours in multiparas. It is frequently associated with excessive analgesia, relative cephalopelvic disproportion, and breech presentation. Methods of treatment of prolonged latent phase are difficult to evaluate because the condition may resolve spontaneously despite attempts at treatment. Sedation and analgesia are generally the most successful forms of treatment. Morphine sulfate, 10 to 15 mg intramuscularly, will afford optimal analgesia from painful contractions and permit a period of rest which is frequently followed by active-phase labor. The use of oxytocics or amniotomy in prolonged latent-phase labor is generally less successful. If treatment fails, delivery by cesarean section may become necessary to avoid further prolongation of labor with its attendant fetal and maternal morbidity.

Protracted active phase occurs when the rate of cervical dilatation in the active phase is less than 1.2 cm per hour in nulliparas, and less than 1.5 cm per hour in multiparas. In contrast, the average rate of dilatation during active phase is approximately 3 cm per

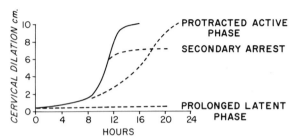

FIGURE 29–17 Labor graph showing the mean cervical dilatation time curve for nulliparas and major labor aberrations. *(After Friedman, 1967.)*

hour for nulliparas and 6 cm per hour for multiparas. This type of dysfunctional labor is associated with relative cephalopelvic disproportion, excessive sedation or analgesia, and conduction anesthesia. Generally the best response to the clinical situation is patience and continued close observation. Amniotomy may be helpful, but oxytocics are usually not, and may produce further deterioration of the patient's condition. Sedation, additional analgesia, or regional anesthesia often further retard the progress of labor, but may be necessary to afford patient comfort. The patient should be given adequate intravenous fluids. Cesarean section may become indicated as a result of deterioration of the maternal or fetal condition.

Secondary arrest of labor occurs when progress of dilatation stops during the active phase of labor. It is most often associated with cephalopelvic disproportion, but may be due to medications or conduction anesthesia. When this pattern is recognized, the patient should be thoroughly evaluated for evidence of cephalopelvic disproportion, and if present, delivered by cesarean section. If there is no evidence of disproportion, treatment by oxytocin stimulation combined with amniotomy is usually successful.

Precipitate labor occurs when there is unusually rapid progress of cervical dilation in labor. This may be defined arbitrarily as rates greater than 10 cm per hour in multiparas or greater than 5 cm per hour in nulliparas. There is a much higher incidence of this dysfunction in multiparas than in nulliparas. It is associated with neurologic damage to the fetus and should be restrained as much as possible by use of conduction anesthesia, avoidance of amniotomy, and carefully controlled delivery.

CEPHALOPELVIC DISPROPORTION

Pelvic contraction refers to a morphologic distortion of the maternal pelvis that will probably be responsible for obstructive labor. It is never absolute, for virtually any pelvis may permit vaginal delivery of a small fetus. The pelvic deformity associated with childhood rickets is rarely encountered at present; however, it was a common pelvic deformity until recent decades. In this deformity there was a marked flattening of the pelvis due mainly to loss of the normal concavity of the sacrum. Currently, pelves with obvious distortion of shape are rarely encountered. Pelvic examination during pregnancy basically gives one an impression of overall size and shape, but rarely suggests absolute contraction. A disparity in the dimensions of the maternal pelvis and fetus is usually not certain prior to observation of clinical progress in labor. It must be remembered that dystocia, or dysfunctional labor, is determined by several factors of which pelvic capacity is but one.

The value of x-ray pelvimetry has recently been subjected to serious reevaluation. The technique, which was formerly widely employed even prior to the onset of labor, generally does not afford clinical evidence of pelvic and fetal relationships that are not readily detected by physical examination. In addition, the increasing general concern for quality of life has focused attention on the potential hazards of diagnostic x-ray. Most authorities agree that there is no entirely safe dose of irradiation. Although ultrasonic techniques now permit detailed evaluation of fetal growth throughout pregnancy, they have not yet proved of value in evaluation of fetopelvic disproportion during labor.

There are many clinical circumstances which suggest the possibility of disproportion between the fetus and maternal pelvis. The classic example is a young primigravida who presents in early labor with the fetal head unengaged. Even when examination reveals apparently normal pelvic capacity and fetal size, any subsequent aberration of normal labor progress strongly suggests disproportion which warrants operative delivery before further deterioration of the clinical situation. If such labors are permitted to continue, there is considerable risk of fetal distress, infection, cord prolapse, lacerations, and a host of other complications. The diagnosis of cephalopelvic disproportion with breech presentation may not become apparent until the fetal head has become hopelessly impaled within the pelvis. If labor is to be permitted with breech presentation, it is imperative that x-ray pelvimetry be used to establish additional evidence of normal pelvic dimensions. Even with adequate pelvic dimensions, the frequency of fetal and maternal complications from vaginal delivery in primigravidas with breech presentation has convinced most obstetricians of the need for cesarean section delivery. X-ray evaluation may occasionally be indicated when it is not otherwise possible to clearly diagnose fetal presentation, but when this becomes necessary, a single exposure will usually suffice. The use of ultrasonic techniques will probably replace any remaining relative indications for x-ray examination during pregnancy.

Fetopelvic disproportion is suggested by abnormal fetal presentation, position, or attitude. Breech and transverse presentations frequently occur when there is obvious pelvic contraction or pelvic tumors distorting pelvic capacity, or when the placenta occupies a position in the lower uterine segment. Although breech, face, and brow presentations are most common with premature labor, they are also associated with pelvic contraction. Lateral deflection of the fetal head, referred to as *asynclitism,* also occurs commonly when there is fetopelvic disproportion. An excessive degree of fetal skull molding or caput succedaneum formation is also suggestive of disproportion.

If labor is permitted to continue despite fetopelvic disproportion, the lower uterine segment becomes progressively longer and thinner, and eventually may rupture. When the ridge on the inner surface of the uterus, referred to as the *physiologic retraction ring,* is higher and more prominent than usual, it is called the *pathologic retracting ring* or Bandl's ring (see Fig. 29–18). The pathologic ring may be evident as an indentation of the uterus and must be differentiated from the hourglass abdominal wall contour caused by the gravid uterus and a distended bladder. Although it may represent a degree of the same abnormality, some have described uterine *constriction rings* as localized thickening of the uterine wall at sites of indentation of the fetal contour. These changes of uterine contour may also occur with protracted labor, especially with prolonged rupture of membranes and in association with intrauterine manipulations.

FIGURE 29–18 Diagram of uterine retraction ring and constriction ring.

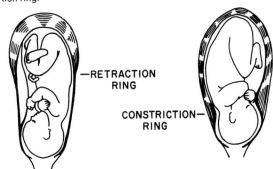

FETAL DISTRESS

The term *fetal distress* implies a condition of fetal jeopardy due to a compromise of the intrauterine environment. In general, fetal distress is produced by a compromise of fetal oxygenation which may vary considerably in its rapidity of onset, severity, and duration. Myers has described experimental models of brain damage in fetal monkeys subjected to partial or total asphyxia. When exposed to total asphyxia, fetal monkeys died within 8 to 10 minutes; however, partial asphyxia over longer periods of time resulted in cerebral cortical lesions similar to the lesions of cerebral palsy in humans. Also working with fetal monkeys, Adamsons and Myers observed that the late deceleration pattern of fetal heart rate developed in response to asphyxia prior to the development of permanent neurologic injury. From our clinical experience in human pregnancy, it is obvious that in most instances of fetal distress, as diagnosed by fetal heart rate patterns, there is no evidence of permanent disability.

Fetal hypoxia may be caused by a variety of fetal, placental, and maternal factors. Of the factors producing fetal distress in labor, the vast majority lead to compromise of placental blood flow. *Placental insufficiency* is a term used to denote a compromise of the functional capacity of the placenta which is typical of diabetes mellitus and hypertensive diseases of pregnancy. Placental function is dramatically disturbed by premature separation of the placenta or rupture of the uterus. The constriction of myometrial vessels during contractions normally produces a temporary disruption of the placental blood flow. The amount of uterine activity that will produce fetal distress depends on all the other fetal, placental, and maternal factors. For example, with placental insufficiency of maternal diabetes mellitus, even mild uterine contractions may produce evidence of fetal distress. On this basis, various functional stress tests may provide early evidence of placental insufficiency. Mild compression of the umbilical cord may produce the variable deceleration pattern; a fetal heart rate response which does not suggest fetal distress but rather a physiologic response to the physical stress. More severe or prolonged compression of the umbilical cord produces fetal hypoxia by compromise of blood flow through the cord. Fetal hypoxia may be due to fetal anemia caused by erythroblastosis, or to the relative maternal hypoxia of anemia or cardiorespiratory distress. Maternal hypotension is a rather common cause of fetal distress which may be due to hypovolemia resulting from hemorrhage, uterine compression of the vena cava occurring in the supine position, or vasodilatation associated with conduction anesthesia.

Diagnosis

In the past, the diagnosis of fetal distress has been vague and tentative, pending further clinical evidence at delivery. The detection of increased fetal movement, fetal heart rate irregularity, or variations above or below arbitrary limits of normal rate frequently did not correlate well with subsequent evidence of fetal compromise. It became quite obvious that intermittent auscultation of fetal heart activity was not an adequate method of diagnosis.

Beginning in 1956, the studies of Hon (1958, 1959, 1960, 1967), Caldeyro-Barcia, and subsequently many others concerning the beat-to-beat fetal heart rate responses to the stresses of labor, led to much of our current understanding of the diagnosis of fetal distress. The promising results of the early studies gave impetus to the development of vastly improved instruments which now permit widespread use of labor monitoring.

This technique affords the clinician continuous information on the ability of the fetus to tolerate the additional stress of labor. The correlation of normal fetal heart rate patterns to good outcome is very high, but the ability of abnormal pattern to predict poor outcome is limited (Schifrin and Dame). In general, the most reliable fetal heart rate sign of developing fetal distress is a loss of base-line variability; however, variability is decreased by most psycholeptic, narcotic analgesic, and sedative drugs, some of which are commonly used in labor. The late deceleration pattern, which represents a response to fetal hypoxia with a contraction, may occur with a number of clinical circumstances which are not related to poor perinatal outcome. For example, this pattern is common when a patient assumes the supine position, in which the gravid uterus compresses the abdominal aorta and vena cava to produce compromise of uteroplacental blood flow. Although the development of late decelerations in this clinical situation suggests fetal distress as a sign of fetal hypoxia, the pattern is easily treated by simply turning the patient to her side. However, when late decelerations are associated with minimal or absent base-line variability, the fetus is usually acidotic, depressed at birth, and does poorly in the neonatal period (Hon et al., 1975). The variable deceleration pattern, which represents a sign of umbilical cord compression, is evidence of potential fetal jeopardy, or fetal distress, yet it is present during second-stage labor in most patients. As with late decelerations, the variable deceleration pattern becomes a more reliable predictor of poor outcome when accompanied by decreased base-line variability. Thus, fetal heart rate patterns are reliable signs of fetal well-being, but they are rather poor predictors of the degree of fetal compromise.

The presence of meconium in amniotic fluid has long been considered a sign of fetal distress. Evidence suggests that hypoxia produces vasoconstriction of the fetal gut which causes hyperperistalsis and sphincter relaxation with passage of meconium. It has also been suggested that vagal activity from cord compression may trigger passage of meconium. Although the presence of meconium in amniotic fluid is associated with increased perinatal mortality, current evidence suggests that the presence of meconium in the amniotic fluid without signs of fetal asphyxia (late decelerations and acidosis) is not a sign of fetal distress and need not be an indication for active intervention. The finding of meconium in amniotic fluid may reflect an earlier hypoxial insult which has resolved spontaneously. Prior to rupture of membranes, an amnioscope placed against the membranes within the cervical os permits detection of meconium in the amniotic fluid (Saling, 1962).

Fetal acidosis develops when there is an accumulation of carbonic acid (respiratory acidosis) with decreased placental exchange, and an accumulation of lactic acid (metabolic acidosis) with anaerobic metabolism of glucose due to hypoxia. The detection of fetal pH and other acid-base data is accomplished by intermittent sampling of fetal scalp blood during labor. Clinical studies (Saling et al., 1967; Beard et al.; Kubli et al.; Wood et al.; Hon et al., 1969; Mendez-Bauer et al.) have established that when fetal pH is below 7.20, there is a high degree of correlation with other signs of fetal distress and with depression of the newborn. Although the fetal pH value may be falsely low due to technical problems or maternal acidosis, the likelihood of a false abnormal (low pH) from this testing procedure is considerably less than the incidence of false-abnormal interpretation of fetal heart rate patterns. Thus, fetal pH determination is a useful method for confirmation of fetal distress suspected from fetal heart rate patterns. The rationale of this approach to fetal diagnosis is further emphasized by the clinical indication that permanent neurologic damage from hypoxia does not occur until after the development of acidosis (Mann). The use of pH monitoring as a primary method of surveillance throughout labor has not been practical due to the potential danger of repetitive scalp wounds for fetal blood sampling. However, a fetal pH electrode for continuous monitoring, developed by Stamm and associates, is currently being tested in the United States (Young et al.).

Management

The management of fetal distress, as diagnosed by fetal heart rate patterns plus fetal acid-base status, is considerably more specific than its diagnosis. The basic actions to be rapidly accomplished are to (1) change maternal position, (2) administer oxygen, (3) decrease uterine activity, (4) correct hypotension if present, and (5) perform a vaginal examination to rule out cord prolapse and determine the status of labor progress. If then the signs of fetal distress do not disappear within 15 to 20 minutes, the fetus should be delivered by the most expeditious and safest method. A change in maternal position from supine to lateral will potentially improve uterine blood supply, relieve supine hypotension, decrease uterine activity, and relieve pressure on the umbilical cord. Administration of oxygen to the patient improves fetal oxygenation and has no known detrimental effects on uteroplacental circulation or fetal status (Khazin et al.). It should be given at a rate of 7 to 10 liters per minute by face mask. The repetitious stress of uterine contractions may be the primary factor producing fetal distress. The fetus will generally benefit from a decrease of uterine activity, which may be accomplished by turning the patient to the lateral position, slowing or stopping the infusion of an oxytocic drug, and possibly the administration of a uterine relaxing agent. Pharmacologic control of uterine activity was first suggested by Caldeyro-Barcia (1969), Poseiro, and co-workers, who successfully inhibited labor in a series of patients with fetal distress using the uterine-inhibiting agent, orciprenaline. After inhibition of labor, fetal acidosis, as detected by periodic scalp sampling, resolved prior to delivery of the patients by cesarean section. At present, there are no compounds available in the United States that are suitable for this potential application; however, several drugs are being tested and may become available in the future. The management of hypotension depends on its etiology, with replacement of whole blood or blood substitutes for hemorrhagic shock, and rapid fluid infusion and lateral displacement of the uterus off the vena cava for hypotension following spinal anesthesia. Vasopressor drugs are initially contraindicated in either circumstance, for they correct hypotension by vasoconstriction of peripheral vessels, including the uterine blood supply, and thus further endanger the fetus. Vasopressors are useful if other treatment fails and hypotension threatens maternal life. While instituting these various actions in response to fetal distress, the appropriate personnel are alerted for possible emergency cesarean section. Vaginal examination should be performed to rule out prolapse of the umbilical cord and determine labor progress. If the cord is palpable, extending through the cervical os, the vaginal examining hand should exert upward pressure on the presenting part until delivery is accomplished by cesarean section. If signs of fetal distress are not corrected within 15 to 20 minutes, the patient is then prepared for an immediate cesarean section delivery, or a vaginal delivery if labor progress permits.

ABNORMAL PRESENTATIONS

BREECH PRESENTATION

This presentation occurs in approximately 3 percent of labors at term but is much more common in earlier pregnancy, with an incidence of about 30 percent at 28 weeks' gestation. Thus, there is a strong association of premature delivery with breech presentation. It is also quite common in multiple pregnancy, with approximately 30 percent incidence of breech presentation of the second twin at delivery.

In early pregnancy there is proportionately more amniotic fluid versus fetal size than in late pregnancy, and the fetus moves freely about in the uterine cavity. In later pregnancy, it is presumed that the fetus normally accommodates itself to the uterine cavity with the larger but less bulky head in the lower segment, and the mobile lower extremities and buttocks in the roomier fundus. Breech presentation is more common if there is distortion of the uterine cavity by a placenta

previa, a lower segment leiomyoma, hydramnios, or relaxation of the uterus in high parity, and if there is relative distortion of fetal shape as in hydrocephalus or multiple pregnancy.

The diagnosis of breech presentation is established on abdominal examination by finding the fetal head in the uterine fundus and the breech in the lower uterine segment. The area in which fetal heart tones are most readily detected is not diagnostic. The diagnosis may be confirmed by palpation of the fetal breech at vaginal examination, or by ultrasonic or x-ray examination. Fetal position is designated by the location of the fetal sacrum in relation to the maternal pelvis (i.e., sacrum left anterior, sacrum right posterior) (see Fig. 29–19). Various fetal attitudes are referred to as *frank* breech when the fetal hips are flexed and the knees are extended with the legs alongside the fetal body, *complete* breech when hips and knees are flexed with feet and buttocks presenting, and *incomplete* breech when one or both feet or knees present below the fetal buttocks. The frank breech attitude is the most common near term.

The most significant feature of breech delivery is the progressively increasing fetal diameters that must negotiate the pelvis. If cephalopelvic disproportion is not diagnosed until the fetal body has been delivered and the head will not descend, the fetal prognosis is extremely grave. In a breech presentation the term *engagement* indicates that the fetal breech has entered the pelvic inlet. The fetal hips descend in one of the oblique diameters of the pelvis until they rotate into the anteroposterior diameter on reaching the pelvic floor. The posterior hip usually delivers first, followed by the anterior hip, legs, and lower body. Next, as the fetal trunk delivers, the fetal shoulders rotate into the anteroposterior diameter for delivery. The fetal head delivers from a flexed attitude with the occi-

FIGURE 29–19 Fetal attitudes in breech presentation.

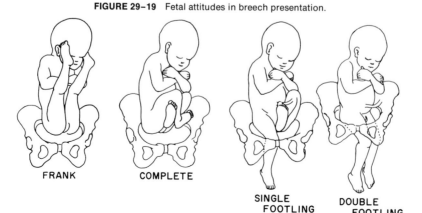

FRANK   COMPLETE   SINGLE FOOTLING   DOUBLE FOOTLING

put anterior and the face delivering across the perineum.

The only methods of avoiding the potential fetal and maternal morbidity associated with breech delivery are antepartum external version or the use of cesarean section. The use of external version for conversion of breech to cephalic presentation is somewhat controversial, and not widely employed in the United States. The procedure is performed in late pregnancy prior to labor, without analgesia or anesthesia, by gentle rotation of the fetal poles to orient the fetal head at the pelvic inlet and the breech in the fundus. The procedure is immediately stopped in the event of patient discomfort that could imply impending uterine rupture. External version is often difficult in primigravidas with their relatively tense abdominal wall, and with frank breech where the fetal legs tend to splint the body. The incidence of uterine rupture with external version appears to be very low. Other complications including premature rupture of membranes, cord prolapse, fetal bradycardia, and placental separation have been reported, but the statistics of their frequency are inconclusive. Critics of the procedure point out that it is frequently followed by reversion to breech, it does not significantly lower the incidence of breech presentation in subsequent labor, and it is an unnecessary risk considering the frequency of spontaneous version.

With the onset of labor in breech presentation, the patient is carefully evaluated to determine the safest mode of delivery. Among factors to be considered are the relative size of the pelvis versus the fetus, fetal attitude, parity, and the gestation of the pregnancy. The aftercoming head does not permit a trial of labor in order to detect possible cephalopelvic disproportion, for the smaller fetal body will deliver through even a very contracted pelvis. Thus, if vaginal delivery is considered, x-ray pelvimetry is performed to establish that pelvic dimensions are average or more. Reasonable limits for minimal acceptable measurements are transverse inlet 11.5 cm, AP (anteroposterior) inlet 10.5 cm, transverse midpelvis 10.0 cm, and AP pelvis 11.5 cm. X-ray pelvimetry films do not permit accurate measurement of the fetal skull, but they do reveal the separation of cranial sutures with hydrocephalus. Measurement of the fetal biparietal diameter is readily accomplished by ultrasonic imaging. Cesarean section delivery is indicated if there is any evidence of possible cephalopelvic disproportion.

The irregular contour of the breech and lower extremities does not fill the pelvis as completely as the fetal head. Thus, the incidence of umbilical cord prolapse is 3 to 4 percent in breech presentation versus about 0.5 percent in cephalic presentations. But because the risk of cord prolapse with frank breech presentation is about comparable to that of cephalic presentation, the incidence is much higher in those with feet presenting (complete and footling). The fetal prognosis with cord prolapse in breech presentation is better than with cephalic presentation, for the irregular presenting part is less apt to severely compress the umbilical cord. The unacceptable fetal risk of cord prolapse in all but frank breech presentations is another reasonable indication for cesarean section delivery.

The attitude of the aftercoming fetal head also influences the judgment of optimal route of delivery in breech presentations. With hyperextension of the aftercoming fetal head by more than 90°, the risk of cervical cord injury during vaginal delivery is as high as 25 percent (Bhagwanani et al.; Abrams et al.; Ballas and Toaff). Some degree of hyperextension occurs in up to 16 percent of breech presentations, but in most instances it is less than 90°. The risk of fetal injury during vaginal delivery with marked hyperextension is a clear indication for cesarean section.

Dysfunctional labor is common with breech presentations, particularly in primigravidae. Augmentation of labor with oxytocin in breech presentations further increases the risk of fetal morbidity (Brenner et al.). Also, many reports of clinical experience have indicated that vaginal delivery of a premature breech presents even more risk of fetal injury than at term. From this and other evidence, many obstetricians conclude that the risk of fetal injury from vaginal delivery in a primigravida or premature breech justifies delivery by cesarean section in early labor.

The incidence of congenital anomalies is approximately 6 percent in breech presenting, in contrast to 2.4 percent in nonbreech presenting fetuses. When diagnosed prior to delivery, only uniformly fatal malformations such as anencephaly should influence the decision for vaginal rather than cesarean section delivery. Zatuchni and Andros described a scoring system to determine the relative risk of vaginal delivery of breech presentations (see Table 29–1). With a possible score of 0 to 11, patients with a score of 3 or less clearly deserve cesarean section delivery.

When vaginal delivery is permitted, the usual method of management is referred to as a *partial or assisted breech extraction*. The fetus is permitted to deliver spontaneously to the level of the umbilicus with support, but with no downward traction of the lower extremities and body. The fetal lower extremities or breech may pass into the vagina prior to com-

TABLE 29-1 Zatuchni-Andros Prognostic Index for Vaginal Delivery in Breech Presentation at Term

	Points		
	0	1	2
Parity	Primigravida	Multipara	—
Gestational age	39 weeks or more	38 weeks	37 weeks or less
Estimated fetal weight	Over 8 lb (3630 g)	7 lb–7 lb 15 oz (3629–3176 g)	Less than 7 lb (3175 g)
Previous term breech	None	1	2 or more
Dilatation (admission)	2 cm	3 cm	4 cm or more
Station (admission)	−3 or higher	−2	−1 or lower

plete cervical dilatation. Awaiting spontaneous delivery to the umbilicus permits time for additional cervical dilatation to accommodate the aftercoming head. If delivery progress is normal, the decomposition of a frank breech should be accompanied only after delivery of most of the body, when the fetal legs may be delivered with ease. With the fetal legs and lower body supported in a towel held by an assistant, the obstetrician should exert gentle downward pressure on the fetal hip, keeping the fetal back in its lateral or oblique position to facilitate descent of the shoulders. No attempt is made to deliver the upper extremity until at least one axilla becomes visible. Generally the posterior presenting arm is easily delivered by inserting a finger over the fetal shoulder to push downward on the anterior surface of the upper arm, thus flexing the elbow and sweeping the arm across the fetal chest until it delivers. The same procedure may then be readily accomplished on the anterior presenting arm. If the fetal arms are extended alongside the head, or are located behind the fetal neck, their delivery may be facilitated by rotation of the fetal trunk toward the back of the arm to be delivered. In this manner, the arm is swept downward and across the fetal chest until it delivers. Often a combination of the two maneuvers most readily accomplishes delivery of the arms. After delivery of the arms, the fetal back should be rotated anteriorly. Regardless of fetal size, delivery of the aftercoming head is generally accomplished with the greatest degree of safety by use of Piper forceps. Prior to their application, the fetal head is guided into the lower pelvis and flexed by gentle suprapubic pressure. The left blade is applied first, followed by the right blade, with the shank of the forceps beneath the towel-supported fetal body. An episiotomy is performed as the perineum starts to distend. Mucus is aspirated from the fetal mouth and nose as soon as they appear across the perineum. The forceps are removed as the head descends through the introitus.

Total breech extraction refers to vaginal delivery of the entire body of fetus by the obstetrician. It substitutes active extraction of the lower extremities and lower body to the umbilicus for spontaneous delivery in partial breech extraction. The success of either form of breech extraction depends on adequate pelvic capacity and cervical dilatation for delivery of the aftercoming head. Attempted delivery through an incompletely dilated cervix frequently produces deep cervical tears and unacceptable fetal morbidity. Total breech extraction is greatly facilitated by inhalation anesthesia producing uterine relaxation. If this is not possible, epidural or subarachnoid regional blocks are generally satisfactory, but pudendal nerve block is inadequate. Total breech extraction is most frequently indicated in delivery of a breech-presenting second twin or when a breech-presenting fetus develops evidence of distress in second-stage labor. In delivery of a complete or incomplete breech by total breech extraction, the obstetrician's entire hand is introduced into the uterus to grasp one or both feet which are pulled downward into the vagina and through the vulva. If only one leg is initially delivered, the obstetrician next reintroduces a hand to grasp the other foot and deliver the leg. In some cases the second foot is not within easy reach because of extension of the fetal knee as in a frank breech. In this circumstance and in frank breech presentation, the fetal foot may be manipulated into reach by pushing the fetal thigh laterally in order to flex the knee and sweep the leg downward across the fetal abdomen (Pinard's maneuver). When this maneuver fails, the frank breech may be pulled downward by flexing a finger in the fetal groin. In this form of delivery the extended fetal legs tend to splint the body, inhibiting the lateral flexion needed for delivery of the body. This may produce a serious problem in delivery of a large fetus, but is generally of no significance in low-birth-weight infants most often encountered in breech deliveries.

The prognosis of breech presentation is generally good for the mother. In contrast, the perinatal death rate is approximately four times that for cephalic presentations, or about 10 to 12 percent. Prematurity is the major factor contributing to this perinatal loss. Other significant factors include birth trauma, prolapse of the umbilical cord, and association with placenta previa. Other serious complications include fractures of the humerus and clavicle produced during manipulations of the arms, brachial plexus palsy due to overstretching the neck, skull or neck fractures, and brain damage due to prolonged asphyxia. As a result of these and other fetal complications, there is a clear trend toward more frequent use of cesarean section delivery to improve fetal prognosis.

TRANSVERSE LIE OR SHOULDER PRESENTATION

This presentation is seen in 0.2 to 0.5 percent of pregnancies at the onset of labor. It usually occurs in conditions that distort the uterine cavity or provide an unusual degree of fetal mobility such as placenta previa, uterine leiomyomas, uterine anomalies, contracted pelvis, multiple pregnancy, hydramnios, premature labor, multiparity, and fetal anomalies. It is encountered most often in multiple pregnancy, occurring in approximately 5 percent of deliveries of second twins. When transverse lie occurs in a primigravida, one should suspect a low-lying placenta or contracted pelvis. It frequently occurs temporarily in earlier pregnancy when fetal mobility is facilitated by the relatively greater proportion of amniotic fluid than at term. *Oblique lie* is a variation of transverse lie in which the long axis of the fetus is more oblique than transverse to the maternal long axis. It occurs most often in association with high parity and usually resolves spontaneously at the onset of labor.

The diagnosis of transverse lie is established by abdominal examination on finding the fetal head in one flank and the breech in the other, and neither fetal pole in the uterine fundus or pelvic inlet. On vaginal examination the presenting part is usually at high station and when palpable may be identified as fetal back, shoulder, or chest wall. In a transverse lie, the fetal scapula (Sc) or acromion (Ac) is arbitrarily used to designate fetal position in relation to the maternal pelvis. The most commonly employed terminology first indicates the side of the maternal uterus in which the fetal head is located as right (R) or left (L), next the landmark acromion (Ac) or scapula (Sc), and finally the orientation of the fetal back as anterior (A),

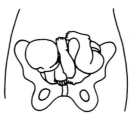
ACROMION RIGHT POSTERIOR

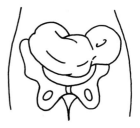
ACROMION LEFT ANTERIOR

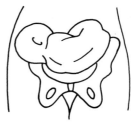
ACROMION RIGHT ANTERIOR

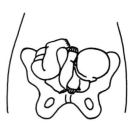
ACROMION LEFT POSTERIOR

FIGURE 29–20 Fetal positions in shoulder presentation.

posterior (P), inferior (I), or superior (S) (see Fig. 29–20).

Vaginal delivery of a fetus in the transverse presentation is mechanically impossible in all but an occasional case of a small fetus in which the head and thorax can simultaneously pass through the pelvis. This situation occurs most often with a macerated, dead fetus. The diagnosis of transverse lie is usually established by abdominal and pelvic examination. When maternal obesity or multiple pregnancy prevents diagnosis by palpation, x-ray or ultrasonic scan techniques may be necessary to substantiate the diagnosis. Any delay in definitive diagnosis and treatment of transverse lie is life-endangering. External version to the cephalic or breech presentation may be attempted if the diagnosis is established in late pregnancy or early labor, prior to rupture of membranes or administration of analgesics. It is generally unsuccessful in primigravidas, but may succeed in multiparas with more abdominal wall relaxation. If version is not successful, preparations should be made for prompt cesarean section delivery. When transverse lie is encountered in the second twin, vaginal delivery is accomplished by *internal podalic version* and complete breech extraction. Internal version is also indicated in the extremely rare situation when initial examination reveals transverse lie, complete cervical dilatation, intact membranes, and an adequate pelvic capacity for vaginal delivery. Internal version, described in management of multiple pregnancy, involves the insertion of the obstetrician's hand into the uterine cavity, relaxed by general anesthesia, to grasp fetal feet and perform a version and breech extraction. Cesarean section delivery is indicated for transverse lie even when the fetus is dead, unless it is quite small and will pass through the pelvis doubled up on itself (*conduplicato corpore*). The procedure of choice is generally a vertical lower segment or classical cesarean section.

When a transverse lie in labor is not promptly delivered by cesarean section, it is referred to as a *neglected transverse lie*. Complications of this situation include umbilical cord prolapse, uterine rupture, infection, fetal death, and maternal death. If transverse lie is diagnosed and properly managed prior to rupture of membranes, the maternal and fetal prognoses are excellent. All fetal and maternal complications dramatically increase following rupture of membranes.

COMPOUND PRESENTATION

This presentation occurs when a fetal extremity prolapses alongside the presenting part so that both enter the pelvic canal simultaneously. The most common variety consists of a fetal arm alongside the head, but rarely involves a fetal leg and head or breech plus upper extremity. The incidence of all varieties is generally less than 0.2 percent. As with other abnormal presentations, compound presentations usually occur with conditions that prevent the fetal presenting part from filling the pelvic inlet, such as

pelvic contraction, small fetal size, uterine or other pelvic tumors, and anterior uterine displacement of high parity. Generally the prognosis is quite good for the mother, but fetal prognosis is poor primarily because of the frequency of prematurity. An attempt to replace the extremity may be complicated by fetal trauma, uterine rupture, intrauterine infection, or cord prolapse. There is no need for interference if labor progress is normal. If labor is abnormal, delivery should be accomplished by cesarean section.

DEFLEXION ATTITUDES OF THE FETAL HEAD

Common in pregnancy prior to the onset of labor, these usually resolve by flexion of the head in early labor. Presentations with increasing degrees of deflexion are designated sincipital, brow, and face (see Fig. 29–21). The etiology of deflexion attitudes is generally factors preventing flexion or favoring extension such as large fetal head, fetal thyroid enlargement, pelvic contraction, anencephaly, placenta or tumor in the lower uterine segment, hydramnios, small fetal size, and uterine displacement associated with multiparity. In general the management of deflexion attitudes consists of careful observation of labor with no interference if there is normal progress. If there is abnormal labor progress or evidence of fetal distress, delivery should usually be accomplished by cesarean section. If the fetus is dead, vaginal delivery may be facilitated by aspiration of cerebrospinal fluid from the ventricles to partially collapse the fetal head. The prognosis for vaginal delivery is improved by low fetal weight.

Sincipital Presentation. This occurs when there is slight deflexion so that the anterior fontanel presents. The occiput is used as a reference point for designation of position. If the fetus is term size and flexion does not occur, the occipitofrontal diameter of ap-

FIGURE 29–21 Deflexion attitudes of fetal head.

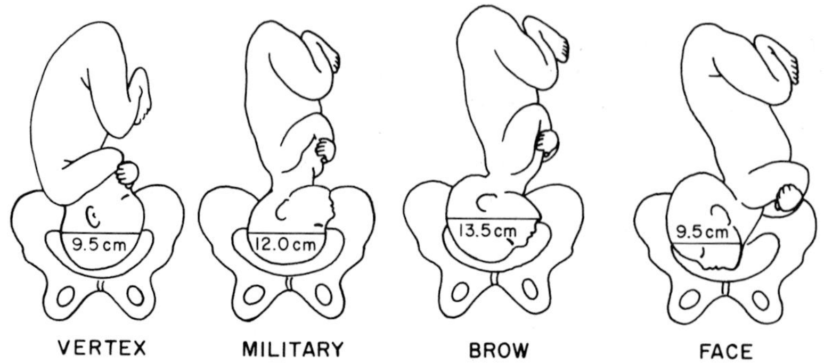

VERTEX   MILITARY   BROW   FACE

proximately 12.0 cm will generally cause cephalopelvic disproportion. In a small fetus this attitude may persist until vaginal delivery.

Brow Presentation. Brow presentation occurs in approximately 0.1 percent of deliveries. The diagnosis is usually established by palpation of the brow, frontal suture, anterior fontanel, and orbital ridges. The brow or bregma is used to designate position. The mechanism of labor depends on fetal size and other factors leading to the deflexion attitude. In a term-size fetus the 13.5-cm occipitomental diameter generally prevents engagement, and flexion or more deflexion to a face presentation is a requisite to further progress of labor. The attitude may persist throughout the labor of a small fetus. Cesarean section delivery is indicated when there is failure of labor progress in a brow presentation. Attempts to convert a brow presentation to vertex or face are often complicated by fetal or maternal trauma and/or by cord prolapse.

Face Presentation. This type of presentation occurs in approximately 0.2 percent of deliveries. Vaginal palpation reveals the facial features which are often quite distorted by edema and may simulate the fetal breech. Position is designated by the orientation of the chin, or mentum. In a face presentation the trachelobregmatic diameter, measuring approximately 9.5 cm in a term fetus, must negotiate the maternal pelvis. This generally occurs without significant obstruction if the fetal chin is anterior, permitting the head to flex as it negotiates the pelvic passage. If the chin is posterior, the fetal head is usually unable to further extend during descent, producing obstructive labor. In about two-thirds of mentum-posterior positions there is spontaneous rotation to mentum-anterior during labor. Thus, the prognosis for vaginal delivery is better in a face presentation than a brow presentation. If fetal size is small, a persistent mentum-posterior may deliver through the vagina.

PERSISTENT OCCIPITOPOSTERIOR POSITION

A potential cause of labor dystocia, particularly in second stage, this presentation persists in approximately 1 to 2 percent of labors. In the remainder of the 10 to 15 percent of patients who start labor with an occipitoposterior position, there is spontaneous rotation to an occipitoanterior position during labor. Persistent posterior position frequently occurs with relative contraction of the midpelvis. The diagnosis is established by palpation of the fetal head topography, locating the posterior fontanel in the posterior

pelvis. Abdominal contour may reflect the fetal position by an indentation of the suprapubic area overlying the fetal chest and abdomen in contrast to the prominence of the shoulders and back in anterior positions of the fetal head. First-stage labor is usually normal with a persistent occipitoposterior position, but second-stage labor tends to be prolonged even when the patient vigorously contracts abdominal wall muscles during contractions. In many cases spontaneous vaginal delivery will eventually occur, but the condition of the mother and fetus may deteriorate during the prolonged labor. If conduction anesthesia prevents voluntary pushing efforts during second-stage labor, spontaneous vaginal delivery is generally not possible. In the majority of cases, the maternal and fetal best interests are served by attempting vaginal delivery after a moderate prolongation of second-stage labor. This arbitrary time limit should be about 30 minutes for a multipara and 90 minutes for a primigravida. After the patient is prepared for delivery, with adequate regional anesthesia, it is often possible to convert the fetal head to an anterior position by manual rotation. If the obstetrician's hand is large, initial use of forceps rotation is preferable. The optimal forceps for this maneuver have minimal or no pelvic curve, e.g., Kielland's forceps (see the section describing forceps below). Rotation generally requires upward movement of the fetal head to facilitate the maneuver and thus produces some risk of fetal and maternal injury. In some patients, vaginal forceps delivery as a persistent posterior will be the least traumatic form of delivery. The posterior position is frequently associated with a mild degree of cephalic deflexion, with the larger diameter requiring a generous episiotomy to avoid lacerations or uncontrolled extension of a smaller episiotomy.

FETAL ABNORMALITIES PRODUCING DYSTOCIA

Of the many abnormalities producing dystocia, the most important are described below.

Excessive Development of the Fetus

This cause of dystocia is usually associated with maternal diabetes mellitus, large size of parents, and multiparity. Fetal weight is directly influenced by maternal weight gain during pregnancy, as well as prepregnancy weight (Eastman, Jackson). There is a tendency for fetal weight to increase with subsequent pregnancies, so that despite previous vaginal deliveries, excessive fetal weight may be a primary cause of dystocia in a multigravida. Prolonged gestation is typically associated with fetal weight loss due to placental insufficiency rather than excessive fetal size. Koff and Potter found the gestational age of large infants similar statistically to those of average weight.

Although the estimation of fetal weight by palpation is quite inaccurate, the ultrasonic measurement of the fetal biparietal diameter has become a useful method for determining fetal head size prior to delivery (Thompson et al.). As with cephalopelvic disproportion primarily due to pelvic contraction, that associated with excessive fetal size may be suspected when in clinical labor the fetal head remains unengaged, with excessive molding and formation of caput succedaneum.

The prognosis is generally rather poor for large infants owing to many factors, including the infant's deterioration during prolonged labor, birth trauma, and the metabolic problems associated with maternal diabetes mellitus. If the latter is diagnosed, preterm delivery is generally indicated to avoid intrauterine fetal death in late pregnancy. In other cases of excessive fetal development, delivery by cesarean section may become necessary to avoid the dangers of labor and attempted vaginal delivery.

Hydrocephalus

The accumulation of excessive cerebrospinal fluid in the cerebral ventricles is termed *hydrocephalus;* it occurs in approximately 0.05 percent of fetuses and accounts for about 10 percent of the major anomalies found at birth. It is frequently associated with spina bifida and other major anomalies. The fetal skull may contain several hundred milliliters of fluid or the condition may be very subtle. The fetus frequently assumes a breech presentation with the large head in the uterine fundus. Hydrocephalus generally produces gross cephalopelvic disproportion.

The diagnosis of hydrocephalus may be obvious by abdominal palpation of the grossly enlarged head, frequently located in the uterine fundus or above the pelvic inlet. The excessive diameter of the fetal head may be confirmed by ultrasonic scan or x-ray; however, there may be difficulty interpreting fetal head size by x-ray in breech presentations where there is considerable variation of distance from the fetal head to the film. X-ray may reveal thin skull bones and widening of the sutures and fontanels to confirm the diagnosis of hydrocephalus. On vaginal examination, the fetal head is generally at very high station, but if palpable, it has widening of sutures and fontanels and a thin indentable cranium. In breech presenta-

tion, the diagnosis may not become obvious until the fetal body has delivered and the head remains above the pelvic inlet. The diagnosis of hydrocephalus should be suspected if spina bifida is encountered in a breech delivery since they often are concomitant malformations.

If appropriate management is not instituted for hydrocephalus, there is considerable danger of uterine rupture and maternal death. Fetal mortality is about 70 percent in even the mildest forms; thus, the treatment is basically aimed at minimizing maternal morbidity and mortality. In most instances, vaginal delivery is preferable to cesarean section. The volume of the fetal head may be reduced by inserting a needle through a fontanel or suture in cephalic presentations, or through the foramen magnum or roof of the mouth in the aftercoming head of a breech. Aspiration of the excessive fluid generally produces a reduction of head size to permit vaginal delivery. An occasional fetus may survive this procedure.

Double Monsters

This anomaly is an extremely rare cause of labor dystocia. Treatment should be directed toward maternal safety as neonatal survival is rare even with atraumatic delivery. As in other forms of multiple pregnancy, labor commonly occurs prior to term, and vaginal delivery may occur without obstruction. If the diagnosis is established in late pregnancy, delivery by cesarean section is generally the treatment of choice.

UMBILICAL CORD PROLAPSE

The incidence of cord prolapse in labor is approximately 0.5 percent, occurring primarily in clinical circumstances where the fetal presenting part does not fill the lower uterine segment during labor or where there is unusual mobility of the cord. It is frequently encountered with breech presentation, multiple pregnancy, hydramnios, transverse lie, small and large fetal weight, premature rupture of membranes, and cephalopelvic disproportion; it is more common in patients of high parity than in primigravidas. The incidence of cord prolapse may be minimized by avoiding artificial rupture of membranes until the fetal presenting part is well applied to the cervix. Cord prolapse occurs after the membranes have ruptured with the umbilical cord prolapsing into the vagina and possibly through the introitus. In contrast, occult prolapse of the cord occurs when the cord is alongside the presenting part, but not through the cervical os, and a cord or funic presentation is present when the cord lies ahead of the presenting part within the intact membranes.

Cord prolapse usually occurs coincident with rupture of membranes; thus it is judicious to perform a vaginal examination immediately after spontaneous rupture of membranes to determine its presence. The diagnosis is established by palpation of the umbilical cord on vaginal examination or by visualization of the cord protruding through the introitus. If labor monitoring is employed at the time of cord prolapse, compression of the cord often leads to fetal distress evidenced by severe variable decelerations, late decelerations, and bradycardia. When fetal death occurs, it may be confirmed by the absence of umbilical cord pulsation. Occult prolapse of the cord is often first diagnosed when the cord is found in the lower uterine segment at cesarean section being performed for fetal distress.

The management of cord prolapse is directed to sustaining fetal life until delivery may be accomplished by the most expeditious method. The only threat to maternal safety in cord prolapse is imposed by the potential actions of the obstetrician. Initially, vaginal examination is performed to determine if pulsations of the cord are present and the status of the presenting part and cervix. If the cord is not pulsating or the fetus is of previable gestation, there is no urgency, and subsequent vaginal delivery may be anticipated. If the fetal presenting part is irregular and poorly applied to the cervical os, as in complete or incomplete breech presentation, there is less urgency for prompt delivery than when it fills the lower uterine segment to compress the cord, as in cephalic or frank breech presentations. Any attempt to replace the cord within the uterine cavity must involve manipulation of the cord and displacement of the presenting part which produce further fetal jeopardy and risk of uterine rupture. Immediate vaginal delivery is indicated if the cervix is fully dilated and the presenting part is engaged. Otherwise, preparations should be made for emergency delivery by cesarean section. Compression of the umbilical cord by the presenting part may be minimized by maintaining upward pressure against the presenting part by vaginal examining fingers and by placing the patient in the knee-chest or Trendelenburg position. If an oxytocic agent is being infused, it should be discontinued to minimize uterine activity. Maternal administration of oxygen by face mask should be started to improve fetal oxygenation. Optimal anesthesia for cesarean section due to cord prolapse should allow rapid induction, adequate oxygenation, and uterine relaxation, and should avoid hypotension. Inhalation anesthesia is generally more suitable than regional block techniques.

The fetal prognosis with cord prolapse is most dependent on presentation, gestational age, and the timing of diagnosis and management. When the fetal presenting part is irregular and high, and if infection does not complicate the situation, the fetus may survive hours or days after prolapse of the cord. In contrast, if there is severe compression of the cord, the fetus may survive for only a few minutes after prolapse of the cord. The perinatal mortality associated with prolapse of the cord is about 25 percent. The high incidence of prematurity with cord prolapse strongly contributes to this rate.

RUPTURE OF THE UTERUS

This very serious complication of pregnancy and labor severely threatens maternal and fetal life. It occurs in about 1 of 1500 pregnancies in the United States, but is more frequent where obstetric care is of poor quality. Rupture of the uterus generally refers to rupture after fetal viability, or 20 weeks' gestation, and does not describe rupture associated with abortion or ectopic pregnancy. It may be spontaneous or traumatic and occur before or during labor.

The most common cause of uterine rupture is a defect of the myometrial wall resulting from a previous cesarean section. When classical cesarean sections were generally employed, there was an incidence of uterine rupture in subsequent pregnancies of about 1 percent prior to labor and 1 percent during labor. With the almost exclusive use of lower-segment cesarean section at present, the incidence of uterine rupture in subsequent pregnancies has been reduced to almost zero prior to labor and to about 0.5 percent during labor. Uterine rupture may also occur in association with uterine scars of previous myomectomy, metroplasty, curettage, or previous rupture, operative deliveries such as forceps rotation or version and extraction, and uterine trauma from contusion or wounds. Approximately 50 percent of cases of uterine rupture during labor are not associated with a uterine scar (Pedowitz, Perell; Delfs, Eastman). Uterine rupture which is not associated with a uterine scar or obstetric manipulations is referred to as spontaneous rupture of an intact uterus. It is generally associated with obstructive labor, excessive uterine activity, or high parity. The use of oxytocic drugs is frequently implicated in production of excessive uterine activity associated with uterine rupture. The threat of uterine rupture is of particular significance when oxytocics are employed in patients of high parity.

The term *uterine rupture* must be differentiated from *uterine dehiscence* or *occult rupture* and *incomplete rupture*. The term uterine rupture implies a complete communication between the uterine and peritoneal cavities which occurs suddenly to produce an obvious clinical picture of pain, shock, and fetal distress as the fetus extrudes into the peritoneal cavity. The terms dehiscence and occult rupture are used synonymously in reference to partial or complete rupture of the uterine wall with at least membranes intact and the fetus remaining in the uterine cavity. With an incomplete rupture, at least the visceral peritoneum remains intact; the tear may be into the broad ligament, and the fetus remains in the uterine cavity. Occult rupture generally occurs gradually and without pain or hemorrhage. It is diagnosed at cesarean section performed for other indications.

The typical clinical picture of uterine rupture in labor consists of severe abdominal pain and a tearing sensation developing during a strong contraction. Labor subsequently stops, but the brief repose is soon replaced by constant abdominal pain, loss of fetal heart activity, and development of shock. Vaginal examination may reveal uterine hemorrhage, upward displacement of the fetal presenting part, and the site of the rupture. There is rapid development of severe hypovolemic shock which may lead to maternal death unless its cause is promptly reversed by appropriate therapy. The diagnosis of complete uterine rupture is essentially self-evident. The major differential diagnosis is premature separation of the placenta (abruptio placentae) which typically produces constant abdominal pain, shock, uterine hemorrhage, and fetal demise, but does not expulse the fetus out of the uterine cavity. Incomplete rupture is diagnosed only when the uterine cavity is carefully examined following delivery.

Treatment of complete uterine rupture consists of immediate laparotomy to control hemorrhage, and treatment of shock by replacement of fluid and blood. Bilateral ligation of the hypogastric arteries is often the most expeditious method of controlling uterine hemorrhage. Hysterectomy is generally indicated, but wound closure may be selected for patients in whom future pregnancy is highly desirable. If occult rupture is diagnosed at cesarean section, the fetus is delivered through the defective area, the wound edges are freshened, and closure of the uterine wall is performed in the usual manner. When incomplete or complete rupture of the uterus is diagnosed by intrauterine examination after vaginal delivery, laparotomy should be performed to repair the uterine wall defect.

The prognosis for the fetus in complete uterine rupture is quite poor with very rare survivals. Maternal mortality following complete rupture varies from 5 percent with prompt treatment to over 50 percent when treatment is delayed. Primarily as a result of the incidence of uterine rupture after cesarean section, and its dismal prognosis, a previous cesarean section is the most common indication for cesarean section in the United States. But there are many centers there and in other parts of the world where patients with previous cesarean section, not for pelvic contraction or other recurrent indications, are delivered vaginally in subsequent pregnancies. In considering the two modes of management, it is clear that even an occasional rupture of a scarred uterus during labor will likely produce worse maternal and perinatal morbidity and mortality than that of repeat cesarean section. The optimal operative conditions which may be achieved for repeat cesarean section are primarily responsible for extremely low maternal morbidity and mortality rates. In the past a major complication of elective repeat cesarean section has been neonatal morbidity due to prematurity. Current utilization of amniotic fluid analysis for evidence of fetal pulmonary maturity, and ultrasonic measurement of the fetal biparietal diameter, promise to improve the accuracy of clinical estimation of fetal maturity prior to elective cesarean section. It must be concluded that optimal patient safety is generally provided by the practice of repeat cesarean section to avoid the risk of uterine rupture.

BLEEDING DISORDERS DURING LABOR

Hemorrhage is a leading cause of maternal morbidity and death during pregnancy and the puerperium. The various conditions associated with vaginal bleeding during the antepartum and postpartum periods are considered in other sections of this book. In this discussion we shall consider the potential causes of vaginal bleeding during labor.

The onset of labor is typically associated with the appearance of blood-tinged vaginal discharge, or "bloody show." Bloody vaginal discharge generally persists throughout labor and often becomes progressively heavier during the phase of active dilatation. It is usually heavier in labor prior to term. The source of this bleeding is primarily the cervix, with some contribution from decidua of the lower uterine segment. It must be differentiated from vaginal bleeding due to complications such as uterine rupture, abruptio placentae, placenta previa, vasa previa, vaginal or cervical erosion or lacerations, laceration of the vaginal septum, carcinoma of the cervix, condyloma acuminatum, vaginal varicosities, or a coagulation disorder. When vaginal bleeding is due to a pathologic source, it is generally heavier than normal and accompanied by other clinical evidence of the disorder. Patients with placenta previa (see Chap. 28) generally have episodic vaginal bleeding prior to the onset of labor, but on occasion the first episode occurs during active labor. The diagnosis should be suspected whenever a patient presents in clinical labor with the fetal presenting part displaced out of the pelvis. The diagnosis is usually confirmed by ultrasonic visualization of the location of the placenta. Digital examination through the cervical os will confirm the diagnosis but usually produces heavier bleeding. Such an examination should only be performed in an operating room with all preparations for immediate cesarean section. Vaginal bleeding that is associated with abruptio placentae (Chap. 30) or uterine rupture is generally accompanied by severe abdominal pain, fetal distress or death, and hypovolemic shock. In uterine rupture the fetus may be expressed from the uterus into the peritoneal cavity so that the presenting part is no longer palpable on vaginal examination. With abruptio placentae the fetus remains within the uterus. Labor stops with uterine rupture, but accelerates following premature separation of the placenta. When the source of bleeding is uncertain, vaginal speculum examination is indicated to permit visualization of the cervix and vagina. If cervical or vaginal lesions are the typical granular-textured, pedunculated lesions of condyloma acuminatum, no specific treatment is indicated until after delivery. When a cervical laceration is found, it probably represents incomplete uterine rupture which should be repaired after delivery by cesarean section. Cervical erosion is the most common source of excessive vaginal bleeding during labor. If a cervical lesion resembles carcinoma, immediate biopsy and histologic examination are indicated to rule out malignancy. When a malignancy is diagnosed, delivery should be accomplished by cesarean section, for maternal progress is worsened by vaginal delivery through the lesion. When a laceration is found in a vaginal septum, further division of the septum may be necessary to facilitate vaginal delivery. In most cases, delivery may occur around the septum. Vaginal varicosities may rupture during labor to produce vaginal bleeding, but the bleeding from them is generally quite minimal. If local sources of vaginal bleeding are not apparent, a coagulation disorder should

be considered and investigated by appropriate hematologic studies, including determination of bleeding and clotting times and fibrinogen level.

A very rare cause of vaginal bleeding in labor is a *vasa previa* in which the source of bleeding is rupture of fetal vessels lying across the cervical os as they pass through the membranes from a velamentous insertion of the cord to the placenta. The vessels may be visible or palpable within the cervical os, but the source of bleeding is usually not discovered until after delivery. When suspected, the fetal source of bleeding may be established by examination of a blood smear showing the frequent nucleated erythrocytes of fetal blood, or by use of the Apt test, which is based on the resistance of fetal hemoglobin to alkali, in contrast to adult blood (Israel). In this test, 2 mL of blood is mixed with 2 mL of water, centrifuged for 2 minutes, then the supernatant is decanted and mixed with one-fifth its volume of 0.25 N sodium hydroxide. If the resulting solution is red, it is fetal blood; if it is yellow-brown, it is maternal blood.

LABOR COMPLICATED BY INFECTION

When labor is complicated by fever, the source is usually found to be intrauterine or urinary tract infection; however, any febrile illness may on occasion occur coincident with labor.

When urinary tract infection becomes clinically evident in labor, there is often a history of similar illness earlier in pregnancy, plus typical symptoms and signs of acute pyelonephritis. Appropriate antibiotic therapy should be instituted after collection of urine for culture and antibiotic sensitivities. At present, ampicillin is generally the drug of choice, for it may be given parenterally, without apparent effects on the fetus, and is usually effective against the offending organisms.

Intrauterine infection develops most often after prolonged rupture of the membranes and presents a major threat to the fetus. When membranes rupture prior to the onset of labor, approximately 80 percent of patients at term develop labor within 24 hours, with a lower incidence of spontaneous labor occurring in earlier pregnancy. In those patients in whom labor does not begin, the incidence of intrauterine infection rises sharply after 24 hours. Lebherz and coworkers reported data of a collaborative study of 25,427 deliveries accomplished at 18 participating naval hospitals. Membranes ruptured prior to the onset of labor in 2934 of these patients. The perinatal mortality rate in patients with premature rupture of membranes was 28 per 1000 in contrast to 16 per 1000 for the 22,493 patients with intact membranes at the onset of labor. Neonatal death was associated with infection in 25 percent of cases with premature rupture of membranes, in contrast to less than 1 percent of cases with intact membranes. These results are supported by general obstetric experience, so that when labor fails to develop within 24 hours after premature rupture of membranes, and the fetus has reached term gestation, induction of labor is usually indicated. However, when the pregnancy is preterm, the obstetrician must weigh the dangers of prematurity against those of intrauterine infection.

The risk of perinatal infection related to premature rupture of membranes has prompted consideration of prophylactic therapy. When intrauterine infection develops, the offending organisms are generally a combination of gram-negative and gram-positive organisms which are normal inhabitants of the vagina. It is not possible to determine clinically if the pathogen was the cause of premature rupture of membranes or invaded the uterus after membranes ruptured. Examination of the placenta and membranes after delivery reveals chorioamnionitis. The affected neonate usually has a severe respiratory infection. The clinical management of patients with premature rupture of membranes includes avoiding vaginal examinations that might introduce pathogens from the vagina into the uterine cavity and induction of labor when it does not develop spontaneously and fetal weight is adequate.

The frequency of rupture of membranes prior to labor and prolonged rupture of membranes during labor, with the related increase of perinatal morbidity and mortality, has prompted evaluations of prophylactic antibiotics. Typical results were obtained in the double-blind study of Lebherz and coworkers, in which the use of tetracycline prior to delivery, plus penicillin and streptomycin given to the newborn, did not lower infant mortality associated with premature rupture of membranes but did significantly lower maternal postpartum morbidity due to endometritis and pyelonephritis. Since the incidence of these infections was not related to the condition of membranes at the onset of labor, the study suggested that prophylactic antibiotics would lower postpartum maternal morbidity regardless of the membrane status. In most clinical circumstances, the relatively low incidence (1 to 2 percent) of postpartum endometritis, and its favorable response to antibiotic therapy, discourages the use of prophylactic antibiotics for maternal indications. If, however, an investigation of maternal fever in labor reveals uterine tenderness and purulent discharge from the cervical os, one should culture the discharge and institute appropriate antibiotic therapy.

PREMATURE LABOR

The incidence of birth weight from 500 to 2500 g is approximately 10 percent of over 3 million annual births in the United States. Low birth weight is the major contributing factor to neonatal morbidity and mortality. There is an alarming incidence of cerebral palsy, mental retardation, and death due to respiratory distress syndrome among infants weighing less than 1500 g at birth. Although medical advances of recent years have led to considerable reduction of maternal morbidity and mortality rates, there has been no significant decrease in the incidence of premature labor or its sequelae.

Despite our growing knowledge of the biophysical mechanisms of labor onset, the pathogenesis is uncertain in approximately 50 percent of premature labors. It is clear that the incidence of premature labor is highest in patients of low socioeconomic status, which may involve factors of nutrition, bacterial flora, coital frequency, multiparity, genetic factors, and inadequate prenatal care (Abramowicz, Kass). In the past, there has been a 10 to 15 percent incidence of low birth weight associated with elective cesarean section or induction of labor. The appropriate use of the techniques of ultrasonic measurement of the fetal biparietal diameter and biochemical studies of amniotic fluid for fetal gestational age should virtually eliminate these iatrogenic factors. Improving prenatal care of all patients will likely reduce the influence of obstetric complications such as toxemia, multiple pregnancy, placenta previa, Rh isoimmunization, urinary tract infection, and incompetent cervix, which are strongly associated with premature labor.

In addition to the potential reduction in the incidence of premature labor by improving prenatal care, recent emphasis has been directed toward identification of a specific method for inhibition of clinical premature labor. There are several inherent problems in such studies. Premature labor is commonly confused with "false labor," or uterine contractility which does not produce progress of labor. The evaluation of any treatment is confused by the influence on "labor" of bed rest or the effect of "treatment" on the psychologic factors associated with the threat of premature labor. The use of specific treatment of premature labor should be tempered by an evaluation of the intrauterine milieu. If conditions are present which are life-endangering to the fetus or mother, termination of pregnancy will be advantageous to both. Such a threat is usually present with abruptio placentae, intrauterine infection, or severe toxemia. However, other conditions may be self-limiting or correctable with appropriate management, so that temporary inhibition of uterine contractility may prevent delivery prior to full term.

Threatened premature labor is often controlled only by bed rest in the lateral position, which promotes maximal blood flow to the uterus. In controlled studies of various drug therapies of premature labor, bed rest alone was effective in about 50 percent of patients (Wesselius-de Casparis et al.; Zlatnik, Fuchs). The most commonly employed drug therapies are the beta-adrenergic agents which produce accumulation of intracellular cyclic adenosine monophosphate to promote cellular relaxation, and intravenous ethanol which is thought to inhibit labor by blocking pituitary release of oxytocin. The interested reader is referred to review articles on this subject (Barden; Zuspan et al.).

PROLONGED GESTATION

It is difficult to compute the incidence of prolonged gestation because of the frequent lack of correlation of presumed gestation with the condition of the cervix, probably resulting from errors of menstrual history. When pregnancy is prolonged, there is danger of either excessive development of the fetus as a cause of dystocia, discussed above, or typical "postmaturity" in which progressive placental dysfunction seriously compromises fetal status. A number of studies of postmaturity have confirmed a significant correlation with increased perinatal mortality (Nesbitt; Walker; Bach; Browne). A typical postmature infant has scant, meconium-stained amniotic fluid, appears malnourished, and has pale, wrinkled, peeling skin, minimal vernix caseosa, long nails, minimal lanugo hair, and long scalp hair. Most obstetricians in the United States consider the typical postmature infant quite rare, and are reluctant to induce labor for prolonged gestation unless the condition of the cervix is favorable. The management of prolonged gestation is based on a careful review of menstrual history and pregnancy events related to gestation (onset of fetal movement or heart tones, previous ultrasonic testing), evaluation of placental function (estriol excretion), fetal maturity (amniotic fluid indices), and signs of fetal condition (antepartum fetal heart rate testing, the finding of meconium in amniotic fluid).

DELIVERY

NORMAL VAGINAL DELIVERY

Spontaneous Delivery

Specific preparations for delivery should be started at a time appropriate to the patient's parity, her labor progress, fetal presentation, labor complications, anesthesia management, and the available facilities. In most obstetric suites, the delivery room is physically separate from the labor room which necessitates movement of the patient prior to final preparations for delivery. Particularly when there are labor complications, the movement of the patient tends to disrupt the continuity of labor monitoring and other patient care. As a result, some obstetric facilities are currently evaluating the efficiency of combination labor and delivery rooms, especially in high-risk patients. If labor progress has been normal, a nullipara should be moved to the delivery room when a small amount of caput, or fetal scalp, becomes visible at the introitus during contractions of second-stage labor. A multiparous patient should be transferred to the delivery room on the basis of her labor progress, when the cervix is 6 to 9 cm dilated, for her second-stage labor may be quite brief. If a multipara is not transferred until she is completely dilated and involuntarily contracting abdominal muscles in a bearing-down effort, there will be very little, if any, time remaining for preparations in the delivery room.

Upon arriving in the delivery room, the patient is moved to the delivery table. If subarachnoid lumbar block anesthesia is to be employed, it is administered as soon as vaginal examination reveals that the patient is ready for delivery with the cervix completely dilated and the fetal head on or near the pelvic floor. Lumbar subarachnoid block is most readily administered with the patient sitting on the delivery table. The lateral decubitus position is preferable if the fetal head is crowning and subject to pressure with the patient sitting. After an appropriate time interval for proper distribution of the anesthetic agent in the cerebrospinal fluid, the patient is placed in the lithotomy position in preparation for delivery. The legs of the anesthetized patient should be placed in the stirrups very carefully to avoid potential nerve injury or other trauma. Fetal heart rate should be checked at frequent intervals throughout the preparations for delivery. Although the lithotomy position is generally used for vaginal delivery in the United States, many obstetric centers in other parts of the world use a lateral position or partial sitting position. The use of the lateral position virtually eliminates the common problem of supine hypotension following spinal anesthesia.

With the patient in position for delivery, her entire vulva, perianal region, and medial thighs are thoroughly scrubbed with surgical soap for an appropriate length of time. Simultaneously the obstetrician and assistants scrub their hands and arms as for a major surgical procedure. All persons in the delivery room should wear face masks and hair coverings. Those who will touch the patient, infant, or instruments also wear sterile gloves and a gown. Sterile drapes are placed over the patient's legs and lower trunk, leaving an opening at the vulva. Although commonly used in the past, catheterization of the bladder is now considered unnecessary and potentially dangerous through introduction of pathogens. A vaginal examination is performed to determine the status of the cervix and fetal presenting part. When pudendal block or local perineal block anesthesia is used, it is administered at this time. Obstetric forceps may then be applied. The technique of their use is considered in a subsequent section of this chapter. For spontaneous vaginal delivery, the obstetrician should then wait until the fetal head almost crowns, distending the vaginal introitus to about 5 to 7 cm during contractions. Fetal heart rate should be checked frequently. In virtually all nulliparous and many multiparous patients, an episiotomy should be performed in order to prevent lacerations and facilitate delivery of the fetal head. Episiotomy techniques are considered in a subsequent section.

To deliver the fetal head, a sterile towel is placed over the obstetrician's hand which is then pressed against the perineal-anal region to exert anterior and downward pressure on the fetal chin in order to promote extension of the head (see Fig. 29–22). The other hand is placed on the fetal occiput to control its descent so that the head gradually slips through the vaginal introitus. This technique of controlling fetal head delivery is referred to as the *modified Ritgen maneuver*. When properly executed, the maneuver protects the fetal head from potential trauma of sudden delivery, as well as favoring delivery of the smallest diameters of the head to prevent maternal lacerations. As the fetal head delivers, the soiled towel used over the anal region is dropped away from the area. The fetal head undergoes external rotation as the shoulders turn into the anteroposterior axis for delivery. A DeLee suction catheter is passed through the nares to the level of the nasopharynx to permit aspiration of any mucus or meconium. Next, the mouth and hypopharynx are aspirated. This simple proce-

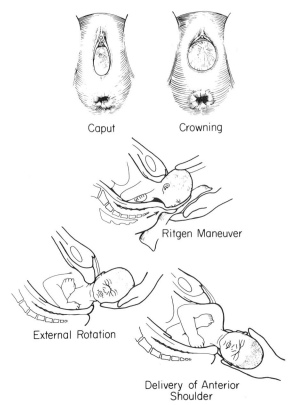

Caput   Crowning

Ritgen Maneuver

External Rotation

Delivery of Anterior
Shoulder

FIGURE 29–22 Assisted vaginal delivery with cephalic presentation.

dure obviates the need for extensive tracheal irrigation if meconium is found in amniotic fluid, and it will reduce the incidence of the life-threatening meconium aspiration syndrome to almost zero (Ting, Brady; Carson et al.). If fetal color is good, the obstetrician should wait for the next contraction, and then gently displace the fetal head posteriorly to facilitate delivery of the anterior shoulder. The fetal head is then held anteriorly to facilitate delivery of the posterior shoulder. Then the remainder of the fetal body is slowly delivered by gentle traction on the shoulders. The time of birth, end of second stage, and beginning of third stage occur as the entire infant delivers. The fetal nose and mouth are again gently aspirated of mucus. If the infant's condition appears good, it may be placed either on the seated obstetrician's lap or on the maternal abdominal wall as the cord is clamped and cut. There is considerable controversy over the optimal management of the infant prior to clamping the cord. The basic problem involves understanding whether there is an advantage for the infant if it receives additional blood from the placenta prior to clamping. Yao and Lind confirmed that the level at which the infant is held in relation to the placenta after delivery determines the volume of blood transferred to the infant. They measured residual blood in the placentae of a series of patients to conclude that about 80 mL of blood is transferred to the infant held at or below the level of the introitus. Others believe that the same transfer of blood may be affected by stripping the cord from the introitus toward the infant. Advocates of these techniques believe that the additional blood protects the infant from anemia and is generally beneficial, while critics are concerned that it may produce hypervolemia, especially in premature infants, and promote hyperbilirubinemia, especially in infants with other conditions producing abnormal levels of bilirubin.

The cord may be clamped or tied by a variety of techniques, none having a particular advantage except the ease of application of the newer plastic clamps. The cord should be clamped about 2 to 3 cm from the infant, leaving an adequate stump for possible umbilical vessel catheterization. The infant is handed to the waiting neonatal attendant for further care. The initial evaluation and resuscitation of the infant are discussed in a subsequent section. A blood sample is collected from the placental end of the umbilical cord for determination of infant serology.

Management of Third Stage

The placental, or third, stage of labor begins when the infant is entirely delivered and ends at delivery of the placenta. It generally lasts only 5 to 10 minutes, but despite its brevity, maternal safety is very dependent on its proper management. If left to spontaneous mechanisms, third-stage labor is frequently complicated by retention of the placenta, uterine hemorrhage, and infection.

The placenta begins to separate from the uterine wall during delivery of the fetus in second-stage labor. As the volume of the uterine cavity decreases, the placenta increases in thickness, buckles, and cleaves from the uterine wall through the decidua spongiosa layer of attachment. As the placenta separates from the uterine wall, there is formation of a retroplacental blood clot which may further promote separation. After the placenta has separated, uterine contractions force it downward into the more flaccid lower segment and vagina, where it generally remains until it is further expressed by pressure over the fundus by contraction of the patient's abdominal muscles, or by the hand of the obstetrician.

Immediately following delivery of the infant, the uterus generally assumes a flattened, or discoidal shape, with the placenta continuing to occupy a portion of the fundal cavity. The uterine contractions of third-stage labor are of greater intensity and similar in frequency to those of late second stage, except when they are inhibited by inhalation anesthetic agents. With contractions, the fundus becomes firm and globular, tending to rise anteriorly. When the placenta separates completely and moves into the lower uterine segment and vagina, the globular shape of the fundus persists between contractions, there is usually a gush of blood from the vagina, and an additional length of cord passes out of the introitus.

The basic management of the third stage consists of effecting delivery of the placenta and secundines by the safest method within a reasonable period of time to avoid complications. As previously noted, lack of action often leads to complications of placental retention, hemorrhage, and infection. Repair of an episiotomy or lacerations should usually be deferred until after delivery of the placenta, for its delivery may disrupt the suture line. After delivery of the infant, the obstetrician's hand is placed gently over uterine fundus in order to detect subsequent contractions and changes of uterine contour. Uterine massage is avoided, for it tends to interfere with the normal mechanism of placental separation and promotes additional bleeding. Unless uterine activity is inhibited by inhalation anesthesia, placental separation occurs during the first or second subsequent contraction. The fundus becomes more prominent and globular as the placenta moves into the lower segment, the cord advances, and there is often a gush of blood escaping into the vagina from behind the separating placenta and membranes. It is usually then possible to express the placenta into the vagina by firm downward pressure on the uterine fundus, in the direction of the pelvic inlet. Care must be taken to avoid trauma to the uterus or adjacent structures by too forceful manipulations. When simple expression fails, delivery of the placenta may be facilitated by holding the umbilical cord taut while using the other hand to push the uterine corpus upward and away from the placenta. As the placenta descends into the vagina, it is easily grasped within the obstetrician's hand and delivered into a shallow basin held at table level (see Fig. 29–23). The aftercoming membranes are gently teased out of the vagina by gradually lowering the basin to permit the weight of the placenta to effect their final separation.

When patients are adequately anesthetized, many obstetricians prefer manual extraction of the placenta to the method of expression. Although some patients are able to tolerate extraction of the placenta

EXPRESSION

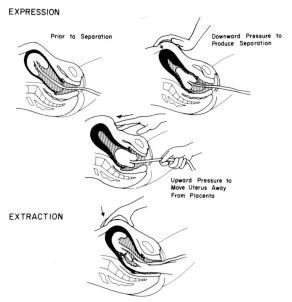

FIGURE 29–23 Delivery of placenta by expression or extraction.

without anesthesia, most require general inhalation or regional spinal block anesthesia. Manual extraction is accomplished by inserting the entire hand into the uterine cavity to grasp and gently pull the placenta downward into the vagina. If the placenta remains attached, separation may be facilitated by placing the hand into the area of attachment and spreading the fingers to complete the separation of the placenta from the decidua spongiosa. After delivery of the placenta, the uterine cavity is explored with the hand, or hand covered by a piece of gauze, in order to locate remaining pieces of membranes or placenta and to detect deformities or lacerations. The major concern with this procedure is the possibility that pathogens will be carried from the vagina into the uterus, or that manual removal of the placenta may produce a laceration. Complications of the procedure are apparently quite rare.

The placenta and membranes should be carefully inspected as soon as they are delivered in order to direct evidence of pathology or missing portions. If there are torn vessels on the fetal surface of the placenta, one should suspect that a succenturiate lobe has been retained. The placental cotyledons should fit together without torn areas. Membranes should appear intact except for the opening through which the infant was delivered. Manual exploration of the uterine cavity should be performed whenever there is suspicion of retained secundines. The placenta is then handed to an assistant who records its weight.

Oxytocic drugs are widely employed in a routine prophylactic manner to minimize maternal blood loss with delivery. Their use is of relatively minimal importance in uncomplicated vaginal delivery. Hemorrhage from the placental site is normally controlled by compression of vessels with closure of spaces between interlacing bundles of myometrium as the uterus contracts after delivery of the placenta. A prompt and sustained postpartum contraction of the uterus may be encouraged by use of drugs such as synthetic oxytocin (Pitocin, Syntocinon), ergonovine maleate (Ergotrate), and methylergonovine (Methergine). Although many obstetricians advocate use of oxytocic drugs during delivery of the infant, intrapartum administration may lead to fetal distress, especially when multiple pregnancy is undiagnosed, or may complicate third-stage labor if the uterus contracts before separation of the placenta. A commonly employed technique of administration consists of 10 units of oxytocin injected intramuscularly at delivery of the placenta. If the uterus does not contract normally during the next few minutes, the uterine cavity is manually explored for retained secundines, and the patient is given ergonovine or methylergonovine, 0.2 mg intramuscularly. If the uterus does not then remain well contracted, oxytocin is given by intravenous infusion of 20 to 50 milliunits per minute as the uterus is gently massaged.

Serious complications may result from injudicious use of oxytocic drugs. Administration of ergonovine and methylergonovine, especially by the intravenous route, commonly produces transient hypertension which may be dangerously additive to existing hypertension. Hendricks and Brenner reported that rapid intravenous injection of oxytocin frequently produces transient hypotension and increased heart rate which may be life-endangering if there is preexisting hypotension due to hemorrhage. Large doses of oxytocin may produce severe antidiuresis which may lead to water intoxication. Massive doses of oxytocin (16,000 milliunits per minute) administered by intravenous infusion produce an initial period of hypotension followed by sustained hypertension (Bieniarz). It is concluded that ergonovine and methylergonovine can safely be used only by intramuscular injection, and oxytocin should be used only by intramuscular injection or slow intravenous infusion.

As soon as the placenta is delivered, and before starting to repair the episiotomy, the entire birth canal should be inspected for lacerations. By manual depression of the posterior vaginal wall, the anterior lip of the cervix becomes visible. It is gently pulled downward by using a ring forceps which is moved laterally to permit inspection of its lateral and posterior aspects. Cervical and vaginal lacerations should be repaired before repair of an episiotomy. At the conclusion of repair of lacerations or episiotomy (see Episiotomy below), it is of particular importance to remove any gauze packing from the vagina and perform a rectal examination to confirm the integrity of the rectal sphincter. If there is any evidence of separation of the rectal sphincter, it should be repaired at this time.

Forceps

Obstetric forceps are instruments used to facilitate delivery of the fetus (see Fig. 29–24). They are generally designed as a pair of interlocking components consisting of blades for application to the fetal head with handles for traction and possible rotation. Each component of the instrument has a blade, shank, lock, and handle. The major exception to the paired design is a single-bladed lifting forceps used in delivery of the fetal head at cesarean section. During the past three centuries, hundreds of varieties of obstetric forceps have been described and usually named for their designers. The most commonly used types of forceps at present are the Simpson's forceps, used for rotation and extraction procedures, the Kielland's forceps, used for rotation procedures, and Piper's forceps, used for delivery of the aftercoming head in breech presentations.

Forceps operations are designated as *low forceps* when application is made to the fetal head in the occiput anterior position on the pelvic floor and *mid forceps* when applied to the fetal head which has engaged, but not yet rotated to occipitoanterior and descended to the pelvic floor. *High forceps* is an obsolete term referring to the application of forceps to the fetal head prior to engagement, a procedure which is never indicated in modern obstetrics. Forceps are currently used in approximately 30 percent of deliveries in the United States. The use of forceps is usually elective in order to minimize the maternal and fetal hazards of longer second-stage labor. The procedure is considered indicated when performed for fetal distress, prolonged second-stage labor, or hemorrhage, or when spontaneous delivery is unlikely because of regional or general anesthesia. The basic prerequisites to forceps delivery in cephalic presentation are complete dilatation of the cervix, engagement of the fetal head, fetal position which permits vaginal delivery, and pelvic dimensions adequate for vaginal delivery. The procedure is facilitated by adequate anesthesia.

The blades of all obstetric forceps are designed to fit the fetal head in the occipitomental diameter.

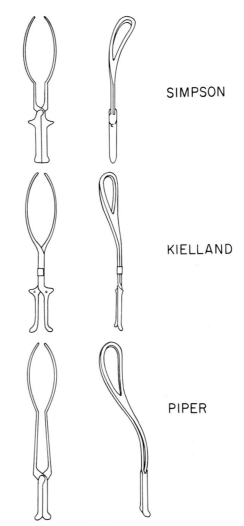

SIMPSON

KIELLAND

PIPER

FIGURE 29–24 Obstetric forceps.

With the exception of the straight shank of rotating forceps, most forceps are designed with a pelvic curve of the shank so that there is a right and left component to the pair. In application of low forceps, the left blade is applied to the left side of the fetal head, positioned in the left side of the maternal pelvis, and gently guided into place by the obstetrician's right hand. The right blade is then applied to the right side of the fetal head so that its shank is superior to the shank of the left, which in most varieties of forceps facilitates interlocking (see Fig. 29–25). Prior to closure of the blades, examination should confirm that the blades are applied in the occipitomental diameter, perpendicular to the plane of the midline, without cervix, fetal extremities, or umbilical cord beneath the blades. The obstetrician should be seated in order to avoid

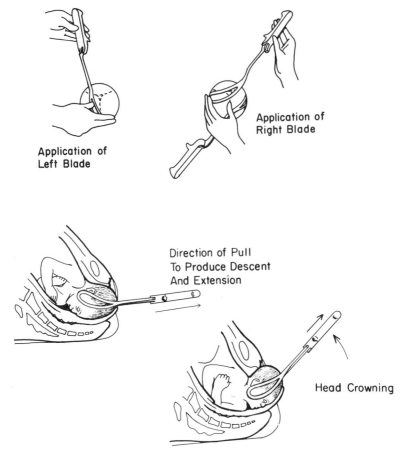

Application of
Left Blade

Application of
Right Blade

Direction of Pull
To Produce Descent
And Extension

Head Crowning

FIGURE 29–25 Application of outlet forceps.

excessive force of traction. With the handles held in one hand, using arm and shoulder muscles only, intermittent traction is applied to simulate the periodic uterine contractions. The force of traction is applied in a horizontal direction until the perineum begins to distend, at which time an episiotomy may be performed when indicated. With further traction and descent the traction is gradually directed upward to facilitate extension of the fetal head. As soon as the head is crowning, the forceps are removed in reverse order of their application, and the infant is delivered as in a spontaneous delivery.

Mid forceps operations are commonly used when fetal descent and rotation are retarded by the patient's inability to use abdominal muscles in second-stage labor after regional anesthesia or to expedite delivery due to fetal or maternal complications. As with outlet forceps, complete dilatation of the cervix is a prerequisite. It is also imperative that position of the fetal head be definitely established prior to appli-

cation of forceps. When diagnosis of fetal position is not clear from palpation of the fetal skull, it is helpful to further insert the examining hand into the posterior pelvis in order to palpate a fetal ear. When the fetal head is in a transverse or anterior oblique position, it is generally advisable to initially insert the posterior blade, being certain that the tip does not cover a portion of cervix. The other branch of the forceps is then inserted into the lateral aspect of the opposite side of the pelvis and gently glided over the surface of the fetal head into proper position opposite the first blade. If Simpson's forceps are used, and if because of the sequence of application in occiput left positions the left blade is now above the right, it is necessary to cross the branches before the lock will properly articulate. The obstetrician, seated, exerts rotary and slightly downward-to-horizontal traction on the forceps, simulating intermittent uterine contractions. The fetal head is rotated to occipitoanterior position and pulled horizontally until it distends the perineum. An episiotomy may be performed before the head is further extended to crowning and delivery.

When it becomes necessary to perform a mid forceps operation on a fetus in an occipitoposterior position, it may be most readily accomplished by delivery of the head as an occipitoposterior, or by rotation to occipitoanterior before delivery. It is often feasible to manually rotate the fetal head to an occipitoanterior position. If this is not possible, it is generally advisable to deliver most infants in the occipitoposterior position. If the size of the fetus and pelvis are likely to produce relative disproportion in delivery of the fetus as an occipitoposterior, delivery may be more readily accomplished by mid forceps rotation. But if the obstetrician lacks experience and skill in this procedure, optimal fetal and maternal safety may be better achieved by cesarean section delivery. For forceps rotation the obstetrician may use either a single or double application technique.

The Kielland's forceps, which lack a pelvic curve in the shank, permit application to the fetal head in a posterior position, rotation to occipitoanterior, and delivery without the need for removal and reapplication. The Simpson's forceps, or similar ones with a pelvic curve, require double application, first for rotation of the fetal head to a transverse position, then removal and reapplication of the forceps for further rotation to occipitoanterior and delivery.

The term "trial forceps" implies an attempt to deliver the fetus when cephalopelvic disproportion is suspected. If a reasonable attempt to accomplish delivery by forceps fails, it is referred to as "failed forceps."

Vacuum Extraction

A vacuum extraction operation consists of traction applied on the fetal head by application of a suction cup to the scalp. The procedure became popular after introduction of the Malmström vacuum extractor in 1954 (Malmström). Subsequent use of the method produced considerable controversy over its relative efficacy and safety. Some advocate its use before complete dilatation of the cervix, but many believe that use of a vacuum extractor in first-stage labor is unsafe. The technique is rarely used in the United States because of numerous reports of its use leading to fetal cephalhematomas, scalp lacerations, intracranial hemorrhage, and retinal hemorrhages (Ahuja et al.; Aqüero, Alvarez; Plauché).

In contrast, advocates of the vacuum extraction technique indicate the ease and comfort of application, which requires less patient cooperation or anes-

thesia and is less apt to produce maternal or fetal injury than forceps operations.

Episiotomy

An episiotomy is an incision of the posterior vaginal wall and a portion of the pudenda which enlarges the vaginal introitus to facilitate delivery and prevent lacerations. It may be made in the midline of the perineum (median) or in an obliqueposterior direction (right or left mediolateral). The incision of a median episiotomy is in the central tendon of the perineal body, while that of a mediolateral episiotomy is through the bulbocavernosus muscle, the superficial transverse perineal muscle, and in some cases involves the lower portion of the bulborectalis muscle.

An episiotomy tends to spare maternal supporting structures, helps to minimize trauma to the fetal head, substitutes a straight incision for an irregular laceration, and generally heals more readily than a traumatic laceration. Most obstetricians agree that an episiotomy should be performed whenever possible in delivery of a primigravida, and is indicated in multiparas unless the vaginal introitus is very patulous. A median episiotomy is usually preferable to the mediolateral type, for it is easier to repair and heals readily with minimal discomfort. The only disadvantage of a median episiotomy is the possibility of third-degree extension through the sphincter ani muscle. This complication is most likely when the perineum is short, the fetal head is large, or with the manipulations of a mid forceps operation. If separation of the rectal sphincter is recognized and properly repaired, there is minimal or no morbidity. Failure to repair the rectal sphincter often leads to anal incontinence and the possibility of a rectovaginal fistula. A mediolateral episiotomy avoids most of the danger of third-degree extension but often is very painful during healing, and may lead to postpartum dyspareunia.

The timing of an episiotomy is important so that it precedes trauma to maternal tissues of the fetus but avoids excessive blood loss before delivery. The incision may be made using scissors or a scalpel. When used in conjunction with forceps delivery, the episiotomy should be performed after the fetal head has begun to distend the perineum and become visible as caput at the introitus. With breech delivery, episiotomy may be performed as the fetal buttocks distend the vulva, but often is not necessary until delivery of the head.

Episiotomy repair should restore anatomy and achieve adequate hemostasis, with a minimum of suture material (see Fig. 29-26). It is preferable to per-

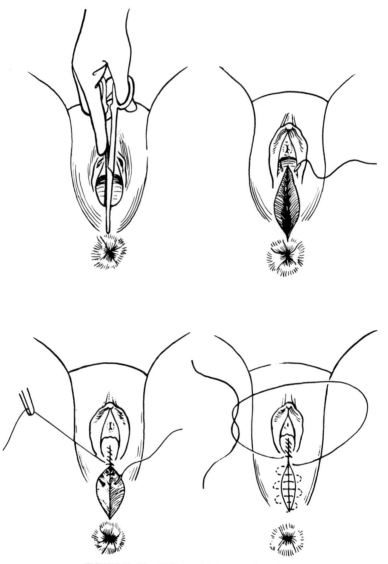

FIGURE 29–26 Midline episiotomy and repair.

form the closure after delivery of the placenta and the possible manual exploration of the cavity, for the manipulations of third-stage labor may disrupt a previous closure. Because there is virtually no tension on the closed wound, most obstetricians use 000 chromic catgut suture on a relatively large atraumatic needle. A commonly employed technique consists of initial closure of the vaginal mucosa, using a continuous suture from the apex to the mucocutaneous junction, leaving the end of the suture untied. Next, the deeper perineal muscles are reapproximated by a series of interrupted sutures. The more superficial layers are closed by a continuous suture leading to subcuticular skin closure ending at the mucocutaneous junction and tied to the end of the vaginal mucosa suture. During the closure, it is helpful in maintaining a dry field to insert a large gauze pack in the vagina. Leaving a tail or portion of the pack outside the vagina helps remind the obstetrician to remove the pack after the repair. With a laceration of the rectal sphincter, the cut ends should be carefully reapproximated using several interrupted sutures. When rectal mucosa is also lacerated, it is closed using a continuous suture starting at the apex of the wound. Many obstetricians prefer to use a submucosal stitch to avoid the possibility of a fistula developing in the site of a suture wound.

The most frequent early complication of an episiotomy is development of a hematoma due to inadequate hemostasis. If recognized within a few hours of repair, the wound may be resutured after evacuation of the hematoma and ligation of the bleeding vessels. When recognition and treatment are delayed, secondary infection often develops in the wound. Optimal treatment then consists of adequate drainage and antibiotics, rather than secondary closure. Blood transfusion may be necessary to replace excessive loss into a hematoma. Postpartum episiotomy pain is usually controlled by analgesics and application of local heat or sitz baths. Infection of an episiotomy wound is a rare complication and responds readily to adequate drainage and appropriate antibiotic therapy.

COMPLICATIONS

Lacerations (See Fig. 29–27)

Injuries of the birth canal due to vaginal delivery may or may not be apparent by examination after delivery. Perineal and vaginal lacerations are quite obvious, cervical and other uterine lacerations may be diagnosed by adequate examination, but damage of the supporting structures of the birth canal are generally not recognized at the time of delivery. The extent of these hidden injuries becomes apparent as evidence of pelvic relaxation appears in future years. Most lacerations are preventable by the use of good obstetric techniques, including the appropriate use of cesarean section, forceps, and episiotomy. Factors which may cause lacerations include excessive fetal size or pelvic inadequacy, abnormal presentations, prolonged labor, obstetric manipulations, and uncontrolled delivery. Some lacerations occur despite every precaution against them.

Perineal lacerations are classified as four types on the basis of their depth. First-degree lacerations involve only perineal skin and vaginal mucosa. In second-degree lacerations there is involvement of the underlying muscles of the perineal body, but not of the sphincter ani. Third-degree lacerations involve the sphincter ani, and fourth-degree lacerations also involve the anterior wall of the rectum. Lacerations may also occur in the labia minora and the enclosed vestibule, especially near the urethral meatus. Perineal and vulvar lacerations should be repaired im-

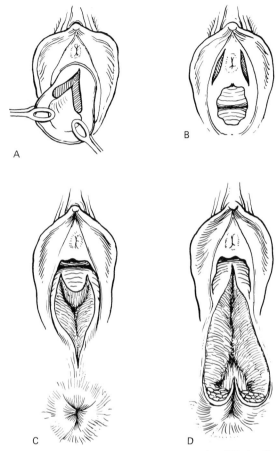

FIGURE 29–27 Lacerations: *A* Cervical laceration. *B* Periurethral laceration. *C* Second-degree perineal laceration. *D* Third-degree perineal laceration.

mediately after delivery of the placenta and inspection of the remainder of the birth canal. As with an episiotomy, the repair should achieve hemostasis and anatomic reconstruction of the area. It is especially important to recognize and repair a laceration of the sphincter ani muscle.

Vaginal and cervical lacerations are diagnosed at vaginal examination, which should routinely follow delivery of the placenta. The cervix may be visualized by gentle downward traction with a ring forceps applied to various segments of its circumference. Visualization for repair is facilitated by use of vaginal wall retractors. Cervical lacerations should be closed with interrupted 000 chromic catgut sutures. Vaginal lacerations are readily closed by a continuous suture. If manual exploration of the uterine cavity reveals a laceration extending through all or most of the wall, exploratory laparotomy should be performed to assess the extent of the injury and to facilitate its further treatment.

Shoulder Dystocia

This condition occurs when the fetal head has delivered but the shoulders will not pass through the pelvic outlet. The complication is generally caused by excessive fetal size rather than pelvic contraction, which usually occurs throughout the pelvis and interferes with descent of the fetal head. Shoulder dystocia frequently occurs with vaginal delivery of large infants of diabetic mothers. Efforts to deliver the shoulders should be started as soon as shoulder dystocia is recognized, for despite a clear airway, the fetus is unable to breathe adequately because of compression of the chest, and umbilical cord circulation is also compromised.

The obstetrician should first attempt to deliver the posterior arm, which, if accomplished, will permit the anterior shoulder to slip beneath the symphysis. It is usually possible to produce flexion of the posterior arm by pushing the upper arm toward the fetal back

until the forearm and hand sweep downward across the fetal chest. Then the hand is grasped and pulled downward to deliver the posterior shoulder. The shoulder girdle then moves posteriorly, and the anterior shoulder moves beneath the symphysis (see Fig. 29–28). If delivery of the posterior shoulder is not possible in this manner, it may be possible to rotate the fetal shoulder girdle 180° so that the posterior shoulder delivers as it is rotated anteriorly and downward in a corkscrew fashion. When other maneuvers have failed, the infant's life may be spared by intentional fracture of one or both clavicles to permit delivery of the shoulder girdle. This is accomplished by the obstetrician inserting a finger beneath the fetal clavicle and forcing an outward fracture to avoid injury to the lung.

Third-Stage Abnormalities

Third-stage labor is usually rather brief, lasting only 5 to 10 minutes. Any complications that develop during this portion of the delivery are generally resolved by expeditious delivery of the placenta, followed by re-

FIGURE 29–28 Maneuvers for shoulder dystocia: *A* Delivery of posterior arm. *B* Rotation of shoulders.

A-I Flexion of Post. Arm

A-2 Delivery of Post. Arm to Permit
Delivery of Ant. Shoulder

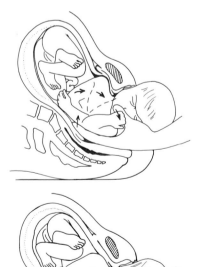

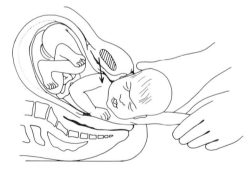

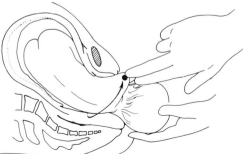

B-I Rotation of Post. Shoulder

B-2 Delivery of Rotated Shoulder

pair of lacerations or of an episiotomy. On rare occasions the placenta fails to separate because of abnormal adherence to the uterine wall. *Placenta accreta* refers to adherence of all or a portion of the placenta to myometrium due to defective decidua which permits direct adherence of trophoblasts to the myometrium. In *placenta increta* chorionic villi penetrate into the myometrium, and in *placenta percreta* they penetrate the entire thickness of the myometrium. The abnormal adherence of the placenta to the uterine wall leads to failure of separation with minimal bleeding. The diagnosis becomes apparent with failure of attempts to manually separate and extract the placenta. The treatment is immediate hysterectomy.

On occasion, the lower uterine segment contracts prior to delivery of the placenta. If there is active bleeding, the placenta should be extracted manually as soon as uterine relaxation is produced by general anesthesia. When hemorrhage does not prompt immediate intervention, attempts to extract the placenta should be continued for 20 to 30 minutes before administration of general anesthesia for manual removal.

Inversion of the uterus is a rare complication of third-stage labor which occurs most often with vigorous attempts to deliver an adherent placenta. The inversion may be complete or incomplete. It usually produces severe pain and shock, but neither may be present. If the complication is recognized promptly and the placenta is not adherent, it may be repositioned with no sequelae. If the placenta is adherent, initial reposition should be followed by hysterectomy after treatment of shock. When the complication occurs after delivery of the placenta, and vaginal replacement is not possible, laparotomy may be necessary in order to incise the constriction ring that prevents reposition. If future pregnancies are not desired and the patient's condition permits, hysterectomy may be the treatment of choice.

Postpartum Hemorrhage

This is usually defined as loss of more than 500 mL of blood during the first 24 hours following delivery. It is a poor definition that should be revised, for studies have indicated that average blood loss at delivery exceeds 500 mL (Pritchard et al.; Newton). A blood loss in excess of 1000 mL would be a more realistic value for hemorrhage. The diagnosis of abnormal loss is further confused by the tendency of obstetricians to grossly underestimate blood loss despite the frequent admixture of blood with amniotic fluid or urine. Unfortunately, there is no practical means of measuring actual blood loss during and after delivery. Odell and Seski reported that the average blood loss from an episiotomy is 253 mL.

Hemorrhage is the primary cause of approximately 15 percent of maternal deaths at childbirth in the United States. Postpartum hemorrhage due to uterine atony is the most common form of life-endangering hemorrhage associated with pregnancy, occurring more often than hemorrhage from abortion, placenta previa, abruptio placentae, ectopic pregnancy, or uterine rupture. In addition to uterine atony, postpartum hemorrhage may occur due to lacerations, retained placental fragments, bleeding from uterine myomata, or coagulation disorders. Postpartum uterine atony is commonly associated with overdistention of the uterus due to a large fetus, multiple pregnancy, or hydramnios, high parity, prolonged labor, rapid delivery, intrauterine manipulations such as internal version, and general anesthesia producing uterine relaxation. The risk of postpartum hemorrhage with multiple pregnancy is particularly high due to the overdistention of the uterus, high parity, and use of general anesthesia and internal version.

Maternal death from postpartum hemorrhage is rarely caused by sudden exsanguination, but generally occurs over a period of several hours. Beecham reported from a series of maternal deaths that the average time from delivery to death from hemorrhage was over 5 hours. Profound shock may develop despite minimal vaginal bleeding when blood accumulates within the uterine cavity, or in the peritoneal cavity. The ultimate effect of hemorrhage is dependent on the patient's general condition and especially her previous blood volume. Her reserve may be seriously depleted by anemia or dehydration. Modern obstetric care should serve to minimize risk and provide prompt recognition and treatment of postpartum hemorrhage.

The diagnosis of postpartum hemorrhage is usually evident by excessive vaginal bleeding leading to signs of impending hypovolemic shock. Uterine atony is apparent by the relaxed condition of the uterine fundus, which should be examined at frequent intervals during the early postpartum period. If bleeding persists, or signs of shock are developing despite a firm fundus, a laceration is the probable source of the bleeding. If the uterus remains atonic following massage and administration of oxytocic drugs, an examination of the uterine cavity is indicated to rule out retained placental fragments or a laceration of the uterine wall. When postpartum hemorrhage is not apparently due to uterine atony, a laceration, or a retained placental fragment, it may be caused by a coagulation disorder. This diagnosis may be confirmed by observation of the clotting and lysis behavior of venous blood.

Optimal obstetric care will decrease the incidence of postpartum hemorrhage very significantly. Maternal anemia should be corrected prior to onset of labor. During labor, adequate hydration should be maintained by administration of intravenous fluids, which is continued for at least 8 to 12 hours postpartum. The blood type of every patient should be known before labor, and when conditions that favor postpartum hemorrhage are present, blood should be crossmatched during labor. Every effort should be made to avoid prolonged labor by careful observation of labor progress and aggressive intervention when it is prolonged. General anesthesia should be avoided whenever possible, and particularly when other conditions favor postpartum hemorrhage. Delivery of the fetus should be performed slowly to permit the uterus to contract firmly over its decreasing contents. Mid forceps operations should be avoided when not clearly indicated. An episiotomy should not be performed earlier than necessary, and its repair should be accomplished as soon as possible after delivery of the placenta. Forceps operations should be performed with skill to avoid unnecessary lacerations. No attempt should be made to deliver the placenta until there is evidence of separation. The placenta should be carefully examined for evidence of missing cotyledons or torn vessels that might have led to a succenturiate lobe. The fetal membranes should also be inspected for any evidence of missing portions. Oxytocic drugs should be administered prophylactically to patients who are likely to experience uterine atony.

A careful examination of the birth canal for lacerations should be performed routinely after delivery of the placenta. Every patient should receive intensive care, comparable to that during labor, for the first 24 hours after delivery. Maternal vital signs, the amount of vaginal bleeding, and the condition of the uterine fundus should be checked every 15 to 30 minutes for the first 8 hours postpartum. If abnormal bleeding persists, the patient should be promptly returned to the delivery room for exploration of the uterine cavity for retained placental fragments or lacerations.

If postpartum hemorrhage is apparently due to uterine atony, oxytocic drugs should be administered if they were not given prophylactically within the previous 15 to 30 minutes. Synthetic oxytocin is given by intravenous infusion of 20 to 50 milliunits a minute. This dosage is comparable to 30 to 75 drops per minute of a solution of 10 units of oxytocin in 1000 mL of 5% dextrose in water. Simultaneously, the patient is given ergonovine or methylergonovine, 0.2 mg intramuscularly. The uterine fundus should be firmly compressed to express contained blood clots and then gently massaged to stimulate a sustained, firm contraction. At the first evidence of postpartum hemorrhage, blood should be crossmatched for possible transfusion. If estimated blood loss exceeds 1000 mL and the situation has not been resolved, the first unit of whole blood should be started as soon as it becomes available. If the uterus remains atonic, the patient should be prepared for immediate exploration of the uterine cavity. Obstetricians generally agree that compression of the uterus is a more effective method for controlling hemorrhage than insertion of an intrauterine pack. The latter tends to prevent firm contraction of the uterus and may encourage further bleeding, as well as frequently leading to intrauterine infection. The uterus may be compressed by either firm compression of the corpus against the back by abdominal wall pressure or bimanual compression between a vaginal fist and the other hand through the abdominal wall. If these measures fail to control hemorrhage, blood transfusion should be continued as the patient is prepared for exploratory laparotomy. In occasional cases, hemorrhage may be controlled only by performing bilateral ligation of hypogastric arteries or hysterectomy.

The term *late postpartum hemorrhage* refers to excessive vaginal bleeding occurring during the puerperium, but after the first 24 hours. It occurs infrequently, and is most often due to retained placental fragments or subinvolution of the placental site. The treatment consists of replacement of whole blood and uterine curettage. Retained placental fragments may have undergone necrosis with deposition of fibrin to form a *placental polyp. Subinvolution of the placental site* is evidenced by microscopic features such as an increase of elastic tissue around thrombosed blood vessels, an increase of fibrous tissue elements, congestion, and edema. Curettage is generally curative, but when it fails, a hysterectomy may be necessary to control uterine hemorrhage.

Amniotic Fluid Embolism

A rare and frequently fatal complication of labor, amniotic fluid embolism is confirmed only by finding amniotic fluid particulate matter in the maternal lungs at postmortem examination. It is not clear how amniotic fluid enters the maternal circulation. The condition occurs most often in a Caucasian, para II or III, at term or slightly past term, with ruptured membranes, in late labor, stimulated by oxytocin, and progressing rapidly (Kistner et al.). The typical clinical course is sudden development of dyspnea, cyanosis, and shock, with death in a few minutes. When death does not occur initially, hypofibrinogenemia usually develops, producing uterine hemorrhage. If the patient recovers, there is no means of establishing the diagnosis. Treatment is usually ineffective, but should include administration of oxygen, digitalization, vasopressors, whole blood, and appropriate treatment of the specific coagulation disorder with clotting factors or heparin.

SPECIAL CONSIDERATIONS

PREMATURITY

Approximately 9 percent of deliveries in the United States involve infants weighing less than 2500 g. In most series, about 15 percent of these low-birth-weight infants die during the neonatal period, with prematurity a major contributing factor in over 75 percent of neonatal deaths. The etiology, prevention, and treatment of premature labor were considered earlier in this chapter under Premature Labor. During labor, analgesic medications which may produce neonatal depression should be used with caution. The use of electronic fetal heart rate monitoring has been found to be of particular value in reducing perinatal mortality of low-birth-weight infants (Paul, Hon). Epidural or other regional block techniques are preferable to systemic medications or general anesthesia. If labor is stimulated with an oxytocic, it should be given with caution to avoid excessive uterine activity that could be injurious to the fetus. At delivery, the fetal head is protected by use of an episiotomy and gentle delivery with low forceps. The cord is promptly clamped to avoid excessive transfusion from the placenta which may be poorly tolerated by the premature cardiovascular and hepatobiliary systems. The premature neonate should be handled very gently and protected from excessive heat loss.

MULTIPLE PREGNANCY

Although about 1 percent of pregnancies are multiple, they are associated with a significantly higher incidence of numerous complications including abnormal presentations, cord prolapse, dysfunctional labor, and postpartum hemorrhage. These pregnancies are frequently complicated by toxemia, which probably combines with the excessive size of the uterine contents, and in some cases hydramnios, to produce the typical onset of labor at about 37 weeks' gestation. Labor should be managed with minimal use of systemic drugs that may produce depression of the neonates, who will generally weigh less than 2500 g each. The presentations of the fetuses should be definitely established early in labor, for in the occasional instance in which the presenting fetus is in a transverse lie, the pregnancy should be delivered by immediate cesarean section. X-ray, or ultrasonic visualization, should be utilized when necessary to diagnose fetal presentations. Because of the frequency of postpartum uterine atony and hemorrhage, blood should be crossmatched for potential transfusion. It is of particular importance to have an intravenous infusion running at delivery. Labor monitoring should be employed as fully as possible, ideally using a separate monitor for each fetus. The occurrence of breech presentation in one or both fetuses in approximately 45 percent of twin pregnancies in labor is probably the major factor contributing to a high incidence of cord prolapse. Patients should be carefully examined for evidence of cord prolapse immediately after rupture of membranes.

Delivery of a multiple pregnancy should be consistent with delivery of any premature infant. Analgesia and anesthesia should permit spontaneous delivery without producing neonatal depression. Elective forceps and episiotomy are used to minimize fetal head trauma. As soon as the first infant is delivered, its cord is doubly clamped and cut. Blood is not permitted to drain from the cord, for there may be transplacental communication with the circulation of the second fetus. Following delivery of the first infant, the presentation of the second should be confirmed by abdominal and vaginal examinations. The heart rate of the second fetus should be checked, and if there is bradycardia, an amniotomy should be performed and followed by a total breech extraction or mid forceps delivery in cephalic presentation. If the fetal heart rate is normal, the obstetrician should wait for the next few uterine contractions to produce further descent of the fetal presenting part. Then the membranes should be ruptured artificially. Delivery may then occur spontaneously, or be easily accomplished by partial breech extraction or by the use of forceps in cephalic presentations. If the second fetus presents as a transverse lie, it is often possible to perform an external version to either a cephalic or breech presentation prior to artificial rupture of membranes and delivery. If this is not possible, the patient should be given a general anesthetic for uterine relaxation, and the fetus should be delivered by internal podalic version and total breech extraction. In multiple pregnancies of three or more fetuses, management of the subsequent infants is merely repetition of the procedures used for the second twin.

Following delivery of the placentas, prophylactic oxytocic drugs should be used to protect against uterine atony. If internal version and extraction were used for delivery, the uterine cavity should be manually explored for evidence of a laceration. Careful gross and microscopic examination of the placentas and membranes may help to establish the zygosity of the infants. Single-ovum twins are confirmed by finding a single amniotic sac that encloses both fetuses, or a septum between the chambers that consists of a double amnion and no chorion. In every instance of double-ovum twins, regardless of the separate or fused relationship of the placentas, each fetus is enclosed in its own membranes composed of an inner amnion and outer chorion. However, the same anatomic conditions may be present in single-ovum twins if there was early division of the egg.

CESAREAN SECTION

Cesarean section is an abdominal hysterotomy for delivery of the infant. In contrast to its previous use as a last resort to save the mother's life, cesarean section has become a method of delivery used for a variety of maternal and fetal indications, with very little more risk than with vaginal delivery. The relative safety of cesarean section has increased dramatically because of improved surgical techniques, methods of anesthesia, blood transfusion procedures, and the availability of antibiotics. At present, maternal mortality following a cesarean section is approximately 0.1 percent, or 10 per 10,000, which is about 20 times that encountered after vaginal delivery. However, maternal deaths following cesarean section are frequently related to life-endangering complications which developed prior to delivery. Despite its relative safety at present, delivery by cesarean section produces maternal morbidity not associated with uncomplicated vaginal delivery. The incidence of cesarean section varies widely among hospitals, but generally is between 10 and 20 percent. During recent years there has been a definite increase in cesarean section delivery for breech presentation and fetal distress.

Cesarean section may be indicated for maternal, fetal, or a combination of factors that produce unacceptable risk for labor and vaginal delivery. At present, in the United States, approximately 30 percent of cesarean sections are performed because of a previous cesarean section scar. The rationale for this practice is to avoid rupture of low-segment scars in about 0.5 percent of these patients during labor, who in turn would experience about 3 percent maternal mortality and 75 percent fetal mortality. Some obstetricians in the United States, and most in other parts of the world, permit at least some patients to deliver vaginally in subsequent pregnancies. The most frequent indication for primary cesarean section is labor dystocia, which includes 35 percent for fetal-pelvic disproportion, 10 percent for fetal malpresentation, and 10 percent for uterine dysfunction. Other less common indications include toxemia, abruptio placentae, placenta previa, fetal distress, prolapsed cord, and carcinoma of the cervix. Many of these factors are interrelated, and quite often several indications are present. There is a definite trend toward more frequent use of cesarean section in breech presentation, particularly in primigravidas. The indications may be quite relative, as in an elderly primigravida, a diabetic, or an Rh-sensitized patient, where vaginal delivery would be preferable, but owing to the condition of the cervix or the status of the fetus, labor would require too much time for optimal safety of the mother and fetus.

There are no absolute contraindications to cesarean section. It is rarely indicated when the fetus is dead or too small for probable survival. Cesarean section should never be used as an elective procedure for the convenience of the patient or the obstetrician. The procedure should not be performed if there are inadequate facilities or personnel, or if the procedure will obviously jeopardize the mother's life.

Cesarean section may be performed through either the thick upper segment or the thin lower segment (see Fig. 29–29). The classical cesarean section, employing a vertical incision through the easily accessible upper segment, was the basic technique employed until it became largely replaced by the lower-segment technique during the past four decades. The classical technique is still useful when the lower segment is poorly developed or covered by dense adhesions, with transverse lie, and in anterior placenta previa. At present the lower uterine segment technique is usually the operation of choice. It is much less subject to rupture in subsequent pregnancies, the wound is easier to repair with less bleeding, and it is routinely covered by peritoneum during closure to prevent adhesions and reduce the incidence of infection. The procedure consists of a transverse incision in the visceral peritoneum just below its firm attachment to the anterior wall of the uterus. The blad-

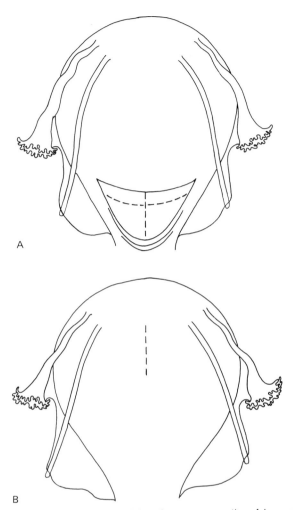

FIGURE 29-29 Uterine incisions for cesarean section: *A* Lower segment. *B* Classical.

der and its reflection of peritoneum are pushed downward to expose the lower uterine segment. A transverse or vertical incision is made through the lower segment, and the fetus is delivered through the wound. Following delivery of the fetus, the placenta and membranes are easily extracted from the uterine cavity. The uterine wound is closed in two layers, and the visceral peritoneum is closed over the uterine wound. The abdominal wound is closed in appropriate layers. An alternate technique, extraperitoneal cesarean section, has been recommended when there is evidence of intrauterine infection (Imig, Perkins). By avoiding the peritoneal cavity. the procedure may serve to reduce postoperative morbidity.

A sterilization procedure by bilateral tubal ligation or bilateral salpingectomy is easily performed in conjunction with cesarean section. Although there is no limitation to the number of pregnancies a patient may deliver by repeat cesarean sections, most obstetricians recommend that sterilization be considered with the third cesarean section. This recommendation is based primarily on the repeated risk of cesarean section delivery in contrast to the same number of pregnancies delivered vaginally. There are no data that indicate a significant increase of uterine rupture or other serious complications with the fourth or subsequent cesarean section. Some obstetricians prefer cesarean hysterectomy to tubal ligation for sterilization. Cesarean hysterectomy involves cesarean section followed by a total hysterectomy; thus, the patient's uterus is removed to eliminate the possibility of future malignancy and other diseases. Critics of the procedure consider as unacceptable the additional blood loss and postoperative morbidity of cesarean hysterectomy in contrast to cesarean section and tubal sterilization.

ALTERNATIVE FORMS OF OBSTETRIC CARE

During recent years, the United States has experienced a growing interest in home or homelike delivery programs. Advocates of home delivery are critical of the overutilization of medications and technology in the hospital environment. They encourage labor with no medications, participation by the father, and intimate contact with the newborn. In general, such programs attempt to exclude patients who are at high risk of complications. Critics of the home birth experience warn that approximately 25 to 30 percent of patients considered low risk prior to labor become high risk by virtue of labor complications (see Hobel et al.). Despite the similarities of philosophy toward childbirth among home birth programs, they tend to differ considerably in screening criteria, qualifications of personnel, and services available in the event of a complication. In response to the growing public interest in homelike delivery, many hospitals have created "birth room" facilities within the hospital. If a complication is recognized during labor, adjacent facilities are immediately available for the appropriate form of emergency care. When feasible, there is little or no technological intervention and the birth room is used for delivery as well as labor, with support and participation by the father, and intimacy of the family after the birth.

Although obstetricians are uniformly in favor of

atraumatic, gentle birth, the concept of "birth without violence," as presented by Leboyer has received considerable attention in the United States during recent years. The technique involves a minimum of light and extraneous noise during the birth, minimal or no suction of mucus, cutting the umbilical cord only after pulsations have stopped, placing the infant on the mother's abdomen for warmth and massage, and finally bathing the infant in warm water. At present there is no valid scientific data that the technique is either beneficial or harmful.

THE NEWBORN

INITIAL EVALUATION AND CARE

The condition of the infant at birth may be anticipated from the status of the mother during pregnancy, as well as events of labor and delivery. Any of a host of maternal, placental, or fetal factors which produce fetal hypoxia and acidosis may be responsible for depression at birth. The effects of some of these factors may be amenable to partial improvement by good obstetric care, but others are essentially unavoidable accidents of pregnancy. Control of maternal glucose metabolism and proper timing of delivery tend to minimize the adverse effects of maternal diabetes mellitus. Other factors such as chronic malnutrition may not respond well during a relatively short period of improved nutrition during pregnancy. Factors such as cord prolapse and abruptio placentae are generally sudden in onset without premonitory signs. However, cord prolapse may occur as a result of artificial rupture of membranes before the fetal presenting part fills the pelvis, or abruptio placentae may occur with injudicious use of oxytocic drugs. Neonatal depression may result from administration of analgesics during labor, or the use of inhalation anesthesia at delivery; avoidance of these factors tends to improve the outlook for the neonate. The most useful measures of fetal condition prior to birth include the reflection of fetal-placental health in maternal estriol excretion, ultrasonic studies of fetal and placental configuration, fetal heart rate characteristics, and data of fetal acid-base status. Despite the many clues afforded by the clinical situation, the ultimate determination of the infant's condition awaits delivery.

As soon as the infant delivers, the obstetrician aspirates mucus from the nasopharyngeal airway, looks for gross malformations, prepares to ligate and cut the umbilical cord, and evaluates the infant's needs for possible resuscitation. The Apgar scoring system is the most widely employed method of initial evaluation (Apgar et al.). By the criteria of heart rate, respiratory effort, muscle tone, reflex irritability, and color, infants are evaluated 1 minute after delivery. Apgar scores of 7 to 10 indicate no depression, 4 to 6, moderate depression, and below 4, severe depression. As soon as the cord is severed, the infant is gently dried, placed in a heat-retaining plastic bag under a radiant-heat source, in Trendelenburg's position, with a slight lateral tilt and moderate head extension. If necessary, the infant's nasopharynx is again gently aspirated with a bulb suction apparatus. Many neonatologists recommend that a nasogastric tube be passed to empty the stomach as prophylaxis against aspiration of stomach contents. Heart rate is monitored at frequent intervals. If the infant's condition continues to be good, nothing further is required, and Apgar scoring is repeated at 5 and 10 minutes.

RESUSCITATION

An understanding of the pathophysiology of depression in the first few minutes of life helps one to appreciate the need for rapid and effective treatment. Hypoventilation quickly leads to cardiovascular depression, leading to slowing of heart rate, which is the most sensitive sign of infant status. In utero, oxygen-rich blood from the placenta reaches the right side of the heart and is predominantly shunted around the vascular bed of the unexpanded lung. At birth, the lung expands; there is a dramatic decrease in pulmonary vascular pressure; oxygen-poor blood arriving in the right heart is oxygenated as it circulates through the lung; and the ductus arteriosus closes as oxygen tension rises. If the lung does not expand, hypoxia develops from inadequate pulmonary oxygenation, the ductus arteriosus remains patent, pulmonary resistance remains abnormally high, and systolic blood pressure falls because of the effects of hypoxia on the myocardium. Anaerobic metabolism quickly leads to metabolic acidosis. which further weakens respiratory and cardiac muscles to compound the problem of depression. The cycle is broken only by producing normal expansion and ventilation of the lungs.

It is imperative that every obstetric unit be properly equipped and provided with trained personnel for infant resuscitation. The necessary equipment should include a worktable on which the infant may be conveniently placed in Trendelenburg's position, with source of radiant heat, suction, oxygen, bag and infant face masks, a supply of infant laryngoscopes, spare batteries, suitable endotracheal tubes, an apparatus to administer intermittent positive pressure ventilation, and a stethoscope. The equipment should be constantly ready for immediate use. There should be a supply of medications such as epinephrine, sodium bicarbonate, 10% calcium gluconate, naloxone (Narcan), Plasmanate (plasma protein fraction, human, a Cutter product), normal saline, and 5% dextrose in water.

If evaluation at 1 minute reveals mild depression, an infant usually responds favorably to gentle stimulation by slaps across the soles of the feet or brief exposure to oxygen by mask. More vigorous stimulation by backslapping or analsphincter dilation is not indicated because they are usually ineffective and may result in trauma or shock. Artificial ventilation and other resuscitation measures are indicated immediately if the heart rate falls below 100 beats per minute, or within a few minutes if the infant fails to respond to gentle stimulation.

Artificial ventilation requires a relatively clear airway. Drainage of fluid from the upper respiratory tract is facilitated by placing the infant on a surface with the head declined about 30° and extended over a rolled towel under the shoulders. Aspiration may be performed using a bulb suction aspirator or a suction trap apparatus operated by the resuscitator rather than mechanical suction. Prolonged or deep suction may produce trauma, bradycardia, laryngospasm, or reflex apnea. The infant's pharynx should be aspirated first, for initial stimulation of the nose may produce reflex inhalation of secretions in the pharynx. The catheter should also be gently passed into the stomach to empty it of fluid that might be regurgitated and aspirated, as well as to check for patency of the esophagus. Normal respiratory activity may be stimulated by these manipulations of the infant, obviating the need for mechanical ventilation. If it is not possible to establish a clear airway by suction, and in every case of meconium-contaminated amniotic fluid that the fetus might have inspired, the trachea should be aspirated under direct visualization through a laryngoscope.

If the infant is moderately depressed with Apgar score of 4 to 6 at 1 minute, and with heart rate over 80 beats per minute, ventilation should be performed using a bag and mask apparatus for intermittent positive pressure insufflation. An oropharyngeal airway may be helpful in preventing obstruction of the airway by the infant's tongue. The bag and mask devices

(Ambu, Penlon, Hope, Kreiselman, or Emerson) permit control of pressure and volume of insufflated gas. They consist of a mask, a nonrebreathing valve, and a self-inflating bag. Some are equipped with a pressure gauge. When connected to a source of 100 percent oxygen, they deliver a high percentage of oxygen to the infant. In use of the face mask, it is important to avoid occluding the airway while supporting the infant's mandible with the fingers. The initial inflating pressure should be just enough to cause the infant's upper chest to rise gently. In the first few respirations, the pressure required to overcome resistance of the respiratory tract may exceed 50 cm of water pressure, while subsequent expansions require 5 to 15 cm of water pressure. The value is more of academic than clinical interest, for the pressure of each insufflation should produce only a mild movement of the chest. Each insufflation is maintained for 1 to 2 seconds, with intervals of expiration of similar length by recoil of the elastic chest wall.

The effectiveness of the artificial ventilation is assessed by observation of chest movements and by auscultation of breath sounds. If the infant is probably depressed by a narcotic analgesic given to the mother during labor, the infant should be given the narcotic antagonist, naloxone (Narcan), 0.1 mg intravenously or 0.2 mg intramuscularly. This treatment is of no value if depression is due to barbiturates. If meperidine or morphine was administered to the mother in labor, the peak activity occurs about $1\frac{1}{2}$ hours after intravenous, and 3 hours after intramuscular, administration. When depression has not improved within 2 minutes after starting artificial ventilation, the infant may benefit from administering 0.5 mL of epinephrine, 1:10,000, into the umbilical vein or injected at the base of the tongue. Depression may be caused by magnesium sulfate used in treatment of toxemia. An effective antidote is 10% calcium gluconate. If ventilation by bag and mask is continued for more than 3 or 4 minutes, the infant's stomach often fills with air, preventing full expansion of the lungs by pressure against the diaphragm. The stomach should again be emptied by insertion of a nasogastric tube.

Endotracheal intubation is indicated immediately when evaluation of the infant at 1 minute reveals severe depression, or whenever it is not possible to maintain a clear airway by other methods. The most important element in success of the procedure is proper positioning of the infant (see Fig. 29–30). The air passages are aligned by placing a folded towel under the infant's shoulders, producing moderate extension of the infant's neck. The head is held steady by the right hand as the laryngoscope, held in the left

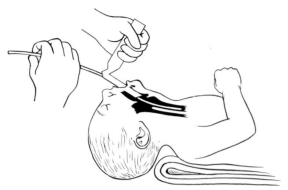

FIGURE 29–30 Endotracheal suction through a laryngoscope.

hand, is introduced at the right corner of the mouth. As it is advanced, it is moved toward the midline, pushing the tongue to the left of the blade. It is advanced until the tip of the blade is between the base of the tongue and the epiglottis. The glottis is seen as a vertical dark slit, just anterior to the pink arytenoid cartilages. Meconium or thick mucus should be gently aspirated from the area. An endotracheal tube is gently inserted through the cords and the laryngoscope is withdrawn. Artificial ventilation through the endotracheal tube is started immediately. If it is properly placed, breath sounds are heard in both lungs, with minimal sound over the stomach. The endotracheal tube should be removed after the infant begins to breath spontaneously, the heart rate is over 100 beats per minute, and the infant's color is normal.

Cardiac massage is indicated immediately when there is no heart rate at birth or when cardiac arrest occurs during resuscitation. It should be started only after the lungs have been initially expanded. Cardiac massage is performed by vigorous compression of the midsternum with both thumbs at a rate of 100 to 120 beats per minute. Combined with artificial ventilation, it is performed alternately, three heart beats to one insufflation. Cardiac massage should be stopped briefly every 30 seconds for evidence of spontaneous activity of the heart. Intracardiac injection of medications is not indicated because of ineffectiveness and potential trauma.

When resuscitative measures have included the need for endotracheal intubation, cardiac massage, the administration of epinephrine and Plasmanate, it must be presumed that severe acidosis is present. After confirmation of its presence, acidosis is treated by sodium bicarbonate, 2 to 3 meq/kg, diluted in an equal volume of water, infused slowly through the umbilical vein. Correction of acidosis increases myocardial responsiveness to sympathetic amines, de-

creases pulmonary vascular resistance, and shifts the oxygen dissociation curve back to the left.

The infant is transferred to the nursery as soon as breathing is well established, where, if necessary, ventilation is continued by a mechanical ventilator. The orotracheal tube may be replaced by a nasotracheal tube for convenience in care of the infant. Further care is greatly facilitated by insertion of a catheter in the umbilical vein or artery. Use of the artery permits monitoring of blood pressure and blood gases, while use of the vein is easier technically and permits more rapid distribution of drugs. Administration of plasma expanders should be considered if the infant appears pale, has tachycardia, or is hypotensive. Blood pressure below 50/30 is significant hypotension in a term infant. Shock may be treated with Plasmanate, 10 mL/kg intravenously.

FURTHER EVALUATION AND CARE

Care of Eyes

There is a general consensus that every infant's eyes should be treated prophylactically against gonorrheal ophthalmia, a potential cause of blindness. The original description of this treatment by Crede in 1884 is still commonly employed with instillation of a drop of 1% silver nitrate solution in each eye. It is performed immediately after ligation and section of the umbilical cord, or during the subsequent delivery-room care of the infant. The use of silver nitrate solution commonly produces a chemical conjunctivitis, but no permanent damage to the eyes. The incidence of conjunctivitis may be decreased somewhat by flushing the eyes with saline after 2 minutes. Many prefer to use penicillin or tetracycline ointment, which do not produce conjunctivitis as commonly, but may induce drug sensitivity. The use of silver nitrate is required by law in a number of states.

Identification

A complete system of identification of each infant should be completed before transfer from the delivery room to the nursery. The primary method of identification consists of a wrist or ankle band on which is written the mother's full name, the infant's sex, and the time and date of delivery. The band is attached around the infant's extremity by a secure clip or rivet. The use of lettered beads for identification is more apt to lead to confusion due to similar or identical names of mothers. Most obstetric units also use a system of maternal fingerprints and infant footprints, which are often required by existing laws. The value of dermatoglyphics rests on the quality of the prints, which varies considerably among personnel.

Physical Examination

An initial physical examination of the infant in the delivery room should determine general cardiorespiratory status, neuromuscular responsiveness, apparent sex, and presence of gross anomalies or injuries. Weighing the infant in the delivery room or on admission to the nursery, permits anticipation of related morbidity, calculation of drug dosages, and compilation of statistics related to birth weight. Traditionally infants weighing less than 2501 g have been considered *premature,* while those weighing more than 2500 g have been categorized as *term.* In recent years there has been widespread use of gestational age scoring, based on a variety of neuromuscular and physical maturity criteria (Farr et al.; Ghosh, Daga; Amiel-Tison; Dubowitz et al.) (see Fig. 29–31). From this experience it is clear that prematurity is more accurately determined by gestational age less than 38 weeks than it is by birth weight under 2501 g. It is estimated that approximately one-third of infants weighing less than 2501 g at birth have gestational age of 38 weeks or more. At any given weight, these "small for dates" infants are at less risk than infants of premature gestational age, but their postnatal development is retarded for several years in contrast to infants of appropriate weight for gestational age (Paton, Fisher; Babson, Benson).

In addition to its use for gestational age scoring, a thorough physical examination of the infant is performed as soon as feasible after birth in order to detect the presence of more subtle anomalies which may require subsequent treatment. The parents of the infant should be promptly informed of any abnormal findings and their probable significance. The general appearance of infants varies by gestational age, but physical findings that are generally consistent among normal newborns during the first hour of life include some degree of cyanosis of the lower extremities, possible discoloration and edema of the presenting part, a flat but open anterior fontanel, ears properly placed, lack of sternal or intercostal retraction with respirations, bilateral breath sounds, heart rate often higher than during labor, patent nares, esophagus, and anus, liver palpable 1 to 3 cm beneath the costal margin, and movement of all extremities. It is of utmost importance that this examination disclose any ambiguity of genitalia to permit early additional evaluation and information to the parents. Female external genitalia are usually hypertrophied because of antepartum stimulation by maternal estrogen. The same stimulus generally produces slight breast hypertrophy in both sexes. In the male infant, testes are usually in the scrotum, but may retract upward by stimulation of the cremaster muscle during the examination.

Birth Injuries

Despite improved obstetric techniques, including more liberal use of cesarean section delivery to prevent difficult vaginal delivery, birth trauma is still an important factor contributing to neonatal deaths. If the term *birth injury* is considered to represent any fetal damage which occurs during labor or delivery, it must include fetal brain damage due to hypoxia, trauma, or other factors. At present, the incidence of subtle brain damage due to labor and delivery is not known, but clinical evidence suggests that it is not uncommon. There is convincing evidence that sublethal lesions of the fetal brain due to hypoxia in labor are frequently associated with cerebral palsy and mental retardation, conditions diagnosed in approximately 125,000 infants born in the United States each year. The increasing utilization of labor-monitoring techniques for early detection and treatment of fetal distress (see Labor Monitoring and Fetal Distress) promises to reduce the incidence of brain damage due to fetal hypoxia and asphyxia during labor.

Intracranial Hemorrhage. Intracranial hemorrhage is responsible for approximately 10 percent of neonatal deaths. It may occur because of trauma, hypoxia, or both. When associated with trauma, there may be tears of dural septums and subdural hemorrhage. Brain hemorrhage occurs almost equally among infants of low birth weight and those of excessive size. Clinical factors commonly associated with its occurrence are difficult forceps delivery, shoulder dystocia, breech delivery, and precipitate delivery. Signs of brain damage in the neonate are quite variable, ranging from restlessness and irritability to lethargy, and often including weak cry, refusal to nurse, pallor, cyanosis, vomiting, dyspnea, and convulsions. Treatment is generally supportive with relief of intracranial pressure by lumbar puncture.

Cephalhematoma. A subperiosteal hemorrhage, cephalhematoma occurs over one or both parietal bones but is limited by the midline attachment of the periosteum to the skull. It must be differentiated from a caput succedaneum (see Pelvic Examination above) which usually overlies the midline. Cephal-

Assessment of Gestational Age

Neuromuscular Maturity

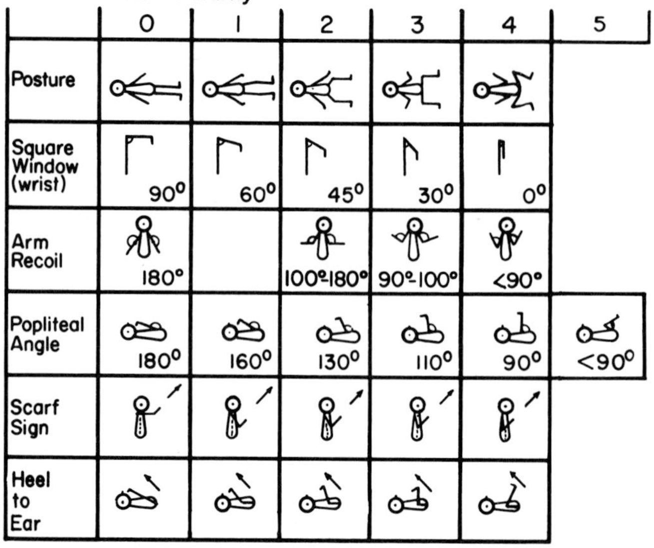

	0	1	2	3	4	5
Posture						
Square Window (wrist)	90°	60°	45°	30°	0°	
Arm Recoil	180°		100°-180°	90°-100°	<90°	
Popliteal Angle	180°	160°	130°	110°	90°	<90°
Scarf Sign						
Heel to Ear						

Physical Maturity

Skin	gelatinous red, transparent	smooth pink, visible veins	superficial peeling, &/or rash few veins	cracking pale area rare veins	parchment deep cracking no vessels	leathery cracked wrinkled
Lanugo	none	abundant	thinning	bald areas	mostly bald	
Plantar Creases	no crease	faint red marks	anterior transverse crease only	creases ant. 2/3	creases cover entire sole	
Breast	barely percept.	flat areola no bud	stippled areola 1-2mm bud	raised areola 3-4mm bud	full areola 5-10mm bud	
Ear	pinna flat, stays folded	sl. curved pinna; soft c̄ slow recoil	well-curv. pinna; soft but ready recoil	formed & firm c̄ instant recoil	thick cartilage ear stiff	
Genitals ♂	scrotom empty no rugae		testes descending few rugae	testes down good rugae	testes pendulous deep rugae	
Genitals ♀	prominent clitoris & labia minora		majora & minora equally prominent	majora large minora small	clitoris & minora completely covered	

Adapted from: Devel. Med. Child. Neurol. 8:507-511, 1966
Arch. Dis. Child. 43:89-93, 1968
J. Ped. 77:1, 1970
By: J. Ballard, M.D. August, 1971
Revised: February, 1972

Apgars____ I min____ 5min

Age at Exam _____ hrs

Race _____ Sex _____

B.D. _____

LMP _____

EDC _____

Gest. age by Dates ____ wks

Gest. age by Exam ____ wks

B.W. _____ gm. ____ %ile

Length ____ cm. ____ %ile

Head Circum. ____ cm. ____ %ile

Clin. Dist. None__ Mild____
Mod.__ Severe__

MATURITY RATING

Score	Wks.
5	26
10	28
15	30
20	32
25	34
30	36
35	38
40	40
45	42
50	44

FIGURE 29-31 Assessment of gestational age.

hematomas are commonly associated with an underlying skull fracture or a fetal blood dyscrasia. Aspiration of a cephalhematoma is contraindicated by the danger of infection.

Scalp Trauma. Fetal heart rate monitoring with a scalp electrode and/or acid-base monitoring for fetal scalp blood samples are responsible for small wounds of the fetal scalp. In general, these wounds heal uneventfully, but they deserve careful observation for evidence of inflammation and/or abscess.

Facial Trauma. Generally, pressure from obstetric forceps causes facial trauma. The marks are often quite obvious for several days, but they gradually heal without permanent sequelae.

Facial Nerve Injury. This trauma is usually associated with forceps injury of the facial nerve after it emerges from the stylomastoid foramen. The resulting facial paralysis, or Bell's palsy, is characterized by failure of closure of the eyelid on the affected side and distortion of the mouth toward the unaffected side. The eye should be protected by antibiotic ointment, but otherwise treatment is expectant and nerve function generally returns within a few days.

Brachial Plexus Injury. This injury may occur from lateral traction of the head or downward traction on the shoulder or arm during delivery. The resulting paralysis of the arm, known as Erb's or Duchenne's palsy, is due to injury of the lower cervical and upper thoracic nerve roots producing variable degrees of paralysis of the arm. When only the lower roots are damaged, paralysis is limited to the hand, referred to as Klumpke's paralysis. Treatment should involve appropriate physiotherapy and protection of the arm. Full recovery usually occurs within 2 years, but there are occasional cases of permanent paralysis of the arm.

Spinal Cord Injuries. Such injuries may occur from excessive traction or compression, with or without vertebral fractures. Towbin has reviewed this subject to conclude that spinal cord injury contributes to over 10 percent of neonatal deaths in the United States. Spinal cord injury has been specifically related to vaginal delivery of a breech-presenting fetus with hyperextension of the head (see Breech Presentation). The clinical signs of these lesions vary from early neonatal death or survival with permanent paralysis to minor nerve deficits, epilepsy, or mental retardation.

Fractures of the Clavicle. Occasionally vaginal delivery of large infants is associated with fractures of the clavicle. As noted earlier, in Shoulder Dystocia, intentional fracture of the clavicle may be necessary to accomplish delivery in certain cases of shoulder dystocia. There is usually minimal or no disability, and recovery is spontaneous.

Fractures of the Humerus. Fractures of this kind are not unusual and are generally associated with difficult delivery of the arms with shoulder dystocia or breech presentation; with appropriate immobilization, the fracture heals without sequelae.

Fractures of the Femur. These fractures are rare and are usually associated with breech delivery; if recognized early, they heal well with appropriate traction and immobilization.

Visceral Injuries. These injuries, particularly of the liver and spleen, are most often associated with the trauma of breech delivery or with vigorous resuscitation efforts. They are generally diagnosed at autopsy.

Sternocleidomastoid Injury. This may occur by lateral flexion of the neck, particularly during breech delivery. Scar formation in the muscle may eventually lead to torticollis.

THE PUERPERIUM

NORMAL COURSE AND MANAGEMENT

The puerperium is the period from delivery of the placenta until return of the reproductive organs to their normal nonpregnant morphologic state, which generally lasts for 6 to 8 weeks. Its conclusion is usually simultaneous with a return to the nonpregnant physiologic state of cyclic function, but this may be delayed by lactation or other endocrinologic factors.

Following delivery of the placenta, the entire birth canal should be inspected for lacerations. The techniques of laceration and episiotomy repair, and the prophylactic use of oxytocic drugs, were discussed previously. The uterus continues to contract periodically with the uterine fundus assuming a position about midway between the umbilicus and the symphysis. The cervix is generally patulous at the external os, but the internal os soon closes with contraction of the muscular uterus. The obstetrician's primary concern during the early puerperium should be toward prevention of postpartum hemorrhage. This may be accomplished by judicious use of oxytocic drugs (see Management of Third Stage above), careful inspection of the placenta and membranes for evidence of missing portions, identification and repair of lacerations (see Lacerations above), and continued close observation of the patient after she is moved from the delivery room.

Numerous complications may first become evident during the next few hours. It is clearly ill advised to place a patient in relative isolation with sedation for rest. Her state of physical relief and relative exhaustion will generally promote very adequate rest in an active recovery area. Her vital signs, the height and consistency of the uterine fundus, and the character of vaginal bleeding should be checked frequently for several hours. During this period, she should be catheterized if her bladder becomes moderately distended and she is unable to void. The intravenous infusion of the maintenance fluids started during labor is continued for 6 to 8 hours, or until the patient is alert and able to tolerate fluids by mouth.

It is common for the patient to have a slightly elevated temperature and moderate leukocytosis during the first 12 to 24 hours postpartum. Temperature over 38°C (100.4°F) generally signifies postpartum infection. Complications which may become manifest during the early puerperium include eclampsia, thromboembolic disease, infections, and unrecognized lacerations or retained placental fragments. Their diagnosis and management are discussed in Chap. 31.

Uterine involution progresses very rapidly in the early puerperium so that the fundus is no longer palpable above the symphysis by the tenth day. It is now recognized that the dramatic atrophy of myometrium through this period predominantly involves decreasing size of individual cells rather than death of cells. Uterine weight decreases from approximately 1000 g immediately postpartum to less than 100 g by 6 weeks postpartum. Through the period of involution, the uterus contracts periodically, which may produce "afterpains" requiring an analgesic. These painful contractions are particularly prevalent in multiparas and nursing mothers, but they tend to subside within the first few days of the puerperium.

The placenta normally separates through the decidua spongiosa layer, which in part remains in the uterus. The superficial portion of this tissue is sloughed as a constituent of the lochia of the early puerperium, while the deeper layer remains to generate new endometrium and facilitate repair of the site of placental implantation. The process requires up to 6 weeks for completion.

The uterovaginal discharge of the puerperium is referred to as *lochia*. During the first 2 or 3 days it is predominantly blood mixed with decidua and is referred to as *lochia rubra*. Except for an occasional small blood clot, the presence of clots in this discharge is abnormal and often is due to abnormal involution of the uterus. By the third or fourth day the discharge becomes more admixed with serum to produce a pale, watery substance, still colored with blood, called *lochia serosa*. It is gradually replaced over the next 1 or 2 weeks by creamy, white *lochia alba,* which consists of epithelial cells and leukocytes. Thus, the average patient experiences bloody discharge in decreasing amounts for about three or four weeks postpartum. Generally it is most convenient and comfortable for the patient to wear vulvar pads while the flow is heavy, but as the lochia decreases in quantity, she may prefer to use vaginal tampons. In nonlactating patients, the first menses usually occurs between 6 and 8 weeks postpartum, but there is considerable variation among patients.

The trend to early ambulation after delivery has clearly reduced the incidence of postpartum thromboses and embolism. Patients should begin ambulation by 24 hours postpartum and thereafter avoid long periods of immobility. There are no specific limitations of diet in the puerperal period. Lactating mothers are encouraged to consume additional protein and avoid foods that adversely affect the infant's state of alertness or bowel function. There is a general consensus that continued use of prophylactic iron and vitamins is helpful during the puerperium. Some patients require periodic catheterization of the urinary bladder for a day or two in order to avoid painful overdistention. Bowel function usually resumes without specific measures, but especially when the patient is experiencing episiotomy-site discomfort, the initial bowel movement is facilitated by the use of a mild cathartic or stool softener. Afterpains and episiotomy discomfort are generally responsive to mild analgesics such as aspirin compound or codeine. Application of local heat by a heat lamp or a warm sitz bath generally provides relief of episiotomy pain. The application of local anesthetic solutions by aerosol spray is usually helpful, but may be complicated by allergic or irritative reactions. Bathing during the puerperium may be by tub bath or shower, as there is no evidence that bath water enters the vagina or contributes to the development of infections.

Patients, physicians, and hospitals vary in their preferences of infant-mother rooming-in or nursery care of the infant. With rooming-in, the infant remains in the room or immediate vicinity of the mother between feedings. The advantages of rooming-in include the early establishment of a psychologic relationship of infant and mother, and the preparation of the mother for home care of the infant. Some mothers prefer the relative freedom of infant care afforded by nursery care during hospitalization. There is no evidence that the incidence of febrile morbidity is influenced by the use of rooming-in.

Visitors should be permitted in moderation during the immediate puerperium in the hospital and at home. Early involvement of the father serves to establish a healthy father-child relationship and provides a psychologic lift to the mother confronted by new responsibility of infant care. Ideally, the patient should be able to somehow regulate the variety and length of stay of her visitors. If she is fatigued, a long-winded visitor may be quite annoying. Perceptive hospital personnel may provide her a means of discouraging lengthy visitation by their thoughtful interruption and suggestion of needed rest. Visitors with clinical infections should be prohibited during the early puerperium, although a father with an upper respiratory infection might wear a surgical mask while visiting. Generally, the infant's passive immunity provides moderate protection against common infections.

A patient without complications may be discharged from the hospital after 3 to 5 days, depending primarily on her comfort and ability to assume more complete care of the infant. At home, she should continue to rest with only moderate ambulation. If there are other children, it is very helpful if relatives or friends provide help in their care. As during hospitalization, an effort should be made to avoid over-solicitous visitors. The patient should gradually resume normal activities during the puerperium, initially leaving home for a short ride or walk after 10 days. It is quite beneficial to her psychologic state to be temporarily relieved of her primary responsibility for infant care for brief periods during her recuperation. Her relatives and friends are usually most anxious to provide such help.

The resumption of coitus has traditionally been discouraged until after 6 weeks postpartum. There is no evidence that coitus earlier in the puerperium is harmful except that it may lead to pregnancy if practiced without adequate contraception. Early coitus might also lead to disruption of a partially healed episiotomy. Many patients experience a decrease of libido during this period which may be due to the dramatic hormonal changes and the various psychologic adjustments imposed during the puerperium. The same factors are thought to be responsible for the common development of psychologic depression.

The physician should offer support and encouragement during this difficult period of adjustment.

The care of patients after delivery by cesarean section is essentially the same as after vaginal delivery except for abdominal wound care. The period of hospitalization is usually extended to 7 days to afford additional time for recuperation. Skin sutures are conveniently removed prior to discharge. The postpartum care of patients with obstetric or medical complications of pregnancy is directed by the nature and severity of the complications (i.e., toxemia, diabetes mellitus, heart disease), which are discussed elsewhere in this text.

Patients who do not have complications during the puerperium should return for a complete physical examination in 3 to 6 weeks. By 6 weeks, abdominal or vulvar wounds are usually well healed, and the uterus has involuted to a nonpregnancy size. There is often evidence of mild cervicitis which may be treated by appropriate local antibiotic therapy or cautery at this time. A thorough discussion of family-planning techniques is an important component of this visit (see Chap. 33). Subsequent visits should be scheduled at 6 and 12 months postpartum.

CARE OF THE BREASTS AND LACTATION

Currently, the majority of women in the United States prefer not to breast-feed their infants. Despite the urging of its many advocates, there is no convincing evidence that lack of breast-feeding significantly deprives an infant of either adequate nutrition or needed psychologic support. If no specific measures to suppress lactation are initiated following delivery, the watery colostrum discharge persisting from late pregnancy is replaced by bluish-white lacteal secretion on the second to fourth postpartum day. Simultaneously, the breasts become larger, firm, and uncomfortable. Without the stimulation of breast-feeding, the engorgement and symptoms usually subside within 48 hours. The exact neurohormonal physiology of lactation remains uncertain, but apparently involves a number of events which include the preparation of breasts for lactation by progesterone, estrogen, and placental lactogen during pregnancy, their prompt withdrawal at delivery, and the neurohypophyseal release of prolactin and oxytocin after delivery. (See Chap. 7.)

Suppression of breast engorgement and lactation may be accomplished with various degrees of success by a variety of physical and hormonal methods. A readily available method consists of tight breast binder applied immediately after delivery, with the addition of ice bags and analgesics as needed for discomfort. Formerly, the synthetic estrogen stilbestrol was widely used for its apparent inhibition of lactation. Recent studies by Turnbull and Tindall have indicated an increased incidence of thromboembolic disease after use of estrogens to suppress lactation. In recent years, the most commonly employed methods have been either an intramuscular injection of testosterone, 360 mg, and estradiol valerate (Deladumone), 16 mg, given in late labor or immediately after delivery of the placenta, or oral chlorotrianisene (Tace), 25 mg twice daily for 3 days. In comparative studies (Womack et al.; Morris et al.) the testosterone-estradiol valerate injection method proved to be most effective, but its use may on occasion produce temporary acne and facial hair growth. If severe breast engorgement develops despite these methods, temporary relief may be obtained by partially emptying the breasts with a breast pump and applying a firm binder and ice packs. Repeated use of a breast pump will simulate infant feeding and tend to promote the establishment of lactation.

When the patient desires to breast-feed, it is advisable to provide adequate support of the breasts and to have the patient wash the nipples and areolae with soap and water prior to each feeding. Nursing may be started as soon as the patient has adequately rested following delivery. The initial colostrum feedings should be brief, lasting about 3 minutes but increasing to about 10 minutes per breast as lactation is established. Feeding may be on a scheduled interval or demand basis. Sore nipples may be treated with a protective preparation containing lanolin, or in extreme cases by use of a nipple shield for a few days. Fissured nipples should be treated with a local antibiotic ointment and nipple shield until fully healed. The adequacy of breast-feeding may be judged by the infant's progressive weight gain or loss. Patients who breast-feed tend to experience more pronounced afterpains than their bottle-feeding counterparts, but they also tend to have less lochia rubra. Menses usually do not resume until after breast-feeding is stopped, but ovulation may occur prior to the first menses. Human milk is generally adequate nourishment for human infants until they are 4 or 5 months old. Weaning the infant is readily accomplished by gradual or abrupt cessation of breast-feeding, and rarely is accompanied by bothersome engorgement requiring a breast binder or analgesics.

CONTRACEPTION

The puerperium is an ideal time for the physician to counsel a patient on family-planning techniques. The subject should be initially discussed during her hospitalization for delivery and further expanded at the time of her postpartum examination. The various techniques, their efficacy, and limitations are discussed in Chap. 33.

STERILIZATION

During recent years, elective sterilization procedures performed in the immediate postpartum period have become a common operative procedure in the majority of hospitals in the United States. The procedure is most often accomplished by bilateral partial salpingectomies performed through a small laparotomy wound or at cesarean section. The subject is discussed more fully in Chap. 33.

COMPLICATIONS OF THE PUERPERIUM

Chapters 30 and 31 cover a variety of medical and obstetric conditions which may persist into the puerperium; however, this section will consider several complications which are relatively unique or prevalent in the recent parturient.

Endometritis

No other subject in medical history shares the illustrious history of childbed fever. Its elucidation and control spanned much of the nineteenth and twentieth centuries, from the brilliant observations of Oliver Wendell Holmes and Ignaz Philipp Semmelweis to the development of antibiotics.

The term *puerperal infection* refers to any infection of the genital tract during the puerperium. It is the most common, but not the exclusive, cause of *puerperal morbidity,* which is defined as a temperature of 38.0°C (100.4°F) or higher on any 2 of the first 10 days postpartum, exclusive of the first 24 hours. In addition to the infections of the genital tract, puerperal morbidity may be due to infections of the urinary tract, breasts, respiratory tract, or other sites. Puerperal infection most commonly manifests as endometritis, but frequently it also involves vulvovaginitis, cervicitis, salpingitis, and pelvic peritonitis.

The infection may be due to organisms which are normal inhabitants of the genital tract or others introduced from exogenous sources. Most often the physician transmits organisms from his nasopharynx, hands, or by contaminated instruments, but the organisms may originate from the hospital environment, other personnel, or even from the hands of the patient herself. The process begins as a wound infection of a laceration or other area denuded of epithelium by the birth process and spreads by surface extension or along blood or lymph vessels to involve other structures. Puerperal infection is quite unusual in healthy patients delivered without complications, but it is very prevalent in association with general debilitation, hemorrhage, anemia, premature rupture of membranes, prolonged labor, or traumatic delivery. Therefore, we may anticipate a decreasing incidence of this complication as a result of improving general health and obstetrical care of patients.

Most of the organisms responsible for puerperal infection are common inhabitants of the birth canal, such as anaerobic streptococcus, coliform organisms, aerobic nonhemolytic streptococcus, and staphylococcus (Wierdsma, Clayton). In addition, there is some evidence that *Clostridium perfringens,* a rare cause of puerperal infection, may at times be present in the birth canal of healthy women (Sadusk, Manahan). *Bacteroides* and enterococcus, normal inhabitants of the gastrointestinal tract, are occasionally cultured in puerperal infection (Pearson, Anderson; Slotnick et al.). *Neisseria gonorrhoeae* is rarely the cause of puerperal infection.

Clinical evidence of endometritis typically develops on the third postpartum day with onset of fever, malaise, uterine tenderness, and abnormal vaginal discharge. Because of the variety of pathogens that may be responsible for endometritis, lochia may or may not have a foul odor, but it usually is more profuse than normal. There is a moderate leukocytosis, often not significantly higher than that of the normal puerperium. Abdominal and pelvic findings vary from only mild uterine tenderness to evidence of generalized peritonitis.

Management of endometritis should include initial cultures of lochia for aerobic and anaerobic organisms, sensitivity studies, preliminary broad-spectrum antibiotics, analgesics, and adequate fluid intake. The use of an oxytocic drug, such as ergotrate, tends to improve uterine tonus and to slow excessive lochia. As in the treatment of pelvic inflammatory disease, maintaining the patient in Fowler's position, with the head and upper body elevated, promotes

pelvic localization if the infection spreads from the endometrial cavity. When the results of cultures and sensitivities become available, more specific antibiotic therapy should be considered unless the response to the previous treatment has been favorable.

When infection has spread from the endometrium to the pelvic supporting structures, the resulting pelvic cellulitis is typically characterized by a sustained fever and pelvic adnexal tenderness and thickening. The process is slow to respond to antibiotic therapy and may lead to pelvic abscess which requires surgical drainage. Puerperal infection may lead to pelvic thrombophlebitis which is characterized by an intermittent spiking fever and severe chills, but minimal pelvic examination findings. On occasion, pulmonary embolism may occur and lead to maternal death. The treatment of pelvic thrombophlebitis consists basically of antibiotics and prophylactic anticoagulant therapy to prevent embolism.

The diagnosis and treatment of *N. gonorrhoeae* or *C. perfringens* infections during the puerperium are not unlike treatment in their more frequent occurrence following abortion, and are discussed in Chap. 11.

Urinary Tract Infections

Many factors contribute to the relatively high incidence of urinary tract infections during the puerperium. Asymptomatic bacteriuria is found in approximately 6 percent of patients during pregnancy (Kass); therefore, many puerperal patients have potential pathogens preexisting in the urinary tract. Normal vaginal delivery is commonly associated with trauma of the bladder which, although minor, may lead to a clinical infection. The postpartum bladder is relatively hypotonic, especially if conduction anesthesia has been employed during labor or delivery, which leads to overdistention and residual urine after voiding. In addition, the relative atony of the ureters which developed during pregnancy persists for several weeks postpartum. The practice of catheterization prior to delivery, although not advocated at present, is still widely employed and undoubtedly contributes to the other factors associated with puerperal urinary tract infection.

Urinary tract infections usually become manifest during the first day or two after delivery, but the clinical diagnosis is often difficult because of the normal presence of urinary distention, mild fever, leukocytosis, and even mild pyuria. The infection often leads to progressively more severe dysuria, urinary frequency, or even the inability to urinate. Urinalysis reveals bacteria and leukocytes in clumps. As the infection ascends to involve the upper urinary tract, the patient develops fever, chills, general malaise, and has typical costovertebral angle tenderness. Urine culture most often reveals *Escherichia coli* or other coliforms. Management consists of appropriate antimicrobial drug therapy, bed rest, and support of fluid intake.

Late Postpartum Hemorrhage

Occasionally, postpartum hemorrhage initially develops several days or weeks after delivery. With late onset, it is most often due to subinvolution of the placental site or a retained piece of placenta. This subject was discussed earlier in this chapter (see Postpartum Hemorrhage).

Mastitis

Inflammation of the breasts usually presents clinically after several weeks of lactation. It is generally unilateral and associated with marked engorgement, fever, and pain. The inflammation may be generalized or confined to a local area of the breast, with induration, tenderness, and erythema of the involved area. In more advanced cases there may be local abscess formation.

Mastitis is usually caused by *Staphylococcus aureus* which enters fissures of the nipple from the infant's mouth or nose during nursing. On occasions, other organisms are involved which have probably been carried to the breast by the patient's hands. The infection is usually parenchymatous, predominantly involving the lactiferous ducts and glands, and is thus localized to a functional unit of the breast. But it may be more generalized, involving the supporting structures of the breast. If the initial infection is not aborted by appropriate therapy, either type of infection will eventually progress to abscess formation and more severe systemic manifestations. On occasion, an epidemic of mastitis may develop when the organisms are transmitted among nursery personnel and infants to several mothers. Such an epidemic may be managed by use of a bacterial interference technique in which all infants are inoculated with a nonvirulent strain of *S. aureus* on admission to the nursery; this serves to block the continued spread of the virulent strain (Light et al.).

The prevention of mastitis must include measures directed toward eliminating virulent organisms from nursery personnel and infants, as well as providing optimal care of breasts during lactation. Nursery personnel should be periodically screened by nasal culture and phage typing for virulent organisms. Sus-

pect infants should be promptly isolated and given appropriate antibiotic therapy. Breasts should be cleansed prior to nursing, and when fissures develop, they should be treated by application of tincture of benzoin, lanolin preparations, or the temporary use of a nipple shield.

With diagnosis of mastitis, a culture should be taken from the milk, the patient and her infant should be isolated, and the patient should discontinue breast-feeding. Symptomatic relief may be afforded by use of a breast binder, ice packs, and analgesics. The choice of antibiotics should be appropriate to the current antibiotic-resistant behavior of staphylococcus. Thus, although penicillin is usually effective, the prevalence of penicillin-resistant organisms favors the use of other antibiotics such as erythromycin or kanamycin. The drug should be continued for 10 days even though the symptoms may resolve after 2 or 3 days. Abscess formation is evidenced by continued fever, becoming remittent. An abscess should be drained, after it becomes fluctuant, through an incision made in a radial fashion in order to avoid incision of a lactiferous duct. The procedure should be performed under inhalation anesthesia. Loculations of the abscess cavity should be manually disrupted, and the cavity should be loosely packed, with smaller packs inserted each day until the cavity heals from its base.

Thromboembolic Disease

The frequency of occurrence of thromboembolic disease is greater during the puerperium than during pregnancy. Factors contributing to this incidence include trauma to vessels associated with delivery, stasis of blood in the lower extremities due to immobility, and the coagulation alterations of pregnancy and the puerperium. Its decreasing incidence in recent decades is presumably due to the increasing emphasis on early ambulation in the puerperium and to the decreasing incidence of traumatic delivery. Tindall reported that the incidence of puerperal thromboembolism is increased threefold when estrogen is used to inhibit lactation. There is clearly a higher incidence of thromboembolic disease in patients with varicosities of the lower extremities.

Although some distinguish between phlebothrombosis and thrombophlebitis, both processes tend to involve venous inflammation and are similar clinically. Thrombosis may occur in superficial or deep vessels. Superficial thrombophlebitis is seldom complicated by embolism, but if not promptly treated, it is apt to progress to deep-vessel involvement which is life-threatening. Pelvic vein thrombophlebitis is generally associated with other evidence of puerperal infection (see Endometritis above).

With superficial thrombophlebitis there is pain and elevation of skin temperature over the involved vessel. There may be edema of the extremity and mild systemic fever. Examination reveals erythema, induration, and tenderness over the vessel. Involvement of deep vessels is evidenced by pain in the leg on dorsiflexion of the foot (Homans' sign) or pain with forward leg raising while the knee is extended (Bancroft's sign).

Treatment of superficial thrombophlebitis consists of bed rest with slight elevation of the legs and local heat until pain has subsided, followed by active ambulation with elastic support of the lower extremities. In deep vein thrombophlebitis, anticoagulant therapy is indicated because of the threat of embolism. It should consist of heparin given intravenously in doses of 5000 to 10,000 units every 4 to 6 hours to maintain the clotting time at approximately twice the control value. Many prefer to simultaneously start oral bishydroxycoumarin (Dicumarol) or sodium warfarin (Coumadin), drugs which inhibit the synthesis of vitamin K–dependent clotting factors, reflected by prolongation of the prothrombin time. They have a much slower onset of anticoagulant activity than intravenous heparin, but by their oral administration they are more conveniently used in long-term maintenance therapy. The dosage of bishydroxycoumarin is 300 mg initially, 200 mg the second day, and thereafter a daily maintenance dose of less than 100 mg in order to maintain prothrombin activity at 20 percent of normal. Warfarin is somewhat faster acting, requiring 30 to 50 mg initially, 10 to 20 mg the second day, and 5 to 10 mg daily for maintenance. Anticoagulant therapy is continued for at least 7 days after the resolution of symptoms.

In recent years, the use of intravenous Dextran has emerged as an alternate form of therapy to anticoagulants. Dextran is a high-molecular-weight polysaccharide which is thought to produce antithrombotic effects by coating the vessel walls and blood elements to reduce contact factors which are known to trigger coagulation. The clinical results of Dextran therapy are quite promising (Wallach).

Pulmonary embolism typically produces dyspnea, chest pain, cough, and hemoptysis, but the symptoms are relatively nonspecific. The most common physical findings are tachypnea, tachycardia, and accentuation of the pulmonary second sound. Some patients have cyanosis, a pleural friction rub, hypotension, pleural effusion, and signs of conges-

tive heart failure. The most specific diagnostic procedures are either radioisotope lung scanning or pulmonary angiography. There is usually a moderate decrease of arterial oxygen tension, and lactic dehydrogenase is often elevated, but this may be due to recent pregnancy. There may be electrocardiogram evidence of right ventricular strain. Chest x-ray is usually normal.

The treatment of pulmonary embolism should consist of rapid anticoagulation, supportive measures, and prophylaxis against further embolization. Symptoms may be relieved by analgesics, sedatives, and oxygen inhalation. Ligation of the vena cava and ovarian veins may be lifesaving if pulmonary or other embolism occurs despite anticoagulant therapy.

Psychiatric Disorders of the Puerperium

Mild postpartum depression occurs commonly, often without clinical recognition or specific therapy. A patient's reaction to pregnancy and new motherhood is influenced by many factors in her emotional structure. The loss of the pregnancy, or the acquisition of the infant, may seriously compromise her former psychic defenses. Her potential inability to adjust to a new role may be anticipated and averted by a perceptive physician who strives to prepare her during pregnancy. In the puerperium, the depressed patient most often withdraws to relative isolation, and an attempt to treat her symptoms with sedation may only compound her state of depression. The situation responds most readily to efforts of the physician through verbalization to enforce her sense of accomplishment. Mild tranquilizers may be helpful, but do not substitute for compassion.

Postpartum psychosis is not a specific entity, but rather it generally represents the emergence of preexisting mental illness in response to the psychic and physical adjustments imposed by pregnancy, parturition, and the puerperium. Infrequently, puerperal psychoses occur as results of organic disease or toxic states. The psychosis generally manifests as depression, often involving rejection of the infant, and at times a threat of suicide. Psychiatric consultation is indicated on recognition of hallucinatory, paranoid, or other psychotic behavior. The responses to treatment and prognosis are not specifically influenced by the postpartum state.

Relationship to Family

The puerperium is a period of many potential conflicts of the patient and her family. Her responses may range from rejection of her relatives as annoying intruders to encouragement of their oversolicitousness. Her emotional state is generally quite vulnerable, and subtle conflicts with her relatives may emerge for the first time. The role of the obstetrician clearly extends into the puerperium through efforts to help her toward a normal adjustment. During hospitalization the obstetrician may help her regulate the traffic of visitors or otherwise adjust to hospitalization but, of more significance, remains available to her for counsel after she returns home.

Even when the patient's husband has not been intimately involved during labor and delivery, it is of immeasurable benefit for him and the obstetrician to have a thorough discussion of the situation during the early puerperium. It may become quite apparent that he is in a state of psychic turmoil and requires more support than his wife.

REFERENCES

Abramowicz M, Kass EH: Pathogenesis and prognosis of prematurity. *N Engl J Med* 275:878, 1966.

Abrams IF et al.: Cervical cord injuries secondary to hyperextension of the head in breech presentations. *Obstet Gynecol* 41: 369, 1973.

Adamsons K, Meyers RE: Late decelerations and brain tolerance of the fetal monkey to intrapartum asphyxia. *Am J Obstet Gynecol* 128: 893, 1977.

Ahuja GL et al.: Massive subaponeurotic haemorrhage in infants born by the vacuum extractor. *Br Med J* 3: 743, 1969.

Alvarez H, Caldeyro-Barcia R: Contractility of the human uterus recorded by new methods. *Surg Gynecol Obstet* 91: 1, 1950.

Amiel-Tison C: Neurological evaluation of the maturity of newborn infants. *Arch Dis Child* 43: 89, 1968.

Anderson GG, Steege JF: Clinical experience using intraamniotic prostaglandin $F_2\alpha$ for midtrimester abortion in 600 patients. *Obstet Gynecol* 46: 591, 1975.

Apgar V et al.: Evaluation of the newborn infant: Second report. *JAMA* 168: 1985, 1958.

Agüero O, Alvarez H: Fetal injury due to vacuum extraction. *Obstet Gynecol* 19: 212, 1962.

Babson SG, Benson RC: *Management of High-Risk Pregnancy and Intensive Care of the Neonate*, St. Louis: Mosby, 1971, pp. 167–182.

Bach HG: Postmaturity syndrome, prolonged pregnancy and perinatal mortality. *Gynaecologia* 150: 197, 1960.

Ballas S, Toaff R: Hyperextension of the fetal head in breech presentation: Radiological evaluation and significance. *Br J Obstet Gynaecol* 83: 201, 1976.

Barden TP: The management of premature labor, in *Controversy in Obstetrics and Gynecology,* Philadelphia: Saunders, 1979.

Beard RW et al.: pH of foetal capillary blood as an indicator of the condition of the foetus. *J Obstet Gynaecol Br Commonw* 74: 812, 1967.

Bhagwanani SG et al.: Risks and prevention of cervical cord injury in the management of breech presentation with hyperextension of the fetal head. *Am J Obstet Gynecol* 115: 1159, 1973.

Bieniarz J: Cardiovascular effects of high doses of oxytocin, in *Oxytocin,* eds. R Caldeyro-Barcia, H Heller, Oxford: Pergamon, 1961, pp. 80–83.

Bishop EH: Pelvic scoring for elective induction. *Obstet Gynecol* 24: 266, 1964.

Booth JH, Kurdyak VB: Elective induction of labour: A controlled study. *Can Med Assoc J* 103: 245, 1970.

Brazelton TB: Effect of prenatal drugs on the behavior of the neonate. *Am J Psychiatry* 126: 1261, 1970.

Brenner WE et al.: The characteristics and perils of breech presentation. *Am J Obstet Gynecol* 118: 700, 1974.

Browne JCM: Postmaturity. *Am J Obstet Gynecol* 85: 573, 1963.

Caldeyro-Barcia R, Alvarez H: Abnormal uterine action in labour. *J Obstet Gynaecol Br Commonw* 59: 5, 1952.

———et al.: A better understanding of uterine contractility through simultaneous recording with an internal and seven channel external method. *Surg Gynecol Obstet* 91: 641, 1950.

———: Normal and abnormal uterine contractility in labour. *Triangle* 2: 41, 1955.

———: Treatment of acute intrapartum fetal distress, in *Perinatal Factors Affecting Human Development,* Pan American Health Organization, 1969, p. 248.

———, Poseiro JJ: Physiology of the uterine contraction. *Clin Obstet Gynecol* 3: 386, 1960.

———, Sereno JA: The response of the human uterus to oxytocin throughout pregnancy, in *Oxytocin,* eds. R Caldeyro-Barcia, H Heller, New York: Pergamon, 1961.

Carson BS et al.: Combined obstetric and pediatric approach to prevent meconium aspiration syndrome. *Am J Obstet Gynecol* 126: 712, 1976.

Cibils LA, Hendricks CH: Effect of ergot derivatives and sparteine sulfate upon the human uterus. *J Reprod Med* 2: 147, 1969.

Collea JV et al.: The randomized management of term frank breech presentation: Vaginal delivery vs. cesarean section. *Am J Obstet Gynecol* 131; 186, 1978.

Csapo AI, Sauvage J: The evolution of uterine activity

during human pregnancy. *Acta Obstet Gynecol Scand* 47: 181, 1968.

Delfs E, Eastman JF: Rupture of the uterus (an analysis of 53 cases). *Can Med Assoc J* 52: 376, 1945.

Dubowitz LMS et al.: Clinical assessment of gestational age in the newborn infant. *J Pediatr* 77: 1, 1970.

DuVigneaud V et al.: *Biol Chem* 205: 949, 1953.

Eastman JF, Jackson E: Weight relationships in pregnancy. *Obstet Gynecol Surv* 23: 1003, 1968.

Farr V et al.: The definition of some external characteristics used in the assessment of gestational age in the newborn infant. *Dev Med Child Neurol* 8: 507, 1966.

Freeman RK et al.: Fetal cardiac response to paracervical block anesthesia. pt. 1 *Am J Obstet Gynecol* 113: 583, 1972.

Friedman EA: *Labor, Clinical Evaluation and Management,* New York: Appleton-Century-Crofts, 1967.

————et al.: Relation of prelabor evaluation to inducibility and the course of labor. *Obstet Gynecol* 28: 495, 1966.

————: Evolution of graphic analysis of labor. *Am J Obstet Gynecol* 132: 824, 1978.

Gauss CJ: Geburten in künstlichem dammerschlaf. *Arch Gynaekol* 78: 579, 1906.

Ghosh S, Daga S: Comparison of gestational age and weight as standards of prematurity. *J Pediatr* 71: 173, 1967.

Gonzalez-Ponizza VH et al.: The fate of injected oxytocin in the pregnant woman near term, in *Oxytocin,* eds. R Caldeyro-Barcia, H Heller, New York: Pergamon, 1961, pp. 347–357.

Goodno JA et al.: In vitro and in vivo effects of sparteine sulfate on human uterine contractility: An objective evaluation. *Am J Obstet Gynecol* 86: 288, 1963.

Hendricks CH: Use of intranasal oxytocin in obstetrics. II. A clinical appraisal. *Am J Obstet Gynecol* 79: 789, 1960.

————: Inherent motility patterns and response characteristics of the nonpregnant human uterus. *Am J Obstet Gynecol* 96: 824, 1966.

————, Brenner WE: Cardiovascular effects of oxytocic drugs used post partum. *Am J Obstet Gynecol* 108: 751, 1970.

Hobel CJ et al.: Prenatal and intrapartum high-risk screening I. Prediction of the high-risk neonate. *Am J Obstet Gynecol* 117: 1, 1973.

Hon EH: The electronic evaluation of the fetal heart. *Am J Obstet Gynecol* 75: 1215, 1958.

————: Observations on "pathologic" fetal bradycardia. *Am J Obstet Gynecol* 77: 1084, 1959.

————: The diagnosis of fetal distress. *Clin Obstet Gynecol* 3: 860, 1960.

————et al.: Biochemical studies of the fetus. II. Fetal pH and Apgar scores. *Obstet Gynecol* 33: 237, 1969.

————, Quilligan EJ: The classification of fetal heart rate. II. A revised working classification. *Conn Med* 31: 799, 1967.

———— et al.: The neonatal value of fetal monitoring. *Am J Obstet Gynecol* 122: 508, 1975.

Imig JR, Perkins RP: Extraperitoneal cesarean section: A new need for old skills. *Am J Obstet Gynecol* 125: 51, 1976.

Israel R: Vasa previa in binovular twins. Report of a case. *Obstet Gynecol* 17: 691, 1961.

James LS et al.: The acid-base status of human infants in relation to birth asphyxia. *J Pediatr* 52: 379, 1958.

Karim SMM: Appearance of prostaglandin $F_2\alpha$ in human blood during labour. *Br Med J* 4: 618, 1968.

Kass EH: Bacteriuria and pyelonephritis of pregnancy. *Arch Intern Med* 105: 194, 1960.

Keettel WC et al.: The hazards of elective induction of labor. *Am J Obstet Gynecol* 75: 496, 1958.

Khazin AF et al.: Effects of maternal hyperoxia on the fetus. I. Oxygen tension. *Am J Obstet Gynecol* 109: 628, 1971.

Kistner RW et al.: Pulmonary embolism by particulate matter of the amniotic fluid. *Obstet Gynecol Surv* 5: 629, 1950.

Koff AK, Potter EL: The complications associated with excessive development of the human fetus. *Am J Obstet Gynecol* 38: 412, 1939.

Kubli FW et al.: Observations on heart rate and pH in the human fetus during labor. *Am J Obstet Gynecol* 104: 1190, 1969.

Lamaze F: *Painless Childbirth: The Lamaze Method,* Chicago : Regnery, 1970.

Lebherz TB et al.: Double-blind study of premature rupture of the membranes. *Am J Obstet Gynecol* 87: 218, 1963.

Leboyer F: *Birth Without Violence,* New York: Knopf, 1975.

Light IJ et al.: Use of bacterial interference to control a staphylococcal nursery outbreak. *Am J Dis Child* 113: 291, 1967.

Little B, et al.: Study of Ketamine as an obstetric anesthetic agent. *Am J Obstet Gynecol* 113: 247, 1972.

Malmström T: The vacuum extractor, an obstetrical instrument. *Acta Obstet Gynecol Scand Suppl* 4: 33, 1954.

Mann L: Intrapartum fetal monitoring: Scalp blood pH is a useful tool. *Contemp Ob Gyn* 11: 25, 1978.

Mendelson CL: Aspiration of stomach contents into the lungs during obstetric anesthesia. *Am J Obstet Gynecol* 52: 191, 1946.

Mendez-Bauer C et al.: Relationship between blood pH and heart rate in the human fetus during labor. *Am J Obstet Gynecol* 97: 530, 1967.

Miller FC, et al.: Significance of meconium during labor. *Am J Obstet Gynecol* 122: 573, 1975.

Morris JA et al.: Inhibition of puerperal lactation. *Obstet Gynecol* 36: 107, 1970.

Myers RE: Two patterns of perinatal brain damage and their conditions of occurrence. *Am J Obstet Gynecol* 112: 246, 1972.

———: Experimental models of perinatal brain damage: Relevance to human pathology, in *Intrauterine Asphyxia and the Developing Fetal Brain,* ed. L Gluck, Year Book, 1977, pp. 37–97.

Nesbitt REL Jr: Prolongation of pregnancy. *Obstet Gynecol Surv* 10: 311, 1955.

Newman JW, Hon EH: Induction of labor with transbuccal oxytocin. *Obstet Gynecol* 21: 3, 1963.

Newton M: Postpartum hemorrhage. *Am J Obstet Gynecol* 94: 711, 1966.

Nyirjesy I et al.: Hazards of the use of paracervical block anesthesia in obstetrics. *Am J Obstet Gynecol* 87: 231, 1963.

Odell LD, Seski A: Episiotomy blood loss. *Am J Obstet Gynecol* 54: 51, 1947.

Paton JB, Fisher DE: Dysmaturity, in *Obstetrics and Gynecology Annual; Nineteen Seventy-three,* ed. RM Wynn, New York: Appleton-Century-Crofts, 1973, pp. 205–227.

Paul RH, Hon EH: Clinical fetal monitoring. V. Effect on perinatal outcome. *Am J Obstet Gynecol* 118: 529, 1974.

——— et al.: Clinical fetal monitoring. VII. The evaluation and significance of intrapartum baseline FHR variability. *Am J Obstet Gynecol* 123: 206, 1975.

Pearson HE, Anderson GV: Bacteroides infections and pregnancy. *Obstet Gynecol* 35: 31, 1970.

Pedowitz P, Perell A: Rupture of the uterus. *Am J Obstet Gynecol* 76: 161, 1958.

Plauché WC: Vacuum extraction, use in a community hospital setting. *Obstet Gynecol* 52: 289, 1978.

Plentl AA et al.: Sparteine sulfate. *Am J Obstet Gynecol* 82: 1332, 1961.

Poseiro JJ: Causes of fetal distress in labor. *Int J Obstet Gynecol* 8: 913, 1970.

Pritchard JA et al.: Blood volume changes in pregnancy and the puerperium. II. Red blood cell loss and changes in apparent blood volume during and following vaginal delivery, cesarean section and cesarean section plus total hysterectomy. *Am J Obstet Gynecol* 84: 1271, 1962.

Ralston DH, Shnider SM: The fetal and neonatal effects of regional anesthesia in obstetrics. *Anesthesiology* 48: 34, 1978.

Renou P et al.: Autonomic control of fetal heart rate. *Am J Obstet Gynecol* 105: 949, 1969.

Reynolds SRM: *Physiology of the Uterus,* 2d ed., New York: Hoeber-Harper, 1949.

——— et al.: *Clinical Measurement of Uterine Forces in Pregnancy and Labor,* Springfield, Ill.: Charles C Thomas, 1954.

Roberts RB, Shirley MB: The obstetrician's role in reducing the risk of aspiration pneumonitis with particular reference to the use of oral antacids. *Am J Obstet Gynecol* 124: 611, 1976.

Rogers RE: Fetal bradycardia associated with paracervical block anesthesia in labor. *Am J Obstet Gynecol* 106: 913, 1970.

Rutland A, Ballard C: Vaginal prostaglandin E_2 for missed abortion and intrauterine fetal death. *Am J Obstet Gynecol* 128: 503, 1977.

Sadusk JF, Manahan CP: Observations on the occurrence of *Clostridium welchii* in the vagina of pregnant women. *Am J Obstet Gynecol* 41: 856, 1941.

Saling E: Amnioscopy, a new method for diagnosis of conditions hazardous to the fetus when membranes are intact. *Geburtschilfe Frauenheilkd* 22: 830, 1962.

——— et al.: Microanalysis of foetal blood. A critical study of the method. *Ger Med Mon* 12: 315, 1967.

Schifrin BS, Dame L: Fetal heart rate patterns. Prediction of Apgar score. *JAMA* 219: 1322, 1972.

Schulman H, Ledger W: Sparteine sulfate: A clinical study of 711 patients. *Obstet Gynecol* 25: 542, 1965.

Shnider SM, Gildea J: Paracervical block anesthesia in obstetrics. *Am J Obstet Gynecol* 116: 320, 1973.

Slotnick IJ et al.: Microbiology of the female genital tract. IV. Cervical and vaginal flora during pregnancy. *Obstet Gynecol* 21: 312, 1963.

Smyth CN: The oxytocin sensitivity test for surgical induction of labor. *Triangle* 3: 150, 1958.

Stamm O et al.: Development of a special electrode for continuous subcutaneous pH measurement in the infant scalp. *Am J Obstet Gynecol* 124: 193, 1976.

Stander RW et al.: Continuous intrauterine pressure recordings in the evaluation of sparteine sulfate. *Am J Obstet Gynecol* 86: 281, 1963.

Taylor G, Pryse-Davies J: The prophylactic use of antacids in the prevention of the acid-pulmonary aspiration syndrome (Mendelson's syndrome). *Lancet* 1: 288, 1966.

Thompson HE et al.: Fetal development as determined by ultrasonic pulse echo techniques. *Am J Obstet Gynecol* 92: 44, 1965.

Tindall VR: Factors influencing puerperal thromboembolism. *J Obstet Gynaecol Br Commonw* 75: 1324, 1968.

Ting P, Brady JP: Tracheal suction in meconium aspiration. *Am J Obstet Gynecol* 122: 767, 1975.

Towbin A: Spinal cord and brain stem injury at birth. *Arch Pathol* 77: 620, 1964.

Turnbull AC: Puerperal thromboembolism and the suppression of lactation. *J Obstet Gynaecol Br Commonw* 75: 1321, 1968.

Walker J: Prolonged pregnancy syndrome. *Am J Obstet Gynecol* 76: 1231, 1958.

Wallach RC: Dextran therapy for pregnancy-associated deep thrombophlebitis. *Am J Obstet Gynecol* 112: 613, 1972.

Wesselius-de Casparis A et al.: Results of a double-blind study with ritodrine in premature labor. *Br Med J* 3: 144, 1971.

Wierdsma JG, Clayton EM: The effects of certain antibiotics on the normal postpartum intrauterine bacteriologic flora. *Am J Obstet Gynecol* 88: 541, 1964.

Womack WS et al.: A comparison of hormone therapies for suppression of lactation. *South Med J* 55: 816, 1962.

Wood C et al.: Fetal heart rate and acid-base status in the assessment of fetal hypoxia. *Am J Obstet Gynecol* 98: 62, 1967.

Yao AC, Lind J: Effect of gravity on placental transfusion. *Lancet* 11: 505, 1969.

Young BK et al.: Continuous fetal tissue pH measurement in labor. *Obstet Gynecol* 52: 533, 1978.

Zatuchni GI, Andros GJ: Prognostic index for vaginal delivery in breech presentation at term. *Am J Obstet Gynecol* 93: 237, 1965.

————: Prognostic index for vaginal delivery in breech presentation at term. *Am J Obstet Gynecol* 98: 854, 1967.

Zlatnik FJ, Fuchs F: A controlled study of ethanol in threatened premature labor. *Am J Obstet'Gynecol* 112: 610, 1972.

Zuspan FP et al.: Premature labor: Its management and therapy. *J Reprod Med* 9: 93, 1972.

30

Diseases Specific to Pregnancy

TERRY HAYASHI*

*Assisted by Drs. Marvin C. Rulin, Daniel I. Edelstone, James H. Harger, Eberhard Mueller-Heubach, and Steve N. Caritis, all of the Department of Obstetrics and Gynecology, University of Pittsburgh School of Medicine.

Chronic hypertension with superimposed
preeclampsia or eclampsia
Chronic hypertensive disease
Unclassified hypertensive disorders

DISORDERS OF THE OVUM

ABORTION

INTRODUCTION

Approximately 15 percent of all recognized pregnancies terminate in spontaneous abortion, but the true incidence is probably much higher if all fertilized ova lost without sufficient symptoms to attract the attention of the patient or physician are included. The problem of early pregnancy loss, therefore, is one of considerable magnitude. Spontaneous abortion is defined as the noninduced separation of the products of conception through natural causes at any time before the fetus has attained viability—that is, the capacity to survive outside of its mother. The medically accepted limit of nonviability in the United States is 20 to 24 weeks from the last normal menstrual period or a fetal weight of 500 g. However, many countries accept the 1966 World Health Organization definition which sets the period of viability as the 28th week of fetal life. Health department regulations, which are important in reporting statistics, differ in individual states. Since pregnancies which terminate after the time limit established by a particular state or nation are recorded as births, such nonstandardized reporting can result in significant and erroneous differences in perinatal mortality rates unless the discrepancies are carefully corrected. In most states, abortions are processed pathologically in the same way as any other tissue specimen, but stillborn fetuses or liveborn infants who subsequently die are subjected to the same regulations regarding autopsy and burial that apply to an adult death. Much of the lay public associates the word abortion with a willful act and uses the term miscarriage to denote a spontaneous or involuntary early pregnancy loss. In dealing with many patients it is still prudent to use the term miscarriage to avoid misunderstandings.

ETIOLOGY

A majority of spontaneous abortions result from chromosomal anomalies. The recognized incidence has increased with better karyotyping techniques and now stands at approximately 60 percent. About one-half of these are autosomal trisomies, and another 40 percent are equally divided between monosomy X and polyploidy. The principal mechanism leading to monosomy and trisomy is meiotic nondisjunction, which seems to occur more frequently in oocytes than in spermatocytes. Mitotic nonreductions which cause triploidy or tetraploidy may be of maternal or paternal origin. There is no significant difference in the sex ratio of abortuses when cases of 45X are excluded.

What are the factors which predispose to the chromosomal anomalies described? One hypothesis states that delayed fertilization is responsible, whether it be pre- or postovulatory overripeness of the ovum, or aging of the spermatozoa in the female genital tract. All of these possibilities have been shown to cause numerical chromosomal anomalies in animals but are difficult to prove in humans. Guerrero and Rojas, studying basal body temperature and coital records of 965 patients, showed an increased spontaneous abortion rate when coitus occurred more than 4 days before or 2 days after ovulation. Less than 1 percent of parents of abortuses have chromosomal abnormalities. However, there are a few mothers, as yet undiagnosable, who seem to be at special risk to conceive abnormal fetuses. This is suggested by Alberman's observation that the frequency of Down's syndrome among viable siblings of trisomic abortuses is ten times higher than the expected rate. Parental age seems to be a factor in trisomic abortions but not in monosomy or polyploidy.

Radiation can cause damage to chromosomes in human cells. Comparing the past cumulative dosage of radiation in mothers of abortuses with a matched control group, Alberman et al. found a significantly higher amount of radiation in the abortion group, especially those with abnormal chromosomes. Although this difference seems to suggest damage to maternal gametes, it may merely reflect the state of health of patients who abort. Those in relatively poor health would have had more diagnostic x-rays taken. The preimplanted embryo is sensitive to the lethal effects of radiation but not to developmental abnormalities. Based on animal comparisons, the implanted embryo theoretically should be able to withstand an intrauterine dose up to 25 roentgens, clearly far more than the exposure one might receive from an upper and lower GI (gastrointestinal) series and an intravenous pyelogram combined.

Infections have been implicated as a cause of abortion. Although it is well established that herpes, rubella, and cytomegaloviruses cause developmental abnormalities in the fetus, there is no convincing evidence that they cause chromosomal anomalies. Mycoplasmas were found more frequently in spontaneously aborted tissue than in a control group of induced abortions, but the finding may represent secondary invasion of the abortuses rather than a causal relationship. When a group of women having chromosomally abnormal abortuses were compared with a group having karyotypically normal abortuses, there was no difference in antibody titers against *Mycoplasma hominis* or *M. fermentans,* indicating that mycoplasma is not mutagenic. Lauritsen also showed no significant difference in the frequency of chromosomally abnormal abortuses in women who suffered from nonspecific virus infections early in pregnancy or near the time of conception.

Drugs and environmental chemicals may cause chromosomal damage and probably are responsible for some abortions. Carr, in 1970, found that women who conceived within 6 months of discontinuing oral contraceptives had a significantly higher frequency of triploid abortuses, but subsequent studies by Lauritsen and also by Boué et al. have failed to confirm this finding. Reviewing all of the evidence to date, it seems very unlikely that oral-contraceptive users are at increased risk of having chromosomally abnormal offspring or abortions.

Vinyl chloride monomers are suspected but have not been proved to be causative agents. Several studies have shown that operating room nurses and anesthetists have a higher rate of spontaneous abortion. Whether this is a direct effect of anesthetic gases, the emotional pressure of the operating room, or other factors is not known. The cancer chemotherapeutic agents are variable in their effects. Anomalies and abortion have been induced with folic acid antagonists while alkylating agents and nitrogen mustard compounds seem to produce little or no effect. Since the thalidomide catastrophe, all tranquilizers have been subject to question regarding teratogenicity, but no evidence exists that they cause abortion.

The role of the immune response in rejecting pregnancy has been extensively studied. ABO incompatability is in dispute as a cause of chromosomally normal spontaneous abortions. Incompatibility in the other red cell and HLA systems is not known to be a factor.

It is extremely difficult to dislodge a normally implanted, healthy embryo by any form of indirect trauma. Hertig and Sheldon in 1943 reported only one case in 1000 abortions that was caused by trauma; recently Lauritsen attributed 8 out of 288 karyotypically normal abortions to trauma. Three followed laparotomy, and five were secondary to major traffic ac-

cidents. The mechanical act of intercourse is no threat to a pregnancy, but the physiologic consequences of orgasm present some questions since the uterus undergoes contractions during orgasm. However, the uterus normally contracts and relaxes throughout pregnancy and most women remain sexually active and orgasmic without any adverse effect.

Several other maternal factors should be considered. Congenital anomalies of the uterus cannot cause chromosomal abnormalities and probably do not cause first-trimester abortions, but can precipitate late abortion or premature delivery. Debilitating systemic diseases may cause abortion if they result in a poor intrauterine environment. Included in this category are anoxic heart disease, severe nutritional deficiencies, metabolic disorders, and chronic disease states. One might expect the endocrine system to have a major role, but endocrine disturbances more commonly cause infertility since they inhibit ovulation. The corpus luteum is essential for maintaining pregnancy during the first 3 weeks following conception and then gradually loses its effectiveness over the next 2 weeks. Jones has reported luteal phase defects as a cause of *recurrent* abortions in 28 percent of cases in her highly selective series.

Since the hypothalamus is intimately involved in the entire reproductive process, psychic stress, acute or chronic, is often implicated as a cause of abortion. As with most psychosomatic conditions, proof is difficult to come by, but a vast folklore of case histories exists supporting this hypothesis.

Threatened Abortion

To assist in the management and the assessment of prognosis, abortion has been classified into separate clinical stages, the earliest of which is threatened abortion. The typical symptom complex includes a missed or delayed period and vaginal bleeding of varying degree, with or without mild cramps. The cervix remains closed. Pelvic examination is not harmful and is essential to rule out other causes of amenorrhea and vaginal bleeding, such as persistent corpus luteum cysts, ectopic pregnancy, and the multitude of problems that can inhibit ovulation. Approximately one-third of all pregnant patients will have some degree of bleeding in the first trimester. Of these, one-half will abort. In the other half, pregnancy progresses to viability but the eventual outcome varies considerably in several studies. The most consistent findings are a twofold increase in prematurity, a small but significant increase in placenta previa, abruptio placentae, and perhaps congenital anomalies. Since the overwhelming majority of patients go on to full-term delivery of normal infants, there is no value in applying these reported statistics to an individual patient.

In the past we have relied on clinical findings to attempt to predict which pregnancy would remain intact. Increasing cramps or bleeding, disappearance of nausea or breast fullness, and a small-for-dates uterus were correctly interpreted as discouraging signs. Conversion of a positive pregnancy test to negative was even more ominous. Today ultrasonic B scanning has become a valuable tool in evaluating the status of the early embryo. With this technique, if the following signs of a normal pregnancy are present, the prognosis for successful outcome is greater than 90 percent. An intact gestational sac can be detected as early as 3 weeks following conception and should be apparent up to 8 weeks of amenorrhea. From 8 to 11 weeks, fetal echoes can be discerned within the sac, and after 12 weeks echoes of a fetal head are visible. Sonographic characteristics of severely disorganized growth or death of the embryo, which are incompatible with normal progress, include loss of definition or fragmentation of the gestational sac, absence of a fetal echo after 9 weeks, and, later, absence or failure of the fetal head to grow.

If sonography is unavailable, the treatment of threatened abortion is entirely expectant. Some limitation of activity for 48 hours may be helpful, but more prolonged bed rest is unnecessary and can be quite disruptive to the family unit. A clear explanation of what is happening and what can be expected is important. Sexual activity is discouraged until the condition becomes stabilized. Since 85 percent of spontaneous abortions occur in the first trimester of pregnancy, progressive growth of the uterus beyond the 12th week of amenorrhea is a very favorable sign. The empiric use of drugs such as tranquilizers or hormones is condemned. Progestogens, once widely used, are of limited therapeutic value; they have been associated with a small increase in the incidence of limb reduction defects and can cause virilization of the external genitalia of female offspring.

Incomplete Abortion

Incomplete abortion means that a portion of the products of conception has been expelled while part is retained within the uterus. When such tissue remains in utero, the uterus cannot contract completely; therefore blood vessels leading to the placental site cannot be compressed by uterine muscle fibers, and excessive bleeding results. Infection is another complication of retained tissue. Beginning, and usu-

ally ending, as endometritis, it can (rarely) progress to septicemia, peritonitis, or septic thrombophlebitis. Oxytocin is helpful in management of these patients since it stimulates uterine contractions, but definitive therapy depends upon evacuation of the uterus by sharp curettage or vacuum aspiration under local, regional, or general anesthesia. Paracervical block has gained wide acceptance since it can be performed on an outpatient basis and is associated with less blood loss and lower morbidity.

Inevitable Abortion

Even though tissue may not have been passed, an abortion is deemed inevitable when the cervix is dilated in the presence of pain and bleeding, or when the membranes are ruptured, or when bleeding is so profuse as to require transfusion. Sonography may confirm the presence of a gestational sac in a dilated lower uterine segment. Treatment is the same as for incomplete abortion.

Complete Abortion

A complete abortion is one in which the products of conception have been totally expelled. If the uterus is empty, curettement is not necessary. However, the clinical recognition of small fragments of placental tissue is often difficult; therefore, in cases of doubt, a curettage should be performed. Complete abortion is most frequently observed with very early abortions.

Missed Abortion

A missed abortion is one in which the embryo dies but is not expelled for 6 weeks. The loss of subjective symptoms of pregnancy such as nausea, breast tenderness, and urinary frequency may occur. The uterus remains unchanged or decreases in size. A positive pregnancy test becomes negative if the placenta also dies, since gonadotropin production ceases. The characteristic sonographic findings of abortion have already been described. An infrequent danger of missed abortion is the development of coagulation defects secondary to hypofibrinogenemia. The etiology of the coagulation defect, though not clearly understood, is probably related to the release of thromboplastin from the degenerating decidua, with subsequent development of disseminated intravascular coagulation (DIC). With time these patients will show a decrease in fibrinogen as well as factor V and factor VIII. Other manifestations of DIC also become apparent. The process takes at least 30 days to become clinically significant, so there is no danger in waiting a month to confirm the diagnosis. After careful hematologic workup, the pregnancy should be evacuated utilizing an oxytocin drip, curettage, intraamniotic injection of hypertonic saline or prostaglandin $F_{2\alpha}$. Recent experience has also demonstrated the efficacy of prostaglandin $F_{2\alpha}$ in the form of vaginal suppositories.

Counseling Following Abortion

Once a woman has had a spontaneous abortion, what is her reproductive prognosis? If there is no history of previous abortion, the possibility remains at 15 percent. If there has been a previous abortion, the risk doubles to 30 percent, and increases to 45 percent if the karyotype of the abortuses was *normal*. Summarizing eight studies of recurrent abortions, balanced translocations were found in one parent in only 4 percent of the total number of cases. Perhaps paradoxically, it can be concluded that recurrent or habitual abortions are less likely to be caused by chromosomal abnormalities than are single or random abortions. A careful investigation of the environmental and maternal causes of abortion is therefore clearly indicated.

Because spontaneous abortions occur so commonly, medical personnel tend to take them for granted. However, for most patients, regardless of their level of intellectual sophistication or whether the pregnancy was planned, abortion represents a real loss. There is almost always an element of guilt and depression which follows, often not expressed. Anticipation of this reaction is extremely important in order to reassure the patient that abortions are extremely common, completey unavoidable, and not related to any physical activity that might have taken place. Furthermore, the patient should be reassured that a miscarriage does not jeopardize her chances of having children. After a first-trimester abortion, there is no need to put off a subsequent pregnancy beyond the first normal menstrual period.

Incompetent Cervix

A separate and uncommon cause of abortion is the incompetent cervix. Occurring in approximately 1 in 500 pregnancies, this distinct clinical entity is only one of several causes of second-trimester abortion. Spontaneous dilatation of the internal os of the cervix occurs, rendering it incapable of supporting the increasing weight and pressure of the growing pregnancy. The cervix dilates without perceivable contractions and the pregnancy is expelled in the second or very early third trimester. A history of painless dil-

atation with recurring pregnancy losses is classical. The patient may present either with a dilated cervix and bulging membranes or with spontaneous rupture of the membranes and a dilated cervix, followed by rapid labor and delivery. If pain or bleeding has occurred, the diagnosis should not be made since other factors are probably involved. Often there is a past history of cervical trauma such as lacerations from a previous obstetrical delivery or dilatation and curettage (D&C). However, congenital cervical incompetence may result in women having this problem in their first pregnancy.

The treatment of choice was developed by Shirodkar. The cervix is reinforced surgically by tunneling a nonabsorbable, heavy ligature submucosally around the cervix at the level of the internal os. At times a heavy silk purse-string suture suffices, the McDonald procedure. When the patient reaches term, or labor begins or bleeding occurs, the suture should be cut and labor allowed to progress. Once the problem has occurred, it will recur in subsequent pregnancies. Surgical treatment can prevent subsequent pregnancy losses, but generally should not be performed until after the 12th or 13th week in case early spontaneous abortion should occur, since this would not be caused by an incompetent cervix. The patient should be examined weekly or twice weekly for painless effacement or dilatation. If the past history is highly suggestive, it may be preferable to empirically perform the surgery at less than 14 weeks' gestation to prevent dilatation, rather than wait for the problem to become manifest.

Cervical cerclage is not a panacea for all second-trimester aborters. A favorable success rate is related directly to care in selection of patients. A typical history is most important. Other causes of second-trimester abortion, including congenital anomalies of the uterus, the presence of submucous myomas, and all of the problems associated with first-trimester abortion, should be ruled out whenever possible.

ECTOPIC PREGNANCY

Ectopic pregnancy is the implantation of a fertilized ovum outside the endometrial cavity. The various abnormal sites are depicted in Fig 30–1. Ninety-eight percent of ectopic gestations occur in the fallopian tube, most often in the ampullary portion. Tubal pregnancy has serious consequences of rupture and intraabdominal hemorrhage, accounting for approximately 60 deaths per year in the United States, or 10 percent of all maternal deaths. Three-fourths of these

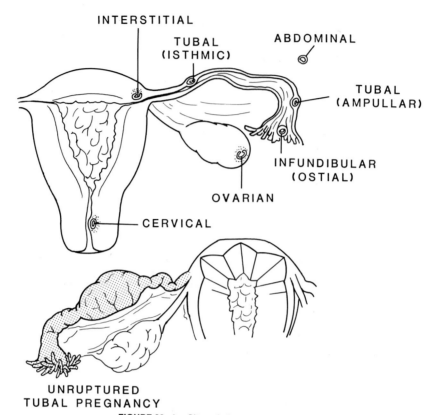

INTERSTITIAL

TUBAL
(ISTHMIC)

ABDOMINAL

TUBAL
(AMPULLAR)

INFUNDIBULAR
(OSTIAL)

OVARIAN

CERVICAL

UNRUPTURED
TUBAL PREGNANCY

FIGURE 30-1 Sites of abnormal pregnancy.

deaths can be prevented by early diagnosis and prompt treatment. It is therefore imperative to consider the possibility of an ectopic pregnancy and rule it in or out whenever clinical findings are suggestive.

ETIOLOGY

Tubal pregnancy occurs approximately once in every 100 to 200 pregnancies; its incidence is affected by a variety of factors. The most important are conditions which narrow the lumen of the fallopian tube, permitting upward migration of sperm but interfering with transport of the larger fertilized ovum. It is more common in patients who have a history of pelvic inflammatory disease, tubal sterilization by any means, tuboplasty, and perhaps endometriosis. Aberrant tubal physiology, as yet undefined, must be an important factor; delayed ovulation has also been implicated. The incidence of tubal pregnancy also increases with increasing maternal age and gravidity.

The role of contraceptives in ectopic pregnancy has been thoroughly studied. The incidence of ectopic pregnancy is not increased in women who use oral or barrier contraceptives, but is ten times greater in those who conceive with an IUD in place, whether the IUD is medicated or not (e.g., with copper or progesterone). This is not an absolute increase in total tubal gestations but a relative increase in incidence, since the IUD more effectively prevents intra-uterine gestation. Several small studies also show an increased relative incidence among patients using oral contraceptives containing progestagen only.

CLINICAL COURSE

Although one-third of tubal pregnancies are self-limiting, either by regression or tubal abortion, the other two-thirds result in various degrees of rupture. Fully one-half of these patients present with hemoperitoneum, some with hypovolemic shock on their initial visit, while the other one-half undergo periodic or slowly progressive leakage of blood through the damaged tubal wall, with subsequent hemoperitoneum. Pain occurs in nearly all cases, but amenorrhea or irregular vaginal bleeding is present 80 percent of the time. Although most tubal pregnancies become symptomatic 6 to 10 weeks after the last menstrual period, the presenting signs and symptoms and the clinical course depend largely on the location of the ectopic gestation. If implantation occurs in the roomier, more distensible, infundibular portion of the tube, pain and tenderness will be a later manifestation, and tubal abortion rather than rupture may occur. If the implantation is either in the ampullary or the narrow isthmic portion, distention and trophoblastic erosion of the tubal wall account for an earlier manifestation of pain, followed by rupture into the peritoneal cavity, or less often into the broad ligament. Interstitial pregnancies often progress beyond 12 weeks' gestation without significant symptoms and appear indistinguishable from a normal intrauterine pregnancy, but then suddenly rupture with massive intraperitoneal hemorrhage.

Amenorrhea occurs because chorionic gonadotropin sustains the corpus luteum, producing in some cases a full decidual reaction, including Arias-Stella phenomenon in the endometrium. Since the vascular supply to the tube is usually inadequate to sustain pregnancy, the placenta degenerates, gonadotropin production declines, the corpus luteum regresses, and endometrial sloughing occurs. The resultant vaginal bleeding is seldom heavy enough to constitute a problem per se, but sometimes an entire decidual cast may be expelled and can be mistaken for a spontaneous abortion.

DIAGNOSIS

A diagnosis of ectopic pregnancy should be considered in anyone with a history of lower abdominal discomfort and amenorrhea or irregular vaginal bleeding. Shoulder pain may occur if intraperitoneal bleeding produces diaphragmatic irritation. Hypovolemia may be manifested by syncope, hypotension, or tachycardia. Body temperature rarely exceeds 38°C (100.4°F). Abdominal examination may include hypoactive bowel sounds, distention, and/or rebound tenderness, but positive findings can be minimal. Vaginal examination often reveals fullness or tenderness in the adnexa or cul-de-sac. If the tubal pregnancy is unruptured, a distinct, unilateral, tender, oblong mass may be present. Most observers report a moderate degree of uterine enlargement.

The diagnosis should be suspected on the basis of clinical history and can be confirmed in several ways. Culdocentesis, aspiration of the cul-de-sac, offers a rapid means of detecting intraperitoneal bleeding and should be performed whenever the diagnosis is considered. A positive result, consisting of obtaining blood or bloody fluid that does not clot, mandates surgical exploration of the pelvis. If clear peritoneal fluid is obtained, one has not ruled out an unruptured tubal pregnancy. A "dry tap" or a yield of fresh blood that clots readily neither rules out nor substantiates hemoperitoneum.

Standard latex and hemagglutination pregnancy tests, although helpful, are not diagnostic since gonadotropin titers may be too low to be detected. Positive tests, when present, can be confused with intrauterine pregnancy. The recently developed radioreceptor assay (RRA) for HCG (human chorionic gonadotropin) is highly sensitive and can detect the low levels of HCG present in abnormal pregnancies. A rapid modification of the radioimmune assay has also been developed.

As described earlier in this chapter, ultrasonography is highly accurate in detecting and assessing early intrauterine gestational sacs. It is also useful in evaluating adnexal masses. Therefore the combined use of radioreceptor assays and ultrasonography offers a noninvasive, new dimension in accurately diagnosing tubal pregnancy at an early stage. A positive RRA and an empty uterus are strong indicators of an ectopic pregnancy.

Surgical intervention is often necessary to confirm one's diagnostic suspicion, especially when the clinical picture and laboratory tests are equivocal or conflicting. Posterior colpotomy and culdoscopy still have a role in diagnosis but are rapidly being replaced by laparoscopy.

TREATMENT

The treatment of tubal pregnancies is surgical. Although the surgery can sometimes be accomplished through a colpotomy incision, exploratory laparotomy is usally preferred and is often carried out immediately following diagnostic laparoscopy. Blood and fluid replacement are essential in surgical management. Once the abdomen has been opened, careful exploration of both adnexa should be carried out before a definitive procedure is performed. If the opposite tube appears normal, salpingectomy is the procedure of choice. The need for cornual resection of the tube once widely practiced, is doubtful.

If exploration of the pelvis reveals a damaged or absent contralateral tube, either salpingostomy or a process of milking the contents of the tube out through the fimbria can be performed to preserve potential fertility, but the chances of a repeat tubal pregnancy are significantly increased. If the affected tube is not salvageable and the opposite tube is absent or badly damaged, hysterectomy may be considered, but should not be carried out unless this possibility has been thoroughly discussed with the patient prior to surgery. Also, if the patient's general condition has been compromised by excessive blood loss, a more extensive procedure such as hysterectomy should not be undertaken.

Nontubal Ectopic Pregnancies

Ovarian pregnancies constitute 1 percent of all ectopic gestations and result either from intraovarian fertilization or retrograde extrusion of the fertilized ovum with subsequent implantation into the ovarian cortex. They behave clinically much like tubal pregnancies and can only be diagnosed at the time of laparotomy with histologic confirmation. Treatment is salpingo-oophorectomy.

Cervical pregnancy is the rarest of ectopic gestations. As the villi begin to degenerate and separate, profuse hemorrhage occurs since the cervix cannot contract around the open sinusoids. After separation of all placental fragments, bleeding may be controlled by suturing and packing of the placental site, but hysterectomy is often necessary.

Most abdominal pregnancies probably begin in the tube but reimplant somewhere in the abdominal cavity if a tubal abortion occurs while the conceptus is still viable. Sites of reimplantation include the broad ligament, pelvic wall, intestine, mesentery, or omentum. In contrast to tubal gestations, abdominal pregnancies may progress to viability. Clinically there is often a history of transient abdominal pain and vaginal bleeding followed by progressive asymptomatic enlargement of the abdomen. Vague gastrointestinal or urinary symptoms or increasing abdominal discomfort may develop. The diagnosis should be suspected if the fetal parts feel very superficial, especially in the presence of a deflection attitude or malpresentation. Careful pelvic examination should reveal a normal-sized uterus. The diagnosis can then be confirmed by hysterogram, ultrasonography, or by the failure of oxytocin stimulation to produce uterine contractions.

The great risk of uncontrollable hemorrhage from placental separation mandates prompt exploratory laparotomy and termination of the pregnancy regardless of the gestational age at which the diagnosis is made. After the amniotic sac is opened, the umbilical cord should be carefully ligated and the fetus extracted so the placenta is not disturbed. The area of placental attachment should be gently delineated. If the blood supply to the placental site can be controlled, appropriate ligatures should be placed and the placenta removed. If not, the placenta can be left in place to gradually degenerate, eventuating in a prolonged postoperative course, complicated by repeated chorionic cysts, possible sepsis, intestinal obstruction, or intraabdominal bleeding. This is still preferable to the massive and potentially fatal hemorrhage which can occur if the placenta is dislodged from an area where the blood supply cannot be controlled.

MULTIPLE PREGNANCY

Pregnancies in which more than one fetus is produced are a relatively frequent finding in the human species. Nevertheless, pregnancies with multiple fetuses should not be considered normal because numerous maternal and fetal complications can occur during the antepartum, intrapartum, and postpartum periods. Common maternal complications include preeclampsia, eclampsia, anemia, hemorrhage, as well as a variety of intrapartum complications. Perinatal mortality is 2 to 3 times greater for twin births than for single births primarily because of prematurity, prolapsed umbilical cord, and asphyxia (Naeye).

Twin pregnancies are the most common form of multiple gestation. Although triplet, quadruplet, and quintuplet multiple gestations are less common, the maternal and fetal problems associated with them are basically the same as those for twin pregnancies.

INCIDENCE

Greulich reported the following incidences of pregnancies with multiple fetuses: twins, 1:85; triplets, 1:7629; and quadruplets, 1:670,734. Monozygotic (monovular, identical) twins occur at a frequency of approximately 1:250 pregnancies, independent of heredity or other factors. The development of dizygotic (diovular, nonidentical, fraternal) twins is influenced by several factors, including race, heredity, maternal age and parity, and the administration of various drugs that induce ovulation.

Multiple gestation occurs more frequently in blacks than in whites, and is less frequent in the oriental races. The chance of a twin gestation in black women is approximately 30 percent greater than in white women; this racial difference is even more striking for triplets. A strong maternal history for multiple births is important. Women who themselves were the product of a dizygotic twin pregnancy give birth to twins more frequently than women whose husbands were one of dizygotic twins (White, Wyshak). Increasing maternal age and parity also result in greater frequency of twinning. The use of ovulation-inducing drugs such as pituitary gonadotropins or clomiphene citrate has increased the incidence of multiple gestation. Pituitary gonadotropin therapy results in multiple fetuses in 20 to 40 percent of pregnancies while clomiphene citrate is associated with 4 to 8 percent incidence of twinning. All of these differences in the incidence of multiple gestation relate entirely to variations in the occurrence of dizygotic twins.

Monozygotic twin gestations account for approximately 20 to 30 percent, while dizygotic twins provide the remaining 70 to 80 percent. Dizygotic twins result from the release from the ovary of two oocytes with fertilization of both by different spermatozoa. Since both zygotes have different genetic material, dizygotic twins are no more alike than any two siblings in a family. Monozygotic twins, however, result from fertilization of one ovum with one spermatozoa and the subsequent division of the fertilized zygote into two equivalent and separate zygotes.

Monozygotic twins can arise from separation of the fertilized ovum into two zygotes at various stages of development (Langman).

1. *Separation at the two- to eight-cell stage (morula).* Two separate zygotes develop within one zona pellucida. Both implant separately and each embryo has its own amnion and chorion; thus this pregnancy is diamnionic, dichorionic. There may be two distinct placentas or a single fused placenta. Approximately 33 percent of all monozygotic twins are in this category.
2. *Separation early in the blastocyst stage.* The inner cell mass divides into two separate groups of cells located within one blastocyst. There is a single placenta and a single chorionic cavity, but each fetus has its own amnionic sac. Thus this pregnancy is diamnionic, monochorionic. Approximately 66 percent of all monozygous twins are in this group.
3. *Separation of the zygote at the stage of the bilaminar germ disc, before the appearance of the primitive streak, but after the establishment of the amnion.* This results in a monozygotic twin pregnancy that is monoamnionic and monochorionic with a common placenta. It occurs in less than 1 percent of twin pregnancies.
4. *Separation of the zygote after the primitive streak has developed.* This may result in an abnormal or incomplete splitting of the germ disc with formation of conjoined (Siamese) twins. It occurs in less than 1 percent of twin pregnancies.

Dizygotic twins implant individually in the uterus. Each twin has its own placenta, its own amnion, and its own chorion. Occasionally, the two placentas will fuse if they are closely situated. Despite the close approximation of the two placentas, communication of the placental blood vessels of one twin with vessels of the other twin never occurs (Benirschke, Kim).

FETAL DEVELOPMENT

At birth each twin is generally smaller than a single fetus of the same gestational age. More than 50 percent of newborn twins weigh less than 2500 g at delivery (Farooqui). Although small differences in size are not important, large differences in the size of the twins suggest the presence of the twin-twin transfusion syndrome. This syndrome results from the existence of vascular communications (artery-artery, artery-vein, or vein-vein) between the placentas of monozygotic twin fetuses (Benirschke). Artery-artery anastomoses may result in hypervolemia in one twin with hypovolemia in the other especially during labor and delivery. Artery-vein anastomoses may be significant enough to affect the size of both fetuses at birth. One twin may be considerably smaller than the other as a consequence of chronic intrauterine underperfusion and undernutrition. The larger twin is plethoric, edematous, and polycythemic while the smaller one is pale, anemic, and dehydrated. The difference in size between twins generally relates to the quantity and caliber of the arteriovenous anastomoses present. In rare circumstances, a considerable number of anastomoses result in failure of one of the twins to develop (fetus papyraceus).

DIAGNOSIS

The obstetrician should think of multiple gestation whenever the pregnant uterus seems too large for the estimated length of gestation. The presence of an excessive amount of amniotic fluid or the palpation of numerous small fetal parts or of more than one head should all suggest the diagnosis of multiple gestation, as should a positive maternal family history of twins. Nonetheless, in one-quarter of cases, multiple pregnancy is not diagnosed until after the first fetus has been delivered. Differential diagnosis in cases in which the uterus appears larger than gestational age include inappropriate menstrual history, polyhydramnios, hydatidiform mole, uterine myomas, adnexal masses, and elevation of the uterus by a distended maternal bladder.

Definitive diagnosis of multiple gestation can be

made with sonography or radiography. Sonography can diagnose multiple gestation with safety and reliability as early as the sixth week after the last menstrual period. Early in pregnancy, diagnosis depends on the the identification of more than one gestational sac; later in pregnancy (after 15 weeks) diagnosis requires the identification of more than one fetal skull. Roentgenological examination of the abdomen can also reliably confirm a clinical impression of multiple pregnancy. This procedure should generally be performed late in pregnancy because of the risks to the embryo and fetus associated with exposure to ionizing radiation. Palpating two distinct fetuses as well as simultaneously recording two different fetal heart rates can also support the diagnosis of a twin gestation. In triplet, quadruplet, and quintuplet pregnancies, the clinical findings are exaggerated when compared with the findings in twin gestation. Sonographic or radiographic examination will ascertain the number of fetuses present within the uterus.

MANAGEMENT OF PREGNANCIES WITH TWIN FETUSES

The early diagnosis of pregnancy with multiple fetuses is invaluable because it enables the obstetrician to carefully evaluate the mother and her fetuses during the remainder of her pregnancy. Frequent prenatal examinations throughout pregnancy will help detect maternal complications such as preeclampsia and premature labor. The patient should be instructed in a diet containing ample amounts of iron, folic acid, vitamins, and protein to guard against the potential complications of iron- and folate-deficiency anemias.

Most fetal complications in multiple pregnancies relate to the frequent occurrence of premature labor and of intrauterine growth retardation. Although the etiology of premature labor in twin pregnancies is unclear, bed rest has been beneficial, particularly after the 32d week of gestation. Jouppila et al. showed that prolonged bed rest in hospital resulted in an increase in the birth weight of each twin and a reduction in perinatal morbidity and mortality. Jeffrey et al. showed that twin fetuses of mothers who had considerable bed rest after the 30th week weighed more than did twin fetuses of similar gestational age in whom the mothers were not kept at bed rest. Serial measurements of the biparietal diameter by ultrasound allow the obstetrician to detect intrauterine growth retardation in pregnancies with multiple fetuses. If abnormalities of fetal growth are detected, fetal activity tests, and in some cases oxytocin chal-

lenge tests, can be performed on both fetuses to determine whether fetal distress is present.

LABOR

Twin pregnancy has little effect on the length of labor in either primigravidas or multigravidas, but dysfunctional labor is more common in multiple pregnancy than with singletons. Premature labor may be treated with bed rest and mild sedation and with infusions of ethanol or magnesium sulfate in an attempt to decrease uterine contractility. The value of ethanol in treating the premature labor of multiple pregnancy has not been clearly established.

Once labor begins, the fetal presentations should be determined either clinically or by roentgenologic examination. Possible fetal presentations include (Guttmacher):

1. Vertex–vertex (47%)
2. Vertex–breech (30%)
3. Breech–vertex (7%)
4. Breech–breech (9%)
5. Vertex–transverse (5%)
6. Breech–transverse (2%)
7. Transverse–transverse (< 1%)
8. All others (< 1%)

When the fetuses are small, the presentations may include compound, face, brow, and footling breech presentations. Prolapse of the cord is more common in these circumstances.

Even though labor is generally normal in twin gestations, two common complications include (1) rupture of the membranes without effective labor, and (2) prolonged, inefficient labor with or without previous rupture of the membranes. These problems may best be treated with cesarean section, although in certain circumstances the administration of oxytocin in dilute concentrations may initiate or stimulate labor.

Analgesia and Anesthesia for Labor and Delivery

The choice of analgesia and anesthesia will depend considerably on the presence or absence of various maternal or fetal complications such as prematurity, maternal hypertension, or labor inertia. Furthermore, if there is need for operative delivery (e.g., internal podalic version and extraction of the second twin), then specific analgesia and anesthesia may be necessary. It is best to administer the fewest possible analgesics and anesthetics to the pregnant woman with a twin gestation. For vaginal delivery, pudendal block anesthesia will provide sufficient analgesia for spontaneous vaginal delivery. If intrauterine manipulation is necessary to deliver the second twin, uterine relaxation is best achieved with halothane inhalation anesthesia. For cesarean section, it is best to avoid subarachnoid block or epidural or caudal anesthesia because of the risks of maternal hypotension due to the supine hypotensive syndrome.

Methods of Delivery

There are few problems with delivery of the first twin when the vertex presents (Farooqui). The first twin may be delivered spontaneously or by low outlet forceps. When the first fetus presents as a breech, however, several potential problems arise. In the unusually large or small fetus, there is considerable risk of fetal asphyxia in delivery of the aftercoming head. There is also the potential for umbilical cord prolapse. Cesarean section is preferred when the breech presents in other than a frank breech position, when the breech is unusually large or small, or when there is suspicion that there will be locking of twins. Otherwise, labor is allowed to continue when the breech presents. Other indications for cesarean section are the same as with singleton presentations.

The complication of interlocked twins occurs in approximately 1:1000 twin gestations (Fox et al.). Locking only occurs in breech-vertex presentations. With descent of the first fetus (breech), both fetal chins interlock. If unlocking cannot be effected, cesarean section or decapitation of the first fetus must be performed. In any case, fetal mortality is extremely high.

The type of delivery planned for the second twin depends on the fetal presentation. A mother in whom the second twin presents as a vertex or breech can generally deliver the second twin spontaneously (Guttmacher). Fetal membranes should be ruptured only after the presenting part enters the pelvis; moderate fundal pressure can be applied to maintain the presenting part in the pelvis. The best outcome for the second twin is obtained when delivery occurs between 3 and 20 minutes after delivery of the first twin. After 20 minutes, the risks of premature separation of the placenta and of umbilical cord prolapse increase; both of these complications can quickly result in fetal asphyxia. If the second twin presents as a transverse or oblique lie, or cannot be guided into the pelvis as a breech or vertex presentation, general anesthesia is administered to the mother to relax the uterus. The

obstetrician then determines the precise position of the fetus by placing the examining hand in the uterus. The operator then grasps both fetal feet, ruptures the fetal membranes, and performs an internal podalic version with delivery of the fetus by breech extraction.

In very rare circumstances (e.g., an unusually large second twin, or a transverse fetal lie with the back down), the operator is unable to perform an internal podalic version safely. In these instances, cesarean section may be necessary for delivery of the second twin. Cesarean section is more likely when there has been undue delay following delivery of the first twin. It should be emphasized that there are very few circumstances in which the time of delivery from first to second twin should exceed 20 minutes; delay can only be justified when the second twin is a vertex or breech presentation.

Following delivery of both twins, manual removal of the placenta is immediately performed. A dilute concentration of oxytocin is administered intravenously to hasten and enhance contraction of the uterus and to decrease the postpartum blood loss associated with twin pregnancies.

DISORDERS OF PLACENTA AND MEMBRANES

PREMATURE RUPTURE OF MEMBRANES AND CHORIOAMNIONITIS

The incidence of spontaneous rupture of placental membranes prior to the onset of labor is about 10 percent at term and may be as high as 20 percent before 34 weeks' gestation. The term *premature rupture of membranes* (PROM) is ambiguous because it may refer to spontaneous amniorrhexis (rupture of membranes) prior to fetal maturity or prior to the onset of labor, or both. The interval, or latent period, between amniorrhexis and onset of labor required for the definition of PROM in term pregnancy varies from author to author, ranging from 1 to 12 hours. The major importance of PROM is the loss of a major host-defense mechanism against chorioamnionitis, although microorganisms can occasionally be cultured from intact amnionic sacs as well. Amniorrhexis may result from infection of the intact membranes, which causes uterine irritability and contractions, or it may allow ascent of endogenous vaginal flora into the uterus in numbers sufficient to cause fetal and uterine infection. Amniorrhexis may also increase the risk of these infections by allowing the escape of antibacterial factors in amnionic fluid, factors characterized by Galask as the zinc-dependent polypeptide system, lysozyme, peroxidase, transferrin, complement, and immunoglobulins (Galask, Snyder; Larsen, Galask). Appropriate management of PROM is reasonably clear in normal term pregnancies but has been addressed in very few prospective studies of premature gestations (Townsend et al.; Sacks and Baker; Bauer et al.). Recent advances in the care of the premature neonate have made previous prognostic data obsolete. Current studies, therefore, are sorely needed to determine optimum management of the problem with early third-trimester pregnancies.

TERM GESTATION

In term gestations, the significant complications of PROM are generally related to, and increased by, increasing duration of the latent period. In Gunn's studies at the University of California at Los Angeles, perinatal mortality rate was 0.5 percent when the latent period was less than 24 hours but was 2 percent when the latent period exceeded 24 hours. Eastman and Hellman give a 1.7 percent perinatal mortality rate among 2615 term infants delivered less than 48 hours after PROM but a perinatal mortality rate of 6.8 percent with latent periods over 48 hours. Further, Huff indicates that delivery within 24 hours of PROM was associated with a 19 percent incidence of puerperal endomyometritis in 215 women, but a latent period of 24 to 48 hours was related to a 22 percent incidence; a latent period longer than 48 hours was associated with a 50 percent incidence of endomyometritis. Bryans studied a predominantly medically indigent black population in Georgia and found that amnionitis occurred in 6.4 percent of those who delivered within 24 hours after PROM but occurred in 30.7 percent of women whose latent period exceeded 24 hours.

The development of clinical signs and symptoms of chorioamnionitis is associated with a less favorable fetal prognosis. In Lanier's series, 50 percent of neonatal deaths occurred with evidence of clinical chorioamnionitis, while 32 percent of neonatal deaths in Bryans' report occurred with chorioamnionitis; in the study by Russell and Anderson, 47 percent of the neonatal deaths were associated with chorioamnionitis. The diagnosis of clinical chorioamnionitis is difficult because uterine tenderness may result from either contractions or infection and because leukocytosis may also result from labor or from infec-

tion. Maternal and fetal tachycardia are often observed but are somewhat nonspecific. Fever rarely develops early in the course of the disease unless the infection is caused by beta-hemolytic streptococci.

In term pregnancies, reduction of perinatal morbidity and mortality and of maternal puerperal endomyometritis is best accomplished by delivery within 24 hours of amniorrhexis. Antibiotic therapy has been suggested; but in a large cooperative study of prophylactic dimethylchlortetracycline by Lebherz et al., fetal morbidity and mortality did not improve although the incidence of puerperal endomyometritis was reduced. Huff similarly demonstrated a profound reduction in the frequency of puerperal endomyometritis with penicillin/kanamycin prophylaxis, although no benefit for the fetus could be shown. Burchell supported these findings in a retrospective review of 1788 women with PROM in Chicago. Prophylactic penicillin and streptomycin reduced the incidence of puerperal fever from 3.9 to 0.6 percent when the latent period was less than 48 hours and from 11.7 to 7.1 percent with a latent period greater than 48 hours. He further argued that perinatal mortality rates improved with this antibiotic prophylaxis from 42.9 per 1000 live births to 34.5 per 1000 with latent periods less than 48 hours and from 87.4 per 1000 live births to 66.7 per 1000 with latent periods over 48 hours. The arguments given against use of antibiotic prophylaxis include (1) risk of allergic reactions, (2) risk of alteration of the patient's bacterial flora, (3) cognizance of the increasing percentage of antibiotic-resistant hospital strains of bacteria, and (4) possible interference by the antibiotics with cultures of the potentially infected neonate. Other studies of antibiotic prophylaxis in gynecology have indicated that, while febrile morbidity may be reduced, the frequency of serious infections or pelvic abscesses is not at all diminished (Mead and Clapp).

PRETERM GESTATION

Spontaneous rupture of membranes prior to fetal maturity has always been a clinical problem involving more questions than answers. Antepartum corticosteroid therapy and improvement in pediatric management have reduced the morbidity and mortality associated with hyaline membrane disease and have made previous statistics about this problem obsolete. Immaturity of fetal kidneys, liver, intestine, central nervous system (CNS), and immunologic system now assumes relatively greater significance. Current data are needed to determine optimum management at each week of gestation.

Diagnosis of amniorrhexis is very important in preterm gestation, for the diagnosis may set in motion drastic action or prolonged hospitalization. Observation by speculum exam of amniotic fluid escaping from the cervix or pooling in the posterior vaginal fornix is most helpful; the fluid should display ferning on microscopic examination. Amniotic fluid gives an alkaline reaction to litmus paper, but cervical mucus may yield the same reaction. Staining of the amniotic fluid with Nile blue sulfate yields orange-colored fetal squamous cells. Once spontaneous rupture of membranes is confirmed by these methods, ultrasonic measurement of fetal biparietal diameter helps to establish approximate gestational age.

The duration of the latent period is greater in preterm gestation than in term pregnancies, allowing the possibility of delaying delivery to permit further maturation of several fetal organ systems. In term pregnancies, about 80 percent of women with PROM will commence labor within 4 hours, but only 35 to 50 percent of preterm gestation patients will begin labor in 24 hours. In fact, labor begins spontaneously after 72 hours' latent period in 95 percent of term pregnancies but in only 70 percent of preterm pregnancies. Some 10 percent of preterm patients do not begin labor spontaneously even in 14 days. Perinatal mortality may increase with an increased latent period, since Gunn et al., found that 10.2 percent of infants weighing 1000 to 2500 g died if latent period was less than 24 hours but 22.5 percent of these infants died if latent period exceeded 24 hours. At gestational ages of 28 to 32 weeks, however, perinatal mortality is so high (about 45 percent at 28 weeks and around 10 percent at 32 weeks) that delaying delivery may improve fetal maturity without significantly increasing the incidence of chorioamnionitis. A study is needed to answer this question satisfactorily.

Following the original suggestion by Liggins and Howie, Mead and Clapp report that betamethasone therapy reduces the risk of hyaline membrane disease with PROM in the preterm pregnancy, and found no increase in the risk of chorioamnionitis. Their study was small and retrospective, however, and betamethasone has no proven effect on CNS, hepatic, intestinal, or renal maturity. Even if pulmonary immaturity can be alleviated, the immaturity of other organs is so harmful that there are potential advantages to waiting until labor begins spontaneously because the gain of several days to a few weeks may permit sufficient maturation of these other organs to make the difference between neonatal survival and death. Of course, the significant risk of chorioamnionitis to mother and child might be increased by this delay. Previous articles by Russell and Anderson in 1962 and by Webb in 1967 implicate PROM and chorioamnionitis in maternal deaths from sepsis, which caused 5.2 percent of 1054 maternal deaths in Webb's series from California over an 8-year period. Although we surmise that, with current knowledge of microbiology and antibiotic therapy, expectant management of the preterm patient with PROM is reasonably safe, no study has proved a neonatal benefit which offsets fetal and maternal risk.

Further complicating this problem is the evidence that PROM in preterm gestation is associated with a higher incidence of fetal malpresentation. Contrast the 3 to 4 percent incidence of breech presentation in term gestations in labor with the 10 to 20 percent incidence of breech presentation associated with PROM in preterm pregnancies (Huff). If cesarean section is employed to deliver these fetuses with their proportionately larger heads, thus avoiding the perinatal morbidity and mortality of head entrapment during vaginal delivery, then further maternal risk is added. Many authors have found that PROM prior to cesarean section increases the risk of puerperal endomyometritis and that the longer the latent period, the greater the risk of infection. Expectant treatment of the preterm pregnancy with PROM may therefore increase maternal morbidity substantially. Studies performed with random patient selection are essential to determine the correct management of this problem.

PLACENTAL ABRUPTION

DEFINITION

Placental abruption, also known as premature separation of the normally implanted placenta, or abruptio placentae, or ablatio placentae, is the detachment of the placenta from the uterine wall at any time between the 20th week of pregnancy and the end of labor. Placental separation prior to the 20th week of gestation is not classified as a separate clinical entity, but it is considered a cause of spontaneous abortion.

Premature separation of the normally implanted placenta is one of the most serious complications of pregnancy for both mother and fetus. Although 85 to 90 percent of all cases of placental abruption are of the mild to moderate variety, 10 percent of all cases represent the more severe form of premature separation. This severe form has a maternal mortality rate as high as 10 percent (Krupp et al.). Mortality has generally been related to hemorrhagic shock in association with renal failure and pituitary insufficiency. In patients managed with aggressive blood replacement, the maternal mortality rate approaches zero.

Placental abruption may be complete if the placenta is completely detached from the uterine wall, or partial if a portion of the placenta still retains its connection to the uterus. Abruptions, whether complete or partial, may or may not be associated with vaginal bleeding. Some of the blood lost with placental abruption can appear externally by passing between the membranes and the uterus and out through the cervix and vagina (Fig. 30–2). Less often, however, blood does not appear externally but is retained between the placenta and the uterus (concealed abruption). A concealed abruption is associated with greater maternal morbidity because the extent of the hemorrhage cannot be accurately gauged.

INCIDENCE

Placental abruption complicates approximately 1 to 2 percent of all deliveries. The higher incidence figures usually include cases of rupture of the marginal sinus. Although marginal sinus rupture was formerly considered a separate clinical entity, currently it denotes placental separation limited to the margin of the placenta. Approximately 50 percent of placental separations occur before the onset of labor and fully 15 percent are diagnosed only during routine examination of the placenta after delivery of the fetus. Placental abruption severe enough to compromise the fetus occurs less than once in 420 deliveries (Pritchard et al.). Fetal hypoxia or even fetal death generally depends on the amount and duration of placental separation as well as the degree of maternal hypotension and hypovolemic shock. With complete placental

FIGURE 30–2 Bleeding in placental abruption.

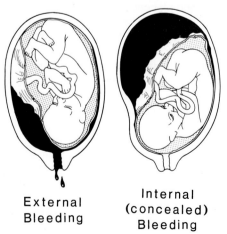

External
Bleeding

Internal
(concealed)
Bleeding

abruption, fetal mortality rates are as high as 95 percent.

ETIOLOGY

The primary cause of placental abruption is unknown but several factors are thought to play a role in its development. These factors include acute and chronic hypertension, sudden decompression of the uterus, partial or complete occlusion of the inferior vena cava, and older maternal age or high parity. Acute and chronic hypertensive diseases are present in one-third to one-half of women who develop complete placental separation (Pritchard et al). Of hypertensive women with placental abruptions severe enough to kill the fetus, one-half have chronic hypertensive cardiovascular disease; the remainder have acute hypertension associated with preeclampsia. The risk of severe placental abruption also increases with parity. Since the risk of chronic hypertensive vascular disease increases with age and parity, it is difficult to determine which predisposing factor is more important. Hibbard has shown that a woman with a previous severe placental abruption is more likely to develop the same complication in a subsequent pregnancy.

Howard et al. suggested that the supine hypotensive syndrome was important in the etiology of premature placental separation. They postulated that compression of the inferior vena cava by the weight of the pregnant uterus increased the venous pressure below the occlusion. The resulting increase in blood pressure in the intervillous space resulted in local hemorrhage and placental separation. In support of this theory, Mengert et al. were able to produce premature placental separation by compressing the vena cava before opening the uterus at the time of cesarean hysterectomy. Nevertheless, placental separation due to inferior vena caval compression is a rare complication because of the extensive collateral circulation in and around the uterus that prevents excessive pressure from developing within the choriodecidual space.

Mechanical factors associated with premature separation are rare (less than 5 percent). These include sudden decompression of the uterus such as occurs with delivery of the first twin, with rupture of the membranes in patients with polyhydramnios, or in association with traction on a short umbilical cord.

Two other factors, folic acid deficiency and acute trauma, have also been suggested as causes for abruptio placentae, but more recent investigations have not confirmed these initial observations. However, folate deficiency may be an indication of nutritional deprivation, which is probably associated with placental separation.

PATHOPHYSIOLOGY

Degeneration and necrosis of the decidua basalis produce the earliest uterine lesion associated with placental abruption. The vascular lesion associated with this degeneration and necrosis is an acute degenerative arteriolitis. The extent of placental separation is determined by the amount of decidual bleeding. With extensive bleeding part or all of the placenta may be dissected off the uterine wall, leaving a thin layer of decidua basalis adherent to the myometrium. Blood may accumulate behind the placenta (concealed abruption) or may dissect its way between membranes and the uterine wall to appear externally (external hemorrhage). In severe abruptio, blood may superficially infiltrate the myometrium or may involve the entire uterine musculature. A uterus with this characteristic mottled, ecchymotic appearance is commonly referred to as a Couvelaire uterus. Considerable blood may also extravasate into the broad ligaments and into the pelvic retroperitoneal space.

Without prompt therapy for the abruption, a consumption coagulopathy or disseminated intravascular coagulation can develop. This is more likely with a complete separation, but some alterations in clotting may develop with less severe forms of abruption. The clotting defect is caused by an abnormal activation of the normal coagulation mechanism (Pritchard, Berkken). Thromboplastin from abnormal subplacental decidua, from the disrupted placenta, or from serum in the subplacental clot can enter the circulation through open blood vessels at the placental site. This thromboplastin ultimately converts fibrinogen to fibrin. As more thromboplastin is generated and released into the circulation, more fibrinogen and clotting factors (factors V and VIII and platelets) are utilized. The blood then becomes incoagulable, and abnormal bleeding occurs. (For DIC see Chap. 21).

SYMPTOMS AND SIGNS

In general, the clinical findings with abruptio correspond to the amount of placental separation. With small degrees of separation, there may be a small amount of external hemorrhage of either bright or dark blood. There may be little or no uterine tenderness, minimal uterine irritability, and no evidence of fetal distress. Premature labor may be present but is not likely unless the fetal membranes have also ruptured.

Approximately one-third of all placental separations are mild and produce few or no symptoms; many of these are not detected until the placenta is inspected postpartum. Moderate placental abruptions are associated with uterine hypertonus; the fetus may or may not be dead; the mother is not usually in shock, and generally there is no coagulation defect. The most severe abruptions present with uterine tetany, sudden severe uterine pain, maternal hypotension, fetal death, and a consumptive coagulopathy. If there is a concealed abruption, the uterus will gradually enlarge as blood collects within the cavity and infiltrates the muscular wall; DIC may also develop gradually.

The quantity of vaginal bleeding may be disproportionate to the gravity of symptoms and the degree of hypovolemic shock. It has long been thought that the shock seen with severe placental abruption is out of proportion to the amount of hemorrhage. Schneider showed that large doses of thromboplastin, injected intravenously into experimental animals, could cause profound shock. Despite Schneider's observations, most current evidence indicates that the intensity of shock is directly related to maternal blood loss. Pritchard measured blood loss in gravidas with severe placental abruption and fetal death and found blood loss often to be greater than one-half of the normal blood volume during pregnancy.

Differential diagnosis must consider placenta previa, rupture of the uterus with abdominal pregnancy, torsion of the uterus, a ruptured uterine varix, and various acute surgical conditions such as cholecystitis with cholelithiasis, acute appendicitis with rupture, and intraabdominal traumatic injuries. Making the distinction between abruptio placentae and placenta previa is usually easy, but occasionally difficulties may be encountered. Mild abruptions may present initially with painless vaginal bleeding. Conversely, some patients with placenta previa may present with uterine irritability and tenderness. Diagnostic ultrasound evaluation of the placental site is especially valuable because placenta previa can be diagnosed or excluded with a considerable degree of accuracy with ultrasound. Furthermore, the occasional identification of a retroplacental clot will support the diagnosis of abruptio placentae (Fig. 30–3).

TREATMENT

Placental abruption with its associated hemorrhage and hypovolemia must be treated rapidly and aggressively. *It is imperative that an effective circulation be restored by the intravenous administration of appropriate fluids, particularly whole blood.* In instances in

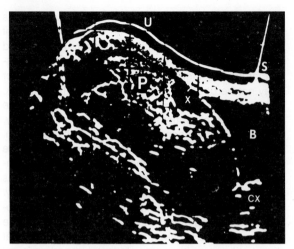

FIGURE 30-3 Placental abruption, 27 weeks. A retroplacental blood clot is represented by the clear space (*x*) between the placental basal plate and the uterine wall. Other abbreviations: *P*–placenta, *B*–bladder, *CX*–cervix, *U*–umbilicus, and *S*–symphysis. *(From DI Edelstone, in Diagnostic Ultrasound Applied to Obstetrics and Gynecology, Harper & Row, 1979)*

consumptive coagulopathy which results in hypofibrinogenemia (Beller). The platelet count (platelets per cubic millimeter of blood) may also be decreased but need not be, even in instances of severe placental abruption. With extensive placental abruption, fibrin degradation products are almost universally found in the blood; therefore their measurement provides little help in the management of these patients. The clot observation test is the quickest, simplest, and most valuable clinical test for determining the presence of a coagulation defect. When the patient with a possible placental abruption is admitted to the hospital, a blood sample for clot observation should be obtained. Within 8 to 12 minutes of the drawing of the blood sample, a clot should form and should remain stable during the next hour. If a clot has not formed, a major coagulopathy is present. If a blood clot initially forms but partially or completely disintegrates within 30 minutes, a milder clotting defect is likely to be present.

Therapy with fibrinogen (cryoprecipitate) in cases of placental abruption may occasionally be necessary. Although theoretically the administration of fibrinogen may make DIC worse by resulting in deposition of fibrin in the microcirculation of such vital organs as the kidney and brain, in practical terms intravenous administration of 4 to 8 g of fibrinogen will not complicate the management of a patient with severe hypofibrinogenemia. Conversely, hemostasis may be improved. Fibrinogen treatment prior to delivery by cesarean section is helpful, as is strict attention to the ligation of all bleeding points at the time of abdominal incision. Therapy with individual clotting factors and platelets is almost never necessary. In addition, there are few if any indications for the use of heparin to prevent or treat the DIC of placental abruption (Beller). In many instances, the administration of fresh blood is the best treatment of all.

METHOD AND TIMING OF DELIVERY

As soon as maternal hypovolemia has been corrected, the first step toward delivery is artificial rupture of the fetal membranes. This procedure will minimize hemorrhage and also has the theoretical advantage of reducing the possibility of DIC or the development of an amniotic fluid embolism. Furthermore, it enables the obstetrician to directly monitor intrauterine pressure and fetal heart rate. Artificial rupture of the membranes, in association with induction or stimulation of labor with oxytocin infusion, will ensure that labor progresses rapidly and uninterrupt-

which the fetus is still alive but distressed, rapid delivery should follow stabilization of the mother's circulation. Delivery will almost always be by cesarean section. In situations in which the fetus is dead, vaginal delivery is preferred unless the hemorrhage is so severe that it cannot be controlled by adequate blood and fluid replacement.

In many instances the quantity of blood lost cannot be measured accurately. Therefore, the degree of hypovolemia should not be underestimated and hemorrhage should be treated with enough whole blood and balanced salt solution (lactated Ringer's solution) to maintain a hematocrit of at least 30 percent and a urinary output of at least 30 mL per hour. Insertion of a catheter for the measurement of central venous pressure may be helpful in monitoring fluid replacement. The pregnant woman should also be closely evaluated for pulmonary congestion (cough, dyspnea, rales) because central venous pressure measurements may not detect early pulmonary edema caused by fluid overload.

Abnormalities in coagulation generally occur within the first few hours after placental abruption and generally do not worsen except in relation to the dilutional effects of vigorous transfusions with stored whole blood (which lacks many clotting factors) and lactated Ringer's solution. The most common coagulation defect in patients with placental abruption is a edly. An attempt at vaginal delivery is indicated if the degree of placental separation is limited and the fetus can be evaluated for signs of distress. In most cases of moderate to severe abruptio, delivery should occur within 6 to 12 hours of the diagnosis of placental separation. This recommendation is related to the observation that maternal morbidity and mortality rates diminish when delivery is achieved rapidly (Page et al.). Recent studies, however, have indicated that the outcome depends more on the adequate management of the patient's blood loss than on the time from diagnosis to delivery. Brame et al. showed that women with severe placental abruption experienced no greater complication rate when delivery was delayed for 18 hours or more if an adequate central blood volume and urine output were maintained.

In patients with mild degrees of placental separation and in whom the fetus is very premature by gestational age, expectant management may be used in carefully selected cases.

Complications

Acute renal failure may complicate severe placental abruption and is directly related to delayed or incomplete treatment of hypovolemia. Renal failure may be a result either of cortical or tubular necrosis. These renal lesions are probably produced by severe renal arteriolar vasospasm secondary to hypovolemic shock often complicated by fibrin deposition in the kidney following DIC. Yet, even in the presence of severe placental abruption complicated by intravascular coagulopathy, aggressive measured treatment of the hypovolemia with blood and balanced salt solution often prevents acute renal failure.

The possibility of renal cortical or tubular necrosis must be considered when oliguria or anuria persist after the intravascular blood volume has been restored. In these instances, the intravenous administration of 50 mL of 20% mannitol may be helpful in determining which patients are still hypovolemic. If oliguria or anuria persists after mannitol administration, renal necrosis is likely and fluid intake and output must be carefully balanced. Intermittent peritoneal dialysis or hemodialysis will be necessary either acutely or chronically depending on the diagnosis. Patients with renal tubular necrosis may recover if the damage is not too severe, but those with cortical necrosis inevitably develop chronic renal failure.

Postpartum pituitary insufficiency (Sheehan's syndrome) may also complicate the care of patients with severe placental abruptions. The development of pituitary insufficiency is related to the degree of antepartum hypovolemia.

PLACENTA PREVIA

DEFINITION AND INCIDENCE

In normal pregnancies, the placenta generally implants in the upper uterine segment. If the placenta implants in the lower uterine segment and partially or completely covers the cervical os, this constitutes placenta previa. Placenta previa complicates approximately 0.3 to 0.5 percent of all pregnancies (Hibbard; Crenshaw et al.). The occurrence of placenta previa increases with advancing maternal age and parity. Age, however, appears to be the more significant factor. Women over the age of 35 are approximately three times more likely to have placenta previa than are women under age 25, irrespective of parity (Hibbard). Approximately 80 percent of patients with placenta previa are multigravidas and the remaining 20 percent are primigravidas.

Placenta previa has been classified in different ways, based on the relationship of the placenta to the cervix either prior to labor or at specific times during labor. Prior to labor, a placenta may be classified as a complete placenta previa if it covers the entire internal cervical os; a partial placenta previa if the os is incompletely covered; or a low-lying placenta (but not a previa) if the placenta is located in the lower uterine segment but does not obstruct the cervical os (Fig. 30–4). During labor, effacement and dilatation of the cervix can change the relationship of the placental edge to the cervix. Nevertheless, the definition of placenta previa still depends on finding placenta obstructing the cervical os, whether this is diagnosed before or during labor.

ETIOLOGY

The cause of placenta previa is unknown, and speculations as to why the placenta implants in the lower uterine segment vary. Atrophic or inflammatory changes in the decidua may be related to the development of placenta previa. If decidual abnormalities were the major etiologic factor, however, then placenta previa would be likely to repeat more frequently in subsequent pregnancies. Yet the recurrence rate for placenta previa is generally less than 5 percent.

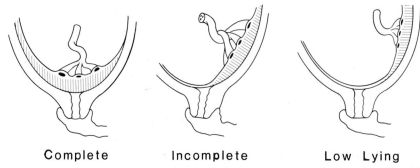

Complete   Incomplete   Low Lying

FIGURE 30–4   Types of placenta previa.

Placenta previa may develop because of the need for an excessively large surface area for effective exchange of oxygen and nutrients between mother and fetus. In this case, the placenta would tend to develop asymmetrically in relation to the site of implantation. Therefore the umbilical cord should be marginally inserted in a placenta that ultimately becomes a placenta previa. Indeed, marginal insertion of the umbilical cord is not uncommon in patients with placenta previa.

Other factors are known to be associated with the development of placenta previa. A low cervical cesarean section scar increases the incidence of placenta previa by a factor of 3. Since cesarean sections tend to be repeated, the chance of a subsequent occurrence of placenta previa in a patient with a previous cesarean section also increases. Rarely, placenta previa is associated with placenta accreta. This is thought to be related to the poor development of the decidua that is present in the lower uterine segment. Although placenta accreta (see below) is a rare complication of pregnancy, it is frequently found in association with placenta previa (Weekes, Greig).

The cause of the hemorrhage is understood when one considers the changes that take place in the lower uterine segment and cervix in the latter weeks of pregnancy. The rapid expansion of the lower uterine segment before labor and the dilatation of the cervix during labor will ultimately result in separation of placental attachments from the lower uterine segment; separation is followed by hemorrhage from uterine sinuses. Extensive bleeding results because of the limited ability of the uterine musculature of the lower segment to contract.

SIGNS AND SYMPTOMS

Painless vaginal bleeding is the single most reliable symptom of placenta previa. The initial episode of vaginal bleeding may be slight or may be extensive enough to cause hypovolemic shock. Bleeding can occur as early as the middle of the second trimester. Typically the bleeding is unrelated to trauma or unusual activity and there is no history of abdominal pain or tenderness. The earlier in pregnancy the bleeding is first noted, the more extensive is the degree of placenta previa. The initial bleeding is rarely if ever profuse enough to prove fatal to the mother. Vaginal bleeding usually has decreased or stopped entirely by the time the patient arrives at the hospital. A subsequent episode of vaginal bleeding, however, can be extremely heavy and can recur when least expected.

DIAGNOSIS

The diagnosis of placenta previa is suggested by the onset of painless uterine bleeding in the latter half of pregnancy. Abnormal fetal presentations may coexist with placenta previa in as many as 15 to 20 percent of instances (Hibbard; Crenshaw et al.). Thus a transverse, breech, an oblique fetal lie, or a shoulder presentation, recognized during the third trimester in an otherwise asymptomatic patient, should suggest the possibility of placenta previa.

Localization of the placenta is of considerable help in determining if placenta previa is present in the patient with third-trimester vaginal bleeding. There are several methods available for placental localization. These include soft tissue placentography, arteriography, isotope placentography, and placental localization by ultrasonography. Soft tissue placentography is by far the easiest to perform, yet the information obtained is frequently unsatisfactory (Badria, Young). With this method, the uterine outline appears as a soft tissue shadow around the fetus, and the placenta is visualized as a crescent shadow between fetus and uterus. The radiodensity of the placenta is slightly greater than that of amniotic fluid; this may be partly related to calcium deposits scattered within the placenta. With soft tissue placentography, there may be confusing placenta-like shadows in pregnancies under 32 weeks in duration or in pregnancies complicated by hydramnios (in which amniotic fluid volume is large compared with fetal volume). Furthermore, an abnormal fetal presentation such as a transverse or an oblique lie can present similar diagnostic difficulties. Unfortunately, these clinical conditions are those under which placenta previa is usually seen and in which accurate localization of the placenta is essential.

Arteriography can accurately define the limits of the placenta, although the technique is potentially dangerous for the mother (Sutton). Complications relate to the insertion of a catheter into a maternal femoral artery for the injection of a water-soluble contrast material. Nevertheless, the accurate localization of the placental site can be ascertained more than 95 percent of the time.

Isotope placentography requires the intravenous injection of a radioisotope that will remain in the maternal circulation for several minutes (Russell). By placing a scintillation counter over the maternal abdomen, the radiologist detects increased radioactivity over the highly vascular placental site. In isotope placentography, unlike soft tissue placentography, an abnormal fetal presentation or the presence of polyhydramnios does not influence the accuracy of placental localization. Occasionally, however, it is difficult to determine whether the placenta is located on the anterior or the posterior uterine wall.

More recently, placental localization by ultrasonography has become the technique of choice because of its reliability, accuracy, and safety (Kohorn et al.). The principal advantages of ultrasound localization of the placenta, when compared with the radiographic techniques previously described, include the following. (1) Mother and fetus are not exposed to ionizing radiation; (2) placental localization can be performed at any time after the ninth week of pregnancy; (3) the entire placenta can be visualized; and (4) the limits of the lower uterine segment and the site of the internal cervical os can be clearly defined. This latter point is extremely important because the relationship between the lower placental margin and the cervix is of utmost importance in accurately diagnosing placenta previa.

Sonography is accurate in diagnosing previa more than 97 percent of the time. The ultrasound diagnosis depends on observing placental tissue covering all of the cervix—complete placenta previa

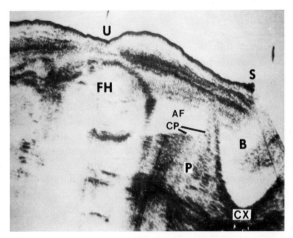

FIGURE 30–5 Complete placenta previa, 36 weeks. Placental tissue *P* displaces fetal head *FH* and amniotic fluid *AF* from the bladder and sacral promotory. Placenta completely obstructs the cervix *CX*. *CP*–chorionic plate. (From DI Edelstone, in *Diagnostic Ultrasound Applied to Obstetrics and Gynecology,* Harper & Row, 1979)

(Fig. 30–5) or part of the cervix—partial placenta previa. When placental tissue is located within the lower uterine segment but does not cover the cervix, these placentas are low-lying but are not previas. The lower uterine segment for diagnostic ultrasonography is arbitrarily defined as that area below the line that joins the sacral promontory with the pubic symphysis (the pelvic inlet). This is obviously an approximation since the lower uterine segment increases from 1 cm at 20 weeks to approximately 10 cm by term (Morrison). The finding of placental tissue located in the lower uterine segment is definitely abnormal. It is usually unnecessary to differentiate a low-lying placenta from a partial placenta previa because the management of the patient depends on the clinical condition of the patient, not on the ultrasound diagnosis alone.

Because of the high degree of accuracy of ultrasound for placental localization, vaginal examination of the patient who is suspected of having placenta previa is generally unnecessary and may only result in further vaginal bleeding. Occasionally, however, vaginal examination is necessary when the diagnosis of placenta previa is uncertain. *It must be stated most emphatically that vaginal examination of the patient with a suspected placenta previa is never permissible unless the patient is in an operating room and all preparations have been made for immediate cesarean section should torrential hemorrhage result from vaginal examination.*

MANAGEMENT

The management of patients with placenta previa may be divided into two main groups: (1) patients who present early in the third trimester before fetal maturity has been reached and in whom there has been some vaginal bleeding, not severe enough to require immediate delivery; and (2) patients in whom the fetuses are mature, or in whom labor has ensued, or in whom severe hemorrhage demands immediate delivery. In the past, patients with placenta previa were generally delivered immediately with disregard for the state of maturity of the fetus (Crenshaw et al.). Perinatal mortality rates were as high as 50 to 80 percent and were usually directly related to the degree of fetal prematurity. In an attempt to decrease perinatal mortality, expectant management has been used in patients with premature fetuses in whom the diagnosis of placenta previa has been made. With expectant management, the obstetrician is attempting to increase the length of pregnancy and fetal maturity, while at the same time keeping the risks from maternal hemorrhage to a minimum (Hibbard; Crenshaw et al.). Expectant management is appropriate for patients with gestation of less than 34 to 35 weeks in whom vaginal bleeding has stopped or is minimal, and in whom the degree of placenta previa is not major. These patients are generally hospitalized and kept at bed rest until fetal maturity is attained.

Fetal maturity is evaluated by measuring the biparietal diameter serially with ultrasound. Measuring the lecithin-sphingomyelin ratio in amniotic fluid will indicate when fetal pulmonary maturity has occurred. In pregnancies of less than 32 weeks, the short-term administration of the glucocorticoid betamethasone has been used to accelerate pulmonary maturation in fetuses that are at considerable risk of hyaline membrane disease (Liggins, Howie). The efficacy and safety of this medication is not entirely established.

An additional complication of placenta previa is premature labor. In selected patients, it is permissible to attempt to inhibit premature labor for at least 24 hours while the patient receives betamethasone to accelerate fetal pulmonary maturation. In these selected instances, it is essential that the diagnosis of abruption be excluded.

The goal of expectant management of the patient with placenta previa is to prolong pregnancy until fetal maturity is reached. Management of each patient is individualized; considerations include the severity of the symptoms as well as the degree of placenta previa as diagnosed by ultrasound. Once fetal maturity is attained (documented by a mature lecithin-sphingomyelin ratio at approximately 36 weeks), patients with placenta previa are generally delivered by cesarean section.

In addition, as part of expectant management of the patient with placenta previa, it is essential to repeat the ultrasound localization of the placenta at approximately 34 weeks. In some patients with presumed partial placenta previas or low-lying placentas, the placenta may be normally implanted at this time. This "change" in placental position relates to the rapid growth of the lower uterine segment during the third trimester, which results in an increase in the distance between the placental edge and the cervix. If a normal implantation site is identified at 34 weeks, these patients are allowed to go into labor and to deliver vaginally.

Liberal use of cesarean section for delivery of patients with placenta previa, when combined with expectant management, has decreased fetal mortality and morbidity over the last decade (Crenshaw et al.). Perinatal mortality has been reduced to less than 8 percent, while the rate of cesarean section has increased to more than 70 percent. Cesarean section in patients with placenta previa results in a decrease in antepartum bleeding and a reduction in the likelihood of cervical and lower uterine segment lacerations. In earlier reports on maternal mortality, deaths from placenta previa were directly related to bleeding from lower uterine segment and cervical lacerations associated with vaginal delivery. Clearly cesarean section is used for placenta previa to safeguard the life of the mother. Thus cesarean section is occasionally necessary when the fetus is dead, because vaginal delivery of a dead fetus can also result in cervical and lower uterine segment injuries.

Immediate postpartum hemorrhage often accompanies placenta previa because the placental implantation site in the lower uterine segment does not contract well after delivery of the placenta. Postpartum infection may also occur because of the closeness of the antepartum placental site to the cervix and vagina, from which organisms may be introduced directly into the uterus.

PLACENTA ACCRETA

DEFINITION

Placenta accreta is the abnormal adherence of placenta to myometrium due to focal or diffuse lack of decidua basalis between the placental trophoblast and myometrium. Placenta accreta may display as (1) placenta accreta: chorionic villi minimally invade the myometrium; (2) placenta increta: villi invade part of the myometrium but do not extend through the full thickness of the uterus; and (3) placenta percreta: villi penetrate through the myometrium and serosa.

Placenta accreta is an extremely rare disorder, complicating from 1:1000 to 1:30,000 pregnancies (Weekes, Greig; Millar). Approximately 20 percent of placenta accretas occur in patients with a placenta previa. The true incidence of the disorder may be higher because in its milder forms placenta accreta may go unnoticed or unreported.

PREDISPOSING FACTORS

Placenta accreta is associated with defective decidua at the site of implantation (Millar). Such defects may be related to trauma from previous endometrial curettage or to destruction of endometrium from previous infection. An accreta is more likely in a patient with placenta previa or in a patient with a previous pregnancy that required manual removal of the placenta (Weekes, Greig).

DIAGNOSIS AND MANAGEMENT

Diagnosis of placenta accreta is generally made postpartum when the placenta fails to completely separate from the uterine wall. When manual removal of the placenta is attempted, postpartum hemorrhage frequently results. Conservative management (manual removal of the placenta) is associated in some studies with maternal mortality rates higher than 50 percent, and thus the treatment of choice is total abdominal hysterectomy (McHattie). This is especially true when the diagnosis is placenta previa accreta. Even with hysterectomy, maternal mortality rates have been reported as high as 6 percent. Mortality is generally related to excessive blood loss with delay in definitive therapy.

POLYHYDRAMNIOS

Amniotic fluid volume throughout pregnancy has been determined by dilutional techniques and by direct measurement at time of hysterotomy (Fuchs; Queenan, Gadow). The mean volume of amniotic fluid increases from approximately 250 mL at 15 to 16 weeks to a peak of approximately 1000 mL in the late third trimester. In the last weeks of pregnancy, the volume of amniotic fluid is reduced and in the postterm pregnancy the volume of amniotic fluid is approxi-

Table 30–1 Associated Conditions in Cases of Polyhydramnios

Maternal
Diabetes mellitus
Preeclampsia
Anemia
Acute pyelonephritis
Hypertension
Fetal and Placental
Congenital anomalies
Multiple gestation
Rh sensitization
Placental chorioangioma

mately 550 mL (Queenan, Gadow). Strictly defined, polyhydramnios should indicate an excessive quantity of amniotic fluid for the stage of pregnancy under consideration. At term, most investigators have defined polyhydramnios as an amniotic fluid volume in excess of 2000 mL (Queenan et al.; Jacoby, Charles; Kramer). Clinically the diagnosis of polyhydramnios is suspected whenever the size of the uterus is in excess of that expected for the period of amenorrhea. If space-occupying masses or multiple fetuses are absent, then the uterine enlargement can be attributed to excessive amniotic fluid. The diagnosis of polyhydramnios can be confirmed antenatally by ultrasound or abdominal roentgenography; however, the former is more desirable because it eliminates the fetal exposure and risk of x-rays. The incidence of polyhydramnios varies from 0.13 to 3.2 percent of all pregnancies (Stevenson) and is greatly increased in certain maternal and fetal conditions (Table 30-I). The wide range in incidence may merely reflect differences in the definition. Polyhydramnios may be acute in onset but most often it is a chronic condition. Acute polyhydramnios commonly occurs in late second trimester and usually results in premature delivery with fetal or neonatal death (Pitkin). Chronic polyhydramnios usully occurs in the third trimester, and fetal outcome is determined more by the associated fetal conditions than by gestational age alone.

ETIOLOGY

Hutchinson and his associates have quantified by tracer techniques the transfer of water between mother, fetus, and amniotic fluid in normal and hydramniotic patients. In normal-term pregnancies, the fetus contributes up to 30 mL per hour and removes up to 175 mL per hour from the amniotic fluid. Large fluxes (3600 mL per hour) of water exist between mother and fetus. Smaller amounts of water (300 mL per hour) are exchanged between mother and amniotic fluid. In patients with hydramnios the exchange of water between mother and fetus is markedly reduced.

The fetus adds urine and possibly tracheal effluent to the amniotic fluid, and fetal deglutition reduces amniotic fluid volume. Fetal renal agenesis, pulmonary hypoplasia, absent or reduced deglutition, and gastrointestinal obstruction produce abnormal amniotic fluid volume. Fetal deglutition may be reduced in cases of central-nervous-system abnormalities, but polyhydramnios in such cases may also be due to increased passage of water across the exposed meninges. Placental pathology may influence the transfer of water between fetus and mother and may also affect the fluxes between mother and amniotic fluid.

MANAGEMENT

The management of women with polyhydramnios is determined by the condition of the fetus, concurrent maternal disease, the degree of uterine enlargement, and the gestational age at the time of diagnosis. In approximately 33 percent of cases with polyhydramnios, the fetus is normal and there are no associated maternal complications. In 20 to 35 percent of cases of polyhydramnios, congenital abnormalities of the fetus are present. Maternal diabetes is present in as many as 25 percent of cases; other conditions such as toxemia, erythroblastosis, and multiple gestation constitute the remainder of cases (Jeffcoate, Scott; Moya et al.).

In suspected cases of polyhydramnios, fetal evaluation for obvious anomalies is necessary. The commonest fetal anomalies detected in cases of polyhydramnios are listed in Table 30–2. By far the most frequent anomaly is anencephaly, occurring in as many as 60 percent of cases with congenital malformation. Anomalies of the central nervous system such as anencephaly, encephalocele, and myelomeningocele can be diagnosed by ultrasound. Additional information about fetal development may be gained by the use of amniography. Abnormalities of the gastrointestinal tract of the fetus can be diagnosed by amniocentesis and/or amniography. The regurgitation of bile acids and bilirubin pigments into the amniotic fluid because of gastrointestinal obstruction will result in an increase in the $\triangle OD_{450}$ value of amniotic fluid as well as an increase in amniotic fluid bile acids. Injection of 15 mL of radiopaque dye

TABLE 30–2 Common Congenital Anomalies in Cases of Polyhydramnios

Anencephaly
Hydrocephaly
Gastrointestinal obstruction
Tracheoesophageal fistula
Diaphragmatic hernia
Cleft palate
Omphalocele
Congenital cardiac disease
Partial obstructive uropathies

into the amniotic fluid should result in opacification of the lower gastrointestinal tract of the fetus within 24 hours. Absence of dye in the gastrointestinal tract indicates either an abnormality in fetal deglutition, obstruction in the fetal gastrointestinal tract, or a severely depressed fetus.

If anencephaly or other severe central-nervous-system abnormalities incompatible with life are diagnosed antenatally, no attempts should be made to maintain the pregnancy; many have suggested that pregnancy should be terminated either by amniotomy or oxytocin induction. If polyhydramnios in such cases is severe, removal of amniotic fluid by amniocentesis will not only improve maternal respiratory embarrassment but may also be helpful in initiating labor.

Management of the patient with polyhydramnios whose fetus does not appear to have a severe central nervous system abnormality depends on the degree of uterine enlargement and the gestational age of the fetus. If uterine enlargement is not producing excessive discomfort, only symptomatic measures are indicated. Bed rest in the lateral recumbent position should be encouraged to reduce the edema of the lower extremities which is common in this condition. Since increased uterine contractility occurs in patients with polyhydramnios, the risk of premature labor must be considered in the management of these patients. In cases of severe uterine enlargement early in pregnancy, repeated amniocentesis can be utilized to provide maternal relief and reduce the risk of premature labor. Volumes of amniotic fluid as great as 12 L have been removed over a 6-week period without adverse effects on mother or fetus. The rate of removal of amniotic fluid must be slow enough to reduce the risk of placental separation and increased uterine activity that might follow a rapid reduction in amniotic fluid volume. A rate of removal of less than 500 mL per day has been suggested.

The fetal risk in pregnancies complicated by polyhydramnios is related to the increased incidence of congenital anomalies incompatible with life, the increased incidence of maternal disease such as diabetes, and the increased incidence of malpresentation, particularly breech positions. These risks must be considered during the intrapartum management of a woman with polyhydramnios. In addition to the risks enumerated for the fetus, the mother is at increased risk for postpartum hemorrhage and cesarean section because of fetal malpresentation and cord prolapse.

OLIGOHYDRAMNIOS

A less than normal quantity of amniotic fluid is termed oligohydramnios. A reduction in amniotic fluid volume can be seen in pregnancies beyond term and in women with chronic amniotic fluid leakage. Oligohydramnios in the absence of prolonged gestation or ruptured membranes is commonly associated with fetal congenital abnormalities, particularly renal agenesis, either singly or combined with pulmonary hypoplasia (Kramer; Jeffcoate; Potter). Lower-limb deformities, low-set ears, depressed nose, micrognathia, and webbed neck are also frequently seen. These latter features are part of the typical "Potter's facies." Intrauterine growth retardation is a prominent feature in many cases of oligohydramnios so that intrauterine fetal demise, meconium aspiration, and intrapartum asphyxia are frequent complications. In many cases of oligohydramnios, examination of the placenta at delivery indicates the presence of amnion nodosum. These small grayish-yellow nodules are located on the fetal aspect of the amnion and may be the result of desquamated fetal epithelium.

Oligohydramnios may be diagnosed prenatally by physical examination. A uterine fundus small relative to the gestational age of the fetus is noted, and the diagnosis of oligohydramnios may be confirmed by roentgenography or by ultrasound. Roentgenographic examination demonstrates an absence of amniotic fluid and apparent fetal compression. Commonly, extreme flexion of the spine and crowding of the fetal skeleton toward the pelvic cavity are noted. Ultrasound may be utilized to demonstrate the absence of amniotic fluid and in some cases the presence or absence of the fetal kidneys.

The management of women with oligohydramnios depends entirely on the condition of the fetus. Confirmation of congenital abnormalities of the fetus is difficult. Frequently when fetuses present with fetal distress, a cesarean section is undertaken which discloses that a severe anomaly incompatible with life is present.

DISORDERS OF THE UTERUS (UTERINE TRAUMA)

RUPTURE OF THE UTERUS

Among obstetric emergencies, rupture of the uterus is an infrequent occurrence; however, it presents one of the most serious problems. The incidence varies widely and relates to the quality of obstetric care. In underdeveloped countries where home deliveries are common, uterine rupture is more frequent than in countries where deliveries occur in well-attended maternity hospitals. In teaching hospitals in the United States, the incidence is about one in 2000 deliveries (Claiborne and Schelin). Over the past decades, maternal and fetal mortality related to uterine rupture have decreased considerably, but the maternal mortality is still between 5 and 10 percent and fetal mortality between 14 and 55 percent in various studies (Beacham et al.; Yussman and Haynes).

Uterine ruptures can be classified as (1) spontaneous ruptures with or without previous uterine surgery, and (2) traumatic ruptures.

SPONTANEOUS RUPTURES

Rupture of the unscarred uterus before the onset of labor is extremely rare. Predisposing factors for rupture of the intact uterus before labor are uterine anomalies such as bicornuate uterus, placental abnormalities such as placenta accreta or percreta, previous curettage, previous endomyometritis, and adenomyosis (Felmus et al.). During labor, rupture of the unscarred uterus is favored by grand multiparity, cephalopelvic disproportion, hydrocephalus, and tumors obstructing the birth canal. Uterine rupture due to such conditions can be avoided in most instances. Careful examination of the patient will reveal a contracted pelvis, fetal malpresentation, or the presence of a tumor obstructing the birth canal. If necessary, x-ray pelvimetry will give further information about pelvic dimensions. Radiographic or ultrasonographic examination can frequently verify the presence of a hydrocephalic fetus. Rupture of the uterus resulting from the use of oxytocic agents can be largely prevented by administering the drug intravenously as a dilute solution by means of an infusion pump and by continuous recording of uterine activity, preferably with an intrauterine catheter. The increased risk of uterine rupture in grand multiparas is due to an increase in fibrous tissue in the myometrium after each pregnancy. Therefore, induction or stimulation of labor in grand multiparas carries a higher risk of uterine rupture and should be avoided if possible.

RUPTURE OF UTERINE SCAR

The desirability of vaginal delivery following previous uterine surgery (cesarean section, myomectomy, unification of bicornuate uterus) has been the subject of debate for decades. Whether the approach "once a cesarean section always a cesarean section" produces less maternal and fetal morbidity and mortality than the occasional rupture of the scarred uterus during labor is an unsettled question. Nevertheless, the risk of uterine rupture during labor is several times greater when a classical cesarean section has been done compared with a low-segment transverse cesarean section. The prognosis of a uterine rupture after classical cesarean section is more grave than after low-segment transverse cesarean section. Accordingly, classical cesarean section should be reserved for specific indications (e.g., transverse lie) and vaginal delivery following classical cesarean section should be an exception. Conversely, uterine rupture following low-segment transverse cesarean section is rare (less than 1 percent) and usually without major hemorrhage, maternal or fetal mortality. No maternal deaths due to uterine rupture were seen in a series of 1115 patients delivering vaginally after previous cesarean section (Douglas). Under certain conditions, vaginal delivery following previous low-segment transverse cesarean section may be justified. A variety of conditions should be fulfilled when vaginal delivery is contemplated. The indication for the previous cesarean section has to be nonrecurrent, the use of oxytocic agents should be avoided, the patient should not be a grand multipara (five or more previous children), and she should carry a singleton fetus of normal size without polyhydramnios.

Uterine rupture following previous myomectomy, unification operation, cervical cerclage, or cervical stenosis due to surgery are rare occurrences and can generally be avoided by use of cesarean section.

TRAUMATIC RUPTURE

Imprudent obstetric interference accounts for most traumatic ruptures of the uterus; thus, it should be rare in contemporary obstetrics. Version and extraction, high forceps delivery or high vacuum extraction, excessive fundal pressure, and, rarely, manual removal of the placenta are the main causes of traumatic rupture of the uterus. During curettage of the postpartum uterus, the soft myometrium may be perforated. Accidents in which strong forces are exerted on the pregnant abdomen may produce traumatic rupture of the uterus. Uterine rupture following use of oxytocic agents is also classified as a form of traumatic rupture.

Clinical Features

Pain, cessation of uterine contractions, bleeding, possibly shock, change in abdominal contour, and greater ease in palpating fetal parts abdominally are the main clinical features of uterine rupture. Although the full-blown picture of rupture is easily recognized, there are instances where symptoms and signs are nonspecific and diagnosis is difficult and delayed. Pain is often described as continuous with a sudden feeling of tearing, followed by cessation of uterine contractions. These symptoms can be obscured when regional anesthesia has been administered. Vaginal bleeding varies greatly in amount and can lead to a suspicion of placental separation or abruption or postpartum uterine atony. Internal bleeding may be slight or may be severe enough to lead to sudden development of surgical shock. An alteration in abdominal contour and easier abdominal palpation of fetal parts occur whenever the fetus has been partly or completely extruded from the uterine cavity. On pelvic examination the presenting fetal part will no longer be palpable. Since rupture of the lower uterine segment may involve the bladder, patients may have blood in their urine. Whenever the patient develops shock of undetermined origin, postpartum exploration of the uterus is necessary in order to evaluate the possibility of uterine rupture.

Treatment

Immediate correction of hypovolemia followed by surgery is necessary in all cases of uterine rupture. After the abdomen has been opened and fetus and placenta are delivered, the surgical approach to the uterus can be either total or subtotal hysterectomy or repair of the rupture site. The choice of procedure depends upon location and extent of the rupture as well as on age and parity of the patient. Total hysterectomy is indicated when a large fundal rupture has occurred; subtotal hysterectomy should be reserved for patients in poor surgical condition. In young patients of low parity with rupture of a low-segment transverse cesarean section scar, repair of the wound may be possible. Similarly, small fundal perforations may be sutured. Agüero and Kizer have reported favorably on a series of 684 ruptures in which the wound was repaired.

During the postoperative period, blood replacement, antibiotic therapy, and careful follow-up of fluid and electrolyte balance are mandatory.

INVERSION OF THE UTERUS

The incidence of inversion of the uterus has been variously reported from 1 in 5000 to 1 in 23,000 deliveries. Although rare, it is a serious and life-threatening complication. Uterine inversion is classified as *incomplete* when the uterine fundus is inverted but has not descended beyond the cervix, and as *complete* when the uterine fundus has passed through the cervix.

ETIOLOGY

Forceful management of the third stage of labor is almost always a prerequisite for uterine inversion; rarely does it occur for no apparent reason. Strong fundal pressure and traction on the umbilical cord before the placenta is separated may lead to inversion. A fundal implantation of the placenta as well as a certain degree of uterine atony is necessary to allow inversion of the uterus.

SYMPTOMS AND DIAGNOSIS

The severity of symptoms depends upon the degree of inversion of the uterine fundus. Incomplete inversion may only cause mild hemorrhage and pain but complete inversion will lead to rapid development of shock. Occasionally the inverted uterus protrudes through the vaginal introitus. The uterus cannot be palpated abdominally, but the diagnosis of uterine inversion can be made by vaginal examination.

MANAGEMENT

Treatment of shock and correction of the inversion as soon as possible are essential to prevent maternal mortality (Kitchin et al.; Lee et al.). If the uterus cannot be replaced easily because of tightness of the cervix, halothane anesthesia should be administered—with care in view of the hypotensive effect of halothane. Replacement is begun at the site which inverted last.

After replacement is completed, oxytocic agents should be administered to prevent recurrence of the inversion.

Whenever manual replacement of the uterus is unsuccessful, surgical intervention is necessary. Following laparotomy, either the uterus is reinverted by traction with clamps applied stepwise to the inverted fundus or the cervical ring is incised to relieve the tight cervical stricture and allow replacement of the uterine fundus. The latter approach is also indicated in cases of chronic inversion when the diagnosis has been delayed. Vaginal approaches to the cervical ring either through the anterior or posterior fornix have also been described.

ACCIDENTS

Blunt or sharp force may lead to trauma of the uterus. Penetrating stab wounds or bullet wounds require surgical exploration. Severe falls or automobile accidents may lead to rupture of the pregnant uterus. Seat belts with a lap and shoulder part are recommended to prevent uterine rupture upon impact. The belt should be drawn tight and the lap part should be worn as low as possible on the protruding abdomen.

DISORDERS OF THE FETUS

FETAL MATURITY AND INTRAUTERINE GROWTH

Maturity may be defined in terms of gestational age, birth weight, or a combination of the two. Birth weight and gestational age are independent variables influencing neonatal risk. Therefore, the use of both variables in defining maturity is inherently more accurate than the use of either variable alone. According to gestational criteria, infants delivered prior to 36 completed weeks are considered preterm; infants delivered after 41 completed weeks of pregnancy are considered postterm. Infants delivered at term (37 to 41 weeks) have the lowest perinatal mortality rates. Infants delivered prior to term are at increased risk for perinatal death, and this risk is inversely related to gestational age. Hyaline membrane disease, asphyxia neonatorum, intraventricular hemorrhage, and necrotizing enterocolitis are commonly responsible for the high death rate among infants born prematurely (Tudehope, Sinclair). Although they make up only 8 percent of the total births annually, premature infants account for an overwhelming majority of the cases of perinatal morbidity and mortality.

Infants delivered after 41 completed weeks are also at increased risk of perinatal death for reasons which are not fully understood. Prolonged gestation is observed with increased frequency among anencephalic fetuses although the vast majority of fetuses delivered postterm are not anencephalic. Fetal adrenocortical insufficiency has been reported in cases of prolonged gestation (Nwosu et al., 1975). Since the fetus is believed to play an important role in the initiation of labor, it has been suggested that prolonged gestation is due to inadequate fetal cortisol production. Support for this theory can be found in studies in which postterm pregnancies were experimentally but successfully terminated by injection of corticosteroids into the amniotic fluid (Nwosu et al., 1976).

The appropriateness of intrauterine growth is judged by both birth weight and gestational age. Three patterns of fetal growth are statistically defined according to these variables (Tudehope, Sinclair). At any given gestational age, if the birth weight of an infant is within 2 standard deviations of the mean, the growth of that infant is considered to be appropriate. (Actually the 10th and 90th percentiles are used to define the lower and upper limits of weight.) If at any given gestational age, the birth weight of the infant is greater than 2 standard deviations above the mean, the infant is termed large for gestational age (LGA). Similarly, infants whose birth weight is more than 2 standard deviations below the mean for their gestational peers are considered to be growth retarded or small for gestational age (SGA). This definition of growth is applicable irrespective of actual gestational age.

Fetal and neonatal outcome are strongly affected by the pattern of intrauterine growth. The neonate who is large for gestational age is more prone to the consequences of fetal and pelvic disproportion, e.g., trauma from shoulder dystocia and difficult forceps delivery, and is at increased risk of delivery by cesarean section. The newborn who is small for gestational age is commonly the product of a pregnancy complicated by severe hypertension, preeclampsia, or poor maternal nutrition. These growth-retarded babies are at increased risks throughout the perinatal period. Antepartum fetal demise is common; intrapartum asphyxia, meconium aspiration, neonatal hypoglycemia, and intraventricular hemorrhage are also commonly seen in this group of infants. Animal studies have indicated that the growth-retarded fetus may have a reduced number of brain cells and later in life may exhibit learning disabilities. Similar findings have been reported in human subjects; however, the data are still inconclusive.

ASSESSMENT OF FETAL GROWTH AND MATURITY

Serial measurements of the fetal biparietal diameter by ultrasound appear to be the most accurate method of assessing fetal growth. The fetal biparietal diameter can be measured very accurately with an error of less than 1 mm. The diagnosis of intrauterine fetal growth retardation may be entertained whenever the growth of the biparietal diameter is less than expected for the stage of pregnancy under consideration. The expected growth of the fetal biparietal diameter is 3.5 mm per week between 13 and 30 weeks' gestation, 2.2 mm per week between 30 and 34 weeks, and approximately 1.5 mm per week thereafter (Campbell). (See Fig. 15–22, Chap. 15, Fetus and Newborn.)

Measurements of fundal height by the same examiner can also be helpful in assessing fetal growth. Serial measurements can detect severe cases of intrauterine fetal growth retardation. Although this technique is ignored by many physicians, the performance of the measurement is justified since it draws the clinician's attention to the growing fetus.

The lecithin/sphingomyelin (L/S) ratio is the most accurate method of assessing fetal pulmonary maturity (Gluck et al.). Since the major cause of death in the preterm infant is hyaline membrane disease, determination of the state of pulmonary maturity provides the most accurate means of predicting neonatal outcome. Other tests of fetal maturity are not accurate in predicting the neonatal risk for hyaline membrane disease. The major surface-active phospholipid in amniotic fluid is lecithin. A dramatic rise in the production of lecithin occurs at approximately 34 to 35 weeks, and it is at this point that the neonatal risk of hyaline membrane disease is greatly reduced. Sphingomyelin is another phospholipid with surface-active properties and it is included in the L/S determination to correct for differences in amniotic fluid volume. A L/S ratio greater than 2.0 in amniotic fluid indicates that the fetus is at very low risk for developing or dying from hyaline membrane disease. If the L/S ratio is less than 2.0, the risk of death from hyaline membrane disease is increased. Several studies have reported an acceleration of fetal pulmonary maturation in cases of chronic fetal stress, such as severe diabetes with vascular complications, intrauterine fetal growth, and third-trimester bleeding. Other studies have failed to substantiate this pulmonary accelerative effect from fetal stress. The L/S ratio value can be altered by the presence of meconium or blood in amniotic fluid. Placental localization prior to amniocentesis greatly reduces the risk of blood contamination of the amniotic fluid.

The foam stability (shake test) is also based on the fact that the lecithin possesses surface-active properties. Aliquots of amniotic fluid are mixed with increasing amounts of 95% ethanol and water in small test tubes. The tubes are gently agitated and the presence or absence of stable bubbles at the air/liquid interface is noted. Amniotic fluid with sufficient quantities of surface-active material will foam, resulting in a complete circle of bubbles at the top of the liquid. Dilutions of the amniotic fluid allow semiquantatitive assessment of the surface-active material. The test is interpreted as positive if bubbles are present in all dilutions, negative if absent in all dilutions, and intermediate if present only at the lowest dilution. False positive shake tests are infrequent, and a positive test usually indicates that pulmonary maturity exists; however, the incidence of false negative tests is high; therefore, prediction of fetal pulmonary immaturity by the shake test is unreliable. Contaminants such as meconium or blood invalidate the test.

The concentration of creatinine in amniotic fluid may also be utilized to estimate gestational age (Pitkin, Zwirek). Amniotic fluid creatinine increases progressively throughout pregnancy and by the 37th week the concentration exceeds 2.0 mg per 100 mL in a majority of cases. The test is of value whenever the L/S ratio or shake test cannot be performed or the results obtained are questionable as, for example, in cases of blood or meconium staining of the amniotic fluid.

Previously, radiographic study of the fetal skeleton was an important method of gestational age assessment. Since the introduction of the L/S ratio, fetal radiography is not used except when tests of pulmonary surfactant are unavailable. The hazards of radiation and the lack of specificity of fetal radiography make it a less-than-ideal method of assessing gestational age.

Other tests have been utilized to evaluate fetal maturity such as amniotic fluid cytology and urinary or serum estriol determinations, but these are much less accurate in predicting neonatal risk than the surfactant tests. In disorders of fetal growth, serum and urinary estriol determinations and human placental lactogen may provide supportive information but should not be used as primary modalities of diagnosis.

OTHER DISEASES

HYPERTENSIVE STATES OF PREGNANCY

The Committee on Terminology of the American College of Obstetricians and Gynecologists has recommended that "pregnancy toxemias" be replaced by a more appropriate designation of hypertensive states of pregnancy. The new classification includes:

1. Mild disorders
   a. Gestational edema
   b. Gestational proteinuria
   c. Gestational hypertension
2. Acute disorders
   a. Preeclampsia-eclampsia
   b. Chronic hypertension with superimposed preeclampsia or eclampsia
3. Chronic hypertensive disease of whatever cause
4. Unclassified hypertensive disorders with insufficient information to classify the hypertensive state

Gestational Edema. Gestational edema is the excessive accumulation of fluid greater than +1 edema after 12 hours of bed rest, or weight gain of 5 pounds or more in 1 week. A certain amount of dependent edema is present among all pregnant women, but excessive fluid retention is more frequently encountered among patients who gain an inordinate amount of weight during pregnancy. Formerly these patients were incorrectly described as a fluid-retention group. Obesity is their major problem, and weight control is the treatment of choice, although it is rarely successful. In spite of gross weight gain and edema, patients otherwise have normal pregnancies and offspring.

Gestational Proteinuria. Gestational proteinuria is the presence of proteinuria in the absence of hypertension, edema, renal infection, or intrinsic renovascular disease. The condition is rare but is seen in clinical practice. A few writers have described the transient nephrosis of pregnancy (Wallace, Smedley), which may include this group of patients. However, by definition, gestational proteinuria alone does not affect the fetus.

Gestational Hypertension. Gestational hypertension is the development of hypertension during pregnancy, or within the first 24 hours postpartum, in a previously normotensive woman. The blood pressure returns to normotensive levels within 10 days following parturition. Gestational hypertension is frequently observed among younger women, especially those with a family history of hypertension. The hyperreactive response in all probability reflects the extreme sensitivity to the renin-angiotensin system among young people. When gestational hypertensive patients are followed for a number of years, they often develop essential hypertension.

PREECLAMPSIA-ECLAMPSIA

Preeclampsia is the development of hypertension with proteinuria, edema, or both, after the 20th week of gestation. It may develop earlier in cases of hydatidiform mole. If preeclampsia progresses without proper treatment, patients may eventually develop eclamptic convulsions.

Throughout the world population, preeclampsia-eclampsia is primarily a disease of the indigent primigravida who has received little or no prenatal care. In spite of a vigorous search for a deficiency of a single food substance, vitamin, or trace element, a specific absence or inadequacy of food material has never been demonstrated. It is interesting to note that eclamptic patients in their succeeding pregnancies usually have either normal or mild preeclamptic pregnancies indicating that there are other factors operating besides dietary ones.

Preeclampsia is considered severe if any one of the following signs or symptoms is found:

1. Blood pressure of 160 mmHg or more systolic, or 110 mmHg or more diastolic on at least two occasions at least 6 hours apart, with the patient resting in bed
2. Proteinuria of 5 g or more in 24 hours (3 or 4+ quantitative)
3. Oliguria (500 mL or less in 24 hours)
4. Cerebral or visual disturbances
5. Epigastric pain
6. Pulmonary edema or cyanosis

Preeclampsia-eclampsia is an important complication of pregnancy since eclampsia still is one of the frequent causes of maternal death in certain sections of this country. The overall maternal mortality rate from eclampsia is 3 to 5 percent; the fetal mortality is 17 to 20 percent.

Etiology

In discussions of preeclampsia and eclampsia, the two disorders are regarded as a single clinical entity since eclampsia represents the finite end of severe preeclampsia. Many theories have been proposed to explain the disease, but no hypothesis has been able to fulfill all the nuances of this condition. The placenta appears to be centrally involved since the absence of the fetus, as in hydatidiform mole, often results in the development of preeclampsia. Whether the trophoblastic cells specifically are involved has not been determined. Certainly placental ischemia, resulting from uteroplacental insufficiency, appears to be characteristic of this disease although it may well be a secondary effect rather than a primary cause. The possibility that immunologic antigen-antibody reactions between maternal and fetal tissues produce fibrin deposits in the body is a tantalizing etiological thought, but the question is not resolved fully (Scott, Beer; Scott, Jenkins; Petrucco et al.). Other studies have cited the vasoconstrictive properties of prostaglandin as the important etiological factor (Speroff; Demers, Gabbe).

The role of salt in the etiology of preeclampsia has been an interesting and perplexing problem. For preeclamptic patients with edema, additional salt intake is obviously contraindicated, but in the early stages of preeclampsia, no study implicates salt as the sole putative agent. Nor has anyone objectively demonstrated the efficacy of diuretics in lowering the incidence of preeclampsia; actually, they are contraindicated among preeclamptic patients since diuretics further reduce blood volume and plasma proteins.

Pathophysiology

Generalized vasospasm is characteristic of preeclampsia and can be readily observed in the retinal arterioles. The resulting increase in peripheral resistance then produces hypertension. There is an associated increase in vascular sensitivity to pressor substances such as angiotensin II, norepinephrine (Talledo et al.), and vasopressin (Browne). There may be increased sensitivity to infusion of angiotensin prior to the clinical manifestation of preeclampsia in certain cases (Gant et al.), but the results may not be so well defined in other patients (Morris et al.). Sodium retention has been noted in preeclampsia, and in severe preeclampsia or eclampsia there is, in addition, a marked reduction in size of the vascular compartment with extravasation of fluid into the extra-cellular spaces. In such patients central venous pressure readings are extremely low.

As a result of systemic vasospasm, there is decreased circulation to vital organs, namely the brain, liver, kidney, and placenta. Although the actual cerebral blood flow is not altered, the cerebral resistance is measurably increased (McCall). The decreased oxygenation of the brain resulting from vasospasm and cerebral edema produces cerebral irritability and may eventuate in seizures. Furthermore, the systemic vasospasm causes metabolic dysfunction in the kidney, liver, and placenta. The decreased perfusion of the placental cotyledons may produce small infarcted placentas and place the fetus in jeopardy of circulatory and nutritional deficits.

Renal function studies, including renal plasma flow, glomerular filtration rate, and uric acid clearance, are all decreased with preeclampsia (Bucht, Werkö; Hayashi). One must remember that in normal pregnancy renal clearances are all increased; all renal function studies must therefore be evaluated in terms of normal pregnancy changes. Unfortunately, in such evaluations there is relatively poor correlation between the degree of renal depression and the clinical severity of preeclampsia because of wide fluctuations of values in both normal and abnormal pregnancies.

Histologic changes in the kidney have shown enlarged glomeruli with swollen endothelial cells (Sheehan). With electron microscopy, investigators in recent years have described a specific renal lesion as glomerular capillary endotheliosis with subendothelial deposits (Spargo et al.). A high correlation was reported between the degree of renal pathology and its clincal severity. Our own studies on renal biopsies from 57 cases, reviewed by two experienced renal pathologists who did not know the clinical status of the patients, did not show a similar degree of correlation (Paul et al.). In addition, no diagnosis of primary renal disease was made in spite of five cases so diagnosed clinically. These results suggest that the kidney changes are not pathognomic but in all probability are secondary changes, albeit very important ones. The findings also attest to the protean nature of the disease.

Placental perfusion is thought to be decreased in preeclampsia although it is exceedingly difficult to accurately measure uterine blood flow in pregnant women. The problem is further compounded by the lack of reliable animal models on which to perform such measurements. Since the conversion of admin-istered labeled dehydroepiandrosterone sulfate (DHS) to 17β-estradiol largely by the placenta appears to correlate with placental perfusion, Gant and coworkers have reported decreased placental perfusion in patients with preeclampsia by demonstrating decreased conversion of DHS to estradiol.

The involvement of the renin-angiotensin system has been an intriguing problem in preeclampsia. The infusion of angiotensin into nonpregnant women or into preeclamptic patients elicits a hypertensive response, whereas similar infusion into normal pregnant women produces a blunted response. Studies have shown that the renin substrate, renin-activating system, and angiotensin are all augmented to the highest degree in the normal pregnant woman and to a lesser degree in preeclamptic patients, with the nonpregnant woman demonstrating the lowest values (Helmer, Judson; Gordon et al.; Symonds, Anderson; Massani et al.). The hypertensive response in the preeclamptic patient is a result of attenuated peripheral vasomotor response, its cause so far undetermined.

Diagnostic Management

In the management of preeclamptic patients after admission to the hospital, an attempt should be made to evaluate the clinical severity of the maternal disease and relate it to the maturity/immaturity and well-being/illness of the fetus. With a severe unremitting preeclamptic or eclamptic patient at 32 weeks, delivery is the treatment of choice although there are advocates of more conservative treatment (Anderson, Harbert). However, with a milder case, the pregnancy should be allowed to progress until either the fetus matures or preeclampsia becomes worse. Combined clinical observation and laboratory tests are useful in judging the clinical status of preeclamptic patients. Clinical studies should include:

1. Vital signs including blood pressure and pulse. Persistent or increasing hypertension after bed rest for 24 hours in left lateral position indicates impending problem.
2. Total input and output. Decreased urinary output is always an ominous sign.
3. Daily weight. Continued weight gain, especially after bed rest, indicates continued fluid retention and signals the seriousness of the condition.
4. Measurement of deep tendon reflexes to ascertain the hyperreactive state.
5. Observation for impending symptoms of severe preeclampsia including headache, vertigo, scoto-

mata epigastric pain, and especially nausea and vomiting.
6. Fetal evaluation should include amniocentesis for L/S ratio, fetal monitoring including stress or non-stress tests, and serial sonography for biparietal diameters (BPD) measurements as needed.

Unfortunately, eyeground examinations are not particularly helpful since retinal vessels demonstrate only arteriolar narrowing and slight alteration in A/V (arteriovenous) ratio—an evaluation that is too subjective to assess accurately, although retinal separation is associated with severe preeclampsia.

Laboratory Studies

Besides the usual admission laboratory tests, additional studies should include:

1. Urine protein over 24 hours. This is the single most reliable laboratory test to ascertain the severity of preeclampsia and should be run frequently. Values over 0.5 g per 24 hours are considered abnormal. During the 24-hour collection period, qualitative check periodically by dip test is extremely helpful.
2. Urinalysis and urine culture. Occasionally, the clinical status of a preeclamptic patient is complicated by an occult pyelonephritis. The proper treatment of such an infection will improve the patient's preeclamptic status.
3. Blood urea nitrogen (BUN). Normally decreases markedly during pregnacy due to expanded blood volume, enhanced renal clearance, and anabolic state of protein metabolism. Values such as 15 to 18 mg per 100 mL in the last trimester of pregnancy signify definite renal decompensation. BUN may occasionally be elevated due to dietary changes (Hayashi et al., 1963).
4. Serum creatinine. Represents an adjunctive test to BUN to evaluate renal function. Normal values should be less than 1 mg per 100 mL.
5. Blood uric acid. Normally during the third trimester, the blood uric acid is less than 4 mg per 100 mL because of augmented blood volume, increased renal clearance, and decreased catabolism of purines. Hyperuricemia is the most characteristic blood change in preeclampsia, resulting from decreased renal clearance, lacticacidemia, and increased placental catabolism (Chesley; Handler; Hayashi et al., 1956).
6. Platelet count. Thrombocytopenia is often associated with preeclampsia, and to some degree the extent of platelet count depression correlates with clinical severity (Kennan, et al.). The hematologic changes are different from the DIC observed after amniotic fluid embolism. Abnormal RBCs (red blood cells) and fibrin split products, though reported, are relatively rare. The etiology of the thrombocytopenia still remains obscure.
7. Liver enzyme studies including SGOT (serum glutamic oxaloacetic transaminase), LDH (lactate dehydrogenase) and CPK (creatine phosphokinase) are all elevated in serious cases of preeclampia. Periportal necrosis and liver capsular hemorrhage have been observed and indicate hepatic involvement in this disease. Alkaline phosphatase is markedly elevated in normal pregnancy due to the presence of phosphatase in placenta.

Other studies, such as serum electrolytes, protein and A/G (albumin/globulin) ratio, and cholesterol, are less helpful in following the progress of preeclampsia. In spite of enthusiastic advocates, we do not find urinary estriol, alkaline phosphatase, and HPL mandatory in the practical management of hypertensive disorders of pregnancy.

In the management and treatment of preeclampsia-eclampsia, there are several broad concepts to keep in mind:

1. The only finite treatment is the delivery of the fetus and the placenta.
2. The mother is young; once delivered alive, she still will have many reproductive years remaining.
3. Bed rest in the hospital must be an integral part of the conservative management of the preeclamptic patient. The best treatment for a preeclamptic patient is bed rest lying on her side; it promotes active diuresis.
4. In the total treatment, the severity of the preeclampsia is balanced against the prematurity and viability of the infant. The final judgment is based on the synthesis of all the clinical findings and laboratory tests.

Treatment

Severe Preeclampsia-Eclampsia. The greatest danger in severe preeclampsia and in eclampsia is the development or the continuation of eclamptic seizures; thus, anticonvulsant therapy is the most important part of treatment. Currently, the basic anticonvulsant agent is magnesium sulfate which depresses interneuronal and myoneuronal junctions, but the exact mechanism of the anticonvulsant effect is unknown.

The initial treatment should consist of 2 to 4 g of magnesium sulfate given slowly intravenously, followed by maintenance dose of approximately 1 to 2 g per hour via infusion pump. An alternative method is intramuscular administration of magnesium sulfate (10 g as a 50% solution) into the buttocks although the injection is painful even with the addition of a local anesthetic agent (1% procaine). Overmedication with magnesium sulfate may be detected by decreased respirations or the disappearance of the knee jerk. The antidote is intravenous calcium which should always be available.

Generally, other anticonvulsants and sedatives have not been as effective as magnesium sulfate. Pritchard has reported the successful treatment, using magnesium sulfate, of 154 consecutive eclamptic patients without a single maternal mortality.

For eclamptic patients, proper airway should be maintained and tongue depressors should be kept handy to prevent mouth injuries. Oxygen therapy should be administered in the fashion most comfortable to the patient. Measures should be taken so that the patient does not injure herself with repeated convulsions. All physical stimuli should be minimized to provide maximal rest.

The effect of magnesium sulfate upon blood pressure is unpredictable. At times a marked hypotensive response is observed; in other cases, there will be no change in the blood pressure. Many eclamptic patients have borderline blood pressure readings of 145 to 160 mmHg systolic and 80 to 90 mmHg diastolic pressures. However, in the unusual patient with blood pressure readings of 200 mmHg systolic and 110 mmHg diastolic pressure or greater, antihypertensive therapy should be instituted. The drug of choice is hydralazine (apresoline) given intravenously and titrated against the blood pressure response. (See next section for details.)

Once the patient has been stabilized on anticonvulsant therapy, a decision has to be reached concerning delivery. Generally with pregnancy at 32 weeks or more, medical induction should be undertaken by amniotomy with or without intravenous oxytocin. The management of earlier-dated pregnancies must be individualized. Severe preeclamptic and eclamptic patients respond surprisingly well to induction in spite of prematurity and the use of magnesium sulfate, which inhibits uterine contraction. The anesthesia of choice for vaginal delivery is pudendal block since it is least disturbing to the body system and does not affect blood pressure. For the 20 to 30 percent of patients who do not respond to induction, cesarean section must be performed to effect delivery. Furthermore, there appears to be an increase in the cesarean-section rate in recent years, perhaps because of an increase in the use of fetal monitoring and fetal scalp blood pH analyses. Weingold et al. have reported an increased incidence of fetal cardiac decelerations among preeclamptic patients with the use of oxytocin.

After delivery is accomplished, severe preeclamptic and eclamptic patients must be observed closely in the postpartum period. Magnesium sulfate along with phenobarbital sedation should be continued during this period. A decrease in pulse pressure during the immediate puerperium is an ominous sign of impending seizure, and vigorous anticonvulsant therapy should be instituted immediately. During the first 12 to 14 hours after delivery, patients with severe preeclampsia or eclampsia do not always have diuresis immediately but display minor to moderate degrees of oliguria from 20 to 40 mL per hour. It is important not to overhydrate the patients with intravenous fluids during this period of body fluid adjustments lest serious pulmonary edema result. After a latent period of 12 to 14 hours, a marked diuresis usually occurs associated with a gradual rise in central venous pressure. Diuresis of 300 to 600 mL per hour is not unusual.

CHRONIC HYPERTENSION WITH SUPERIMPOSED PREECLAMPSIA OR ECLAMPSIA

Clinical

These patients have had definite hypertension prior to pregnancy and after 20 weeks of pregnancy develop an even greater rise in blood pressure accompanied by definite proteinuria. Patients tend to be older, multiparous, and with a strong family history of hypertension. In contrast to preeclamptic patients, the typical superimposed preeclamptic patient does not gain an excessive amount of weight nor develop edema. She tends to be slight and nervous with very small total weight gain. The superimposed preeclamptic patient actually demonstrates enhanced excretion of a sodium load in direct contrast to preeclamptic patients who retain sodium (Willson et al.). Moreover, chronic hypertensive patients display augmented excretion of sodium even in the nonpregnant state. The only group of patients with superimposed preeclampsia who develop edema and show excessive weight gain are the obese women whose hypertension is related to their obesity.

Intrauterine growth retardation and intrauterine fetal demise are definite and serious risks in this group of patients. Stillborn rate in the past has been reported as high as 40 to 60 percent. Because each succeeding pregnancy tends to become even more severely involved, an unusually heavy premium is placed upon the fetus in utero. Maternal mortality is not as high as in the eclamptic patients, probably because the high incidence of intrauterine fetal death ameliorates the preeclamptic condition.

Blood pressure readings may be markedly elevated in cases of superimposed preeclampsia. Patients who develop superimposed eclampsia often display exaggerated hypertension in the range of 250/110 to 260/130. Placental abruption may occasionally develop among such severely hypertensive patients.

Treatment

Since the patient is older and the vascular system is not as resilient as in the younger preeclamptic patient, it is rational to provide antihypertensive therapy to decrease peripheral resistance, especially in patients with elevated diastolic pressure. The antihypertensive drug for acute superimposed preeclampsia is hydralazine (Apresoline) administered intravenously as a single initial dose of 5 to 10 mg, or as slow continuous infusion of 20 mg in 1 L of glucose or Ringer's lactate titrated against the blood pressure response. With severely elevated blood pressure readings, the antihypertensive therapy should be delivered to lower the blood pressure only partially, not as a resort to obtain near-normal values. Persistence in pursuing low values often results in sudden and serious hypotensive episodes.

In severe superimposed preeclampsia with hyperreactive reflexes, or in superimposed eclampsia, anticonvulsant therapy with magnesium sulfate should be provided in addition to antihypertensive medication. The rest of the treatment is comparable to the management of severe preeclampsia and eclampsia, with special emphasis on careful monitoring of the fetus at all stages of pregnancy. The more aggressive management of superimposed preeclampsia with liberal use of cesarean section has benefited fetal salvage in recent years. The improved fetal survival has resulted not only from the earlier delivery but from the remarkable advances in neonatology in managing small premature infants.

For chronic hypertensive patients with superimposed preeclampsia requiring prolonged antihypertensive therapy, oral medications are utilized, such as hydralazine, methyldopa, and reserpine. In our experience, methyldopa appears to be the most reliable with minimal side effects; however, it is difficult to assess any beneficial effect of such antihypertensive agents in improving fetal survival.

CHRONIC HYPERTENSIVE DISEASE AND UNCLASSIFIED HYPERTENSIVE DISORDERS

These two conditions represent hypertensive states that persist through pregnancy but without additional complications; they therefore require no special therapy.

REFERENCES

Agüero O, Kizer S: Suture of the uterine rupture. *Obstet Gynecol* 31:806, 1968.

Alberman E et al.: Previous reproductive history in mothers presenting with spontaneous abortions. *Br J Obstet Gynecol* 82:366, 1975.

Anderson WH, Harbert GM Jr: Conservative management of pre-eclamptic and eclamptic patients: A re-evaluation. *Am J Obstet Gynecol* 129:260, 1977.

Badria L, Young GB: Correlation of ultrasonic and soft tissue x-ray placentography in 300 cases. *J Clin Ultrasound* 4:403, 1976.

Bauer CR et al.: Prolonged rupture of membranes associated with a decreased incidence of respiratory distress syndrome. *Pediatrics* 53:7, 1974.

Beacham WD et al.: Rupture of the uterus at New Orleans Charity Hospital. *Am J Obstet Gynecol* 106:1083, 1970.

Beller FK: Disseminated intravascular coagulation and consumption coagulopathy in obstetrics, in *Obstetrics and Gynecology Annual,* ed. RM Wynn, New York: Appleton-Century-Crofts, 1974.

Benirschke K, Kim CK: Multiple pregnancy. *N Eng J Med* 288:1276, 1973.

Block MR, Rahal DK: Cervical incompetence, a diagnostic and prognostic scoring system. *Obstet Gynecol* 47:3, 1976.

Boué J and Boué A: Anomalies chromosomiques dans les avortements spontanes, in A Boué and C Thibault, eds.: *Chromosomal errors in relation to reproductive failure,* Paris: Inserm, 1973.

Brame RG et al.: Maternal risk in abruption. *Obstet Gynecol* 31:224, 1968.

Breen JL: A 21 year survey of 654 ectopic pregnancies. *Am J Obstet Gynecol* 106:7, 1970.

Browne FJ: Sensitization of the vascular system in preeclamptic toxemia and eclampsia. *J Obstet Gynaecol Br Common* 53:510, 1946.

Bryans CL Jr: Discussion of Lanier et al. *Am J Obstet Gynecol* 93:398, 1965.

Bucht H, Werkö L: Glomerular filtration rate and renal blood flow in hypertensive toxaemia of pregnancy. *J Obstet Gynaecol Br Common* 60:157, 1953.

Burchell RC: Premature spontaneous rupture of the membranes. *Am J Obstet Gynecol* 88:251, 1964.

Campbell S: Ultrasonic and radiological examination in the placenta and the maternal supply, ed. P Gruenwald, Baltimore: University Park Press, 1975, pp. 281-306.

Carr DH: Chromosome studies in selected spontaneous abortions: 1. Conception after oral contraceptives. *Can Med Assoc J* 103:343, 1970.

Chesley LC: Simultaneous renal clearance of urea and uric acid in the differential diagnosis of the late toxemia. *Am J Obstet Gynecol* 59:960, 1950.

Claiborne HA, Schelin EC: Rupture of the gravid uterus. *Am J Obstet Gynecol* 99:900, 1967.

Crenshaw C Jr et al.: Placenta previa: A survey of twenty years experience with improved perinatal survival by expectant therapy and cesarean delivery. *Obstet Gynecol Surv* 28:461, 1973.

Deleze G et al.: Determination of bile acid concentration in human amniotic fluid for prenatal diagnosis of intestinal obstruction. *Pediatrics* 59:647, 1977.

Demers LM, Gabbe SG: Placental prostaglandin levels in pre-eclampsia. *Am J Obstet Gynecol* 126:137, 1976.

Douglas RG: Pregnancy and labor following cesarean section, in *Controversy in obstetrics and gynecology*, eds. DE Reid, TC Barton, Philadelphia: Saunders, 1969, p. 308.

Eastman NJ, Hellman LM: *Williams Obstetrics,* 13th ed., New York: Appleton-Century-Crofts, 1966.

Farooqui MO et al.: A review of twin pregnancy and perinatal mortality. *Obstet Gynecol Surv* 28:144, 1973.

Felmus LB et al.: Spontaneous rupture of apparently normal uterus during pregnancy; review. *Obstet Gynecol Surv* 8:155, 1953.

Foster HW, Moore DT: Abdominal pregnancy—Report of twelve cases. *Obstet Gynecol* 30:249, 1967.

Fox RL et al.: Interlocking twins: Experience with four cases and suggested management. *Obstet Gynecol* 46:53, 1975.

Fuchs F: Volume of amniotic fluid at various stages of pregnancy. *Clin Obstet Gynecol* 9:449, 1966.

Galask RP, Snyder IS: Antimicrobial factors in amniotic fluid. *Am J Obstet Gynecol* 106:59, 1970.

Gant NF et al.: A study of angiotensin II Pressor response throughout primigravid pregnancy. *J Clin Invest* 52:2682, 1973.

_____: A sequential study of the metabolism of dehydroisoantrosterone sulfate in primigravid pregnancies. *Endocrinology,* International Congress Series, *Excerpta Medica* 273:1026, 1972.

Gluck L et al.: Diagnosis of the respiratory distress syndrome by amniocentesis. *Am J Obstet Gynecol* 109:440, 1971.

Gordon RD et al.: Plasma renin activity, plasma angiotensin and plasma and urinary electrolytes in normal and toxemic pregnancy including a prospective study. *Clin Sci Molec Med* 45:115, 1973.

Greulich WW: The incidence of human multiple births. *Am Natural* 64:142, 1930.

Guerrero R, Rojas OI: Spontaneous abortion and aging of human ova and spermatozoa. *N Eng J Med* 293:573, 1975.

Gunn GC et al.: Premature rupture of the fetal membranes. *Am J Obstet Gynecol* 106:469, 1970.

Guttmacher AF, Kohl SG: The fetus of multiple gestations. *Obstet Gynecol* 12:528, 1958.

Handler JS: The role of lactic acid in the reduced excretion of uric acid in toxemia of pregnancy. *J Clin Invest* 39:1526, 1960.

Hayashi T: Uric acid and endogenous creatinine clearance studies in normal pregnancy and in toxemias of pregnancy. *Am J Obstet Gynecol* 71:859, 1956.

_____ et al.: Simultaneous measurement of plasma and erythrocyte oxypurines. I. Normal and toxemic pregnancy. *Gynec Invest* 3:221, 1972.

_____: Effects of diet and diuretic agents in pregnancy toxemias. *Obstet Gynecol* 22:327, 1963.

Helmer OM, Judson WE: Influence of high renin substrate levels on renin-angiotensin system in pregnancy. *Am J Obstet Gynecol* 99:9, 1967.

Hertig AT, Sheldon WH: Minimal criteria required to prove prima facie cause of traumatic abortion or miscarriage. An analysis of 100 spontaneous abortions. *Ann Surg* 117:596, 1943.

Hibbard BM: Abruptio placentae, pre-eclampsia, and essential hypertension. *J Obstet Gynecol Br Common* 69:282, 1962.

_____, Jeffcoate TNA: Abruptio placentae. *Obstet Gynecol* 27:155, 1966.

Hibbard LT: Placenta previa. *Am J Obstet Gynecol* 104:172, 1969.

Howard BK et al.: Supine hypotensive syndrome in late pregnancy. *Obstet Gynecol* 1:371, 1953.

Huff RW: Antibiotic prophylaxis for puerperal endometritis following premature rupture of the membranes. *J Reprod Med* 19:79, 1977.

Hutchinson DL et al.: The role of the fetus in the water exchange of the amniotic fluid of normal and hydramniotic patients. *J Clin Invest* 38:971, 1959.

Jacoby HE, Charles D: Clinical conditions associated wtih hydramnios. *Am J Obstet Gynecol* 94:910, 1966.

Jeffcoate TN, Scott JS: Polyhydramnios and oligohydramnios. *Can Med Assoc J* 80:77, 1959.

Jeffrey RL et al.: Role of bed rest in twin gestation. *Obstet Gynecol* 43:822 1974.

Jones QS: Luteal phase defects, in *Progress in Infertility,* 2d ed., eds. SJ Behrman, RW Kistner, 1975. Little, Brown, Boston

Jouppila P et al.: Twin pregnancy: The role of active management during pregnancy and delivery. *Acta Obstet Gynecol Scand (Suppl)* 44:14, 1975.

Kaiser IH: Pregnancy wastage in operating room personnel. *Obstet Gynecol* 41:930, 1973.

Kennan AL et al.: The pathologic physiology of the clotting mechanism in eclampsia. *Am J Obstet Gynecol* 74:1029, 1957.

Kitchin JE et al.: Puerperal inversion of the uterus. *Am J Obstet Gynecol* 123:51, 1975.

Kohorn EI et al.: Placental localization. *Am J Obstet Gynecol* 103:868, 1969.

Kramer EE: Hydramnios, oligohydramnios and fetal malformations. *Clin Obstet Gynecol* 9:508, 1966.

Krupp PG et al.: Maternal mortality. *Obstet Gynecol* 35:823, 1970.

Landesman R, Saxena BB: Results of the first 1,000 radioreceptor assays for the determination of human chorionic gonadotropin. *Fertil Steril* 27:351, 1976.

Langman J: *Medical Embryology,* 3d. ed., Baltimore: Williams & Wilkins, 1975.

Lanier LR et al.: Incidence of maternal and fetal complications associated with rupture of the membranes before onset of labor. *Am J Obstet Gynecol* 93:398, 1965.

Larsen B, Galask RP: Host resistance to intraamniotic infection. *Obstet Gynecol Surv* 30:675, 1975.

Lauritsen JG: Genetic aspects spontaneous abortion. Dan Med Bull. 24:169, 1977.

Lebherz TB et al.: Double-blind study of premature rupture of the membranes. *Am J Obstet Gynecol* 87:218, 1963.

Ledger WJ et al.: Guidelines for antibiotic prophylaxis in gynecology. *Am J Obstet Gynecol* 121:1038, 1975.

Lee WK et al.: Acute inversion of the uterus. *Obstet Gynecol* 51:144, 1978.

Liggins GC, Howie RN: A controlled trial of antepartum glucocorticoid treatment for prevention of respiratory distress syndrome in premature infants. *Pediatrics* 50:515, 1972.

Massani ZM et al.: Angiotensin blood levels in normal and toxemic pregnancies. *Am J Obstet Gynecol* 99:313, 1967.

McCall ML: Cerebral blood flow and metabolism in toxemias of pregnancy. *Surg Gynecol Obstet* 89:715, 1949.

McHattie TJ: Placenta praevia accreta. *Obstet Gynecol* 40:795, 1972.

Mead PB, Clapp JF: The use of betamethasone and timed delivery in management of premature rupture of the membranes in the preterm pregnancy. *J Reprod Med* 19:3, 1977.

Mengert WF et al.: Observations on the pathogenesis of premature separation of the normally implanted placenta. *Am J Ostet Gynecol* 66:1104, 1953.

Millar WG: A clinical and pathological study of placenta accreta. *J Obstet Gynaecol Br Commonw* 66:353, 1959.

Morris JA et al.: Vascular reactivity to angiotensin II infusion during gestation. *Am J Obstet Gynecol* 130:379, 1978.

Morrison J: The development of the lower uterine segment. *Aust NZ J Obstet Gynaecol* 12:182, 1972.

Moya F et al.: Hydramnios and congenital anomalies. *JAMA* 173:110, 1960.

Naeye RL et al.: Twins: Causes of perinatal death in United States cities and one African city. *Am J Obstet Gynecol* 131:267, 1978.

Nwosu U et al.: Initiation of labor by intraamniotic cortisol instillation in prolonged human pregnancy. *Obstet Gynecol* 47:137, 1976.

_____: Possible role of the fetal adrenal glands in the etiology of postmaturity. *Am J Obstet Gynecol* 121:366, 1975.

Page EW et al.: Abruptio placenta: Dangers of delay in delivery. *Obstet Gynecol* 3:385, 1954.

Paul RE et al.: Evaluation of renal biopsy in pregnancy toxemia. *Obstet Gynecol* 34:235, 1969.

Petrucco OM et al.: Immunofluorescent studies in renal biopsies in preeclampsia. *Br Med J* 1:473, 1974.

Pitkin RM: Acute polyhydramnios recurrent in successive pregnancies. *Obstet Gynecol* 48 (Suppl 1): 425, 1976.

_____, Zwirek SJ: Amniotic fluid creatinine. *Am J Obstet Gynecol* 98:1135, 1976.

Potter EL: Bilateral absence of ureters and kidneys. *Obstet Gynecol* 25:3, 1965.

Pritchard JA: Standardized treatment of 154 consecutive cases of eclampsia. *Am J Obstet Gynecol* 123:543, 1975.

_____, Brekken AL: Clinical and laboratory studies on severe abruptio placentae. *Am J Obstet Gynecol* 97:681, 1967.

_____ et al.: Genesis of severe placental abruption. *Am J Obstet Gynecol* 108:22, 1970.

Queenan JT et al.: Polyhydramnios: Chronic versus acute. *Am J Obstet Gynecol* 108:349, 1970.

_____, Gadow EC: Amniotic fluid volumes in normal pregnancies. *Am J Obstet Gynecol* 114:34, 1972.

Russell JGB: Radiology in Obstetrics and Antepartum Paediatrics, London: Butterworth, 1973.

Russell KP, Anderson GV: The aggressive management of ruptured membranes. *Am J Obstet Gynecol* 83:930, 1962.

Sacks M, Baker TH: Spontaneous premature rupture of the membranes. *Am J Obstet Gynecol* 97:888, 1967.

Schneider CL: Obstetric shock: Some interdependent problems of coagulation. *Obstet Gynecol* 4:273, 1954.

Schneider J et al.: Maternal mortality due to ectopic pregnancy. *Obstet Gynecol* 49:557, 1977.

Scott JR, Beer AA: Immunologic aspects of pre-eclampsia. *Am J Obstet Gynecol* 125:418, 1976.

Scott JS, Jenkins DM: Immunogenetic factors in aetiology of pre-eclampsia/eclampsia. *J Med Genet* 13:200, 1976.

Sheehan HL: Pathological lesions in the hypertensive toxaemias of pregnancy, in *Toxaemias of Pregnancy Human and Veterinary,* eds. J Hammond et al., Philadelphia: Blakiston, 1950, p. 16.

Spargo BH et al.: Glomerular capillary endotheliosis in toxemia of pregnancy. *Arch Pathol* 68:593, 1959.

Speroff L: Toxemia of pregnancy. Mechanism and therapeutic management. *Am J Cardiol* 32:582, 1973.

Stevenson AC: Association of hydramnios with congenital malformations. *Ciba Foundation Symposium on Congenital Malformations,* Boston: Little, Brown, 1960, p. 241.

Sutton D: Arterial placentography and placental previa. *Br J Radiol* 39:47, 1966.

Symonds EM, Anderson GJ: The effect of bed rest on plasma renin in hypertensive disease of pregnancy. *J Obstet Gynaecol Br Commonw* 81:676, 1974.

Talledo OE et al.: Renin-angiotensin system in normal and toxemic pregnancies. *Am J Obstet Gynecol* 100:218, 1968.

Tatum HS, Schmidt, FH: Contraceptive and sterilization practices and extrauterine pregnancy: A realistic perspective. *Fertil Steril* 25:4, 1977.

Townsend L et al.: Spontaneous premature rupture of the membranes. *Aust NZ J Obstet Gynaecol* 6:226, 1966.

Tudehope DI, Sinclair JC: Birth weight, gestational age, and neonatal risk, in *Neonatal-Perinatal Medicine,* 2d ed., ed., RE Behrman, St. Louis: CV Mosby, 1977, pp. 116-127.

Wallace MR, Smedley MG: The transient nephrotic syndrome of pregnancy. *NZ Med J* 71:208, 1970.

Webb GA: Maternal death associated with premature rupture of the membranes. *Am J Obstet Gynecol* 98:594, 1967.

Weekes LR, Greig LB: Placenta accreta: A twenty-year review. *Am J Obstet Gynecol* 113:76, 1972.

Weingold AB et al.: Fetal heart rate response in the pre-eclamptic hypertensive patient during spontaneous and oxytocin stimulated labor. *J Reprod Med* 5:35, 1970.

White C. Wyshak G: Inheritance in human dizygotic twinning. *N Eng J Med* 271:1003, 1964.

Willson JR et al.: Hypertonic saline infusions for the differential diagnosis of the toxemias of pregnancy. *Am J Obstet Gynecol* 73:30, 1957.

Varma RT: Value of ultrasonic B scanning when bleeding is present in early pregnancy. *Am J Obstet Gynecol* 114:5, 1972.

Yussman MA, Haynes DM: Rupture of the gravid uterus: A 12-year study. *Obstet Gynecol* 36:115, 1970.

31

Diseases Complicating Pregnancy

JOSEPH J. ROVINSKY

Gestational polyneuritis
Carpal tunnel syndrome
Meralgia paresthetica
Subarachnoid hemorrhage
Intracranial vascular disorders
Cerebral thrombosis
Multiple sclerosis
Management
Brain tumors
Management
Myasthenia gravis
Management

DISORDERS OF THE SKELETAL SYSTEM AND SKIN

Skin diseases related to pregnancy
Prurigo gestationis
Herpes gestationis
Impetigo herpetiformis
Skin diseases complicated by pregnancy
Psoriasis
Pemphigus
Discoid lupus erythematosus
Melanoma
Condyloma acuminata
Skeletal disorders
Osteogenesis imperfecta
Chondrodystrophy

INFECTIOUS DISEASES

Bacterial infections
Pneumonia
Gonorrhea
Viral infections
Rhinoviruses
Influenza viruses
Rubeola (measles)
Rubella (German measles)
Mumps
Poliomyelitis
Coxsackieviruses
Cytomegalovirus
Herpes simplex
Varicella (chickenpox)
Variola (smallpox) and vaccinia
Spirochetal and protozoal infections
Syphilis
Toxoplasmosis
Malaria

PREGNANCY AND CANCER

Carcinoma of the breast
Other malignant diseases

Carcinoma of the thyroid
Carcinoma of the cervix
Effect of maternal malignancy on the fetus

Pregnancy is an intercurrent, transient, and sometimes repetitive event which periodically may intersect and significantly modify a woman's longitudinal health course. In addition to diseases which may result from or are specific to pregnancy, the gravida may be subject to any of the ailments or conditions which may occur in nonpregnant women in the reproductive years. In the presence of pregnancy, one must deal with two patients: the pregnant woman, who is undergoing significant physiologic and functional alterations, and the fetus. Three important considerations arise which are not present in the nongravid patient: (1) the pregnancy may modify the disease process; (2) the disease itself may have a significant influence on the course of pregnancy; and (3) either the disease process or the therapy required may have serious deleterious effects on the fetus in utero or on the neonate. Each disease complicating pregnancy must be examined in the light of these considerations, and decisions made about the advisability of undertaking pregnancy, continuation of a pregnancy already conceived, management of the patient antepartum and postpartum, and the conduct of labor and delivery. In addition, the physician who cares for pregnant women assumes important responsibilities for interconceptional care, including patient education about long-term fertility and reproductive potential, discussion and implementation of either contraception or sterilization, and appropriate referral for medical or surgical treatment.

DISORDERS OF THE CARDIOVASCULAR SYSTEM

CARDIAC DISEASE

The problems presented by cardiac disease as a complication of pregnancy have changed consonant with changes and improvements in methods of diagnosis and medical and surgical treatments of cardiac disorders. Where once rheumatic heart disease accounted for over 90 percent of cases of cardiac disease complicating pregnancy, today congenital heart disease is encountered with increasing frequency, ranging up to 44 percent in some reports. This change results from years of successful prophylaxis of rheumatic fever, as well as increased survival and longevity of infants born with congenital cardiac defects. Hypertensive cardiovascular disease and arteriosclerotic heart disease occur infrequently in women of reproductive age but present more serious consequences when they do occur (Ueland).

As the incidence of maternal mortality from toxemia, hemorrhage, and infection has decreased, cardiac disease has become one of the leading causes of maternal death, accounting for almost one-fourth of all maternal mortalities in some areas. Cardiac patients who have only limited functional capacity, particularly those who are older or who have a history of cardiac decompensation, face the gravest maternal risk. Active myocarditis, atrial fibrillation, and coexisting disorders such as infection, severe anemia, or hypertension magnify the maternal hazard. Depending on the general condition of the patient, on the accuracy of the cardiac diagnosis, and on the adequacy of medical management through the antepartum, intrapartum, and puerperal course, the mortality rates for pregnant patients with severe cardiac complications may reach 10 to 20 percent. On the other hand, under optimal conditions of diagnosis and modern medical management, there is almost no cardiac complication so severe as to mandate interruption of the pregnancy to preserve the life of the mother.

The management of cardiac disease in pregnancy is complicated by the fact that physiologic cardiovascular alterations in the gravid woman may interfere with accurate diagnosis and may mask or simulate the manifestations of cardiac disease. (Refer to Chap. 9 for a discussion of alterations in cardiovascular hemodynamics in pregnancy.) Labor and delivery impose transient, but very severe, additional cardiac stress on the mother. Cardiac work requirements are even higher immediately postpartum and do not return to nongravid levels for at least 2 weeks.

CARDIOVASCULAR SIGNS AND SYMPTOMS

The diagnosis of existing organic cardiac disease may be obscured by cardiopulmonary manifestations which are normal for pregnancy (Ueland et al.). The pregnant woman may have shortness of breath on exertion and an increased respiratory rate. She may complain of dyspnea while recumbent, simulating the orthopnea of congestive heart failure. She may exhibit tachycardia and palpitations at the slightest exertion or even at rest. Both clinically and radiographically, there is apparent cardiomegaly. Pedal edema frequently is encountered, particularly in the latter half

of gestation. Functional cardiac murmurs may arise secondary to an overactive heart, increased blood velocity, or the "physiologic anemia" of pregnancy. Preexisting functional murmurs may be accentuated as pregnancy progresses. Because of increased pulmonary blood flow and elevated pulmonary artery pressures, there may be accentuation of pulmonic heart sounds with transmission to the vessels in the neck, simulating aortic valvular murmurs (Marcus et al.).

The signs and symptoms of organic heart disease therefore must be differentiated from the manifestations of normal pregnancy. Objective evidence of pulmonary congestion or distended neck veins is useful. X-ray of the chest can confirm the presence of pulmonary congestion or cardiomegaly. Congestive heart failure may be excluded by determinations of venous pressure and circulation time. A careful clinical evaluation of the cardiovascular system is very important in the pregnant patient.

Anemia, either antecedent or newly developed during pregnancy, may pose a difficult problem in diagnosis. The patient may have shortness of breath, fatigue, tachycardia, extrasystoles, and increased blood velocity; these signs and symptoms may be exaggerated by exertion. A loud functional hemic murmur may be present. At times, the patient's cardiovascular status may be clarified only after correction of the anemia.

RHEUMATIC HEART DISEASE

The incidence of rheumatic heart disease in pregnancy has increased in recent decades because of improved survival rates for patients with rheumatic fever, better methods of management of bacterial endocarditis, and decreased utilization of abortion. At the same time, maternal mortality from rheumatic heart disease has declined from 30 per 100,000 deliveries in 1941 to our own experience of 4 per 100,000 deliveries in the past 20 years.

A number of factors are responsible for this reduction in maternal mortality. Most important have been the improvements in medical diagnosis, supervision, and cardiac surgery. In all reported series, the mortality for unregistered patients is two to four times higher than that for registered patients with cardiac disease of the same severity who received continuous antepartum obstetric and medical care. Adequate medical supervision includes not only meticulous cardiac care but also prompt hospitalization of patients requiring additional diagnostic studies or intensive control of cardiac function. In patients with severe disease, hospitalization for the duration of pregnancy may be required.

Patients with rheumatic heart disease tend to develop congestive failure with increasing age, irrespective of parity. Also, congestive heart failure is observed more frequently in multiparas than in primigravidas at any stated age. In these patients, the prevention of congestive heart failure is essential, since congestive failure in pregnancy carries a maternal mortality rate of 33 percent.

Other factors affect maternal mortality as well. The incidence of congestive heart failure varies directly with the duration of the rheumatic process, the interval from the first clinical manifestations of rheumatic heart disease to the onset of the current pregnancy. The degree of cardiomegaly also determines prognosis; the patient without cardiac enlargement is a better risk than one with massive cardiomegaly. As an exception, patients with mitral stenosis are predisposed to the development of pulmonary edema even if there is no cardiac enlargement. Poor prognosis also is presaged by a history of recent attacks (within 1 year) of rheumatic fever or of prior congestive failure, particularly if the latter was present during a prior pregnancy despite adequate medical management.

The most significant basis for determining prognosis of the cardiac patient in pregnancy is her functional capacity. Functional capacity may be difficult to determine during pregnancy and may vary with duration of gestation; interconceptional functional capacity, determined prior to the onset of pregnancy, correlates well with observed clinical results. The functional criteria established by the New York Heart Association (Table 31-1) furnish a valuable index of cardiac functional capacity: patients in classes I and II have an excellent prognosis in pregnancy and require little more than routine prenatal care; patients in classes III and IV have a much higher incidence of complications and mortality and require meticulous medical supervision. The maternal risk is markedly increased in any class in older patients, patients with marked cardiomegaly or arrhythmias, or women with a previous history of congestive heart failure.

Fetal wastage in patients with cardiac disease merits consideration, and often may be affected by the medical management. Perinatal mortality in patients with severe cardiac disease has ranged between 30 and 50 percent. A correlation has been demonstrated between maternal arterial oxygen saturation and pregnancy outcome; all pregnancies in mothers with arterial oxygen saturation less than 80 percent terminated in abortion, premature labor, or the delivery of "small for dates" infants. Prevention or proper management of congestive heart failure, by diminishing maternal hypoxia and venous congestion, has reduced this fetal wastage.

With the possible exception of patients with the most severe forms of rheumatic heart disease, pregnancy in the cardiac patient carries acceptable risks of maternal and fetal morbidity and mortality, as long as medical management is continuous and meticulous. There is no evidence that one or more pregnancies affect adversely the patient's normal life expectancy in view of her cardiac disability; the patient's long-term prognosis relates primarily to the progression and severity of her underlying cardiac lesion (Burch).

Evaluation of the Pregnant Cardiac Patient

An accurate evaluation of the pregnant patient's cardiac status must be made as early in gestation as possible. A thorough medical history must be taken, with special attention to points which the patient herself may not relate to the presence of cardiac disease. A complete physical examination should be performed, all valvular, rhythmic, or other cardiac defects noted, and an etiologic diagnosis established, if possible. A functional classification should be determined. An attempt must be made to determine

TABLE 31-1 Functional Cardiac Classification

Functional class	Definition
I	Patients with a cardiac disorder without limitation of physical activity. Ordinary physical activity causes no discomfort.
II	Patients with a cardiac disorder with slight to moderate limitation of physical activity. Ordinary physical activity causes discomfort.
III	Patients with a cardiac disorder with moderate to marked limitation of physical activity. Less than ordinary physical activity causes discomfort.
IV	Patients with a cardiac disorder who are unable to carry out any physical activity without discomfort.

whether cardiac murmurs present are functional or organic. Organic systolic murmurs frequently are harsh and of high intensity; diastolic murmurs almost always are organic. Women who have a documented history of rheumatic fever but in whom no reliable diagnosis of organic murmurs can be made during pregnancy present a difficult diagnostic problem. Fortunately, from a functional point of view, these patients almost always have minimal (class I) cardiac involvement and usually have no difficulty during pregnancy. Other criteria of organic heart disease, such as significant arrhythmia (atrial fibrillation or heart block), loud mitral or aortic systolic murmurs, or marked cardiomegaly, should be documented. Electrocardiographic abnormalities may be significant. Radiographic and cardiac catheterization studies may be necessary to establish an etiologic diagnosis, but should be reserved for patients in pregnancy who are extremely ill or refractory to routine medical management and in whom either interruption of the pregnancy or cardiac surgical intervention begins to assume an important role.

Specific Valvular Lesions

In general, mitral valve disease occurs more frequently than aortic valve disease, and this is especially true in women of childbearing age. Two-thirds of patients with mitral valve disease have combined mitral stenosis and insufficiency. Of solitary valvular defects, mitral stenosis composes 60 to 70 percent; mitral regurgitation, 25 percent; aortic regurgitation, 10 percent; and aortic stenosis, approximately 1 to 2 percent.

Mitral stenosis is the lesion encountered most frequently in pregnancy, its incidence greater than that of all other valve lesions combined. Because many of the clinical findings of mitral stenosis are masked by normal, physiologic cardiovascular alterations in pregnancy, the severity of the lesion often must await postpartum evaluation. Patients with mitral stenosis are at high risk for developing acute congestive heart failure and pulmonary edema during pregnancy because of the physiologically elevated cardiac rate, increased pulmonary artery and left atrial pressures, and pregnancy hypervolemia. Vigilant observation throughout pregnancy for evidence of impending pulmonary congestion is mandatory, and prompt, intensive therapy should be initiated if the patient exhibits increased dyspnea at rest, tachycardia, cough, hemoptysis, or pulmonary rales.

The diagnosis of organic mitral insufficiency in pregnancy may be difficult because of the frequency of functional apical systolic murmurs. The degree of clinical disability from mitral insufficiency depends on the amount of regurgitation and the extent of cardiac enlargement. Pulmonary edema is rare in mitral insufficiency. Except for patients with far-advanced disease, pure mitral insufficiency usually does not carry a great risk for the pregnant patient.

Aortic insufficiency, with regurgitation of blood through the aortic valve, is accompanied by characteristic signs: Corrigan's (collapsing) arterial pulse, widened pulse pressure, and left ventricular hypertrophy. Pure aortic insufficiency, except for far-advanced disease, does not carry a high risk for the pregnant patient.

Aortic stenosis as a clinically significant solitary lesion is very rare during the childbearing years. In severe cases, the cardiac output is diminished, resulting in low systolic and diminished pulse pressures, angina pectoris, and often attacks of syncope. Congestive heart failure is an unusual complication of aortic stenosis.

Management of the Pregnant Rheumatic Cardiac Patient

The principles of management of rheumatic heart disease in pregnancy are identical to those employed in the nongravid patient. Factors which might precipitate heart failure, such as infection, nutritional deficiency, anemia, or undue physical stress, must be avoided or eliminated. Excessive fluid retention and venous congestion must be reduced. The management during pregnancy is complicated by the increased blood volume, elevated cardiac output, and increased venous pressures which accompany normal pregnancy.

The most important prophylactic and therapeutic measure for the pregnant patient with cardiac disease is *limitation of activity*. The pregnancy itself imposes demands on functional cardiac reserve which the normal heart can meet with relative ease but which may tax the damaged heart unduly. The stress on the gravida's cardiac reserve best can be reduced by minimizing physical activity. The patient's functional classification is a fairly accurate guide to the limitation of activity which must be imposed. Patients in cardiac classes I and II need not be restricted severely; frequent rest periods during the day and assistance in performing household chores are desirable. Working away from home during pregnancy should be interdicted in all but class I cardiac patients. Patients in cardiac class III require greater restriction of physical activity and, together with patients in cardiac class

IV, may require complete bed rest or even hospitalization for the duration of pregnancy. In addition to ensuring limitation of physical activity, complete bed rest in the supine position effectively reduces the return of blood to the heart, and hence cardiac stress, in the later stages of gestation.

The dietary intake of the pregnant cardiac patient should be controlled, preventing excess weight gain by a low caloric intake and excessive fluid retention by salt restriction. Excessive weight gain predisposes the patient to hypertension, toxemia, venous stasis, edema, and dyspnea, increasing the stress on an already overburdened heart. The degree of sodium restriction requires individualization. The severity of the cardiac lesion and its effect on renal tubular function exaggerate the physiologic salt and water retention of normal pregnancy. Patients in cardiac class I require only slight restriction of sodium intake. Patients in cardiac classes II and III usually require moderate to severe sodium and fluid restrictions. The availability of safe and potent diuretics has simplified this aspect of management and permitted liberalization of dietary restrictions.

All patients with moderate or advanced cardiac disease or who show excessive weight gain, fluid retention, venous congestion, or edema should be placed on oral diuretic therapy. Most frequently prescribed are the thiazide derivatives, whose pharmacologic action is based upon the inhibition of enzyme systems in the proximal and distal renal tubules, blocking reabsorption of sodium, chlorides, and water, with a concomitant increase in potassium excretion. The potency of the thiazides is not decreased with prolonged administration. Potassium depletion is an important problem during long-term therapy, and the patient must have adequate supplemental intake of potassium salts. Side effects and toxic reactions may occur but usually are mild; these include gastrointestinal irritation, skin rashes, leg cramps (secondary to profuse diuresis and salt loss), and hypotensive reactions, which are indications for reducing dosage or temporarily discontinuing the drug. Patients with gout may develop hyperuricemia; patients with latent diabetes, hyperglycemia. After prolonged administration, particularly in patients whose dietary sodium intake has been restricted severely, persistent elevation of the blood urea nitrogen may occur, mandating discontinuation of the drug. Thiazides cross the placental barrier and appear in breast milk; occasionally, they may cause fetal hyperbilirubinemia, thrombocytopenia, or altered carbohydrate metabolism. The problem of potassium depletion is magnified in patients receiving digitalis preparations,

since lowered potassium levels may potentiate the digitalis effect and produce myocardial irritability or other signs of digitalis toxicity. In such patients, the dietary intake of potassium should be increased with foods such as citrus fruits and juices, meat, bran, and milk; administration of supplemental potassium salts may be advisable.

Digitalis is the single most important drug in the treatment of the failing heart, increasing cardiac efficiency and output. During pregnancy, digitalis should be administered promptly whenever the earliest manifestations of congestive heart failure appear. Usually, digitalization should be carried out over a period of several days to avoid gastrointestinal side effects; however, in acute cardiac failure and pulmonary edema, digitalization should be accomplished as rapidly as possible with the intravenous administration of rapidly acting digitalis preparations. The responses of edema and pulmonary congestion are the best clinical guides to adequate digitalization and maintenance dosage. Temporary increments in digitalis dosage may be required during periods of increased cardiac stress, as during labor and delivery and in the immediate puerperium. Once class III and IV cardiac patients are digitalized, they should be maintained on digitalis therapy throughout pregnancy and probably into the puerperium. The need of class II patients for continued digitalis therapy once the circulatory overloading of pregnancy is removed must be individualized.

Digitalis glycosides pass the placental barrier and often accumulate in higher concentration in the fetus than in the mother. Nevertheless, when employed in ordinary therapeutic dosage, digitalis glycosides do not precipitate either fetal or neonatal disturbances in heart rate or electrocardiogram.

The prophylactic use of digitalis in pregnant cardiac patients has been a matter of some controversy. Near term, maternal physiologic alterations begin to resemble the manifestations of incipient congestive heart failure—tachycardia, elevated pulmonary artery and end-diastolic right atrial pressures, and edema; there is thus some theoretic basis for administration of digitalis to the pregnant patient with severe cardiac disease before the development of overt congestive failure. In our clinics, class II and III cardiac patients have been digitalized prophylactically during pregnancy if they had a previous history of congestive failure, moderate cardiac enlargement, or severe mitral stenosis. Digitalization is started during the midtrimester before the circulatory adjustments of pregnancy reach their peak, or at least several weeks before the anticipated delivery. Digitalis maintenance is continued postpartum for at least 6 weeks. Prophylactic digitalization is accomplished very slowly in ambulatory patients to minimize the risk of toxicity.

The most serious complication of cardiac disease in pregnancy is the development of acute pulmonary edema, which may incur a maternal mortality rate of 30 to 50 percent. Acute pulmonary edema rarely occurs in patients under close medical control. Early manifestations of pulmonary congestion, such as dyspnea at rest, nocturnal paroxysmal dyspnea, orthopnea, or basal pulmonary rales, require immediate hospitalization and treatment with bed rest, digitalis, diuretics, and dietary salt restriction; almost always, gross pulmonary edema can be averted. Should pulmonary edema supervene and the patient present with acute dyspnea, orthopnea, wheezing respirations, frothy, blood-tinged sputum, cyanosis, and moist, bubbling rales in all lung fields, energetic therapy must be applied to preserve both the pregnancy and the life of the patient; oxygen administration, narcotics and sedatives, digitalis, diuretics, aminophylline, rotating tourniquets, phlebotomy, and antibiotics all play a significant role in management.

In any patient with organic heart disease, anemia must be treated promptly and vigorously. Large doses of iron and vitamins should be prescribed, and folic acid supplementation should be routine. Only the unreliable or uncooperative patient may require parenteral iron therapy. In cardiac patients in whom severe anemia presents as an emergency, marked improvement may be achieved by the infusion of packed erythrocytes.

Intercurrent upper respiratory tract or pulmonary infection is the most frequent precipitating cause of cardiac failure in pregnancy. At the first signs of respiratory tract infection, pregnant cardiac patients should be hospitalized promptly and treated with appropriate antibiotics. Determinations of venous pressure and circulation time will serve to distinguish between respiratory tract infection and congestive heart failure; if the distinction is not clear, the patient should be treated as if congestive failure were present.

Patients with rheumatic heart disease are predisposed to the development of acute, recurrent carditis and of subacute bacterial endocarditis when exposed to infection by streptococci. Prophylactic antibiotic therapy may be administered to all pregnant patients with rheumatic heart disease regardless of age or the interval since the last rheumatic infection. In addition, prophylactic antibiotic therapy is indicated for patients without rheumatic valvular disease who have

had acute rheumatic fever within the past 10 years, and all patients with congenital heart lesions. One method of prophylaxis is the monthly injection of benzathine penicillin G (Bicillin), 1.2 million units intramuscularly; later in gestation, when patient visits are closer together, 600,000 units of benzathine penicillin G may be injected every 2 weeks. If the patient's reliability is established, oral penicillin, 200,000 units twice daily, is equally effective. Patients allergic to penicillin should receive alternative antibiotics either parenterally or orally.

With the onset of labor, prevention of subacute bacterial endocarditis requires additional attention. Susceptible patients are at special risk during labor, delivery, and the immediate puerperium, since bacillemia occurs in almost every parturient. Starting with the onset of labor and continuing for 1 week postpartum, all patients with known valvular disease or congenital cardiac defects should receive penicillin, 1.2 million units, and streptomycin, 1.0 g, intramuscularly daily. If clinical evidence of perineal or uterine infection develops, more intensive antibiotic therapy, culture-sensitivity specific, should be substituted. Patients allergic to penicillin should receive alternative, broad-spectrum prophylactic antibiotics.

Should subacute bacterial endocarditis develop during gestation, prompt and intensive therapy is indicated. Pregnancy does not alter either the therapy or the prognosis of subacute bacterial endocarditis. If the bacterial endocarditis occurs in early gestation, interruption of the pregnancy may be considered; the indication for interruption, however, should be based upon the severity of the underlying heart disease rather than the presence of infection. The underlying valvular lesion may be aggravated even though the bacterial endocarditis responds to therapy. In the nonpregnant patient, pregnancy should be deferred for approximately 6 months after cure of subacute bacterial endocarditis, to permit adequate stabilization of cardiac reserve and reevaluation of cardiac functional capacity.

Management during Labor and Delivery

The stress imposed on the heart of a woman in labor has been discussed in detail in Chap. 9. Nevertheless, the mode of delivery should be determined by the obstetric situation and not be based upon the presence of a cardiac lesion. *There is no cardiac indication for cesarean section.* Cardiac stress is no less severe and cardiac complications no less frequent with abdominal than with vaginal delivery. Operative procedures carry the additional risks of surgical stress, infection, protracted anesthesia, greater blood loss, and higher incidence of thromboembolic complications. On the other hand, if there is an obstetric indication for delivery by cesarean section, maternal cardiac disease is not a contraindication to operation.

Cardinal principles in the management of labor in patients with cardiac disease are relief of pain, distress, and apprehension (all contributing to tachycardia); avoidance of hypotension; and adequate oxygenation of both mother and fetus. Analgesic and sedative drugs may be employed, care being taken to avoid depression of respiratory and vasomotor centers in the mother or reduction in maternal alveolar ventilation. The use of amnesic agents such as scopolamine should be avoided, since they may increase the patient's restlessness, hyperactivity, and tachycardia. Oxytocin has no direct myocardial or vasopressor effects and may be utilized as necessary, as long as the problem of possibly excessive intravenous fluid administration is borne in mind.

It is advisable to shorten the second stage of labor by forceps delivery once full cervical dilatation has occurred and the leading point of the fetal vertex has descended low in the maternal pelvis. Premature forceps intervention, leading to traumatic delivery with increased risk of hemorrhage and shock, is by far a greater hazard to the patient with heart disease than additional time in the second stage of labor.

All principal modes of anesthesia are suitable for use during delivery of the pregnant cardiac. Intravenous barbiturates may be employed safely either alone or to supplement inhalation or regional anesthesia. Inhalation anesthesia per se is a safe technique, as long as adequate oxygenation of the mother is ensured. Local anesthesia, such as perineal infiltration or pudendal block, is appropriate for the severely ill patient with significant respiratory embarrassment and for whom regional anesthesia is not possible. Regional anesthesia, i.e., spinal, caudal, or epidural, provides excellent analgesia as well as anesthesia, and probably is the best technique for managing a pregnant cardiac patient, as long as care is taken to avoid hypotension.

Management of the Puerperium

The maternal heart may be under greater stress during the immediate postpartum period than at any other time. Rigid cardiac management should not be relaxed during this interval, and all measures used antepartum should be continued. Cardiac complications after delivery are best prevented by intensive antepartum and intrapartum care.

CONGENITAL HEART DISEASE

The second most frequently encountered cause of cardiac disability in pregnancy is congenital heart disease. The diagnosis of a congenital cardiac defect may be made for the first time when a young patient appears for obstetric care. If the patient is asymptomatic and has no history of cardiac difficulties, specialized diagnostic techniques to define the cardiac diagnosis, such as angiocardiography and cardiac catheterization, may be deferred until after the pregnancy.

Patients with severe congenital heart disease often do not remain in adequate physical condition for reproduction or even survival into the childbearing years. Less severe lesions which are compatible with maternal longevity therefore account for most of the cases encountered. The major hemodynamic disturbance affecting the fetus of a pregnant congenital cardiac patient is the degree of maternal oxygen unsaturation. Patients with trivial shunts or purely stenotic lesions may undergo pregnancy without apparent ill effect on the fetus. Pregnancies in severely cyanotic patients frequently terminate in abortion. Less severe oxygen unsaturation may be associated with premature delivery or intrauterine growth retardation. Amelioration of the cyanotic state by palliative or reconstructive cardiac surgery before or during pregnancy improves the obstetric performance and reduces the fetal risk. In the absence of maternal complications, such as heart failure, pulmonary hypertension, bacterial endocarditis, or cerebrovascular accidents, simple left-to-right shunts and purely stenotic lesions offer no specific fetal hazard.

The distribution of congenital cardiac lesions reported in association with pregnancy is given in Table 31–2, and the associated maternal mortality is indicated (Stevenson). Several reports have agreed that infants born to mothers with congenital heart defects have themselves an increased incidence of congenital cardiac defect (approximately 2 percent) and that the infants' cardiac lesions may be either concordant or discordant with those of the mothers. Since an increase in noncardiac congenital anomalies has not been reported in these same children, it may be assumed that hereditary factors rather than intrauterine environment probably are responsible in most instances (Buemann, Kragelund).

TABLE 31–2 Distribution of Congenital Cardiac Defects in Pregnancy

Defect	Percentage of cases	Maternal mortality, %
Patent ductus arteriosus	25	0.6
Atrial septal defect	20	1.9
Coarctation of aorta	18	4.3
Ventricular septal defect	15	2.7
Pulmonic stenosis	9	0.0
Tetralogy of Fallot	5	4.2
Eisenmenger syndrome	3	27.0
Ebstein's anomaly	1	0.0
Others*	4	

*Dilatation of pulmonary artery, disturbances of rhythm and conduction, undiagnosed defects, dextrocardia, transposition of great vessels, truncus arteriosus, and mixed lesions, each less than 1.0 percent.

Patent Ductus Arteriosus

The most frequently encountered congenital cardiac defect during pregnancy is patent ductus arteriosus. Many women who have had a patent ductus arteriosus have been treated surgically before becoming pregnant and may be considered as perfectly normal patients.

The presence of a patent ductus arteriosus is suggested by a typical to-and-fro "machinery" murmur in the pulmonic area, prominent pulmonary artery segment and pulmonary vascular markings on chest x-ray, and a normal or left ventricular strain pattern on electrocardiogram. Often the diagnosis may be made on purely clinical grounds, but sometimes cardiac catheterization may be required for confirmation. The usual shunting of blood in a patent ductus arteriosus is from the left to the right side of the circulation. High pulmonary artery pressure or hypotension in the systemic circulation may result in reversal of shunt flow. Most patients with patent ductus arteriosus do well during pregnancy with proper medical supervision. Subacute bacterial endocarditis is a constant threat, and prophylactic antibiotic therapy is recommended. Surgical correction of a patent ductus may be deferred until after completion of gestation, unless heart failure develops and is refractory to medical treatment or subacute bacterial endarteritis becomes established despite prophylactic administration of antibiotics.

A sudden drop in blood pressure and peripheral vascular collapse may precipitate reversal of shunt flow, and must be avoided in patients with patent ductus arteriosus. Patients with severe pulmonary hypertension are at special risk for this complication; early termination of pregnancy and interconceptional surgical correction of the defect are advised.

Atrial Septal Defect

In many patients, an atrial septal defect is compatible with minimal physical disability until the third or fourth decades of life, and therefore may be diagnosed for the first time during pregnancy. The typical patient presents with a systolic murmur in the third left interspace, an accentuated pulmonic second heart sound, and on fluoroscopy increased pulmonary vascular markings and "hilar dance." Electrocardiography may show right ventricular hypertrophy or right bundle branch block. The diagnosis may be established definitively by cardiac catheterization.

Medical management during pregnancy is sufficient for patients who have had little cardiac disability. A strict cardiac regimen (as described above) should be followed to reduce the possibility of congestive failure. If cardiac disability already is severe and there is evidence of pulmonary hypertension and possible congestive failure, the pregnancy may have to be aborted. At delivery, every precaution must be taken to avoid postpartum hemorrhage and secondary systemic hypotension, which may precipitate reversal of shunt flow. Surgical correction of atria septal defect has been accomplished successfully during pregnancy; nevertheless, it probably is best performed in the nongravid state, either following abortion or after delivery.

Ventricular Septal Defect

The prognosis for a patient with an interventricular septal defect depends on the size of the communication between the two ventricles. In most patients, the diagnosis has been made before pregnancy. There is a characteristic harsh, loud, systolic murmur best heard in the third or fourth left intercostal space. Electrocardiographic and x-ray findings vary with the size of the shunt, the amount of pulmonary blood flow, and changes in the pulmonary vessels. Cardiac catheterization can establish the definitive diagnosis by demonstrating an increased right ventricular oxygen content and increased pulmonary blood flow. Selective angiocardiography also may be useful.

In patients with interventricular septal defect who are asymptomatic or have only mild cardiac disability, routine cardiac management will permit successful pregnancy. Patients with a large interventricular septal defect and pulmonary hypertension secondary to increased pulmonary blood flow and elevated pulmonary vascular resistance cannot tolerate the cardiovascular stress of pregnancy; cardiac failure during pregnancy has been reported in approximately 10 percent of such patients, despite optimal medical management. These patients also are at risk for subacute bacterial endocarditis, and antibiotic therapy should be administered prophylactically. Hypotension and severe blood loss at delivery must be prevented, and peripheral vasomotor collapse promptly corrected.

Surgical correction of interventricular septal defects is best accomplished when the patient is not pregnant.

Tetralogy of Fallot

The tetralogy of Fallot consists of pulmonic stenosis, ventricular septal defect, an overriding aorta, and right ventricular hypertrophy. Patients with this lesion are cyanotic from birth, and survival to childbearing age without surgical correction of the lesion is rare. Clinically, the patient presents with cyanosis, clubbing of the terminal phalanges, polycythemia, marked fatigability, and marked intolerance to exercise. X-rays show right ventricular hypertrophy and diminution of the pulmonary vascular markings. The electrocardiogram shows right ventricular hypertrophy. Cardiac catheterization and angiocardiography are diagnostic.

In the patient not treated surgically, results of pregnancy are poor; the maternal mortality rate ranges between 5 and 13 percent, and fetal wastage is approximately 40 percent. Earlier surgical procedures (Blalock and Potts' operations) could not attack the basic anatomic problems directly, but simply created an artificial communication between the systemic and pulmonic circulations (artificial patent ductus arteriosus) to increase pulmonary blood flow, improve arterial oxygen concentration, and decrease cyanosis. Recently, these lesions have been approached by open-heart techniques, combining repair of the interventricular septal defect and pulmonary valvotomy or excision of the pulmonary infundibular stenosis. In a few instances, such procedures have been successful during pregnancy.

Pregnancy in patients with a surgically corrected tetralogy of Fallot does not present a significant hazard. If pregnancy should occur in a patient with an uncorrected lesion, abortion should be recommended. If termination of pregnancy is refused, strict cardiac management should be instituted, including frequent observation, avoidance of excess weight gain, prompt treatment of cardiac failure, administration of oxygen during labor and immediately postpartum; prophylactic antibiotic therapy, and avoidance of hypoxia and hypertension during labor and delivery. Neither palliative nor corrective cardiac surgery should be attempted during pregnancy.

Pulmonic Stenosis

An increasingly frequent diagnosis with improved diagnostic techniques, pulmonic stenosis may occur either at the pulmonic valve itself or in the infundibular portion of the right ventricle. The patient complains of fatigue, dyspnea, syncope, and dizziness; ultimately, right-sided heart failure ensues. Patients may continue to be symptom-free into adulthood and may present without prior diagnosis in pregnancy. The lesion is suggested by a characteristic harsh systolic murmur best heard in the second and third left intercostal spaces, and by radiologic evidence of diminished pulmonary vascular markings, prominence of the pulmonary artery conus (secondary to poststenotic dilation), and right ventricular hypertrophy. Cardiac catheterization reveals a systolic pressure gradient across the pulmonic valve, elevated right ventricular pressure, and normal or low pulmonary artery pressures. Although the patient may present without cardiac symptoms in early pregnancy, she must be considered predisposed to congestive failure in view of the increased cardiac output required by pregnancy; congestive failure supervenes in approximately 10 percent of patients.

Pulmonic stenosis can be corrected or alleviated by pulmonary valvotomy, which carries a low operative mortality. A patient's prognosis for long-term survival without surgical intervention is poor. Pregnancy is best deferred until after surgical correction. Should an asymptomatic patient with pulmonic stenosis become pregnant, the pregnancy may be carried to term with appropriate cardiac care, and surgical intervention deferred until after the puerperium. If a patient with pulmonic stenosis becomes pregnant while having severe cardiac disability or develops cardiac problems after pregnancy has begun, abortion followed by surgical correction of the defect is advisable. Although surgical therapy during pregnancy has been reported, the procedure probably is best performed interconceptionally.

CORONARY ARTERY DISEASE

Coronary atherosclerosis is infrequent in women of childbearing age, and the precise incidence of this complication is difficult to establish. It probably accounts for 1 to 2 percent of all cardiac diseases complicating pregnancy, and should be considered in patients particularly predisposed, i.e., with diabetes, preexisting hypertension, obesity, or familial hypercholesterolemia.

In patients with established coronary artery disease, the increased cardiac output required by pregnancy must stress additionally a myocardium already burdened by coronary insufficiency. Hypothetically, there may be some improvement of myocardial blood flow as a result of pregnancy-induced vasodilatation. The effect of pregnancy on patients with coronary artery disease is variable, but some reports indicate a maternal mortality rate of approximately 20 percent.

The management of angina pectoris in pregnant patients is the same as in the nongravid state, except that even more severe limitation of activity must be imposed. Routine activities must be strictly limited, and frequent periods of rest during the day recommended. All emotional stress should be minimized, and mild sedation is useful in this regard. Coronary vasodilators may be employed as necessary.

Acute myocardial infarction has been reported during pregnancy, immediately preconception, and in the puerperium (Curry, Quintana; Ginz). The prognosis for these patients depends more upon the extent of the infarction than upon the medical management provided. The maternal mortality rate for patients who sustain myocardial infarction during pregnancy is between 25 and 33 percent; the prognosis is poor for patients in whom the infarction occurred during labor or in the very early puerperium. The earlier a myocardial infarction has antedated pregnancy, the better the maternal prognosis. The management of myocardial infarction during pregnancy is the same as in the nongravid state. Treatment consists of limitation of activity, maintenance of coronary artery blood flow, analgesia for cardiac pain, administration of oxygen, treatment of cardiac failure (if present), and anticoagulation. If the myocardial infarction occurred before conception or in early pregnancy, allowing adequate time for clinical con-

valescence, vaginal delivery may be permitted if obstetrically feasible. If the myocardial infarction occurred in late pregnancy, the mode of delivery selected must be individualized. Vaginal delivery is the mode of choice in the multipara in whom a reasonably uneventful and rapid labor and delivery can be anticipated. For the primigravida or the patient in whom a difficult, protracted labor is anticipated, there may be less hazard from delivery by cesarean section.

In view of the high maternal mortality reported in patients with myocardial infarction, pregnancy is not advisable. The question of abortion in such patients must be individualized.

HYPERTENSIVE HEART DISEASE

Cardiac problems secondary to long-standing hypertension are not rare in the childbearing years and are very difficult to manage during pregnancy. Whether the underlying disease state is essential hypertension, renal disease, adrenal tumor, or coarctation of the aorta, the pregnancy may be complicated by toxemia in about one-third of patients, and the risk to both mother and fetus is severe. Maternal mortality rates are approximately 2 percent, the most frequent causes of death being cardiac failure and toxemia. Perinatal mortality is increased markedly, primarily by placental abruption, toxemia, and chronic placental insufficiency.

The manifestations of hypertensive cardiac disease include elevated diastolic and systolic blood pressures; tachycardia with incipient failure; electrocardiographic evidence of left ventricular hypertrophy; radiologic evidence of left ventricular enlargement; and symptoms of left-sided cardiac failure: fatigability, exertional dyspnea, orthopnea, and paroxysmal nocturnal dyspnea. Development of congestive failure may be associated with albuminuria and edema, duplicating the clinical triad of toxemia of pregnancy; the differential diagnosis may be established by determinations of venous pressure and circulation time. At times, this differential diagnosis may be impossible, or congestive failure may complicate toxemia which is superimposed on underlying hypertensive disease. This problem has little clinical importance, management would be identical in either case.

The prime aim of management of hypertensive disease in pregnancy is prevention of cardiac failure. To this end, measures are aimed at alleviation of the hypertensive state and control of fluid and electrolyte retention. Thiazide diuretics are a major weapon in management because of their combination of diuretic and antihypertensive effects. Dietary restriction of salt and water intake is recommended. The use of antihypertensive agents significantly will improve the maternal prognosis, but at times at the expense of reduced fetal salvage. Patients with cardiac enlargement secondary to hypertensive cardiovascular disease should be digitalized prophylactically during pregnancy.

If congestive failure develops, the usual management of that complication should be undertaken. Patients with hypertensive cardiovascular disease are refractory to management of congestive failure and pulmonary edema, and the prognosis is grave once this complication develops.

CARDIAC ARRHYTHMIAS

Sinus Tachycardia

Mild tachycardia during pregnancy and episodes of tachycardia during labor and delivery are physiologic. On the other hand, in patients with organic heart disease increasing tachycardia may be the earliest manifestation of cardiac decompensation. Any unusual tachycardia, unrelated to heart disease, should be investigated for underlying infection, pulmonary embolization, hyperthyroidism, or concealed hemorrhage. Purely sinus tachycardia requires no specific treatment.

Sinus Bradycardia

During pregnancy sinus bradycardia seldom occurs, ordinarily presents no clinical problem, and requires no special treatment. Relative bradycardia in the early puerperium is physiologic.

Heart Block

First-degree heart block (i.e., prolongation of the PR interval) may occur in inactive rheumatic heart disease, acute rheumatic fever, reactivation of a preexisting carditis, nonspecific myocarditis, and digitalis toxicity. The major clinical significance of this electrocardiographic finding is the possibility of acute rheumatic fever, whose presence may be masked during gestation by the physiologic alterations in heart rate, erythrocyte sedimentation rate, and leukocyte count. If the patient with first-degree heart block is taking digitalis, reduction of drug dosage is indicated.

Partial or complete heart block usually is associated with congenital heart disease, rheumatic heart disease, or, in older patients, with arteriosclerotic heart disease. Clinical manifestations may range from asymptomatic bradycardia to Stokes-Adams attacks secondary to ventricular standstill. The prognosis depends upon the cause of the heart block and the associated cardiac disease. Patients with congenital heart block usually do well. Patients with heart block secondary to rheumatic heart disease usually have a slower cardiac rate and associated myocardial or valvular lesions. Theoretically, bradycardia handicaps the pregnant patient who must maintain a high cardiac output and predisposes her to congestive failure.

The treatment of heart block during pregnancy does not differ from that in the nongravid state. No specific treatment is recommended if the heart rate is normal or at least above 50 beats per minute. With more severe bradycardia or with symptoms of dizziness or faintness, administration of isoproterenol (Isuprel), atropine, or ephedrine sulfate may help to increase the heart rate. Patients with Stokes-Adams attacks should be hospitalized and their cardiac rhythms constantly monitored during treatment; a cardiac pacemaker must be available immediately in the event of cardiac standstill during treatment. Recently, implantation of cardiac pacemakers has been of value in these patients and has not interfered with the course of pregnancy or the development of the fetus (Middleton, Lee).

Premature Cardiac Beats

The incidence of premature extrasystoles during pregnancy, labor and delivery, and the puerperium is increased. Predisposing factors in the pregnant patient may be elevation of the diaphragms, vagal or gastrocardiac reflexes, and anxiety or emotional stress. Premature beats almost *never* are associated with underlying organic heart disease. Management consists of reassurance and mild sedation. Occasionally, a patient may require quinidine for suppression of atrial or ventricular extrasystoles, or procainamide for ventricular extrasystoles; in the doses usually required, these drugs have no untoward effect on the fetus or the uterus.

Paroxysmal Tachycardia

Supraventricular tachycardia usually is unaccompanied by organic heart disease but may also be a complication of rheumatic, congenital, or hypertensive cardiac disease. The same predisposing factors are present which were enumerated under premature extrasystoles (see above). The morbidity of supraventricular (nodal or auricular) tachycardia depends on the rapidity and duration of the paroxysm of tachycardia and the severity of any underlying cardiac disease. In patients with rheumatic heart disease, uncontrolled tachycardia leads to congestive heart failure in approximately 15 percent of patients.

The management of supraventricular tachycardia during pregnancy is the same as in the nongravid state: sedation, reassurance, and carotid sinus or eyeball pressure. Rapid digitalization is indicated if these preliminary measures fail. If there is no response to digitalization, quinidine therapy may be utilized. In selected patients without underlying severe cardiac disease or hypertension, the intravenous administration of phenylephrine hydrochloride (Neo-Synephrine) as a primary therapy, prior to either digitalization or the use of quinidine, may result in prompt reversion to normal rhythm in approximately 50 percent of patients.

Ventricular tachycardia is more serious and almost always is a complication of severe cardiac disease. Prompt, vigorous therapy with either quinidine or procainamide is essential. In patients with impending shock or incipient congestive failure, procainamide may be administered intravenously. If drug therapy is not successful promptly, direct current countershock therapy should be considered.

Atrial Fibrillation

This arrhythmia may be paroxysmal or chronic. Paroxysmal atrial fibrillation is rare during gestation; most frequently, it is associated with rheumatic mitral stenosis under conditions of stress, such as delivery, infection, or after cardiac surgery. In the absence of underlying cardiac disease, paroxysmal atrial fibrillation should suggest the possibility of hyperthyroidism. Management consists of sedation and prompt digitalization. Even if the arrhythmia remains refractory, this treatment slows the cardiac rate and controls symptoms of congestive failure. If atrial fibrillation persists after adequate digitalization, quinidine or direct current countershock therapy may be indicated. In the patient with hyperthyroidism, atrial fibrillation will remain refractory to treatment until antithyroid therapy is added.

Chronic atrial fibrillation in the childbearing years almost always is a sequel of rheumatic heart disease, particularly with mitral stenosis. This arrhythmia is pathognomonic of underlying cardiac disease of such severity that major cardiac complications may be anticipated during pregnancy in almost two-thirds of the patients, and abortion should be considered seriously. Secondary embolic phenomena occur in as many as 25 percent of these patients, and anticoagulation almost is mandatory. The combination of chronic atrial fibrillation with rheumatic heart disease during pregnancy has yielded a reported maternal mortality rate of 20 percent.

PERIPARTUM CARDIOMYOPATHY

This is a disorder of cardiac muscle presenting clinically with the onset of congestive failure in the last month of pregnancy or during the first 5 months postpartum, in the absence of a determinable etiology for the cardiac failure and without demonstrable heart disease prior to the last month of pregnancy. Etiology and pathogenesis of this disorder are unknown. Data to support the etiologic relationships of malnutrition, excessive alcoholic intake, viral infection, autoimmune mechanisms, hormonal changes, genetic disorders, and toxemia are not conclusive. Peripartum cardiomyopathy occurs with greatest frequency during the first 3 postpartum months (82 percent) and less frequently during the last month of pregnancy (7 percent) (Demakis, Rahimtoola).

Pathologically in such patients, the heart is soft and enlarged, with dilatation of all four cardiac chambers. Almost all cases present with mural thrombi, but there is no evidence of coronary artery, valvular, or pericardial disease. Histologically, the findings in peripartum cardiomyopathy do not differ significantly from those in other forms of primary congestive cardiomyopathy.

Invariably, the patient with peripartum cardiomyopathy presents with the signs and symptoms of left congestive failure; peripheral edema and hepatomegaly are present in 50 percent of cases as well. A ventricular gallop rhythm almost always is present. X-ray confirms the presence of cardiomegaly and pulmonary congestion. The electrocardiogram shows left ventricular hypertrophy and nonspecific ST and T-wave abnormalities.

Patients with peripartum cardiomyopathy in their first episode of congestive failure respond readily to conventional therapy and rapidly improve symptomatically. Long-term prognosis is related to the rapidity with which the heart returns to normal size. Approximately 50 percent of patients have return of heart size to normal within 6 to 12 months; patients who maintain cardiomegaly for 6 months or longer have an extremely poor prognosis, including recurrent episodes of congestive failure leading to death within a few years. Women who have had one episode of peripartum cardiomyopathy are likely to have recurrences in subsequent pregnancies; there is difference of opinion as to whether patients whose hearts have returned to normal size and are asymptomatic from the cardiac standpoint must avoid subsequent pregnancy.

The management of peripartum cardiomyopathy must be purely symptomatic. Digitalization is employed in congestive failure; these patients are unusually sensitive to digitalis. Because of a high incidence of pulmonary and systemic emboli, anticoagulation is recommended for the duration of the cardiomegaly. Prolonged bed rest, often as long as cardiac enlargement persists, is an important factor. Other forms of congestive cardiomyopathy must be considered in the differential diagnosis.

CARDIAC SURGERY AND PREGNANCY

Advances in techniques of cardiac surgery have improved the prognosis for many cardiac patients with respect to pregnancy. Cardiac surgical procedures principally are divided into those which can be performed with closed-heart techniques and those which require open-heart techniques using pulmonary bypass and pump oxygenators. Both open-heart and closed-heart techniques can be employed in the cardiac patient during pregnancy with acceptable fetal and maternal results.

Whether cardiac surgery *should* be performed during pregnancy because it *can* be is not resolved simply. An attitude which is more conservative toward cardiac surgery during pregnancy, although possibly less conservative of pregnancy, may be more in the patient's best interest. The decision to proceed with cardiac surgery in a gravid patient requires much judgment and skill. It seems more reasonable to reserve cardiac surgery during pregnancy for those patients in whom signs of cardiac decompensation, pulmonary congestion, and edema have persisted despite meticulous medical management, and *in whom the risk of termination of pregnancy is greater than the risk of cardiac surgery.*

Patients with mitral stenosis may be managed medically throughout pregnancy, and mitral valve surgery performed in the nongravid state if indicated. If the patient's cardiac status is poor and she is at high risk during pregnancy, or if there is evidence that medical management will not be sufficient (i.e., history of pulmonary edema during a previous pregnancy), the pregnancy probably should be aborted

early, mitral valve surgery carried out interconceptionally, and another pregnancy undertaken once cardiac convalescence is adequate and cardiac reserve restored. Mitral commissurotomy during pregnancy may be considered if the pregnancy is of particularly high value to the patient (i.e., long history of infertility or elderly primigravida) or abortion is rejected on moral or religious grounds. Valvotomy during pregnancy is necessary only in patients who develop severe and intractable pulmonary edema early in pregnancy but refuse abortion, and those for whom obstetric procedures for the termination of pregnancy may carry greater risk than cardiac surgery.

Surgical procedures for the correction of mitral insufficiency or aortic valve disease currently require "open heart" surgical techniques and often the installation of an artificial valve prosthesis. Under optimal conditions, surgical mortality for these procedures approximates 15 percent. Such patients probably are best managed medically throughout pregnancy, and surgery deferred until at least 6 months postpartum. If the patient's cardiac status will not permit such delay, the pregnancy should be interrupted.

Cardiac surgery is best performed when the patient is in optimal physical condition. Since the normal, physiologic alteration of pregnancy imposes sustained and excessive cardiac stress on the mother, cardiac surgical intervention probably best is deferred, if at all possible, until this additional burden has been eliminated. After cardiac surgery of any type, pregnancy may be undertaken and carried to term successfully if the degree of functional cardiac improvement is adequate. Special problems arise in patients in whom an artificial valve prosthesis has been implanted, in view of their predisposition to thrombosis and the need for continued anticoagulation; there is some evidence that Coumadin anticoagulation during the first trimester may be teratogenic (Casanegra et al.; Limet et al.). Even in such patients, however, successful pregnancies have been reported (Tejani).

ADVISABILITY OF PREGNANCY IN THE CARDIAC PATIENT

The prognosis for the cardiac patient who undertakes pregnancy depends upon the following points:

1. Severity of the cardiac disease
2. Age of the patient (increased risk over age 35)
3. Stage of the cardiac disease
4. Past history of the cardiac disease (i.e., history of

cardiac failure before pregnancy or during a previous pregnancy)
5. Type of medical management during pregnancy

Cardiac patients inquiring about the advisability of pregnancy may be classified into three groups: mild, moderately severe, and advanced. Mild cardiac disease includes functional class I and some class II patients; moderately severe disease includes some class II and most class III patients; advanced disease includes some class III and all class IV patients.

Patients categorized as having "mild" disease usually have normal cardiac reserve despite the presence of organic heart disease. There is no cardiac enlargement, no significant arrhythmia, and no history of significant cardiac disability. Pregnancy in such patients entails little risk, few complications are to be expected, and there should be no maternal mortality as a result of the cardiac disease.

Patients categorized as having "moderately severe" disease have functionally significant valvular lesions, some cardiac enlargement, and moderately impaired cardiac reserve. Signs of congestive failure occur with stress; dyspnea and tachycardia appear with exercise. These patients present a definite risk of cardiac decompensation at any point during pregnancy, labor and delivery, and the puerperium, and require constant supervision and cardiac management during gestation. With advances in therapy, the majority of these patients can be carried through pregnancy successfully. However, it may be necessary to hospitalize some of these patients for the greater portion of pregnancy to ensure restriction of physical activity and daily medical supervision. In this category, the patient's desire for pregnancy carries great weight. The patient and her family should be presented with the medical facts, insofar as they are known, and the theoretic degree of risk, so that a rational decision can be reached.

Patients categorized as having "advanced" disease are very few in number, present with dyspnea at rest or on only mild exertion, paroxysmal nocturnal dyspnea, pulmonary congestion, cardiac enlargement, and often chronic atrial fibrillation. In this group, acute heart failure or pulmonary edema occurs frequently in pregnancy. With disease of this severity, patients should be advised to avoid pregnancy; this advice must be accompanied by expert contraceptive instruction and education, or it will be of no value to the patient. If pregnancy does occur, prompt and early abortion should be recommended. If the patient insists on becoming pregnant and refuses the option of abortion, a successful pregnancy may be accomplished with rigorous medical supervision and frequently long-term hospitalization in the majority of these patients. That such a medical feat *can* be accomplished is not sufficient reason for subjecting patients with cardiac disease of this severity to the life-threatening risks of gestation.

VASCULAR DISEASES

COARCTATION OF THE AORTA

This condition is a focal narrowing of the aorta located almost exclusively in the first portion of the aortic arch near the insertion of the ductus arteriosus. The lesion occurs either as an isolated malformation of the aorta or in association with other cardiovascular anomalies. The resultant hemodynamic manifestations include prolonged arm-to-leg circulation time, decreased blood flow to the kidneys and lower extremities, and massive collateral circulation; there is slight to marked hypertension in the arms without concomitant hypertension in the legs.

Patients with coarctation of the aorta may remain symptom-free for many years and hence may be diagnosed for the first time in pregnancy. This occurs much less frequently today; since 1944, surgical correction of coarctation has been feasible technically, and the condition has been assiduously sought in young children and promptly alleviated. Once surgical correction of pure coarctation of the aorta has been accomplished, the patient may be considered to have a normal cardiovascular status. The present incidence of undiagnosed and unoperated coarctation of the aorta in pregnancy is in the range of 1 per 10,000 pregnancies (Deal, Wooley).

Coarctation of the aorta is beset by three principal complications: bacterial endocarditis, congestive heart failure, and rupture of the aorta (or some other proximal vessel). Bacterial endocarditis should be eliminated as a problem in pregnancy by the prophylactic administration of antibiotics. The physiologic increase in cardiac work in pregnancy contributes to a relatively high incidence of congestive heart failure in patients with coarctation of the aorta. It further is theorized that pregnancy produces structural changes in blood vessel walls and therefore predisposes to catastrophic aortic rupture. Until recently, the reported maternal mortality in patients with uncorrected coarctation of the aorta was approximately 10 percent; with improved medical management, this mortality rate can be reduced substantially.

The patient with uncorrected coarctation of the

aorta, who first presents when pregnant, is best managed in accord with the general medical principles discussed under cardiac disorders above. The prognosis for the infant is good, and vaginal delivery can be effected if obstetrically feasible. Increase in degree of hypertension in the last trimester or during labor can be managed with antihypertensive agents. In spite of reports of successful repair of coarctation of the aorta during pregnancy, surgery should be deferred until after the puerperium or carried out after an early termination of pregnancy interconceptionally.

Abortion should be recommended only if the patient's history or status in early gestation indicates the presence of intractable congestive failure despite optimal medical management. Sterilization is not indicated medically in any patient in whom surgical correction of the aortic defect is considered feasible.

ARTERIAL ANEURYSMS

That aneurysms present an increased risk during pregnancy was documented centuries ago. The contribution of vascular wall changes during pregnancy to rupture of an aneurysm remains unclear. Congenital aneurysms of the iliac, renal, and splenic arteries usually manifest themselves by fatal rupture near term or in labor. Fusiform aortic aneurysms carry a maternal mortality rate during pregnancy of only 40 percent; dissecting aortic aneurysms, a maternal mortality rate of over 97 percent (Pedowitz, Perell).

In general, the stress of labor plays a minor role in aneurysm rupture, and hypertension was found to be only a precipitating and not causal factor. The frequency of aneurysmal rupture parallels the physiologic alterations in cardiac output and blood volume, reaching a peak at the beginning of the third trimester (Cohen et al.). If the diagnosis of an aneurysm can be suspected or is made during pregnancy and before rupture, the pregnancy should be ignored and surgical treatment of the aneurysm undertaken; if necessary, the pregnancy should be terminated to permit an adequate surgical exposure. Once rupture has occurred, intervention becomes a desperate and heroic measure, frequently doomed to failure. In any patient who undergoes sudden cardiovascular collapse, the question of ruptured thoracic or intraabdominal vessels must be kept constantly in mind, for only immediate surgical intervention may preserve the mother's life.

The successful use of synthetic arterial prostheses for repair of either ruptured or unruptured aneurysms is a recent advance in vascular surgery and creates new problems for the obstetrician. Very little

has been reported about pregnancy, labor, and delivery in a patient with an arterial prosthesis, and the degree of risk cannot be evaluated. Whether the vascular changes in pregnancy or the expulsive efforts in vaginal delivery might cause rupture of the arterial prosthesis or result in separation of the suture lines cannot be ascertained from experience. Similarly, the risk of thrombosis in the graft site during pregnancy remains undetermined. In view of the great risks to life and limb in such cases, the successful implantation of a synthetic arterial graft probably should be followed by the recommendation that the patient undergo permanent sterilization.

ESSENTIAL HYPERTENSION

With or without superimposed toxemia of pregnancy, essential hypertension is encountered in almost 1 percent of pregnant patients. This disorder sometimes starts in early adulthood and may produce no signs or symptoms except for high blood pressure for many years. It is due to an increase in arteriolar tone, which may be intermittent at first and later produce structural changes in the smaller arteries, particularly in the brain, heart, eyes, and kidneys. Hypertension first may be revealed by routine measurement in pregnancy or may be brought to clinical prominence by the stress of pregnancy. The frequency with which a family history of hypertension can be obtained probably approaches 40 percent (Welt et al.).

Diagnosis

The persistent finding of an arterial blood pressure of 140/90 or above is pathognomonic of hypertension. All other causes of hypertension must be excluded before a diagnosis of essential hypertension can be established. Some patients who are normotensive at the onset of pregnancy may develop hypertension in the latter half of gestation without other evidence of toxemia; these women may be regarded as having latent essential hypertension which has been exposed by pregnancy, in whom permanent essential hypertension probably will develop later in life.

Effect on Pregnancy

Indirect evidence shows that patients with essential hypertension experience reduction in effective blood flow through the uterine wall and placenta; this reduction is more marked when albuminuria also is present. As a result, the placenta may be small or become infarcted late in pregnancy, with deleterious effects on the fetus. In about 50 percent of patients with essential hypertension, a fall in blood pressure occurs during the middle trimester, which may be indicative of good placental circulation. Fetal salvage is greater in patients who show this midtrimester blood pressure reduction than in patients who do not; a rise of maternal blood pressure in the second trimester is highly indicative of placental insufficiency and is associated with very poor fetal salvage. Failure of a hypertensive mother to gain weight normally during the last trimester suggests probably placental insufficiency and retardation of intrauterine fetal growth, as does failure of maternal urinary estriol excretion to follow normal progressively increasing patterns.

Whatever the initial blood pressure, most women with essential hypertension show blood pressure elevation toward the beginning of the third trimester, and almost one-third develop albuminuria. Despite the best prenatal care, the incidence of superimposed toxemia ranges between 15 and 30 percent—or three to five times the incidence in normotensive patients. In these women, superimposed toxemia tends to develop earlier, be more severe, and have more serious consequences for the fetus.

Effect on Fetus

In the presence of severe maternal hypertension, the fetus fails to grow normally and faces increased perinatal risk. The rate of congenital malformations is not increased. Fetal risk is related directly to the degree of hypertension and the presence of superimposed toxemia. Numerous reports have correlated the degree of maternal hypertension with decreased birth weight and placental weight, fetal loss by spontaneous abortion, and stillbirth and neonatal death rates. Premature labor is not a significant factor. Fetal oxygen deprivation has been demonstrated to be the main cause of fetal morbidity and mortality; autopsies on stillborn infants of hypertensive mothers show findings consistent with anoxic death.

In brief, the following factors correlate with a poor prognosis for the fetus: (1) an elderly mother with hypertension of long duration; (2) maternal blood pressure exceeding 180/110 at the beginning of pregnancy, particularly if accompanied by albuminuria; (3) failure of the maternal blood pressure to fall during the middle trimester of pregnancy; (4) large increase in blood pressure in the last trimester; (5) failure of the mother to gain weight normally in the latter half of gestation; (6) falling or persistently low urinary estriol excretion during the last 6 weeks of pregnancy; and (7) development of proteinuria and toxemia before the 35th week of gestation.

Effect of Pregnancy on Hypertensive Mother

Maternal mortality among mothers with essential hypertension is less than 1 percent. If maternal death supervenes, it usually follows sudden increase in hypertension accompanying preeclampsia or eclampsia and is secondary to cerebral hemorrhage, left ventricular failure, or malignant hypertension. In patients with moderate levels of hypertension, the disease is not exacerbated by pregnancy unless the gestation is complicated by toxemia. When toxemia is superimposed, particularly in women over 35 years of age, the maternal blood pressure after pregnancy may never return to prepregnancy levels, or may drop temporarily in the puerperium to show a secondary, permanent rise some weeks later. Occasionally, superimposed toxemia in women with essential hypertension may induce the rapid development of malignant hypertension, manifested by headache, vomiting, papilledema, and albuminuria. Women with essential hypertension should therefore be encouraged to complete their reproductive careers as early in life as possible.

Management

The course of pregnancy complicated by essential hypertension is so unpredictable early in gestation that therapeutic abortion rarely is justified. Even a very severely hypertensive patient *may* have an uneventful pregnancy and deliver a normal infant. On the other hand, in patients with the handicap of advanced age (over 30), initial blood pressure readings of over 180/110, evidence of cardiac enlargement, advanced retinal changes, or albuminuria, the probability of the salvage of a viable infant is small and must be weighed against the increased maternal risk. In the rare patient with malignant hypertension, pregnancy should be interrupted early.

The management of patients with essential hypertension in pregnancy involves the meticulous application of general principles of prenatal care, frequent observation, and prompt hospitalization should signs of blood pressure elevation or superimposition of toxemia appear. The basic treatment for all types of hypertension in pregnancy is bed rest; often, objective evidence of the beneficial effect of bed rest can be observed in resumption of fetal growth or in reversal of maternal urinary estriol excretion decrements. Other routine treatment includes sedation, dietary restriction, and judicious use of diuretics.

The use of hypotensive drugs in the treatment of

hypertension during pregnancy has been disappointing. Maternal blood pressure levels readily can be controlled, but there is no evidence of improved choriodecidual circulation, increased maternal urinary estriol excretion, or improved fetal salvage rates. To the contrary, there is some evidence that uteroplacental circulation, and hence fetal prognosis, may be affected adversely by such symptomatic treatment. If hypotensive agents are to be used during pregnancy, their potential hazards must be considered. Reserpine acts centrally to decrease sympathetic tonus and peripherally blocks the passage of sympathetic nerve impulses by depleting stores of norepinephrine; the depletion of norepinephrine may persist for about 2 weeks after administration of the drug has stopped, and may result in alarming acute hypotension during the stress of labor or under anesthesia. Methyldopa prevents the biosynthesis of epinephrine and norepinephrine, also depleting the peripheral stores of catecholamines, and its use should be subject to the same precautions as reserpine. Both reserpine and methyldopa have some hypotensive effect even when the patient is recumbent and may be particularly useful in combination with bed rest in pregnancy. Ganglionic blocking agents (mecamylamine, hexamethonium, and phentolamine) exert essentially a postural hypotensive effect and have little practical use in pregnancy; in addition, these agents cross the placenta and may cause paralytic ileus in the neonate. Adrenergic blocking agents (guanethidine, hydralazine) have relatively inconsistent effects on maternal blood pressure during pregnancy, particularly with the patients at bed rest, and in effective dosages have a number of unpleasant side effects. In general, the indication for the use of hypotensive agents during pregnancy is maternal: acute and marked elevation of systolic and/or diastolic pressures, threatening vascular integrity or cardiac failure; there is little indication for the chronic use of hypotensive agents to improve fetal salvage.

In the absence of acute exacerbation of hypertension in the mother or in the development of superimposed toxemia, the major problem faced near term in hypertensive mothers is evaluation of the integrity of the fetoplacental unit and reduction of the risk of intrauterine demise secondary to placental insufficiency. This may be accomplished by serial determinations of maternal urinary estriol excretion and maternal serum estriol levels or by nonstress and stress monitoring of the fetus in utero. In view of the chronic intrauterine relative fetal distress in such pregnancies, fetal lung maturity may be accelerated to a surprising degree. In any event, the indications for termination of pregnancy are fetal rather than maternal; often the greatest safety for the compromised fetus may be expeditious delivery despite the risk of respiratory distress syndrome (Tejani et al.).

THROMBOEMBOLIC DISEASE

This term encompasses the disease entities of thrombophlebitis, phlebothrombosis, and pulmonary embolization; problems of disseminated intravascular coagulation, with deposition of fibrin in the microcirculation and a concomitant consumption coagulopathy ordinarily are not considered in this context.

Thrombophlebitis

An inflammatory reaction in or around a venous channel, usually peripheral but occasionally within the pelvis, is the initiating event in this disease. Vascular wall injury at the site of inflammation attracts the aggregation of platelets, resulting in the development of a firmly adherent platelet thrombus containing little apposition material and hence relatively firm. Theoretically, there should be little risk of embolization in such circumstances; actually, the platelet thrombus may extend along the venous channel, resulting in a secondary phlebothrombosis.

Phlebothrombosis

In this disease, a thrombus forms in a deep venous channel, usually in the lower extremity, and may extend into larger venous channels such as the common femoral vein, the iliac vessels, and infrequently into the inferior vena cava itself. Primarily, this is a coagulation thrombus with a "white" base consisting of platelet aggregates and a "red" tail consisting of fibrin in which blood elements are trapped. This tail grows by apposition, undergoes retraction, and floats freely in the lumen of the vessel. The soft and irregular structure of this apposition thrombus readily disrupts and frequently is the source of pulmonary emboli. After several days, the floating thrombus may attach lengthwise to the vessel wall, resulting in a secondary inflammatory reaction which may be the first clinical manifestation of disease. Opinions differ concerning the time necessary for such a thrombus to undergo organization, which apparently may take weeks, months, or even years.

Thrombosis and Pregnancy

Thrombosis in the pelvic veins and in the deep veins of the lower extremity is a specific risk during pregnancy, and even more frequently during the puerperium, because of maternal physiologic changes, including increase in blood coagulation factors, stagnation of blood in the pelvis and lower extremities (pressure effects), and local trauma or infection during delivery (Aaro, Juergens). The incidence of deep venous thrombosis in the puerperium is approximately 0.3 percent; during pregnancy, 0.09 percent (Howie).

Management

Superficial thrombophlebitis often develops during pregnancy, particularly in the third trimester and in multiparous patients, in varicose veins. The superficial varicosity becomes firm, knotty, and tender to palpation, and exhibits symptoms of inflammation: redness, swelling, pain, and local elevation of temperature. Usually, the only treatment required is circulatory support with an elastic bandage and occasionally the administration of mild analgesics. The patient may remain ambulatory. Anticoagulation is necessary only when deep vein involvement is suspected. The administration of anti-inflammatory drugs (i.e., Butazolidin) is recommended by some; rarely are such agents necessary in what essentially is a self-limiting process of short duration, and they carry significant risk of adverse reactions. Definitive management of varicosities should be deferred until after the puerperium.

The diagnosis of deep vein thrombosis is more difficult to establish, yet the hazards of the disease are much greater (Guril et al.). The frequency of pulmonary embolization makes each case potentially fatal; in one diagnosed but untreated series, the incidence of fatal pulmonary embolization was 2.5 percent! Often, the clinically silent phlebothrombosis first becomes manifest by the appearance of a pulmonary embolus. Repeated small pulmonary emboli may result in chronic pulmonary hypertension. The diagnosis must be made with careful observation and repeated clinical examination. Standard laboratory tests are of little value. Various radioisotope techniques, venography, and some blood coagulation studies effectively can establish the diagnosis but pragmatically are not available for routine clinical screening.

The first requirement for diagnosis is a high index of suspicion, particularly in patients with a history of prior thromboembolic disease, varicose veins of unusual severity, obesity, or multiparity; every patient with puerperal fever of unknown etiology must be suspect. Presenting symptoms may include aching or pain in the thighs, calves or feet, possibly with slight unilateral edema. Examination should include careful search for tenderness in the extremities, lower abdomen, and pelvis; palpation of the venous channels on the inside of the thigh and calf from the groin to the plantar area of the foot (Rielander's sign); pain on pressure over the inner side of the foot (Payr's sign) or on dorsiflexion of the foot with the knee extended (Homans' sign); and compression of the calf with the fingertips against the tibia-fibula. The higher thrombophlebitis extends up the lower extremity, the more venous drainage will be obstructed and the greater the likelihood of edema, increased circumference of the affected extremity, engorgement of the superficial veins, and cyanosis of the foot on the affected side. Often the diagnosis cannot be established definitively, and the signs and symptoms remain equivocal. Because of the potential danger, the patient should receive full therapy even if the diagnosis remains in doubt (Ramsey).

The medical management of thrombosis, in pregnancy or otherwise, is anticoagulation. Two major groups of pharmacologic agents are available to induce anticoagulant activity: heparin, which acts immediately and directly, and coumarin derivatives, which affect the coagulation system slowly and indirectly (Hirsh et al.).

Heparin is a mucopolysaccharide-polysulfide ester with a molecular weight between 12,000 and 17,000. It inhibits tissue thromboplastin and coagulation factors VII and IX, combines with a plasma protein to form an antithrombin, and impairs platelet aggregation. It may be administered by continuous or intermittent intravenous infusion, or by intramuscular or subcutaneous injection. The dose employed must be individualized and determined by the anticoagulant effect—the clotting time, as measured by the Lee-White method, should become three to four times longer than normal approximately 1 hour before the next dose. The toxicity of heparin is low, and pyrogenic and allergic reactions extremely rare. Alopecia occurs in 25 to 75 percent of patients, is dose-related, becomes apparent 5 to 8 weeks after initiation of therapy, and is spontaneously reversed. Heparin is inactivated rapidly by protamine sulfate in a ratio of 1.5 mg of protamine sulfate for each 1.0 mg of heparin. Heparin does not cross the placenta nor affect the fetus, and its administration need not be discontinued or its action reversed prior to vaginal delivery (Hill, Pearson).

The coumarin derivatives inhibit the synthesis of coagulation factors II, VII, IX, and X in the maternal liver, and at least 20 hours are required to increase the prothrombin time significantly. A variety of agents are available for clinical treatment. Coumarin drugs may be used for prophylaxis and for long-term anti-coagulation maintenance in the nongravid patient. They are administered orally, and the daily mainte-nance dose depends on an assessment of the cumu-lative effect of therapy by daily estimations of pro-thrombin times. Allergic reactions to coumarin drugs are rare. A specific deleterious side effect is hemor-rhagic necrosis, which may develop with relation to the duration of therapy, and usually occurs in the thighs, breasts, or lower extremities. The etiology of this complication of treatment is unknown. After de-marcation of the areas of hemorrhagic necrosis, large ulcerations develop which may require months to heal; immediate administration of heparin in the acute phase is helpful in limiting demarcation and progres-sion of the lesions. Administration of vitamin K (Kon-akion, Mephyton) intravenously causes the prothrom-bin time to revert to normal within 6 to 8 hours. During pregnancy, coumarin drugs may be contraindicated except in most unusual circumstances. Coumarin de-rivatives have a low molecular weight and traverse the placenta readily. Hemorrhagic death of the fetus has been reported even with low-dose treatment of the mother and in the absence of bleeding compli-cations in the patient; bleeding complications in the fetus apparently are not dose-related. In addition, coumarin derivatives may have teratogenic potential in the first trimester of pregnancy (Raivio et al.; Shanl et al.).

The treatment of thrombophlebitis is both symp-tomatic and specific. The involved extremity should be elevated to an angle of approximately 30° to im-prove venous return and reduce edema and conges-tion. Local application of wet packs helps to relieve discomfort. Antibiotics rarely are indicated except in cases with frank infection; they should be adminis-tered routinely, however, in postpartum pelvic throm-bophlebitis. The one essential and specific treatment is immediate anticoagulation with heparin. This has changed the course of the disease dramatically, and almost has eliminated the long-term sequelae of *phlegmasia alba dolens*. Absolute bed rest must be imposed not only through the acute, painful phase but for 7 to 10 days thereafter to ensure firm adhesion and organization of the thrombus. During pregnancy, an-ticoagulation should be maintained with heparin alone; once the required dose has been established, the patient may be taught successfully to self-admin-ister the required three to four daily injections (Bon-nar). Anticoagulation should be continued up to and through labor and delivery. Three to four days after delivery, a coumarin derivative regimen may be sub-stituted. In puerperal thrombophlebitis, heparin should be used until subsidence of the acute, painful

phase of the disease, and coumarin derivatives sub-stituted thereafter. Anticoagulation postpartum should be maintained for from 3 to 6 months to elimi-nate completely the risk of pulmonary embolization.

Pulmonary Embolism

Pulmonary emboli arise as thrombi in the peripheral venous system and pass into the pulmonary circula-tion by way of the inferior vena cava. This may occur as massive pulmonary embolization, with sudden vascular collapse and death, embolism in medium-sized lobar or sublobar vessels, or chronic small ves-sel embolization resulting ultimately in chronic cor pulmonale. It has been well documented that 30 to 50 percent of pulmonary emboli may be asymptomatic, or not diagnosed clinically, and are discovered only upon autopsy. Some patients die within the first few minutes after massive pulmonary embolization has occurred; almost 50 percent die within the first 24 hours. Although, because of the difficulty of establish-ing the diagnosis, the precise incidence of pulmonary embolus in pregnancy or the puerperium is difficult to estimate, the risk of maternal death from this compli-cation ranges between 0.014 and 0.017 percent (ap-proximately 1 death in every 7000 deliveries) (Bis-sell).

The patient with thrombophlebitis must be ob-served carefully for evidence of pulmonary emboli-zation, but it must be remembered that almost 50 per-cent of fatal pulmonary emboli occur in previously asymptomatic women. Clinical symptoms (Table 31–3) and findings on physical examination (Table 31–4) are not definitive. The electrocardiogram may show disturbances of rhythm (atrial fibrillation, ec-topic beats, or heart block), enlargement of P waves, ST-segment depression, T-wave inversion, or other

TABLE 31–3 Symptoms of Pulmonary Emboli

Symptom	Medium and large emboli, %	Small emboli, %
Dyspnea	94	77
Pleuritic chest pain	44	100
Cough	56	77
Hemoptysis	38	54
Syncope	31	0
Diaphoresis	31	0
Angina-like chest pain	19	0

Source: Adapted from Romhilt et al.

TABLE 31-4 Signs of Pulmonary Emboli

Signs	Medium and large emboli, %	Small emboli, %
Tachypnea	81	69
Tachycardia	56	77
Pulmonary rales	63	46
Right-sided gallop rhythms	69	15
Thrombophlebitis	50	23
Fever	44	31
Shock	19	8
Distended neck veins	13	8
Fixed splitting S_2	13	0
Friction rub	6	23
Cyanosis	6	0
Right ventricular "heave"	6	0
Pulsus paradoxus	6	0

Source: Adapted from Romhilt et al.

evidence of "right heart strain"; unfortunately, a single electrocardiographic tracing may be normal, or suggestive but not diagnostic. Characteristic serum enzyme studies include elevated serum lactic dehydrogenase and serum bilirubin with normal serum glutamic oxaloacetic transaminase levels; the report of these studies, however, usually is far too late for the initiation of treatment. In the acute phase, routine chest x-ray may not be at all helpful. The arteriographic demonstration of abruptly occluded pulmonary arterial branches is diagnostic. Pulmonary "scan" studies with radioiodinated macroaggregates of human serum albumin are useful, although abnormal tracings may be observed whenever pulmonary blood flow is altered, regardless of cause, as in atelectasis, lung abscess, bronchiectasis, and lobar pneumonia.

Treatment is supportive, symptomatic, and specific. Vasomotor collapse, with altered tissue perfusion and metabolic acidosis, requires prompt treatment. The administration of parenteral fluids must be controlled strictly by use of a central venous pressure monitor to regulate the amounts infused. Significant elevations of pulmonary artery pressure follow embolization, resulting in acute cor pulmonale; these patients may present one of the few indications for the use of vasopressor agents in the treatment of shock. The value of the administration of anticholinergic drugs such as atropine has not been established. Positive pressure oxygen should be administered, particularly in the face of pulmonary edema. Analgesic agents such as meperidine (Demerol) may be re-

quired for relief of pain and to decrease anxiety and hyperpnea. Specific therapy entails immediate anticoagulation with high doses of heparin, utilizing at least 20,000 units intravenously initially, and 40,000 to 80,000 units daily. Large concentrations of heparin, far in excess of the dose required to block the thrombin-fibrinogen interaction, seem to inhibit postembolic bronchoconstriction and improve patient salvage. With heparin doses in this range, it has been reported that all patients who did not succumb to their embolus within the first 15 minutes have survived (Duncan et al.; Henderson et al.).

Surgical intervention is rarely necessary but should always be kept in mind. Pulmonary embolectomy for massive embolization requires cardiopulmonary bypass equipment and occasionally, when immediately available in a large medical center, may be lifesaving (Cohn, Shumway). Peripheral intervention, such as femoral vein ligation or ileofemoral thrombectomy, has not been demonstrated to be superior to simple anticoagulation. Under appropriate indications, inferior vena cava ligation has been of great value. The indications are strict and infrequent: recurrent embolization despite proper heparinization; contraindications to anticoagulation; and/or suppurative thrombophlebitis. In such patients, either during pregnancy or in the puerperium, ligation of the inferior vena cava must be accomplished fairly promptly, utilizing either the transperitoneal or retroperitoneal approach. Near term, the uterus may require evacuation to permit surgical access to the inferior vena cava; the fetus then must be sacrificed in the interests of the life of the mother. There is no evidence that ligation of the inferior vena cava with preservation of the pregnancy predisposes the patient to the risk of placental abruption. *In patients with pelvic thrombophlebitis and recurrent pulmonary emboli, inferior vena cava ligation must be accompanied by bilateral ovarian vein ligation if the disease process is to be contained.*

Patients with a prior history of thrombophlebitis and/or pulmonary embolization are at high risk for recurrence during subsequent pregnancies, should not take hormonal contraceptive agents, and might be considered for prophylactic heparin anticoagulation if pregnancy is desired. Unless there is evidence of recanalization, the patient with antecedent inferior vena cava ligation is not at risk for pulmonary embolization in subsequent pregnancies.

VARICOSE VEINS

Varicosities of the lower extremity usually result from saphenofemoral insufficiency, short saphenopopliteal insufficiency, or incompetent perforators. The varices are most prominent along the courses of the long or short saphenous veins, unless there are atypical "blowouts."

The varices of pregnancy, however, present an entirely different and distinct pattern. They usually appear during the second or third month of gestation and increase progressively in size until term. They may be unilateral or bilateral, and frequently involve the vulva. Several factors predispose the pregnant patient to the formation of these varices: the vascular effect of hormonal changes, increased volume of blood flow within the pelvis, and pressure changes imposed by the enlarging uterus. Nevertheless, although 20 percent of pregnant women are troubled by this complication, the majority do not develop significant varicosities, so that there must be some anatomic or physiologic predisposition in susceptible patients.

The varices of pregnancy usually appear in the first trimester, have a characteristic scattered distribution, and give the clinical picture of multiple incompetent perforators. Often, the varices produce no symptoms. As the venous distention becomes larger, the patient may complain of "heaviness" or fatigability. Marked, bluish discoloration develops, especially in the lower leg and ankle; true "pain" occurs only if the veins become inflamed. The symptoms as well as the size of the varicosities gradually increase through the last trimester of gestation. Within a few hours or days after delivery, there is marked regression of the varices, but some may persist. With a subsequent pregnancy, the varices appear earlier in gestation and usually become much larger.

The treatment of varices in pregnancy is conservative. There has been some advocacy of surgical or injection (sclerosing) therapy during pregnancy. Arguments in favor of more conservative therapy include the following: to a large extent, the varices recede spontaneously after delivery; distortion of the veins during pregnancy makes intervention more difficult; active treatment yields superior results when carried out interconceptionally; and, in almost every case, effective compression of the varicosities with elastic supports during pregnancy alleviates all symptoms and prevents complications.

Patients with varices are instructed to avoid prolonged dependency of the lower extremities and to sit or lie down and elevate their legs every few hours during the day. Leg exercises (rising up on tiptoe repeatedly and flexing and extending the feet) are effective in stimulating blood flow when used in conjunction with proper supports. Elastic bandages are used to compress all varices from the time of their appearance until after delivery. The bandages must be applied from the toes upward, avoiding any tourniquet effect, when the patient first awakens in the morning and is still in bed. Elastic stockings tend to lose effective elasticity after some use and are expensive to replace. Special supports have been devised and are available for the compression of vulvar varicosities (Veltmann, Ostergard). These supports should be worn from early morning until bedtime, and from early pregnancy through labor and delivery and into the early puerperium. Their use during labor and delivery and early ambulation postpartum will minimize the possibility of thrombophlebitis.

Complications of pregnancy varices include thrombophlebitis (see above), hemorrhage, and dermatologic conditions. Hemorrhage may occur following even minimal trauma to a friable varix. Treatment consists of immediate elevation of the affected extremity and application of firm pressure over the site of hemorrhage. After cessation of the bleeding and application of an elastic support, the patient may be fully ambulatory. Rarely is active surgical intervention necessary to control the bleeding. Dermatologic complications appear in cases of neglected varicosities with chronic venous congestion and discoloration of the skin over the malleoli. Eczema and ulceration usually originate around the ankle and spread to adjacent areas. The essence of treatment is the elimination of venous stasis, not the application of a host of dermatologic medicaments. The application of a gelatin-paste boot consisting of zinc oxide, glycerine, and gelatin (Medicopaste bandage) has proved to be very effective in such patients. The boot is simple to apply, controls venous stasis, and soothes the local inflammation. The patient remains fully ambulatory. The boot is changed once weekly. After healing of the skin lesions, continued use of elastic bandages will inhibit recurrence.

Shortly after delivery, the transient varices of pregnancy disappear, and the true extent of residual varicosities can be determined. If there is no evidence of valvular insufficiency and treatment is indicated, local injections of sclerosing solution may be employed. If there are persistent varicose veins and evidence of sphenous vein insufficiency as well, preferred treatment involves high ligation and stripping of the saphenous vein and local ligation of isolated varicosities. Surgical treatment is recommended even though additional pregnancies may be planned. Despite adequate surgical treatment interconceptionally, new varices may develop during subsequent pregnancies. With prior treatment of the major venous channels, these secondary pregnancy varices almost always will become clinically insignificant following delivery. Occasionally, huge, widespread varicosities may present an indication for surgical sterilization.

DISORDERS OF THE RESPIRATORY SYSTEM

TUBERCULOSIS

The incidence of tuberculosis in the general population has decreased in recent years. Forty years ago, according to data accumulated from postmortem examinations, almost the entire population of the United States was infected with some form of tuberculosis before the age of 20. Today, with widespread tuberculin skin testing, only 20 percent of young adults in the United States have a positive reaction to tuberculin, and the incidence of active and clinically significant disease is very much less.

The incidence of tuberculosis in pregnancy nevertheless has remained constant for several decades, ranging between 1 and 3 percent. The reported incidences vary by geographical location and by the socioeconomic status of the population surveyed. Extrapulmonary tuberculosis is much rarer, with an incidence of approximately 0.1 percent.

DIAGNOSIS

Tuberculosis is a disease with protean manifestations, and both routine screening techniques and a high index of suspicion are necessary to ensure its detection. The onset of tuberculosis in a young woman often is insidious. It is not unusual for early, unsuspected tuberculosis to be detected during routine prenatal care. Routine x-ray examination of the chest had been the recommended screening technique for all pregnant women. More recently, in view of the falling rate of positive reactions to tuberculin testing, the suggestion has been made that all antepartum patients have routine tuberculin skin testing, and only patients with positive reactions be subjected to x-ray investigation.

Clinically, the diagnosis of maternal tuberculosis is exceedingly difficult, and often occurs only serendipitously. X-ray examination of the chest remains the primary diagnostic medium in this disease. Single x-ray films may be equivocal, and the disease best is detected and followed by serial examinations. X-ray findings must, however, be related to the entire clinical picture to permit intelligent management of the patient. Bacteriologic confirmation of tuberculous activity either by smear or culture of sputum or gastric washings is desirable before committing the patient to extended therapy, but is not always possible.

The diagnosis of tuberculosis in pregnancy should be established as early in gestation as possible, and a decision reached about the activity of the disease process. The disease process may be of long standing and inactive at the moment, or it may be active currently. The best parameter of activity is *change*, whether progression or regression, of a tuberculous lesion on x-ray. Other diagnostic techniques are at best only of some assistance in reaching a conclusion about activity. There is a great difference between the management of active and inactive tuberculosis in pregnancy, and an early distinction is very important. In making this distinction, a certain degree of physician error is unavoidable, should be anticipated, and the patient protected from its possible consequences.

EFFECT OF TUBERCULOSIS ON PREGNANCY

In the early stages of the disease, ovulation and menstruation are normal and pregnancy easily is achieved; only with pelvic tuberculosis is infertility a specific problem. Patients with inactive or early active disease go through pregnancy without ill effect. In far-advanced disease, the effect upon the pregnancy is determined by the general physical and metabolic condition of the mother, not by the specific disease entity itself. Although theoretically possible, transplacental infection of the fetus with *M. tuberculosis* practically is of no importance.

EFFECT OF PREGNANCY ON TUBERCULOSIS

There is no evidence extant that any causal relationship exists between pregnancy and the onset of tuberculosis, or that the pregnant state consistently brings about progression of the disease process (Wilson et al., 1973). In general, the prognosis of the tuberculous infection is determined by the general and individual host resistance, the extent and type of pathologic changes, the treatment administered, and the social conditions under which the patient lives, regardless of the presence or absence of pregnancy. Exacerbations of tuberculosis during the puerperium are related more to the increased stress and responsibility faced by the new mother than to any specific effect of the puerperal state. The psychic and physical stresses of pregnancy, similarly, may result in nonspecific aggravation.

MANAGEMENT

Therapy of tuberculosis in pregnancy rests upon several principles. (1) *Urgency is paramount*. Because of the relatively short term of pregnancy, the imminent delivery of a very susceptible infant, and problems of infectiousness related to delivery, the diagnosis of tuberculosis and the determination of the state of activity must be accomplished as early in gestation as possible; treatment must be instituted promptly even where these diagnoses and determinations remain equivocal. (2) Modifications of obstetric management may be indicated. (3) Patients with tuberculosis in pregnancy require special care of their disease. (4) The care of the newborn infant must be modified.

Active Tuberculosis

Modern treatment rests upon the cornerstone of chemotherapy of *M. tuberculosis*. Once the diagnosis of active tuberculosis is made or very strongly suspected in pregnancy, chemotherapy should be instituted immediately. The mainstays of treatment have been isoniazid, streptomycin or dihydrostreptomycin, and *p*-aminosalicylic acid (PAS). Combined chemotherapy, using either two or all three drugs, should be employed. Isoniazid always is employed, in a dose of approximately 5 mg/kg per day, usually given as 100 mg tid for the patient of average weight. Where higher doses are necessary, or in some susceptible patients, pyridoxine, 50 to 100 mg daily, may be added to the regimen to minimize the possible occurrence of isoniazid-induced neuropathy. PAS is prescribed in doses as high as the patient will tolerate, often up to 15 g per day. Since gastrointestinal intolerance to PAS is frequent and patients have a tendency to omit the drug, routine urine tests with either ferric chloride or Ehrlich's reagent will confirm PAS ingestion. An infrequently noted side effect of PAS is reversible hypothyroidism during treatment; if this occurs, particularly during gestation, exogenous thyroid supplementation is indicated and the drug should be discontinued. Streptomycin is administered intramuscularly in doses of 1.0 g three times weekly for 4 to 6 months, then twice weekly. Both streptomycin and dihydrostreptomycin are ototoxic, but streptomycin is preferred in treatment because dihydrostreptomycin is more vestibulotoxic than cochleotoxic, and compensatory mechanisms to replace hearing diminution are more satisfactory than any to replace the sense of balance.

Combined chemotherapy in active disease is initiated as soon as the diagnosis is established or strongly suspected. Once begun, the minimum course of therapy is 1 year, and usually the duration of therapy is closer to 2 to 3 years. Often streptomycin is discontinued after 6 to 12 months in the face of a satisfactory response, PAS after 2 years, and isoniazid is continued alone for a longer period.

Other chemotherapeutic agents can be utilized. Various analogues and derivatives of isoniazid are available. Other antituberculous chemotherapeutic agents such as cycloserine, viomycin, ethionamide, and kanamycin may be employed.

Accessory therapeutic measures are prescribed when indicated. Hospitalization and strict bed rest rarely are necessary today. Resectional surgery and thoracotomy collapse are not contraindicated in pregnancy. Pneumoperitoneum or pneumothorax may be induced or maintained but is seldom necessary in the face of the stabilization produced by the elevation and relative fixation of the diaphragms with advancing gestation. Obstetric management should proceed on obstetric indications solely, but every attempt should be made to withhold major operative interference as long as reasonably possible to permit at least the initiation of control of the disease by chemotherapy (de March).

Inactive Tuberculosis

The aim of therapy in these cases is prophylaxis, the prevention of reactivation of presumably quiescent lesions under the stress of gestation. Single-drug isoniazid prophylactic therapy has been found to be effective, safe, and readily tolerated by most patients. It should be instituted as early in gestation as the diagnosis is made and continued through the first two to three postpartum months.

Obstetric Management

Modifications of obstetric care are of less importance with adequate chemotherapy than heretofore. Tuberculosis is not an indication for either termination of pregnancy or for delivery by cesarean section. The conduct of labor and delivery may be based upon obstetric considerations. Interdictions against the use of morphine or scopolamine in tuberculous patients are outmoded, since bronchial secretions are markedly and rapidly reduced once chemotherapy is instituted. The choice of anesthesia may be individualized. Although conduction anesthesia seems preferable, general anesthesia is permissible. *The presence of pulmonary tuberculosis must be made known to the anesthesiologist.*

EFFECT OF TUBERCULOSIS ON THE NEONATE

The fetus rarely contracts tuberculosis prenatally, but is exposed in utero to the effects of drugs used in treatment of the mother. All chemotherapeutic agents used in tuberculosis cross the placental barrier and may affect the fetus. Infants born to mothers who have received streptomycin occasionally are found to have diminished hearing acuity in later life. Fetal neurotoxicity theoretically may result from the maternal use of isoniazid, which appears in higher concentrations in fetal blood and amniotic fluid than in maternal blood. If these problems occur, they are rare; there are no controlled studies on this problem.

Postnatal exposure to the disease poses a much greater threat to the infant of a tuberculous mother. No patient with presumably active disease should have contact with her child in the postpartum period until sufficient time has elapsed to provide both bacteriologic and radiologic proof of continued regression of the disease process and noninfectiousness of the mother. In practice, this means that the child must be isolated from the mother and from her immediate family and environment for at least 3 months, and until surveys have demonstrated that both or either carry no risk for the baby. If the mother has inactive disease, she need not be separated from the baby and may breast-feed if she desires, but she and the immediate home environment still are suspect and must be kept under observation. The cooperation of local public health authorities is of assistance in investigating the patient's home environment and the members of her immediate family.

The clinical and laboratory manifestations of early neonatal tuberculosis are vague and nonspecific. In the more severe cases, there is overwhelming sepsis and rapid death. In less severe cases, there are multiple complications, including osteitis, meningitis, and pulmonary cavitation (Kendig). Prior to the advent of chemotherapy, infant mortality from this cause was 100 percent; even today, the mortality rate is significant (5 percent), and many infants are left with long-term unfavorable sequelae. The management of the uninfected infant born to a tuberculous mother thus becomes very important, even if isolation from the suspect environment can be accomplished. To this end, several suggestions have been made: (1) The infant should be observed every 3 months with repeated tuberculin testing and treated promptly if conversion from a negative to a positive reaction occurs; in practice, this frequency of follow-up seldom can be maintained. (2) If the newborn returns to a suspect environment, the prophylactic administration of

isoniazid, 10 to 20 mg/kg per day, should be instituted and continued for at least 1 year. (3) Infants born to mothers with pulmonary tuberculosis may receive bacillus Calmette-Guérin (BCG) vaccination before leaving the newborn nursery, and should be kept either in the hospital or in a foster home until tuberculin conversion has occurred. Extensive experience indicates that such infants then are protected from the more severe hazards of tuberculous infection and may be returned to their homes with relative safety. Neonatal BCG vaccination does not decrease the incidence of clinical tuberculosis in adolescents and young adults, and its value lies exclusively in its ability to prevent primary pulmonary disease in the highly susceptible neonate. Of the three methods of management, the last probably is the most useful.

ADVISABILITY OF PREGNANCY IN THE TUBERCULOUS PATIENT

A patient with inactive tuberculosis who has been followed for at least 2 years without evidence of reactivation may be permitted to undertake pregnancy without incurring significant risk. If a patient's disease deteriorated during a previous pregnancy despite adequate chemotherapeutic cover, bacterial resistance should be suspected and subsequent pregnancies discouraged. Patients with known sensitivity to isoniazid, PAS, or streptomycin should be cautioned against becoming pregnant, since control of the disease process would be unreliable.

A patient with active tuberculosis should be advised to defer pregnancy until her disease has been controlled and has remained quiescent for at least 2 years.

There is no real indication for therapeutic abortion for purely medical grounds in most cases of pregnancy complicating tuberculosis. Exceptions might be demonstrated bacterial resistance to standard chemotherapy or patient sensitivity to the drugs required, or the patient with far-advanced, extensive, active disease with cavitation and impaired pulmonary function. Sterilization may be indicated when therapeutic abortion is carried out. Otherwise, indications for abortion or sterilization are unrelated to the tuberculous process.

BRONCHIECTASIS

Bronchiectasis is a chronic, progressive disease of the lungs resulting from a combination of chronic infection and bronchial obstruction; the end stages of the disease include obstructive emphysema and right heart failure because of fibrotic obstruction and bronchospasm throughout the lung fields. Patients with clinically significant bronchiectasis give a history of many recurrent pulmonary infections and present with a persistent cough and the expectoration of large quantities of thick, yellowish sputum. On auscultation, wheezes, loud moist rales, and diminished breath sounds are heard over both lung fields, with some tendency to segmental or lobar distribution. The diagnosis often can be confirmed on routine chest x-ray examination; at times, the diagnosis must be made by bronchography. The presence of concomitant tuberculosis must be ruled out.

Bronchiectasis occurs in women of childbearing age with all the sequelae of chronic respiratory disease and the incidence during pregnancy has been reported between 0.03 and 0.04 percent. Early cases of bronchiectasis, in which the pulmonary parenchyma has not had the chance of becoming rigid, benefit to some extent from "collapse" therapy, and the same benefit may be derived by the patient during an incumbent gestation. The decrease in residual air volume which is physiologic in normal pregnancy tends to improve somewhat the respiratory efficiency of the patient with emphysema. In actuality, however, these beneficial effects of pregnancy on the course and clinical picture of bronchiectasis and emphysema are slight and evanescent. The effect of bronchiectasis on pregnancy, except in the very far-advanced, terminal stages, is trivial. Patients severely incapacitated by dyspnea before conception usually can carry a pregnancy successfully to term, provided they are relieved of their usual activities. Labor usually does not evoke undue dyspnea, even in patients whose vital capacities have been severely reduced. Because the diaphragmatic component of respiration is decreased in the latter half of gestation, patients in the late stages of bronchiectasis and with emphysema, whose ribs are elevated permanently into an inspiratory position, may experience considerable respiratory distress. Nevertheless, there is almost no indication for therapeutic abortion because of bronchiectasis or emphysema. On the other hand, because of the chronicity and progressive nature of the pulmonary disorder, which terminates with the patient a respiratory "cripple" with a shortened life expectancy, there is every reason to recommend surgical sterilization.

MANAGEMENT

Treatment of bronchiectasis during pregnancy essentially is supportive and symptomatic. Pulmonary function tests should be performed before and repeated during pregnancy. The activity of the patient should be restricted purely for her own comfort. Smoking should be discouraged, since this may increase the amount of cough, sputum, and dyspnea, and predispose to pulmonary collapse and infection. (This is aside from the well-documented deleterious effect of maternal smoking on the fetus, which results in an increased incidence of abortions, stillbirths, and neonatal deaths, and a significant reduction in mean birth weights in the infants of smoking mothers.) Acute upper respiratory infections should be avoided or treated promptly and vigorously. There is justification in these patients for long-term antibiotic prophylaxis. Specific medical respiratory therapy to increase bronchial drainage and facilitate respiratory exchange should be employed.

The mode of delivery should be determined by obstetric considerations only. Increased respiratory distress during the second stage of labor may be alleviated by forceps delivery as soon as obstetrically feasible. Conduction anesthesia is preferred to inhalation anesthesia; in either event, the anesthesiologist must be prepared for endotracheal intubation and endobronchial aspiration of secretions, and to assist the patient's respiratory efforts. Inhalation of oxygen by mask may help relieve respiratory distress during labor; in the chronically hypoxic patient, however, the administration of high concentrations of oxygen may result in apnea because of CO_2 narcosis. Heavy opiate sedation should be avoided because of the risk imposed by even minimal depression of the respiratory center in these women.

There is no indication for lobectomy or segmental resection during pregnancy in patients with advanced, localized bronchiectasis. Following pulmonary resection, the patient should have a thorough evaluation of pulmonary competence. If the results of pulmonary function tests are satisfactory and the patient exhibits adequate work tolerance, there is no contraindication to subsequent pregnancy.

SARCOIDOSIS

Sarcoidosis is a systemic, granulomatous disease which may affect the lymph nodes, liver, spleen, eyes, and lungs. The etiology of the disorder is unknown, but the pathologic picture bears a close resemblance to tuberculosis, histoplasmosis, and coccidioidomycosis. Next to lymphatic involvement, pulmonary disease is the most frequent manifestation, with an incidence in the childbearing population of about 0.04 percent.

In the lungs, the interalveolar walls are infiltrated

by granulomatous changes, which are replaced by fibrosis as the lesions heal. The diagnosis usually is based on pulmonary symptoms, and the typical x-ray findings of bilateral hilar and bronchial lymph node enlargement and some degree of pulmonary infiltration. Tuberculosis must be ruled out; the tuberculin test should be negative. A positive Nickerson-Kveim test is more specific. Often, the diagnosis must be confirmed by biopsy of the liver or of a palpable lymph node. There is no known specific therapy for sarcoidosis.

The disease has no deleterious effect on pregnancy, and is not transmitted to the fetus in utero. The effect of pregnancy on the course of sarcoidosis is variable; both exacerbations and remissions of the disease have been reported during gestation (O'Leary). Patients who are free of symptoms require no treatment during pregnancy. In patients with symptoms of respiratory changes, exertional dyspnea, and orthopnea, supportive therapy and limitation of activity are indicated. Remission of progressive disease may be induced by the administration of corticosteroids. Careful observation of the patient must continue into the puerperium, because exacerbation of the disease may occur within a few months after delivery.

Sarcoidosis presents almost no indications for either therapeutic abortion or sterilization.

RESPIRATORY TRACT ALLERGY

Respiratory tract allergy, usually manifest as bronchial asthma or asthmatic bronchitis, is not influenced by pregnancy. The severity and frequency of asthmatic attacks are unchanged in most gravidas (Simms et al.). Emotional factors play a large role in asthmatic attacks, over and above the patient's reaction to offending antigens, and her attitude toward pregnancy undoubtedly influences the course of the asthma. In this respect, an unwanted pregnancy may precipitate quite severe exacerbations of the disease, and therapeutic abortion may be indicated. The effect of respiratory tract allergy on pregnancy is negligible. Occasionally, fetal death has been reported as a result of a severe asthmatic attack in the mother, probably as a result of hypoxia. Otherwise, these patients are not predisposed to either spontaneous abortion or premature delivery (Gordon et al.). A high proportion of the infants of asthmatic mothers develop some allergic complaints before the age of 10 years.

MANAGEMENT

Treatment of respiratory tract allergy is the same whether or not the patient is pregnant. The patient should continue the use of bronchodilator drugs, antihistamines, and mild sedation. In acute attacks, the intravenous administration of aminophylline, 250 to 300 mg, may break the bronchospasm rapidly. In the severe attack of asthma which fails to respond rapidly to routine therapy, and in the patient subject to frequently repeated attacks, treatment should move promptly to corticosteroids and/or corticotropins. Any possibly precipitating upper respiratory tract infection should be treated promptly with antibiotics.

The value of desensitization during pregnancy is open to question. If a desensitization regimen already has been initiated prior to conception and can be continued at a slow rate to minimize allergic reactions, it may be continued during gestation. Acute allergic reactions, which may occur during desensitization procedures, liberate large amounts of histamine, and are alleged to result in uterine contractions and possibly premature labor. If desensitization is not already under way, it probably is best deferred until after delivery.

Conduct of labor and delivery may be based upon obstetric considerations. Heavy opiate sedation should be avoided lest the respiratory center suffer even mild depression. Regional anesthesia is preferred to inhalation techniques. There is little indication for therapeutic abortion or sterilization.

CYSTIC FIBROSIS

Cystic fibrosis no longer is an invariably fatal disease of infancy and childhood, and therefore is being encountered more frequently in pregnancy. Patient longevity has improved because of increased understanding of the pathophysiology of the disease, improved diagnostic techniques, and more effective therapeutic measures. The pilocarpine iontophoresis method ("sweat test") is diagnostic (Rosenow, Lee).

The pregnant patient may be adversely affected by her pulmonary condition. The characteristic functional defect is interference with oxygen diffusion from the alveolus to the pulmonary capillary, which results in diminished arterial oxygen saturation in the mother and possibly chronic hypoxia for the fetus. Pancreatic insufficiency or diabetes mellitus may be a complicating factor, but immediate maternal morbidity or mortality usually results from pulmonary insufficiency.

Treatment of patients with cystic fibrosis includes postural drainage, antibiotics, intermittent positive pressure breathing, and administration of potassium iodide and aminophylline; all these agents may be continued during gestation. The management of labor and delivery may be based upon obstetric considerations. Heavy sedation should be avoided, and conduction anesthesia is preferred to inhalation techniques.

Therapeutic abortion may be indicated in the woman with severe respiratory distress antedating conception. Sterilization should be considered in patients requiring therapeutic abortion and might be discussed with other patients with cystic fibrosis on the basis of the reduced maternal life expectancy and the recessive hereditary nature of the disease.

DISORDERS OF THE URINARY SYSTEM

URINARY TRACT INFECTION

BACTERIURIA

Asymptomatic bacteriuria is defined arbitrarily as the presence of 100,000 bacteria per milliliter of urine, usually obtained from a midstream voided specimen. This finding is reduplicable in successive urine specimens in over 90 percent of cases. Asymptomatic bacteriuria has been reported in 5 to 7 percent of all pregnant women. The bacterium cultured from over 80 percent of cases has been *Escherichia*. Bacteriuria of this degree is completely dissociated from pyuria (the presence of leukocytes in the urine) in over 50 percent of patients studied.

Asymptomatic bacteria has significance both for the mother and for the fetus. Over 30 percent of women found to have bacteriuria in early pregnancy and thereafter untreated developed symptomatic urinary tract infections during the pregnancy, as compared with a risk of pyelonephritis of under 3 percent in women with asymptomatic bacteriuria who received treatment or patients without bacteriuria. Early detection and treatment of asymptomatic bacteriuria thus can prevent subsequent attacks of clinically significant pyelonephritis and cystitis.

Of even greater importance is the possible relationship of asymptomatic bacteriuria to fetal welfare. It has been claimed that the presence of bacteriuria is associated with an increased rate of prematurity

(24 percent) and that adequate treatment of the bacteriuria reduced the prematurity rate to the normal range (approximately 6 percent). This is contested by reports which find no relation between bacteriuria and prematurity, and by reports which find an association between bacteriuria and prematurity but cannot alter that association by treatment (Kincaid-Smith). The latter reports suggest that the association might not be between prematurity and bacteriuria but between prematurity and the underlying renal disease which results in bacteriuria; the variability in fetal outcome reported thus might depend on the severity of the underlying renal disease in the different series (Heineman, Lee). There is similar difference of reports and opinion concerning the relationship between bacteriuria and perinatal loss. There is no evidence of transplacental transmission of the bacilli or that the premature babies which survive are compromised in any special way.

The necessity of making the diagnosis of asymptomatic bacteriuria and of treating the pregnant women with this complication is unquestioned. Two weeks of active antibiotic/chemotherapeutic therapy, utilizing a variety of agents including sulfonamides, ampicillin, and nitrofurantoin, have resulted in clearing of bacteriuria in approximately 70 percent of patients; in a small series, treatment with a combination of sulfonamide and trimethoprim cleared the urine of bacteria in 90 percent.

Careful follow-up of patients, with repeated urine colony counts and cultures throughout pregnancy, is essential. In about 30 percent of patients, repeat colony counts and cultures several days after initiation of therapy will reveal the presence of resistant organisms, and other antibiotics can be substituted. The same procedures can be followed if bacteriuria recurs after successful treatment and response. After successful treatment and clearing of the urine, and in patients harboring organisms which are resistant to all the commonly used antimicrobial agents, maintenance of the patient for the duration of pregnancy on methenamine mandelate, 4 to 12 g daily, has been suggested as a means of controlling recurrence or exacerbation of infection with minimal risk to the patient. Caution must be exercised with regard to long-term antimicrobial use. The use of sulfonamides during the last few weeks of pregnancy is contraindicated, because of documented interference in the neonate with bilirubin transport and possible potentiation of kernicterus. Chloramphenicol administered to the mother during the last month of gestation may precipitate the neonatal "gray syndrome." Tetracyclines should not be used during the latter half of gestation because of their deposition at the metaphyseal plates of the long bones and in enamel of the fetus; in addition, in susceptible gravidas, large doses of tetracycline may result in hepatic degeneration. The administration of methenamine mandelate, and its excretion in the maternal urine, makes the detection of maternal urinary estriol excretion levels chemically impossible. Nevertheless, it is the consensus that an active approach to asymptomatic bacteriuria not only is desirable but is necessary (Marchant).

CYSTITIS

Although bladder hypotonicity promotes urinary stasis and increases the risk of infection, cystitis alone without infection of the upper urinary tract is rare during pregnancy. The incidence of cystitis is markedly increased, however, during labor and delivery and in the immediate puerperium. The parturient patient hardly can escape urethral catheterization either before, during, or after delivery; the incidence of significant bacteriuria following urethral catheterization is 2 to 4 percent. In addition, trauma to the base of the bladder may occur during labor or delivery and form a focus for infection. Every effort should be made to avoid urethral catheterization in this susceptible group of patients.

Acute cystitis is manifest by urinary urgency, frequency, dysuria, and occasionally stranguria. Systemic reactions such as fever may or may not be present; pyuria is always found, and occasionally hematuria as well. The offending organism usually is a gram-negative coliform bacillus, and antimicrobial therapy should be instituted pending reports of bacterial cultures and sensitivities, to reduce the possibility of ascending infection of the upper urinary tract and the risk that continued bladder tenesmus will precipitate an autonomic "storm" that may initiate premature uterine contractions in the gravid patient.

PYELONEPHRITIS

Acute pyelonephritis is a serious complication of pregnancy. It occurs in 1 to 2 percent of all gravidas, with a marked predilection for primigravidas, and often is preceded by asymptomatic bacteriuria or cystitis. The pathogenesis of the infection usually is an ascending spread of bacteria from the bladder via the ureteral lumina or the periureteral lymphatic channels; as an alternative, the renal parenchyma may become infected by the hematogenous route.

Acute pyelonephritis usually presents with urinary urgency, frequency, and dysuria; pain and tenderness in the affected flank(s); chills and high fevers (up to 104°F); and anorexia, vomiting, and malaise. The diagnosis usually can be made by urinalysis and urine culture. The differential diagnosis may have to consider lobar pneumonia, acute appendicitis, cholecystitis, and ureteral calculus. The severe maternal hyperpyrexia is associated with increased fetal wastage: spontaneous abortion, premature labor, and stillbirth.

Treatment should entail hospitalization, bed rest, hydration (parenterally or per os, as indicated), and prompt administration of large doses of a broad-spectrum bactericidal antimicrobial, such as ampicillin, while awaiting the results of urine cultures and sensitivity testing. Cautions with regard to antibiotic therapy in pregnancy have been discussed previously. At times, despite appropriate antibiotic therapy, the disease remains unchecked. Usually this results from ureteral blockage by calculus, edema, or simply positional kinking; treatment cannot be effective unless adequate drainage of the affected renal pelvis and ureter is assured. In some patients, this may be accomplished by elevating the foot of the bed and placing the patient in Trendelenburg's position, permitting the kidneys to drop cephalad and unkinking the elongated ureters. Other women may require the placement of indwelling ureteral catheters for several days to ensure adequate drainage; such urologic manipulation carries its own risk of inducing premature uterine contractions, and should be avoided if possible, but not unduly delayed if necessary.

Patients with chronic pyelonephritis may be first diagnosed during pregnancy, presenting with an acute exacerbation. Or the episode of pyelonephritis which occurs during pregnancy may be the initial infection which may progress over the years to chronic disease. Of patients presenting with pyelonephritis in pregnancy, approximately 80 percent had recurrent urinary tract infections after the pregnancy was over, and almost 40 percent subsequently had radiologic evidence of renal abnormality. The conclusion is clear: an episode of pyelonephritis during pregnancy, no matter how acute or how easily and completely "cured," cannot be considered as an isolated event. These patients must have prolonged, careful follow-up with repeated urinalyses and urine cultures, and should have radiologic investigation of their urinary tracts interconceptionally.

Indications for therapeutic abortion and/or sterilization depend entirely on the status of the renal function. In patients with poor renal function, fetal salvage is very low. Exacerbation of acute pyelonephritis in impaired renal function, particularly if refractory to antimicrobial therapy, may lead to progressive oliguria and azotemia, and prompt termination of pregnancy at whatever stage may be lifesaving.

RENAL TUBERCULOSIS

At one time, tuberculosis of the kidney was associated with progressive destruction of the renal parenchyma, eventuating in azotemia and death. The tubercle bacilli reach the kidneys, almost always bilaterally, by the hematogenous route from the lung or mediastinum. The renal lesions may remain dormant for long periods of time or undergo rapid caseation and dissemination. The incidence of renal tuberculosis in pregnancy is less than 0.1 percent. The disease presents with the signs and symptoms of chronic pyelonephritis, and a high index of suspicion is necessary if the diagnosis is to be made during pregnancy, when radiologic studies of the urinary tract usually are deferred. The diagnosis must be established by smear and culture for *M. tuberculosis.*

The prognosis for pregnancy in patients with renal tuberculosis depends entirely upon the state of renal function present. The patient with active disease should receive triple chemotherapy (see Pulmonary Tuberculosis above); a patient with inactive disease, isoniazid prophylaxis. In either case, therapy should be instituted as early in gestation as possible and continued well into the puerperium, or at least 2 years after all evidence of activity has disappeared.

Except in the end stages of the disease, the prognosis for control of the tuberculosis and arrest of parenchymal destruction by medical management is good, and there is no indication for either therapeutic abortion or sterilization. If the renal disease is unilateral and refractory to therapy, or if the destruction of renal parenchyma has progressed to the point where systemic hypertension results, the management is surgical, i.e., nephrectomy.

URINARY TRACT CALCULI

Urinary tract calculi usually present problems after the childbearing age, and the incidence of their coexistence with pregnancy is no more than 0.1 to 0.3 percent. Ureteral stones occur twice as frequently as renal stones (Harris, Dunnihoo). Although stasis and infection in the urinary tract predispose to the development of calculi, these conditions are transient during pregnancy and usually do not exist long enough for significant calculi to be laid down.

The patient may present only with symptoms of renal infection. Renal calculi most frequently occupy the lower calyx of the affected kidney and cause varying degrees of intrarenal hydronephrosis. Ureteral calculi often are silent during pregnancy, perhaps because of the hypotonicity and dilatation of the ureter, and their presence may be detected serendipitously in the investigation of refractory pyelonephritis. In other patients, the calculus is arrested in its passage down the ureter at an area of ureteral constriction: the ureteropelvic junction, the sites where the iliac and ovarian vessels cross over the ureter, or at the ureterovesical orifice. Symptoms of an impacted ureteral calculus include severe costovertebral angle colicky pain often radiating down the ureter and into the groin, urgency, frequency, and hematuria. These symptoms remit when the calculus is passed. Vesical calculi are extremely rare in young women, and may present with hematuria, stranguria, and pain at the end of micturition.

Calculous disease in pregnancy has little effect on the pregnancy or on fetal outcome if treatment is instituted before renal damage occurs (Coe et al.).

MANAGEMENT

Patients with manifestations of urinary tract calculi should be hospitalized for investigation. Radiologic investigation of the urinary tract is necessary, despite the existence of a pregnancy. While every means should be employed to minimize radiation exposure of the fetus, intravenous pyelography and possibly retrograde pyelography may be essential. Included in the work-up should be a search for disease which might predispose to calculus formation: homocystinuria, oxaluria, hypercalcemia, gout, etc.

Several factors govern the management of calculous disease in pregnancy: (1) the stage of the pregnancy, with special consideration of the viability of the fetus; (2) the location of the stone; (3) the presence and degree of obstruction and/or infection; and (4) the state of renal function. A patient in early gestation with a stone in the lower ureter and minimal obstruction usually can be treated conservatively and expectantly, with administration of analgesics as necessary, and the stone be permitted to pass spontaneously. With complete ureteral obstruction and declining renal function, cystoscopic manipulation and ureteral catheterization may be successful in facilitating passage. Usually, only stones in the distal third of the ureter are approached by intraureteral manipulation. Later in pregnancy, if necessary, retroperitoneal ureterolithotomy can be performed. Closer to term, time may be gained for increased fetal maturation by placement of indwelling ureteral catheters to permit drainage, and uretero- or nephrolithotomy subsequently carried out at the time of delivery by cesarean section.

Vesical calculi usually do not require treatment during pregnancy and can be crushed and removed through the urethra in the puerperium.

GLOMERULONEPHRITIS

ACUTE GLOMERULONEPHRITIS

This condition is an extremely rare complication of pregnancy. The patient usually presents with generalized edema, particularly in the periorbital regions. aching in the flanks, dyspnea, and macroscopic hematuria. Upon examination, she usually has an elevated venous pressure and hypertension. Her urine contains albumin; the urinary sediment, many casts and erythrocytes. A history suggestive of streptococcal infection approximately 2 weeks prior to the acute episode may be elicited, and antistreptolysin titers usually are elevated.

Both the course of the illness and its effect on pregnancy depend in large measure on the rapidity with which the disorder is recognized and treated, which determines in turn the duration and degree of hypertension (O'Dwyer, Montgomery). If treatment is initiated within 24 to 48 hours of the onset of acute glomerulonephritis, the patient usually experiences a brisk diuresis, a fall in arterial and venous blood pressures, becomes edema-free, and shows marked decrease in albuminuria and hematuria. In such patients, the pregnancy usually proceeds normally to term, and there is no evidence of placental insufficiency and retardation of intrauterine growth.

The longer treatment is delayed, the more slowly acute glomerulonephritis responds, and the higher the patient's blood pressure levels go. In these cases, abortion, stillbirth, or premature labor may ensue. These differences in the initiation of treatment probably account for the variety of opinions extant about the effect of acute glomerulonephritis on coexistent pregnancy.

About 5 percent of patients with acute glomerulonephritis fail to respond to treatment and progress to renal failure, cardiac failure, and death. It is possible, although by no means proved, that the presence of a pregnancy may, in these few patients, contribute to the maternal deterioration. Therapeutic abortion therefore may merit consideration in the patient who

fails to respond satisfactorily to medical management within 10 to 14 days. In patients with illness of this severity, however, spontaneous abortion or premature onset of labor probably will have occurred before this. The differential diagnosis must consider periarteritis nodosa and systemic lupus erythematosus.

Management

Once the diagnosis is established, the patient should be placed at bed rest and prescribed a low-salt diet. A course of antibiotic therapy should be administered to eradicate any residual streptococci; cultures of the nose and throat serve to monitor this problem. Hypotensive agents should be administered to control the blood pressure; hydralazine has been effective in this regard. In patients with compromised renal function and oliguria, the administration of furosemide (Lasix) has initiated diuresis. After the episode of acute glomerulonephritis has begun to subside, the patient should be maintained on prophylactic antibiotic therapy, preferably with penicillin, for the duration of pregnancy to prevent recurrence of streptococcal infection and exacerbation of the renal problem.

A patient with healed glomerulonephritis and normal renal function may undertake pregnancy without any increased risk to herself or the fetus, provided there is no residual maternal hypertension. If hypertension persists after the acute stage of the nephritis is over, the prognosis for future successful pregnancy is poor, even worse than it would be for a patient with essential hypertension of the same degree. There is no evidence of nephritis in infants born of pregnancies during which the mothers suffered acute glomerulonephritis.

CHRONIC GLOMERULONEPHRITIS

About 10 percent of patients with acute glomerulonephritis fail to recover completely and pass into a chronic stage of the disease. Such patients present with persistent albuminuria and occasional bouts of hematuria, and usually are symptom-free. The incidence of this complication in pregnancy is less than 0.05 percent. In a mild case, especially with the patient presenting late in pregnancy, diagnosis may be difficult. The differentiation from toxemia of pregnancy or chronic pyelonephritis may require renal biopsy; in the third trimester of pregnancy; it may be impossible to distinguish the severity of the renal lesion from the effect of superimposed toxemia clinically. The absence of a history of acute glomerulonephritis is of no diagnostic value.

The maternal and fetal prognoses in chronic glomerulonephritis depend on the extent of renal impairment. If the only abnormal finding is albuminuria, without hypertension or evidence of azotemia, the prognosis for successful pregnancy is good, although superimposed toxemia is not infrequent; a fetal survival rate of 90 percent can be anticipated. In these mild forms of the disease, pregnancy causes no exacerbation of the course of chronic glomerulonephritis. If maternal hypertension also is present, the prognosis for pregnancy and fetal salvage is markedly reduced. Toxemia of pregnancy may occur in as many as 75 percent of patients, despite optimal medical and obstetric management, and fetal wastage may range from 33 to 75 percent. The higher the maternal blood pressure at the time of conception, the worse the prognosis for the fetus. In the presence of retinopathy in the mother, fetal wastage is almost 100 percent. In about half of patients with chronic glomerulonephritis and hypertension, pregnancy leads to permanent deterioration of the maternal condition. Increasing nitrogen retention correlates closely with maternal mortality. The renal function of patients with chronic glomerulonephritis should be evaluated periodically throughout pregnancy, with serial measurements of creatinine clearance, quantitative urinary protein, and blood urea nitrogen included in the evaluation. Therapeutic abortion is indicated for the patient with progressive renal failure, increasing hypertension, and azotemia. In patients refusing abortion and who carry the pregnancy into the third trimester, perinatal mortality still is around 50 percent. Maternal urinary estriol excretion levels often are of no value in predicting impending fetal loss in such patients, but instead never show the usual rise beyond 35 weeks' gestation, an indication of chronic distress of the fetoplacental unit.

Management

There is no known treatment which can alter significantly the course of chronic glomerulonephritis. Moderate restriction of activity throughout pregnancy is advisable. Any acute infection should be treated promptly. Dietary restrictions are indicated in the patient with azotemia.

The major contribution to management is the decision about continuation of pregnancy. In patients with albuminuria alone, the chance of obtaining a living baby is only slightly less than in the normal patient, and the pregnancy may be permitted to continue. At the first evidence of maternal deterioration, as manifest by increasing hypertension, albuminuria, or edema, the pregnancy should be terminated, since fetal survival is negligible and the risk of accelerating the maternal disease is considerable.

If the maternal blood urea nitrogen is above 50 mg per 100 mL before pregnancy, the probability of obtaining a living baby is so small that conception is contraindicated; if conception occurs, abortion should be recommended (Mackay). If the patient chooses to continue her pregnancy despite medical advice, long-term hospitalization may be in order, and the pregnancy termination recommended again at the first sign of maternal deterioration. In the case of patients with hypertension and azotemia, rigorous contraception or sterilization should be recommended.

NEPHROSIS

The nephrotic syndrome is a symptom complex characterized by massive proteinuria (more than 5.0 g per 24 hours), lipiduria, hypoalbuminemia, hypercholesterolemia, and massive edema. Nephrosis is rare during pregnancy, with an incidence less than 0.1 percent, and may occur as a result of chronic glomerulonephritis, systemic lupus erythematosus, diabetes mellitus, amyloidosis, syphilis, renal vein thrombosis, and reactions to drugs or insect venom. The etiology of the syndrome is not well understood. Deposition of immunoglobulins and complement on the renal basement membrane has been described. Serum complement usually is decreased, and eosinophilia increased. The presence of edema and proteinuria in early pregnancy, without hypertension, is suggestive of the diagnosis.

Proper management depends upon accurate diagnosis, and renal biopsy may be necessary. Proper evaluation is required to minimize the complications of renal biopsy, which may vary from transient hematuria to massive hemorrhage. Contraindications to biopsy include a hemorrhagic diathesis, increasing azotemia, severe hypertension, and a unilateral kidney. Renal biopsy technically is easier and is best performed before 30 weeks of gestation.

Maternal and fetal prognoses in nephrosis depend upon the nature and severity of the underlying renal disease (Fisher et al.). Hypoproteinemia results in a decrease in colloid osmotic pressure, with secondary hypovolemia. A patient with nephrosis therefore is susceptible to thrombosis and infection, and tolerates hemorrhage very poorly. Pregnancy in nephrosis usually does not cause progression of the underlying renal disease.

MANAGEMENT

A pregnant patient with the nephrotic syndrome should be hospitalized, placed at bed rest, and prescribed a high-protein, low-salt diet. Baseline laboratory studies to be obtained before initiation of therapy include creatinine clearance, quantitative urine protein, serum proteins with albumin/globulin ratio, and blood urea nitrogen. Corticosteroids often are effective in decreasing protein loss through the kidneys. Urinary tract infection and venous thrombosis occur relatively frequently in patients with nephrosis, and should be treated promptly and specifically.

Most patients with nephrosis tolerate pregnancy well. Therapeutic abortion is indicated only in patients with deteriorating renal function (Makker, Heymann).

ACUTE RENAL FAILURE

Acute renal failure is defined as a decrease in urine excretion to less than 500 mL per 24 hours. Early renal failure may be associated with no structural abnormalities in the renal parenchyma. However, with persistent failure, acute tubular and cortical necroses supervene. The primary etiology is obstetric hemorrhage, leading to maternal hypovolemia and hypotension, and renal ischemia and lack of perfusion. It is probable that cortical necrosis is a further stage of tubular necrosis, occurring when ischemia is particularly severe and prolonged. Other etiologic factors may be septic shock, clostridial infection, severe preeclampsia and eclampsia, and disseminated intravascular coagulation. In the latter instances, renal ischemia can develop in the absence of maternal systemic hypotension because of local renal vasoconstriction or blockage (Chugh et al.).

The primary sign of renal failure is decreased urine output; high-output renal failure is possible but exceedingly infrequent. Progressive deterioration in renal output may be accompanied by maternal increased neuromuscular irritability, acidosis, hyperpnea, and convulsions. The maternal and fetal prognoses are related directly to the rapidity of diagnosis and institution of effective therapy. The lesions in early renal failure are focal and almost entirely reversible; prompt diagnosis and treatment often result in return of almost normal renal function. Conversely, prolonged renal failure and progression to renal cortical necrosis carry a much more serious prognosis.

MANAGEMENT

The best management of acute renal failure is prevention. The extent of obstetric hemorrhage may be underestimated, or the renal arteriolar involvement in toxemia not appreciated. In any patient where acute renal failure is even a remote possibility, the urine output must be monitored hourly and continuously by indwelling bladder catheter, at the same time that other therapeutic measures, including adequate parenteral fluid and blood replacement (guided by central venous pressure readings), are carried out. Should the hourly rate of urine production fall below 25 mL per hour (i.e., approximately 600 mL per 24 hours), in the face of adequate fluid and blood replacement and the maintenance of maternal blood pressure, impending renal failure is near. Prompt stimulation of urine excretion and renal blood flow may reverse the pathophysiologic process. The intravenous administration of mannitol or furosemide (Lasix) has been helpful in this regard.

The other etiologic factors which precipitated the acute renal failure must be treated vigorously. Infection should be treated with large doses of appropriate antibiotics; ampicillin and penicillin can be administered safely in patients with oliguria, while streptomycin and kanamycin can be used only with caution. Prompt treatment of toxemia of pregnancy is essential. Progressive oliguria in the face of adequate medical management of toxemia of pregnancy mandates evacuation of the uterus by the most expedient route. The appearance of hematuria in such patients is a poor sign, being indicative of developing cortical necrosis. Where disseminated intravascular coagulation is suspected, intravenous administration of heparin may prevent the formation of microthrombi in the renal capillaries.

Once renal failure has developed in a pregnant patient, the management is the same as in the nongravid. The kidneys will pass through the same stages of oliguria and diuresis. In the former phase, restriction of fluid intake, low-protein diet, management of hyperkalemia, and alleviation of azotemia are necessary. The maternal prognosis has been related to the duration of the anuric phase. There is increasing evidence today that prompt and repeated hemodialysis results in very significant improvement in mortality figures.

NEOPLASTIC DISEASES

Malignancy of the urinary tract is a rare complication of pregnancy. Only some 20 cases coincident with pregnancy have been reported in the medical literature; conversely, series of deliveries numbering over 20,000 have been reported without a single case of urinary tract malignancy (Fetter, Koppel).

The management of urinary tract malignancy complicating pregnancy revolves around two factors, diagnosis and treatment. Hematuria is the major presenting symptom in urinary tract malignancy and requires careful evaluation despite the presence of the gestation; too frequently, delay in the diagnostic investigation of hematuria during pregnancy contributes to delay in treatment of a malignancy and to the poor prognosis. The differential diagnosis of hematuria includes calculus, neoplasia, tuberculosis, and infection. Occasionally, hematuria during pregnancy may result from bleeding from varicosities at or near the renal pyramids or from engorged veins in the region of the bladder trigone. Despite customary studies, the cause of hematuria in a particular case may remain undetermined.

If the diagnosis of tumor is made, therapy should be concerned with the treatment of the neoplastic disease and ignore the presence of pregnancy. Pregnancy itself is little influenced by tumors of the urinary tract, and in some cases surgical excision of these tumors can be accomplished without interfering with the incumbent gestation; this certainly is the case with renal tumors. Carcinoma of the bladder, on the other hand, requires termination of pregnancy to ensure adequate treatment, whether surgery or radiotherapy be employed (Fehenbaker et al.).

The important principle is not to delay diagnosis or defer treatment in an attempt to preserve a pregnancy.

ANOMALIES OF THE URINARY TRACT

UNILATERAL RENAL AGENESIS

This condition, also termed *solitary kidney,* is found in about 0.2 percent of all women according to information from postmortem examinations, but is diagnosed during life even less frequently. Although the incidence of associated genital tract anomalies is high, pregnancy may occur. Renal function should be assessed prior to pregnancy; if function is normal, maternal and fetal prognoses are good.

Consideration of pregnancy, however, is complicated by intercurrent infection. Often, unilateral renal agenesis is discovered during investigation of pyelonephritis. Evidence of chronic or recurrent pyelo-

nephritis in the unilateral kidney would be a severe contraindication to pregnancy.

The same precautions and considerations apply to the patient who has undergone unilateral nephrectomy prior to the onset of pregnancy. After nephrectomy, the contralateral kidney undergoes hypertrophy and after 12 to 28 months can safely bear the burden of one or more pregnancies, *provided it does not have any underlying disease.*

ECTOPIC KIDNEY

The incidence of ectopic kidney complicating pregnancy is about 0.2 percent. Over half of all ectopic kidneys are situated in the pelvis and are secured there by anomalous vascular attachments. Pelvic kidneys usually are rotated on their axis and have short ureters. Other pelvic structures may be compressed by the ectopic kidney, resulting in a variety of symptoms. Pyelonephritis and hydronephrosis are more frequent in patients with ectopic kidney.

The diagnosis of ectopic kidney usually is made by intravenous pyelography in a patient presenting with a pelvic mass. A pelvic kidney may obstruct labor directly because of its size or position, or may interfere with vaginal delivery by causing fetal malpresentation. In such patients, delivery by cesarean section should be accomplished early, before any injury to the ectopic kidney may ensue; it must be borne in mind that the ectopic kidney may be a solitary kidney. In such an instance, elective cesarean section may be the most prudent course. Pelvic ectopic kidney alone is not an indication for either abortion or sterilization.

URETEROPELVIC OBSTRUCTION

Congenital ureteropelvic stricture, either alone or in association with large, aberrant vessels, may be asymptomatic, and may first attract attention during pregnancy by virtue of superimposed infection, by the size of the concomitant hydronephrosis, or even by rupture of the renal pelvis. Once discovered, surgical management may be deferred until after delivery if the condition of the affected kidney permits. If intervention is urgently necessary, nephrostomy during pregnancy and later definitive surgery should be considered.

POLYCYSTIC KIDNEY DISEASE

This kidney disease occurs in about 0.025 percent of all women, and is inherited as an autosomal dominant. The condition usually remains latent and undiagnosed for many years, and 80 percent of affected women may be asymptomatic at the time of initial conception. The affected patient may present with a history of intermittent costovertebral angle pain, hematuria, or pyuria. Palpation may reveal enlarged and irregular kidneys, but the diagnosis usually is made on intravenous pyelography. On x-ray examination, the renal calyces are elongated and distorted, and multiple cystic areas may be visible in the renal parenchyma.

The risk of pyelonephritis is high in affected women, and vigorous antibiotic therapy should be initiated at the earliest suspicion of urinary tract infection. Fetal and maternal prognoses are related to the level of renal function. In the asymptomatic, normotensive patient with good renal function, fetal outcome usually is excellent. In a pregnant patient with polycystic kidney disease who suddenly develops hypertension and proteinuria, early termination of pregnancy may be advisable. Pregnancy does not adversely affect the course of the renal disease.

In view of the chronic and progressive nature of the deterioration of renal function in affected patients, women with a family history of polycystic kidney disease should be encouraged to have their families at an earlier age, if possible. Associated anomalies in patients with polycystic kidney disease include hepatic cysts and cerebral basilar artery aneurysms. Women who have a family history of polycystic kidney disease or who have delivered an infant with that condition should be referred for preconceptional genetic counseling.

PREGNANCY AFTER RENAL TRANSPLANTATION

Increasingly, the modern treatment of chronic renal failure, the end result of a variety of renal diseases, has become the renal homograft. Since young patients with chronic renal failure are selected preferentially for kidney transplantation, the question of subsequent reproductive function is important.

Women with chronic azotemia usually are amenorrheic. The recovery of menstrual function after transplantation was related directly both to the frequency and severity of rejection episodes and the reestablishment of adequate renal function. Menses generally resumed within 6 months of successful transplantation. All recipients were treated with prednisone, azathioprine, and some with heterologous antilymphocyte globulin as well (Merkatz et al.).

In male recipients, sexual function and spermatogenesis was restored as renal function improved, and conception, where desired, resulted in successful pregnancies and the delivery of normal infants. Successful male recipients of renal homografts may be advised that their subsequent reproductive potential is excellent.

For female renal homograft recipients, the picture is not as clear (Davison et al.; Popoff et al.). Of approximately 300 women of childbearing age who have received renal homografts, there have been 12 who attempted at least one pregnancy. All these patients had had excellent recovery of renal function prior to conception, and, if receiving antilymphocytic globulin, this medication was stopped several months before conception. The fetal salvage in these pregnancies was good, and there was no evidence of serologic problems between mother and infant nor of any teratogenic influences of therapy. There was evidence of adrenocortical insufficiency in almost one-third of the neonates, which responded to therapy.

The fact that normal pregnancies may ensue in female recipients of successful renal homografts does not mean that pregnancy should be advised for such patients. In addition to the possible teratogenic potential of maternal maintenance therapy, other factors must be considered: the increased incidence of hepatitis in these patients, possibly more serious during gestation; interference with function of the renal transplant because of pregnancy-induced diseases such as toxemia; and the risks of renal infection inherent in pregnancy. In all, the patient whose life depends on a single, transplanted kidney probably should avoid pregnancy, should be offered effective means of contraception or surgical sterilization, and abortion should be recommended if conception should occur.

HEMATOLOGIC DISORDERS IN PREGNANCY

PHYSIOLOGIC ALTERATIONS

During pregnancy, maternal blood volume increases by approximately 30 to 40 percent. This represents an increase both in red cell mass and in plasma volume. The increase in plasma volume is somewhat greater in degree and more constant, resulting in hemodilution and a relative "physiologic anemia of pregnancy." In the normal, nongravid female, accepted normal values include: hemoglobin concentration, 12.0 g per 100 mL; hematocrit, 40 percent; and erythrocyte count, 4.5 million per cubic millimeter. During pregnancy, mean reported levels were lower: hemoglobin concentration, 11.4 g per 100 mL; hematocrit, 34 percent; and erythrocyte count, 3.7 million per cubic millimeter.

Pregnancy is associated with a relative leukocytosis of 5000 to 12,000 per cubic millimeter rising to 25,000 per cubic millimeter during labor and delivery. There is an associated lymphocytopenia. The platelet count is elevated slightly, but plasma viscosity is not altered.

The plasma fibrinogen level is increased during pregnancy and into the puerperium. Other bloodclotting factors whose activity is increased during gestation include factor II (prothrombin), factor VII (proconvertin), factor VIII (antihemophiliac globulin), factor IX (plasma thromboplastic globulin), and factor X (Stuart-Power factor). An increase in fibrinolytic activity near term and during labor also has been reported.

ANEMIA IN PREGNANCY

Anemia is the most frequently encountered complication of pregnancy, and may be found in as much as 80 percent of a given gravid population. In the United States, a patient is considered mildly anemic during pregnancy if her hemoglobin concentration falls below 11.0 g per 100 mL, and moderately to severely anemic if below 10.0 g per 100 mL. Anemia aggravates many obstetric problems, such as concomitant heart disease. Anemic patients have an increased incidence of abortion, premature labor, infection, and toxemia of pregnancy. Maternal anemia may affect the fetus deleteriously, resulting in intrauterine growth retardation and elevated perinatal mortality and morbidity rates.

IRON-DEFICIENCY ANEMIA

Because of increased maternal and fetal demands for iron (Chap. 23), iron-deficiency anemia is the most frequent cause of anemia in pregnancy. It is encountered more often in multiparous than primigravidous patients, particularly when repeated pregnancies have followed in rapid succession. The anemia usually becomes manifest during the last trimester of pregnancy. The patient may be asymptomatic and the anemia detected only by routine laboratory determination, or she may present with weakness, dyspnea,

fatigability, and nail-bed and conjunctival pallor. At this point, hemoglobin levels usually are below 10.0 g per 100 mL, with a corresponding reduction in erythrocyte count. Blood smear will show varying degrees of anisocytosis, poikilocytosis, hypochromia, and microcytosis. The total serum iron binding capacity is elevated (normal in pregnancy), but the iron content is low, usually between 20 and 50 μg per 100 mL. Examination of the bone marrow reveals normoblastic hyperplasia, with little or no iron reserves demonstrable.

Management

Because of the documented iron requirements during pregnancy and high probability that women enter pregnancy with depleted iron stores if not with actual iron-deficiency anemia, all gravid patients should receive iron supplementation therapy throughout pregnancy, or at least from the beginning of the second trimester. The recommended daily dose is 0.6 g of ferrous sulfate, or its equivalent in elemental iron. It has been demonstrated that the "physiologic anemia of pregnancy" does not occur in patients who have received adequate supplementation of iron intake during gestation.

Once iron-deficiency anemia has developed, it can be reversed rapidly by the administration of iron. A rise of 1.0 g per 100 mL in hemoglobin concentration represents the utilization of at least 25 mg of elemental iron. The oral route of administration is preferred because of its simplicity and relative safety. Many satisfactory oral iron preparations are available; the dosages vary because of differential absorption from the gastrointestinal tract (see Table 31–5). The limiting factor for oral iron therapy is gastrointestinal irritation, manifest as nausea, vomiting, abdominal cramps, diarrhea, or constipation. After initiation of adequate oral iron therapy, maximal reticulocyte response may be expected within 5 to 10 days, and a gradual increase in hemoglobin concentration thereafter, returning to normal levels in 2 to 3 months. Failure to observe this response has one of two implications: either the patient is not taking the medication as prescribed (probably because of gastrointestinal side effects) or the etiology of the patient's anemia was not purely iron deficiency.

Effect on the Fetus

To satisfy its prenatal needs, the fetus is dependent entirely upon the transfer of iron across the placenta. The fetus accumulates iron throughout gestation at a

TABLE 31–5   Gastrointestinal Absorption of Iron Supplements

Compound	Daily doses, g	Metallic iron, mg	Daily absorption, mg
Ferrous sulfate (anhydrous)	0.5	180	27
Ferrous carbonate	2.0	330	25
Ferric ammonium citrate	6.0	1000	23
	3.0	500	20
	1.0	170	19
Reduced iron	3.5	3000	23

rate directly proportional to fetal weight gain, maintaining a relatively constant iron content of approximately 75 mg per kilogram of body weight. The bulk of the iron transfer takes place during the last trimester which is the period of greatest fetal mass accumulation. The fetus parasitizes maternal iron stores regardless of the state of the mother's iron metabolism. The mean neonatal hemoglobin concentration does not vary signficantly whether the mother is anemic or not anemic.

There is controversy about the effect of maternal iron-deficiency anemia on the infant's hematologic status. Some suggest that the infant born of a mother with untreated iron-deficiency anemia has reduced iron stores which contribute to the development of iron-deficiency anemia some months after birth (Sisson, Lund). By this thesis, premature infants regularly develop iron-deficiency anemia because fetal iron stores largely are filled in the last 8 weeks of gestation. Other, apparently equally valid, work denies this thesis, and holds that the mother's status with regard to iron has no appreciable effect on the infant's iron homeostasis either at birth or during the first year of life (Lanzkowsky). The lack of postnatal dietary iron intake is held to be responsible for anemia during the first year, and the more severe anemia in premature infants based on their relatively greater postnatal growth rather than depleted iron stores.

FOLIC ACID AND VITAMIN B_{12} METABOLISM

At the cellular level, folic acid, vitamin B_{12}, and ascorbic acid interact intimately and play important roles in the synthesis of nucleic acids. Normal nucleic acid and nucleoprotein synthesis is required for hematopoiesis. Any deficiency in folic acid, vitamin B_{12}, or ascorbic acid therefore results in a megaloblastic erythropoietic disturbance.

Folic acid plays an important role in pregnancy, whose precise limits have not been defined as yet. Maternal ingestion of antifolic acid drugs in early gestation may inhibit progesterone activity, cause fe-

tal death, or result in significant fetal malformation; these results occur, however, only with a true folic acid deficiency state, which is exceedingly rare in nature. Fetal growth and development are not significantly impaired by the degree of folic acid deficiency which results from an inadequate maternal dietary intake, nor does the degree of maternal insufficiency affect the infant's survival or ability to maintain normal hematologic function (Pritchard et al.). Other pregnancy complications have been ascribed to folic acid deficiency, including abruptio placenta, antepartum hemorrhage, toxemia of pregnancy, and spontaneous abortion; the evidence to date is insufficient to indict folic acid etiologically in these complications (Hibbard, Jeffcoate; Scott et al.; Hall). In normal pregnancy, maternal folic acid levels are high during pregnancy and fall after parturition; folic acid is transferred preferentially to the fetus, so that serum folic acid levels at birth are higher in the fetus than in the mother.

Vitamin B_{12} is derived principally from foods of animal origin, although some may be synthesized endogenously by gastrointestinal tract bacteria, and is absorbed in the ileum. Intrinsic factor, produced in the corpus of the stomach, is essential for the absorption of physiologic amounts of vitamin B_{12} in human beings; there is no change in intrinsic factor production throughout pregnancy. Nevertheless, during the latter half of gestation there is decreased maternal absorption of vitamin B_{12}, and serum B_{12} levels are low. The fetus draws on maternal B_{12} stores, and cord serum B_{12} levels are about twice those of maternal serum levels. There is no evidence that infants born to mothers with vitamin B_{12} deficiency have an overt avitaminosis or tend to develop pernicious anemia in early infancy, although they may have limited vitamin B_{12} stores.

MEGALOBLASTIC ANEMIA

Megaloblastic anemia of pregnancy may appear at any age during the childbearing years and tends to recur with increasing severity during successive pregnancies. The patients usually are multiparas living in deprived socioeconomic circumstances. Megaloblastic anemia may have either an acute or insidious onset, and clinical symptoms usually arise in the third trimester or in the puerperium. Presenting symptoms may include, inconstantly, one or more of the following: diarrhea; soreness or atrophy of papillae of the tongue; slight pedal edema; pearly-white coloration of the skin (as distinguished from the lemon-yellow pallor seen in true pernicious anemia); hepato- and splenomegaly; purpura and mucous membrane and retinal hemorrhages; and predisposition to pyrexia and septic complications.

Hematologic findings in peripheral blood are variable (Rae, Robb). The erythrocytes may be normocytic or macrocytic; if there is a coexistent iron deficiency, the cells may be hypochromic. The most constant erythrocyte change is macroovalocytosis. Nucleated red cells of normoblastic or megaloblastic types are difficult to demonstrate on peripheral blood smears; occasionally, there may be macrogranulocytes, hyper- or nonsegmented neutrophils, and macrometamyelocytes. As a rule, the reticulocyte count is normal, and platelet counts may be normal or slightly decreased. Bone marrow examination reveals increased cellularity with a mixed megaloblastic-normoblastic picture. Macrogranulocytes almost always are present. Occasionally, the classic megaloblast cannot be seen, and the marrow cannot be distinguished from that in pernicious anemia. Achlorhydria almost never is present, and maternal serum vitamin B_{12} levels are normal.

Management

Almost invariably, megaloblastic anemia of pregnancy and the puerperium is related to folic acid deficiency and very rarely results from lack of vitamin B_{12}. Patients therefore should respond promptly to therapeutic doses of folic acid in some form: folic acid, 30 mg daily orally, or sodium folate, 30 mg daily intramuscularly, administered daily for 10 days and then three times weekly. The clinical response is slower than in iron-deficiency anemia and may take from 2 to 6 weeks; response is more rapid postpartum than antepartum. Clinical improvement may be accompanied by a leukemoid reaction. If untreated, spontaneous remission often occurs after delivery.

In obstetric patients from lower socioeconomic groups or having culturally imposed dietary limitations, folic acid deficiency is almost endemic (Fletcher et al.). For some patients, a raw diet adequate in folic acid loses its value after excessive cooking. For such groups, the prophylactic administration of folic acid, 1.0 mg per day orally, should be prescribed as a routine supplementation in pregnancy, in addition to iron. Failure of a patient to respond quickly to this prophylactic treatment, or the development of megaloblastic anemia despite prophylaxis, mandates a rigorous investigation for possible vitamin B_{12} deficiency and pernicious anemia. Patients with pernicious anemia treated with folic acid alone are predisposed to the rapid development of neurologic changes related to vitamin B_{12} deficiency (van Nagell et al.). If maternal serum vitamin B_{12} levels are less than 100 μg per 100 mL, treatment must include vitamin B_{12}, 100 μg daily intramuscularly for a period of 10 days, followed by 50 μg intramuscularly three times weekly.

APLASTIC ANEMIA

Also known as refractory anemia, this condition is manifest by a significant diminution in all three formed blood elements, i.e., erythrocytes, leukocytes, and platelets. The association of aplastic anemia with pregnancy is rare, and in most instances its etiology in pregnancy does not differ from that in the nongravid patient (Collins et al.). The majority of cases are secondary in nature, resulting from exposure to any of a large variety of drugs or chemicals, an early stage of undiagnosed leukemia, or bone marrow depression from chronic infection or renal failure. Although many hematologists feel that primary aplastic anemia in adults represents merely an inability to determine the cause of the bone marrow depression, a small number of cases have been described in which gravid women develop an anemia or pancytopenia aplastic to all hematinic drugs and undergo spontaneous remission several months after delivery. Some patients who have this aplastic anemia in one pregnancy exhibit the same hematologic picture in subsequent pregnancies, and there is some suggestion that therapeutic abortion will alleviate the condition.

The diagnosis of aplastic anemia is suggested by greatly reduced numbers of erythrocytes, leukocytes, and platelets in the peripheral blood. The bone marrow shows extensive fatty replacement and initially a tendency toward hyperplasia, followed by hypoplasia. Serum and bone marrow iron stores are normal.

Management

The first step in the management of aplastic anemia, both in and outside of pregnancy, is a search for and removal of any possible precipitating factors. Endogenous factors include chronic nephritis, tuberculosis, rheumatoid arthritis, and aleukemic leukemia; of these, chronic pyelonephritis is by far the most frequently encountered, and the development of aplastic anemia during pregnancy mandates an investigation of the patient's renal function. Exogenous factors include drugs, chemicals, and particularly cosmetics, hair dyes, and permanent wave solutions. Success in this initial step does not assure bone marrow regeneration or even eventual recovery from the disease.

Management usually is supportive, keeping the patient alive while awaiting regeneration of the hematopoietic tissues. No known hematinic agents are of value. Antibiotics are used to combat infection. Corticosteroids are administered in an attempt to control hemorrhagic tendencies, but their use has not been encouraging. Blood transfusions are administered as necessary. Prior to delivery, the transfusion of platelets will reduce the probabilities of hemorrhagic complications.

In recent years, the administration of androgenic hormones in large doses has been part of the treatment of aplastic anemia, in an attempt to stimulate bone marrow regeneration. During pregnancy, this therapy carries the obvious risk of masculinization of the female fetus, and should be deferred until after delivery, if possible. Bone marrow transfusions create problems of tissue rejection and probably have no place in treatment during pregnancy.

Whether therapeutic abortion will interrupt the progress of aplastic anemia remains a matter of debate. In a very small number of patients, the course of the disease suggests that pregnancy produces an inhibitory effect on hematopoietic function. For most other patients with aplastic anemia, however, the pregnancy is purely coincidental. Usually, the interruption of pregnancy is based upon the patient's general physical condition. Provided the patient can be supported adequately through pregnancy, there will be no deleterious effect on the newborn.

HEMOLYTIC ANEMIA

This form of anemia occurs rarely in conjunction with pregnancy. In the majority of cases, hemolysis is associated with obvious factors such as malaria, infection with *Clostridium welchii,* or a variety of hemoglobinopathies (to be considered separately below).

Congenital spherocytosis is transmitted as an autosomal dominant and causes recurrent exacerbations of hemolytic anemia. Pregnancy appears to increase the frequency of these hemolytic episodes.

Occasionally, splenectomy may be indicated during pregnancy.

Another group of congenital hemolytic disorders are the results of red cell enzyme deficiencies: glucose 6-phosphate dehydrogenase (G6PD) and glutathione. G6PD deficiency is a sex-linked characteristic and is incompletely dominant. It has been estimated that 13 percent of American blacks carry this deficiency, transmitted by the X chromosome; the homozygous female patient is exceedingly rare. G6PD deficiency sensitizes the erythrocyte to hemolysis upon exposure to oxidizing agents, including sulfone drugs, salicylates, nitrofurantoin, and some vitamin K analogues.

Acquired hemolytic anemias may result from environmental factors such as autoimmune hemolytic disease, paroxysmal (cold) nocturnal hemoglobinuria, and ingestion of various toxic substances: phenylhydrazine, benzene, saponin, aniline, toluene, and phenacetin.

Hemolytic anemia apparently also may develop acutely during gestation for no apparent reason; this group of cases has been characterized as Lederer's anemia. Some cases are associated with the presence of circulating hemolysins or autoagglutinins, and may represent acquired hemolytic anemias of obscure etiology. In others, however, the Coombs' test is negative, and no explanation for the hemolytic episode can be found. Several patients have been reported who develop severe hemolytic anemia, requiring blood transfusions, in successive pregnancies, but whose hematologic status was normal interconceptionally.

Acute hemolysis presents with fever, headache, and backache, usually accompanied by anorexia, vomiting, and diarrhea. The liver and spleen become enlarged, the patient develops jaundice, and excessive urobilinogen appears in her urine. If intravascular hemolysis is very severe, there may also be hemoglobinuria. Anemia develops extremely rapidly, with hemoglobin levels dropping to 4 to 9 g per 100 mL. A blood smear shows anisocytosis, possibly spherocytosis, polychromasia, and many normoblasts. Reticulocytosis ranges around 10 to 25 percent. The bone marrow is normoblastic.

Management

The treatment of congenital spherocytosis is unrewarding. Meticulous prenatal care is necessary, iron and folic acid supplements should be prescribed, and blood transfusions administered as necessary. Splenectomy usually brings about a reversal of the hemolytic processes.

Other cases of hemolytic anemia can be divided into those with and without a positive Coombs' test. In patients with a negative Coombs' test, repeated blood transfusions are the mainstay of therapy. When the Coombs' test is positive, administration of corticosteroids and/or ACTH is a useful adjuvant to transfusion. The question of interruption of pregnancy must be highly individualized.

HEMOGLOBINOPATHIES IN PREGNANCY

In these disorders, the amount of normal hemoglobin A in the patient's red blood cells is diminished, either because the body cannot produce the globin necessary to form hemoglobin A (as in thalassemia) or because hemoglobin A is replaced by an abnormal hemoglobin (as in sickle-cell disease).

The hemoglobin molecule consists of two pairs of polypeptide chains, α and β, attached to a heme group which has the property of combining reversibly with oxygen. More than 20 abnormal hemoglobins are known; different types are caused by substitution of specific amino acids in either the α or β chains. In all cases, the heme portion of the molecule remains unaltered, and the oxygen-carrying capacity of the hemoglobin is unaffected. Hemoglobin A is electrophorectically normal hemoglobin. Hemoglobin F is alkaliresistant or "fetal" hemoglobin, normally found in large amounts in the fetus and newborn and in small amounts (up to 2 percent) in normal adults; in various hemoglobinopathies, hemoglobin F is present in increased amounts. Hemoglobin A_2 is a normal variant of hemoglobin A, separable on starch-block electrophoresis, and is increased significantly in patients with thalassemia minor. In hemoglobin S, substitution of a hydrophobic amino acid radical, valine, for a hydrophilic amino acid radical, glutamic acid, in the sixth position on the β chain of a normal hemoglobin molecule profoundly modifies the physical characteristics of the hemoglobin and is responsible for the clinical feature of "sickling." In hemoglobin C, the same glutamic acid radical in the β chain is replaced by lysine. Hemoglobins C and S are alleles of each other, and probably also of the thalassemia gene. All of the abnormal hemoglobins as well as the thalassemia gene are inherited as dominants, but other types of hemoglobin, including D, E, G, H, and others, are not necessarily alleles of C and S. In thalassemia, there is complete failure to synthesize either the α or β peptide chains from which the globin of hemoglobin A is formed, resulting in two types of thalassemia;

α-thalassemia, found primarily in southeast Asia, and β-thalassemia primarily distributed in the Mediterranean littoral. Thalassemia major occurs in the homozygous patient, while thalassemia minor is the heterozygous form of the abnormality.

Various genetic combinations of the abnormal hemoglobins are possible. It is generally agreed that the older clinical nomenclature should be replaced by a designation of the hemoglobinopathies in terms of the hemoglobin types and concentrations present in the individual patient. Thus, sickle-cell disease becomes hemoglobin SS disease; sickle-cell trait, hemoglobin AS (because the carrier usually has more A than S hemoglobin); sickle-cell hemoglobin C disease, hemoglobin SC disease; and sickle-cell β-thalassemia, β-thal SA disease. Different genetic combinations result in clinical disease of varying severity (see Table 31–6).

HEMOGLOBIN SS DISEASE

Hemoglobin SS disease (sickle-cell disease) is inherited as an autosomal dominant, transmitted equally by males and females, and may be found in an estimated 25,000 to 50,000 people in the United States, almost exclusively in the black population. In the affected homozygous individuals who have inherited an HbS gene from each parent, as much as 75 to 95 percent of hemoglobin is in the form of HbS, the remainder often being HbF. Heterozygous individuals (sickle-cell trait) usually have about 35 percent HbS, the remainder being HbA. There is no clear evidence that individuals with hemoglobin AS (trait) suffer any impairment of longevity or experience any abnormality either in pregnancy or in the nongravid state. These individuals are asymptomatic carriers of the genetic trait, and their number in the United States may be around 2 million. Identification of individuals with hemoglobin AS can be accomplished only with hemoglobin electrophoresis; sickle-cell screening tests ordinarily employed do not identify the heterozygote patient and are useless as a basis for genetic counseling (Fort).

HbS has the unique attribute that its reduced form has only about 1 percent of the solubility of oxyhemoglobin S and at the lower ranges of tissue oxygen tensions, 35 to 40 mmHg, it crystallizes out of solution. The exact mechanisms by which sickling results is not known but may be largely the effect of abnormally polymerized hemoglobin molecules pressing against and stretching the cell membrane; there also may be an intracellular gelation phenomenon involved, as well as other as yet undetermined factors. Once sickling occurs, the blood becomes increasingly viscid,

TABLE 31–6   Clinical Syndromes in Hemoglobinopathies

Disease	Clinical severity	Hemolytic crises	Splenomegaly	Severity of anemia
SS	+++	+++	±	+++
AS	±	−	−	−
SC	± to ++	− to ++	− to ++	+ to ++
SE	+	−	±	+
CA	−	−	−	−
CC	+	−	± to ++	+
EE	+	−	±	+
Thalassemia major	+++	−	+++	+++
Thalassemia minor	− to +	−	− to +	− to +
Thal-S	++	+	− to ++	++
Thal-C	+ to ++	−	− to +	− to ++
Thal-E	+ to +++	±	+++	+ to +++

and multiple intracapillary thromboses occur, particularly in the bones, spleen, gastrointestinal tract, and kidneys. The erythrocytes are mechanically, but not osmotically, very fragile, and are rapidly removed from the circulation by the phagocytes of the reticuloendothelial system; a chronic hemolytic-type of anemia results. The rate of hemoglobin synthesis may be five times greater than normal, resulting in secondary folic acid deficiency (Anderson).

The symptoms of hemoglobin SS disease usually start in infancy, and the natural history of the disease is a state of chronic ill health with mild hemolytic anemia, interrupted from time to time by acute hemolytic or painful crises precipitated by hypoxygenation, stasis of blood flow, or infection (reducing blood pH levels). The patients often are tall and thin, with elongated extremities and chronic ulceration of the legs. Early in life, there may be splenomegaly; later, after multiple infarctions and fibrosis, the spleen is shrunken. A blood count shows a normocytic, orthochromic anemia, with polychromasia indicative of constant reticulocytosis. The majority of patients become adjusted to their anemia and remain relatively free of symptoms with hemoglobin levels around 8.0 per 100 mL.

Crises are precipitated by any type of infection or decreased oxygenation. In the *hemolytic* crisis, anemia develops with great rapidity, there is marked leukocytosis, and jaundice is present. Fever may reach 103°F (39.4°C). A *painful* crisis is caused by sludging of sickled cells in various organs, with resultant capillary thromboses and infarctions, and may present with pain in the lower back or long bones, abdominal pain and vomiting, hemoptysis from pulmonary in-

farction, hematuria, or central nervous system signs and symptoms. Frequently, both types of crises occur together. Death may occur during a crisis from heart failure or infarction in the heart or brain.

Effect of Hemoglobin SS Disease on Pregnancy

Women with hemoglobin SS disease have reduced fertility potential. The incidence of hemoglobin SS disease is about 1 in 600 among American blacks, while its incidence in pregnancy is far less, in the range of 1 in 1500 to 1 in 3000 among black patients. Some patients with hemoglobin SS disease die before reaching the reproductive years. Others are so incapacitated that they are incapable of normal sexual function or elect not to conceive. Some undoubtedly pass through pregnancy without detection of the disease. Finally, women with hemoglobin SS disease who reproduce have fewer pregnancies than the mean (Perkins).

Pregnant patients with hemoglobin SS disease have a higher incidence of abortion, stillbirths, neonatal death, and premature labor (Hendrickse et al., 1972a). Overall fetal wastage is approximately 36 percent. The cause of this perinatal loss is not known; examination of the placentas has failed to demonstrate damage from sickling or infarction. There is no increase in the incidence of congenital anomalies, although there is some tendency to intrauterine growth retardation. Although the infants of mothers with hemoglobin SS disease must be considered "high-risk" infants, only intensive newborn care can be recommended (Dajani et al.)

Patients with hemoglobin AS (trait) have normal fertility and no problem during pregnancy. It has been suggested that they may be subject to a higher incidence of urinary tract infections, but this is not definitively demonstrated. The pregnancies do not result in an increased incidence of abortion, stillbirth, prematurity, or congenital anomaly, and the newborn infants are unaffected (Platt).

Effect of Pregnancy on Hemoglobin SS Disease

Pregnancy and hemoglobin SS disease are a hazardous combination. Maternal death may occur suddenly during the last trimester, during labor, and in the puerperium, with a rate as high as 10 percent. Patients tend to have at least one crisis during gestation, most frequently during the third trimester or after delivery. Maternal mortality seems to increase with each successive pregnancy, but the increasing age of the mother and the natural life history of the disease process may be factors in this.

The patient with hemoglobin SS disease has an irreversible, hereditary, and ultimately fatal disorder which not only compromises her reproductive ability but also interferes with her capability of caring for children. Surgical sterilization should be available if desired, and abortion permitted if requested (Fort et al.).

Management

The primary problem is the detection of the patient with HbSS disease. To this end, all patients theoretically at risk presenting in pregnancy should be screened for sickling, and all pregnant women with chronic anemia should have hemoglobin electrophoresis as part of their hematologic evaluation. These patients must be seen frequently throughout gestation, and hospitalized and treated intensively at the earliest sign of infection or crisis. Air travel during pregnancy in unpressurized aircraft should be avoided.

Iron deficiency is not a characteristic of HbSS disease, and administration of iron will not influence the anemia present (Anderson). Because of the increased rate of hemopoiesis, however, there usually exists a folic acid deficiency which may become more severe as the pregnancy progresses. Patients with HbSS disease should receive prophylactic folic acid supplementation, 5.0 mg daily, throughout gestation (Freeman, Ruth).

Currently, there is no standard treatment for HbSS disease other than supportive measures. Several agents alleged to minimize or eliminate the sickling phenomenon have been tested in small groups of nongravid patients; these include infusions of urea and potassium cyanate. The success of this therapy during pregnancy and the possible effects on the fetus have yet to be determined.

The place of transfusion in the treatment of HbSS disease in pregnancy also remains moot. Previously, the role of blood transfusion was reserved to the maintenance of the patient's hemoglobin level at around 7.0 to 8.0 g per 100 mL, the level to which the patient has become accustomed; it had been suggested that blood transfusion beyond this level might worsen the condition and even precipitate an aplastic anemia. Current thinking has been more aggressive therapeutically. Exchange transfusions with packed red cells containing HbA, replacing 2000 mL or more of the patient's blood and elevating hemoglobin and hematocrit levels to normal, have been remarkably successful (Edwards, Saáry). In theory, the patient's flawed erythrocytes are replaced with normal adult red cells which will remain in the maternal circulation for 2 to 3 weeks, while at the same time the patient's normal hematopoiesis is suppressed and the creation of new HbSS-containing erythrocytes diminished. To maintain this effect, the patient requires multiple transfusions during the course of gestation, a procedure which has inherent risk in itself. It has been suggested that only intensive and aggressive prenatal care, including exchange transfusions, heparinization, antibiotic prophylaxis, and folic acid and iron supplementation, can reduce both maternal mortality and fetal wastage in patients with HbSS disease (Hendrickse, Watson-Williams).

HEMOGLOBIN CC DISEASE

Very few cases of hemoglobin CC disease have been reported in association with pregnancy. Hemoglobin C is found in approximately 2 to 3 percent of American blacks, and the frequency of hemoglobin CC disease is about 1 in 6000 in that population. The symptoms of the disease are mild. The hemolytic anemia usually is well compensated; splenomegaly may be a significant clinical problem. The patient's erythrocytes characteristically appear as target cells on blood smear.

With HbCC disease, fertility and life-span are not diminished. Maternal mortality and fetal wastage are not increased significantly. Management during pregnancy is limited to usual prenatal care, plus iron and folic acid supplementation (Hendrickse et al., 1972b).

HEMOGLOBIN SC DISEASE

The combination of hemoglobins C and S occurs in approximately 0.05 percent of American blacks and presents a clinical picture similar to HbSS disease, including chronic hemolytic anemia, tissue infarction, and sequestration of erythrocytes. Patients with HbSC disease usually become symptomatic later in life, often survive the childbearing years, have normal fertility, and show only slightly increased fetal wastage (Freeman, Ruth).

The course of gestation in patients with HbSC disease often is complicated by anemia, bone pain, pulmonary infarction, urinary tract infection, and toxemia of pregnancy. The number of hemolytic crises may increase markedly in the last trimester. The fetus of a mother with HbSC disease has a decreased chance of survival in utero, lower birth weight, and increased neonatal mortality; all three risks are lesser in degree than that found in HbSS disease (Hendrickse et al., 1972b).

Management during pregnancy is identical with that discussed for HbSS disease.

THE THALASSEMIAS

A genetically determined disorder, the thalassemias are characterized by a depressed rate of synthesis of one of the component polypeptide chains of hemoglobin. Homozygous α-thalassemia results in the depressed production of all three normal hemoglobins; most of the hemoglobin mass exists as tetramers of gamma chains (hemoglobin Bart's). Affected individuals give the clinical and pathologic appearance of hydrops fetalis at birth and generally die in late pregnancy or in the early neonatal period. Homozygous β-thalassemia results in diminished production of beta chains, decrease in HbA concentration, and increased concentrations of HbA_2 and HbF. The affected patient presents with severe anemia (Cooley's anemia), in which circulating hemoglobin levels adequate to maintain life can be achieved only by multiple, periodic transfusions, and rarely survives into the reproductive years (Freedman). Pregnancy in patients with thalassemia major (homozygous thalassemia) has not been reported.

Heterozygous thalassemia (thalassemia minor) is not as serious a condition. The thalassemia gene may combine with a normal gene for HbA, or with any of the genes for abnormal hemoglobins (that is, S, C, or E). In patients with thalassemia minor, the erythrocytes contain hemoglobin A, hemoglobin F, and up to 10 percent of hemoglobin A_2. Chronic hemolytic ane-

mia is present; the erythrocytes are hypochromic and unusually thin, and are mechanically but not osmotically more fragile. The patient does not exhibit iron deficiency; hypochromia results from failure to produce sufficient hemoglobin A to utilize the iron already present. The peripheral blood picture includes a hypochromic, microcytic anemia, with anisocytosis and poikilocytosis, stippling, polychromasia, and target cells. The bone marrow, in attempting to maintain normal hemoglobin levels, is actively normoblastic.

Patients with heterozygous thalassemia have normal fertility and little difficulty during pregnancy. They are subject to neither excessive maternal mortality nor undue fetal wastage (Pakes et al.). Treatment of the chronic anemia with iron is unnecessary and useless, and even may lead over long periods of time to hemochromatosis. Folic acid supplementation always should be administered, because of the increased rate of erythropoiesis.

Thalassemia-S disease results from the combination of the thalassemia gene with the gene for HbS and carries the same maternal and fetal risks in pregnancy as does HbSC disease (see above) (van Enk et al.). The very rare combination of thalassemia with HbC results in a pregnancy prognosis similar to that in HbCC disease (see above).

THROMBOCYTOPENIC PURPURA

Purpura is a term applied to a generalized intra- or subdermal extravasation of blood, a feature of a variety of hematologic disorders including defects in capillary hemostasis, coagulopathies, and platelet disorders in either number or function.

Idiopathic thrombocytopenic purpura (ITP) is characterized by purpuric skin lesions, easy bruising, and hemorrhages from body orifices, associated with a reduction in the number of blood platelets. The disease occurs most frequently in young females, in both acute and chronic forms. The acute form of ITP usually occurs in children, often preceded by an upper respiratory infection. The chronic form has a gradual onset and occurs more frequently in adults. The Rumpel-Leede test always is positive. The history must exclude recent drug ingestion, exposure to noxious substances, allergies, recent infections, toxemia of pregnancy, or evidence of any other disease. Hematologically, the patient's peripheral blood shows a platelet count of 100,000 per milliliter or less, prolonged bleeding time, clot retraction time, and prothrombin consumption time, but normal clotting time; and normal plasma clotting factors and cell counts.

Bone marrow biopsy shows normal or increased numbers of megakaryocytes.

ITP results from a decrease in the rate of platelet formation from megakaryocytes because of splenic inhibition, from an increased rate of platelet destruction by the spleen, or from a combination of these factors. The pathogenesis of the disease is related to autoimmune mechanisms, to a deficiency of factors needed for platelet formation, and to platelet suppression by metabolites or splenic dysfunction. Circulating platelet auto- or isoagglutinins have been demonstrated in maternal blood. These antibodies damage or cause agglutination of platelets, which then are removed from the circulation by the spleen; the occurrence of transient ITP in infants born to mothers with ITP further supports this pathogenetic mechanism. The reason for the concomitant capillary fragility in this disorder is not known.

EFFECT OF PREGNANCY ON ITP

ITP does not decrease fertility potential, and the natural course of the maternal disease is not altered appreciably by pregnancy.

EFFECT OF ITP ON PREGNANCY

The presence of maternal ITP adds formidable complications to pregnancy, and in particular to delivery (Heys). There have been some reports of excessive antepartum hemorrhage. There is increased risk of hemorrhage and hematoma formation during delivery and the postpartum period primarily at the sites of lacerations or incisions. Myometrial contractility provides adequate hemostasis at the placental site, and uterine hemorrhage is almost never a problem. The reported maternal mortality is increased (approximately 5.5 percent), but only in patients who have not undergone splenectomy prior to gestation, or in whom splenectomy was attempted during pregnancy or the puerperium. Women with splenectomy prior to pregnancy apparently are not subject to this increased risk (Goodhue, Evans).

EFFECT OF ITP ON THE FETUS

Approximately 65 percent of infants born to patients with ITP experience signs and symptoms of platelet deficiency. The development of ITP in the newborn results from the placental transfer of maternal platelet antibody to the fetus. The process in the newborn is self-limiting, and subsides as the acquired antibody globulin dissipates. Labor and delivery are critical

periods for the affected infant, intracranial hemorrhage being the most frequent cause of death. Fetal scalp blood samples can detect the infant with deficient platelets in utero. The risk of bleeding from obstetric trauma is minimized by early cesarean section. (Ayromlooi). Once this period of obstetric trauma is passed without serious hemorrhage, the probability of subsequent life-threatening bleeding is minimal. Purpura or thrombocytopenia may appear at birth or during the first few months of life; usually, if purpura will develop, it appears during the first neonatal day. Some infants may develop rectal bleeding, cephalohematomas, and/or intracranial bleeding. The severity of the neonatal thrombocytopenia bears no relationship to the state of the maternal disease. Neonatal purpura has been observed in infants born many years after the last clinical or laboratory evidence of maternal ITP!

In the majority of affected infants, no treatment is necessary, and the bleeding tendency resolves in 2 to 3 months. Administration of steroids to the newborn may be helpful in minimizing clinical manifestations of the disease. Platelet transfusions may be necessary in severe cases, but also may sensitize the infant to foreign platelets. Theoretically, exchange transfusion would be a reasonable treatment.

A second origin of neonatal platelet depression must be borne in mind. In about 20 percent of cases, the mother does not have, and never has had, ITP, but has become isoimmunized to platelet antigens by virtue of past infusion with blood products or by transplacental transfusion with fetal platelets. In such cases, the mother is clinically and immunologically normal and produces antibodies not against her own, but only against foreign platelets. In these patients with transient *isoimmune thrombocytopenic purpura,* the neonatal care is similar to that described for ITP (Pearson et al.).

MANAGEMENT

The management of ITP is the same regardless of pregnancy. Administration of ACTH and/or corticosteroids diminishes capillary fragility, reduces the bleeding time, slows the destruction of platelets, and may even enhance platelet production. Splenectomy eliminates an organ which is responsible for the removal from the circulation of damaged but possibly still viable and functional platelets, may be a source of production of platelet antibodies, and may exercise an inhibitory effect on the production of platelets from megakaryocytes. The individual response to splenectomy is variable; a good therapeutic response seems to occur primarily in patients in whom a platelet antibody can be demonstrated. Finally, platelet transfusions are valuable as short-term measures, remaining in the recipient's circulation only for a few hours. In patients with platelet antibodies, the survival of transfused platelets is brief; in the absence of platelet antibodies, platelet transfusion may dramatically stop severe hemorrhage in minutes. A platelet transfusion may be administered prophylactically to the mother during labor, anticipating episiotomy or perineal lacerations (Territo et al.).

Patients with ITP who desire to become pregnant should be advised to undergo splenectomy before attempting conception. When maternal ITP appears for the first time during pregnancy, management depends on the severity of the maternal status. In the face of severe thrombocytopenia or bleeding, steroid therapy should be started at once. Prednisone, 40 to 60 mg daily, or its equivalent should be administered for 1 to 2 weeks, and then the dosage reduced gradually to 10 to 20 mg daily. If there is no rise in platelets over a period of 4 to 6 months, splenectomy must be considered. Some have suggested that splenectomy should be performed if indicated, irrespective of the presence of a pregnancy; more recent evidence proscribes this operation during pregnancy or the immediate puerperium because of attendant maternal and fetal mortalities. In general, if the platelet count is above 40,000 to 50,000 per cubic millimeter and there is no excessive bleeding, the patient should be maintained on steroid therapy during pregnancy, and splenectomy performed 3 to 6 months postpartum. Vaginal delivery is the route of choice, but cesarean section, although extremely hazardous, should be carried out for proper obstetric indications. ITP, properly treated, is not an indication for surgical sterilization, and the risk of abortion may approximate the risk of carrying the pregnancy to term.

COAGULOPATHIES IN PREGNANCY

Normal blood is unique in its ability to remain fluid while circulating in blood vessels and yet to clot firmly within 10 minutes of coming into contact with a foreign surface. This solidification of the blood results from the transformation of the soluble protein, fibrinogen, into a web of insoluble fibrin in which are enmeshed erythrocytes, leukocytes, and platelets. Many factors involved in the coagulation process have been identified and their contributions assessed. For a review of current theories of coagulation mechanisms, see Chap. 9.

CHANGES IN BLOOD COAGULATION DURING PREGNANCY

Both fibrinogen and factor VIII show progressive increases from the end of the first trimester to term, when the fibrinogen level may be twice, and the factor VIII level three times, above normal. In addition, the stress of labor may cause a further increase in factor VIII level, which persists for 7 to 10 days postpartum. Significant increases also have been reported during pregnancy in factors V, VII, IX, and X. The cause of the increase in concentration of these blood coagulation factors is not known, but probably is related to the hormonal state of the gravid woman; similar changes are reported in women taking hormonal contraceptive drugs. However, the relationship between in vitro tests of blood coagulation and in vivo coagulation and thrombosis is not simple, and the elevated levels of blood coagulation factors cannot be considered purely as a state of hypercoagulability. Toward term, there also occur increases in circulating plasminogen and proactivator substances.

The blood of the normal newborn usually is deficient in factors II, VII, IX, and X, and the levels of these factors fall still lower in the first few days of life, rising to normal adult levels in about 2 weeks. The deficiency of these vitamin K–dependent clotting factors results principally from immaturity of the newborn liver and poor stores of vitamin K. Spontaneous bleeding from the gastrointestinal tract or the umbilical stump may occur if the bleeding diathesis is severe enough. The bleeding state may be eliminated by the administration to the mother of vitamin K_1 prophylactically during the week preceding delivery. Also, vitamin K_1, 1 to 2 mg, may be administered intramuscularly to the neonate on the first day of life. If full-blown hemorrhagic disease develops, vitamin K_1, 1 to 2 mg, should be administered intramuscularly daily until the laboratory tests have returned to normal; occasionally, blood or plasma transfusions may be required to replace hemoglobin or blood coagulation factors.

Unlike the vitamin K–dependent clotting factors, factor VIII is present in normal amounts in the newborn infant's blood, but not at the elevated maternal level near term. Very little factor VIII crosses the placenta from the mother to the fetus.

CONGENITAL COAGULATION FACTOR DEFICIENCIES

Defects in the blood coagulation process usually are due to a lack of one of the essential clotting factors, although occasionally some inhibitory substance may interfere with the reactions between clotting factors. Only a deficiency of factor XII (Hageman factor) is not associated with a clinical hemorrhagic disorder. In the congenital bleeding states, usually only one factor is deficient. In general, treatment consists of raising the blood concentration of the missing clotting factor to a level compatible with hemostasis by intravenous infusion of a substance rich in the requisite factor (see Table 31–7) (Biggs, MacFarlane).

Factor VIII Deficiency (Hemophilia)

Classical hemophilia is a sex-linked, recessive bleeding disorder resulting from a congenital deficiency of factor VIII and accounts for more than 90 percent of cases of hereditary bleeding. Males are affected primarily, although there are a few reports of females involved. Deficiency of factor VIII may be partial or complete, and there is good correlation between the blood level of factor VIII and the severity of the bleeding manifestation. Because of a lack of factor VIII, there is a failure of formation of the intrinsic activator of prothrombin, delayed and impaired conversion of prothrombin to thrombin, and delayed fibrin formation. Treatment consists of replacing the missing factor.

Factor IX Deficiency (Christmas Disease)

The condition clinically cannot be distinguished from hemophilia, and also is a sex-linked congenital bleeding disorder.

Factor I (Fibrinogen) Deficiency

This condition is extremely rare, and only 30 cases have been described. Because of the absence of fibrinogen, the blood is completely incoagulable even upon the addition of massive amounts of thrombin. Both males and females have been affected; several of the patients described have been born of consanguineous marriages. The hemorrhagic manifestations may be severe and may include bleeding from the umbilicus at birth, hemarthroses, bleeding from lacerations and sites of venipuncture, and subcutaneous hemorrhages. Despite the complete absence of fibrinogen from the blood, the bleeding episodes usually are less severe than those found in hemophilia; women with this condition rarely have menorrhagia. The minimum levels of fibrinogen replacement required for hemostasis are thought to be 50 to 100 mg per 100 mL.

Factors II, V, VII, and X Deficiencies

Isolated congenital absences of these factors have been described. Either sex may be affected, and the hereditary factors seem to be autosomal recessive genes. The clinical bleeding diatheses usually are mild. Occasionally, in an affected female, menorrhagia may be troublesome and usually can be controlled by hormonal contraceptive agents.

Factor XI (PTA) Deficiency

This deficiency is familial, is attributed to an autosomal recessive gene, and affects both sexes equally. Bleeding is not very severe and usually follows serious trauma or surgery. Epistaxis and hematuria are reported, and menorrhagia is encountered frequently.

Factor XII (Hageman Factor) Deficiency

Patients with factor XII deficiency do not present a clinical problem and rarely bleed excessively, although their blood may take hours to coagulate in vitro. At present, these patients remain a coagulation hypothesis enigma.

Factor XIII (Fibrin Stabilizing Factor) Deficiency

In affected patients, both the blood fibrinogen level and its conversion to fibrin are normal, but the fibrin plugs formed are weak and easily disrupted. As a result, the patient presents with severe bleeding after injury, delayed healing, and abnormal scar formation.

Von Willebrand's Disease

This condition originally was defined as a bleeding tendency affecting either sex transmitted as an autosomal dominant and characterized by a prolonged bleeding time, normal clotting time, and normal platelet count. The more severely affected patients have low levels of factor VIII, and there is a correlation between the degree of factor VIII deficiency and the severity of the bleeding diathesis. More recent evidence also suggests that these patients have abnormal platelet function. Although both conditions are based on factor VIII deficiency, the similarities and differences between von Willebrand's disease and hemophilia have formed the basis for fundamental coagulation research.

Clinically, the affected patient shows easy bruisability, bleeding from superficial lacerations and from mucous membranes, epistaxis, gastrointestinal hemorrhage, and often severe menorrhagia. Postpartum hemorrhage has been a problem, but may be minimized in some patients by the naturally occurring increase in factor VIII concentration in late gestation (Noller et al.). Treatment consists of the infusion of factor VIII–rich materials and packing the bleeding site if accessible. Menorrhagia may be controlled by the administration of hormonal contraceptive agents; curettage of the uterus to control bleeding rarely helps and may make the blood loss worse (Evans, 1971).

ACQUIRED COAGULATION FACTOR DEFICIENCIES

While in the congenital coagulation factor deficiencies almost always only one coagulation factor is lacking, in acquired bleeding disorders several factors are usually deficient. Treatment again depends on raising the blood levels of the missing coagulation factors (Table 31-7), and if possible elimination of the cause of the coagulation defect.

Factors II, VII, IX, and X Deficiencies

The most frequent cause of acquired hemorrhagic diathesis is hepatic dysfunction resulting either from hepatocellular damage (i.e., cirrhosis) or lack of vitamin K. Fibrinogen and factors II, VII, IX, and X (and possibly also factor V) are produced in the liver, and factors II, VII, IX, and X require vitamin K for their synthesis. In hepatocellular disease, synthesis of the above clotting factors may be impaired despite the presence of adequate amounts of vitamin K. The combined deficiencies result in a bleeding diathesis

TABLE 31-7 Treatment of Coagulation Disorders

Factor deficient	Therapeutic materials
I	Fresh-frozen plasma
	Fibrinogen concentrate
II	Fresh-frozen plasma
	Plasma concentrates
V	Fresh-frozen plasma
VII	Fresh-frozen plasma
	Plasma concentrates
VIII	Fresh-frozen plasma
	Cryoprecipitated fibrinogen fraction of human plasma
	AHG concentrates (human plasma)
	AHG concentrates (animal plasma)
IX	Fresh-frozen plasma
	Plasma concentrates
X	Fresh-frozen plasma
	Plasma concentrates
XI	Fresh-frozen plasma
XII	Fresh-frozen plasma
XIII	Fresh frozen plasma

which may be severe and may be exaggerated by concurrent hypersplenism and/or thrombocytopenia.

Vitamin K deficiency may result from failure of vitamin K production by the intestinal flora (as in hemorrhagic disease of the newborn or with the use of broad-spectrum antibiotics), failure of absorption of vitamin K from the intestine (as in steatorrhea or obstructive jaundice), or functionally by inhibition of vitamin K activity by a coumarin-type anticoagulation drug. Bleeding due to vitamin K deficiency usually can be controlled by the administration of vitamin K or its analogues.

Factor I Deficiency (Defibrination Syndrome)

This is an acquired bleeding disorder in which there is depletion of various clotting factors as well as thrombocytopenia. The onset usually is acute, and the hemorrhagic diathesis severe. The blood is completely incoagulable even with the addition of large amounts of thrombin; hence the name *defibrination syndrome.* The etiologic factors are complex, and at least two important mechanisms, are implicated in the development of this syndrome.

1. Intravascular coagulation may be initiated by the release into the circulation of tissue or tissue fluids, with resulting generation of thromboplastin in the circulating blood. This activates the extrinsic coagulation process, converts prothrombin to thrombin, and then fibrinogen to fibrin, as well as depleting factors V and VIII. This chain reaction places the patient in double jeopardy: not only does a coagulopathy develop but simultaneously multiple microemboli form in the circulation and may lodge in the small vessels of the liver, kidney, or brain (McKay).

2. Activation of the fibrinolytic system may result in the destruction of coagulation factors, including fibrin, fibrinogen, factor V, and factor VIII. The hemorrhagic diathesis which develops further is complicated by the fact that some breakdown products of fibrinogen act as antithrombins or as inhibitors of fibrin polymerization, adding an anticoagulant effect to the clinical picture. The fibrinolytic system may be activated by a variety of factors, including disseminated intravascular coagulation.

The defibrination syndrome occurs with moderate frequency in patients with amniotic fluid embolism, septic abortion, hydatidiform mole, missed abortion, and toxemia of pregnancy. It also is associated with surgical procedures on the lung, prostate, and pancreas, mismatched blood transfusion, the use of an extracorporeal pump, and is seen as a component of the generalized Schwartzman reaction. Management consists of replacing the depleted clotting factors by transfusions of fresh-frozen plasma and fibrinogen, blocking the intravascular coagulation process by the administration of heparin, rarely by the infusion of an antifibrinolytic agent such as ϵ-aminocaproic acid, and, where possible, by elimination of the precipitating cause.

Circulating Anticoagulants

Occasionally, a hemorrhagic diathesis may be caused by the appearance in the blood of substances which interfere with coagulation by inactivating or destroying one of the coagulation factors or by inhibiting some reaction between factors. The most frequently encountered are substances which act against factor VIII. These may develop in hemophiliacs who have received numerous transfusions of factor VIII–rich materials, and are thought to represent an immune response. Circulating inhibitors of factor VIII also may arise in women following childbirth, and in association with rheumatoid arthritis, regional ileitis, and penicillin allergy. The presence of this inhibitor results in a hemophilia-like state which is difficult to treat, since infused factor VIII rapidly is destroyed (Marengo-Rowe et al.).

Patients with disseminated lupus erythematosus sometimes develop inhibitors which interfere with the reaction between factors VIII and IX, or between factors V and X. These inhibitors may be one of the abnormal proteins produced in this disease.

MYELOPROLIFERATIVE DISORDERS

THE LEUKEMIAS

The leukemias are proliferative, neoplastic disorders of the blood-forming tissues. Any of the different types of blood cells may be involved in the neoplastic process. The disease may be acute or chronic; in the former, the course of the disease may be measured in weeks or months. Myeloid leukemia is the most frequently encountered form, both in the acute and chronic categories. Usually the patient is known to have the disease before conception occurs, but occasionally it first is diagnosed during pregnancy in the investigation of splenomegaly or a refractory anemia.

Effect of Pregnancy on Leukemia

Pregnancy has no direct effect on the course of leukemia. Interruption of pregnancy does not affect the progress of the disease in any way. Pregnancy is never a reason to proscribe or delay the application of standard therapeutic measures to the patient with acute leukemia; the risk to the mother is so great that the presence of a fetus must be ignored (Bhoopathi et al.). In a patient with chronic leukemia or leukemia in remission, the risks to the fetus of maternal therapy may merit more consideration.

Effect of Leukemia on Pregnancy

The coexistence of pregnancy with acute or chronic leukemia is rare (Yahia et al.). Except in the patient with acute disease in whom infiltration of the uterus and ovaries has reduced fertility potential, leukemia does not interfere with conception. The incidence of spontaneous abortion is increased in acute leukemia, but near normal in the chronic disease. The course of pregnancy may be stormy, complicated by anemia, bleeding, infections, and drug toxicity (Ewing, Whitaker). Many physiologic changes additionally may burden the gravid patient: jaundice, renal failure, electrolyte imbalance, and general mental and physical ill health. There is a fetal loss of approximately 30 percent, resulting from stillbirth and prematurity. The maternal mortality from leukemia during pregnancy has been reduced markedly by the development and application of more effective therapy (Willoughby).

Effect of Leukemia on the Fetus

Effects of this disorder on the fetus depend in great measure on the mother's status. If the mother survives to deliver at or near term, the infant is at no increased risk. Maternal leukemia does not result in intrauterine growth retardation; low birth weight infants frequently are encountered, however, as a result of premature labor and delivery. Congenital anomalies in infants of untreated mothers have been deemed coincidental. Two major considerations which merit further discussion are the possibility of transmission of the disease to the fetus and the fetal effects of maternal therapy.

Theoretically, there is little to protect the fetus against intrauterine transmission of maternal leukemia. The placental barrier is incomplete, and both normal and malignant blood cells easily may gain access to the fetal circulation. The fetus has an immature immunologic system, particularly in early gestation, and the possibility of fetal tolerance of foreign cells is increased. Fetal cells have a prolonged exposure to the same (unknown) etiologic agents which have produced the disease in the mother. Finally, a constitutional predisposition to the development of leukemia might be transmitted from mother to infant. The question remains moot. At least three such cases have been reported, but must represent rare exceptions (Wintrobe). Furthermore, it is a fact that in the rare cases of congenital leukemia recorded, the mothers never themselves suffered from the disease during pregnancy or for at least 2 to 3 years thereafter.

Cytotoxic agents form the basis for the treatment of leukemia. Alkylating agents such as Myleran, triethylenemelamine, chlorambucil, and cyclophosphamide are not particularly harmful to the embryo (Hardin). Antimetabolites, such as Aminopterin, methotrexate, and mercaptopurine have disastrous effects on the fetus; abortion, fetal resorption, and massive fetal anomalies have been reported following the use of these agents in the first trimester. The risk of fetal injury is decreased after the period of maximum organogenesis is passed.

Management

The pregnant patient with leukemia should be treated for her disease as if the pregnancy did not coexist. Immediate control of the patient's hematologic problems is crucial, and steroids, alkylating agents, and antimetabolites should be administered as indicated. For both the mother and the fetus, uncontrolled leukemia is more dangerous than any of the therapeutic agents to be employed. Unless antimetabolites are employed in the first trimester of gestation, induced abortion is not necessary; if folic acid antagonists have been used during the first trimester, abortion is recommended because of the high incidence of fetal anomaly resulting. The question of termination of pregnancy, however, rests on other bases as well as on medical indications: for instance, the likelihood of orphaning an infant born to a mother destined for early incapacitation or death. The patient and her family obviously must participate in this decision.

If the pregnancy continues, the fact that the alkylating agents and antimetabolites used in treatment of the mother may produce myelosuppression, anemia, and even megaloblastosis must be borne in mind. Adequate dietary supplements of iron and folic acid should be prescribed for the mother, and maintenance of hemoglobin levels by transfusion may become necessary. Delivery should be accomplished in accord with obstetric indications, with due regard for possible maternal thrombocytopenia and hemorrhagic tendencies.

HODGKIN'S DISEASE

Hodgkin's disease differs from other forms of lymphomas in its granulomatous nature and the occurrence of toxic states with fever. The disease has a bimodal age distribution, the first mode occurring between 15 to 34 years, the second over 50 years of age. Hodgkin's disease is the most frequent primary lymph gland disorder encountered during pregnancy, occurring in approximately 1 in 6000 deliveries. Onset of the disease usually is manifest with the onset of adenopathy, with or without systemic signs or symptoms. Painless, progressive enlargement of superficial lymph nodes may be followed by malaise, anorexia, weight loss, nausea, vomiting, fever, and/or pruritus. The cause of the disease remains unknown. Definitive diagnosis of Hodgkin's disease must be made before the institution of therapy and can only be made by biopsy. The clinical course of the disease is characterized by great variability, and many patients survive in relatively good health for many years.

Effect of Pregnancy on Hodgkin's Disease

Pregnancy does not adversely affect the course of the maternal disease nor shorten the mean survival time. Exacerbations of the disease during pregnancy or in the puerperium occur no more frequently than in the nongravid patient (Barry et al.).

Effect of Hodgkin's Disease on Pregnancy

Early in the course of the disease, the patient's general health is relatively good, and there is no decrease in fertility potential nor increase in rates of abortion, prematurity, or perinatal loss. Pregnancy wastage later in the course of the maternal disease, manifest by increased rates of abortion and fetal death in utero, depends primarily on the state of the mother's general health.

Effect of Hodgkin's Disease on the Fetus

One report in the medical literature records two cases in which the maternal disease was transmitted to the fetus (Kasdon). There has been no corroboration of this occurrence in several hundred other cases reported.

Management

Each case of Hodgkin's disease must be managed individually. If the patient's condition permits delay in instituting therapy, this should be deferred until after the first trimester of pregnancy (Lacher, Geller). On the other hand, if the patient with chronic disease is on chemotherapy when she becomes pregnant, abortion is recommended only if antimetabolites have been employed. X-ray therapy may be employed during therapy if provisions can be made to shield the fetus (D'Angio, Nisce). In other respects, all necessary supportive measures must be taken to ensure the patient's general well-being.

POLYCYTHEMIA

Polycythemia vera (erythremia) is a disease of unknown cause, insidious onset, and slow, chronic course. Only less than 10 percent of affected patients are less than 40 years of age. Affected males predominate over females in a ratio of 2:1. Hence the association of polycythemia with pregnancy should be rare; the paucity of reports on the combination, however, raises questions about possible impairment of fertility in affected patients.

The diagnosis of polycythemia vera depends on an elevated hematocrit in the absence of a discernible cause for secondary polycythemia, such as chronic heart disease, pulmonary disability, extreme obesity, chronic renal disease, or erythropoietin-producing tumors. Among affected patients, 20 percent have concomitant thrombocytopenia, and 60 to 70 percent have splenomegaly (Centrone et al.).

From the few cases reported, only suggestions as to the possible interaction of pregnancy and polycythemia can be derived. Pregnancy did not have an unfavorable influence on the course of the maternal disease. In almost all patients, the erythrocyte count remained in good control throughout pregnancy without therapy; it is the consensus that this represents a hemodilution effect rather than suppression of erythropoiesis. Hemodilution also may account for the absence of reports of thrombosis in these cases. A fetal salvage rate of only 53 percent is given, secondary to an increased rate of early abortion, and elevated perinatal mortality related to premature delivery. There is no evidence of effect of the maternal disease on the surviving fetus.

Management

Theoretically, maintenance of hematocrit below 50 percent will decrease the risk of abnormal bleeding and thrombosis and permit increased tissue perfusion and oxygenation by reducing blood viscosity. Since various forms of radiotherapy are best avoided during pregnancy, the lower hematocrit may be achieved by phlebotomy as indicated (Ruch, Klein). There is no medical indication for abortion or surgical sterilization. Because increased pulmonary resistance and decreased pulmonary elasticity are by-products of increased blood viscosity and volume, resulting in decreased maximum breathing capacity and vital capacity, the patient with polycythemia requires special care during the administration of anesthesia for delivery. General anesthesia is hazardous, and regional, conduction techniques are preferred.

DISORDERS OF THE ENDOCRINE SYSTEM

DIABETES MELLITUS

CARBOHYDRATE METABOLISM IN PREGNANCY

During pregnancy, maternal carbohydrate metabolism undergoes important alterations. The human fetus utilizes primarily glucose for its energy requirements, an allegation supported by many disparate observations: a respiratory quotient of approximately 1.0 in newborn infants; the ready movement of glucose across the placenta; large arteriovenous differences in glucose concentrations in umbilical cord blood in the primate fetus; poor mobility of fatty acids in traversing the placenta; and the inability of fetal and neonatal muscle to utilize fatty acids efficiently in vitro. The maternal organism spares glucose and transfers some of its energy requirements to the oxidation of fats. This occurs from a combination of several mechanisms.

Human placental lactogen (HPL, somatomammotropin) is a protein hormone immunologically similar to human growth hormone (HGH), and is produced by the syncytiotrophoblast. Among its other effects, HPL mobilizes and raises circulating blood levels of free fatty acids and exerts an "antiinsulin" effect by interfering with the peripheral utilization of glucose, both influences which can be termed "diabetogenic." In addition to the lipolytic effect and the insulin antagonism of HPL, the human placenta contains an active proteolytic enzyme system capable of degrading insulin. To maintain homeostasis in the face of insulin antagonism and increased insulin degradation, the pancreatic beta cells are stimulated to increased insulin production. Maternal circulating insulin (or insulinlike activity) is slightly higher as pregnancy progresses and fasting blood sugar levels are slightly lower (Spellacy).

Pregnancy thus represents a stress on pancreatic beta cell reserves. As a result, minor inborn deficiencies in insulin production capability, ordinarily of no clinical significance in the nongravid patient, become overt. This mechanism is confirmed by the decreased or absent hypoglycemic effect of tolbutamide in normal pregnancy. The major, if not only, action of tolbutamide is to stimulate the synthesis and release of endogenous insulin. Tolbutamide is not hypoglycemic in a patient without pancreatic beta cells or in a pregnant patient whose beta cells already are overstimulated.

CLASSIFICATION OF MATERNAL DIABETES

To standardize descriptions, facilitate evaluations of various methods of treatment, and simplify prognostic determinations, White's classification of maternal diabetes has been adopted (Table 31–8).

The definition of diabetes mellitus purely as an abnormality of glucose tolerance is outdated. Anatomic and metabolic aberrations pathognomonic of diabetes may occur long before there is clinical manifestation of a carbohydrate metabolic defeat, and even in the presence of a normal glucose tolerance test. Retinopathy, neuropathy, and nephropathy, once considered complications of long-standing disease, may precede any evidence of hyperglycemia and/or glycosuria. The present concept of diabetes mellitus is that of a lifelong diabetic diathesis which progresses slowly from preclinical, latent, or prediabetes to overt disease with the usual clinical manifestations.

Prediabetes can be converted into clinical diabetes by certain stress phenomena, such as pregnancy, administration of steroids, infection, trauma, or myocardial infarction. Once the stress situation has passed, the clinical manifestations of diabetes may subside, but they may persist as well. The class A diabetic gravida is a woman with no prior diagnosis of diabetes in whom the stress of pregnancy has produced an abnormal glucose tolerance curve. In most cases, the curve will revert to normal after the pregnancy is over; in some, the curve will remain abnormal, and other symptoms and signs of diabetes may appear, after delivery. Even if the glucose tolerance abnormality disappears after pregnancy, the patient has demonstrated that she is a "prediabetic" with diminished beta cell reserves; that she is subject to a return of the glucose tolerance abnormality with sub-

sequent stress situations; and that she is predisposed to the eventual development of clinical diabetes mellitus.

TABLE 31–8 Classification of Maternal Diabetes in Pregnancy

Class	Definition
A	Chemical diabetes (gestational diabetes, prediabetes). Diagnosis made during pregnancy solely on basis of abnormal glucose tolerance test; fasting blood sugar normal. No therapy with hypoglycemic agents.
B	Clinically overt diabetes with maturity onset (age over 20), duration less than 10 years, and no vascular lesions.
C	Disease of moderate duration, without vascular lesions.
C_1	Age 10–19 at onset.
C_2	10–19 years' duration.
D	Disease of long duration or evidence of vascular complications.
D_1	Under age 10 at onset.
D_2	Over 20 years' duration.
D_3	Benign retinopathy (microvascular disease).
D_4	Calcification of leg vessels (macrovascular disease).
D_5	Hypertension.
(E)	(Eliminated).
F	Nephropathy.
G	Prior obstetric failures.
H	Cardiopathy.
R	Proliferative retinopathy.
T	Renal transplantation (Tagatz et al.).

Source: Adapted from White.

EFFECT OF PREGNANCY ON DIABETES MELLITUS

The incidence of diabetes complicating pregnancy has increased in the past half century, until now it occurs in almost 2 percent of all gestations. This increased incidence is the result of several factors. First, with the introduction of insulin maintenance, the young diabetic patient survives into the reproductive years and retains normal fertility potential. Second, the diabetic diathesis is hereditary, and one result of successful reproduction in diabetic patients is a spread of the defect through the genetic pool. Finally, greater efforts have been expended and more sophisticated techniques employed to discover mild cases which previously were not recognized (Tyson, Felig).

The pregnant diabetic patient undergoes changes in glucose tolerance and alterations in insulin utilization, and has an increased tendency to ketosis. The stable, "adult" type of diabetes may be converted into the brittle, "juvenile" form. Insulin requirements in any given patient usually increase during gestation and decrease markedly after delivery. Complications of pregnancy such as toxemia and pyelonephritis, and the lowered renal threshold for glucose which may occur, complicate the management of the diabetic patient during gestation (Shea et al.). Progressive degenerative changes related to diabetes may be accelerated during pregnancy; however, the postpartum status of such patients does not differ markedly from their preconceptional condition (Burt, Weaver). In general, with modern management, maternal mortality is less than 1 percent, as compared with 25 percent before the insulin era.

EFFECT OF DIABETES MELLITUS ON PREGNANCY

Diabetes exerts a deleterious influence on pregnancy. The incidence of spontaneous abortion in the pregnant diabetic does not differ from that in the nondiabetic population. Polyhydramnios is present in about 10 percent of diabetic pregnancies but rarely is of any clinical importance. Only occasionally will the degree of polyhydramnios be so great as to result in premature labor or in postpartum uterine atony and hemorrhage. Toxemia of pregnancy occurs in approximately 25 percent of cases. The incidence of urinary tract infection is increased, probably because of persistent glycosuria.

The placenta of the diabetic patient grossly is normal, although it may be slightly enlarged. In some cases, but not all, diabetic vascular lesions can be seen.

EFFECT OF DIABETES MELLITUS ON THE FETUS

Perinatal mortality is increased significantly in diabetes mellitus (Table 31–9). With the best management, perinatal mortality rates of 15 to 20 percent, distributed equally between stillbirth and neonatal death, have been reported heretofore. The causes of fetal death, which occurs most frequently in the last month of gestation, may be vascular placental insufficiency, cardiac arrest secondary to myocardial glycogen deposits, or remain unexplained in most cases. The neonatal losses are attributable mainly to respiratory distress syndrome and to congenital anomalies.

Infants of diabetic mothers have a threefold increase in the incidence of major congenital anomalies, 6 to 9 percent as compared with 2 to 3 percent in control groups. This rate apparently increases with the severity of the maternal diabetes, and has been reported as high as 15 percent in infants born to mothers with class F diabetes (Pedersen et al.). The frequency of congenital anomalies is not related to the use of insulin, which has teratogenic qualities in some lower species, nor to maternal hypo- or hyperglycemia. Diabetic acidosis or coma in the mother is lethal for the fetus in utero. One anomaly frequently reported in diabetic pregnancy is sacral agenesis, but all systems have been involved.

Macrosomia is a frequent complication for the fetus in a diabetic pregnancy. Excessively large infants, with birth weights of 10 pounds or more (4500+ g), are born in almost 30 percent of diabetic pregnancies, or more than 10 times the expected incidence. The infants have a characteristic facies, with prominent jowls and swollen cheeks, and appear plethoric. The excessive birth weight mainly is the result of obesity and organomegaly, rather than fluid re-

TABLE 31–9 Outcome of Pregnancy in Diabetes Mellitus

	Class A	Class B	Class C	Class D to R
Perinatal death rate (per 1000)	19	42	53	63
Birth weight				
>4000 g	20%	24%	29%	6%
<25000 g	4%	7%	8%	16%
Neonatal morbidity*	24%	61%	74%	78%
Congenital anomalies	5%	6%	8%	16%

*Hypoglycemia, hyperbilirubinemia, and/or hypocalcemia.
Source: Adapted from Gabbe et al., 1977a, 1977c.

tention or edema. The cause of this excessive weight probably is overutilization of glucose in utero; to some extent, fetal size may be controlled by not permitting excessive maternal hyperglycemia. The macrosomia has several important consequences in the management of diabetic pregnancies. First, estimation of gestational age by fetal size is even less reliable in diabetic pregnancies than it usually is. Second, problems of dystocia in labor and an increased incidence of birth trauma may be anticipated, even with a normal maternal bony pelvis. Third, an obstetric history of the past delivery of a large infant whose birth weight was over 9 pounds (4000+ g) should alert the physician to the possible presence of a maternal diabetic diathesis. Finally, the absence of macrosomia or the detection of intrauterine fetal growth retardation is an indication of relatively severe vascular disease and impaired placental transfer.

Neonatal problems similarly are based on the intrauterine diabetic milieu. The increased incidence of respiratory distress syndrome in babies born to diabetic mothers is related not to the diabetic diathesis but to the empiric obstetric decision to deliver these babies prematurely to minimize the risk of intrauterine demise in the last month of gestation. With modern methods of management, this will be a decreasing problem.

The fetus of a diabetic gravida is exposed in utero to excessive amounts of glucose, supplied by facilitated diffusion across the placenta from maternal hyperglycemia. As a result, the beta cells of the fetal pancreas hypertrophy and produce excessive amounts of insulin. This tendency toward hypersecretion of insulin does not abate abruptly with birth, but the hyperglycemic environment is terminated. The neonate thus tends to develop hypoglycemia in the nursery, which if undetected and untreated can lead to structural brain damage, neurologic disorders, or death (McCann).

MANAGEMENT OF DIABETES MELLITUS IN PREGNANCY

The basic principles of management of diabetes in pregnancy and of pregnancy complicated by maternal diabetes include (1) diagnosis, careful evaluation, and classification of the diabetic woman before or as early as possible in pregnancy; (2) meticulous and constant management of the diabetes through pregnancy, labor and delivery, and the puerperium; (3) termination of pregnancy at the optimal time, as indicated by tests of fetal maturity and fetoplacental function; and (4) immediate and intensive neonatal observation and care of the baby (Ayromlooi et al.).

The obstetrician often is in a particularly advantageous case-finding situation, and the incidence of diabetes complicating pregnancy, especially class A disease, depends on the diligence with which the diagnosis is pursued. As an initial screening technique, a diabetic diathesis should be suspected and sought in all pregnant patients presenting with (1) glycosuria or giving a history of (2) diabetes in the mother's family, (3) previous unexplained stillbirths, (4) previous delivery of an infant weighing 4000+ g, (5) habitual abortion, (6) delivery of an infant with multiple congenital anomalies, or (7) excessive maternal obesity. For initial screening, a blood sugar determination 2 hours after the ingestion by the patient of 100 g glucose has been effective. A fasting blood sugar level frequently is normal in early or latent diabetes, and a full glucose tolerance test may be impractical as a screening procedure on large volumes of patients. When the 2-hour post-100-g glucose blood sugar level is at all doubtful or abnormal (by the standards of the local laboratory), a standard glucose tolerance test should be performed. If the test in early pregnancy is normal, it should be repeated early in the third trimester, as increasing stress may highlight the diabetic diathesis. An oral glucose tolerance test may be considered abnormal if blood sugar levels are abnormal at two or more points on the curve. The curve may show a higher peak value and a slower fall—a "shift to the right" which has been attributed to delayed gastrointestinal absorption during pregnancy. The intravenous glucose tolerance test obviates these objections, with the 15-minute, 30-minute, and 1-hour blood sugar levels corresponding to the 1-, 2-, and 3-hour levels in the oral test. Pragmatically, either test has sufficed to make the diagnosis during gestation.

MANAGEMENT OF DIABETIC PREGNANCY

Class A Diabetes

Patients with class A diabetes mellitus rarely suffer intrauterine fetal death and their perinatal mortality rate should approach that of the nondiabetic population. Nevertheless, because of possible errors in precise definition of class A status, monitoring of the condition of the fetus in utero and of fetal pulmonary maturation should be carried out as classes B to R (see below), and decisions about delivery individualized accordingly.

The class A diabetic patient can be managed with dietary control alone. The patient should be observed at 2-week intervals throughout pregnancy until 34 weeks' gestation and at weekly intervals thereafter. The prescribed diet should be limited to 2000 to 2500 cal daily and increased only if acetonuria develops, which poses a risk for fetal intellectual development (Stehbens et al). Fasting blood sugar levels should be determined at each visit. If the fasting blood sugar level becomes abnormal, the patient is considered to have class B disease with regard to possible intra-uterine fetal death and neonatal morbidity and usually will require insulin therapy. Fetal size should be evaluated toward the end of pregnancy by ultrasonography. When fetal macrosomia is detected and fetal weight is estimated at over 4000 g, delivery by cesarean section is advisable because of the increased risk of traumatic morbidity with vaginal delivery. Whether there is benefit to be derived from the treatment of class A diabetic gravidas with insulin (Roversi et al.; Coustan et al.) or with pyridoxine (Spellacy et al.) remains unsettled.

Class B to R Diabetes

The patient in an advanced category of diabetes must have preconceptional counseling, if possible, concerning the medical risks, the financial cost, and the emotional stress that pregnancy will create for her and her family. As far as feasible, the patient's reproductive career should be planned in advance, and conception should be encouraged as early in the life history of the disease as possible and before vascular complications have developed.

Once pregnant, such a patient requires meticulous antepartum care. Weekly visits throughout the latter half of pregnancy are in order, with immediate hospitalization at the least suggestion of difficulties with diabetic management or the appearance of any intercurrent medical or surgical disease, such as upper respiratory or urinary tract infection, which might compromise diabetic control (Gyves et al.).

The hallmark of good management of diabetes in pregnancy is the maintenance of *euglycemia*. Fasting plasma glucose levels should be kept at 100 to 110 mg per 100 mL, and postprandial levels at 140 to 150 mg per 100 mL. Diabetic control that is acceptable in the nongravid state may not be sufficient during pregnancy; evidence has accumulated that hyperglycemia alone may be very detrimental for the fetus (Whitelaw). All of these patients will require insulin, often in divided doses during a 24-hour period and of differing types. In assessing insulin requirements, fractional urine tests are of no value in pregnancy; serial, multiple blood sugar determinations are required. It should be kept in mind that insulin requirements may increase progressively in about two-thirds of pregnant patients, so that frequent reassessment of diabetic control is necessary as pregnancy advances. Insulin does not cross the placenta or affect the fetus.

A fairly rigid diabetic diet should be encouraged, offering approximately 30 cal per kilogram of body weight, with 50 percent of the calories in carbohydrates and 25 percent each in protein and fat. The total daily food intake should be divided into multiple small feedings during the day, i.e., three meals and two or three snacks, the purpose of which, in conjunction with divided dose insulin therapy, is to maintain stable blood glucose levels. The importance of strict dietary control must be reemphasized to the patient, who is probably accustomed to a freer dietary regimen when not pregnant.

The diabetic gravida's status must be assessed thoroughly: urine culture, creatinine clearance, and base-line pelvic ultrasound examination should be accomplished as early in gestation as possible and repeated every 6 weeks. Ophthalmologic funduscopic evaluation is important to assess vascular status, and retinal photographs are helpful in detecting and following possible progression of disease.

Precise monitoring of the intrauterine status of the fetus becomes crucial once potential fetal viability is reached, from the 28th week of gestation onward. Weekly nonstressed monitoring of fetal reactivity is an excellent, noninvasive means of assessing fetal well-being; any abnormality in the nonstressed monitoring should be evaluated further by contraction stress testing. This nonstressed monitoring should be performed biweekly after the 34th week of gestation.

A biochemical means of assessing fetal well-being is the serial measurement of maternal urinary estriol (E_3) excretion (Goebelsmann et al.). The level of estriol is a measure both of fetal health and placental function. Normally, the excretion of maternal urinary estriol rises throughout pregnancy, more rapidly in the last 10 weeks. Absolute values vary with the method used. Low estriol levels or failure of levels to rise sharply in the last 10 weeks of gestation is indicative of diseases of the fetus and/or placenta. False low values may result from incomplete 24-hour urine collection (there is marked diurnal variation in excretion), bacterial degradation of urinary estriol, maternal adrenal suppression with corticosteroid therapy, maternal renal disease which interferes with estriol excretion, or contamination of the urine by agents that interfere with determination of estriol levels, such as methamine mandelate (Mandelamine), ampicillin, and *glucose*. Twenty-four-hour urine collections should be checked for estriol content weekly beginning at 30 weeks' gestation, biweekly at 34 weeks' gestation, and at least every other day from the beginning of the 36th week. A low or falling estriol excretion pattern usually indicates that the fetus is in jeopardy; a normally rising pattern is reassuring but does not invariably guarantee fetal survival in the diabetic mother. Some of the problems of urinary estriol excretion testing may be obviated by techniques that measure maternal plasma levels of estriol.

In current practice, the biochemical and biophysical techniques described above are used concurrently. Superiority of one over the other has not been documented at this point.

The progression of fetal growth is another important variable to be observed. Serial ultrasonic scans for estimation of fetal size and weight should be performed every 2 weeks from the 28th week of gestation onward. In patients with advanced maternal disease, intrauterine growth retardation is more frequent than macrosomia and may influence decisions about management.

In view of the increasing risk of fetal death near term, the timing of delivery at a point where the combined risks of stillbirth and of prematurity are at a minimum is critical. Just as better techniques have been developed to evaluate the risk of fetal death, so can fetal maturity be better assessed than previously. Radiographic attempts to estimate fetal bone age and ultrasonic estimation of gestational dates by measurement of fetal biparietal diameter have followed the clinical estimation of fetal weight by palpation into obsolescence. Biochemical tests of amniotic fluid for fetal maturity have been useful: percentage of fetal cells in amniotic fluid that stain for lipids with Nile blue stain; amniotic fluid bilirubin concentration; and amniotic fluid creatinine level. However, the maturation of specific fetal organs and/or enzyme systems is related only statistically to gestational age. Since the major cause of neonatal death in premature infants is the respiratory distress syndrome, the study of amniotic fluid lecithin concentration (or lecithin/sphingomyelin ratio) which correlates with the development of fetal pulmonary surfactant and the absence of neonatal respiratory distress syndrome has been of greatest value (Roberts et al.; Mueller-Heubach et al.). In diabetic pregnancy, amniocentesis should be carried out at 5- to 7-day intervals, starting at about 35 weeks' gestation.

The analysis of amniotic fluid has been modified and refined after recognition that the respiratory distress syndrome still may occur in infants born to diabetic mothers, despite adequate levels of lecithin, because of the delayed appearance in these infants of phosphatidyl glycerol, which is necessary to stabilize the surfactant complex in the neonatal lung (Cunningham et al.; Gluck). When lecithin levels are adequate and phosphatidyl glycerol is present, the incidence of respiratory distress syndrome is equal to or less than that in the nondiabetic neonate population (Gabbe et al., 1977b).

The parameters useful in selecting a delivery point are indicated in Table 31–10. The decision to effect delivery depends on a judgment that balances maternal status and fetal status against fetal maturity factors. The neonatal morbidities of hypoglycemia, hypocalcemia, and hyperbilirubinemia indicate that maturation of the fetal lung is not the only factor, albeit perhaps the most important. Delivery should be delayed until all evidence of fetal maturity is present *unless prior uterine evacuation is forced by deterioration of the maternal or fetal status*. The administration of corticosteroids to accelerate fetal pulmonary maturation may impair maternal diabetic control and be detrimental to fetal pancreatic function (Colle, Goldman).

The method for accomplishing delivery, once the determination is made that delivery is indicated and is safe for the fetus, should be chosen on obstetric indications. If the cervix is "favorable," induction of labor may be attempted even weeks before term. With the onset of uterine contractions, any sign of fetal distress, such as meconium in the amniotic fluid, abnormal fetal heart rate patterns, or evidence of fetal acidosis in scalp blood samples, is an indication for immediate cesarean section. If the cervix is deemed to be "unfavorable," or attempts to induce labor are not successful within a reasonable interval (12 to 24 hours), delivery by cesarean section should be ac-

TABLE 31–10 Timing of Delivery in Diabetic Mothers

Maternal clinical factors	
Degree of maternal diabetic control	
Presence and severity of preeclampsia	
Previous obstetric history	
Other factors conferring special risk	
Fetal well-being	
Nonstress/stress test fetal monitoring	
Maternal urinary or plasma estriol levels	
Indications of fetal growth or growth retardation	
Fetal maturity (amniotic fluid)	
Creatinine	2.0 mg/100 mL or higher
Lecithin	5.0 mg/100 mL or higher
Lecithin/sphingomyelin ratio	2 or higher
Bilirubin concentration (Δ_{450})	0
Phosphatidyl glycerol	+ (present)
Phosphatidyl inositol	− (absent)

complished expeditiously. Prolonged attempts at induction of uterine contractions and protracted labor should be avoided, since control of the maternal diabetic state can deteriorate during this interval (West, Lowy; Yeast et al.). Vaginal delivery of a macrosomic infant (4000 g or more) should be avoided. A liberal approach to cesarean section can be employed in these high-premium, high-risk infants.

Neonatal Care

The newborn infant must have intensive pediatric care from birth. Cord blood levels of electrolytes, glucose, and calcium should be obtained as base lines. The infant must be observed for respiratory distress, hypoglycemia, hyperbilirubinemia, hypocalcemia, and congenital anomalies. The routine aspiration of gastric contents in such infants has been abandoned.

THYROID DISORDERS

THYROID METABOLISM IN PREGNANCY

The increased levels of estrogens in pregnancy result in an increased production of alpha and beta globulins by the liver, among which is thyroxine-binding globulin (TBG). In order to maintain a euthyroid state in the face of increased levels of TBG and increased proportions of globulin-bound thyroxine, thyroid gland activity in pregnancy is increased. Thyroid uptake of radioiodine is elevated markedly, reflecting an increased clearance of iodine by the thyroid gland but not clinical hyperactivity. The serum protein-bound iodine (PBI) and butanol-extractable iodine levels rise sharply as early as the first trimester to levels of 8 to 10 μg per 100 mL, (nongravid levels rarely

are above 7.5 μg per 100 mL), demonstrating that increased amounts of globulin-bound and therefore inactive thyroxine are circulating in the mother. Clinically, there is moderate thyromegaly during pregnancy, secondary to glandular hyperplasia and increased vascularity, both regressing almost totally postpartum. The basal metabolic rate of the mother increases progressively throughout pregnancy, reaching a peak of approximately + 15 percent near term, reflecting the sum of maternal and fetal metabolic activities. Functionally, the gravida remains euthyroid (Souma et al.).

Thyroid function tests must be interpreted with an understanding of these physiologic alterations in pregnancy. In many aspects, thyroid activity as depicted by standard thyroid function tests in the normal pregnant woman mimics hyperthyroidism (Table 31–11).

Iodine and antithyroid drugs pass readily through the placenta. Human fetal thyroid tissue can accumulate radioactive iodine as early as the end of the first trimester. Thyroxine readily crosses the placenta. Thyroid-stimulating hormone (TSH, thyrotropin) probably does not cross the placental barrier, but the delivery of thyrotoxic and exophthalmic infants to mothers with thyrotoxicosis is evidence that long-acting thyroid-stimulating hormone (LATS) can cross.

HYPERTHYROIDISM AND PREGNANCY

Severe hyperthyroidism often is associated with amenorrhea and infertility and thus is encountered only rarely in pregnancy. Conception is not infrequent, however, in patients with minor degrees of hyperthyroidism. The incidence of hyperthyroidism in pregnancy is about 0.04 percent. The initial onset of hyperthyroidism during pregnancy is coincidental.

TABLE 31–11   Changes in Thyroid Function Tests*

Thyroid function tests	Euthyroid nongravid	Euthyroid gravid	Hyperthyroid	Hypothyroid
BMR	←→ (−20 to + 10%)	↑ (+25%)	↓ (>+20%)	↓ (<−20%)
PBI	←→ (4−8 μg/100 mL)	↑ (6−12 μg/100 mL)	↑ (>8 μ/100 mL)	↓ (<4 μg/100 mL)
BEI	←→ (3.5−7.5 μg/100 mL)	↑ (5.5−11.5 μg/100 mL)	↓ (>7.5 μg/100 mL)	↓ (<3.5 μg/100 mL)
¹³¹I uptake	←→ (15−45%)		↑ (>45%)	↓ (<15%)
T_3 uptake†	←→	↓	↑	↑
Free T_4†	←→	←→	↑	↓

*←→, normal or unchanged; ↑, increased; ↓, decreased.
†Values vary with method used.

Effect of Hyperthyroidism on Pregnancy

Pregnancy in a patient with severe and uncontrolled thyrotoxicosis is complicated by increased frequencies of abortion, premature labor, and toxemia of pregnancy (Prout). Mild hyperthyroidism has little effect on the course of pregnancy. If the thyrotoxicosis is adequately controlled by treatment, the prognosis for successful pregnancy outcome is good.

Effect of Pregnancy on Hyperthyroidism

Pregnancy does not exacerbate maternal hyperthyroidism or change the life history of the disease process. There is no indication for therapeutic abortion. Some patients with thyrotoxicosis undergo mild remission during gestation, possibly as a result of increased binding of thyroxine to globulin and a fall in the levels of free thyroxine.

Effect of Maternal Hyperthyroidism on the Fetus

The fetus is not affected ordinarily by the maternal disease process, and is much more susceptible to influence by the treatment to which the mother is subjected (see Management below). Some infants are born with transient, neonatal hyperthyroidism, manifest by loss of weight, hyperkinesis, tachycardia, and diarrhea, and sometimes even exophthalmos. This condition regresses within 3 to 4 weeks of birth, and is attributable to the transplacental transmission of LATS, an IgG globulin originating in maternal lymphocytic tissues (McKenzie). This substance may be present, and the fetus affected, in mothers whose own thyrotoxicosis was treated successfully years before the current gestation.

Management

The management of hyperthyroidism in pregnancy requires a delicate balance between the effect of treatment on the mother and possible deleterious effects of the treatment on the fetus. In general, treatment should aim at bringing the mother toward the euthyroid state but avoiding the hypothyroid state with its significant fetal effects.

In mild cases, no treatment may be required beyond increased rest and mild sedation with barbiturates. If the patient's sleeping pulse rate consistently is under 80 beats per minute, it is unlikely that antithyroid drugs will be required.

The treatment of more severe maternal thyrotoxicosis depends on either medical or surgical control of the disease. Therapy with radioactive iodine is contraindicated during pregnancy (Green et al., 1971). Inorganic iodine (Lugol's solution) has the paradoxic effect of blocking thyroid activity when administered in pharmacologic doses for short periods of time. When the disease is encountered late in gestation, such a regimen may suffice until delivery can be accomplished; otherwise, treatment with iodides is reserved for preoperative preparation of patients destined for surgical treatment of their disease.

There are three drugs currently in use which diminish the production of thyroid hormone: carbimazole and methylthiouracil or propylthiouracil, which by enzyme inhibition prevent the incorporation of iodine into the tyrosine nucleus, and potassium perchlorate, which interferes with the iodine-trapping mechanism of the gland. All these agents pass freely across the placenta and may affect fetal thyroid gland function, resulting in congenital goiter which usually is transient and regresses spontaneously after 3 to 4 weeks, but may be large enough to cause dystocia at delivery or neonatal respiratory obstruction. Excessive exposure to the drugs also may result in fetal hypothyroidism and mental retardation (Burrow et al.). The drugs also are excreted in breast milk and contraindicate breast-feeding. Treatment doses are as follows: propylthiouracil, initial treatment with 100 mg three times daily; as soon as symptoms are controlled (6 to 8 weeks), the dose may be halved; when the euthyroid state is reached, the dose is reduced further to 50 mg per day. Carbimazole has an initial treatment dose of 15 mg three times daily, reduced to 10 mg three times daily when symptoms are controlled and to 5 mg three times daily in the euthyroid state. With potassium perchlorate, the initial dose is 250 mg three times daily until the patient is euthyroid, and then 300 mg daily for maintenance. Because the judgment of the state of thyrotoxicosis is confused by normal pregnancy changes, antithyroid drug therapy is more difficult to regulate and carries a higher risk of complications during pregnancy than in the nongravid state.

It has been recognized that a level of free thyroxine is essential for the normal development of the fetus, which starts to produce its own thyroxine about the middle of gestation; without this, there may be impairment of cortical brain development (cretinism) which cannot be reversed by treatment after delivery, as well as fetal thyromegaly secondary to excessive fetal TSH production and release. The human placenta is relatively impermeable to thyroxine, and the amount available to the fetus may be insufficient if the fetal production of hormone as well is suppressed by antithyroid drug therapy. Thus, one current approach to the use of antithyroid drugs in the management of thyrotoxicosis in pregnancy includes the administration of full thyroid hormone replacement to the mother (Selenkow). A balanced thyroid state compatible with normal pregnancy results, and both mother and fetus are protected from the deleterious effects of hypothyroidism and from the side effects of antithyroid drug therapy. The development of fetal goiter is prevented, and the futher enlargement of the maternal gland is inhibited.

The surgical management of thyrotoxicosis requires partial or total thyroidectomy. Pregnancy does not increase the risk of the surgical procedure. Preoperatively, the patient is prepared with the administration of antithyroid drugs and/or iodides. The procedure is accomplished best during the middle trimester of pregnancy. Following thyroidectomy, thyroid hormone substitution should be routine, to avoid the risk of hypothyroidism. Surgical management avoids the fetal hazards of antithyroid drug therapy, is definitive treatment for a patient who may require thyroidectomy at a later stage of her disease, and is particularly applicable to a patient deemed unreliable or unable to cooperate with the detailed medical regimen required (Cunningham, Slaughter). Perinatal survival rates are the same with either medical or surgical management. The surgical procedure entails the usual risks of thyroid surgery, including the possibility of postoperative hypoparathyroidism or injury to the recurrent laryngeal nerve. Treatment of the individual patient will depend on the features of the case, the judgment of the responsible physician, and the capability of the medical center where therapy is undertaken. As understanding of thyroid hormone production and function has grown, there has been a decreasing need to utilize surgery for hyperthyroidism during pregnancy (Burrow).

The neonate born to a thyrotoxic mother who has been under treatment rarely shows signs of hyperthyroidism. The appearance of clinical disease in such infants may be delayed until the third or fourth post-delivery day. All babies born to affected mothers must be observed for signs of the disease, primarily tachycardia and irritability. The infant may be treated, if necessary, with iodides or thioamides.

HYPOTHYROIDISM AND PREGNANCY

The clinical syndrome of hypothyroidism (myxedema) is encountered infrequently in pregnancy because its development usually occurs after the reproductive age, and because it is associated with marked impairment of fertility and loss of libido. The diagnosis of myxedema during pregnancy may be suspected on clinical grounds, or by the fact that expected increases in various thyroid function tests during gestation do not occur. Whether maternal hypothyroidism is related etiologically to increased rates of abortion or fetal death in utero is unclear. If the diagnosis is made promptly and treatment instituted, the pregnancy will progress without difficulty (Kennedy, Montgomery).

The fetus of a mother with untreated myxedema often is a cretin or becomes mentally retarded. The pituitary-thyroid axis of the fetus develops independently from that of the mother, however, and hypothyroid, untreated mothers have delivered normal infants. Nevertheless, early diagnosis and thyroid hormone replacement therapy are recommended. In view of the previously discussed physiologic changes in thyroid hormone balance during gestation, hypothyroid patients already on thyroid replacement therapy who become pregnant should have their maintenance dose of thyroxine increased by at least 0.1 mg per day.

The analysis of amniotic fluid obtained at amniocentesis for T_4 derivatives has been reported (Hollingsworth, Austin). In a few patients, the levels of amniotic fluid T_4 and PBI predicted correctly the status of the neonate. This approach may be useful in monitoring the status of the fetus and the efficacy and safety of therapy in both hyper- and hypothyroid mothers.

PARATHYROID DISORDERS

HYPERPARATHYROIDISM

This disorder may be either primary or secondary. Primary disease results from a solitary parathyroid adenoma, multiple parathyroid adenomas, glandular hyperplasia, or carcinoma of the parathyroid gland. In each case, there is excessive secretion of parathyroid hormone and a consistent elevation of the serum calcium level well above the normal value of 10 mg per 100 mL. Usually, hypercalcinuria is present (unless there is impairment of glomerular filtration), and three-fourths of patients affected have calcium and phosphate renal calculi. The clinical syndrome may include adynamic ileus, muscular weakness, and psychosis. Almost all patients have hypophosphatemia, and characteristic bone changes, secondary to mobilization of calcium from bony tissue, are present in 25 percent of cases. A similar clinical picture may result from secondary hyperparathyroidism, which may occur with chronic renal insufficiency or osteomalacia.

Hyperparathyroidism is an extremely rare complication of pregnancy, only some 40 cases appearing in the medical literature. Unless the patient has a history of renal colic or renal infection suggestive of calculus formation, the condition may be asymptomatic during pregnancy, becoming manifest only when the newborn infant develops hypocalcemia, tetany, and/or convulsions. These conditions in an otherwise normal infant should raise the question of possible maternal hyperparathyroidism (Jacobsen et al.).

From the limited experience reported, it appears that the treatment of choice in primary hyperparathyroidism is prompt parathyroidectomy. Preoperative administration of phosphates or calcium disodium edetate, a chelating agent with a strong affinity for calcium and other metallic ions, may be helpful in binding calcium and removing it from the serum and alleviating hypercalcemic toxicity. Pregnancy is not an indication to delay surgical intervention because control of the hyperparathyroidism may improve the chances for fetal salvage, while the renal changes incurred by delay in treatment (nephrocalcinosis and chronic pyelonephritis) are irreversible (Johnstone et al.).

Indications for therapeutic abortion depend entirely on the patient's renal status. Bone changes and clinical symptoms are rapidly reversible after successful treatment, while chronic renal impairment subjects both mother and fetus to significant pregnancy risks.

HYPOPARATHYROIDISM

Deficiency of parathyroid hormone rarely may be encountered in pregnant women who have been subjected to thyroidectomy and accidental excision of the parathyroid glands. Serum calcium levels are lowered in normal pregnancy, probably secondary to the physiologic decrease in serum albumin concentration. In untreated hypoparathyroidism, there is a decreased urinary excretion of phosphorus, resulting in elevated serum phosphorus levels and correspondingly decreased serum calcium levels.

The most frequent manifestation of hypoparathyroidism is tetany, secondary to hypocalcemia. The differential diagnosis must include rickets, osteomalacia, steatorrhea, hyperventilation, ingestion of alkali, pernicious vomiting, and renal insufficiency with phosphate retention. The crucial parameter, the serum concentration of ionized calcium, varies with serum pH, total calcium concentration, and the protein-binding of calcium.

Hypoparathyroidism is controlled by supplying adequate amounts of calcium. In an acute emergency, the intravenous injection of calcium gluconate is effective. Oral administration of calcium gluconate or lactate also is useful, but acts more slowly. Long-term management of the disorder requires a diet high in calcium and low in phosphates, calcium supplementation, and vitamin D, in doses of 50,000 to 200,000 units per day. During pregnancy, there is the added requirement of supplying calcium for fetal needs; the supplementation of 250 mg of calcium daily is necessary during the third trimester.

With proper treatment, the pregnant hypoparathyroid patient shows no significant changes in calcium dynamics, and her serum and urine calcium and phosphate levels remain within normal levels. With well-controlled hypoparathyroidism, there is no increase in fetal wastage (Bolen). The major fetal problems occur neonatally. Hypocalcemia in the newborn can be a serious complication, resulting in tetany or convulsions. Another neonatal hazard associated with hypocalcemia is heart block, which presents pathognomonic electrocardiographic patterns. Both situations respond readily to the administration of calcium gluconate.

PITUITARY DISORDERS

PHYSIOLOGIC CHANGES IN PREGNANCY

During normal pregnancy, there is enlargement of the anterior pituitary gland to approximately twice normal size. Both acidophilic and basophilic cells show evidence of increased activity, resulting from increased production and release of pituitary hormones and depletion of hormones stored. A cell whose morphologic appearance is intermediate between acidophilic and basophilic has been described as characteristic of the pregnant state and named the "pregnancy cell." The gonadotropin content of the gland is low during gestation. There is no pregnancy-induced hypertrophy of the posterior lobe. All pregnancy changes in the pituitary gland revert to normal within a few months after delivery.

ACROMEGALY

This disorder is caused by an eosinophilic adenoma of the anterior lobe of the pituitary, resulting in increased secretion of growth (somatotropic) hormone.

The disease is characterized by thickening and enlargement of the bones of the patient's extremities and skull; the jaw and supraorbital ridges particularly become prominent. There may be excessive hair growth, and glucose tolerance usually is impaired. Although most patients with acromegaly do not menstruate, pregnancy may complicate this rare disease.

Acromegaly does not affect pregnancy adversely, nor does pregnancy exacerbate the course of acromegaly. The disease must be differentiated from physiologic pregnancy changes: increased production of somatotropic hormone (by either the pituitary or the placenta) may lead to a transient acromegaly-like syndrome manifest by nonedematous thickening of the features and extremities, and increased pituitary size occasionally may produce transient bitemporal hemianopsia. Neither therapeutic abortion nor sterilization is indicated. Usually, the patient will have been treated preconceptionally. No treatment is necessary during pregnancy unless signs and symptoms of a rapidly expanding pituitary tumor appear. If necessary in such circumstances, radiotherapy to the sella turcica can be applied safely during pregnancy and without interfering with normal metabolic function.

Maternal acromegaly has no effect on the fetus or neonate.

BASOPHILISM

Excess activity of the basophilic cells of the anterior lobe of the pituitary may result from basophilic hyperplasia or adenoma, with secondary stimulation of the adrenal cortex from increased secretion of ACTH, and the development of Cushing's syndrome. There may be no localizing pituitary signs; the tumor, if present, often is very small. The differential diagnosis from adrenal cortical hyperplasia or tumor, masculinizing ovarian tumor, or hypothalamic disease may be very difficult.

Treatment of the pituitary tumor may be delayed until after the pregnancy is over, unless there is evidence of rapid increase in pituitary size. Radiotherapy is the treatment of choice. The management of the clinical picture is discussed under adrenal gland hyperactivity below.

CHROMOPHOBE ADENOMA

Although very rare in pregnancy, this is the pituitary tumor most frequently seen. The patient presents with signs and symptoms of increased intracranial pressure: headaches, nausea, and vomiting. If the tumor enlarges enough to encroach upon the optic chiasm,

visual disturbances occur. There may be radiologic evidence of destruction of the sella turcica. Treatment should be individualized; radiotherapy may be accomplished during pregnancy. There is no evidence that pregnancy and chromophobe adenoma have any mutual interaction. There is no indication either for termination of pregnancy or for sterilization.

DIABETES INSIPIDUS

This is a chronic disorder resulting from an inability of the kidneys to conserve water, usually because of a deficiency of antidiuretic hormone (ADH). There is a nephrogenic form of diabetes insipidus, extremely rare, which is caused by an inability of the kidneys to respond to ADH. Normally, ADH is elaborated in the supraoptic and paraventricular nuclei of the hypothalamus, moves through the pituitary stalk to the posterior lobe of the pituitary gland where it is stored, whence it subsequently is released. Anything which interferes with this process, such as damage to the stalk or hypothalamus by thrombosis, tumor, or infection, can result in the disorder; occasionally, diabetes insipidus accompanies pituitary necrosis (Sheehan's syndrome) (Beernink, McKay). The clinical picture is that of polydipsia and polyuria, with the production of urine of fixed low specific gravity.

The pituitary type of diabetes insipidus responds to maintenance therapy with exogenous ADH, usually in the form of injections of vasopressin (Pitressin). These patients do well during pregnancy, and there is no increased risk to the fetus (Oravec, Lichardus; Cobo et al.). There is no indication for therapeutic abortion or for sterilization. Paradoxically, the nephrogenic form of diabetes insipidus is treated with thiazide diuretics; the depletion of sodium over a 3- to 4-day period decreases glomerular filtration rates to the point that polyuria diminishes (Burstein, Chen).

PANHYPOPITUITARISM

Hypofunction of the entire anterior pituitary gland may result from postpartum pituitary necrosis (Sheehan's syndrome), neoplasia, or hypophysectomy. Untreated, there is failure of release of all pituitary trophic hormones, with secondary clinical manifestations of adrenal, thyroid, and ovarian failures: amenorrhea, decreased size of breasts, atrophic vulva, loss of pubic and axillary hair, myxedema, mental apathy, chronic fatigue, and poor reaction to stress. Treatment involves adequate replacement therapy with appropriate hormones. Without such therapy, conception and pregnancy are impossible.

If the treated patient does achieve a pregnancy,

there is no indication for abortion and every prospect for a favorable pregnancy outcome. The increased requirements for hormonal replacement because of the physiologic change in pregnancy and the stress of labor and delivery must be kept in mind. There is no effect on the fetus or neonate.

ADRENAL DISORDERS

PHYSIOLOGIC CHANGES IN PREGNANCY

Measurement of secretion products of the maternal adrenal gland confirm increased function during pregnancy. Free and bound cortisol both are increased, with a diminution in diurnal variation. Adrenal androgen production similarly is increased. Aldosterone secretion is elevated, partly because of increased activity of the renin-angiotensin system, and partly to compensate for the increased natriuretic effect of progesterone. In spite of these functional changes, the maternal adrenal does not undergo morphologic change or hypertrophy. Further, there is no consistent increase in the activity of adrenal hormones in the gravid patient, probably because of increased globulin levels and protein binding.

ADRENAL CORTICAL HYPERFUNCTION

A variety of clinical syndromes may result from adrenal cortical hyperfunction, depending on the category of hormone elaborated.

Cushing's Syndrome

This is a clinical complex consisting of hirsutism, characteristic ("buffalo-hump") obesity, abdominal striae, hypertension, a plethoric complexion, "moon" facies, polycythemia, resorption of bone, and impaired glucose tolerance. The disease results from adrenocortical hyperfunction secondary to hyperplasia, adenoma, or carconima of the adrenal cortex, or to pituitary basophilism. Although there is increased secretion of 11-oxysteroids and 17-ketosteroids, and amenorrhea and infertility occur early in the course of the disease, the clinical picture results primarily from the hypersecretion of glucocorticoids. Pregnancy may occur early in the course of the disease, or the disease may appear first during a pregnancy; the combination is rare (Grimes et al.).

The major threat to pregnancy from adrenal cortical hyperfunction is chronic hypertension, predisposing to the acute problems of superimposed tox-

emia and the long-term problems of possible placental insufficiency (Wieland et al.). In general, early treatment of the patient with Cushing's syndrome is recommended to forestall the development or progression of serious cardiovascular and skeletal abnormalities. The treatment varies with the specific diagnosis, which is difficult to establish during gestation, and may involve bilateral adrenalectomy or pituitary irradiation. Where possible, definitive treatment should await the end of gestation, when the differentiation between hyperplasia, adenoma, or carcinoma can be made with greater security, and the risks of adrenal surgery are less.

Patients who have had successful treatment for adrenal hyperfunction, such as bilateral adrenalectomy, and are receiving appropriate hormonal replacement therapy, may anticipate return of fertility and relatively uncomplicated pregnancies. Their management is discussed with that of adrenal cortical hypofunction below.

Only infants born to mothers with untreated Cushing's syndrome run the risk of neonatal adrenal insufficiency, secondary to intrauterine pituitary suppression by the maternal hormonal blood levels (Kreines, DeVaux). The neonate's condition may deteriorate within the first 24 hours of life, with the development of hyponatremia, hyperkalemia, hypoglycemia, and vascular collapse. Treatment requires correction of electrolyte and fluid balance with parenteral infusions, and hormonal replacement. Cortisol succinate, 50 to 100 mg, should be added to the first day's fluids. Cortisol, 25 mg daily and DOCA, 1 to 2 mg daily, should be administered intramuscularly. In the absence of continuing stress, the medication may begin to be tapered after 1 to 2 weeks, reducing the administered doses by one-half every 4 to 5 days.

Adrenogenital Syndrome

This condition results from the overproduction of androgens by the adrenal cortex. The most frequent cause, congenital virilizing adrenal hyperplasia, results from one of several inborn errors of metabolism of adrenal steroids (Table 31-12). Because of the steroid deficiency caused by the enzymatic block, the pituitary gland secretes excess ACTH, resulting in secondary adrenal hyperplasia and hyperfunction.

Under the influence of the excess androgenic hormones, the external genitalia and secondary sex characteristics become altered in females. The degree of masculinization depends on the age of the individual and the level of androgenic activity. Exposure of a female fetus during the first 12 weeks of in-

TABLE 31–12 Enzymatic Defects in Adrenogenital Syndrome

Enzyme lack	Effect on fetus and neonate
17-Hydroxylase	Virilization of female; ±salt losing; advanced bone age; rapid somatic growth; premature isosexual development in males.
11-Hydroxylase	Virilization in females; ±hypertension; advanced bone age; rapid somatic growth; premature isosexual development in males.
3β-Hydroxysteroid dehydrogenase	Virilization in females; salt losing; male fetus may be incompletely virilized (cryptorchidism, hypospadias).
17-Hydroxylase	Male fetus incompletely virilized; hypertension; absent secondary sex characteristics; ±hypokalemia; alkalosis.
Desmolase	Male fetus incompletely virilized; ±salt losing.

trauterine existence disrupts totally normal development of the female external genitalia and results in fusion of the labia and incomplete development of the vagina and vaginal introitus. Androgenic stimulation later in fetal life results in enlargement of the labia majora and clitoris, leading to the diagnosis at birth of female pseudohermaphroditism. In prepubertal girls, the clinical picture includes clitoral hypertrophy, precocious growth of pubic hair, and rapid somatic growth. In postpubertal women, the syndrome is manifest by amenorrhea, clitoral enlargement, hirsutism, and masculinization of features and voice. In all these situations, the ovaries, fallopian tubes, and uterus are normal, and the possibility of pregnancy after treatment is not excluded.

The principal therapeutic agent is cortisone, which inhibits secretion of ACTH by the anterior pituitary. Often, surgical correction of anatomic abnormalities is required: amputation of the clitoris and/or correction of vaginal and vulvar fusion. Several examples of pregnancy in patients who had been treated for the adrenogenital syndrome are reported, and the prognosis for a favorable outcome is good. Corticosteroid administration is maintained at pre-

pregnancy levels throughout gestation without fetal effect. Steroid supplementation during labor and delivery is customary. The newborn infants should be observed closely for possible adrenal insufficiency.

There are several cases on record in which the presence of the adrenogenital syndrome in the fetus was detected by the presence of excessive amounts of pregnanetriol in the maternal urine.

Primary Aldosteronism

This is an infrequent condition caused by an aldosterone-secreting adenoma of the adrenal cortex. This disease state is characterized by hypertension, elevated aldosterone secretion, decreased plasma renin activity, hypokalemia, and normal renal function. Treatment is surgical excision of the adenoma.

Pregnancy in affected patients is influenced deleteriously by the maternal hypertension and gestational complications secondary thereto (Crane et al.). The tumor should be suspected in the presence of hypertension and hypokalemia (without diuretic therapy). Spontaneous remission may occur during gestation, as elevated progesterone levels counteract aldosterone function. Administration of spironolactone successfully may suppress aldosterone secretion by the adenoma, but care must be exercised to avoid abrupt changes in blood pressure (Biglieri, Seaton). If there is no improvement, surgical excision of the adenoma is required, and the presence of the pregnancy must be disregarded.

ADRENAL CORTICAL HYPOFUNCTION

This condition may by primary (spontaneous or secondary to destruction by disease) or secondary to surgical excision (as for Cushing's syndrome). Its association with pregnancy is rare, but its frequency is increasing with the greater availability of hormonal replacement therapy.

Clinically, in the untreated state, fertility potential is depressed, although menstruation may be maintained. The signs and symptoms of adrenal insufficiency, nausea and vomiting, weight loss, weakness, easy fatigability, increased pigmentation, hypotension, syncopal attacks, vertigo, and hypoglycemia, may be dismissed as exaggerations of the complaints of normal pregnancy if the diagnosis has not been made preconceptionally. The diagnosis may become apparent only after an unusual stress or an adrenal crisis at delivery. Prior to hormonal replacement therapy, maternal mortality in gestation was in the range of 75 percent.

Treatment consists of replacement of gluco- and mineralocorticoids. Additional salt must be included in the diet. Hydrocortisone, 20 mg daily, is the usual maintenance dose for glucocorticoids. Deoxycorticosterone acetate (DOCA) can be supplied by the subfascial implantation of two 120-mg pellets, a dose sufficient to maintain salt metabolism throughout pregnancy. Hydrocortisone dosage may be increased to 40 to 50 mg daily just prior to, during, and after delivery, and then gradually tapered back to the maintenance dose. Postpartum, implantation of additional DOCA may be indicated. A patient with diagnosed adrenal insufficiency and under adequate therapy incurs no excess risk of morbidity or mortality during gestation.

Maternal treatment has brought fetal salvage and perinatal mortality in infants born to affected mothers into the range of normal. Neither maternal disease nor treatment increases the risk of fetal malformation (Khunda). The neonate should be observed closely for evidence of transient adrenal insufficiency secondary to pituitary suppression in utero.

PHEOCHROMOCYTOMA (ADRENAL MEDULLARY HYPERFUNCTION)

Pheochromocytoma is a rare tumor of the adrenal medulla (and other sites) which is particularly dangerous if encountered during gestation. The incidence of the tumor in the general population is estimated at 0.1 to 0.5 percent; in patients with hypertension, 2 percent (Shenker, Chowers). It is surprising that the disorder has been reported in only 95 patients during pregnancy.

The tumor arises from chromatin cells present in the adrenal medulla and other sympathetic nervous system tissue, and secretes dopamine, norepinephrine, and epinephrine, all through a tyrosine metabolic pathway. Dopamine is converted to norepinephrine by hydroxylation; norepinephrine is converted to epinephrine by methylation. Methylation occurs only in the adrenal medulla, and tumors originating there secrete both norepinephrine and epinephrine, as distinguished from extramedullary tumors which usually secrete only norepinephrine. Occasionally, these tumors may be malignant.

The clinical manifestations are variable and overlap with other hypertensive diseases in pregnancy: hypertension, tachycardia, sweating, headaches, blurred vision, nausea and vomiting, proteinuria, and syncope. The major differential diagnosis is with toxemia of pregnancy (el-Minawi et al.). The hypertensive pattern of pheochromocytoma frequently is paroxysmal, but may be sustained, and occasionally is sustained with paroxysmal exacerbations. The diagnosis may be made by assay of 24-hour urine collections for catecholamines and their metabolites (Brenner et al.). Vanillylmandelic acid (VMA) is elevated in 90 percent of patients with pheochromocytoma, but may be normal in 10 percent; false positives may result from diet or drugs. Urinary catecholamines always should be assayed as well; the ratio of norepinephrine to epinephrine may help determine the location of the tumor (Simanis et al.). Provocative tests using histamine or tyramine are dangerous, since they may provoke a hypertensive crisis. Blockade with phentolamine is safer, but the positive response, a drop in blood pressure of 35 mmHg (systolic) or 25 mmHg (diastolic) may compromise uterine circulation and the fetus. Radiologic diagnostic studies (intravenous pyelography and arteriography) all carry additional risk in pregnancy, but should be accomplished.

The maternal mortality from pheochromocytoma in pregnancy is approximately 50 percent; fetal wastage is at least equally high. If delivery intervenes prior to treatment, labor and vaginal delivery should be avoided because massive discharge of catecholamines may follow mechanical disturbance of the tumor; cesarean section probably is safer, and can be performed concurrently with definitive treatment of the tumor (Sprague et al.).

Treatment of pheochromocytoma is surgical removal. Preoperative treatment for 7 to 10 days with adrenergic blocking agents will minimize the possibilities of hypertensive crisis and cardiac arrhythmia during manipulation of the tumor. Beta-receptor blockade with drugs such as propranolol should be imposed before and during surgery. Postoperative follow-up with urinary assays of catecholamines is mandatory.

The risk of maternal death is such that the pregnancy at any stage must be ignored and definitive treatment for the pheochromocytoma instituted (Schenker, Luttwak). Thus, there is no indication for either abortion or surgical sterilization.

OVARIAN DISORDERS

FUNCTIONAL OVARIAN TUMORS

Unilateral ovarian enlargement may be detected upon pelvic examination in early pregnancy. If the ovary is free, mobile, round, cystic, smooth, and less than 6 cm in diameter, it probably is a physiologic corpus luteum of pregnancy. The management should be conservative, with repeated examinations at 2- to 4-week intervals. The presumptive diagnosis will be confirmed in the absence of further increase in ovarian size, and a return of the ovary to normal size postpartum.

It is uncertain whether the corpus luteum of pregnancy is essential to the maintenance of gestation in human beings. Although purposeless resection of the corpus luteum of pregnancy should never be performed, it is important to know that its surgical removal in very early gestation, without hormonal replacement, does not result in abortion (Csapo et al., 1972, 1973).

OVARIAN NEOPLASMS

The presence of an ovarian neoplasm ordinarily does not disturb the menstrual cycle or inhibit fertility. In addition, an ovarian neoplasm may arise de novo during pregnancy. Nevertheless, the incidence of ovarian neoplasms complicating pregnancy is low, having been estimated at about 0.1 percent.

An ovarian tumor in pregnancy frequently is asymptomatic. Usually, there is delay in diagnosis; pelvic examination is performed routinely on the first prenatal visit (usually in the first trimester), and not repeated until near term unless upon specific indication. Further, as the gravid uterus enlarges beyond the first trimester, the ovaries are drawn out of the pelvis into the maternal abdomen. A large ovarian tumor may be palpated abdominally, but a tumor of only moderate size may remain masked by the gravid uterus throughout gestation. Ovarian tumors have been mistaken for gravid uteri or have been responsible for alleged increase in uterine size out of proportion to gestational dates; hypertonic saline has been instilled into ovarian tumors to induce "abortion," and patients with large cystic tumors have been administered oxytocin in an attempt to "induce labor." It is obvious, therefore, that an ovarian tumor in gestation may grow insidiously to rather large proportions before the diagnosis is made.

There is an increased frequency of acute accidents for ovarian tumors complicating pregnancy: torsion, hemorrhage, suppuration, and tumor previa with dystocia. The frequency of torsion, hemorrhage, or rupture of ovarian tumors in the immediate puerperium is as high as 40 percent. In view of these complications, and always with the thought in mind that the histologic nature of the tumor is unknown, surgical exploration is indicated for all ovarian neoplasms.

Cystic Tumors

The cystic tumors most frequently encountered during gestation are dermoid, serous or pseudomucinous, paraovarian, and endometrial cysts. The benign cystic teratomas (dermoid cysts) make up from 25 to 40 percent of the total, but it is important to note that fully one-third of these tumors are serous or pseudomucinous cystadenomas, with significant potential for malignant transformation.

Solid Tumors

The incidence of solid tumors complicating pregnancy is about 0.01 percent, but two-thirds of such tumors are malignant. In one series of 36 solid ovarian tumors complicating pregnancy, the distribution by tumor type was as follows: dysgerminoma, 25.0 percent; Brenner tumors, 13.9 percent; fibroma, Krukenberg's tumor, and arrhenoblastoma, each 11.1 percent; granulosa cell tumor, 8.3 percent; theca cell tumor and sarcoma, each 5.6 percent; and fibromyoma, lymphosarcoma, and adenocarcinoma, each 2.8 percent (Dougherty, Lund). Because of the size and weight of the solid tumors, their cellularity, and their proliferative potential, the incidence of accidents such as torsion, degeneration, or rupture is 50 percent, almost double the rate of similar accidents in cystic ovarian tumors.

Feminizing ovarian tumors rarely are diagnosed clinically during gestation, since their hormonal contribution is masked by the effects of pregnancy. Granulosa or theca cell tumors which are hormonally active are associated with hyperestrinism, oligoamenorrhea or menometrorrhagia, anovulation, and infertility; coexistence of these tumors with pregnancy suggests either minimal hormonal activity or development of the tumor after conception.

A masculinizing ovarian tumor (arrhenoblastoma) results in virilization of the patient (see above, under Adrenogenital Syndrome) and in amenorrhea and infertility, so that its existence prior to conception is unlikely. With development of such a tumor during gestation, there will be virilizing effects upon the gravida, and androgenic stimulation of the fetus may result in pseudohermaphroditic changes in the external genitalia of the female neonate (Novak et al., 1970). The malignant potential of arrhenoblastoma makes immediate surgical intervention mandatory.

Theca Lutein Cysts

Theca lutein, large, often multilocular cysts are a benign, exaggerated ovarian response to excessive gonadotropic stimulation. They frequently are associated with hydatid mole or choriocarcinoma, may be found as well in patients with multiple gestation, occur infrequently in otherwise single gestation, and may complicate new hormonal techniques for the induction of ovulation. Except for acute accidents such as torsion or hemorrhage, surgical intervention is not necessary if the diagnosis can be established with good probability; almost irrespective of size attained, the ovaries return to normal size within a few weeks, once the abnormal gonadotropic stimulus is removed.

Management

The differential diagnosis of ovarian tumors depends in part on the stage of gestation. The possibilities which must be considered include the following: in the first trimester, ectopic pregnancy or pedunculated, subserous fibroid; in the second trimester, acute appendicitis, ureteral colic, pyelonephritis, degeneration of a fibroid, twisted adnexa, ectopic kidney, double uterus, or rudimentary uterine horn; and in the third trimester, degenerated fibroid, abruptio placentae, multiple gestation, or polyhydramnios. Considerable information about ovarian cysts or pelvic masses can be obtained by ultrasonography.

The optimal time for surgical intervention for ovarian tumors is the second trimester of gestation, when the possibilities of both spontaneous abortion (first trimester) and premature onset of labor (third trimester) are least. When an apparently benign, cystic ovarian neoplasm is discovered in the first trimester, surgery may be deferred until after the fourteenth week of gestation unless an acute accident supervenes. If cesarean section is anticipated for other, obstetric indications and the cyst can be kept under observation, its removal might be deferred until laparotomy for delivery. Any acute complication such as torsion or hemorrhage mandates immediate intervention. If the tumor is solid, bilateral, or in any other way is suggestive of possible malignancy, no delay in surgical extirpation should be tolerated.

Ovarian tumors discovered in the midtrimester can be removed promptly. Delay only increases the chance of abdominal crisis.

Tumors discovered in the third trimester and deemed benign should be observed, and extirpated in the immediate puerperium after accomplishing vaginal delivery. If there is any possibility of tumor previa and the tumor cannot be displaced from the posterior cul-de-sac by gentle pressure (with the patient in the knee-chest position), cesarean section and ovarian surgery should be accomplished promptly. Both a trial of labor and aspiration of the contents of a cystic tumor through the vaginal vault are contraindicated.

If the ovarian lesion is discovered to be malignant at the time of operation, treatment should be definitive and radical, and the presence of the pregnancy completely disregarded.

The postoperative treatment of patients subjected to ovarian surgery during pregnancy involves only the usual supportive measures. No specific advantage to the postoperative administration of progesterone has been demonstrated. The most important factor in minimizing the premature onset of uterine contractions is gentle handling of the uterus during surgery.

CONNECTIVE TISSUE DISORDERS

SYSTEMIC LUPUS ERYTHEMATOSUS

Systemic (visceral) lupus erythematosus (SLE) is a collagen disease with variable clinical manifestations and is ultimately fatal. Characteristic findings include skin eruption, intermittent fever, arthritis, arthralgia, renal damage (proteinuria and renal failure), anemia, leukopenia, and thrombocytopenia. A specific diagnostic feature of the disease is the presence, both in peripheral blood and bone marrow, of a pathognomonic lupus erythematosus (LE) cell.

The etiology of lupus erythematosus is not known. Recent theory holds that an abnormal autoimmune process develops gamma globulin antibodies which are active against the patient's own tissues. There is some evidence that lupus erythematosus may have a heredofamilial tendency.

Lupus erythematosus is encountered most frequently between the ages of 15 and 40, and 85 percent of cases reported have been in women. It therefore can be expected to occur in association with pregnancy, although the incidence of the combination is very low. The clinical manifestations of systemic lupus erythematosus are manifold and may be confusing. Frequently, exacerbation of the disease process results from administration of antibiotics and sulfonamides, acute infection, routine skin testing, or exposure to sunlight. An almost universal finding is joint pain, and 30 percent of affected patients have an associated arthritis. The diagnosis should be suspected when a female in the childbearing years develops fever, joint pain, arthritis, or chest pain with unknown etiology. In the absence of the pathognomonic LE cell, the differential diagnosis may include such disparate entities as toxemia of pregnancy, rheumatoid arthritis, subacute bacterial endocarditis, glomerulonephritis, idiopathic thrombocytopenia, or hemolytic anemia.

EFFECT OF PREGNANCY ON SLE

The influence of pregnancy on the course of SLE, to judge from published reports, must be quite variable. Both amelioration and exacerbation of the disease by pregnancy have been noted, as well as initial onset during pregnancy and exacerbation in the puerperium. With the advent of steroid therapy for SLE, the situation has improved; with steroid maintenance therapy throughout gestation, any exacerbation usually can be controlled very effectively. There is no indication for either therapeutic abortion or surgical sterilization (Zurier, 1975).

EFFECT OF SLE ON PREGNANCY

Fertility in patients with SLE is not impaired, except in the end stages of the disease. Fetal wastage is greatly increased, both in terms of spontaneous early abortion (25 percent) and premature labor (approximately 20 percent), and this poor result is not modified significantly by steroid therapy. In patients with significant renal and vascular involvement, problems of superimposed toxemia of pregnancy and intrauterine fetal growth retardation arise (McGee, Makowski).

EFFECT OF MATERNAL SLE ON THE FETUS

The "LE factor" circulating in the maternal blood, presumably an abnormal gamma globulin, is capable of transplacental transmission to the fetus (Berlyne et al.). Cord bloods of neonates born to mothers with SLE are capable of inducing the formation of LE cells when incubated with normal leukocytes. This capability diminishes with time and disappears within 6 to 8 weeks of life. A few cases of congenital SLE have been reported, as well as instances of neonatal neutropenia or pancytopenia (Seip).

Management

The modern treatment of systemic lupus erythematosus consists of the administration of corticosteroids in doses adequate to control the manifestations of the disease. Adequate corticosteroid dosage may be ad-

ministered throughout gestation with relative safety for mother and fetus. Care must be taken in adjusting the steroid dosage for the stress of labor and delivery, to continue the higher doses of corticosteroid through the puerperium to prevent exacerbation of disease, and to observe the neonate for possible secondary adrenal suppression and hypofunction (Zurier, 1978).

RHEUMATOID ARTHRITIS

Rheumatoid arthritis is a diffuse collagen disorder in which the principal symptoms and tissue changes affect the joints and juxtaarticular connective tissue. This disease is chronic and may result in permanent, severe joint deformities. The etiology of the disease is unknown; a heredofamilial predisposition has been postulated. Since the disease (except in the spinal form) occurs three times more frequently in females, and the age of onset ranges between 25 and 40, its association with pregnancy can be expected.

The onset of rheumatoid arthritis may be acute and fulminant or nonspecific and insidious. On the one hand, the patient may present with signs of an acute febrile illness and acute inflammatory changes in the joints. On the other hand, nonspecific constitutional symptoms (anorexia, malaise, fatigability) may be followed over a period of time by parasthesias and numbness of the extremities, fleeting, aching pains in the muscles and joints, and migratory polyarthritis.

EFFECT OF PREGNANCY ON RHEUMATOID ARTHRITIS

That pregnancy can result in amelioration of the symptoms of rheumatoid arthritis, and that exacerbations of the disease may occur in the puerperium are clinical observations of long standing. This association led Hench to the consideration of steroid therapy for rheumatoid arthritis, although the supposition that pregnancy results in a state of corticosteroid hyperactivity was shown to be unfounded (Pitkin). Any amelioration of the disease by gestation is only of very short duration (Persellin). A few cases have been reported in which the disease either started in or became worse during gestation.

EFFECT OF RHEUMATOID ARTHRITIS ON PREGNANCY

The disease has no effect on fertility, pregnancy, or the fetus and neonate. Occasionally, deforming arthritis of the spine, hips, or lower extremities may interfere with the usual procedures employed for delivery. For example, inability of the mother to abduct the hips may be so severe as to preclude access to the perineum; if the delivery cannot be accomplished in lateral Sims' position, cesarean section may be necessary. There is no indication for abortion or sterilization on purely medical grounds.

MANAGEMENT

All methods of treatment for rheumatoid arthritis are empiric, and should be administered in pregnancy as in the nongravid state in order to alleviate symptoms. Reducing the usual maintenance dosage may be possible during gestation in view of the ameliorating influence of pregnancy on the disease. In general, the aim of therapy is relief of pain, preservation of motion of affected joints, and prevention of deformity. The antenatal management of pregnancy is unaffected. Drug therapy may include salicylates, corticosteroids, phenylbutazone (Butazolidin), gold salts, and chloroquine. Aspirin, in large doses, has been implicated as a cause of a neonatal hemorrhagic diathesis. Chloroquine has been implicated as a possible cause of VIII cranial nerve deafness. Chrysotherapy has been administered without reported ill effect on the fetus. Phenylbutazone crosses the placenta easily and carries such a battery of potential maternal complications (especially leukopenia and thrombocytopenia) that its use during gestation is best avoided.

SCLERODERMA

Scleroderma is a diffuse collagen disease characterized clinically by focal or generalized induration of the skin. The focal form runs a benign clinical course. The generalized form involves many organ systems, including the esophagus, other portions of the gastrointestinal tract, the kidneys, the heart, and the lungs. The etiology of the disease is unknown. The diagnosis is established by biopsy of affected sites. Treatment is nonspecific and not curative.

The association of scleroderma with pregnancy is rare, and it is difficult to draw conclusions about pregnancy effects from the relatively small number of cases reported. In one large series (36 cases), pregnancy exerted no influence on the course of scleroderma in approximately 40 percent of cases, and produced amelioration in 20 percent and exacerbation in another 20 percent. Scleroderma appeared *de novo* in about 20 percent (Johnson et al.). There is evi-

dence of increased pregnancy wastage from spontaneous abortion, premature labor and delivery, fetal death in utero, and neonatal death. Any indicated treatment may be pursued throughout gestation; there is no evidence that treatment can alter the poor fetal outcome, or that pregnancy modifies the course of scleroderma.

MARFAN'S SYNDROME

Marfan's syndrome is a congenital form of mesodystrophy, characterized by cardiovascular anomalies (especially diffuse or dissecting aneurysm of the ascending aorta), ocular abnormalities (ectopia lentis), anomalies of the skeletal system (excessive length of long bones, "spider feet," and arachnodactyly), and pulmonary disease (often congenital cystic disease of the lungs). The disease has a heredofamilial tendency, probably based upon a single Mendelian autosomal dominant gene, but also may arise de novo.

This syndrome is the major cause of dissecting aneurysm in patients under 40; fully one-half of all cases of dissecting aneurysm reported in women under 40 years of age have occurred in pregnancy. Thus the association between Marfan's syndrome and pregnancy may be particularly lethal: women with the vascular anomalies of Marfan's syndrome have a greatly increased risk of fatal dissecting aneurysm during pregnancy.

The diagnosis of Marfan's syndrome can be suspected from observation of the patient's body habitus. Affected individuals are tall and thin and have markedly elongated extremities. Ocular examination shows a subluxation of the lens, redundancy of the suspensory ligaments, a tremulous iris, and hypotonia of the dilator pupillae muscles; occasionally, retinal detachment may occur. Angiocardiogram may disclose aneurysms of the ascending aorta or of the aortic sinuses of Valsalva.

In view of the high fatality rate of dissecting aneurysm, pregnancy should be proscribed for women with Marfan's syndrome. As soon as the diagnosis of Marfan's syndrome is made, surgical sterilization should be recommended. Therapeutic abortion should be carried out if pregnancy occurs. If the pregnancy is carried to term, every effort must be made to avoid increases in intravascular pressure. Continuous caudal or epidural anesthesia and prompt low-forceps delivery will minimize the Valsalva maneuvers required of the gravida during the second stage of labor. Despite all obstetric and medical management, a cardiovascular accident still may be unpreventable (Novell et al.).

PERIARTERITIS NODOSA

Periarteritis nodosa is a rare, necrosing angiitis. The characteristic lesion is a fibrinoid necrosis of medium-sized muscular arteries in which there is inflammation of all layers of the vessels. Clinical manifestations depend on which vessels are involved; classically, this is a progressive disease with myalgia, neuropathy, gastrointestinal disorders, hypertension, and renal disease. The disease is uniformly fatal when there is renal or cardiac involvement.

Few cases of periarteritis nodosa complicating pregnancy have been reported. All pregnant patients with the disease had hypertension and renal involvement, and all died soon after delivery. Pregnancy had no effect on the course of the disease. The fetal outcomes in five reported cases were good; one patient had a therapeutic abortion. The number of cases is too small to infer risks from these data (Varriale et al.).

Corticosteroids are the mainstay of therapy for periarteritis nodosa, but there is little evidence that they do more than provide symptomatic relief or can alter the course of the disease.

DISEASES OF THE GASTROINTESTINAL SYSTEM

HEPATIC DISORDERS

VIRAL HEPATITIS

Viral (acute infectious) hepatitis is an acute, inflammatory disease of the liver caused by infection with any of several hepatotoxic viruses, particularly hepatitis virus A (infectious hepatitis) and hepatitis virus B (serum hepatitis). Hepatitis virus A is transmitted by the ingestion of infected feces or fecally contaminated products and has an incubation period of from 2 to 7 weeks. Hepatitis virus B is transmitted primarily (but not exclusively) by the injection of blood products and has an incubation period of from 1 to 6 months. The period of viremia in hepatitis virus A infection is limited to the incubation period and to the first few days of active disease. Viremia after infection with hepatitis virus B may persist for a number of years; it has been estimated that 0.2 to 0.5 percent of

the population carries hepatitis virus B in the blood despite no prior clinical symptoms of hepatitis (Krugman, Giles).

The diagnosis of hepatitis depends on history, clinical findings, laboratory evidence of hepatic involvement, and the demonstration of hepatitis virus B antigen. The hepatitis virus B antigen [also known as Australian antigen, serum-hepatitis (SH) antigen, HBsAg, or hepatitis-associated antigen] has been demonstrated in the serum of patients with hepatitis virus B infection. The antigen appears to be specific for this infection. In patients with serum hepatitis, the antigen is detectable for varying periods of time. In some patients, it appears before there is any biochemical evidence of liver disease, and may disappear before the peak of biochemical abnormalities is reached. In other patients, the antigen may persist for years or even throughout life. More recently, a separate antigen has been identified in the serum of patients with hepatitis virus A infection (Milan antigen), which seems to be short-lived and disappears within 4 weeks of the onset of symptoms.

Effect of Hepatitis on Pregnancy

The incidence of hepatitis complicating pregnancy in the United States has ranged between 1 and 3 per 10,000 deliveries; the incidence in countries such as Israel or India is 30 to 60 times higher. Inadequate nutrition, poor general health, absent sanitation, and population crowding are contributory factors to increased prevalence of hepatitis. Hepatitis does not impair fertility. The reported effects of hepatitis on pregnancy, maternal mortality, and fetal wastage differ widely by geographical area and population studied. Maternal mortality, under ideal circumstances, probably does not exceed the risk of death from hepatitis in the nongravid population, about 0.4 percent. The incidences of spontaneous abortion, premature labor, and perinatal death depend on the state of maternal health, and invariably are increased above normal expectations (Cossart).

Effect of Pregnancy on Hepatitis

The symptoms of hepatitis during pregnancy are the same as in the nongravid state. Except in epidemic circumstances, the diagnosis tends to be made clinically only in jaundiced patients, which comprise less than half of patients with viral hepatitis. The prodromal stage of the disease preceding the development of icterus lasts up to 2 weeks. Presenting symptoms include fever, malaise, lethargy, and nausea.

Additional findings after the icteric phase develops include light-colored stools, dark urine, enlarged, tender liver, anorexia, vomiting, and/or diarrhea. In the absence of jaundice, it is obvious that many of these presenting symptoms might be mistaken for symptoms of pregnancy.

Pregnancy does not increase susceptibility to or severity of hepatitis. Mortality rates in pregnancy are the same as in the nongravid population (Borhanmanesh et al.). If general health is poor, nutrition inadequate, and supportive care not available, maternal mortality may range from 33 to 50 percent. Hepatitis usually resolves within 3 months, and the patient shows full recovery of hepatic function. In less than 5 percent of cases, however, the disease progresses to chronic hepatitis, posthepatitic cirrhosis, and fatal liver failure.

Effect of Hepatitis on the Fetus

In areas with poor sanitation and inadequate nutrition, the incidence of fetal wastage is very high, mainly from early abortion, premature labor, and perinatal death. Even under ideal circumstances, fetal wastage is increased in affected pregnancies as compared with uncomplicated controls. It has been suggested, but not confirmed elsewhere, that hepatitis in the first trimester of gestation carries a marked teratogenic potential (Mansell).

The mode of transmission of HBsAg between mother and infant has been debated (Holzbach; Cossart et al.). Clearly, infection seems to occur more frequently neonatally than in utero. Some of the variations reported may result from differences in the infectivity of the hepatitis virus. The presence of an e-antigen which seems to be associated with Dane particles (the presumptive virus) is related to a high degree of infectivity and to transplacental transmission (Okada et al., 1975), while the presence in maternal serum of antibody to e antigen seems to offer protection to perinatal infection (Okada et al., 1976). Infected infants tend to carry HBsAg chronically, and it is not known what proportion of such infants ultimately may develop chronic liver disease (Schweitzer et al.). It may prove possible to protect infants in utero and perinatally from infection by the administration to e antigen—positive mothers of gamma globulin rich in e antigen antibody, thus interrupting the chain of vertical transmission.

Women who are carriers of hepatitis virus B antigen do not excrete the antigen in breast milk. There are no studies of hepatitis virus A antigen in relation to breast milk (Gerety et al.).

Management

No specific treatment can be offered for maternal hepatitis, nor can prevention be ensured. Avoidance of blood transfusions and nonmedical drug injections would prevent the majority of cases of hepatitis virus B infection. After known exposure to hepatitis virus A infection, the administration of human gamma globulin (0.01 to 0.03 mL per pound of body weight) will provide some passive immunity to the mother and ameliorate the symptoms of hepatitis, but whether this will influence the degree of viremia is not known. Supportive treatment is the requisite: adequate nutrition, bed rest, and avoidance of further hepatic insults. Intravenous alimentation or fluid therapy rarely is necessary. Drugs only impose additional stress upon the liver and should be employed only where absolutely essential. Stool and needle isolation precautions should be used for both types of hepatitis.

There is no indication for therapeutic abortion in maternal hepatitis. Indeed, since the strain of surgical procedures may increase the possibility of the development of posthepatitic syndromes and chronicity of the disease, obstetric intervention, whether for abortion or induction of labor, should be deferred as long as possible, and the liver disease treated as if the pregnancy did not exist (Hieber et al.).

ACUTE YELLOW ATROPHY

Acute obstetric yellow atrophy is a rare complication of pregnancy, first characterized by Sheehan in 1940 as an entity distinct from hepatitis. The syndrome presents with severe jaundice, epigastric pain, vomiting, and headache starting acutely in the last trimester of gestation, frequently associated with the delivery of a stillborn fetus within 7 to 12 days, and often with maternal death a few days after delivery (Breen et al., 1970). At autopsy, the liver is small. The lobular architecture is not destroyed. Usually, there are gross fatty changes affecting the hepatic lobule, with a sharply defined rim of normal cells around the portal tract. Physical signs and the biochemical profile are compatible with acute liver failure; the pathologic picture, with severe toxic hepatitis. The etiology of the condition is unclear. The fatty infiltration may be the result of a metabolic injury which interrupts the conversion and mobilization of fat through inhibition of an enzyme system or impairment of the transmethylation function of the liver. The concurrent presence of fatty infiltration within the renal tubules and the occasional association of acute pancreatitis suggest a possible nutritional deficiency. For some authorities, acute obstetric yellow atrophy continues to be a manifestation of an unusually severe viral or toxic hepatitis occurring during pregnancy (Cano et al.).

Treatment is nonspecific. There is no indication for therapeutic termination of pregnancy (Breen et al.). The anticipated maternal mortality rate is approximately 85 percent (Hatfield et al.).

RECURRENT JAUNDICE OF PREGNANCY (CHOLESTATIC HEPATOSIS)

This condition is characterized by pruritus and jaundice, with mild elevations of serum alkaline phosphatase, bilirubin, and serum glutamic oxalacetic transaminase. Most reported cases have occurred in the last half of gestation, and the syndrome has resolved within 2 weeks postpartum. Anicteric pruritus is a milder form of the same condition. At times, the patient also complains of anorexia, nausea, vomiting, epigastric pain and/or diarrhea. The prothrombin time is low in approximately one-third of affected patients. Histologically, the liver shows bile duct proliferation and periportal inflammatory cell infiltrates (Rencoret, Aste).

The pathogenesis of this syndrome derives from altered bile metabolism and hepatocyte excretory function secondary to increased levels of estrogens and progesterone in pregnancy. Usually, the additional steroid load presented to the liver in gestation results only in the stimulation of the microsomal system and some competition for enzyme sites, manifested clinically by an excess of both free and esterized cholesterol in the blood, elevated serum phospholipid and lipoprotein levels, and slight impairment of the ability of the liver to handle bilirubin. When the enzyme system is overstressed by excessive steroid substrate or diminished hepatocyte capacity, which may be caused by an inborn genetic determinant or nonspecific injury (i.e., toxin or infection), this physiologic function decompensates. The clinical condition of cholestasis develops as a result of a primary hepatocellular alteration in the secretion of micelles containing bile salts. Abnormal micellar excretion causes biliary sludging in the bile canaliculi, decreased fluid content of bile, and diminished biliary tree excretory rate. The patient becomes predisposed to the inflammatory sequelae of cholestasis.

The diagnosis of recurrent jaundice of pregnancy depends on ruling out other liver diseases such as hepatitis, drug toxicity, and cholelithiasis. The syndrome recurs with successive pregnancies in the affected individual, and can be provoked by the administration of exogenous steroids such as hormonal contraceptives (Rannevik et al.).

Treatment is mainly symptomatic. The disease has a benign, self-limited course, and results in no demonstrable effects on pregnancy or on the fetus. The pruritus may be controlled by the administration of cholestyramine (an ion-exchange resin which absorbs bile salts), 8 to 20 mg orally per day. A low prothrombin time indicates the need for parenteral supplementation of vitamin K.

CIRRHOSIS OF THE LIVER

Below the age of 30, cirrhosis of the liver occurs infrequently, and it is a very rare complication of pregnancy. It is probable that unless the patient's cirrhosis is well compensated, with adequate return of hepatic function, fertility is impaired.

For the compensated cirrhotic with no unusual symptoms, no ascites, no esophageal varices, and laboratory evidence of adequate liver function, pregnancy presents no additional hazards, and the prognosis for the fetus is excellent. There is no evidence that the underlying liver disease is aggravated by pregnancy (Borhanmanesh, Haghighi, 1970).

The decompensated cirrhotic with jaundice, ascites, esophageal varices, and laboratory evidence of impaired liver function faces severe problems. The metabolic load of pregnancy may be difficult to accommodate, raising the possibility of hepatic coma. The hypervolemia of pregnancy may add to preexisting portal hypertension, increasing the risk of hemorrhage from esophageal varices (Evans el al., 1972; Salam, Warren).

Patients with cirrhosis should be discouraged from attempting pregnancy unless the disease is in remission and there is laboratory evidence of liver function approximating normal; pregnancy should be proscribed completely in the patient with portal hypertension, unless treated successfully with a portacaval shunt procedure (Niven et al.). If conception occurs in a patient with signs of progressive cirrhosis or portal hypertension, therapeutic abortion is indicated. Pregnancy in the well-compensated cirrhotic should be permitted to continue to term, with every expectation of good maternal and fetal results (Verma et al.).

The usual nonspecific supportive treatment should be continued through gestation: high-carbohydrate, normal-protein, low-fat diet; vitamin supplementation, especially of vitamin K; and avoidance of additional liver insults such as drugs, anesthetics, toxins, and infections.

CHOLECYSTITIS AND CHOLELITHIASIS

Gallbladder disease and gallstones are prevalent among women, and pregnancy is alleged to be a contributing factor thereto. The etiologic factors in gallbladder disease which arise in pregnancy include biliary tree hypotonia and decreased emptying time, hypercholesterolemia, and the changes in bile excretion described above (see Recurrent Jaundice of Pregnancy). Despite these predisposing conditions, the incidence of acute cholecystitis in pregnancy is only 0.02 percent; 90 percent or more of patients with cholecystitis in pregnancy have cholelithiasis as well.

The symptoms of gallbladder disease during pregnancy include epigastric distress and typical attacks of biliary colic: right upper quadrant colicky pain with radiation to the homolateral subscapular area. The development of acute cholecystitis and hydrops is associated with fever, tachycardia, and the presence of a tender, globular mass in the right upper quadrant of the abdomen. Occasionally, jaundice may develop. Usually, there is an associated significant leukocytosis.

Pain relief can be obtained by the administration of meperidine, which acts not only as an analgesic but as a smooth-muscle relaxant in relieving biliary colic. Cholecystography is of no value in making the diagnosis in an acute, obstructive episode. Ultrasonography is a valuable diagnostic aid. The management consists of stopping oral intake, administration of appropriate intravenous fluids, antispasmodics, anticholinergics, antimicrobials, and constant nasogastric suction. On this conservative regimen, most patients with acute cholecystitis improve within 48 hours.

Surgery of the biliary tract is best avoided during pregnancy, because it is technically more complicated as a result of the enlarged, gravid uterus. Nevertheless, failure of the patient to respond to conservative therapy, the development of empyema, impending rupture of the gallbladder, or continued obstruction of the common duct by stone may mandate surgical intervention. Despite the duration of gestation, there should be no hesitation in proceeding to surgery in the indicated case, since rupture of the gallbladder and resultant peritonitis carry a maternal mortality of well over 50 percent! No attempt should be made to carry out definitive surgery at this time. Frequently, a cholecystostomy will suffice to relieve the acute episode, and cholecystectomy can be deferred into the puerperium.

Patients with known, chronic gallbladder disease should be maintained on a bland, relatively low fat diet and on antispasmodics during pregnancy. Patients who have had attacks of gallbladder disease during gestation should have radiographic studies of their biliary tract, despite complete absence of symptoms, 3 to 4 months postpartum, when a more accurate evaluation of the disease can be made. Cholecystectomy will be necessary in more than 25 percent of these women, and should be carried out interconceptionally.

PANCREATITIS

Acute pancreatitis presents the same clinical picture in pregnancy as in the nongravid state. It has been suggested that the onset of symptoms in women suffering from pancreatitis frequently is related to pregnancy or the puerperium, but possible etiologic factors are unknown. Frequently, the condition coexists with disease of the biliary tree and becomes manifest during the last trimester or in the puerperium (Montgomery, Miller).

The onset of acute pancreatitis is characterized by sudden severe upper abdominal pain and vomiting. The signs and symptoms include fever, upper abdominal tenderness, distention, decreased bowel sounds, and obstipation. Muscle guarding and rigidity are infrequent, which helps to differentiate acute pancreatitis from other intraabdominal crises. Occasionally, the patient will complain of a severe, boring pain radiating through to the midback. The symptoms and findings may simulate those of a ruptured viscus, particularly of a perforated peptic ulcer. The presence of an enlarged uterus often makes it impossible to localize the findings to the region of the pancreas.

The most important factors in the diagnosis of pancreatitis in pregnancy are a high index of suspicion and a serum amylase level taken at the time of the acute onset. Serum amylase usually is elevated markedly within a few hours of the onset of pain but returns to normal within 24 to 72 hours. Serum lipase increases more slowly and tends to remain elevated longer. The concentrations of these enzymes may be elevated in other acute abdominal conditions, such as peritonitis or perforated peptic ulcer, but usually not to as high a level. X-ray examination of the abdomen frequently reveals a "sentinal loop" or pattern of ileus. The serum calcium may be lowered, which is indicative of a very severe, necrotizing pancreatitis (Storch et al.).

It is desirable to avoid surgical exploration in acute pancreatitis. The purpose of medical treatment is to achieve complete rest for the pancreas. This management includes nothing by mouth; continuous nasogastric suction; anticholinergic medication to decrease the stimulation·of secretion release by acid gastric contents [i.e., atropine, 0.4 mg every 2 to 3 hours; or propantheline bromide (Pro-Banthine), 30 mg every 2 to 4 hours]; and antibiotics to control associated infection. A broad-spectrum antibiotic is preferred, such as ampicillin or cephalothin, since bacterial peritonitis almost invariably follows the initial chemical peritonitis. Relief of pain usually requires the use of narcotics: meperidine hydrochloride (Demerol), 75 to 100 mg every 3 to 4 hours, is particularly useful; occasionally, paravertebral, sympathetic, or epidural block may be required. To meet the large fluid deficits which occur in acute pancreatitis and to maintain an effective circulating blood volume, blood, human serum albumin, plasma, dextran and other volume expanders, and electrolytes must be administered parenterally. The amount of fluid administered should be monitored by a central venous pressure catheter and by maintenance of urine output, with good specific gravity, at 40 to 60 mL per hour. Impairment of respiratory reserve is supervised by measurement of arterial blood pH, oxygen tension, and CO_2 tension.

Should the disease be encountered during exploratory laparotomy, opinions differ as to whether the abdomen should be closed promptly or biliary drainage instituted. Stones obstructing the pancreatic ducts should be removed; otherwise, only the simplest palliative surgery, such as cholecystostomy, should be contemplated. Drainage of the peritoneal cavity is indicated only in patients with extensive necrosis and abscess or pseudocyst formation.

Most patients will survive an acute attack of pancreatitis if managed conservatively. Recurrent attacks may be expected. The chances for fetal survival after an attack of acute pancreatitis are good. There is no indication for therapeutic abortion; conversely, any surgical intervention, including induction of labor, should be delayed as long as possible while medical treatment is under way (Corlett, Mishell).

DISORDERS OF THE ALIMENTARY TRACT

THE ORAL CAVITY

Pregnancy can have an effect on tissues in the oral cavity. The most obvious and severe changes are inflammatory in nature and particularly affect the gin-

givae surrounding the teeth. Early recognition of oral lesions and referral for treatment are essential if permanent damage is to be avoided. The incidence of periodontal disease (pyorrhea) in some form is almost 100 percent; gingivitis and periodontitis make up over 90 percent of this problem. The estimated incidence of dental caries in the United States is 98 percent. Although pregnancy does not play an etiologic role in dental disease, it may serve as an exacerbating factor in preexisting periodontal disease. Thus, the early detection of disorders of the oral cavity in pregnant women is an important aspect of prenatal care (Marder).

Gingivitis

An enlargement of the free gingivae caused by edema fluid may be the first manifestation of gingivitis. The free gingivae and interdental papillae appear glossy smooth rather than dull, enlarged, tend to bleed easily, and may pit upon application of pressure. The signs of gingivitis may begin as early as the second month of gestation. If untreated, the condition deteriorates progressively to term. Near term and postpartum, there is sudden, dramatic improvement in the gingival condition, which reverts clinically to the state antedating gestation. This hyperreactivity of gingival tissues during pregnancy to local irritating factors has been ascribed to increased levels of circulating steroid hormones (Lindhe et al.). If dental treatment interrupts the progressive morbidity and good oral hygiene is reinstituted, the gingivitis may resolve completely regardless of the stage of gestation. Alternatively, regular dental and home care will prevent the development of pregnancy gingivitis.

Pregnancy Epulis (Pregnancy Tumor, Angiogranuloma)

A pregnancy epulis is a local, exaggerated gingival response to irritative factors which occurs in less than 2 percent of gravidas. These pregnancy tumors usually occur in the midtrimester. If untreated, the tumor will either disappear or regress in size postpartum, but will recur in subsequent pregnancies (Lindhe et al.). The tumor appears as a discrete, soft mass, red to magenta in color, with a smooth, glistening surface. In the absence of secondary infection or trauma, pain or bleeding are not significant presenting symptoms. Histologically, the tumor is composed of fibroblasts, inflammatory cells, and a large number of thin-walled capillaries. Treatment of the tumor depends upon its location. If it interferes with normal oral function or can be traumatized during such function, or if its presence creates cosmetic or psychologic problems, complete excision under local anesthesia can be accomplished at any stage of gestation without risk to either mother or fetus.

Dental Caries

Most dental research supports the contention that pregnancy per se does not cause an increased incidence of dental caries. The number of decayed, missing, or filled teeth (DMF index) increases with age regardless of parity. Minerals are not withdrawn from teeth during pregnancy to fill fetal needs, nor are maternal teeth affected adversely by breast feeding and lactation. The incidence of caries in pregnancy may increase in a caries-susceptible woman if proper oral hygiene procedures are deferred—as in hyperemesis—but the same circumstances would apply as well to the nongravid state.

Dental Treatment during Pregnancy

Dental treatment for the alleviation of oral disease during pregnancy may be emergency, essential, or elective. In general, an uncomplicated pregnancy is not a contraindication to necessary dental therapy. Emergency treatment must be carried out as the need arises, regardless of the stage of gestation, and includes the management of acute dentoalveolar or periodontal abscesses, pulpitis, and tooth or jaw fractures. With proper radiographic equipment and shielding of the maternal abdomen, dental x-rays may be taken when indicated. The instillation of local anesthetic agents is safe for mother and fetus. Drugs should be prescribed only after consultation between dentist and obstetrician.

Essential treatment includes management of caries and gingivitis, and should be accomplished routinely during gestation. Purely elective procedures, including advanced gingival and osseous surgery, major oral rehabilitation and restorative treatment, and the removal of asymptomatic teeth, best are deferred until the late puerperium.

HEARTBURN

Heartburn (pyrosis) is one of the most frequently encountered complaints during pregnancy, being experienced by at least 60 percent of patients. Heartburn usually begins during the second trimester and becomes progressively worse as pregnancy advances. The patient complains of an uncomfortable burning sensation in the epigastrium or substernal area.

The cause of pyrosis is not known definitively. It seems to be unrelated to motor disorders of the esophagus. Factors in pregnancy which may contribute to gastroesophageal reflux include an elevated intraabdominal pressure, decreased tone of the lower esophageal sphincter, and temporary loss of the valve-like action of the intraabdominal segment of the esophagus. Usually, in affected patients, no disease can be demonstrated. Esophagitis may occur, especially in patients who vomit excessively. Continued reflux of hydrochloric acid and pepsin may lead to ulceration, hemorrhage, or stricture formation. Patients with hiatal hernia usually have pyrosis during pregnancy, but most women with pyrosis during gestation do not have hiatal hernia. Pyrosis does not result from excessive gastric acidity per se, but may be associated with achlorhydria as well.

Management

The symptoms of esophageal reflux are worse after heavy meals, and are exacerbated by lying down flat or by bending forward. Management therefore consists of prescription of small meals taken at frequent intervals and modifying posture, particularly for sleeping. The patient is instructed to sleep supported by several pillows or to elevate the head of the bed on blocks, and to relieve pyrosis by drinking liquids and ingesting effective antacids. Anticholinergic medication provides little relief of symptoms.

HIATAL HERNIA

This form of hernia can be demonstrated in 2 to 5 percent of the general population, perhaps more frequently in multiparous women. The hernia is of the "sliding" type, with the esophagogastric junction lying outside the abdomen at the apex of the herniated mass in 75 percent of cases; in the remaining 25 percent, the herniated mass is paraesophageal. Mucosal inflammation usually is found in the distal 1 to 5 cm of the esophagus. Erosions, hemorrhage, and fibrosis of the esophagus may be present. In addition to congenital or traumatic enlargement of the diaphragmatic hiatus, the causes of hiatal hernia include any condition which increases intraabdominal pressure or relaxes the muscular and ligamentous supports of the diaphragm and stomach, both factors present in pregnancy.

Most hiatal hernias are asymptomatic. The patient may present with complaints of dull, retrosternal, postprandial fullness, often associated with belching or hiccups. This discomfort may be aggravated by lying down or exertion after meals and by orange juice or sweet liquids. The pain may radiate to the back, jaws, shoulders, and arms. The diagnosis is made upon x-ray demonstration of a hiatal hernia. Esophagoscopy may reveal distal mucosal inflammation.

Management

The symptoms of hiatal hernia are controlled by avoiding overdistention of the stomach with large meals, elevating the head of the bed during sleep, reducing gastric acidity with antacids, and reducing intraabdominal pressures. Recommendations usually include multiple small meals consisting of bland foods and the interval use of aluminum hydroxide, magnesium trisilicate, or magnesium hydroxide. Surgical correction of the hiatal defect rarely is necessary, although it must be kept in mind that incarceration of a hiatal hernia is a surgical emergency.

ACHALASIA

True achalasia of the esophagus is rarely encountered in pregnancy. The principal symptom, dysphagia, is insidious in onset, may be intermittent, and varies in severity. Severe, prolonged achalasia is associated with significant weight loss. Chronic pulmonary infection and pneumonia may result from aspiration of the esophageal contents, especially during sleep.

The etiology of the disorder is not known. The peristaltic activity of almost the entire esophagus is diminished, and the lower esophageal sphincter fails to relax with advance of the peristaltic wave. The condition usually is chronic and progressive, and its course is unchanged by gestation.

Management

Therapy involves altering the esophagogastric sphincter by dilation or rupturing of muscle fibers to permit passage of food into the stomach by gravity. Pneumatic or hydrostatic dilation is effective in relieving symptoms in 75 percent of cases; esophageal myotomy rarely is necessary during pregnancy.

PEPTIC ULCER

The secretion of hydrochloric acid by the stomach is decreased during pregnancy. Pepsinogen secretion is unchanged during the first two trimesters, increases in the third trimester, and reaches a peak in the early puerperium. Simultaneously, pregnancy results in a prolongation of gastric emptying time. As a result, the development of peptic ulcer disease during gestation is extremely rare, and women with preexisting disease usually experience relief of symptoms during pregnancy.

The true incidence of peptic ulcer disease in pregnancy is not known. Although remission of symptoms during gestation is the usual course, pregnancy is not a cure for peptic ulcer. Complications, including perforation, hemorrhage, and death, have occurred during pregnancy. Exacerbation of symptoms in the puerperium is to be anticipated, as the ameliorating effects of gestation are removed; furthermore, lactation appears to be associated with an increase in gastric secretion.

The classic signs of perforation of a peptic ulcer frequently are altered during late pregnancy, and the diagnosis of peptic ulcer disease is complicated by an overlay of gestational digestive complaints and the reluctance to utilize radiologic diagnostic techniques. Nevertheless, the diagnosis must be pursued and may be facilitated by newer endoscopic techniques.

The treatment of uncomplicated peptic ulcer disease during gestation is medical, and usually is effective. The therapeutic regimen includes the liberal use of sodium-free antacids, frequent feedings of a bland diet, antispasmodic and anticholinergic medications, and mild sedatives. The hemorrhaging ulcer may require supportive blood transfusions, and perforation and pyloric or duodenal obstruction mandate surgical intervention. Many of the fatalities secondary to ulcer complications in pregnancy have resulted from reluctance to intervene surgically in equivocal cases, and this tendency should be reversed.

APPENDICITIS

Inflammation of the vermiform appendix is the most frequent acute surgical condition encountered in pregnancy. The frequency of acute appendicitis in pregnancy is the same as in the nongravid population of the same age group, but the hazards are much greater. The greatest risk in acute appendicitis occurring during pregnancy is the increase in maternal and fetal mortality and morbidity associated with delay in diagnosis and treatment. Most instances of acute appendicitis occur during the last trimester, labor, or the puerperium, and diagnosis is complicated by the overlay of pregnancy gastrointestinal symptoms, the physiologic leukocytosis of pregnancy, displacement of the appendix from its position in the right lower quadrant of the abdomen by the enlarging uterus, and the inability of the abdominal musculature to provide the classic responses to peritoneal irritation (i.e., muscle spasm, rigidity and guarding, etc.). Abdominal distress may be attributed to the onset of labor or to severe afterpains in the puerperium. Delay in diagnosis permits the disease to proceed to appendiceal rupture and peritonitis. During pregnancy, walling off of the infection is inhibited by the inability of the omentum to return to the right lower quadrant; often, the uterus and right adnexa are involved in localization of the infection and walling off of the appendiceal abscess. Peritoneal irritation stimulates the onset of labor, and with delivery and consequent change in size and position of the uterus, the appendiceal abscess may rupture, and widespread peritonitis may follow.

The diagnosis of peritonitis rests upon a high index of suspicion and careful attention to the patient's history, no matter how trivial the abdominal complaints may seem to be. The only significant physical finding may be localized tenderness to deep pressure over the site of the appendix—which, in pregnancy, may be above the right iliac crest, near the umbilicus, or even in the right flank. Because of the upward displacement of the cecum, the value of vaginal or rectal examinations in detecting the disease is diminished. The differential diagnosis includes urinary tract disease, adnexal pathology, and degeneration of uterine myomata. At times, the diagnosis of appendicitis cannot be confirmed without exploratory laparotomy. The hazard of appendectomy is so small, and the risk of delay in diagnosis and treatment so great, that *exploratory laparotomy should be undertaken in every suspected case, more readily in the gravida than in the nonpregnant patient!*

Management

The treatment of appendicitis is surgical. Vigorous antibacterial therapy is indicated in all cases, but only as an adjuvant to the removal of the appendix. The usual McBurney's incision should be avoided; better exposure of the displaced organ will be achieved with a high right perirectus incision near the point of maximal tenderness. Abdominal or cul-de-sac drainage may be required if an appendiceal or pelvic abscess is encountered. *Under no circumstances should delivery by cesarean section be attempted in the presence of appendiceal disease!* Regardless of the type of incision used, and even if appendectomy is performed during the first stage of labor, the wound will not disrupt as a result of vaginal

delivery. If appendicitis is suspected during the latter part of labor, appendectomy might await, and be performed immediately after, vaginal delivery.

REGIONAL ILEITIS

Also known as regional enteritis and Crohn's disease, this is a granulomatous, transmural, inflammatory disease of the small intestine, frequently involving the terminal portion of the ileum, but affecting all parts of the small bowel. The cause of the disease is not known. The characteristic clinical manifestations include diarrhea, abdominal cramps, progressive weight loss, anemia (secondary to intestinal bleeding), fever, and sometimes an abdominal mass in the right lower quadrant of the abdomen.

Regional ileitis does not affect fertility or influence the outcome of pregnancy deleteriously; there is no increase in the rates of abortion or fetal death (Norton, Patterson). Pregnancy does not influence the course of ileitis when the disease is quiescent, but may exert an unfavorable effect on the disease if the ileitis is active at the time of conception. The course is likely to be severe when ileitis arises for the first time during pregnancy. Exacerbation during the puerperium may occur in about half of the affected patients. When ileitis occurs for the first time within several months after pregnancy, the course of the disease usually is comparatively mild.

Management

In pregnancy, management of regional ileitis is symptomatic and supportive, as in the nongravid patient. If medical management is unsuccessful in achieving remission of the disease, surgical intervention may become necessary; if at all possible, this should be postponed until after the pregnancy is completed. Immediate surgical intervention is required in the face of complications such as intestinal obstruction, perforation, or abscess formation. There is no indication for either therapeutic abortion or surgical sterilization.

INTESTINAL OBSTRUCTION

Intestinal obstruction or ileus represents an inability of the intestinal tract to propel its contents toward the rectum. It may result from absence of peristaltic movement of the intestinal musculature (adynamic ileus, pregnancy ileus) or from mechanical obstruction of the intestinal lumen. The obstruction may arise in the lumen of the bowel (i.e., foreign body, intussusception), within the intestinal wall (i.e., constricting carcinoma), or from an extrinsic source (i.e., adhesions, hernia, or extrinsic mass).

Adynamic ileus of pregnancy is rare and accounts for only 6 percent of intestinal obstruction in pregnancy. The most frequent cause of intestinal obstruction associated with pregnancy is mechanical obstruction, often related to post-cesarean section adhesions. In order of frequency, other organic causes of ileus are volvulus, intussusception, strangulated hernia, and obstructing tumor.

There are three periods of increased frequency of occurrence of adynamic ileus in pregnancy: the middle trimester; at term; and immediately postpartum and during the puerperium. The same hormonal factors which decrease ureteral and gallbladder tone during gestation probably are involved here also; reflex adynamic ileus may develop in association with conditions such as severe pyelitis.

With adynamic ileus, the presenting symptoms are similar to those for large-bowel obstruction, but no organic cause can be demonstrated. The ileus usually involves the sigmoid colon and largely is confined to the large bowel. X-ray examination reveals large-bowel distention, and fluid levels can be demonstrated. Surgical intervention is unnecessary, and medical, conservative treatment is effective in restoring intestinal function: nasogastric suction to decompress the intestinal tract, enemas, and stimulation of peristalsis with parasympathomimetic agents such as neostigmine bromide (Prostigmin) or acetylocholine bromide.

In organic mechanical obstruction of the intestine, the patient's abdomen is distended and tympanitic. Characteristic of mechanical obstruction are hyperactive peristaltic sounds which are concurrent with spasms of colicky abdominal pain. As the bowel becomes more distended with gas and fluid, the peristaltic sounds become more high pitched and "tinkling." These evidences of peristaltic activity are in marked contrast to the inactivity found in adynamic ileus; the disappearance of peristaltic sounds in a patient with mechanical intestinal obstruction is a sign of impending necrosis or perforation. Abdominal tenderness appears only late in the course of the disease, with intestinal strangulation or impending perforation. If obstruction continues without relief, necrosis of the intestine may ensue, followed by peritonitis, septic shock, and often maternal mortality.

In pregnancy, intestinal obstruction may result from compression, torsion, or incarceration of intestines by the enlarging uterus, particularly in the presence of intraperitoneal adhesions which limit bowel mobility. The immediate puerperium, when the post-partum uterus abruptly has returned to a smaller size, is another time of increased risk, particularly for volvulus of the sigmoid colon. Mechanical obstruction, with its accompanying systemic complications of dehydration and electrolyte imbalance, is an acute surgical emergency in pregnancy, and intervention should not be delayed no matter what the stage of gestation (Weston, Lindheimer). Relief of the obstruction and removal of the cause (i.e., lysis of adhesions) usually is adequate therapy; only rarely will evacuation of the uterus be necessary to accomplish this result. If intraperitoneal suppuration occurs, abortion or premature onset of labor is probable, and fetal wastage will be increased. As with other intraperitoneal inflammatory processes requiring surgical intervention, pregnancy is an indication for earlier operation rather than procrastination if better maternal and fetal results are to be achieved.

CONSTIPATION

Irregular bowel habits are a frequent complaint during pregnancy and probably are related to the generalized smooth muscle hypotonia which is physiologic in pregnancy and to the pressure of the enlarged uterus upon the colon and rectum. Constipation may be exacerbated by inadequate intake of fluids and bland bulk. As a result of prolonged intestinal tract transit time, the stool may become excessively dry and hard (scybalous); elimination of such hard fecal matter requires straining and usually is painful.

The management of pregnancy constipation in women with previously normal bowel habits includes emphasis upon maintenance of regular gastrocolic reflex habits; dietary supplementation with large amounts of fluid and bulk (i.e., fresh, canned, or cooked fruits and vegetables); and a planned program of light exercise and moderate physical activity. If symptoms continue, mild laxatives such as milk of magnesia or stool-softening agents may be employed. In the face of very severe symptoms, enemas and rectal instillations of oil may become necessary, and infrequently manual release of impacted feces is required. Prevention is much more to be sought than cure.

ULCERATIVE COLITIS

This inflammatory and ulcerative disease of the colon and rectum has both acute and chronic manifestations. Clinically, it is characterized by rectal bleeding, diarrhea, abdominal discomfort, fever, weight loss, malaise, anorexia, and a wide variety of local and systemic complications. The disease further is characterized by unpredictable exacerbations and remissions, and by long periods of freedom from symptoms. The cause of ulcerative colitis is unknown. Local complications may include hemorrhage, toxic dilatation of the colon, perforation and peritonitis, polyp formation, and malignancy. Systemic complications include erythema nodosum, pyoderma gangrenosum, pericholangitis and biliary cirrhosis, nephrolithiasis, nonspecific polyarthritis, hypoproteinemia, and malnutrition.

The disease may begin at any age, but in the female usually develops before or during the reproductive years. There is no consensus about the factors which aggravate or ameliorate the disease, but emotional disturbances play a major role in the pathogenesis. In most adult females with mild or moderate ulcerative colitis, the menses are normal and fertility is not impaired, and the disease does not have an adverse effect upon pregnancy or the fetus. Very severe ulcerative colitis may be associated with oligomenorrhea and relative infertility, probably related to the patient's general state of debilitation.

Pregnancy frequently results in an exacerbation of ulcerative colitis, the disease most frequently becoming worse during the first trimester or in the puerperium. Patients with ulcerative colitis should defer conception until at least several years after remission of an acute episode. Ulcerative colitis developing initially during gestation tends to be very severe, and occasionally follows a fulminating course which may terminate fatally. Patients who have had total colectomy and ileostomy for ulcerative colitis have an excellent prognosis for uneventful pregnancy and normal vaginal delivery, obstetric factors permitting.

There is great individual variation in response to the disease process both in the nongravid state and in relation to pregnancy. Many patients remain in good health and report excellent control of the ulcerative colitis during gestation; in others, there may be exacerbation of bloody diarrhea, fever, and toxic symptoms. The extent of the disease process and its activity must be considered in evaluating the advisability of conception. Pregnancy during acute ulcerative colitis is a serious problem, and there is no assurance that the disease will be ameliorated by abortion, which may instead result in exacerbation. Colitis may remain quiescent during gestation only to flare up, or to appear for the first time, in the puerperium. In any event, the eventual impact of pregnancy upon ulcerative colitis may be an accentuated disease process (Goligher et al.).

Management

The medical management of ulcerative colitis includes a bland, high-calorie, high-protein, low-residue diet; multiple vitamin supplementation; sedation and adequate rest; reassurance and supportive psychotherapy; antidiarrheal drugs; corticosteroids and/or ACTH; antibiotics; and iron supplements or transfusions as necessary. Therapy is directed toward the maintenance of general good health and adequate nutrition.

If the patient fails to respond to medical management, surgery may become necessary. If operation during pregnancy is unavoidable, temporary ileostomy should be performed, and colectomy delayed until after delivery, when the procedure technically is easier. If colectomy can be deferred, it may be accomplished during gestation without disturbing the pregnancy or the incumbent fetus.

Unless obstetric indications for cesarean section exist, patients with ulcerative colitis should be delivered vaginally. Elective cesarean section should be considered for the patient in whom chronic disease has caused extensive scarring or fistula formation in the perineal area or rectovaginal septum.

If corticosteroid therapy was necessary for control of ulcerative colitis prior to conception, it should be continued through the pregnancy, although possibly a reduction in dose may be accomplished. Similarly, initiation of treatment with corticosteroids is not contraindicated in pregnancy if necessary for medical management of the disease process, and dosage is monitored in terms of clinical symptoms. Corticosteroid therapy may be instituted or increased in the puerperium in an attempt to ameliorate the anticipated exacerbation of the disease.

NEOPLASMS OF THE GASTROINTESTINAL TRACT

Malignancies of the gastrointestinal tract are relatively rare during pregnancy, with a reported incidence of 0.01 percent (1 per 100,000 deliveries). The majority of these lesions involve the descending colon and rectum. Except as it affects the general condition of the mother, the disease does not affect the course of pregnancy. Isolated cases of metastatic disease to the placenta and to the fetus have been reported (Rothman et al.).

The initial manifestation of a bowel malignancy in pregnancy may be intestinal obstruction, perforation of the bowel, or even the appearance of tumor previa as a cause of dystocia. Delay in the diagnosis of the neoplasm is constant, since the earlier manifestations of bowel cancer may mimic physiologic alterations in bowel function during pregnancy. Intractable or recurrent hematemesis, melena, rectal bleeding, abdominal cramps, diarrhea alternating with constipation, or partial intestinal obstruction mandate thorough investigation of the gastrointestinal tract. Radiologic diagnostic procedures may be necessary regardless of the stage of gestation. Endoscopic examination of the rectum and sigmoid colon is possible and permissible at all stages of pregnancy, and suspicious mucosal lesions should be biopsied.

Management

Treatment of malignancies of the gastrointestinal tract usually requires surgery no matter what the stage of gestation. Rarely does upper abdominal surgery require hysterectomy or evacuation of the uterus technically to facilitate the operation. Treatment of lesions of the lower bowel may vary with the extent of the tumor and the duration of pregnancy. Treatment of the malignancy must not be deferred on account of an incumbent pregnancy. In the first and second trimesters, the technical problems usually are simple; the uterus is not so large as to interfere mechanically with any indicated operative procedure, and there is sufficient time for complete healing to occur before parturition. The operative procedure usually consists of an adequate bowel resection with primary anastomosis if the lesion lies above the peritoneal reflection, and abdominoperineal resection for rectal lesions. In the third trimester, management must be individualized. If labor is imminent and the bowel tumor does not present pelvic dystocia, labor should be induced and definitive surgery carried out in the puerperium. If labor is not imminent, or if the tumor presents an obstructive problem, delivery should be accomplished by cesarean hysterectomy, and definitive bowel surgery carried out at the same time. If the tumor is inoperable or has distant metastases, the fetus should be considered of primary importance in deciding upon management. If tumor complications arise, the pregnancy must be disregarded and the complication treated: transverse colostomy for obstruction may be accomplished without interfering with the gestation.

Successful pregnancy and vaginal delivery have been reported after abdominoperineal resections. There is no contraindication to pregnancy once late recurrence has been excluded by the usual clinical evaluations (Lea).

ANORECTAL DISORDERS

Hemorrhoidal disease is a special problem which may originate during or be aggravated by pregnancy. Hemorrhoids are vascular dilatations of the internal or external venous plexuses of the anus, or both. Hemorrhoids cause only moderate discomfort, if any, unless accompanied by complications such as thrombosis, strangulation, prolapse, or necrosis. Hemorrhoids may appear or become exacerbated during pregnancy because of the vascular and structural weaknesses and hormonal changes which develop, especially during the last trimester, the physiologic problems with constipation, the increased venous pressure which results from the presence of the gravid uterus, and the straining during and traumatic injuries which may result from delivery. Usually, hemorrhoids which appear during gestation recede appreciably after delivery, but tend to recur during succeeding pregnancies. Treatment is determined by the patient's symptomatology and by the findings on examination. Soft, perianal hematomas (external thrombosed piles), in the absence of sphincter muscle spasm, should be treated conservatively with external moist heat and analgesics as required. Large, painful, thrombosed hemorrhoids best are managed by excision of the overlying skin with extrusion of the thrombi. If possible, hemorrhoidectomy should be deferred until after the patient has completed her reproductive career.

The patient with hemorrhoids will benefit from a diet with a minimum of coarse residue and which results in a soft, easily passed stool. Constipation and straining at stool should be avoided. Relief of symptoms from a thrombosed anorectal vessel, with local swelling and pain, may be achieved with application of cold witch hazel packs, bland anesthetic ointments or suppositories, sitz baths, and rest. Recurrent prolapsing hemorrhoids or rectal mucosa should be replaced digitally by the patient whenever prolapse occurs. Injection of hemorrhoids with sclerosing solutions should not be attempted during pregnancy.

DISORDERS OF THE NEUROMUSCULAR SYSTEM

EPILEPSY

Idiopathic epilepsy, either grand mal or petit mal, occurs in about 0.4 percent of the population, and the incidence of epilepsy in association with pregnancy is about 0.15 percent. The frequency of the association is increasing with greater efficacy of treatment and better lay understanding of the disorder.

Idiopathic epilepsy is associated with a paroxysmal cerebral dysrhythmia which is present in all patients during a seizure and which in 90 percent of affected individuals may be detected electroencephalographically at some time between seizures. Conversely, although the electroencephalographic abnormality is present in 10 percent of the population, only 1 in 25 of these individuals suffers from a seizure disorder. The dysrhythmia, which may be considered an epileptic diathesis, probably is an inherited trait, occurring in 60 percent of relatives of known epileptics. Affected individuals tend to respond with convulsions to a variety of stimuli which affect the cerebral cortex: trauma, fever, toxins, drugs, and chemical substances.

The risk that the child of an epileptic mother will develop seizure disorders on a hereditary basis is less than 2 percent, with a good probability that the disorder may be limited to a few seizures during childhood. Many cases of seizure disorders are secondary to organic brain damage or hypoxia sustained during the pre- or perinatal periods; in such cases, there is no hereditary tendency.

EFFECT OF PREGNANCY ON EPILEPSY

There is no definite pattern to the behavior of epilepsy during gestation. The effect of pregnancy on the frequency and intensity of seizures is unpredictable, and may vary in the same patient from pregnancy to pregnancy. Why epileptic seizures should become worse in some pregnant patients is not known; it is postulated that increased water retention during pregnancy, a physiologic phenomenon, may increase cerebral irritability.

Epilepsy may appear for the first time during gestation and continue unabated after parturition. Patients with this type of "gestational epilepsy" must be examined very carefully for evidence of intracranial neoplasms, which tend to become edematous during pregnancy.

EFFECT OF EPILEPSY ON PREGNANCY

Epilepsy has no deleterious effect on gestation. Abortion and premature labor are not the result of seizures under ordinary circumstances. The prognosis for normal labor is excellent. The gravida has a lowered threshold for seizures and may have a higher incidence of eclampsia with even mild degrees of hypertension and fluid retention (Knight et al.).

MANAGEMENT

If an epileptic patient has infrequent seizures and is not taking anticonvulsant medication in the nongravid state, there is no need a priori to initiate such therapy merely because of supervening gestation.

The anticonvulsant regimen followed in the nonpregnant state should be continued into pregnancy, with adjustments in dosage only if there is an increase in either the frequency or the intensity of seizures. The doses of drugs are regulated by seeking a balance between minimizing seizures and avoiding a soporific effect. Control of seizures with drugs may be affected adversely during gestation because of decreased absorption from the gastrointestinal tract (especially with nausea and vomiting) or increased protein binding; the latter is particularly applicable to diphenylhydantoin and phenobarbital. During pregnancy, serum anticonvulsant levels must be monitored and adjusted carefully if increased seizure frequency is to be avoided or reversed. The pregnant woman also should receive supplementary folic acid, since most of the major anticonvulsants, especially diphenylhydantoin, may induce folic acid deficiency.

Every effort must be made to reduce water retention, manifest by rapid weight gain and edema. A low-sodium diet may be adequate; often, intermittent use of diuretics is necessary.

If, in spite of treatment, seizures increase in frequency as pregnancy progresses, the patient must be hospitalized for more intensive therapy. If status epilepticus is threatened, recourse may be had to diazepam (Valium), 10 mg intravenously as an initial dose, followed by an infusion of 100 mg of diazepam in 500 mL of saline solution, adjusted to deliver 20 to 40 mg of diazepam an hour until the seizures are controlled, and then decreased very gradually. The patient's airway must be ensured, oxygen administered, serum electrolytes monitored, and supportive measures applied as necessary.

Treatment is directed solely to control of the seizure disorder. Idiopathic seizure disorders that can be controlled medically are not an indication for immediate delivery, premature evacuation of the uterus, therapeutic abortion, or sterilization. The presence of an idiopathic seizure disorder in either parent is not an adequate reason for advising against conception. Idiopathic seizure disorders do not alter the course of labor and delivery. The possible fetal consequences of maternal anticonvulsant therapy must be discussed with the parents preconceptionally if possible or early in gestation.

FETAL EFFECT OF MATERNAL ANTICONVULSANT THERAPY

Acute Problems

When central-nervous-system depressants are used during labor or shortly before delivery, fetal intoxication may result. The management of such acute toxicity in the neonate is similar to that in the adult: adequate pulmonary ventilation and hydration. The administration of analeptics to the newborn has not proven to be of much value.

Infants exposed to diphenylhydantoin or barbiturates in utero may show evidence of depressed clotting factors and even neonatal hemorrhage (Bleyer, Skinner). The administration of 5.0 mg of water-soluble vitamin K (menadiol sodium) to the mother at least once weekly during the last month of gestation prevents such clotting factor depression; the same agent, administered to the affected infant, is therapeutic.

Chronic Problems

An unusual complication of long-term maternal anticonvulsant therapy is a seizure or "jitteriness" in the newborn because of "withdrawal" of the central-nervous-system depressant. Management requires medication of the infant with the respective anticonvulsant and institution of a regimen of gradual withdrawal. Since convulsions may be precipitated by the sudden withdrawal of *any* central-nervous-system depressant, even in the adult, such a reaction in the newborn infant does not presage the development of a convulsive disorder.

A more serious problem is the question of teratogenicity. There is evidence of an increased risk of congenital heart disease and cleft palate in infants born to mothers with epilepsy, most of whom have been taking anticonvulsant drugs (Smith; Shapiro et al.). It is unclear if this increased risk of malformation results from epilepsy in general (or any one particular form of epilepsy), from a common genetic predisposition to epilepsy *and* the malformation, from a maternal or fetal genetic difference in pharmacokinetics and drug utilization, from one specific anticonvulsant agent, or from deficiency states in the mother or fetus induced by the anticonvulsant agent. The risk of all

anomalies in infants born to women with epilepsy is in the range of 4 to 5 percent, approximately twice that in the general population. Diphenylhydantoin is the drug most frequently associated with this problem. In addition, isolated reports have suggested that about 10 percent of infants exposed to diphenylhydantoin in utero may show an ill-defined "fetal hydantoin syndrome," which includes intrauterine growth retardation, postnatal growth deficiency, microcephaly, and mental retardation. The present consensus is that this syndrome has *not* definitively been linked to drug exposure, but existing data are scanty. Information on fetal malformations associated with maternal ingestion of barbiturates is even less conclusive; data on the effects of other anticonvulsant medications are minimal or nonexistent.

There is agreement about the following principles:

1. No woman should receive anticonvulsant medication unnecessarily; if the patient has been free of seizure for a long period, attempts should be made to withdraw the anticonvulsant medication prior to conception.
2. Women with a seizure disorder requiring anticonvulsant medication for control who seek advice about conception must be fully informed of the risks described above.
3. Women on anticonvulsant medication who first are seen after conception should be informed about the same risks. There is no absolute medical indication for abortion, and the data may be reassuring. Drug therapy should be continued throughout pregnancy for maternal welfare. There is no reason at present to switch from diphenylhydantoin or phenobarbital to another anticonvulsant drug about which even less may be known.
4. Most anticonvulsant agents present in therapeutic levels in the mother also are present in breast milk, but in concentrations so low that demonstrable effects on the infant are unlikely. There is nothing to suggest that a puerpera on anticonvulsant medication either must avoid breast-feeding or must discontinue the medication.

CHOREA GRAVIDARUM

Chorea gravidarum is synonymous with Sydenham's (rheumatic) chorea occurring in a pregnant patient and is not a neurologic disorder specific to pregnancy. Of women affected by chorea gravidarum, 60 percent have suffered from chorea or rheumatic fever in childhood, and over one-third have clinical rheumatic heart disease. With the decreasing frequency of chorea and rheumatic fever in childhood, the incidence of chorea gravidarum similarly has diminished.

Chorea gravidarum occurs most frequently in young primigravidas. It seems that pregnancy predisposes to a recurrence of chorea in a woman who once has suffered from it, but the relapse rate is only about 4 percent (Zegart, Schwartz). Usually, the choreic movements begin early in pregnancy, in the first trimester in over half of the cases, and continue throughout gestation, modified but not abolished by treatment. Only slightly more than 10 percent of cases start in the third trimester, when the condition must be differentiated from eclampsia; rarely, chorea gravidarum first becomes manifest in the puerperium.

Pregnancy and labor are unaffected by chorea, except in the most severe cases in which abortion, premature labor, or intrauterine fetal demise may occur. The disorder usually disappears after delivery or after termination of pregnancy.

MANAGEMENT

Management is mainly supportive, ensuring adequate rest, proper dietary intake (by intragastric or parenteral routes if necessary), and protection against self-injury. Medications may include barbiturates, acetylsalicylic acid, and phenothiazine tranquilizers. Termination of pregnancy may be indicated in very severe cases, when violent movements interfere with sleeping and exhaustion sets in, or when the patient becomes maniacal and hallucinatory. In any obstetric or surgical intervention, it must be borne in mind that the patient may have concurrent active rheumatic carditis; 80 percent of patients who died of the disease showed pathologic changes of rheumatic carditis at postmortem examination. Maternal mortality usually has resulted from cardiac failure, exhaustion, or hyperpyrexia (Lewis, Parsons).

TETANY

Paresthesias of the hands and tongue and bouts of abdominal pain are early symptoms of tetany. These are followed by attacks of carpopedal spasm and laryngismus stridulus (laryngeal spasm, with crowing inspiration and cyanosis). Chvostek's sign, spasm of the facial muscles when the facial muscles or branches of the facial nerve are tapped, and Trous-

seau's sign, muscular spasm when pressure is applied over large arteries or nerves, are positive. The serum calcium levels are below 7.5 mg per 100 mL.

Transfer of calcium from mother to fetus may result in maternal tetany, if for any reason the gravida's serum calcium levels already are low. Symptoms and signs of tetany thus may become manifest during gestation or during lactation in patients with underlying osteomalacia, steatorrhea, or hypoparathyroidism (see above under Hypoparathyroidism). Hysterical hyperventilation during pregnancy, or overventilation during the first stage of labor (which may occur with some "natural childbirth" regimens), may produce a respiratory alkalosis and transient tetany, but the patient's total serum calcium remains normal.

Tetany is a symptom and not a disease. Clinical manifestations can be relieved immediately by the injection of 20 to 30 mL of a 10% solution of calcium gluconate. Long-term treatment must be directed toward identification and management of the underlying disorder.

OBSTETRICAL PARALYSIS

Maternal obstetrical paralysis, or traumatic neuritis of the puerperium, is characterized by paralysis of some of the muscles of the lower extremities, accompanied by various degrees of parasthesias and loss of sensation. The syndrome develops during pregnancy or labor or shortly after delivery. It is different from the paralysis which occasionally follows compression of the common peroneal nerve between the head of the fibula and the obstetric stirrup. Severe cases of the syndrome are extremely rare.

The disorder usually occurs in a primigravida who may or may not give a history of preexisting backache or sciatica. The onset may be late in pregnancy, but more frequently occurs during labor when the fetal head engages in the maternal pelvis. When the condition arises early in the puerperium, its true onset may have been obscured by the sedation and analgesia administered during the course of labor. Usually, the labor has been difficult, with relative cephalopelvic disproportion and deep transverse arrest of the fetal head.

The patient complains of pain in the back and in one or both legs, usually with radiation to the backs of the calves; occasionally, the pain is in the distribution of the anterior crural nerve over the front of the thigh. The pain has a stabbing quality, and is exacerbated by each uterine contraction. Examination reveals weakness of the dorsiflexors of the foot and toes and of the peroneal muscles of the affected limb; occasionally, plantar flexors of the foot also may be affected. Careful testing often reveals a wider distribution of paresis; the quadriceps, adductors of the thigh, iliopsoas, and gluteus muscles all may be involved. The patellar reflex frequently is diminished, while the ankle jerk is unaffected; Babinski's sign is negative (flexor response). Straight leg raising may cause severe pain. Loss of sensation does not correspond to the cutaneous distribution of any branch of the sciatic plexus.

Two suggestions have been made as to the pathogenesis of this syndrome: first, pressure by the fetal head on the lumbosacral trunk as it overlies the sacroiliac joint; second, acute herniation during pregnancy or labor of a lumbar intervertebral disk, usually between the third and fourth or fourth and fifth lumbar vertebrae. It is possible that each of these mechanisms is responsible at times for the neurologic syndrome, and the precise cause in a given case cannot always be determined (Hill).

MANAGEMENT

Treatment involves complete bed rest for 3 to 6 weeks, with measures to prevent deformities in the lower extremity affected. Massage of the muscles involved and galvanic stimulation will assist in maintaining muscle tone and restoration of power. The patient should not be permitted to become ambulatory until she is free from pain and there is objective evidence of nerve regeneration. Cases which may be caused by a prolapsed intervertebral disk require additional neurologic and radiologic evaluation, and eventually may come to surgical removal of the prolapsed disk.

PERIPHERAL NEUROPATHIES

GESTATIONAL POLYNEURITIS

This polyneuritis is encountered most frequently in the primigravida, although it may occur in successive pregnancies. It almost always accompanies or follows severe hyperemesis, and usually becomes manifest in the second trimester; occasionally, it may accompany lactation. The first symptoms are paresthesias in the lower extremities, followed by weakness of the legs (with foot drop), the progressive weakness of the arms and legs proceeding proxi-

mally. The deep tendon reflexes initially are unusually brisk but then are lost. Eventually, a full lower motor neuron syndrome develops, with muscular wasting and degeneration. It is rare for the bladder and rectum to be affected. The cranial nerves are involved at times, and in severe cases there may be mental confusion and deterioration into a mental status resembling Korsakoff's psychosis.

The etiology of gestational polyneuritis is a deficiency of vitamin B complex intake. Specific treatment, in addition to the usual neuromuscular supportive measures, is the administration of thiamine, 50 to 100 mg daily, parenterally. With the discovery of the etiology of this syndrome, its prevention and management have been so satisfactory that it has markedly decreased in incidence and no longer is an important clinical problem in obstetrics.

CARPAL TUNNEL SYNDROME

The carpal tunnel syndrome results from compression of the median nerve under the carpal ligament at the wrist. The syndrome may appear initially during pregnancy, or previously present symptoms may be aggravated during pregnancy. Onset usually is in the third trimester; the symptoms may continue into the puerperium and recur in subsequent pregnancies. Occurrence of the syndrome during pregnancy has been attributed to unusual manual activity and domestic duties, and to an increase in volume of the contents of the carpal tunnel resulting from physiologic fluid retention during gestation. The symptoms characteristically occur at night, the patient being awakened by severe pain and paresthesias in the hands radiating proximally to the elbow, and sometimes even to the shoulder. The pain is aching in quality, occasionally extremely severe, and is accompanied by a sensation of tingling or burning in the affected digits. Shaking or massaging the hand and clenching and unclenching the fist may afford some relief. In the morning, the hands feel numb and useless until movements of the wrists and fingers have been initiated. The pain rarely is a problem during the day. The diagnosis usually is easy; when atypical features are present, x-ray examination of the cervical spine is indicated to rule out cervical spondylitis or narrowing of the intervertebral foramina (Nicholas et al.).

Management

In the majority of cases, signs and symptoms disappear soon after labor and delivery. It is not necessary to consider surgical relief unless the symptoms are extremely severe, were present before the onset of pregnancy, or persist after delivery. Work which involves prolonged use of the hands and fingers is proscribed. Fluid retention may be minimized by the judicious prescription of thiazide diuretics. Sometimes relief of symptoms may be obtained by injection of hydrocortisone, 25 to 50 mg, into the carpal tunnel.

Surgical treatment consists of division of the carpal ligament and almost always is successful.

MERALGIA PARESTHETICA

In this syndrome, paresthesias and objective loss of sensation occur over the anterolateral aspect of the thigh. The etiology is compression of the lateral cutaneous nerve of the thigh, arising from the second and third lumbar roots and coursing either through or under the inguinal ligament. The symptoms are initiated by walking or prolonged standing, and are eased by sitting or lying down. The condition usually develops in obese gravidas, and is thought to be due to stretching of the nerve as a result of the increased lumbar lordosis of pregnancy.

Management

Mild cases require only rest and simple analgesics; spontaneous remission will ensue after the pregnancy is over. If the symptoms are severe, the nerve may have to be exposed at the inguinal ligament and freed from the constricting fasciculi of the ligament.

SUBARACHNOID HEMORRHAGE

Subarachnoid hemorrhage is not an infrequent medical emergency during adult life. The hemorrhage seldom is related to exertion or physical strain. Subarachnoid hemorrhage is not more frequent during pregnancy, and does not seem to be precipitated by pregnancy or labor (Amies, 1970a).

In about 90 percent of cases, the hemorrhage results from rupture of a congenital "berry" aneurysm. These aneurysms may be multiple, and occur more frequently in women than in men. In the childbearing years, hemorrhage from a cerebral angioma is more frequent than in older patients, and may account for as many as 10 to 15 percent of cases.

The clinical picture consists of the sudden onset of severe occipital headache, vomiting, and coma, occasionally with associated convulsive seizures. If not unconscious, the patient may manifest photophobia and mental irritability. On examination, there are nucchal rigidity, bilateral Babinski reflexes, sometimes retinal hemorrhages, and occasionally papilledema. The definitive diagnosis may be confirmed by examination of the cerebrospinal fluid.

Management

The management of subarachnoid hemorrhage during gestation is the same as in the nongravid state. Immediate discomfort may be eased with analgesics. The patient must be hospitalized immediately under expert neurologic care. If the patient survives the stage of immediate shock and cerebral vasospasm, cerebral angiography may be performed without increased risk during pregnancy. If a lesion or site of bleeding which is amenable to surgery is demonstrated, the indicated neurosurgical procedures should be carried out regardless of the stage of gestation, and usually incur no additional risks to the pregnancy; prolonged hypothermia, often required for such procedures, has been shown not to influence gestation deleteriously (Robinson, Sedzimir). If no operable lesion can be demonstrated radiographically, treatment consists solely of prolonged bed rest; after 6 to 8 weeks, the risk of recurrent bleeding is somewhat reduced. Computerized axial tomography (CAT scan) is of great help in making the diagnosis.

The physical exertion of labor has not been implicated in the etiology of subarachnoid hemorrhage. When a vascular lesion has been demonstrated and corrected surgically, pregnancy should be permitted to continue to term, and normal vaginal delivery anticipated if obstetric factors permit. If no operable lesion is found or no surgical treatment accomplished, the mode of delivery must be individualized (Poole). If labor is anticipated within 6 to 8 weeks after occurrence of the subarachnoid hemorrhage, the lesion will not have had adequate time for firm healing, and delivery by elective cesarean section probably is safest. There is no indication for cesarean section after an adequate convalescent period has followed the hemorrhagic episode.

Toxemia of pregnancy, with hypertension and fluid retention, may not be instrumental in initiating subarachnoid hemorrhage, but effectively may increase the amount of bleeding and therefore the extent of cerebral damage. When subarachnoid hemorrhage occurs in a patient who has toxemia of pregnancy, termination of the pregnancy should be considered as soon as obstetrically and medically feasible.

When subarachnoid hemorrhage is extensive and seems to be proceeding toward a maternal mortality, concentration on salvaging the fetus, if viable, is indicated, and cesarean section should be accomplished before the fetus has been damaged irreparably by prolonged maternal hypoxia.

If subarachnoid hemorrhage occurs during labor, the labor should be terminated promptly by the most expeditious method, and that which involves the patient in the least strain or risk of hypertension.

There is no evidence that pregnancy is more likely to cause recurrence of subarachnoid hemorrhage than other activities of normal life, so there is no absolute medical indication for surgical sterilization or abortion. On the other hand, patients who have had one subarachnoid hemorrhage statistically are at higher risk for a recurrence and have a lessened life expectancy; the patient and her husband may take this into consideration when contemplating subsequent conception or possible abortion.

INTRACRANIAL VASCULAR DISORDERS

CEREBRAL THROMBOSIS

Thrombosis of the cerebral cortical veins or of the dural sinuses is a rare complication of pregnancy or the puerperium; when it occurs, it is associated with a high maternal mortality. Usually, the thrombosis occurs within several weeks of the delivery and is unassociated with dehydration or either localized or generalized infection. Some have suggested that cerebral thrombosis in these patients is secondary to embolic thrombi which pass from the pelvic veins cephalad along the vertebral venous system. Others postulate, as causative factors, stasis of blood in the cerebral venous sinuses during the straining during labor, plus the hypercoagulability of blood which occurs normally in the early puerperium (Amies, 1970b).

Initial symptoms usually include vomiting, stupor, speech disturbances, mental confusion, and headaches which may be either generalized or unilateral. Depending on the vessel affected, there may follow focal or generalized convulsions, and hemi- or monoparesis, the arm more frequently involved than the lower extremity. Aphasia, hemianopsia, or sensory disturbances may occur. As a rule, the patient retains consciousness; development of coma presages a fatal outcome. If the sagittal sinus is involved, symptoms may be bilateral and papilledema develops. As the thrombosis spreads to adjacent vessels, symptoms are progressive slowly over several days.

Cerebral venous thrombosis must be differentiated from postpartum eclampsia, which rarely develops after the first few postpartum days. Distinction from subarachnoid hemorrhage is facilitated by the absence of blood from the cerebrospinal fluid. Other factors which must be considered in the differential diagnosis are cerebral arterial thrombosis and intracranial neoplasm.

Management

Unless the signs and symptoms suggest that the thrombosis is extending, deferring anticoagulation therapy is probably best in order to avoid possible bleeding from ruptured tributaries of the affected vein. Treatment consists of sedation with barbiturates and control of convulsions with intravenous diazepam (Valium). Rehabilitative treatment will be necessary during the phase of recovery from paresis.

Maternal mortality is reported as from 30 to 50 percent, but these figures probably are exaggerated because the diagnosis is not made accurately in cases of minor degree. In patients who survive the initial episode, the degree and rapidity of recovery are remarkable (Cross et al.).

MULTIPLE SCLEROSIS

Multiple sclerosis is characterized by exacerbations and remissions which are unpredictable and by an involvement of the central nervous system which is uniquely erratic. Its etiology and pathophysiology are unknown. The onset is insidious, the course slowly progressive, and the average life expectancy after the initial diagnosis approximately 12 years. In clear-cut cases, there is involvement of many parts of the central nervous system in erratic succession, with great variation in the severity of the disease from time to time.

Pregnancy is not responsible for the onset of multiple sclerosis, and exacerbations and remissions of the disease observed during pregnancy are coincidental (Novak, Johnson). There is no medical indication for therapeutic abortion or surgical sterilization. On the other hand, progression of the disease to the point of severe disability may contraindicate conception and maternity.

MANAGEMENT

Since there is no specific treatment for multiple sclerosis, symptoms which occur during gestation must be treated as in the nongravid state, on a mainly supportive and rehabilitative basis. The disease does not affect the mechanisms of labor and delivery, nor does it inhibit the discomfort associated therewith. The mode of delivery depends exclusively upon obstetric indications. The disease has no deleterious effects upon the fetus or neonate (Schapiro et al.).

BRAIN TUMORS

Brain tumors are an infrequent complication of pregnancy, both primary and metastatic lesions being rare in the reproductive age groups. Pregnancy tends to highlight the clinical recognition of latent brain tumors, especially of angiomata. Meningiomas, neurofibromas, and some hemangiomas undergo rapid growth during pregnancy, increased proliferation being associated with the more immature cell lines (i.e., glioblastomas). In addition, relatively benign tumors may increase in size as a result of fluid retention, and have been demonstrated to be edematous when excised; in such cases, the symptoms and signs may improve dramatically following delivery.

Meningiomas grow rapidly during pregnancy, not only because of edema and increased vascularity but also as an effect of hormonal alterations (Bickerstaff et al.). The glioblastoma multiforme is affected severely by pregnancy; in the rare event of a "cure" of this highly malignant lesion, further pregnancies must be proscribed. Oligodendrogliomas are least affected by gestation.

MANAGEMENT

Brain tumors must be extirpated surgically as soon as the diagnosis is made, in view of the mother's poor chances of survival. Only the location and type of tumor must be considered in evaluating therapy; the presence of pregnancy must be ignored. If the fetus is viable, pregnancy may be terminated by elective cesarean section before attacking the intracranial neoplasm. The strain of labor may increase intracranial pressure with disastrous effects. In earlier gestation, the diagnosis of brain tumor is an indication for excision of the tumor, not for abortion.

MYASTHENIA GRAVIS

Myasthenia gravis is a chronic neuromuscular disorder. It affects mostly young women in the reproductive age group. Symptoms include weakness and easy fatigability of striated muscles and appear most fre-

quently in the third decade of life. Muscles innervated by cranial nerves usually become involved first, followed by bulbar and skeletal muscle involvement. Although almost any variation of onset and course may be seen, the usual progression of symptoms is diplopia, ptosis, oculomotor palsies; difficulties of articulation, mastication, swallowing, speech, facial expression, and neck control; and finally, weakness of the muscles of the trunk and limbs. Remissions and exacerbations of the disease occur without specific pattern. Throughout, smooth, cardiac, and uterine muscles function normally.

The pathogenesis of this disease has been clarified. Older theories postulated insufficient production of acetylcholine, rapid dissipation of acetylcholine by excessive amounts of cholinesterase, and circulation of curare-like substances. Evidence now strongly suggests that myasthenia gravis is an autoimmune disorder, in which a muscle antigen-antibody reaction interferes with neuromuscular function (Oosterhuis et al.). Another hypothesis suggests that an autoimmune reaction in the thymic medulla releases a humoral substance which is responsible for the neuromuscular block; thymomas have been found in 10 percent of affected patients. The number of muscle acetylcholine receptors is decreased in these patients (Fambrough et al.), and acetylcholine receptor antibodies have been demonstrated (Appel et al.).

The clinical course of myasthenia gravis is one of remissions and exacerbations; as a result, the effect of pregnancy on the disease process is difficult to establish. The frequency of exacerbations and remissions does not appear to differ significantly between the pregnant and nonpregnant population (Plauché).

The effect of myasthenia gravis on pregnancy is more serious. There is an increased frequency of abortion during myasthenic crises, but no increased frequencies of stillbirth and neonatal death. Smooth muscle activity is not affected, so that uterine inertia does not present a problem. Total body fatigue may occur if labor is strenuous or prolonged. Thymectomy and/or anticholinesterase drug therapy have not altered pregnancy outcome.

Infants born to mothers with myasthenia gravis may show myasthenic symptoms in the neonatal period. They behave as if some humoral substance with a half-life of 20 to 30 days had been transmitted transplacentally from the affected mother (Namba et al.). The symptomatic period usually lasts less than a month, and with prompt and adequate cholinergic therapy the infants recover completely. Infants with transient myasthenia have been born to mothers on treatment or on no treatment, in relapse and in remission, and both before and after thymectomy. Patients with transient neonatal myasthenia must not be confused with those exhibiting the congenital form of juvenile myasthenia gravis, who are not born of myasthenic mothers, have the disease for life, and are encountered much less frequently.

MANAGEMENT

Rest restores strength at least partially. Anticholinesterase drugs such as neostigmine methylsulfate (Prostigmine) and pyridostigmine bromide (Mestinon Bromide) effectively control the symptoms in most patients. The dose of anticholinesterase medication may require adjustment throughout pregnancy. The adequacy of anticholinesterase dosage the patient is receiving may be evaluated by the Tensilon test, which indicates whether a greater or lesser dose is required.

Affected neonates usually will show symptoms within the first few hours of life. Almost uniformly, they feed poorly, swallowing function is inadequate to handle even normal oropharyngeal secretions, regurgitation occurs frequently, and suckling is weak. The neonate may have an expressionless face and dropping jaw. The cry usually is poor or absent. Body tonus may be diminished markedly, but rarely are reflexes obtunded. Seldom are ptosis and oculomotor palsies evident. The condition is self-limited, resolving spontaneously within 1 month (Wise, McQuillan). During the symptomatic stage, however, there is a significant risk of respiratory death. Treatment with neostigmine methylsulfate (0.125 mg IM every 4 to 6 hours) or pyridostigmine bromide (0.15 mg IM as an initial dose) provides symptomatic relief until spontaneous remission occurs. During the first day of life, anticholinesterase drugs carried over from maternal therapy may still be in the neonate's circulation, and caution must be exercised in treatment. The dosage and frequency of administration of medication to the infant must be determined by the clinical response. Atropine sulfate, 0.01 mg per kilogram of body weight, effectively counteracts overdosage. Thymectomy has no place in the treatment of transient neonatal myasthenia gravis.

DISORDERS OF THE SKELETAL SYSTEM AND SKIN

A host of epidermal changes occur as a physiologic consequence of pregnancy. These are well described in Chap. 9.

SKIN DISEASES RELATED TO PREGNANCY

PRURIGO GESTATIONIS

This persistent, papular eruption occurs toward the end of the first trimester, usually appearing first on the abdomen, thighs, and buttocks or on the dorsal surfaces of the hands or feet; as pregnancy progresses, the lesions may spread to the extensor surfaces of the forearms and to the shoulders and chest. The individual lesions are discrete and small, and often are bloody because of scratching; sometimes, there is an urticarial component. Usually the onset is gradual and the eruption disappears rapidly after delivery, leaving areas of hyperpigmentation. The associated pruritus may be very disabling. The disease has a tendency to recur in subsequent pregnancies. The etiology of the disorder is unknown. Treatment is purely symptomatic, including antipruritic lotions with or without corticosteroids, antihistamines, and sedatives.

HERPES GESTATIONIS

This is a rare complication of pregnancy. The condition usually is heralded by severe pruritus and burning sensations. The earliest lesions are erythematous patches which appear on the extremities or trunk, followed by vesicles which present in crops (like herpes) and are distributed in rings or arcs of circles. These vesicles coalesce, forming tense, thick-walled bullae of various sizes which may become pustular or hemorrhagic. The eruption may spread to other areas, and eventually the entire body may be involved. The involvement of mucosal surfaces is rare. The lesions slowly regress and heal, leaving areas of hyperpigmentation. Constitutional symptoms such as fever, chills, vomiting, and albuminuria may accompany the eruption. There may be marked eosinophilia, reaching as high as 50 percent, and eosinophils are found in the blister fluid. As pregnancy progresses, there may be remissions and exacerbations of the disease, with final remission in the first few days after delivery. A few fatal cases have been reported in the older literature, but generally the prognosis for the mother is good. Associated fetal wastage, mainly in terms of abortion or stillbirth, is alleged to be about 25 percent; recent reviews have not supported this finding (Greenbaum).

The cause of the disease is unknown (Katz et al.). Similar lesions may be produced artificially with progestational steroids, suggesting that herpes gestationis may be a response to altered hormonal environment. This is the only noninfectious erythematobullous eruption which may be manifest both in the mother and fetus; the neonates of affected mothers will present similar skin lesions in about 10 to 20 percent of cases. The condition is self-limited in the infant and disappears in about 1 week. Once manifest, the disease tends to recur in subsequent pregnancies. The eruption must be differentiated from pemphigus, erythema multiforme, ordinary urticaria, and dermatitis herpetiformis. Herpes gestationis has no relation to the herpes virus, and is synonymous with pemphigus gravidarum, dermatitis multiformis gestationis, and pemphigus pruriginosus, names which have been applied to this eruption in the past.

Treatment essentially is supportive, including maintenance of adequate fluid and caloric intake, and a diet rich in protein and vitamins. Electrolyte balance must be monitored, and blood transfused as indicated. Sedatives and antihistamines may alleviate the severe pruritus. Prevention of secondary infection is paramount; systemic antibiotic therapy is recommended for this purpose, since topical applications have great risk of sensitization. Some patients benefit from administration of corticosteroids. In very severe cases, it may become necessary to consider termination of pregnancy (Carruthers).

IMPETIGO HERPETIFORMIS

This is an inflammatory condition of the skin associated with severe constitutional symptoms, such as fever, chills, vomiting, and delerium. The eruption consists of groups of minute pustules which appear on normal skin. The etiology is unknown. The pustules are arranged in groups or rings and contain pus from the moment of their appearance; no vesicular stage exists. The eruption spreads by peripheral extension, leaving yellowish crusts covering a red, oozing surface and resembling exudative eczema. Itching is not a prominent symptom. Blood cultures and contents of the pustules are sterile bacteriologically. Mucosal surfaces frequently are affected, interfering with oral alimentation.

The maternal prognosis has been reported to be poor, with as high a maternal mortality rate as 70 to 80 percent; this has improved in recent years with corticosteroid therapy. Fetal wastage is high, particularly if the disease occurs in early gestation.

Impetigo herpetiformis is resistant to most forms of treatment. The most reliable therapies include administration of ACTH and cortisone. General supportive measures are important. If the diagnosis can be established with some certainty in early gestation, therapeutic abortion may be considered. If the mother survives the pregnancy, exacerbations of the disease in subsequent pregnancies may be anticipated, and surgical sterilization should be considered.

SKIN DISEASES COMPLICATED BY PREGNANCY

PSORIASIS

This is a chronic, recurring skin disease characterized by the development of dry, scaly patches covered by silvery white, piled-up scales distributed widely over the body. The effect of pregnancy on preexisting psoriasis is unpredictable. Psoriasis seldom arises de novo during gestation, and generalized lesions tend to improve. Localized lesions, particularly flexural psoriasis, tend to be aggravated during pregnancy. Postpartum exacerbation occurs frequently and seems to be unrelated to pregnancy changes. Psoriasis has no effect on either pregnancy or the fetus (Church). The usual dermatologic treatments should be maintained during gestation.

PEMPHIGUS

This name refers to a group of chronic, bullous skin diseases which are relapsing and usually terminate in a fatality. Less than 15 cases during pregnancy have been reported in the medical literature. In this condition, in contrast to the thick-walled bullae of herpes gestationis, the bullae are thin-walled, arise on normal skin, and are not polycyclic in arrangement. Mucosal involvement usually is present and may be severe. Pruritus is not a characteristic feature of pemphigus. Nikolsky's sign (the outer layer of skin easily is rubbed off by slight mechanical injury) is present in pemphigus but not in herpes gestationis.

Pemphigus fluctuates in severity during pregnancy and may be either relieved, exacerbated, or unaffected. There are several reports of bullous eruptions in newborns born to affected mothers (McElin, Cromer).

Treatment with ACTH and corticosteroids may produce cures of this potentially fatal disease and must be continued throughout gestation and into the puerperium. Intensive antibiotic therapy is necessary to prevent secondary infections. There is no indication for therapeutic abortion; in view of the chronicity of the condition, surgical sterilization may be considered.

DISCOID LUPUS ERYTHEMATOSUS

This is an inflammatory skin disorder characterized by pinkish or reddish macular lesions which upon subsiding leave whitish, atrophic scars. The lesions occur predominantly across the malar eminences, bridge of the nose, earlobes, mastoid areas, and scalp. The etiology is unknown. The disease is chronic, capricious, and erratic in its course. Modern treatment includes mainly corticosteroids. The course of discoid lupus erythematosus is unaffected by pregnancy.

MELANOMA

This is a highly malignant tumor arising from the melanocytes of the skin. Although rare in women during the reproductive years, it occurs in 1 of every 50,000 women in the general population. Melanomas produce excessive amounts of melanin and melanin-precursors, which may result in increased pigmentation of the skin (melanosis); intermediary metabolites may be excreted in the patient's urine (melanuria). During normal gestation, there is an increase in melanoblast activity because of hormonal stimulation; the skin pigment deepens and nevi also may darken. Nevertheless, it cannot be demonstrated that this predisposes the gravida to either the development of malignant melanoma or a more virulent course of the disease. Treatment involves both surgery and radiation; 5-year survival is less than 50 percent (George et al.).

Malignant melanoma has distinguished itself as the tumor with the greatest potential for transplacental transmission (Rothman et al.). In all reported cases, metastatic disease was identified in the placenta, and the fetal liver was the primary metastatic focus in the infant. Metastasis to the placenta has been reported without involvement of fetus or neonate. Infants of mothers with melanoma should be observed closely for the first few years of life for evidence of tumor. The placenta must be examined carefully in all such cases; the absence of placental metastases almost ensures a good prognosis for the newborn.

CONDYLOMA ACUMINATA

These are warty excrescences which may present as moist, vegetating masses on the external genitalia, perianal region, and perineum; less frequently, they involve the vaginal mucosa and even the portio vaginalis of the cervix. The condylomata flourish and spread in a moist medium, and often grow rapidly during pregnancy; they may attain a size which re-

sults in dystocia (Gorthy, Krembs). They are held to be of virus origin, are both contagious and autoinnoculable, and may be transmitted venereally.

Management

Scrupulous personal cleanliness is essential. Small lesions require no treatment and usually regress spontaneously after delivery. Podophyllin resin in a variety of vehicles has been the most widely used treatment for larger lesions; systemic absorption of this agent may have serious teratogenic effects in pregnancy (Chamberlain et al.). During gestation, therefore, large lesions probably are best treated by surgical excision or electrocauterization under general anesthesia (Young et al.).

SKELETAL DISORDERS

OSTEOGENESIS IMPERFECTA

This is a hereditary disease arising from defects in osteoblastic function which result in faulty matrix formation and subnormal deposition of bone salts. The disease may arise in intrauterine life, predisposing the fetal bones to fracture in utero and during delivery. Because of the fragile bones, great care must be exercised during delivery to protect both mother and infant. Surgical sterilization is indicated in the affected female because of her disabilities, usually multiple by adulthood.

CHONDRODYSTROPHY

This condition, also known as achondroplasia, begins in fetal life and results in failure of the long bones to achieve normal length. A genetic factor is assumed to be responsible, although cases lacking a hereditary background have been recorded. The result of this disproportion in membranous and cartilagenous bone is a form of dwarfism in which the trunk may be of relatively normal proportions and size. The patient often has dorsal kyphosis and marked lumbar lordosis, with a backward-tilted sacrum. In chondrodystrophy, cephalopelvic disproportion is the rule, and delivery by cesarean section almost universal.

INFECTIOUS DISEASES

Maternal infection in pregnancy presents a threefold problem: management of the infection in the mother, the effect of the infection upon the course of gestation, and the influences on the fetus not only of the maternal infection but also of the therapy applied.

Maternal infections have great potential for involving the fetus. The exact mechanisms by which certain bacteria, viruses, and protozoa cross from the maternal to the fetal side of the placenta remain unknown. It is probable that bloodstream sepsis with bacteria or protozoa results in a nidus of infection in the placenta, which permits penetration to the fetal circulation. The mode of transmission of viruses across the placenta is unknown.

Maternal infection during pregnancy may result in a variety of untoward fetal effects: abortion, fetal death and stillbirth, premature labor and delivery, congenital malformation, nonfatal fetal infection, and retarded intrauterine growth. In general, abortion, fetal death, and premature delivery may occur even in the absence of fetal infection. This occurs in a number of diseases which have in common high fever and/or maternal hypoxia: typhoid fever, bacterial pneumonia, malaria, influenza, measles, mumps, chickenpox, bulbar poliomyelitis, serum hepatitis, and variola (smallpox). Abortion and fetal death also may result from direct invasion of the conceptus by microorganisms, as in congenital syphilis, toxoplasmosis, cytomegalic inclusion disease, varicella (chickenpox), variola, and occasionally in herpes simplex.

BACTERIAL INFECTIONS

PNEUMONIA

Antibiotic therapy has reduced maternal mortality and morbidity of this complication of pregnancy. Because of maternal hypoxia, the fetal risk in unrecognized and untreated maternal pneumonia is high, and premature delivery and fetal death may occur (Oxorn).

Management

A high index of suspicion of maternal infection is required. Early hospitalization, complete rest, oxygen supplementation, and intensive antibiotic therapy are essential. Active intervention reduces the incidence of maternal complications. Failure to respond to treatment suggests the appearance of secondary problems such as pulmonary abscess or empyema.

GONORRHEA

Infection with *Neisseria gonorrhoeae* currently is occurring with increasing frequency during pregnancy and without regard to socioeconomic class of the patient (Kraus, Yen). The maternal infection may involve the cervix, vagina, or vulva, but rarely, except in the early puerperium, the fallopian tubes or parametria. The diagnosis is based upon finding characteristic gram-negative intracellular diplococci in smears of purulent exudates, and on specific identification of the organism on suitable culture media.

Management

Penicillin remains the drug of choice in the treatment of gonorrhea, although progressively higher doses have been recommended as drug-resistant strains of gonococci have appeared. The treatment currently recommended is procaine penicillin G in aqueous suspension, 2.4 million units intramuscularly in each buttock at one sitting (total dose of 4.8 million units). Alternative treatments include tetracycline, oxytetracycline, or erythromycin, 2.0 g initially and then 0.5 g four times daily orally for 5 days; doxycycline hyclate (Vibramycin), 200 mg initially and 100 mg two times daily orally for 5 days; ampicillin, 3.5 g, or amoxicillin, 3.0 g, either with probenecid, 1.0 g, orally or with spectinomycin, 2.0 g, in an intramuscular injection. In almost all areas of the country, the disease must be reported to the local health officials for contact followup. There must be a high index of suspicion of concurrent luetic infection (Rudolph).

Gonococcal ophthalmia neonatorum remains a serious problem in infants born to mothers with untreated gonorrhea. A high index of suspicion is required, and appropriate smears and cultures of the conjunctival discharge must be obtained (Friendly). Topical prophylaxis for neonatal ophthalmia is not adequate treatment for infants born to mothers with proven or suspected gonococcal infection. Such neonates require, in addition, a single intravenous or intramuscular injection of aqueous crystalline penicillin G, 50,000 units. Should clinical ophthalmia develop in the newborn, additional treatment must be administered. Since untreated gonococcal ophthalmia is highly contagious, the infant must be isolated upon suspicion and for 24 hours after initiation of treatment. Management includes aqueous crystalline penicillin G, 50,000 units per kilogram of body weight per day in two divided doses, intravenously, for 7 days. Saline irrigation of the eyes should be carried out as necessary; topical antibiotic therapy is neither adequate nor necessary (Center for Disease Control).

VIRAL INFECTIONS

Viral infections are of special importance during gestation. Not only do they represent disease in the mother but they may result in defective fetal organogenesis and clinical disease in the fetus or newborn. Viruses readily cross the placenta without demonstrable morphologic change in the trophoblast (Table 31–13.).

There has been considerable investigation of the teratogenic effects of viruses (Blattner et al.). For example, herpes simplex, vaccinia, and influenza A viruses consistently cause microcephaly in the early chick embryo; this teratogenic effect of the influenza virus can be prevented by neutralization of the virus with specific antiserum. The teratogenic effect of viruses in human beings has been much more difficult to evaluate. At present, only the rubella virus and the cytomegalovirus unequivocally have been shown to produce congenital anomalies in human beings. It has been suggested but not proved that other viruses, such as serum hepatitis virus, influenza virus, and vaccinia virus may be teratogenic during fetal organogenesis. Clinical investigations of the possible teratogenic effects of viral diseases are difficult to interpret. Retrospective reports often are not specific about the time in pregnancy when a viral infection oc-

TABLE 31–13 Viral Infections and the Fetus

Viruses causing intrauterine congenital defects
  Rubella
  Cytomegalovirus (CMV)
  Varicella zoster
  Herpesvirus hominis
  Lymphocytic choriomeningitis (LCM)
Viruses associated with (but not proved to cause) congenital defects
  Influenza
  Mumps
  Enteroviruses
  Hepatitis A
Viruses causing perinatal infection
  Herpesvirus hominis
  Varicella zoster
  Coxsackievirus B
  Poliomyelitis
  Hepatitis B
  Variola
  Vaccinia

curred, a crucial factor in fetal susceptibility to malformation. Prospective studies pose great practical difficulties.

A viral etiology for congenital malformations is an attractive theory and has several bases: the two established disease models of rubella and cytomegalovirus, the ubiquity of viruses, the fact that maternal viral infection may be occult, and the propensity of viruses to multiply in rapidly dividing cells. Clinical support of this theory is difficult to establish (Carlström).

First, the teratogenic potential of a given virus may be related inversely to its pathogenicity. Rubella has a low pathogenicity for the cells it invades; it damages some of the cells engaged in organogenesis but does not kill the fetus. Other viruses of greater pathogenicity may kill the embryo and cause abortion rather than congenital malformations; this may explain the high incidence of spontaneous abortion in mothers who contract smallpox or measles.

Second, the importance of viruses in the causation of congenital anomalies easily can be underestimated since the acute viral infection may escape clinical notice (Marx 1973a, 1973b). Recent studies indicate that the human fetus can form antibodies when infected. Antibody production may begin in utero in response to antigenic stimulation as early as the twentieth week of gestation. In the fetus, antibody response of the dominant immunoglobulin, IgM, is prolonged and may persist to delivery and beyond. In an adult, the initial response to an antigen is in the IgM fraction of serum proteins, but within a week IgG activity prevails. Thus, specific IgM antibody detectable in cord serum or serum collected in the first few days of life reflects intrauterine fetal infection which may have occurred as early as the first half of gestation. The demonstration of increased amounts of nonspecific serum IgM antibody suggests that an unidentified intrauterine infection had supervened (Silverstein). The amount of IgM antibody found in cord serum may depend upon differences in the nature of the pathogens (antigenic hierarchy), duration of infection before delivery, the quantity of pathogen generated, and the distribution of the pathogen in fetal tissues. Preliminary surveys indicate that almost 20 percent of neonates in some series have elevated IgM globulin levels. Of these, 10 percent show characteristic clinical manifestations of the underlying infection, 60 percent show nonspecific signs of infection, and 30 percent remain clinically normal.

Nonfatal intrauterine infection may appear in one of three forms: the infant may be born with healed lesions of an infectious course passed entirely in utero; it may be born with active evidence of current infection; or it may develop clinical infection within a few days of birth.

RHINOVIRUSES

There is no evidence that rhinoviruses (acute coryza, common cold) cause intrauterine death or fetal disease, or that pregnant women are predisposed to infection with these agents. However, upper respiratory tract infections are prolonged and may be more severe during pregnancy because of the physiologic respiratory changes of late pregnancy. Treatment consists of rest, avoidance of secondary infection, and maintenance of a good fluid intake. Salicylates may give some symptomatic relief. Antibiotic therapy will have no effect on the viral infection; however, evidence of secondary bacterial infection should be treated promptly and actively.

INFLUENZA VIRUSES

Influenza is an acute, communicable disease usually occurring in epidemics which appear periodically in fairly regular sequence. Influenza viruses are subdivided into a number of antigenic categories; their heterogeneity and antigenic instability account for the persistence of the disease as a clinical problem. The characteristic influenza lesions found in the lungs include peribronchial infiltrations and epithelial necrosis in the finer bronchioles and alveoli. Although viral pneumonia itself may prove fatal, death usually results from superimposed bacterial infections.

Pregnant women are at special high risk during influenza epidemics. In the influenza pandemic of 1918, the maternal mortality rate from influenza was 27 percent; if bacterial pneumonia supervened, the mortality rate rose to 50 percent. Pregnancy wastage was approximately 25 percent, but rose to 50 percent in the presence of pneumonic complications. The maternal mortality rates and pregnancy wastage have been much lower in more recent epidemics, but the increased risk to the gravida remains (Greenberg et al.).

Management of influenza during pregnancy includes symptomatic therapy, protection from exposure to bacterial pathogens, and vigorous antibiotic treatment if there is any evidence of superimposed infection. Because of the degree of maternal and fetal risk in this circumstance, prophylactic antibiotic therapy may be considered. During an outbreak of influenza, pregnant women should be considered prime candidates for immunization, provided type-specific vaccine is available. The antigenic response to im-

munization during pregnancy is the same as in the nongravid state. Immunization even in the first trimester of gestation is successful in providing protection without apparent harm to the fetus.

Congenital malformations and fetal wastage are not increased appreciably by influenza (Wilson, Stein). In seriously ill patients, the fetus is always in jeopardy from either maternal hypoxia or the onset of premature labor (Griffith et al.).

RUBEOLA (MEASLES)

Rubeola is a common childhood disease with an incubation period of approximately 2 weeks and a characteristic clinical course. Measles epidemics occur every few years, and it is estimated that 90 percent of susceptible children develop the disease. An attack of measles usually confers lifelong immunity. The almost universal prevalence in children, and recent advances in active immunization against this disease, make rubeola in women of childbearing age rare.

The effect of measles on pregnancy is unclear. Some reports have suggested that rubeola virus may be responsible for congenital anomalies and increased fetal wastage. Others have documented that maternal viremia does occur and that the virus can cross the placenta and infect the fetus, but have not documented an increased incidence of fetal malformation (Siegel). Occasionally, the neonate may show the typical skin lesions of rubeola at birth or develop the disease in the immediate neonatal period (Siegel et al.).

Management consists of supportive care of the mother, guarding against secondary bacterial infection, and, if possible, passive immunization with immune globulin within 7 days of exposure to the disease. Measles in pregnancy does not present a problem for the patient who previously has had either infection with or active immunization against the rubeola virus.

RUBELLA (GERMAN MEASLES)

Rubella is a common childhood disease with an incubation period of 16 to 18 days and a characteristic clinical picture, including mild, constitutional symptoms, low-grade fever, a maculopapular rash, and posterior cervical adenopathy. Thrombocytopenia and arthritis frequently are encountered. The clinical manifestations are exceedingly mild, and the infection may pass entirely unnoticed in the mother. The effect of rubella virus on the fetus, however, has been a major problem.

The marked teratogenic effect of the rubella virus has been documented repeatedly (Tartakow) (Table 31–14). If rubella infection occurs during the period of formation of the eye, the incidence of congenital ocular defects ranges between 15 to 75 percent, and the defects themselves vary from cloudiness of the cornea to total blindness. Cardiac anomalies, sometimes not apparent at birth, may be a cause of death in infancy. Brain damage may vary from abnormal behavior patterns to mental retardation and cerebral palsy. A wide variety of fetal and neonatal findings have been reported in addition: intrauterine and postnatal growth retardation, violaceous birthmarks, hepatosplenomegaly, hepatitis and jaundice, generalized lymphadenopathy, bone lesions of the extremities, cleft palate, anemia and leukopenia, pneumonia, myocarditis, encephalitis, and abnormal fingerprints, palmar creases, and other skin patterns (Sallomi).

The prognosis for the fetus depends upon the stage of gestation during which the maternal infection occurred. The peak incidence of malformations re-

TABLE 31–14 Abnormalities Associated with Congenital Rubella

Common
  Growth retardation
  Deafness or impaired hearing
  Cardiovascular lesions
    Patent ductus arteriosus
    Pulmonary artery hypoplasia
  Eye lesions
    Cataracts
    Retinopathy
  Hepatosplenomegaly
Less frequent
  Thrombocytopenic purpura
  Interstitial pneumonitis
  Central-nervous-system defects
  Psychomotor retardation
  Meningoencephalitis
  Radiolucencies of long bones
  Micrognathia
  Coarctation of aorta
  Myocardial necrosis
  Microphthalmia
  Jaundice
Rare
  Microcephaly
  CNS calcifications
  Chronic, progressive panencephalitis
  Cardiac septal defects
  Glaucoma
  Genitourinary tract anomalies
  Hepatitis
  Humoral immunologic defects

sults during the first 12 to 14 weeks of gestation. Intrauterine infection later in pregnancy still has a significant deleterious effect on the fetus. Infants born after intrauterine rubella infection may continue to excrete the virus in their urine, throat secretions, and tears for as long as 6 months.

One attack of rubella ordinarily confers a lifelong immunity. In the past, it had been recommended that females be exposed deliberately to rubella infection during childhood or adolescence; active immunization with attenuated, living rubella virus has replaced this approach. Because of the theoretic possibility of affecting the fetus, the pregnant woman should not be vaccinated with live virus. To date, all evidence indicates that this is not a real problem. Neither accidental maternal immunization during pregnancy nor exposure of a gravida to virus shed by recently immunized children has resulted in fetal infection (Bolognese et al., 1972). Immunization immediately preconceptionally also carries theoretic risks, and women should be instructed to defer pregnancy for several menstrual cycles after immunization (Chin et al.).

The management of a gravida newly exposed to rubella infection still is a clinical problem. In view of the mild clinical course, a history of rubella infection in infancy is subject to both positive and negative error. Only determination of maternal rubella antibody titers permits an accurate evaluation of maternal susceptibility and fetal risk. The antibody response develops simultaneously with the appearance of the rash. The presence of appreciable titers of rubella antibody shortly after exposure, or upon the initial appearance of the xanthem, documents prior rubella infection and eliminates need for current concern. To prove that a current infection indeed is rubella requires either isolation of the virus or demonstration of a sharp rise in maternal antibody titers in blood specimens drawn 2 to 3 weeks apart, the initial specimen no later than the initial appearance of a clinical rash. If rubella infection is documented in the nonimmune pregnant patient, the problems concerning the fetal risk should be explained, and therapeutic abortion considered. The administration of immune globulin to pregnant women exposed to infection by rubella virus is not effective in preventing maternal or fetal infection, and confuses the issue by masking the maternal disease.

MUMPS

Infection with mumps rarely complicates pregnancy. The disease is of theoretic interest because neonates born with endocardial fibroelastosis show a positive skin reaction to mumps antigen. The mumps virus, however, can cross-react serologically with a number of other viruses, and no etiologic association has been established (Gersony et al.).

Abortion and stillbirth have occurred after mumps infection in pregnancy, characteristically following the onset of mumps infection within 2 weeks (Siegel et al., 1966). On the basis of available data, mumps virus is not implicated as a teratogen (Siegel, 1973).

POLIOMYELITIS

Effective, active immunization against the three serologic types of poliomyelitis virus virtually has eliminated the disease as an obstetric complication.

The unimmunized gravida is particularly susceptible to poliomyelitis, especially of the bulbar form (Siegel, Greenberg). The diagnosis rests on clinical findings, serologic tests, and virus isolation. Management of the acute phase of the disease is concerned mainly with supportive measures, prevention of deformities, and anticipation and treatment of complications. Maintenance of adequate maternal ventilation, to minimize fetal hypoxia and acidosis, is of prime importance. Tracheostomy to permit adequate tracheobronchial toilet may be lifesaving.

The fetus may become infected during the course of the maternal disease and either exhibit paralytic manifestations in utero or neonatally or show intrauterine growth retardation (Schaeffer et al.). There is no increased incidence of congenital anomaly or abortion. The poliomyelitis virus has been isolated from the feces of infected mothers and neonates for as long as 8 weeks postpartum, making special isolation techniques in the newborn nursery mandatory in such cases.

Only killed virus vaccine (Salk) should be used for immunization during pregnancy. Following vaccination with live attenuated virus, 40 percent of gravidas show significant viremia; Sabin vaccine therefore should be deferred until after the pregnancy is over.

COXSACKIEVIRUSES

These viruses are divided into two groups, A and B; there is cross-antigenicity between group A coxsackieviruses and some echoviruses. Group A coxsackievirus infection results in short episodes of nonspecific febrile illness accompanied by pharyngitis, gastroenteritis, or aseptic meningitis. Group A coxsackievirus infection is of no clinical importance for either mother or fetus.

Group B coxsackievirus infection produces serious and often fatal illness in the fetus or results in rapid neonatal deterioration and death, the primary pathology being myocarditis and encephalomyelitis (Bates). There is no indication of maternal predisposition to infection by Group B coxsackievirus and maternal mortality is zero. Perinatal mortality of affected infants is almost 40 percent; surviving infants may exhibit evidence of hepatitis, interstitial pneumonitis, pancreatitis, and adrenal necrosis (Benirschke, Pendelton). The diagnosis depends upon a high index of suspicion. Treatment consists of general supportive care and digitalization for cardiac failure or severe tachycardia. Surviving infants show no long-term sequelae.

CYTOMEGALOVIRUS

Cytomegaloviruses (CMV) are the most frequent cause of congenital infection in the United States. The CMV can be isolated from the cervix or urine of 3 to 5 percent of pregnant women (Hildebrant et al.). The majority of infected women are asymptomatic. The infection is best documented by the development of specific antibody. Congenital infection occurs in 0.5 to 1.5 percent of all births but is more frequent in the lower socioeconomic groups. The effects on the infant of such infection are detailed in Table 31–15. Children with normal neurologic findings at 2 years of age generally have a good prognosis.

Fetal infection results from transplacental spread from the mother. Infection in the neonate can be documented by isolation of the virus from the urine or nasopharynx and by the demonstration of specific IgM CMV antibody titers. Infected children shed the virus for many months, and spread of infection from the baby to other family members has been documented. For this reason, infected neonates must be isolated in the neonatal nursery, although they may be permitted to go to the mother. Nursery personnel who are CMV antibody–negative are at risk of infection.

The treatment of infants with congenital cytomegalic inclusion disease has been unsatisfactory. Agents such as cytosine arabinoside and adenosine arabinoside effectively decrease the amount of virus shed during therapy, but the virus frequently rebounds after treatment is halted. The drugs may produce undesirable side effects, including bone marrow suppression. No currently available treatment improves the long-term prognosis for the infected in-

TABLE 31–15 Manifestations of Intrauterine CMV Infection

	Incidence, %
Short-term	
Hepatomegaly	64
Splenomegaly	58
Jaundice	49
Purpura	29
Long-term	
Cerebral palsy	25
Microcephaly	19
Intracerebral calcifications	12
Hyperactivity	12
Conduction deafness	12
Epilepsy	10
Visual defects	10
Sensorineural defects	8
Speech defects	7
Nonspecific retardation	3

*Multiple defects common.

fants. Immunization against CMV disease is still in the early experimental stages.

HERPES SIMPLEX

Herpes simplex virus (HSV) has been divided into two types: type 1 usually affects the oral mucosa, and type 2 usually involves the genitalia. The type may be determined by serologic and virologic (cell culture) techniques. Antibodies against the two types cross-react, but the presence of antibody of one type does not prevent infection by the other type. It has been suggested that transplacental infection might occur only in patients who have antibodies to neither type. Type 2 HSV appears to be more important than type 1 HSV in prenatal infection and teratogenicity.

The major clinical problem presented by HSV in pregnancy is the development of herpes genitalis. In lower socioeconomic groups, the incidence of this complication may be as high as 1 percent. There is little question that the disease is transmitted venereally, and pregnant women should avoid sexual contact with men who have penile herpes. Herpes genitalis may be hard to diagnose during pregnancy, only about one-third of affected patients showing typical herpetic bullae or ulcerations on the cervix or vulva. Accurate diagnosis is possible only with cytologic and/or serologic techniques.

In early gestation, maternal herpes genitalis carries a threefold increase in abortion rate, a rate which rises to over 50 percent if the maternal infection is primary rather than recurrent (Naib et al.). Whether this is due to transplacental infection, ascending infection, or a nonspecific maternal systemic response is not known. Studies of aborted material do not show clear evidence of viral invasion but do suggest a lethal effect on the conceptus. If conception occurs immediately after the development of herpes genitalis, the risk of abortion is even higher (Florman et al.).

The development of herpes genitalis in the midtrimester has a variable influence. Infection prior to 20 weeks' gestation cannot be shown to have a deleterious effect on either the pregnancy or the fetus. Infection after 20 weeks' gestation is associated with a premature labor rate of 14 percent in recurrent disease and 35 percent in patients with primary infection.

The major problem of maternal herpes genitalis is in late pregnancy, when generalized herpetic infection of the newborn becomes a serious and even lethal complication (Nahmias et al.; Amstey). The risk of neonatal infection near term is highest in infants born to mothers with primary genital herpes, i.e., without HSV antibodies to either type. The route of infection probably is by direct contact of the infant with the infected birth canal, as may occur during vaginal delivery or during a prolonged latent period following premature rupture of the membranes. There is little evidence of transplacental infection in human beings, although that this occurs in rare cases cannot be denied (Gagnon). The preferred management of pregnancy near term complicated with herpes genitalis is delivery by cesarean section if labor ensues while the virus still is present or if membranes rupture prematurely (Flanders et al.). It has been documented that virus still is being shed while herpetic lesions are visible and for 4 to 6 weeks thereafter (Bolognese et al., 1976). No antiviral therapy currently is available which can eradicate the virus from the infected genital tract.

Herpes simplex virus has not been shown to have teratogenic capabilities in humans.

VARICELLA (CHICKENPOX)

This infection is characterized by a vesiculopapular rash, mild constitutional symptoms, and symptoms referable to the respiratory tract, with an incubation period of 10 to 18 days. Ordinarily, bacterial superinfection is the major maternal problem, although maternal death secondary to pneumonitis has been reported.

Varicella does not have teratogenic capabilities (Siegel, 1973). Transplacental infection may occur during the viremia stage which immediately precedes the appearance of the rash. Fetal infection therefore lags 2 to 3 weeks behind that of the mother. The infant may be born with evidence of healed or healing intrauterine infection, or may develop clinical varicella in the first few weeks after birth (Cutter, Hansman).

VARIOLA (SMALLPOX) AND VACCINIA

Variola is a rare disease in the United States, probably as a result of compulsory vaccination. The incidence of endemic variola infection *plus* the risk of importation of the disease from less well-protected countries is less than the rate of complications from vaccination; as a result, compulsory vaccination is under reconsideration.

Congenital infection of the fetus with variola virus may occur whether or not the mother has had the disease or has been vaccinated. Maternal immunity to variola is cellular and not humoral, so viremia and transplacental transmission can occur although the mother remains clinically well. If the mother does manifest clinical disease, the fetus and mother will exhibit the same stage of infection simultaneously.

Vaccination for smallpox with living vaccinia virus carries its own inherent risks. Revaccination of a pregnant woman is safe, but primary vaccination during pregnancy may result in fetal death or delivery of an infant showing clinical vaccinia infection (Kaplan et al.). The risk of transplacental transmission of vaccinia virus is present at all stages of gestation. The fetus becomes infected during the maternal incubation period, and the pregnancy usually terminates several weeks later, the embryo or stillborn fetus showing the characteristic skin lesions of generalized vaccinia and a specific form of bronchopneumonia (Green et al.).

Because of this documented risk, pregnant women should not have primary vaccinia vaccination electively, although revaccination is safe. Vaccination will protect the mother but not the fetus against variola infection, so that even immunized gravidas must avoid exposure to variola.

SPIROCHETAL AND PROTOZOAL INFECTIONS

SYPHILIS

Despite the availability of adequate and effective therapy, sensitive diagnostic procedures, and regulations for mandatory luetic testing, the incidence of maternal syphilis and congenital infection of the fetus seems to be increasing.

In pregnant women with primary luetic infection, invasion of the fetus by spirochetes occurs after the sixteenth to eighteenth weeks of gestation if no therapy has been administered to the mother. Approximately 25 percent of fetuses thus infected die in utero, and an equal number of infected neonates die in the immediate puerperium. Of the damaged infants who survive, 40 percent develop late symptomatic syphilis. Adequate treatment of the infected gravida even after 16 to 18 weeks' gestation will cure the infected fetus, but the fetal damage and stigmata incurred before therapy was administered will remain. Mucous membrane, skin, and skeletal lesions are most characteristic in the fetus and neonate (Holder, Knox).

Prenatal examination affords an opportunity to detect the disease in the pregnant patient. An accurate history is essential. A complete and careful examination is required. The primary lesion frequently is missed; if present, the chancre usually presents as a hard-rimmed ulceration about 1 cm in diameter on the labia or in the lower vagina. A suspension made from scrapings of the ulcer (or, in later secondary syphilis, from aspiration of involved lymph nodes) will be positive on dark-field examination for *Treponema pallidum*. Failure to demonstrate the spirochete from a suspect lesion may mean that the lesion is not luetic in origin, that the patient has received antiluetic drugs systemically or locally, that too much time has elapsed since the appearance of the lesion, or that the lesion is that of late lues.

More frequently, the diagnosis is made by serologic testing. The most frequently employed serologic test is the VDRL (Venereal Disease Research Laboratory) test, a test for the presence of nonspecific antibodies (reagins) which may be falsely positive. Tests for specific antitreponemal antibodies are more selective, and should be utilized where a conventional serologic test is reactive and a biologic false positive reaction is suspected. A positive antitreponemal antibody test, such as the fluorescent treponemal-antibody absorption (FTA-ABS) test, is a specific indication of past or present infection by spirochetes, and should never be used as a test of cure (Sparling).

Syphilis may be acquired during pregnancy and after a negative serologic test antepartum; in high-risk populations, the serologic tests should be repeated at the beginning of the third trimester and at delivery.

Penicillin is the drug of choice for the treatment of syphilis. For primary, secondary, and early latent syphilis, including syphilis in pregnancy, benzathine penicillin G (Bicillin), 2.4 million units, is administered intramuscularly twice with an interval of 1 week, for a total of 4.8 million units. For late syphilis (late latent, cardiovascular, or neurosyphilis), benzathine penicillin G, 2.4 million units, is administered intramuscularly four times at weekly intervals, for a total dose of 9.6 million units. If a patient is known to have been exposed to syphilis, it is a fallacy to await the development of clinical or serologically reactive disease; preventive treatment is benzathine penicillin G, 2.4 million units, administered intramuscularly once. Treatment of congenital syphilis, when the patient is less than 2 years of age, requires benzathine penicillin G, 75,000 to 100,000 units per kilogram of body weight, divided into two injections with an interval of 1 week between injections, for a total dose of 300,000 to 1.5 million units. Other forms of penicillin also may be used in the treatment of syphilis. Procaine penicillin G in oil or procaine penicillin G aqueous are effective but require more frequent injections and higher total dosages. Treatment with these forms of penicillin is more costly and inconvenient and increases the probability of patient lapse from treatment.

When penicillin is contraindicated because of a history of sensitivity, alternative treatments are possible (Allyn). In the first 4 months of gestation, erythromycin, 500 mg, may be administered orally four times daily for 20 days, for a total dose of 40 g. During this period, infection of the fetus is unlikely, and one need be concerned solely with treatment of the mother; erythromycin has relative difficulty in crossing the placental barrier. After the fourth month of gestation, one must be concerned as well with adequate fetal serum concentrations of drug. Effective are tetracyclines (tetracycline, oxytetracycline) which traverse the placenta more readily but may adversely affect fetal bones and teeth. The dose of tetracycline is 500 mg orally four times daily for 20 days, for a total dose of 40 g. The risk of congenital lues must be balanced in such cases against the probability of treatment complications in the fetus.

Syphilis is a reportable disease, and epidemiologic follow-up by local health authorities is mandatory. The neonate born to a mother with syphilis, treated or not, must be observed carefully for at least 6 months and treated actively if there is any clinical evidence of disease. Positive serologic tests at birth result from placental passage of antibodies, and an uninfected infant should show decreasing antibody titers on follow-up (Saxoni et al.).

Once luetic therapy has been completed, ensuing pregnancies may be undertaken without risk to an incumbent fetus. If there is any doubt about the status of an infected pregnant patient, retreatment should be instituted to protect the fetus (George, 1971).

TOXOPLASMOSIS

Maternal infection with *Toxoplasma gondii* frequently is asymptomatic. In the United States, there is no reliable estimate of the incidence of toxoplasmosis in pregnant women; in France, the risk of maternal infection during pregnancy has been estimated at 5 percent. Often the diagnosis in the mother is established only by seroconversion. During the phase of maternal parasitemia, *Toxoplasma* may establish a focus of infection in the placenta and be disseminated thence to the fetus. The source of initial maternal infection is unclear.

The fetus almost always becomes infected only during acute, primary disease in the mother, and there is little evidence that women with chronic toxoplasmosis transmit the parasite in successive pregnancies; siblings of affected infants rarely manifest the disease. There is considerable controversy about the role of chronic toxoplasmosis in repeated abortion (Sharf et al.). In the acute phase of maternal infestation, treatment with pyrimethamine and sulfadiazine may be useful. There is no evidence that this therapy is effective in the chronic form of the disease. If there is evidence of acute maternal toxoplasmosis during pregnancy, therapeutic abortion should be considered; the possibility of transmission of the disease to the fetus has been estimated at 37 percent, and in infected infants the risk of significant cerebral or ocular defects is about 27 percent (Hume; Ruoss, Bourne).

The effects of congenital toxoplasmosis may be very severe (Kimball et al.). All clinical signs of disease result from chronic destructive infection of fetal and neonatal tissues. The consequences of infection, usually cerebral or ocular, may continue to appear years after active infection can no longer be demonstrated. Toxoplasmosis is not teratogenic in the true sense of the word; indeed, it is doubtful that fetal infection can occur during the period of organogenesis and before the formation of the placenta. The hydrocephalus or microcephalus which results from prenatal infection arises from chronic, destructive meningoencephalitis.

Clinical manifestations of congenital toxoplasmosis may be diverse. The classic triad includes chorioretinitis, hydrocephalus, and cerebral calcifications; but the complete classic triad is found in only a small percentage of cases. Infants affected acutely may have a rash, hepatosplenomegaly, jaundice, and meningoencephalitis with hypertonicity and convulsions. To date, there is no specific therapy which, administered postnatally, seems to be effective in preventing or reversing central nervous system or ocular manifestations.

Prevention of maternal toxoplasmosis is not yet possible, particularly since the mode of infection is not clear. Chemotherapy to the mother during gestation to prevent prenatal infection has not been tested in controlled situations for either efficacy or safety.

MALARIA

Any one of the four *Plasmodium* species, *P. falciparum, P. ovale, P. malariae,* and *P. vivax,* causes malaria. The disease is transmitted by the bite of an infected *Anopheles* mosquito or, more frequently in this country, by the transfusion of blood from an infected donor or the use of a common syringe and needle among drug addicts. An acute, febrile attack of malaria in early pregnancy may result in abortion. Transplacental infection of the fetus may occur. The protection afforded the fetus is related directly to the degree of maternal immunity. Prenatal infection of the fetus may result in stillbirth, retardation of intrauterine growth, and/or persistent neonatal infection (Smith, 1972; Lewis et al.).

The diagnosis is based upon the laboratory identification of *Plasmodium* organisms within erythrocytes. Treatment consists of chloroquine, 1.5 g orally followed by 0.5 g daily for an additional 3 days; suppressive therapy should be continued throughout gestation, in a dose of 0.5 g weekly.

PREGNANCY AND CANCER

Malignant tumors are encountered not infrequently in women of childbearing age. If this maternal disease complicates pregnancy, it or the treatment required may jeopardize the fetus and neonate and significantly impair the mother's ability to care for her child (McGowan).

Although uncommon, the coexistence of cancer with pregnancy is not rare, the incidence being estimated at 0.1 percent (Phelan). Each case must be individualized not only in terms of the patient but also for the type of malignancy encountered. There is general agreement, however, upon a series of questions which are applicable to the broad spectrum of tumors:

1. Does pregnancy alter the prognosis for the patient?
2. Will the patient benefit by termination of pregnancy?
3. Will the patient benefit from castration?
4. After successful treatment of the malignancy, may the patient have subsequent pregnancies?
5. Will the malignancy affect the fetus of the current pregnancy?
6. Will therapy for the malignancy affect the fetus?
7. When should therapy be started?

These questions may be applied to some of the more frequently encountered malignancies which may complicate gestation. It is accepted that, with the exception of choriocarcinoma, pregnancy per se does not cause malignant disease.

CARCINOMA OF THE BREAST

The incidence of carcinoma of the breast complicating pregnancy and the puerperium ranges in different reports from 0.1 to 2.0 percent. Conversely, pregnancy complicates less than 2 percent of all cases of breast carcinoma.

As in the nongravid patient, the presenting complaint in 95 percent of cases of carcinoma of the breast complicating pregnancy is the discovery of a breast mass. Usually the patient herself first is aware of the abnormality, but the obstetrician shares the responsibility of detection in the gravida. Examination of the breasts should be routine not only on the first antepartum visit but at regular intervals throughout gestation, after delivery, and into the puerperium. Benign breast masses, especially fibrocystic disease, far outnumber malignancies in pregnant and lactating patients. This should not lead, however, to any delay in diagnosis. Mammography and thermography may assist in elucidating the diagnosis; needle aspiration may reveal galactoceles; ultimately there is no substitute for excision biopsy. In most series reported, there is inordinate patient as well as physician delay in making this diagnosis in the gravida, a fact which must worsen her prognosis.

In a recent study of breast cancer in pregnancy, the prognosis for pregnant women was compared with that for the nongravid, a matched group of women under 40 years of age, comparing comparable stages of disease at the time of diagnosis (Mausner et al.). Five-year survival rates were the same in both groups of patients treated by radical mastectomy when no axillary nodes were involved. Women who were pregnant or lactating and had axillary involvement when first treated had a 5-year survival rate of 30 percent, as compared with 48 percent in the control group. The reason for this difference is not clear. Once the disease has spread to the regional lymph nodes, this "barrier" may be less effective in containing tumor during pregnancy or lactation than at other times. If hormones are responsible for increased activity of breast cancer during pregnancy, this effect has not been documented clearly in human beings. In the series reported above, the disease remained localized and without axillary metastases in the same proportion of women whether gravid, lactating, or nongravid.

In view of these data, therapeutic abortion should not influence the prognosis for the patient with breast cancer who is adequately and promptly treated for her disease. The beneficial effect of immediate castration has been equally difficult to justify. A patient with breast carcinoma who has received definitive treatment and has remained free from disease for at least 3 years may undergo pregnancy without significant risk of reactivation of dormant metastases.

Data suggest that mothers who breast feed their babies are two to three times less at risk of developing carcinoma in later life (Peters, Meakin). Recently, caution has been voiced against breast feeding by mothers with a family history of breast cancer or whose breast milk may contain viruslike particles. The transmission of mammary cancer via a milk virus (Bittner's virus) to suckling offspring has been documented in certain strains of mice. While it has not been shown that this form of transmission of breast cancer is applicable to human beings, the demonstration of viruslike particles in the breast milk of some nursing mothers is at least alarming. It has been suggested that if such particles are demonstrable, the mother should not breast feed and should be watched closely thereafter for possible development of breast carcinoma herself (Dmochowski). To date, this attitude is purely theoretical and very controversial.

OTHER MALIGNANT DISEASES

Other malignant diseases have been discussed in detail in previous sections of this chapter: malignant melanoma, leukemias, Hodgkin's disease, malignancies of the gastrointestinal tract, and tumors of the central nervous system.

CARCINOMA OF THE THYROID

This is rare in pregnancy, but several small series have been reported. In no instance did pregnancy appear to have an adverse effect upon the course of the maternal disease. The treatment of thyroid cancer during pregnancy is the same as in the nonpregnant patient, total thyroidectomy and removal of the lymph node draining tissue. Abortion is of no therapeutic value in most instances, but should be considered if radioiodine therapy for metastatic disease is contemplated. There is no reason that pregnancy should be proscribed for a patient adequately treated and free of disease for a reasonable interval after therapy.

CARCINOMA OF THE CERVIX

In pregnancy this presents a special problem. There is no evidence that cervical cancer either dedifferentiates or becomes more rapidly invasive under the influence of pregnancy or hormones. In several series, the 5-year survival rates for patients with invasive cervical carcinoma treated before the middle of the last trimester were equivalent stage for stage to those of nongravid controls. The maternal prognosis worsened materially after the 34th week of gestation and was deteriorated markedly if labor supervened. The treatment of invasive cervical carcinoma is radical in all phases of gestation, without regard to the state of the fetus (Lutz et al.).

EFFECT OF MATERNAL MALIGNANCY ON THE FETUS

Tumors that are active metabolically by the production of hormones or abnormal metabolites will have much the same effect on the fetus as on the mother. Once removed from the abnormal metabolic influences at delivery, the infant's metabolic milieu will return to normal. Residual effects may persist, as in the case of pseudohermaphroditism in female offspring of women with arrhenoblastomas.

Patients with malignancies frequently are treated with radiation or potent antimetabolites which specifically attack rapidly dividing cells. The property of rapid cell division is common to both neoplastic tissue and to fetal embryonic tissue. Both chemotherapeutic and radiologic treatments of malignant disease are potentially hazardous for the fetus. Specific problems have been discussed above.

Of major theoretic concern is the transmission of neoplastic disease from the mother transplacentally to the fetus. There have been reports of 36 cases of maternal malignancy with placental or fetal involvement: 11 patients with malignant melanoma, 8 with leukemia-lymphoma, 6 with breast carcinoma, 3 with carcinoma of the bronchus, 2 with gastric carcinoma, and single instances of colonic carcinoma, myxosarcoma of the thigh, carcinoma of the adrenal gland, and malignancies of the ethmoid bone, ovary, and liver (Rothman et al.). In each case, the mother had disseminated disease during the pregnancy and died either of her disease or of obstetric complications. In only two patients was tumor demonstrated at every metastatic level: maternal nonplacental lesion, placenta (including maternal and fetal sides), and the fetus. Fetal involvement was documented either histologically or clinically in 11 of the 36 cases, all among the malignant melanomas or leukemia-lymphoma group. The evidence suggests that intervillous involvement of the placenta by tumor without invasion of the villi indicates that the fetus may be relatively secure from the malignancy; conversely, however, violation of this placental barrier does not result inevitably in fetal or neonatal disease.

REFERENCES

Aaro LA, Juergens JL: Thrombophlebitis associated with pregnancy. *Am J Obstet Gynecol* 109:1128, 1971.

Allyn G: Adequate treatment for syphilis. *Arch Dermatol* 103:462, 1971.

Amies AG: Cerebral vascular disease in pregnancy. 1. Hemorrhage. *J Obstet Gynaecol Br Commonw* 77:100, 1970a.

———: Cerebral vascular disease in pregnancy. 2. Occlusion. *J Obstet Gynaecol Br Commonw* 77:312, 1970b.

Amstey MS: Management of pregnancy complicated by genital herpes virus infection. *Obstet Gynecol* 37:515, 1971.

Anderson MF: The iron status of pregnant women with hemoglobinopathies. *Am J Obstet Gynecol* 113:895, 1972.

Appel SH et al.: Acetylcholine receptor antibodies in myasthenia gravis. *N Engl J Med* 293:760, 1975.

Ayromlooi J: A new approach to the management of idiopathic thrombocytopenic purpura in pregnancy.

——— et al.: Modern management of the diabetic pregnancy. *Obstet Gynecol* 49:137, 1977.

Barry RM et al.: Influence of pregnancy on the course of Hodgkin's disease. *Am J Obstet Gynecol* 84:445, 1962.

Bates HR: Coxsackie virus B$_3$ calcific pancarditis and hydrops fetalis. *Am J Obstet Gynecol* 106:629, 1970.

Beernink FJ, McKay DG: Pituitary insufficiency associated with pregnancy and panhypopituitarism and diabetes insipidus. *Am J Obstet Gynecol* 84:318, 1962.

Beller FK: Thromboembolic disease in pregnancy. *Clin Obstet Gynecol* 11:290, 1968.

Benirschke K, Pendelton ME: Coxsackie virus infection. *Obstet Gynecol* 12:305, 1958.

Berlyne GM et al.: Placental transmission of the lupus erythematosus factor. *Lancet* 2:15, 1957.

Bhoopathi B et al.: Acute promyelocytic leukemia in pregnancy. *Obstet Gynecol* 41:275, 1973.

Bickerstaff ER et al.: The relapsing course of certain meningiomas in relation to pregnancy and menstruation. *J Neurol Neurosurg Psychiatry* 21:89, 1958.

Biggs R, MacFarlane RG: *Treatment of Haemophilia and Other Coagulation Disorders,* Oxford: Blackwell, 1966.

Biglieri EG, Seaton PE: Pregnancy and primary aldosteronism. *J Clin Endocrinol* 27:1628, 1967.

Bissell SM: Pulmonary thromboembolism associated with gynecologic surgery and pregnancy. *Am J Obstet Gynecol* 128:418, 1977.

Blattner RJ et al.: The role of viruses in the etiology of congenital malformations. *Prog Med Virol* 15:1, 1973.

Bleyer WA, Skinner AL: Fatal neonatal hemorrhage with maternal anticonvulsant therapy. *JAMA* 235:626, 1976.

Bolen JW: Hypoparathyroidism in pregnancy. *Am J Obstet Gynecol* 117:178, 1973.

Bolognese RJ et al.: Herpesvirus hominis type II infections in asymptomatic pregnant women. *Obstet Gynecol* 48:507, 1976.

———: Rubella vaccination during pregnancy. *Am J Obstet Gynecol* 112:903, 1972.

Bonnar J: Long-term self-administered heparin therapy for prevention and treatment of thromboembolic complications in pregnancy, in *Heparin— Chemistry and Clinical Usage,* eds. VV Kakkar et al., London: Academic Press, 1976.

Borhanmanesh F, Haghighi P: Pregnancy in patients with cirrhosis of the liver. *Obstet Gynecol* 36:315, 1970.

———— et al.: Viral hepatitis during pregnancy. *Gastroenterology* 64:304, 1973.

Breen KJ et al.: Idiopathic acute fatty liver of pregnancy. Gut 11:822, 1970.

————: Uncomplicated subsequent pregnancy after idiopathic fatty liver of pregnancy. *Obstet Gynecol* 40:813, 1972.

Brenner WE et al.: Pheochromocytoma. Serial studies during pregnancy. *Am J Obstet Gynecol* 113:779, 1972.

Buemann B, Kragelund E: Morbidity and mortality among infants born to mothers with heart disease. *Acta Obstet Gynecol Scand* 41:80, 1962.

Burch GE: Heart disease and pregnancy. *Am Heart J* 93:104, 1977.

Burrow GN: Hyperthyroidism during pregnancy. *N Engl J Med* 298:150, 1978.

Burrow GN et al.: Children exposed in utero to propylthiouracil. *Am J Dis Child* 116:161, 1968.

Burstein PN, Chen CM: Diabetes insipidus, nephrogenic type, complicating pregnancy; a case report *Am J Obstet Gynecol* 108:1292, 1970.

Burt RL, Weaver RG: Proliferative diabetic retinopathy in pregnancy. *Obstet Gynecol* 40:199, 1972.

Cano RI et al.: Acute fatty liver of pregnancy. *JAMA* 231:159, 1975.

Carlström, G: Viral infections and birth defects. *Acta Obstet Gynecol Scand* 67 (suppl):21, 1977.

Carruthers JA: Herpes gestationis: Clinical features of immunologically proved cases. *Am J Obstet Gynecol* 131:865, 1978.

Casanegra P et al.: Cardiovascular management of pregnant women with a heart valve prosthesis. *Am J Cardiol* 36:802, 1975.

Center for Disease Control, U. S. Public Health Service, Department of Health, Education, and Welfare: *Treatment Schedules for Gonorrhea.* January 1979.

Centrone AL et al.: Polycythemia rubra vera in pregnancy. *Obstet Gynecol* 30:657, 1967.

Chamberlain MJ et al.: Medical memoranda. Toxic effect of podophyllum application in pregnancy. *Br Med J* 3:391, 1972.

Chesley LC, Duffus GM: Posture and apparent plasma volume in late pregnancy. *J Obstet Gynaecol Br Commonw* 78:406, 1971.

Chin J et al.: Avoidance of rubella immunization of women during or shortly before pregnancy. *JAMA* 215:632, 1971.

Chugh KS et al.: Acute renal failure of obstetric origin. *Obstet Gynecol* 48:642, 1976.

Church R: The prospect of psoriasis. *Br J Dermatol* 70:139, 1958.

Cobo E et al.: Low oxytocin secretion in diabetes insipidus associated with normal labor. *Am J Obstet Gynecol* 114:861, 1972.

Coe FL et al.: Nephrolithiasis in pregnancy. *N Engl J Med,* 298:324, 1978.

Cohen SG et al.: Spontaneous rupture of a renal artery aneurysm during pregnancy. *Obstet Gynecol* 39:897, 1972.

Cohn LH, Shumway NE: Pulmonary embolectomy during pregnancy. *Arch Surg* 106:214, 1973.

Colle E, Goldman H: Effects of glucocorticoids on insulin release from human fetal islets. *Diabetes* 25 (suppl. I):359, 1976.

Collins DJ et al.: Aplastic anemia in pregnancy. *Obstet Gynecol* 39:884, 1972.

Corlett RC Jr., Mishell DR Jr.: Pancreatitis in pregnancy. *Am J Obstet Gynecol* 113:281, 1972.

Cossart YE: The outcome of hepatitis B virus infection in pregnancy. *Postgrad Med J* 53:610, 1977.

———— et al.: Australia antigen and the human fetus. *Am J Dis Child* 123:376, 1972.

Coustan DR et al.: Insulin therapy for gestational diabetes. *Obstet Gynecol* 51:306, 1978.

Cramblett HG et al.: Leukemia in an infant born of a mother with leukemia. *N Engl J Med* 259:727, 1958.

Crane MG et al.: Primary aldosteronism in pregnancy. *Obstet Gynecol* 23:200, 1964.

Cross N et al.: Cerebral strokes associated with pregnancy and the puerperium. *Br Med J* 2:214, 1968.

Csapo AI et al.: The significance of the human corpus luteum in pregnancy maintenance. I. Preliminary studies. *Am J Obstet Gynecol* 112:1061, 1972.

————: Effects of lutectomy and progesterone replacement therapy in early pregnant patients. *Am J Obstet Gynecol* 115:759, 1973.

Cunningham MD et al.: Incomplete surfactant phospholipid complex formation: absence of phosphatidyl glycerol. *Gynecol Invest* 8:76, 1977.

Cunningham MP, Slaughter DP: Surgical treatment of disease of the thyroid gland in pregnancy. *Surg Gynecol Obstet* 131:486, 1970.

Curry JJ, Quintana FJ: Myocardial infarction with ventricular fibrillation during pregnancy treated by direct current defibrillation and fetal survival. *Dis Chest* 58:82, 1970.

Cutter BG, Hansman D: Neonatal varicella. *Med J Aust* 1:411, 1968.

Dajani RM et al.: Urinary estriol excretion and hemoglobinopathies of pregnancy. *Am J Obstet Gynecol* 110:125, 1971.

D'Angio GJ, Nisce LZ: Updated Hodgkin's disease. C. Advanced disease and special problems. Problems with the irradiation of children and pregnant patients. *JAMA* 223:171, 1973.

Davison JM et al.: Planned pregnancy in a renal transplant recipient. *Br J Obstet Gynaecol* 83:518, 1976.

Deal K, Wooley CF: Coarctation of the aorta and pregnancy. *Ann Intern Med* 78:706, 1973.

Demakis JG, Rahimtoola SH: Peripartum cardiomyopathy. *Circulation* 44:964, 1971.

de March P: Tuberculosis and pregnancy. Five-to-10 year review of 215 patients in their fertile age. *Chest* 68:800, 1975.

Dmochowski L: Viruses and breast cancer. *Hosp Prac* 7:73, 1972.

Dougherty CM, Lund CJ: Solid ovarian tumors complicating pregnancy. *Am J Obstet Gynecol* 60:261, 1950.

Duncan ID et al.: Management and treatment of 34 cases of antepartum thromboembolism. *Obstet J Gynaecol Br Commonw* 78:904, 1971.

Editorial: Safety of immunizing agents in pregnancy. *Med Lett Drugs Ther* 12:23, 1970.

Edwards RF, Saáry M: Emergency maternal exchange transfusion for sickle-cell anemia complicating twin pregnancy. *J Obstet Gynaecol Br Commonw* 78:751, 1971.

el-Minawi MF et al.: Pheochromocytoma masquerading as pre-eclamptic toxemia. Current concepts of diagnosis and treatment. *Am J Obstet Gynecol* 109:389, 1971.

Evans IMA et al.: Bleeding esophageal varices in pregnancy. *Obstet Gynecol* 40:377, 1972.

Evans PC: Obstetric and gynecologic patients with von Willebrand's disease. *Obstet Gynecol* 38:37, 1971.

Ewing PA, Whitaker JA: Acute leukemia in pregnancy. *Obstet Gynecol* 42:245, 1973.

Fambrough DM et al.: Neuromuscular junction in myasthenia gravis: decreased acetylcholine receptors. *Science* 182:293, 1973.

Fehenbaker LG et al.: Transitional cell carcinoma of the bladder during pregnancy: Case report. *J Urol* 108:419, 1972.

Fetter TR, Koppel MM: Urologic malignancy associated with pregnancy. *Clin Obstet Gynecol* 6:1010, 1963.

Fisher KA et al.: Nephrotic proteinuria with preeclampsia. *Am J Obstet Gynecol* 129:643, 1977.

Flanders RW et al.: Is herpes simplex infection of the newborn preventable? The possible role of cesarean section in minimizing risk. *Clin Pediatr* 11:293, 1972.

Fletcher J et al.: The value of folic acid supplements in pregnancy. *J Obstet Gynaecol Br Commonw* 78:781, 1971.

Florman AL et al.: Intrauterine infection with herpes simplex virus. Resultant congenital malformations. *JAMA* 225:129, 1973.

Fort AT: Sickle cell disease and trait in pregnancy. *Obstet Gynecol Annu* 5:189, 1976.

——— et al.: Counseling the patient with sickle-cell disease about reproduction: Pregnancy outcome does not justify the risk. *Am J Obstet Gynecol* 111:324, 1971.

Freedman WL: Alpha and beta thalassemia and pregnancy. *Clin Obstet Gynecol* 12:115, 1969.

Freeman, MG, Ruth GJ: SS disease, SC disease, and CC disease—obstetric considerations and treatment. *Clin Obstet Gynecol* 12:134, 1969.

Friendly DS: Gonococcal conjunctivitis of the newborn. *Clin Proc Child Hosp DC* 25:1, 1969.

Gabbe SC et al.: Management and outcome of class A diabetes mellitus. *Am J Obstet Gynecol* 127:465, 1977a.

———: Lecithin/sphingomyelin ratio in pregnancies complicated by diabetes mellitus. *Am J Obstet Gynecol* 128:757, 1977b.

———: Management and outcome of pregnancy in diabetes mellitus, classes B to R. *Am J Obstet Gynecol* 129:723, 1977c.

Gagnon RA: Transplacental inoculation of fetal herpes simplex in the newborn. *Obstet Gynecol* 31:682, 1968.

George PA et al.: Melanoma and pregnancy. *Cancer* 13:854, 1960.

George RP Jr.: Therapy for syphilis during pregnancy. *N Engl J Med* 284:1271, 1971.

Gerety RJ et al.: Viral hepatitis type B during pregnancy, the neonatal period, and infancy. *J Pediatr* 90:368, 1977.

Gersony WM et al.: Endocardial fibroelastosis and the mumps virus. *Pediatrics* 37:430, 1966.

Ginz B: Myocardial infarction in pregnancy. *J Obstet Gynaecol Br Commonw* 77:610, 1970.

Gluck L: Evaluating functional fetal maturation. *Clin Obstet Gynecol* 21:547, 1978.

Goebelsmann U et al.: Estriol in pregnancy. II. Daily urinary estriol assays in the management of the pregnant diabetic woman. *Am J Obstet Gynecol* 115:795, 1973.

Goligher JC et al.: Ulcerative colitis and pregnancy. *Lancet* 2:595, 1965.

Goodhue PA, Evans TS: Idiopathic thrombocytopenic

purpura in pregnancy. Report of a case and review of the literature. *Obstet Gynecol Survey* 18:671, 1963.

Goodwin JF: Peripartal heart disease. *Clin Obstet Gynecol* 18:125, 1975.

Gordon M et al.: Fetal morbidity following potentially anoxigenic obstetric conditions. VII. Bronchial asthma. *Am J Obstet Gynecol* 106:421, 1970.

Gorthy RL, Krembs MA: Vulvar condylomata acuminata complicating labor. *Obstet Gynecol* 4:67, 1954.

Green DM et al.: Generalized vaccinia in the human foetus. *Lancet* 1:1296, 1966.

Green HG et al.: Cretinism associated with maternal iodide I^{131} therapy during pregnancy. *Am J Dis Child* 122:247, 1971.

Greenbaum CH: Herpes gestationis. *Arch Dermatol* 103:218, 1971.

Greenberg M et al.: Maternal mortality in the epidemic of Asian influenza, New York City, 1957. *Am J Obstet Gynecol* 76:897, 1958.

Griffith GW et al.: Influenza and infant mortality. *Br Med J* 3:553, 1972.

Grimes EM et al.: Cushing's syndrome in pregnancy. *Obstet Gynecol* 42:550, 1973.

Guril N et al.: Peripheral venous thrombophlebitis during pregnancy. *Am J Surg* 121:449, 1971.

Gyves MT et al.: A modern approach to management of pregnant diabetics. A 2-year analysis of perinatal outcomes. *Am J Obstet Gynecol* 128:606, 1977.

Hall MH: Folic acid deficiency and congenital malformations. *J Obstet Gynaecol Br Commonw* 79:187, 1972.

Hardin JA: Cyclophosphamide treatment of lymphoma during third trimester of pregnancy. *Obstet Gynecol* 39:850, 1972.

Harley JMG: Essential hypertension complicating pregnancy; factors affecting the foetal mortality. *Proc R Soc Med* 59:535, 1966.

Harris RE, Dunnihoo DR: The incidence and significance of urinary calculi in pregnancy. *Am J Obstet Gynecol* 97:720, 1967.

Hatfield AK et al.: Idiopathic acute fatty liver of pregnancy. Death from extrahepatic manifestations. *Am J Dig Dis* 17:167, 1972.

Heineman HS, Lee JH: Bacteriuria in pregnancy. A heterogeneous entity. *Obstet Gynecol* 41:22, 1973.

Henderson SR et al.: Antepartum pulmonary embolism. *Am J Obstet Gynecol* 112:476, 1972.

Hendrickse JP de V et al.: Pregnancy in homozygous sickle-cell anemia. *J Obstet Gynaecol Br Commonw* 79:396, 1972a.

————: Pregnancy in abnormal hemoglobins CC, S-thalassemia, SF, CF, double heterozygotes. *J Obstet Gynaecol Br Commonw* 79:410, 1972b.

————, Watson-Williams EJ: The influence of hemoglobinopathies upon reproduction. *Am J Obstet Gynecol* 94:739, 1966.

Heys RF: Child-bearing and idiopathic thrombocytopenic purpura. *J Obstet Gynaecol Br Commonw* 73:205, 1966.

Hibbard BH, Jeffcoate TNA: Abruptio placenta. *Obstet Gynecol* 27:155, 1966.

Hieber JP et al.: Hepatitis and pregnancy. *J Pediatr* 91:545, 1977.

Hildebrant JR et al.: Cytomegalovirus in the normal pregnant female. *Am J Obst Gynecol* 98:1125, 1967.

Hill EC: Maternal obstetric paralysis. *Am J Obstet Gynecol* 83:1452, 1962.

Hill WC, Pearson JW: Outpatient intravenous heparin therapy for antepartum ileofemoral thrombophlebitis. *Obstet Gynecol* 37:785, 1971.

Hirsh J et al.: Anticoagulants in pregnancy: A review of indications and complications. *Am Heart J* 83:301, 1972.

Holden TE, Sherline DM: Hepatitis and hepatic failure in pregnancy. *Obstet Gynecol* 40:586, 1972.

Holder WR, Knox JM: Syphilis in pregnancy. *Med Clin North Am* 56:1151, 1972.

Hollingsworth DR, Austin E: Thyroxine derivatives in amniotic fluid. *J Pediatr* 79:923, 1971.

Holzbach RT: Australia antigen hepatitis in pregnancy. Evidence against transplacental transmission of Australia antigen in early and late pregnancy. *Arch Intern Med* 124:195, 1972.

Horger EO III: Sickle-cell and sickle cell-hemoglobin C disease during pregnancy. *Obstet Gynecol* 39:873, 1972.

Howie PW: Thromboembolism. *Clin Obstet Gynaecol* 4:897, 1977.

Hume OS: Toxoplasmosis and pregnancy. *Am J Obstet Gynecol* 144:703, 1972.

Jacobsen BB et al.: Neonatal hypocalcemia associated with maternal hyperparathyroidism. New pathogenetic observations. *Arch Dis Child* 53:308, 1978.

Johnson TR et al.: Scleroderma and pregnancy. *Obstet Gynecol* 23:467, 1964.

Johnstone RE 2d et al.: Hyperparathyroidism during pregnancy. *Obstet Gynecol* 40:580, 1972.

Kaplan JP et al.: Congenital vaccinia: Some doubts. *Pediatrics* 50:971, 1972.

Kasdon SC: Pregnancy and Hodgkin's disease. *Am J Obstet Gynecol* 57:282, 1949.

Katz SI et al.: Herpes gestationis: Immunopathology

and characterization of the HG factor. *J Clin Invest* 57:1434, 1976.

Kendig EL: Prognosis of infants born of tuberculous mothers. *Pediatrics* 26:97, 1960.

Kennedy AL, Montgomery DAD: Hypothyroidism in pregnancy. *Br J Obstet Gynaecol* 85:225, 1978.

Khunda S: Pregnancy and Addison's disease. *Obstet Gynecol* 39:431, 1972.

Kimball AC et al.: Congenital toxoplasmosis; a prospective study of 4,048 obstetric patients. *Am J Obstet Gynecol* 111:211, 1971.

Kincaid-Smith P: Bacteriuria and urinary infection in pregnancy. *Clin Obstet Gynecol* 11:533, 1968.

Knight AH et al.: Epilepsy and pregnancy: A study of 153 pregnancies in 59 patients. *Epilepsia* 16:99, 1975.

Kraus GW, Yen SSC: Gonorrhea during pregnancy. *Obstet Gynecol* 31:258, 1968.

Kreines K, deVaux WD: Neonatal adrenal insufficiency associated with maternal Cushing's syndrome. *Pediatrics* 47:516, 1971.

Krugman S, Giles JP: Viral hepatitis, a new light on an old disease. *JAMA* 212:1019, 1970.

Lacher MG, Geller W: Cyclophosphamide and vinblastine sulfate in Hodgkin's disease during pregnancy. *JAMA* 195:486, 1966.

Lanzkowsky P: The influence of maternal iron-deficiency anemia on the haemoglobin of the infant. *Arch Dis Child* 36:205, 1961.

Lea AW: Pregnancy following radical operation for rectal carcinoma. *Am J Obstet Gynecol* 113:504, 1972.

Lewis BV, Parsons M: Chorea gravidarum. *Lancet* 1:284, 1966.

Lewis R et al.: Malaria associated with pregnancy. *Obstet Gynecol* 42:696, 1973.

Limet R et al.: Cardiac valve prostheses, anticoagulation, and pregnancy. *Ann Thorac Surg* 23:337, 1977.

Lutz MH et al.: Genital malignancy in pregnancy. *Am J Obstet Gynecol* 129:536, 1977.

Lindhe J et al.: Changes in vascular proliferation after local application of sex hormones. *J Periodont Res* 2:226, 1967.

McCann MI: Infants of diabetic mothers. *Pediatrics* 45:887, 1970.

McColleem RW: Epidemiology of infections with type B virus. *Am J Dis Child* 123:364, 1972.

McElin TW, Cromer DW: Pemphigus vulgaris complicated by pregnancy. *Am J Obstet Gynecol* 92:1122, 1965.

McGee CD, Makowski EL: Systemic lupus erythematosus in pregnancy. *Am J Obstet Gynecol* 107:1008, 1970.

McGowan L: Cancer and pregnancy. *Obstet Gynecol Survey* 19:285, 1964.

McKay DG: *Disseminated Intravascular Coagulation*, New York: Hoeber-Harper, 1965.

MacKay EV: Pregnancy and renal disease. *Aust NZ J Obstet Gynaecol* 3:21, 1963.

McKenzie JM: Studies of the thyroid activator of hyperthyroidism. *J Clin Endocrinol* 21:635, 1964.

Makker SP, Heymann W: Pregnancy in patients who have had the idiopathic nephrotic syndrome in childhood. *J Pediatr* 81:1140, 1972.

Mansell RV: Infectious hepatitis in the first trimester of pregnancy and its effect on the fetus. *Am J Obstet Gynecol* 69:1136, 1955.

Marchant DJ: Urinary tract infections in pregnancy. *Clin Obstet Gynecol* 21:921, 1978.

Marcus FI et al.: The effect of pregnancy on the murmurs of mitral and aortic regurgitation. *Circulation* 41:795, 1970.

Marder MZ: Responsibility of the physician toward oral care of the pregnant patient. *Am J Obstet Gynecol* 103:437, 1969.

Marengo-Rowe AJ et al.: Hemophilia-like disease associated with pregnancy. *Obstet Gynecol* 40:56, 1972.

Marx JL: Slow viruses (I): Role in persistent disease. *Science* 181:1351, 1973a.

———: Slow viruses (II): The unconventional agents. *Science* 182:44, 1973b.

Mausner JS et al.: Breast cancer in Philadelphia hospitals, 1951–1964. *Cancer* 23:260, 1969.

Merkatz IR et al.: Resumption of female reproductive function following renal transplantation. *JAMA* 216:1749, 1971.

Middleton EB, Lee YC: Pregnancy associated with cardiac pacemaker generator implanted in abdominal wall. A case report. *Obstet Gynecol* 38:272, 1971.

Montgomery WH, Miller FC: Pancreatitis and pregnancy. *Obstet Gynecol* 35:658, 1970.

Mueller-Heubach E et al.: Lecithin/sphingomyelin ratio in amniotic fluid and its value in the prediction of neonatal respiratory distress syndrome in pregnant diabetic women. *Am J Obstet Gynecol* 130:28, 1978.

Nahmias AJ et al.: Perinatal risks associated with maternal genital herpes simplex virus infection. *Am J Obstet Gynecol* 110:825, 1971.

Naib ZM et al.: Association of maternal genital herpetic infection with spontaneous abortion. *Obstet Gynecol* 35:260, 1970.

Namba T et al.: Neonatal myasthenia gravis: Report of 2 cases and review of the literature. *Pediatrics* 45:488, 1970.

Nicholas GG et al.: Carpal tunnel syndrome in pregnancy. *Hand* 3:80, 1971.

Niven P et al.: Pregnancy following the surgical treatment of portal hypertension. *Am J Obstet Gynecol* 110:1100, 1971.

Noller KL et al.: Von Willebrand's disease in pregnancy. *Obstet Gynecol* 41:865, 1973.

Norton RA, Patterson JF: Pregnancy and regional enteritis. *Obstet Gynecol* 40:711, 1972.

Novak DJ, Johnson KP: Relapsing idiopathic polyneuritis during pregnancy. Immunological aspects and literature review. *Arch Neurol* 28:219, 1973.

—— et al.: Virilization during pregnancy. Case report and review of the literature. *Am J Med* 49:281, 1970.

Novell HA et al.: Marfan's syndrome associated with pregnancy. *Am J Obstet Gynecol* 75:802, 1958.

O'Dwyer EM, Montgomery D: Pregnancy and acute nephritis. *J Obstet Gynaecol Br Commonw* 61:454, 1964.

Okada K et al.: e Antigen and anti-e in the serum of asymptomatic carrier mothers as indicators of positive and negative transmission of hepatitis B virus to their infants. *N Engl J Med* 294:746, 1976.

——: Hepatitis B surface antigen in the serum of infants after delivery from asymptomatic carrier mothers. *J Pediatr* 87:360, 1975.

O'Leary JA: Ten year study of sarcoidosis and pregnancy. *Am J Obstet Gynecol* 84:462, 1962.

Oosterhuis HJGH et al.: Muscle antibodies in myasthenic mothers and their babies. *Lancet* 2:1226, 1966.

Oravec D, Lichardus B: Management of diabetes insipidus in pregnancy. *Br Med J* 4:114, 1972.

Oxorn H: Changing aspects of pneumonia complicating pregnancy. *Am J Obstet Gynecol* 70:1057, 1955.

Pakes, JB et al.: Studies on beta thalassemia trait in pregnancy. *Am J Obstet Gynecol* 108:1217, 1970.

Pearson HA et al.: Isoimmune neonatal thrombocytopenic purpura—clinical and therapeutic considerations. *Blood* 23:154, 1964.

Pedersen LM et al.: Congenital malformations in newborn infants of diabetic women. Correlation with maternal diabetic vascular complications. *Lancet* 1:1124, 1964.

Pedowitz P, Perell A: Aneurysms complicated by pregnancy. I. Aneurysms of the aorta and its major branches. *Am J Obstet Gynecol* 73:720, 1957.

Perkins, RP: Inherited disorders of hemoglobin synthesis and pregnancy. *Am J Obstet Gynecol* 111:120, 1971.

Persellin RH: The effect of pregnancy on rheumatoid arthritis. *Bull Rheum Dis* 27:922, 1977.

Peters MV, Meakin JW: The influence of pregnancy in carcinoma of the breast. *Prog Clin Cancer* 1:471, 1965.

Phelan JT: Cancer and pregnancy. *NY State J Med* 68:3011, 1968.

Pitkin RM: Autoimmune diseases in pregnancy. *Semin Perinatol* 1:161, 1977.

Platt HS: Effect of maternal sickle cell trait on perinatal mortality. *Br Med J* 4:334, 1971.

Plauché WC: Myasthenia gravis in pregnancy. *Am J Obstet Gynecol* 88:404, 1964.

Poole JL: Treatment of intracranial aneurysms during pregnancy. *JAMA* 192:209, 1965.

Popoff P et al.: Pregnancy in renal transplant recipients; report of 2 successful pregnancies in a patient with impaired renal function. *Can Med Assoc J* 117:1288, 1977.

Pritchard JA et al.: Infants of mothers with megaloblastic anemia due to folate deficiency. *JAMA* 211:1982, 1970.

Prout, TE: Thyroid disease in pregnancy. *Am J Obstet Gynecol* 122:669, 1975.

Rae PG, Robb PM: Megaloblastic anemia of pregnancy; a clinical and laboratory study with particular reference to the total and labile serum folate levels. *J Clin Pathol* 23:379, 1970.

Raivio KO et al.: Fetal risks due to Warfarin therapy during pregnancy. *Acta Paediatr Scand* 66:735, 1977.

Ramsey DM: Thromboembolism in pregnancy. *Obstet Gynecol* 45:129, 1975.

Rand RJ et al.: Maternal cardiomyopathy of pregnancy causing stillbirth. *Br J Obstet Gynaecol* 82:172, 1975.

Rannevik G et al.: Effect of oral contraceptives on the liver in women with recurrent cholestasis (hepatosis) during previous pregnancies. *J Obstet Gynaecol Br Commonw* 79:1128, 1972.

Rencoret R, Aste H: Jaundice during pregnancy. *Med J Aust* 1:167, 1973.

Roberts MF et al.: Association between maternal diabetes and the respiratory distress syndrome in the newborn. *N Engl J Med* 294:357, 1976.

Robinson JL, Sedzimir CB: Subarachnoid hemorrhage in pregnancy. *J Neurosurg* 36:27, 1972.

Romhilt DW et al.: Mimicry in pulmonary embolism. *Geriatrics* 27:73, 1972.

Rosenow EC, Lee RA: Cystic fibrosis and pregnancy. *JAMA,* 203:227, 1968.

Rothman LA et al.: Placental and fetal involvement by maternal malignancy: A report of rectal carcinoma and review of the literature. *Am J Obstet Gynecol* 116:1023, 1973.

Roversi GD et al.: Insulin in gestational diabetes, in

Early Diabetes in Early Life, eds. RA Camerini-Davalos, HS Cole, London: Academic Press, 1975, p. 469.

Ruch WA, Klein PL: Polycythemia vera and pregnancy. *Obstet Gynecol* 23:107, 1964.

Rudolph AM: Control of gonorrhea. *JAMA* 220:1587, 1972.

Ruoss CF, Bourne GL: Toxoplasmosis in pregnancy. *J Obstet Gynaecol Br Commonw* 79:1115, 1972.

Salam AA, Warren WD: Distal splenorenal shunt for treatment of variceal bleeding during pregnancy. *Arch Surg* 105:643, 1972.

Sallomi SJ: Rubella in pregnancy. A review of prospective studies from the literature. *Obstet Gynecol* 27:252, 1966.

Saxoni F et al.: Congenital syphilis: A description of 18 cases and re-examination of an old but ever-present disease. *Clin Pediatr* 6:687, 1967.

Schaeffer M et al.: Intrauterine poliomyelitis infection. *JAMA* 155:248, 1954.

Schapira K et al.: Marriage, pregnancy, and multiple sclerosis. *Brain* 89:419, 1966.

Schenker JG, Luttwak E: Pregnancy and delivery after bilateral adrenalectomy for pheochromocytoma. Case report and review of the literature. *J Obstet Gynaecol Br Commonw* 77:1031, 1970.

Schweitzer IL et al.: Viral hepatitis B in neonates and infants. *Am J Med* 55:762, 1973.

Scott DE et al.: Maternal folate deficiency and pregnancy wastage. II. Fetal malformation. *Obstet Gynecol* 36:26, 1970.

Seip M: Systemic lupus erythematosus in pregnancy with hemolytic anemia, leucopenia, and thrombocytopenia in the mother and her newborn infant. *Arch Dis Child* 35:364, 1959.

Selenkow HA: Antithyroid-thyroid therapy of thyrotoxicosis during pregnancy. *Obstet Gynecol* 40:117, 1972.

Shanl WL et al.: Multiple congenital anomalies associated with oral anticoagulants. *Am J Obstet Gynecol* 127:191, 1977.

Shapiro S et al.: Are hydantoins (phenytoins) human teratogens? *J Pediatr* 90:673, 1977.

Sharf M et al.: Latent toxoplasmosis and pregnancy. *Obstet Gynecol* 42:349, 1973.

Shea MA et al.: Diabetes in pregnancy. *Am J Obstet Gynecol* 111:801, 1971.

Shenker JG, Chowers I: Pheochromocytoma and pregnancy. *Obstet Gynecol Survey* 26:739, 1971.

Siegel M: Congenital malformations following chickenpox, measles, mumps, and hepatitis. Results of a cohort study. *JAMA* 226:1521, 1973.

——— et al.: Comparative fetal mortality in maternal virus diseases (a prospective study on rubella, measles, mumps, chickenpox, and hepatitis). *N Engl J Med* 274:768, 1966.

———, Greenberg M: Poliomyelitis in pregnancy. *N Engl J Med* 253:845, 1955.

Silverstein AM: Fetal immune responses in congenital infection. *N Engl J Med* 286:1413, 1972.

Simanis J et al.: Unresectable pheochromocytoma in pregnancy. Pharmacology and biochemistry. *Am J Med* 53:381, 1972.

Simms CD et al.: Lung function tests in bronchial asthma during and after pregnancy. *Br J Obstet Gynaecol* 83:434, 1976.

Sisson TRC, Lund CJ: The influence of maternal iron deficiency on the newborn. *Am J Clin Nutr* 6:376, 1958.

Smith AM: Malaria in pregnancy. *Br Med J* 4:793, 1972.

Smith DW: Teratogenicity of anticonvulsant medications. *Am J Dis Child* 131:1337, 1977.

Souma JA et al.: Comparison of thyroid function in each trimester of pregnancy with the use of triiodothyronine uptake, thyroxine coline, free thyroxine, and free thyroxine index. *Am J Obstet Gynecol* 116:905, 1973.

Sparling PF: Diagnosis and treatment of syphilis. *N Engl J Med* 284:642, 1971.

Spellacy WN et al.: Vitamin B_6 treatment of gestational diabetes. *Am J Obstet Gynecol* 127:599, 1977.

———: Insulin, in *Endocrinology of Pregnancy,* eds. F Fuchs, A Klopper, New York: Harper & Row, 1971, pp. 197–215.

Sprague AD et al.: Pheochromocytoma associated with pregnancy. *Obstet Gynecol* 39:887, 1972.

Stehbens JA et al.: Outcome at age 1, 3, and 5 years of children born to diabetic women. *Am J Obstet Gynecol* 127:408, 1977.

Stevenson RE: *The Fetus and Newly Born Infant,* St. Louis: Mosby, 1973, pp. 332–336.

Storch MP et al.: Hyperlipoproteinemia and acute hemorrhagic pancreatitis complicating pregnancy. *Am J Obstet Gynecol* 129:343, 1977.

Tagatz GE et al.: Pregnancy in a juvenile diabetic after renal transplantation (Cass T diabetes mellitus). *Diabetes* 24:497, 1975.

Tartakow IJ: The teratogenicity of maternal rubella. *J Pediatr* 66:380, 1965.

Tejani N: Anticoagulant therapy with cardiac valve prosthesis during pregnancy. *Obstet Gynecol* 42:785, 1973.

Tejani SN et al.: Modern management of hypertensive disorders of pregnancy. *Obstet Gynecol* 51:648, 1978.

Territo M et al.: Management of autoimmune thrombocytopenia in pregnancy and the neonate. *Obstet Gynecol* 41:579, 1973.

Tyson JE, Felig P: Medical aspects of diabetes in pregnancy and the diabetogenic effect of oral contraceptives. *Med Clin North Am* 55:947, 1971.

Ueland K: Cardiovascular diseases complicating pregnancy. *Clin Obstet Gynecol* 21:429, 1978.

——— et al.: Cardiorespiratory response to pregnancy and exercise in normal women and patients with heart disease. *Am J Obstet Gynecol* 115:4, 1973.

van Enk A et al.: Benign obstetric history in women with sickle cell anaemia associated with thalassemia. *Br Med J* 4:524, 1972.

van Nagell JR et al.: Preventable anemia and pregnancy. *Obstet Gynecol Survey* 26:551, 1971.

Varma RR et al.: Pregnancy in cirrhotic and non-cirrhotic portal hypertension. *Obstet Gynecol* 50:103, 1976.

Varriale P et al.: Polyarteritis nodosa in pregnancy. Report of a case. *Obstet Gynecol* 25:866, 1965.

Veltman LL, Ostergard DR: Thrombosis of vulvar varicosities during pregnancy. *Obstet Gynecol* 39:55, 1972.

Welt SI et al.: Concurrent hypertension and pregnancy. *Clin Obstet Gynecol* 21:691, 1978.

West TET, Lowy C: Control of blood glucose during labor in diabetic women with combined glucose and low-dose insulin infusion. *Br Med J* 1:1252, 1977.

Weston PV, Lindheimer MD: Intermittent intestinal obstruction simulating hyperemesis gravidarum. *Obstet Gynecol* 37:106, 1971.

White P: Classification of obstetric diabetes. *Am J Obstet Gynecol* 130:228, 1978.

Whitelaw A: Subcutaneous fat in newborn infants of diabetic mothers. An indication of quality of diabetic control. *Lancet* 1:15, 1977.

Wieland RG et al.: Cushing's syndrome complicating pregnancy. *Obstet Gynecol* 38:841, 1971.

Willoughby MLN: Blood and neoplastic diseases: acute myeloblastic leukemia. *Br Med J* 4:337, 1974.

Wilson EA et al.: Tuberculosis complicated by pregnancy. *Am J Obstet Gynecol* 115:526, 1973.

Wilson MG, Stein AM: Teratogenic effects of Asian influenza. An extended study. *JAMA* 210:336, 1969.

Wintrobe, MM: *Clinical Hematology,* Philadelphia: Lea & Febiger, 1974, p. 1454.

Wise GA, McQuillan MP: Transient neonatal myasthenia. Clinical and electromyographic studies. *Arch Neurol* 22:556, 1970.

Yahia C et al.: Acute leukemia and pregnancy. *Obstet Gynecol Survey* 13:1, 1958.

Yeast JD et al.: The use of continuous insulin infusion in the peripartum management of pregnant diabetic women. *Am J Obstet Gynecol* 131:861, 1978.

Young RL et al.: Treatment of large condylomata acuminata complicating pregnancy. *Obstet Gynecol* 41:65, 1973.

Zegart KN, Schwartz RH: Chorea gravidarum. *Obstet Gynecol* 32:24, 1968.

Zurier RB: Systemic lupus erythematosus. Management during pregnancy. *Obstet Gynecol* 51:178, 1978.

———: Systemic lupus erythematosus and pregnancy. *Clin Rheum Dis* 1:613, 1975.

32

Genetic Counseling

ALBERT B. GERBIE   MORRIS B. FIDDLER   HENRY L. NADLER

EVALUATION OF THE GENETICS PATIENT
Diagnosis
Initial assessment of the genetics patient
Content of the genetic counseling session
Follow-up to genetic counseling

PRENATAL DIAGNOSIS OF GENETIC DEFECTS
Amniocentesis and amniotic fluid analysis
Fetal visualization
Indications for intrauterine diagnostic studies

PREVENTION AND TREATMENT OF CONGENITAL DEFECTS

SOME LEGAL AND ETHICAL DIMENSIONS OF GENETIC COUNSELING

SUMMARY

Advances in the identification and understanding of hereditary disease processes have provided the foundation for improved management of affected patients. These advances have made it possible to provide information to individuals and their families on the prognosis and risks of recurrence of genetic disorders. These areas have become the domain of genetic counseling. Professionals who provide input to the delivery of genetic counseling include physicians, geneticists, biochemists, and cytologists. Obstetricians, as members of this group, have an important role in case finding, diagnosis, follow-up, and management. Because of their intimate role with families, obstetricians should be prepared to provide genetic information and the family counseling which often accompanies it; these responsibilities may be performed directly by the informed obstetrician or indirectly through referral to one of an increasing number of genetic centers.

Genetic counseling is generally defined as the delivery of information regarding the risk(s) of occurence or recurrence of a genetic disease or trait. Genetic counseling may be categorized as retrospective or prospective. Most people seeking counseling fall into the retrospective group. They already have a child or a relative with a genetic disease; they wish to know the risk of recurrence and, in many cases, want more information about the disorder than a physician in general practice has been able to provide. Prospective counseling, on the other hand, attempts to deliver information to individuals who, by virtue of their family or ethnic background, exposure to certain drugs or chemicals, or their age, may be at risk for having a child with a genetically determined condition, although it has not shown up in prior generations. Large-scale screening programs for heterozygotes of Tay-Sachs disease, sickle-cell anemia, or chromosome abnormalities are examples of prospective genetic counseling methods.

EVALUATION OF THE GENETICS PATIENT

Although genetic counseling is by no means practiced in a uniform manner, guidelines and procedures are evolving as this aspect of health care delivery becomes more common. The indications for a genetic analysis of an individual include: (1) presence of familial congenital abnormalities, developmental delay, or mental retardation; (2) a familial history of an inborn error of metabolism; (3) congenital anomalies consistent with an abnormal chromosome constitution; (4) a history of two or more early miscarriages; (5) a history of exposure to environmental agents which can cause chromosome damage (eg., drugs, x-rays, infections); (6) an identifiable genetic syndrome; and (7) infertility or intersex problems.

The workup of a genetic case may be conveniently divided into four parts (1) diagnosis; (2) initial assessment; (3) the counseling itself; and (4) follow-up.

DIAGNOSIS

Accurate diagnosis is the foundation of good genetic counseling. The information which leads to an accurate diagnosis can come from a medical history, a complete physical examination, special laboratory tests (e.g., of chromosomes, enzymes, metabolites, results of x-ray examinations) and, frequently, from autopsy reports, or even from photographs of presumably affected individuals. It is important to realize that genetic disorders can be mimicked by the effect of environmental factors. The latter situation, known as a phenocopy, is not an inheritable one and may be difficult to distinguish from true genetic causation. An examination of the family history and a review of literature reports are the usual ways to make the distinction. Mental deficiency, growth disorders, and cardiac anomalies raise the question of phenocopy versus genetic phenotype.

In addition to discerning possible phenocopies, the diagnostic workup must take into account various kinds of heterogeneity among genetic disorders. Heterogeneity in the clinical course, in biochemical abnormalities, or in patterns of inheritance of genetic diseases may confuse the diagnosis, and information should be obtained which can sort out these complexities. For example, Hurler and Hunter syndromes are both mucopolysaccharidoses which present in clinically similar fashion. However, Hurler syndrome is inherited as an autosomal recessive condition while Hunter syndrome is usually X-linked; thus a family history and detailed physical examination may help to distinguish the two. Individuals with Hurler syndrome tend to develop corneal opacities and severe skeletal dysplasias; those with the Hunter syndrome do not have corneal clouding and their skeletal problems tend to be less severe. Furthermore, the enzyme deficiencies in these clinically similar disorders are significantly different and can be determined by appropriate laboratory studies.

Finally, the need for a complete diagnostic workup may be underscored when the physician attempts to determine whether a patient has an isolated congenital defect or a syndrome in which that defect is only one feature. Cleft lip/cleft palate (CL/CP) usually occurs by itself, but it may also occur in conjunction with other anomalies. Some of these anomalies have a subtle presentation but exist as syndromes with a mendelian mode of inheritance, or they may result from a chromosomal aberration. The isolated CL/CP, however, is generally a multifactorial situation. The implications for counseling and management may be very different, depending on the complete diagnosis.

INITIAL ASSESSMENT OF THE GENETICS PATIENT

The first step after the physical examination and diagnostic workup is the recording of a family physiologic pedigree. Although this information may help establish a diagnosis, it has additional importance in the calculation of risk figures, identification of other family members who may benefit from genetic counseling, and establishment of an inheritance mode where ambiguities exist. Although it is helpful to include information on three generations, it is usually not possible to get documentation on more than two. Standard questions in a genetic interview should elicit information about the age, sex, ethnic background, state of health, miscarriages, fetal deaths, and consanguinity from the patient and spouse and their first- and second-degree relatives. Some genetic conditions, particularly those inherited as dominant traits, will show varying degrees of severity or heterogeneity in their clinical expression; this phenomenon is referred to as *variable expressivity*. Minor or subtle manifestations of a disorder of family members should be probed for both during their physical examination and in questioning while compiling a pedigree. A similar situation regarding subtle or preclinical symptoms arises when dealing with disorders that show an age dependence in their development of manifestations (e.g., Huntington's disease).

Once a pedigree has been established, the calculation of risk figures for occurrence or recurrence of the condition in a family can be made; in addition, those individuals who should be tested for heterozygote status can be identified. As shown in Chapter 6, genetic disorders may be transmitted as single-gene defects (autosomal or X-linked dominant, autosomal or X-linked recessive) or multiple-gene loci (polygenic). In addition, they may arise from chromosomal aberrations. The risk of recurrence of the single-gene defects follows mendelian laws. If a couple has given birth to a child with an autosomal recessive disorder, each subsequent child has a 25 percent chance of also having the disorder. If the disorder is an autosomal dominant, each subsequent child has a 50 percent chance of being similarly affected if one of the parents exhibits the condition. A careful physical examination of the parents (or grandparents) may reveal the presence of the dominant gene and support the calculation of a 50 percent risk to future children. If no manifestations can be detected either in the parents or in at-risk relatives (sibs, grandparents), then the possibility of a new mutation should be considered. The presence of a new mutation in a child would not place subsequent children at a higher risk than the general population for having the disorder. For example, Apert's syndrome (a combination of craniosynostosis, midface hypoplasia, syndactyly, and broad distal phalanx of thumb and big toe) is often the result of a fresh mutation; thus unaffected parents have a negligible risk of having another child with this syndrome, but the offspring of the affected individual have a 50 percent chance of also having Apert's syndrome.

X-linked recessive disorders may pose special problems in determining the risk figures. In some cases, female heterozygotes may be detected by biochemical or clinical examinations; if this is possible, each son of a heterozygous female has a 50 percent chance of inheriting the gene and being affected, but daughters have only a 50 percent probability of becoming *carriers* of the gene, and are not affected. Some heterozygous females may exhibit symptoms of the disorder because of X-chromosome inactivation, or Lyonization (Chapter 6), and this becomes a consideration in explaining the risks during the counseling session. It is not possible to predict the proportion of X chromosomes bearing the mutant allele that will not be inactivated. Lyonization is a random process and follows a normal distribution curve. Thus, heterozygous mothers should be told that although their daughters have a 50 percent chance of also being heterozygotes, the daughters may show signs of being affected by the disorder in question if a significant majority of X chromosomes bearing the mutant allele remain active. This phenomenon appears to have been seen in X-linked hemophilia and Fabry's disease (a lipid storage disorder).

If an X-linked trait cannot be detected in the female carrier, however, the estimation of a risk figure may be complicated. Figure 32-1 illustrates a pedigree for an X-linked trait which is not detectable in heterozygous females. The risk that the consultor (i.e., the person seeking genetic counseling) will have an affected son would appear to be 1 in 4. The fact that she already has one normal son, however, contributes information to this calculation and alters the probability to 1 in 6. This kind of calculation integrates both the possibility that she is a carrier and has one normal son and the possibility that she is not a carrier and has a normal son in determining the risk to future sons. Although even larger differences in apparent versus actual risk figures can be illustrated with more complex pedigrees, the point of this example is that this much information from the pedigree should be utilized in analyzing risk figures. Of course, had the consultor's son been affected, the risk to each future son would have been 50 percent.

The determination that a defect or disorder is the result of a multifactorial process usually means the genetic counselor will have to rely on empirical data in estimating a risk figure. In the absence of adequate

FIGURE 32-1 Pedigree for an X-linked trait not detectable in heterozygous females.

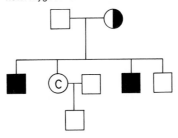

predictive models to explain the mechanisms of polygenic inheritance, the use of data from family and population studies is the only recourse. Some caution should be exercised in the use of such data. Although the risk that a mother at age 25 to 29 with no previous children will have a child with anencephaly is approximately 1 in 400, this figure can be significantly different for women of other age groups, of other parity, and, for unknown reasons, of specific social classes. Parents of the "lowest" social class have been reported to have a 1 in 259 chance of having an anencephalic child whereas those of the "highest" social class have an approximately 1 in 9100 risk. Some question has been raised, however, about the validity of these figures.

As a rule of thumb, the risk of recurrence of a multifactorial disorder if one child is already affected is the square root of the frequency of the disorder or defect in the general population (determined from large population studies). This number usually turns out to be 2 to 4 percent; the results of empiric studies on various congenital heart defects have demonstrated a good correlation between the observed risk and that predicted by the above calculation. Again, however, attention must be paid to the specifics of the sample from which the empiric figure is derived. For example, as the number of affected sibs increases, the recurrence risk also increases, generally increasing to 6 to 10 percent (for two affected sibs) or 12 to 15 percent (three affected sibs). Sex differences in recurrence risks may also be found, as for CL/CP (male/female ratio is approximately 1.7:1 for Caucasians) or pyloric stenosis (approximately 4:1).

Although reports may indicate that a condition is multifactorial, it might present as a single-locus entity in some families and this possibility should be considered, particularly in families with more than one affected individual. Hydrocephalus, for example, may be inherited as a multifactorial defect or an X-linked recessive disorder.

The assessment of risk figures for chromosomal abnormalities depends on the nature of the aberration. Most chromosomal abnormalities are the results of meiotic nondisjunction or some other error during cell division which results in a congenital disorder which is not hereditary. The recurrence risk, however, is considered to be slightly higher than the frequency of aneuploid births in the general population. While the frequency of trisomy 21 Down's syndrome is approximately 1 in 600 births, the risk of recurrence to a couple who both have normal karyotypes and who already have had a child with Down's syndrome is ap-

proximately 1 in 100. This figure may also be altered by the data which demonstrate an increase in all chromosomal abnormalities, particularly for Down's syndrome, with increasing maternal age, especially after age 35.

When the chromosomal abnormality is a translocation and one of the parents is a balanced translocation carrier, the theoretical risk of having a child with an abnormal chromosome constitution is 33 percent. Again, however, empiric data have been collected which provide the actuarial risk figures. If the mother, for example, is a carrier of a D/G translocation, the risk of having a child with Down's syndrome is 11 percent; if the father carries the translocation, the risk is 2 to 3 percent. The reasons for these differences are unknown.

In addition to the analysis of the family pedigree and the determination of risk figures, the initial assessment phase of genetic counseling should include two other features: (1) an evaluation of the psychosocial status of the consultor(s); and (2) an identification of the specific questions and concerns which the consultor would like answered or discussed.

The former consideration will affect the depth of information which should be presented during the counseling session, the areas of inquiry which the counselor may pursue regarding reproductive alternatives, care, and management of an affected individual, and the emotional reactions which may be anticipated to the content of the counseling session. The second point, the identification of specific concerns, will affect the content of the session, allowing the counselor to research the answers, if necessary, and ensuring that the consultor has the opportunity to discuss even the most tangential issues. Often the counselor will need to raise questions and issues beyond those presented by the consultor, but it is important that the genetic counselor spend time with the issues which appear most pressing during the initial assessment.

CONTENT OF THE GENETIC COUNSELING SESSION

The genetic counseling procedure itself first offers a clear explanation of genetics to the parents (or other consultors) and a presentation of occurrence or recurrence risk figures. The risk figures must be presented so that they can be clearly understood. Some people readily grasp the concept of an independent probability for each pregnancy; others may benefit from illustrative examples of chance situations such as dice or card games. The assessment of the consultor's educational and/or intellectual level during the initial assessment should indicate the level at which the counseling can be initiated. Although several frames of reference will probably be used to explain probability odds, the actual presentation of the risk may color both understanding of and reaction to the figure. Instead of presenting a 5 percent recurrence risk of a central nervous system anomaly, one can just as honestly give a 95 percent probability that a child will not have the anomaly. It often takes considerable time to adequately explain the risk figures and help the patient see that the risk of a child being born with a birth defect is approximately 5 percent.

In addition to presenting risk figures and clarifying their meaning, often through an explanation of the genetic principles from which those figures are derived, the counseling session may identify sibs or other relatives of the consultor who are at risk of being affected or having a child with the condition. Although it is not the province of the genetic counselor to contact these individuals, the importance of passing on the genetic information to relatives may be stressed so that potential at-risk individuals may seek genetic counseling themselves.

If the consultors are being seen for a diagnostic workup on themselves or child, the prognosis and future course of the disease which has been identified should be discussed. Classification of a group of symptoms or anomalies into a syndrome may not result in the identification of a course of therapeutic action, but it will often provide a basis for describing the natural history which can be expected as the individual ages. Issues such as mental retardation, deterioration processes, medical complications, etc., should be dealt with openly and honestly. Suggestions for referrals to special social or paramedical services should be made when appropriate. The impact which the diagnosis of genetic disease can make on the family may be considerable. A spectrum of reactions can be anticipated including anger, fear, denial, shame, blame, and guilt. The latter may be particularly true for X-linked disorders in which the mother of an affected child is a carrier of the gene. Although extensive psychological counseling is not possible during genetic counseling nor appropriate for an untrained counselor, these issues and feelings can be raised and discussed as an integral part of genetic counseling. It should be explained that these reactions are natural and the suggestion may be made that the consultor(s) seek help from a family counselor, clergyman, groups composed of parents in similar situations, or the family physician to deal with these critical issues. The consultor(s) should be encouraged to ask any open-ended questions, and answers should be honestly provided by the counselor.

Finally, it may be helpful to the patients to introduce the subject of reproductive options, including birth control and prenatal diagnosis. The latter will be discussed more thoroughly later in this chapter.

Once the relevant facts have been presented, the ultimate decision regarding the use of genetic information rests with the family. Very frequently, couples will ask the obstetrician/genetic counselor for recommendations or the course of action which the counselor would take. It is important to remain objective and emphasize that the decision-making responsibility rests with the consultor, particularly when it comes to reproductive options. The experiences of the genetic counselor regarding relative risk and consequences of a disease will almost unavoidably color the presentation of genetic information; however, the role of the counselor should remain one of providing as much information as possible, not directly participating in the decisions which will be made on that information.

Finally, it is most effective to close a genetic counseling session with a review of what has been discussed, either through repetition by the counselor or through having the patients feed back the information to the counselor. A brief written summary with diagrams may be helpful for the consultor to take home.

FOLLOW-UP TO GENETIC COUNSELING

Following the actual genetic counseling, a letter summarizing the information which was discussed should be sent both to the consultor and the physician who made the referral. This letter should restate the risk figures and their derivation, the prognosis if necessary, information regarding future prenatal diagnosis, and any other specific recommendations for care and management of the affected individual(s). Other follow-up material may include referral suggestions, pertinent literature, or a request to see the patients again at some future date. The followup letter acts as a record of the genetic counseling session and as a source of information for the parents to draw upon when their recollection of the details of the genetic information fades.

PRENATAL DIAGNOSIS OF GENETIC DEFECTS

AMNIOCENTESIS AND AMNIOTIC FLUID ANALYSIS

The prenatal detection of genetic disorders is probably the most important adjunct to genetic counseling today. Several technological advances have emerged which, in conjunction with tissue culture and cytogenetic and biochemical methodologies, make the intrauterine diagnosis of over 130 metabolic and virtually all chromosomal defects possible. They further demonstrate the feasibility of adding many other congenital anomalies to this list in the near future.

The primary tool used in prenatal diagnosis is transabdominal amniocentesis. This procedure provides ready access to fetal cells and metabolites in amniotic fluid. The procedure appears to be very reliable and relatively safe in the hands of an experienced obstetrician. Although the risks of amniocentesis performed after the 20th week of gestation have been documented, the risks of the procedure during the second trimester are only beginning to emerge. Potentially, these risks include maternal bleeding, infection, blood group sensitization secondary to disruption of the fetomaternal circulation, spontaneous abortion, and puncture or induced malformations of the fetus. Various studies have estimated the extent of fetal loss related to amniocentesis, and it now appears that this risk is not significantly different from fetal loss in all mid-trimester pregnancies. The patient should be informed of the potential complications and that a repeat amniocentesis may be needed because of failure to obtain fluid or to cultivate an adequate number of cells for analysis. The total frequency of these problems is approximately 2 percent while the total reliability of obtaining a diagnosis following an amniocentesis, including repeated taps, is 97 to 98 percent.

Amniocentesis should be performed between the 14th and 16th week of gestation. Most frequently, the procedure is preceded by an ultrasonic localization of the placenta; ultrasound is also used to determine

gestational age and the presence of twins, a complicating factor in making a prenatal diagnosis. Methods to circumvent the diagnostic problem of twins have been suggested, including the injection of a water-soluble dye into one amniotic sac followed by an attempt to obtain clear fluid from the other. The amniocentesis itself is performed under strict aseptic conditions using a 22-gauge, $3\frac{1}{2}$-inch spinal needle. This is inserted through the abdominal wall in the midline, directed at the correct angle toward the middle of the uterine cavity. After puncture, the stylet is removed and a sterile plastic syringe is used to withdraw 10 to 25 mL of amniotic fluid, after which the needle is swiftly withdrawn. Fetal heart tones should be determined by a Doppler apparatus before and after this procedure. The patient may feel some cramps after the procedure and any discomfort, fluid loss, bleeding, or fever should be evaluated for complications resulting from the amniotic tap.

Amniotic fluid offers three possible sources for diagnostic analysis: the fluid itself, amniotic fluid cells, and cultivated amniotic fluid cells. The amniotic fluid, separated from the suspended cells by centrifugation, may be analyzed for amino acids, hormones, metabolites, and enzymes. The analysis of enzymes or enzymic activities, however, may be complicated because of the current lack of knowledge regarding their origin; studies have shown that some enzymes in cell-free amniotic fluid may be of both fetal and maternal origin.

Uncultivated amniotic fluid cells offer a second, direct source for prenatal diagnosis. These cells originate primarily from the amnion or from desquamation of fetal skin, buccal mucosa, vaginal epithelium, umbilical cord, and fetal urine. These cells may be examined for Y-chromosome fluorescence to detect fetuses at risk for X-linked disorders. The cells may also be analyzed histochemically to detect accumulating substrates associated particularly with lysosomal storage diseases. Some attempts have also been made to utilize the uncultivated cells for enzyme determinations; however, the presence of many nonviable cells makes this a highly questionable approach to the detection of inborn errors of metabolism.

The most important material for analysis is cultivated amniotic fluid cells. The use of amniotic fluid in this manner requires extensive experience in tissue culture techniques. Once cultivated, amniotic fluid cells may be used for cytogenetic studies in the antenatal diagnosis of chromosome abnormalities and for biochemical studies in the diagnosis of metabolic defects. It is important to realize, however, that the growing of cells in culture may alter some biochemical properties as a function of growth medium, duration of cultivation, extent of confluency, and gestational age; therefore, conditions for using cultivated amniotic fluid cells should be standardized in order to obtain reliable results. In general, it takes approximately 3 to 4 weeks to obtain a sufficient number of cells to perform diagnostic tests, although more rapid diagnoses on a limited number of cells have been attempted. Most of the disorders are rare, with frequencies less than 1 in 20,000 live births; however, taken as a group of detectable, (infantile) lethal disorders, the impact of prenatal diagnosis can be appreciated, particularly because the list in Table 32–1 will certainly continue to grow rapidly in the next decade.

Theoretically, it is possible to diagnose prenatally any metabolic defect for which there is a reliable enzyme assay or system which will detect the abnormal accumulation of a metabolite. The normal enzymic activity or metabolic pathway must be demonstrable in cultured amniotic cells from normal individuals. Table 32–1 lists some of the metabolic disorders which either can be or have been prenatally diagnosed. The majority of these rely on enzyme determinations for the diagnosis, although in some instances characterization of abnormal levels of substrates has provided supportive information. In at least one case, cystinosis, in which the primary lesion is not understood, accumulation of radioactive L-cystine provided the basis for determining the presence of an affected fetus. In all cases, confirmatory studies

on the aborted fetus should be carried out; this was done in most of the prenatally diagnosed disorders listed in the table.

In addition to cytogenetic and biochemical analyses of amniotic fluid components for direct evidence of an inherited congenital defect, recent work has provided the capacity to diagnose neural tube defects. This diagnosis relies on the measurement of α-fetoprotein in amniotic fluid. This protein is synthesized in early fetal development by normal embryonic liver, yolk sac, and the fetal gastrointestinal tract, and has been recognized to be a fetal specific α-globulin although its function is unknown. It is now well documented that significant elevations of α-fetoprotein levels in second-trimester amniotic fluid are highly correlated with the presence of a severe "open" neural tube defect. "Closed" or small open neural tube defects are not marked by elevated levels of this protein in the amniotic fluid. The significant lesions can be detected currently with 90 to 95 percent accuracy, and many centers are including this determination as a routine part of their analyses of amniotic fluid obtained by amniocentesis.

The diagnosis of neural tube lesions by α-fetoprotein determination is not, however, without other limitations. Increased levels of this protein have also been reported in patients with congenital nephrosis, intrauterine fetal death, severe Rh isoimmunization, congenital esophageal atresia, omphalocele, and hydrocephalus. These other associations should be clarified to couples receiving genetic counseling for

TABLE 32–1 Some Inborn Errors of Metabolism Which Can Be Diagnosed Prenatally

Amino acid and organic acid disorders	GM$_1$ gangliosidoses
Arginosuccinicaciduria	GM$_2$ gangliosidoses
Branched-chain ketoacidosis	Krabbe's disease
Citrullinemia	Metachromatic
Cystinuria	leukodystrophy
Cystinosis	Niemann-Pick disease
Methylmalonic aciduria	Wolman's disease
Other storage disorders	Others
Fucosidosis	Acid phosphatase
Glycogenoses types II, III, IV	deficiency
Mannosidosis	Adenosine deaminase
Mucopolysaccharidoses types I, IIA,	deficiency
III, VIA	Hypercholesterolemia type II
Mucolipidosis type II	Hypophosphatasia
Lipid storage disorders	Lesch-Nyhan syndrome
Fabry's disease	Thalassemia
Gaucher's disease	Xeroderma pigmentosum

prenatal diagnostic studies, although in many instances the information will not affect their decision regarding termination of pregnancy.

Recent data also suggest that open neural tube defects may be associated with elevated maternal serum α-fetoprotein levels early in pregnancy, particularly during the 13th to the 21st week of gestation. Although the reliability of this association is at present only 65 percent, its observation may provide the basis for mass screening of all pregnant women to identify a majority of those carrying a fetus with such an anomaly.

FETAL VISUALIZATION

Although amniocentesis, with subsequent cultivation and analysis of the amniotic fluid cells, is the most prevalent tool for prenatal diagnosis, significant developments have been made in techniques for visualization of the fetus. These techniques are most applicable to disorders with anatomic (e.g., skeletal and central nervous system) malformations. Four methods have been used to detect congenital defects by visualization: roentgenography, fetography (or amniography), ultrasonic scanning, and fetoscopy.

X-ray examination of the fetus has made possible the antenatal diagnosis of several malformations including anencephaly, hydrocephalus, microcephaly, encephalocele, myelomeningocele, achondroplasia, osteogenesis imperfecta congenita, ectromelia, symelia, and bilateral cleft palate. However, in most cases the accurate diagnosis of these defects can be made only in the last trimester. Roentgenograms can also diagnose the thrombocytopenia which includes absent triradii syndrome because of the associated phocomelia, Fanconi's anemia, Holt-Oram syndrome, and other malformation syndromes. The drawbacks here are the danger of radiation exposure to the fetus (probably small) and the inability to exclude a diagnosis if the x-rays are normal (probably large).

Amniography is an extension of the classic radiographic approach. In this procedure, the amniotic fluid is made opaque with a contrast medium injected during an amniocentesis. The amniotic fluid is then either displaced by fetal soft tissue abnormalities (e.g., myelomeningocele, extrophy of the bladder) or swallowed by the fetus resulting in an outline of the gastrointestinal tract. This permits the diagnosis of esophageal atresia, tracheoesophageal fistula, diaphragmatic hernia, or atresia of the GI tract.

Amniography can also indicate fetal distress or death.

Fetography differs from amniography in that an oil-soluble medium instead of a water-soluble contrast medium is used. This technique has advantages over amniography because the oil-soluble medium has an affinity for the vernix caseosa and limited diffusion into the amniotic fluid. These features permit a better outline of the fetus. Since the use of fetography is governed by the presence of the vernix caseosa, the optimal time for the procedure is 28 to 38 weeks, a distinct drawback to its more widespread application. Fetography has, however, been shown to demonstrate fetal neck tumors, anencephaly, the Pierre Robin anomaly, lymphangioma, meningocele, and sacral teratomas. Fetography has also been used to successfully diagnose trisomy of an E-group chromosome based on the characteristic hand malformation. It is possible that this procedure may be applicable to intrauterine diagnosis at an earlier stage of pregnancy.

Ultrasonic scanning is a probably highly safe procedure that has been used for many years to localize the placenta during the third trimester of pregnancy. The conversion of electrical energy to sound waves which can be reflected by tissues and reconverted to electrical energy permits the visual projection of an anatomic cross section of examined tissues. Ultrasonography has permitted the prenatal detection of anencephaly and polycystic kidneys in the last trimester and anencephaly during the second trimester. This technique, in conjunction with amniography, has also been used for the intrauterine detection of duodenal atresia. The use of ultrasound should continue to be of increasing value in the prenatal diagnosis of malformations, particularly neural lesions.

Probably the most exciting advancement in intrauterine visualization is fetoscopy. A series of developments in optics, particularly fiberoptics, has made the direct visualization of the fetus a feasible technique for the prenatal detection of congenital anomalies. In addition to visualization, which is currently limited by the small visual field and by difficulty in orientation following insertion of the fiberoptic, fetoscopy is providing a means to draw fetal blood samples from placental veins. These samples, together with sensitive techniques to analyze various types of hemoglobins, have provided the material to detect prenatally a variety of hemoglobinopathies, including sickle-cell anemia, the thalassemias (see Chap. 25), and muscular dystrophy. Furthermore, small skin biopsies may be obtained for cultivation and analysis. Because these procedures have the potential to cause hemorrhage or otherwise put both mother and fetus at risk for induced tissue damage, they should still be considered highly experimental techniques. Their promise for future contributions to intrauterine diagnosis, however, is considerable.

INDICATIONS FOR INTRAUTERINE DIAGNOSTIC STUDIES

The indications for prenatal diagnosis are continually changing. Today they include maternal age (> 35 years old), a previous child with a chromosomal abnormality or inborn error of metabolism, the determination that both parents are heterozygotes for an enzyme deficiency, a previous child or a parent with a neural tube malformation, or a child at risk for X-linked recessive disorder. The proportion of prenatal cytogenetic studies will probably decrease as methods to detect biochemical disorders, such as the hemoglobinopathies, continue to develop.

Education, lay articles, and mass screening programs for various disorders will increase the number of people seeking prenatal studies. As was previously stated for genetic counseling in general, data obtained from antenatal analyses and transmitted to consultors should not be contingent upon any prior commitment to abortion if a congenital defect is detected. Intrauterine diagnosis is an available procedure for providing information which couples (or individuals) can draw on in considering reproductive options.

PREVENTION AND TREATMENT OF CONGENITAL DEFECTS

Health care delivery is optimal when it can be preventive. For the most part, genetic counseling and individual choice regarding reproductive options are the only approaches available to control the effects and frequency of genetic diseases. Increased public education, the capacity to diagnose chromosomal abnormalities and an increasing number of metabolic and other congenital anomalies prenatally and screening programs which focus on groups of individuals at high risk for genetic disorders represent genetic contributions to preventive medicine. The

number of individuals and couples at risk for having children with genetic diseases or congenital malformations who will be seeking genetic counseling, both prospectively and retrospectively, will probably increase dramatically in the coming years through the dissemination of both technological and educational information. Screening programs such as we now have for Tay-Sachs disease (for the Jewish population) and sickle-cell anemia (for the black population) will probably serve as models for the detection of other conditions, for instance, the hyperlipidemias and cystic fibrosis. Neonatal screening programs, often mandated through state legislation, can be expected to continue for the purpose of early therapeutic intervention. These programs will have increasing impact on the demand for counseling services.

More recent efforts to cope with genetic diseases and to expand the benefits of genetic counseling have been directed at various forms of therapeutic intervention. The understanding of genetic mechanisms has provided the framework for several different strategies to treat inherited disorders. The ideal "cure" for a genetic disease is direct gene replacement; this is not yet a feasible approach, although the technology which may lead to its accomplishment is beginning to develop. Prophylaxis of the manifestations of metabolic disease, however, may now be accomplished, particularly following early diagnosis. Dietary restriction of substrates, cofactor supplementation (particularly vitamins), and metabolite replacement have proved successful in treating some inborn errors of metabolism. Phenylalanine restriction in phenylketonuria, vitamin B_{12} administration to restore normal enzymic activity in some forms of methylmalonic aciduria, and steroid replacement in the adrenogenital syndrome exemplify these strategies. The restoration of normal methylmalonic acid metabolism has even been accomplished prenatally by administration of B_{12} to a mother carrying an affected fetus. Enzyme-replacement therapy is being evaluated as treatment of some storage diseases and may prove effective in the future. In addition to therapeutic approaches at the biochemical level, surgical techniques have provided satisfying lives to many individuals with malformations such as congenital cataracts, congenital dislocation of the hip(s), many congenital heart defects, facial clefts, tracheoesophageal fistulas, and pyloric stenosis. The number of genetic disorders being treated by a variety of approaches is increasing, and continual survey of reviews and recent articles is a part of the genetic counselor's responsibility.

SOME LEGAL AND ETHICAL DIMENSIONS OF GENETIC COUNSELING

Although genetic counseling as the vehicle for delivering information in a nondirective manner about the risks and consequences of birth defects would appear to be a relatively straightforward process, given sufficient knowledge and experience of the genetic counselor, a number of legal and ethical questions are arising, both from the experiences of practitioners and from theoretical legal considerations. Many of these issues are complex and cannot be dealt with in sufficient detail here; however, several examples should illustrate points of importance to genetic counselors.

Confidentiality of information transmitted during genetic counseling should be maintained as in any other professional-client relationship. The application of this principle, however, may not always be clearcut. In counseling a family with an X-linked or a dominant disorder (particularly one with variable expressivity), relatives of the consultor may be identified who are also at-risk as carrier or affected individuals. The consultor, for a variety of reasons, may not wish to contact these individuals so that they may seek an appropriate workup. The counselor is restricted from contacting these people in deference to the right of privacy of the initial consultor. The question may be asked, however, whether the counselor by not transmitting the information to the relatives is being negligent, particularly since the relatives' health or the health of the relatives' children may be placed in unnecessary jeopardy.

The problem of the right of privacy may also be raised when a counselor discovers, through heterozygote testing, for example, that the father of a child affected with a recessive disorder is not really the husband of the woman being counseled, but the husband is unaware of the wife's extramarital liaison. To ignore the situation results in providing a recurrence risk significantly higher than exists; to confront the issue may invade the privacy of the wife and lead to marital difficulties for which few counselors would like to take responsibility. This kind of situation may be further aggravated if the couple requests amniocentesis, and the risks of the prenatal procedure are greater than the risks of having an affected child.

Another general area of difficulty comes from the problem of informed consent. This topic has raised much controversy in all areas of medical care; considering the complexity of genetic information, what constitutes sufficient evidence that an individual or couple satisfactorily comprehends relative risks and prognosis? The decisions which consultors make as a result of genetic counseling often concern abortion, long-term reproductive behavior, and marital compatibility. The counselor's role is particularly complicated when counsel is being given to individuals with mild mental retardation who have difficulty in dealing with abstract concepts such as probabilities, genes, or even the implications of child-bearing.

Mass screening programs for genetic diseases, both pre- and postnatally, have undergone a series of criticisms and revisions in the last decade. Several issues regarding their implementation have been raised, particularly for the mandatory programs. These have been reviewed in detail (Milunsky and Annas) because of legislative excesses in some states where testing of all black individuals for sickle-cell-anemia carrier status, even at elementary school age in some instances, has been mandated. At the present time, the recommendation is to ensure voluntary participation and informed consent of prospective parents or neonates. Those programs which are provided for by state legislation should retain provisions to ensure voluntary participation, with parents acting as agents in the case of neonatal screening.

It is also becoming increasingly clear, however, that physicians, particularly obstetricians, have an obligation to inform patients that they are at risk for having a child with a genetic disorder by virtue of age, ethnic background, or medical history. The physician also has an obligation to provide information regarding the availability of screening programs or testing options. It is probable that the courts will continue to extend physicians' responsibilities as a result of malpractice suits and decisions regarding the role of genetic counseling in the delivery of good health care.

SUMMARY

A well-trained obstetrician can participate in genetic counseling if he or she will follow these basic guidelines: (1) make an accurate diagnosis, utilizing a complete family history, laboratory procedures where applicable, and referral services; (2) understand the principles of genetics and realize where complexities in their application and interpretation apply; (3) transmit the proper risk figures in a manner which the consultor(s) will understand, and confirm their understanding by appropriate questions or supplementary written materials; (4) know the indications and limitations of antenatal diagnosis; (5) be aware of the psychosocial impact which genetic counseling may have on a family, particularly regarding the effects of a diagnosed disease and the responsibilities they may feel for its occurrence; and (6) refer to a genetics specialist or center those patients who require counseling when appropriate facilities (e.g., cytogenetic, biochemical, consultative services) are not available. Genetic counseling takes time.

In the past few years, techniques have been developing to successfully detect heterozygotes and to diagnose over 130 inborn errors of metabolism as well as virtually all chromosomal aberrations prenatally. These capabilities will continue to grow as will methods to detect abnormalities of morphogenesis prenatally and to treat genetic disorders antenatally. The approaches for diagnosis and treatment of genetic diseases appear to be limited only by the ingenuity of the scientist.

REFERENCES

Bergsma, D (ed.): *Birth Defects: Atlas and Compendium,* Baltimore: Williams and Wilkins, 1973.

deGrouchy, J, Turleau, C: *Clinical Atlas of Human Chromosomes,* New York: John Wiley, 1977.

Gerbie, A. B. (ed.) *Amniocentesis. Clinics in Obstetrics and Gynecology,* London, Saunders, April, 1980.

Gorlin, RJ et al.: *Syndromes of the Head and Neck,* 2d ed., New York: McGraw-Hill, 1976.

McKusick, VA: *Mendelian Inheritance in Man. Catalogs of Autosomal Dominant, Autosomal Recessive, and X-linked Phenotypes,* 4th ed., Baltimore: Johns Hopkins University Press, 1975.

Milunsky, A: *The Prevention of Genetic Disease and Mental Retardation,* Philadelphia: Saunders, 1975.

Milunsky, A, Annas, GJ (eds.): *Genetics and the Law,* New York: Plenum Press, 1976.

Murphy, EA, Chase, GA: *Principles of Genetic Counseling,* Chicago: Year Book Med Pub, 1975.

Nadler, HL: Prenatal detection of genetic defects. *Adv Pediatr* 22:1, 1976.

Smith, DW: *Recognizable Patterns of Human Malformation. Genetic, Embryologic, and Clinical Aspects,* 2d ed., Philadelphia: Saunders, 1976.

Stanbury, JB, et al. (eds.): *The Metabolic Basis of Inherited Disease,* New York: McGraw-Hill., 1978.

Yunis, JJ (ed.): *New Chromosomal Syndromes,* New York: Academic Press, 1977.

33

Birth Control, Abortion, and Sterilization

MARY JANE GRAY   DAVID A. GRIMES

BIRTH CONTROL

From very early times a variety of customs and practices ranging from continence and late marriage to abortion and infanticide have been employed to limit population growth and prevent births. General demographic considerations are covered in Chap. 3, while the measures used by individuals for birth control are presented here. These can be divided into contraceptives, i.e., methods and devices which prevent conception, postcoital measures which prevent implantation (sometimes referred to as *interception*), abortion, which is the disruption of the already implanted embryo, and sterilization.

Of the old methods, coitus interruptus made the woman dependent upon the control of her partner, breast-feeding made her dependent on the steady presence of a nursing child, and abortion in the preantiseptic era endangered her life. More recently, the diaphragm and condom have been associated with a 3 to 15 percent risk of pregnancy. Only with the advent of the oral contraceptive pill has the woman been able to separate sex completely from reproduction if she so desires. This ability, together with new methods of abortion and new laws permitting their use, has led to a gradual change in the way men and women regard sex, and also to a falling birthrate despite an increasing incidence of premarital and extramarital coitus. Because recommendations regarding the contraceptive use of hormones and intrauterine devices (IUDs) change so rapidly, the book *Contraceptive Technology,* revised annually by Hatcher et al., is suggested for those who wish to keep up to the minute in this area.

The advantages and disadvantages of the various techniques of birth control are considered in this chapter along with those social and psychologic factors which limit their use.

GENERAL CONSIDERATIONS

MOTIVATION

Motivation for contraception and abortion varies from the individual's concern for the direction of his or her own life to a concern for world problems. Family planning clinics estimate the cost of providing contraceptive services at $100 per patient per year, which is low when compared with the overt and hidden cost of unwanted children. Current estimates place the direct and indirect costs of rearing a child in the United States at more than $100,000. Children born to women who have been refused abortion show an increased incidence of academic, emotional, and social problems.

Beyond individual and social indications for contraception are public health figures clearly relating maternal and infant morbidity and mortality to maternal age, parity, and birth interval (Perkins). The risk of maternal death is increased in the teenager, minimal

between 20 and 24, and progressively rises to four to five times the minimum rate beyond the age of 40. Maternal risk increases with parity, independent of age, after the third pregnancy. The risks of prematurity, infant death, and congenital defects roughly parallel the maternal mortality rate in these groups. Birth intervals of less than 12 months are associated with a prematurity rate that is double the average. The lowest fetal mortality rates are correlated with birth intervals of 3 to 4 years. An increased risk of death for the offspring of women having closely spaced pregnancies continues throughout childhood (Day).

Although 98 percent of young couples report the use of contraception at some time during their marriage (Westoff and Jones, 1977a), it is known that far fewer succeed in having only wanted pregnancies at planned intervals. Among the factors responsible for inadequate contraception are lack of available clinics, physicians' attitudes, religious dogma, cultural bias, psychologic motives, and method failure.

Cultural Factors

Religious teachings on birth control have been of importance in the past and continue to be in some parts of the world, but despite the official Roman Catholic stand prohibiting any method except periodic continence (rhythm), 90 percent of young Catholic women in the United States use nonapproved methods (Westoff and Jones, 1977b). Some young people have turned to "natural" methods as part of their protest against chemical pollution of the human body and the environment.

The accusation of "genocide" has been raised by young American black males against family planning clinics, but despite this, black women use these clinics according to their personal needs. A classic study by Rainwater of contraceptive practices among lower-class couples has examined some of the cultural factors which interfere with effective birth control.

Psychologic Factors

Knowledge of methods of contraception does not ensure use. Psychologic factors involved in misuse and rejection of contraceptives, as identified by Sandberg and Jacobs, include the following:

1. Denial
   a. That pregnancy may occur.
   b. That contraceptives work.

  c. That individuals are responsible for the consequences of their actions.
2. Love—equated with total surrender, self-sacrifice, and risk-taking.
3. Guilt
  a. Pregnancy is normal and interference is wrong.
  b. Pregnancy is punishment for coitus.
4. Shame—fear of discovery by others.
5. Coital gamesmanship—especially related to control of partner.
6. Sexual identity conflicts—pregnancy confirms feminity for women and virility for men.
7. Hostility—pregnancy is a way of "getting even" with partner or parents.
8. Masochism—pregnancy is a way of proving the unworthiness of self.
9. Eroticism—related to risk-taking.
10. Nihilism—the helplessness and hopelessness of the poor and depressed.
11. Fear and anxiety
  a. Concerning adverse effects of contraceptive method.
  b. Concerning inability to control sexual impulses.
13. Opportunism—using coitus for immediate advantage.
14. Iatrogenesis—negative attitudes or ambivalence on the part of the physician.

In addition, *ambivalence* on the part of the woman and her partner toward the desirability of pregnancy, childbirth, and parenthood may prevent effective contraception. Careful counseling with attention to psychologic factors and cultural attitudes, and a supportive concern for the well-being of the couple will reduce the incidence of unwanted pregnancy. The importance of finding a method that a couple will *use* therefore outweighs the absolute reliability of any particular method.

RISK VS. EFFECTIVENESS

Ideal Contraceptive

The characteristics of the "ideal" contraceptive are that it is (1) 100 percent effective; (2) safe—has no side effects; (3) simple to use—minimum level of education or intelligence required; (4) inexpensive; (5) removed from the act of intercourse; (6) completely reversible; and (7) easily obtainable.

It is apparent that different methods fulfill some of these criteria but that no method presently available or soon to be released comes close to fulfilling all. Currently, about 34 percent of couples in this country use a contraceptive pill, 30 percent have been sterilized (half by vasectomy and half by tubal ligation), 11 percent use condoms, 9 percent use IUDs, and 4 percent use diaphragms (Westoff and Jones, 1977a).

Practical Evaluation

In evaluating methods of contraception, the factors of greatest concern are the medical *risks* including the risk of death and the *effectiveness* in preventing conception. When considering risks, the risk of death associated with pregnancy must also be considered. When evaluated this way, *any* form of contraception is safer than *no* contraception, and even rhythm becomes a method with a substantial risk (Fig. 33–1). The minimum number of deaths would theoretically occur if a no-risk method of contraception such as the diaphragm or condom were backed up by legal abortion. In practice, such a plan could lead to careless use of primary contraception.

Effectiveness can be reported in two ways as the *theoretical effectiveness* in which the method, under ideal conditions, is thoroughly understood and always used correctly, and *use effectiveness* which considers the results under actual conditions of use.

Older terminology referred to *method failure* and *patient failure* in comparing methods of birth control. Traditionally, results are reported according to Pearl's formula as pregnancies per hundred woman-years of exposure. Cumulative life-table statistical evaluations, as used by life insurance companies, are also employed, and are often considered the preferred way of reporting.

Reflected in the figures on use effectiveness are such factors as convenience, cost, separation of method from the sex act, the reliability, sobriety, and motivation of the user, and inhibitions about touching the genitalia. Furthermore, complications and side effects of the contraceptive pill and the IUD, as well as fear of these methods, cause a high proportion of users to drop out in the months and years following initiation of the method, although at a decreasing rate relative to time. Thus, although the oral contraceptive is almost 100 percent effective, only about 50 percent of women electing this method will remain on it after 2 years. Continuation rates in some series are higher for women using IUDs. Lippes and Feldman have found comparable continuation rates for the two methods.

Table 33–1 attempts to compare the effective-

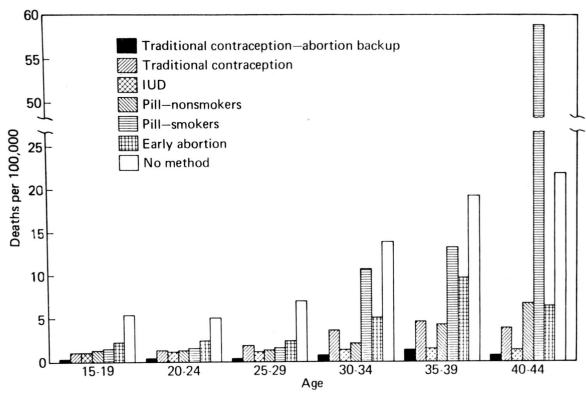

FIGURE 33–1 Annual mortality associated with control of fertility. *(From Jain.)*

TABLE 33–1 Relative Effectiveness of Various Methods of Fertility Control Expressed as Pregnancy Rate per 100 Woman-Years

	Theoretical effectiveness	Use effectiveness*
Chance	80	80
Rhythm		
Calendar	14	35–40
Symptothermal	1.4	22
Coitus interruptus	3	15–23
Foam or jelly alone	3	20
Condom	3	3–15
Diaphragm and jelly	3	3–13
Condom and spermatocide	1	5
Intrauterine device	2	5
Oral contraceptives	0.1	1– 4
Progestin alone	1	3
Vasectomy	0	<0.15
Tubal ligation	0	0.4
Hysterectomy	0	0.0001
Abortion	0	0.1

*Use effectiveness does not include failures due to discontinuation of the method.

ness of the various methods of contraception in common use. The oral contraceptives and the IUD have been meticulously studied over a long period of time. Recently studies with good follow-up have reported better use effectiveness for diaphragms and condoms than was previously thought possible. Some combinations such as condoms and foam which are theoretically effective have never been studied in a controlled fashion. Failures are easy to document, but the number of people using a nonmedically acquired method can only be estimated.

AGE FACTOR

Contraception for the Adolescent

More women at risk of pregnancy are receptive to contraception postpartum than at any other time. Nonetheless, prevention of the *first* pregnancy in the *unwed teenager* is of great importance, and this group has more difficulty getting and accepting contraception than any other. Although the change in teenage sexual activity has not been revolutionary, it constitutes a problem which society attempts to deny. In 1976, 55 percent of unmarried women in the United States had had intercourse by the age 19 (Zelnik and Kantner).

Fear of the law has prevented physicians from helping adolescents obtain contraception. Many states are now passing laws to permit physicians to treat teenagers for venereal disease and to prescribe contraceptives. Some physicians fear that contraceptives will encourage promiscuous sexual behavior; many studies, however, have shown that the young girls who became pregnant were using *no* method of birth control at the time. For most young couples intercourse precedes the use of contraception. Pregnancy rates among teenagers remain high; the term birthrate has decreased slightly, reflecting an increasing use of abortion. Sex education which includes information about contraception and affords opportunity for discussion of the problems of early coitus as it relates to premature childbearing, marital stability, and individual fulfillment is much needed. Early childbearing is strongly associated with decreased educational attainment (Moore and Waite).

Adolescents often begin the use of contraception with readily available but less effective methods such as coitus interruptus, foam and condoms, and only later seek medically prescribed methods. Because of the emotional and physical hazards of pregnancy in the young adolescent and the ease of administration of the pill, most clinics have relied on oral contraceptives in this age group. Concern by physicians about the effect of hormones on early menstrual cycling and on epiphyseal closure may be justified, but there is little evidence to support these fears. Young women, however, have heard that the pills are dangerous and discontinuation rates among adolescents are very high, ranging upward of 50 percent in the first year.

The IUD is often painful to insert and thus a poor choice for the first pelvic examination. Furthermore, the teen population is at high risk for gonorrhea and the presence of an IUD appears to increase the risk of pelvic inflammatory disease. Although the teenager is often thought to be too unsophisticated to use the diaphragm, Lane was able to teach the use of the diaphragm to many in this age group. She found an 80 percent continuation rate after 1 year and a 2 percent unplanned pregnancy rate. More time than usual was spent counseling these patients. If other clinics can do as well, this method may gain in popularity with the adolescent.

Contraception for the Older Woman

Although the woman over 30 has been found to practice contraception more effectively than the younger woman, part of her advantage is decreasing fecundity. Data correlating complications of oral contraceptive pills with advancing age suggest that these agents should be used infrequently by the older woman (Fig. 33–1), particularly by the smoker!

Pregnancy, however, also presents her with increased physical and emotional problems. The diaphragm and IUD can be used with a high degree of effectiveness by these women. Once the decision is reached that no further pregnancies are desired, sterilization of either the man or woman is a rational step.

HORMONAL METHODS

ORAL CONTRACEPTIVE PILLS

The concept that the corpus luteum prevents ovulation during pregnancy was postulated by Beard in 1897. Research during the ensuing years demonstrated that estrogen, progesterone, and testosterone were all able to inhibit ovulation in animals. The search for an orally active synthetic progestational compound with this capability led to the synthesis of norethynodrel and norethindrone by separate research teams in the early 1950s. Rock, Garcia, and Pincus demonstrated the effectiveness of these preparations in preventing ovulation in women when used with mestranol, the 3-methyl ether of ethinyl estradiol. The estrogen was found to *stabilize* the endometrium, allowing more regular menstrual bleeding. The first commercially available preparation was a combination of norethynodrel, 10 mg, and mestranol, 150 μg and was called Enovid. This preparation was dubbed "the pill," and all subsequent oral hormonal preparations designed to achieve contraception have been lumped together under this all-encompassing title.

The theoretical effectiveness of the combination oral contraceptive pill approaches 100 percent with a use effectiveness reported from 85 to 99 percent. Because of this high degree of protection from pregnancy, use of the pill has spread around the world with approximately 100 million women currently using this method of birth control. Nonetheless, the discontinuation rate in the first 2 years ranges from 50 to 70 percent. As the physiologic and long-term effects of the oral contraceptives on various organ systems of

FIGURE 33–2 Estrogens present in oral contraceptives commercially available in 1979.

the body have become better known, decisions regarding their use have become difficult for both patient and physician.

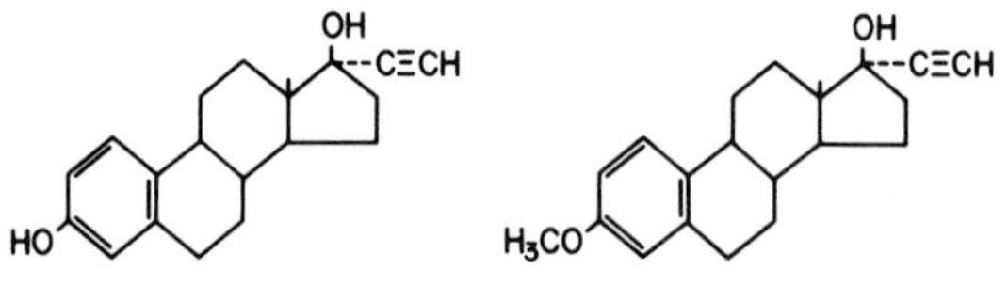

Chemistry

The estrogenic component of oral contraceptives is either ethinyl estradiol or its 3-methyl ether, mestranol (Fig. 33–2). Biologically, 17β-estradiol is the most potent of the natural estrogens but, like most natural

TABLE 33–2 Oral Contraceptives Available in the United States in 1979

Combination pill: type of progestin	Progestin: estrogen	Trade name, MANUFACTURER
Ethynodiol diacetate	1 mg:100 μg MEE*	Ovulen SEARLE
	1 mg:50 μg EE†	Demulen SEARLE
Norethindrone	10 mg:60 μg MEE	Ortho-Novum 10 g ORTHO
	2 mg:100 μg MEE	Norinyl 2 mg SYNTEX
		Ortho-Novum 2 mg ORTHO
	1 mg:80 μg MEE	Norinyl 1+80 SYNTEX
		Ortho-Novum 1/80 ORTHO
	1 mg:50 μg MEE	Norinyl 1+50 SYNTEX
		Ortho-Novum 1/50 ORTHO
		Ovcon-50 MEAD JOHNSON
	1 mg:35 μg EE	Ortho-Novum 1/35 ORTHO
	0.5 mg:35 μg EE	Modicon ORTHO
		Brevicon SYNTEX
	0.4 mg:35 μg EE	Ovcon-35 MEAD JOHNSON
Norethindrone acetate	2.5 mg:50 μg EE	Norlestrin 2.5 mg PARKE DAVIS
	1 mg:50 μg EE	Norlestrin 1 mg PARKE DAVIS
	1.5 mg:30 μg EE	Loestrin 1/30 PARKE DAVIS
	1 mg:20 μg EE	Loestrin 1/20 PARKE DAVIS
Norethynodrel	5 mg:75 μg MEE	Enovid 5 mg SEARLE
	2.5 mg:100 μg MEE	Enovid-E SEARLE
Norgestrel	0.5 mg:50 μg EE	Ovral WYETH
	0.3 mg:30 μg EE	LoOvral WYETH
Progestin alone		
Norethindrone	0.35 mg	Micronor ORTHO
		Nor-Q-D SYNTEX
Norgestrel	0.075 mg	Ovrette WYETH

*MEE, mestranol.
†EE, ethinyl estradiol.

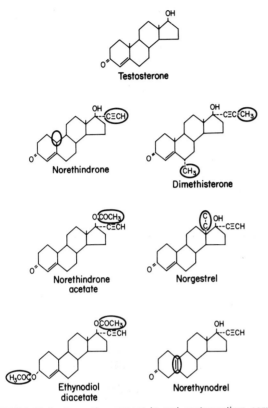

FIGURE 33-3 Progestins present in oral contraceptives commercially available in 1979, compared with testosterone.

The progestational potency of the contraceptive preparations is variable. The most commonly used measure of progestational activity is the delay of menses test, where in the minimum dose of a progestin which will maintain the endometrium and prevent break-through bleeding for a specific period of time is determined. Other tests measure gonadotropin suppression, fetal masculinization, conversion to estrogen, antiestrogenic properties, and anabolic effects. Masculinization in female infants has been reported following treatment with norethindrone and to a lesser degree with norethindrone acetate. All progestins can be converted to estrogen; however, only norethynodrel and ethynodiol diacetate are considered to have estrogenic activity of clinical importance. The remaining progestins are considered to be somewhat antiestrogenic.

The potencies of ethinyl estradiol (EE) and mes-

steroids, it has little activity when taken orally. The addition of the 17-ethinyl group imparts high oral potency to both these components.

Many compounds with progestational activity have been investigated but only a few have been marketed. The chemical structures of the progestins listed in Table 33-2 are shown in Fig. 33-3. All but dimethisterone, a derivative of testosterone, are missing an angular methyl group at the 19 position and thus are classed as 19-nortestosterone derivatives. Both the absence of the angular methyl group and the addition of the acetate radical increase progestational potency. The presence of the 17-ethinyl group is largely responsible for potency when taken orally.

Biologic Properties

Several authors have attempted to classify the biologic characteristics of the oral contraceptives as either estrogenic or progestational (Dickey). Table 33-3 summarizes those properties about which there is general agreement.

TABLE 33-3 Symptoms Generally Attributed to Estrogen and Progestins

Estrogen

Nausea, bloating
Cyclic weight gain, edema
Nervousness, irritability, premenstrual tension
Venous or capillary engorgement
Headaches
Breast tenderness or cystic change
Chloasma (melasma)
Mucorrhea, cervical erosion, or polyposis
Fibroid growth
Hypermenorrhea
Dysmenorrhea
Changes in carbohydrate metabolism
Hypertension
Thrombophlebitis
Suppression of lactation

Progestins

Amenorrhea or oligomenorrhea
Acne
Hirsutism
Breast regression
Increased appetite and steady weight gain
Depression and change in libido
Fatigue
Moniliasis
Early spotting and breakthrough bleeding
Oily scalp and loss of hair

Source: Dickey.

tranol (EE3ME) are similar. Ethinyl estradiol is slightly more effective in preventing ovulation, while mestranol is more potent in preventing breakthrough bleeding and in causing major estrogenic side effects. Fig. 33–4 attempts to relate the relative estrogenic and progestational strengths of the current oral contraceptive pills (OCPs). Dickey has classified the various OCPs on the basis of their clinical side effects. He then attempts to reverse or enhance specific side effects by changing to preparations which are theoretically more or less estrogenic in order to reduce these side effects. Berger and Talwar (1978) found these properties to be poorly defined in 50-μg pills.

Mechanism of Action

The various oral contraceptives are thought to work through one or more of the following mechanisms:

1. Inhibition of ovulation, probably at the hypothalamic level
2. Interference with normal tubal transport of the zygote

FIGURE 33–4 Relative potency of estrogens and progestins in currently available oral contraceptives. (From Hatcher et al.)

Potency Units (progestin)	PROGESTINS (mg)		Product	ESTROGENS (mcg)	Potency Units (estrogen)
.3	NORETHINDRONE .35 mg	(1)	NOR-QD MICRONOR		
2.2	NORGESTREL .075 mg	(2)	OVRETTE		
2	NORETHINDRONE ACETATE 1 mg	(3)	LOESTRIN 1/20 ZORANE 1/20	ETHINYL ESTRADIOL 20 mcg	.7 .8
1	NORETHINDRONE 1 mg	(4)	ORTHO-NOVUM 1/50 NORINYL 1/50	MESTRANOL 50 mcg	1.0
9	NORGESTREL .30 mg	(5)	Lo-OVRAL	ETHINYL ESTRADIOL 30 mcg	1.0 1.2
3	NORETHINDRONE ACETATE 1.5 mg	(6)	LOESTRIN 1.5/30 ZORANE 1.5/30	ETHINYL ESTRADIOL 30 mcg	1.0 1.2
.4	NORETHINDRONE 0.4 mg	(7)	OVCON 35	ETHINYL ESTRADIOL 35 mcg	1.2 1.4
5	NORETHINDRONE 0.5 mg	(8)	MODICON/BREVICON	ETHINYL ESTRADIOL 35 mcg	1.2 1.4
1	NORETHINDRONE 1 mg	(9)	ORTHO-NOVUM 1/80 NORINYL 1/80	MESTRANOL 80 mcg	1.6
1	NORETHINDRONE 1.0 mg	(10)	OVCON 50	ETHINYL ESTRADIOL 50 mcg	1.7 2
2	NORETHINDRONE ACETATE 1 mg	(11)	NORLESTRIN 1 ZORANE 1/50	ETHINYL ESTRADIOL 50 mcg	1.7 2
2	NORETHINDRONE 2 mg	(12)	ORTHO-NOVUM 2 mg NORINYL 2	MESTRANOL 100 mcg	2
2.7	NORETHYNODREL 2.5 mg	(13)	ENOVID-E	MESTRANOL 100 mcg	2
5	NORETHINDRONE ACETATE 2.5 mg	(14)	NORLESTRIN-2.5	ETHINYL ESTRADIOL 50 mcg	1.7 2
15	NORGESTREL 0.5 mg	(15)	OVRAL	ETHINYL ESTRADIOL 50 mcg	1.7 2
15	ETHYNODIOL DIACETATE 1 mg	(16)	DEMULEN	ETHINYL ESTRADIOL 50 mcg	1.7 2
15	ETHYNODIOL DIACETATE 1 mg	(17)	OVULEN	MESTRANOL 100 mcg	2

15 10 5 0
POTENCY UNITS

0   1   2
POTENCY UNITS

THE RELATIVE POTENCY OF PROGESTINS EXPRESSED IN THIS TABLE IS BASED ON A "DELAY OF MENSES" TEST. (See Greenblatt, R.B. "Progestational Agents in Clinical Practice," Med. Sci. 18:37, 1967). OTHER MEASURES OF POTENCY CAN BE USED BUT THESE GIVE DIFFERENT RELATIVE STRENGTHS THAN SHOWN HERE.

THIS TABLE IS AN ADAPTATION OF A TABLE DEVELOPED BY HEINEN, GERT. "The Discriminating Use of Combination and Sequential Preparations in Hormonal Inhibition of Ovulation." Contraception 4:393 (1971).

3. Creation of an abnormal endometrial lining which is unfavorable for implantation
4. Creation of unfavorable cervical mucus which acts as a barrier to penetration by spermatozoa.

The original oral contraceptives were almost 100 percent effective in inhibiting ovulation. Those with 50 μg of estrogen or less probably depend on other, chiefly progestational, effects (Table 33–4).

Physiologic and Pathologic Effects

In general, the physiologic effects of the oral contraceptive agents depend on their estrogenic and progestational effects and, therefore, resemble the changes during the menstrual cycle and pregnancy. These agents affect not only the reproductive tract, but also other organ systems. These physiologic effects underlie the side effects and complications seen in women using the oral contraceptives and will be considered by organ systems.

Cardiovascular Effects. The first serious complication attributed to the OCP was thromboembolic disease, linked causally in 1968 (Inman, Vessey). Almost 10 years later an increase in deaths from all cardiovascular causes was found to be associated with prior use of the pill (Mann; Vessey; Beral). Three physiologic changes underlie these complications:

Effect on clotting. The estrogenic component of the pill increases blood clotting factors VII, VIII, IX, and X,

decreases antithrombin activity and increases non-epinephrine-induced platelet aggregability. These effects together with venous dilatation are thought to be responsible for the increased risk of death from pulmonary embolus (1.4 per 100,000) in women taking oral contraceptives, compared with nonusers of OCPs (0.2 per 100,000). The risk seems to be less with low estrogen pills, but recent British studies, as analyzed by Jain, indicate that the risk increases greatly in women on contraceptive pills with increasing age and with smoking (Table 33–5). Thrombosis may involve cerebral, optic, coronary, and mesenteric vessels, as well as those of the legs. The risk of postoperative thromboembolic phenomena is also increased in women who are on the OCP. The incidence of thromboembolic disease is disproportionately high in women with blood type A. Because the index of suspicion is high, thromboembolic disease tends to be overdiagnosed in women on the OCP.

Effect on vascular reactivity. In 1967 Laragh reported an association between the use of oral contraceptives and hypertension. In susceptible women (approximately 5 percent of those taking the pill) renin substrate levels increased followed by lesser increases in renin and aldosterone activity and the development of hypertension. Blood pressure usually returned to normal levels within 3 to 6 months after the OCP was discontinued. Similar increases in plasma renin activity have been found in normotensive pill users. The Walnut Creek Study (Fisch and Frank) suggests that

TABLE 33–4   Mechanism of Action of Oral Contraceptive Components

Oral contraceptive components	Effect on			
	Ovulation	Tubal transport	Endometrium	Cervical mucus
Estrogen	Inhibits	Accelerates	Prevents nidation in large doses	Produces clear, watery mucus of low viscosity, favorable to penetration by spermatozoa
Progestin	Usually prevents	No effect	Causes regression of proliferative phase, rapid progression through progestational phase to mixed phase	Produces scanty, cellular mucus of raised viscosity; unfavorable to penetration by spermatozoa
Estrogen-progestin combinations	Tend to follow the action of the progestin, but this depends on the degree of estrogenic or progestational dominance			

TABLE 33-5 Estimated Annual Mortality Rate per 100,000 Women from Myocardial Infarction and Thromboembolism by Use of Oral Contraceptives, Smoking Habits, and Age (in Years)

	Myocardial Infarction				Thromboembolism			
	Women aged 30-39		Women aged 40-44		Women aged 20-34		Women aged 35-44	
Smoking habits	Users	Nonusers	Users	Nonusers	Users	Nonusers*	Users	Nonusers
All smokers	10.2	2.6	62.0	15.9	1.6	0.2	4.1	0.6
Heavy	13.0	5.1	78.7	31.3	4.4	0.2	11.4	0.6
Light	4.7	0.9	28.6	5.7	0.7	0.2	1.9	0.6
Nonsmokers	1.8	1.2	10.7	7.4	1.4	0.2	3.6	0.4
Smokers and nonsmokers	5.4	1.9	32.8	11.7	1.5	0.2	3.9	0.5

*Estimated rates for smokers and nonsmokers were 0.24 and 0.16, respectively. Rates appear the same because of rounding.
Source: Jain.

most women sustain a slight elevation in blood pressure while on the pill. The exact mechanism remains obscure and since there are no means of predicting which women will develop significant hypertension, blood pressure should always be checked 2 to 3 months after OCP therapy is begun.

Vascular hyperreactivity is also noted in women with migraine headaches. Fifty percent report worsening of attacks while using the pill (Dalton). Because an excess of deaths due to strokes has been found in pill users (Bauer et al.), migraine headaches are considered a relative contraindication to the use of oral contraceptive agents. Small bowel ischemia and infarction are rare but appear to be increased by use of the OCP.

Effect on lipid metabolism. Mean cholesterol levels increase only 5 percent in women on oral contraceptive agents but mean plasma triglyceride levels are up 48 percent in women 20 to 24 years old, and levels beyond the normal range occur five times as frequently in the pill user as in the nonuser (Wallace et al.). These changes are thought to predispose to the development of arteriosclerosis.

Part but not all of the effects of the pill on the cardiovascular system may be due to smoking. Jain (Table 33-5) has clarified the effect of smoking and age on the pill-induced risk of cardiovascular deaths, and Berger (1977) has evaluated other risk factors. The cardiovascular risk appears to be negligible for the young nonsmoker, but is 78.7 per 100,000 for the heavy smoker over the age of 40.

Gastrointestinal Tract. Nausea and vomiting of pregnancy are generally considered to be estrogen effects. These symptoms were frequent in the first cycles of women on the early high-estrogen pills, but are now reported to be as low as 3 percent in the first cycle and with decreasing frequency thereafter. When the symptom is troublesome, patients may be instructed to take the medication just before going to sleep.

Liver. Alterations in liver function tests have long been reported in women on the pill and are considered to be dose related, reversible, and due to the estrogen. BSP retention is increased, serum glutamic oxaloacetic transaminase and alkaline phosphatase levels may be slightly elevated, and excretory function is reduced. Cholestatic jaundice, similar to the jaundice of pregnancy, occurs rarely as an idiosyncratic reaction soon after the pill is started.

The risk of developing gallbladder disease is doubled in women who have been on the pill 2 years or longer. This risk is approximately 1 in 6000 users. Hepatitis appears to be increased threefold in women on the pill (Morrison et al.).

A serious pill complication first noted in 1972 is the development of liver dysplasia, hepatic adenomas, and, very rarely, malignant tumors (Nissen et al.). It is postulated that the reduced efficiency of the liver in excreting drugs, secondary to the effect of the steroids in the pill on liver cells, may be a factor in the development of these tumors. Death may occur as a result of rupture and intraperitoneal hemorrhage, a risk increased during pregnancy following OCP use. The risk of hepatocellular adenoma, approximately 0.2 per 100,000 users, increases with age, estrogen dose, and duration of pill use. More than 7 years of continuous pill usage is related to a 500-fold increased risk in women over 30 (Center for Disease Control, 1977). The tumors tend to regress with discontinuation of the pill. The diagnosis should be considered in women with right upper quadrant pain or mass. Liver scans and sonography may help confirm the diagnosis.

Endocrine Glands. *Adrenals.* There is apparently no interference with the normal pituitary-adrenal axis. A reduced response to the metyrapone test has been reported, suggesting a lack of compensatory increase in pituitary ACTH.

Thyroid. There is an increase in thyroxine-binding globulin under the influence of estrogen, leading to an increase in protein-bound iodine (PBI), butanol-extractable iodine (BEI), and T_4 and a decrease in T_3. The basal metabolic rate (BMR), cholesterol, ^{131}I, and free thyroxine levels are all normal, and the response of TSH (thyroid stimulating hormone) is maintained, indicating that the functional state of the thyroid is unchanged. The abnormal test results return to normal 2 to 4 months after the pill is discontinued. There is no evidence that either hypo- or hyperthyroid states or adenomatous change are caused by oral contraceptive agents.

Pancreas and carbohydrate metabolism. The combination oral contraceptives increase fasting blood sugar in 10 to 25 percent of patients. In addition, some 20 percent of patients will show an abnormal glucose tolerance test (GTT) immediately after starting the pill. Neither the oral nor the intravenous GTT continues to be abnormal after 3 months on the pill. There is a relative state of hyperinsulinism and a threefold increase in human growth hormone (HGH). This suggests that normal patients will respond to estrogen in oral contraceptives, or from other sources, with an elevated HGH and a compensatory increase in plasma insulin which then maintains a normal GTT. In patients with impaired beta-cell function, an altered GTT may be expected.

The only contraindication to the use of oral contraceptives in the insulin-dependent diabetic is concern about their effect on an already impaired cardiovascular system. Medical control of the diabetes may be more difficult, just as it is in pregnancy. The population at risk is made up of potential diabetics whose compensatory production of insulin may be impaired.

Pituitary: postpill amenorrhea. The mechanism by which the OCP inhibits ovulation is probably mediated through the hypothalamus and pituitary. Within 60 days of stopping the pill, 89 percent of women resume normal cycles, with 2 to 3 percent continuing to have amenorrhea at 6 months. Late onset of men-arche, low body weight, and a history of oligomenorrhea seem to predispose to postpill amenorrhea. Some investigators claim that the occurrence of amenorrhea after discontinuation of the pill is no more frequent than in a similar untreated group of women. If the condition continues for more than 6 months, a search for other causes should be conducted. When galactorrhea is associated with the amenorrhea, up to 32 percent of patients have been found to have prolactin-secreting pituitary tumors (Campenhout et al.).

Other Effects. *Lactation.* High doses of estrogen have long been used to inhibit lactation. The low-dose OCPs do not prevent lactation when used for postpartum contraception, but there is a significant decrease in the quality of milk as evidenced by the need for more supplemental feedings and by a lower weight gain for the infants. Protein, fat, and the inorganic constituents of milk, sodium, potassium, calcium, and magnesium, are all decreased. There appears to be no significant effect on the infant except for the occasional need for supplement. Progestin-only pills appear to have little if any effect on breastfeeding. As a general rule, however, OCPs should not be used in the lactating woman.

Skin. Melasma, or chloasma, has been reported in 29 percent of users of oral contraceptives. It is especially likely to occur in patients with prolonged exposure to sunlight. Chloasma may decrease slightly after stopping pills, but unlike the melanoderma of pregnancy, it does not go away entirely. In one study, 87 percent of patients having melasma after the use of oral contraceptives also had had melanoderma during pregnancy. This effect in pregnancy may be used as an indicator in detecting the susceptible individual. Estrogen also causes a decrease in sebaceous gland activity. Some patients using the more androgenic preparations have noted an increase in acne. By contrast, estrogen-dominant pills are occasionally prescribed to treat this condition. There have been isolated case reports of erythema nodosum, erythema multiforme, and photodermatitis.

Emotional Factors. Problems of depression and decreased libido are probably more common in pill users than originally suspected, but one should not assume that the hormonal components of the pill are solely responsible. Mood and sexual interest may change in either direction, but there are few objective data available regarding the role of the pill. Some studies discount a significant change in libido, and some suggest that the progestational component may decrease premenstrual symptoms. Because of the capability of the pill to separate intercourse from pregnancy, the woman on the pill may feel relief, guilt, freedom, anxiety, or may even entertain fantasies of promiscuity (Sheehan and Sheehan). It is not surprising, therefore, that a variety of psychologic changes have been attributed to the use of the contraceptive pill.

Nutrition. Weight gain was commonly reported following use of the higher-dose contraceptive pills. Estrogens lead to sodium retention as do the synthetic progestins. In some preparations the anabolic effect of the progestins is a significant factor contributing to weight gain. With the pills containing 30 μg of estrogen, weight gain is negligible (Woutersz).

A relative deficiency of vitamin B_6 and folic acid has been reported for women taking OCPs (Prasad et al.). Supplementation of these factors has been suggested.

Genetic Effects. Any medication used by women of childbearing age must be scrutinized for possible effects on the developing fetus. Although chromosomal abnormalities have been reported in the fetuses of women who have been on the pill and have aborted spontaneously, the differences are probably not significant. Sex ratio and birth weights in pill users do not differ from nonusers although twinning is slightly more frequent (Rothman). In women who receive female sex hormones during early pregnancy, cardiovascular and other birth defects are found to be slightly increased in the offspring (Nora and Nora). It is recommended that oral contraceptives be discontinued 3 months before conception is attempted.

Neoplasia. The possible carcinogenicity of oral contraceptives has been of concern throughout their clinical use, since excessive doses of estrogen can cause cancer of the ovary, breast, pituitary, and uterus in a variety of laboratory animals.

Cancer of the cervix in humans is not influenced by female sex hormones, so it is consistent to find no change in incidence in women on the pill. Confusion resulted from early studies which were not controlled for age of initial coitus and number of partners, both important factors in the incidence of cervical cancer. A recent prospective study suggests that steroid contraception speeds the progress of cervical dysplasia to cancer in situ (Stern et al.). This remains to be confirmed.

In contrast, a connection between estrogen stimulation of the endometrium and subsequent cancer of the endometrium has long been known. Synthetic progestins are used to treat endometrial cancer and the combination pills do not increase this neoplasm, but the use of sequential agents has been found to be associated with an increased risk of carcinoma of the endometrium and these have now been removed from the market (Silverberg and Malcowski). Ovarian cancer has not been linked at all with OCPs.

The hormonal dependence of some carcinomas of the breast has directed attention to the possible relationship of breast problems to use of the pill. Several studies have shown a decreased incidence of benign breast disease in women on the pill. The long-term incidence of carcinoma of the breast is unchanged, but a slightly increased rate has been found 2 to 4 years after initiating OCP therapy. This suggests that the hormones in the pill may stimulate growth of subclinical malignancies (Fasal and Paffenbarger).

The relationship of hepatic neoplasm and the very rare liver malignancies to long-term OCP use has been discussed.

Effects on Laboratory Tests. The effects of OCPs on the results of laboratory tests are of great practical concern to the clinician. Thyroid and liver function tests are among those affected. Miale and Kent have compiled a table of some 100 tests where results are either increased or decreased by OCP.

Choice of Agents

Currently available oral contraceptives include combination pills with an estrogen content from 20 to 100 μg and the progestin - only pills (Table 33 – 2). There is no accurate way to predict which women will do best on which formulations of the pill. It seems reasonable to start women on combination pills with estrogen in the range of 30 to 35 μg, minimizing the risk of estrogen-related complications. These preparations are associated with breakthrough bleeding or spotting in 15 to 20 percent of initial cycles, dropping to 5 to 10 percent after 3 months. Patients who continue to have irregular bleeding can be switched to a 50-μg estrogen pill. The 20-μg pills have a slightly increased pregnancy rate and higher incidence of irregular bleeding than the 30-μg pills.

Side effects can often be related to either the estrogen or progestin component of the pill (Dickey), and changes made accordingly (Table 33–3). Talwar and Berger correlated pill symptoms in a ratio of drug to body weight and suggested that weight be taken into account in selecting the agent to be used.

The progestin-only pills, often called minipills, are associated with continuing irregular periods in a high proportion of women. They should be chosen only for women with a history of headaches, hypertension, chloasma, or nausea (conditions made worse by estrogen), who wish to use an oral contraceptive and who can tolerate irregular periods. The theoretical pregnancy rate with the minipill is about 2 per 100 woman-years, only slightly higher than the combination pills.

Contraindications. As of 1979, it is recommended that oral contraceptives not be used in women with the following conditions:

1. Thrombophlebitis or thromboembolic disorders
2. A past history of deep-vein thrombophlebitis or thromboembolic disorders
3. Cerebral vascular or coronary artery disease
4. Known or suspected carcinoma of the breast
5. Known or suspected estrogen-dependent neoplasia
6. Undiagnosed abnormal genital bleeding
7. Known or suspected pregnancy
8. Hepatic adenoma.

Relative contraindications include:

1. Smoking if over the age of 30
2. Liver or gallbladder disease
3. Hypertension
4. Depression
5. Breast-feeding
6. Severe renal or heart disease
7. Migraine or other vascular headaches
8. Prediabetes or diabetes
9. Sickle-cell or sickle-C disease
10. Anovulatory or infrequent periods
11. Elective surgery scheduled within 1 month

Drug interactions have been reported with rifampin, ampicillin, barbiturates, diphenylhydantoin and primidone. Use with these drugs may lead to bleeding and/or pregnancy.

Favorable Effects. Use of the OCPs reduces the length and amount of menstrual bleeding, decreases dysmenorrhea, increases predictability of periods, and decreases premenstrual tension. The incidence of rheumatoid arthritis is reduced in women on the OCP (Wingrave). These effects, as well as the almost total protection against pregnancy afforded by the agents, may be very important to the women who take them.

OTHER APPROACHES TO HORMONAL CONTRACEPTION

The use of hormonal steroids for contraception has been restricted largely to the oral contraceptives. Because these require daily patient motivation, efforts to discover better preparations and better modes of administration continue. The following approaches to hormonal contraception have undergone clinical trials, but none of them is currently considered superior to the standard OCPs.

Once-a-month pill. Quinestrol, 17α-H-ethinylestradiol 3-cyclopentyl ether is a long-acting, orally effective estrogen. Its prolonged activity relates to its storage in and later release from body fat. The progestin, quingestanol acetate, is a 3-cyclopentyl enol ether derivative of norethindrone acetate with similar biologic activity but with twice the potency of norethindrone acetate. Both hormones are administered orally every 4 weeks regardless of the bleeding pattern. The pregnancy rate is 4 per 100 woman-years of use, and menstrual cycle control is good. Side effects are similar to those for conventional oral contraceptives. This pill has not been released for general use.

Postcoital contraception. Intercourse frequently precedes concern about the consequences. Aref and Hafez recently reviewed postcoital contraception. Morris and van Wagenen first demonstrated in human beings that large doses of estrogen taken for 5 days after unprotected intercourse are effective in preventing implantation. They described this as *interception.* There were 29 pregnancies in over 9000 treatment cycles which represents a Pearl index of 4.0. If the figures are corrected to exclude those who received inadequate treatment, the Pearl index for method failures becomes 0.4 (Aref and Hafez).

Successful therapy is dose related. Optimal treatment consists of 50 mg of diethylstilbestrol (DES), 3 to 5 mg of ethinyl estradiol, or 25 mg of conjugated estrogen daily for 5 days starting within 72 hours of unprotected intercourse. Therapy should be undertaken only if exposure to pregnancy occurs near the time of ovulation. Of these estrogens, only DES had limited Food and Drug Administration (FDA) approval as a morning-after pill.

The mechanism of action appears to be on the endometrial implantation site. The principal side effects are nausea and vomiting. While there may be some variation in the next cycle, at least 40 percent of patients noted no change in their menstrual pattern. There is no evidence of an increase in abnormal fetuses either in human beings or in other primates studied, but the role of stilbestrol in the production of vaginal tumors in young girls suggests that therapeutic abortion be considered if a pregnancy ensues. Long-range effects are unknown.

Prostaglandins have been used as vaginally administered postconceptional agents to interrupt very early pregnancies. These agents have been associated with a high rate of success and moderate side effects. Prostaglandins affect tube transport and disrupt ovarian hormonal synthesis. The method is still experimental (Bygdeman et al.).

Long-lasting injectable contraception. Medroxyprogesterone acetate has been administered in doses of 150 mg every 90 days and has proved an effective and convenient contraceptive particularly suited to those women who cannot or do not wish to take a daily pill (Toppozada). The pregnancy rate is comparable with that for oral contraceptives and side effects are similar. The principal adverse effects are irregular bleeding and amenorrhea. There is an occasional delay in fertility for as long as 3 years after stopping treatment. Use of medroxyprogesterone acetate in

this fashion has not been approved by the FDA on the ground that the drug is associated with mammary tumors in dogs, occupies no unique role relative to contraception, has significant side effects, and poses a potential risk to the fetus.

Progestational devices. Several devices have been developed in an attempt to solve the problem of continuous administration of low doses of progesterone for contraception. The progesterone-containing IUD is discussed in the section on IUDs later in this chapter. Most of the other progesterone-releasing devices have utilized the unique property of silicone rubber which allows the hormones impregnated in the silastic to be released at a constant rate.

Clinical trials have been carried out using progestin-impregnated capsules buried in subcutaneous tissue. A silastic device has been designed to be placed in the endocervical canal as well as a silastic vaginal pessary which can be inserted or removed by the patient at will. These methods are limited by the lower contraceptive effectiveness of progestins alone and the irregular pattern of bleeding which may occur. None has yet been released for general use.

FIGURE 33–5 Contraceptive devices: A condom and diaphragm pictured together with four IUDs available in 1979. These are, from left to right, the Lippes Loop, the Saf-T Coil, the Copper-7, and the Progestasert.

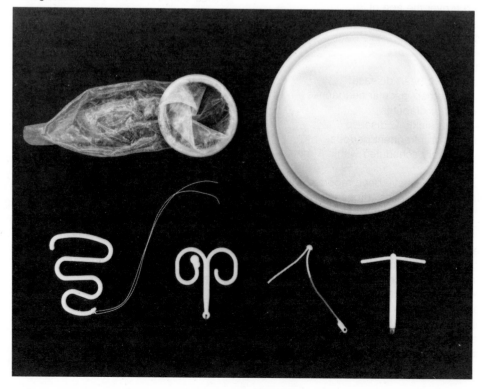

NONHORMONAL APPROACHES TO CONTRACEPTION

Common contraceptive devices currently in use include condoms, diaphragms, and intrauterine devices, pictured in Fig. 33–5. Additional methods to be considered are vaginal foams, creams, and suppositories, and the "natural" techniques of coitus interruptus and rhythm. Table 33–1 compares the theoretical and use effectiveness of these contraceptive measures.

INTRAUTERINE DEVICES

History

The modern placement of substances in the uterus to prevent pregnancy dates from the use of silkworm gut rings by a Polish physician, Richter, in 1909, followed by Grafenberg's use of a ring of German silver (copper, nickel, and zinc alloy). The latter in 1930 reported 1 to 6 percent pregnancies in 600 placements. Occasional severe intrauterine infections were reported, and the method was widely condemned. Interest revived in 1959 with reports by Oppenheimer and Ishihama on the long-term safe use of intrauterine rings (Davis).

Margulies and Lippes developed plastic devices with "memories" which retained their shape after being briefly straightened into hollow cannulas for easy insertion. These were followed by a plethora of devices which were tested in an attempt to find a design that would prevent pregnancy while having minimal side effects, few expulsions, and rare major complications. Many of the early designs have been discontinued. The plastic tip of the Margulies Gynecoil caused penile lacerations and the expulsion rate was high. Closed devices such as the Birnberg bow could incarcerate loops of bowel causing intestinal obstruction if the uterus was perforated and the device entered the abdominal cavity; these devices have been removed from the market. The Majzlin

spring of stainless steel wire was well retained and had a low (2.2) pregnancy rate, but tended to embed in the myometrium, leading to difficult removals and pelvic infections. It has been abandoned. The Dalkon Shield has been associated with a higher rate of uterine infection than other devices and has also been removed from the market.

Current Devices

The four IUDs currently in use are pictured in Fig. 33–5. The Lippes Loop is an early device which has stood the test of time; it is easy to insert and remove and is available in four sizes (Somboonsuk, Rosenfield). The Saf-T-Coil is a modification using a double coil which is inserted much like the loop (Caraway and Vaughn). A small coil is available for the nulliparous woman.

Zipper et al. first showed that intrauterine copper prevents pregnancy in the rabbit. The Copper-7 is a simple device which relies on copper rather than on surface area to reduce pregnancy rates to 2 to 3 per 100 and is well tolerated by most patients. The Copper-T, not yet approved for use in the United States as of 1979, is much like the Copper-7. The Progestasert is a T impregnated with progesterone and relies on the local effect of the hormone on the endometrium to reduce pregnancy rates. This device must be replaced annually.

Pregnancy and complication rates for the devices mentioned above are given in Table 33–6. In most cases rates have been quoted as claimed by the inventors of the devices and are generally better than those obtained in routine clinic use. There are no good randomized series in which these devices have been compared under carefully controlled conditions. It should be noted that although pregnancy rates are low, only about 80 percent of women electing to use the IUD continue with the method at the end of a year because of expulsions and removals for medical problems. Tatum (1977) reviewed clinical aspects of intrauterine contraception in detail.

TABLE 33–6 Events per 100 IUD Users during the First Year

Device	Pregnancies		Expulsion	Medical removals	Continuations
	Nullipara	Multipara			
Lippes	8.0	1.8	5.1	10.1	80.1
Saf-T-Coil	2.8	1.3	11.9	15.4	80.0
Copper T	1.8	1.5	5.3	7.2	83.2
Progestasert	2.5	1.9	3.1	9.7	79.1
Copper-7	2.0	1.5	6.0	12.0	80.0

Mechanism of Action

Local Effects. Despite much speculation and a large body of data based on animal research, the precise mechanism of action of the IUD is still unknown. That the effect is probably local rather than systemic was demonstrated by the finding that a silk suture placed in the lumen of the uterine horn of the rat prevents pregnancy in that horn but has no effect on the other. Surgical anastomosis of the horns, however, allows the contraceptive effect to spread to the opposite horn. The theory that increased tubal and uterine motility causes the fertilized egg to reach the endometrium before conditions are favorable for implantation has not been substantiated.

Inflammatory and Immune Reaction. A local inflammatory effect on the endometrium has been postulated. Although some bacteria are introduced at the time of insertion, cultures taken 1 month later are sterile. A small but increasing incidence of endometritis can be demonstrated with the passage of time, but this is not the basis of effectiveness. Sagiroglu found that macrophages are attracted to the surface of the IUD, causing phagocytosis of spermatozoa.

Increased immunoglobulin G and M levels in women with IUDs in place have supported an immunologic antifertility mechanism, substantiated by the reduction of antifertility action if immunosuppressive agents are used, but the exact nature of the local effect remains unclear (Tatum, 1977).

Effects of Copper. The addition of copper to the T and the loop as well as the "7" has been associated with an additional reduction in pregnancy rates. Copper interferes with migration of spermatozoa as well as with implantation, probably by disrupting sulfhydryl groups in the endometrium and in spermatozoa (Oster and Salgo). It is of interest that the early German silver IUDs had a high proportion of copper.

Because the copper in IUDs may be absorbed systemically, all copper-bearing IUDs have been subjected to regulation by the FDA. Detailed studies of serum copper levels suggest that systemic effects are probably not significant. Most of the copper is lost vaginally in cervical mucus and menstrual discharge (Tatum, 1973).

Advantages of the IUD

The greatest advantage of the IUD is that once the device is in place, no further motivation, effort, or equipment is required for continuing contraception. Many women are delighted by this, and for those in whom there are no failures, no side effects, and no complications, the method is highly satisfactory. The IUD is particularly valuable to those who, for whatever reason, have trouble following directions or remembering to use a method. The lack of systemic effects appeals to some, although major complications including death have been reported. The IUD, like most contraceptives, is used with greatest long-term success in older women who have already achieved their desired family size (Lippes, Feldman).

Disadvantages of the IUD

Disadvantages of the IUD relate to (1) pain and difficulty associated with insertion; (2) side effects; (3) failures; and (4) complications.

Pain on Insertion. Insertion in the nulligravida is frequently painful and may be associated with bradycardia, syncope, nausea, and other vagal responses. Rarely, convulsions occur. Insertion in a uterus sounding less than 6 cm is not advised. Thus, the IUD is usually not the first method offered the young woman just beginning sexual activity. Paracervical block and premedication with atropine have been advocated to reduce symptoms in this group.

Side Effects. Cramps and bleeding are common immediate side effects of insertion but diminish with time. In 2 to 20 percent of women, these symptoms will necessitate removal. The medical removal rate is influenced by the attitudes of the physicians. The cause of any abnormal bleeding should be diagnosed and treated before an IUD is inserted.

Failures. The pregnancy rate of 2 to 5 percent makes the IUD one of the most effective methods of birth control, but the pill or sterilization should be offered the woman who needs total protection from pregnancy.

Complications. The more serious complications of the IUD are considered in a later section.

Contraindications. Pregnancy or the suspicion of pregnancy should stop the insertion of an IUD until the question is resolved. Some physicians have used the IUD as a means of postcoital contraception, but this has not been widely accepted. Any recent acute or chronic pelvic infection is an absolute contraindication to insertion of the device because a flare-up of the infection may follow. An IUD should not be used in any woman who has heart disease which is associated with an increased risk of endocarditis.

Mechanical considerations make women having

congenital anomalies of the uterus or with myomata distorting the endometrial cavity poor candidates for this method. Undiagnosed irregular bleeding is a contraindication until the cause can be ascertained. Great care must be taken after an IUD has been inserted in attributing irregular bleeding to the presence of the IUD.

Blood loss during menses will usually increase with an IUD in place (Table 33–7) (Tatum, 1973). A history of very heavy periods or documented anemia should preclude the use of an IUD. Similarly, dysmenorrhea increases with an IUD, and women who already require more than aspirin for menstrual cramps are not usually good candidates for the IUD.

A previous ectopic pregnancy is a relative contraindication because of the increased incidence of ectopics in association with this method of contraception. Stenosis of the cervical canal or a uterus which sounds to less than 6 cm may prevent the insertion of an IUD.

Insertion of the IUD

When an IUD is the contraceptive method selected by a given woman, a Pap smear and culture for gonorrhea should be obtained since cancer and gonorrhea are contraindications to the use of the IUD. The patient should then be scheduled for insertion *during* a menstrual period for the following reasons:

1. The cervix is slightly softened and dilated at the time of menses, and therefore insertion is easier.
2. Insertion is often followed by bleeding which is unnoticed by the menstruating woman.
3. This timing avoids the problem of placing an IUD in a uterus which is already pregnant. There are

better ways of inducing an abortion if such is desired, and there is an increased risk of serious infection in the pregnant uterus with an IUD in place.

A pelvic examination is performed to ascertain the size and position of the uterus. Significant enlargement is a contraindication to the IUD. *It is imperative to know whether the uterus is anteflexed or retroflexed before insertion is attempted.*

A vaginal speculum is inserted, exposing the cervix which is painted with an antiseptic solution and grasped with a tenaculum. Traction on the cervix straightens the axis of the uterus and makes insertion easier. Sterile technique involving all instruments which go into the uterus is essential. All IUDs marketed in this country come in presterilized packages. Most must be placed into the introducer just before insertion so that the plastic will not lose its "memory."

The uterus is sounded and the direction and depth of the cavity noted. The exact method of insertion will vary with the type of device used. The string attached to the device is left long enough to make it easy for the patient to check and to facilitate future removal. High fundal placement is necessary for optimal effectiveness.

Pain and syncope immediately after insertion are not uncommon. Paracervical blocks may be used to prevent this. Atropine and analgesics will help afterward. Most patients will be able to leave the examining room within 15 minutes.

IUDs can be inserted immediately postpartum, but the high expulsion rate makes this impractical except in those patients who are unlikely to be seen again. An experimental device called the Antigon is said to have a relatively low expulsion rate postpartum (Wiese, Osler). If the insertion is not carried out

TABLE 33–7 Average Menstrual Blood Losses per Cycle in Patients Having Different Contraceptive Methods

Method	No. women	Average menstrual blood loss, mL per cycle	Relative blood loss*
None	145	36.7 ± 0.57	1.0
Copper IUD Copper-T 200 Copper-7	91	49.8 ± 1.47	1.4
Lippes Loop	50	78.0 ± 2.76	2.1
Combination contraceptive pill	50	20.1 ± 1.83	0.6

*Based on an index blood loss of 36.7 mL per cycle for women without contraceptive.
Source: Tatum 1973.

immediately, it is recommended that it not be performed until 6 or 8 weeks postpartum since an increased incidence of perforation has been reported between 2 and 6 weeks postpartum, attributed to postpartum involution of the uterus. Immediate postabortal insertion appears to be safe (Goldsmith et al.).

Instructions to the Patient

1. Pain and/or bleeding following insertion is normal and will gradually diminish. Irregular spotting may occur for the first 2 or 3 months.
2. Cramps and bleeding may be increased with menstrual periods.
3. The IUD string should be located and checked weekly at first and then after each period.
4. Report to the doctor if you are unable to locate the string, if the solid portion of the IUD is felt, or if the device is expelled. You are *not* protected in these circumstances.
5. Supplemental vaginal foam for the first 2 months will reduce the chance of pregnancy.
6. If you suspect pregnancy, call your doctor.
7. Copper and progesterone-bearing devices must be replaced at intervals depending on the device.
8. Unusual discharge, pelvic pain or tenderness, or any suspicion of pelvic infection may be indicative of a serious problem. You should consult your physician immediately.

Complications

Bleeding. Transient bleeding will occur in most women in the first 2 months after insertion and will persist in up to 40 percent. Continued spotting or heavy periods account for most medical removals. The attitude of the patient and physician toward abnormal bleeding as well as the type of device will influence the removal rate, which varies from 2 to 20 percent. Incompatibility between the size and shape of the device and of the endometrial cavity may be partially responsible for irregular bleeding, especially in the nulligravida.

The occurrence of unusual bleeding in a previously asymptomatic woman should suggest the possibility of intrauterine pathology or infection, and its persistence indicates that the device should be removed for evaluation of the problem. Ober et al. have shown that of the 20 percent of women who develop symptoms after 26 months, 40 percent will show a significant inflammatory reaction of the endometrium compared with 2.5 percent of asymptomatic women.

Bleeding does not appear to be caused by the calcium deposits on the IUD.

Pregnancy. The pregnancy rate with an IUD in place is about 2 to 3 per 100 women-years with the devices in current use (Tatum, 1976). Because the mode of action is local, intrauterine but not ectopic pregnancies are prevented, and the latter thus constitute a significant proportion of the total. Deaths have been reported from ruptured ectopic pregnancy in women with an IUD in place, and this possibility must always be considered (Erkkola, Liukko). The FDA reports data indicating an increased risk of ectopic pregnancy with the Progestasert compared to other IUDs.

Although intrauterine pregnancies can continue normally to term with an IUD lodged between the membranes and the uterine wall, 48 percent will abort (Alvior). This can be reduced to 30 percent if the device is removed in early pregnancy. The woman must be warned of the possibility of abortion in either case. Infection is more likely if the woman aborts or delivers with the IUD in place. Infections causing death of the premature infant have been reported. Several maternal deaths have been reported in association with second-trimester septic abortions when the IUDs were left in place. The risk of death is 50 times as great if the woman continues a pregnancy with an IUD in place than if it is removed (Cates et al.). Although most involved the Dalkon Shield, the problem may occur with any IUD. The current recommendation is to remove the IUD as soon as pregnancy is diagnosed and offer therapeutic abortion to those patients who desire it. All patients should be warned of this potentially serious problem.

Expulsion. Expulsion rates vary from 1 to 15 percent (Tatum, 1977). They are higher in nulligravidas and with small devices. Most expulsions occur shortly after insertion or during a menstrual period. Patients should be instructed to check the cervix for the string after each period. Partial expulsion may be detected by a change in the length of the string or by palpating the plastic portion of the device in the cervical os.

Pain. Pain with insertion and increase in menstrual cramps are to be expected. Increasing pelvic pain and uterine tenderness after a pain-free interval may indicate endometritis, and appropriate measures should be taken to diagnose and treat this.

Perforation. One of the most potentially serious complications of insertion of the IUD is perforation. The incidence varies with the skill of the operator and the type of device used but averages about 1 in 1000 insertions. The accident should be suspected when the string disappears and expulsion has not been noted. Some perforations are first recognized when a pregnancy occurs. Confirmation is by x-ray, sometimes combined with hysterosalpingogram or by ultrasound. Closed devices such as the ring or bow may catch a loop of bowel, causing intestinal obstruction. The use of such devices is no longer recommended, and if one is found in the abdominal cavity, its removal is mandatory. This may be attempted by laparoscopy, but, depending on the location of the device, laparotomy may be necessary. Removal of open devices is less urgent, but reports of conversion of the Lippes Loop into a closed device and the development of inflammatory reactions around the copper devices suggest that removal should be planned.

A slightly different type of perforation has been reported in association with the Copper T in which the stem of the device penetrates the cervix and vaginal mucosa. Perforation of the uterus by the arms of the T has also been reported.

Infection. In 1968, Scott published a survey of IUD complications in which 7 to 10 deaths of women using the IUD involved overwhelming pelvic infections which occurred 6 days to 24 months after insertion and involved organisms other than *Neisseria gonorrhoeae*. A total of 369 other severe nonfatal infections were reported. Other deaths have been reported since. Infections occurring just after insertion correlate with Mishell's finding that all endometrial cavities are contaminated at insertion (Mishell, Moyer). In his series all were again sterile within a month. Most clinically significant infections occur after the device has been in place several months.

Although it is convenient to attribute all pelvic infections to gonorrhea, an analysis of the organisms cultured and the histories of the women with fulminating infection suggest that the IUD itself either causes an infection or makes one worse. Faulkner, Ory, and others have found the incidence of PID (pelvic inflammatory disease) to be five times as high in women with IUDs as controls. Young nulliparous women with multiple partners are at high risk and should be discouraged from this method of contraception, if possible.

Burnhill has reported a syndrome of progressive endometritis in women with IUDs in place. This consists of a progression in symptoms from foul-smelling leukorrhea, metrorrhagia, and menorrhagia to frank endometritis and finally pelvic peritonitis. Removal seems indicated if the previously asymptomatic woman develops uterine pain and bleeding. If there is evidence of acute infection, removal should take place after antibiotic coverage has been established. Pelvic abscesses including the previously infrequent unilateral pelvic abscess are now recognized as sequelae of IUD infections (Scott). Many of these eventually require surgery. Pelvic actinomycosis has recently been associated with IUD use.

Other Complications. Various mechanical problems are occasionally seen with IUDs including fracture of the devices in utero or loss of the string from the IUD. These can usually be treated by removal in the office, although anesthesia may be required in some cases. No relationship with cancer has been found.

Removal and Replacement of the IUD

Removals, whether for symptoms or because pregnancy is desired, are generally easier than insertions and can be performed at any time in the cycle. Some devices such as the Dalkon Shield and the Majzlin spring tend to embed in the myometrium if left in place a long time. These devices should always be removed as soon as possible.

If a device is removed because of infection, the infection should be treated and the device not replaced until several months after all signs of infection have disappeared.

Copper and progesterone-bearing devices must be replaced according to the manufacturer's instructions. Any device should be removed if pregnancy ensues. No standard policy for removal and replacement of other devices with time has evolved. Fractures and calcium deposits on devices suggest that they should not be retained indefinitely. Certainly all devices producing severe symptoms should be removed.

DIAPHRAGM

The contraceptive diaphragm was developed in 1882 and was one of the mainstays of birth control for many years. Use waned as the oral contraceptives gained popularity. There are now increasing numbers of women who cannot or will not use the pill or an IUD and are therefore turning to the diaphragm as the best of the remaining alternatives. Some recent studies show that highly motivated women can use the diaphragm with a failure rate of only 2 to 5 pregnancies per 100 woman-years of use (Lane et al.; Vessey, Wiggins). The diaphragm consists of a flexible ring covered by a thin rubber membrane which covers the cervix and most of the anterior vaginal wall when in place. A modification, the cervical cap, has not been widely used in this country.

Some reasons for renewed interest in the diaphragm are (1) the safety of the method; (2) the availability of menstrual extraction or abortion as a backup for method failure; (3) the increasing sophistication of women regarding their own anatomy and the use of tampons for menstruation have made women more accepting of the manipulation required; (4) the desire for a reliable interim method of contraception; and (5) the realization that the diaphragm, unlike foams and condoms, *need not be immediately related to coitus.*

Contraindications to Diaphragm Use

Medical. As a practical matter there are no medical contraindications. The rare sensitivity to the cream or jelly can almost always be solved by a change in spermicide used.

Anatomic. Anatomic contraindications include a damaged pelvic floor or pelvic relaxation which interferes with the snug fit of the diaphragm behind the symphysis, a short anterior vaginal wall, a prolapsed uterus or severe cystocele or rectocele, a small cervix which prevents proper fit of the distal rim of the diaphragm in the posterior fornix, and any condition which prevents the patient from identifying her cervix.

Psychologic, Social, and Educational. These contraindications include disgust with the need to touch the genitalia, inability to learn the method, lack of privacy for insertion and removal, and pressure from the sexual partner.

Failure Rate. Although the failure rate with the diaphragm is often reported as being about 15 percent, Lane et al. reported a large series of patients with a pregnancy rate of only 2 per 100 woman-years and Vessey and Wiggins 2.4 per 100 woman-years. Many unplanned pregnancies among diaphragm users are the result of patient failure. To be effective, the diaphragm must be used with every coital experience. If a patient assumes she is "safe" because her period is due or has just finished and does not bother with the diaphragm, she becomes subject to the same 35 percent failure rate as in the rhythm method.

Other common causes of failure are:

1. Improper fit or type of diaphragm. The diaphragm may be too small because the patient was tense at the time of examination. She may have been given a rigid arcing spring type of diaphragm when she needed a soft flexible coil spring type or vice versa.

2. Lack of appropriate teaching and follow-up.
3. Displacement during coitus especially with multiple mounting and orgasm (Johnson et al.).

Type of Diaphragm

The soft flexible *coil spring diaphragm* is most comfortable but requires well-developed anatomic architecture to stay in place.

The *flat spring diaphragm* will fit below the symphysis even with women who have a shallow notch behind the symphysis.

The *arcing spring diaphragm* is best where there is any significant pelvic abnormality or if the uterus is retroverted. Its firmness and arcing design make it easier to handle and insert, a particular advantage to the novice user.

Fitting and Instruction

Adequate time should be allowed for fitting the diaphragm and for patient education. The diaphragm should be the largest size that fits easily behind the symphysis without sensation for the patient when in place. It should not move inside nor protude when the patient strains down, and neither the patient nor her partner should be aware of it during intercourse regardless of position. She should be instructed to put one or two strips of cream or jelly in the dome of the diaphragm and to spread additional spermicide around the rim with her finger.

A model should be used to demonstrate how to hold and insert the diaphragm with the sides compressed and leading edge of the diaphragm sliding along the posterior wall of the vagina until it is past the cervix when it is allowed to flatten out (Fig. 33–6). Removal is accomplished with one or two fingers hooking the forward rim down and out from behind the

FIGURE 33–6   Self-examination of diaphragm position.

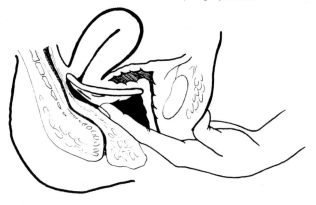

symphysis. If the patient bears down slightly, both insertion and removal may be easier.

Ideally, the patient should practice insertion and removal in the office with a final check for position after she has inserted it. If this is impractical, she may be sent home to practice and to return within the week with the diaphragm in place for a check, but the method should not be used for contraception until after the follow-up visit. Written instructions should always be sent along with the patient for review.

Some practical points to remember:

1. The diaphragm can be inserted any time prior to intercourse and does not have to be "coitus related." Many women find routine insertion at bedtime most satisfactory.
2. If intercourse does not occur for 3 or 4 hours after insertion or if it is repeated prior to removal, additional spermicide should be added without removing the diaphragm.
3. The diaphragm must be left in place for at least 6 to 8 hours after intercourse but need not be removed until it is convenient.
4. The diaphragm should be washed with warm water and mild soap and stored dry with cornstarch or a nonmedicated powder.
5. The diaphragm should be rechecked for holes or deterioration before use by holding it up to light and stretching the rubber along the rim.
6. With proper care, a diaphragm should last 2 to 3 years, but the size should be checked if there is a weight change of more than 15 pounds, a pelvic infection, pelvic surgery, or a pregnancy.

CONDOM

The condom (prophylactic, sheath, safe, rubber, skin) is reported to be the most frequently used contraceptive in the world, and the second most widely used method in the United States (Diller and Hembree). In spite of this, there has been little written about condoms and almost no promotional effort or research carried out. This is due in part to restrictive laws in some states regarding the sale, advertising, and display of condoms, and the apparent assumption by researchers, physicians, and manufacturers that a condom is a condom and there is nothing to improve but quality. Potts and McDevitt, in a poorly controlled series testing spermicidally lubricated condoms, reported only 0.83 pregnancies per 100 woman-years.

The advantages of condoms are many. They require no prescription, are easy to understand and simple to use, cause no side effects, and require no sophisticated regimen. In addition, they protect against venereal disease (VD). The main drawbacks of the condom are the decreased sensation, the need to interrupt foreplay, and the lower effectiveness as compared with the pill or the IUD. Rigorous FDA standards for quality have resulted in condoms made in the United States being two to three times the thickness of Japanese brands. In cultures where the condom is widely used, the placing of the condom is included as an erotic part of the total coital experience. In Japan, oral contraceptives and IUDs are illegal so that more than two-thirds of the contraceptive-using population use condoms as their primary contraceptive technique. They have approached the usual disadvantages with imagination by producing condoms which are thinner and thus more sensitive and in addition have explored a variety of shapes, textures, colors, and lubricants in an attempt to make the method more acceptable. Recently, a plastic sheath has been developed which is 0.02 mm thick as compared with condoms made in the United States, which are 0.05 to 0.09 mm. Some condoms produced in Japan, England, and the United States are shown in Fig. 33–7.

Condoms may be opaque or clear, and as the use of color has increased, there appear to be definite preferences expressed by both men and women. Lubricants may be moist or dry (silicone). These lubricated condoms are hermetically sealed to protect them from dirt and abrasion when they are carried for a prolonged period prior to use. Other innovations include small plastic disposal bags, more attractive packaging, and the experimental use of perfumes, spermicides, lubricants, and hormones.

The condom is a major form of contraception which deserves a greater emphasis than it has received. It should be made more acceptable and more available for the younger population in which VD control is so vital and where the use of the pill or the IUD

FIGURE 33–7 Types of condoms available in various parts of the world. *(From PD Harvey: Condoms—A new look. Fam Plann Perspect 4:27, 1972, by permission.)*

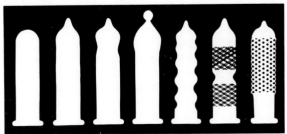

may present special problems for the immature reproductive system.

VAGINAL CHEMICAL METHODS

Foams, creams, and gels are designed to be used just prior to intercourse and are moderately effective, simple methods which may be used as a routine, as a supplement, or as a temporary type of contraception. Each forms a chemical barrier to the cervical os. Cream and foam spread more uniformly than the gels (Johnson et al.). As they mix with semen, they release an immobilizing spermicide, The aerosol foams expand immediately to cover all folds of the vagina and then, like vanishing creams, seem to disappear, leaving a long-lasting invisible coating which inhibits movement of the sperm into the uterus. The gels or creams require a few minutes' time to spread over the vaginal surface. The gels offer greater lubrication, while the creams are preferred by those who need little or no additional lubrication. A repeat application is essential for each coital act regardless of the time interval.

In addition to the more commonly used foams, creams, and gels, there are vaginal suppositories, foam tablets, and sponge and foam preparations. Although suppositories have been recently marketed with claims of 98 percent effectiveness, data from which to substantiate these claims are not currently available and there is no reason to believe that they differ greatly in effectiveness from other forms of vaginal foam.

RHYTHM

Rhythm involves periodic abstinence during the fertile or "unsafe" portion of the menstrual cycle. Physiologically, spermatozoa are usually only capable of fertilization for 2 days after ejaculation. The egg may be fertilized within 24 hours of ovulation. Theoretically, therefore, conception could result from coitus occurring anytime from 2 days before ovulation through the day following ovulation. By abstaining during this 4-day unsafe period, a couple should be able to avoid pregnancy. Unfortunately, the practical use of the method requires rather extensive modification of this theory.

Since ovulation precedes the next menstrual period by 14 ± 2 days in almost all ovulatory cycles, it is possible to estimate the approximate time of ovulation by examining the length of all the menstrual cycles for several months and allowing for as much variation as the maximum difference in cycle length. The greater the variation in cycle length, the longer the period of observation must be. A full year is optimal. A patient should take her shortest cycle during the preceding year and subtract 18 days to find the start of her fertile period, then subtract 11 days from the longest cycle to determine the end of her fertile period. For example, 26 − 18 or day 8 would be the start of the unsafe period, and 32 − 11 or day 21 would be the end of the fertile period for a patient whose cycles varied from 26 to 32 days during the preceding 12 months.

Additional problems with the rhythm method arise from the fact that spermatozoa have been known to survive as long as 7 days in the female reproductive tract, that almost all women will occasionally and unpredictably have a period which is more than 1 week early or late, and that most women have occasional anovulatory cycles. Ovulation may occur at *any* time after an episode of anovulatory bleeding. There is thus *no* time during the menstrual cycle that is 100 percent safe.

In an attempt to identify ovulation more accurately, a patient may keep a basal body temperature (BBT) chart. When properly maintained, the BBT should show a sustained rise of more than 0.5°F following ovulation. When the temperature has been elevated for 3 consecutive days, the "safe" period has begun. Restriction of intercourse to the postovulatory half of the cycle as determined by BBT cuts the pregnancy rate to 6 per 100 or less.

Recently the Billings method which depends on changes in cervical mucus to pinpoint ovulation has gained popularity. Although women can be taught to detect these changes themselves, a viscometer has been devised to measure the properties of cervical mucus.

Although the rhythm method is purported to be an absolutely safe method of birth control, it has its own risks which relate to fertilization of an "overripe" egg. Studies in animals and in man indicate that fertilization of overripe eggs is associated with an increased incidence of early embryonic death, fetal developmental abnormalities, and chromosome defects. Because this hazard is related to conception other than at the expected time of ovulation, rhythm method failures are likely to fall into this category.

COITUS INTERRUPTUS

Withdrawal or coitus interruptus is the oldest method of birth control and, outside the United States, may still be used by more people than any other method. For some couples who practice this, the method seems to be satisfactory. For others, it clearly is not. The essential requirement is for the male to anticipate the start of ejaculation in time to withdraw his penis from the vagina before emission occurs. This may present a problem in that ejaculation can occur in an interrupted fashion with little or no sensation at the beginning. In addition, some spermatozoa may be present in the urethra when erection occurs which can then leak out at the beginning of coitus. There is considerable theory but few data on the possible harmful effects of this practice for either the man or the woman. Whatever the pros and cons concerning its routine use, it costs nothing and is always available so that couples should be aware of its usefulness for those situations in which no other method is available.

LACTATION

The effect of lactation on ovulation and the effect of contraception on lactation are important factors in world health. Elevated prolactin levels postpartum in association with breast-feeding appear to inhibit ovulation despite rising levels of follicle-stimulating hormone (FSH). On the average, ovulation is resumed 6 weeks postpartum in the nonnursing mother and sometime after 10 weeks in those nursing (Perez et al.). Some effect of lactation on ovarian function persists longer, reflected in a 9-month pregnancy rate of 74 percent in noncontraceptive-using, nonlactating women compared with 6 percent in those who are nursing.

The OCPs inhibit lactation in most women, the high-dose pills being more deleterious than the lower ones. Progestin-only pills have been reported not to influence quantity or quality of milk but this is disputed.

MALE CONTRACEPTION

Many people are concerned about the relative lack of male contraceptives. This overlooks the historical perspective that the methods available for the female have been developed relatively recently, while the two oldest and most widely used methods, coitus interruptus and the condom, are methods used by the male (Diller, Hembree).

One of the reasons for the recent emphasis on female contraception is the woman's desire to control conception since she bears the consequence of failure. From the scientific standpoint the reasons are more compelling. In the female, it is necessary to prevent only a single egg from being fertilized and successfully implanted once each month. By contrast, in the male it is necessary to prevent each of several hundred million spermatozoa from getting through the cervix to the egg every time coitus takes place. These differences are summarized by Segal in Fig. 33–8.

The areas in the male where reproduction may be controlled are spermatogenesis in the testes, maturation of spermatozoa in the epididymis, transport of spermatozoa in the vas deferens, and composition of seminal fluid (Segal).

Suppression of Spermatogenesis. There has been extensive research in the suppression of spermatozoa production using the bis(dichloroacetyl)-diamines. Unpleasant side effects and the production of abnormal sperm showed these agents to be unsuitable. Testosterone and progestins inhibit spermatogenesis in many animals including man. Much more testing is required before the safety and practicality of these agents can be established.

Interference with Seminal Fluid Biochemistry. Seminal fluid is essential to the normal activity of human spermatozoa. Although it has not been possible to interfere with fertility by removing any one of the major components of seminal fluid, it may be possible to alter the fluid by the addition of a chemical which will be picked up by the semen.

Interference with Transport of Spermatozoa. Interference with transport of spermatozoa has been the principal area of success with male contraception. In addition to the barrier methods, there has been extensive use of male sterilization through vas ligation or occlusion. These methods are highly successful in preventing conception, although they are not as reversible as might be desired.

FUTURE DIRECTIONS IN CONTRACEPTION

Research in human reproduction will probably lead to new concepts in fertility control as well as to improvements in available techniques. Numerous substances are being investigated as potential luteolytic or antiprogesterone agents; such substances, when used during the second half of the menstrual cycle, might prevent implantation even if fertilization has occurred. Other types of antiimplantation agents are being sought as well.

Immunologic approaches to fertility control may

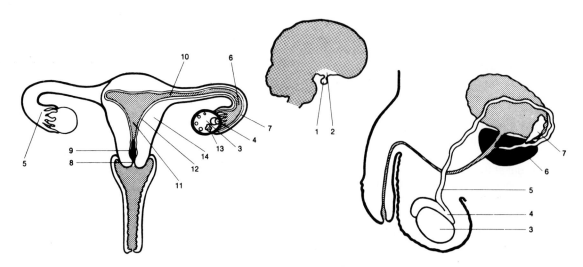

Female

OVULATION

Steroid negative feedback (1 & 2)
Central nervous system drugs (2)
Gonadotropin antagonists (3)
Local action on follicle (4)

OVUM TRANSPORT

Ovum pickup by fimbria (5)
Cilia activity (6)
Tubal fluid secretion (6)
Tubal musculature (7)

SPERM TRANSPORT

External os of cervix (8)
Cervical mucus (9)
Utero-tubal junction (10)

FERTILIZATION

Shedding of zona pellucida of ovum (6)
Sperm capacitation (11)
Sperm penetration of egg membrane (6)
Pronuclei fusion (6)

ZYGOTE TRANSPORT

Tubal fluid secretion (6)
Tubal musculature (7)

PREVENTION OF IMPLANTATION

Estrogen binding (12)
Corpus luteum function (13)
Progesterone binding (12)

PLACENTATION

Trophoblast formation (12)
Chorionic gonadotropin production (12)

MAINTENANCE OF PREGNANCY

Embryogenesis (12)
Placental function (12)
Myometrial activity (14)

Male

Pituitary control (1)
Steroid negative feedback (1 & 2)
Sperm formation in testis (3)
Sperm maturation in epidydimis (4)
Sperm transport in vas (5)
Seminal fluid biochemistry (6 & 7)

FIGURE 33–8   Potential sites of interruption of the reproductive process. *(From Segal.)*

offer attractive alternatives. In addition, to evaluate vaccines against human chorionic gonadotropin (HCG), investigators are searching for inhibitors of follicular maturation and sperm motility.

ABORTION

INCIDENCE

Abortion is one of the most prevalent methods of fertility control throughout the world today. Between 30 and 55 million abortions are performed worldwide each year (Grimes and Cates). In the United States, legal abortion has become an important component of the health care of women. Over a million American women underwent legal abortions in 1976, making this one of the nation's most frequently performed operations. Because abortion remains a controversial means of fertility control, it has attracted intense scru-

tiny. As a result, more is known about abortion than any other operation.

LEGAL BACKGROUND

Prior to 1973, state regulations governing the practice of abortion in the United States varied greatly. In January 1973, the Supreme Court ruled that government cannot interfere with a pregnant woman's decision to terminate or continue her pregnancy (*Roe v. Wade; Doe v. Bolton,* 1973). The Court ruled that during the first trimester of pregnancy the government cannot regulate abortions at all, except to require that licensed physicians perform them. During the second trimester and before the stage of fetal viability, the government may regulate abortions to protect the health of the woman. These regulations such as licensing of medical facilities, cannot interfere with the decision to choose abortion.

Regarding consent of the spouse, the Supreme Court ruled in 1976 that since the government has no authority to veto an abortion, a husband should not have that authority either (*Danforth v. Planned Parenthood of Central Missouri,* 1976). Thus, the abortion decision rests with the woman. Concerning parental consent for abortion, the Court ruled that mandatory parental consent laws that apply to all teenagers are unconstitutional. The Court left room for regulation however. States may be able to require that an "immature" minor consult with or notify her parents, who may decide that abortion is not in her "best interests." This presents the questions of determining which minor is immature and whether the parents are acting in the immature minor's best interests (*Danforth v. Planned Parenthood; Baird v. Bellotti,* 1976).

Concerning public funding of abortion, the Supreme Court decided in 1977 that states are not constitutionally bound to pay for nontherapeutic abortions for poor women even though childbirth expenses are covered through Medicaid programs (*Beal v. Doe; Maher v. Roe,* 1977). This does not, however, prohibit states from funding such abortions. In *Poelker v. Doe,* the Court also ruled that public hospitals are not required to provide nontherapeutic abortions. The Court's interpretation of what constitutes a "therapeutic" abortion remains unclear (Chaps. 4 and 5).

COUNSELING

The wide range of attitudes toward abortion currently held in our society creates problems for the woman contemplating an abortion. It is important for a counselor to help her explore the values she holds, the feelings she is experiencing, and the choices that are available. If these issues are considered before the abortion, it is unlikely that the woman will be seriously upset by the procedure. She may regret the situation that led to the problem pregnancy, but she will feel comfortable with her choice. The very young, those with previous psychiatric problems, and those who feel abortion is wrong require extra help in arriving at the best decision.

TYPES OF PROCEDURES

Most techniques of legal abortion can be grouped into five general categories: (1) curettage procedures, (2) intrauterine instillation of abortifacients, (3) hysterotomy and hysterectomy, (4) intrauterine mechanical devices, and (5) extrauterine administration of abortifacients. Curettage abortions are the most

important type because they are not only the most frequently used but also the safest. Curettage procedures can be further divided into four classes: (1) "menstrual regulation," (2) sharp curettage, (3) suction curettage, and (4) midtrimester dilatation and evacuation.

CURETTAGE PROCEDURES

Menstrual Regulation

Menstrual regulation (endometrial aspiration or "miniabortion") is a relatively new technique for suction abortion within the first few weeks after a missed menses. Designed to minimize the risk of uterine trauma, a flexible plastic cannula evacuates the uterine contents. A 50-cc syringe with a self-retaining lock on the plunger provides a convenient source of suction. Because of the small diameter of the cannula, cervical dilatation usually is not required. Two problems that occur more frequently with this technique than with later suction abortions are failure to abort the pregnancy and performance of the procedure on a woman not pregnant (Population Reports, 1974).

Sharp Curettage

Sharp curettage was for many years the predominant method used for first-trimester abortions. This technique entails cervical dilatation, usually by metal dilators, followed by uterine evacuation by means of ovum forceps and a sharp curette. With the development of suction curettage, sharp curettage accounted for a smaller percentage of abortions each year in the United States until 1976 (Fig. 33–9). The increase in sharp curettage abortions in that year may have been caused by increasing numbers of midtrimester dilatation and evacuation abortions being reported as "sharp curettage."

Suction Curettage

Suction curettage is the most widely used method of abortion in the United States. After having dilated the cervix, the operator inserts a suction cannula to evacuate the uterine contents. The cannula is usually connected to an electrically powered vacuum source by clear, flexible tubing. With rotary motions of the cannula, the operator aspirates the uterine contents. In general, the cannula diameter in millimeters should approximate the gestational age in weeks from last menstrual period, e.g., a 9-mm cannula for a 9-week pregnancy.

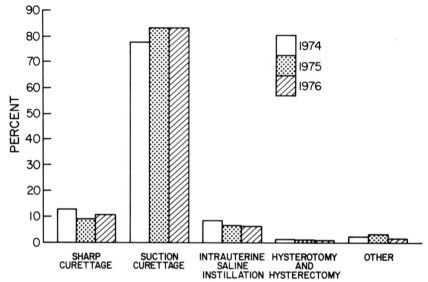

FIGURE 33-9 Distribution of legal abortions by type of procedure 1974-76. *(From Center for Disease Control, 1978.)*

Dilatation and Evacuation

Dilatation and evacuation (D&E) is a generic term encompassing instrumental removal of the products of conception. When used in the midtrimester, D&E is an extension of first-trimester sharp and suction curettage used to evacuate the larger volumes of tissue encountered in later pregnancies. Because the cervix must be dilated to greater diameters, some operators use overnight placement of intracervical laminaria. Laminaria are hygroscopic sticks of dried seaweed which expand slowly when exposed to moisture. Other physicians dilate the cervix with large-caliber metal dilators. After adequate dilatation has been achieved, the fetus and placenta are removed with forceps, sharp curettage, suction curettage, or a combination of these (Grimes et al., 1977b). This is the predominant method of abortion used in the United States between 13 and 15 menstrual week's gestation, and the second most frequently used method thereafter (Center for Disease Control, 1978).

INTRAUTERINE INSTILLATION

Intrauterine instillation of solutions capable of initiating the abortion process accounts for most terminations of pregnancy performed at 16 weeks or later. Hypertonic saline is the most widely used agent, followed by prostaglandin $F_{2\alpha}$ (Center for Disease Control, 1978). To induce an instillation abortion, the physician performs an amniocentesis under local anesthesia and confirms free flow of amniotic fluid. No further fluid need be withdrawn. The physician then injects the abortifacient into the amniotic fluid. While prostaglandin $F_{2\alpha}$ acts directly to induce uterine contractions, hypertonic solutions such as saline or urea work indirectly. First, the hypertonic agents cause fetal death. Labor usually ensues, although the mechanism initiating contractility is not known. The use of hypertonic solutions plus small doses of prostaglandin $F_{2\alpha}$ as an augmenting agent is increasing (WHO Prostaglandin Task Force).

SURGICAL PROCEDURES

Prior to the development of safer means of midtrimester abortion, hysterotomy and hysterectomy were important abortion techniques. Hysterotomy is analogous to a cesarean section performed on a smaller uterus. Because the morbidity and mortality of major operations for abortion are prohibitive, these operations are infrequently used for this purpose today. In 1976, hysterotomy and hysterectomy together accounted for fewer than 0.5 percent of abortions in the United States (Fig. 33-9).

INTRAUTERINE FOREIGN BODIES

Insertion of a foreign body into the uterus is one of the oldest and least desirable methods of abortion. Devices used have included catheters, bougies (large, soft rubber catheters), balsa, laminaria, and metreurynters (inflatable rubber bags similar to a Foley catheter). All of these mechanical methods share the disadvantages of long abortion times and high infection rates.

EXTRAUTERINE ABORTIFACIENTS

Although a number of different agents have been administered by many routes, few have shown promise as abortifacients. One exception is the group of prostaglandins. Prostaglandin E_2 vaginal suppositories have been approved by the FDA for abortions at 13 weeks' gestation or later, and in cases of fetal death in utero through 28 weeks. Other prostaglandins have been used successfully by other routes, such as intramuscular and extraovular. Cytotoxic drugs, antimetabolites, and high doses of oxytocin or ergot derivatives are all both dangerous and ineffective.

MORBIDITY AND MORTALITY

Legal abortion has emerged as not only one of the most frequent operations in contemporary practice but also one of the safest. Two large multicenter prospective studies in the United States since 1970 have documented an incidence of major complications of only 0.7 per 100 abortions among over 125,000 healthy women without concurrent sterilization (Grimes and Cates). Moreover, the death/case ratio for legal abortions in the United States from 1972 through 1976 was only 3.0 per 100,000 abortions of all types (Center for Disease Control, 1978).

Two predominant factors influence the safety of abortion, gestational age and method of abortion. From a nadir at 7 to 8 weeks' gestation, the complication rate for legal abortion increases with advancing gestational age (Table 33–8). As shown in this table, abortion complication rates should be thought of as a continuum; there is no gestational age threshold beyond which rates increase exponentially. In general, earlier abortions are safer abortions.

The second important variable influencing complication rates from abortion is the type of procedure used (Table 33–9). Curettage abortions are the safest, with suction curettage being safer than sharp. Instillation abortions have a higher total complication rate than curettage abortions, much of the difference the result of minor complications. On the other hand, major abdominal operations for abortion have high rates for both total and major complications.

TABLE 33–8 Total and Major Complication Rates for Abortions by Gestational Age

Gestational age (weeks from LMP)	Complications per 100 abortions	
	Total	Major
≤ 6	7.2	0.36
7–8	4.7	0.27
9–10	5.6	0.45
11–12	8.2	0.77
13–14	17.0	1.37
15–16	33.1	1.91
17–20	39.9	2.16
21–24	36.1	2.26
Total	12.3	0.80

Source: Grimes et al. 1977a.

Hemorrhage, infection, retained products of conception, and cervical injury are among the more frequent complications encountered. The incidence of hemorrhage is difficult to determine, since definitions of hemorrhage vary widely. If one uses transfusion of blood as an index of clinically important blood loss, then rates of hemorrhage range from 0.06 per 100 abortions by suction curettage to 1.53 per 100 abortions by $PGF_{2\alpha}$ (Grimes, Cates). Local anesthesia is associated with lower rates of hemorrhage than general anesthesia, and use of oxytocics significantly decreases blood loss during suction curettage.

Rates of infection, manifested by a temperature of ≥38°C for 1 or more days, range from less than 1.0 per 100 abortions by suction curettage to 10.8 per 100 abortions by $PGF_{2\alpha}$ (Grimes, Cates). As with other gynecologic infections, the organisms generally responsible are those found in the vagina, with the important exception of *N. gonorrhoeae*. Risk factors

TABLE 33–9 Total and Major Complication Rates for Abortions by Type of Procedure

Type of procedure	Complications per 100 abortions	
	Total	Major
Suction curettage	5.0	0.4
Sharp curettage	10.6	0.9
Intrauterine instillation	42.7	1.9
Hysterotomy	49.4	14.9
Hysterectomy	52.9	16.1
Total	12.3	0.8

Source: Grimes et al. 1977a

TABLE 33–10 Death/Case Ratios for Abortions by Weeks of Gestation, United States, 1972–1976

Weeks of gestation (weeks from LMP)	Ratio*	Relative risk†
≤ 8	0.6	1.0
9–10	1.7	2.8
11–12	2.8	4.7
13–15	7.8	13.0
16–20	16.1	26.8
≤ 21	26.8	44.7
Total	3.0	

*Deaths per 100,000 abortions.
†Relative risk based on an index rate for ≤ 8 weeks gestation of 0.6 per 100,000 abortions.
Source: Center for Disease Control, 1978.

for infection include nonprivate patient status, preexisting untreated endocervical gonorrhea, instillation abortion techniques, and instillation-to-abortion times greater than 48 hours. The advisability of prophylactic antibiotics remains controversial, but one large study has suggested that oral tetracycline may be of value.

Retained products of conception can lead to bleeding, infection, or both. This problem is especially troublesome with instillation abortions, where the placenta may not be expelled with the fetus in as many as 40 per 100 abortions. With saline abortions, removal of the placenta is indicated if it has not been passed within 2 hours after the fetus.

Cervical trauma is a relatively common but usually minor complication. Cervical injury associated with suction curettage most often occurs during dilatation, when the tenaculum may tear loose. Such lacerations may require direct pressure or suturing. Lacerations caused by dilators may be more serious. Formation of cervicovaginal fistulas has emerged as

a problem of instillation abortions, especially those induced by PGF$_{2\alpha}$. Concurrent use of laminaria may decrease the risk of trauma associated with cervical dilatation from dilators or uterine contractions.

Death/case ratios for abortion parallel ratios for morbidity. As shown in Table 33–10, gestational age is the most important factor determining the risk of death from abortion. Delays of any origin, whether caused by a woman's ambivalence, medical custom, or administrative procedures, increase the risk of death. For example, delaying an abortion from 8 to 16 menstrual weeks increases the risk of death 27 times. Mortality rates are lowest for curettage abortions and highest for major operations, with instillation procedures intermediate (Table 33–11). These figures can be compared to the risk of death from pregnancy and childbirth; in this country from 1972 to 1975 it was 14.0 per 100,000 live births (Grimes, Cates).

The preceding tables suggest ways of reducing complications from abortion. Women requesting abortion need prompt service. Once abortion has been elected the choice of method then becomes an important determinant of risks. Suction curettage appears to be the method of choice through 12 menstrual weeks. In the 13- to 20-week interval, D&E abortions performed by experienced operators appear significantly safer than saline abortions (Grimes et al., 1977b). This observation awaits confirmation by appropriate clinical trials. Of the two most frequently used abortifacients, saline appears safer but slower than prostaglandin F$_{2\alpha}$ as demonstrated in both large randomized (WHO Prostaglandin Task Force) and nonrandomized prospective studies (Grimes et al., 1977c).

Ancillary measures may also help prevent complications. For curettage abortions local rather than general anesthesia may reduce the risk of hemorrhage and uterine trauma while oxytocin may reduce

TABLE 33–11 Death/Case Ratios for Abortions by Type of Procedure, United States, 1972–1976

Type of procedure	Ratio*	Relative risk†
Curettage/dilatation and evacuation	1.7	1.0
Intrauterine instillation	15.5	9.1
Hysterotomy/hysterectomy	42.4	24.9
Other	9.9	5.8
Total	3.0	

*Deaths per 100,000 abortions
†Relative risk based on an index rate for curettage/dilatation and evacuation of 1.7 per 100,000 abortions
Source: Center for Disease Control, 1978.

blood loss. Treatment of preexisting endocervical gonorrhea should minimize the risk of postabortal endometritis since untreated gonorrhea is associated with a threefold increased risk of this complication. Pratt dilators are preferable to Hegar dilators for abortion. The former dilate the cervix with less force and thus provide better control.

For saline instillation abortions, the use of oxytocin shortens abortion time; this, in turn, may reduce the risk of infection. On the other hand, oxytocin administration increases the risk of coagulation defects, water intoxication, and uterine rupture. If the placenta has not delivered within 2 hours after the fetus, its instrumental removal appears to lower complication rates. Finally, all Rh-negative women not previously sensitized should be given Rh immunoglobulin after abortion; new lower doses of Rh immunoglobulin designed for use after abortions in the first 12 weeks of pregnancy should lower costs for this service.

EFFICACY

Abortion is an effective means of birth control. Curettage abortions have the highest rate of success. In the Joint Program for the Study of Abortion under the auspices of the Center for Disease Control, the failure rate for curettage abortions was 0.1 per 100 abortions. Menstrual regulation procedures have higher rates of failure to evacuate the pregnancy; rates from 0.3 to 40 per 100 abortions have been reported (Population Reports, 1974). Instillation abortions tend to be less effective than curettage abortions. A recent report encompassing 8662 saline abortions described a failure rate of 2.5 per 100 abortions (Grimes et al., 1977b). Prostaglandin $F_{2\alpha}$ produces faster abortions than saline; hence, proportionately more women expel the fetus within specified intervals of time. By 72 hours, however, failure rates are similar.

SUMMARY

Legal abortion is a widely used means of fertility control in the United States and throughout the world. Suction curettage in the first trimester accounts for most such abortions. Gestational age and type of procedure are the two most important factors determining the safety of abortion. Suction abortion in the first eight weeks of pregnancy carries a risk of death similar to that of an injection of intramuscular penicillin. While the debate concerning the ethics of abortion will continue in the years ahead, the safety and public health benefits of legal abortion have been clearly established.

STERILIZATION

INCIDENCE

The most dramatic change in contraceptive practice among American couples in recent years has been the growing popularity of surgical sterilization. As of 1975, among continuously married white couples, sterilization closely rivaled oral contraception as the predominant method of birth control. Among couples married 10 or more years, sterilization was the single most popular method (Westoff, Jones, 1977a). In 1975, approximately 674,000 and 639,000 contraceptive sterilizations were performed on women and men, respectively, in the United States (Association for Voluntary Sterilization). This section will provide an overview of current sterilization procedures for both women and men.

INDICATIONS

Indications for sterilization may be grouped into two broad categories, medical and contraceptive. Until recently medical and psychiatric illnesses, obstetric conditions including grand multiparity, and genetic abnormalities prompted most sterilizations in the United States. Formulas were developed which restricted sterilization services to women of advanced age or high parity (e.g., age times parity must equal 120).

In the past decade, however, because of concern over the safety of temporary contraception, rising economic goals, and expectations of greater personal fulfillment, many couples in their twenties and early thirties have been seeking permanent contraception. As a consequence contraception has emerged as the principal justification for sterilization. Still other factors underlying the increased reliance upon sterilization include female emancipation, earlier marriage and completion of childbearing, reduction in perinatal and childhood deaths, and the need for extended periods of highly effective contraception. Rising educational achievement may also play a role since, in general, the prevalence of contraceptive sterilization in the United States is correlated with level of education (Shepherd).

FEMALE STERILIZATION

TUBAL OCCLUSION PROCEDURES

Two methods of female contraceptive sterilization predominate: tubal occlusion techniques and hysterectomy. Ovarian ablation, either by radiation or operation, is not justified as a sterilization technique because it induces premature menopause. Both tubal techniques and hysterectomy can be further categorized by the surgical approach, temporal relationship to pregnancy, and technical differences. Tubal sterilization accounts for the majority of female sterilizing operations undertaken primarily for contraception. Of the two surgical approaches to the tube, the abdominal is used far more frequently than the vaginal.

Puerperal Laparotomy

Puerperal tubal ligation by laparotomy remains a popular, safe, and effective sterilization technique. A subumbilical incision provides access to the tubes in the early postpartum period. Among the various techniques devised for occluding the tubes, the Pomeroy method and its modifications are probably the most widely used. In the Pomeroy technique the operator elevates a knuckle of tube, then ligates the knuckle with a single suture of plain catgut. A segment of the ligated knuckle is then excised. In several days the suture is absorbed, and the cut ends separate and reperitonealize. Other less often used methods include the Irving and Uchida techniques. With the Irving technique each tube is divided, the cut ends ligated, and the proximal stump buried in the myometrium, thus creating a blind loop. With the Uchida method the tubal serosa is ballooned by an injection of saline and epinephrine. After the tube has been severed and ligated, the proximal stump is closed within the serosal pouch, isolating it from the peritoneal cavity.

Minilaparotomy

For sterilization in women not recently pregnant ("interval" sterilization) a modified laparotomy has been used recently with favorable initial results. The "minilaparotomy" entails a 1.5- to 3-cm suprapubic incision in which a miniature speculum or proctoscope can be inserted for retraction. By means of an intrauterine manipulator, the operator elevates the uterus to the incision and then occludes the tubes in a conventional manner.

Laparoscopy

Widespread use of laparoscopy has revolutionized female sterilization in the United States. Laparoscopic tubal sterilization has emerged as a safe, convenient, and relatively inexpensive outpatient procedure. Local anesthesia suffices in many cases. Laparoscopic sterilization can be performed using either a double-puncture or single-puncture approach; with the latter, the laparoscope contains an operating channel.

The most popular technique of tubal occlusion by laparoscope is coagulation of the tubes, with or without division of the tubes thereafter. Most authors advise dividing the tubes after coagulation, although others report equally good results with several contiguous burns alone (Yuzpe et al.). Because of the risk of electrical burns to intraperitoneal contents during laparoscopic coagulation, investigators have developed alternative means of occluding the tubes via the laparoscope. Hulka and Clemens (Hulka et al.) have pioneered the spring-loaded clip which can be applied to the tubes via an operating laparoscope. Similarly, Yoon (Yoon et al.) and Lay independently developed a silastic band that is applied to a knuckle of tube via a single- or double-puncture approach. With bipolar coagulation the electric current passes only through the tube rather than through the woman's body to a base plate. Preliminary reports suggest that a battery-powered thermal cautery may also provide safe and effective sterilization via the laparoscope.

Vaginal Tubal Ligation

Interval or postabortal sterilizations can also be performed vaginally. Most authors describe the use of a conventional colpotomy incision through which a Pomeroy procedure or fimbriectomy can be performed. Some authors, however, advocate the combined use of colposcopy or laparoscopy with colpotomy.

Hysteroscopy

With the development of improved fiberoptics, the hysteroscope has recently attracted renewed interest as a transvaginal means of tubal sterilization. Operators using the hysteroscope can coagulate the cornual areas of the uterus under direct visualization. This method must still be considered experimental.

MORBIDITY AND MORTALITY

Assessment of the relative safety of tubal sterilization techniques is difficult because of the paucity of well-controlled prospective studies. Most reports describe the results of a single technique in a single institution. Moreover, definitions of complications and lengths of follow-up vary widely between reports. Thus, few conclusions can be drawn.

Total complication rates appear related to timing of the procedure, with the highest rates from sterilizations performed in conjunction with cesarean section or abortion, intermediate rates from puerperal abdominal ligations, and the lowest from interval abdominal operations (Table 33–12). These findings should be interpreted with caution, however, because few studies identify the risk attributable to the sterilization itself as compared with that of the concurrent event. The available studies disagree on the safety of combined abortion and sterilization. Several found that the risks of abortion and concurrent sterilization were no greater than the sum of both independent procedures (Cheng, Rochat; Fishburne et al.) while others found the risks were potentiated by combining the abortion and sterilization (Hernandez et al.). Tubal ligation at the time of cesarean section does not appear to influence the morbidity of the latter (Shepherd). Contrary to previous thinking, the time interval between delivery and postpartum tubal ligation does not seem to influence febrile morbidity rates, at least within the first 5 days after delivery.

A multicenter prospective study (Brenner et al.) comparing laparoscopic sterilization using coagulation, spring-loaded clips, and silastic bands found the clips to have significantly more technical problems, largely related to the prototype clip applicator. Rates of operative and early postoperative complications were not significantly different. A double-blind study comparing the comfort of coagulation versus silastic band laparoscopic sterilization has revealed the former to be significantly less painful after operation (Pelland).

Complications of laparoscopy have received much attention in recent years. The most common problem appears to be uterine perforation by the intrauterine manipulator; this usually does not require treatment. Abdominal wall emphysema secondary to failed pneumoperitoneum seems to be the next most common problem. Serious complications, however, are rare. According to the American Association of Gynecologic Laparoscopists (AAGL), the incidence of bowel burns is 0.5 per 1000 cases and the incidence of mesosalpingeal tears necessitating laparotomy is 1.8 per 1000 cases.

The principal disadvantage of vaginal tubal ligation is that its morbidity rate is higher than other methods of tubal sterilization. Both hemorrhage and infection appear to be more common than with abdominal approaches. As with abdominal techniques, concurrent abortion involves higher overall morbidity rates than with sterilization alone. Experience with hysteroscopy for sterilization is too limited to compare morbidity rates.

TABLE 33–12   Selected Composite Data for Sterilization Procedures, 1968–1974

Procedure	No. of patients	Operative complication rate*	Infectious morbidity rate*	Failure rate*
Puerperal abdominal ligation	6,717	1.9	8.4	0.2
Cesarean section ligation	1,739	10.3	19.7	0.3
Interval abdominal ligation	1,115	5.6	3.6	0.6
Interval laparoscopic procedure	16,997	1.3	0.6	0.3
Interval vaginal ligation	3,706	3.7	6.9	0.3
Hysteroscopic procedure	335	3.3	0	2.3
Interval vaginal hysterectomy	895	22.1	36.7	0

*Per 100 sterilization procedures
Source: Shepherd

The risk of death from tubal sterilization is small. The mortality rate is cited as approximately 0.25 per 1000 cases (Shepherd).

EFFICACY

Two important factors influence, failure rates of sterilization, correct identification of the tubes and the management of the tubes once identified. The first large-scale study to measure pregnancy rates by the life-table method (Center for Disease Control, 1977) suggests that ligation by minilaparotomy is significantly more effective than three alternative methods. The minilaparotomy approach used a modified Pomeroy ligation; the other three techniques studied included culdoscopic excision of a portion of the tubal ampulla, vaginal fimbriectomy, and laparoscopic coagulation. Virtually all failures occurred within 24 months of operation.

Combined data from recent reports suggest a cumulative failure rate from puerperal abdominal tubal ligation of approximately 2 per 1000 cases (Shepherd). The Pomeroy technique was the predominant technique used in these studies. Because they isolate the proximal tubal stump from the peritoneal cavity, the Irving and Uchida procedures have very low failure rates (less than 1 per 1000 cases). Alternative tubal techniques such as the Madlener, Aldridge, and single ligature have largely been abandoned because of unacceptably high failure rates.

Timing of sterilization in relation to pregnancy may influence failure rates. For example, higher rates of failure may be associated with interval procedures (Table 33–12). In contrast to prior thinking, failure rates of ligations associated with cesarean section and the puerperium are not significantly different.

With interval laparoscopic sterilization, a common cause of failure is sterilization of a woman in the postimplantation stage of pregnancy. Data from AAGL reveal intrauterine pregnancy rates of 2 per 1000 sterilizations by coagulation and division, 2 per 1000 by silastic band, and 7 per 1000 by the spring-loaded clip. Of note is the finding that the rate of ectopic pregnancies with the band appears higher than the intrauterine pregnancy rate associated with this technique. In prospective randomized studies, however, pregnancy rates associated with various laparoscopy techniques have not been significantly different.

Data are inadequate to evaluate the efficacy of vaginal tubal ligation since most reports lack this information. The Pomeroy technique, however, is the most frequently described method. Preliminary experience with hysteroscopy has revealed high failure rates with present techniques.

HYSTERECTOMY

The legitimacy of elective hysterectomy for sterilization remains one of the most controversial topics in modern gynecology. Types of procedures include interval vaginal or abdominal hysterectomy, abortion-sterilization by vaginal or abdominal removal of a pregnant uterus, and cesarean section combined with hysterectomy.

Since all hysterectomies are sterilizing, the incidence of hysterectomy for purely contraceptive reasons is difficult to establish. Nevertheless, the incidence of elective hysterectomy for sterilization appears to be increasing (Shepherd).

The morbidity and mortality of this major operation raise the most serious ethical questions about the justification for elective hysterectomy. Examining data on vaginal and abdominal hysterectomies for various indications from the Professional Activity Study (Ledger and Child) found that 33 out of 100 women had fevers of 38°C or more, and 17 per 100 received blood transfusions. The average length of stay in hospital was 10 days, while the death-to-case rate was 1.6 per 1000 operations. While the morbidity and mortality of purely elective hysterectomy would be expected to be lower, the rates would probably still exceed those of tubal sterilization cited previously (Table 33–12).

The efficacy of hysterectomy for sterilization is exceeded only by that of bilateral oophorectomy. Niebyl has reviewed 21 reported cases of pregnancy after hysterectomy. These ectopic pregnancies were attributable to preimplantation gestations at the time of operation or to fistulous tracts from the vaginal apex allowing sperm access to the tubes or peritoneal cavity.

Advocates of vaginal hysterectomy for sterilization cite as its advantages the avoidance of a visible scar, less postoperative discomfort, and the opportunity to perform a concurrent colporrhaphy. On the other hand, the complication rate for abdominal hysterectomy is lower in most reports. Hysterectomy for combined abortion and sterilization does not appear to have a significantly increased incidence of morbidity over interval hysterectomy. Hysterectomy for sterilization has the advantages of high efficacy, elimination of dysmenorrhea, and prevention of subsequent uterine disease but the disadvantages of greater risk, higher cost, more frequent psychologic sequelae, and longer recuperation. Certainly the advantages and disadvantages should be made clear to the woman involved so that she can make a truly informed choice.

MALE STERILIZATION

Surgical interruption of the vas deferens within the scrotum has become one of the safest, least expensive, and most effective means of contraception. Some of its recent popularity may stem from increasing public awareness of the potential complications of female contraception and sterilization procedures.

Vasectomy for sterilization is a frequently performed operation in the United States. In 1975, vasectomies accounted for 49 percent of sterilization procedures in the United States (AVS). Striking racial differences exist as to which partner obtains sterilization. Among white sterilized couples, vasectomies and female sterilizations are nearly equally represented. On the other hand, among black couples, the woman is the partner sterilized in over 90 percent of cases (Westoff, 1976).

TYPES OF PROCEDURES

Vasectomy is a simple office procedure requiring only local anesthetic in most cases. The operator may use either a single midline or two incisions, one over each vas. After each vas has been identified, the operator cuts the vas, sometimes removing a segment. The optimal management of the cut ends remains unclear, with some operators ligating, cauterizing, or applying clips. Some physicians turn and ligate the cut ends in a 180-degree arc, while others interpose the sheath of the vas between the cut ends to serve as a fascial barrier.

In order to determine that men are sterile after vasectomy, one or more sperm counts are customarily obtained ranging from 6 to 12 weeks after operation. The time required for residual sperm to be cleared from the ejaculate is a function of the number of ejaculates since operation. A period of 5 days to 6 months may be required before the semen becomes aspermic although the majority of men are free of viable sperm after 20 ejaculates. Some operators irrigate the vas during operation in an attempt to reduce the postoperative sperm count, but this practice is not widely used.

MORBIDITY AND MORTALITY

Vasectomy is a safe operation. Only one death in the United States has been reported. Complication rates range from 2 to 4 per 100 in large studies (Population Reports, 1975). The most frequent complication is local trauma to the scrotum manifested by ecchymoses and edema. More serious complications include hematoma, granuloma, infection, or epididymitis. Approximately 50 of every 100 men who undergo vasectomy will develop antibodies to sperm. This occurrence has not been associated with the subsequent development of immunologic diseases in men.

EFFICACY

Vasectomy is an effective sterilization procedure. Failure rates are approximately 0.15 per 100 person-years (Population Reports, 1973). The most common cause of failure is spontaneous recanalization. Division of the wrong structure, inadequate occlusion of the cut ends, unprotected intercourse prior to aspermia, and duplication of the vas account for most other failures. Use-effectiveness is lower in nonmonogamous cultures.

SUMMARY

Vasectomy provides many unique advantages. The operation is effective, safe, technically simple, rapid, and relatively inexpensive. On the other hand, infertility is not immediate, and for men who equate masculinity with fertility this method has little appeal.

In conclusion, voluntary sterilization has become a social decision rather than a medical one. The physician's role should be to counsel the couple about risks and benefits of available procedures, their effectiveness, and their cost.

Vasectomy should usually be offered to couples seeking sterilization. If, however, female sterilization is selected, then tubal sterilization is the method of choice. During the puerperium the preferred method appears to be a subumbilical laparotomy. For interval sterilizations or those combined with suction curettage abortion, laparoscopic sterilization appears preferable to other tubal procedures by the abdominal or vaginal routes.

If preexisting gynecologic pathology necessitates operation, hysterectomy is indicated. When vaginal relaxation is present, the vaginal approach is preferred. Elective cesarean hysterectomy for sterilization appears unjustified because its complication rates, especially hemorrhage and trauma to the urinary tract, are prohibitively high.

REFERENCES

Contraception

Alvior GT: Pregnancy outcome with removal of intrauterine device. *Obstet Gynecol* 41:894, 1973.

Aref I, Hafez ESE: Postcoital contraception: Physiological and clinical parameters. *Obstet Gynecol Surv* 32:417, 1977.

Bauer R et al.: Oral contraception and increased risk of cerebral ischemia or thrombosis. Collaborative group for the study of stroke in young women. *N Engl J Med* 288:871, 1973.

Beard J (quoted by SA Asdell): The growth and function of the corpus luteum. *Physiol Rev* 8:313, 1928.

Beral V: Mortality among oral-contraceptive users. *Lancet* 2:727, 1977.

Berger GS: Oral contraceptives and myocardial infarction. *NC Med J* 38:323, 1977.

―――― **Talwar PP:** Oral contraceptive potencies and side effects. *Obstet Gynecol* 51:545, 1978.

Billings JJ: *National Family Planning: The Ovulation Method,* 3d ed., Collegeville, Minn.: Liturgical Press, 1975.

Burnhill M: Syndrome of progressive endometritis associated with intrauterine contraceptive devices. *Adv Plan Parent* 8:144, 1973.

Bygdeman M et al.: Outpatient postconceptional fertility control with vaginally administered 15(S)15-methyl-PGF$_{2\alpha}$-methyl ester. *Am J Obstet Gynecol* 124:495, 1976.

Campenhout J et al.: Amenorrhea following the use of oral contraceptives. *Fertil Steril* 28:728, 1977.

Caraway AF, Vaughn BJ: Florida's five years experience with the double coil IUD. *J Reprod Med* 10:170, 1973.

Cates WJr et al.: The intrauterine device and deaths from spontaneous abortion. *N Engl J Med* 295:1155, 1976.

Center for Disease Control: *Morbid. Mortal. Weekly Rep. Increased Risk of Hepatocellular Adenoma in Women with Long-Term Use of Oral Contraception,* U.S. Dept. of Health, Education, and Welfare/Public Health Service 26:293, 1977.

Dalton K: Migraine and oral contraceptives. *Headache* 15:247, 1976.

Davis HJ (ed.): *Intrauterine Devices for Contraception: The IUD,* Baltimore: Williams & Wilkins, 1971.

Day RL: Factors influencing offspring. *Am J Dis Child* 113:179, 1967.

Dickey R: Diagnosis and management of patients with oral contraceptive side effects. *JCE Ob/Gyn,* 20:19, 1978.

Diller L, Hembree W: Male contraception and family planning: A social and historical review. *Fertil Steril* 28:1271, 1977.

Erkkola R, Liukko P: Intrauterine device and ectopic pregnancy. *Contraception* 16:569, 1977.

Fasal E, Paffenbarger RS Jr: Contraceptives as related to cancer and benign lesions of the breast. *J Natl Cancer Inst* 55:767, 1975.

Faulkner WL, Ory HW: Intrauterine devices and acute pelvic inflammatory disease. *JAMA* 235:1851, 1976.

Fisch IR, Frank J: Oral contraceptives and blood pressure. *JAMA* 237:2499, 1977.

Goldsmith A et al.: Immediate postabortal intrauterine contraceptive device insertion: A double-blind study. *Am J Obstet Gynecol* 112:7, 1972.

Hatcher RA et al.: *Contraceptive Technology 1978–1979,* 9th ed., New York: Irvington-Halsted Pub., 1978.

Inman WHW, Vessey MP: Investigation of deaths from pulmonary, coronary, and cerebral thrombosis and embolism in women of childbearing age. *Br Med J* 2:193, 1968.

Jain AK: Mortality risk associated with the use of oral contraceptives. *Stud. Fam. Plann.* 8:49, 1977.

Johnson VE et al.: Factors in failure, in *Manual of Family Planning and Contraceptive Practice,* ed. MS Calderone, Baltimore: Williams & Wilkins, 1970, p. 232.

Lane ME et al.: Successful use of the diaphragm and jelly by a young population: Report of a clinical study. *Fam Plann Perspect* 8:81, 1976.

Laragh JH: Oral contraceptive-induced hypertension—nine years later. *Am J Obstet Gynecol* 26:141, 1976.

Lippes J, Feldman J: A five year study of loops and orals, Adv. Plan. Parent 7:111, 1972.

Mann JI et al.: Oral contraceptive use in older women and fatal myocardial infarction. *Br Med J* 2:445, 1976.

Miale JB, Kent JW: The effects of oral contraceptives on the results of laboratory tests. *Am J Obstet Gynecol* 120:264, 1974.

Mishell DR, Moyer DL: Association of pelvic inflammatory disease with the intrauterine device. *Clin Obstet Gynecol* 12:179, 1969.

Moore KA, Waite J: Early childbearing and education attainment. *Fam Plann Perspect* 9:220, 1977.

Morris JM, van Wagenen G: Interception: The use of postovulatory estrogens to prevent implantation. *Am J Obstet Gynecol* 115:101, 1973.

Morrison AW et al.: Oral contraceptives and hepatitis. *Lancet* 1:1142, 1977.

Nelson JH: Selecting the optimum oral contraceptive. *J Reprod Med* 11:135, 1973.

Nissen ED et al.: Etiologic factors in the pathogenesis of liver tumors associated with oral contraceptives. *Am J Obstet Gynecol* 127:61, 1977.

Nora JJ, Nora AH: Birth defects and oral contraceptives. *Lancet* 1:941, 1973.

Ober WB et al.: Polyethylene intrauterine contraceptive device: Endometrial changes following long term use. *JAMA* 212:765, 1970.

Ory HW: A review of an association between intrauterine devices and acute pelvic inflammatory disease. *J Reprod Med* 20:200, 1978.

Oster G, Salgo MP: The copper intrauterine device and its mode of action. *N Engl J Med* 293:432, 1975.

Perez A et al.: First ovulation after childbirth: The effect of breast-feeding. *Am J Obstet Gynecol* 114:1041, 1972.

Perkins GW: Indications: Establishing priorities for intensive contraceptive care, in *Manual of Family Planning and Contraceptive practice,* 2d ed., ed. MS Calderone, Baltimore: Williams & Wilkins, 1970.

Potts M, McDevitt J: A use-effectiveness trial of spermicidally lubricated condoms. *Contraception* 11:701, 1975.

Prasad AS et al.: Effect of oral contraceptives on nutrients III. Vitamins B_6, B_{12} and folic acid. *Am J Obstet Gynecol* 125:1063, 1976.

Rainwater L: *And the Poor Get Children,* Chicago: Quandrangle, 1960.

Rock J, Garcia CR, Pincus G: Effects of certain 19-norsteroids on the normal human menstrual cycle. *Science* 124:891, 1956

Rothman KJ: Fetal loss, twinning and birth weight after oral-contraceptive use. *N Engl J Med* 297:468, 1977.

Sandberg EC, Jacobs RI: Psychology of the misuse and rejection of contraception. *Am J Obstet Gynecol* 110:227, 1971.

Scott RB: Critical illnesses and deaths associated with intrauterine devices. *Obstet Gynecol* 31:322, 1968.

Scott WC: Pelvic abscess in association with intrauterine contraceptive device. *Am J Obstet Gynecol* 131:149, 1978.

Segal SJ: Contraceptive research: A male chauvinist plot? *Fam Plann Perspect* 4:21, 1972.

Sheehan DV, Sheehan KH: Psychiatric aspects of oral contraceptive use. *Psych Ann* 6:500, 1976.

Silverberg SG, Makowski EL: Endometrial carcinoma in young women taking oral contraceptive agents. *Obstet Gynecol* 46:503, 1975.

Somboonsuk A, Rosenfield AG: Experiences with the Lippes Loop 1965–71. *Int J Gynaecol Obstet* 11:16, 1973.

Stern E et al.: Steroid contraceptive use and cervical dysplasia: Increased risk of progression. *Science* 196:1460, 1977.

Talwar PP, Berger GS: Side effects of drugs: The relation of body weight to side effects associated with oral contraceptives. *Br Med J* 1:1637, 1977.

Tatum HJ: Clinical aspects of intrauterine contraception: Circumspection 1976. *Fertil Steril* 28:3, 1977.

_____: Metallic copper as an intrauterine contraceptive agent. *Am J Obstet Gynecol* 117:602, 1973.

_____ et al.: Management and outcome of pregnancies associated with the Copper T intrauterine contraceptive device. *Am J Obstet Gynecol* 126:869, 1976.

Toppozada M: The clinical use of monthly injectable contraceptive preparations. *Obstet Gynecol Surv* 32:335, 1977.

Vessey M, Wiggins P: Use-effectiveness of the diaphragm in a selected family planning clinic population in the United Kingdom. *Contraception* 9:15, 1974.

Vessey MP et al.: Mortality among women participating in the Oxford/Family Planning Association Contraceptive Study. *Lancet* 2:731, 1977.

Wallace RB et al.: Altered plasma-lipids associated with oral contraceptive or estrogen consumption. *Lancet* 2:11, 1977.

Westoff CF, Jones EF: Contraception and sterilization in the United States, 1965–1975. *Fam Plann Perspect* 9:153, 1977a.

_____, _____: The secularization of U.S. Catholic birth control practices. *Fam Plann Perspect* 9:203, 1977b.

_____: Trends in contraceptive practice: 1965–1973. *Fam Plann Perspect* 8:54, 1976.

Wiese J, Osler M: Immediate post-partum insertion of the Antigon. *Acta Obstet Gynecol Scand* 56:509, 1977.

Wingrave SJ: Reduction in incidence of rheumatoid arthritis associated with oral contraceptives. *Lancet* 1:569, 1978.

Woutersz TB: Three and one-half years' experience with a lower-dose combination oral contraceptive. *J Reprod Med* 16:338, 1976.

Zelnik M, Kantner JF: Sexual and contraceptive experience of young unmarried women in the United States 1976 and 1971. *Fam Plann Perspect* 9:55, 1977.

Zipper J et al.: Suppression of fertility by intrauterine copper and zinc in rabbits. *Am J Obstet Gynecol* 105:529, 1969.

Abortion

Center for Disease Control: *Abortion Surveillance 1976,* Aug 1978.

Grimes DA, Cates W Jr: Complications of legally induced abortion: A review. *Obstet Gynecol Surv* 34:177,1979.

_____ et al.: Mid-trimester abortion by dilatation and evacuation. A safe and practical alternative. *N Engl J Med* 296:1141, 1977b.

_____ et al.: Mid-trimester abortion by intraamniotic prostaglandin $F_{2\alpha}$. Safer than saline? *Obstet Gynecol* 49:612, 1977c.

_____ et al.: The joint program for the study of abortion/CDC: A preliminary report, in *Abortion in the Seventies,* eds. WM Hern, B Andrikopoulos, New York: National Federation, 1977a, p. 41.

Population Reports: *Menstrual Regulation Update,* seri. F, No. 4, May 1974.

World Health Organization Prostaglandin Task Force: Comparison of intraamniotic prostaglandin $F_{2\alpha}$ and hypertonic saline for induction of second-trimester abortion. *Br Med J* 1:1373, 1976.

Sterilization

American Association of Gynecologic Laparoscopists: *1977 AAGL Complications Committee Report: The Prevention and Management of Laparoscopic Complications,* Dec., 1977.

Association for Voluntary Sterilization: *AVS News,* Sept, 1976.

Brenner WE et al.: Laparoscopic sterilization with electrocautery, spring-loaded clips, and silastic bands: Technical problems and early complications. *Fertil Steril* 27:256, 1976.

Center for Disease Control: *Morbid and Mortal Weekly Rep, Pregnancy rates following sterilization procedures — Singapore.* 26:137, 1977.

Cheng MCE, Rochat RW: The safety of combined abortion-sterilization procedure. *Am J Obstet Gynecol* 129:548, 1977.

Fishburne JI et al.: Outpatient laparoscopic sterilization with therapeutic abortion versus abortion alone. *Obstet Gynecol* 45:665, 1975.

Hernandez IM et al.: Postabortal laparoscopic tubal sterilization. Results in comparison to interval procedures. *Obstet Gynecol* 50:356, 1977.

Hulka JF et al.: Spring clip sterilization: One year follow-up of 1,079 cases. *Am J Obstet Gynecol* 125:1039, 1976.

Lay CL: The new improved silastic band for ligation of fallopian tubes. *Fertil Steril* 28:1301, 1977.

Ledger WJ, Child MA: The hospital care of patients undergoing hysterectomy: An analysis of 12,026 patients from the Professional Activity Study. *Am J Obstet Gynecol* 117:423, 1973.

Niebyl JR: Pregnancy following total hysterectomy. *Am J Obstet Gynecol* 119:512, 1974.

Pelland PD: Patient acceptance of laparoscopic tubal fulguration versus Falope-ring banding. *Obstet Gynecol* 50:106, 1977.

Population Reports: *Vasectomy — Old and New Techniques,* ser. D, no. 1, U.S. Bureau of the Census, December 1973.

_____: *Vasectomy — What Are the Problems?* ser. D, no. 2, U.S. Bureau of the Census, January 1975.

Shepherd MK: Female contraceptive sterilization. *Obstet Gynecol Surv* 29:739, 1974.

Westoff CF, Jones EF: Contraception and sterilization in the United States, 1965–1975. *Fam Plann Perspect* 9:153, 1977a.

Yoon IB et al.: A two-year experience with the Falope ring sterilization procedure. *Am J Obstet Gynecol* 127:109, 1977.

Yuzpe AA et al.: Laparoscopic tubal sterilization by the "burn only" technic. *Obstet Gynecol* 49:106, 1977.

34

Sexual Counseling

HAROLD I. LIEF

THE SEXUAL SYSTEM ("SEXUALITY")
Biological sex
Sexual identity
Gender identity
Gender role behavior

THE PHYSIOLOGY OF SEXUAL RESPONSE
Stages of sexual response
Similarities and differences of male and female
responses

THE SINGLE FEMALE
Adolescent psychosexual development
Adolescent sexual problems
The never-married woman
Problems of homosexuality

THE WOMAN WHO MARRIES
Sexual concerns of the woman who marries
The married woman and her family
Working-class marriages
Sexual attitudes and behavior: class and race

**OBTAINING SEXUAL DATA IN A MEDICAL
HISTORY**

**COMMON SOURCES OF SEXUAL
DYSFUNCTION**
Pregnancy
Aging

TYPES OF SEXUAL PROBLEMS
Masked sexual problems
Sexual problems masking marital and other
problems
Sexual responsivity
Sex drive and interest

OTHER PROBLEMS OF SEXUAL BEHAVIOR
Vaginismus and dyspareunia
Infidelity
Problem pregnancies
Problems of the separated, divorced, or widowed
woman
Illness, ablative surgery, and sexual functioning
Sexual aspects of infertility

SEXUAL DYSFUNCTION TREATMENT
General considerations
Taking a sexual history preparatory to
dysfunction treatment
Sex counseling
  Inhibition of sexual desire
  Inhibition of sexual excitement
  Orgasmic dysfunction
  Failure to achieve orgasm during coitus
  Vaginismus and dyspareunia
Other treatment approaches to sexual inadequacy

**THE PLACE OF SEX COUNSELING IN
GYNECOLOGIC PRACTICE**

Many physical symptoms brought to the attention of doctors mask underlying sexual and/or marital difficulties. Examples are pelvic pain, dysmenorrhea, vaginal discharge, backache, and fatigue. Burnap and Golden found that when physicians initiated discussion of sexual functioning, 15 percent of the problems presented to practicing gynecologists had their origins in sexual and marital dysfunction. Pauley and Goldstein found that over 66 percent of the physicians who routinely obtain a sexual history from their patients identify significant sexual problems in at least half of their patients.

It is fair to say that the frequency of sexual and/or marital problems in one's practice depends on the physician's (1) alertness in looking for them, (2) willingness to initiate discussion in those areas, and (3) comfort in dealing with them.

But the question remains, should the gynecologist treat sexual and marital problems or refer them to other specialists? What Vincent (1968) says about the general physician applies to the gynecologist, as today *the* doctor for many women is the gynecologist:

The theoretical position that the physician cannot or should not engage in any marriage or sexual counseling becomes meaningless when the patients expect this role of their physician and when their illnesses have sexual and marital implications—if not origins. The majority of physicians literally have no choice; even to do and say nothing in response to the patient's questions and/or presentation of symptoms in the sexual and marital areas is, by default, one form of counseling.

Fortunately, medical schools have responded to this new reality. In 1960, only three had formal programs of education in human sexuality. In 1968, when the Center of the Study of Sex Education in Medicine was formed in Philadelphia, approximately 30 medical schools were offering such courses. Almost every medical school now includes such courses in the curriculum. Half of them have developed clinical facilities for sex counseling and therapy.

In this chapter, the sexual consequences of marital or relational dysfunction are of concern, not the psychosomatic symptoms or syndromes, unless they have sexual underpinnings. The chapter begins with a discussion of the factors responsible for the sexual orientation of human beings, followed by a description of normal sexual physiology. After a discussion of the sexual development and problems of the teenager and unmarried woman, there is a review of the typical milestones in the life of the woman who marries, including a look at her family satisfactions and problems, for who can understand the sexual life of the married woman without knowing what goes on in her family? With this groundwork laid, the reader is better placed to appreciate the subsequent discussions of sexual dysfunction likely to be presented to the gynecologist who considers a sexual history a normal part of medical care. Finally the treatment situation is described, including interviewing and the various degrees of intervention–education, counseling, and therapy–within the scope of the gynecologist who undertakes treatment of sexual dysfunction.

THE SEXUAL SYSTEM ("SEXUALITY")

The discussion of normal and abnormal sexual functioning in the sections that follow will be aided by describing women's sexuality in terms of a system analogous to the circulatory or respiratory system (Lief, 1979). The components of the sexual system are set forth in Table 34–1.

Sexual behavior of the human being results from interaction between the phenotype and the environment, but even prior to birth the fetal environment may have a profound effect on sexual development. In the human being there is extreme plasticity in sexual development. With rare exceptions, the sex assigned during rearing will override the biological programming of the organism, provided that the sex assigned during early life by the child's parents and other caretakers is clear-cut and definite. Even ambiguous anatomical sexual characteristics will not prevent unambiguous sexual and gender identity later on, provided there is concurrence and certainty on the part of the parents and other meaningful adults.

BIOLOGICAL SEX

In the female, inheritance of the XX chromosome will lead to normal ovarian development and function. Un-

TABLE 34–1 The Sexual System (Sexuality)

Biological sex—chromosomes, hormones, primary and secondary sex characteristics
Sexual identity (sometimes called core-gender identity)—sense of maleness and femaleness
Gender identity—sense of masculinity and femininity
Gender role behavior: sex behavior—behavior motivated by desire for sexual pleasure, ultimately orgasm (physical sex); gender behavior—behavior with masculine and feminine connotations.

less there are abnormal amounts of androgen, the fetus will develop into a phenotypic female. The primordial fetus is always female and will develop as a female unless androgen is added. Even the XY fetus will develop in a female direction if there is failure of fetal testicular function or androgen insensitivity. Presumably, there is a critical period in fetal life when the sexual programming of the brain, primarily the hypothalamus and connecting neural circuits, takes place, supposedly between the sixth and twelfth weeks after conception. Seemingly, human development is like that of many animal species, for which a large amount of data indicate that androgen, or lack of it, in fetal life programs the brain for later appropriate sex-linked behavior. Normal female development can be changed by introducing excessive androgen. For instance, girls born of mothers who were given progestational agents during pregnancy to prevent spontaneous abortion often turn out to be tomboys. Male development can also be modified by the blocking of androgen uptake. Ward has reported that maternal stress has a demasculinizing effect on some male offspring. The hypothesis is that under stress the mother's adrenals secrete an androgenlike steroid which competes for receptor sites in the "sexual center" of the developing brain, preventing the action of testosterone in completing the "male behavior" programming of the fetus' brain.

Genetic or constitutional faults may create abnormalities in biological sex which may be minor or major. Major abnormalities create problems of intersexuality. If not corrected early in life, they may lead to conflicts in sexual or gender identity.

In brief, a deficiency or excess of internal hormones, as well as viral infections, trauma, toxicity, nutritional deficiency, or maternal stress may adversely affect the fetus even before the environment can become effective after birth.

SEXUAL IDENTITY

Sexual identity is sometimes referred to as "coregender identity" (Stoller). It may be defined as the person's inner feeling of maleness or femaleness over time, a feeling that is reinforced by the ways in which people, notably parents, react. Blue or pink is an early manifestation of sex assignment. Ordinarily, the presence of appropriate external genitals is the strongest reinforcer, except in children with ambiguous sexual morphology who have been subjected to ambiguous sex rearing, and transsexuals, who are convinced that they belong to the opposite sex and may reject their body appearance. Normal psychosexual develop-

ment leads to a secure sense of maleness or femaleness by the age of 3.

GENDER IDENTITY

This refers to the broader, vaguer concepts of masculinity and femininity. In the stereotype, masculinity is associated with assertive, even aggressive behavior, competitiveness, strength, sexual prowess, rational thinking, financial success, and so forth, while femininity means passive-receptive stance, gentleness, nurturance, and seductiveness. The individual learns masculine or feminine identity by a series of experiences which reinforce or extinguish certain gender-linked attitudes and behavior. In our culture, sexual "scoring" is a masculine reinforcement for adolescent boys, and social popularity is the chief reinforcer for adolescent girls. Doubts and conflicts about gender identity are almost universal in United States culture. Serious disturbances lead to sex deviation such as transvestism, fetishism, voyeurism, and exhibitionism. Homosexuality is a special variation of gender identity in that homosexuals do not doubt their maleness or femaleness, that is, their sexual identity.

In milder disturbances of gender identity, reparative efforts at reassurance cover a wide spectrum from compulsive promiscuity to competitiveness in sports, or by dress and appearance. Inhibitory or avoidance responses are equally common. Attitudes and behavior toward the opposite sex are strongly influenced by the sense of security or insecurity about one's gender identity. Most of the problems in marriage that are played out in the battle of the sexes have their roots in gender insecurity. There are strong societal influences which cause many women to regard themselves as inferior. Males are not exempt from insecurity because of the great pressure placed on performance and achievement. The ultimate symbol of masculine achievement is erection and intromission hence the frequent impotence caused by nonsexual competitive failures. Paralleling impotence is the failure of women to become aroused and responsive in sexual situations because of inner doubts about femininity caused by nonsexual threats to feminine self-esteem, e.g., the reaction to hysterectomy.

GENDER ROLE BEHAVIOR

Gender role behavior is divided into sex behavior and gender behavior. *Sex behavior* is physical sex in all of its aspects, based on the desire for sexual pleasure, ultimately orgasm; *gender behavior* is behavior with masculine and feminine connotations. (It is difficult to think of any behavior that does not have *some* gender implication, but there is enormous variation in degree.) The sexual response cycle and sexual dysfunctions come under the category of sex behavior; sexual relatedness or relationship comes under the category of gender behavior. Gender behavior was once handed down or assigned by tradition; today roles are negotiable, and problems may become serious if negotiation is impossible because of faulty communciation. In turn, communication often breaks down because of disturbed perception, the fear of compromise, or conflicts over rights and privileges.

One may separate sexual behavior and gender behavior for the purposes of analysis and study, but in actual functioning, sex and sexuality are intimately connected. With rare exceptions, sexual relations and relationships are different facets of a mosaic, with complex patternings and interfaces.

THE PHYSIOLOGY OF SEXUAL RESPONSE

Through the pioneering efforts of Robert Latou Dickenson we obtained information about human sexual anatomy and, to a lesser extent, physiology. For example, his anatomical atlas of drawings demonstrates the shape and size (range up to 20 mm) of the clitoris in its flaccid and erect states in great detail. At the turn of the century, the Chicago gynecologist Denslow Lewis had described the role of the clitoris and had even described the retraction of the clitoris under its hood. But we are indebted to Masters and Johnson for their basic research in human sexual physiology, especially in the female. Since the publication of their work in 1966, it seems unnecessary to repeat the details of their description of the four stages of sexual response: excitement, the plateau, orgasm, and resolution.

STAGES OF SEXUAL RESPONSE

Sexual Motive Stage

There is, however, a preparatory psychological stage that exists prior to excitement. Through anticipatory arousal, a person develops a "sexual motive stage." As the individual anticipates the approach of a sexual situation, excitement often begins before there is any tactile stimulation. This anticipatory state of arousal may occur many minutes before the start of actual physical contact. This state normally decreases with age, or with repeated experiences with the same partner. Some people have such an intense sexual inhibition that anticipatory arousal is blocked and, instead, anticipatory anxiety takes over. If this happens, there is a strong likelihood that no part of the mechanism of arousal will occur, and the stage of excitement will be stopped before it can begin. There are therapeutic implications relating to the level at which inhibition occurs—at the level of early arousal, during the stage of excitement, and at the level of orgasm—the three primary levels of psychic inhibition.

Major emphasis will be given to the stages of response in the female, augmented by a discussion of some of the major differences between male and female sexual arousal.

Excitement

Sexual excitement results in local and genital vasocongestion of the skin including the beginning of mottling; myotonia; swelling of the breasts; erection of the nipples; beginning vaginal lubrication; vasocongestion of clitoris; enlargement of the uterus which rises in the pelvis; beginning of the ballooning of the vaginal barrel.

The Plateau

Increased mottling of skin; swelling and coloration of labia minora; rising of the uterus anteriorly; lumen of the outer one-third of the vagina reduced in size; formation of "orgasmic platform" (Masters and Johnson's term for the vaginal and perivaginal muscles that contract during orgasm) in the lower portion of the vagina; retraction of clitoris just prior to orgasm.

Orgasm

At orgasm, reflex rhythmic contractions of the circumvaginal and perineal muscles and swollen tissues of the orgasmic platform occur at 0.8-second intervals. In the female, multiple orgasms may occur seconds after she has achieved the first orgasm.

Resolution

Heart rate, blood pressure, respiration, and skin vasodilatation are decreased during resolution; clitoris returns to normal position within seconds; the "sex skin" of the labia minora loses its deep coloration within 10 to 15 seconds; detumescence of the orgasmic platform occurs; cervical os closes in 20 to 30 minutes; uterus descends to its usual position.

The pleasure sensations of the female are probably derived in part from the pacinian corpuscles, which mediate deep pressure and proprioception. These receptors are most numerous in the clitoris and, to a somewhat lesser extent, in the mons veneris and the labia. They are absent or almost completely absent in the vagina. From a histologic standpoint, the vagina is completely anesthetic, although the vaginal musculature contains the deep pressure receptors.

From an anatomic and physiologic standpoint, it seems clear that the clitoris is the primary site of erotic arousal, whether stimulated directly by finger or tongue, or indirectly during coitus by the pull on the preputial hood. In addition to the pacinian corpuscles described above, the clitoris is also richly supplied with sensory nerve endings sensitive to touch. In fact, it may be so exquisitely sensitive that direct tactile stimulation of the area may be, for some women at some times, intolerable, especially when not lubricated. The outer one-third of the vagina is reported as highly pleasurable and erotic by many women, although these sensations are of a different kind from the sensations experienced when the clitoris is stimulated. Although most women report they respond to a combination of vaginal and clitoral sensation, the majority state the clitoral stimulation makes the more important contribution to orgasm. Fewer than 10 percent state that vaginal stimulation is the more significant dimension of the experience (Fisher).

In brief, no matter what the source of the stimulation, orgasm is probably almost always evoked by clitoral stimulation. (There are a few women who have an orgasm either through fantasy or breast stimulation alone.) Whatever the source of stimulation, however, orgasm is always expressed by certain circumvaginal or orgasmic-platform muscle discharge. The reflex orgasm thus has a sensory and a motor component, the clitoris being the essential factor in the sensory component, and the circumvaginal muscles in the motor (Kaplan). Facilitation and inhibition are both caused by stimuli from the higher neural centers acting through a spinal reflex center, thus accounting for low or high thresholds of erotic arousal for different women, or for the same woman at different times.

In ordinary experience, most men can come to the point of ejaculation much more rapidly than women can come to the point of orgasm. This is, however, apparently the result of either inadequate preparation by the male partner, or a psychic inhibition. Most responsive women attain their orgasm within 8 minutes during coitus. However, many women with inhibition of coital orgasm can achieve orgasm through masturbation within 2 minutes. This indicates that probably psychologic factors are even more important than physiologic ones in inhibiting coital orgasm. Nonetheless, it is important to recognize that men and women react differently to anxiety. If anxiety does not cause failure in erection, it is apt to cause a quick ejaculation, while in the female it is more apt to retard orgasm. Thus, if anxiety is present in both partners, coital orgasm is much less likely to occur.

SIMILARITIES AND DIFFERENCES OF MALE AND FEMALE RESPONSES

In many ways the male response is parallel to that of the female: vasocongestion, myotonia, and ejaculation are comparable phenomena to those taking place in the female, with the exception that the female does not ejaculate. The number and frequency of contractions are the same. Similarly, both excitement and orgasm in male and female carry analogous mechanisms of autonomic-nervous-system discharge. There is a complex interplay between the sympathetic (adrenergic) and parasympathetic (cholinergic) systems, with one dominant in one phase and the other dominant in the other. In the male, vasocongestion and erection seem to be governed by the parasympathetic system, and ejaculation by the sympathetic nervous system. (Emission results from a somewhat different mechanism than does ejaculation.) In the female, lubrication and arousal seem to be under the control of the parasympathetic system, while the muscular contractions of orgasm are under the control of the sympathetic system (Kaplan). It is possible, then, to make a sharper clinical differentiation between impotence and premature ejaculation, as well as retarded ejaculation in the male, and between failure in arousal and failure to have an orgasm in the female. These seem to be parallel phenomena.

The most striking difference between males and females is the capacity of the female to have multiple orgasms. In view of the attitude expressed in the past that woman either do not enjoy sex or are essentially passive and should follow the lead of the male who has the higher sexual drive, it is ironic to recognize that, biologically, the orgastic potential of the female is limited only by physical exhaustion. She does not have a refractory period, as does the male.

Additional evidence that the female's role in sex may be much more initiatory than reactive has been reported by Persky et al. (1977). Couples in their twenties were studied through three successive ovulatory menstrual cycles (31 ovulating cycles). The investigators found that testosterone levels in the males peaked at the same time in the cycle the females' levels peaked, namely at ovulation and approximately a week later. How this information is transmitted from the female to the male is not known.

THE SINGLE FEMALE

ADOLESCENT PSYCHOSEXUAL DEVELOPMENT

During the variable period of adolescent psychosexual development, psychological and social responses to puberty are shaped by biological, cultural, and psychological influences. The biological aspects of puberty and adolescence are discussed in Chapter 17. The preadolescent child shows increasing emotional lability, partly due to the rising production of sex hormones influencing behavior even before the physical signs of puberty appear. Among girls, homoerotic play peaks between the ages of 9 and 11, and through age 13 remains more common than heterosexual play. Under the influence of increasing amounts of sex hormones, erotic play increases, more safely carried out with same-sex peers than with the less familiar members of the opposite sex.

Part of the early adolescent's struggle for independence and self-reliance relates to her need to distance herself emotionally from the parent of the opposite sex and to focus her growing sexual interests on a boy outside the family. The pull toward and away from her parents is a principal factor in the turbulence of this period of life. This becomes a period of intense preoccupation with self in the context of exploring sexual feelings and behaviors. By the time they reach the senior year in high school, about 50 percent of girls have experimented with masturbation; the eventual cumulative incidence approaches 80 percent by the age of 25 (Miller, Lief).

Early adolescence gradually evolves into later adolescence without a sharp point of demarcation. It occurs about the age of 16 in girls, and a year or two later in boys. Self-centered sexual preoccupation develops into a greater concern with relationships and their meaning, the implications of caring and sharing, the risks and rewards of being emotionally involved.

Of 21 million adolescents in the United States, about 11 million are coitally active. By the end of high school, in most areas 50 percent or more of the males have had coitus and the proportion is often higher among girls. The trend toward almost universal premarital intercourse, as in Sweden, is definite; Zelnik and Kantner (1977) reported it to be 80 percent. By the end of their teens, a clear majority of adolescents have experienced intercourse at least once.

Emotional readiness for active sexuality, especially for coitus with its attendant risks of pregnancy and venereal disease, varies greatly. There is no evidence that sexual intercourse per se is damaging. The reward in emotional growth or, on the other hand, the cost to the teenage girl, is derived from the consequences of coitus and the emotional significance of the relationship. The gynecologist has a splendid opportunity to be helpful in counseling the teenager about relationships, as well as about the prevention of pregnancy and venereal disease. The key to good counseling is the development of a "therapeutic alliance" with a patient, an alliance which is in turn dependent on developing an empathic and trusting relationship. Such a relationship is created by the physician's ability to listen, to tactfully inquire, to understand, to label feelings honestly and, above all, to be comfortable with sexual topics.

Many gynecologists are now prepared to prescribe contraceptives to unmarried minors; in the past they were reluctant to do so. Their new attitude has been created by the following factors: (1) About half of the states now have laws which permit minors to obtain medical attention, contraceptives and abortion without their parents' permission. (2) Studies show that by age 19 the majority of teenage unmarried girls have had coital experience. (3) It has become widely understood that most teenage girls ask for contraceptive services after, rather than before, beginning coital activity, so the gynecologist has little reason to think that prescribing a contraceptive method will be a license for sexual activity. (4) The often devastating effects of becoming a teenage unmarried parent on the educational, vocational, and emotional aspects of life have been well documented. (5) The ultimate risks of marital strife and divorce among those who marry after becoming pregnant are extremely high— the divorce rate is close to 80 percent.

ADOLESCENT SEXUAL PROBLEMS

Since sexual problems during adolescence are discussed in Chapter 17, only a brief review is included in this section. Guilt over masturbation, while decreasing, has not entirely disappeared. Although the cumulative incidence of masturbation in females has increased from 63 percent (Kinsey et al.) to 78 percent (Miller, Lief), only 57 percent of females masturbated prior to the age of 19, indicating that the inhibitory effects of societal repression have not been eliminated, despite the "sexual revolution." (Paradoxically, 19 percent of females stated they had masturbated prior to the age of 10.) Only occasionally does guilt over masturbation create clear-cut symptoms, physical or mental. Masturbatory guilt, however, may influence the adolescent girl's reaction to the gynecologist's sexual interviewing or the physical examination itself. A more significant factor is the influence of masturbatory guilt in creating sexual inhibition which interferes with the capacity for orgasm in heterosexual play or coitus. Other problems during adolescence discussed in Chapter 17 are unwanted pregnancy, venereal disease, and pelvic inflammatory diseases such as vaginitis and cystitis, which may affect sexual functioning.

The gynecologist is apt to be consulted about several other problem areas revolving around conflicts in relationships and sexual performance. Even though there has been a vast liberalization of attitudes toward premarital sexual behavior, many adolescent girls are still concerned about virginity; "how far to go" is an age-old problem that still persists. Even if the girl herself does not feel that premarital intercourse is wrong, she may be torn between her need for sexual expression, her desire for intimacy, and the fear that there will be parental and social disapproval. Although petting to orgasm is a norm among high school girls, many are still fearful of that degree of sexual behavior, since they are uncertain of their capacity to control themselves or their partners. Some girls have little difficulty about accepting intercourse as desirable behavior but have qualms about engaging in coitus with a particular male; it isn't the sex act itself but the relationship that may be the major concern. In helping the teenager with relationship problems, the ability of the gynecologist to listen, to inquire, understand, and label the feelings of the young woman is probably more helpful than direct advice. The "bottom line" of the physician's task is to sum up the advantages and disadvantages of the various alternatives, enhancing the capacity of the adolescent to make responsible decisions. Certainly, the sexually active young woman should be aware of her contraceptive responsibilities. The clear-cut correlations between adolescent girls who "always" or "sometimes" or "never" use contraceptives and the number who become pregnant have been established by the studies of Zelnik and Kantner (1978). Pregnancies in always-users is 10.9 percent, in sometimes-users 23.9 percent, and in never-users 58 percent.

Adolescent girls do have concerns about performance. This is particularly true of those who are cohabiting. An ongoing relationship with a steady boyfriend brings to the fore concerns about capacity for sexual excitement and orgasm. If the relationship is sufficiently stable, especially if a long-term relationship is contemplated, the couple should be treated in the same way that one would treat a married couple. If the relationship is a troubled one, the gynecologist's attention should usually be directed toward the relationship instead of the sexual difficulties per se, since the latter may very well be a consequence of the disturbed relationship.

It should be recalled that 50 percent of nonvirgins had coitus only with a fiance and that many other nonvirgins had only one partner during the previous year. Those adolescents who had four, five, or more partners are at risk not only for pregnancy and venereal disease, but on occasion for premalignant or malignant lesions of the cervix. It is also possible that sexually active adolescent girls may be at greater risk of developing antisperm antibodies and infertility when they have intercourse with a number of peers since preliminary studies indicate that an immunosuppressant in the male ejaculate that prevents an autoimmune reaction to spermatozoa is absent in males under the age of 20 (Rauh, Burket).

Another relationship problem area is the fear of a young woman that she is developing an erotic interest in females. This may lead to difficulty in defining her own gender identity and a sense of isolation from many of her peers, frequently accompanied by an intense internal struggle heightened by actual or anticipated parental and societal disapproval or rejection. The gynecologist should adopt a neutral, noncondemnatory, nonjudgmental approach. Too quick an acceptance of the patient's "lesbianism" may increase the young woman's anxiety for she may be far from certain of her sexual preferences. On the other hand, a judgmental, censorious attitude will make her too uncomfortable to remain in treatment. It may take considerable time for the gynecologist to help the patient reach some sense of sexual direction, and then to help her with the social skills necessary to achieve a degree of intimacy, either heterosexual or homosexual. If her preference is for lesbianism, the physician may also be called on to help the patient deal realistically with her parents and, possibly, with school authorities.

THE NEVER-MARRIED WOMAN

Spurred by the drive for sexual equality and the liberalization of sexual attitudes, there have been striking changes in courtship patterns, in premarital coital sex, and in heterosexual "bonding" arrangements.

Courtship

Courtship has changed from the premarital "bundling" of the early settlers in the United States to "going steady" and, for approximately 20 to 25 percent of college students, "living together." The latter is the most visible of all the new forms of courtship. With the decrease in colleges of the policy of in loco parentis as well as the freedom of young people from adult supervision of any kind, premarital heterosexual living together is likely to increase in the next few decades. A striking feature of this form of cohabitation is the attitude toward having children. These couples use modern contraceptive methods, usually the pill, in order to avoid pregnancy. If pregnancy occurs, the couples are apt to resort to abortion or to marriage. If a prime function of marriage is to legitimatize the offspring of that union, this type of cohabitation is not an alternative to marriage, but a more open sexual affair between people who are emotionally involved with each other (Reiss, 1976). While cohabitation may be increasingly endorsed by society, it is unlikely to become a substitute for marriage. The tax, inheritance, and legal difficulties encountered by couples who are not married probably will preclude the substitution of this form of relationship for the institution of marriage. However, the increase in premarital heterosexual living together is reducing the marriage rate and increasing the age at marriage for females. It may be playing a minor role in the reduced birthrate as well. In any case, the relationship is based on the exchange of affection, and intimacy remains a dominant theme.

Premarital Sexual Relations

Demographic data now make it clear that there have been two periods of very rapid attitudinal and behav-

ioral change in the 20th century in the United States. The first period was approximately from 1915 to 1920, the second from approximately 1965 to 1970. In the first period the proportion of females nonvirginal at marriage doubled from 25 to 50 percent; in the second period the increase rose from 50 percent to a current rate between 75 and 80 percent. It is of interest that those were times of rapid social change in all our major social institutions. In the first period, the major social change was urbanization; in the second period, demands for civil rights legislation and women's rights were the signs that society's concerns had shifted from production of goods to equitable distribution of goods and services. With these changes has come an increase in the capacity to make sexual choices, accompanied by a rise in the divorce rate and a rise in premarital pregnancy. The latter two are unfortunate consequences of the increased freedom of choice. The search for equity is altering our marriage and family relations, as well as our sexual relations, and more flexible male and female role models in and outside of marriage are in the process of development.

Sexual Problems of the Never-Married Woman

Sexual problems of the never-married woman are in two major categories: (1) sexual dysfunctions and (2) relationship problems.

Sexual dysfunctions include inhibition of sexual desire, excitement, and orgasm, and are discussed in detail later in this chapter. If the woman has a quasi-permanent relationship with a man, even if she is not living with him, treatment by the physician differs little from the treatment of a married couple. Ambivalence about commitment to the relationship may modify the attitude of either the woman or her partner toward sex counseling. Resistance to treatment may occur because of conflicts about the nature of the relationship. These attitudes also occur in marriages, but are apt to be more frequent in cohabiting couples. If the woman does not have an ongoing quasi-permanent relationship with a man, the gynecologist should try to determine whether her essential difficulty is in establishing intimacy, or if she is a woman who has the capacity to develop an ongoing relationship but nevertheless has one or more sexual problems. In other words, does she have a discrete sexual problem or a personality problem with sexual manifestations? If it is a personality problem, referral to a mental health therapist is probably the course of action taken by most gynecologists. If it is a specific sexual problem which does not respond to education and counseling in approximately six counseling sessions, referral to a sex counselor or therapist is indicated.

Some women are poor "pair-bonders." Their relationship problems are related to conflicts over intimacy. Some women are frightened of close relations. They may be schizoid or so-called "borderline patients" who manifest suspiciousness and fear of dependency (despite being overly dependent) because of an underlying fear of being abandoned. At the same time they are frightened of loneliness and have little capacity to enjoy their own company. They flit from relationship to relationship. For these women sexual problems are a manifestation of a more basic fear of intimacy. If the gynecologist diagnoses this form of personality difficulty, referral to a psychiatrist or other mental health therapist is indicated.

In treating single women, the gynecologist's role often focuses on contraceptive counseling, counseling for unplanned pregnancies, and the treatment of venereal disease. Since the gynecologist is the primary-care physician for approximately 85 percent of the female population, both married and unmarried, it is likely that this percentage is even higher for unmarried women. (For married women the primary-care physician is sometimes the physician who also treats the husband.) The single woman may bring mental and emotional as well as nongynecological physical problems to the gynecologist for treatment. For this reason the gynecologist often plays the role of "first contact" psychotherapist. The gynecologist's diagnostic skills are essential in making certain that the patient has appropriate treatment or referral for emotional, including sexual, problems.

Problems of Homosexuality

Long-standing relationships are more frequent among female than among male homosexuals. Kissing, fondling, and mutual masturbation are the primary sources of sexual gratification. Lesbian patients are less likely to complain of sexual dysfunction than of problems of their total relationship. They are more likely to seek out a female than a male gynecologist. In many instances, the physician will not be able to distinguish the unmarried lesbian from a heterosexual woman who has never married. There are far fewer obvious "male" or "butch" lesbians than is commonly believed. Between 60 and 70 percent of lesbians are exclusively homosexual in their current sexual behavior, leaving a sizable minority who maintain some heterosexual contacts (Bell, Weinberg).

A married woman who is homosexual and comes to the physician to remedy her sexual conflicts is best referred tactfully to a psychiatrist.

THE WOMAN WHO MARRIES

The strains on the contemporary marital pair are enormous. The traditional pattern of family formation, involving the creation of an intimate, heterosexual, couple relationship in which the couple establishes a household and forms a nuclear family (parents and children without other kinfolk) puts great psychic strain on the members of the marital unit. The nuclear family, often relatively isolated from friends and relatives and from a variety of support systems in the community such as church, fraternal orders, and clubs, demands that each partner meet most of the other's emotional needs—in fact, to be, almost, the other's psychotherapist. In addition, the partner is expected to provide stimulation and excitement, to share in the economic responsibilities and social tasks, and to raise a family. The extended family of several generations back provided more emotional support, as well as surrogate parents, giving the husband and wife greater freedom. It is a common estimate that four of every ten marriages end in divorce, and of the remaining six marriages, three are chronically unhappy.

The stress does not fall equally upon the husband and wife. More wives than husbands report marital problems and consider their marriages to be unhappy, consider separation or divorce, or have regretted their marriages. The mental health hazards for married women are far greater than for married men. More married women than married men have felt they were about to have a nervous breakdown; more experience psychological and physical anxieties; more demonstrate a variety of psychiatric symptoms and, as Bernard points out, marriage protects men more than women against suicide: "only about half as many white married as single men commit suicide; almost three-fourths as many married women as single women do."

It might be thought that this is simply a sex difference, and that women in general are "sicker" than men. However, when one examines the differences between married and unmarried women, one finds that married women are more severely damaged psychologically than are unmarried women. Whether one chooses to compare them on the basis of symptoms of psychological dysfunction such as anxiety, phobias, depression, social inhibitions, discontent with work, fear of death, hypochondriasis, or psychosomatic symptoms, married women are affected far more than unmarried women. In addition, unmarried women are healthier than unmarried men: they show less than the expected frequency of psychological distress and are less often depressed. If one uses social indices, one finds that single women are more educated, have higher average incomes, and are in higher occupations than are single men. Single women are "spectacularly better off so far as psychological distress symptoms are concerned" than are married men, "suggesting that women start out with an initial advantage, which marriage reverses" (Bernard).

It has been postulated by some social scientists that the shock of marriage is greater for the bride than for the bridegroom. The wife ceases to be looked after and pampered and becomes the one who has to nurture her husband. Many wives also come to realize that their overidealization of their husbands during courtship leads to disillusionment. If the woman acquires the status of her husband, it is a reflected status that does not create self-esteem.

Working women do not suffer from the above-cited complaints to the same degree as nonworking married women. The complaints of the "unemployed" married woman have been referred to as the "housewife syndrome." The woman who is relatively well-educated and is unable or unwilling to make use of her education often becomes a bored, middle-aged housewife with a variety of psychosomatic complaints including headache, backache, vaginal discharge, dysmenorrhea, or other ailments. These women often go from physician to physician in order to find the magic potion which will relieve their stress when, in fact, their problems are the result of a particular lifestyle and the difficulties it creates.

Working mothers tend to be much healthier and better off than housewives. Fewer of them have nervous breakdowns and fewer of them suffer from nervousness, insomnia, nightmares, fainting, headache, and dizziness. Forty-two percent of married women are in the work force; conversely, 60 percent of working women are married.

This dismal picture is offset in cases in which the nonworking married woman takes great satisfaction in running her household, rearing the children, and helping her husband.

Highlights of some of the major aspects are needed if the gynecologist is to have the perspective required to treat marital sexual problems. Following Erikson, the tasks of the young adult are seen as the capacity to establish intimacy and to attain an occupational identification; both taken together form the nucleus of a person's "ego identity." An individual's self-concept is based on one's competence and effectiveness, especially in work and the ability to elicit love from significant others. Intimacy involves not only the capacity to share affection and sexual pleasure with another, but also includes the ability to share joys, pains, triumphs, and defeats with the loved person, and it means the capacity to subordinate one's own needs and expectations to the needs of the marital unit, without being so submissive that one becomes a self-sacrificing cipher or serves only as an appendage of the partner. In our society, this is more difficult for the female than for the male. The traditional marriage is male dominated, with sexual specialization and tasks within the house assigned by tradition; the female tends to subordinate herself for the family's survival. Individual growth and the pursuit of autonomy are often sacrificed for the husband's career and the welfare of the family. It is against this traditional format that the women's liberation movement delivers many of its criticisms.

If the woman has aspirations for an occupational identification other than "housewife," these difficulties are often augmented. Social sanction as well as approval by the mate may not solve the problem because she has been programmed to adopt the traditional attitudes (conformity, emotionality, submissiveness, coquettishness, etc.) and stereotyped sex roles of her mother and grandmother, potentially setting up an internal conflict. If she pursues outside activities, she is filled with guilt; if she gives them up, she is filled with resentment. Juggling an occupational identification along with a household is apt to result in frustration, internal conflict, or conflict with her husband, her parents, and with social attitudes in general.

If she is successful in lasting through these stages of psychosocial development with a good ego identity and sense of worth, she is well prepared for the next stage—that of "generativity." For a woman whose primary tasks are within the household, this usually involves the creating of new life and the caring for and of her offspring. Generativity may, of course, include creative activities in the professional world, or in the expression of artistic or athletic skills, etc. For the woman who is dissatisfied with motherhood but has no ready access to other creative activities, or inhibits these because of internal or external conflict, significant trouble in her marriage may result.

The woman who has attained a feeling of creativity and generativity generally has little difficulty in dealing with the anticipation of old age and death. For those who feel unfulfilled, the prospects of aging and of death often create an intense feeling of despair.

Within this broad overview of the life cycle, biologic events which have significant consequences, not only for the marriage but for the woman's sex life, include pregnancy, childbirth and childrearing, the effects of the menstrual cycle, the menopause, and infertility. The aging process leads to certain physiologic changes which affect sexuality. In addition to these biologic events—including illnesses—social events leave their mark. Stressful experiences include new jobs, moving from one locality to another, deaths in the family, economic loss or threats, divorce, etc. The inquisitive gynecologist will be alert to these life-cycle events and the effects they may have on the feelings, attitudes, and behavior of patients.

SEXUAL CONCERNS OF THE WOMAN WHO MARRIES

The Premarital Stage

During the premarital examination, patients may want sex education and sex counseling in addition to the usual physical examination and venereal-disease testing (Nash, Louden). This, unfortunately, is rarely included, often because of an unconscious collusion of silence between the physician and the premarital couple. Generally, the couple are seen separately, but even if they are seen together, the typical physician is uncomfortable about asking about their sexual hopes and fears, let alone their actual sexual behavior. The couple, each blinded by the overidealization of the mate, may hide their fears and concerns. The wife is worried about her inexperience and fears about being hurt or, if she is already experienced, she wonders if her sexual life will be changed by marriage. But she may be reluctant to reveal this to her partner, let alone the physician. The bridegroom may be hiding his concerns about sexual incompetence, such as premature ejaculation, or he may be worried that the change in their general relationship will adversely affect their sexual relationship as they shift from a dating-and-courting arrangement to one in which they will be together far more often than heretofore. This presents an excellent opportunity for preventive medical intervention; a few moments of appropriate listening and counseling may prevent unnecessary anguish later. Not to discuss family planning including contraceptive care at this juncture is almost unethical, yet it seems that this opportunity is often lost.

Early Marriage

Despite the increase in premarital coitus, inexperience still plays a role in sexual nonresponsivity during the first years of marriage. If the husband is having trouble with potency and his bride is unable to help him, he becomes resentful, worries about his masculinity, and withdraws. Similarly, the bride who is tense and finds intercourse either painful or disappointing may avoid coitus. Even if the couple continues to have intercourse on a fairly regular basis, the built-up resentment creates further difficulties in sexual performance.

The physician is apt to respond to sexual concerns mentioned in the early months of marriage by telling the patients, "This is a phase, and it will pass." This is sometimes true, and the couple may work things out on their own. But if they are greatly disappointed and cannot effectively talk with each other about it, and if anger builds up, considerable marital strife may result.

During his twenties, the husband is generally concerned with his occupational identification, attempting to get ahead, while his wife is at home, perhaps taking care of their young children and the household. Resentment may occur if the husband no longer gives his wife the attention that he had given her during the courtship or early years of marriage. If she does little to develop new interests, she may become boring to her husband. Frequently he suggests that she go back to school or find some outside occupation. The wife may resent this, not only because of her own inner conflicts, but because she recognizes that often he wants this for his own convenience rather than for her development.

The conflict of interests between husband and wife may reach a crescendo in their late twenties. A transition point is reached between the ages (approximate) of 28 and 32, when people subconsciously review their lives, including their marriages, work, and life-styles, and decide on additional commitment or change. Change may include infidelity and/or separation from each other as the "7 year itch" becomes an open, painful, festering wound. It is at this point that many people seek marriage counseling (Berman, et al.). Along the way many men have had their first extramarital relationship during the wife's first pregnancy.

If the marriage continues and if the couple passes through this normative transition (not always a crisis) in good shape, commitments deepen both to job and to marriage. And yet, satisfaction with marriage too often goes downhill because there is continuing disillusionment as the early expectations of both the husband and the wife are not fulfilled.

Mid-Marriage

Another crisis period occurs between the late thirties and early forties in what might be called the "midlife transition," when there is an attempt to assess what has gone on before in terms of what one can expect in the future. This reappraisal by the male often creates a period of depression in his early forties, which may affect his potency. Much of the spark may go out of the marriage and, unless there is adequate communication and an attempt to find sufficient variety in their sexual expression, apathy may set in. If the marriage again sustains these normative periods of crisis, it is apt to take a satisfying turn during the couple's forties. The two people have taken stock and have recognized they will not achieve everything they have hoped for, nor can they expect complete understanding from the spouse nor the satisfaction of all their needs. If this happens in a realistic fashion, their sexual life is apt to be a fairly satisfactory one for both partners.

During her forties and early fifties, the woman has to face two other normative crises. The children leave home, and she goes through the menopause. Her adjustment is dependent on two factors: (1) the degree of security in her feminine identity; and (2) whether her emotional interests have been almost entirely within the household, or whether there had been sufficient interests outside the home. If her feelings about her feminine identity have been based on physical beauty and her capacity to bear children rather than on her feeling of worth as a person and the satisfaction she has had in the variety of roles she has played, she may face depression. Insecurity and depression often create sexual problems with a decreased interest in sex and a decreased capacity to respond in a woman who previously had enjoyed sex.

Later Years

After the age of 60, sexual activity drops off quite sharply, but does not decrease as much for the woman who has an available partner and who has had pleasurable sexual experiences during midlife. The most significant difference between sexual activity for men and women over 60 is the unavailability of partners for many women who outlive their men. The need for companionship and physical contact can of-

ten be as important as the release of sexual tensions. The wise physician can help by advising older women wherever possible about suitable living arrangements, so that these gratifications may be more readily obtained. Society makes it difficult for older women without partners to have even a modicum of male companionship, let alone sexual gratification.

On a biologic level, with the decrease and eventual cessation of ovarian function, estrogenic replacement is necessary in order to prevent the vaginal mucosa from becoming dry and paper-thin. Whether steroid replacement therapy is oral, local, or a combination of both, or whether it should be used at all, in view of the possibility of cancer, is a matter of clinical judgment (see Chap. 35).

THE MARRIED WOMAN AND HER FAMILY

The pressures on the marital unit and hence on the family have been described in the preceding section. Despite the push for new life-styles, the nuclear family is a stable pattern which is likely to be retained for the rest of this century. Changes will occur, giving women a greater degree of equality and autonomy, but within the same nuclear family system. It should be borne in mind, however, that the proportion of families consisting of the stereotypical two parents and one or more young children (under age 18) with no one else in the household has been declining since 1970. In 1970 it was 40 percent; in 1977, 35 percent. In other societies, as they move toward urban industrial development, the nuclear family is becoming the dominant pattern, in which there are fewer ties with distant relatives, and there is much greater stress on the father, mother, and their children.

If there is a romantic view of marriage in our culture, there is still greater romanticism with regard to the role of parent. Inadequate as may be the preparation for marriage, it is much better than preparation for parenthood. The shift from a two-person to a three-person group is a normative crisis. An addition to the family might be similar psychologically to the loss of a key person in the family. In one study, 38 of 46 couples reported that the birth of the first child precipitated severe crisis (LeMasters). The women reported loss of sleep, loss of social activity, additional work, and increased worry. The men reported less sexual response from their wives, more economic pressures, and more work.

Other studies, however, have failed to confirm LeMasters' view that first parenthood was a crisis.

Other researchers concluded that the advent of the first child was a significant transition point in the maturation of the marital relationship, but that for most couples the new triadic system was more rewarding than the old dyadic one. In general, beginning parenthood was no worse than moderately stressful for 80 to 95 percent of the subjects who were studied. Findings, however, consistently indicated that more difficulty was experienced by mothers than by fathers. In a representative sample of couples, over 90 percent of the subjects reported that prior to the birth of their child, their marriages were happy and satisfying and that most problems which arose after the birth of the first child were resolved. It seems safe to generalize that if a marriage has been unrewarding and troubled, the advent of the first child increases frustration and conflict, but if the marriage has been a satisfying one, the marital relationship is enhanced by the coming of the first child.

The romantic myths about becoming a parent increase the disillusionment of women, most of whom suffer from some variant of "postpartum blues" and then feel guilty about it. This is succeeded by a period in which there may be a severe loss of energy and excessive fatigue. All of this tends to diminish the woman's interest in sexual activity. Feldman found that the advent of children led to a decrease in both marital communication and marital satisfaction. For most couples, the joys of parenthood soon outweigh the immediate crisis situation. However, an unstable marital relationship with mutual dissatisfaction will be adversely affected by parenthood. The impact of children on marital and especially on sexual gratification varies from family to family. For some marriages, children increase the feeling of intimacy, but for others they serve as a force separating husband and wife (Rollins and Feldman).

About 10 percent of all marriages remain childless, with about 30 percent of those being by design. There is a trend developing toward an increase in purposely childless marriages. The proportion of families consisting of childless couples has been increasing (from 28 percent in 1970 to 30 percent of all families in 1977). This is, of course, a time-related statistic, because two out of three of these families will eventually have children. While divorce for childless couples is more common than among those with children, when the marriage survives, it is apt to be a happier one. The wave of the future, however, does not seem to be childlessness, but families with fewer children. Families with many children are prone to increased stress. There is more ill health in parents with large families, especially mothers. An inverse rela-

tionship exists between marital adjustment and family size; that is, the more children, the worse the adjustment. Having more than one child early in marriage is also correlated with a poorer marital adjustment, and the poorest marital adjustment is found among couples with unwanted children.

Studies of marital satisfaction through the life cycle indicate that the nadir of general marital satisfaction occurs when children are between the ages of 6 and 14. This stage seems to be especially hard on the wives. Positive companionship is at its lowest level, as is satisfaction with the children. While the husband is devoting most of his energies to his work, the wife is swamped by demands from all sides. Many women go through a developmental crisis of their own as they struggle for autonomy in the face of family pressures. Rearing of teenagers often creates friction between husband and wife, which has its negative effect on sex relations. Despite the pressures that lead to the "empty-nest" syndrome, studies indicate that marital satisfaction *increases* when the children leave home.

It can easily be seen that to understand the sexual life of a patient, a gynecologist should attempt to obtain additional information about what is going on in her family.

WORKING-CLASS MARRIAGES

Black "blue-collar" marriages have not been studied as intensively as have marriages of white couples in this social class, so the following discussion is confined to white marriages.

Sexual problems are frequent in white working-class marriages. Prominent are conflicts over frequency, oral sex, sexual experimentation, and orgasm in the females. These conflicts stem from the different ways in which working-class men and women are socialized. Men frequently have difficulty expressing their feelings except in sex, while the woman's development encourages the expression of emotions in all phases of life other than the sexual one (Rubin).

Working-class women want their men to be affectionate and to share their feelings about many things with them; then they feel like making love. Men feel that the only way they can express feelings is by making love, so husbands and wives frequently misunderstand each other. Men want sex much more frequently than do their wives, the women resist, and a battle for control ensues. Sharpest of all the conflicts are those over oral sex. Women have been programmed to think of it as nasty; indeed, for many of them only coital sex, usually in the missionary position, is "natural" and "normal." The woman is frequently nonorgasmic; even when she is able to reach orgasm, she often resents the husband's attitude which seems to convey the message that her orgasm is important mostly because it validates his masculinity rather than because it is a source of pleasure for her. Paradoxically, when a preorgasmic woman becomes orgasmic, some husbands lose interest in sex or even become impotent because their control and power are threatened by the wife's new-found equality in bed. The dominant form of sexual behavior for the wife of a blue-collar worker, however, is to engage in sex out of a sense of obligation or as a way to coerce the husband into giving her some of the things she wants. Used in these ways, sex is rarely a pleasurable event for the woman.

SEXUAL ATTITUDES AND BEHAVIOR: CLASS AND RACE

Most students of human sexuality have believed that the greater sexual permissiveness observed among blacks is a social-class phenomenon, i.e., that class accounts for the differences between whites and blacks rather than race per se. This turns out to be an inaccurate hypothesis, for when black and white lower classes are compared with respect to sexual permissiveness (Reiss, 1976), it is found that lower-class blacks are even more permissive in their attitudes than are whites of the same social class. Lower-class black men accept premarital coitus much more readily than white men of the same social class, and black women more than white women. Black-white differences are also reflected in the sexual behavior reported by Zelnik and Kantner (1978). Of black young women aged 15 to 19, 43 percent never used contraceptives, compared with 28 percent of white young women, indicating a lesser sense of personal responsibility. In their original study Zelnik and Kantner (1972) reported that 23 percent of the white teenagers and 54 percent of the black teenagers were nonvirginal.

The hypothesis set forth by Reiss (1976) is that

> black lower-class people, even more than white lower-class people, may believe they have little control over their future, and therefore take a more hedonistic approach to sex and love. Also, the relative advantage of the marriage institution over the nonmarital state as a place for sexual relationships may be even more mini-

mized in the black lower-class than it is in the white lower-class . . . thus, the marital state does not look so advantageous, and a freer sex ethic regarding sex outside of marriage may emerge.

To some extent this hypothesis is contradicted by the original Zelnik and Kantner (1972) report that sexually active black teenagers tended to have fewer partners than did sexually active white girls, at least when comparing those having had four or more partners. Moreover, an interesting finding in Zelnik and Kantner's (1978) data is that when black young women used contraception at all, they were much *less* likely to become pregnant than were white women. Unfortunately, the data do not reveal the social class of these respondents, and one can only guess that this may be more of a middle-class phenomenon. Zelnik and Kantner (1972) did find that higher-educated black teenagers reported less premarital coital experience. Middle-class blacks as a group tend to be even more conservative in their sexual attitudes and behavior than are middle-class whites.

OBTAINING SEXUAL DATA IN A MEDICAL HISTORY

Many physicians feel awkward about introducing the topic of sex into the medical history. Clumsy questions such as, "How is your sex life?" should be avoided. As Vincent (1973) points out:

> Such questions usually appear to bother the patient, not necessarily because they deal with sex, but because they are so nonspecific as to be unanswerable. The patient would undoubtedly be just as confused and uncomfortable if the physician would ask, "How is your urinary life?" or "How is your defecation life?"

There are natural ways to introduce the topic of sexuality into history taking. Should the details of the present illness suggest a contributory sexual problem, inquiry may begin at this point. Or it can come as part of the discussion of menstruation, or when the topic of the menarche is brought up. The patient's attitude toward her first period can lead to questions about other aspects of her sexual life. It is often easy to talk about a woman's marriage, and then to ask, "How do your feelings about your marriage affect your sexual relationship with your husband?" When interviewing an unmarried woman, the gynecologist may move from the discussion of the menarche to a discussion of relationships, and any sexual experience the patient may have had. As the Group for the Advancement of Psychiatry's "Guide to Interviewing" states:

> Often it is easier to uncover the patient's attitudes than to learn about his personal experiences. Indeed, attitudes may be more important than actual behavior. The physician may remark, "There are a lot of questions these days about oral-genital sex. How do you feel about it?" This approach is based on the principle that it is easier to talk about anything the physician suggests is universal, or at least common, than to talk about something that may be unusual or suspect. For example, the patient is more likely to reply negatively to the question "Did you ever masturbate?" but usually acknowledges the practice readily when asked, "How young were you when you started to masturbate?" This approach unlocks the information when, how often, and with what fantasies and guilt the patient masturbates. However, a matter-of-fact attitude is not necessarily conveyed by abruptness or tactlessness. Through sensitivity and tact the physician transmits the feeling to his patient that there is very little about human life which cannot be discussed between them.
>
> Another useful technique is to ascertain what expectations the patient had about certain experiences before actually undergoing them. After the first question, "What kind of sexual satisfaction did you expect when you got married?" the second follows easily: "How have your actual experiences matched your expectations?" This is another approach that generally unlocks the information sought.

With increasing ease and experience in counseling, the physician will find that it is a rare patient who resists tactful questioning about her sexual attitudes, feelings, and behavior. Inquiry by the physician about the patient's sexual functioning is sanctioned by the role given the physician by society and expected by patients.

Reassurance about confidentiality may be necessary, although most patients assume confidentiality as an aspect of the trust they place in their physician. If the interviewer senses anxiety about confidentiality, it is better to bring it out into the open.

The issue of sexual material appearing in hospital records may be troublesome, because hospital records have become more and more readily available to insurance companies and social agencies and may even be subpoenaed in legal matters. If concern is warranted, the physician should keep sepa-

rate records in the office files. (For a much more complete discussion of ethical issues in sex counseling and therapy, see Masters et al.).

COMMON SOURCES OF SEXUAL DYSFUNCTION

PREGNANCY

Three studies of sexual responsivity during pregnancy report a decline in sexual interest and activity as the pregnancy progresses, with the most pronounced trend during the third trimester. These three studies do not confirm the original findings of Masters and Johnson (1966) that there is an increase in all major parameters of sexual behavior during the second trimester. However, it seems that the decline in sexuality occurs mainly among primiparas, while sexual responsivity and satisfaction increase among multiparas. A logical hypothesis was confirmed by one of these studies (Pasini), namely, that women who had a positive attitude toward pregnancy maintained or improved an already good sexual relationship, while women who held negative feelings toward their pregnancy had a decrease in sexual satisfaction. There is some evidence that there may be a social-class factor that influences sex drive during pregnancy, with middle- and upper-class women continuing to show the same degree of interest that they had shown prior to pregnancy and lower-class women demonstrating a marked drop in interest. One clear-cut change during pregnancy is the increased desire of the woman for physical closeness. This desire is apparently a basic ingredient of the affectionate system. There is a return to a more fundamental dimension of human sexuality as the more complex sexual response is compromised during pregnancy.

It is difficult to exclude the influence of physicians on the attitudes and behavior of women during pregnancy, because until recently obstetricians cautioned their patients not to have intercourse for 6 weeks prior to the anticipated delivery date and for 6 weeks after delivery. This advice was based upon beliefs handed down from one generation of obstetricians to another: The thrust of the penis against the cervix or the uterine contractions of orgasm would induce labor; coitus can rupture the membranes, heightening the probability of infection within the womb; the sex act itself is physically uncomfortable for the majority of women during the last few weeks of pregnancy. If women literally followed this advice and refrained from intercourse for 6 weeks after delivery, it would mean that they would abstain from intercourse for 3 months. Based on the findings of Pugh and Fernandez and Masters and Johnson (1966), who noted the absence of ill effects among women who had had sexual intercourse during the final weeks of pregnancy, physicians have been modifying their recommendations.

Masters and Johnson also report that when husbands are "put on the shelf for two or three months," many of them stray "from the marital bed for the first time under these circumstances." Of 79 husbands whom they questioned, 18 reported that during the period of enforced abstinence from marital sexual activity before and after childbirth, they had had extramarital coital encounters, some for the first time. Another effect of the interdiction of coitus during pregnancy is that couples disregard their physician's advice, continue to have sexual activity, but feel guilty.

After delivery there is no reason to prohibit intercourse, once the vaginal bleeding has stopped and any incisions or tears in the introitus have healed. Of course, the woman should be psychologically ready to resume intercourse.

Most instructors of obstetrics now teach that intercourse is permissible, as long as it is comfortably acceptable to both partners, during the entire pregnancy period until labor begins, except in the presence of ruptured membranes or uterine bleeding. Another reason for prohibiting intercourse would be the occurrence of vaginal or abdominal pain in association with coitus. Experimentation by the couple for comfortable positions or the use of noncoital techniques of achieving orgasm is generally sufficient to take care of the problem of physical comfort. During the last weeks of pregnancy, cunnilingus should be avoided because of the possibility, however slight, of air embolism caused by air blown into the vagina finding its way through the cervix and into the placenta then into the general circulation.

The physician should be aware that the psychologic balance between husband and wife may be sufficiently modified during pregnancy to create interpersonal problems which are reflected in their sexual adjustment. The wife's increased dependency and need for nurturance may be a burden to the husband, who perhaps himself feels threatened by the incipient rival for his wife's affections. On occasion, the husband's perception of his wife changes drastically. The wife-mother no longer becomes the object of his passionate feelings, as old incest taboos interfere with the delicate balance between lust and love. These men may find a sudden and decided drop in their sexual arousal during the wife's pregnancy or following childbirth. On her part, the wife may turn her attention to the child and withdraw from affectionate contact with her husband.

During the first 6 months after delivery, there may be a period of marked psychological stress. Many couples report a disruption of their previous sexual pattern during this 6-month period after the birth of their baby, especially after the first baby. The 6-week postpartum consultation should include not only a discussion of contraception, but of the wife's reactions to, or her anticipation of, sexual relations with her husband. Both the husband and wife need more educative counseling during pregnancy, enabling them to anticipate some of the difficulties and adjustments not only during pregnancy, but in the postpartum period.

Newton has pointed out the similarities between undisturbed, undrugged childbirth and sexual excitement in bodily characteristics such as breathing, vocalizing, facial expressions, uterine reactions, cervical reactions, abdominal muscle reactions, sensory reactions, and emotional responses. In some women clitoral engorgement begins about the time the cervix is 8 or 9 cm dilated. Similarly, Masters and Johnson reported on 12 women who, during the second stage of labor, described sensations which they had identified with orgasm.

Many women who breast-feed their infants report sexual stimulation by the infant and some have reported orgasm. Although many women are free enough to enjoy this sensation, there are some who find the sensation unpleasant because of feelings of guilt, based on their lack of understanding that this is a normal response. During breast-feeding, uterine contractions and nipple erection occur. The vascular changes of the skin during breast-feeding and coitus are quite similar. (In some women sexual excitement triggers the milk-ejection reflex.) In addition, there seems to be a correlation between an accepting attitude toward breast-feeding and an accepting attitude toward sexuality. Masters and Johnson noted that the highest level of sexual interest in the first 3 months after delivery was reported by nursing mothers. Conversely, feelings of aversion for the breast-feeding act appeared to be related to dislike of nudity and sexuality. Newton points out that coitus, parturition, and lactation are all based on closely related neurohormonal reflexes and that they all trigger "care-taking behavior" which is an essential and important part of mammalian reproduction.

AGING

The sexual drive of women peaks between the ages of 25 and 35, a decade after men. Although there is some decline in sexual frequency during the mid-years, the woman who has had an active and satisfying sex life should have no interruption of that during her menopause. Some women even report an increase in sexual interest and capacity to respond after the onset of menopause because they no longer fear pregnancy. Any inhibition in sexual activities is due to changes in self-image and worth as the woman reluctantly relinquishes her capacity to bear children. Her new infertility, along with body changes that decrease her sense of attractiveness to men, provide a threat to her femininity. Psychologic and symbolic factors, not physiologic ones, create sexual inhibition. Estrogen replacement therapy should take care of any of the physiologic problems, and a still-interested husband will make it possible for the woman to enjoy coital activity into the seventh or eighth decade. Indeed, the woman is capable of multiple orgastic response, essentially without a refractory period, throughout life. Aging seems to have its primary effect on the ejaculatory aspect of male orgasm, rather than on erectile capacity. This difference in orgastic capacity promotes the female's potentially greater sexual responsiveness than the male's in later years.

Without a regular sexual opportunity, however, there is a definite drop in sexual interest. Aside from this, there is a slow, gradual decline in sex drive (in contrast to responsivity) after the age of 65. For women, aging does have some biologic effects. During orgasm, contractions decline from five or six at age 30 to two or three at age 70. Erotic sensations tend to be less intense. Nevertheless, 25 percent of 70-year-old women still masturbate. The gynecologist should be on the lookout for those couples of whom the woman is still very responsive in her sixties and seventies, but there is decreasing frequency of sexual intercourse as her husband feels threatened because his wife's continued interest and responsivity are greater than his own. He may withdraw from much sexual activity with his wife, leaving her frustrated.

TYPES OF SEXUAL PROBLEMS

MASKED SEXUAL PROBLEMS

Sexual frustration or sexual conflict or both may lie behind a wide variety of complaints brought to the attention of the physician. These may be fatigue, loss of appetite, insomnia, constipation, backache, abdominal pain, pelvic pain, dysmenorrhea, and vaginal discharge. At times the woman is fully aware of the underlying nature of her difficulties, but is reluctant to reveal these to the physician because of shame and fear of the physician's ridicule, or the fear of opening for further exploration her marital problems, or a combination of these. At other times, the woman is only partially aware of the underlying nature of her problems; it is "preconscious," rather than either fully conscious or unconscious. When the link is suggested to her, she readily agrees to the connection. More often, however, the patient has completely cut the associations between her sexual frustrations and conflict and the complaints with which she presents herself in the physician's office. In the first type, in which the woman is fully conscious of the connections, the physician's tactful, comfortable questioning will soon put the patient at ease, and the connections will become clear. The second type—the patient who is only dimly aware of the nature of her difficulties—is also readily handled by gentle, suggestive questioning. The third type of patient—the woman who does not associate her symptoms with sexual frustrations—may be more resistant to uncovering techniques. More "organized" psychosomatic syndromes such as primary amenorrhea, repeated spontaneous abortions, very severe dysmenorrhea, and severe premenstrual tension may all have an underlying sexual problem. These are apt to be associated with conflicts about feminine identity, involving strong fears about assuming an adult feminine role (Ludwig et al.; Filler, Lief). These cases stubbornly resist the usual methods of treatment, and if the gynecologist determines that there is a severe personality disorder, joint treatment by the gynecologist and a psychiatrist is indicated.

In addition to the fear of making a connection between a sexual conflict and frustration and bodily symptoms and distress, additional psychologic mechanisms are at work. The normal reaction to sexual frustration is anger. If a woman blames her husband for her sexual difficulties, she may find that her anger produces no change in him. If she assigns blame to herself, or is unable to express her anger for any number of reasons, depression will follow. Some of the symptoms such as loss of appetite, insomnia, and constipation are really manifestations of depression. Depression itself decreases sexual drive. A depressed state lowers the capacity for arousal, possibly because of the decrease in androgens which accompanies depression. Many of the symptoms, therefore, are nonspecific reactions to anger turned back against oneself with consequent loss of self-esteem as the woman tries to deal with the failure of sexual functioning. On the other hand, some of the symptoms may be symbolic representations of underlying conflict. A striking example is the condition of pseudocyesis. Secondary amenorrhea may also have symbolic sexual meaning, whether or not it occurs in conjunction with pseudocyesis. If the gynecologist suspects that these are really conversion phenomena, hysterical in nature, referral to a psychiatrist is indicated. In less-severe cases, once the underlying sexual dysfunction is brought to light, appropriate treatment should be offered (see later discussion).

SEXUAL PROBLEMS MASKING MARITAL AND OTHER PROBLEMS

In approximately two out of five situations in which the woman complains of a sexual dysfunction, the difficulty is an interpersonal one with her husband; the sexual problem is not compartmentalized but is a manifestation of other areas of marital dysfunction. Sometimes the sexual dysfunction created marital disharmony in the first place, and then spread to other areas of the marriage. The counselor may still have to deal with these areas before returning to the sexual problem. Two people who are intensely angry or bored with each other cannot make effective sexual partners. A reasonable amount of clinical acumen is required to be able to separate the situations which will be amenable to sex counseling from those which have to be referred to a marriage counselor.

A host of pseudoproblems exist in which the woman mistakenly thinks that some aspect of normal functioning is really abnormal. This may involve some aspect of behavior, some bodily sensation, fantasy, etc. Reassurance by the physician that these behaviors, feelings, or fantasies are within the broad range of normality will relieve the patient's anxiety.

Clinicians report that some cases of hypersexuality may be based on vaginitis, or possibly cystitis,

or both. The irritation of the clitoris and labia may simulate the sensation of arousal, and create a state of hypersexuality. These same conditions may cause dyspareunia and have the opposite effect. I once treated a patient who, for 20 years, had had "honeymoon" cystitis with recurrent episodes of dyspareunia. Vigorous treatment by a urologist cleared up a situation in which intercourse had been so infrequent that this union verged on being an "unconsummated marriage."

SEXUAL RESPONSIVITY

The inhibition of sexual excitement or orgasm has many possible causes. Among them are localized illness such as endometriosis or pelvic inflammatory disease. A pervasive psychiatric disorder such as depression may be a cause. Systemic illness such as hypothyroidism or pituitary dysfunction may be responsible. The same is true of illness that affects the neurologic apparatus required for sexual responsivity, or disease that interferes with muscle tone and contractility. In general, however, even illnesses such as multiple sclerosis and diabetes affect the male before the female. They cause impotence far more frequently than they cause so-called "frigidity."[1]

Most cases of dysfunction of excitement and orgasm, however, are consequences of (1) ineffective sexual preparation, (2) marital conflict, and (3) sexual conflicts, fears, and guilt that the woman brought into her marriage. In this regard, the perspectives of the psychiatrist or marriage counselor and of the gynecologist may differ, because the marriage counselor and the psychiatrist will tend to see cases in the last two categories, while the gynecologist is apt to see a larger number of cases of the first type, in which ignorance and ineffective preparation of the woman by her partner are the major factors responsible for her inability to experience orgasm.

In this section the discussion will be confined to those cases in which inadequate preparation, marital conflict, or sexual inhibition based on faulty learning in childhood are the primary causes in the sexual dysfunction. Understanding the cause is complicated by the fact that ignorance itself may be the surface manifestation of a deeper conflict, in which

---

[1]"Frigidity" is not only a pejorative term but also a confusing one. Patients and physicians alike use it to cover a wide range of symptoms, from actual vaginal anesthesia to merely the loss of the ability to have multiple orgasms. Used in so many ways, the term loses all specificity and is best eliminated from the medical vocabulary.

psychic inhibitions prevent an individual from acquiring the necessary information enabling her to secure sexual pleasure.

Whatever the past or remote causes, there are always immediate factors that contribute to the lack of sexual pleasure and satisfaction. These are (1) "spectatoring," (2) performance anxiety, (3) avoidance of sex, or ineffective arousal, (4) rationalization for the ineffectiveness of erotic arousal, and (5) disturbance in communication.

The amount of ignorance concerning the genitalia and the patterns of erotic arousal is at first astonishing to the physician, but such lack of knowledge is by no means uncommon. Many couples have no knowledge of the clitoris or, if they have heard of it, do not know where it is located. There is equal ignorance about the patterns of erotic arousal and the techniques of effective stimulation. The male often effects penetration as soon as he obtains an erection and the woman has had hardly any preparation for coitus. Many women are afraid to complain, either because they are afraid of irritating their husbands and provoking his rejection, or because they have no basic knowledge which would help them assess their own reactions. Women may think their own lack of responsivity is normal, or if they think there is something wrong, they may blame themselves for not responding, not realizing they have not had adequate preparation.

Other couples make love in a mechanized fashion, always using the same pattern. The lack of variety eventually dulls the capacity to respond. Partners may not say anything to each other because of modesty, the fear of being rejected, or because of the fear of hurting the partner. The need to protect oneself or the partner is frequently the cause of silent suffering that may go on for years.

If the ignorance is based on underlying fear or guilt which has interfered with learning, resistance to therapy will become evident. This will be described in the section on Sexual Dysfunction Treatment.

Whatever the underlying cause of orgasmic dysfunction, invariably *performance anxiety* is present. Performance anxiety is composed of three elements: fear of failure, pressure to perform, and overconcern about pleasing the partner. After several failures, the woman begins to observe herself or to become a spectator at her own performance. Her "observing self," rather than her "participating self," takes over and as she begins love play she wonders, "Will I have an orgasm?" "Will I take too long?" "Will my partner become angry?" The combination of observing herself, or "spectatoring," and her anxiety about perfor-

mance are sufficient to inhibit orgastic response and often sufficient to inhibit much in the way of erotic arousal. With the anxiety comes a great pressure to succeed, and thoughts such as "I *must* come this time," "I *can't* fail him again," increase the pressure, and tension. She may be so concerned about pleasing her partner that she becomes insensitive to her own bodily sensations, effectively turning off her own mechanism of erotic arousal.

If these patterns go on for any length of time, they often result in a collusion between the husband and wife to avoid intercourse; or when they do have sex, they fall into a pattern which eventuates in ineffective sexual arousal. The husband may mechanically stimulate the clitoris in the same fashion—he may not be aware of the signs of her readiness, and may go on to have intercourse even when there is insufficient or no lubrication. If he develops premature ejaculation, which occurs in approximately half the cases in which the woman is nonorgasmic, he may be afraid to have his wife touch his penis, for fear of having his ejaculation before entrance. The entire sequence becomes a series of "no-nos." The woman whose husband is suffering from premature ejaculation may try to avoid continuing frustration by speeding up the entire sexual act, "to get it over with." This makes it certain that she will not be sufficiently arroused, inhibiting the sexual excitement phase and, of course, orgasm.

These difficulties are often rationalized on the basis of fatigue, or preoccupation (which can, in fact, be important contributing factors, but are often used as rationalizations), or illness. Communication begins to break down either in a conspiracy of silence or in a torrent of angry words or by the woman's silent crying. Each partner begins to second-guess the other, trying to figure out what the other is thinking or feeling, which leads to an increase in misperceptions. Poor communication generally does not cause sexual difficulties as much as it becomes a contributing factor to a vicious cycle, interfering with what might be natural, reparative efforts on the part of the couple to deal with initial difficulties. In dealing with the immediate causes of sexual dysfunction, attention must be given to the patterns of communication, and these become a central focus of counseling (see the later discussion of communication under Sexual Dysfunction Treatment).

Underlying causes of the failure of effective sexual functioning have two basic roots: (1) marital unhappiness and (2) inhibitory emotions due to faulty learning during childhood and adolescence. Marital discord probably accounts for about half of these problems. It is difficult to respond sexually when one is angry with one's partner, of if one feels guilty. This is not invariably true, since there are people who have the capacity to separate their sexual responses from the rest of their reactions to their mates. At times, a husband and wife who are on the edge of separation and divorce still continue to have very satisfactory sex relations with each other. Although a sadomasochistic element may account for this paradoxical situation, even sadomasochism does not always explain the compartmentalization of sexual activity. One may see an unhappy couple responding passionately to each other, holding on, as it were, to the last vestiges of mutual pleasure.

Although there are exceptions, in the vast majority of people sexual responsivity is very much influenced by the emotional reactions to one's partner. Generally speaking, if there are love and trust between the man and woman, there is much greater chance of erotic arousal and orgasm. One of the treatment tasks is to augment these "welfare" emotions of hope, pride, joy, love, and trust, and to decrease the so-called "emergency" emotions of fear, rage, guilty fear, and guilty rage. Sustained rage becomes hatred. The emergency emotions inhibit erotic arousal; the welfare emotions facilitate the mechanism of erotic arousal. The sources of emergency emotions are varied and are too complex to describe in detail in this chapter. Often, they relate to the need to control the partner (and the fear of being controlled), the anger at failure to gratify needs and expectations (which, of themselves, may be unrealistic or even altogether irrational), and the need to provoke damaging relations by the fear of closeness and intimacy. Linked to these emotions is the fear some women have that if they respond with pleasure, they will be that much more under the control of the husband. Pleasure itself may augment the guilt that they always associate with sexuality, but even in the absence of guilt, there may be fear of the pleasurable responses because of the wife's increased dependency on her husband.

There are many women who bring emergency emotions into their marital sex lives and would have these reactions with any partner. Sex, for them, has become either frightening or guilt-ridden or both. On occasion, this reaction may be related to a single traumatic event in the woman's early life, but much more often it is related to the atmosphere surrounding sexual functioning, or to a series of traumatic events such as incestuous relations. Even in the absence of actual incest, unconscious incestuous fantasies can be as damaging as the real thing. While many of these cases will not respond to counseling by the gynecologist, it is strange that even some of the cases with deep-rooted causes for sexual dysfunction will respond to the form of reeducative and behavioral therapy that will be described later under Sexual Dysfunction Treatment.

SEX DRIVE AND INTEREST

There are many reasons other than the release of sexual tension why a woman may desire sexual activity. She may feel the need for closeness, the need to please her partner, the need for reassurance about being loved, the need to prove her femininity, a desire for play, etc. Because these needs are so varied, it is difficult to correlate sexual activity with a definite subjective feeling of sexual tension.

Despite the multiple reasons for sexual activity, recent evidence indicates that there is a correlation between the plasma testosterone level at midcycle and the degree of sexual activity in young women. Not only is *frequency* correlated with testosterone level, so also is the degree of *sexual gratification,* which was found to be significantly related both to the average testosterone level across the entire menstrual cycle and to a woman's average base-line testosterone level (Persky et al., 1978).

Problems about sex drive can be placed into the following categories: (1) an avoidance reaction, (2) disparity with the partner's needs. The woman may avoid sex entirely or engage in it infrequently because of previous unsatisfactory reactions. She may have been blamed by her partner for being nonresponsive; she herself may feel inadequate; or there may have been insufficient pleasure in previous sexual activities in different degrees up to and including dyspareunia.

A problem arises if one partner wants sex more frequently than the other and places incessant demands for additional sex. Although this is more often the male's demands for greater frequency, in one-sixth of the cases studied, the woman desires sex more frequently than does her husband. If one compares their perceptions of frequency with the actual frequency of sex relations, one often finds that there is quite a difference. There is a tendency to under- or overestimate the frequency, depending upon whether one desires more or less sex. Sometimes the partner is unable to say "no," and in a self-sacrificing fashion attempts to please the spouse, albeit with considerable resentment. This may eventuate in a failure to become sufficiently aroused to attain orgasm. More often, when the partner goes along with the other's request, he or she finds that within a few minutes it becomes pleasurable and no problem arises. If there is chronic resentment at the partner's not complying with one's wishes, or compliance occurs but with resentment, the situation may require therapeutic intervention.

The more specific types of sexual dysfunction, inhibitions of excitement and orgasm, are discussed in the section on treatment later in this chapter.

OTHER PROBLEMS OF SEXUAL BEHAVIOR

Occasionally there are disagreements between the woman and her husband about some aspects of foreplay, coital positions, and sexual variations, usually stemming from difficulties in communication because one of the partners is unable to let the other one know what he or she really likes. Occasionally, however, there are clumsy efforts at stimulating the clitoris, or the woman may be reluctant to touch the penis. Arguments sometimes ensue over oral-genital sex, with one of the partners liking it very much and the other partner finding it distasteful. The same is true of quasi-sadomasochistic "bits" of behavior such as biting and spanking.

Differences with regard to coital positions may also be present. There may be different needs for experimentation, and different likes which have to be dealt with in some fashion. For example, some women will not tolerate the woman-above position because it is associated with aggression, which they reject. Similarly, some men may reject the same position because it does not seem to be sufficiently "masculine" for them.

VAGINISMUS AND DYSPAREUNIA

Vaginismus always causes pain during intercourse. It is characterized by a conditioned spasm of the muscles surrounding the vaginal orifice and represents the woman's unconscious attempt to ward off penetration. This may be associated with inhibition of erotic excitement, but on occasion these women are very responsive to, and orgastic with, clitoral stimulation.

This is one sexual condition that must be confirmed by direct pelvic examination. The woman will have an involuntary spasm of the vaginal outlet during the pelvic examination. An avoidance reaction is sometimes seen just in anticipation of the examiner's approach.

Vaginismus is generally the most frequent finding in cases of unconsummated marriage. Masters and Johnson point out that it is often associated with primary impotence of the male partner; sometimes vaginismus does not occur until there have been several unsuccessful attempts at coitus due to the failure of erection. Masters and Johnson reported that "religious orthodoxy" was a factor in 12 of 29 cases. In addition to the prominence of guilty fear about sex, there may be more specific fears of penetration accompanied by fantasies of bodily damage. In some of these cases, there has been a history of rape which was more than usually traumatic.

On occasion, vaginismus has developed in patients who had first had severe dyspareunia. The latter may result from laceration of the broad ligaments, endometriosis, cystitis, etc., but the most frequent cause of dyspareunia is lack of adequate vaginal lubrication during sexual arousal. Thus it is mostly a response to ineffective stimulation.

The presence of persistent pain during or after intercourse should alert the gynecologist to do a thorough pelvic and rectal examination. A careful history should be taken to obtain a full and exact description of the pain, since this may vary from a mild postcoital vaginal irritation to a sensation of lacerating pain with pelvic thrusting. Examination should include looking for vaginal scarring, probably a residual of episiotomies, clitoral adhesions, irritation of the glans of the clitoris, infection of the vaginal barrel. allergic reactions to chemicals in contraceptive creams, jellies, etc. In the postmenopausal woman the loss of elasticity of her vagina and the loss of lubrication may be responsible for pain during intercourse. If not supported by replacement steroids, the vaginal mucosa becomes thin and atrophic. Radiation reactions in the vagina will produce similar effects.

Not infrequently the pelvic examination reveals no abnormality, and the gynecologist is left with choosing between inadequate lubrication as the cause of the dyspareunia or trying to figure out whether indeed the woman is exaggerating some mild discomfort in order to avoid sex. She may have learned that if she complains of pain, this will prevent her husband from attempting sex, except at very infrequent intervals. Obtaining a good description of the pain will frequently enable a choice between those two possibilities. Treatment of vaginismus and dyspareunia is described in the section on Sexual Dysfunction Treatment.

INFIDELITY

Extramarital sex may cause sexual difficulties. A woman whose husband is "cheating" may respond with sexual jealousy and anger, leading to a decrease in her sexual responsivity. On the other hand, if it is her own extramarital affair that is creating the problem, she may respond with guilt, which will have a similar effect on her sexual performance. A woman may be very responsive with her lover, but nonorgasmic with her husband. Thus, a thorough sexual history is necessary, for without a history of the extramarital relationship, the counselor may find therapeutic efforts undermined by the woman who is concealing a crucial bit of information.

Not always is extramarital sex a cause of sexual difficulty. Sometimes the outside relationship serves to keep the marriage together and, on occasion, even permits a greater tolerance and higher responsivity in a woman who otherwise would be much less interested in her husband. On the other hand, an extramarital relationship may be a cry for help and a calling card for therapeutic intervention. It may be the couple's first recognition that their marriage is in trouble. People who are happily married are much less apt to have sex outside of their marital relationship; therefore, an outside relationship is at least presumptive evidence that there is something wrong in the marriage. At times women will seek help because they are suddenly tempted to have an extramarital relationship and feel "alive," perhaps for the first time in their lives, as they experience an erotic "turn-on" with someone other than their husband. These women become very disturbed as they recognize, perhaps for the first time, what they have been missing. If the wife has the courage to be open about this with her husband, and if he has the ability to deal with what he may perceive as a blow to his masculine pride, the husband and wife have a chance to achieve a sexual relationship that is far more satisfactory than before.

PROBLEM PREGNANCIES

For the single woman, the options in the case of pregnancy are whether to carry the baby to term and keep it or give it up for adoption versus legal abortion.

Legalized abortion has increased the range of options considerably. The majority of women experience an abortion with marked relief from anxiety and depression, but a few suffer severe guilt and must be screened out beforehand. Not infrequently, women who are prone to a guilty reaction have had similar responses to contraception.

This issue of marriage has to be explored, keeping in mind that 80 percent of "forced" marriages end in divorce. Whether the woman is unmarried or married (and far more unwanted pregnancies occur to married than to single women), the interaction between the patient and her partner is a critical factor. The attitude of her partner may push her toward an alternative that is against her best interests and may create a serious problem in the relationship regardless of her choice. There will be her resentment if she later feels she has capitulated to pressure against her true wishes, and his resentment if she declines the alternative he favors. The same possibility exists for a teenage girl and the pressure of her parents. Counseling is directed toward finding out the genuine desires of the patient. In this clinical situation, it is useful for the gynecologist to interview the husband, sexual partner, or parents either alone or conjointly (interviewing strategies are discussed later under Treatment of Sexual Dysfunction).

PROBLEMS OF THE SEPARATED, DIVORCED, OR WIDOWED WOMAN

Two out of three divorcees will remarry. The majority of them continue to have sexual intercourse, and many will have more sexual activity than they had during the last stage of marriage. About 15 percent have multiple partners. The increase is not only in sexual activity but also in the experience of orgasm, presumably in reaction to a decrease in frequency during the latter period of the unhappy marriage, as well as the relief of anxiety and pain once the unhappy situation has been resolved.

Prior to physical separation, the woman getting a divorce goes through an emotional crisis. This "emotional divorce" usually carries with it a decreased interest in sex and responsivity, and often an increase in extramarital relations. The separation crisis is followed by a divorce crisis in which sexual activity is often unpredictable. Sex is used for the relief of loneliness, to prove one's attractiveness—which may reassure the woman that she is not really responsible for the breakup of the marriage—or as an expression of her desire for another mate, etc. Sex is used for a variety of reparative purposes, and not merely for the relief of sexual tension.

The ratio of widows to widowers is 4 to 1, with the majority of widows being over the age of 60. Their sexual needs are compounded by the frequent occurrence of a grief response which, with its attendant depression, generally decreases sexual interest. There is often a moratorium on sexual activities, much more so than among divorcees. Fewer widows remarry than do divorcees, presumably because of the older age of widows. This brings with it the problems of sexual gratification among the aged and the many problems faced by women who are not able or willing to find available and willing sexual partners.

The gynecologist should be alert to the possibility of sexual problems in the separated, divorced, and widowed resulting from their needs for sexual gratification, affection, and companionship. The gynecologist often becomes the target of the emotional needs of such women, when the usual transference fantasies are heightened because of their difficulty in finding partners. At the same time, the gynecologist should be sensitive to the benefits of initiating discussion of sexual functioning in these women, and not assume that their nonmarital state indicates an absence of interest.

ILLNESS, ABLATIVE SURGERY, AND SEXUAL FUNCTIONING

Psychiatric disorders may interfere with sexual functioning. In schizophrenic women, there is no consistent pattern of interference with arousal or orgasmic response; on the other hand, patients with schizophrenia frequently exhibit patterns of chaotic sexuality in which fluctuations from compulsive promiscuity to complete abstinence may be seen in the same person. For the practicing gynecologist, however, the most important psychiatric disturbance is depression. Characteristically, as a consequence of depressive moods, sexual interest is decreased. It is still unclear whether psychological factors by themselves are the primary cause of a decreased sex drive, or whether the psychophysiologic responses to depression are the more important etiologic factors. Along with a decreased interest in sex, there is usually a decreased capacity to enjoy pleasurable activities of any kind, even eating. While a mild depression may increase the desire for food, more severe depressive reactions generally are accompanied by anhedonia, of which anorexia is a prominent symptom. A psychophysiologic response characterized by a drop in androgen levels accompanies these states. Even though blood testosterone levels are lower in females, variations in these levels seem to be even more significant than they are in men.

Emergency emotions evoked by a stressful life situation usually result in some decrease in sexual activity. Clearly, preoccupation with stressful life circumstances will decrease a person's interest in sex. On the other hand, as in depression, psychophysiologic responses may be important. Presumably, the hypothalamus inhibits the pituitary's secretion of gonadotropins, which in turn leads to decreased androgen production. The cortical steroids, increased in stress, may also exert an antiandrogen influence. Even if the psychophysiologic mechanisms are imperfectly understood, the clinical response is almost always that of a decreased libido. Under the influence of stress some people, however, need the reassurance of emotional support, and this reassurance may be gained through coital contact with a loved person.

Of all the systemic illnesses that interfere with sexual function, diabetes takes first place. Although its impact on the male is much more clear-cut, recent evidence indicates that diabetes may also inhibit the arousal mechanism in the female. Other systemic illnesses which tend to produce depression, such as hepatitis, or to interfere with the excretion of bodily substances, such as renal disease, may decrease sexual drive. Since sexual response is dependent on an intact nerve and vascular supply to the genitalia, diseases which interfere with the innervation of the pelvis may also affect sexual functioning.

The clinician should always inquire about medication. Oral contraceptives have been mentioned before; their effect seems variable, with most women not reporting any significant drop in sexual functioning. The exceptions are frequent enough, however, for this possibility to be kept in mind. Similarly, antihypertensive medications, although more clearly implicated in impotence than in interference with the arousal mechanism in the female, should be evaluated as well. Tranquilizers have a variable effect; if anxiety is decreased, sexual functioning may be improved. On the other hand, large doses of tranquilizers tend to inhibit sexual interest and behavior. As it counteracts the effects of depression, antidepressive medication may enhance sexual functioning.

In ablative surgical procedures, the physician should keep in mind not only the possibility of anatomical defects and their impact on sexual functioning, but the psychological implications of the procedure as well. It is clear that hysterectomy should have no effect whatsoever on the capacity for arousal and orgasm; yet women who feel that their femininity has been curtailed, perhaps even destroyed, may no longer be as responsive. The effect of mastectomy on body image may also be so devastating as to have a profound effect on sexual behavior. There is often a decrease in the response to breast stimulation, and hence an avoidance of it. About 50 percent of the women who have had a mastectomy report this decrease. There is also a marked decrease in those who can undress in front of their partners and also a decrease in nudity during sex. In these instances, withdrawal from sexual activity is the most frequent response, but sometimes a kind of compulsive attempt to reassure oneself about one's attractiveness and femininity creates heightened sexual drive—sometimes accompanied by decreased responsivity.

Any operation on the vagina that entails some degree of multilation should be counteracted by appropriate plastic surgical procedures, not only for anatomical functioning but for impact on the woman's view of herself. When both ovaries and adrenals are removed, sexual interest disappears almost entirely, presumably due to the absence of androgen.

When contemplating any ablative surgery, the surgeon should consider carefully the discussion of the implications of the surgery not only on sexual functioning but on the woman's attitude toward her feeling of being an attractive and "whole" person. While anxiety about cancer may preoccupy the minds of many women, once the acute anxiety is removed, these other concerns lie not far behind. Much psychic disability can be prevented by discussion prior to surgery, if appropriate, or soon thereafter, once the acute anxiety about the surgical procedure itself has passed.

SEXUAL ASPECTS OF INFERTILITY

While a thorough review of the sexual aspects of infertility is out of place in this chapter, some of the more significant associations with sexual activity should be mentioned. Careful history taking is essential. It is not unusual to find that a couple actually avoids sex during the time of maximum fertility. Behind this may be fears of pregnancy, childbirth, or parenthood. Psychophysiological responses, even when coital activity occurs when conception might occur, are related to unconscious fears of pregnancy which, in turn, may mask fears of childbirth or the capacity to be an adequate parent. These fears may lead to spasm of the fallopian tubes or some other unknown intermediate mechanisms by which conception is prevented.

The woman who wants to become pregnant above all else and makes demands on her husband for sexual performance may be creating sufficient marital stress to provoke an avoidance response in her husband. Stress may also decrease the capacity for conception, although the mechanisms are by no means clear.

Treatment carries with it some disadvantages for adequate sexual functioning. The need for coitus around the time of ovulation sets up a demand situation in which sex is regarded as a treatment. When that happens, the male occasionally becomes impotent or develops premature or retarded ejaculation, and the woman, although continuing to engage in sex, may no longer be orgasmic. If the couple reports this kind of emotional response, the clinician may have to modify the therapeutic regimen.

SEXUAL DYSFUNCTION TREATMENT

GENERAL CONSIDERATIONS

When confronted with a woman with a sexual problem, the gynecologist will ask himself or herself many questions. Is this patient's problem one that I am competent to handle, or must I refer the patient to a sex therapist, a marriage counselor, or a psychotherapist? Is this a problem that can be managed by counseling the woman alone, or must I see the couple? If I do see the couple, to what extent should I deal with the destructive aspects of the relationship? Or should I deal only with the specific sexual problem?

The answers to these questions depend on the competence of the gynecologist in treating sexual dysfunction. Over time, clinicians generally discover those kinds of situations in which they can be helpful, and those that demand more training and experience than they themselves have received. A reasonably safe rule to follow is this: if, after six sessions, no improvement is noted, referral is indicated.

Treatment can be divided into three somewhat overlapping dimensions, namely, education, counseling, and therapy. (See Table 34–2.) Every treatment situation involves some education or transmission of new information to the patient. *Counseling* adds specific interventions aimed at increasing sexual functioning. *Therapy* includes education and counseling but, in addition, involves the capacity to deal explicitly in a more sophisticated fashion with problems of interaction between the partners and individual psychopathology. In this perspective the gynecologist should, at the very least, be a good sex

TABLE 34–2 The Physician's Roles and Tasks in Sex Counseling and Therapy

Level of diagnosis of sexual problem	Patient need	Professional task	Professional role
Sexual ignorance	To know	To provide accurate information	Inquirer-educator
Situational discomfort-anxiety	To relax	To reduce or eliminate immediate causes of sexual dysfunction	Counselor
Interpersonal distance-conflict	To reorient the relationship	To reshape dyadic system	Marital therapist
Historical intrapsychic conflict	To explore tension between intrapsychic and interpersonal systems	To explore the interface between historical conflict and sexual discomfort-dysfunction	Psychotherapist
All of the above	Flexible use of new repertoire of sexual behaviors	Formulating hierarchy of patient needs and incorporating them into a sequence of treatment	Sex therapist

Source: H. Lief, 1978.

educator; many of them ought to be competent counselors; a few of them will be skillful sex therapists.

When there is a sexual problem, there is no uninvolved partner. Consequently, gynecologists should consider the option of interviewing the sexual partner, either together with the woman, or alone if indicated. Even if the gynecologist has had no specific training in marriage counseling, the male partner's views will increase the counselor's information about the etiology of the problem and about his capacity to participate effectively in the planned treatment. It is one thing to find a very cooperative partner who will do whatever is necessary to help the woman overcome her sexual inadequacy, and another to find a male so angry or so intent on destroying the relationship or, for reasons of his own, so needful of maintaining the woman's dysfunction, that referral becomes the only course of action.

The target of treatment should be the relief of sexual symptoms, and this usually becomes the criterion for termination. The counselor must be certain that the gains will be maintained, so it is wise to have built-in follow-ups at 3 and 6 weeks, and again at 3 and 6 months after the removal of symptoms. Occasionally the symptom removal changes the equilibrium between the couple so drastically that there are difficul-

ties in other areas of the relationship and/or the male develops sexual problems of his own. Only follow-up will determine whether the gains at the end of treatment have been maintained. If other problems have occurred, it is again up to the gynecologist to decide whether to deal with them or to refer the couple elsewhere for therapy.

The nature of the problem generally determines the indications for treatment. Ignorance about sexual functioning is enormous, and the counselor can do a great deal by correcting misinformation and dispelling myths. Sexual inhibitions are so pervasive and negative conditioning in childhood so long-lasting, that it is not unusual to see college-educated women who have marked distortions in their knowledge of sexual anatomy and little awareness of the role of the clitoris in sexual arousal. Many college-educated males share this ignorance. More often than not, couples have very inadequate information about what constitutes erotic arousal and have poor information about their own "sensate focus," as described by Masters and Johnson, as well as that of their partners. Many men, quick to erotic arousal, are unaware that their wives may require a setting of the mood earlier in the day, and longer periods of preparation for intercourse. People seem generally unaware that the partner's sexual response is itself potent in sexual arousal. Add to these the misconceptions about age and sex, myths about the dangers of masturbation, the effect of hysterectomy or the menopause on sexual functioning, gross misinformation about contraception, etc., and it can be seen that the clinician has a wide field for transmitting information that will make patients more effective sexually.

In addition to dispelling myths and misconceptions and teaching correct anatomic and physiologic facts, education includes two other facets: letting patients know something about behavioral norms and reducing undue expectations. Many patients are overly concerned about whether their behavior is "normal". Their questions may include items such as the frequency of intercourse, aspects of foreplay such as oral-genital sex, coital positions, length of intromission, etc. Of course, the wise clinician wants to know the implications of these questions, before offering information. The question, "What are your concerns?" about a particular item under discussion may bring the interviewer valuable information about attitudes, if not about explicit behavior.

Undue expectations are the cause of much unnecessary misery. Demands for simultaneous orgasm or even single orgasms 100 percent of the time demonstrate some examples of expectations that can hardly be realized. The woman who declares herself to be "frigid" because she can no longer obtain multiple orgasms represents such a "problem".

Every instance of sexual dysfunction is accompanied by ineffective communication. As was stated previously, the need to protect one's self-esteem or the fear of injuring the partner often leads to withdrawal and the silent nursing of frustration and angry feelings, usually preceded by outpourings of vindictive anger. Since emotions are contagious, anger provokes anger and a vicious cycle of escalating anger ensues. Communication in this instance can be accurate, but is hardly effective because in most people anger inhibits erotic arousal. (To be sure, there are some for whom anger is a potent erotic stimulus, but these people are unlikely to seek help for sexual difficulties.)

Often the nonorgasmic woman is uncertain if her response is normal, yet is reluctant to discuss this openly with her partner for fear of his ridicule or because she is concerned that he may regard this as his failure and be deeply hurt. She has not learned to signal what it is that she needs to be sexually turned on, and sometimes does not even recognize that she has a right to convey her sexual needs to the man. To compound the problem, failure of communication in the bedroom generally extends to an inability to effectively communicate in the living room or the kitchen. Every phase of the relationship may be affected by this breakdown in communication.

The clinician must understand that communication is more than verbal. There are people with very effective and pleasurable sexual relations who never discuss sex with each other at all, yet they are effective communicators. Their nonverbal forms of communication through facial expression, body language, intonation, and other aspects of vocalization convey signals to the mate which are readily understood. Whether cause or consequence, faulty communication and sexual dysfunction are involved in an escalating vicious cycle. It is for these reasons that Masters and Johnson state flatly:

> The cotherapists are fully aware that their most important role in reversal of sexual dysfunction is that of catalyst to communication.

Adequate communication in teaching the mutual pleasuring of "sensate focus" becomes the first step in sexual reeducation (see later under Sex Counseling).

Teaching a couple to communicate their physical pleasures and irritations without anger and recriminative hostility is one of the principal tasks of therapy. Unfortunately, effective communication is usually undermined in the beginning of therapy by the same kinds of emergency emotions that existed before treatment. Anger, guilt, and anxiety interfere with communication and inhibit erotic arousal. It is the therapist's task to diminish these negative emergency emotions and gradually replace them with the welfare emotions of love, hope, pride, joy, and trust. These latter emotions speed communication and make possible effective arousal and responsivity.

The gynecologist who wishes to engage in sex counseling has to recognize that this takes time. Although the skillful clinician can be helpful in a 10- or 15-minute interview, this amount of time is generally inadequate, especially in the early stages of treatment, when eliciting a history and preparing the patient for specific sexual-behavior tasks are the prominent missions of the counselor. Many gynecologists find it rewarding to set aside 1 or 2 half-days a week in which appointments are made specifically for sex counseling. Sessions generally last from 30 to 50 minutes, depending on the nature and stage of the case. The gynecologist who dislikes counseling because of antipathy toward this role, sexual inhibitions, or greater interest in other areas of gynecology should recognize this and should not attempt it. Instead, such gynecologists should listen carefully to those patients who give them clues that they are troubled by sexual concerns and honestly tell the patient that a colleague is better equipped to handle this particular problem.

After having set aside time for counseling, the clinician must set the proper atmosphere, inviting communication from the patient, who is usually somewhat embarrassed and inhibited when talking about sexual problems.

In selecting cases for counseling, the gynecologist must decide whether this is a fairly healthy person with a sexual problem or a person with psychopathology sufficient to warrant referral to a psychiatrist. Next is the decision whether the difficulty lies within the relationship or within the patient herself. If the interaction between the sexual partners is the primary reason for their sexual difficulty, the gynecologist has the task of deciding whether the problem is one best handled by a marriage counselor or a sex therapist. It is often difficult to make this decision at the first interview. In many instances, it is a good idea to see the couple for a number of sessions while attempting to make the decision as to whether the problem can be handled without referral.

Since most gynecologists have not been trained to do conjoint counseling and many of them rarely see the male at all, treating the couple may represent a considerable departure from the usual practice. There are many reasons why it makes sense: first, the couple's interaction itself may be the most important reason for the woman's sexual problems; second, the partner's cooperation is often essential for the success of the treatment; third, even if the original cause of the problem lies within the woman herself, the interaction with the male may maintain or even increase her sexual dysfunction. Since the male invariably suffers from the woman's sexual failures, he is always involved to some extent.

In essence, the gynecologist has to decide (1) whether education itself will be sufficient; (2) whether counseling the individual patient will be sufficient; or (3) whether conjoint marital counseling is essential for therapeutic success.

TAKING A SEXUAL HISTORY PREPARATORY TO DYSFUNCTION TREATMENT

The clinician must obtain specific detailed information about the patient's sexual life. Not only must information be obtained about behavior, such as the usual "scenario" adopted in the couple's sexual intercourse, but also the patient's feelings about erotic arousal and coitus itself. Furthermore, do the couple discuss their likes and dislikes about lovemaking? Is she worried about criticism from him? Is she embarrassed about nudity? How does she think her partner responds to the sight of her nude body? What does she think her partner's feelings are about her passivity or her strong pelvic thrusting movements? What turns her on and off?

If the gynecologist does conjoint counseling, similar questions will be asked of the man. (I believe the most difficult step for the gynecologist is overcoming inhibition about asking the partner these questions; yet ease in doing so is the single most important point in successful treatment.)

A basic plan for eliciting information and making an adequate appraisal is essential, provided the interviewer does not keep to a schedule in a mechanical, impersonal way. Questions should be specific but open-ended, as described in the earlier section on history taking. Important information is also elicited by observing the patient's nonverbal behavior, including the way she speaks, her facial expressions, and her body language. Particular attention must be paid to the interaction of doctor and patient, for this provides valuable clues about the attitudes of the patient and potential transference responses.

Motivations for change should begin in the first interview. The clinician is not only obtaining information but is starting in motion a process that may end in the alleviation of the patient's distress and dysfunction. In this process, the physician's attitude is all-important.

The physician's task becomes more delicate when there is an ethnic, racial or social-class difference between physician and patient. The patient's descriptive terms for sexual activity or body parts may be unfamiliar. The use of vernacular speech should be avoided, as it may be construed by the patient as condescension. Furthermore, women from a different subculture may be reluctant to give sexual information which they may think the physician will consider aberrant behavior.

Although errors are constantly made even by skilled interviewers, they are not serious unless the physician is unaware of them. Errors that are perceived from the patient's response can lead to adjustments helpful to the physician and the patient.

SEX COUNSELING

The major job of sex counseling is the assignment of behavioral tasks. This begins after setting an atmosphere in which the patient can speak freely and after dissemination of correct information. Tasks are best given to the couple together, but if that is impossible, the woman can pass along instructions to her sexual partner. The tasks are divided into three stages and were named "sensate focus" exercises by Masters and Johnson, who devised this method of therapy. They are carried out in private by the couple in the nude.

The man and woman gently caress and stroke each other's bodies with fingers or lips. Generally the man does so first. Beginning with the woman turned face down, the man strokes her head, hair, back of neck, ears, and works his way down to her buttocks, legs, and feet. When she has had enough of this she turns on her back and he caresses the front of her body, again from top to bottom, but avoiding her nipples and genitals. Then the woman strokes the man in the same way. The caresser concentrates on what it feels like to caress; the partner on the sensations of being caressed. The person receiving caresses is told to tell what things please or displease, without talking too much; to tell what strokes are too rough or too gentle, and when the pace is too slow or fast.

The second stage repeats the caressing of the first stage but with the addition of the genitals and breasts. The couple is asked not to use the stimulation that would ordinarily produce orgasm. The entire experience is done without demand for orgasm or coitus. Indeed, coitus is prohibited. The object is to remove the concern for performance, hence the "spectatoring" and much of the anxiety. As a result, the couple learn more effective sexual communication.

Eventually, in the third stage, coitus is reached. Before this, the clinician must deal with the reactions to the first two stages of the sensate-focus exercises. Most people report a positive response to the first stage and, often, erotic stimulation. However, negative reactions do occur, and these indicate resistance to the treatment based on individual psychological problems or problems in the marriage or relationship. Often a detailed analysis of the reaction will give clues about the nature of the problem.

There may be an inhibition of sexual excitement because of guilt, or such intense anger or distrust of the partner that they cannot go through with the assignment. Or there may be fear of closeness and intimacy. The gynecologist must decide whether to treat patients who have a negative response or to refer them to someone with greater psychotherapeutic skill.

Each type of sexual dysfunction has some specific treatment. Inhibition of sexual responsivity may

occur at several stages. At the level of the "sexual motive state" the woman has little or no desire for sex, nor does she easily allow herself to be put in a situation in which sex follows naturally, for the pleasurable anticipation of sex found in most people is absent or minimal; inhibition can affect the process of vasocongestion leading to lubrication, dilatation of the vagina, and the establishment of the orgasmic platform; or the inhibition may prevent orgasm. If the inhibition is very severe, spasm of the perivaginal musculature creates vaginismus.

TREATING INHIBITION OF SEXUAL DESIRE

The clinician must determine whether inhibition of sexual desire, which affects a third of all women with sexual dysfunctions, is primary or secondary. Has the woman been uninterested in sex from adolescence, or is she reacting as a consequence of angry or fearful feelings toward her partner? The latter may be a reflection of the general relationship, or may be more specifically due to repeated sexual failures in the past. If the inhibition of sexual desire is primary and has existed for years, referral for individual psychotherapy is the treatment of choice. If it is secondary, i.e., based on the partnership or marital interaction, again the gynecologist must make an assessment of whether to undertake therapy or whether to refer the patient to a marriage or sex counselor. If the interference with sex interest is primarily a response to repeated sexual failures in the past, the gynecologist has the best chance for effective intervention. The treatment techniques will be the same as those described for the second category—the inhibition of sexual excitement, described in the following secion.

INHIBITION OF SEXUAL EXCITEMENT

Diagnosis of inhibited sexual excitement is based on a recurrent and persistent failure, partial or complete, to attain or maintain the lubrication-swelling response of sexual excitement until completion of the sexual act. The diagnosis should be made only for the woman who, in the clinician's judgment, is receiving stimulation that is adequate in focus, intensity, and duration. If she is not receiving adequate stimulation, the diagnosis should be held in abeyance until the condition can be corrected by couple-counseling, perhaps including sensate-focus exercises.

Thus, the first question that should come to the mind of the counselor is: "Is this woman receiving adequate stimulation?" Since each woman's sensate focus is as individual as fingerprints, has she been able to communicate her pattern of stimulation to her husband effectively? She may think that her sexual activity ought to be under the male's direction and that she should be a passive recipient of his desires and behavior. Even if she does not believe in this myth, stated as "fact" in the old textbooks of gynecology, she may be afraid of his reaction if she becomes explicit about her sexual preferences. On the other hand, she may be able to communicate effectively, but her husband may be so tuned in to his own sensations and either unaware or unconcerned about his wife's needs that the entire sexual encounter may be guided by his urges, rather than by concern over whether his wife is receiving sufficient arousal. Answers to these questions come through the feedback from the sensate-focus exercises previously described.

As mentioned previously, in the first two stages of the sensate-focus exercises, coitus is prohibited. There should be no demand for performance. In cases of inhibition of sexual excitement, it may be wise to have the wife perform the caressing first. This reduces her guilt from being on the receiving side as well as her fear of not responding. She learns the lesson of "giving to get." Eliminating the need to perform and to please her husband may produce dramatic results. For the first time she may begin to really feel the full intensity of erotic arousal. The husband's willingness to defer orgastic gratification is another expression of his desire to help his wife. This, in turn, may have a salutary effect on their interaction. If the response to the nongenital or first stage of sensate focus is positive and pleasurable, they can move on to the second stage. If there are negative reactions, these have to be discussed in great detail, so that the sources of resistance or inhibition are made clear.

The second stage in which the breast and genitals are stimulated, should produce a sharp increase in her sexual responsiveness. When the husband is considerate and affectionate and unthreatened by this experience, there should be mutual pleasure, even enthusiasm for the second stage of the sexual "tasks."

The third stage, which involves coitus, should be under the control of the woman. She should initiate coitus when she feels she is ready. Generally, it is helpful if the woman is on top so that she has control of the thrusting. The man is instructed to be essentially passive while she focuses her attention on her sensations as she slowly thrusts while contracting her pubococcygeal muscles.

If the husband feels that he cannot control his ejaculation, the couple can be advised to stop thrusting and to use the "stop and start" technique, in which they stop for 15 to 20 seconds to allow some decrease in the man's excitement, and then to resume thrusting, repeating several times until the woman herself feels like continuing this cycle to the point of orgasm, which she then communicates to her husband.

The entire sequence of events is aimed at the woman's erotic pleasure, not the husband's. The whole sexual encounter is under her control. If, while this is going on, she senses that her husband is enjoying the experience and she does not feel rejected, orgasm becomes probable.

ORGASMIC DYSFUNCTION

The preorgasmic woman does not abandon herself to her reflex response; despite adequate vasocongestion, she "holds back." The woman who has never achieved an orgasm from any source is a special problem. The whole issue of masturbation should be raised with the patient in a tactful manner. Some patients are so turned off by the idea that without an extensive series of interviews it is unlikely that one can suggest masturbation without running the risk of the patient's abandoning treatment.

In many homes, sexual curiosity, exhibitionism, and masturbation are prohibited by parents, so that feelings of guilt and shame are extremely common among adults reared in such homes. Many people are unable to achieve a balance between control over their sexual impulses and the capacity to fully enjoy their bodies, either by masturbation or with another person. Seemingly, girls are subject to more sexual prohibitions, for studies previously mentioned show the cumulative incidence of masturbation in women is close to 80 percent, compared with 97 percent in males. Kinsey discovered that in women as well as men, experience with masturbation and sexual adjustment in marriage are positively correlated.

Masturbation, which begins at an early age, may go on through the life cycle, and in many older women with increased frequency after age 65, when there may not be an available sexual partner. The majority of women have experimented with masturbation, but in cases of orgasmic dysfunction, without success. When this is true, the woman should be instructed to contract her abdominal and perineal muscles during masturbation at what she feels to be the peak of her sexual tension. This not only adds to her sexual tension, but probably distracts her from the feeling of guilt and the fear of abandonment previously inhibiting her orgastic release. If manual masturbation is insufficient, she may be instructed to use a vibrator. The clinician must be mindful of the fact that the intense stimulation produced by the vibrator may create a situation in which the patient depends on a vibrator for orgastic release and cannot achieve it by any other means. Sole reliance on the vibrator is to be encouraged only if nothing else works. The use of the vibrator, contraction of the muscles, and the use of fantasy, if necessary, generally produce an orgasm in a previously preorgasmic woman, although, as in every other form of therapy, there are failures. Once a woman has attained orgasm and has practiced sufficiently with masturbation manually or with a vibrator, she can then be treated in the same way as those who have had orgasm but have not been able to achieve it with a male partner.

FAILURE TO ACHIEVE ORGASM DURING COITUS

We have just been discussing the woman who has never had an orgasm from any source, including masturbation. Countless women are able to masturbate to climax, either alone or in the presence of the partner, and respond to the partner's stimulation, sometimes with a high level of arousal, and can achieve orgasm with clitoral stimulation but cannot experience orgasm during coitus. If approximately 90 percent of women eventually experience orgasm, perhaps 75 percent on a fairly regular basis, more than 50 percent of the women who have achieved orgasm are unable to achieve it during coitus. This means that more than half of all women are found in this group. Because this is such a large group, the question is whether we are dealing with a pathological entity, a form of inhibition, or whether this is a normal variation. Some women are content with this state of affairs and do not experience any sense of frustration. On the other hand, some feel that they have been cheated out of an experience to which they are entitled, and complain angrily to the gynecologist about their inability to have an orgasm during intercourse. As mentioned earlier, it may be the husband who is the primary complainant.

The sensate-focus exercises often serve to increase sexual communication between the partners and heighten arousal during foreplay. This may be sufficient to produce coital orgasm, although in many women who are relatively responsive with clitoral stimulation, the sensate-focus exercises do not help in achieving coital orgasm, even though they increase communication. The woman who cannot "let go" or abandon herself to her own sensations has to learn to concentrate on these premonitory sensations

just prior to orgasm and to decrease her concern about her performance and about pleasing her partner. The use of fantasy during this premonitory stage can be very helpful. Contracting her pubococcygeal muscles can also be an aid.

Coitus can be augmented by clitoral stimulation, either by the woman or the man. When the woman learns to "receive" the premonitory symptoms just prior to orgasm, she can begin to thrust actively while she contracts her vaginal and abdominal muscles. The rhythmic contraction and relaxation of perineal muscles are an aid to many women in facilitating coital orgasm. Of course, intromission should start only when the woman is close to the orgasm she ordinarily has during clitoral stimulation.

In summary, the points used in sexual reeducation are: (1) waiting until the woman is close to orgasm before instituting coitus; (2) the use of fantasy; (3) the contraction of the perineal and abdominal muscles; (4) the stop-start technique; (5) the adjunctive use of clitoral stimulation during coitus; and (6) the woman's rapid thrusting when she feels an impending orgasm. By distracting the woman from thoughts which separate her from her sensations, these "tasks" help the woman to reach orgasm even more than their "physiological" input.

Clinicians do not report uniform success in treating women who are orgastic with clitoral stimulation but are not orgastic during coitus. It may be easier to help a woman who has never been orgastic to achieve orgasm either through self-stimulation or through clitoral stimulation by her partner than it is to take her from the range of clitoral orgasm to coital orgasm. Nonetheless, these techniques work often enough to warrant their use with those women who are frustrated by their inability to achieve coital orgasm. If these techniques fail, the woman and her husband can be reassured that there are millions of women who achieve orgasm only with clitoral stimulation and not during intercourse, and that this should be regarded as a normal variant.

If the woman still remains frustrated at the lack of coital orgasm, referral to a psychiatrist or marital therapist for "therapy" rather than counseling is the final step. Therapy aimed at removing intrapsychic and interpersonal conflicts may bring success. If not, she may be helped to accept her limitations in this as in other areas.

VAGINISMUS AND DYSPAREUNIA

Once all painful conditions such as infections have been corrected, the persistence of vaginismus calls for techniques to eliminate the conditioned spasm of the muscles guarding the vaginal entrance. Masters and Johnson (1970) have advocated the use of graduated dilatation, moving from a wire-thin catheter to the next larger size, etc. Both rubber and glass catheters have been used with success. After the patient is able to tolerate the insertion of the larger catheters without discomfort, she can attempt intercourse, guiding the penis with her hand. During the process of dilatation she should be able to insert her own fingers into her vagina (which for many women is surprisingly difficult).

There are other methods for treating vaginismus, which probably have their specific place in specialized sex-therapy clinics or for those who specialize in sex therapy.

The gynecologist is best advised to use a combination of dilatation augmented between office sessions by the woman and then her husband inserting a finger in the vagina after she has examined her vagina with the aid of a hand mirror. In women with vaginismus, ignorance about anatomy is enormous and, in many instances, this ignorance is shared by the husband. The self-examination in the husband's presence serves to reduce the phobic element and facilitates the insertion of the catheter at the next visit to the gynecologist's office. Instructing the woman to contract and relax her vaginal muscles also gives her a sense of voluntary control over the vaginal entry. During the entire process, the patient must be able to tolerate some anxiety and tension and continue with the tasks despite her unpleasant feelings.

In general, dyspareunia can be cured by dealing with the physical factors that create it, or by making certain that the woman waits until she is adequately lubricated before intercourse is attempted. If vaginismus is a factor in her dyspareunia, the treatment then follows the methods just described.

OTHER TREATMENT APPROACHES TO SEXUAL INADEQUACY

Allusion has been made to the use of behavioral therapy in a more formal sense than the sexual-reeducation techniques of Masters and Johnson (1970), as well as the use of hypnosis by sex therapists. These methods, however, are not generally employed by gynecologists.

The use of erotic films in treatment has been developed by a few centers. More recently a rapid method for the treatment of sexual dysfunction using erotic films and group discussions following the initial workup of the couple has been described by Powell et al. Members of the treatment team include a gynecologist, a psychiatrist, a clinical psychologist, and a social worker.

Group methods may cut down the total professional time, create additional sources of influence on patients, and decrease the costs of treatment. Selection of cases for these different methods is always the key issue.

THE PLACE OF SEX COUNSELING IN GYNECOLOGIC PRACTICE

Sex counseling can become one of the most rewarding aspects of gynecologic practice. Symptoms are usually definite, and the therapeutic outcome with symptom alleviation unambiguous. Even if other marital problems come to light as a result of successful treatment of sexual inadequacy, opportunity for working these out may be provided by referral for marital therapy, enhancing the couple's potential for growth and productive living.

REFERENCES

Bell AP, Weinberg MS: *Homosexualities,* New York: Simon & Schuster, 1978.

Berman EM et al.: The age 30 crisis and the 7-year-itch. *J Sex Marital Therapy* 3: 197, 1977.

Bernard J: *The Future of Marriage,* New York: World Pub., 1972.

Burnap DW, Golden JS: Sexual problems in medical practice. *J Med Educ* 42: 673, 1967.

Dickenson RL: *Atlas of Human Sex Anatomy,* 2d ed., Baltimore: Williams & Wilkins, 1949.

Erikson E: The problem of ego identity. *J Am Psychoan Assoc* 4:56, 1956.

Feldman H, Feldman M: The family life cycle: Some suggestions for recycling. *J Mar Family* 37:277, 1975.

Filler W, Lief HI: A psychological approach to the gynecological patient, in *The Psychological Basis of Medical Practice,* eds. HI Lief et al., New York: Hoeber/Harper & Row, 1963, pp. 449-460.

Fisher S: *The Female Orgasm,* New York: Basic Books, 1973.

Group for the Advancement of Psychiatry: *Assessment of Sexual Function: A Guide to Interviewing, GAP*

Report No. 88, Committee on Medical Education, New York: GAP, 1973.

Kaplan HS: *The New Sex Therapy,* New York: Brunner/Mazel, 1974.

Kinsey AC et al.: *Sexual Behavior in the Human Female,* Philadelphia: Saunders, 1953, p. 397.

LeMasters E: Parenthood as crises. *Marriage and Family Living* 19:352, 1957.

Lief HI: Medical aspects of sexuality, in *Cecil Textbook of Medicine,* 15th ed., eds. P. Beeson, W. McDermott, Philadelphia: Saunders, 1979.

Lief HI: Sex education in medicine: Retrospect and prospect, in *Sex Education of the Professional,* eds. N Rosenzweig and FP Pearsall, New York: Grune and Stratton, 1978.

Ludwig A et al.: *Psychosomatic Aspects of Gynecological Disorders,* Cambridge: Harvard University Press, 1969.

Masters W, Johnson V: *Human Sexual Response,* Boston: Little, Brown, 1966.

————, ————: *Human Sexual Inadequacy,* Boston: Little, Brown, 1970.

———— et al.: *Ethical Issues in Sex Therapy and Research,* Boston: Little, Brown, 1977.

Miller W, Lief HI: Masturbatory attitudes, knowledge, and experience: Data from the Sex Knowledge and Attitude Test (SKAT). *Arch Sex Behav* 5:447, 1976.

Nash EM, Louden L: Premarital medical examination: With patients' desire. *JAMA* 210:2365, 1969.

Newton M: Interrelationships between sexual responsiveness, birth, and breastfeeding, in *Contemporary Sexual Behavior: Critical Issues in the 1970's,* eds. J Zubin, J Money, Baltimore: Johns Hopkins Univ. Press, 1973, pp. 77–98.

Pasini W: Sexuality during pregnancy and postpartum frigidity, in *Handbook of Sexology,* eds. J Money, J Musaph, Amsterdam: Excerpta Medica, 1977, p. 887.

Pauley ID, Goldstein SF: Physicians' perception of their education in human sexuality. *J Med Educ* 45:745, 1970.

Persky H et al.: Reproductive hormone levels and sexual behaviors of young couples during the menstrual cycle, in *Progress in Sexology,* eds. R Gemme, CC Wheeler, New York: Plenum Publ., 1977.

———— et al.: Plasma testosterone level and sexual behavior of couples. *Arch Sex Behav* 7:157, 1978.

Powell LC, et al.: Rapid treatment approaches to human sexual inadequacy. *Am J Obstet Gynecol* 119:89, 1974.

Pugh WE, Fernandez FL: Coitus in late pregnancy. *Obstet Gynecol* 15:449, 1960.

Rauh JL, Burket RL: Adolescent sexual activity and resultant gynecologic problems. *Med Aspects of Human Sexuality,* in press.

Reiss IL: *The Family System in America,* New York: Holt, Rinehart, Winston, 1971, p. 407.

————: *The Family System in America,* 2d ed., Hinsdale, Ill.: Dryden Press, 1976, p. 88.

Rollins BC, Feldman H: Marital satisfaction over the family life cycle. *J Mar and Family* 32:2028, 1970.

Rubin LB: *Worlds of Pain: Life in the Working-Class Family,* New York: Basic Books, 1976.

Stoller RJ: *Sex and Gender,* New York: Random House, 1968.

Vincent CE (ed.): *Human Sexuality in Medical Education and Practice,* Springfield, Ill.: Charles C Thomas, 1968.

————: *Sexual and Marital Health: The Physician as a Consultant,* New York: McGraw-Hill, 1973, p. 4.

Ward I: Prenatal stress feminizes and demasculinizes the behavior of males. *Science* 175:82–84, 1972.

Zelnik M, Kantner JF: Sexuality, contraception and pregnancy among young unwed females in the United States, in *The United States Commission on Population Growth and The American Future, Demographic and Social Aspects of Population Growth, Vol. 1,* 1972.

————, ————: Sexual and contraceptive experience of young unmarried women in the United States, 1976 and 1971. *Fam Plann Perspect* 9:55, 1977.

————, ————: Contraceptive patterns and premarital pregnancy among women aged 15–19 in 1976. *Fam Plann Perspect* 10:135, 1978.

35

Physiology and Pathophysiology of Menstruation and Menopause

HOWARD L. JUDD   DAVID R. MELDRUM

THE PHYSIOLOGY OF MENSTRUATION

It is frequently forgotten in the presence of modern methods of hormone measurement that one of the most common gynecologic events is uterine bleeding, and yet the mechanisms of normal and abnormal bleeding at the level of the endometrium are not undergoing the same degree of study as was true years ago. Under normal circumstances, women bleed only during the menstrual period. Menstrual endometrium is that which has gone through a physiologic cycle of estrogen proliferative stimulation followed by a progesterone secretory effect. The slough of menstrual endometrium leaves a basal endometrium which is repaired and then proliferates once again. The first day of bleeding is the first day of a cycle, which is usually 28 days in length; the first day of bleeding of the subsequent period thus represents the end of the cycle. Successive phases of the cycle correspond to histological changes taking place in the endometrium, and these changes can be identified in endometrial biopsy material by experienced pathologists.

The endometrium proliferates for about 14 days under the influence of estrogen, primarily 17β-estradiol. During this phase, the glands are straight and mitoses can be seen. The glands are parallel and are lined up in a regular manner equidistant from each other. Some interstitial fluid accumulates. Accurate dating of the endometrium in the proliferative phase requires a knowledge of the normal cyclic changes. In studying endometrial biopsies, these changes are compared with the known day of the cycle (i.e., days since the last menstrual period). It should be remembered that the cycle being biopsied is a new cycle, unrelated to the last menstrual flow, and whereas the luteal phase is constant, the length of the proliferative phase may vary. Therefore, the duration of the menstrual cycle must ultimately be determined from the day of onset of the next cycle. For example, if a biopsy is taken on day 17 and the next menstrual period occurs on day 35, ovulation would have taken place on day 20 or 21, and the day 17 endometrium would then be expected to have the appearance of a late proliferative phase rather than that of a day 17 endometrium from a normal 28-day cycle. The latter endometrium has a rather characteristic appearance which includes the presence of subnuclear vacuoles in the columnar glandular epithelial cells. Since it is variable, dating in the proliferative phase is rarely planned clinically, and for this reason, the endometrium is usually described as being in the early, mid, or late proliferative stage. However, proliferative endometrium may also be encountered when not expected, such as in association with anovulation. In these and other instances, it is most helpful to relate the appearance of the endometrium to the actual clinical dates.

The arcuate artery is a branch of the uterine artery which runs in an arc about the uterus, sending off smaller branches to the basilar portion of the endometrium. These basilar branches, in turn, give rise to the spiral arterioles which support the proliferating stroma and which are responsible, by their eventual constriction, for the sloughing of the endometrium during the menstrual flow.

Progesterone begins to be secreted 2 to 3 days before ovulation, and the classical marker of early ovulation is endometrium from day 16 to day 18. Characteristic basal or subnuclear vacuolation is seen in the glandular epithelium beginning 36 to 48 hours following ovulation, and this progresses on to later secretion into the glandular lumen. Eventually, as the phase comes to a close, this secretion becomes inspissated and a predecidual reaction begins to appear around the vessels. Decidua is so named because, like the deciduous tree, it is shed; however, the shedding of decidua occurs, not in autumn, but during the postpartum period. Decidua is a pregnancy-associated change of the endometrium produced by a combination of estrogen and progesterone stimulation. It is characterized by plump, eosinophilic stromal cells which have a pavement-like, polygonal appearance. Their distinct cell borders create a reticulum. This reticulum is presumably a glycoprotein, as it is amylase resistant. Other areas of decidualization which also result from estrogen and progesterone stimulation and which develop on the ovary and tube in relation to both term pregnancy and ectopic pregnancy are called pseudodecidua. Thus, the reddish, friable areas seen on the ovary at the time of cesarean section are pseudodecidual in nature and need not be biopsied. The true decidua (like menstrual endometrium) is shed from the endometrial cavity following delivery when the estrogen and progesterone secretions fall and are no longer able to support its growth. Decidua, therefore, is a major component of lochia, the reddish, blood-containing secretion that is produced in the first few postpartum days and that later becomes clear (see Chap. 15).

The characteristics of the secretory endometrium from the luteal phase of the cycle are very reproducible, and, therefore, specific days of the cycle between ovulation and menstruation can be identified. Endometrial biopsy during the luteal phase can be of great value in the infertile patient, where one significant problem may be an inadequate luteal phase (see Chap. 27). Under such circumstances, a biopsy on day 23 may show a variance of greater than 2 days from normal and may thus be diagnostic of such a deficit. If, for example, on day 23 the endometrium shows only day 20 histologic characteristics *and* the subsequent menstrual period still begins 5 days later on day 28, as expected, the diagnosis is made. A knowledge of the endometrium and its dating can also be invaluable in the management of dysfunctional uterine bleeding. If endometrial biopsy is coupled with a knowledge of the normal hormonal levels throughout the ovarian cycle, many problems of both abnormal bleeding and infertility can be intelligently handled.

As the menopause approaches, inadequate secretion of estrogen begins, and ovulation may or may not occur. The endometrium may reveal a varied appearance of incomplete proliferation and/or inadequate luteal effect. In part, this endometrial change may protect the mature woman from pregnancy after the age of 40. As the perimenopausal years approach, endometrial hyperplasia, either cystic, adenomatous, or combined, may occur. Finally, as ovarian ovulatory function ceases, the endometrium becomes atrophic. With mild inflammation or erosion into a vessel, such postmenopausal endometrium may unexpectedly bleed (atrophic endometritis).

Normal menstruation is the result of cessation of estrogen and progesterone secretion at the end of the menstrual cycle. As estrogen and progesterone levels fall, the spiral arterioles contract and remain physiologically constricted. The resulting ischemia allows the endometrium to slough efficiently. Fortunately, the endometrium does not slough off all at once, a situation that could result in a social disaster, but rather sloughing occurs gently in different areas. First, there is a little ischemia, followed by some bleeding and sloughing of tissues. This is followed by a more general response. Thus, normal menstruation cannot occur without appropriate preparation, which is principally hormonal in nature.

Not only does bleeding occur from secretory endometrium as in menstruation, but it can occur at any time from endometrium which is incompletely or improperly stimulated. Thus, bleeding may occur from proliferative endometrium or from premenstrual endometrium. The bleeding from proliferative endometrium usually occurs as the result of a fall in estrogen secretion and as the result of the failure of ovulation and the absence of progesterone secretion.

Changes take place in the biochemical composition of the endometrium which allow it to slough off readily following the secretion of progesterone. In addition, as estrogen and progesterone levels fall, the endometrium becomes first hypoxic, then ischemic. The cells previously altered begin to degenerate next. The mucopolysaccharide-rich ground substance of the endometrium, predominant during the proliferative phase, is gradually dissolved, presumably by alteration initiated by progesterone secretion. Ultimately, the altered estrogen and progesterone metabolism lead to an instability of the cellular lysosomes. These in turn release active catalytic enzymes into the cytoplasm of the endometrial cells. Phospholipase acts to free arachidonic acid from its ester. The cyclo-oxygenase (also called prostaglandin synthetase) released activates the prostaglandin system. Endoperoxides are formed (prostaglandin G and H), followed by prostaglandin E_2 and $F_{2\alpha}$. It is not presently known if thromboxanes are biosynthesized in the endometrium, and if so what effect these might have. The prostaglandins will affect uterine contractions and the vascular spasm of the uterine vessels.

Enzyme activity takes place in the endometrium under estrogen stimulation during the preovulatory phase. During the proliferative phase to ovulation, alkaline phosphatase, β-glucuronidase, glucose-6-phosphatase, nonspecific esterases, diphosphopyridine nucleotide diaphorase, and glucose 6-phosphate dehydrogenase are predominant. Presumably, these enzymes prepare the endometrium for implantation augmented by the brief activation of those enzymes which predominate early in the luteal phase.

Acid phosphatase dominates in secretory endometrium with the accumulation of glycogen mucopolysaccharides and lipids. Such accumulation plays a role in nutritional support of the implanted fertilized egg. It is presumed that the proliferative phase of the endometrium is dominated by anaerobic glycolysis and the luteal phase by aerobic glycolysis. The important enzyme in this change is lactic dehydrogenase. The acid hydrolases, presumably also released from the lysosomes are responsible for the initiation of menstruation.

Endometrial cells are capable of metabolizing steroid hormones, there being present both 17β- and 20α-steroid dehydrogenase as well as 5α-oxidase. Specific protein receptors for steroids, both estrogen and progesterone, have also been identified in the endometrium. Currently, estrogen is thought to stimulate the accumulation of progesterone receptors, while progesterone inhibits and reduces the concentration of the estrogen receptors. Progesterone concomitantly induces 17β-estradiol steroid dehydrogenase which also, through metabolic effects, reduces estrogen action. The receptors are presently being studied in relationship to the development of cancer of the endometrium.

The release of prostaglandin into the bloodstream may be associated with dysmenorrhea. Increased concentrations have been observed both in the uterus and peripherally in women with severe dysmenorrhea.

Normal sloughing of endometrium represents a complex series of biochemical and enzymic events. Bleeding from proliferative endometrium, as in anovulatory bleeding, has no such preceding course. The endometrium does not slough, it may be hyperplastic, and the spiral arterioles do not turn off efficiently. Bleeding, which may be profuse, is from the surface of the endometrium. With inappropriate sloughing or stimulation, polyps may be formed, which makes the ultimate management more complex.

PREMENSTRUAL TENSION AND DYSMENORRHEA

Physiological disruptions which occur during the menstrual cycle and lead to subjective discomfort and emotional disturbance have been subject to an unusual degree of disdain by both male and female physicians. These complaints have been attributed to underlying emotional difficulties, to faulty attitudes about female function instilled by parents, and to various environmental stresses. Because of this negative view, there has been remarkably little discriminating research into the underlying pathophysiology of these symptoms. In the following sections, recent advances that point to an organic basis of these disturbances will be presented. These studies provide new insight into these frequent and perplexing symptoms. However, an appreciation of the effect of emotional illness and situational stresses on the perception of these discomforts is still an important aspect of their treatment. Supportive treatment and psychiatric referral should be utilized when appropriate, but this should not detract from attempts to understand the underlying mechanisms.

PREMENSTRUAL TENSION

During the latter part of the luteal phase a wide variety of physical discomforts are experienced throughout the body. These may be limited to a mild mood change, breast tenderness, and abdominal bloating; such symptoms are often referred to as molimina. These symptoms commonly accompany ovulatory menses and are considered to be physiological. In some women these complaints are so severe that they impair the individual's ability to function. Additional changes which are commonly experienced are weight gain, emotional instability, increased appetite, lower abdominal discomfort, headaches, changes in libido, fatigue, generalized aches and pains, nausea, and vomiting (Timonen, Procope).

Epidemiological studies have documented that these changes can represent a definite danger to women. Dalton has shown that women are involved in more accidents and commit more crimes in the premenstrual and menstrual days of the cycle (Dalton). Admissions to psychiatric hospitals and suicides are similarly related to this phase of the menstrual cycle. Studies on intellectual performance have shown conflicting results, with one study reporting no difference in college scores during various quarters of the cycle, while another study showed lower marks during the 4 days preceding and the 4 days following the start of menses in schoolgirls. The syndrome is extremely common if mild symptoms are included. In one study of 748 female students, 67 percent experienced "tension"; 52 percent, nervousness; 23 percent, headaches; 10 percent, nausea; and 35 percent, depression. It has been estimated that one-third of all women experience moderate irritability and that 10 percent

have severe irritability. Thus, the psychosocial impact of the syndrome is considerable.

Premenstrual tension has been correlated with increasing age in most studies. In the patients studied by Dalton over 80 percent were 30 years of age or older. The syndrome has also been related to parity, with only 19 percent of patients being nulliparous and 54 percent having two or more prior pregnancies (Dalton). Coppen and Kessel did not find a relationship to age or parity in studying the incidence in the general population (1963). These conflicting results may be related to the small number of patients with severe symptoms in the latter study. The syndrome has been correlated with the occurrence of dysmenorrhea, suggesting a common etiology. In 40 percent of women with both complaints, the pelvic pain preceded menses, whereas in women with dysmenorrhea alone, only 22 percent had premenstrual pain (Coppen, Kessel).

A relationship has also been observed between psychiatric disturbances and the premenstrual syndrome (Coppen, Kessel; Rees), suggesting that the symptoms are more likely to be severe in certain predisposed individuals. Rees found moderate to severe symptoms in 62 percent of psychiatric patients as compared with 21 percent in normal persons (1953). The symptoms correlated with a variety of neurotic complaints and with maladjustment and neurosis in general. Although this association has been observed, it is not inevitable. The premenstrual syndrome often occurs in entirely normal women, and many severely neurotic women have no premenstrual symptoms.

Investigation of the etiology of premenstrual tension has centered mainly on the serial measurement of estrogens, progesterone, gonadotropins, prolactin, and various hormones with fluid-retaining properties in patients with the syndrome. To date, these studies have been unable to establish a definitive pattern of abnormal hormonal secretion which could explain the occurrence of the symptoms. The finding of an increase in the capillary filtration coefficient, reflecting increased capillary permeability, suggests that the associated edema results in part from local vascular changes rather than from fluid retention alone.

Different lines of study have suggested other possible etiological factors. For instance, hypoglycemia has been implicated in the occurrence of depression, headache, and fatigue during the premenstrual period. A higher incidence of hypoglycemia and increased glucose tolerance has been observed with a return of glucose tolerance to normal after menses. A craving for food or sweets has been correlated with tension, depression, and fluid retention. Animal studies have suggested that the period of estrogen and progesterone withdrawal is associated with changes in monoamine levels within the brain and the uptake of dopamine and serotonin into brain tissue. These observations have been of interest, but, again, have provided no unified concept of the etiology.

Recently, it has been suggested that prostaglandins may play a role in the occurrence of premenstrual tension. It is known that the levels of prostaglandins in the endometrium increase during the luteal phase of the cycle. The widespread effects of these compounds on the brain, kidney, cardiovascular system, gastrointestinal tract, and glucose metabolism could explain the wide range of complaints experienced. The forementioned correlation of the premenstrual syndrome with dysmenorrhea suggests a common etiology, and mounting evidence indicates that these compounds are responsible for many, if not all, of the symptoms experienced during menses in dysmenorrheic women. The relationship of the premenstrual syndrome to parity could relate to the well-known development of the uterine blood supply with pregnancy, allowing increased absorption of these compounds into the circulation. Finally, it has been observed empirically that hysterectomy can relieve severe premenstrual symptoms in some patients. Although this is an attractive hypothesis, further support is required to substantiate the relationship.

To date, treatment of the premenstrual syndrome has been unsatisfactory. It has been customary to treat the most obvious physical manifestation, fluid retention, in the hope that other symptoms would also be relieved. Diuretics are effective in reducing edema, but controlled trials have shown no additional effect on psychological disturbances beyond that obtained with placebo (Mattson, Schoultz). This finding reinforces the conclusion that central-nervous-system symptoms are not secondary to edema.

As a result of the observation of elevated prolactin levels in patients with the premenstrual syndrome, bromocriptine has been investigated for a possible therapeutic effect. An initial finding of symptomatic relief in a small double-blind study has not been confirmed by two larger, controlled trials, with the exception of a beneficial effect on mastodynia. Since the dosage and duration of treatment were not the same in the above studies, a specific effect of bromocriptine cannot be entirely ruled out. The prominent placebo effect documented in these and other reports indicates the necessity for double-blind trials in the investigation of this symptom complex.

Pyridoxine has been reported to be effective, but a double-blind trial did not confirm a specific effect. Lithium, which is effective in psychiatric disorders with cyclic mood swings, has not shown benefit over placebo aside from a mild diuretic effect. Exercise has been suggested because of a negative correlation of the syndrome with physical activity. This treatment remains speculative. Recently, it has been observed that prostaglandin inhibitors provide relief of the premenstrual syndrome. This uncontrolled observation needs to be confirmed but does provide another link between these hormones and the occurrence of this symptom complex.

One of the most frequently suggested treatment modalities has been the use of progesterone, by either injection or suppository. The finding of a low progesterone/estradiol ratio in patients whose principal symptom was premenstrual anxiety supports such a consideration (Backstrom et al.). However, a double-blind trial in patients with premenstrual depression showed no benefit from progesterone therapy. This raises the possibility that the reputed benefit of progesterone on premenstrual tension is also a placebo response.

DYSMENORRHEA

Dysmenorrhea refers to pelvic pain associated with menses, generally beginning within 1 day prior to the onset of menstrual flow and terminating during or at the end of bleeding. Dysmenorrhea is termed primary when it occurs in the absence of pelvic disease and secondary when it occurs in association with diseases known to cause painful menstruation.

Primary dysmenorrhea generally begins shortly after menarche, when ovulatory periods become established. It is characterized by episodic central lower abdominal pain radiating to the lower back and upper thighs. It is often associated with nausea, vomiting, diarrhea, headache, and dizziness. Psychological symptoms of irritability, tension, and depression are commonly experienced. In a large survey, Coppen and Kessel found an incidence of severe dysmenorrhea of 12 percent and moderate to severe symptoms of 45 percent (1963). Dysmenorrhea occurs less frequently with increasing parity, being only half as frequent following the birth of the first child. This symptom complex is a significant cause of absenteeism from work and school.

Greater understanding of factors controlling uterine contractility has led to a new appreciation of the pathophysiology of this disturbance. Menstruation is associated with release of prostaglandins in the menstrual fluid. These compounds are potent stimulators of the myometrium. Local application reproduces the hypercontractility and increased tonus found in primary dysmenorrhea. The concentration of prostaglandins increases in the endometrium during the luteal phase. The luteal phase concentration is markedly increased in patients with dysmenorrhea (Willman et al.). In controlled studies, prostaglandin inhibitors have been found to relieve primary dysmenorrhea with a high degree of success, and the effect of these agents in reducing uterine contractions and endometrial prostaglandins has been documented. Finally, exogenous administration of prostaglandins produces nausea, vomiting, diarrhea, and cardiovascular changes—all of the systemic symptoms which accompany primary dysmenorrhea. Thus, the uterine cramps of dysmenorrhea and the associated systemic symptoms may relate to enhanced synthesis of prostaglandins in the endometrium and to the release of these hormones into the circulation or to a possible local effect on the bowel from retrograde flow of menstrual fluid.

The actual production of pain has been generally assumed to be ischemic in origin, because of the role of high resting uterine tonus in the production of pain and the beneficial effect of parity, with its concomitant development of uterine vascularity.

Diagnosis of primary dysmenorrhea depends upon a typical history of onset shortly after menarche. Onset and progression later in life should prompt thorough investigation to rule out secondary causes such as endometriosis, uterine myomata, adenomyosis, endometrial polyps, pelvic inflammatory disease, and cervical stenosis. Even with a typical history and an apparently normal pelvic examination the possibility of a uterine anomaly or endometriosis should be considered.

Recently, the most frequent mode of therapy has been the use of oral contraceptives in the form of combination estrogen and progestin preparations. Since sequential pills were associated with less relief of menstrual pain, it is believed that oral contraceptives do not relieve pain just by inhibiting ovulation. Instead, they work by decreasing the amount of bleeding and tissue slough. In addition, reduced concentrations of prostaglandins and their metabolites have been shown in the endometrium of treated patients, and a decreased response of the myometrium to prostaglandins has also been demonstrated in women taking oral contraceptives. The high degree of effectiveness of the combination pill supports its use in symptomatic women who desire contraception.

In women who do not need contraception or should not take oral contraceptives, the use of specific inhibitors of prostaglandin synthesis appears to hold the most promise for relief. For example, in women with severe dysmenorrhea, mefenamic acid (Ponstel) produced complete relief during 67 of 75 cycles (Pulkkinen, Kaihola). No relief was experienced in only four cycles. Other prostaglandin inhibitors such as flufenamic acid, indomethacin, and naproxen have also been shown to be highly effective, but are either not available in the United States or are officially indicated solely for the treatment of arthritis. Mefenamic acid is indicated for the relief of mild to moderate pain of short duration and is effective. Ibuprofen (Motrine) is also highly effective and recently has been approved for use in dysmenorrhea. Use of such agents requires a familiarity with their contraindications and potential side effects and complications. In view of the concern over the widespread metabolic effects of oral contraceptives, the use of antiprostaglandins should be considered for dysmenorrhea as an alternative to oral contraceptives even in women who do need contraception.

If the patient fails to respond to oral contraceptives or prostaglandin inhibitors, then prompt reevaluation should be undertaken for a secondary cause of the pain. Laparoscopy should be considered to rule out endometriosis. In conjunction with hysterosalpingogram or hysteroscopy, uterine anomalies and other causes may be ruled out.

If specific relief is not obtained and no etiology is found on thorough evaluation, a psychological cause should be considered. However, the lack of relationship of primary dysmenorrhea to emotional illness (Cloppen, Kessel) and the specific response to therapy suggest that such an etiology is infrequent.

MENOPAUSE

The cessation of ovarian function spontaneously or surgically presents a woman and her physician with a constellation of problems concerning her medical and psychological well-being. At issue is the question of whether the hormonal changes resulting from ovarian failure are of sufficient liability to necessitate replacement therapy. This question takes on overwhelming significance because of the number of women faced with the problem and the recent association of estrogen therapy with endometrial cancer.

In the United States census of 1970 there were 104 million females in this country, 27 million being 50 years of age or older. Women who live to age 50 have an average life expectancy of 78 years. These figures indicate that a large minority of our population has undergone ovarian failure and will live more than one-third of their lives after its occurrence. As the older members of our society increase in number, the magnitude of this problem will also increase. Consequently, it is essential that physicians who treat women have understanding of the hormonal and metabolic changes associated with the menopause and an appreciation of the potential benefits and risks of replacement therapy. Some of these considerations are reviewed in this section.

MECHANISM OF THE MENOPAUSE

In the human female, oogenesis begins in the fetal ovary around the third week of gestation (Ross, Vande Wiele). Primordial germ cells appear in the yolk sac of the embryo and by the fifth week migrate to the germinal ridge, where they undergo successive mitotic cellular divisions to give rise to oogonia. It has been estimated that the fetal ovaries contain approximately 7 million oogonia at 20 weeks' gestation. From then until the menopause there is a reduction in the number of germ cells in the ovaries. After 7 months' gestation no new oocytes are formed. At birth there are approximately 2 million oocytes, and by puberty this number has been reduced to 300,000. There is continued reduction in the number of oocytes during the reproductive years. Two general processes are responsible for this reduction in germ cells: ovulation and atresia. Nearly all oocytes vanish by atresia, with only 400 to 500 oocytes being ovulated. Very little is known about oocyte atresia. Animal studies have shown that estrogens prevent and androgens enhance the process.

Menopause apparently occurs in the human female because of two processes. First, there is the disappearance from the ovary of oocytes which are responsive to gonadotropins. Isolated oocytes are present in postmenopausal ovaries and can be seen on very careful histological evaluation. Some of the remaining oocytes have shown some development, but these are usually atretic. Second, the remaining primordial follicles show no signs of development despite excess gonadotropin secretions. This suggests that the few remaining follicles are not responsive to gonadotropins (Costoff, Mahesh).

THE PERIMENOPAUSAL PERIOD

Reproductive life is characterized by generally regular menses with a slow, steady decrease in cycle length. In a large population, Treloar et al. (1967) observed the mean cycle length to be 28 days at age 35, 30 days at age 25, and 35 days at age 15. By analysis of basal body temperature records, Vollman (1977) was able to show that the decreased cycle length was due to shortening of the interval from menses to the thermal shift (follicular phase) and that luteal phase length was constant in women with regular menses, regardless of age. This observation was confirmed in a small group of women (Fig. 35–1) by measurement of serum gonadotropins, estradiol (E_2), and progesterone (P) levels throughout the menstrual cycle (Sherman, Korenman).

In women over age 45 who are still menstruating regularly, the cycle is quite distinct from that seen in younger subjects. First, the cycle is significantly shorter, and again the follicular phase is the shortened interval. Second, E_2 levels do not rise as high

FIGURE 35–1 The mean and ranges of serum LH, FSH, estradiol, and progesterone in five women, aged 40 to 41, are compared with the mean ± 2 SEM in 10 cycles in women aged 18 to 30. Note shorter follicular phases of older subjects. *(From Sherman, Korenman.)*

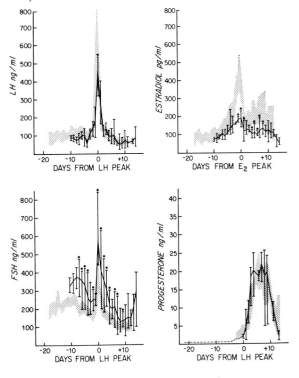

during either follicular maturation or corpus luteum formation. Third, FSH concentrations are strikingly elevated during the early follicular phase, the midcycle peak, and the later portion of the luteal phase. LH levels throughout the cycle and corpus luteum function appear to be similar to that seen in younger women (Sherman, Korenman).

The mechanisms responsible for these changes in menstrual function in older cycling women have not yet been established. Of particular interest is the early elevation of FSH levels. Evidence that FSH is more sensitive than LH to the suppressive effects of exogenous estradiol suggests the increase in FSH is not due only to decreased effective estrogen concentration. In addition, FSH and LH appear to change proportionally when estrogen is given. These observations have prompted Sherman and Korenman (1975) to question if another ovarian hormone may be regulating FSH secretion. Such a factor, analogous to the inhibin postulated to exist in men, would be reduced with age consequent to a reduced number of follicles. A loss of inhibin secretion would explain the elevated follicular phase concentrations of FSH in older women with relatively normal E_2 levels. Consistent with this hypothesis is the preliminary study which identified a nonsteroid, inhibinlike material in bovine follicular fluid (De Jong, Sharpe).

The transition from regular cyclic function to the permanent amenorrhea of menopause is characterized by a phase of marked menstrual irregularity (Treloar et al.). The duration of this transition varies greatly among women. Women who experience the menopause at an early age have a relatively short duration of cycle variability before amenorrhea ensues. By contrast, later menopause is accompanied by a steadily lengthening phase of menstrual irregularity characterized by unusually long and short intermenstrual intervals and an overall increased mean cycle length and variance.

The hormonal characteristics of this transitional phase are of special interest and importance and have been well described by Sherman and Korenman (1975). The irregular episodes of vaginal bleeding in perimenopausal women represent the irregular maturation of ovarian follicles with or without hormonal evidence of ovulation. The potential for hormone secretion by these remaining follicles is diminished and variable. Menses may be preceded by follicular maturation with normal E_2 and P secretion or may be preceded by maturation of a follicle with limited secretion of both E_2 and P. Vaginal bleeding also occurs after a rise and fall in E_2 levels without a measurable increase in P levels. This bleeding is compatible with anovulatory menses. Nevertheless, one can see how the potential for conception could exist even during this transitional phase of reproductive life.

HORMONAL METABOLISM AFTER THE MENOPAUSE

The menopause is associated with marked reduction of ovarian estrogen production. Numerous studies have measured levels in postmenopausal women and found the mean E_2 concentration to be between 12 and 20 pg/mL, a level that is much lower than that seen in premenopausal women (Judd). The E_2 metabolic clearance rate is approximately 900 L per day, which results in a production rate between 10 and 20 μg per day. In older women, estrone (E_1) levels are higher than E_2 concentrations, with most investigators reporting mean levels of approximately 30 pg/mL. The metabolic clearance rate of E_1 is 1600 L per day, resulting in an average production rate of approximately 45 μg per day.

The sources of these circulating estrogens have only been partially clarified. After the menopause ovarian secretion is essentially absent. Several groups have shown no reduction of estrogen levels (Fig. 35–2) or production after castration and the step-up found in the ovarian veins is minimal (Fig. 35–3). Thus, the adrenal glands play the major role. Bilateral adrenalectomy is associated with a reduction to approximately 5 and 12 pg/mL for E_2 and E_1, respectively (Veldhuis et al.). Whether the low levels of circulating estrogens that are present after adrenalectomy and oophorectomy represent real steroid or only the limits of assay detectability has not been established.

The adrenal glands could contribute to the estrogen pool by either direct glandular secretion or peripheral conversion from precursor steroids. For E_2 the relative role of each process has not been established. Limited studies have looked at adrenal vein concentrations of E_2. These studies have been complicated by inadequate E_2 assay sensitivity (Baird, Guevara), questionable adequacy of adrenal vein sampling (Greenblatt et al.), and distortion of circulating estrogens by endocrine-active ovarian tumors (Wiel and et al.). Peripheral conversion of precursor steroids to E_2 is limited. The conversion of E_1 (5 percent) and testosterone (T) (0.1 percent) to E_2 could account for only a portion of the E_2 found in postmenopausal women. More is known about the source of E_1. Limited direct adrenal secretion of E_1 was reported in two patients by Baird, while Judd et al. (1976) did not

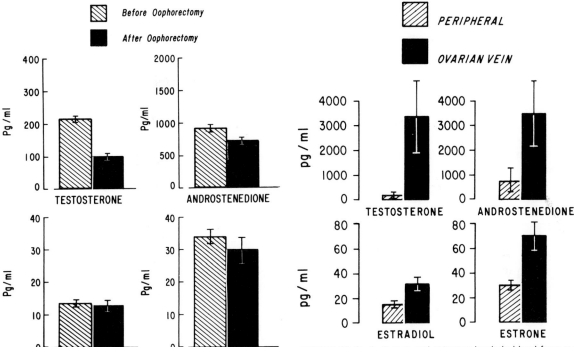

FIGURE 35–2 Mean ± SE serum testosterone, androstenedione, estradiol, and estrone levels in 16 postmenopausal women before and 6 to 8 weeks after bilateral ovariectomy. *(From Judd.)*

FIGURE 35–3 Androgen and estrogen levels in blood from peripheral and ovarian veins in 10 postmenopausal women. *(From Judd et al.: Endocrine function of the postmenopausal ovary: Concentration of androgens and estrogens in ovarian and peripheral vein blood. J Clin Endocrinol Metab 39:1020, 1974.)*

observe a step-up in the adrenal vein in two women with androgen-secreting ovarian tumors. With the use of blood-urine and blood-blood techniques to evaluate peripheral aromatization of androgens, it has been found that the principal source of E_1 is the peripheral conversion of androstenedione (A) (Siiteri, MacDonald; Longcope et al., 1969). This peripheral conversion is enhanced with increasing body weight, age, liver disease, and hyperthyroidism (Edman, MacDonald). The conversion has been shown to occur in fat, muscle, brain, skin, and liver cells (Longcope et al., 1978). To what extent each cell type contributes to total conversion has not been established, but Longcope and coworkers suggested fat cells contribute only 30 to 40 percent (Longcope et al., 1978).

The menopause is also associated with significant changes in ovarian androgen secretion. In older women, A levels (approximately 900 pg/mL) are about one-half the concentration seen in intact premenopausal women and are similar to the levels found in younger patients after ovariectomy (Judd). There is no difference in the clearance rate (1800 L per day) of this hormone in older and younger sub-

jects. Thus, the average production rate is approximately 1.5 mg per day. In postmenopausal subjects ovariectomy results in a small but significant decrease in circulating A.

For T the mean concentration is minimally lower (approximately 250 pg/mL) than that found in premenopausal women, and is distinctly higher than the level observed in younger women after gonadectomy (Judd). The metabolic clearance rate of T (600 L per day) does not change with the menopause (Calanog et al., 1976). Thus the production rate of T is approximately 150 μg per day. Ovariectomy is associated with a significant decrease of circulating T in older subjects (Fig. 35–2). Fifteen percent of circulating A is converted to T (Calanog et al., 1977). The small simultaneous fall in A following ovariectomy could account for only a limited amount of the total decrease in T. The remainder presumably represents direct ovarian secretion and is larger than the amount secreted directly by the premenopausal ovary. Large increases of T in the ovarian veins of older women (Fig. 35–3) is consistent with the hypothesis that the postmenopausal ovary secretes more T directly than does the premenopausal gonad (Judd).

For years it has been suspected that the post-menopausal ovary continues to produce steroids, particularly androgens. By means of in vitro incubation methods, it has been shown that postmenopausal ovaries can convert radioactive precursors to T, A, and dehydroepiandrosterone (Mattingly, Huang). With the use of histochemical studies the presence of steroid-specific enzymes has also been documented in hilus cells and stromal theca cells (hyperthecosis) of postmenopausal ovaries (Judd). These cells have been shown to be capable of producing androgens in premenopausal women and presumably could do so in postmenopausal subjects. A proposed mechanism for the increased ovarian T production by postmenopausal ovaries is stimulation of gonadal cells capable of androgen production by excess endogenous gonadotropins, which, in turn, are increased because of reduced estrogen production by the ovaries. This increased ovarian T secretion, coupled with a reduction of estrogen production, may explain, in part, the development of symptoms of defeminization, hirsutism, and even virilism seen in some postmenopausal women.

GONADOTROPINS

In postmenopausal women, both LH and FSH levels are significantly elevated over the concentrations seen in premenopausal women, with FSH usually higher than LH (Judd). The higher FSH levels are thought to be caused by the slower clearance of this gonadotropin. The reason for the marked increase in circulating gonadotropins is the absence of the negative feedback of ovarian steroids and possibly inhibin on gonadotropin release. As in younger women the levels of both gonadotropins are not steady but show random oscillations. These oscillations are thought to represent pulsatile secretion by the pituitary. In older women these pulsatile bursts occur every 1 to 2 hours, a frequency similar to that seen during the follicular phase of premenopausal subjects. Although the frequency is similar, the amplitude is much greater. This increased amplitude is thought to be secondary to increased release of the hypothalamic hormone called gonadotropin-releasing hormone (GnRH) and enhanced responsiveness of the pituitary to GnRH as a result of the low estrogen levels. The presence of prominent pulsatile secretion of GnRH in the hypophyseal portal blood of castrated rats is consistent with increased pulsatile release of the hormone after the menopause (Eskay et al.). The large pulses of gonadotropin in the peripheral circulation are believed to maintain the high levels of the hormones that are found in postmenopausal women.

METABOLIC ALTERATIONS ASSOCIATED WITH THE MENOPAUSE

Numerous metabolic alterations occur in women at the time of the menopause. The above-mentioned changes of ovarian function have been implicated in the etiology of many of these functional alterations. These include hot flashes, atrophy of the reproductive tract, osteoporosis, altered incidence of cardiovascular disease, loss of skin integrity, and psychological problems. Some of these are clearly due to altered ovarian function and can be corrected by estrogen therapy, i.e., vaginal atrophy. The relationship of the other alterations to the menopause is less clear. The following sections review the evidence for and against these relationships.

HOT FLASHES

The hot flash is by far the most common symptom of the menopause that leads patients to seek medical attention. Three-fourths of all women experience the symptom during the physiological menopause or following ovariectomy. In one-fourth of the cases, these hot flashes will persist for more than 5 years. The symptom complex is described as a sudden feeling of warmth and flushing over the chest, neck, and face, followed rapidly by perspiration. The subjective event lasts only 3 to 4 minutes (Fig. 35–4). Extensive temperature recording throughout the body by Molnar (1975) in one postmenopausal woman showed that the disruption is more generalized than was previously appreciated. He observed marked increases of finger and toe temperatures at the time of the subjective hot flash. This suggested that a generalized cutaneous vasodilatation accompanies the event. Hot flashes occur on the average of once per hour, with the minimum interval being about 25 minutes. It has been stated that flashes are more severe after a surgical than natural menopause, but this observation has not been documented.

Although hot flashes are a frequent reason for older women to seek medical attention, remarkably little is known about their pathogenesis. It is clear that reduced ovarian hormone production is directly or indirectly responsible for their occurrence. The lack of hot flashes in prepubertal children and in hypogonadal individuals who have not been exposed to exog-

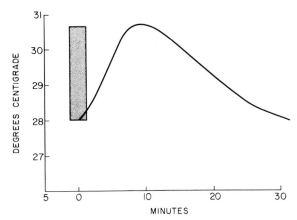

FIGURE 35–4 Mean characteristics and typical configuration of finger temperative fluctuations associated with hot flashes. The shaded area delineates the period from the mean and beginning to completion of subjective flushing. *(From Meldrum et al.)*

enous estrogen suggests that it is the reduction rather than the absence of ovarian function that triggers the events.

Until recently, attempts to relate hot flashes to endocrine function have not been fruitful. It was observed that LH and FSH levels correlated with a vasomotor score following ovariectomy, with both increasing to a maximum 6 weeks after surgery (Aksel et al.). A negative correlation of vasomotor score and total estrogen levels was also observed, although the decrease of estrogen was very rapid following surgery, while the vasomotor score continued to rise for several more weeks. Recently, Tataryn and coworkers measured continuous finger temperature and serum LH and FSH levels at frequent intervals for 8 hours in six postmenopausal women with hot flashes. These investigators observed a close temporal association of hot flashes and the pulsatile discharge of LH but not FSH. These data suggest that hot flashes are related to pulsatile LH secretion or factors which trigger its release. The observation that flushes occur after hypophysectomy suggests that the mechanism is not caused directly by LH release (Mulley et al.). As mentioned previously, GnRH fluctuates significantly in hypophyseal portal vein blood in animals (Eskay et al.). These fluctuations are thought to represent pulsatile secretion and are believed to be responsible in part for episodic LH release from the pituitary. It is possible that GnRH, or the hypothalamic factors responsible for its release, may somehow alter the heat-regulating centers of the hypothalamus, resulting in a new set point for triggering integrated thermoregulatory events. The close proximity of some of the GnRH neurons with the heat-regulating centers in the preop-

tic hypothalamus is consistent with this view (Reaves, Hayward; McCann et al.). The observation that catecholamines play a role in central thermoregulatory function and GnRH release is also consistent with this hypothesis (Cox, Lomax; Simpkins, Kalra). Further studies are necessary to determine the exact nature of the relationship between these two central functions.

The hallmark of the treatment of hot flashes has been the use of estrogens. Estrogens block the occurrence, not just the perception of the event, since the number of finger temperature elevations is significantly reduced in symptomatic postmenopausal women receiving estrogen therapy (Meldrum et al.). Injections of medroxyprogesterone acetate have also been shown to decrease subjective hot flashes in a double-blind prospective study (Bullock et al.). Several other compounds are also said to be effective but either have not been studied critically or conflicting results have been reported. Critical evaluation of medications said to relieve hot flashes is essential, since a large placebo effect has been noted in several studies.

OSTEOPOROSIS

Osteoporosis is the single most important health hazard associated with the menopause. It is a disorder characterized by a reduction in the quantity of bone without changes in its chemical composition (Nordin). Loss of trabecular bone is more marked and develops earlier than it does for cortical bone, with a 50 percent and 5 percent loss of trabecular and cortical bone, respectively, occurring with aging. Loss of mineral content of bone occurs in all individuals during aging, with women losing bone mass after age 30 and men after age 45 to 50. In women this reduction of bone mass is accentuated by the loss of ovarian function (Meema et al.). Osteoporosis is more prevalent in women than in men. The problem is particularly severe in women who have been castrated early or have gonadal dysgenesis. Bone loss appears to be rapid during the first 3 to 4 years after the menopause, with the rate of loss being about 2.5 percent per year. After this, the rate decreases to approximately 0.75 percent per year until death. In addition to a sexual difference, there is also a racial difference, with whites having the highest incidence, then Orientals, and finally blacks. Smoking is believed to enhance the development of osteoporosis (Daniell). Slender women also seem more susceptible to the condition, with the classic subject being a little old white woman who is hunched over and walks with a cane (Daniell).

In itself the loss of bone mass produces no symptoms but does lead to reduced skeletal strength. Thus, osteoporotic bones are more susceptible to fractures. The vertebral body is the most common site of fracture resulting from menopausally related osteoporosis, but fractures of other bones are also enhanced, including the humerus, upper femur, distal forearm, and ribs. With cross-sectional studies 25 percent of white women in northern European countries have vertebral fractures by age 65, and 50 percent have them by age 75 (Gallagher et al., 1964). There is a tenfold increase of Colles' fractures in women from age 35 to 65 (Knowelden et al.). A similar increase is not seen in men. The incidence of hip fractures also increases with age in women, rising from 0.3 per 1000 to 20 per 1000 from ages 45 to 85 (Knowelden et al.). This latter fracture is of particular concern. The mortality secondary to it remains high. Between 15 and 20 percent of patients will succumb as a result of the fracture or its complications within 3 months, and one-third will die within 6 months of the injury (Meyn et al.). Many of the remaining patients are permanently disabled and remain invalids for the rest of their lives.

The cause of menopausal osteoporosis has not been completely established. Initially, Albright suggested it was due to decreased bone formation (Albright et al.). However, most subsequent data have implicated increased bone resorption coupled with normal bone formation (Jowsey et al.). This increase in bone resorption results in a net loss of calcium of approximately 100 g between ages 50 and 70 years, or 15 mg per day.

Currently, it is believed that reduction of ovarian estrogen production plays a key role in the genesis of menopausal osteoporosis. Short-term estrogen replacement has consistently brought about a reduction in bone resorption and of calcium loss as measured by bone density (Lindsay et al., 1976). These studies have now been extended to 8 years of treatment, and still the loss of calcium from bone has been inhibited with estrogen therapy (Lindsay et al., 1978). Second, endogenous estrogen production shows a negative correlation with parameters of bone resorption. A negative correlation between circulating E_2 levels and urinary calcium excretion (an index of bone resorption) has also been reported (Lindsay et al., 1977). Frumar et al. (1979b) extended this observation to show a negative correlation between E_1 and E_2 levels and calcium excretion. These investigators also noted a negative correlation between body weight or excess fat and calcium excretion. It is well recognized that slender women have a greater incidence of osteoporosis. It is possible that body fat, with its effect on endogenous estrogen metabolism, may influence bone resorption so that obese women resorb less calcium than slender subjects.

Attempts to look at endogenous estrogen levels in postmenopausal women who do or do not have osteoporosis have resulted in inconsistent findings. Riggs and coworkers (1973) found no difference between total estrogen levels in women with and without osteoporosis who were matched for age, while Marshall and coworkers (1978) found lower E_1 and A levels in postmenopausal women with osteoporosis. The reasons for these inconsistent findings are not readily apparent.

Parathyroid hormone (PTH) also appears to play a central role in the genesis of the condition. PTH is the principal hormone which stimulates bone resorption. In animal and human studies osteoporosis does not develop in the absence of PTH, confirming its key role in the process (Houssain et al.). To date, attempts to determine whether PTH levels are elevated in patients with osteoporosis have revealed inconsistent results. In general, levels have been found to be low or normal (Gallagher et al., 1977). If this is correct, it suggests that bone may become more sensitive to PTH after the menopause. The role of estrogen in the altered sensitivity of bone to PTH is not clear. In vivo animal studies have shown that estrogens do indeed decrease the effect of PTH on bone (Gallagher, Williamson), but in vitro data are not as convincing. Atkins and Peacock (1975) found a decrease in the responsiveness of bone tissue cultures to PTH in the presence of high concentrations of estrogens. Other investigators concluded that these effects were nonspecific and found that physiological levels of estrogens would not inhibit PTH action (Caputo et al.). These latter observations are enhanced by the inability of investigators to document the presence of estrogen receptors in bone (Chen, Feldman). Current dogma on the mechanism of action of estrogen indicates that cytosol receptors for estrogen are obligatory for the hormone to have effects in a target issue.

If estrogen receptors are not present in bone, then estradiol has to exert its action on bone resorption indirectly. Currently, two theories have been suggested as possible mechanisms. First, estrogens may act on bone by regulating the 25-hydroxycholecalciferol-1-hydroxylase enzyme in the kidney, thus modulating the synthesis of 1,25-dihydroxycholecalciferol, the active metabolite of vitamin D (Tanaka et al.). One problem with this mechanism is that vitamin D deficiency results in osteomalacia and not osteoporosis. Second, estrogens may enhance calcitonin secretion (MacIntyre). Since calcitonin is a potent inhibitor of bone resorption, enhanced secretion of this hormone could inhibit calcium loss from bone and possibly the future development of osteoporosis. More studies are needed to substantiate these concepts.

In summary, a growing list of publications indicate that the menopause and the associated reduction of endogenous estrogens play a major role in the development of osteoporosis in older women. The mechanism by which estrogens exert this action has not been defined. However, this problem is responsible for the most serious complications resulting from the loss of ovarian function and represents the major reason to contemplate replacement therapy.

CARDIOVASCULAR EFFECTS

It is well known that in the United States heart disease is less prevalent in women than in men before the age of 55 (Ryan). The chance of a man dying of heart disease is five to ten times greater than a woman before this age. Not only is heart disease less frequent but it is also less severe in younger women. Because of these observations, a popular opinion has developed that ovarian estrogen production is protective against heart trouble and that the increased risk of coronary disease after the menopause is related to the decline in ovarian hormones. New data have been published, and the relationship between cardiovascular disease and ovarian function has been partially clarified. The following is a review of the information for and against the association.

In general the incidence of death from coronary heart disease increases with age in all populations and both sexes. There is much less heart disease in younger women. This sex difference is not consistent in all countries. In nations where the incidence of heart disease is high, the sex difference is marked, while in countries where the incidence is low, the sex difference is not apparent. In the age group between 25 and 55 the ratio of deaths from heart attacks between men and women varies from 5:1 in the United States, to 2:1 in Italy, to 1:1 in Japan (Ryan). When present, the sex difference disappears with age, so that by age 85 the ratio is unity. This change results from reduction in the incremental death rate in men. For each decade after age 55, there is a twofold increase in deaths from heart attacks in men and a threefold increase in women.

Two types of studies have been utilized to determine whether cessation of ovarian function increases the incidence of heart disease. In the first type, the Framingham study has reported the results of biannual exams for 24 years on nearly 3000 women (Kannel et al.; Gordon et al.). These data reveal there indeed is an increased incidence of heart disease in women following the menopause that is not just age-related. Based on these studies the impact of the menopause appears to be substantial and relatively abrupt, and increases afterwards only slowly, if at all. In this study population it was unusual to see heart disease in premenopausal women, and when present the disease was usually mild, being just angina pectoris. Serious heart disease, such as myocardial infarcts, was not observed.

Second, case control studies have been performed comparing the degree of coronary heart disease or the incidence of myocardial infarcts in women undergoing early castration with age-matched premenopausal controls (Gordon et al.). Some of these studies have found an increased risk of cardiovascular disease in the castrated subjects, while others did not. All of these studies have been criticized because of patient selection bias, particularly the controls. For example, one of the largest studies compared the incidence of coronary heart disease in women undergoing hysterectomy and bilateral oophorectomy with controls undergoing hysterectomy alone (Ritterband et al.). No difference was found in the incidence of cardiovascular disease between the groups, but both groups had a higher incidence than has been reported in unoperated patients. This observation took on special meaning when the Framingham study observed a greater incidence of coronary heart disease in women undergoing hysterectomy with or without ovariectomy (Gordon et al.).

Although heart disease appears to increase with cessation of ovarian function, the use of replacement estrogens does not seem to decrease the risk. With large doses of estrogen an increase of recurrent heart disease was observed in a large series of men treated with 5 mg of conjugated estrogens, while no reduction in deaths was noted in patients treated with 2.5 mg of the same estrogen over placebo (Coronary Drug Project Research Group). In postmenopausal women treated with usual replacement doses a doubling of the incidence of coronary heart disease was observed, although the total mortality was not changed (Gordon et al.; Rosenberg et al.). The increase was in the incidence of angina pectoris. The incidence of myocardial infarcts was the same as that of the control population. Thus, current estrogen replacement does not seem to reduce but to actually increase the already enhanced incidence of coronary heart disease that occurs with the menopause.

Several factors could be involved with the increase in heart disease associated with the menopause and estrogen therapy. These factors are known to increase the incidence of heart disease in all populations and are influenced by cessation of ovarian function, estrogen therapy, or both.

It is well recognized that increased circulating levels of cholesterol are associated with an increased risk of heart attacks. An elevation of only 40 mg per 100 mL will increase the risk three- to fivefold (Ryan). The menopause is associated with a rise of cholesterol of approximately 16 mg per 100 mL. Normal replacement doses of estrogens have little effect on cholesterol, while higher doses will reduce the concentration.

High triglyceride levels are also a putative risk factor for coronary heart disease. No data are available about the effect of the menopause on this parameter, but it is well recognized that estrogens in normal replacement dosages will increase triglyceride concentrations (Stern et al.).

Lipoproteins are also a risk factor for coronary heart disease. The menopause is associated with an increase of all lipoprotein fractions, with a decrease in the ratio of the high- to low-density fractions (Gordon et al.). Estrogens tend to increase the cholesterol in high-density lipoproteins and decrease it in the low-density fraction. However, estrogens have effects on the protein moiety of high-density lipoproteins as well as on just cholesterol.

Hypertension enhances susceptibility to coronary heart disease fivefold (Ryan). After age 45, hypertension apparently is more important than hyperlipidemia as a cause of heart disease. Hypertension practically obliterates the sex advantage in women and probably accounts for the higher vulnerability of both black men and women to heart disease at an earlier age. The menopause does not appear to be associated with a systematic change in either systolic or diastolic blood pressure. However, estrogen therapy does influence these parameters, with small increases of both diastolic and systolic blood pressure being observed (Stern et al.). To date, the use of estrogen replacement in postmenopausal women has not been associated with an increased risk of stroke. The mechanism thought to be responsible for the increase in blood pressure with estrogen therapy involves the renin-angiotension-aldosterone system. Estrogen stimulates hepatic synthesis and secretion of the protein renin substrate, resulting in enhanced production of angiotensin I and II and aldosterone. These agents promote vasoconstriction and fluid retention resulting in mild increases in blood pressure.

Diabetes is another risk factor for heart disease,

with the risk of myocardial infarction being twice as much in patients with the disease (Ryan). To date, an effect of the menopause on carbohydrate metabolism has not been established. The actions of estrogen therapy on carbohydrate metabolism are unclear; some investigators have found no effect, while others have observed a decrease of glucose tolerance without an accompanying increase in insulin secretion. The alterations of carbohydrate metabolism observed with oral contraceptives appear to be related mainly to the progestins in the pills.

There are a variety of other risk factors for heart disease, including smoking, obesity, heredity, and lack of exercise. The menopause and sex hormone therapy appear to have little, if any, effects on these factors in comparison with socioeconomic and cultural variables.

From this review of the risk factors for coronary heart disease, it is obvious that several are influenced by the menopause and estrogen therapy. However, the increase in the incidence of cardiovascular disease which occurs with the menopause cannot be explained by the changes recorded in any of the above risk factors, either singly or in combination. Some other feature of the menopause must account for this increased risk. Whatever this feature is must account for the fact that hysterectomy without ovariectomy apparently leads to the same increased risk of heart disease as is observed with bilateral oophorectomy.

REPRODUCTIVE TRACT ALTERATIONS

Estrogen functions as the principal growth factor of the reproductive tract in women. At the time of the menopause the reduction of estrogen results in atrophic changes throughout the reproductive organs. The atrophic changes occurring in the vagina are responsible for many of the symptoms referable to the reproductive tract of postmenopausal women. Vaginal atrophy results in vaginitis, vaginal dryness, dyspareunia, and occasionally vaginal obliteration. Vaginal bleeding can also occur secondary to vaginal infection. These symptoms are related specifically to reduced ovarian estrogen production and respond to estrogen therapy. The medication can be given locally or systemically, and symptoms are reduced with either type of administration.

Atrophic changes also appear in the endometrium, resulting in cessation of menstruation. On biopsy, atrophic endometrium is found in the majority of postmenopausal women. In some older subjects vaginal bleeding occurs. On biopsy, proliferative or hyperplastic endometrium may be present. In some cases adenocarcinoma of the endometrium is found and is of particular concern. The presence of hyperplastic rather than atrophic endometrium suggests enhanced endogenous estrogen production, or exposure to exogenous steroid may have occurred. Based on a variety of evidence, it has been suggested that continuous estrogen stimulation of the endometrium, unopposed by progesterone, can produce a progression of changes from benign proliferation to cystic hyperplasia, adenomatous hyperplasia, and varying degrees of anaplasia, including invasive adenocarcinoma. Extensive reviews for and against this association have been reported (Lucas).

Recent work has shed considerable light on the relationship of estrogens and the development of endometrial hyperplasia or adenocarcinoma in older women. As mentioned earlier the principal source of estrogens in older women is the peripheral aromatization of circulating androgens. Thus, increased endogenous estrogen production can occur secondary to three mechanisms: (1) enhanced production of precursor androgens, (2) increased rate of peripheral aromatization, and (3) enhanced production of estrogens directly. Enhancement of each of these mechanisms has been observed and has been associated with an increased incidence of endometrial cancer.

Androgen-secreting tumors are usually responsible for enhanced precursor production, resulting in secondary estrogen excess (Aiman et al.). Endometrial hyperplasias or adenocarcinomas have been associated with these tumors. These neoplasms can be classical androgen-secreting tumors or so-called nonendocrine ovarian neoplasms. These latter tumors are associated with ovarian stromal hyperplasia. The excess androgens, which are secreted by the hyperplastic stroma, are aromatized in peripheral tissues, leading to chronically elevated estrogen levels.

A variety of conditions are associated with enhanced peripheral aromatization resulting in chronically elevated estrogens. These include obesity, liver disease, and hyperthyroidism (Siiteri, MacDonald; Edman, MacDonald). The association between obesity and endometrial cancer has been known for years (Lucas).

Granulosa–theca-cell tumors of the ovary are capable of estrogen secretion directly. Numerous reports have associated this tumor with adenocarcinoma of the endometrium; some authors have disputed the association, however, citing bias as a result of a selective concentration of these relatively unusual tumors into those centers reporting a significant association (Lucas).

The exact relationship between endogenous estrogen metabolism and the development of endometrial cancer has not been established. It is quite clear that obese, postmenopausal women have greater endogenous estrogen production than slender subjects. Both E_1 and E_2 production rates are enhanced. This has been shown by the measurement of circulating E_1 and E_2 levels, the peripheral conversion ratios of A to E_1, and the production rate of E_1 (Judd; Siiteri, MacDonald). These findings provide a plausible explanation for the common association of endometrial cancer and obesity. What is not clear is whether patients with this tumor have some other common abnormality of estrogen metabolism. Published comparisons of various indices of estrogen metabolism in postmenopausal women with and without endometrial cancer have reported conflicting findings. Judd et al. (1976) found no difference between E_1 and E_2 levels in 16 postmenopausal women with endometrial cancer and 10 age- and weight-matched controls, (Fig. 35–5), while Benjamin and Dentsch (1976) reported higher concentrations of the same estrogens in 20 cancer patients than in 30 control subjects. However, the latter controls were not matched to the cancer patients for weight and age. A few studies have compared the metabolic clearance rate and the

FIGURE 35–5 Serum androgens and estrogens in postmenopausal women with and without endometrial cancer. *(From Judd.)*

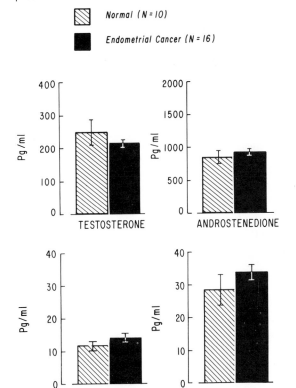

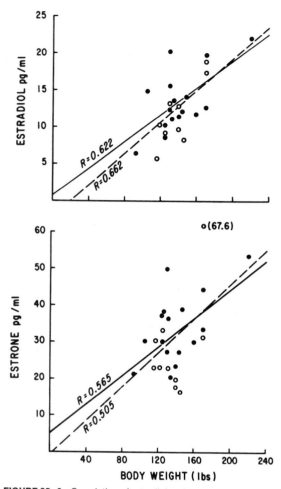

FIGURE 35–6 Correlation of estradiol and estrone levels with excess fat in postmenopausal patients with endometrial cancer (•) and without endometrial cancer (o). Dashed regression line is for all patients, while solid line is for cancer patients only. *(From Judd et al.: Serum 17β-estradiol and estrone in postmenopausal women with and without endometrial cancer, J Clin Endocrinol Metab 43:272, 1976.)*

androgen-to-estrogen conversion ratio in patients with and without this tumor. Most of them described a limited number of patients or used inappropriate controls. Hausknecht and Gusberg (1973) found higher A-to-E_1 conversion in 21 cancer patients than in controls, but the weights of the subjects were not given. Rizkallah et al. (1975) measured A-to-E_1 conversion in 10 cancer patients but did not compare the results to those found in control subjects. Calanog et al. (1976, 1977) observed similar clearance and production rates of A and T but higher A-to-E_1 conversion ratios in 14 cancer than in 5 control patients matched for

age but not weight. The most extensive and best-conceived study was reported recently by MacDonald et al. (1978), who found similar A-to-E_1 conversion ratios in 25 cancer patients and an equal number of controls matched for both weight and age. Thus, the two studies, which used control subjects matched to the patients with endometrial cancer for both age and weight, reached similar conclusions (Judd; MacDonald et al.). There appears to be no difference of estrogen metabolism in patients with adenocarcinoma of the endometrium and in appropriately selected controls. In addition, enhanced endogenous estrogen production, which is associated with obesity, appears to be a risk factor for the development of this tumor (Fig. 35–6).

The role of estrogen therapy in the development of endometrial cancer has been and continues to be one of the most highly charged issues related to the menopause. Although some older studies did not find an association, many early reports implicated exogenous estrogen administration as a factor in the genesis of endometrial hyperplasia and adenocarcinoma both in postmenopausal women and in patients with gonadal dysgenesis (Lucas). These observations were strengthened by the recent report of six case control studies which observed an increased incidence of estrogen usage in patients with endometrial cancer as compared with matched controls (Antunes et al.). The risk ratios varied between 3.1 and 8.0 (Table 35–1). All replacement estrogens were implicated, with no one preparation being of greater risk. Increased risk was associated with larger dosage and prolonged use. Inconsistent findings were reported concerning the effect of a medication-free interval on the risk ratios.

Several of these studies have been criticized because they were retrospective, used inappropriate controls, contained mainly early lesions, and did not have independent review of the pathological specimens. One of the groups criticizing these studies reported their own series as showing no increased in-

TABLE 35–1 Relative Risk of Endometrial Cancer with Use of Exogenous Estrogen

Study	Risk ratio
Ziel et al., 1975	7.6
Smith et al., 1975	7.5
Mack et al., 1976	8.0
McDonald et al., 1977	7.9
Gray et al., 1977	3.1
Antunes et al., 1979	6.0

cidence of estrogen use in patients with endometrial cancer as compared with women with other gynecological diseases (Horwitz, Feinstein). This latter paper was contested in an editorial of the same journal for its choice of control subjects (Hutchison, Rothman). With the exception of the retrospective nature of these case control studies, many of the above criticisms have now been answered by subsequent reports. Recently, it was pointed out by Doll et al. (1977) that risk ratios of the magnitude found in these retrospective studies are almost always confirmed when examined prospectively.

Another factor suggesting that exogenous estrogen use is associated with the development of this tumor is the rising incidence of the tumor, which parallels the known increase of estrogen use in the United States (Greenwald et al.). Several tumor registries have now reported significant increases of endometrial cancer during the past few years. During a similar time there has been at least a fourfold increase in the use of estrogen in this country. These observations have been enhanced by the recent report of a decreased incidence of endometrial cancer in the Seattle area, which parallels the drop in estrogen use resulting from the initial report associating estrogens and endometrial cancer (Jick et al.). The increasing incidence of endometrial cancer in the United States has been attributed to factors other than just estrogen use. These include better reporting, closer follow-up of patients receiving estrogens, and changes in pathological classifications. A telling factor against any real increase of endometrial cancer during the last few years is the lack of an accompanying increase in mortality from the tumor.

In summary, a rapidly accumulating body of data is being reported that suggests an association between enhanced endogenous estrogen production or exogenous estrogen administration and the development of adenocarcinoma of the endometrium. Although this relationship continues to be contested, most physicians now recognize the possibility and advise their patients accordingly.

SKIN ALTERATIONS

As people age, noticeable changes of the skin occur. There is a generalized thinning with an accompanying loss of elasticity, resulting in wrinkling. These changes are particularly prominent in the areas exposed to light, i.e., the face, neck, and hands. Wrinkling around the mouth in a "purse string" fashion and around the eyes is characteristic. Skin changes on the dorsum of the hands are particularly noticeable.

The skin in this area may be so thin as to appear transparent, with the details of the underlying veins easily visible. The skin is loose and inelastic, and its surface is smooth.

Histologically, the epidermis is thinned and the basal layers become even with age. Dehydration is typical. Reduction in the number of blood vessels to the skin is also seen. Degeneration of elastic and collagenous fibers in the dermis also appears to be part of the process of aging.

These skin changes are of cosmetic importance, and women have related them to the occurrence of the menopause. It is commonly stated that women undergoing estrogen replacement look younger, and the cosmetic industry has been placing estrogens in skin creams for years for precisely this purpose. However, little work has been accomplished that addresses either the role of the menopause or the effect of estrogen therapy on these age-related skin alterations.

The possibility that estrogens may have effects on skin was suggested by the recent demonstration of the uptake of radiolabeled estradiol into the nuclei of both dermal and epidermal cells of mice (Stumpf et al.). The radiolabeled estrogens were found to be concentrated in the nuclei of the basal cell layers of the epidermis and fibroblasts of the dermis. There were differences in estrogen-binding affinities in different regions of the epidermis, with the perineal epidermis showing the greatest binding. These results suggest that the skin, or, more specifically, certain structures of the skin have the capacity to concentrate and retain estradiol in a fashion characteristic of more classical target tissues for estrogen such as the uterus, vagina, and mammary gland. This study gives credence to the hypothesis that estrogens can affect skin.

Very little work has been reported on the effect of the menopause on skin. Skin circulation has been found to be decreased in women after castration. [^{3}H]Thymidine incorporation (an index of new DNA metabolism) was also observed to decrease during the several months following ovariectomy (Punnonen).

The effect of estrogen on skin has been studied by only a few investigators. In animals, estrogens have been shown to increase the mitotic rate (a reflection of growth) of skin in some studies (Punnonen). Estrogens appear to alter the vascularization of skin. They have also been shown to change the collagen content of the dermis as reflected by mucopolysaccharide incorporation, hydroxyproline turnover, and alterations of the ground substance. In addition, dermal synthesis of hyaluronic acid and dermal water content are enhanced. The effects of estrogen on human skin have been studied very little and the reports have been conflicting (Shahrad, Marks). Some investigators have found epidermal atrophy after prolonged estrogen use, while others observed antiwrinkling effects secondary to thickening of the epidermis and collagenous fibers. Oral estrogens have been found to enhance [^{3}H]thymidine incorporation and dermal thickness using in vivo studies, while in vitro experiments yielded conflicting results (Punnonen; Shahrad, Marks).

It is obvious that critical assessment of this important aspect of the menopause has yet to be performed. With the quantities of estrogen-containing skin creams that are in current use and their potential for adverse side effects, studies of this nature are essential.

PSYCHOLOGICAL PROBLEMS

There is a common belief that the menopause may be associated with major alterations of psychological function. This has led to the recommendation of hormonal replacement therapy in older women experiencing emotional difficulties. However, the role of ovarian failure in the initiation of psychiatric disease is not clear. Numerous stresses occur at the time of the menopause, such as adjustment to aging and loss of the maternal role, and these may lead to psychological disturbances only coincidentally related to ovarian failure. In addition, there are prominent responses of these symptoms to placebo. These factors have contributed to the creation of misleading information based on poorly controlled studies.

Little information is available to define whether increased psychiatric morbidity occurs with ovarian failure, and conflicting findings have been reported. Ballinger (1975) found increased morbidity in the year following the menopause but also observed more psychiatric problems in women in the 45- to 49-year age group apparently independent of menopausal status. Ballinger (1976) also observed no characteristic symptom related to ovarian failure but found patients with morbidity were more likely to have had previous psychological problems. This is consistent with the view that the menopause may be a stress which brings out psychopathology in a vulnerable subgroup. Conversely, Winokur (1973) found the same rate of occurrence of depressive episodes within 3 years of the menopause as in other years. However, it should be noted that objective testing of

psychological function was not employed in the above studies.

This type of testing has been used to assess the effect of castration on psychological function by Rauramo and coworkers (1975). Comparisons were made between untreated oophorectomized women and women who had undergone hysterectomy only or who where oophorectomized and given estrogen. Results showed a decline in well-being and more negative feelings in the untreated oophorectomized patients. They complained of being more nervous, tired, tense, distressed, irritable, dejected, and more inclined to cry than the other subjects. However, there were no changes in anxiety score, memory, logical thinking, or reaction time in the oophorectomized patients before and after surgery. Such a study suffers from the deficiency that the patients' and investigators' expectations may be influenced by the known change in hormone status.

Another approach to investigating the link between psychological changes and the menopause has been to ascertain the response of various complaints to estrogen replacement therapy. This must be carried out using a controlled, preferably double-blind study design to provide any meaningful information. The following is a review of the few studies which meet these criteria. In a single-blind study, Utian (1972) noted improved "mental tone" by objective testing, but found no effect on mood or depression over placebo. A double-blind study by Thomson (1977) found no effect on anxiety or depression, but did document increased sleep duration. Vanhulle and Demol (1976) showed a significant improvement of attention, alertness, and subjective estimations of state of health with estriol treatment over placebo, but did not observe effects on visual or auditory memory, concentration, or learning ability. Campbell (1976) studied the largest group of patients to date, using a double-blind cross-over design and subjective and objective indices of psychometric function. Sixty-four patients with severe menopausal symptoms were studied for 4 months. Conjugated estrogens, 1.25 mg, resulted in a significant reduction of hot flashes, insomnia, irritability, headaches, and anxiety and enhancement of memory, good spirits, and optimism. Sixty-one patients with less severe symptoms were studied for 1 year. The same dose of estrogen reduced only hot flashes and insomnia and improved poor memory. Effects on mood were no greater with estrogen than with placebo. Thus, it appears that estrogen replacement may influence certain aspects of brain function. Additional large studies are needed to critically evaluate these potentially important therapeutic effects.

Basic investigations are now beginning to substantiate biochemical mechanisms through which ovarian activity could influence brain function. Increased monoamine oxidase (MAO) activity and greater EEG driving responses have been found in premenopausal women who are depressed, as compared with controls. Both indices return to normal with estrogen treatment (Klaiber et al.). Increased MAO levels have also been observed in postmenopausal women, and significant reductions toward the levels seen in premenopausal controls again have been reported with estrogen treatment (Klaiber et al.). These data are consistent with the hypothesis that depression may be associated with decreased brain catecholaminergic function and that under certain circumstances estrogen deficiency and estrogen treatment may have affects on central catecholamine metabolism.

Changes in indole amine metabolism also have been postulated to be related to affective disorders in perimenopausal patients (Aylward). Free plasma tryptophan levels have been found to have a highly significant inverse correlation with objective measurements of depression and a strong positive correlation with circulating estrogen levels. Estrogen treatment has been shown to increase free tryptophan levels and decrease the depression score in a group of women manifesting menstrual disturbances in the perimenopausal period. Similar relationships have been confirmed in women who are clearly postmenopausal. Because of these observations, it has been postulated that estrogen increases free plasma tryptophan and consequently the metabolism of serotonin in the brain.

Although these findings appear to suggest a physiologic role of estrogen in brain serotonin and catecholamine metabolism, it is also possible that the apparent effects of endogenous estrogen are merely coincidental or that the effect of treatment is pharmacologic. Nevertheless, there appear to be indications of neuropharmacologic mechanisms whereby estrogen deficiency could influence brain function. More research is needed in this critical area.

TREATMENT OF THE MENOPAUSE

The preceding discussion has documented that hormonal replacement of ovarian function is a very complex issue. There are advantages as well as liabilities associated with estrogen replacement. Adding to this complexity is the fact that the role of ovarian hormones on the metabolism of other organ systems is not completely defined. Until this is accomplished the issue of hormonal replacement will remain controversial. In spite of this, physicians are continually confronted with patients seeking care for their menopausal symptoms, and decisions for or against replacement must be made now! What factors can be considered to ascertain which patients should receive replacement, and how should this replacement be given to reduce the chance of side effects?

Generalized guidelines for all patients cannot be made. Each patient needs to be evaluated individually, and her symptoms and risk factors must be considered.

Current replacement therapy should be directed toward the relief of hot flashes and vaginal atrophy and the prevention of osteoporosis. The other suggested indications for replacement are less clearly defined and should be approached cautiously until better data are available to substantiate a beneficial effect. This includes the treatment of osteoporosis that has already been established.

For hot flashes and vaginal atrophy the severity of the symptoms is important. If disabling, then replacement should be considered. If symptoms are minimal or absent, the need for treatment is reduced. For the prevention of osteoporosis, other clinical criteria may be considered. As already indicated, reduced body fat, Caucasian race, history of smoking, and early castration are all factors which have been associated with an increased incidence of osteoporosis. Thus, obese black women who do not smoke may have a reduced need for estrogen replacement to prevent osteoporosis.

The reason for therapy will also dictate how replacement should be given. Hot flashes can be treated for finite periods of time with progressive reduction in dosage. Prevention of osteoporosis with estrogen appears to require lifelong treatment. After 8 years of follow-up Lindsay and coworkers (1978) found the same reduction in bone density in women treated for only the initial 4 years as compared with women who were untreated during the duration of the study.

If estrogens are given, there are certain factors which seem to influence the incidence of complications. It does not appear to make any difference which estrogen preparation is utilized. Synthetic estrogens, naturally occuring steroids, or nonsteroidal estrogens have been incriminated in the genesis of side effects, particularly endometrial cancer (Antunes et al.). Dosage is apparently an important consideration. There is a reduced risk of endometrial cancer when lower amounts of medications are utilized. Length of treatment also appears to be an important factor, with longer usage being associated with an increased incidence of tumor formation (Antunes et al.). Data are inconsistent concerning continuous versus interrupted administration, with one study reporting a reduced risk with interrupted therapy (Mack et al.) and another finding no difference between the two types of administration (Antunes et al.). It should be noted that the latter study reviewed a much larger patient population. Combination estrogen-progestin therapy has certain theoretical advantages over estrogen administration alone. These include interruption of endometrial growth and induction of organized endometrial shedding. This form of therapy has been associated with a reduced incidence of endometrial cancer formation but results in periodic vaginal bleeding, a condition which is unacceptable to many postmenopausal patients (Hammond et al.). The dosage of estrogen and progesterone can be reduced sufficiently to avoid vaginal bleeding, but the benefit of regular endometrial shedding is lost. To date, it is not known if this form of therapy is safer than estrogen administration alone. When considering combination estrogen-progestin administration, it must be remembered that complications of estrogen therapy are not limited to the effects on the endometrium. For some of the other side effects the combined use of progestins does not prevent the action of estrogen. The complications associated with oral contraceptives are examples of this. Thus, the use of combination replacement has potential advantages but does not prevent all adverse effects of estrogen therapy.

The route of administration of hormonal replacement also appears to be a factor that could contribute to complications of replacement therapy. Oral administration of most estrogens necessitates passage of the hormone through the portal vessels and liver prior to entry into the general circulation. A portion of the estrogen is metabolized and inactivated by the liver before exposure to the rest of the body. It is possible that differential effects of estrogen on hepatic function as compared to other organ systems may occur. Since the action of estrogen on liver function is responsible for many of the side effects of the drug, this differential effect may significantly enhance the chance of complications. The recent finding of Frumar and coworkers (1979a), showing greater actions of oral estrogens on liver function than on sites of systemic action, is consistent with this concept.

Another drawback of oral therapy is that the gastrointestinal tract and liver can alter the medications in unexpected ways. The recent demonstration of conversion of micronized estradiol to estrone with oral but not vaginal administration is an example of this problem (Riggs et al.).

Systemic therapy also has potential drawbacks. Subcutaneous implants provide constant and sustained estrogen exposure. This may or may not turn out to be a problem. Injections necessitate the use of large hormonal dosages to lengthen the time interval between repeat administrations. Thus, no ideal route of administration has been identified. Fortunately, several groups of investigators are now examining this question.

The presence of certain diseases can preclude the use of estrogen. These include estrogen-dependent tumors; active acute or marked chronic liver disease with abnormal function; undiagnosed uterine bleeding; congenital hyperlipidemia; and a past history of thrombophlebitis, thromboembolism, or thrombotic disease; including a cerebrovascular accident. Relative contraindications include uterine leiomyomata, endometriosis, and hypertension. When these conditions are present, other forms of therapy or no treatment should be contemplated. For example, intramuscular injections of medroxyprogesterone acetate have been shown in a prospective double-blind study (Bullock et al.) to effectively relieve the subjective occurrence of hot flashes. Other compounds are said to relieve hot flashes but have not been studied as critically or inconsistent results have been reported. For prevention of osteoporosis, calcium carbonate, in a dose of 2.6 g per day, has been shown to significantly reduce the loss of calcium from bone (Recker et al.). Other forms of therapy are being recommended for the prevention of osteoporosis but have not been evaluated in a prospective double-blind study.

If a decision is reached to use estrogens, our current recommendations are to employ either conjugated equine estrogens, 0.3 to 0.625 mg per day, or ethinyl estradiol, 0.01 or 0.02 mg per day for 3 weeks with a 1-week rest period. The higher dosage of ethinyl estradiol is equivalent to the amount of mestranol which is being utilized by Lindsay and coworkers (1978) to prevent loss of calcium from bone. If the patient's uterus is intact, daily administration of progestin can be added during the last week of estrogen administration. Larger doses of estrogen may be required to decrease the occurrence of hot flashes, but attempts to reduce the dosage should be entertained as early as possible. Finally, a thorough dialogue between the patient and her physician should occur, so that an understanding of the therapeutic limits of estrogen replacement therapy and its advantages and disadvantages is clearly established in the patient's mind.

REFERENCES

Aiman J et al.: The origin of androgen and estrogen in a virilized postmenopausal woman with bilateral benign cystic teratomas. *Obstet Gynecol* 49:695, 1977.

Aksel S et al.: Vasomotor symptoms, serum estrogens, and gonadotropin levels in surgical menopause. *Am J Obstet Gynecol* 126:165, 1976.

Albright F et al.: Post menopausal osteoporosis. *Trans Assoc Am Physicians* 55:298, 1940.

Antunes CMF et al.: Endometrial cancer and estrogen use. *N Engl J Med* 300:9, 1979.

Atkins D, Peacock M: A comparison of the effects of the calcitonins, steroid hormones and thyroid hormones on the response of bone to parathyroid hormone in tissue culture. *J Endocrinol* 64:573, 1975.

Aylward M: Estrogens, plasma tryptophan levels in perimenopausal patients, in *The Management of the Menopause and Postmenopausal Years,* ed. S Campbell, Lancaster, England: MTP Press, 1976.

Backstrom J et al.: FSH, LH, TeBG-capacity, estrogen and progesterone in women with premenstrual tension during the luteal phase. *J Steroid Biochem* 7:473, 1976.

Baird DT, Guevara A: Concentration of unconjugated estrone and estradiol in peripheral plasma in nonpregnant women throughout the menstrual cycle, castrate and postmenopausal women and men. *J Clin Endocrinol Metab* 29:149, 1969.

Ballinger CB: Psychiatric morbidity and the menopause: clinical features. *Br Med J* 31:1183, 1976.

———: Psychiatric morbidity and the menopause: Screening of general population sample. *Br Med J* 3:344, 1975.

Benjamin F, Dentsch S: Plasma levels of fractionated estrogens and pituitary hormones in endometrial carcinoma. *Am J Obstet Gynecol* 126:638, 1976.

Bullock JL et al.: Use of medroxyprogesterone acetate to prevent menopausal symptoms. *Obstet Gynecol* 46:165, 1975.

Calanog A et al.: Androstenedione metabolism in patients with endometrial cancer. *Am J Obstet Gynecol* 129:553, 1977.

———: Testosterone metabolism in endometrial cancer. *Am J Obstet Gynecol* 124:60, 1976.

Campbell S: Double-blind psychometric studies on the effects of natural estrogens on postmenopausal women, in *The Management of the Menopause and Postmenopausal Years,* ed. S Campbell, Lancaster, England: MTP Press, 1976.

Caputo CB et al.: Failure of estrogens and androgens to inhibit bone resorption in tissue culture. *Endocrinology* 98:1065, 1976.

Chen TL, Feldman D: Distinction between alpha-fetoprotein and intracellular estrogen receptors: Evidence against the presence of estradiol receptors in bone. *Endocrinology* 102:236, 1978.

Coppen A, Kessel N: Menstruation and personality. *Br J Psychiatr* 109:711, 1963.

Coronary Drug Project Research Group: The coronary drug project; initial findings leading to modifications of its research protocol. *JAMA* 214:1303, 1970.

Castoff A, Mahesh VB: Primordial follicles with normal oocytes in the ovaries of postmenopausal women. *J Am Geriatr Soc* 23:193, 1975.

Cox B, Lomax P.: Pharmacologic control of temperature regulation. *Annu Rev Pharmacol Toxicol* 17:341, 1977.

Dalton K: *The Premenstrual Syndrome and Progesterone Therapy,* Chicago: Year Book, 1977.

Daniell HW: Osteoporosis of the slender smoker. *Arch Intern Med* 136:298, 1976.

De Jong FH, Sharpe RM: Evidence of inhibin-like activity in bovine follicular fluid. *Nature* 263:71, 1976.

Doll R et al.: Hormone replacement therapy and endometrial cancer. *Lancet* 1:745, 1977.

Edman CO, MacDonald PC: Effect of obesity on conversion of plasma androstenedione to estrone in ovulatory and anovulatory young women. *Am J Obstet Gynecol* 130:456, 1978.

Eskay RL et al.: Relationship between luteinizing hormone releasing hormone concentration in hypophysial blood and luteinizing hormone release in intact, castrated and electro-chemically-stimulated rats. *Endocrinology* 100:263, 1977.

Frumar AM et al.: Biological effects of estrogen at different sites of action in postmenopausal women. *Proc 26th Annu Meeting Soc Gynecol Invest,* San Diego, 1979a, abstract 109.

———: Urinary calcium-creatinine ratio and estrogen status in postmenopausal women. *Proc 26th Annu Meeting Soc Gynecol Invest,* San Diego, 1979b, abstract 17.

Gallagher JC, Williamson R: Effect of ethinyl estradiol on calcium and phosphorus metabolism in postmenopausal women with primary hyperparathyroidism. *Clin Sci Mol Med* 45:785, 1973.

——— et al.: Aging and immunoreactive parathyroid

hormone in normal and osteoporotic subjects. *Clin Res* 25:562A, 1977.

———: The crush fracture syndrome in osteoporosis. *J Clin Endocrinol Metab* 2:293, 1973.

Gordon T et al.: Menopause and coronary heart disease. *Ann Intern Med* 89:157, 1978.

Greenblatt RB et al.: Ovarian and adrenal steroid production in the postmenopausal woman. *Obstet Gynecol* 47:383, 1976.

Greenwald P et al.: Endometrial cancer after menopausal use of estrogens. *Obstet Gynecol* 50:239, 1977.

Hammond CB et al.: Effects of long-term estrogen replacement therapy. *Am J Obstet Gynecol* 133:537, 1979.

Hausknecht RU, Gusberg SB: Estrogen metabolism in patients at high risk for endometrial carcinoma. *Am J Obstet Gynecol* 116:981, 1973.

Horwitz RI, Feinstein AL: Alternative analytic methods for case-control studies of estrogens and endometrial cancer. *N Engl J Med* 299:1089, 1978.

Houssain M et al.: Parathyroid activity and postmenopausal osteoporosis. *Lancet* 1:809, 1970.

Hutchison GB, Rothman KJ: Correcting a bias. *N Engl J Med* 299:1129, 1978.

Jick H et al.: Replacement estrogens and endometrial cancer. *N Engl J Med* 300:218, 1979.

Jowsey J et al.: Quantitative microradiographic studies of normal and osteoporotic bone. *J Bone Joint Surg* 47A:785, 1965.

Judd HL: Hormonal dynamics associated with the menopause. *Clin Obstet Gynecol* 19:775, 1976.

Kannel WB et al.: Menopause and risk of cardiovascular disease. *Ann Intern Med* 85:447, 1976.

Klaiber EL et al.: Plasma monoamine oxidase activity in regularly menstruating women and in amenorrheic women receiving cyclic treatment with estrogens and a progestin. *J Clin Endocrinol Metab* 33:630, 1971.

Knowelden J et al.: Incidence of fracture in persons over 35 years of age. *Br J Prev Soc Med* 18:130, 1964.

Lindsay R et al.: Bone response to termination of oestrogen treatment. *Lancet* 1:1325, 1978.

———: The effect of endogenous oestrogen on plasma and urinary calcium and phosphate in oophorectomized women. *Clin Endocrinol* 6:87, 1977.

———: Long-term prevention of postmenopausal osteoporosis by oestrogen. *Lancet* 1:1038, 1976.

Longcope C et al.: Aromatization of androgens by muscle and adipose tissue in vivo. *J Clin Endocrinol Metab* 46:146, 1978.

———: Conversion of blood androgens to estrogens in normal adult men and women. *J Clin Invest* 48:2191, 1969.

Lucas WE: Causal relationships between endocrine-metabolic variables in patients with endometrial carcinoma. *Obstet Gynecol Surv* 29:507, 1974.

McCann SM et al.: Gonadotropin-releasing factors. Sites of production, secretion and action in the brain, in *Anatomic Neuroendocrinology*, ed. W Stumpf, LD Grant, Basel: Karger, 1975, p. 192.

McDonald PC et al.: Effect of obesity on conversion of plasma androstenedione to estrone in postmenopausal women with and without endometrial cancer. *Am J Obstet Gynecol* 130:448, 1978.

Mack TM et al.: Estrogens and endometrial cancer in a retirement community. *N Engl J Med* 294:1262, 1976.

MacIntyre I: The action and control of the calcium-regulating hormones. *J Endocrinol Invest* 1:277, 1978.

Marshall DH et al.: The relation between plasma androstenedione and oestrone levels in untreated and corticosteroid-treated post-menopausal women. *Clin Endocrinol* 9:407, 1978.

Mattingly RF, Huang WY: Steroidogenesis of the menopausal and postmenopausal ovary. *Am J Obstet Gynecol* 103:679, 1969.

Mattson B, Schoultz B: A comparison between lithium, placebo, and a diuretic in premenstrual tension. *Acta Psychiatr Scand* 255 (suppl.):75, 1974.

Meema HE et al.: Loss of compact bone due to menopause. *Obstet Gynecol* 26:333, 1965.

Meldrum DR et al.: Elevations in skin temperature of the finger as an objective index of postmenopausal hot flashes: Standardization of the technique. *Am J Obstet Gynecol* 135:713, 1979.

Meyn MA Jr et al.: Fracture of the hip in the institutionalized psychotic patient. *Clin Orthoped* 122:128, 1977.

Molnar GW: Body temperatures during menopausal hot flashes. *J Appl Physiol* 3:499, 1975.

Mulley G et al.: Hot flushes after hypophysectomy. *Br Med J* 2:1062, 1977.

Nordin BEC: Clinical significance and pathogenesis of osteoporosis. *Br Med J* 1:571, 1971.

Pfeffer RI, Van den Noort S: Estrogen use and stroke risk in postmenopausal women. *Am J Epidemiol* 103:445, 1976.

Pulkkinen MO, Kaihola HL: Mefenamic acid in dysmenorrhea. *Acta Obstet Gynecol Scand* 56:75, 1977.

Punnonen R: Effect of castration and peroral estrogen therapy on the skin. *Acta Obstet Gynecol Scand Suppl*, vol. 21, 1977.

Rauramo L et al.: The effect of castration and peroral estrogen therapy on some psychological functions, in *Estrogens in the Postmenopause, Frontiers in Hormone Research,* Basel: Karger, 1975.

Reaves TA, Hayward JM: Hypothalamic and extrahypothalamic thermoregulatory centers, in *Body Temperature: Regulation, Drug Effects and Therapeutic Implications,* ed. P Lomax, E Schonbaum, New York: Dekker, 1979, p. 39.

Recker RR et al.: Effect of estrogens and calcium carbonate on bone loss in postmenopausal women. *Ann Intern Med* 87:649, 1977.

Rees L: Psychosomatic aspects of the premenstrual tension syndrome. *J Ment Sci* 99:62, 1953.

Riggs BA et al.: Absorption of estrogens from vaginal creams. *N Engl J Med* 298:195, 1978.

————: Serum concentrations of estrogen, testosterone and gonadotropins in osteoporotic and nonosteoporotic postmenopausal women. *J Clin Endocrinol Metab* 36:1097, 1973.

Ritterband AB et al.: Gonadal function and the development of coronary heart disease. *Circulation* 27:237, 1963.

Rizkallah TH et al.: Production of estrone and fractional conversion of circulating androstenedione to estrone in women with endometrial carcinoma. *J Clin Endocrinol Metab* 40:1045, 1975.

Rosenberg L et al.: Myocardial infarction and estrogen therapy in postmenopausal women. *N Engl J Med* 294:1256, 1976.

Ross GT, Vande Wiele RL: The ovaries, in *Textbook of Endocrinology,* ed. RH Williams, Philadelphia: Saunders, 1974, p. 423.

Ryan KJ: Estrogens and atherosclerosis. *Clin Obstet Gynecol* 19:805, 1976.

Shahrad P, Marks R: A pharmacologic effect of estrogen on human epidermis. *Br J Dermatol* 97:383, 1977.

Sherman BM, Korenman SG: Hormonal characteristics of the human menstrual cycle throughout reproductive life. *J Clin Invest* 55:699, 1975.

Siiteri PK, MacDonald PC: Role of estraglandular estrogen in human endocrinology, in *Handbook of Physiology,* vol. 2, ed. RO Greep, EB Astwood, Washington DC: Am Physiol Soc, 1973, p. 615.

Simpkins JW, Kalra SP: Central site(s) of norepinephrine and LHRH interaction. *Fed Proc* 38:1107, 1979.

Stern MP et al.: Cardiovascular risk and use of estrogens or estrogen-progestagen combinations. *JAMA* 235:811, 1976.

Stumpf WE et al.: Estrogen target cells in the skin. *Experientia* 30:196, 1974.

Tanaka Y et al.: Control of renal vitamin D hydroxylases in birds by sex hormones. *Proc Natl Acad Sci* 73:2701, 1976.

Tataryn IV et al.: LH, FSH, and skin temperature during the menopausal hot flash. *J Clin Endocrinol Metab* 49:152, 1979.

Thomson J: Double-blind study of the effect of oestrogen on sleep, anxiety and depression in perimenopausal patients. *J Endocrinol* 72:395, 1977.

Timonen S, Procope B: The premenstrual syndrome: Frequency and association of symptoms. *Ann Chir Gynaecol Fenn* 62:108, 1973.

Treloar AC et al.: Variation of the human menstrual cycle throughout reproductive life. *Int J Fertil* 12:77, 1967.

Utian WH: The true clinical features of postmenopause and oophorectomy, and their response to estrogen therapy. *S Afr Med J* 46:732–737, 1972.

Vanhulle G, Demol R: A double-blind study into the influence of estriol on a number of psychological tests in postmenopausal women, in *Concensus on Menopause Research,* eds. PA Van Keep, RB Greenblatt, M Albeaux-Fernet, Lancaster, England: MTP Press, 1976, pp. 94–99.

Veldhuis JD et al.: *60th Annu Meeting Endocrine Soc,* Miami, June 1978, abstract 254.

Vollman RF: *The Menstrual Cycle.* Philadelphia: Saunders, 1977, p. 193.

Wieland AJ et al.: Preoperative localization of virilizing tumors by selective venous sampling. *Am J Obstet Gynecol* 131:797, 1978.

Willman EA et al.: Studies in the involvement of prostaglandins in uterine symptomatology and pathology. *Br J Obstet Gynecol* 83:337, 1976.

Winokur G: Depression in the menopause. *Am J Psychiatry* 130:92–93, 1973.

36

Sexually Transmitted Diseases

AUDREY J. MCMASTER

DEMOGRAPHY AND GENERAL DISCUSSION
Age
Marital status
Education
Race
Developmental attitudes and beliefs
Life-style and economics

THE TOP FIVE TRADITIONAL STDs
Gonorrhea
    Upper-reproductive-tract involvement—
    salpingitis
    Upper abdominal involvement
    Disseminated gonorrheal infection
Syphilis
    Lesions specific to the lower reproductive tract
    Upper-genital-tract disease
Lymphopathia venereum
Chancroid (soft chancre)
Granuloma inguinale

OTHER PROBLEM STDs
Herpes genitalis
Condyloma acuminatum
Candidiasis
Trichomoniasis
Cytomegalovirus (CMV) infection
Pediculosis pubis (pubic lice)
Genital scabies

CONCLUSIONS

Every 10 seconds, a sexually transmitted disease (STD) occurs in the United States. Therefore, all physicians providing care to women must be knowledgeable about STDs and must understand the role which the host, the host's environment, and the organism play in the natural history of these diseases.

Among the top 12 STDs, five have been traditionally and legally termed venereal diseases: gonorrhea, syphilis, chancroid, lymphopathia venereum, and granuloma inguinale. Only gonorrhea and syphilis are prevalent in the United States. Lymphopathia venereum, granuloma inguinale, and chancroid occur most frequently in the developing nations. The remaining seven diseases, herpes genitalis, trichomoniasis, cytomegalovirus, moniliasis, condyloma acuminatum, pubic lice, and scabies, are also sometimes, but not always, transmitted by sexual contact. Therefore, the term STD includes many diverse organisms that cause health problems. Their patterns of distribution, sites of infection, complications, and management are shared by many, some by all, of the STDs.

DEMOGRAPHY AND GENERAL DISCUSSION

The true incidence of STDs in the United States is unknown. If one allows for underdiagnosing and underreporting of disease, gonorrhea is the leading communicable disease in the United States, with an estimated 3 to 4 million new cases annually. Of these reported cases, 17 percent will develop pelvic inflammatory disease, making gonorrhea also the leading cause of sterility in the United States. Syphilis ranks as the third most common communicable disease with 75,000 to 85,000 new cases reported per year. Of the remaining top seven STDs, an estimated 6.8 million cases occur annually. Herpes genitalis is estimated at 300,000 cases per year and trichomoniasis at 3 million cases detected annually.

Epidemiologic data suggest that early reproductive maturity with a longer sexual life-span, amount and type of individual sexual activity, infection status of sex partner, age, marital status, education, ethnic background, developmental attitudes and beliefs, life-style, and economics all play important roles in determining which individuals are at risk of STDs. The diverse interrelationships of these parameters make it difficult to select any one given factor or group of factors as a cause. However, some understanding of the contribution each makes to the spread of STDs can be of value in the prevention, treatment, and control of the diseases.

The most important individual risk factor in the acquisition of STD is the number of sexual encounters with an infected partner. The partner one chooses is of more importance than the number of partners or the number of encounters.

AGE

Individuals, single by choice or age, separated, divorced, or widowed, and the handicapped members of our society, regardless of age, in many instances experience sexual expression by chance only. Regular sexual relationships with steady partners are not available to them nor sanctioned by society. This situation fosters multiple, casual encounters which result in a group of individuals at high risk of STDs. At present, adolescents and young adults, aged 15 to 25 years, have the highest reported STD rate. The infection rate for children under 15 is unrecognized and unreported. Most studies indicate that it is far from rare. The most important aspect of age as a high-risk factor is the time of encounter not the actual age.

MARITAL STATUS

Couples with marital and/or sexual problems are vulnerable to extramarital sexual encounters. Couples who are separated for short or long periods of time by job requirements, by military assignment, illness, and/or incarceration may seek casual sexual liaisons. Both partners then become high risks for STDs, either from the outside contact or through transmission of infection by the spouse.

EDUCATION

Individuals with higher educational status tend to (1) establish regular sexual outlets with steady partners, thus lowering the incidence of risk with infected partners; (2) take advantage of health services in order to effectively control gonorrhea and syphilis, and, however inadequately, to control other bacterial, viral, and fungal infections; (3) frequently utilize prophylaxis; (4) possess a wide variety of nonsexual activities; and (5) tend not to depend upon a sexual outlet during periods of stress.

RACE

Ethnic background, when combined with the other parameters outlined above, can be helpful in defining high-risk groups in certain communities or geographic locations. By itself, race offers no predictability.

DEVELOPMENTAL ATTITUDES AND BELIEFS

Misinformation and myth permeate our society's attitudes about health and disease, about when to seek treatment, about who is responsible and for what, about medical advice, contact tracing, and follow-up. The belief, for example, that masturbation is abnormal, harmful, or shameful may prevent individuals from practicing it in preference to seeking casual partners or prostitutes. Clearly, irrational beliefs and attitudes may contribute to STDs.

LIFE-STYLE AND ECONOMICS

Wide-ranging, inexpensive travel, increased leisure time, higher standards of living, and greater life stresses have created new opportunities for sexual encounters. Homosexuality and prostitution continue, as they have always, to create at-risk subgroups. Homosexual behavior, as an example, is responsible for

40 to 70 percent of reported cases of syphilis in the United States. Prostitution in Western countries, especially in lower socioeconomic populations, is becoming a major source of infection.

The apathy of the general population and of the medical profession in dealing with diseases shrouded by social stigma fosters a "tolerance" which makes our society a prime target and source for perpetuation of STDs.

THE TOP FIVE TRADITIONAL STDs

GONORRHEA

Definition

Gonorrhea is a communicable bacterial disease that can involve any mucosal structure of the body. Severe forms of the disease can invade the bloodstream, speading the disease to joints, tendons, meninges, and endocardium.

Etiology

The bacteria of gonorrhea is a gram-negative intracellular diplococcus termed *Neisseria gonorrhoeae*, first described by Neisser in 1879. Accurate recognition of this bacteria in females requires culture identification. A group of organisms termed *Mimmina*, commonly found in the genital tract, are also gram-negative intracellular diplococci which on differentially stained smears are indistinguishable from *Neisseria gonorrhoeae*.

Natural History

Direct physical contact with an infected host or inanimate object is the method of disease spread. Direct sexual contact is the most common mode of transmission. However, indirect spread by instruments, linens, etc. does occur. Drying, heat, and washing with an antiseptic solution effectively kill the bacteria, making indirect spread of the disease rare.

Clinical Manifestations

From 3 to 21 days following exposure, the endotoxin produced by the gonococcus causes redness and swelling at the site of contact. The disease process may limit itself to a localized area of inflammation, but if tissue destruction occurs, a purulent exudate develops with the potential for abscess formation or a chronic disease process. By direct tissue extension, bloodstream invasion, or both, the gonococci can spread to other organ systems within the same host or become accessible to new host contact.

Local Manifestations

Urethra. A primary site of gonorrheal contact is the exposed urethra. The patient complaint, "Doctor, I think I have a bladder infection," may be the sole clue to its presence. Pain on urination, frequency of urination, and involuntary loss of urine may be experienced by the patient within the first few days of contact. The symptoms may spontaneously resolve because of the short length of the urethra and the acid composition of the urine. If the patient delays care for even a few days, the organisms may be absent, or so few in number that physical findings and diagnostic tests are inconclusive. If the discharge gains access to the periurethral ducts or glands, the organism may remain without patient symptoms or physical findings. If the periurethral duct becomes obstructed by swelling, drainage of the gland is impaired, causing a periurethral abscess. The urethra may be deviated from its midline position by the enlarged gland. A painful, fluctuant mass and urinary retention are the usual complaints of patients. Digital compression of the urethra and periurethral glands should be done at the time of examination to express any exudate present for culture evaluation. Treatment should be started on the basis of the patient's history, whether exam or laboratory findings are confirmatory or inconclusive. Failure to provide treatment can lead to urethral stenosis and chronic skenitis.

Vulva. The intact squamous epithelium of the healthy adult vulva is resistant to penetration by the gonococcus. This resistance may be lowered or absent in females prior to puberty, after menopause, or in the presence of coexistent disease or debilitating conditions.

If exudate drains from the infected adjacent genital structures to the warm, moist vulva, which is normally subjected to garment friction and constriction, swelling, redness, excoriation, maceration, and adhesions can develop. Itching, burning, and pain frequently compel the patient to seek medical attention. Vulvitis of gonorrheal origin is most severe in the prepubertal female.

Vagina. The vaginal mucosa is an uncommon site of gonorrheal infection. Absence or low levels of estrogen in the prepubertal or menopausal female may prevent or alter the normal stratification of vaginal epithelium. This allows invasion of the gonococci into the mucosal surface, producing engorgement, redness, swelling, and a profuse vaginal discharge. In children, the vagina is the primary site of infection. The profuse discharge which is produced drains to the vulva, causing severe vulvitis.

Bartholin's Gland. Infection in the Bartholin's duct or gland is still considered pathognomic of *Neisseria gonorrhoeae* by most physicians, despite culture evidence that supports streptococci, *E. coli,* and staphylococci as the most frequently cultured organisms. When *Neisseria* gonococci are the causative factor, the infection is usually an extension of urethral or periurethral disease. If the duct is obstructed, the gland becomes abscessed. As the abscess enlarges, tension on adjacent tissue structures produces a reddish-purple discoloration of the overlying tissue and pain. The abscess will eventually resolve by spontaneous rupture but surgical incision and antibiotic therapy are necessary for prompt symptomatic relief and the prevention of a chronic, recurrent cystic or abscess state.

Cervix. The specificity of the gonococci for the endocervical mucous membrane provides a silent reserervoir to harbor and proliferate the gonococcus and allows for its direct extension to the upper genital tract structures. The clinical appearance of the cervix infected with gonorrhea is not unlike the redness, erosion, or swelling produced by other cervical diseases. A profuse, irritating discharge may be the only physical finding or patient complaint. Patients who are asymptomatic and who therefore fail to seek treatment become asymptomatic carriers and are the primary source for new host contacts.

Rectum. Approximately 78 years before Neisser isolated and identified the gonococcus, Hecter described the clinical findings recognized today as rectal gonorrhea. The extent of its presence today is unknown. Physicians' reluctance to obtain a sexual history, patients' embarrassment and fear at divulging their sexual behavior, and the failure to obtain rectal cultures contribute to our lack of knowledge. Schroeter and Reynolds reported in 1972 that 60 percent of infected females have rectal gonorrhea. Whether by rectal coitus or the flow of infected vaginal discharge to the perineum, rectal involvement does occur. If unrecognized and untreated, anal crypt abscesses, rectal stenosis, and septicemia can result.

Pharynx. Though considered rare by many and seldom discussed in textbooks, the oral cavity is a site

of gonorrheal infection. Zilz in 1911 reported cases of gonococcal stomatitis in patients who had had oral-genital contact. A decline in preference for vaginal intercourse in pregnancy has increased the prevalence of pharyngeal gonorrhea in pregnant women. If only endocervical or rectal cultures are done, as many as one-third of gonococcal infections in pregnancy will be missed. In one study, 35 percent of patients had positive pharyngeal cultures; in another, 15 percent had positive cultures, but only 1 percent had positive endocervical cultures. Social stigma and moral judgments against oral sexual intercourse have limited our ability to obtain the information essential in evaluating the oropharynx as a site of gonorrheal infection.

If infected discharge comes into contact with the moist mucous membrane of the oropharynx, gonococcal pharyngitis or tonsillitis can occur. If the possibility of a gonorrheal infection is not considered, it will be missed, as the clinical findings of edema and a beefy red color at the posterior pharynx are not unlike those seen with streptococcal pharyngitis. If the tonsillar bed is involved, a purulent exudate similar to follicular tonsillitis is present. Since the *Neisseria* species is a common inhabitant of the oropharynx, the diagnosis of gonorrhea must be confirmed by sugar-fermentation tests. If a history of oral-genital contact is obtained and the patient has physical findings suggestive of pharyngitis, the patient should be treated before laboratory confirmation has been obtained. A case of gonococcal arthritis complicating primary gonococcal pharyngitis was reported by Metzger in 1970. Delay in treatment can permit the organism to spread to other organ systems and be the source of a new host contact.

Diagnosis of Local Disease

The patient's history is the most accurate diagnostic tool we have in the detection of any STD. A physician not only must "see it to believe it" but "believe it in order to see it." A tactful, nonjudgmental discussion of the patient's sexual behavior at the time of routine evaluation can provide information as to whether the possibility of STD exists. It is obvious that other infections can produce the same complaints and physical findings. An accurate history will be helpful in determining the possible source of infection. The patient's presenting complaint may be misleading and the physical findings may be absent or difficult to interpret.

A culture of the endocervical canal should be obtained routinely. Unfortunately, many physicians still do not examine menstruating patients and an opportune time to screen patients for gonorrhea is lost. There is an increased diagnostic yield at the time of menses in women at high risk for STDs. Many patients with newly developed or increased dysmenorrhea or intramenstrual bleeding have positive cultures for gonorrhea. The use of Thayer-Martin media will provide approximately 85 to 90 percent accuracy. Routine cultures of the rectum, urethra, and pharynx will increase the ability to diagnose asymptomatic disease. Kellogg has reported a 5 to 6 percent incidence of positive rectal cultures in women with negative cultures taken from the cervix and urethra. If there is a history of oral-genital intercourse, the oropharynx should be cultured. In Holmes' experience, 10 to 20 percent of females with positive cervical cultures have a positive pharyngeal culture.

For optimum return in detecting gonorrhea by culture, the following steps in obtaining a culture should be observed: (1) use a nonlubricated speculum; (2) place a cotton swab in the site to be cultured and allow enough time for the swab to absorb any organisms present; (3) streak the tip of the swab directly onto the culture medium; and (4) immediately place the culture in a candle jar or CO_2 incubator. Trans-gro and Clinicult medium can be used if laboratory facilities are not readily available. A delay of more than 48 to 72 hours will decrease the viability of the organisms.

Sugar-fermentation tests must be carried out when pharyngeal and rectal cultures are obtained, as the *Neisseria* species found at these sites will also grow on each medium. Cultures obtained specifically to exclude or document gonorrhea should be labeled as such to reduce the time and exploration of other organisms by the laboratory, thereby decreasing their work load and the cost to the patient. In women, gram stains to identify the gram-negative intracellular diplococci provide unreliable information and should not be done.

Treatment of Local Sites

Treatment of the organism, its host, and the host's environment is essential for successful therapy.

The Organism. Penicillin is still the drug of choice in the treatment of *Neisseria* gonorrhea, regardless of its site or extent of involvement. Sensitivity to penicillin is an obvious exception. Uncomplicated gonorrheal infection involving the urethra, periurethral duct and glands, Bartholin's gland, vulva, vagina, cervix,

rectum, and pharynx is effectively treated with the administration of 4.8 million units of aqueous procaine penicillin G in divided doses in one visit. This establishes prompt high blood levels of antibiotic necessary for effective treatment. Probenicid 1 g given orally 30 minutes prior to the antibiotic injection prevents rapid excretion of penicillin by the urinary tract, permitting maintenance of high blood levels of the antibiotic. Initial penicillin therapy should be followed by oral ampicillin 500 mg four times per day for 10 days. Individuals with penicillin sensitivity should be treated with tetracycline hydrochloride 1.5 g initially followed by 0.5 g four times per day for 10 days. Spectinomycin 2 g intramuscularly should be restricted to those infected with documented penicillinase-producing organisms and their sexual partners, and those whose cultures remain positive after initial therapy with penicillin, tetracycline, or ampicillin. If the disease is associated with pregnancy, erythromycin 0.5 g four times per day for 5 days (a total dosage of 10 g) is the treatment of choice. The low prevalence of penicillinase-producing gonococci in the United States does not necessitate any change in the current treatment recommendations. A greater emphasis on testing cure cultures for all patients is encouraged.

Many new drugs have recently been advocated as specific in the treatment of this disease but have not demonstrated an increased treatment effectiveness. Their side effects are still relatively unknown and the cost may be unwarranted when compared to penicillin or tetracycline. No therapeutic agent is 100 percent effective or without possible side effects. Organism resistance does occur. If adequate follow-up with repeat examination and culture is done, resistant disease can be documented and treatment effected. Anaphylactic reactions do occur with penicillin; however, the amount of drug and its mode of dispensing bear no relationship to the severity of the reaction. Small doses of antibiotics over a longer period of time will not obviate a reaction but can reduce the effectiveness of the antibiotic. The patient should be observed for at least 30 minutes following the administration of penicillin, as most reactions will occur within that time period. Equipment and support facilities must be readily available to treat any untoward reactions.

Women with a history of gonorrheal contact but without clinical documentation should receive the same treatment as those known to have the disease. In the treatment of children, the amount of antibiotic used should be calculated on the basis of known scales for the amount of drug per kilogram of body weight.

A word of caution: since organisms, their host, and host's environment are ever-changing, any treatment schedule printed today may be outdated by the time it is needed. Therefore, physicians must keep current in their knowledge about the varying drugs used in treatment, their dosage, and appropriate methods of follow-up.

The Host. An individual should never be told that gonorrhea is present unless a positive culture for the disease is available. The psychologic and social stigma that persists relative to this disease may obviate continued rapport with the patient, making appropriate treatment and follow-up impossible and legal action likely. Treatment should not be withheld, however, until a proven culture is available. If by history and clinical evaluation the possibility of the disease exists, the patient should be told that an infection is present and that the specific organism must await culture determination. Treatment can be instituted and at a later date the patient can be informed of the organism found. Reevaluation and further treatment can then be discussed.

Additional supportive therapy is indicated if swelling, redness, excoriation, and maceration are present. The itching, burning, pain, and discharge experienced by the patient may be more incapacitating and of greater concern to her than the disease itself. Gentle cleansing of the vulva and perineal area can be accomplished with a warm tap-water sitz bath or a potassium permanganate 1:10,000 sitz bath three or four times per day. This will assist in cleansing the infected, irritated tissue. If the periurethral duct or gland or Bartholin's gland or duct is involved, moist heat will encourage drainage and/or provide early localization of the infected site so surgical incision and drainage can be accomplished. Following cleansing, a cream such as iodochlorhydroxyquin with hydrocortisone can be applied to the affected external tissues in order to relieve the subjective symptoms of itching and burning. The addition of an oral antihistamine such as diphenhydramine hydrochloride 25 to 50 mg every 6 hours by mouth, or tripelennamine 25 to 50 mg by mouth can be an adjunct to therapy. These agents also provide a mild sedative action that helps prevent scratching, which most frequently occurs at night.

In the prepubertal or postmenopausal female, the addition of an estrogen cream or suppository will allow for cornification of the vaginal epithelium, frequently eradicating the organism. This, however, does not obviate the use of appropriate antibiotic therapy. In the reproductive female, if vaginitis is present, the use of Aci-Jel to achieve optimum pH and/or broad-spectrum antibiotic suppository or cream can be of assistance in resolving the secondary trauma to the vaginal mucosa.

If the infection is associated with menses, the trauma of a perineal pad can lead to further irritation and excoriation by its friction, moisture, and heat. The use of a vaginal tampon should be considered. Synthetic materials used in most undergarments frequently increase or exacerbate local irritations and excoriations. They are less absorbent and retain more body heat. Cotton undergarments provide better absorption and are cooler and more comfortable. Soap, washcloths and towels, deodorant sprays, and powders and douches commonly used by the patient in self-treatment should be discouraged: they can aggravate the symptoms and spread the disease.

The potential for pregnancy also exists when gonorrhea is present or suspected. Therefore, pregnancy screening, the option of abortion, and methods of family planning should be made available to the patient when indicated. Instruction of the patient in the use of condoms by the sexual partner is important. If sexual activity occurs before treatment of the patient and her partner has been completed, the use of condoms can prevent the spread of disease or reinfection.

The Host Environment. An optimum time and method for public education about venereal disease has not has not yet been achieved. Once a patient acquires gonorrhea, she is a captive audience. Therefore, the physician must educate the patient and, when possible, her partner about the disease in order to effect cure and, it is hoped, prevent future exposures. Partner involvement in treatment and education may be a delicate and traumatizing dilemma for the physician. The patient can be of significant assistance if given factual information and the responsibility to contact her partner. This can provide him with appropriate knowledge and assist him in obtaining treatment. In situations where the partner is married and the disease is acquired outside marriage by the woman or her husband, it is obvious that other marital concerns are present. The acute problem may serve as an initiative to other problem solving. The physician must be of support to both individuals in the evaluation and treatment of the acute disease. Avoiding the initiative the situation demands or the patient requires creates apathy and continues ignorance about the disease, implying to the patient and the public that our profession does not choose to deal with this problem and that the situation is tolerable. Public health agencies can be of assistance and should be called upon for their expertise.

UPPER-REPRODUCTIVE-TRACT INVOLVEMENT—SALPINGITIS

When a localized lower-tract site of gonorrhea is undiagnosed, untreated, resistant to treatment, or inadequately treated, the disease can spread by direct extension through the endocervical canal to the endometrial cavity, fallopian tubes, and peritoneal cavity. This is facilitated at the time of menstruation when the endocervical canal becomes dilated, the mucous plug disintegrates, and the availability of necrotic tissue and serum from the endometrial cavity enhances propagation of the organism. However, several cases of gonorrheal peritonitis in prepubertal females have been reported, making menstruation as a prerequisite for peritoneal involvement questionable. Intrauterine infection, when present, is usually transient. It becomes clinically significant when a recent delivery or surgical procedure precedes the infection. The organism quickly spreads by direct extension to the mucosal lining of the fallopian tube which is patent at its internal os at the time of menstruation. The previously described tissue reactions begin. The exudate produced drains from the distal opening of the fallopian tube into the peritoneal cavity causing varying degrees of pelvic peritonitis. The virulence of the organism, the innate tissue resistance of the host, and the availability of treatment are decisive factors in the arrest or progression of the disease at this stage. If the disease progresses, the tubes may become thickened, leading to occlusion and inability to drain. An abscessed cavity is the usual result. Microscopically, the tubal plicae become swollen and infiltrated with neutrophilic leukocytes with evidence of tissue destruction. The adjacent blood vessels are engorged and the surrounding tissues are hyperemic. With severe infections, the muscular and serosal layers become involved. The presence of plasma cells and lymphocytes indicates a chronic disease process.

The functional capacity of the tube following an infection is difficult to predict. Residual effects may be absent if treatment is early and adequate. However, even in mild infections where adequate treatment has been instituted, sufficient alteration in tubal physiology can produce a potential for ectopic pregnancy, infertility, and/or a chronic disease process. These complications are to be anticipated with increased virulence, extensive tissue involvement, and abscess formation.

Subjective Symptoms

The normal anatomic relationships within the pelvis become distorted when inflammation, obstruction, or abscess formation occurs, producing a variety of patient complaints, clinical findings, and laboratory data. The symptoms of upper-tract gonorrheal involvement are not unlike those of many other inflammatory disease processes within the abdominal cavity. When a history of recent sexual contact followed by menses is obtained and there is no apparent history of bowel, bladder, or kidney disease, the possibility of gonorrhea should be considered by the physician.

Pain is the universal complaint. It is usually present in both lower quadrants, as involvement of the fallopian tube is rarely a unilateral process unless one tube is absent or obstructed. Palpation of the abdominal wall and manipulation of the uterus at the time of pelvic examination will usually elicit the most probable site of involvement but it may be vague and unrevealing. The pain may be dull, cramping, and intermittent, or it may be persistent, severe, and incapacitating. A temperature of 102°F or greater with the presence of nausea or vomiting indicates peritoneal involvement or abscess formation. Abdominal distention and muscular rigidity are apparent at examination. If the infected process progresses, the pulse rate may increase, the patient's symptoms and physical findings may extend to the upper abdomen. When the infections occurs near or at the time of a menstrual period, the flow may be increased in amount and prolonged in number of days due to transient involvement of the endometrium. A low hemoglobin and hematocrit may be present if the amount of blood lost at the time of the period has been significant. Blood specimens may reveal a leukocytosis with increased neutrophils and elevated sedimentation rate.

Diagnosis of Salpingitis

Subacute salpingitis is the most common form of upper-reproductive-tract involvement. It is the most frequently misdiagnosed stage of the disease because of its similarity to findings present in urinary tract infections, appendicitis, ruptured ovarian cysts, and uterine and menstrual dysfunctions. The symptoms may be so minimal that the patient may not seek treatment, or often treatment for other suspected conditions has begun and when unsuccessful, the diagnosis may then be reconsidered. If a recent uterine curettage, tubal ligation, or vaginal delivery has occurred, the gonococcal organism may enter the uterine lymphatics and veins, permitting the organism to spread to parametrial tissues, causing pelvic cellulitis and/or pelvic thrombophlebitis.

Complications of Salpingitis

Today, acute and chronic salpingitis is the most common reason for major gynecologic surgery. Exacerbations or reinfections may require surgical intervention to relieve the patient's symptoms of chronic pelvic pain or menstrual abnormalities. In the acute disease with no response to antibiotic therapy, an emergency total abdominal hysterectomy and bilateral salpingoophorectomy may be necessary to cure the disease.

The incidence of infertility secondary to subacute and/or chronic salpingitis in the United States is unknown. In Scandinavia, 15 to 40 percent of patients in a controlled series with a single acute episode of salpingitis developed infertility. One might speculate that the incidence would either be equal or higher in the United States.

Ectopic pregnancy as a result of salpingitis has never been studied with objective data. Therefore, to attribute ectopic pregnancy directly to previous salpingitis is difficult. It is considered by most, however, to be strongly correlated.

Treatment of Salpingitis

Subacute salpingitis should be treated as previously described under uncomplicated local infections. However, the patient should be reevaluated in 24 to 36 hours. If she is responding to therapy, a second injection should be administered or oral ampicillin 0.5 g four times a day for 10 days. If the patient's reliability to follow-up is questionable, or if there is no response to treatment, the patient should be hospitalized. The most important treatment is antibiotic therapy. Higher antibiotic dosages over a longer period of time are indicated with increased severity of the disease. A dosage of 10 to 20 million units of intravenous aqueous penicillin per day should be instituted until the patient's symptoms either subside or the acuteness of the illness diminishes. The patient can then be put on intramuscular procaine penicillin or oral penicillin in the outline previously recommended. Complications such as bacteremia, arthritis, pericarditis, meningitis, etc. must be individualized. The efficacy of alternate antibiotic therapy is yet unproved. If concomitant infections are present or suspected other forms of antibiotic therapy such as an amminoglycoside may need to be added or replace the penicillin regime.

Intravenous fluids for hydration are important when peritoneal signs are present and the patient is febrile. Once these symptoms have subsided, diet can be given as desired by the patient. If a pelvic mass is demonstrated on examination, best rest in a semi-Fowler's position may be of help in localizing the abscess to the cul-de-sac area and may prevent upper abdominal contamination. Incision and drainage of the abscess should be done when localization has occurred. This can usually be accomplished through the vagina. Douching is contraindicated.

Other supportive measures such as sitz baths, whirlpool, etc., may make the patient more comfortable subjectively, but there is little documentation that they assist in the resolution of the disease process.

On discharge from the hospital or clinic the patient should be instructed in the abstinence from sexual intercourse until her pelvic examination and her culture evaluation return to normal. The need for family planning methods should be explored.

With the widespread use of intrauterine contraceptive devices, many have questioned whether the device should be removed at the time the disease is diagnosed. In patients whose fever remains elevated on antibiotics or who subjectively do not respond to therapy, the intrauterine device is removed and the patient is placed on an alternative method of birth control. Reinsertion of the device should await a negative culture and a normal pelvic examination.

Contamination of the neonate at delivery has been documented, with the classical infection being ophthalmia neonatorum and with organisms also being found in the oral and anal cavities. If there has been a prolonged rupture of the amniotic sac, there appears to be an increased risk of this infection in the neonate. Pneumonia and meningitis have been documented in 12 infants. Therefore an appropriate history, physical exam, and treatment are indicated in the antepartum period or at the time of labor and delivery if the disease is suspected.

Postpartum endometritis is frequently accepted as a nongonococcal infection. However, the gonococcus, as an offending organism, has increased. The disease may be present and unrecognized at the time of labor and delivery, or the patient may become infected after discharge from the hospital prior to her return for postpartum evaluation. The postpartum uterus is an ideal incubator for the gonorrheal organism.

UPPER ABDOMINAL INVOLVEMENT

If purulent exudate from the pelvic area spreads to the upper abdomen, the Fitz-Hugh–Curtis syndrome or gonococcal perihepatitis must be considered. Acute cholecystitis must be ruled out, as the patient's presenting symptoms and physical findings may be similar.

DISSEMINATED GONORRHEAL INFECTION

In several series, 60 to 70 percent of patients with disseminated infections were women. The onset of the symptoms was related to either a recent menstrual period or pregnancy. The subjective symptoms were rash, fever, and polyarthritis of the wrists, ankles, knees, hands, and feet. The infection is usually asymmetrical and presents like a tenosynovitis with swelling at the site of the joint involvement. In approximately two-thirds of the cases, the characteristic skin lesion of hemorrhagic papules is identified on the hands, arms, or legs (Fig. 36–1). A gram stain or fluorescent antibody stain of the discharge from these papules may demonstrate the gram-negative intracellular diplococci. Blood cultures during the first few days of acute symptoms are usually positive for *Neisseria* gonorrhea. If the infection is not treated, the symptoms may resolve spontaneously or may progress to joint areas with the development of a purulent synovial fluid. Unfortunately, joint aspiration and staining of synovial fluid has had low yield in the identification of this organism. Rapid destruction of the joint occurs if treatment is delayed or unrecognized. Endocarditis, meningitis, toxic hepatitis, myocarditis, and pericarditis have all been reported, although the incidence is usually less than 3 percent. The treatment for disseminated infection is the same as previously outlined in local and upper reproductive tract disease.

For the physician whose practice includes the evaluation and treatment of couples with infertility, it is important to recognize that gonorrhea may be transmitted by artificial insemination. Fiumara has reported a case of gonorrheal infection in the recipient following infected donor insemination. Physicians must be aware of this as a possible epidemiologic source of new disease. All donors should be evaluated for the possibility of gonorrhea in order to prevent acute infection in the recipient, possible permanent sequelae, and legal action.

SYPHILIS

It was not until the fifteenth or sixteenth century that syphilis became a disease of significance prompting medical concern. Viewed as a skin complaint, it was treated with mercury or decoctions of mercury.

Natural History

As an infectious systemic disease, syphilis is a continuous pathologic process initiated when the anaerobic *Treponema pallidum* interacts with its host. This continuum of organism-host interaction permits discussing the natural history of this disease by its stages.

The incubation period begins when the *Treponema pallidum* invades any intact, moist mucosal surface or is transmitted to the bloodstream. It spreads throughout the body within 24 hours of contact and remains without subjective or objective signs and symptoms for 10 to 60 days.

Within 2 or 3 weeks of exposure a sharply defined ulcer known as a *chancre* erupts at the site of contact in the vulva, vagina, or cervix. It may appear as an area of traumatic erosion or as a punched-out ulcer with rolled edges. Extragenital lesions on fingers, lips, tongue, and nipples may exhibit varying degrees of discomfort due to secondary infection or local trauma, causing the patient to seek medical treatment (Figs. 36–2 and 36–3). The diagnosis is frequently unsuspected and the condition frequently is misdi-

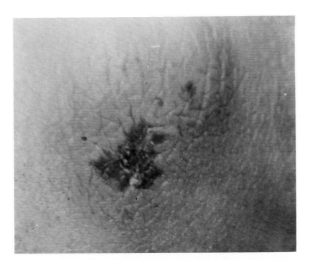

FIGURE 36–1 Gonococcemia: hemorrhagic lesion on elbow. *(Courtesy Department of Dermatology, University of Oklahoma College of Medicine.)*

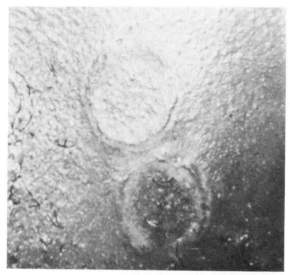

FIGURE 36-2 Primary syphilis: annular chancre of the face. *(Courtesy Department of Dermatology, University of Oklahoma College of Medicine.)*

agnosed by the physician when it is seen distant from the genital tract. Ulcerations of the cervix or vagina often escape detection. Untreated primary lesions will heal spontaneously within 3 to 9 weeks of exposure. Unless the patient seeks medical evaluation for other genital tract problems within that time, the disease will go undiagnosed and untreated.

Secondary syphilis begins approximately 2

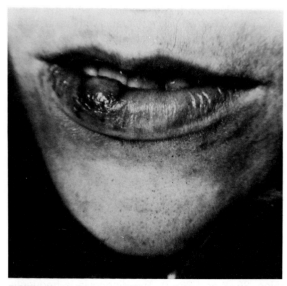

FIGURE 36-3 Primary syphilis: lower lip chancre. *(Courtesy Department of Dermatology, University of Oklahoma College of Medicine.)*

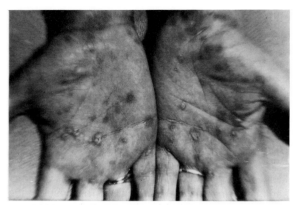

FIGURE 36-4 Secondary syphilis: skin lesions. *(Courtesy Department of Dermatology, University of Oklahoma College of Medicine.)*

months after exposure. A flulike syndrome of malaise, headache, and anorexia may be its only manifestations. The conspicuous appearance of a generalized skin rash with local vegetative lesions on mucous membranes makes this stage highly contagious. The maculopapular skin lesions, when present, are found in follicular groups in the anogenital area, oral cavity, and on palms and soles of the feet (Fig 36–4). Their lack of pruritus typifies the eruption. Patchy alopecia, pharyngitis, and iritis occasionally coexist.

Tertiary syphilis begins when secondary syphilis resolves spontaneously or is inadequately treated. Benign tertiary syphilis manifests itself as a nodular or ulcerative lesion of the skin known as "gumma." Whether the lesion is nodular or ulcerative depends on the degree of sensitivity of the host to the organism. Visible lesions will occur within a 1- to 10-year period following initial exposure. Induration, tissue destruction, scarring, and hyperpigmentation are basic manifestations of this stage. Since the lesion at this stage is not unlike those lesions found in at least 20 other disease entities, a dark-field examination is mandatory to make the diagnosis of benign tertiary syphilis in any patient with a characteristic lesion and a reactive serologic test for syphilis.

The late findings of syphilis appear clinically 8 to 10 years following the initial contact and continue until the death of the patient if untreated or inadequately treated. Any anatomic structure or body tissue can be a focus for late syphilitic involvement. The skeletal system, urinary tract system, upper respiratory tract, gastrointestinal tract, central nervous system, cardiovascular system, and the eye are all documented foci. The subjective symptoms and objective findings will be dependent on the site and extent of involvement.

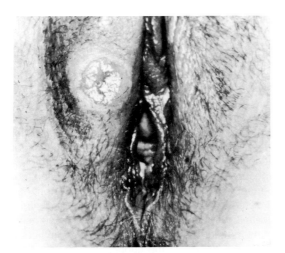

FIGURE 36-5 Primary syphilis: chancres of labium majus. *(Courtesy Center for Disease Control.)*

LESIONS SPECIFIC TO THE LOWER REPRODUCTIVE TRACT

Primary Syphilis

Single or multiple chancres may erupt at the site of contact. The chancre is a punched-out ulcer crater (Fig 36–5). Induration in adjacent tissues is readily palpable but pain is uncommon unless secondary infection or secondary trauma has occurred. Regional lymph-node enlargement is common but it may be difficult to demonstrate clinically as many nodes are not accessible to direct palpation (e.g., deep pelvic nodes which drain the cervix and upper vagina).

Primary vaginal chancres are rare but when

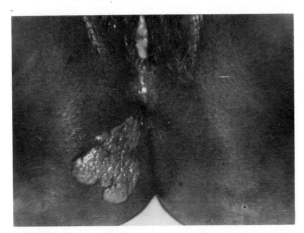

FIGURE 36-6 Condyloma latum: perianal lesion. *(Courtesy Department of Dermatology, University of Oklahoma College of Medicine.)*

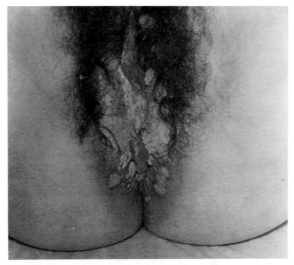

FIGURE 36-7 Condyloma latum: vulvar and perianal lesion. *(Courtesy Department of Dermatology, University of Oklahoma College of Medicine.)*

present appear as a leukoplakial lesion or as a soft, irregular-shaped sore which is flush with the adjacent mucosa.

Cervical lesions are usually diagnosed by accident. Their appearance may be indistinguishable from cervical erosion or other cervical pathology. They may clear spontaneously before examination. Syphilis should be suspected when lesions of the cervix are isolated from the os by an area of normal epithelium or when lesions fail to respond to usual treatment methods.

Secondary Syphilis

Condyloma latum is the characteristic genital lesion of secondary syphilis. These lesions are broad-based exophytic excrescences that ulcerate and produce a foul discharge which is highly contagious. The entire anogenital area can be involved, as may any other site which comes in contact with the infected discharge (Figs. 36–6 and 36–7).

UPPER-GENITAL-TRACT DISEASE

In pregnancy, syphilis can be transmitted to the fetus in utero through the placenta. The *Treponema pallidum* is rarely found in fetal tissue prior to the 18th week of gestation. It has been speculated that Langhans' layer of the chorion (cytotrophoblast), which is present until the 16th week of pregnancy, creates a barrier to the spirochete. If adequate treatment of the mother is carried out before the 18th week of gestation, the potential of congenital syphilis is decreased. However, spirochetes are capable of survival despite appropriate antibiotic therapy. The site of infection, the type of cell involved, and the virulence of the organism may alter its response to therapy. Consequently, repeated serologic testing of the mother throughout pregnancy is imperative. The newborn must be evaluated by serologic testing to rule out the presence of disease and to prevent irreversible sequelae.

Diagnosis

As pointed out in the discussion on gonorrhea, a physician must not only "see it to believe it" but "must believe it in order to see it." Before definitive diagnostic tests for syphilis can be carried out, the possibility of the disease must be entertained. The first step in diagnosis is an adequate patient history relevant to her sexual behavior.

Specific Tests

Serology. *Nontreponemal tests.* The VDRL (Venereal Disease Research Laboratory) and Kolmer's tests represent flocculation and complement fixation determinations of nonspecific antibodies directed against the lipoidal antigens of the treponema or the antigen formed by the interaction of the host and treponema. Their simplicity and minimal cost have established them as standard screening tests in diagnosis and response to treatment. Both tests become reactive within 1 to 2 weeks after the appearance of the primary lesion, or 4 to 5 weeks following the initial infection. Quantitative titers rise rapidly thereafter. The highest dilution in a patient's serum that remains positive is the reported figure. A titer of 1:8 or below may signify either a false-positive reaction or the presence of disease. A repeat titer should be obtained and a specific treponemal antigen test should be employed. Titers of 1:32 or higher signify the presence of disease and the addition of an antigen-specific test is usually unnecessary. However, the reported titer gives no indication as to the infectiousness of the disease or its stage. Antibiotic treatment of a patient for other disease entities during the incubation period or within the first few weeks of primary syphilis will delay the appearance of a reactive titer, particularly if penicillin has been used in the treatment regimen. Therefore, clinical data obtained from the patient are necessary to interpret test results. Of greater importance is a fourfold or greater rise in subsequent test samples. Weakly reactive tests may represent laboratory error. They should be repeated and a specific anti-body test should be employed. It has been estimated that 3 to 40 percent of quantitative serology testing will produce a false-positive reaction. Pregnancy, aging, drug abuse, collagen diseases, pneumococcal pneumonia, measles, and other diseases have been associated with false-positive reactions.

Treponemal tests. Methods to test for specific treponemal antibodies were introduced by Nelson and Mayer in 1949. The *Treponema pallidum* immobilization test (TPI) is costly and difficult; therefore its widespread use is limited. The Reiter protein-complement fixation test is cheaper and easier but has a 50 percent chance of error in cases of late syphilis and may be falsely positive in 0.1 to 0.2 percent of normal patients tested. With the advent of immunofluorescent techniques, the fluorescent treponemal antibody test (FTA) was developed. Modifications and refinements of this test have led to the fluorescent treponema antibody-absorption test (FTA-ABS) presently used by most laboratories. It is currently the most sensitive clinical test available to diagnose all stages of syphilis. Although false-positive reactions do occur, they are infrequent. Other disease entities where increased or abnormal globulins are present (e.g., collagen disease, alcoholic cirrhosis, pregnancy, etc.) may account for these false-positive reactions. Additional patient information and further clinical evaluation with a repeat FTA-ABS test should be carried out in these instances. Here a TPI test may be of some help in clarifying any false-positive reactions.

The non-*Treponema pallidum* tests (VDRL, Kolmer) are usually employed in the follow-up examination of all patients after treatment. Repeat testing should be done monthly for 6 months, followed by testing every 3 months for 1 year. If the patient was adequately treated before the serology became positive, the test will remain negative on repeat evaluation. If treatment followed a positive serologic test, follow-up evaluation will remain positive for several months but should reveal no rise in titer. Approximately 90 percent of positive titers will revert to negative within 12 months. In secondary syphilis, follow-up titers may be positive from 12 to 18 months. Any patient with a rise in titer during follow-up evaluation may have acquired a new infection and a specific treponemal antibody test should be performed and the patient retreated. Any patient whose titer remains positive after 12 months should have a lumbar puncture for cerebral spinal fluid evaluation. When syphilis has been present for several years before diagnosis or treatment, the serology may remain positive for the life of that patient, but without a rising titer.

The diagnosis of congenital syphilis in the newborn who presents without typical clinical findings can be difficult. If the infant's VDRL is reactive at birth, it may only signify the passively transferred VDRL antibody from the mother. However, the infant's titer should be no higher than the titer in the mother's serum and it should decline rapidly in the first 2 to 3 months of life. A negative VDRL in the newborn infant does not necessarily mean absence of disease. If syphilis was acquired by the mother late in her pregnancy, passively transferred VDRL antibodies may be absent, and clinically the newborn will not demonstrate clinical lesions until 1 to 2 months following birth. Thus, the physician must either delay treatment until several serologic titers have been done, await the onset of clinical lesions in the infant, or treat newborn infants without documented syphilis. The IgM (gamma-M globulin) FTA-ABS test currently in experimental use appears promising. It has been shown that IgM, when present in the umbilical cord or fetal blood, correlates well with active fetal infection. Total IgM is often increased in congenital syphilis. Fluorescein-labeled antihuman IgM to detect treponemal IgM antibodies may prove to be a specific test for congenital syphilis in the future.

Dark-Field Examination

Demonstrable *Treponema pallidum* from a lesion on dark-field examination permits an absolute and immediate diagnosis of syphilis. The lesion from which the specimen is to be obtained must be free of topical medications and exudate. Saline soaks to the lesion or abrasion of the lesion with a gauze sponge until bleeding occurs will permit collection of serum which is necessary for dark-field examination. A glass slide is then applied directly to the site of collection. A cover slip whose edges have been coated with petroleum jelly should then be applied over the serum to prevent drying of the specimen before interpretation.

The inaccessibility of this test to most practicing physicians and the physician's lack of training and experience in collection of specimens and morphologic identification of the organism make its clinical use quite limited. However, when the test is available, it offers an immediate evaluation and positive identification of the disease. It is of value in patients whose serology is negative but who present with a history and/or clinical findings compatible with syphilis. Dark-field evaluation enables the physician to begin specific therapy at an earlier stage in the disease and obviates the clinical confusion that frequently arises

when false-positive tests in either the nontreponemal or treponemal serologic tests occur.

Biopsy

Dark-field examination of the lesion, when available, is more reliable than biopsy because the diagnosis of syphilis may not be evident on biopsy material. A biopsy is of benefit when used to assist in the differential diagnosis of other or coexisting diseases (Fig. 36–8). Vasculitis, endothelial proliferation, and swelling of small vessels with adjacent paravascular inflammatory reactions and a predominance of large mononuclear cells and plasma cells are suggestive of syphilis. These findings, however, bear no relationship to the stage of the disease or the organ site. Any lesion which fails to heal with appropriate treatment should be biopsied to rule out the presence of coexistent disease.

Differential Diagnosis

In the space allotted, a detailed descriptive differential diagnosis is not possible. However, a summary of the diseases to be considered in the differential diagnosis of syphilis should be (1) primary syphilis—

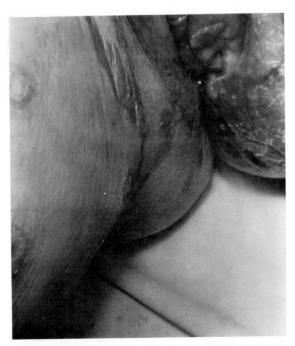

FIGURE 36–8 Secondary syphilis: chancres of inner thigh and vulva with cancer of vulva. Biopsy can assist the differential diagnosis of the two diseases. *(Courtesy of Department of Dermatology, University of Oklahoma College of Medicine.)*

drug eruptions, herpes, trauma, carcinoma, chancroid, tuberculosis, lymphogranuloma venereum, granuloma inguinale; and (2) secondary syphilis—drug eruptions, fungal infections, various exanthemata, infectious mononucleosis, seborrheic dermatitis, pityriasis rosea, and erythema multiforme. When extragenital lesions are present, herpes, tuberculosis, sporotrichosis, cat-scratch fever, and amelanotic melanoma must be considered.

Treatment

The recommendations of the U.S. Public Health Service for the treatment of syphilis are as follows: In documented primary or secondary syphilis, a single intramuscular injection of 2.4 million units of benzathine penicillin G is curative in the majority of cases. The alternative schedule is procaine penicillin G in a dose of 600,000 units intramuscularly daily for 8 to 10 days; or procaine penicillin G with 2% aluminum monosterate in a dose of 2.4 million units intramuscularly on the first day, and an additional 1.2 million units in each of the two subsequent injections 3 days apart can be used. Knowledge about the patient's reliability is of essence in the use of this treatment regimen. Either of the above regimens should be instituted in patients with known or suspected syphilitic contact. Patients who are allergic to penicillin should be treated with tetracycline hydrochloride 0.5 g four times a day for 15 days 1 hour before, or 2 hours after meals, or with erythromycin 0.5 g four times a day for 15 days.

Syphilis of more than 1 year's duration (latent, intermediate, cardiovascular, late benign, or neurosyphilis) should be treated with benzathine pencillin G 7.2 million units total, 2.4 million units intramuscularly weekly for 3 weeks, or with aqueous procaine penicillin G 9.0 million units total, 600,000 units intramuscularly daily for 15 days. Treatment dosage appropriate for the stage of syphilis should be the same during pregnancy.

Treatment of congenital syphilis can be accomplished with aqueous crystalline penicillin G, 50,000 units per kilogram intramuscularly or intravenously daily in divided doses for a minimum of 10 days, or aqueous procaine penicillin G, 50,000 units per kilogram intramuscularly daily for 10 days.

As previously stated, treatment must be carried out in conjunction with follow-up serologic testing. Any elevation in titer during or following treatment is indicative of reinfection and retreatment is indicated. Although other antibiotics have been used with suc-

cess in the treatment of syphilis, penicillin is the drug of choice unless the patient is allergic to penicillin.

It is appropriate to reemphasize that when one STD is present, another may coexist. Therefore, evaluation for the presence of other STDs is mandatory. If coexistent STD is documented or suspected, both diseases need to be treated as though they were separate entities. This is done in order to achieve treatment success and prevent carrier states or long-term sequelae.

The appropriate public health authority should be notified of all cases of syphilis diagnosed and/or under treatment so appropriate epidemiologic investigations can be carried out. Evaluation and treatment of contacts must be considered as important as the patient under treatment.

When the disease is documented, the patient's treatment should include education about the disease, its method of transmission, and the importance of appropriate follow-up. The importance of disease that persists despite appropriate treatment schedules cannot be accurately assessed without the full cooperation of the patient. Accurate diagnosis, treatment, and follow-up will provide those in research a better understanding of the biology of the organism and its interaction with its host.

The search for a vaccine which will cause a protective antibody response but without infectious lesions has been pursued for decades.

In 1969 Thatcher reported studies demonstrating that infection with one of the treponemas of pinta, begel, yaws, or syphilis provided a degree of immunity to infection with some or all of the other treponemas. This spectrum of natural attenuation might afford protection from one disease to another. However, no one has yet been able to culture the *Treponema pallidum* in vitro, and therefore infected animals are the only currently available source of vaccine material. The variety of immunologic effects such as serum antibodies and transplantation reactions is yet unknown in humans. At least a direction for further study is now available that may be fruitful in the prevention of syphilis by immunization.

LYMPHOPATHIA VENEREUM

A viruslike organism, *Miyagawanella lymphogranulomatosis,* is the pathogen responsible for lymphopathia venereum. It is highly contagious, with an affinity for lymphatic structures.

Natural History

From 1 to 4 weeks after the initial contact, the patient may develop generalized muscle aching, headache, fever, and nausea. The lymph nodes above and below the inguinal ligament become swollen and painful. The inguinal buboes frequently described in males are an uncommon finding in the female, but direct lymphatic spread to the deep nodes of the perianus and rectum is extremely common in females.

Lymphopathia venereum is frequently a chronic, progressive disease causing vulvar ulcerations, elephantiasis, proctocolitis, and anal or rectal strictures. Fistulas, abscesses, secondary infections, and obstruction and destruction of bowel cause the patient varying degrees of discomfort and incapacitation.

Diagnosis

Eighty percent of patients with lymphopathia venereum will have a positive reaction to the Frei test within 10 to 40 days after the appearance of a primary lesion. The current commercial preparation used is Lygranum S.T. (Squibb).

Differential Diagnosis

Lymphopathia venereum must be differentiated from other granulomatous diseases such as granuloma inguinale, syphilis, chancroid, and carcinoma before a definitive diagnosis is made and specific treatment is started.

Treatment

Tetracycline, oxytetracycline, or chlortetracycline 500 mg orally every 6 hours for 10 to 15 days will cure most patients. Sulfadiazine, 1 g orally every 6 hours for 14 to 21 days may be used in patients with treatment failures, recurrent disease, or in the presence of coexistent disease or any allergies to the above medications.

If buboes are present, they may be aspirated for patient discomfort, but incision and drainage are contraindicated.

Patients with rectal strictures or fistulas may require dilatation, colostomies, or pull-through procedures. A simple vulvectomy may relieve the embarrassing and uncomfortable symptoms of vulva elephantiasis. Since poor healing can be expected in these areas, the patient should be treated with chemotherapy prior to any planned surgical procedure and during the postoperative period.

Lotions, ointments, and sprays should be avoided, but the addition of warm water sitz baths or potassium permanganate sitz baths in a 1:10,000 solution can assist in cleansing the disease site, prevent secondary infections, and provide the patient local comfort.

CHANCROID (SOFT CHANCRE)

Chancroid is found in tropical or subtropical countries.

Natural History

Unlike *Neisseria* gonococcus and *Treponema pallidum*, Ducrey's bacillus, which is responsible for chancroid, will not penetrate a healthy, intact epithelial surface.

Following an incubation period of 3 to 5 days, a small papule appears at the site of entry, which rapidly breaks down to form a shallow, circular ulcer with a halo of redness and swelling. The suppurative ulcer base is a dirty-gray color, malodorous, painful to the touch, and highly contagious. Regional lymph-node involvement with suppuration and/or bubo formation is not uncommon. When untreated, multiple ulcerations can occur by autoinoculation with subsequent destruction of large tissue areas. Chronic nonhealed ulcers can persist for years, permitting continued contagion. The vulva, groin, and inner thigh are the most common sites of involvement but the cervix and vagina may also be affected.

Diagnosis

The gram-negative, plump, short, round-ended bacillus on a smear is the basis of diagnosis. Bacteriologic cultures on blood agar approach 75 percent accuracy. Material aspirated from buboes permits more accurate detection.

Differential Diagnosis

Dark-field examination and serologic testing are mandatory to rule out lymphopathia venereum, granuloma inguinale, and syphilis.

Systemic Treatment

Sulfadazine or triple-sulfa preparations in 1-g doses four times daily for 7 to 10 days is the usual treatment schedule.

When sensitivity to sulfa exists, tetracycline, Aureomycin, or Terramycin can be used effectively in doses of 250 mg orally, four times per day, for 7 to 10 days. Treatment with these drugs should be withheld, however, until diagnostic tests for syphilis have been completed.

Lymph-node involvement usually necessitates long-term treatment. Buboes lesions when painful or about to rupture can be aspirated but should not be incised as autoinoculation will be likely to occur.

Persistent lesions, after adequate therapy, warrant further evaluation.

GRANULOMA INGUINALE

Donovania granulomatis is the causative organism of granuloma inguinale. It is uncommon outside India, New Guinea, and the Caribbean. Age of occurrence is 20 to 40 years; the ratio is 10:1 black to white.

Natural History

The disease can be described by its clinical stages. The first stage occurs eight days to 12 weeks following the initial contact. A papule appears at the site of contact and rapidly ulcerates. With autoinoculation, multiple ulcer sites develop in the perianal area, the vagina, and the cervix. Since this stage of the disease is usually painless, the patient employs self-treatment and fails to seek medical evaluation.

The second stage begins when existing lesions become secondarily infected.

Fibrosis, scarring, depigmentation, and keloid formation characterize the third stage of the disease. The scar tissue that forms during the healing process creates variable degrees of lymphatic obstruction which lead to elephantiasis and stenosis of the vaginal and/or anal orifices.

Extragenital lesions of the nose, mouth, pharynx, uterus, ovary, and bone disseminated granuloma inguinale have been reported in pregnant patients with cervical lesions.

Diagnosis

Donovan bodies in tissue smears stained with Giemsa's stain are necessary to make the diagnosis of granuloma inguinale.

Differential Diagnosis

The presence of carcinoma, lymphopathia venereum, chancroid, syphilis, and other diseases must be ruled out as primary or coexistent diseases.

Treatment

Tetracycline, oxytetracline, or chlortetracycline given orally in doses of 500 mg every 6 hours for 10 to 21 days is the treatment of choice.

Healing occurs within a period of 6 weeks. In those cases unresponsive to therapy, a longer course of treatment, a change in antibiotic, or a reevaluation of the lesion to rule out the possibility of coexistent disease is necessary.

OTHER PROBLEM STDs

HERPES GENITALIS

Definition

The second most common STD, genital herpes, produces a variety of clinical manifestations and involves the mouth, eyes, skin, urogenital tract, and brain.

Etiology

Herpes genitalis is a viral disease of the lower reproductive tract caused most commonly by herpes simplex virus type 2; type 1 more commonly involves the mouth or face. However, increased oral-genital practices and more infections spread by hands mean both types can be passed to either area.

Natural History

Transmission is most frequently by sexual contact, but not always. A wide variety of stresses, temperature change, drug therapy, and sunlight have been implicated in recurrent disease because of the persistence of the virus in the nerve cells of the host. Chronic herpes with disseminated infection can lead to a fatal outcome; it occurs primarily in immunoincompetent patients and in the newborn.

Clinical Manifestations

After an incubation period of 2 to 20 days (usually 6 days following exposure), symptoms of pain, tenderness, and pruritus of the genital area occur, associated with generalized malaise, headache, and fever. Single or multiple raised blisters develop on the vulva, perineum, vagina, or cervix. Inguinal adenopathy occurs frequently. With traumatic or spontaneous rupture of the blisters, painful, shallow uclers and labial edema occur which may produce considerable pain on urination. The ulcers may persist for 1 to 3 weeks depending upon the severity of the infection and the immune state of the host. Following the initial episode, the virus goes into a latent phase and antibodies develop. Recurrent infections are characterized by more localized lesions with fewer generalized symptoms. The course of the recurrent disease is shorter; the antibody titer remains unchanged.

Diagnosis

The variability of clinical presentation may make the diagnosis difficult in some patients.

Cytologic studies correlated with clinical findings will verify the presence of the disease. The finding of multinucleated giant cells in a smear, especially a vaginal smear, always suggests a herpetic infection.

Serum antibody titers that reveal a rise in titers during the convalescent phase are considered evidence of a primary infection. A titer which is sustained at the same level in the convalescent period is indicative of recurrent infection.

Unlike other viruses, the herpesvirus grown in tissue culture (human embryo lung or fibroblasts, rabbit or monkey kidney cells) permits identification of the virus in 24 to 48 hours.

Differential Diagnosis

Primary or coexistent chancroid, granuloma inguinale, and primary or secondary syphilis must be ruled out.

Treatment

No safe, effective systemic treatment is yet known. Therefore, treatment is directed at relief of pain and prevention of secondary infection. Oral analgesics, topical anesthetics, wet compresses, sitz baths, antiseptics, and antibiotics will assist in pain relief, improve hygiene, and decrease infection. Sexual contact should be avoided until all lesions have completely healed.

Photoinactivation, levamizole, BCG (bacillus Calmette-Guérin), 5-IUDR (idoxuridine), and Ara-A are still controversial approaches to treatment.

Complications

An association has been demonstrated between herpes infection and cervical cancer. AG-4, an antigen and an active piece of the herpesvirus type 2, has been found in cervical tumors and in the blood of 86 percent of women with invasive cervical cancer; it has been found in a smaller percentage of women in the early stages of cancer. Perhaps a future screening test in conjunction with a Pap smear will facilitate early cancer detection in this high-risk group.

The most severe complication of herpes type 2 is infection of the newborn at birth. Infants exposed to an actively infected birth canal by vaginal delivery or to ruptured membranes for more than 4 hours have a 5 to 50 percent chance of getting the disease; up to 60 percent of those who get the disease will die. Weekly Pap smears taken 1 month prior to delivery and/or viral cultures at weekly intervals in the ninth month will establish the presence or absence of active disease. If there is active disease at the time of labor or ruptured membranes, a cesarean section is the delivery method of choice. This may reduce the likelihood of neonatal infection.

CONDYLOMA ACUMINATA

Definition

Condyloma acuminata are squamous papillomas which characteristically occur on moist mucocutaneous regions of the genitalia.

Etiology

A papovavirus, the causative organism, presents as a cauliflowerlike lesion that may vary in size from a few millimeters to many centimeters.

Natural History

The lesions may be spread by sexual contact, but they are of low infectivity so that repeated exposures, persistent moisture, and trauma may be necessary before the lesions are acquired. An incubation period of 1 to 3 months is usual if transmission is from an infected partner. Disfigurement, recurrence, and possible malignancy can result.

Clinical Manifestations

Verrucous papillary or sessile growths, ranging from a few millimeters to many centimeters, are localized to the urethra, vulva, vagina, cervix, perineum, or anus. They are similar to common skin warts and occur singly or in multiple growths. They may be pink, indurated, and moist with a cauliflowerlike texture or be hard and yellow-gray. Depending upon their location, they may be subject to chronic irritation and secondary infection, and they may obstruct urinary or defecation processes, or the vaginal canal at delivery.

Differential Diagnosis

Condyloma latum, cancer, chancroid, granuloma inguinale, and lymphopathia venereum must be ruled out as primary or coexistent lesions.

Treatment

Podophyllin 25% in tincture of benzoin, electrocautery, cryosurgery, and surgical excision have all been used. Podophyllin is the most popular therapy. Because of its caustic properties, it should be used in small quantities. Contact with adjacent tissues should be avoided and these sites can be protected with Vaseline.

Since condyloma acuminatum has a propensity to proliferate in pregnancy and is more difficult to eradicate at that time, treatment is sometimes difficult. The toxic potential of podophyllin to both mother and fetus in pregnancy contraindicates its use. Cesarean section may be necessary for delivery if either obstruction of the vagina or hemorrhage due to trauma is likely.

Cervical and intravaginal lesions are a challenge. Podophyllin may create ulceration, hemorrhage, and scarring as can cryosurgery, especially of the vagina. Although douching has not been shown to be effective, improvement of vaginal hygiene by alternating use of sulfa and estrogen vaginal creams twice daily while external lesions are treated has been of benefit in some patients. Surgical excision may be the treatment of choice when large or multiple lesions are present. Fortunately, spontaneous resolution frequently occurs following pregnancy.

Condoms should be used to prevent transmission or recurrence.

CANDIDIASIS

Definition

Candidiasis is a fungus found in 50 percent of healthy individuals. The mouth, intestine, and vagina are the most common sites.

Natural History

The proliferation of candidiasis, with its associated clinical symptoms, occurs when competing organisms at the specified site are altered. Changes in body heat, moisture, the use of antibiotics and steroids, systemic conditions which lower the host resistance, such as diabetes, cancer, chronic infection, and pregnancy, are all implicated. It can be spread sexually, by oral or genital contact.

Etiology

This mycotic infection is caused by a fungus of the species *Candida albicans*.

Clinical Manifestations

Candida may produce a variety of symptoms, but its most common is vaginitis. A thick, white, curdy, adherent discharge with associated severe pruritus is the usual clinical picture. Women harboring fungi at delivery can transmit the organism to the fetus born through the vagina or by hand contact with the infant after birth. Oral candidiasis (thrush) is the result.

Diagnosis

Identification from vaginal or oral secretions of the hyphae or mycelia of *Candida albicans* on wet prep or potassium hydroxide (KOH) wet prep plus the clinical manifestations previously described establish the diagnosis.

Treatment

Antifungal agents such as gentian violet, Nystatin vaginal suppositories, or Micronazole cream are effective. Nystatin applied locally can be used in the neonate.

Complications

Persistent or recurrent candidiasis may be an early symptom of other disease states, and the patient should be evaluated for the predisposing factors previously mentioned. There is no known deleterious effect on pregnancy, but pregnancy may provoke a persistent or recurrent infection.

TRICHOMONIASIS

Definition

Trichomoniasis is a protozoan infection of the lower genital tract.

Etiology

Trichomonas vaginalis, a protozoan parasite, is the causative organism.

Natural History

The organism may exist, without symptoms, in the lower genital tract of the female. Symptoms rarely occur in men, but the infection may be carried and sexually spread by them. With alterations in normal vaginal flora caused, for example, by douching, feminine hygiene products, other systemic diseases or their treatment, subjective and clinical symptoms occur.

Clinical Manifestations

A thin, frothy, vaginal discharge which stains undergarments and produces an offensive odor is the usual beginning symptom. Inflammation, severe itching, and edema of the vagina, vulva, and perineum follow. Coitus frequently aggravates the symptoms and often precludes further coital activity.

Diagnosis

The presence of *Trichomonas vaginalis* on a wet prep of the vaginal discharge, and inflammation, petechiae, and edema of the involved tissues verify the diagnosis.

Treatment

The best treatment is a single oral dose of 2 g of metronidazole. Since the sexual partner is frequently a source of reinfection, both should be treated even though the male may have no signs or symptoms of the disease.

In pregnancy, metronidazole is contraindicated in the first trimester. Furazolidone vaginal suppositories may be used in its place. If treatment is deferred or is indicated following delivery, metronidazole should be avoided if the patient is breast-feeding as the drug is excreted in breast milk. However, if the newborn develops an infection from vaginal contact or transmission by hands, oral metronidazole may be used to treat the infant.

Complications

There are no known serious complications.

CYTOMEGALOVIRUS (CMV) INFECTION

Definition

CMV is a viral infection, generally asymptomatic except in immunoincompetent patients or in the newborn.

Etiology

This medium-sized virus belongs to the herpesvirus family and is similar to the hepatitis virus B. It grows in human fibroblast and myometrial tissue culture.

Natural History

CMV, considered a sexually transmitted virus, can be carried asymptomatically or can present as a systemic disease. Breast milk, blood, and saliva are potential vehicles for transmitting the virus. It is observed most commonly during first pregnancies of young women.

In contrast to the herpesvirus, CMV during delivery does not seem to damage the newborn child, although intrauterine infection may cause serious damage to the fetus from the fourth week to the third trimester, probably because of hematologic spread.

Clinical Manifestations

The maternal illness may present as a mononucleosis with no or mild symptoms. The results may be fatal in those patients with immunity system deficiencies.

In the fetus, the period of greatest susceptibility is when the central nervous system is developing. Microcephaly and mental retardation are the likely outcome. A wide range of teratogenic defects have been identified including congenital cardiac disease, liver and hematologic manifestations, central-nervous-system malformations other than those previously mentioned, abdominal wall defects, clubbed feet, brachial arch syndrome, and arched palate.

Diagnosis

Virologic, serologic, and cytologic findings of the virus after body fluids have been inoculated into the appropriate tissue culture establish the diagnosis. Since the diagnostic cells within intranuclear inclusion bodies are shed intermittently, it must be remembered that adenoviruses produce similar findings and may cause confusion in the diagnosis.

Treatment

As with most viral STDs, there is no known cure for CMV. Treatment in the neonate is essentially symptomatic. Vaccines for prevention and antiviral agents for treatment are being used experimentally, but their efficacy has not been adequately determined.

Complications

One percent of all newborns in the United States are effected by CMV in utero. Of these fetuses, 5 to 15 percent have overt central-nervous-system abnormalities. The option of abortion is recommended by some physicians for women who acquire this infection during the first trimester of pregnancy.

PEDICULOSIS PUBIS (PUBIC LICE)

Definition

This infection is transmitted by sexual contact and by inanimate objects such as linen and clothing.

Etiology

Pediculosis pubis is caused by *Phthirius pubis*, a blood-sucking louse 1 to 4 mm in length.

Natural History

The louse, transmitted by close contact with infected persons or clothing, rarely survives off the host after 24 hours.

Clinical Manifestations

Eggs deposited by the louse hatch from 7 to 9 days after contact. Although the infection may be asymptomatic, slight to intolerable itching of the pubic area is the most common symptom.

Diagnosis

The diagnosis is made by seeing the parasite with the naked eye or a hand lens.

Treatment

Gamma benzene hexachloride or benzyl benzoate applied to the affected area will effect cure. To prevent reinfestation, thorough cleansing of clothing and other linens must not be forgotten.

GENITAL SCABIES

Definition

This infection is usually transmitted by nonsexual contact although, in Western society, sexual contact spreads the infection.

Etiology

Genital scabies are caused by the mite *Sarcoptes scabiei*.

Natural History

The gravid female mite burrows into the skin to deposit eggs and feces.

Clinical Manifestations

In 1 to 3 months, itching begins and a red raised lump appears. The itching increases when the patient is in bed, becomes warm, or after bathing. Scratching may lead to secondary infection.

Diagnosis

Visualization of the mite on the skin of the affected site or under the microscope confirms the diagnosis.

Treatment

Gamma benzene hexachloride or benzyl benzoate applied to the affected area will effect cure.

CONCLUSIONS

As previously stated, anyone who engages in sexual activity with an infected partner may acquire an STD. However, the risk of acquiring disease is directly related to the infection status of the sexual partner. The number of sexual acts with an infected partner is the most important factor.

Hart has stated that human behavior is the dominant reason for the STD epidemic. The community and its leaders provide priorities, funds, and other resources for disease control. Health personnel manage the diseases with varying degrees of competence and may exert a positive or negative influence on a patient's behavior. Perhaps the most important behavior is of individuals who are at risk of contracting STDs.

Any patient or couple who acquires an STD or is at personal risk should consider (1) discretion in choice of partners and consistency in relations with one partner; (2) the use of condoms, of good hygiene habits, including washing the genitalia before and after sexual activity, and urination immediately following coitus; and (3) periodic health examinations. Freedom from symptoms is an unreliable guide to freedom from infection. If and when medical treatment is initiated, the individual and the partner should undergo all the prescribed therapy as well as reexamination and evaluation.

One should always suspect the spectrum of diseases possible in a given patient to avoid the diagnosis of one to the exclusion of others. STDs can coexist with other reproductive tract diseases. Pertinent historical findings and appropriate diagnostic methods will establish the correct diagnosis and permit cure in the majority of patients.

REFERENCES

American College of Obstetricians and Gynecologists, Technical Bulletin: *Sexually Transmitted Diseases (STD)*, No. 51, July 1978.

Amstey MS, Monif RGR: Genital herpesvirus infection in pregnancy. *Obstet Gynecol* 44:394, 1974

Brown WJ: Paper presented at the International Venereal Disease Symposium, St. Louis, Mo., 1971.

Burry Virgil F: Gonococcal vulvovaginitis and possible peritonitis in prepubertal girls. *Am J Dis Child* 121:536, 1971.

Chancroid, donovanosis, lymphogranuloma venereum. U.S. Dept. HEW (CDC) 75–8302 (1975 b).

Chang T, O'Keefe P: Cesarean section and genital herpes. *N Engl J Med* 296:573, 1977.

Darrow William W: Approaches to the problem of venereal disease prevention. *Prev Med* 5:165, 1976.

Fam A et al.: Gonococcal arthritis: A report of six cases. *Can Med Assoc J* 108:319, 1973.

Fiumara NJ: Transmission of gonorrhea by artificial insemination. *Br J Vener Dis* 48:308, 1972.

Fuld Gilbert L: Gonococcal peritonitis in a prepubertal child. *Am J Dis Child* 115:621, 1968.

Jensen T: Rectal gonorrhea in women. *Br J Vener Dis* 29:222, 1953.

Jordan MC et al.: Association of cervical cytomegalic virus infection with venereal disease. *N Engl J Med* 288:932, 1973.

Kaufman RH, Rawls WE: Herpes genitalis and its relationship to cervical cancer. *Cancer J Clin* 24:258, 1974.

Metzger AL: *Ann Intern Med* 73:267, 1970.

Monif GRG et al.: Blood as a potential vehicle for the cytomegalic virus infection. *Am J Obstet Gynecol* 126:443, 1976.

Nahmias Andre J et al.: Infection with herpes-simplex viruses 1 and 2. *N Engl J Med* 289:667, 1973.

Newest strategy for Syphilis Control. *Contemp Ob Gyn* 8:117, 1978.

Nicol CS: Some aspects of gonorrhea in the female with special reference to infection of the rectum. *Br J Vener Dis* 24:26, 1948.

Notkins AL et al.: Workshop on the treatment and prevention of herpes simplex virus infections. *J Infect Dis* 127:117, 1973.

Oriel JD: Natural history of genital warts. *Br J Vener Dis* 47:1, 1971.

Owen RL, Hill LJ: Rectal and pharyngeal gonorrhea in homosexual men. *JAMA* 220:1315, 1972.

Potterat John J et al.: Prepubertal infections with Neisseria gonorrhoeae: Clinical and epidemiologic significance. *Sexually Transmitted Diseases* 5:1, 1978.

Ratnatunga CS: Gonococcal pharyngitis. *Br J Vener Dis* Received for publication February 11, 1972.

Rudolph AH, Price E: Penicillin reactions among patients in venereal disease clinics. *JAMA* 223:449, 1973.

Sabin AB: Misery of recurrent herpes: What to do? *N Engl J Med* 293:986, 1975.

Schroeter AL, Reynolds G: The rectal culture as a test of cure of gonorrhea in the female. *J Infect Dis* 125:499, 1972.

Singh B et al.: Treponema pallidum and Neisseria gonorrhoeae. *Br J Vener Dis* 48:57, 1972.

———et al.: Candida albicans and Trichomonas vaginalis. *Contraception* 5:401, 1972.

Solberg DA et al.: Sexual behavior in pregnancy. *N Engl J Med* 288:1098, 1973.

Sparling PE: Diagnosis and treatment of syphilis. *N Engl J Med* 284:642, 1971.

Stern H, Elek SD: The incidence of infection with cytomegalic virus infection in a normal population. *J Hyg* 63:79, 1965.

Symposium—The gonorrhea epidemic. *Contem Ob Gyn* 1:2, 1973.

Syphilis vaccine may be one step closer. *JAMA* 217:1174, 1971.

Thatcher RW: The search for a vaccine for syphilis. *Br J Vener Dis* 45:10, 1969.

U.S. Dept. of Health, Education, and Welfare: *Infection with Herpes-Simplex Viruses 1 and 2,* Washington, Pub. no. 00–2585, 1973.

———: *Penicillinase-Producing Neisseria gonorrhea: Results of Surveillance in the United States*, Washington, Committee on Disease Control, Pub. no. 00–2954, 1978.

———: *Sexually Transmitted Diseases (STDs) Clinics*, Washington, Committee on Disease Control, Pub. no. 00–3226, 1978.

Wiesner PJ et al.: Clinical spectrum of pharyngeal gonococcal infection. *N Engl J Med* 288:181, 1973.

Willcox RR: A world-wide view of venereal disease. *Br J Vener Dis* 48:163, 1972.

Youmans John B (guest ed.): Syphilis and the venereal diseases. *Med Clin North Am* 48:1964.

Zilz J: Ost-ung. (1911) *Vischr. Zahn heillk, :*27, 1974.

37

Endometriosis

JAMES A. MERRILL

Endometriosis is a unique disease of protean nature, occurring commonly, accounting for many days of disability, and responsive in diverse ways to gonadal steroid. It demonstrates certain characteristics of malignancy as well as inflammation. Although lesions of endometriosis were described as early as 1860 or 1889, it was not until Sampson's series of publications, beginning in 1921, that endometriosis received clinical attention and scientific investigation of its natural history and treatment.

DEFINITION

Endometriosis is a benign disease characterized by the presence and proliferation of endometrial tissue in sites outside the endometrial cavity. The ectopic endometrium demonstrates the ability to grow, infiltrate, spread, and even disseminate in a manner similar to malignant tissue. However, histologic changes of malignancy are rare. Only when they occur is endometriosis truly malignant in the sense of interfering with vital functions or causing death. Indeed, endometriosis is reversible and may regress following removal of ovarian activity and possibly under the influence of pregnancy. The ectopic endometrial tissue is usually responsive to the hormonal variations of the menstrual cycle, and the subsequent menstrual-type bleeding is important in pathology and symptomatology of the disease.

An *endometrioma* is a cystic lesion, usually found in the ovary, lined by functioning endometrium. In addition to the symptoms of endometriosis, such endometrial cysts may produce symptoms and findings similar to those of other ovarian cysts and tumors.

Adenomyosis is a benign disease of the uterus, characterized by endometrial glands and stroma found deep within the myometrium. In the past, adenomyosis has sometimes been referred to as *endometriosis interna*. This is an unfortunate choice of terms. While adenomyosis has certain morphologic similarities to endometriosis, it is not, in the author's opinion, actually related to endometriosis, nor should it be considered a part of the endometriosis complex. The histogenesis, clinical picture, and natural history are different. Adenomyosis is not found commonly in association with endometriosis.

INCIDENCE AND IMPORTANCE

There is great variation from one hospital to another in the reported incidence of endometriosis. The diagnosis is made with accuracy only at operation or endoscopy. It is a pathologic finding in about 20 percent of all gynecologic operations, with a range from 0.9 to 29 percent. Moreover, there is disagreement between the operative and pathologic diagnoses in about 8 percent of cases. Some place the disagreement rate much higher. At least one investigator has stated that the operative diagnosis is not confirmed pathologically in more than 40 percent of cases. Endometriosis is a *significant* finding in only about one-third of the patients in whom it is found at surgery. Associated pelvic pathology is commonly reported and is often the reason for surgery. Myomata may be present in as many as one-third of the cases, and uterine cancer is not rare. The exact incidence of endometriosis is difficult to determine because the disease exists in many patients without causing symptoms, and the indications for surgery in women with no or minor symptoms vary greatly in different institutions.

Active endometriosis is found most commonly between the ages of 30 and 40. It is rarely found in patients under 20, and in those patients congenital anomalies of the genital tract which favor retrograde menstruation are commonly reported (Schifrin et al.). Although endometriosis is rarely found in postmeno-

pausal patients, Kempers reported 136 such patients. In 29 percent of these patients, the endometriosis was clinically significant by virtue of producing symptoms or a palpable pelvic mass.

Many gynecologists state that endometriosis is more prevalent among private patients than among indigent patients. It has been suggested that this can be accounted for by late marriage and late childbearing in the high-income groups (Meigs). Others have questioned the reliability of these impressions. It may be asked if the pressure for attention among people in higher socioeconomic classes is not responsible for earlier and more frequent diagnoses. In a study of 646 patients with proven endometriosis, it was found that these patients married and became pregnant just as early as a comparable control series without endometriosis. Also, there was no difference based on social or economic status. There is at least one report of equal incidence rates for endometriosis in black and white patients (Ridley). It is possible that selectivity accounts for the great variation in reported incidence of endometriosis in different hospitals and among different socioeconomic classes.

Ranney has suggested a hereditary tendency in the development of endometriosis. Of 350 women operated on for endometriosis, 153 reported family histories of the condition. This finding has not been confirmed by other investigators.

It is frequently stated that endometriosis is a common cause of infertility. The fertility rate of patients with endometriosis is stated to be 66 percent, as opposed to 88 percent for the general population. Again, it is possible that selectivity and sampling errors account for the apparent relationship between endometriosis and infertility. Infertile patients are likely to receive the careful evaluation, including surgical exploration or endoscopy, leading to a diagnosis of endometriosis more often than fertile patients with the disease.

Since endometriosis is usually responsive to cyclic ovarian hormones, the lesions commonly regress following suppression of ovarian activity artificially, or naturally at the menopause. However, there are well-documented cases of endometriosis becoming active and even symptomatic many years following the menopause. The author has seen a 74-year-old patient with symptomatic endometriosis of the sigmoid colon. Ten percent of endometriosis of the bowel is diagnosed in postmenopausal women.

It has been stated often that endometriosis improves during and following pregnancy. However, it is impossible to document this impression, and there

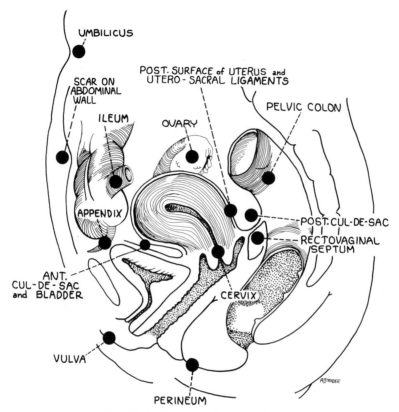

FIGURE 37–1 Various locations of endometriosis.

have been cases in which there has been active growth during pregnancy, even requiring surgery. MacArthur and Ulfelder reviewed the literature and concluded that the impression that pregnancy exerts a consistent curative effect is not supported and appears to be ill-founded. Patients with permanent regression following pregnancy were less common than patients with persistent disease. The behavior of endometriosis during pregnancy was extremely variable.

LOCATION OF LESIONS

The majority of lesions are limited to the pelvis, although endometriosis has been described in unusual and remote sites in the body (see Fig. 37–1). The ovary is the most common site, and involvement is usually bilateral. The next most common site is the peritoneum of the cul-de-sac of Douglas. Such lesions may extend to involve the rectovaginal septum and, rarely, the vagina. The uterosacral ligaments may be involved with or without involvement of the peritoneum of the cul-de-sac. The round ligaments, oviduct, and peritoneal surfaces of the uterus and bladder reflection are next in frequency. The rectosigmoid can be involved either as an isolated lesion or as an extension from ovarian or uterosacral lesions. Bowel involvement occurs in 3 percent of patients with endometriosis.

Far less common sites for endometriosis are isolated lesions of the ileum, cecum, appendix, bladder, ureter, cervix, and vagina. Endometriosis is not uncommon in the pelvic lymph nodes of patients with pelvic endometriosis. Unusual sites of endometriotic involvement include the umbilicus, laparatomy scars, episiotomy scars, inguinal canal, spinal canal, kidney, pleura, lung, arm, hand, thigh, and spleen (Ridley).

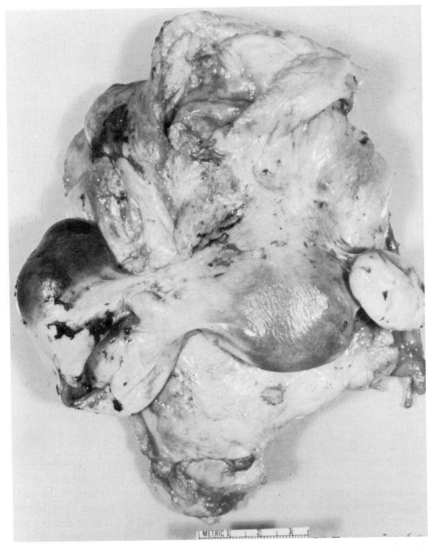

FIGURE 37–2 Gross appearance of the pelvic viscera with endometriosis. One ovary is replaced by a blood-filled cyst. The other ovary and peritoneal surfaces exhibit puckered hemorrhagic foci and scars.

PATHOLOGY

GROSS APPEARANCE

Early lesions of endometriosis appear as multiple tiny, puckered, hemorrhagic foci or minute bloodfilled cysts referred to as "mulberry spots" or "powder-burn spots." They are usually surrounded by stellate scars and are commonly associated with dense adhesions.

The degree of fibrotic reaction is variable. However, the adhesions associated with endometriosis are far more dense than the adhesions associated with pelvic gonorrhea or other pelvic inflammatory disease. In the ovary, lesions may present as endometrial cysts or endometriomas. These are rarely larger than 10 cm and are filled with material that looks like chocolate syrup but is composed of blood and blood pigment. These are the so-called "chocolate cysts of the ovary" (Fig. 37–2). Not all blood-filled cysts of the ovary are endometriosis, but chocolate cysts most commonly

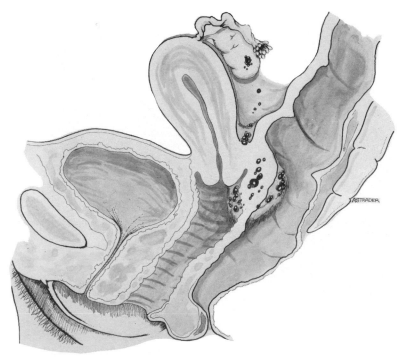

FIGURE 37–3 Endometriosis of the ovary and the cul-de-sac. Bluish red nodules involve the recto-vaginal septum and the posterior fornix of the vagina. This location may cause dyspareunia.

are. Because of the dense pelvic adhesions, endometrial cysts are often ruptured during surgical removal.

Involvement of the peritoneum of the cul-de-sac of Douglas consists of puckered bluish-red nodules. The surrounding scar tissue often makes them large enough to be palpated by rectovaginal examination (Fig. 37–3). Lesions in this location may obliterate the posterior cul-de-sac, fixing the uterus in retroversion. As the lesions advance, they may become completely scarred and lose their blue hemorrhagic appearance. Dense adhesions involving the posterior surface of the broad ligament and uterus should suggest the probability of endometriosis to the physician, even in the absence of blood-filled cysts or puckered hemorrhagic spots.

Lesions present in the large bowel rarely penetrate the mucosa. The main pathologic change is fibrotic thickening of the outer coats of the bowel, sometimes associated with stricture formation. In this location, endometriosis is easily mistaken for carcinoma or diverticulitis of the rectosigmoid. The presence of more than one lesion helps to distinguish endometriosis from cancer. The rare small-bowel involvement usually consists of subserosal fibrosis

and scarring. With extensive pelvic endometriosis, multiple loops of small bowel may be involved in the fibrous adhesions.

In addition to the small lesions present in the peritoneum overlying the bladder, endometriosis may produce fibrotic nodules in the wall of the bladder. The lesions are usually subserosal but rarely they protrude into the lumen as a hemorrhagic nodule. In uncommon sites, fibrotic scars or tiny blood-filled cysts are grossly visible.

MICROSCOPIC APPEARANCE

Microscopically, the lesions of endometriosis reveal endometrial epithelium, endometrial glands, and stroma, frequently with hemorrhage into the stroma and adjacent tissue (Fig. 37–4). Such hemorrhage may result in accumulation of large numbers of hemosiderin-laden macrophages. Endometrial glands and stroma usually show a morphologic response to the hormonal changes of the menstrual cycle comparable to that of uterine endometrium. Sometimes the endometriosis shows poor secretory response to progesterone. During pregnancy, there may be a typ-

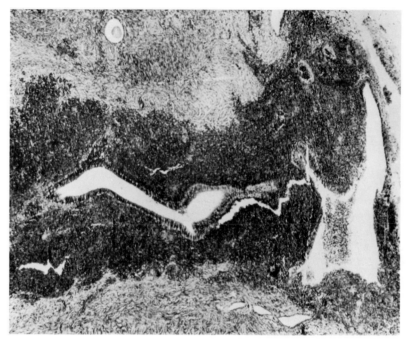

FIGURE 37–4 Microscopic appearance of endometriosis of the ovary. At the cortex of the ovary the lesion consists of endometrial gland, endometrial stroma, and hemorrhage.

ical decidual response of pelvic endometriosis. However, the finding of extrauterine decidua alone is not diagnostic of endometriosis. Such decidua often is only a mesenchymal response to pregnancy hormones.

Hemorrhage, particularly into the lumen of an endometrial cyst, frequently results in pressure atrophy and obliteration of recognizable endometrial epithelium. Such lesions may be lined only by granulation tissue, hemosiderin-laden macrophages, or cholesterol-crystal clefts with giant-cell foreign body reaction. The presence of endometrial stroma alone is diagnostic of the disease, particularly when associated with old or recent hemorrhage and fibrous reaction.

There may be a remarkable degree of fibrous proliferation surrounding endometriosis lesions. In the bowel, this may take the form of an annular constriction. Because of this reactive fibrosis, there are many cases of unquestioned gross endometriosis seen at the operating table in which the removed tissues show no evidence of microscopic endometriosis. Microscopic confirmation of gross endometriosis may be increased if the lesions are marked with a suture by the surgeon before they are removed.

ETIOLOGY AND HISTOGENESIS

ETIOLOGY

Although the theory that peritoneal mesothelium is stimulated to undergo metaplasia into functioning endometrium was one of the first ideas regarding the pathogenesis of this disease, a more commonly held theory is that of Sampson. He believed that viable fragments of endometrium, regurgitated in a retrograde fashion through the oviducts during menstruation, were subsequently *implanted* on the ovaries or the pelvic peritoneum. Such theories are easy to apply to the usual cases of pelvic endometriosis, but do not readily explain endometriosis found in such unusual sites as the spinal canal, kidney, or the palm of the hand. Over 20 cases of thoracic endometriosis have been reported (Yeh). Of the cases with pleural or diaphragmatic endometriosis, the majority had pelvic-abdominal endometriosis. However, of the cases with involvement of the lung, bronchus, or heart, none had definite evidence of peritoneal endometriosis but each had a history of prior gynecologic surgery. In the former, it was suggested that endometriosis was disseminated directly across the diaphragm, and in the latter it was suggested that vascular transportation occurred as a result of the surgical trauma.

Endometriosis is a disease occurring essentially only in patients with endometrium. It is rare or nonexistent in the absence of menstruation. In fact, improvement of endometriosis has been observed following hysterectomy. A notable exception is one recorded case of endometriosis in the bladder of a *male* who received long-term estrogen therapy for cancer of the prostate (Oliker and Harris).

Meyer and others postulated that inflammation, particularly inflammation of the pelvic peritoneum, was important in the etiology of endometriosis. Most now believe that the inflammatory reaction is secondary rather than primary. However, observations in the rhesus monkey, where endometriosis is a spontaneous disease, suggest that irritation or inflammation from radiation may contribute to the development of endometriosis. Disseminated endometriosis has been observed in animals receiving total body radiation (McClure et al.).

The concept that endometriosis is more common among women who voluntarily limit their childbearing to the late reproductive years is difficult to document or accept. It is equally difficult to confirm the possibility of a hereditary tendency to the development of endometriosis.

HISTOGENESIS

Essentially there are three major theories of histogenesis: (1) transportation, (2) formation in situ, and (3) a combination of these.

TRANSPORTATION

Sampson's theory is that endometriosis arises by retrograde tubal flow of menstrual fragments, *implantation* and growth on the ovary and peritoneal surfaces, followed by secondary seedings from the new foci. Reliable observations indicate that transportation of endometrial fragments, naturally or experimentally, is associated with the development of endometriosis. Endometriosis is more common in deformities of the uterus, congenital or acquired, which favor menstrual regurgitation. Menstrual fragments have been observed in the lumen of the oviduct as well as the peritoneal cavity, and endometrial fragments appear in

lymphatic and venous channels of the uterus. The continued viability of menstrual endometrium is supported by the observation of tissue-culture growth of menstrual endometrium. The fact that endometrial tissue is found in lymphatics and pelvic lymph nodes is widely accepted. The hematogenous spread of endometrial fragments offers the best explanation for the rare distant sites of endometriosis. In animals, transplantation of fragments of endometrium is followed by endometriosis, as is diversion of menstrual flow into the peritoneal cavity or anterior abdominal wall. Even human endometriosis has been observed following experimental subcutaneous injection of menstrual discharge. Direct transplantation and growth of endometrium has been suggested by the observation of endometriotic lesions in incisional scars following surgery involving the uterus and in vaginal incisions such as episiotomies.

A composite theory of the histogenesis of endometriosis includes (1) direct extension into the myometrium or endosalpinx, (2) exfoliation and implantation of endometrial cells at menstruation or during curettage, (3) lymphatic spread, (4) venous spread and hematogenous metastasis to distant organs, and (5) secondary lesions from foci already established.

FORMATION IN SITU

Metaplasia or differentiation of coelomic epithelium to endometrial epithelium, possibly triggered by inflammatory or hormonal alterations, was suggested by Meyer and Novak as the histogenesis of endometriosis. This theory gains support from embryologic studies, observations of differentiation of surface epithelium of the ovary into the various cell types of the Müllerian duct, and the decidual reaction seen frequently in tissue beneath the pelvic peritoneum during pregnancy. Endocervical and tubal epithelium has been observed in lesions of endometriosis (Lauchlan). Inflammation is observed to result in growth of coelomic epithelium with invagination into the cortex of the ovary and the subsurface connective tissues of the mesosalpinx and broad ligament. The inflammatory or irritating effect of radiation has been observed to produce decidual (endometrial stroma) reaction in the surface of the ovary and broad ligament in nonpregnant and even postmenopausal women. Disseminated peritoneal endometriosis has been observed in monkeys following total body radiation (McClure et al.).

There is little doubt that multiple irritants may trigger growth and metaplasia of the coelomic epithelium. The somewhat related theory of embryonic cell rests has largely been abandoned.

COMBINATION (INDUCTION)

Hertig and Gore have stated that the development of human endometriosis could include the formation of a fibrinopurulent exudate, its organization by subperitoneal stroma, and resultant formation of glandlike spaces lined by pelvic peritoneum or coelomic epithelium. They remind us of the known Müllerian potential of the coelomic epithelium and subperitoneal connective tissue and the presence of endometrial stroma in a regional distribution comparable to that of endometriosis. They believe the sequence could be due to the irritating, probably inductive, factors inherent in the menstrual discharge. A theory of induction has been proposed, in which chemical-inducing substances may be liberated from endometrium, activating undifferentiated mesenchyme to the formation of endometrial epithelium and stroma. Such a combination theory encompasses both the transportation and formation in situ theories.

Merrill has reported a series of experiments supporting this theory of induction. Endometrial tissue was observed to develop in connective tissue adjacent to cell-free extracts of endometrium and adjacent to diffusion chambers containing autologous or heterologous endometrium. Such chambers prevent escape of any cellular material but permit diffusion of noncellular material from the degenerating endometrium. Endometrial tissue also developed in connective tissue adjacent to diffusion chambers which contained endometrium from donors histoincompatible with the recipient. Absence of nuclear sex chromatin was observed in the endometrial tissue which developed in experiments where male animals were the recipients, further indicating that induction occurred. Although there are many observations and experiments which strongly support the idea that transportation of endometrial fragments by one means or another is important in the development of endometriosis, none of these observations or experiments conclusively proves that endometriosis arises from *growth* of such transported endometrial fragments. It is equally possible that they degenerate and, in the process, induce differentiation in the adjacent mesenchyme. The potential is well documented as previously indicated.

At present, it seems likely that no one theory satisfactorily explains all of the lesions of endometriosis, that each may play a role, and that this interesting entity may arise from a combination of influences.

SYMPTOMS

The symptoms of endometriosis are extremely variable. This has led some investigators to suggest that endometriosis is usually an asymptomatic disease, contrary to the more commonly held opinion. There may be extensive endometriosis without any symptoms whatsoever. The frequency and degree of symptoms are poorly related to the extent of disease. Indeed, many patients with very small lesions appear to be severely disabled. The symptoms are related to the functional state of the endometriosis.

Pelvic pain is the most significant symptom of endometriosis. In many women, this takes the form of *acquired dysmenorrhea* beginning in the late twenties or early thirties and gradually progressing in severity. The pain is described as a dull aching, or cramping, lower abdominal or back pain, occurring with menstruation and diminishing gradually after the onset of flow. Not all patients have pain that is related to menstruation. Many complain of vague aching, cramping, or a bearing-down sensation in the pelvis or low back, which may be constant or intermittent and may not become worse during the menstrual period. Some patients are somewhat relieved following menstruation. The necrosis and hemorrhage occurring in areas of endometriosis may account for pelvic pain by irritation of the peritoneum or distention of tissue. Pelvic pain and dysmenorrhea may be related to hemorrhagic distention of an endometrial cyst which is restricted by fibrosis or to the escape of bloody discharge into the peritoneal cavity. Dysmenorrhea may be related to increased local concentration of prostaglandins produced by ectopic endometrium.

Endometrial cysts may rupture producing intraabdominal bleeding and signs of acute peritoneal irritation. Such emergency circumstances have been reported to occur in from 1 to 15 percent of patients with proven endometriosis. The reports are conflicting with respect to the time of the menstrual cycle when spontaneous rupture of endometrial cysts is more likely to occur (Pratt; Ranney). Hemoperitoneum may occur with bleeding from small peritoneal lesions.

Abnormal uterine bleeding is the presenting symptom of patients with endometriosis almost as often as pain. It has no specific pattern and may be excessive, prolonged, or frequent. When actually caused by endometriosis, it may be due to involvement of the ovaries by the endometriotic lesions, causing alteration in hormonal function. The cause possibly may be the frequent association of other pelvic pathology, such as myomas.

The symptoms of pelvic pain and abnormal uterine bleeding are obviously associated with a variety of pelvic disorders and cannot be considered specific for endometriosis. Somewhat less often, but more significantly, patients complain of *dyspareunia,* particularly when the uterus is fixed in retroversion and when endometriotic lesions are present in the rectovaginal septum, the posterior fornix of the vagina, or the uterosacral ligaments (Fig. 37–3). Upon direct questioning, one may obtain a history of *pain with defecation* during menstruation, particularly if the lesions involve the area of the rectovaginal septum. Although the mechanism of pelvic pain is not always clear, dyspareunia and pain with defecation are clearly related to pressure upon distended lesions or the stretching of adhesions.

Infertility may bring a patient with endometriosis to the physician. It is impossible to determine the true incidence of infertility in patients with endometriosis and difficult to explain exactly how endometriosis may interfere with fertility. The oviducts are usually patent and ovulation usually is not interrupted (Devereux; Soules et al.). However, it is possible that endometriosis is associated with at least a relative infertility. Kinking or fixation of the oviducts by adhesions may be significant. Kelly and Rock reported endometriosis of the pelvis producing tubal adhesions in only 34 cases out of 417 infertile patients who underwent culdoscopic examination. Pain associated with cul-de-sac endometriosis may prevent deep intromission during coitus. Fixation of the uterus in a retroverted position may interfere with adequate placement of semen at the cervical os. Investigation into possible relationships between endometriosis and altered fertility reveals a small but significant incidence of anovulation in infertile patients (Dmowski and Cohen; Soules et al.). In one histologic study of 87 cases of ovarian endometriosis with salpingectomy, 33 percent of the removed oviducts showed chronic salpingitis. Tubal obstruction, however, was demonstrated in only one of these cases (Czernobilsky and Silverstein). Meldrum has studied peritoneal fluid in patients with endometriosis and found that it contained dramatically elevated levels of prostaglandin $F_{2\alpha}$. Prostaglandin $F_{2\alpha}$ stimulates smooth muscle activity in human oviducts. Whether prostaglandin re-

lease by lesions of endometriosis causes altered tubal function and an antifertility effect is unknown. It is also possible that the apparent relationship between infertility and endometriosis is an example of sampling error related to the frequency with which infertile patients are evaluated by laparotomy or endoscopy.

The rare sites of endometriosis produce uncommon and unusual clinical situations. Symptoms related to the involvement of the gastrointestinal tract or urinary tract may occur from obstruction or interference with function of these organs. Patients have been reported with cyclic hematuria resulting from endometriosis in the bladder, and cyclic renal colic resulting from endometriosis involving the ureter (Bergman and Friedenberg). Ureteral lesions may enlarge at the time of menstruation because of bleeding into the focus of endometriosis with resultant ureteral obstruction. Patients with intestinal endometriosis may have significant gastrointestinal symptoms in about one-third of the cases. Those with endometriosis involving the appendix rarely do. The most common gastrointestinal symptoms are abdominal pain and constipation. Rectal bleeding occurs in 20 percent of patients with intestinal endometriosis (Panganiban and Corwog). Intestinal endometriosis is rarely diagnosed preoperatively. Lombardo reported the case of a patient with repeated episodes of subarachnoid hemorrhage from endometriosis in the spinal canal at the level of T1. The patient bled coincident with her menstrual periods. Recurrent spontaneous pneumothorax has been reported in a patient with thoracic endometriosis (Kovarik and Toll). Hemoptysis occurring at the time of menstruation has been described in the rare cases of endometriosis involving the lung or bronchus (Rodman and Jones). Pain, tenderness, swelling, redness, and occasional bleeding have been observed in patients with endometriosis in the umbilicus or abdominal and vaginal scars.

PHYSICAL FINDINGS

Multiple tender nodules palpable along the uterosacral ligaments or in the rectovaginal septum of the posterior fornix of the vagina are significant specific clinical findings of endometriosis. These nodules are noted to enlarge and become more tender during menstruation. Reexamination of a patient with suspected endometriosis during menstruation thus will be helpful. The uterus may be fixed in retroposition. Attempts to move it are accompanied by severe pain. Thickening and nodularity of the adnexa may be similar to, and suggestive of, pelvic inflammatory disease. Endometrial cysts of the ovary present as irregular enlargement of the ovary. These are rarely movable and usually closely adherent to the uterus with adjacent induration and tenderness. Endometrial cysts are rarely larger than 10 cm in diameter. Intraabdominal bleeding diagnosed by cul-de-sac aspiration may be present with spontaneous rupture of an endometrial cyst. In rare cases, blue cystic areas may be seen at the umbilicus, in abdominal wound scars, on the cervix or vagina, or elsewhere. These appear or enlarge during menstruation. The lesions of endometriosis have been seen during cystoscopy but are rarely observed during proctosigmoidoscopy. Even more rarely, the hemorrhagic lesions of endometriosis have been observed during bronchoscopy.

DIAGNOSIS

The diagnosis of endometriosis can be made only by visualization of the lesion. This may be accomplished directly with external lesions or by laparotomy or various types of endoscopy for internal lesions. A clinical diagnosis is established on the basis of history and physical findings. There are no laboratory studies which are of particular value in the diagnosis of this disease. The clinical impression of endometriosis is often in error and this is especially so if only cases with significant extent of disease are considered. Endometriosis should be considered in a young woman with acquired progressive dysmenorrhea, intermittent or constant pelvic pain, dyspareunia and menstrual abnormality who has a tender, fixed, retroverted uterus and palpable nodules in the retrovaginal septum or the region of the uterosacral ligaments. Endometriosis should be considered in patients with similar symptoms who have unilateral or bilateral adnexal thickening or adnexal masses. Laparoscopy with visualization of the typical foci may be of great value in confirming the diagnosis. Such an attempt at establishing a positive diagnosis is important if expensive and long-range hormone therapy is to be contemplated. Biopsy of externally visible lesions on the cervix or vagina or those seen at cystoscopy, proctoscopy, or bronchoscopy will establish the diagnosis.

Endometriosis should be part of the differential diagnosis of such diverse lesions as ovarian cancer, chronic salpingo-oophoritis, cancer of the rectum and colon, diverticulitis, intestinal obstruction, tumors of the umbilicus, inguinal swellings, causes of hematuria, intraabdominal bleeding with signs of peritoneal irritation, and acute abdomen. Endometriosis may prove to be the accurate diagnosis in patients who have been observed and followed for long periods of time with a presumed diagnosis of psychosomatic pelvic pain. The diagnosis is often made at laparotomy done for another indication. The possibility of endometriosis should be entertained when hemorrhagic or fibrotic lesions are encountered on the pelvic viscera in women in the reproductive ages. It is impossible to palpate all small endometriotic lesions, but remembering the protean manifestations of endometriosis may increase the frequency (approximately 20 percent) with which an accurate diagnosis is made.

TREATMENT

The treatment of endometriosis will depend upon the manifestations of the disease, the complaints and desires of the patient, and the method of diagnosis. Endometriosis found incidentally at surgery for another reason may be treated differently from endometriosis found or suspected in the course of an infertility workup, or from endometriosis thought to be the cause of incapacitating pelvic pain. The treatment of endometriosis must be influenced by a recognition that it is predominantly a disease of women in the childbearing age, infertility is often the presenting complaint, and an accurate diagnosis is difficult to make without surgical exploration. Since endometriosis is to some extent responsive to cyclic ovarian hormones, removal of the ovaries will result in symptomatic relief in a majority of patients. Such may be the case with removal of the uterus only. However, such treatment is not compatible with future childbearing and can be recommended only in those patients near the menopause. For young patients, treatment should be designed to produce a maximum of symptomatic relief with a minimum of interference with childbearing function, or it should actually increase fertility.

The evaluation of different methods of treatment is complicated by the difficulty in accurate diagnosis and by the inherent selection of patients. It is, for example, difficult to compare the results of surgical therapy and hormonal therapy where the diagnosis of patients treated surgically has been established by pathologic examination but the diagnosis of patients treated with hormones has been based only on clinical findings, with possibly an 80 percent chance of being inaccurate. Similarly, it is difficult to assign a fertility-promoting effect to therapy when the only patients under study are women under the age of 30 who seriously desire pregnancy, who have limited endometriosis which allows conservative therapy, and who have no other cause of sterility. Such selection, which is common in the management of endometriosis, must be recognized when evaluating therapy.

Further, adequate comparison of different methods of treatment is complicated by the varying extent of the disease in the patient populations studied. Several investigators have described methods of classifying endometriosis based upon the extent of the disease. The factors used which progressively increase the degree of severity are (1) adhesions, (2) scarring and retraction, (3) endometrial cysts, (4) fixation of pelvic structures, and (5) obliteration of the cul-de-sac. Acosta and Garcia have both shown a direct relationship between the extent of the endometriosis and the success of subsequent pregnancy following therapy. Spangler, however, showed no relationship between extent of disease and rate of pregnancy following therapy. None of the several suggested systems of classifying extent of disease has been commonly utilized by investigators in this field.

In general, treatment consists of (1) observation and symptom palliation, (2) surgery, and (3) hormone therapy.

OBSERVATION

Observation, reassurance, and mild analgesia are effective in many patients and should be the initial management of young patients whose symptoms are not severe or incapacitating. If the lesions are small and multiple and are producing few symptoms, it is wise to leave them alone. Indeed, they sometimes become inactive after a while. Time is often helpful and some procrastination is justified. Education and reassurance of the patient that a life-threatening or health-threatening process does not exist are often successful in relieving minor or moderate symptoms of pain and in permitting a patient to accept and live with minor discomfort. The value of education and reassurance should not be underestimated.

It is also important to defer active measures in young women attempting pregnancy. Many gynecologists feel that pregnancy may result in relief of symptoms or in permanent cure. An expectant course should *not* be followed if masses are palpated, if the differential diagnosis includes more significant pathology, or if long-standing infertility is the primary complaint. A clinical diagnosis of endometriosis is often inaccurate.

SURGERY

Surgery is often employed in the management of patients with endometriosis and may be of a "radical" or "conservative" nature depending upon whether or not the surgical procedure preserves the childbearing function. When symptoms are severe, incapacitating, or acute, surgery is indicated. Surgery is indicated if symptoms become worse under observation or medical management or if infertility persists and no cause other than endometriosis is found. Endometrial cysts of the ovary are indications for operation if they are larger than 6 to 8 cm in diameter. When surgery is undertaken, efforts should be made to accomplish a conservative procedure which will preserve the opportunity for childbearing function if this is desired. The extent of surgery will also depend upon the extent and location of the lesions and the surgeon's judgment concerning the safety of removal of such lesions.

RADICAL SURGERY

Endometriosis in a symptomatic patient may be dealt with "radically" if the woman is approaching the menopause or has no desire to continue childbearing and menstruation. This is the more common surgical approach used. The endometriotic lesions together with adjacent fibrosis and adhesions should be removed along with the uterus, oviducts, and ovaries. Efforts to remove endometrial cysts and to separate adhesions often result in rupture of endometrial cysts with escape of the old blood contents. It may be impossible to remove all of the endometriotic lesions without causing undue injury to normal adjacent structures. Bilateral salpingo-oophorectomy and hysterectomy alone will relieve symptoms without the risk of injury to bowel or other structures that may follow attempts to excise every fragment of endometriosis. Even constricting lesions of the bowel or urinary tract may regress following this therapy. On the other hand, isolated endometriotic lesions of the intestine may be treated by bowel resection with or without treatment of the pelvic lesions.

Hysterectomy alone may relieve symptoms while

maintaining ovarian function, even in the presence of residual areas of endometriosis. Ablation of cyclic menstruation and repeated regurgitation of menstrual fragments may possibly result in quiescence of remaining areas of endometriosis. Endometriosis is rarely, if ever, observed to develop in patients without endometrium. Thus, hysterectomy with removal of as many foci of endometriosis as is easily possible, but preservation of all or part of the ovarian tissue, is recommended for the young woman who does not desire future childbearing but wishes to retain cyclic ovarian function. There is also evidence that the cyclic administration of estrogen in patients who have had the uterus and ovaries removed may be accomplished without aggravation of endometriosis and such estrogen is more readily altered than endogenous ovarian estrogen.

CONSERVATIVE SURGERY

"Conservative" surgery is indicated for those patients desiring further children. This usually involves excision of all gross endometriosis with preservation of the uterus and as much ovarian tissue as possible. This may include unilateral oophorectomy, resection of endometrial cysts of one or both ovaries, excision of peritoneal lesions, release of adhesions, and resection of portions of rectal or bladder wall. It is possible to excise even fairly large endometrial cysts and conserve adequate functioning ovarian tissue. Small peritoneal lesions, particularly those in the cul-de-sac, may be destroyed by electrocauterization. Some gynecologists recommend suspension of the uterus and presacral neurectomy in patients undergoing conservative surgery for endometriosis.

The results of conservative surgery are generally good with regard to relief of symptoms. Progression is possible, however, when there is residual endometriosis and continuing ovarian function. The incidence of reoperation varies from 2 to 46 percent and is proportional to the frequency with which conservative surgery is the first chosen treatment. Among patients complaining of infertility the average pregnancy rate is 35 percent. Recently, several authors report pregnancy rates as high as 50 percent (Green; Spangler et al.) and Ranney reported a 60 percent pregnancy rate which was correctable to 87 percent. The mechanism by which fertility is improved is certainly not clear. Spangler reported no differences in the pregnancy rate following surgery related to the factors of age, duration of infertility, extent of endo-

metriosis, previous parity, or accomplishment of uterine suspension. Moreover, one-third of patients treated had such minimal endometriosis that none was removed for pathologic examination.

HORMONE THERAPY

Since endometrium is highly responsive to ovarian steroid hormones and endometriosis often shows a similar responsiveness, it was natural that hormone therapy would be advocated in the treatment of endometriosis (Eisnefeld; Green; Hammond). The use of hormones has been recommended for patients with symptoms not relieved by reassurance and mild analgesia who desire subsequent pregnancy and in whom surgery is either contraindicated or not acceptable to the patient, and in patients with recurrence of symptoms following "conservative" surgery. Estrogens, androgens, and progestins in various dose schedules have been administered. Recently, antigonadotropins have been used in preference to those steroids. It is noteworthy that almost all reported doses and combinations of hormones have been successful in the hands of their advocates. Almost all report relief of symptoms in approximately 80 percent of cases. This is about the same percentage of success obtained in selected patients who have not received specific treatment. In the majority of cases, the relief is reported to be temporary and the medication has been associated with annoying side effects.

The long-term use of hormonal medication, which may be expensive, should not be undertaken without an accurate diagnosis.

ESTROGEN

Estrogen, in the form of diethylstilbestrol, has been recommended in small doses (5 mg per day for 30 days) for the purpose of ovulation suppression and in large doses (1 mg per day increasing to 100 mg per day for 6 months or increasing to 400 mg per day for 3 to 9 months) for the purpose of producing "pseudopregnancy" and the beneficial effects which have been reported sometimes with pregnancy (Karnaky). At present, it is generally agreed that this type of therapy is usually ineffective. The symptoms and objective findings soon return, and intermenstrual bleeding, edema, and nausea may be annoying side effects. In experimentally induced endometriosis in the primate, stilbestrol had no effect upon the morphology of the endometriotic lesions (Scott and Wharton).

ANDROGEN

Testosterone and methyltestosterone have been used and reported to be effective in relieving the symptoms of endometriosis. Methyltestosterone linquets, 10 mg daily, is one recommended dose. This may be reduced to 5 mg daily. The medication is continued for 6 to 12 weeks and, if effective, repeated after 1 to 2 months' rest. The 5-mg dose may be given continuously. Relief of symptoms has been reported to occur in 80 percent of patients, and subsequent pregnancy in 11 to 60 percent of those complaining of infertility. Side effects of hirsutism, acne, and increased libido are reported with androgens, but are rare with the previously mentioned dosage schedules. The effect of androgens is thought to be suppression of ovulation through the hypothalamus, but there must be a direct effect upon the lesion as well. Ovulation is not always suppressed in patients reporting benefit from androgen therapy.

ESTROGEN-PROGESTINS

The most frequently used hormone therapy is synthetic estrogen and progestins. The treatment is based upon ovulation suppression and the production of a state of "pseudopregnancy" (amenorrhea) with decidual reaction in the endometrial stroma, atrophy of glands, and eventual fibrosis and obliteration of the endometriotic lesions. The improvement obtained with the use of estrogen-progestins has been reported to be overestimated when results are correlated with actual surgical findings (Borglin et al.; Scott and Wharton). The degree of change in the epithelial components of the lesion is small. The greatest response has been a reduction of inflammatory reaction and regression of pelvic adhesions.

A variety of synthetic estrogens and progestins have been used. The medication is given continuously in a dose which results in amenorrhea for many months. The estrogen-progestin is increased and the new dose maintained if any bleeding occurs. Norethynodrel combined with ethinylestradiol (Enovid) was an early and extensively used preparation. Enovid was given in gradually increasing doses starting at 2.5 mg daily and increasing to usually 20 mg daily. Occasionally as much as 40 or 60 mg daily was ad-

ministered to complete the 6- to 9-months' course of treatment. More commonly now, however, progestin-estrogen contraceptives have been used in a continuous fashion starting with a dose of 1 tablet daily. This dosage is increased to 2 tablets daily after 2 to 3 weeks. If breakthrough bleeding occurs, the dose is increased by 1 tablet daily and continued.

Improvement in symptoms has been reported in 85 to 89 percent of patients, with pregnancy occurring in infertility patients in 30 to 47 percent (Williams; Green; Kourides and Kistner). A significant number of patients complain of nausea, restlessness, edema, irregular uterine bleeding, and excess weight gain. Remarkable growth of uterine myomas may result. The improvement in the endometriosis following therapy persists for varying intervals, but in many cases the physical findings and symptoms return. Some gynecologists feel that there is no objective evidence that synthetic estrogen-progestins actually cure endometriosis and that the use of such agents should be considered a temporizing measure for specially selected cases. The use of progestins for about 5 to 8 weeks prior to contemplated surgery may make the lesions more easily identifiable and soften the usually dense adhesions.

ANTIGONADOTROPINS

Danazol, a synthetic (2,3-d-isoxazol) derivative of 17 α-ethynyltestosterone has been recently used in conservative treatment of endometriosis (Dmowski and Cohen). This drug appears to suppress gonadotropin release but has little significant estrogenic or progestational activity, although modest androgenicity is present. The treatment thus is an induction of "pseudomenopause," with anovulation and atrophy of endometrial tissue. The current treatment regimen is 200 mg orally 4 times a day, although in some patients 200 mg per day has been adequate. A 6- to 9-month course is usually recommended. The medication is expensive and costs roughly $120 per month.

The results of treatment are difficult to analyze because of the limited number of patients treated. However, 70 to 100 percent symptomatic improvement has been reported as well as overall pregnancy rates of approximately 50 percent. The latter compare favorably with pregnancy rates following conservative surgery. In contrast to pseudopregnancy, relief of symptoms occurs early in the course of therapy. Regression of lesions of endometriosis has been documented by endoscopic examination. Mild side effects include weight gain, muscle cramps, acne, and minimal hirsutism. Danazol therapy has superseded the use of pseudopregnancy as the preferred medical therapy.

RADIATION THERAPY

Radiation therapy has been rarely recommended for the treatment of endometriosis and has no place in primary treatment (Brosset.) In recurrent cases after failure of conservative surgery, radiation suppression of the ovaries may be an effective mode of therapy. The external radiation dose required is not large. If employed, care must be taken to avoid damage to normal structures that are fixed by the dense adhesions. The use of this modality definitely should be restricted to the occasional exceptional case.

SUMMARY OF TREATMENT

There is no agreement regarding the most successful mode of treatment of endometriosis. Each case must be treated individually based on the patient's experience, understanding, and desires. Certainly patients without desire for fertility who have significant symptoms are most effectively treated by hysterectomy and removal of the adnexa and other tissue containing endometriosis. Young patients not currently desiring pregnancy may be satisfactorily managed with observation, reassurance, and mild analgesia. Danazol may be used for this group and also for those with recurrence following conservative surgery. For the young patient with an infertility problem, conservative surgery is most often recommended. Any recommended therapy should be modified by the extent of disease and economic considerations.

MALIGNANCY

True malignancy has been reported in areas of endometriosis (Stevenson). Most patients with cancer arising in endometriosis are postmenopausal and fall in the age range common for ovarian cancer. Criteria for the diagnosis of cancer arising in endometriosis of the ovary were proposed by Sampson in 1925: (1) the ovary must be the site of benign endometriosis, (2) there must be a genuine adenocarcinoma, and (3) a transition from benign to malignant areas must

be demonstrable. If these criteria are used, the diagnosis is *rarely* made. It is possible that more ovarian cancers originate in areas of endometriosis, but at the time of diagnosis, all areas of benign endometriosis have been replaced by tumor. Thus, fewer than 50 cases of carcinoma arising in endometriosis have been reported. The majority of these have been adenocanthomas and others have been endometrioid tumors. Both of these are generally less malignant biologically than the more common ovarian cancers. Endometrioid tumors of the ovary have been emphasized recently. This histologic tumor type may account for 10 to 15 percent of primary ovarian malignancies. The vast majority of the endometrioid tumors appear to arise primarily from the ovary and not as a malignant transformation of endometriosis. Other histologic types of malignancy arising from endometriosis in the ovary include mucinous adenocarcinoma, clear-cell carcinoma, mixed mesodermal sarcoma (Saunders and Price), and carcinosarcoma (Lauchlan). The fact that malignancies composed of various types of Müllerian epithelia have been observed to arise in endometriosis adds some strength to the theory of induced metaplasia of coelomic epithelium. Exceedingly rare cases of malignant change in endometriosis at sites other than the ovary or the pelvic peritoneum have been reported. Adenocarcinoma arising within cervical endometriosis invaded the adjacent vagina (Chang and Maddox). Sarcoma developed simultaneously in areas of pelvic endometriosis and endometriosis of the right pleura (Labay and Feiner). Adenocarcinoma has been reported to arise in endometriosis of the rectovaginal septum and vagina (Young and Gamble). Essentially in each case, the diagnosis of malignancy arising in endometriosis has been established after examination of the surgical specimen and has not been a preoperative diagnosis.

REFERENCES

Acosta AA et al.: A proposed classification of pelvic endometriosis. *Obstet Gynecol* 42:19, 1973.

Bergman H, Friedenberg RM: Endometriosis: Urologic manifestation. *NY State J Med* 72:1152, 1972.

Borglin NE et al.: Roentgenographic observations on the effect of pseudopregnancy in endometriosis. *J Obstet Gynaecol Br Commonw* 72:544, 1965.

Brosset A: Value of irradiation therapy in the treatment of endometriosis. *Acta Obstet Gynecol Scand* 36:209, 1957.

Buttram VC: An expanded classification of endometriosis. *Fert Steril* 28:1008, 1977.

Chang SH, Maddox WA: Adenocarcinoma arising within cervical endometriosis and invading the adjacent vagina. *Am J Obstet Gynecol* 110:1015, 1971.

Czernobilsky B, Silverstein A: Salpingitis in ovarian endometriosis. *Fert Steril* 30:45, 1978.

Deverux WP: Endometriosis: Long term observation, with particular reference to incidence of pregnancy. *Obstet Gynecol* 22:444, 1963.

Dmowski WP, Cohen MR: Antigonadotropin (Danazol) in the treatment of endometriosis. *Am J Obstet Gynecol* 130:41, 1978.

Eisenfeld AJ et al.: Radioactive estradiol accumulation in endometriosis of the rhesus monkey. *Am J Obstet Gynecol* 109:124, 1971.

Garcia C, Sami SD: Pelvic endometriosis: Infertility and pelvic pain. *Am J Obstet Gynecol* 129:740, 1977.

Green TH Jr (ed.): Symposium on endometriosis. *Clin Obstet Gynecol* 9:00, 1966.

Hammond CB, Haney AF: Conservative treatment of endometriosis. *Fert Steril* 30:497, 1978.

Hertig AT, Gore H: *Tumors of the Female Sex Organs.* Parts 2, 3, Washington: Armed Forces Institute of Pathology, 1960, 1961, 1968.

Karnaky KJ: Diagnosis and treatment of endometriosis. *Am J Obstet Gynecol* 111:598, 1971.

Kelly JV, Rock J: Culdoscopy for diagnosis of infertility: Report of 492 cases. *Am J Obstet Gynecol* 72:523, 1956.

Kempers RD et al.: Post-menopausal endometriosis. *Surg Gynecol Obstet* 111:348, 1960.

Kistner RW et al.: Suggested classification of endometriosis. *Fert Steril* 30:240, 1978.

Kourides IA, Kistner RW: Three new synthetic progestins in the treatment of endometriosis. *Obstet Gynecol* 31:821, 1968.

Kovarik JL, Toll GD: Thoracic endometriosis with recurrent spontaneous pneumothorax. *JAMA* 196:595, 1966.

Labay GR, Feiner F: Malignant pleural endometriosis. *Am J Obstet Gynecol* 110:478, 1971.

Lauchlan SC: The secondary Müllerian system. *Obstet Gynecol Surv* 27:133, 1972.

Lombardo L et al.: Subarachnoid hemorrhage due to endometriosis of the spinal canal. *Neurology* 19:423, 1968.

MacArthur JW, Ulfelder H: The effect of pregnancy upon endometriosis. *Obstet Gynecol Surv* 20:709, 1965.

McClure HM et al.: Disseminated endometriosis in a rhesus monkey. *J Med Assoc Ga* 60:11, 1971.

Meigs JV: Endometriosis: Etiologic role of marriage, age and parity; conservative treatment. *Obstet Gynecol* 2:46, 1953.

Merrill JA: Endometrial induction of endometriosis across millipore filters. *Am J Obstet Gynecol* 94:780, 1966.

Oliker AJ, Harris AE: Endometriosis of the bladder in a male patient. *J Urol* 106:858, 1971.

Panganiban W, Corwog JL: Endometriosis of the intestine and vermiform appendix. *Dis Colon Rectum* 15:253, 1972.

Pratt JH, Shamblin WR: Spontaneous rupture of endometrial cysts. *Am J Obstet Gynecol* 108:56, 1970.

Ranney B: Endometriosis I. Conservative operations. *Am J Obstet Gynecol* 107:743, 1970.

_____:Endometriosis II. Emergency operations due to hemoperitoneum. *Obstet Gynecol* 36:437, 1970.

_____: Endometriosis IV. Hereditary tendency. *Obstet Gynecol* 37:734, 1971.

Ridley JH: Histogenesis of endometriosis. *Obstet Gynecol Surv* 23:1, 1968.

Rodman MH, Jones CW: Catamenial hemoptysis due to bronchial endometriosis. *N Engl J Med* 266:805, 1962.

Saunders P, Price AB: Mixed mesodermal tumor of the ovary arising in pelvic endometriosis. *Proc R Soc Med* 63:1050, 1970.

Schifrin BS et al.: Teenage endometriosis. *Am J Obstet Gynecol* 116:973, 1973.

Scott RB, Wharton LR Jr: Effects of progesterone and norethindrone on experimental endometriosis in monkeys. *Am J Obstet Gynecol* 84:867, 1962.

Soules MR et al.: Endometriosis and anovulation: A coexisting problem in the infertile patient. *Fertil Steril* 26:1151, 1975.

Spangler DB et al.: Infertility due to endometriosis. *Am J Obstet Gynecol* 109:850, 1971.

Stevenson CS: Malignant transformation of ovarian endometriosis. *Obstet Gynecol* 36:443, 1970.

Williams BFP: Conservative management of endometriosis: Follow-up observation of progestin therapy. *Obstet Gynecol* 30:76, 1967.

Yeh TJ: Endometriosis within the thorax: Metaplasia, implantation or metastasis? Thoracic and Cardiovascular Surg 53:201, 1967.

Young EE, Gamble C: Primary adenocarcinoma of the rectovaginal septum arising from endometriosis. *Cancer* 24:597, 1969.

38

Gynecologic Urology

GEORGE W. MITCHELL, JR.   MARTIN FARBER

INTRODUCTION

The reproductive and urinary tracts in the human female have in common many embryologic and anatomic characteristics and they share the impact of a large variety of pelvic diseases. So interrelated are the disorders of function, and so ambiguous the resulting symptoms, that gynecologic and urologic histories are necessarily taken together. The diagnostic plan must have sufficient scope to include all possible ramifications of the suspected interaction between the two systems.

The implication is either that urologic techniques are within the gynecologist's purview and must be mastered, or that urologic consultation must be resorted to frequently. From the patient's viewpoint, it is essential that the interrelationships be understood.

The urologic conditions encountered by the gynecologist/obstetrician may be broadly categorized under the headings (1) stasis, (2) infection, and (3) incontinence. Many are not amenable to surgical correction and are often modified indirectly by emotional, medical, and pharmacologic factors. A detailed general history and physical examination are essential in all cases prior to employing specialized diagnostic techniques.

HISTORY AND PHYSICAL EXAMINATION

The history of the present illness must include questions which will not only precisely define the urologic symptom (e.g., the presence of dysuria, frequency, hematuria, pyuria, urgency, enuresis, incomplete emptying, stress or continuous incontinence), but which will also elucidate problems relative to other systems that indirectly affect the urinary tract (e.g., endocrine, neurologic, psychiatric). The past history should include previous surgery, the use of pharmacologic agents, and precise accounts of labors and deliveries. Metabolic diseases (e.g., diabetes, hyperparathyroidism, gout) and other pathologic processes which may be relevant to the presenting symptom must be ruled out.

In the course of the complete physical examination, it is unusual to detect a sign that was not strongly suspected from the history. Normal female urologic organs cannot be inspected (except the external urethral meatus) and are usually not palpable. The lower pole of the right kidney may be palpable in thin women. If the left is palpable, it is because it is pathologically enlarged or dislocated. The ureters are usually not palpable. The bladder can be felt during bimanual examination when it is full or the wall is thickened and the urethra when it is the site of tumor, diverticulum, chronic infection, etc. The urinary tract is best visualized endoscopically and radiographically.

EMBRYOLOGY

The nephrogenic cord is derived from intermediate mesoderm located between the somites and the lateral coelomic mesoderm. The pronephros, mesonephros, and metanephros all arise from the nephrogenic cord. The pronephric tubules appear opposite somites 7 to 14 late in the third week of fetal life. The pronephric duct which connects the tubules with the cloaca is probably never functional. The most craniad pronephric tubules begin to be resorbed at the end of the fourth week. Mesonephric tubules begin to appear in the middle of the fourth week; by the end of the fifth week, they have appropriated the pronephric duct (now designated the mesonephric duct) and extend from the 14th to the 26th somite.

The metanephric duct, the forerunner of the ureter, arises early in the fifth week as an outgrowth of that portion of the mesonephric duct just craniad to its entrance into the cloaca at the level of the 28th somite. Uriniferous tubular formation is induced by contact of the blind cranial terminus (progenitor of the renal pelvis) of the metanephric duct with the metanephrogenic mass. The major and minor renal calyxes and the straight collecting tubules derive from progressive subdivisions of the renal pelvis. Coalescence of the lumina of the uriniferous tubules with the straight collecting ducts to permit excretory function is accomplished by the 11th week. As additional straight collecting ducts arise from their points of junction with the uriniferous tubules and new nephrons are formed about the additional straight collecting ducts, expansion of the major and minor calyxes concomitantly results in resorption of previously formed collecting ducts. The net result is great expansion of the metanephric mass and the ultimate formation of a kidney whose minor calyxes receive papillary ducts (terminal collecting ducts) from a renal lobe derived from the fifth generation of collecting ducts.

The developing metanephros migrates cranially and rotates 90°. Subsequent to more accelerated fetal growth caudal to the metanephros, the kidney assumes its final position at term with the renal pelvis opposite the twelfth thoracic or first lumbar vertebra. Its convex border is directed laterally, having rotated from a dorsal position.

The expanded terminal part of the hindgut, the cloaca, is continuous with the allantois ventrally and receives the mesonephric ducts laterally. During the fourth to the seventh week of gestation, the urorectal septum divides the cloaca into a ventral urogenital sinus and a dorsal anorectal canal. From that portion of the urogenital sinus, craniad to the entries of the mesonephric ducts, the bladder and urethra originate. Absorption of the terminal end of the mesonephric ducts into the wall of the urogenital sinus results in a separate entrance for the metanephric ducts. The mesonephric ducts proximal to the ureteric buds grow caudomedially in a loop. They are partially incorporated into the dorsal wall of the developing urinary bladder to contribute to the formation of the bladder trigone and a portion of the urethra, and they ultimately enter the developing bladder caudal and medial to the entrance of the metanephric ducts (ureters).

The Müllerian ducts, primordia of the vagina, cervix, uterus, and fallopian tubes, arise as infoldings in the coelomic mesothelium on the lateral border of the mesonephros in the seventh week. Distal fusion of the Müllerian ducts with the urogenital sinus at Müller's tubercle occurs at the end of the fifth week, but the caudal migration of the primitive genital ducts is dependent on the presence of the mesonephric ducts which serve as their guides.

ANATOMY

The kidneys are dorsal paired retroperitoneal organs surrounded by fat and loose areolar tissue and extend from the superior border of the twelfth thoracic vertebra to the third lumbar vertebra. Their vertical dimensions (11.25 cm) are about twice their width (5 to 7.5 cm), and their external configurations are bean-shaped with their concavities pointed medially.

The ureter is continuous with the renal pelvis originating retroperitoneally at the level of the spinous process of the first lumbar vertebra and terminating at its insertion in the bladder trigone. This long tortuous course, which ranges from 28 to 34 cm, necessitates its division for anatomic purposes into abdominal and pelvic components. Depending upon peristaltic compression, ureteral diameter ranges from 1 mm to 1 cm. With chronic partial obstruction, it can stretch to 3 cm.

The abdominal ureters rest on the medial aspects of the psoas muscles. The right abdominal ureter, crossed by the right colic and ileocolic vessels, passes dorsal to the terminal ileum to enter the pelvis. The left abdominal ureter, crossed by the left colic vessels, passes dorsal to the sigmoid colon and its mesentery to enter the pelvis.

The pelvic ureters cross the iliac vessels (either the termination of the common or the origin of the external iliac vessels) and run caudally on the lateral pelvic wall, turning medially at the level of the inferior part of the greater sciatic foramen. They are accompanied by the uterine arteries for about 2.5 cm of their medial course in the bases of the broad ligaments, but 2 cm lateral to the cervix they loop under the uterine vessels and run anteromedial to the cervix and upper vagina to terminate in the bladder.

The arterial blood supply to the ureter comes from the renal artery, aorta, and common iliac, internal iliac, and vesical arteries. The innervation is derived from the inferior mesenteric and pelvic plexuses. Histologically, the ureteral mucosa is composed of transitional epithelium surrounded by fibrous connective tissue. This is enveloped by a circular muscle tunic outside of which is a longitudinal muscle layer surrounded by a fibrous adventitia.

The collapsed bladder assumes the shape of a flattened tetrahedron. The fundus is the triangular area dorsally connected to the anterior cervix and upper vagina by loose, relatively avascular, areolar tissue. The superior surface of the bladder is continuous with the fundus and extends in a triangular fashion from a line joining the two ureters to the vertex, which is directed ventrally toward the symphysis pubis. Peritoneum partially covers the superior surface of the bladder, and this part is separated from the anterior surface of the uterus by the uterovesical excavation. The retroperitoneal inferior surface of the bladder is directed toward the symphysis pubis and separated from it by the cavum Retzii.

Internally, the bladder trigone is an equilateral triangle whose sides are about 2.5 cm long. The posterolateral angles are formed by the ureteral orifices and the anterior angle by the internal urethral orifice. Joining the ureteral orifices is an elevated ridge of nonstriated muscle, the torus uretericus, which forms the base of the trigone.

The mucosa of the bladder is composed of transitional epithelium which is loosely attached to the underlying musculature by the submucosa except in the region of the trigone. In the collapsed state the pink mucosa is thrown into folds except in the region of the trigone where the mucosa is closely attached to the muscularis and therefore appears smooth and "fishbelly white" in color. The detrusor muscle is the external longitudinal layer of smooth muscle which surrounds a middle circular layer, internal to which is another longitudinal layer. Innervation is derived from the second, third, and fourth sacral nerves and from the hypogastric plexus. The rich arterial supply is from the superior, middle, and inferior vesical arteries, and branches from the obturator, inferior gluteal, uterine, and vaginal arteries (all derived from the internal iliac artery).

The urethra averages 4 cm in length, extending from the bladder to the external meatus in the vestibule. The mucosa of the superior urethra is a continuum of the transitional epithelium of the bladder, but inferiorly it is lined by stratified squamous epithelium. Submucosally, there is a layer of erectile tissue surrounded by a layer of circular smooth muscle which is continuous with the bladder musculature. The blood supply is derived from the inferior vesical, the middle vaginal, and the pudendal arteries.

ANOMALIES

Congenital absence of the bladder represents failure of development of the superior portion of the ventral cloaca. The ureters terminate in the vestibule of the vagina. Patients having this anomaly complain of infection and incontinence. Failure of complete embryonic obliteration of the distal ventral cloaca produces various urachal anomalies, from complete patency extending from the vertex of the bladder to the umbilicus to partial patency for a variable distance, resulting in a urachal cyst, sinus, or diverticulum. Complete duplication of the bladder and urethra and partial or complete sagittal or frontal bladder septa are very un-

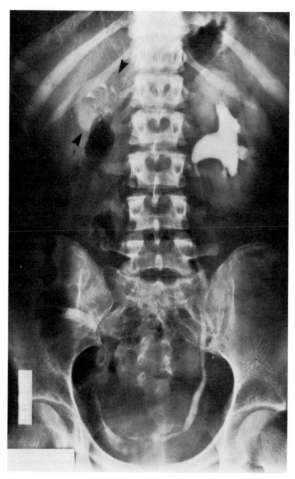

FIGURE 38–2 Intravenous pyelogram demonstrating right renal hypoplasia (arrows).

FIGURE 38–1 Intravenous pyelogram demonstrating right renal agenesis in a patient with the Rokitansky-Kuster-Hauser syndrome. A chain has been placed in the urinary bladder.

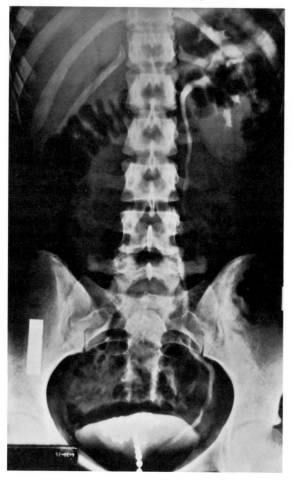

usual. These malformations are commonly associated with vertebral, anal, rectal, and genital malformations.

Among the most common developmental anomalies in women are malformations of the kidneys and ureters. Although patients are frequently asymptomatic, they may present symptoms as diverse as dyspareunia, hypertension, flank pain, abdominal pain, frequency or dysuria. These anomalies may be categorized as abnormalities of renal mass, duplication or position, with or without fusion.

Bilateral renal agenesis with pulmonary hypoplasia, hypertelorism, prominent epicanthal folds ending in a wide semicircle directed downward and then laterally under the lower lid, low-set ears, and nasal flattening and broadening (Potter's syndrome) occurs in 0.3 per 1000 births. Commonly the neonates are small for dates, present by breech, deliver prematurely, and are associated with oligohydramnios.

Unilateral renal agenesis is clinically diagnosed in about 1:1500 patients either when the solitary kidney is chronically infected due to (1) vesicoureteral reflux, (2) relative obstruction by a calculus, or (3) asymptomatic association with anomalous development of the Müllerian ducts. This agenesis may be present with a unicornuate uterus, a double uterus with a single cervix and a unilateral rudimentary, non-communicating, functioning, or nonfunctioning uterine horn, a completely duplicated uterus and vagina with unilateral hematocolpos, and the Rokitansky-Kuster-Hauser syndrome (Fig. 38-1). Ninety percent of patients with unilateral renal agenesis have anomalous Müllerian duct development.

Unilateral renal hypogenesis is commonly associated with hypertension. The diagnosis is made radiographically when the kidney is less than two-thirds normal size (Fig. 38-2). This may be due to a generalized decrease in numbers of nephrons or to segmental renal hypoplasia (Ask-Upmark kidney). In the latter syndrome, the hypoplastic renal segment is externally demarcated by a transverse groove; histologically, it demonstrates glomerular hyalinization and

renal tubular atrophy. Juxtaglomerular apparatus hyperplasia in the adjoining normal renal parenchyma is thought to be responsible for the increased renin activity in venous effluents from these kidneys. There is no increased association with Müllerian anomalies.

Ureteral duplications are the most common anomalies of the urinary tract (Fig. 38-3). Duplication of the ureters occurs in 0.6 percent of the population. It is complete in 33 percent of these, and bilateral in 16 percent. The solitary kidney with a double renal pelvis and variably duplicated ureter is usually asymptomatic but may be associated with pyelonephritis, hydronephrosis, or urinary incontinence. When it is completely duplicated, the ureter from the superior renal pelvis usually crosses under its duplicate and enters the bladder inferior to the entrance of the ureter from the lower renal pelvis. The vesical orifice of the lower pole ureter is frequently incompetent as a result of its short course through the bladder wall. The resulting vesicoureteral reflux causes pyelonephritis of the lower renal pole. The ureter that serves the upper pole may terminate ectopically in the vestibule, urethra, vagina, cervix, uterus, or rectum and can be associated with urinary incontinence and intermittent episodes of normal voiding. The ectopic

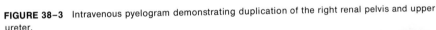

FIGURE 38-3 Intravenous pyelogram demonstrating duplication of the right renal pelvis and upper ureter.

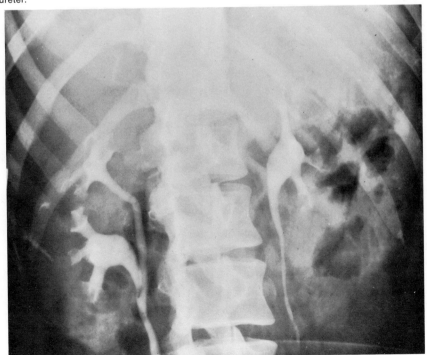

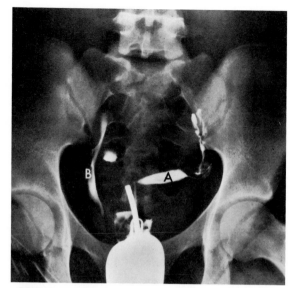

FIGURE 38–4 Hysterosalpingogram of a patient with right renal agenesis demonstrating a left unicornuate uterus (A) and a tubular structure (B) extending from the right cervix to the level of the first sacral vertebra. Histologic examination of the excised right tubular structure proved it to be a chronically infected, blind ending, ectopic ureter.

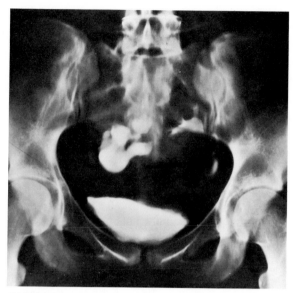

FIGURE 38–5 Intravenous pyelogram demonstrating fused pelvic kidneys.

FIGURE 38–6 Intravenous pyelogram demonstrating low lying, medially displaced kidneys with a horseshoe type of malrotation.

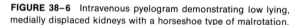

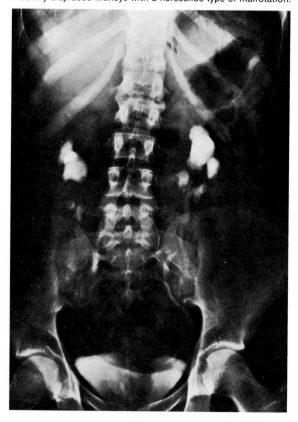

ureter (Fig. 38-4) is susceptible to distal obstruction, and half of these patients present with infection rather than with urinary incontinence.

Renal ectopia results from failure of the fetal kidney to ascend to its normal adult position and is commonly associated with renal fusion, malrotation, and anomalous vasculature. The fused pelvic kidney (lump, discoid, or cake kidney), an unusual anomaly consisting of an irregular fused mass of renal tissue in the pelvis, results from complete bilateral failure of renal ascent and rotation (Fig. 38-5). A horseshoe type of renal malformation results from union of the lower renal pole across the midline by an isthmus of renal parenchyma. Commonly there is an arrest of renal ascent and malrotation, although 40 percent of cases reach the normal adult position (Fig. 38-6). Unilateral renal ectopia or crossed renal ectopia (resulting in a final renal position contralateral to its ureteral origin) are further variations on the same theme. Although many of these anomalies are asymptomatic, their high frequency of association with Müllerian duct anomalies may lead to their detection. Their propensity to become relatively obstructed results in their diagnosis when hydronephrosis, calculi, or pyelonephritis develops. Renal ectopia must always be included in the differential diagnosis of a pelvic mass.

URINARY STASIS

Obstruction of the urinary tract may occur at any point from the renal tubules to the urethral meatus, and the causes range from neuromuscular dysfunction to simple blockage by precipitated drugs, calculi, blood clots, or a variety of gynecologic and urologic diseases. The obstruction is more often partial than absolute, in which case the process may remain symptomatically occult and the serious sequelae may appear quite late. It is therefore important that the possible impact of gynecologic pathology upon the flow of urine be recognized and that the diagnostic procedures which are necessary to evaluate the urinary tract be carried out prior to any attempts at management.

URETERS

As they enter the pelvis overlying the common iliac artery, the ureters are slightly elevated relative to their position above and below this point and are therefore vulnerable to compression or displacement by large tumors, particularly those arising in the pelvis. Uterine leiomyomata and ovarian cystic and solid tumors large enough to rise out of the pelvis may cause obstruction at this point. In the absence of associated tumor extension or inflammatory process, such obstruction is seldom complete. Prior to surgery for these diseases, the upper urinary tracts should be studied by intravenous pyelography to ensure exploration of the affected area.

In the third trimester of normal pregnancy, dilatation of the upper urinary tract on one or both sides is commonly present. This results chiefly from compression by the large uterus as noted above, with the additional component of reduction in the frequency and amplitude of ureteral contractions as a result of secretion of high levels of progesterone. A similar mild type of ureteral atony may be produced by the administration of potent progestational agents for contraception or other purposes.

Involvement of the ureters in pathologic processes at the midpelvic level is less common but is occasionally seen in cases of advanced pelvic inflammatory disease with large tuboovarian abscesses. The infection may be of the primary gonorrheal variety, a result of secondary invasion, or it may follow abortion; thus, a large variety of offending organisms may be involved. Under these circumstances, the ureter may be both compressed and functionally incapacitated as a result of direct invasion of the ureteral sheath and musculature by the organisms. Incomplete clearing of the infection or late fibrosis can cause permanent damage. Operations to relieve the condition may cause additional trauma to the ureters. In postabortal infections, when septic shock may supervene, the differential diagnosis between oliguria resulting from renal shutdown and oliguria resulting from ureteral obstruction can be confusing, and the correct solution may require invasive techniques such as ureteral catheterization.

Cases of ureteral obstruction caused by external endometriosis are sporadically reported, but this eventuality is extremely rare.

A variety of retroperitoneal conditions, most of them uncommon, can affect the pelvic ureter. These include retroperitoneal sarcomas, pseudocysts resulting from radical pelvic surgery, postoperative hematomas, dermoid cysts, lymphomas, and retroperitoneal fibrosis, a disease of uncertain etiology which occasionally follows pelvic irradiation. The presence of any pelvic retroperitoneal mass is an indication for intravenous pyelography.

At its terminal portion, the ureter runs close to the lateral wall of the cervix; just before it enters the bladder, it ducks under the uterine vessels at a distance not more than 2 cm from the endopelvic fascia covering the cervix. This proximity, plus the fact that rich lymphatics follow the vascular channels and envelop the ureter at this point, make it susceptible to the spread of carcinoma of the cervix, carcinoma of the endometrium and ovary to a lesser extent, and also to the injurious effects of ionizing irradiation and surgery used in the treatment of these conditions. For all gynecologic malignancies, the pretreatment evaluation must therefore include intravenous pyelography and cystoscopy; posttreatment follow-up entails the use of these same diagnostic procedures to assess possible injury, treatment failure, or recurrent disease. The presence of hydroureter and hydronephrosis prior to treatment indicates a very poor prognosis. If such a condition is noted for the first time immediately following treatment, it suggests injury; late occurrence usually signifies recurrent disease. Most often the obstruction is in the terminal or isthmic portion of the ureter, but, rarely, enlarged lymph nodes from tumor spread may block the ureter as high as the ureteropelvic junction.

Late carcinomas of the vulva and vagina sometimes behave like cervical carcinomas in obstructing the lower ureters. Carcinomas of the endometrium and ovary may behave similarly but more often involve lymphatic pathways higher in the pelvis, where they are less likely to obstruct.

As has been noted, irradiation may produce fibrosis which may not appear for months or years after the completion of treatment. This type of ureteral entrapment is permanent and must be treated by surgical bypass or diversion. Radical surgery denervates the ureter and deprives it of its blood supply, either of which may cause loss of normal function, stricture, or fistula formation. These conditions must also be treated by appropriate surgical intervention.

Angulation, with resulting partial obstruction of the lower ureters, has been shown to occur in severe forms of uterine prolapse and of cystocele. If these conditions are associated with severe urinary tract infection, which in itself can inhibit ureteral peristalsis, the effect may be considerably more severe.

Simple surgical trauma to the ureters at any point may cause partial or complete urinary obstruction. The most likely points of injury are just below the pelvic brim where the infundibulopelvic ligament containing the ovarian vasculature is clamped or in the lowermost portion of the ureter where the cardinal ligament and the vaginal branches of the uterine vessels must be ligated during hysterectomy. Appropriate steps at the time of operation to avoid these eventualities include ligature of the ovarian vessels as close to the ovary as possible, identification of the ureter below the point of ligature, and the use of an intracapsular approach to the enucleation of the cervix. This involves splitting the endopelvic fascia and clamping the supporting structures inside its envelope. Identification of the ureter below the point of ligature is considered good technique. Such operations are not designed for the removal of malignant disease when greater surgical risks must be accepted to secure a wide margin of safety.

Total occlusion of the ureter by clamp or ligature, unnoticed at the time of surgery, has variable manifestations postoperatively. If uninfected, the kidney may die quietly in the face of acute obstruction, but it may subsequently become infected as a result of bacteremia in later life. If infected at the time of surgery, pyelonephritis and abscess may develop, and immediate intervention may be necessary. Occasionally, the damaged ureter may reopen spontaneously. If the occlusion is partial, the initial effect may be polyuria rather than oliguria. Pyelographic evidence will indicate the extent of the damage and the resulting hydronephrosis. Ureterovaginal fistula may occur, just above the point of obstruction, or there may rarely be an extravasation of urine intra- or retroperitoneally. With partial obstruction untreated, pyelonephritis is almost certain to occur, and the patient will have back pain and tenderness, intestinal ileus, and chills and fever. Early retrograde catheterization of the affected side may be attempted, but open surgical correction is delayed until the patient's condition is stable and the tissues surrounding the injury in good enough condition to permit reanastomosis. In acute instances when the life of the kidney is in danger, temporary diversion by nephrostomy or ureterostomy is indicated. The former can often be accomplished by percutaneous catheterization of the renal pelvis using ultrasonic localization.

BLADDER

Bladder stasis is more often functional than mechanical, although large stones, clots, and debris may block the outflow of urine at the urethrovesical junction. Functional obstruction occurs on a neurologic basis and may be congenital or due to disease or injury. It is an adynamic condition analogous to intestinal ileus. Bladder incapacity of this type is due to defects in innervation either in the bladder wall, the reflex arc, or the centers in the spinal cord. Motor loss as a result of damage to the anterior horn cells of the second, third, and fourth sacral parasympathetic fibers can be caused by a variety of neurologic diseases. Multiple sclerosis is the most common. Neoplasms and trauma, particularly extensive pelvic operations which strip the pelvic nerves as they pass along the posterolateral walls, are also etiologically responsible. Sensory nerve pathways may also be damaged by surgery and by disease, especially diabetes mellitus. In both of these situations, the bladder fails to exert the necessary propulsive effort, in the one case because of lack of power, and in the other because of lack of ability to recognize the need. The bladder becomes overdistended and may attain a very high volume unless appropriate measures are taken to relieve it. Overstretching of the bladder muscle has the secondary effect of damaging its intrinsic nerve supply and compounding the problem. Even though these conditions are often associated with pelvic symptoms including pain and pressure, the possible presence of a pelvic mass due to the distended bladder and the likelihood of overflow or paradoxical incontinence (which must be differentiated from other types of incontinence) make it desirable that their management be in the hands of the neurologist and urologist. The gynecologist must be prepared to recognize the problems.

Retention of urine at the bladder level may also

follow surgical procedures on the vulva, vagina, perineum, and anus. Usually the cause is muscular spasm of the levator ani and superficial perineal muscles as a result of pain following the procedure. Anterior vaginal colporrhaphies and plications of the vesical sphincter for urinary incontinence are commonly thought to occlude the vesical neck because of postoperative edema or the narrowing of the urethrovesical junction by sutures. Postoperative calibration of this area, however usually shows this not to be the case; the problem is more likely to be psychogenic or a result of pain when pelvic musculature is in spasm and intraabdominal pressure is increased.

Judicious use of the catheter to avoid overdistention and consequent damage to the intrinsic nervous system is an essential part of the management of patients with bladder retention. Depending upon the situation, either long-term straight drainage or tidal drainage should be used in attempting to reeducate the bladder. Scheduled intermittent catheterizations are considered by some observers to cause less infection than long-term drainage. If the latter is indicated, suprapubic insertion of an indwelling catheter is probably associated with less infection than the transurethral method.

Occasionally, a large tumor may become impacted in the posterior pelvis and cause obstruction by wedging itself under the urethrovesical junction. This seldom occurs acutely, and by the time the patient discovers she is unable to empty her bladder completely, it may be greatly overdistended. If reflux is present, there may be hydroureter and hydronephrosis. Reflux is a poorly understood condition which is thought to involve dysfunction of the ureterovesical valves allowing retrograde voiding up the ureters. The long-term effects include pyelonephritis and renal scarring. The condition may be present when there is severe back pressure within the bladder but also when there is no obvious stasis.

URETHRA

The urethra seldom suffers complete obstruction. As in the case of the bladder, tumors in the posterior pelvis pressing it against the undersurface of the pubis may cause intermittent or sudden occlusion. Diaphragms and pessaries improperly positioned in the vagina may cause similar difficulty. In the very young or in the mentally defective, the possibility of an intraurethral foreign body must be kept in mind when sudden anuria occurs.

In the past, strictures of the urethra caused by infections such as gonorrhea were quite common in the male but less so in the female. Such strictures rarely occur today as a result of infection, but may be seen following operative procedures such as meatotomy, excision of diverticula, and urethral plications. Once strictures have occurred, they do not lend themselves readily to subsequent surgical management. Further operations in the same area tend to make the situation worse. Repeated dilatations over a long period of time are usually necessary. The injection of corticosteroids directly into the stricture site has been advocated, but its efficacy has not been definitely substantiated.

Congenital obstructions caused by heaped-up folds of mucosa in the posterior aspect of the vesical neck have been termed "congenital obstructions" in female children and some adults. When stasis has been associated, these obstructions have been treated urologically by transurethral resection. This procedure carries with it the very grave hazard of causing permanent urinary incontinence and should be reserved only for extreme cases where definite obstruction can be proved.

Eversion of the urethral mucosa at the meatus is a rather common occurrence, particularly in the elderly. The most likely cause is relaxation in the tone of the external urethral sphincter and of the endopelvic fascia supporting the urethra. Such eversions are usually asymptomatic, do not result in obstruction, and only occasionally cause slight sensitivity. The exposure of the urethral mucosa to the outside, however, not infrequently results in the development of granulation tissue, producing little red polyps which are often referred to as caruncles. These may cause some contact bleeding which may be confused with vaginal bleeding but otherwise are generally asymptomatic. Attempts to treat these lesions by resection or fulguration must be reserved for those cases with definite symptoms. The operations are often unsuccessful and have as a complication a high rate of stricture formation.

Malignant tumors of the urethra are usually classified with tumors of the vulva since they are most often composed of squamous epithelium and are exophytic. They are obstructive, and in preparation for surgical or irradiation treatment it may be necessary to divert the urinary stream. Small benign tumors such as papillomata may occur in the urethral lumen, and there are rare tumors of the urethral wall or cysts of Skene's glands which interfere with micturition. All of these lesions are readily palpable at the time of bimanual examination or can be observed with either the water or carbon dioxide urethroscope.

URINARY INFECTIONS

Although there are a number of mechanisms which serve to protect the urinary tract from infection, the most important is its ability continually to expel urine from the system. Washing out bacteria and other organisms which may have gained entrance is the mechanism of primary importance. Stasis is, therefore, one of the most common causes of urinary infections, especially those that are persistent or recurrent. In order to prevent such infections or combat those which have already occurred, means must be found to eliminate or modify the obstructive conditions discussed in the preceding section. There are other nonpathologic causes of stasis which must be sought in the history. These include voluntarily refraining from emptying the bladder because of embarrassment, lack of facilities, and psychogenic retention. Patients with recurrent urinary infections and women seeking preventive health care should be encouraged to void at regular intervals. Those under treatment for infection should be instructed to arise once during the night to empty their bladders. The chronic use of tranquilizing and narcoleptic drugs, particularly in the high doses used in treating the mentally ill, causes urinary stasis of such a marked degree that it can be demonstrated pyelographically. Should such drugs have to be continued, suppressive antibacterial medication may be necessary. Allusion has been made to the possible static effect of high doses of progestational agents on the urinary tract. Some clinical observations have suggested a higher incidence, and a lower cure rate, of urinary infections in patients taking these drugs. The possible depressing effect of progestins on other host-defense mechanisms, such as macrophage activity, has also been considered. A cause-and-effect relationship between oral contraceptives and urinary infections has not been substantiated nor has the pathophysiologic basis for such an observation been clarified.

As in the case of infections elsewhere, urinary infections may occur as an effect of lowered resistance. This is true in the prepubertal and postmenopausal age groups and in individuals with debilitating medical diseases or those who have been receiving immunosuppressant drugs. In youth and old age, the common factor is the lack of estrogen, which matures and keratinizes the epithelium of the lower urinary tract as it does in the vagina. It maintains the local pH on the acid side, which helps to resist the inroads of pathogenic bacteria.

TRAUMA AND LOCAL DISEASE

Trauma is another important factor predisposing to urinary tract infections. Because of the close anatomic apposition of the vagina and the lower urinary tract and the interlocking network of vascular and lymphatic channels, many women have episodes of urinary infection following coitus. This is especially true of nulliparous individuals whose vaginal supports have not been stretched by childbirth. The use of vaginal tampons, pessaries, diaphragms, and other foreign bodies over a long period of time not only can give rise to infection but may also prevent effective treatment. Even bimanual examinations have been shown to cause bacteriuria. If the urethra is milked to demonstrate infection in the course of such an examination, bacteriuria may be expected within 24 hours in over 30 percent of the cases.

Injury due to surgical procedures, particularly those involving prolonged or frequent catheterizations, is likely to cause infection. Following abdominal or vaginal hysterectomy, and particularly after anterior colporrhaphy, the base of the bladder becomes congested and the mucosa shows erythema and occasionally gross hemorrhage. A catheter indwelling for more than 24 hours allows bacteria to reach this excellent culture medium in over 50 percent of patients. The same result occurs after 72 hours in over 90 percent of patients. Routine postoperative urine cultures are likely to show bacteriuria in 25 percent of the cases; following removal of a catheter which has been used for more than 5 days, bacteriuria is found in 80 percent. In most instances, the bacteriuria is washed out when normal voiding is resumed; in only 2 percent of the cases does it persist long-term. However, patients who have had pelvic surgery or who have had indwelling catheters for long periods of time should have urine cultures at intervals of 6 months to a year as a precaution.

Because of its short, 3- to 4.5-cm length, its anatomic position, the surrounding racemose glands of Skene which empty into it at several points, and a combination of poor hygiene and the fact that its meatus is constantly bathed in discharges coming from the vagina, vulva, and rectum, the urethra, as well as the lower urinary tract, is susceptible to sequences of local infection. Cervicitis and vaginitis must be treated to prevent urinary infections and to clear up those that exist. Patients must be taught to keep the vulvar area clean and to avoid wiping fecal matter toward the urethra.

LOCAL ANATOMY

Marked degrees of uterine descent or prolapse which often tend to carry the bladder downward also cause gradual bladder decompensation. Unable to function normally because of its disadvantaged position, the bladder first develops muscular hypertrophy. The latter condition is recognized cystoscopically as trabeculations bulging beneath the mucosa. Later, inability to empty produces stasis, infection, and even overflow incontinence. The patient may compensate by manually replacing the uterus and potentiating bladder action. However, the condition should not be allowed to persist. The healthy patient can be successfully treated by vaginal hysterectomy and repair of the pelvic floor. The elderly and those with medical conditions precluding surgery may be fitted with a pessary or some occluding device. The extended use of such foreign bodies increases the risk of infection, and they must be cleaned, inspected, and replaced monthly.

Cystoceles per se, even of large size, are seldom the reservoirs of residual urine they have been considered to be, nor are they more likely to be associated with a greater risk of infection. The latter becomes a problem if the anatomic defect is subjected to repair and an indwelling catheter is present. Repair of cystocele to eliminate recurrent urinary infections is unlikely to be successful. If the bladder protrudes beyond the introitus, of course, repair may be necessary to avoid local discomfort, difficulty starting the urinary stream, and injury to the vaginal mucosa.

DIAGNOSTIC TECHNIQUES

In gynecologic practice, urine cultures should be obtained routinely on patients (1) entering the hospital for surgical procedures, (2) prior to discharge, (3) on the first postoperative visit, and (4) at the time of yearly checkups. Urine cultures are done by the clean-catch technique which has only a 5 percent false-positive result if two consecutive specimens indicate bacteriuria with a colony count in excess of 100,000 organisms per milliliter. In addition to routine studies, urine cultures are done when symptoms of urgency, frequency, nocturia, pressure, hematuria, or pyuria suggest the presence of an infection. It is often advisable to treat a patient with any of the above symptoms before waiting for the culture report. The office use of dipsticks, slide tests, microscopic examination of urine sediment for leukocyte clumps,

and the examination of a gram-stained drop of unspun urine are all helpful in confirming the diagnosis since they correlate well with cultures.

In recurrent infections, lower colony counts are sometimes noted because the patient has been under treatment with antibacterial drugs and has been emptying her bladder more frequently. The persistence of the organism in these lower dilutions, however, should suggest that additional treatment is necessary.

Urinary infections encountered by the gynecologist most often involve the lower urinary tract. Because of the likelihood of ascent or descent of the organisms in the urinary stream or through vascular and lymphatic pathways, the possibility of a persistent focus of infection in the renal parenchyma must be kept in mind. In the acute phase, renal infections are associated with flank pain, general malaise, and fever; these symptoms are very uncommon in lower urinary tract infections. In the chronic stage, pyelonephritis may be completely asymptomatic. The introduction of immunofluorescence for detecting antibody-coated bacteria in urinary sediment complexes, which form only in the upper urinary tract, has made it possible to differentiate between the two locales without invasive instrumentation.

In women, the offending organism is *Escherichia coli* in 95 percent of lower urinary tract infections, although different serotypes may be present at the time of recurrence. The presence of other organisms such as *Proteus mirabilis* or enterococcus is usually associated with some obstructive uropathy or is a product of inadequate therapy resulting in the emergence of resistant strains.

The recurrence of lower urinary tract infections at frequent intervals in spite of all attempts to treat appropriately and to eliminate predisposing factors is an indication for more complete evaluation. More than two such recurrences should lead to intravenous pyelography, cystoscopy, and when neurologic problems are suspected, to cystometric studies. Some doubt has recently been cast on the need for intensive investigation of recurrent lower tract infections because of the low yield of positive findings. Some modification of this precept may be in order, but failure to diagnose obstructive uropathy can have serious consequences for patient and physician. When upper urinary tract involvement is suspected, serum creatinine, creatinine clearance, and blood urea nitrogen should be requested. In patients allergic to the intravenous injection of radiopaque material and when an invasive procedure like retrograde pyelography is contraindicated, ultrasonograms are helpful in diagnosing the presence or absence of dilatation of the upper urinary tract. The latter technique can also be useful in determining bladder overfilling and the presence of residual urine after voiding.

URETHROTRIGONITIS (THE URETHRAL SYNDROME)

A common type of inflammation, usually not referred to as an infection because specific etiologic organisms have not been identified, occurs in the lower urinary tract and often gives rise to symptoms similar to those of verified bacterial infection. The patient complains of urgency, often very severe, a feeling of pressure even when the bladder is virtually empty, and a desire to void again immediately upon completion of micturition. Usually the patient is otherwise well. Often she is elderly, and repeated cultures are usually negative. Sometimes the urgency is so severe that it leads to the loss of a few drops of urine (urgency incontinence), which may be followed by some burning. Cystoscopic examination shows erythema which characteristically involves the area of the trigone and proximal urethra. Vascular dilatation may be present locally or throughout the bladder mucosa. White patches indicative of squamous metaplasia may be scattered about the trigone. Occasionally, some white, filmy exudate is seen in the region of the internal sphincter. The sphincter closes readily over the end of the cystoscope as it is withdrawn, but during the procedure, the patient has a constant desire to void, even with only a small volume of water in the bladder. A cystometrogram often shows fluctuations in detrusor activity indicating frequent involuntary contractions. This condition, sometimes in a more generalized form, is often seen in patients with so-called detrusor dyssynergia, those who have incontinence as a result of involuntary voiding, suggesting the possibility that the two conditions may be related. It seems likely that this syndrome is due to specific infectious organisms which have not yet been identified. Recent studies implicating *Chlamydia trachomatis* as one of the causes of nonspecific urethritis in males and their conclusion that such urethritis is venereally contracted suggest that these organisms are active in the female genitourinary tract also. Current routine culture techniques do not attempt to make this diagnosis nor do they identify *Mycoplasma,* viruses, or a host of other agents. Until this diagnosis can be clarified and accurately established, many women will continue to suffer from this benign but incapacitating condition.

MANAGEMENT OF URINARY INFECTIONS

For the first episode of lower urinary tract infection, antibacterial sensitivity studies are not indicated. As noted above, *E. coli* is responsible in the vast majority of cases, and it is sensitive to a variety of antibacterial drugs of which the most commonly used are sulfasoxazole and ampicillin. In the case of the sulfonamide, 2 to 4 g are given daily in divided doses over a period of 10 days. Ampicillin is given in 250-mg doses, four times daily for 10 days. During this time the patient is requested to force fluids and to void frequently. The importance of continuing the drugs well past the time when the patient becomes asymptomatic must be emphasized in order to prevent recurrences. Patients with known upper urinary tract infections must be treated vigorously for much longer periods of time and, unless there is an associated gynecologic problem which needs to be treated, should be under the control of an internist. At the onset of symptoms, patients with upper urinary tract infections should be hospitalized.

When recurrent urinary infections develop, sensitivity studies should be done and the appropriate drug chosen on this basis. If the secondary infection is thought to be a relapse, i.e., persistent infection with the same organism, a period of treatment up to 1 month is indicated. Because of rapid bacterial adaptation to sulfonamides, a drug such as nitrofurantoin is useful for secondary infections. A considerable number of individuals continue to have recurrences in the absence of renal involvement or recognizable predisposing causes. The management problem is sometimes made difficult because of the logistics of obtaining cultures and medical advice on short notice. Those whose problem seems related to coitus should be told to take the drug of choice at a low dosage level prophylactically for 24 hours, or for 24 hours immediately following coitus. In this way, many can control their transient bacteriuria and resulting symptoms. Long-term acidification of the urine by diet and the use of cranberry juice is sometimes helpful, the latter being excreted in the urine as hippuric acid.

Patients who have had gynecologic surgery and whose culture is positive at the time of discharge from the hospital should be treated with a sulfonamide or ampicillin as noted above. Patients with indwelling catheters are not treated until the catheter is removed since the suppression of bacteria which enter the bladder as a result of the catheter is temporary and resistant strains may emerge.

Urethrotrigonitis has no specific treatment other

than attempting to eliminate local infections and improve local hygiene. In patients lacking estrogen, the vaginal application of estrogenic creams or the use of oral estrogen is likely to be beneficial. Instrumentation or operations designed to dilate or enlarge the urethra are not helpful and are actually dangerous in that they may cause superimposed infection or incontinence. Urethral suppositories and intraurethral and intravesical topical applications of caustic drugs are similarly ineffective. Empirical use of tetracycline, effective against *Mycoplasma* and *Chlamydia,* may be considered, but the patient must be given concomitant treatment with antimonilial drugs to prevent vaginal infection with *Candida albicans.*

RADIATION CYSTITIS

During radiation treatment for malignant disease in the pelvis, which usually entails the delivery of 4000 to 6000 rads to the total pelvis, the bladder receives a full share of the dose and can usually sustain this without permanent damage. During treatment, the bladder becomes edematous and erythematous, both of which promote infection. However, symptoms are usually transient and, if the infection is properly treated, no long-term difficulty results. An occasional late effect of irradiation upon the bladder is the development of fibrosis in the bladder wall which interferes with normal function. In combination with the appearance of telangiectases in the bladder mucosa, these effects predispose to infection and cause hemorrhages which can be very severe. In its most severe form, this condition results in a contracted, nonfunctional bladder, and some type of urinary diversion and even cystectomy may be necessary. In the less severe forms, infection may require long-term antibacterial medication and palliative drugs to reduce bladder spasm and pain.

URINARY INCONTINENCE

In the gynecologic patient, the most common application of the term "urinary incontinence" is stress incontinence, which is defined as involuntary loss of urine following increase in intraabdominal pressure. Unfortunately, this simplistic definition and the implication that proper management consists merely of an adjustment at the point of outflow, like shutting off a garden hose by twisting the nozzle, has led to a great

deal of unnecessary or inappropriate surgery. Stress incontinence is a functional derangement of the apparatus of normal micturition and may bear no relationship to the anatomy noted at the time of physical examination. In addition, there are other types of partial incontinence which may be independent of, or associated with, stress but which must be excluded by proper diagnostic techniques prior to treatment.

Initiation of normal micturition depends upon a smoothly occurring sequence of events. As the bladder dilates with an increasing volume of urine, sensory proprioceptive nerve endings in the bladder wall transmit the sensation to the sacral spinal cord. In the newborn, the elderly, and occasionally in those who suffer from severe mental illness or brain trauma, the reciprocal motor impulse travels directly back without cortical control, initiating detrusor contraction and causing so-called reflex voiding. In mature normal individuals, the impulses denoting bladder filling pass upward through the posterior columns of the spinal cord to centers in the thalamus and cerebral cortex. The perception of fullness is relayed to the corticoregulatory centers in the motor cortex which are able to maintain the reflex arc of the bladder in a state of inhibition. If the individual desires to void, the reflex arc can be relieved of this inhibition and detrusor action can begin. By another voluntary action initiated in the motor cortex and traveling to striated muscles through the pudendal nerves, the muscular supports of the pelvic diaphragm, including principally the levator ani muscles, are relaxed, allowing the bladder neck to drop downward slightly. The external sphincter muscle, by contracting, assists in shortening the urethra and pulling open its proximal and midportions. At the same time, the diaphragm is usually set by a short inspiration, thus slightly increasing intraabdominal pressure. Detrusor contraction, beginning in the region of the trigone, passes simultaneously upward over the dome of the bladder and downward to the midportion of the urethra. The resulting involuntary contraction of this continuous sheath of interlocking muscle fibers causes reduction in bladder volume, propelling urine toward the outlet. At the same time, it pulls open the urethrovesical junction and the proximal urethra. Both of these structures together form the controlling so-called sphincter mechanism, converting the lower bladder and proximal urethra into a funnel. The bladder rotates slightly forward toward the pubis, and the net result is optimal contracting force against minimal resistance. As the bladder is emptied and the contraction subsides, normal resting relationships are gradually resumed. It has been noted that many types of pathology, both in the ancillary participating structures and in the end organ, can produce dysfunction in this complicated mechanism. The net effect sometimes results in obstruction, or in incontinence, and sometimes in a combination of the two.

Prolonged partial obstruction of the outflow of urine, whether on a functional or an anatomic basis, leads to overflow or paradoxical incontinence. Small voidings occur while the bladder retains a large volume of residual urine. Retention leads to infection, and the resulting frequency and urgency complicate the picture. Sudden increases in intraabdominal pressure, as by coughing and sneezing, may cause the expulsion of small quantities of urine and point toward a diagnosis of stress incontinence. The proper diagnosis is made by cystometry. Many types of cystometers are in use, but the easiest and least expensive is a simple water drip which permits the filling of the bladder at a measured rate. The pressure in the bladder is recorded through another channel in the catheter on a manometer which is fixed to the same stand as the drip bottle and placed so that the zero mark is on a level with the patient's bladder. The curve of gradually increasing bladder pressure together with the patient's expressed sensation, including first desire to void and feeling of fullness, can be identified as normal or pathologic. Using this technique, bladder innervation and muscular action can be further tested by a stress test using bethanechol chloride (Urecholine) to increase expulsive forces, or a parasympatholytic drug like propantheline bromide (Pro-Banthine) to reduce involuntary contractions and spasms. These techniques are essential to exclude neurologic problems in the diagnosis and management of urinary incontinence and to suggest possible medical regimens for relief.

DETRUSOR DYSSYNERGIA

Another common form of urinary incontinence, often causing complete involuntary bladder emptying, is due to inappropriate and often violent detrusor contractions. It is possible that in some instances these contractions stem from incomplete inhibition at the cortical level. However, the occurrence of the condition after operations for stress urinary incontinence and in association with bladder inflammation and the urethral syndrome suggests that local factors are more often at fault. Cystoscopy and cystometry are both helpful in the diagnosis. Parasympatholytic drugs offer the best chance of control, but the results to date have been only moderately encouraging.

STRESS INCONTINENCE

The patient who states that she loses urine by coughing, sneezing, straining, walking, laughing, or performing any exercise that increases intraabdominal pressure, and in whom the involuntary expulsion of urine may be observed either in the lithotomy position or standing when asked to strain on a full bladder, may be said to have stress incontinence. As has been noted, the condition is often complicated by associated urgency and may therefore have two components which require independent treatment. The infection is always treated first, if this is possible. The stress factor may then become less prominent. Sphincter action occurs in a more normal way and the bladder is less likely to be reflexly triggered.

In making the differential diagnosis, the history is of utmost importance. The patient must be closely questioned regarding (1) frequency of occurrence, (2) severity of leakage, (3) sensation of discomfort, (4) degree of control, and (5) tolerance of the symptoms. Many women have varying degrees of stress incontinence, urgency, and urgency incontinence from time to time without significant interference with their lives. Such individuals are subjects for corrective advice and appropriate drugs but not for corrective surgery. Apart from the local anatomy, other conditions which, by increasing intraabdominal pressure, can lead to stress urinary incontinence include marked obesity, especially when there is a heavy abdominal panniculus, the wearing of tight constricting garments such as corsets or back braces, chronic heavy cough due to smoking or bronchial asthma, occupations and household activities requiring heavy lifting, and strenuous athletics. Alleviation of these conditions by proper counseling can be helpful in treating the incontinent patient.

Pure stress urinary incontinence is classically supposed to be determined by relaxation of the bladder neck as a result of birth injury and the muscular stretching associated with aging. This relaxation allows the bladder neck and proximal urethra to drop away from the undersurface of the pubis, resulting in the loss of the so-called posterior urethrovesical angle. Anatomically, this is perceived by physical examination as a bulging of the anterior vaginal wall toward the introitus. This loss of support and gradual stretching make it difficult for the detrusor to maintain sufficient inhibitory tone to prevent wedges of urine from entering the proximal urethra when sudden pressure is applied from above. Also, by lowering, the bladder neck is brought into more direct alignment with the intraabdominal forces. Continence requires that the proximal urethra maintain a higher differential pressure than the lower bladder, and this relationship is lost as the supporting structures give way. Compensatory voluntary action by the levator ani muscles and, to a lesser extent, by the external urethral sphincter sometimes serves to offset this pathologic imbalance and thus constitutes the basis for the prescription of exercises (Kegel) designed to strengthen the voluntary musculature and restore relative or complete continence. In many instances such exercises, intended to elevate the pelvic floor and strengthen the pubococcygeal muscles, are effective in rehabilitating patients with minor degrees of stress urinary incontinence.

Differing categorizations of stress urinary incontinence have been developed in an attempt to define varying degrees of anatomic disruption and to correlate each of these with an appropriate surgical repair. The categories are determined not so much by physical examination as by x-ray studies designed to show the relationship of bladder and urethra in the resting state and under stress. Cystograms in the anterior/posterior and lateral views and voiding cinefluoroscopy have been used for this purpose. With the aid of differential urethral and bladder pressure studies, the voiding hydrodynamics of the affected patient can be precisely calculated. In spite of these advances, the surgical cure rate for afflicted individuals has not improved significantly during the past generation. Women with no defect that can be determined either by physical examination or by x-ray and laboratory studies may have stress incontinence, and those with obvious abnormalities may be continent. The latter include those with large cystoceles and relatively well-supported urethras. In such situations, vaginal plastic repair may produce stress incontinence when none existed before.

Over many years, a large number of surgical procedures have been developed to correct stress urinary incontinence. Some advocate a vaginal approach while some favor the suprapubic. The general principle involved is restoration of the proximal urethra and bladder neck to a normal position within the pelvis, restoring the normal pressure balance, and elongating the urethra. This must be done without undue constriction of the urethra and bladder neck and without interfering with the detrusor activity so essential for normal micturition. The proximal urethra and bladder neck must rest on a muscular platform which is firm but not restrictive. Marked constriction may seem to alleviate the symptoms for short periods of time, but over the long run may lead to obstruction, infection, and inappropriate detrusor activity.

The 5-year cure rate for reasonable operations for stress urinary incontinence approximates 80 percent. Failures may be due to faulty technique but more often to inappropriate selection of patients for surgery. Recurrent stress urinary incontinence is more difficult to evaluate and to correct since it is often complicated by infection and detrusor dyssynergia. Repeat operations are less likely to be successful since more rigid scar tissue has been laid down and more intrinsic nerve damage has been done.

DIVERTICULA AND FISTULAS

Urethral diverticula are a not uncommon cause of urinary incontinence and also of urgency and recurrent urinary infection. They may be congenital, but more often they are caused by trauma or infection in the paraurethral tissues or in Skene's glands. They may be single or multiple and, if large, are palpable externally. Often they are infected, and pressure beneath them will cause the extrusion of purulent material from the urethral meatus. When they are occult, they can be diagnosed by urethroscopy, the entrance into the urethral lumen usually being easily visible. A urethrogram performed by occluding the vesical neck and the urethral meatus simultaneously and injecting dye directly into the urethra will outline the sac. The patient's symptoms are frequency, urgency, and dribbling of urine, especially when she rises from voiding. Recurrent lower urinary infections are common. The treatment is excision.

Total urinary incontinence occurs when there is diversion of urine from the normal passage into the vagina, uterus, or rectum as a result of injury or disease affecting the ureters or bladder base. The late stages of carcinomas of the cervix, vagina, and bladder may produce a breakdown of the adjacent vesicovaginal tissues. Irradiation designed to treat these conditions may produce the same result. Under these circumstances, urinary diversion at a higher level is usually necessary.

Injuries to the ureters and to the bladder occur as a result of accidents or as complications of gynecologic surgery. The inadvertent application of crushing clamps, cutting instruments, or ligatures directly to the organs or in such a manner as to damage their blood supply may cause extravasation of urine, and if the uterus has been removed concomitantly, the urine usually descends to the sutured cuff of the vagina. These injuries are more likely to occur when difficult or radical surgery is performed, necessitating careful dissection close to the ureters or bladder base. When cesarean section is done, especially repeat section when the attenuated bladder wall must be dissected from the cervix and subsequently refastened to the anterior wall of the uterus, a vesicouterine fistula may develop in a very small proportion of cases.

Possible injuries should be recognized and corrected at the time of surgery. If they are not, fistulas may develop within the first few hours postoperatively or may not appear for as long as 6 weeks. The patient immediately becomes aware of the problem when it occurs and her concern should lead to immediate action. If the urethral or suprapubic catheter has been removed, it should be replaced at once, since smaller fistulas may close spontaneously when the bladder is placed at rest. A trial of 1 week will provide the answer. When constant urinary incontinence persists in spite of drainage, the upper urinary tract must be evaluated by pyelography to ascertain whether the ureters have been damaged. The differential diagnosis between ureterovaginal and vesicovaginal fistulas can be made by instilling dye directly into the bladder and noting extravasation on a vaginal sponge. If this test is negative, and the intravenous injection of dye produces colored vaginal drainage, it is obvious that the ureter is involved. In either case surgical repair is indicated, preferably immediately, or in the event of infection or the poor condition of the patient, at a time when both the patient and her tissues are in good condition. If ureteral damage threatens the existence of one or both kidneys and immediate repair cannot be undertaken, urinary diversion above the point of injury is indicated.

REFERENCES

Benjamin J et al.: Urethral diverticulum in the adult female. *Urology* 3:1, 1974.

Corliss CE: The urogenital system, in *Human Embryology: Elements of Clinical Development,* ed. B Patten, 1st ed., New York: McGraw-Hill, 1976, pp. 342–388.

Dees JE: Prognosis of the solitary kidney. *Urology* 83:550–552, 1960.

Delson B: Ectopic kidney in obstetrics and gynecology. *NY State J Med* 75:2522–2526, 1975.

DiSaia PJ et al.: *Synopsis of Gynecologic Oncology,* New York: Wiley, 1975.

Everett HS, Ridley JH: *Female Urology,* New York: Harper & Row, 1968.

Fallon B, Culp DA: The urologic examination, in *Gynecologic and Obstetric Urology,* 1st ed., eds. HJ Buehsbaum, JD Schmidt, Philadelphia: Saunders, 1966, pp. 51–70.

Farber M, Mitchell GW: Anomalies of the kidneys and ureters. *Clin Obstet Gynecol* 21:831–43, 1978.

Gleason et al.: Urethral compliance and its role in female voiding dysfunctions. *Invest Urol* 2:2, 1973.

Goss CM: The urogenital system, in *Gray's Anatomy,* 28th ed., Philadelphia: Lea & Febiger, 1966, pp. 1265–1298.

Gray SW, Skandalakis JE: The kidney and ureter, in *Embryology for Surgeons: The Embryological Basis for the Treatment of Congenital Defects,* 1st ed., Philadelphia: Saunders, 1972, pp. 443–518.

Green FH: The problem of urinary stress incontinence in the female. *Obstet Gynecol Surv* 23:7, 1968.

Hodgkinson CP, Doub HP: Roentgen study of urethrovesical relationships in female urinary stress incontinence. *Radiology* 61:335, 1953.

Jones SR et al.: Localization of urinary tract infections by detection of antibody-coated bacteria in urinary sediment. *N Engl J Med* 290:591, 1974.

Kass EH (ed.) et al.: The significance of bacteriuria in preventive medicine, in *Progress in Pyelonephritis,* Philadelphia: F. A. Davis, 1964.

Kraft JK et al.: The natural history of symptomatic recurrent bacteriuria in women. *Medicine* 56:55, 1977.

Kunin CM: *Detection, Prevention and Management of Urinary Tract Infections,* Philadelphia: Lea & Febiger, 1972.

Lapides J: Symposium on neurogenic bladder. *Urol Clin North Am* 1:1, 1974.

Long JP, Montgomery JB: The incidence of ureteral obstruction in benign and malignant gynecologic lesions. *Am J Obstet Gynecol* 59:552, 1950.

Marchant DJ et al.: The urinary tract in pregnancy. *Clin Obstet Gynecol* 21:3, 1978.

Marshall JR, Judd GE: Guide for the management of women with symptoms arising in the lower urinary tract. *Clin Obstet Gynecol* 19:247, 1976.

Potter EL: Facial characteristics of infants with bilateral renal agenesis. *Am J Obstet Gynecol* 51:885–888, 1946.

Privett JTJ et al.: The incidence and importance of renal duplication. *Clin Radiol* 27:521–530, 1976.

Robertson JR: *Genitourinary Problems in Women,* Springfield, Ill.: Charles C Thomas, 1978.

Rosenfeld JB et al.: Unilateral renal hypoplasia with hypertension (Ask-Upmark kidney). *Br Med J* 2:217–218, 1973.

Stamey TA et al.: Studies of introital colonization in women with recurrent urinary infections. *J Urol* 114:261, 1975.

Villa Santa U: Complications of radiotherapy for carcinoma of the uterine cervix. *Am J Obstet Gynecol* 114:717, 1972.

Wear JB: Cystometry. *Urol Clin North Am* 1:45, 1974.

39

Disorders of Pelvic Support

RICHARD STANDER

ANATOMY AND DYNAMICS OF SUPPORT

It was long assumed that, as a result of evolutionary events, the human pelvis represented the pelvis of the quadruped after a simple 90° rotation. Closer study, however, reveals that many additional modifications have occurred that assure appropriate function and protection for the pelvic viscera. It is important that the physician who assumes the responsibility for prevention or treatment of disorders of the pelvic supporting structures have a thorough understanding of pelvic anatomy and function of the soft tissue components.

BONY SKELETON

It is notable that although the pelvic girdle of other mammals is a uniformly cylindrical ring carried at right angles to the axis of the vertebrae, in man it is funnel-shaped and meets the vertical axis of the vertebral column at an angle of over 45°. The pelvis has been able to partially maintain its horizontal position because the vertebral column above has acquired two compensatory curvatures that permit the head to be carried directly above the pelvis and in the body axis itself (see Fig. 39–1). Funneling of the bony pelvis has been accomplished by marked lengthening

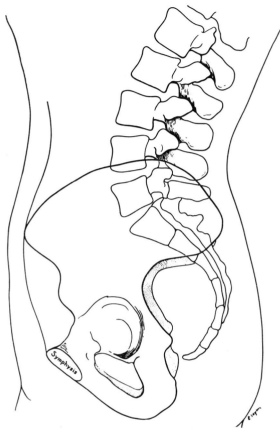

FIGURE 39-1 Tracing from the lateral roentgenogram of a nulliparous living female in the standing position showing lumbar curve of the vertebral column and tilt of pelvic girdle. *(From Ulfelder.)*

and inward bowing of the inferior pubic rami and sacrum. However, the single most effective structural modification has been the shortening of the caudal skeleton and its incorporation into the pelvic floor as the relatively rigid coccyx.

In addition to this direct effect of diminishing the bony outlet's internal diameter, there are several notable anatomic modifications which indirectly offer strong supporting surfaces for heavy organs which would otherwise vector on the outlet itself. The first of these is failure of the pelvis to rotate 90° with the vertebral axis. As a result, the pubic arches and strong central lower-abdominal musculature still underlie the fluid-filled urinary bladder, which in turn bears the weight of the small bowel and omentum. Also as a result of this incomplete rotation of the pelvic axis, the lumbar curve of the spinal column protrudes massively forward: with its strong paravertebral muscle bundles, it provides a shelf on which rest the liver,

spleen, stomach, transverse colon, and other upper-abdominal viscera of considerable bulk and weight. Finally, only in the human does one find the blades of the iliac bones turned both outward and upward in a manner which firmly supports the contents of the iliac fossae, transmitting these forces down the columns of the lower extremities and away from the central cavity.

MUSCLES

As noted in Fig. 39-2, four pairs of muscles originate on the interior circumference of the bony girdle and, with fibers running centripetally and edges slightly overlapping from back to front, insert into the coccygeal sacrum or its continuation as a firm tendinous raphe extending to the anal sphincter. The resultant so-called levator plate provides an effective hammock which occludes all of the outlet area except for *a narrow slot* between the puborectalis components and immediately under the symphysis pubis. It is significant that these same paired muscle sets are found in the quadruped emerging through the outlet and inserting into the root of the tail. Here their action controls the position of the tail, which is fully mobile, relative to the sacrum. In the human, with disappearance of the tail and loss of mobility in its remnant, one would expect that these muscles would also somewhat diminish or become atrophic. In actual fact, the reverse is true--the human *levatores ani* are bigger, thicker, stronger, and more powerful structures than their evolutionary antecedents, and provide support of the pelvic outlet.

The urinary, fecal, and generative tracts as they

FIGURE 39-2 Sketch of pelvic muscular diaphragm from below. *(From Francis, after De Lee. See Ulfelder, Am J Obstet Gynecol 72:857, 1956.)*

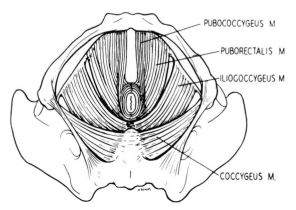

PUBOCOCCYGEUS M.

PUBORECTALIS M.

ILIOCOCCYGEUS M.

COCCYGEUS M.

emerge upon the skin are crowded forward into the slot between the levators. Even so, in the erect posture this would present an area of diminished resistance and potential herniation, were it not additionally reinforced by a structure unique to the human, the *urogenital diaphragm.* This is as a triangular platform of fascias and muscles (see Fig. 39–3), two sides of which attach firmly to the inferior pubic rami from symphysis to the ischial tuberosities. Somewhat more superficially located than the levators, it offers firm support in the area beneath the slot described in the previous paragraph. Penetrated in the male only by the urethral canal, it successfully closes off the last area where bulging might normally occur. In women, it must yield passage for the vaginal canal. The vagina represents a potential site for herniation, and the potential is enhanced by vaginal enlargement resulting from coitus and parturition.

The problem presented by the passage of a hollow viscus through the firmer wall of a body cavity which varies in pressure relative to the atmosphere is how to minimize bulging inward or outward through the aperture around the perforating viscus. Wherever in the body this anatomic dilemma presents as a serious threat, the anatomic solution has always been

the same: the viscus penetrates the barrier on an axis so oblique that pressure exerted at one end cannot impinge on the orifice at the other end of the tunnel. Remarkably, the same solution seems to have been developed in the human pelvis, for under normal circumstances the apex of the vagina is found well back in the hollow of the sacrum, and the axis of the vagina is almost parallel with the plane of the levator plate.

LIGAMENTS

Of particular interest are those paired ligaments, namely uterosacrals, cardinals, pubocervicals, etc., which extend outward from the cervix like the spokes of a wheel (see Fig. 39–4) and blend in peripherally with the fascias and periosteum of the bony ring. These serve chiefly to maintain the cervix in its position in the posterior pelvic cavity where its downward thrust is extended against the coccyx and levator muscles. In the normal adult woman, herniation of the vaginal introitus is actually a small risk since the bladder is fended away from it by an intact urogenital diaphragm and the cervix and uterus are deflected from it by the ligamentous supports. When the vaginal

FIGURE 39–3 The superficial layer of the urogenital diaphragm in the female.

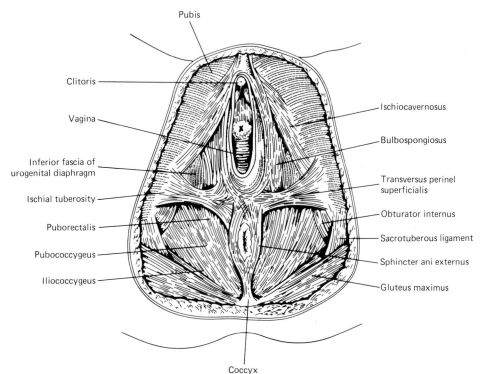

Pubis

Clitoris

Vagina

Inferior fascia of urogenital diaphragm

Ischial tuberosity

Puborectalis

Pubococcygeus

Iliococcygeus

Ischiocavernosus

Bulbospongiosus

Transversus perinel superficialis

Obturator internus

Sacrotuberous ligament

Sphincter ani externus

Gluteus maximus

Coccyx

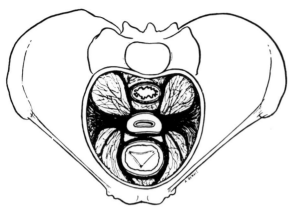

FIGURE 39–4 Diagram of connective tissue supports of the cervix. *(From Francis, after De Lee. See Ulfelder, Am J Obstet Gynecol 72:859, 1956.)*

orifice is enlarged by childbearing with permanent widening and lengthening of the slot between the levators, when the urogenital diaphragm has been partially disrupted, or when the cervix has become hypermobile within the pelvis as a result of ligamentous damage or stretching, a defect exists in the supporting mechanism which cannot oppose the gravitational pull on the anterior vaginal wall structures. If the cervix rests over the unprotected vaginal outlet, its conical leading part and bulk will act as a dilator, seeking to exploit the aperture with every increase in intraabdominal pressure.

TISSUE QUALITIES

Also necessary to the proper management of a vaginal hernia is an understanding of the qualities of the tissues present. There are just four of these: bone, skeletal muscle, smooth muscle, and connective tissue. Bone is the strongest biologic structure with resistance to stress; in fact, that is its most important mission. It is fair to say that evolutionary modifications in the human pelvic skeleton, although originating partly in response to a stubborn and persistent preference for a biped stance and gait, also have achieved significant protection against too facile disruption of the soft parts' outlet structures.

Skeletal muscle is an ideal supporting structure having both strength and contractility. Its chief virtue lies in its property of *tonus,* which is an involuntary response to stretching in an effort to restore optimum length. Smooth muscle, on the other hand, is decep-

tive and disappointing in this regard. Although possessed of strength and contractility, its tonus is a property which responds to distraction by seeking to restore optimum tension within the muscle fibers themselves. When the stretching force is maintained, the muscle cells rearrange themselves gradually into a longer, thinner sheet of tissue which still retains the power to contract and shorten. This facility is ideal for a material which is used to surround viscera of intermittent varying internal pressure, girth, and volume of content, such as the stomach, intestine, uterus, and blood vessels. However when smooth muscle is stretched beyond a certain point, its contractile function ceases and as a supporting structure it quickly becomes incompetent. One illustration of this statement is provided by the former surgical practice of repairing procidentia by abdominal exposure of the pelvic organs and high suspension or fixation of the uterus to the abdominal wall. Many of these patients, with the passage of time, once again noted protrusion of the cervix at the vulva so similar to their original complaint that both patient and surgeon assumed it to be due to disengagement of the repair. This impression is quickly corrected when the surgeon reoperates and finds that the fundus of the uterus is still firmly attached abdominally but the body and cervix have stretched to an overall length of many inches. Thus we see the bulkiest, most compact bundle of smooth muscle in the body utterly incapable of resisting by itself the forces that normally work against the pelvic outlet.

Finally, there is connective tissue which derives its strength from collagen and elastic fibers. These possess no contractility and limited elasticity. When structures formed of this tissue—such as ligaments and fascias—are distracted beyond their elastic limits, rupture will occur either as a gross tear or as multiple tiny losses of continuity. In either case, there is some degree of hemorrhage and repair by granulations and scar. The resultant of these accidents is of little value for long-term support since scar will stretch and cause permanent lengthening of the connective tissue bundle.

It is concluded that restoration of competence to the pelvic supporting mechanism requires the achievement of a reconstructed and repositioned vagina with outlet and canal of approximately normal caliber, lying in an axis across the pelvis with the apex firmly held back in the hollow of the sacrum. Additionally, the posterior vaginal wall must rest on a floor of skeletal muscle and bone. In other words, repair of vaginal hernia is best achieved by reconstructing, insofar as possible, the normal mechanism of support.

SIMPLE UTERINE DISPLACEMENTS

In childhood, the bulk of the uterus is cervix which, as described above, is a relatively immobile central tissue mass at the hub of paired sets of ligamentous spokes. The growth stimulus at the menarche affects chiefly the fundus above, and as the fundus increases in length and bulk, it will inevitably come to lie where intraabdominal viscera and forces direct. In most young women, the fundus is forward and resting on the urinary bladder and anterior vaginal wall. In addition, the axis of the uterus and cervix tends to follow the same straight line, so that the external cervical os or orifice will be found pointing toward the posterior vaginal wall. Abnormal positions of the uterus may consist of displacement of the fundus away from the anterior position, or significant angulation in the uterocervical axis or both. The descriptive terminology involves terms such as *retroversion* and *anteversion* to describe abnormal dislocation of fundus backward or forward (see Fig. 39–5) with qualifications of first, second, or third degree to indicate the severity of the "deformity." The adjective *fixed* is used to indicate apparent immobilization of the fundus in its displaced position. Significant angulation of the canal is referred to as *retroflexion* or *anteflexion*. Familiarity with these considerations is necessary to help an examiner detect significant masses of importance and differentiate them with confidence from the normal uterus or cervix in displacement.

Simple displacements are most often detected in asymptomatic women upon routine examinations. On occasion, displacements may be secondary to pelvic tumors such as uterine myomata or ovarian tumors. When a fixed retroversion is found, one should suspect the presence of an adhesive process such as that associated with endometriosis or chronic pelvic inflammatory disease.

Since uterine displacements are usually asymptomatic, it is very difficult to attribute pelvic symptoms to retroversion and other variations in uterine position. It is unfortunate if the physician attributes such complaints as backache and dyspareunia to simple uter-

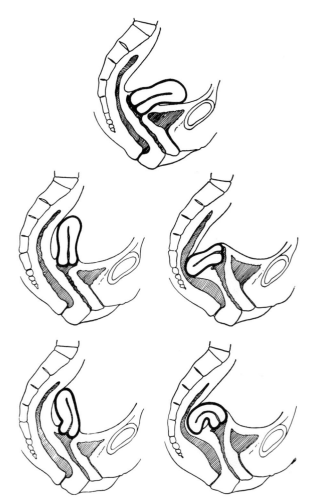

FIGURE 39–5 Degrees of retroposition. Top, normal position of uterus; center left, slight retroversion; center right, marked retroversion; bottom left, slight retroflexion; bottom right, marked retroflexion. *(From Novak et al.: Textbook of Gynecology, 7th ed., Baltimore: Williams & Wilkins, 1965, p. 265.)*

ine retroversion. It is even more unfortunate if surgical correction is recommended without thorough investigation of potential urologic, neurologic, orthopedic and psychosomatic causes for the patient's symptoms. After disorders of other organ systems have been excluded by appropriate consultation and diagnostic studies, a trial of pessary (see Fig. 39–6) may be indicated in the symptomatic patient. Only if the symptoms are relieved after the uterus is brought to a normal position and retained by the pessary and if they recur after removal of the pessary should the physician consider that the patient's symptoms were related to uterine displacement.

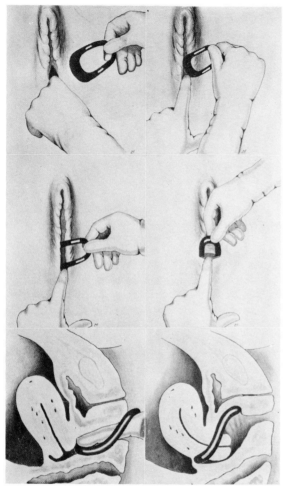

FIGURE 39–6 Diagram showing the successive steps in the introduction of a pessary. *(From CH Davis: Gynecology and Obstetrics, Hagerstown, Md.: W. F. Prior, 1933. See also Novak et al.: Textbook of Gynecology, 7th ed., Baltimore, William & Wilkins, 1965, p. 265.)*

PELVIC RELAXATION

SYMPTOMS AND ETIOLOGY

The term pelvic relaxation may be applied to varying degrees of displacement of one or more of the pelvic organs, including the bladder, urethra, uterus, or rectum. Such displacements generally result from a weakening of the organ's supporting structures. The symptoms are usually of gradual onset, although occasionally the patient will express a specific time at which she first noted symptoms, e.g., following a fall

or some other traumatic episode. Initial symptoms are often expressed as a heaviness in the pelvis or a dragging or bearing-down sensation. The patient may tell the physician that she feels that "everything is falling out." Accompanying symptoms may be backache, nervousness, and irritability.

Symptoms of pelvic relaxation are more pronounced at the end of the day as the forces of gravity accentuate the displacement of pelvic structures. They may be minimal or absent upon arising in the morning. An exacerbation of symptoms often accompanies the vascular congestive changes associated with the premenstrual phase of the menstrual cycle as well as early pregnancy. Seldom is specific, sharp, or localized pain a part of the symptom complex.

Pelvic organ displacement and attendant symptoms advance with age and in many individuals seem to accelerate after the menopause. This may result from decreased output of ovarian hormones with resulting adverse effect on connective tissue integrity. As weakness of pelvic support increases, organ displacement progresses, and the patient may complain of actual protrusion of tissue from the vagina. This may be vaginal mucosa covering the bladder or rectum, or it may be the cervix, depending on the specific defect in support.

In addition to the general feelings of heaviness and bearing down, more specific complaints may be related to displacement of an individual pelvic structure. For example, if there is weakening of support of the bladder and urethra (*cystocele, urethrocele,* or *cystourethrocele*), the loss of the urethrovesical angle may lead to a loss of urine whenever intraabdominal pressure is increased as with laughing or sneezing (see Chap. 38). If the weakness involves primarily the anterior rectal wall, there may be herniation of the rectum into the vaginal introitus when intraabdominal pressure is increased (*rectocele*). Under these circumstances, a patient may complain of increasing constipation and difficulty in defecation. In severe forms of this disorder, that patient may actually have to effect bowel movement by pressing against the posterior vaginal wall with a finger. On the other hand, the main defect may be in the supporting structures of the uterus, and descent of the cervix and uterus into the vaginal canal may be primarily responsible for pelvic symptomatology (*uterine prolapse*). Under advanced conditions, the cervix may protrude from the introitus where it is subject to trauma, irritation, and secondary infection. If uncorrected, these circumstances may lead to a malodorous discharge or bleeding from the cervix.

Most disorders of pelvic support are caused by

repeated childbearing or specific injury to supporting structures during an isolated obstetric episode. The incidence of significant disorders of pelvic support tends to be lower in populations with limited childbearing as well as those populations with the highest level of obstetric care. Familial and racial determinants also seem to be involved. Although rare, severe defects may occasionally be found in a nulligravida. In such instances there is often a strong family history of related or identical disorders. Occasionally, pelvic relaxation may be seen following abdominal or vaginal hysterectomy if the operative procedure has failed to provide adequate support of the vaginal vault or to correct an unrecognized herniation of small bowel through the pouch of Douglas (*enterocele*). In the latter case, continued downward dissection of the peritoneal sac between the rectum and vaginal mucosa may result in pelvic symptoms following the operation.

The symptoms related to pelvic relaxation vary markedly among individuals. Many patients with minimal physical evidence of displacement through weakening of support complain of significant disability because of pelvic discomfort. Conversely, many women with marked displacement of the uterus, bladder, and/or rectum have minimal complaints or are totally without symptoms. Certainly the emotional makeup of the patient, her fears, and her own interpretation of her symptoms are important factors affecting expression to her physician of symptoms related to pelvic relaxation.

A history and physical examination are usually sufficient to detect the cause of the patient's complaints if they are related to loss of support of pelvic structures. It must be remembered, however, that when the patient is being examined in the dorsal lithotomy position, the forces of gravity do not exert the same effect, and organ displacement may be less obvious than when the patient is standing. This is particularly true of uterine prolapse; in such cases, the degree to which the uterus descends into the vagina may be demonstrated by having the patient bear down as if having a bowel movement or by placing gentle traction on the cervix with a single-toothed tenaculum. When the patient coughs, one is able to detect a marked descent of the urethra and/or bladder by depressing the posterior vaginal wall. A rectocele may be detected by using a narrow-bladed retractor to elevate the anterior vaginal wall and again having the patient increase intraabdominal pressure by bearing down or coughing. Under these conditions, the posterior vaginal wall will bulge inward toward the lumen of the vagina and possibly downward toward

the vaginal introitus. Rectocele and enterocele cannot always be differentiated by simple inspection, since both may appear as a bulging of the posterior vaginal wall. In the case of simple rectocele, a finger inserted into the rectum should easily reach the apex of the mass bulging into the posterior aspect of the vagina. If this cannot be accomplished, an intervening enterocele may be present.

During the physical examination, it is important to determine whether or not extragenital disease may be contributing to pelvic organ displacement, e.g., massive ascites or abdominal or pelvic tumors.

SPECIFIC DEFECTS

UTERINE PROLAPSE

On examination, the level reached by the advancing cervix with the patient straining allows quantification of the degree of prolapse. If the cervix comes to the introitus, it is called first-degree prolapse. It is labeled second-degree if the cervix appears to be well outside of the vagina, and third-degree if the entire uterus can be felt in the external protruding mass. This condition is also called procidentia. However, there is considerable variation among patients in the overall length of the cervix and the extent of eversion of the posterior and anterior vaginal walls. Each of these features is presumably related to the nature of the original damage, the size and position of the fundus of the uterus, and the subsequent progression of descent. All of these circumstances are important in management for they signal the location of the pelvic peritoneum in relation to the presenting bulge. In addition, attention to these features will inform the examiner to what extent the urinary bladder, the rectum, and occasionally sigmoid, small bowel, or omentum may be displaced into the hernia. The chronically exteriorized cervix or vagina acquires a hyperkeratinized epithelial surface that is many layers thicker than normal. It will not stain brown with iodide solutions, perhaps because the iodine cannot get into the layer where cells are actively storing glycogen. Often at the point where the presenting bulge chafes against clothing, a flat ulcer will develop which stains the clothes with bloody discharge and heightens the concern about cancer. Just reducing and maintaining reduction by bed rest, pack, or pessary will quickly result in epithelial repair. Failure to achieve this would suggest the presence either of a pathogenic organism or malignant change. If either of these complications is a possibility the lesion should certainly be investigated without delay and before definitive surgery is carried out.

The surgical treatment of prolapse aims to eliminate the herniated mass and repair the defective supporting mechanism which permitted descent in the first place. Of first importance is the delineation of anatomic structures and the decision as to which part of the redundant and bulging protrusion cannot be sacrificed. Certainly these are the considerations for bladder, urethra, ureters, and rectum, and usually with the vagina as a coital passage. When, for childbearing purposes, the uterus also is to be saved, one must face squarely the judgment as to whether surgical alleviation of signs and symptoms warrants the risk of an operation with a significant chance for recurrence following childbirth. Although small series of cases are from time to time reported with apparent high degrees of successful surgical repair and preservation of fertility, the general experience has been to the contrary.

The technical procedures that have been much used for repair of prolapse are numerous. At present, the majority of cases are managed by repair of the anterior and posterior vaginal walls, combined with vaginal hysterectomy. Removal of the uterus is eminently reasonable on the grounds that removal prevents subsequent pregnancy and its risks, and also eliminates one important organ source of potential malignancy. The pistonlike action of the uterus and cervix descending against the repair is also of importance. Questions remain as to whether surgery for prolapse is less safe when hysterectomy is included, and as to whether repair is as successful over the long term.

The risk of operation with and without hysterectomy is essentially the same, although a properly designed evaluation of a comparable large series of the two is not to be found in the literature. Almost the only serious additional hazard with removal of the uterus is related to the fact that the peritoneal cavity is entered, and this hazard is small. Whether repair is equally successful is not known, in part because very few reports that have been published involve long-term evaluation of all patients. Many thousands of women have undergone vaginal hysterectomy for prolapse, and it is regarded by gynecologists as a successful approach to the problem.

Most recurrences after proper repair are some form of enterocele. In other words, the recurrent sac consists of vaginal wall and peritoneum; rarely does bladder or rectum participate in the protrusion except after very long delay and with the inevitable widening of the ring of the defect. One goal of surgical repair at the initial operation, therefore, must be to prevent any area of vagina from being adjacent to peritoneum and in a position to be pressured to bulge into the canal. Initially, only the upper posterior vagina between the uterosacral ligaments is in this situation, but with removal of the uterus, this potential defect is immediately increased by the size of the cervix which is removed. Specific steps must always be taken to eliminate or at any rate minimize this space by attaching the supporting structures to the vaginal apex and by tailoring the vaginal plastic reconstruction so that this area of weakness and potential recurrence comes to lie well back in the hollow of the sacrum. Thus the weight of the viscera is directed away from the reconstructed apex. Over the years, an assortment of procedural steps has been reported which aim to attach the uterosacral ligaments to the vagina and to each other, or to obliterate the pouch of Douglas with mattress or purse-string sutures. The common denominator in all procedures is the attempt to fix the vaginal apex in a secure position which is well posterior in the pelvis and to prevent abdominal contents and pressures from bearing on the area of least strength.

In general, vaginal operations are considered safe and well tolerated, but they are often accompanied by blood loss that would be considered unacceptable in other areas. Observation shows that the bleeding takes place along the incisions through the vaginal wall and during the dissection between vagina and the urinary organs or rectum. The former may easily be diminished by tedious hemostasis, by an over-and-over running stitch along the cut edge, or by the injection of very dilute solutions of vasoconstrictor drugs in the areas where incisions are planned. Bleeding during the development of planes of dissection, here as elsewhere, can be trivial if the patient is positioned to diminish venous back pressure and if anatomic spaces between layers of tissue are faithfully followed.

Anterior and posterior repair with vaginal hysterectomy seldom can be omitted. Only the rare instance of nulliparous prolapse, in which a normal uterus has descended through an unscathed vagina like a piston in a cylinder, lends itself to hysterectomy alone. Here one must be alert to the possibility that congenital enterocele (hernia of the pouch of Douglas) was the primary lesion, with the uterus prolapsing and presenting on the front surface of it. Anterior repair is indicated whenever the presenting bulge includes redundant anterior vaginal wall and urinary bladder. When stress incontinence is a preoperative complaint, or when the supports of the urethrovesical junction are visibly relaxed (urethrocele), special additional steps should be taken to correct the anatomic deficiencies in this area. These consist of deliberate extension of the dissection toward the pubic symphysis to expose and develop the urethra as well as the bladder neck, and then the approximation underneath of sufficient muscle and connective tissue to elevate and support the urinary structures in a position which restores the normal urethrovesical angles (see Chap. 38).

Posterior repair affords the only opportunity to reestablish the normal length and obliquity of the vaginal canal and, at the same time, to attempt to recreate a floor of skeletal muscle that will take the place of the disrupted urogenital diaphragm and widened interlevator gap. All this can usually be accomplished by incision along the posterior rim of the vaginal introitus and by dissection sufficiently high and lateral to separate vagina completely from rectum. Thus, one can identify the fascia-covered medial aspects of both puboccygeus muscles and approximate them— somewhat abnormally but effectively—between the lower rectum and the vagina.

Before vaginal hysterectomy gained wide usage, surgical correction of prolapse utilized some variant of the procedure best known as the Manchester operation. It was in the gynecologic service of the University of Manchester during the leadership of Donald and Fothergill, that the technique was evolved, described, and widely taught. The critical steps are identification and shortening of the stretched cardinal ligaments lateral to the cervix then extensive posterior repair with approximation of the levator muscles. Because these steps tend to produce an apparently longer segment of cervix extending below the vaginal fornices, and because the cervix is often elongated in cases of prolapse, shortening of the cervix by amputation is another feature of this procedure. These steps achieve the desired result of fixing the vaginal apex so that it is posterior in the pelvis, restoring the normal caliber and obliquity of the vaginal canal, and placing a firm, skeletal muscle shelf of support under it all.

Although many formerly popular techniques for repair of uterine prolapse have been abandoned, one procedure of long standing still has its occasional usefulness; this is the operation of colpocleisis, or vaginal obliteration, of LeFort. It consists of denudation of symmetrical facing surfaces of anterior and posterior vagina and their careful approximation by sutures to create a broad bridge across the upper and midvagina, thus preventing descent of the cervix. The indication for this choice of operation is usually an extensive prolapse with symptoms in a woman so el-

derly or debilitated that she should be exposed to the absolute minimum of anesthesia and surgery, and in whom a pessary is ineffectual.

On the rare occasion when a patient is either found unsuitable for colpocleisis or refuses operation, alternate management may include use of a pessary. A variety of pessaries are available, allowing a wide selection of shapes, sizes, and materials. A trial of several pessaries may be necessary before one is found that is suitable for the individual patient. To assure patient comfort, the pessary should lie as high in the vagina as possible and cause minimal vaginal distention. Preferably the pessary should be one that is easily removed by the patient. This allows for periodic cleansing of the device and permits the patient to remove it at night when it is not needed. Such circumstances reduce trauma to the vaginal epithelium. If the patient is unable or unwilling to remove her pessary, the physician should arrange periodic office visits for removal and cleaning of the pessary as well as inspection of the underlying vaginal epithelium.

CYSTOCELE

It is unusual for a vaginal hernia to involve purely one or another of the adjacent structures. The components, however, do lend themselves to identification by a simple descriptive terminology. This is eminently practical and useful; it permits accurate recording of findings at the time of examination, which is the only way physicians can evaluate changes which occur with the passage of time or after treatment (see Fig. 39–7). It also facilitates classification of cases in order to discuss or report them.

Cystocele is weakness and bulging on effort of any part of the anterior vaginal wall between the cervix and the transverse sulcus under the neck of the bladder. Symptoms, aside from the presenting tissue protrusion with its associated pressure sensations, are those associated with interference in normal bladder function. Inability to empty completely at the time of voiding is the result of trapping significant volumes of urine in the dependent sac. The presence of this residual urine leads to a feeling of the need to void again after an unusually short interval. It is easily confirmed when catheterization of the woman after apparently complete voiding shows substantial amounts of urine still present. Urgency and dysuria will also be noted if secondary infection develops. Incontinence of urine is not indicative of cystocele per se but will be noticed if there is loss of normal bladder-neck control. The visible external evidence that indicates this possibility may be relaxation of the normal sup-

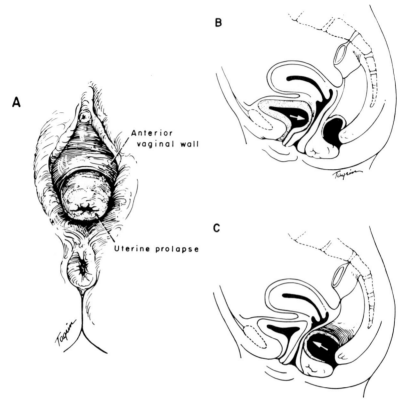

FIGURE 39–7 *A* Uterine prolapse. *B* Cystocele. *C* Rectocele. The typical gross anatomic appearance of each of these common forms of pelvic relaxation is shown individually; actually they frequently coexist. *(From TH Green Jr: Gynecology, 1st ed., Boston: Little, Brown, 1965, p. 390.)*

ports of proximal urethra and bladder neck, a physical change designated as urethrocele. However, in the multiparous woman there may be redundance of vaginal wall at this point without any incontinence whatsoever; conversely, the presence of urethrocele in no way mandates the presence or future appearance of stress urinary incontinence.

In cases where surgical repair is first choice of treatment, it is advisable to accomplish this at the first convenient time for the patient. One most important consideration will be the patient's plans for the immediate future. Surgical repair of any hernia is dependent for its ultimate success on solid healing of tissues in the positions they occupy at the conclusion of the operation. Although prolonged immobilization is now recognized to be more deleterious to the organism as a whole than advantageous to the local process, nevertheless the stresses placed upon the area of the repair should be no greater than required for ordinary physiologic activities for at least 4 to 6 weeks.

Repair of cystocele by dissection of the anterior vaginal wall in layers, imbrication of the base of the bladder, and trimming and closure of the vagina are unlikely to result in more than transient improvement. Reasoning by analogy with hernia repair elsewhere in the body, the procedure just described does no more than get rid of the hernial sac. The weakness or defect which permitted its appearance will not have been identified or corrected, and the fabric of the anterior wall will be no better able to resist gradual stretching and protrusion than in the first instance. One must assume that loss of support by the perineal floor is an integral participant in the genesis of the hernia, and that this is correctable only by the kind of perineal dissection and repair previously described in the management of uterine prolapse.

In the selection of procedure for repair of cystocele, it must be established during the examination under anesthesia that the apparent absence of uterine prolapse is not due chiefly to enlargement or nodularity of the fundus sufficient to prevent its descent below midpelvis. If the ligamentous attachments around the cervix are really quite stretched and relaxed and the woman is just entering into the menopausal epoch, it will be only a matter of time before the fundus shrinks sufficiently for prolapse to be demonstrated and perhaps require reoperation. Cystocele repair is rarely justified as a solitary procedure (see Chap. 38).

RECTOCELE

A rectocele is recognized by a prominent bulging of the posterior vaginal wall, and this herniation contains only large bowel. There is always evidence of previous injury to the perineum. Many authors attribute the development of rectocele solely to thinning of the fascial layer between the vagina and the rectum, but the histologic evidence to support this is tenuous at best. A frequent but often unrecognized contribution to rectocele formation is damage of the vaginal attachments to the lateral vaginal wall. When these are stretched or detached, they permit significant inward bulging of the rectal wall and encroachment upon the vaginal lumen. As the defect progresses, as with advancing age, constipation may also progress, since the anterior rectal wall now yields more readily to increases in intraabdominal pressure than does the anus.

Surgical repair of a rectocele involves the following fundamental approach. A vertical incision is made in the posterior vaginal mucosa beginning at the mucocutaneous junction of the outlet and carried superiorly well above the upper margin of the defect. If a transverse incision has been previously made for a perineal repair, the lower portion of the vertical incision will transect the transverse incision. The rectum is then separated from the vaginal wall throughout the length of the defect. At this point, the surgeon should assure himself that an enterocele is not present before proceeding with repair of the rectocele. The fascia of the rectovaginal septum will be found to be densely adherent to the vaginal mucosa. It should be separated from the mucosa by sharp dissection and mobilized laterally until the fascia covering the medial aspects of the levator muscles is exposed. The mobilized fascia is then approximated in the midline over the rectal wall by several interrupted, absorbable sutures, reducing and supporting the anterior herniation of the rectal wall. Following closure of the fascia, three or four sutures are placed through the fascia of the levators bilaterally and the levator muscles are brought together in the midline, creating additional support (see Fig. 39–8). Finally, the vagi-

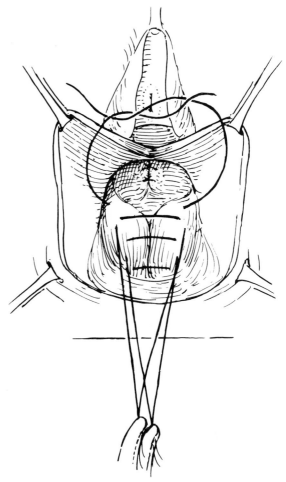

FIGURE 39–8 Surgical repair of rectocele. *(From Parsons, Ulfelder.)*

nal mucosa is trimmed of excess tissue and is closed in the midline by either an interrupted or continuous suture of absorbable material.

ENTEROCELE

A unique variety of vaginal hernia, and the one most like other abdominal hernias, is the enterocele. Although its site of predilection is the upper posterior vagina, its unique characteristic is that the sac consists of stretched-out vaginal wall lined with peritoneum, and its cavity communicates directly with the free pelvic peritoneal space. Within the sac may be found, on occasion, ascitic fluid, omentum, sigmoid, or any other mobile structure. Enterocele has its beginning in the upper posterior vaginal wall between the attachment of the uterosacral ligaments because this is the only point where the space between the vagina and the coelomic cavity contains no interposed organ. In a very real sense, this is a congenital point of weakness which is rarely exploited because it is rarely exposed to increased pressure from within.

Enteroceles divide themselves roughly into three groups according to their predisposing factors. The first of these appears to be a true congenital hernia occurring in women of all ages without regard to marital status or previous surgery. When recognized early, these exhibit a well-defined ring or neck between the uterosacral ligaments and just below the cervix when viewed from above. Extending downward into the rectovaginal septum will be found a fingerlike peritoneal pouch. In every respect the findings resemble the persistent processus vaginalis extending down from the inguinal ring in hernia of congenital origin. With the passage of time and enlargement of the sac and its neck, the characteristics become blurred, and it will appear that the whole pouch of Douglas participates in the protrusion, often with some descent of the rectosigmoid in the manner of sliding hernia elsewhere.

The second type of enterocele is associated with a history of prior pelvic surgery for correction of malposition or descensus. The procedure (whatever its details) always has fixed the fundus of the uterus well forward in the pelvis. When postmenopausal uterine atrophy develops, the cervix perforce moves forward in the pelvis as the uterus shrinks and in some women—perhaps with an exaggerated pelvic tilting —this may suffice to open up the cul-de-sac and expose its walls continuously and directly to the pressures which develop in the abdominal cavity. The weak spot between the uterosacral ligaments undoubtedly gradually gives way in certain circumstances and leads to the appearance of a diffuse bulging enterocele, in this circumstance quite analogous to a direct hernia in the inguinal region.

The third category of enterocele seems to follow vaginal hysterectomy or abdominal hysterectomy in the presence of prolapse. The interval is usually not long; often at the first postoperative visit there is already a suggestion that the vaginal apex descends expulsively on coughing or straining. The mechanism of genesis of enterocele in these cases appears to be dependent on a failure at the time of hysterectomy to diminish redundancy of the vaginal wall, particularly in the upper posterior segment. When the cervix is also removed, there is left an even greater area with only a layer of vaginal wall and one of peritoneum exposed to the pressures from above and within.

This undesirable sequel to hysterectomy has long been recognized and several prophylactic measures described. It is no longer considered appropriate to carry out abdominal hysterectomy for prolapse unless there is another reason for approaching the surgery from above. In indicated instances, specific additional steps are recommended as concomitant vaginal procedures to effectuate the necessary repair and reconstruction. When vaginal hysterectomy is selected, a choice of special steps is available with the objective being to obliterate the "deep" cul-de-sac, or to attach the apex firmly in a position well posterior in the hollow of the sacrum. Perhaps equally important is construction of a solid posterior colporrhaphy with levator approximation and restoration of the perineal body.

As in the case of rectocele, pessaries are usually ineffective for enterocele because the hernia escapes below and behind the device unless it completely fills the vagina under some pressure, an uncomfortable arrangement for the wearer.

In general, the surgical correction of enterocele is somewhat different for the three categories. However, the most important determinants in the choice of method are the size of the defect and the patient's wishes for maintenance of coital potential. Surgery should be recommended because the lesion is inexorably progressive and, although incarceration or strangulation of bowel or omentum is exceedingly rare, the presence of intestine in the sac can be the cause of local discomfort. If there is full-thickness scar somewhere in its wall, the scar is particularly prone to stretch and thin out and very rarely will rupture, with escape of viscera through the vagina.

Operation on enterocele should begin with careful dissection of the posterior vagina from below until the sac is clearly identified. A Valsalva maneuver by the patient, induced by the anesthetist, will sometimes demonstrate a peritoneal sac so closely applied to vaginal wall or rectum that it cannot easily be identified. Further dissection then continues between sac and vagina until the upper margin of the defect is defined. This plane can be followed laterally on either side to establish about three-quarters of the circumference. To free the final rim of the neck of the sac requires careful separation of the sac posteriorly from the rectum. Since the bowel itself is incorporated into the posterior wall of the pouch of Douglas, this dissection can inadvertently lead to tedious effort to free the rectosigmoid of its serosal cover which is, of course, quite unnecessary. Confusion usually is created in cases of large, soft, collapsed vaginal sacs

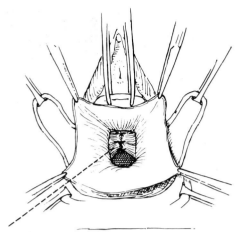

Uterosacral
ligaments

FIGURE 39-9 View through open neck of congenital enterocele showing sutures approximating uterosacral ligaments. *(From Parsons, Ulfelder, p. 265.)*

with defects which occupy the entire available outlet space behind the bladder or the cervix, if the uterus is still present. Often the rectum has been distracted from its posterior attachments to the sacrum and drawn down with the peritoneum of the pouch of Douglas, in which case the bowel actually is part of the sac, exactly as in a sliding hernia anywhere.

The purpose of the procedure up to this point has been to develop the peritoneal component of the hernia in its entirety. Usually, after easily developing the majority of the sac, it is helpful to open it at its presenting point; the rest of the dissection is then carried out with a finger in the peritoneum to help establish the proper planes. Once the entire sac and the size and location of its neck are defined, as in all hernia repair the sac is obliterated and the defect somehow repaired. In early cases of congenital enterocele with the uterus still present and well supported, it will be possible to treat it like an indirect inguinal hernia (see Fig. 39–9). The neck of the sac should be clearly exposed and a purse-string suture laid in place. Several sutures approximating the uterosacral ligaments can usually be placed through the opening, the purse-string tied, redundant sac trimmed away, and a second tie placed on its puckered remnant to be sure to obliterate all traces of a dimple at that point. Reconstruction of the perineum after levator approximation and the trimming away of excess posterior vagina should complete the repair.

Unfortunately, few cases present themselves in this situation. The majority will have extended past the point where a well-defined neck is demonstrable, or will have had a previous hysterectomy, or suspension, or an attempt at repair of enterocele. The peritoneum after dissection will consist of a diffuse, collapsed tent filling the field of operation, and obliteration of the sac will consist at best of transverse closure with imbrication. If uterosacral ligaments of decent texture are identifiable, they should be seized and firmly attached to the corners of the vaginal apex, making sure they pull on the anterior vagina and thus reestablish the axis in its normal position at right angles to the plane of the sacrum. When this is not feasible, it may be desirable to eliminate the deeper aspect of the pouch of Douglas by a series of concentric sutures firmly tied (in the manner of Moschcowitz). This also helps restore the rectum to its normal location and reduces the sliding hernia before the levators are approximated and the perineum rebuilt. It is important to leave no excess of vaginal wall at the apex; otherwise it will at once distend under increased intraabdominal pressure and provide the leading point for a recurrence. If there is any doubt about the quality of the repair, or the axis of the vagina, or the amount of redundant mobile vaginal wall left at the apex to permit coitus, it should be the signal to add laparotomy to the procedure at the same sitting. This will permit additional steps to obliterate the cul-de-sac or to attach the vaginal apex to firm supportive tissue or to some strong, well-tolerated, foreign material like mersilene, which will be in turn solidly fixed to the presacral fascia (see Fig. 39–10).

FIGURE 39–10 Mersilene strap suspension of vaginal apex to presacral fascia. *(From Parsons, Ulfelder, p. 283.)*

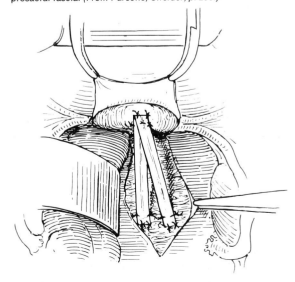

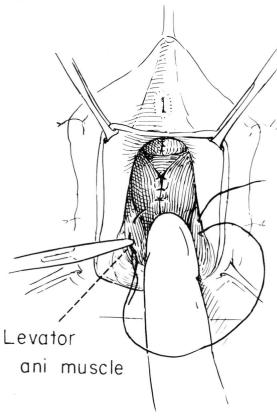

Levator
ani muscle

FIGURE 39–11 Surgical closure of muscular pelvic floor after total vaginal excision. *(From Parsons, Ulfelder, p. 249.)*

Total Vaginal Prolapse

Posthysterectomy vaginal prolapse with extrusion of all or most of the anterior and posterior walls on straining is the most extreme form of the third type of enterocele described above. When the patient desires to retain vaginal function, the operative procedure required will be along the lines described immediately above. It will be helpful, in addition, to tack down the posterior vaginal wall as it is reconstructed to the levator fascia, and it will always be necessary to carry out a laparotomy and attach the vaginal apex to the presacral fascia subperitoneally with fascia lata or mersilene sutures.

However, and this applies to all cases of large recurrent enterocele, the patients should be urged to consider acceptance of vaginal excision with obliteration of the canal. This offers far and away the best chance for permanent cure. Dissection is performed from below as in all cases, but is carried under the vaginal wall circumferentially almost to the introitus and bladder neck. The levators are identified and the

fascias then incised just medial to their reflection onto the rami of the pubic bones. Blunt dissection between muscle and bone will develop a substantial edge of muscle and fascia on both sides which can be approximated up the midline with multiple sutures without tension from the perineum to the bladder neck anteriorly (see Fig. 39–11). This effectively closes the gap between the levators entirely; the vaginal flaps are trimmed away, leaving just enough to come together at a more superficial level. Deep hematoma is the rule in these extensive dissections. Drainage should be provided for the space deep to the levator closure for 24 to 48 hours.

FECAL INCONTINENCE

Absence of tonus and sphincteric control of rectal contents may exist at birth, and if examination shows the anus to be normal in appearance and location, it can be assumed to be due to neurologic anomalies interfering with the normal reflex arc. In like fashion, acquired neuropathy later in life may engender incontinence of feces; the most frequent cause is probably chordotomy performed for the relief of intractable bilateral pelvic pain in cases of advanced and incurable cancer.

By far the majority of cases of incontinence, however, are the result of damage to the sphincter during operation or vaginal delivery. The severity of the complaint will certainly vary with the extent of the injury and the nature of healing which followed it. By and large the local findings suggest more difficulties than actually prove to be the case, evidence perhaps that Malpas is correct when he states that only a few fibers of the voluntary sphincter need remain intact to preserve inhibition of the rectal reflex and apparent good control.

As in the case of urinary leakage, the possibility of fecal fistula must always be borne in mind. The tract between bowel and external opening, however, may occasionally be so tortuous as to defy probing, and injection of fluid under some pressure is more likely to point to the internal orifice than continuation of forcible instrumentation. General principles of repair are considered below.

There is no available means of relieving this symptom other than by surgical repair. The indication will clearly be the finding of anatomic deformity in association with complaints which are continual and accompanied by more than trivial soiling. Properly executed repair in healthy tissue is almost always successful, but failure for a variety of reasons occurs often enough to make it mandatory to explain this possibility to the patient, and to be sure that the existing situation warrants the risk.

During operation, it is prudent to discard no tissue unless absolutely necessary, to establish clearly the planes of dissection around the bowel, and to carry this process sufficiently far to permit comfortable closure of the entire bowel wound in two layers without tension. When it is possible to reestablish continuity of the circumferential sphincter ani muscle, the results appear to be much better. However, when this sphincter has been completely transected, and particularly after the passage of much time, there is retraction of the cut ends which in effect so shortens the muscle that scarcely enough seems left to go around the anus. Nevertheless, it is always indicated to seek out the two ends, hook them securely for purposes of easy handling, and then suture them together. Vaginal wall and perineal skin are comfortably approximated over the raw field; when extensive dissection has been required, this procedure also permits one first to free and bring together the medial edges of the levator muscles as an additional layer.

Attempts to modify or diminish defecation during the first few days are usually carried out, but there is a real doubt whether they are worthwhile if postponement results eventually in the need to pass large firm masses. It is of value to prepare the patient with a residue-free diet and to continue this until spontaneous function appears to have resumed.

REFERENCES

Malpas P: *Genital Prolapse and Allied Conditions,* New York: Grune & Stratton, 1955.

Mattingly RF: *Telinde's Operative Gynecology,* 5th. ed., Philadelphia: Lippincott, 1977.

Nichols DH, Randall CL: *Vaginal Surgery,* Baltimore: Williams & Wilkins, 1976.

Parsons L, Ulfelder H: *An Atlas of Pelvic Operations,* 2d. ed., Philadelphia: Saunders, 1968.

Ridley JH: *Gynecologic Surgery: Errors, Safeguards, and Salvage,* Baltimore: Williams & Wilkins, 1974.

Ulfelder H: The biological mechanics of uterine support in *Progress in Gynecology,* vol. III, JV Meigs, SH Sturgis, eds. New York: Grune & Stratton, 1957.

40
Diseases of the Vulva and Vagina

BENIGN DISEASES
Viral infections
  Herpes genitalis
  Condyloma acuminatum
  Molluscum contagiosum
Behçet's syndrome
Benign tumors
  Solid tumors
  Cystic tumors
Vulva dystrophies
Vaginitis
  Trichomoniasis
  Candidiasis
  Hemophilus vaginalis vaginitis
  Atrophic vulvovaginitis
  Contact vulvovaginitis and allergic
  vulvovaginitis
Dermatoses
Insect bites
Fungal infection
Carcinoma in situ

MALIGNANT DISEASES OF THE VULVA AND VAGINA
Cancer of the vulva
  Squamous-cell (epidermoid) carcinoma
  Melanoma
  Paget's disease
  Bartholin's gland cancer

Other neoplasms
Cancer of the vagina
  Squamous-cell carcinoma
  Adenocarcinoma
  Sarcoma botryoides
  Other neoplasms

BENIGN DISEASES

RAYMOND H. KAUFMAN AND HERMAN L. GARDNER

The vulva lies between the genitocrural folds laterally, the mons pubis anteriorly, and the anus posteriorly (Fig. 40–1). Since it is covered by skin and mucosa, the vulva is subject to those disease processes that affect skin and mucosal surfaces elsewhere on the body; however, the local environment of warmth and moisture is unique to this area and results in alterations of the gross appearance of disease processes that are recognized easily elsewhere in the body. Normal vaginal secretions are within the range of pH 3.8 to 4.2 and usually are not malodorous. Nevertheless, a few women with grossly normal secretions, a normal pH, and a *Lactobacillus* flora still complain of an objectionable odor. Many such patients exercise poor hygiene of the vulva or have increased activity of the apocrine gland system and tend toward hirsut-

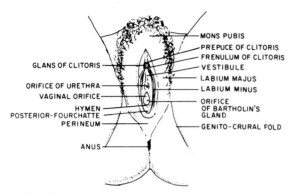

FIGURE 40-1 Principal parts of the vulva.

ism. Additionally, dietary habits may affect the odor of vaginal secretions. The vulva is subject to manifestations of many sexually transmitted diseases (see Chap 36).

VIRAL INFECTIONS

Viral diseases that involve the female genitalia are listed below in the general order of frequency in which they are seen by the practicing gynecologist:

1. Herpes genitalis
2. Condyloma acuminatum
3. Molluscum contagiosum
4. Cytomegalovirus
5. Herpes zoster
6. Vaccinia
7. Hepatitis B, introduced by sexual contact
8. Vulvar manifestations of systemic viral infections

Only the most frequently encountered diseases will be discussed.

HERPES GENITALIS

Herpes genitalis is an acute, inflammatory disease of the genitalia caused in most cases by the herpes simplex virus type 2. About 85 to 90 percent of genital infections are caused by this virus, and 10 to 15 percent by the closely related type 1 virus (Kaufman et al., 1973, 1978). This entity is being seen with increasing frequency, and a gynecologist in private practice probably diagnoses this disease more often than gonococcal infections. In fact, the incidence of

this infection is far greater than is generally suspected. Studies in Houston have indicated that approximately 9 percent of patients seen in the private practice of gynecology and 22 percent of patients seen in the gynecology clinic at a city-county hospital have serologic evidence of prior herpesvirus type 2 infection (Rawls et al., 1970). These studies confirmed the venereal nature of the infection (Rawls et al., 1971) and demonstrated as well the large percentage of women with concomitant *Hemophilus vaginalis* vaginitis, trichomoniasis, and condyloma acuminatum. The studies also indicated that the majority of patients with primary genital herpes infections are teenage girls and unmarried women. The infection is most commonly transmitted by patients with active lesions, but can be contracted from asymptomatic individuals. Virus has been recovered from asymptomatic male carriers (Deardouff et al.) and from the cervix of asymptomatic women (Kaufman et al., 1978).

Clinical Features

The clinical symptoms of primary herpes infections usually appear within 3 to 7 days after exposure to the virus. It is apparent from the number of patients with antibodies against the type 2 virus who demonstrate no history of prior infection that an initial infection may be relatively mild or even completely asymptomatic. Also, investigations by Rawls et al. (1971) and Nahmias et al. (1969) suggest that individuals who have had prior extragenital type 1 herpesvirus infections may have been provided with a degree of protection against subsequent type 2 virus infections. The heterologous nature of the antibodies of herpes simplex viruses may explain the mild or even asymptomatic primary infections. The lesions seen in primary herpes infections are frequently extensive and involve the labia majora, labia minora, perianal skin, and vestibule of the vulva, as well as the vaginal and ectocervical mucosa (Fig. 40-2). Vesicles appear early in the course of the disease but usually rupture quickly, leading to the formation of shallow, painful ulcers. A red areola is frequently present around these areas. Lesions may involve extensive areas of the vulva and perianal skin. Superficial ulcerations may occur on the ectocervix and vagina. On occasion, a fungating, necrotic-appearing mass covers the ectocervix. Inguinal lymphadenopathy is usually present. Many patients run a low-grade fever for several days. The primary lesions may persist from 3 to 6 weeks. When healing occurs, there is no residual scarring or ulceration.

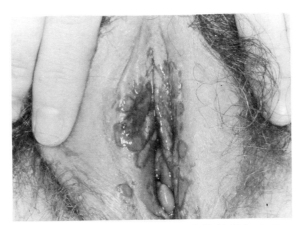

FIGURE 40–2 Vulva, primary herpes genitalis. Multiple, shallow, painful ulcers scattered over the inner labia majora and labia minora are noted.

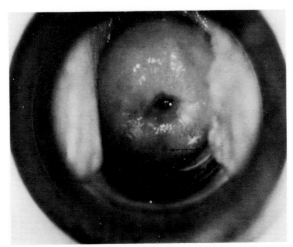

FIGURE 40–3 Cervix, recurrent herpes. Shallow ulcers are noted on the posterior lip of the cervix (arrow).

Mild paresthesia and burning may be experienced before lesions become visible. With the development of the lesions, the patients complain of severe vulvar pain and exquisite tenderness of the infected tissues. Patients may also complain of inguinal pain, as well as pelvic pain related to inguinal and pelvic lymphadenopathy. Urination may be exceedingly painful, and not uncommonly patients develop urinary retention. Urinary symptoms usually occur when the urethra and bladder mucosa become infected (Person et al.)

Recurrent Herpes

Not all patients who have had primary herpes genitalis develop recurrent episodes of this infection; some patients never experience a second infection, whereas others have repeated flare-ups for many years. Approximately 50 percent of women will develop a recurrent infection within 6 months after the primary episode. Factors that are reputed to precipitate recurrences of infection include a febrile episode, emotional disturbance, premenstrual tension, and severe systemic disease. In fact, these conditions and recurrences are unrelated. The cause for the recurrence is unknown. The virus of herpes genitalis is harbored in the dorsal nerve route ganglia that receive sensory fibers from the genital tissues (Stevens, Cook). It is believed to migrate down the nerve fibers to the affected area when the infection recurs.

Recurrent lesions are often inconspicuous and difficult to identify. The infections involve the same sites described for the primary infection. Individual vulvar lesions are vesicular-ulcerative in type; they may vary from 1 to 5 mm in diameter and have an erythematous base. These lesions frequently develop in small, localized patches. The clear, vesicular fluid within the vesicles rapidly becomes turbid, and the vesicles rupture within 24 to 48 hours. Healing usually takes place within 7 to 10 days following onset of the disease and leaves the vulva with a completely normal appearance. Secondary bacterial infection may delay healing and give rise to inguinal lymphadenopathy. Lesions of the cervix and vagina are similar (Fig. 40–3). Patients with recurrent infection complain of burning and pain lasting from 7 to 10 days. Burning on urination may also be a distressing symptom. These symptoms are much less severe than those noted with the primary infection.

Diagnosis

Herpes genitalis should always be suspected in the presence of superficial ulcerated conditions of the vulvovaginal tissues. Cytologic studies can be used to confirm the presence of herpes simplex infection and are frequently useful in the diagnosis of unsuspected cases. The cytologic changes are most pronounced in the cell nuclei. Early in the course of the infection the nuclei enlarge and the chromatin is displaced against the nuclear membrane, which gives the nuclei a glassy appearance. Multinucleated cells are common (Fig 40–4). Acidophilic intranuclear inclusion bodies may be seen. The cytoplasm of the epithelial cells is often vacuolated and occasionally fragmented. The diagnosis of herpes simplex infection can be confirmed most accurately by means of virologic culture studies of the lesions. Cotton-tipped applicators containing samples from the base of the

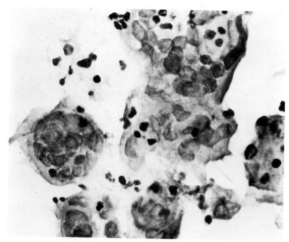

FIGURE 40–4 Cervicovaginal smear, H & E, 450X. Multinucleated giant cells are noted in the presence of herpes infection.

ulcerated lesions and from the cervix should be placed in special virologic culture media (Eagle's media with 5% calves' serum) and transported rapidly to the laboratory. The virus grows on the chorioallantoic membrane of chick embryos and HeLa cultures and produces typical plaques. A rise in neutralizing antibodies may be demonstrated in primary infections with the use of serologic methods.

Herpes Genitalis During Pregnancy

One of the most serious consequences of herpesvirus infection is associated with pregnancy. Primary herpes genitalis during early pregnancy results in increased numbers of abortions and late in pregnancy in an increase in the prematurity rate (Nahmias et al., 1971). Infants delivered through the birth canal in the presence of an active infection are at great risk to develop herpes infections which are usually systemic and may be fatal or leave the infant with severe brain damage. The presence of herpesvirus infection at or near term (primary disease after 34th week) constitutes an indication for cesarean section if the fetal membranes are intact or have been ruptured for less than 4 hours. The risk to the infant is greatest when the mother has a primary infection.

Herpesvirus and Carcinoma of the Cervix

Since the mid-1960s there has been controversial evidence of an etiologic relationship between the presence of herpesvirus 2 and carcinoma of the cervix. Nahmias et al. (1970) and Rawls et al. (1973) have published extensive epidemiologic evidence of

this possible relationship. Patients with antibodies to the herpesvirus type 2 are up to ten times more likely to have invasive carcinoma than women without such viral antibodies. Nahmias et al. (1973) found that cervical dysplasia was present twice as often and carcinoma in situ eight times as often in women who had had genital herpes than in control women.

Treatment

No specific treatment is available for herpes genitalis, and no prophylactic treatment is available to prevent its recurrence. Treatment is directed toward the relief of symptoms through utilizing analgesics, hot sitz baths, and occasionally topical antibiotics to prevent secondary infection of the herpetic lesions. Several new antiviral agents (Phosphonacetic acid, Ribavirin, Vidarabine) are currently under investigation as means of treating this infection.

Efforts should be directed to preventing infection by instructing patients to avoid sexual contact during and for 7 to 14 days after active infection.

CONDYLOMA ACUMINATUM

Condylomata acuminatum, also called venereal or genital warts, are wart papillomata of the genitalia which consist of a fibrous-tissue overgrowth from the dermis, covered with extremely thick epithelium.

Etiology

Condylomata acuminatum, also called venereal or genital warts, are wart papillomata of the genitalia ally. Oriel and Almeda demonstrated the virus particles in human genital warts. They noted that the viral particles were similar to those found in common skin warts. Aside from the local environmental conditions in the region of the vulva, the two lesions are similar.

Clinical Features

The vulva, particularly the vestibule and the labial folds, is the most common site of condylomata acuminatum. Lesions may also be seen on the perianal skin, the mons pubis, the vagina, the cervix, and even on the mucosa of the lower anal canal and urethra. The warts appear first as small discrete papillary structures which may spread and enlarge (Fig. 40–5) and in so doing coalesce to form large, cauliflower-like masses with broad bases. Lesions may become ulcerated and infected and exude a foul odor. Associated vaginal infections, such as trichomoniasis, candidiasis, and gonorrhea, may also be present.

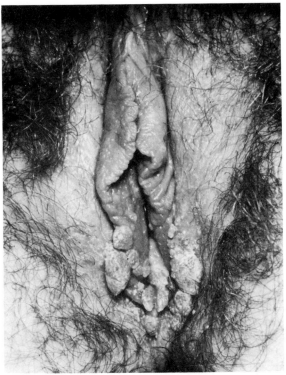

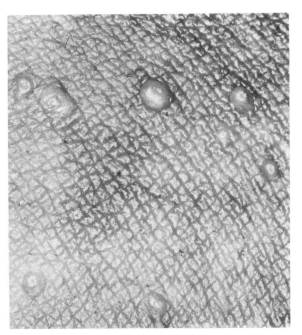

FIGURE 40–6 Vulva, molluscum contagiosum. Multiple dome-shaped papules with central umbilication are seen.

FIGURE 40–5 Vulva, condyloma acuminatum. Multiple wartlike structures are noted over the perineum and lower labia minora and majora.

Histopathology

The basic microscopical appearance of condylomata acuminatum is that of a markedly thickened epithelium forming numerous folds around stalks of connective tissue. Pronounced acanthosis with elongation of epithelial folds and papillomatosis are present. Variable degrees of parakeratosis and inflammatory reaction within the dermis are seen. Cytoplasmic vacuolization of individual cells in the upper half of the epithelium may be conspicuous.

Treatment

The first step in the treatment of condylomata acuminatum should be the eradication of any associated infections that may serve as independent source of leukorrhea. For small lesions, a 20% solution of podophyllin in tincture of benzoin is quite effective in eradicating the lesions. Local application usually causes blanching of the lesions within a few hours and sloughing within 2 to 4 days. Trichloroacetic acid (Nevatol) is equally effective in eradicating isolated lesions. Lesions over 2 cm in diameter are best removed by means of cryocautery, the electric cutting loop, or knife excision. Electrodesiccation followed by curettage of the condylomata may also be utilized effectively in treating large lesions. Occasionally, patients are seen with condylomata acuminatum that are completely refractory to treatment. Powell et al. reported successful results with the use of an autogenous vaccine prepared by grinding up the patient's own warts.

Reportedly, vulvar carcinoma and condylomata are seldom associated, yet Josey et al. feel that there is an association of condyloma acuminatum with carcinoma of the vulva, penis, and anorectum. Although the association of these diseases is not common, the clinician should maintain a high index of suspicion, especially in the patient with long-standing vulvar condylomata.

MOLLUSCUM CONTAGIOSUM

Molluscum contagiosum involves a proliferative process of the skin which resembles a localized neoplasm. The disease usually affects the vulva and is more prevalent than most gynecologists realize. Molluscum contagiosum is caused by a mildly contagious, growth-stimulating pox virus that is limited in its effect to the epithelium. The infection is transmissible by both direct and indirect contact; coital transference is the usual method in the adult.

Clinical Features

The lesions are usually multiple, with individual growths varying in size from a pinhead to 1 cm in diameter. The typical lesion is a dome-shaped papule (Fig. 40-6). Beginning as a seedling 1 to 2 mm in diameter, the lesion grows slowly over a period of many months. Necrosis and infection of the overlying skin may produce umbilication with an opening in the center of the small papules. Pruritus is frequently noted.

Histopathology

The papule is a circumscribed mass of proliferating acanthotic epithelium with hyperkeratosis. During proliferation, downward growth of the epithelium compresses the connective tissue of the dermis to form a pseudocapsule. Many of the epidermal cells undergo degeneration as they advance from the basal layer to the surface. As these degenerated cells are desquamated, a central cavity forms at the surface. Degeneration of the epithelial cells is caused by the formation of cytoplasmic inclusion bodies, referred to as molluscum bodies. The molluscum bodies contain numerous elementary bodies representing the virus. The molluscum bodies compress the nucleus of the individual cells, displacing them to the periphery of the cell and giving them a crescent appearance.

Treatment

Manual expression of the contents from each lesion, followed by the application of carbolic acid or trichloroacetic acid to the cavity, is a simple method of treatment. Another method of therapy consists of removing the individual papules with a small dermal curette. After curettage, the base of the lesion may be desiccated lightly or painted with Monsel's solution.

BEHÇET'S SYNDROME

The "triple-symptom complex" of Behçet is rarely found in the United States. Although the disease complex is characterized chiefly by genital and oral ulcerations and ocular inflammation, disorders of the skin resembling erythema nodosum and erythema multiforme, disturbances of the central nervous system, arthritic disease, and thrombophlebitis are not uncommonly associated with Behçet's syndrome.

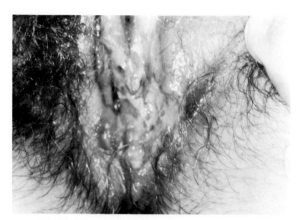

FIGURE 40-7 Vulva, Behçet's syndrome. Large, deep, necrotic-appearing ulcer is present on the lower aspect of the left labia and extends to the perineum. This ulcer had been present for 6 months.

Etiology

This disease used to be considered viral in etiology. Several workers have reported a specific virus to be its cause (Sezer; Evans et al.). Currently, however, most opinions suggest that this is probably one of the so-called "autoimmune" diseases. Its exact cause is unknown.

Clinical Features

The ulcers begin as small vesicles or papules which eventually ulcerate, become craterous, and are usually covered by a gray slough (Fig. 40-7). Lesions of the mouth, eyes, and genitals may appear on separate occasions. The genital lesions may involve the vulva, vagina, and cervix, and healing may be followed by fibrosis, scarring, and labial perforation. Pain and dyspareunia are outstanding symptoms. The oral lesions may also present as painful ulcers. Ocular lesions begin as a superficial inflammation, but at times progress to iridocyclitis and even blindness.

Treatment

Systemic corticosteroids are the most consistently successful treatment. Forty milligrams of Kenalog, IM, repeated in 7 to 10 days, may result in complete regression of the ulcerated lesions. Prolonged use of corticosteroids is not recommended. The local intralesional injection of Kenalog suspension 10 mg/mL diluted 3:1 with normal saline is also frequently of benefit.

Recently "transfer factor" has been successfully utilized in the treatment of this disease.

BENIGN TUMORS

Both solid and cystic tumors occur frequently in the vulva and occasionally in the vagina, with cystic tumors being the more common. A general classification of both groups of tumors is presented, and the more common lesions are discussed.

SOLID TUMORS

Solid tumors of the vulva (Gardner, Kaufman):

Epidermal origin:	Condyloma acuminatum
	Acrochordon
	Seborrheic keratosis
	Nevus
Epidermal appendage origin:	Hidradenoma
	Sebaceous adenoma
	Basal-cell carcinoma
Mesodermal origin:	Fibroma
	Lipoma
	Neurofibroma
	Leiomyoma
	Granular-cell myoblastoma
	Hemangioma
	Pyogenic granuloma
	Lymphangioma
Bartholin's gland origin:	Adenofibroma
Urethral origin:	Caruncle
	Prolapse of urethral mucosa

Each of the above tumors may present as a superficial mass involving the skin or may occur within the dermis. In many instances, such as those of condyloma acuminatum, acrochordon, and intradermal nevus, the diagnosis is usually obvious. When the exact nature of the tumor is unclear, an excision biopsy should be carried out. In most patients, this procedure can be performed in the office under local anesthesia.

Acrochordon

The acrochordon is a polypoid fibroepithelial lesion that frequently appears on the vulva and the adjacent medial aspect of the thigh or in the perianal area; it is usually referred to as a "skin tag." Most so-called papillomata are probably no more than acrochordons. The acrochordon is a soft, flesh-colored, gray-tan, wrinkled polypoid structure devoid of hair which varies in size from several millimeters to one centimeter (Fig. 40-8). Microscopically, the acrochordon is seen to be covered by gentle folds of mature, slightly hyperkeratotic epithelium. The stalk and substance of the tumor are composed of loose, fibrous tissue which

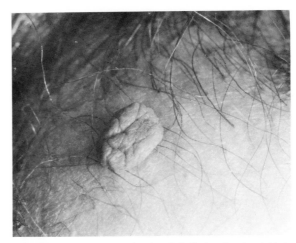

FIGURE 40-8 Vulva, acrochordon. Soft, flesh-colored, wrinkled, polypoid structure is seen.

contains scattered capillaries. The cause of the acrochordon is unknown. Acrochordons do not become malignant; they need not be treated. They may be removed for cosmetic reasons or if they show chronic irritation.

Pigmented Nevus

The chief significance of the pigmented nevus, junctional or compound, is the fact that it may be the starting point for malignant melanoma. Raised or sessile nevi are less likely to develop into malignant melanomas, but owing to their location, they are frequently irritated and annoying to the patient. Therefore, these nevi, as well as all flat dark nevi, should be removed surgically. This procedure can frequently be accomplished when other minor gynecologic surgery is indicated, at the time of delivery, or under local anesthesia in the office.

Basal-Cell Carcinoma

Generally recognized as a locally invasive lesion, this tumor does not represent a carcinoma in the usual sense of the term. No adequately documented, properly treated case of basal-cell carcinoma of the vulva, in which death has occurred due to neoplasm, has been reported. The incidence of basal-cell tumor of the vulva is reported to be between 2 and 4 percent of neoplasms in this site. The tumor arises most often in postmenopausal women. Most investigators support the concept of basal-cell origin of this tumor.

Clinical manifestations of the basal-cell carcinoma include pruritis, burning, and chronic ulceration. Bleeding and discharge may be associated with

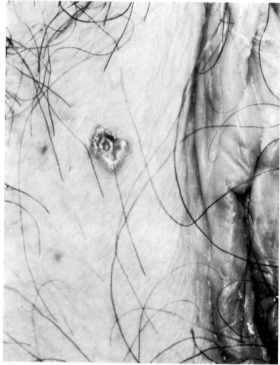

FIGURE 40–9 Vulva, basal-cell tumor. Ulcerated area with raised, curled borders is seen. *(From Gardner, Kaufman.)*

large lesions. Typically, vulvar tumors are slightly raised, slow-growing nodules with central ulcerations that rarely cause annoyance (Fig. 40–9). The base of the ulcers may be covered with a small amount of necrotic debris or small crusts. If untreated, the tumors may erode deeply into the underlying tissues and into the bone of the symphysis pubis.

Histopathologic examination shows that the basal-cell carcinoma is composed of nests of closely packed, uniform cells of oval or fusiform shape. The clusters of cells appear as single or multiple growths arising from the basal layer of the epidermis or from a hair shaft or glandular apparatus. Many of the cell clusters are rimmed by a single layer of cells arranged in a radial pattern which results in peripheral palisading of cells.

These tumors should be excised widely; a wide margin of surrounding normal skin and a considerable depth of underlying tissue should also be removed.

Tumors of Mesodermal Origin

These tumors arise frequently in the vulva and less frequently in the vagina; they may originate in fibrous tissue, fat, smooth muscle, blood vessels, or nerves. In most instances, they should be surgically removed, primarily to establish the diagnosis and occasionally because their presence may cause the patient some discomfort. One of the more interesting varieties of tumors in this category is the granular-cell myoblastoma, which may be found in almost any location in the body. Birch and Sondag found that 35 percent of the lesions involved the tongue, 30 percent occurred in the skin or nearby tissues, and 35 percent at various other sites. Seven percent of the tumors were found on the vulva. Although several origins of this tumor have been hypothesized, recent studies suggest that the granular-cell myoblastoma originates from the nerve sheath (Sobel et al.). The granular-cell myoblastoma is a benign, usually solitary, discrete nodule that tends to infiltrate the adjacent tissues. Tumors may invade deeply into the vulva, but more often they are superficial and elevated and occasionally the overlying skin may be ulcerated. Microscopical study shows irregularly arranged bundles of large, pink-staining, round, and polyhedral cells with indistinct cell borders, the bundles separated by bands of collagen fibers. The cytoplasm of the cells contains numerous eosinophilic granules, 0.1 to 3.0 μm in diameter. The nuclei may be small or large and are usually dark-staining, centrally placed structures that contain one or two nucleoli. The margins of the tumor are irregular; bands of tumor cells extend into the contiguous tissue and follow nerve fibers. Treatment of the tumor consists of wide, local excision. If nests of tumor cells remain, there is a strong possibility that the tumor will recur.

Urethral Caruncles

These lesions appear on the posterior distal urethra in postmenopausal women; they seldom appear during the childbearing years. The urethral caruncle probably develops from ectropion of the posterior urethral wall, secondary to postmenopausal shrinkage of the surrounding tissues. All the subsequent changes in the everted mucosa are caused by altered environmental conditions and trauma.

The urethral caruncle is a benign, red, fleshy tumor noted in the distal portion of the posterior urethral mucosa (Fig. 40-10). Most caruncles are only a few millimeters in diameter, but many grow to 1 cm. Most urethral caruncles are asymptomatic, but occasionally the small growth may be noted by the patient either because she palpates it or because of irritation of the lesion, with associated pain and bleeding.

Histopathology of caruncles shows a core of

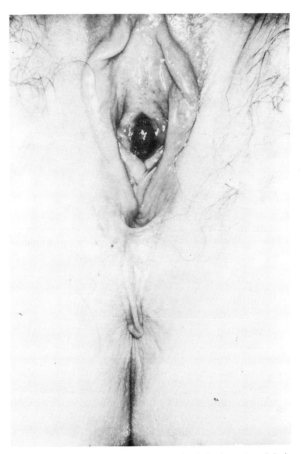

FIGURE 40–10 Vulva, urethral caruncle. A fleshy red nodule is noted extending from the posterior urethra.

of electrocoagulation or cryocautery. Large symptomatic caruncles are best treated by local excision.

CYSTIC TUMORS

Cystic tumors of the vulva:

Epidermal origins:	Traumatic inclusion cyst
	Epidermal cyst
	Pilonidal cyst
Epidermal appendage origin:	Sebaceous cyst
	Hidradenoma
	Fox-Fordyce disease
	Syringoma
Embryonic origin:	Mesonephric (Gartner's) cyst
	Paramesonephric (Müllerian) cyst
	Cyst of canal of Nuck (hydrocele)
	Cyst of supernumerary mammary glands
	Adenosis
	Dermoid cyst
Bartholin's duct cyst and Bartholin abcess	
Urethral and paraurethral origin:	Skene's duct cyst
	Urethral diverticulum
Miscellaneous origins:	Endometriosis
	Cystic lymphangioma
	Liquefied hematoma
	Vaginitis emphysematosa

Epidermal Inclusion Cyst

Viable stratified squamous epithelium, if buried beneath either skin or mucosa, may proliferate, secrete, and desquamate, forming an "inclusion cyst." The epidermal cyst is the most common variety of cyst found in the vulva and probably the most common tumefaction of the vulva. Traumatic inclusion cysts are the most common vaginal cysts; most follow implantation or entrapment of fragments of mucosa incident to repair of an episiotomy or vaginal laceration.

The cysts vary from several millimeters to several centimeters in diameter (Fig. 40–11). The contents of the cysts resemble a thick, purulent exudate. Epidermal cysts arise chiefly in the labia majora, particularly the anterior half. As a rule, they are multiple, grow slowly, and are round, nontender, and deep-seated. Unless these cysts are quite large, they are usually asymptomatic.

Vaginal epidermal cysts are lined with stratified squamous epithelium similar to, but thinner than, vaginal mucosa. The cysts contain masses of desquamated epithelial cells.

loose connective tissue, dilated blood vessels, and inflammatory cells covered by an epithelial layer. The core of loose fibrous tissue contains a heavy infiltration of lymphocytes as well as some plasma cells and an occasional neutrophil. Columns of transitional or squamous epithelium may extend down into the lesion, which makes it difficult at times to differentiate this tumor from carcinoma. The lesion may be covered by a lining of squamous or transitional epithelium, or its surface may be ulcerated and have no surface epithelial covering.

Small asymptomatic caruncles need not be treated. If the nature of the lesion is questionable, a small specimen should be removed for microscopical study to confirm the diagnosis. As a rule, the subjective complaints and bleeding associated with caruncles can be controlled by topical application of estrogen cream to the vagina and urethra or by oral estrogen. Small lesions can be destroyed by means

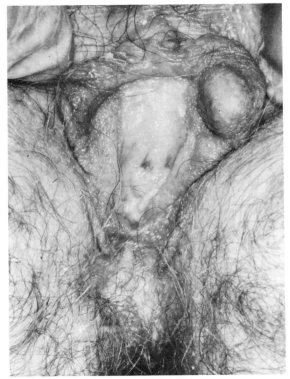

FIGURE 40–11 Vulva, epidermal cyst. A cystic, nontender swelling is noted on the inner aspect of the labia minora. *(From Gardner, Kaufman.)*

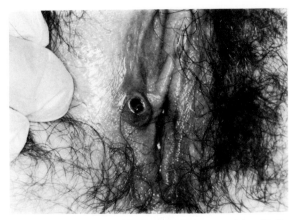

FIGURE 40–12 Vulva, hidradenoma. A tumor nodule with the ventral surface ulcerated and red papillomatous tissue protruding.

Since vaginal epidermal cysts seldom produce symptoms and their presence is thus unknown to the patient, the majority do not require treatment. Their excision is occasionally desirable if they prove to be annoying to the patient on the basis of their presence, pain, or irritation.

Hidradenoma

Although a hidradenoma may be solid, the majority are cystic. This relatively rare, essentially asymptomatic, small tumor arises from the sweat glands of the vulva. For unknown reasons, the tumor occurs almost exclusively in Caucasian women.

The hidradenoma appears chiefly on the labia majora as a sharply circumscribed, elevated nodule only occasionally larger than 1 cm in diameter. The consistency of the tumor varies from hard to soft, and it is usually freely movable beneath the skin. Occasionally, pressure necrosis of the overlying skin results in eruption of the tumor's contents with protrusion of the red granular papillomatous tissue (Fig. 40–12).

Hidradenomata frequently appear to be cystic nodules partially or completely filled with papillomatous growths. They consist of irregular acini and tubules separated by fine connective-tissue septa. The papillary projections are covered by a single layer of epithelial cells, as are many of the acini. The cells are tall columnar or cuboidal, have a pale eosinophilic cytoplasm, and a vesicular nucleus located near the base of the cell. A second layer of myoepithelial cells may lie deep to the secretory cells. Because of the pronounced glandular proliferation, the tumor may be mistaken for an adenocarcinoma.

Local excision is the only treatment required since these lesions are rarely, if ever, malignant.

Fox-Fordyce Disease

Fox-Fordyce disease is exceedingly rare. It is characterized by a chronic pruritic eruption of multiple microcytes (Fig. 40–13). These small cysts are formed by retention of sweat in the apocrine gland ducts following their obstruction by excessive keratinization of follicular epithelium. The disease does not appear until after puberty since apocrine function does not begin until after this phase of life. Numerous discrete, minute papules, 1 to 3 mm in diameter, are closely grouped together in the area of the labia majora, on the thighs, and mons pubis. The axilla may also be involved. Itching is quite intense; it is more severe during the menses and is associated with emotional crises. The pruritus probably results from escape of apocrine secretions into tissues through ruptured apocrine ducts. Biopsy of the lesions reveals small intraepidermal cysts lined by flattened epithe-

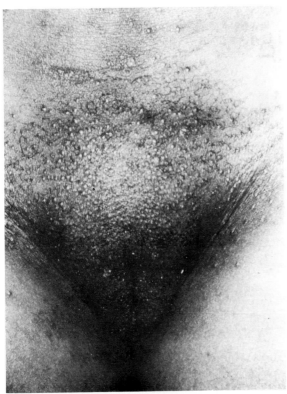

FIGURE 40–13 Fox-Fordyce disease. Typical discrete, minute papules are present over the lower abdomen, mons pubis, labia majora, and inner thighs. *(Courtesy of John M. Knox, Houston, Texas.)*

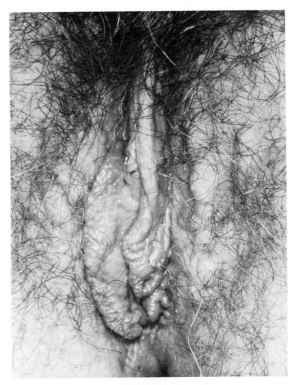

FIGURE 40–14 Syringoma. Multiple small cystic structures seen as papules on the labia majora.

lium. Apocrine excretory ducts are occluded by keratin and enlarged.

The pruritus associated with Fox-Fordyce disease is intense, and until recently an effective means of relieving it was unknown. As already indicated, this is a disease process seen in women during the childbearing years. The use of estrogen-dominant combination birth control pills has proved to be extremely effective in relieving the pruritus. Since the disease primarily affects women with normal hormonal activity, the reason for the beneficial response to this type of hormone therapy is quite confusing.

Syringoma

Syringoma is exhibited by multiple, small, firm papules of cystic structures beneath the skin of the labia majora (Fig. 40–14). Although frequently asymptomatic, it may be associated with pruritus. Biopsy of one of the papules reveals numerous small cystic ducts lined by two layers of epithelial cells. The cells are cuboidal, and the inner layer has a clear, vacuolated appearance.

Cysts of Embryonic Origin

Mesonephric, paramesonephric, and urogenital sinus (mucous) cysts are similar and will be discussed jointly.

True Gartner's duct cysts arise from vestigial remnants of the vaginal portion of the mesonephric (Wolffian) ducts in the female, referred to as Gartner's ducts. These ducts normally become atretic during embryonic development and lose their glandular lining. If parts of the ducts persist and remain functional, secretory activity may give rise to cystic tumors (Fig. 40–15). These cysts arise within the vagina, along the anterior lateral walls. Most of the vaginal cysts referred to as "Gartner's duct cysts" are Müllerian in origin and probably represent areas of adenosis.

A second, more common variety of embryonic cyst arises from vestiges of paramesonephric epithelium. In early embryonic life, the vagina is lined with Müllerian epithelium. Subsequently, the latter is replaced by stratified squamous epithelium that grows

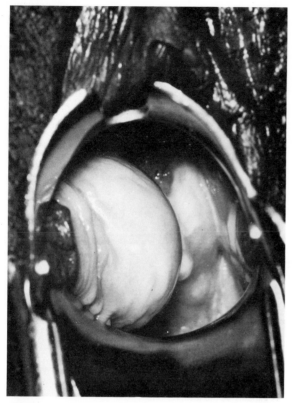

FIGURE 40–15 Vagina, Gartner's duct cyst. A cystic structure can be seen bulging into the vagina from the lateral vaginal wall. *(From Gardner, Kaufman.)*

upward from the urogenital sinus. During this process of upward displacement, islands of Müllerian epithelium may persist in the vaginal wall.

Another type of developmental cyst seen in the vulva is the so-called mucous cyst, which is indistinguishable from cysts of paramesonephric origin. Mucous cysts are believed to derive from epithelium of urogenital-sinus origin.

The gross appearance and symptomatology of the developmental cysts of embryonic origin are not characteristic. Those cysts that are actually of mesonephric origin are located along the route followed by the Gartner's duct, but paramesonephric cysts may arise anywhere in the vagina, and mucous cysts are found primarily in the vestibule, near the clitoris or hymenal ring. Most embryonic vaginal cysts appear in the wall of the vagina; they are usually less than 2 cm in diameter and are asymptomatic. A few cysts reach sufficient size to protrude through the vaginal introitus. Cysts that primarily involve the vulva are

usually solitary, less than 2 cm in diameter, and asymptomatic. The development of carcinoma or infection in the embryonic cyst is extremely rare.

The majority of mesonephric-duct cysts are lined by nonciliated cuboidal or low-columnar epithelium which generally has a demonstrable basement membrane. Occasionally, a partial lining of squamous epithelium is observed. Mesonephric-duct cysts are distinguished from paramesonephric cysts on the basis of histochemical stains. The latter contain substances within the cell cytoplasm that give rise to a positive periodic acid Schiff (PAS) reaction and a positive mucin stain.

Paramesonephric (Müllerian) cysts are mainly of two types, endocervical and tuboendometrial. The endocervical cysts, characterized by tall columnar cells with basal nuclei and a clear cytoplasm, constitute the vast majority of cysts. These characteristics are also present in that group of cysts supposedly of urogenital-sinus origin. The "tuboendometrial" cyst is usually lined by irregular columnar epithelium with both ciliated and secretory cells on a poorly defined or absent basement membrane. The paramesonephric epithelium contains both acid and neutral polysaccharides and mucin, and PAS stains are positive.

Since most of these cysts are small, asymptomatic, and benign, a patient usually requires no treatment. However, if the cyst becomes large and causes mechanical problems or discomfort to the patient, its removal may be indicated.

Several investigators have noted a relationship between the ingestion of diethylstilbestrol (DES) during the first half of pregnancy and the presence of adenosis (Fig. 40–16) and clear-cell adenocarcinoma in the vaginas of female offspring of such pregnancies (Herbst et al.; Stafl et al.). Adenosis may be found in over 30 percent of DES-exposed young women. In such individuals the "original squamocolumnar junction" is frequently found within the vagina rather than in the region of the anatomic external os of the cervix. Islands of columnar epithelium of endocervical or tuboendometrial type are frequently found beneath the squamous epithelium lining of the vagina. These islands of epithelium frequently exit into the vaginal mucosa.

No treatment is required for asymptomatic adenosis. If the patient is troubled by a profuse mucorrhea, the adenosis can be eliminated by electrodessication, cryocautery, or laser beam. The use of the vaginal application of progesterone or acidifying vaginal gel has been reported to be successful in producing

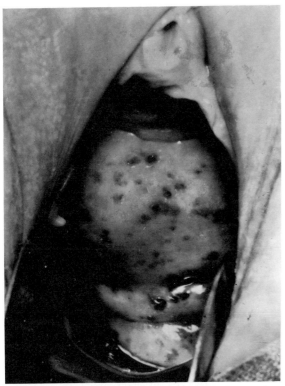

FIGURE 46–16 Vaginal adenosis *(From D Evans, H Hughes, J Obstet Gynecol Br Commonw 68:247, 1961.)*

regression of the lesions. Indeed, spontaneous regression may occur.

Although a very small percentage of DES-exposed females with vaginal adenosis and cervical ectropion develop clear-cell carcinoma of the vagina or cervix, such patients should be carefully examined at regular intervals.

Bartholin Abscess and Bartholin's Duct Cyst

Bartholin's duct cysts arise in the duct system of Bartholin's glands. There is occlusion of some part of the duct system, and the continued secretory activity of the Bartholin's gland results in distention of the duct and formation of the cyst. Most commonly, the occlusion is near the opening of the main duct into the vestibule. When a cyst becomes infected, the contents become purulent and a Bartholin abscess is formed.

Obstruction of the Bartholin's duct is an essential etiologic factor in the development of Bartholin cysts. The cause of this obstruction is usually obscure; ab-

scesses and cysts are sometimes the result of a gonorrheal infection. If primary gonorrheal bartholinitis is present, it becomes a potent factor in the production of occlusion of the duct. Bartholinitis from other microbial agents is uncommon and thus unimportant in the etiology of ductal occlusion and cyst formation. Although a cause-and-effect relationship between Bartholin cysts and abscesses is well established, it is unknown whether obstruction and cyst formation occur more before bartholinitis or after it. Congenital stenosis or atresia of the ducts may play a role in the formation of Bartholin cysts. Another factor that may cause obstruction of the duct is thickened or inspissated mucus near the ductal opening. Mechanical trauma from any cause may also give rise to ductal occlusion.

The chief symptom of Bartholin abscess is a varying degree of pain and tenderness over the infected gland. Some abscesses develop slowly over a week or longer and may give rise to only mild symptoms. This type of smoldering infection may ultimately regress. Most abscesses, however, usually develop rapidly over a period of 2 to 3 days and are associated with exquisite pain and tenderness. Considerable edema of the surrounding tissues is noted, and the abscess usually ruptures spontaneously within 72 hours. The objective signs include unilateral swelling over the site of the infected gland, redness of the overlying skin, and edema of the labia (Fig. 40–17). The abscess is palpable as an extremely tender, fluctuant mass. The size of the lesion may vary from 2 to 3 cm to as large as 5 to 6 cm in diameter.

Local application of heat, preferably by hot wet dressings or sitz baths, promotes spontaneous drainage of the abscess or its development to a stage suitable for incision and drainage. Early treatment of obvious bartholinitis with broad-spectrum antibiotics may prevent the formation of an abscess. If the abscess is fluctuant, incision and drainage should be performed. If a small, inflatable bulb-tipped catheter (Word catheter) is inserted into a small stab incision in the abscess and is left in place for 4 to 6 weeks, it will not only result in drainage of the abscess but will frequently lead to the formation of a new opening for the duct and will prevent recurrence of a Bartholin's duct cyst.

Most patients with a small Bartholin cyst have no symptoms although some may observe minor discomfort on sexual intercourse. If the cyst becomes enlarged or infected, other complaints arise. Extremely large lesions may interfere with walking or coitus. Examination shows the presence of a cystic structure in

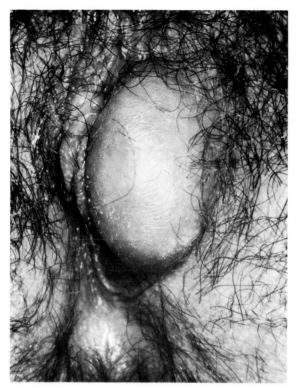

FIGURE 40–17 Vulva, Bartholin abscess. Unilateral swelling with edema distorts the left side of the vulva. *(From Gardner, Kaufman.)*

the region of the Bartholin's gland. The cysts are usually unilateral, nontender, and tense and are situated in the posterior part of the labia majora. The cysts may vary in diameter from 1 to as much as 10 cm.

If the cyst is asymptomatic and small, no treatment is necessary. Cysts that are subject to recurrent abscess formation and those that cause pressure symptoms or introital obstruction require surgical attention. The complications and morbidity associated with removal of Bartholin cysts may preclude total removal of the cyst and gland. Marsupialization of Bartholin cysts is often a preferable manner of treatment. A longitudinal incision approximately 1.5 cm in length is made parallel to and outside the hymenal ring over the cyst. With the use of interrupted sutures, the edges of the cyst wall are sutured to the edges of the skin. Within 2 to 3 weeks the opening shrinks to a fraction of a centimeter and remains as a permanent outlet for secretions of the gland. The insertion of a Word inflatable, bulb-tipped catheter into such a cyst is also highly successful.

VULVAR DYSTROPHIES

Vulvar dystrophies are among the most misunderstood disease processes involving the vulva. The term encompasses what used to be called leukoplakia, leukoplakic vulvitis, kraurosis vulvae, primary atrophy, and atrophic and hyperplastic vulvitis. In the past, the significance of these lesions was their alleged relationship to the development of vulvar carcinoma. We prefer to accept Jeffcoate's recommendation and to designate all these related lesions under the term "chronic vulvar dystrophies." The word dystrophy is defined as "abnormal nourishment" or "defect of nutrition," which means little to the clinician attempting to treat these diseases. Thus, we have classified all the dystrophic lesions, based primarily upon their histopathology, in a manner which we hope will be readily understood by both clinician and pathologist. Further, we believe the older terms alluded to above should be deleted from the nomenclature of the gynecologist and pathologist.

Vulvar dystrophies include, in the classification proposed by the International Society for Study of Vulvar Disease, hyperplastic dystrophy with and without atypia; lichen sclerosus; mixed dystrophy (lichen sclerosus with foci of epithelial hyperplasia) with and without atypia. Most hyperplastic dystrophies fall within the group without atypia (what many dermatologists would call neurodermatitis). All the hyperplastic lesions are associated with epithelial hyperplasia and hyperkeratosis, but the gross appearance may be quite variable. Furthermore, the gross appearance may change from time to time, depending upon the local environment of moisture and heat and the extent to which the patient rubs and scratches the vulvar areas. Lesions may involve labia majora, the interlabial sulci, the outer aspect of the labia minora, the hood of the clitoris, and the posterior commissure. The skin changes may also extend onto the lateral surfaces of the labia majora and the adjacent thighs. Frequently, the areas of dystrophy are localized, elevated, and delineated. On other occasions, the vulvar lesions may be extensive and poorly defined. The vulva may have a red appearance. Under other circumstances, the vulva may contain numerous thick white patches or a combination of red and white areas. The tissues appear thick and lichenified. Fissuring and excoriation may be present as a result of scratching. Examination of biopsies of these lesions shows a variable increase in thickness in the horny

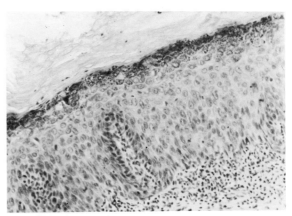

FIGURE 40-19 Vulva, hyperplastic dystrophy with atypia (dysplasia). H & E, 289X. Changes of nuclear variability in size and shape are seen extending almost up to the granular layer. A rare mitosis is noted. There is hyperkeratosis.

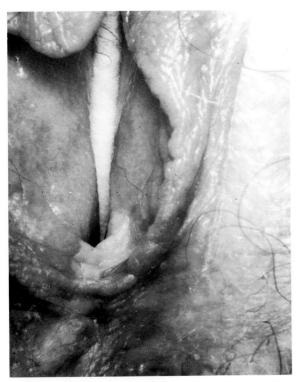

FIGURE 40-18 Vulva, hyperplastic dystrophy with atypia (dysplasia). Sharply demarcated, raised, white area is noted at the lower tip of the white pointer.

layer (hyperkeratosis) and an irregular thickening of the malpighian layer (acanthosis), which results in thickening of the epithelium, lengthening and elongation of the rete pegs, and, frequently, distal clubbing of the rete pegs. A variable inflammatory reaction is present within the dermis. This infiltrate consists primarily of lymphocytes and a small number of plasma cells.

To date, the authors have not seen a single case of carcinoma that has developed in lesions classified as hyperplastic dystrophies without atypia in 55 women studied. These women's cases were followed from several months to 18 years. The vulvar dystrophies exhibiting epithelial atypia have far greater potential for malignancy. Jeffcoate observed such lesions in only a small percentage of the patients he studied, but these lesions proved to be precursors of carcinoma. The majority of such lesions are localized, well dèlineated, and white (Fig. 40-18). Occasionally, they have a red appearance, or both red and white patches may be present. In the presence of mild

atypia, the significant changes are first detected in the deeper layers of the epithelium. The nuclei vary in size and shape, and some are hyperchromatic. Scattered mitoses are noted. As the cellular atypia progresses, changes extend toward the surface and are associated with more pronounced degrees of atypia (Fig. 40-19) and loss of cellular polarity and cytoplasmic maturation. Finally, as these atypical changes extend through the full thickness of the epithelium, the picture of squamous-cell carcinoma in situ is seen.

Lichen sclerosus represents a specific disease entity, even though it is included in the general group of chronic vulvar dystrophies. Lesions identical to those seen on the vulva may be located elsewhere on the body, and thus the development of lichen sclerosus is not so dependent on the local environment of the vulva. The disease may involve the labia majora, the labia minora, the perianal skin, skin folds adjacent to the thighs, and clitoris, frequently in a bilaterally symmetric pattern. In addition, lesions may arise on the neck, on the trunk, on the forearms, under the breasts, and in the axilla. Oberfield observed genital lesions in only 22 of 56 women with lichen sclerosus. Chernosky et al. reported that the lesions were limited to the anogenital region in only 32 percent of their cases in children. Initially, the lesions appear as low, irregularly outlined, flat-topped, white maculopapules which later coalesce and form well-defined plaques. In the well-developed lesion, the skin has a crinkled "cigarette paper" appearance (Fig. 40-20). These changes frequently extend around the anal region in a figure-of-eight, keyhole fashion. Frequently,

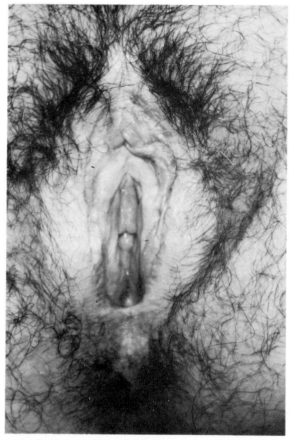

FIGURE 40-20   Vulva, lichen sclerosus. The tissue of the labia minora and perineum has a white, brittle, "cigarette paper" appearance.

narrow band of chronic inflammatory cells may be seen. On occasion, foci of epithelial hyperplasia are mixed within the areas of atrophic epithelial change. The areas of hyperplasia that develop adjacent to an otherwise atrophic lesion may well represent a response of these tissues to the local trauma.

In more than 50 patients with lichen sclerosus followed prospectively, the authors have seen only 1 patient with associated vulvar carcinoma. The woman was first seen with carcinoma of the vulva present without the changes of lichen sclerosus and subsequently was found to have changes of lichen sclerosus associated with the second early invasive carcinoma.

Pruritus is the predominant symptom associated with all the vulvar dystrophies. It is possible that this severe pruritus is associated with degeneration and inflammation around the terminal nerve fibers. The hyperplastic lesions appear to be associated with the most intense itching; in lichen sclerosus it is frequently mild. When pruritus is present, a vicious cycle is established; the itching provokes grattage, which in turn increases the pruritus. Scratching of the vulva frequently results in excoriations and further thickening of the skin and mucosa, which may result in soreness and pain in the vulvar region. Dyspareunia is frequently noted in association with lichen sclerosus secondary to the marked shrinkage of the introitus.

There are certain basic principles of treatment that should be followed. The patient should eliminate the use of all feminine deodorants, douches, perfumes, or other materials foreign to the vulvar area. The vulva and intertriginous areas should be kept dry, which can be accomplished by the elimination of underclothes of synthetic fabrics and of tight, constricting garments. The synthetic fabric in underpants prevents adequate evaporation of moisture, and thus the patient should be instructed either to wear no underpants at all or to wear cotton panties. Nonirritating soap should be used in the area, and the soap should be washed off thoroughly and the tissues thoroughly dried after bathing. Next, proper diagnosis should be made by adequate biopsy of the vulvar disease.

Vulvar biopsy is vital in arriving at the correct diagnosis of many vulvar disease processes. This is especially true in establishing the diagnosis of a vulvar dystrophy as well as intraepithelial carcinoma. A biopsy of the vulva is easily accomplished. The area to be biopsied should be thoroughly cleansed with an antiseptic solution. A 1% solution of lidocaine may be infiltrated into the tissues, but often is not necessary.

severe edema of the clitoral foreskin results in phimosis; subsequently, the foreskin may atrophy and adhere, resulting in complete disappearance of the clitoris from sight. The labia minora may completely disappear as a result of atrophy. Not uncommonly, splitting of the skin in the midline is observed. The introitus may become so stenotic that the opening will barely admit the tip of the small finger. Focal ecchymotic areas and small hematomas may be seen in the skin of the labia majora. This disease process may be seen in children, and the gross appearance of lichen sclerosus is typical. Characteristically, hyperkeratosis and thinning (atrophy) of the epithelium are present. There is flattening of the epithelial folds, and cytoplasmic vacuolization of the basal layer of cells is common. Beneath the squamous epithelium, there is a homogenized, collagenous-appearing zone having a pink acellular appearance. Just below this zone, a

A 4- or 6-mm dermal punch is then twisted into the recently made wheal, and the base of the tissue plug is severed with small scissors. The local application of Monsel's solution followed by pressure is adequate in the majority of cases to control bleeding. If necessary, a single figure-of-eight stitch can be used to close the skin edges. This biopsy specimen should then be bisected, properly oriented, fixed, and sent to the laboratory for evaluation. When carcinoma is suspected, the local application of toluidine blue followed by washing with acetic acid often helps in selecting biopsy sites. In an area where there is hypercellularity with increased numbers of active nuclei, the toluidine blue stain is retained by the cells. However, in areas with pronounced hyperkeratosis overlying areas of atypicality, the toluidine blue stain may not be retained after washing the area with acetic acid.

Since the overwhelming majority of chronic vulvar dystrophies are not premalignant, vulvectomy is not recommended except in highly exceptional circumstances, such as the presence of significant and extensive cellular atypia. The incidence of recurrence of the dystrophies following vulvectomy is so high that, for most lesions of this type, surgical treatment is contraindicated. After a correct diagnosis of a vulvar dystrophy has been established and the malignant potential of the lesion determined (presence or absence of atypia), local measures for the control of pruritus can be instituted. The general measures outlined above should be followed. The hyperplastic dystrophies without atypia are best treated by means of local application of one of the corticosteroid creams. Complete control of the pruritus and burning is no assurance that the lesions will regress.

The hyperplastic lesions, however, may improve to a striking degree or disappear entirely once pruritus is controlled. Richardson and Williams first reported pronounced improvement of the tissues with the use of 500 mg of testosterone proprionate in 10 g of white petrolatum jelly massaged into the vulvar tissues two to three times daily. Other experience has demonstrated that testosterone applied locally to the hyperplastic lesion has been of little value for either controlling symptoms or altering the gross and microscopic changes of the vulvar tissues. It has been effective in the treatment of lichen sclerosus. In the patient with lichen sclerosus, a 2 to 5 percent mixture of testosterone propionate in petrolatum jelly which is massaged thoroughly into the vulva two to three times a day results in relief of pruritus and in a thickening and softening of the vulvar tissues. If the pruritus is severe and is not relieved by the use of testosterone alone, the testosterone can be alternated with the topical application of a corticosteroid cream, or the corticosteroid can be mixed with the testosterone propionate. Once the patient has obtained relief of pruritus, the testosterone should be applied locally once or twice each week indefinitely. The treatment of lichen sclerosus in children is directed primarily to the relief of pruritus and can usually be accomplished with topical corticosteroids. Many lesions in children improve or disappear spontaneously during or after adolescence. Resolution usually leaves normal skin.

If atypical changes are noted within the epithelium, such lesions should be excised widely; it is vitally important that the margins of the excised tissue be studied carefully to confirm that all foci of atypia have been removed.

All patients with a chronic vulvar dystrophy should be examined at regular intervals, and biopsies should be taken from areas of ulceration or excoriation or from foci of retained toluidine blue stain.

VAGINITIS

The three most common types of vaginitis are trichomoniasis, *Hemophilus vaginalis* vaginitis, and candidiasis. The most common symptom associated with vaginal infections is leukorrhea. The various causes of vaginal discharge and the investigation of patients with vaginal discharge are presented in Chap. 24. (For a comprehensive review of all the major causes, see Gardner and Kaufman.)

Cultures are rarely required in the differential diagnosis of vaginitis. The wet mount is reliable in the diagnosis of most cases. The isolation of one of several bacterial agents in culture does not prove an etiologic relationship between the vaginitis present and the organisms isolated. Clinicians must guard against always assigning etiologic significance to bacterial agents enumerated on a laboratory report. In clinical laboratories, as a group, success with cultures for isolating *Trichomonas vaginalis* and *H. vaginalis* is highly variable.

Casman's blood agar (Difco) with 5 percent defibrinated rabbit blood is the best medium for culturing *H. vaginalis* (Dukes, Gardner). Incubation must be in an increased carbon dioxide atmosphere such as that produced in a candle jar. The colonies are minute and have a characteristic appearance when examined under magnification.

TABLE 40–1 Clinical and Laboratory Features of Vaginitis*

Symptoms	Normal	Trichomoniasis	H. vaginalis vaginitis
Discharge	0	1 to 3	0 to 3
Pruritus	0	0 to 3	0
Burning	0	0 to 1	0
Urinary	0	0 to 1	0
Dyspareunia	0	0 to 1	0
Characteristics of discharge			
Amount	0+	1 to 3	0 to 3
Consistency	Curdy	Homogeneous	Homogeneous
Color	White or slate	Gray or greenish (10%)	Gray
Order	0	1 to 3	1 to 3
Frothiness	0	10%	7%
pH	3.8 to 4.2	5.5 to 5.8	5.0 to 5.5
Gross tissue changes, vagina			
Erythema	0	0 to 3	0
Swollen papillae	0	15%	0
Petechiae	0	10%	0
Ulcerations	0	0	0
Gross tissue changes, vulva			
Erythema	0	0 to 2	0
Edema	0	0 to 2	0
Excoriations or ulcers	0	0 to 1	
Laboratory findings			
Wet mount			
Clue cells	0	0	1 to 3
Trichomonads	0		0
Spores and filaments	0	0	0
Leukocytes	0+	4	0+
Parabasal cells	0	1 to 3	0
Bacteria	Large rods	Mixed	Small rods
Stained smears	Lacto-dipth?	Mixed bacteria	Short gram-negative bacilli
Cultures	Lacto or dipth predominate	*Trichomonas vaginalis*	*Hemophilus vaginalis*

*Key: 0 = none, 3 = severe.

Nickerson's medium has proved highly accurate and practical for identifying candidal species. Nevertheless, culturing for *Candida* species (all are not *C. albicans*) is unnecessary if the organisms are identified on a KOH (potassium hydroxide) or saline wet mount. The only vaginal fungus encountered in material from either the vulva or vagina, which shows both spores and filaments, belongs to the genus *Candida*.

Many patients with vaginitis have two or more causes. For example, 25 percent of patients with trichomoniasis also have *H. vaginalis vaginitis,* both of which conditions are examples of minor venereal diseases. Experience shows that patients with one venereal disease are more apt to acquire a second or even a third sexually transmitted infection. Table 40–1 summarizes the clinical and laboratory findings in patients with vaginitis.

Candidiasis	Atrophic vaginitis	Herpes genitalis	Cervicitis
0 to 2	0 to 1	0 to 2	1 to 3
1 to 3	1 to 2	0+	0
1	1	2	0
1	0+	3	0
0 to 2	2	3	0
0 to 2	1	1	1 to 3
Curdy or thrush patches (20%)	Serous or mucopurulent	Serous	Mucoid or mucopurulent
White or slate	Variable	Clear	Clear yellow
0	1	0	0
0	0	0	0
4.0 to 5.0	6.7 to 7.0	Variable	Mucus 7+
0 to 2	1	Variable	None
0 to 1	0 to 1	0	0
0	10%	0	0
0	Occasional	0 to 2	0
1 to 3	0 to 1	1 to 3	0
0 to 3	0 to 0+	0 to 3	0
0 to 1	0−	1 to 3	0
0	0	0	0
0	0	0	0
1	0	0	0
1 to 3	3	2	0 to 2
0	3	0 to 2	0
Large rods	Mixed	Lacto-mixed	Lacto
Lacto-dipth	Mixed	Giant cells	Lacto-mixed
Candida species	Mixed bacteria	Lacto or mixed	Lacto occ. Neissa.

TRICHOMONIASIS

Trichomoniasis, which at one time represented 40 percent of all vaginitis, now accounts for only about 7 percent of vaginitis problems, a decrease that is associated with the introduction of metronidazole (Flagyl). Most infected patients have a gray, homogenous, malodorous discharge, but fewer than half have irritative symptoms. Frothiness, green discharge, and "strawberry vagina" (Fig. 40–21) occur in approximately 10 percent of patients with trichomoniasis, but in only the most acute infections. The amount of discharge varies considerably. During the acute phase of the infection, the discharge may be profuse and associated with some redness and edema in the region of the introitus. If untreated, the symptoms may gradually subside, with the persistence of a small to moderate amount of slightly odoriferous discharge;

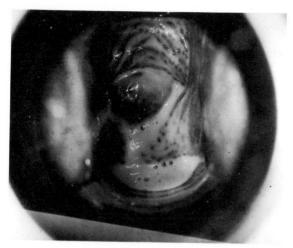

FIGURE 40-21 Trichomoniasis. Focal red punctate hemorrhage gives the appearance of a "strawberry vagina." A frothy, homogeneous discharge is also noted.

the gross appearance of the vulva and vagina may be perfectly normal.

Trichomoniasis (*Trichomonas vaginalis vaginitis*) must be considered a venereal disease since it is most commonly transmitted by sexual contact. The disease can also be transmitted by contact with droplets of discharge from the vagina, but this occurrence is extremely rare.

Diagnosis

A wet-mount preparation of vaginal secretions made with physiologic saline is the most accurate means of diagnosing this infection. The finding of motile trichomonads confirm the diagnosis. This organism is pear-shaped and motile, with obvious flagella that propel the organism through the saline.

Treatment

Since trichomoniasis is both a vaginal and a lower-urinary-tract infection, systemic agents are essential for its cure, and since it is a venereal disease, both sexual consorts must be treated if the infection is to be prevented from recurring. Metronidazole (Flagyl), a systemic agent, is the treatment of choice; the dose which is recommended for both sexes is 500 mg every 12 hours for 5 days. Recently, 2 g given as a single dose over a 30-minute period of time has been reported to be effective.

CANDIDIASIS

Candidiasis, the most common significant vaginitis, accounts for approximately half of all vaginal infections. The cardinal symptom is pruritus rather than discharge. The incidental finding of candidal organisms in vaginal secretions in the absence of signs and

FIGURE 40-22 *A* Spore and filaments of *Candida*. *B* Vaginitis due to *Haemophilus vaginalis*. Clue cells consist of stippling of squamous cells.

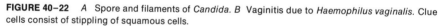

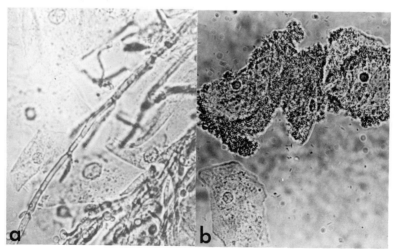

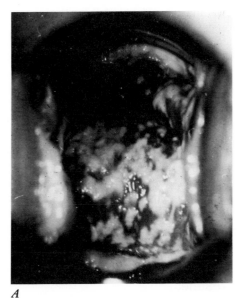
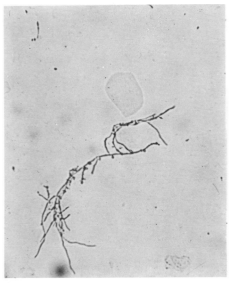

A *B*

FIGURE 40–23 *A* Candidiasis. Vaginal thrush patches are seen. *B* Candidiasis. Candidal organisms in a KOH preparation reveal typical filaments and spore of *Candida.*

symptoms does not constitute an indication for treatment. The associated vaginal secretions are usually of a curdy consistency, with thrush patches evident in only about 20 percent of the patients (Fig. 40–23*A*). Widespread use of antibiotics is directly related to the increased incidence of this infection. Antibiotics not only precipitate individual attacks of infection, but they are related to a marked increase in intestinal colonization which may account for many reinfections. Although oral contraceptives are in themselves not causative, their use may result in difficulty in eradicating an existing candidal infection. There has been some recent evidence to suggest a relationship between the occurrence of persistent candidiasis and a change in the individual's "immune competence."

The prime symptom associated with candidiasis is that of vulvar pruritus. In many instances, the objective findings are minimal. In most cases, however, the region of the introitus, labia majora, and inner aspects of the labia minora appear fiery red and occasionally have white patches of thrushlike material on the surface. A curdy white discharge is present within the vagina in most instances, although this may vary considerably. Not uncommonly, patches of white material are scattered over the surfaces of vaginal and cervical mucosa.

Cutaneous candidiasis may be seen in association with vaginal candidiasis but is also seen as a

primary disease. It is fostered by warm, humid climates in which masceration and other changes of the skin provide a good environment for fungal growth. Obese patients seem particularly susceptible. The primary cutaneous lesions involve the labia majora and the genitocrural folds, the mons pubis, the perianal region, and the inner thighs. The lesions may be beefy red and weeping, with sharply demarcated edges. The older, larger lesions frequently are associated with smaller, discrete satellite lesions (Fig. 40–24). Cutaneous candidiasis is associated with intense pruritus, burning, irritation, and occasionally local pain.

Diabetic vulvitis rightfully should be considered in the context of candidiasis since most of its manifestations are associated with candidal infections of the vulva and vagina. Most physicians consider diabetic vulvitis to be candidiasis in a predisposed patient. However, the term "diabetic vulvitis" is acceptable if the close relationship of the disease to chronic, recurrent candidiasis is understood. The skin changes and symptomatology frequently persist long after the fungal infection has been eradicated. The recurrence of repeated candidal infections leads to persistent vulvar pruritus, which in turn results in chronic scratching of the area. This, in turn, leads to skin changes which are compatible both grossly and microscopically with a neurodermatitis. The cycle of pruritus, scratching, and more pruritus persists until

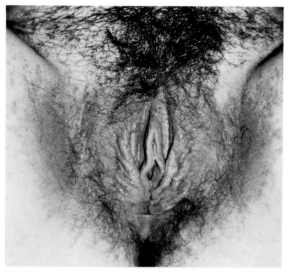

FIGURE 40–24 Vulva, cutaneous candidiasis. Vulva has a beefy red appearance with changes extending to the inner aspect of the thighs. Discrete satellite lesions are noted peripherally.

adequate treatment alleviates the symptoms. The gross clinical features of the vulva and surrounding skin are determined primarily by the presence and duration of candidal infection, obesity, local sensitivity to the substances produced by the candidal organism, hygienic measures, and previous treatment. Frequently, there is extensive involvement of the tis-

FIGURE 40–25 Vulva, "diabetic vulvitis." Tissues of vulva, mons pubis, and the inner aspect of the thighs have a thickened red appearance. A glazed "sugar coated" appearance is noted along the crural folds.

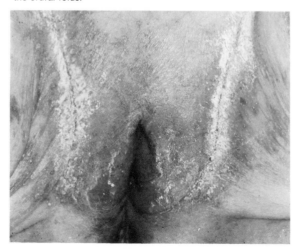

sues including the inner aspect of the thighs, mons pubis, and lower abdomen, perianal skin, and inner aspect of the buttocks. Edema of the tissues is frequently present. Erythema is exhibited by a typical vivid color of the tissues which may vary from a bright, beefy red to a profuse, intense red (Fig. 40–25).

Diagnosis

Wet-mount preparations of vaginal secretions made with both physiologic saline and 20% KOH solution are effective in confirming the diagnosis of candidiasis. Detection of the intact Candida particles is easy (Figs. 40–22A and 40–23B) because the spores and the filaments of candidiasis can be visualized readily. A gram-stained smear is dependable for identification of candidal species.

Treatment

A variety of intravaginal medications are available for the treatment of candidiasis, none of them uniformly successful. Probably the medication used most commonly is vaginal nystatin tablets. Vaginal applications should be used twice daily for a minimum of 15 days. Newer preparations found to be as effective as or more effective than nystatin are clotrimazole suppositories (Gyne-Lotrimin) and miconazole (Monistat) cream.

Control of reinfection is the primary problem associated with the treatment of candidiasis. Apparently the high reinfection rate of many subjects is related to the heavy colonization of the intestinal tract, brought about by large doses of oral antibiotics. No effective solution has been found for this source of infection. Oral nystatin has not proved particularly effective in alleviating this problem.

HEMOPHILUS VAGINALIS VAGINITIS

A gray, homogeneous, malodorous discharge with a pH of 5.0 to 5.5 that does not show trichomonads in the wet smear is most characteristic of *H. vaginalis* vaginitis (Fig. 40–26). Minimal frothiness is present in approximately 7 percent of the cases. Since the causative agent is a surface parasite, it does not cause irritative signs or symptoms of the vulva and vagina. Thus, patients complain primarily of a very malodorous vaginal discharge not associated with significant pruritus or burning. The disease that in past years was referred to as "non-

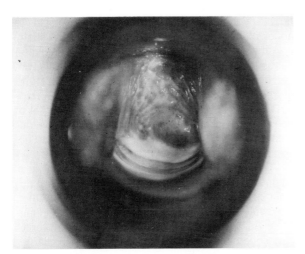

FIGURE 40–26 *Hemophilus vaginalis* vaginitis. A gray, homogeneous, malodorous discharge with a pH of 5.0 to 5.5 is present within the vagina.

specific vaginitis" was probably infection with *Hemophilus vaginalis*.

Diagnosis

The diagnosis is confirmed by the finding of "clue cells" (Gardner, Dukes) (Fig. 40–22B) in the wet mount preparation. The organism parasitizes the cells and causes them to appear as stippled, granular epithelial cells. The gram-stained smears show heavy fields of characteristic short, gram-negative bacilli predominating in the vaginal flora. The organism is so fastidious that many bacteriologic laboratories have difficulty making a positive identification by culture methods.

Treatment

Since *H. vaginalis* vaginitis is a sexually transmitted disease, practically all patients will become reinfected if the sexual consort is not treated effectively at the same time. This treatment is accomplished by the use of 500 mg of ampicillin or cephalexin monohydrate (Keflex), four times daily, for 6 days for both partners; even then, the success rate is not uniform. Recently metronidazole (Flagyl), 500 mg twice daily for 7 days, has been found to be very effective in eliminating this infection (Phiefer et al.). Third-party contacts explain many apparent treatment failures. Regardless of the method of treatment, both the patient and physician often experience frustration because of unexplained treatment failures or reinfections.

ATROPHIC VULVOVAGINITIS

Occasionally one sees atrophic changes of vulvar tissues secondary to estrogen deficiency. There is considerable variation from woman to woman in degree of estrogen deficiency and subsequent atrophic change of the vulva and vagina. The earliest changes noted in atrophy of the vulvovaginal tissues are found in the vaginal mucosa. The vagina loses its normal pink color and assumes a pale, pasty, thin appearance. Vulvar changes become apparent only many months or years after vaginal atrophy is observed. The skin and mucosal surfaces tend to become thin and almost translucent (Fig. 40–27). The tissues are easily traumatized, and occasionally excoriation and fissuring may be noted. The distribution of hair over the labia majora and mons pubis becomes sparse, and the hairs become brittle and coarse. The labia minora shrink in thickness and length and may totally disappear. The glans of the clitoris may atrophy and disappear beneath the prepuce. The introitus may become narrow and rigid so that intercourse is impossible. Symptoms of pruritus, burning, and tenderness

FIGURE 40–27 Vulva, atrophic vulvitis. Skin and mucosal surfaces of the vulva have become thin and almost translucent.

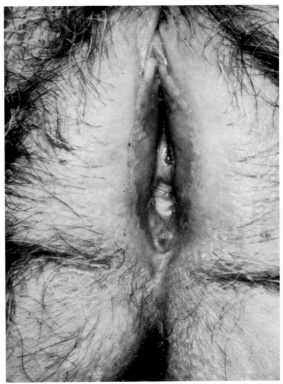

may well be related to bacterial effects upon the atrophic tissues of the vagina and vulva. The extent of pruritus may vary and, in the individual with strictly atrophic changes without secondary infection, this is usually a relatively minor symptom.

Treatment

Local application of estrogen cream to the vagina usually results in thickening of the vaginal mucosa. Half an applicator of estrogen vaginal cream can be applied daily to the vagina until symptoms are relieved and then once or twice weekly as needed. Systemic estrogens also give relief of symptoms and are more effective in relieving symptoms related to vulvar atrophy than is local therapy.

CONTACT VULVOVAGINITIS AND ALLERGIC VULVOVAGINITIS

Contact dermatitis is an inflammatory reaction of the skin due to a primary irritant or allergenic substance. The majority of contact vulvovaginal reactions are induced by agents applied for therapeutic and hygienic purposes. Most individuals having such reactions are merely hypersensitive to the particular irritating agent. Reactions caused by primary irritants are induced by substances such as corrosive chemicals, acids such as those used in douches, potassium permanganate tablets, hygienic sprays, gentian violet, and podophyllin. Allergic contact dermatitis, occasionally called eczematous dermatitis and allergic eczema, is an eruption arising from contact with allergenic substances in susceptible individuals. The allergic reactions may not provoke clinical changes until days or weeks after contact. It is almost impossible to distinguish the local changes in the vulvar tissues caused by primary irritant reactions from those caused by allergenic responses. The local changes usually consist of erythema, edema, and vesicle formation, and possible weeping. Crusting may develop as the lesions dry. The severity of the reaction is influenced by the sensitivity of the person as well as by the environmental conditions at the site of contact. Contact dermatitis of long duration may result in lichenification, scaling, and thickening of the skin with the development of white plaques. Pruritus, pain, burning, and tenderness are common symptoms.

Allergic dermatitis may be seen in response to contact with poison oak or poison ivy. Oleoresins produced by these plants may result in severe local reaction of the skin and mucosa. The allergen is usually transmitted to the vulvar tissues by contaminated hands rather than by direct contact of the plants with the genital area. The period between contact and eruption varies from a few hours to several days. Redness and the development of wheals at the point of contact are usually seen, followed by the development of vesicles in 1 to 2 days. These lesions are associated with severe local pruritus.

Dermatitis medicamentosa (drug eruption) is a cutaneous reaction secondary to allergenic substances circulating throughout the body, rather than the result of their direct contact with the skin and mucosa. As part of a generalized reaction, red pruritic maculopapules may develop on the vulva. Similar reactions may develop locally, following the intravaginal and vulvar application of drugs such as penicillin and sulfa.

Contact and allergic vulvovaginitis resolve rapidly after the causative agent is withdrawn. For severe reactions, the immediate institution of external treatment is usually indicated, even if the responsible agent has been discovered and its use eliminated. The use of remedies that may further aggravate the eruption should be avoided. Wet compresses such as Burow's solution (diluted 1:20) or concentrated boric acid solution may afford considerable immediate relief of symptoms. The topical application of an appropriate corticosteroid preparation often promptly relieves the patient's symptoms and may result in rapid objective improvement.

DERMATOSES

The vulva is not an uncommon site for manifestation of many of the generalized dermatoses such as psoriasis, lichen planus, and seborrheic dermatitis. Two to three percent of the population in the United States suffer from psoriasis. The lesions usually develop in multiple sites and begin at a relatively early age. The disease most often arises in the scalp, behind the ears and over the extensor surfaces of the extremities, the nails, the trunk, and sacral and genital areas. When the latter areas are involved, careful examination of the remaining skin surfaces will reveal characteristic lesions elsewhere. In the genital area, however, moisture, heat, and friction may give rise to lesions that resemble a fungus infection (Fig. 40–28). Seborrheic dermatitis, though an extremely

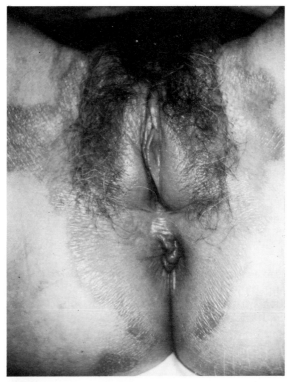

FIGURE 40–28 Psoriasis. Extensive, sharply demarcated lesions are noted. They do not have the same appearance as the more typical lesions elsewhere in this patient.

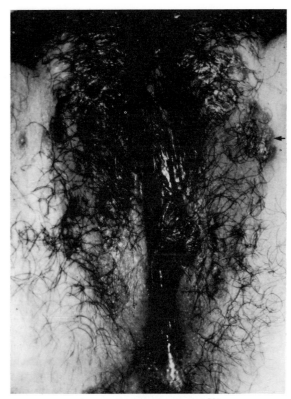

FIGURE 40–29 Seborrheic dermatitis. Lesions are red and greasy with fine scales covering the surface. *(From Gardner, Kaufman.)*

common disease, seldom involves the vulva (Fig. 40–29). When it does, however, characteristic lesions may additionally be seen on the midportion of the face, scalp, and the interscapular regions. These are areas most profusely supplied with sebaceous glands. Lichen planus frequently involves the mucosal surfaces of the lips and mouth in addition to the characteristic sites of predilection on the flexor aspects of the wrists, forearms, back, and nape of the neck. The extremely rare vulvar lesions are seen as slightly elevated, discrete, white papules. As with other dermatoses, involvement of other areas of the body should suggest the correct diagnosis.

INSECT BITES

Pediculosis pubis is an infection of the hair-bearing area of the vulva by the crab louse, *Phthirius pubis* (pediculosis pubis). This organism may be found in all the hair-bearing areas of the body. Careful exami-

nation will reveal nits and parasites at the bases of the hairs. The finding of these ova and parasites is facilitated by the use of a magnifying glass. Any skin lesion present usually consists of a very minute, inflamed maculopapule, on which crusts may form. Itching is a constant symptom. Scratching may induce secondary skin changes such as lichenification, pigmentation, and excoriations.

Scabies of the vulva caused by the mite *Sarcoptes scabiei* is also frequently part of a widespread disease. The female of the species burrows into and deposits her ova and feces in the epidermis, producing a minute papule or vesicle. Itching is essentially the only symptom and is extremely severe. Mosquito, tick, chigger, flea, and bedbug bites may also be responsible for localized areas of vulvar pruritus.

Insect bites of the vulva are treated as insect bites elsewhere. Both pediculosis pubis and scabies can be effectively treated by the use of agents such as Topocide lotion.

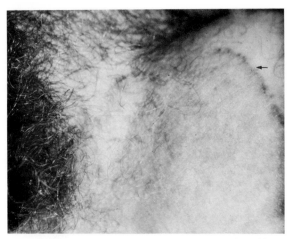

FIGURE 40-30 Tinea cruris. Well-circumscribed lesion with active, vesiculated margins. *(From Gardner, Kaufman.)*

FUNGAL INFECTION

Tinea cruris is a fungal infection of the genitocrural areas. The most common etiologic agents are *Epidermophyton floccosum, Trichophyton mentagrophytes,* and *Trichophyton rubrum*. Identification of the exact fungus is of little value since the signs and symptoms associated with each are identical. The infection begins as a small erythematous patch with vesiculation, crusting, and scale formation. The lesions spread peripherally and coalesce, sometimes healing in the center as they enlarge. They develop most often on the upper inner thighs and usually are erythematous, slightly elevated, and vesiculated (Fig. 40-30). Scaling is minimal on the moist vulvar tissues. The color varies from almost normal to slightly pigmented to red. Mild to intense pruritus is the chief symptom. The infection may be transmitted from person to person at the time of coitus. Scrapings from the active edges of the lesion, when mixed with 20% potassium hydroxide solution, will yield filamentous forms. No conidia, such as those found in candidal infections, are seen.

Tinea cruris may be treated with keratolytic agents such as ointments of salicylic acid (half-strength Whitfield's or Pragmatar), as well as those containing resorcinol. Undecylenic acid ointment 5% (Desenex ointment) is also an effective fungicide. Griseofulvin, given orally, has been accepted with varying degrees of enthusiasm. Usually, 4 to 6 weeks of treatment with this medication is required. More recently the topical application of clortrimazole (Lotrimin) cream has proved an effective treatment.

CARCINOMA IN SITU

The outstanding symptom associated with in situ carcinoma of the vulva is pruritus. A few patients complain of a lesion, and many are asymptomatic. There is considerable variation in both the gross and microscopical appearance of squamous-cell carcinoma in situ of the vulva. It may be seen as a sharply demarcated red patch (Fig. 40-31). On other occasions it may be seen as a sharply demarcated, irregular, thick, white patch (Fig. 40-32). Well-delineated, brown-pigmented papules are also an occasional manifestation of this disease. When located on the inner aspects of the labia minora, the lesion may be seen as a red velvetlike granular lesion. Where the lesion is not covered by a thick keratin layer, it will retain a toluidine blue stain which has been applied to the vulvar tissues and then washed with acetic acid (see Fig. 40-35). (A solution of 1% toluidine blue is applied to the vulva and allowed to dry. The area is then washed with adequate amounts of 1% acetic acid. The dye will be retained in areas of in situ car-

FIGURE 40-31 Carcinoma in situ. A sharply demarcated, full, red, moist patch is seen on the lower labium minus and majus.

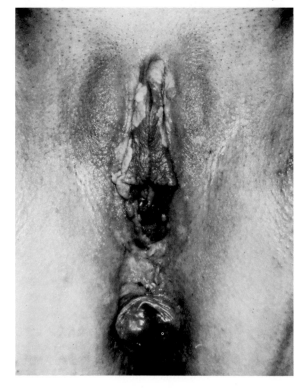

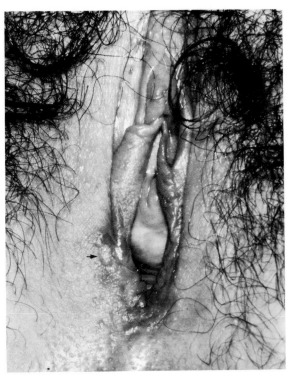

FIGURE 40–32 Carcinoma in situ. Multiple sharply demarcated, thick white patches are seen.

cinoma.) Although the method is often helpful in selecting sites for biopsy, failure to retain the dye does not eliminate the possibility of carcinoma in situ. The microscopical features of in situ carcinoma are also quite variable but consist primarily of epithelium containing cells that lie in complete disorder with enlarged, irregular, plemorphic nuclei. At times hyperchromatic multinucleated cells are noted. Occasionally, cytoplasmic vacuoles may be observed. Individual cell keratinization is commonly found. These changes extend through the full thickness of the epithelium, but an outer hyperkeratinized covering may be present, or an outer surface of cells demonstrating parakeratosis. The basal layer of the epithelium is intact, and the abnormal changes within the epithelium are sharply demarcated from the underlying dermis.

Carcinoma in situ is usually treated surgically. After adequate diagnosis and localization of the disease process, wide local excision or vulvectomy can be performed, depending upon the extent of involvement. When multiple foci of disease are present, the skin of the vulva can be peeled off, followed by the application of a skin graft to the denuded area (Rutledge, Sinclair). Especially in young women, 5% 5-fluorouracil can be applied to the lesions twice daily for 6 to 8 weeks. A pronounced irritation and redness of the treated tissues usually develop, followed by local ulceration. The treatment can be repeated in 6 to 8 weeks if necessary. Of vital importance in the treatment of intraepithelial carcinoma of the vulva is that an associated invasive squamous-cell carcinoma not be missed and inadequately treated. Conservative treatment of carcinoma in situ should be done only if the lesion is localized and the remaining vulva looks healthy and if the patient is young and sexually active.

In 15 to 40 percent of women with in situ carcinoma of the vulva, multicentric manifestation involving in situ or invasive carcinoma of the cervix or vagina will precede the vulvar lesion, be found in association with the vulvar disease, or will be subsequently diagnosed.

MALIGNANT DISEASES OF THE VULVA AND VAGINA

JAMES A. MERRILL

CANCER OF THE VULVA

Cancer of the vulva is uncommon, constituting less than 1 percent of all cancers in women. Because of the external location of these cancers, they should be the most amenable of all female genital cancers to early diagnosis and treatment. Yet such is not the case. Women tend to seek help for vulvar disease late, and physicians tend to delay establishment of an accurate diagnosis. Furthermore, this malignancy is difficult to treat. The majority of women with vulvar cancer are elderly, which often requires compromise in therapy. The diffuse lymph drainage of the area makes extensive surgery mandatory. As in other cancers, the success is directly correlated with the extent of the disease at the time of treatment and thus is correlated with early diagnosis (Merrill, Ross; Franklin; Morley).

Most vulvar cancers are squamous-cell carcinoma. Adenocarcinoma, Paget's disease, basal-cell carcinoma, malignant melanoma, and sarcoma constitute less than 10 percent of vulvar malignancies.

SQUAMOUS CELL (EPIDERMOID) CARCINOMA

Incidence

This carcinoma of the vulva constitutes 3 to 5 percent of genital malignancies in women (Merrill, Ross; Rutledge et al.). There has been an increase in the number of vulvar cancers observed in recent years (Woodruff et al.). This may be related to the fact that women are living to an older age (this is a disease of old women) and that interest in early diagnosis of cancer has increased. The greatest increase has been reported in cases of noninvasive vulvar cancer or carcinoma in situ. Woodruff has asked if this represents a true increase in noninvasive cancer or misdiagnosis. It has been suggested that some cases of morphologic carcinoma in situ or epithelial dysplasia may be the result of an infectious agent—possibly a virus—and that the changes seen may regress spontaneously. Such a concept has a direct influence upon the philosophy of conservative therapy for these early lesions (see Carcinoma In Situ earlier in this chapter).

Age

Vulvar cancer occurs predominantly in postmenopausal women. In the author's experience, 75 percent of patients were 50 years of age or older. The average age of patients with invasive vulvar cancer is 62 whereas the average of patients with carcinoma in situ is 10 years younger, or 52. There is a great age range, and primary vulvar cancer has been described in teenage women and women in their nineties.

Symptomatology

The most common presenting symptom is awareness of a lesion on the vulva. Somewhat less often, the patients complain of pruritus, pain, discharge, or bleeding. It appears that patients are not overly impressed with the significance of these symptoms for they tend to seek care after considerable delay. Various authors report a patient delay of more than a month in 30 to 60 percent of patients. Nor is this delay limited solely to the patient, for a physician delay greater than 2 months has been observed in as many as 18 percent of cases (Merrill, Ross; McKelvey, Adcock; Morley). A greater educational effort relating to vulvar disease obviously is needed for both women and their physicians. Commonly, the lesion is inadequately treated as benign with ointments and topical medications before the actual diagnosis is established. This further emphasizes the need for biopsy of all vulvar lesions before instituting topical therapy of vulvar disease. The technique of vulvar biopsy, as described earlier in this chapter, is simple and can be accomplished easily as an office procedure. It is imperative that physicians encourage patients to report vulvar symptoms and adopt the attitude of biopsying vulvar lesions with the same facility that they have demonstrated in the biopsy of the cervix.

Diagnosis

Diagnosis of vulvar cancer is readily accomplished by pelvic examination and liberal use of biopsy. The lesions involve the labia majora in approximately two-thirds of the cases. In one-third of cases, the lesions involve the labia minora, clitoris, or posterior fourchette (perineum). The majority of lesions are located in the anterior one-half of the vulva. Lesions may be ulcerated or exophytic. Small lesions may present as slightly raised, red, granular foci (Fig. 40–33). Advanced lesions may have a fungating, infected, poly-

FIGURE 40–33 Superficial squamous-cell carcinoma of the vulva. The discrete lesion is slightly raised and velvety.

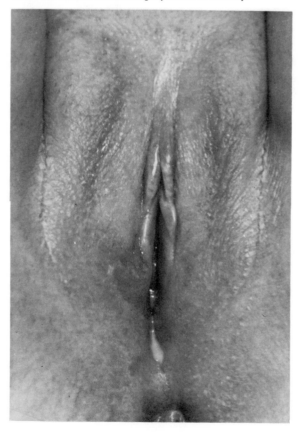

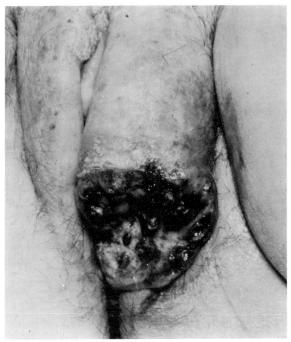

FIGURE 40–34 Carcinoma of the vulva. The large lesion is deeply ulcerated, and the adjacent labium is red and edematous.

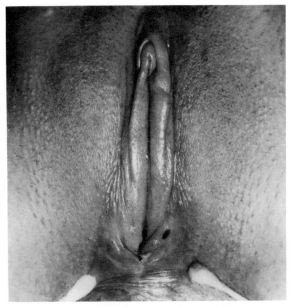

FIGURE 40–35 Carcinoma in situ of the vulva which is apparent because the lesion retains toluidine blue dye after the vulva has been rinsed with acetic acid.

poid surface or may produce an extensive shallow ulcer with indurated rolled borders. In either circumstance, extensive edema may surround the lesion (Fig 40–34). Edema has a bad prognosis, for it indicates the probability of lymphatic extension and obstruction. In our experience, diagnosis of carcinoma in situ of the vulva most usually has been established in asymptomatic patients at the time of routine pelvic examination. The use of toluidine blue, as described earlier in this chapter, to identify appropriate sites for biopsy is important in the early noninvasive lesions (Fig. 40–35).

Associated Diseases

The association of vulvar cancer and other primary malignancies is great. Various authors have reported associated malignancies in 16 to 40 percent of cases of squamous cancer of the vulva (Jimerson, Merrill). Of the associated malignancies, carcinoma of the cervix is the most frequent and, at the University of Oklahoma, has been observed in 35 percent of patients with vulvar cancer. Associated cervical cancer is even more common in patients with carcinoma in situ of the vulva. This makes it especially important that patients who have been treated successfully for cervical cancer be followed, with particular emphasis

on careful examination of the vulva and early biopsy of suspicious lesions. Indeed it has been suggested that cancer of the vulva may be one manifestation of "field" cancerization, in which the carcinogenic influence is expressed in various sites of squamous epithelium in the genital "field" extending from the cervix down to the perineum and perianal skin (Marcus). Certainly the multicentricity of vulvar cancer and the association with other malignancy of squamous epithelium support such a suggestion.

Vulvar dystrophy is commonly found in association with squamous-cell carcinoma of the vulva. Gross or microscopical evidence of vulvar dystrophy or leukoplakia has been observed in approximately 50 percent of cases of vulvar carcinoma (Merrill, Ross; Franklin; Krupp et al.; Morley). This does *not,* however, support a contention that vulvar dystrophies should be considered and treated as premalignant lesions. As indicated earlier in this chapter, the vast majority of these dystrophic lesions pursue a perfectly benign course. Syphilis and granulomatous venereal disease have been found in the history of patients with carcinoma of the vulva and have been suggested as possible predisposing diseases (Krupp et al.; Franklin; Morley). Vulvectomy has been suggested as an appropriate treatment for granulomatous disease of the vulva not only to relieve discomfort but also because of the potential for subsequent malignant change (Krupp et al.). This issue certainly is not agreed upon universally. Seski reports that patients with noninvasive carcinoma were shown to have an underlying defect in cellular immunity which could possibly be related to the development of cancer.

Histology

The microscopical appearance of most carcinoma of the vulva is that of a well-differentiated squamous carcinoma with many foci of epithelial pearls or keratinization. Less well-differentiated tumors occur and are said to be more common in the vestibule and clitoris. Lymphatic and nerve-sheath invasion is seen commonly. Multiple sites of neoplastic development may be seen if multiple sections are taken from a vulvar specimen (Fig. 40–36). These microscopic foci of cancer may exist in areas that appear normal to the naked eye. Furthermore, Woodruff et al. report evidence of altered nucleic acid synthesis in adjacent cell nests that also appear normal microscopically. This emphasizes the necessity of removal of the entire vulva in the treatment of vulvar cancer. The coexistence of granulomatous venereal disease and vulvar cancer may pose a problem in differential diagnosis. This requires that multiple biopsies from various areas of large vulvar lesions be obtained and studied carefully.

Lymphatic Drainage

The lymphatics of the vulva are numerous, diffuse, and tend to cross the midline. The regional lymph nodes include:

1. Superficial inguinal nodes
2. Deep inguinal nodes
3. Superficial femoral nodes
4. Deep femoral nodes (including Cloquet's node)
5. Deep pelvic nodes (including the external iliac, obturator, and internal iliac nodes)

From here, the lymph drainage is to the periaortic nodes. DiSaia has emphasized that the superficial inguinal nodes are the primary nodal group for the vulva and can serve as the "sentinel" nodes of the vulva.

Lymph-node metastasis is observed in approximately one-third of the patients treated surgically (Merrill, Ross; McKelvey, Adcock; Rutledge et al.; Morley). Node metastasis has been reported in 59 percent of patients by Green et al. Although many authors have reported a lack of correlation between the

clinical finding of palpably enlarged lymph nodes in the groin and microscopical lymph-node metastasis, Rutledge and Merrill have both shown a positive correlation. In Rutledge's experience, palpation of enlarged lymph nodes in the groin was 88 percent accurate in predicting nodal metastasis. In Merrill's experience, when lymph nodes were palpable, 76 percent of patients had lymph-node metastasis. When nodes were not palpable, only 14 percent had lymph-node metastasis. It is clear, of course, that failure to palpate enlarged lymph nodes does not ensure the absence of node metastasis. Morley reported 25 percent error in preoperative evaluation of groin nodes. Involved nodes may be bilateral, ipsilateral, or contralateral to the tumor. Metastases have been observed to the cross midline in as many as 71 percent of cases. In patients with lymph-node metastasis, 30 to 40 percent had involvement of the deep pelvic lymph nodes (Merrill, Ross; Dean et al.; Franklin). The frequency with which deep pelvic lymph nodes are involved in the absence of superficial inguinal- or femoral-node involvement is subject to question. Although there have been reports in which deep nodes were involved in the absence of superficial-node involvement, careful pathologic examination of the superficial nodes and especially careful examination of Cloquet's node suggest that deep-node involvement in the absence of superficial-node involvement is extremely uncommon.

Progressive local growth may involve the urethra, vagina, anus, and occasionally the rectum. Although in some instances these structures may be involved early in the course of the disease, their involvement usually reflects significant delay and is associated with regional-node metastases. With a locally advanced disease, there may be communication with vaginal lymphatics draining to the pelvic nodes and the hemorrhoidal system draining to the periaortic nodes.

Clinical Staging

The FIGO (International Federation of Gynecology and Obstetrics) classification is based on the analysis of tumor (T) by size and location, node (N) status by palpation, and distant metastases (M) as determined by palpation of the pelvis and by radiology. This classification is somewhat complex, and most clinicians rely upon a more conventional staging. Clinical staging utilizing both these classifications appears in Table 40-2. Using this staging, Rutledge demonstrated that the 2-cm diameter measurement seems to be a significant point in determining prog-

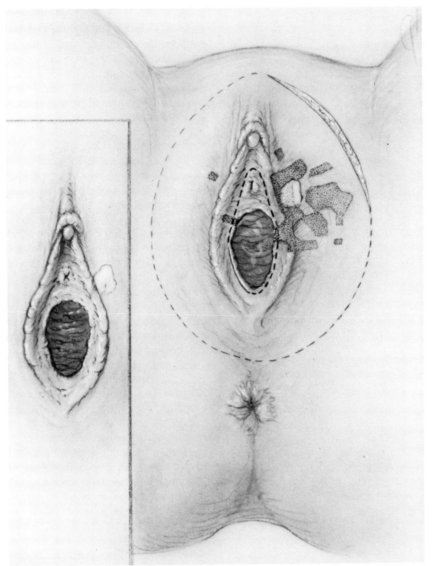

FIGURE 40–36 Multicentric carcinoma of the vulva. The insert shows the gross appearance of the malignant lesion. The shaded areas represent multiple foci of malignant eptihelium found by microscopical examination of the entire vulva.

nosis. Those patients with lesions less than 2 cm in diameter had significantly fewer lymph-node metastases than those whose lesion was greater than 2 cm. Survival is directly related to the clinical stage.

Natural History

In general, carcinoma of the vulva is a slow-growing lesion which spreads to the groin and pelvic lymph nodes and remains localized in these areas for fairly long periods. Pelvic-node metastases may result in ureteral obstruction. Distant metastases are uncommon and usually occur late in the disease process. Local recurrence following treatment may occur in the vulvar area or the groin. Death usually occurs from widespread metastases, bilateral ureteral obstruction and uremia, hemorrhage, or sepsis. Untreated vulvar cancer may result in large, ulcerating, painful infected lesions of the vulva occasionally producing fistulas into the bladder and/or rectum (Fig. 40–37).

TABLE 40–2   Clinical Staging

Stage I	T1 N0 M0 T1 N1 M0	All lesions confined to the vulva, with a maximum diameter of 2 cm or less and no suspicious groin nodes
Stage II	T2 N0 M0 T2 N1 M0	All lesions confined to the vulva, with a diameter greater than 2 cm and no suspicious groin nodes
Stage III	T3 N0 M0 T3 N1 M0 T3 N2 M0 T1 N3 M0 T2 N3 M0 T1 N2 M0 T2 N2 M0	Lesions extending beyond the vulva but without grossly positive groin nodes Lesions of any size confined to the vulva and having suspicious or grossly positive groin nodes Lesions extending beyond the vulva, with grossly positive groin nodes
Stage IV	T3 N3 M0 T4 N3 M0 T4 N0 M0 T4 N1 M0 T4 N2 M0 M1A M1B	Lesions involving mucosa of rectum, bladder, urethra, or involving bone All cases with distant or palpable deep pelvic metastases

Treatment

The treatment for carcinoma in situ has been presented and is quite varied, due to increasing knowledge of the biology of vulvar neoplasia (Dean et al.; Woodruff et al.). Current attitudes favor increased

FIGURE 40–37 Far-advanced, untreated cancer of the vulva.

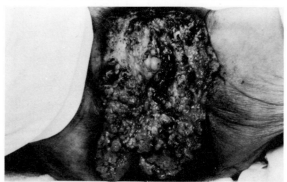

conservatism. The optimum treatment for invasive cancer is radical vulvectomy and bilateral groin dissection. Complete removal of the vulva is necessitated because of the multicentric nature of the disease, and bilateral dissection and removal of the regional lymphatics and lymph-node areas are necessitated because of the frequent bilateral or contralateral spread of disease. With this treatment, survival is reported in 50 to 83 percent of patients (Green et al.; Merrill, Ross; Rutledge et al.; McKelvey, Adcock; Dean et al.; Morley). Dean reported no recurrence in patients with stage I to stage III disease treated in this fashion. The overall success is dependent upon the rate of operability.

The necessity of including bilateral dissection and removal of the deep pelvic lymph nodes, in addition to the inguinal and femoral nodes, is debated. Addition of this portion of the operation increases the operative morbidity and probably accomplishes less than a 2 percent increase in overall salvage. Metastases to the pelvic nodes, without involving the inguinal nodes as well, almost never happen. Thus, the status of the first chain of inguinal nodes is studied carefully as a guide for a concern with deeper nodes. The lowest node of the external iliac group (node of Cloquet), located at the entrance of the femoral canal, has received attention as a focal point for drainage from the inguinal and femoral group. The node is frequently sought but usually not found at the time of surgery. If a frozen section of this node shows metastatic cancer, a deep pelvic lymphadenectomy is indicated. In the author's experience, primary dissection of the deep pelvic lymph nodes should be limited to those cases in which the primary lesion extends beyond the vulva (including the clitoris, vagina, and anus), to those cases with enlarged lymph nodes in the groin, and to patients with histologically positive inguinal, femoral, or Cloquet's nodes. A second stage pelvic lymphadenectomy has been suggested in those cases with metastases to the groin nodes.

The treatment of vulvar cancer should be individualized. There is no justification for a rigid therapeutic dictum. Many patients are poor operative risks. In addition to their age, there is a high incidence of obesity, hypertension, diabetes, arteriosclerosis, and other cardiovascular disease. Success with conservative therapy in these high-risk patients can be anticipated if the cases are selected carefully (Merrill, Ross; Rutledge et al.). If the lesion is less than 2 cm in diameter, if there are no palpably enlarged nodes in the groin, and if microscopical examination shows only limited invasion, a high-risk patient may be treated successfully by vulvectomy alone. DiSaia has recommended a unique conservative approach designed to minimize sexual dysfunction, in the treatment of early invasive cancer in carefully selected young patients. This approach is to sample the superficial inguinal lymph nodes (sentinel) and, if negative, to treat the lesion with local excision. It is too early to judge the wisdom of this innovation.

The en bloc resection of the subcutaneous tissue and fat in the groin often includes a segment of overlying skin. Since these wounds frequently are closed under tension and because of the moist nature of the area, wound breakdown and sepsis are common complications of radical surgery for cancer of the vulva. The hospital stay is long, and wound healing is often by secondary intention, sometimes requiring skin grafting. Another significant complication of this type of radical surgery is bilateral lymphedema of the legs, with swelling and pain.

Advanced carcinoma of the vulva involving the rectum or bladder may require exenteration. This radical operation involves removal of the bladder and/or rectum in addition to the female genitalia and vulva. The value of this type of extensive radical surgery is extremely limited.

Radiation therapy has essentially no place in the treatment of carcinoma of the vulva. The area tolerates radiation poorly, and the success cannot match that achieved with radical surgery. Far-advanced or recurrent vulvar cancer has been treated with high-energy electrons and pelvic irradiation has been used when the groin lymph nodes have shown metastases (Morley).

MELANOMA

Primary malignant melanoma is rare and constitutes less than 5 percent of all vulvar malignancies (Morrow, Rutledge). The gross and microscopical appearance of vulvar melanoma is similar to that of melanomas in other parts of the body. The anterior labia minora are involved most commonly. These tumors are usually very aggressive, and lymph-node metastases are demonstrated frequently. Because of rapid dissemination, both by lymphatics and blood-stream invasion, prognosis for cure is poor—approximately 50 percent. The treatment is essentially that of squamous carcinoma of the vulva, including bilateral deep-pelvic-node dissection.

PAGET'S DISEASE

A superficial neoplasm similar to the lesions found in the breast occurs rarely in the labia majora. Paget's disease appears as a pruritic, bright red, scaling, slightly elevated lesion with scattered white patches. Occasionally pain and bleeding may be present. The skin is thick or indurated, but there is usually no discrete mass.

The microscopical diagnosis is based on the presence of multicentric foci of large clear tumor cells (Paget cells) in the epidermis. In approximately one-third of cases, microscopic foci of adenocarcinoma in underlying apocrine sweat glands may be identified. Paget's disease may be accompanied by invasive epidermoid carcinoma. The differential diagnosis is facilitated by stains (periodic acid Schiff) to identify mucopolysaccharides in Paget cells. The prognosis for patients with tumor limited to the epidermis is good. However, Boehm reports that one-half of those patients with involvement of the adnexal glands had lymph-node metastases. The cure rate of patients with lymph-node metastases is essentially nil. Local recurrences are common.

Therapy should be total vulvectomy. If invasive disease is found on careful examination of the removed specimen, then radical groin dissection should be added as a second-stage procedure. Topical 5-fluorouracil may be effective in treating local recurrences.

BARTHOLIN'S GLAND CANCER

The rare carcinoma of Bartholin's gland presents as a nodule which must be distinguished from a Bartholin cyst or abscess. Commonly the patient is seen first after the surface of the tumor has ulcerated or become necrotic. Chamlin reports that one-half of cases were originally misdiagnosed as cyst or abscess of Bartholin's gland. Approximately half of Bartholin's gland cancers are squamous-cell carcinoma, developing from the duct, and half are adenocarcinoma of a mucoid appearance, developing from the acini of the gland.

Treatment should follow the principles presented for squamous-cell carcinoma of the vulva.

OTHER NEOPLASMS

Rare malignant tumors of the vulva include sarcomas, lymphomas, and metastatic tumors (DiSaia et al.).

CANCER OF THE VAGINA

Cancer of the vagina is extremely rare and constitutes only 1 to 2 percent of all malignant neoplasms of the female genital tract (Merrill, Bender; Herbst et al., 1970). Since it is usually metastatic, it always should be the first consideration in the differential diagnosis of a malignant lesion in the vagina. Carcinoma of the endometrium, choriocarcinoma, and carcinoma of the ovary are the common genital malignancies which metastasize to the vagina. Squamous-cell carcinoma of the cervix may involve the vagina by direct extension. Primary cancer of the vagina is most often a squamous-cell carcinoma. Adenocarcinoma is rare and may arise from remnants of the mesonephric duct or from developmental abnormalities of the lower Müllerian duct.

SQUAMOUS-CELL CARCINOMA

The exact incidence of primary squamous-cell carcinoma of the vagina is unknown. The criteria for its diagnosis are:

1. That the cancer be present in the vagina
2. That the cervix be free of cancer
3. That there be no other suspected source of a primary malignancy

Thus, it is entirely possible that cases classified as cervical cancer are, in fact, primary tumors of the vagina which have involved the cervix.

Clinical Picture

The majority of patients are between the ages of 50 and 60, and almost all are postmenopausal. The early lesion may be asymptomatic. Painless bleeding is the most frequent symptom, and patient delay is common (Merrill, Bender). Other complaints are vaginal discharge, the presence of a mass, pain, and pruritus. The posterior wall of the vagina is reported to be the most common site of primary carcinoma. The results of treatment are better in those patients with involvement of the anterior wall. Most of the lesions are present in the upper one-third of the vagina. The prognosis is worse with lesions in the lower vagina. Vaginal cancer may appear as a fungating exophytic mass, an ulcerative lesion, or as a raised, red, granular lesion (Fig. 40–38). In the upper portion of the vagina, the tumor generally spreads in a manner sim-

ilar to that of cancer of the cervix; in the lower portion of the vagina, the spread is likely to be more nearly that of vulvar cancer. Death is usually the result of urinary-tract obstruction with uremia and/or infection.

Extent

Carcinoma in situ may appear as one of multiple foci of origin when there is carcinoma of the vulva or cervix. This is rarely diagnosed as an isolated lesion, but carcinoma in situ of the vagina should be suspected when carcinoma of the cervix or vulva is present. The areas may be identified by lack of staining with Lugol's solution or by characteristic changes seen with colposcopy. The microscopic pattern is the same as that described for carcinoma in situ of the cervix (see Chap. 41). The clinical extent of vaginal cancer may be staged according to the following classification:

0. Carcinoma in situ
I. Carcinoma limited to the vaginal wall
II. Carcinoma involving the subvaginal tissue but not extended to the pelvic wall
III. Carcinoma extending to the pelvic wall
IV. Carcinoma extending beyond the true pelvis or involving the mucosa of the bladder or rectum

Diagnosis

Diagnosis of vaginal cancer is similar to that of carcinoma of the cervix and includes vaginal cytology in the asymptomatic patient, pelvic examination with careful speculum examination of the vagina, and biopsy of vaginal lesions or suspicious areas.

Treatment

The survival rates following therapy are influenced by the clinical extent (stage) of the cancer at the time of treatment and the size of the primary. In the majority of instances, therapy should consist of irradiation, using external beam and radium systems. Tumors in the upper vagina are usually treated with a modification of the treatment scheme for carcinoma of the cervix. For lesions located further down in the vagina, the radium system is often modified to include an intravaginal tandem or cylinder. Radical surgery may be suitable for lesions located in the outer one-third of the vagina without evidence of distant spread. Exenteration may be necessary for advanced lesions that involve the rectum and the bladder. Even under these circumstances, irradiation therapy should be consid-

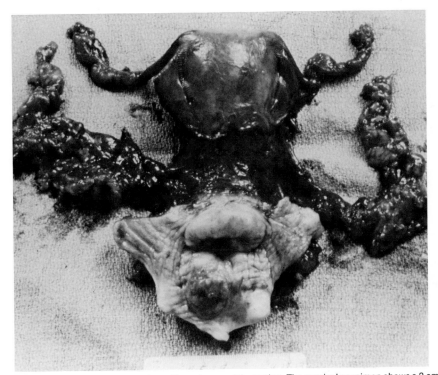

FIGURE 40–38 Primary squamous-cell carcinoma of the vagina. The surgical specimen shows a 2 cm polyploid lesion in the posterior midvagina.

ered and may be successful. Carcinoma in situ may be treated by partial removal of the vagina and immediate placement of a skin graft.

The overall cure rate for cancer of the vagina is in the range of 35 percent (Merrill, Bender; Herbst et al., 1970). There are several reasons for the low salvage rate in this disease. They include:

1. The relative rarity of vaginal cancer, making it difficult for any one center to gain sufficient experience and to develop and perfect a reliable technique of treatment.
2. The anatomy of the vagina, a thin-walled structure, well supplied with lymphatic vessels, and surrounded by loose connective tissue. Not only can widely separated node metastases occur readily, but there is no effective barrier to the local spread of disease.
3. The technical difficulties inherent in accurately applying radium to the lesion in the vagina and in accomplishing radical surgery of the area.
4. The usually advanced stage of the disease when treatment is first sought.

ADENOCARCINOMA

Although most adenocarcinomas found in the vagina are metastatic, rare primary vaginal adenocarcinoma arising from mesonephric-duct remnants, Müllerian-duct remnants, ectopic cervical glands, or even areas of endometriosis have been reported. In general, the clinical picture, diagnosis and treatment are similar to squamous-cell carcinoma.

Clear-Cell Carcinoma

Adenocarcinoma of the vagina of the clear-cell type was described by Herbst (1978) to occur in young females and has received much attention because of its histogenesis. Three hundred cases of vaginal and cervical clear-cell carcinoma had been collected through December 31, 1976. The patients ranged in age from 7 to 27. The incidence curve showed a sharp rise beginning at age 14 with a peak at age 19. Ninety percent were over the age of 12. There is a very frequent association with prenatal exposure to a synthetic estrogen (Diethylstilbestrol) or similar nonste-

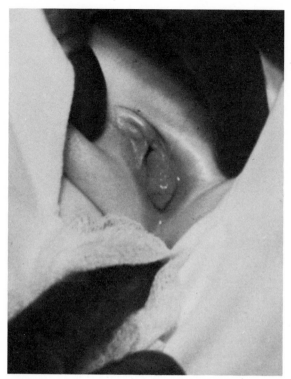

FIGURE 40–39 Sarcoma botryoides presenting at the introitus of an infant.

roidal estrogens. There is a great range in the dose and duration of administration of the hormone during pregnancy, but the probable carcinogenic effect is generally accepted. It is difficult to estimate the risk of clear-cell adenocarcinoma for a female exposed to DES in utero. Reasonable estimates are 0.14 to 0.27 cases of clear-cell carcinoma developing per 1000 DES-exposed females through the age of 24.

Most of the patients had vaginal bleeding or discharge. In 30 cases there was an abnormal cytology report, but many of the smears were negative. Although colposcopy has been advocated, it has not been particularly useful in the detection of clear-cell adenocarcinoma. The diagnosis is made by careful direct inspection and palpation and with biopsies of grossly suspicious lesions. Periodic examination of DES-exposed females should begin at approximately ages 12 to 14.

There is a very common association of vaginal adenosis (see Fig. 40–16) and transverse vaginal or cervical ridges. These are each considered to be DES-related disturbances in the embryonic development of the lower Müllerian tract. Although vaginal adenosis is relatively common in young women whose mothers received DES, clear-cell adenocarcinoma is extremely rare. It is obviously important to examine carefully all young women whose mothers received DES during pregnancy.

Surgery and irradiation have been used to treat clear-cell adenocarcinoma and both have resulted in success in a high proportion of cases. Lymph-node metastases occur in approximately 16 percent of stage I cases. Local surgical excision of a few small tumors has been performed, but is not recommended because of observed lymph-node metastases. Follow-up of most cases is still too brief for meaningful 5-year survival data. Of the 333 cases, 54 have died and 29 are known to have recurrent disease. The results of chemotherapy have been disappointing. In the author's institution, lesions present in the upper one-third of the vagina are treated by radical hysterectomy, partial vaginectomy and lymph-node dissection with ovarian preservation.

SARCOMA BOTRYOIDES

Sarcoma botryoides is a rare, highly malignant tumor arising from the vagina or cervix during the first decade of life (Ober, Edgcomb). The malignancy presents as a grapelike polypoid lesion often distending the vagina and protruding from the vaginal introitus (Fig. 40–39). The surface is pink or gray and glistening. The presenting symptom is often a bloody vaginal discharge noticed by the mother at the time of changing diapers.

The tumor is a type of mixed mesenchymal sarcoma. Microscopically, the polypoid nodules consist of loose scattered stellate cells in a myxomatous stroma. Various types of immature connective-tissue cells may be seen, but striated-muscle cells (rhabdomyoblast) are most common. This tumor must not be confused with benign vaginal polyps.

The prognosis for patients with these tumors is poor. Metastasis occurs early, both by lymphatics to regional nodes and by bloodstream invasion to distant organs. The treatment of choice is surgery which usually involves radical hysterectomy, total vaginectomy, and pelvic lymph-node dissection. Occasionally, some form of pelvic exenteration procedure may be required if the bladder or rectum is involved. Radiation therapy has been used but the success is not great. Recently combinations of radical surgery, chemotherapy and radiation have been reported to be successful (Razek et al.).

OTHER NEOPLASMS

Rare malignant neoplasms of the vagina include leiomyosarcoma, reticulum-cell sarcoma, and malignant melanoma.

REFERENCES

Birch HW, Sondag DR: Granular cell myoblastoma of the vulva. *Obstet Gynecol* 18:443, 1961.

Boehm J, Morris JMcL: Paget's disease and apocrine gland carcinoma of the vulva. *Obstet Gynecol* 38:185, 1971.

Chamlin DL, Taylor HB: Primary carcinoma of Bartholin's gland. *Obstet Gynecol* 39:489, 1972.

Chernosky MD et al.: Lichen sclerosus et atrophicus in children. *Arch Dermatol* 75:647, 1957.

Dean RE et al.: The treatment of premalignant and malignant lesions of the vulva. *Am J Obstet Gynecol* 119:59, 1974

Deardouff SL et al.: Association of herpes hominis type 2 and the male genitourinary tract. *J Urol* 112:126, 1974.

DiSaia PJ et al.: Sarcoma of the vulva. *Obstet Gynecol* 38:180, 1971.

_____: An alternate approach to early cancer of the vulva. *Am J Obstet Gynecol* 133:825, 1979.

Dukes CD, Gardner HL: Identification of *Haemophilus vaginalis vaginitis*. *J Bacteriol* 81:277, 1961.

Evans HD et al.: Involvement of the nervous system in Behçet's syndrome. *Lancet* 2:349, 1957.

Franklin EW III: Clinical staging of carcinoma of the vulva. *Obstet Gynecol* 40:277, 1972.

_____, Rutledge FD: Epidemiology of epidermoid carcinoma of the vulva. *Obstet Gynecol* 39:165, 1972.

_____, _____: Prognostic factors in epidermoid carcinoma of the vulva. *Obstet Gynecol* 37:892, 1971.

Friedrich EG Jr: Relief for herpes vulvitis. *Obstet Gynecol* 41:74, 1973.

_____ Wilkinson EJ: Mucous cysts of the vulvar vestibule. *Obstet Gynecol* 42:407, 1973.

Gardner HL, Dukes, CD: *Haemophilus vaginalis vaginitis*. *Am J Obstet Gynecol* 69:962, 1955.

_____, Kaufman RH: *Benign Diseases of the Vulva and Vagina*. St. Louis: Mosby, 1969.

Green TH Jr et al.: Epidermoid carcinoma of the vulva. *Am J Obstet Gynecol* 76:692, 1960.

Herbst AL et al.: *Intrauterine Exposure to Diethylstilbestrol in the Human*, Chicago: Am. Coll. Ob. Gyn., 1978.

_____ et al.: Primary carcinoma of the vagina. *Am J Obstet Gynecol* 106:210, 1970.

Jeffcoate TNA: Chronic vulvar dystrophies. *Am J Obstet Gynecol* 95:51, 1966.

Jimerson GK, Merrill JA: Multicentric squamous malignancy involving both cervix and vulva. *Cancer* 26:150, 1970.

Kaufman RH et al.: Clinical features of herpes genitalis. *Cancer Res* 33:1446, 1973.

_____ et al.: The vulva dystrophies—an evaluation. *Am J Obstet Gynecol* 120:363, 1974.

_____ et al.: Herpes genitalis treated by photodynamic inactivation of virus. *Am J Obstet Gynecol* 117:1144, 1973.

_____ et al.: Treatment of genital herpes simplex virus infection with photodynamic inactivation. *Am J Obstet Gynecol,* 132:861, 1978.

Krupp PJ et al.: Carcinoma of the vulva. *Gynecol Oncol* 1:345, 1973.

Lever WF: *Histopathology of the Skin,* Philadelphia: Lippincott, 1967.

Marcus SL: Multiple squamous-cell carcinomas involving cervix, vagina, and vulva: The theory of multicentric origin. *Am J Obstet Gynecol* 80:802, 1960.

McKelvey JL, Adcock LL: Cancer of the vulva. *Obstet Gynecol* 26:455, 1965.

Merrill JA, Bender WT: Primary carcinoma of the vagina. *Obstet Gynecol* 11:3, 1958.

_____, Ross NL: Cancer of the vulva. *Cancer* 14:13, 1961.

Morley GW: Infiltrative carcinoma of the vulva. *Am J Obstet Gynecol* 124:874, 1976.

Morrow CP, Rutledge FN: Melanoma of vulva. *Obstet Gynecol* 39:745, 1972.

Nahmias AJ et al.: Perinatal risk associated with maternal genital herpes simplex virus infection. *Am J Obstet Gynecol* 110:825, 1971.

_____ et al.: Antibodies to herpesvirus hominis types 1 and 2 humans: Women with clinical cancer. *Am J Epidemiol* 91:547, 1970.

_____ et al.: Genital infections with type 2 herpesvirus hominis. *Br J Vener Dis* 45:294, 1969.

Ober WB, Edgcomb JH: Sarcoma botryoides in the female genital tract. *Cancer* 7:75, 1954.

Oberfield RA: Lichen sclerosus et atrophicus and kraurosis vulvae: Are they the same disease? *Arch Dermatol* 83:806, 1961.

Person DA et al.: Herpesvirus type 2 in genitourinary tract infections. *Am J Obstet Gynecol* 116:993, 1973.

Pheifer TA et al.: Nonspecific vaginitis. *New Engl J Med* 298:1429, 1978.

Powell LC et al.: Treatment of condyloma acuminata by autogenous vaccine. *South Med J* 63:202, 1970.

Rawls WE et al.: An analysis of seroepidemiological studies of herpesvirus type 2 and carcinoma of the cervix. *Cancer* 33:1477, 1973.

——— **et al.:** Genital herpes in two social groups. *Am J Obstet Gynecol.* 110:682, 1971.

——— **et al.:** Antibodies to genital herpesvirus in patients with carcinoma of the cervix. *Am J Obstet Gynecol* 107:710, 1970.

Razek AA et al.: Combined treatment modalities in rhabdomyosarcoma in children. *Cancer* 39:2415, 1977.

Richardson AC, Williams GA: Topical androgenic hormones and vulvar kraurosis-leukoplakia syndrome. *Am J Obstet Gynecol* 761:791, 1968.

Rutledge F, Sinclair M: Treatment of intraepithelial carcinoma of the vulva by skin excision and graft. *Am J Obstet Gynecol* 102:806, 1968.

——— **et al.:** Carcinoma of the vulva. *Am J Obstet Gynecol* 106::1117, 1970.

Seski VC et al.: Abnormalities of lymphocytic transformation in women with carcinoma of the vulva. *Obstet Gynecol* 52:332, 1978.

Sezer N: Further investigations on the virus of Behçet's disease. *Am J Ophthalmol* 41:41, 1956.

Sobel HJ et al.: Is schwannoma related to granular cell myoblastoma? *Arch Pathol* 95:396, 1973.

Stafl et al.: Clinical diagnosis of vaginal adenosis. *Obstet Gynecol* 43:118, 1974.

Stevens JG, Cook ML: Latent infections induced by herpes simplex viruses. *Cancer Res.* 33:1399, 1973.

Woodruff JD et al.: The contemporary challenge of carcinoma in situ of the vulva. *Am J Obstet Gynecol* 115:677, 1973.

Work B: New instrument for office treatment of cysts and abscesses of Bartholin's gland. *JAMA* 190:777, 1964.

41

The Cervix

PHILIP J. DISAIA

GENERAL CONSIDERATIONS

The uterine cervix is of major interest and importance to every gynecologist-obstetrician. To the gynecological oncologist, it represents the most common focus for the development of malignant tissue. For the obstetrician, it represents the primary barometer in the process of labor and delivery. No organ is as accessible to the gynecologist-obstetrician in terms of both diagnosis and therapy. Its accessibility led to the great strides earmarked by the Papanicolaou smear, resulting in complete reversal of the prognosis in cancer of this organ. Easy access to the cervix led to the skillful application of radiation techniques which have resulted in some of the best overall cure rates for any malignancy.

Benign lesions of the cervix are common entities. A great deal of evidence has suggested that proper treatment of such cervical abnormalities may result in a decrease in the development of invasive carcinoma. Other benign lesions of the cervix and endocervix can be associated with infertility and chronic symptoms. The "incompetent cervix" has been found to be one of the major contributors to the incidence of midtrimester abortion. Surgical techniques which correct this defect have salvaged thousands of fetuses and brought them to viability.

EMBRYOLOGY

Embryological development of the cervix remains in a cloud of controversy. Although it is clearly established as a median primordium, the uterus obtains its characteristic configuration only gradually. At first there is no obvious line of demarcation between that portion of fused Müllerian ducts destined to form the uterus and cervix and that which will give rise to the upper part of the vagina. In the latter part of the third month, the uterine portion begins to be set off by the more robust character of its walls and the beginning of the formation of vaginal fornices adjacent to the cervical portion of the uterus. During the fourth month, the muscular and connective tissue coats of the uterus begin to be suggested by the arrangement of the mesenchymal concentrations. The vagina results from fusion of the urogenital sinus and Müllerian vaginal tube, and the squamous epithelium of the vagina develops from the upward growth of squamous epithelium from the urogenital sinus, which terminates near the external cervical os. Classic teaching states that toward the end of the sixth month, the epithelial lining of the uterus begins to send the primordial buds for the uterine glands into the underlying connective tissue and this process results in columnar epithelium and endocervical glands. Fluhmann postulates that the urogenital squamous epithelium continues its upward growth into the cervical canal with subsequent transformation into columnar epithelium.

This suggests, of course, that the endocervical lining, like that of the vagina, is of entodermal origin. Another opinion expressed by Song suggests that the endocervical columnar epithelium is a product of endocervical mesenchymal cells which have been transformed from endometrial mesenchymal cells at about the 25th week of gestation. From the 28th week until birth, a rapid linear growth of endocervical mucosa results in deep in-folding of surface epithelium to form clefts, or plicae palmatae. It is undoubtedly this rapid proliferation of endocervical mucosa occurring after the 28th week that produces the so-called "congenital erosion" found in a high percentage of newborns and premenarchal females. Recent studies in Australia, confirmed by others in the United States, have established the fact that columnar tissue initially exists on the endocervix in at least 70 percent of pubescent females and extends on to the vagina in an additional 5 percent of these women. Metaplastic transition from columnar to squamous epithelium progresses over many years and is most active during three periods of a woman's life: fetal development, adolescence, and her first pregnancy. The process of metaplasia is enhanced by the acid environment of the vagina and this pH is greatly influenced by estrogen and progesterone production.

The more common congenital abnormalities of the uterus and vagina are the result of variations in the extent or manner of fusion of the Müllerian ducts during their early development. This may result in a double cervix with a septate uterus and double vagina; a double cervix with bicornuate uterus and single vagina; a double cervix with didelphic uterus; or, indeed, a complete atresia of the cervix.

While the vestigial mesonephric (Gartner's) duct is usually just lateral to the cervical duct, its remains are occasionally seen in the form of tubules deep in the cervical substance, and these at times present an adenomatous appearance. For that matter, they may in rare cases constitute the source of adenocarcinoma. It has been noted by Novak and others that these malignant lesions may arise at any portion where the primitive mesonephric duct has been present. Huffman examined serial sections of about 1200 cervices and found remnants of fetal mesonephros in about 1 percent.

ANATOMY AND HISTOLOGY

The cervix (L. *neck*) is a narrow cylindrical segment of the uterus; it enters the vagina through the anterior

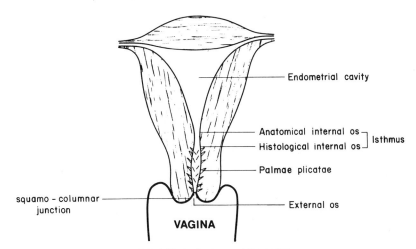

FIGURE 41–1 Anatomy of the cervix.

vaginal wall and lies at right angles to it. It is from about 2 to 4 cm long and it is continuous above with the inferior aspect of the uterine corpus. The point of juncture is known as the *isthmus;* it is marked by an area of slight constriction (Fig. 41-1). Since the cervix pierces the vagina, it can be divided into supravaginal and intravaginal portions. The supravaginal portion lies above the area of vaginal attachment covered with peritoneum posteriorly. Anteriorly, it is separated from the bladder by fatty tissue and is connected laterally with the broad ligament and the parametrium, which contains its blood vessels and lymphatics. The lower intravaginal portion is a free segment which projects into the vault of the vagina and is covered with mucous membrane. The cervix opens into the vaginal cavity through the external os. The os has anterior and posterior lips which are normally in contact with the posterior vaginal wall; this wall ascends to a higher cervical level than does the anterior wall and thus envelops the inferior third of the cervix. In the nullipara, the os is a small transverse slip, the lips of which are smooth and rounded; but in the multipara it is wider, and the lips are quite irregular. The mucous membrane in the canal is raised into medium longitudinal folds both in front and behind, and between these are secondary branching folds which pass upward and laterally. The treelike appearance has been called arbor vitae (rugae or plicae palmatae); these folds are absent after the first pregnancy.

The cervical canal extends from the anatomic external os through the internal os where it joins the uterine cavity (Fig. 41-1). The histologic internal os is an area where there is a transition from endocervical

to endometrial glands. The cervical canal is somewhat fusiform, with a narrowed portion at the level of the histologic internal os. This narrowed portion continues up approximately ½ cm and then enters into the cavernous endometrial cavity. The point at which it enters into the endometrial cavity is called the *anatomical internal os,* and the area from this point to the histologic internal os below is termed the isthmus. The isthmus of the uterus is of importance in the process of labor. The isthmus musculature is thinner than that of the corpus and provides an area in which effacement and dilatation can occur in early labor. This isthmic portion of the uterus is usually referred to as the *lower uterine segment* during the processes of pregnancy and labor.

The portio vaginalis or intravaginal portion of the cervix, also called the ectocervix, is covered with stratified squamous epithelium that is essentially identical with the epithelium of the vagina. The portio supravaginalis contains the cervical canal, and this is lined by endocervical mucosa which displays branching folds (plicae palmatae) and is surmounted by cylindric epithelium. The cervical glands may be visualized as branching clefts formed by ramifications of the endocervical epithelium. The squamocolumnar epithelial junction lies at or near the level of the external os. The narrow zone of the endocervix, abutting the mucosa of the portio vaginalis, is referred to as the transitional zone. The stroma of the cervix are composed of connective tissue, with unstriated muscle fibers and elastic tissue. The elastic tissue is found chiefly around the wall of the larger blood vessels. An area of transition separates the connective tissue of the cervix from the muscle of the lower uter-

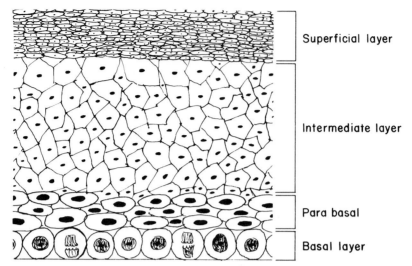

FIGURE 41-2 Histology of squamous cervical epithelium (diagrammatic).

ine segment. This zone is usually about 10 mm in length but occasionally is absent, and the cervical uterine junction is abrupt.

The stratified squamous epithelium of the portio of the cervix is made up of several layers conventionally described as basal, parabasal, intermediate, and superficial (Fig. 41-2). The basal layer consists of a single row of cells and rests on a thin basement membrane. This is the layer wherein active mitosis is seen. The cells are basophilic, the basophilia being enhanced by pregnancy. The parabasal and intermediate layers together constitute the prickle-cell layer analogous with the same layer in the epidermis. The cells of the parabasal layer show cytoplastic basophilia, less in degree than that of the basal layer and decreasing toward the intermediate layer. The intermediate layer is vacuolated, largely due to the presence of glycogen, which either is not stained or is dissolved out in any preparation of the sections. The superficial layer varies in thickness depending upon the degree of estrogen stimulation. It consists of flattened cells showing an increasing degree of cytoplasmic acidophilia in the direction of the surface. The surface cells retain their nuclei until they are cast off into the lumen of the vagina. This desquamation of surface cells goes on constantly, and the epithelium is replenished by mitotic division of the cells in the basal layer and to a lesser extent in the parabasal layer. The superficial and intermediate layers of the epithelium contain a large amount of glycogen. This glycogen serves an important function in maintaining the acid pH of the vaginal content. The glycogen is released by cytolysis of desquamated cells and is then acted upon by glycolytic bacterial flora of the vagina, forming lactic acid. Both the thickness of the epithelium and the glycogen content of the epithelium are increased following estrogen stimulation, thus accounting for the therapeutic effect of estrogens in atrophic vaginitis. The staining of glycogen in the normal epithelium of the portio vaginalis is the basis of the Schiller test.

PHYSIOLOGY

Cervical mucus is produced by the secretory cell of the endocervical gland. The cervical canal contains approximately 100 crypts (plicae palmatae), often referred to as glands. The secretory cells in these crypts secrete mucus into the lumen of the endocervical canal. Under normal conditions, the mucus undergoes both quantitative and qualitative changes depending on the hormonal predominances in the different phases of the menstrual cycle. The cervix also undergoes anatomical changes during the menstrual cycle. The external os progressively widens during the proliferative phase, reaching maximum width just prior to or at ovulation. At the time of maximum widening, cervical mucus can usually be noted to exude from the external os. Following ovulation, the cervical os returns to a smaller diameter and the profuse watery mucus becomes scant and viscid. These cyclic variations have not been noted in the prepubertal, the postmenopausal, or the castrated female. Administration of exogenous estrogen in the castrate usually has an effect on the cervix resembling that observed in a normal female at midcycle. Progesterone does not produce the changes similar to estrogen and is, in effect, inhibitory, causing changes resembling those observed in the luteal phase of the normal cycle. When estrogen and progesterone are given simultaneously, the progesterone seems to counteract the effect of estrogen.

Cyclic variations in cervical mucus have been studied by Davajan. In the immediate postmenstrual phase, the cervical mucus is sparse, viscid, and sticky, and microscopic examination reveals abundant vaginal and cervical cells as well as leukocytes. Beginning on the eighth day and continuing until ovulation, the quantity of mucus increases as well as its viscosity. At midcycle, the mucus is a hydrogel consisting of 98 percent water and 2 percent solids. The spermatozoa must first penetrate and then migrate through this column of hydrogel in order to reach the fallopian tube where fertilization takes place. If this midcycle cervical mucus is allowed to dry on a slide, it is noted to be clear, and when dried it gives the typical fern or palm-leaf pattern (Fig. 41-3). The fernlike pattern of cervical mucus is present only in the first half of the menstrual cycle and during the ovulation period. It is absent after ovulation, during pregnancy, and after menopause, at which time the mucus exhibits only cellular content.

The ferning or arborization test may be of value in the infertility study of a patient for the following purposes: (1) to determine exogenous estrogen activity, (2) to evaluate luteal phase, (3) to approximate the time of ovulation, (4) to diagnose endocervicitis, and (5) to evaluate response of the endocervical glands to exogenous estrogens.

The fern test can be performed by aspirating mucus from the external os using an infant feeding catheter (no. 14 or no. 16) and placing this mucus on a glass slide. The mucus is permitted to dry for approximately 30 seconds and then examined under the microscope at a magnification of about 90×. The presence of blood or other fluid in the aspirate can alter the result and interpretation is not possible. The use of saline must be avoided, since the sodium chloride content may result in an arborization pattern very similar to cervical mucus. A portion of the aspirated mucus in the catheter may be tested for its capacity to be drawn into a thread (spinnbarkeit). With a small hemostat, the catheter segment is pressed against a microscopic slide. The extruding portion of the mucus plug is held against the slide by means of a cover slip. The catheter segment is then elevated to the

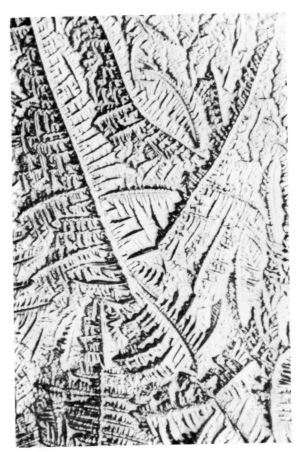

FIGURE 41-3 Cervical mucus fern pattern.

maximum capacity of the mucus threadability. This maximum height is measured with a centimeter ruler positioned vertically behind the slide. A spinnbarkeit of at least 6 cm has been accepted as normal. The ability of mucus to thread (spinnbarkeit) is still the most reliable measurement that can be performed with ease.

ANATOMIC AND PHYSIOLOGIC DEFECTS

STENOSIS

Congenital stenosis of the endocervical canal is an uncommon finding occasionally encountered in the diagnostic investigation of an infertile couple. The diagnosis is made by exclusion and is heralded by failure in attempts to pass a small catheter or probe into the endocervical canal. Stenosis of the cervix may follow chronic cervical infection, treatment of endocervicitis, cauterization of the cervix, cryosurgery of the cervix, radium therapy, and senile atrophy. All of these factors must be excluded when a diagnosis of congenital stenosis is made. Stenosis is usually asymptomatic but may cause abnormal genital bleeding, dysmenorrhea, and infertility. Stenosis can occur following diagnostic conization of the cervix, and cervical patency should be ensured by sounding the cervical canal at postoperative examinations. When stenosis is complete or nearly complete, accumulation of cervical or uterine secretions may cause distention of the uterine cavity, resulting in distention of the uterus with blood (hematometra), fluid (hydrometra), or exudate (pyometra). These conditions which produce a distended fluid-filled endometrial cavity can be confused with adnexal masses of ovarian origin. They may be asymptomatic for prolonged periods of time and on bimanual examination often appear cystic to palpation. The diagnosis can often be confirmed by passing a small uterine sound or probe through the area of cervical stenosis into the fluid-filled endometrial cavity. Other patients must be treated with endocervical dilatation and maintenance of a patent endocervical canal with an indwelling drain.

ABNORMAL MUCUS

Some patients will have thick, yellow-colored, cellular cervical mucus noted at midcycle, prior to the expected basal body temperature rise. Exact etiology of this finding as yet has not been determined. A daily dose of 0.1 mg of diethylstilbestrol (DES) taken every day except when menstruating does change the mucus into normal, watery type of mucus and allows normal sperm penetration to take place. An occasional patient will have very viscid mucus secreted in the lower one-third of the endocervical canal, noted when the mucus plug is aspirated at the external os and a clear watery mucus gushes from behind this thick plug. On occasion these patients have presented with infertility and have successfully responded to removal of the viscid mucus followed by cervical-cup insemination using husband's semen.

An abnormally low quantity of cervical mucus is also seen in other patients, usually with very small endocervical canals. DES therapy may increase the

mucus secretion in some of these patients as it may be a factor in sperm transport.

POLYPS

Cervical polyps vary from a few millimeters to 3 cm in length; they are pedunculated, roughly pearshaped, soft, smooth, and reddish or purplish. The pedicle nearly always rises from the cervical canal (Fig. 41-4) but occasionally from the external surface of the cervix. In the vast majority of instances, only a single polyp is present, but occasionally two or three are found at the same time. They seldom recur after removal. Microscopically, polyps are found to be a hyperplastic condition of the endocervical epithelium. They usually have a large number of blood vessels, especially near the surface. Those polyps present in an edematous and inflamed condition which contributes to their size. The chief symptoms of polyps are menorrhagia and leukorrhea, but women with cervical polyps often have no complaints. Often the polyp is readily felt on bimanual examination, but at other

FIGURE 41-4 Elongated cervical polyp extruding from cervical canal.

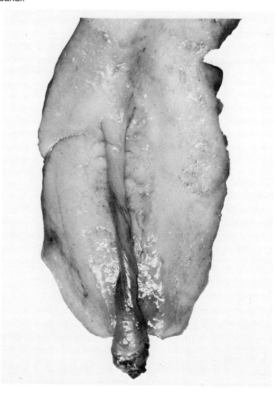

times it may not be evident until a speculum examination is performed. It is difficult to prevent the formation of polyps because their exact etiology is unknown. The treatment of these polyps is usually quite simple. If the polyp is quite large, a clamp can be applied approximately 0.5 cm above the origin of the pedicle. A surgical ligature should be tied between the clamp and the cervix and then the clamp can be removed. The polyp can be excised by cutting along the line of crush or indeed it can be allowed to remain in situ where it will undergo infarction and slough. All tissue removed should, of course, be sent for pathologic review since occasionally a malignancy will arise in these benign-appearing structures.

HYPERPLASIA AND METAPLASIA

Foci of apparently abnormal proliferation of endocervical glands can be found frequently in surgical specimens. The most appropriate designation is *adenomatous hyperplasia*. Fluhmann suggests the name "tunnel clusters" for the same formation. The lesion is suspected when examining a surgical specimen of cervix if there is an endocervical polyp, a series of closely placed cystic glands, or a sessile projection of mucosa of the endocervical surface. It is doubtful whether one could seriously suspect presence of adenomatous proliferation on pelvic examination from physical evidence. Microscopically, the cross section of the cervix displays a localized profusion of small gland spaces somewhat irregularly shaped and crowded tightly together. Most of the time the glands are filled with a mucinous material, indicating that they are not well drained or are occluded altogether. Around the periphery of the area there are normal cervical glands with specific mucous columnar cells, and often a direct origin of the abnormal process may be noted from normal glands. Adenomatous hyperplasia probably represents an imbalance of the hormonal and local response mechanisms which regulate growth of endocervical mucosa under usual conditions. No definite neoplastic potential has been established. In recent years, a lesion termed *polypoid adenomatous hyperplasia* or microglandular hyperplasia of the endocervical glands has been found to be related to the ingestion of oral contraceptive pills. This lesion occurs under the influence of the contraceptive and regresses when the hormone is withdrawn. These lesions are of considerable importance since they can be misinterpreted as a well-differentiated malignancy by an inexperienced pathologist. It is frightening to consider the magnitude of

radical treatment that might be given to one of these young patients and its possible sequelae.

Epidermization is a name given to the process of lateral or horizontal growth of stratified squamous epithelium from its natural position on the portio inward along the endocervical surfaces. The edge of this process as it abuts the endocervical glands is the so-called transformation zone where active physiologic metaplasia takes place. Meyer and Novak believed that this mechanism of epidermization explained the process of "erosion healing." In fact, the descriptions of the process are given in language actually depicting the lateral motion. The epithelium is said to creep along the surface, displacing the columnar cells as it moves. The several inner layers of basal cells and the stratified squamous layer have been described as tunneling under the glandular epithelium both on the surface and down in the endocervical glands. In a typical area of epidermization, the squamous epithelium differs from the normal in that the normal maturation and keratinization are absent, the cell layers are not apparent, and there may be a certain amount of disorganization of architecture. The line of epidermization or the transformation zone is always encountered proximal or cranial to the original squamocolumnar junction, replacing a variable portion of the cervical columnar epithelium which originally occupied the site. Several ectopic sites of metaplastic epithelium can often be identified separate from the main extent.

Squamous metaplasia designates the process of multiplication of cells of the endocervix which normally forms the replacement for the columnar epithelium, this multiplication resulting in production of cells of squamous type. The histologic picture of squamous metaplasia is not generally different from that of epidermization, except possibly that the changes are found higher in the endocervical canal and they are not necessarily contiguous with the portio epithelium. Like the term epidermization, squamous metaplasia describes a mechanism and also names a histologic finding. The most prevalent hypothesis assumes that mature columnar cells do not change into squamous cells. Hence, the progenitors are certainly multipotent cells of the cervical subepithelial tissue. Coppleson and others believe that the cell of origin is the stroma cell of the cervix. Other organs of the genital tract, specifically endometrium and endosalpinx, are able to produce squamous metaplasia. A reasonable hypothesis, therefore, is that squamous metaplasia in the endocervix results from pathologic stimuli as well as constituting part of the picture of "erosion healing."

INFLAMMATORY LESIONS

Inflammation of the cervix, or cervicitis, is so prevalent that one must search long and hard to find a specimen without some indication of either active or chronic inflammation. The cervix is constantly exposed to trauma during the life processes of childbirth, coitus, etc. The abundant mucus secretion of the endocervical glands in conjunction with the bacterial flora of the vagina which bathes the cervix creates a situation which is very conducive to infection. In most women, cervicitis is a microscopic finding of no clinical consequence and only an occasional patient is symptomatic and requires treatment.

ACUTE CERVICITIS

Undoubtedly the most common cause of acute cervicitis is an infection brought about by the gonococcus organism. The organism involves the endocervical glands as it does the glands of the urethra, Skene's glands, and Bartholin's gland. Other organisms such as streptococci, staphylococci, enterococci, and *Hemophilus vaginalis* may also affect the cervix and cause acute cervicitis. Although the inflammatory process is chiefly confined to the endocervical glands, involvement of the squamous epithelium of the portio does occur and has been termed *acute exocervicitis*. The extent of endocervical involvement versus exocervical involvement appears to have some relation to the infecting agent. Gonococcal infections are largely confined to the epithelial lining and the ducts of their racemose endocervical glands located deep in the cervical stroma. The streptococcal and staphylococcal organisms, on the other hand, tend to penetrate deeper into the cervical wall and involve the gland acini themselves. This pathogenesis explains the manner in which streptococcal infections reach the lymphatic channels of the cervix and produce a pelvic cellulitis. Undoubtedly this is the pathway of infection in the septic abortion. In contrast, gonorrhea usually spreads along contiguous mucous membrane surfaces as a superficial infection.

Diagnosis is made by appropriate smears and cultures of the cervix. The cervix, along with the rest of the vaginal canal, is often red, swollen, and edematous, and purulent discharge can be seen exuding from the cervical canal. The primary symptom of acute cervicitis is discharge. The type of discharge varies considerably but may be purulent and profuse, particularly if the cause is gonorrhea. Other symptoms may be backache, bearing-down feeling in the pelvis, dull pain in the lower part of the abdomen, and urinary disturbances, especially frequency and urgency of urination. Some women complain of painful intercourse. There is little in the way of systemic reaction. There may be a slight elevation of body temperature, but most of the symptoms are concentrated in the genitalia. In many instances the only symptom is a profuse discharge.

The treatment of acute cervicitis is simply limitation of pelvic activity and appropriate antibiotic therapy. There is no longer any place for local treatment of this disease. Overenthusiastic attempts to treat local cervicitis by cauterizing agents in the acute phase present a real danger of dissemination of infection to the pelvic lymphatics, resulting in a diffuse pelvic cellulitis.

CHRONIC CERVICITIS

From 90 to 95 percent of parous women have some evidence of chronic cervicitis but this is usually minimal, asymptomatic, and not even critically apparent. The cervix that harbors chronic infection does not offer any constant picture which may be regarded as characteristic. The most common clinical manifestation is the so-called "cervical erosion." Erosion indicates the presence, around the cervical os, of a zone of infected tissue which has a granular angry appearance. It implies the loss of superficial layers of the stratified squamous epithelium of the cervix and overgrowth of infected endocervical tissues. There is usually a yellow mucopurulent discharge which on culture yields organisms such as *Escherichia coli* and *Aerobacter aerogenes*. At times, chronic cervicitis is associated with the formation of a *cervical ulcer,* which is a lesion in which the full thickness of the cervical epithelium is lost and the underlying stroma are exposed and involved in the infection. A predisposing cause to both erosion and cervical ulcer is a condition known as *ectropion,* in which there has been a laceration or dilatation of the external os, usually during previous childbirth, leaving a considerable area of the endocervix exposed to the acid pH and bacterial flora of the vagina. At times, the chronic cervicitis appears as a reddish granulation raised above the surrounding surface and giving the impression of being papillary (Fig. 41-5).

The inflammatory process stimulates a reparative attempt in the form of an upward growth of squamous

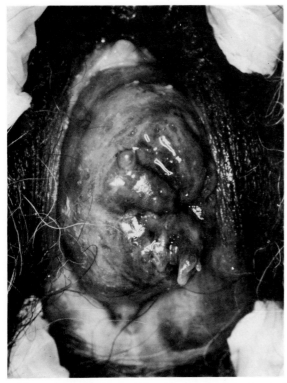

FIGURE 41-5 Chronic cervicitis with cervix prolapsed out of vaginal introitus.

epithelium, causing some of the ducts of the endocervical glands to be pinched off. Retention of mucus and other fluid within these glands results in the formation of *Nabothian cysts*. These cysts are nothing more than endocervical glands which are filled with infected secretions and whose ducts have become occluded secondary to the inflammation and reparative processes. They may be single or multiple and vary considerably in size. Upon drainage they usually emit a clear mucus, but occasionally drainage reveals a mucopurulent material, signaling a recent infection. The symptoms of chronic cervicitis are vaginal discharge, usually yellow/white, thick, and tenacious, and postcoital or postdouche spotting or bleeding. The endocervical epithelium is often swollen, edematous, and exposed; thus, it is readily traumatized, with the result that the patient frequently presents with slight irregular intermenstrual bleeding. This symptom is not unlike that which often heralds a cervical polyp. Backache is a common complaint in the patient who has chronic cervicitis. Other patients with chronic cervicitis complain of urgency and frequency of urination. Cystoscopic examination of these patients may reveal an acute or chronic trigo-

nitis of the bladder. It has been postulated by some that the trigonitis is secondary to spread of the infection from the cervix to the trigone via the lymphatic pathways to the floor of the bladder. Indeed, this is the probable explanation of the so-called "honeymoon cystitis," in which excessive stimulation and trauma to the cervix result in a lowgrade inflammatory process in the cervix which then manifests itself as trigonitis. This condition has traditionally responded well to sexual abstinence, which undoubtedly results in avoidance of trauma to the cervix and decreased inflammation to both cervix and trigone.

The most important consideration in the diagnosis of chronic cervicitis is the exclusion of a malignant process. Before treatment is begun, a careful examination of the cervix (possibly with a colposcope) should be carried out. A Papanicolaou smear should be obtained and areas which appear suspicious should undergo biopsy. It is important to emphasize that the final reports on both cytologic smears and tissue biopsies should be awaited before treatment is instituted. Should the diagnostic procedures result in a positive or doubtful report, further investigation would, of course, be necessary; intervening treatment frequently results in confusion and difficulty with further investigation. Suspicious areas should be biopsied. Suspicious areas are identified by the use of Gram's iodine solution (Schiller's test). This solution is applied liberally to the exocervix and the examiner's biopsies are directed to those areas which do not stain a deep mahogany color. Staining occurs when an adequate amount of glycogen is present in the cells of the epithelium. Glycogen deprivation may be seen in association with multiple benign processes, and therefore a Schiller positive area (nonstaining) is not diagnostic of cervical intraepithelial neoplasia (CIN) but suggests the possibility. Colposcopic examination of the cervix appears to allow greater accuracy in predicting those areas which present with the greatest risk of intraepithelial neoplasia. The final diagnosis, of course, rests with the histologic review of the biopsy specimen.

Treatment of chronic cervicitis and endocervicitis, erosions, and Nabothian cysts is both preventive and curative. Prevention of recurrent infections of the cervix, such as gonorrhea, will eliminate a large portion of the cases, as will optimal obstetric care. Prophylactic measures during labor, such as awaiting spontaneous complete dilatation of the cervix before delivery is attempted and immediate repair of all cervical lacerations, will result in decreasing the incidences of ectropion, erosion, cervical ulcers, and indeed chronic cervicitis. The traditional treatment of

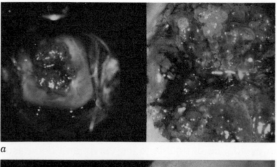

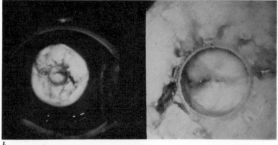

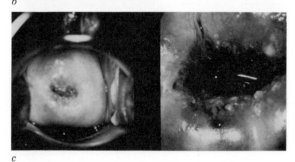

FIGURE 41–6 Cryosurgery for chronic cervicitis. *A.* Before therapy. *B.* Immediately after cryosurgery. *C.* Six weeks after therapy. Left-hand views are with the naked eye. Right-hand views are with colposcope.

this condition has been electrocauterization. In many clinics throughout the world, cryosurgery has replaced electrocauterization for this condition. Following cryosurgery, an enlarged friable cervix will usually be converted into one which more nearly resembles that of a nulliparous woman (Fig. 41-6).

TECHNIQUE OF CRYOSURGERY

Cryosurgery is best performed within 1 week after the cessation of the last menstrual period. This will avoid freezing a uterus with an early pregnancy and permit the most active phase of cervical regeneration to take place prior to the onset of the next menses. Treatment

is performed in the office or clinic without anesthesia or analgesia. Nitrous oxide is the preferred refrigerant for most purposes. A speculum as large as the patient will tolerate is inserted and the blades are fully extended. This provides optimum visualization of the cervix as well as reduced chance of freezing vaginal epithelium. All mucus and cellular debris are removed from the vagina and cervix with cotton balls soaked with 3% acetic acid. The extent of the disease which will be treated should be previously determined. Once the area to be treated has been outlined, that cervical probe which approximates the anatomic configuration of the cervix is attached to the unit. If the lesion is more than 1½ times greater than the surface area of the probe tip, the lesion should be subdivided and each segment individually frozen. The tissue is thoroughly moistened with saline to make sure of proper heat transfer, and the probe tip at room temperature is firmly but gently positioned so that the greatest extent of the lesion is covered. A tenaculum is not used to stabilize the cervix as this can cause excess bleeding and unnecessary pain. The refrigerant is circulated once the probe has been carefully positioned. Ice crystallization initially forms on the back of the probe tip and then spreads laterally from the edge of the probe. The lateral spread of the ice ball usually begins within 10 to 15 seconds after the refrigerant has been circulated. If timing is to be conducted, it is initiated at time of the lateral spread of the ice ball. However, it is more important to make certain that the ice extends at least 4 to 5 mm onto the normal-appearing epithelium. The actual duration of freezing is less important than the extent of the freeze process. When timing has been conducted, we note that the average probe position is about 2 to 3 minutes in duration. During the freezing process, it is unnecessary to know the probe tip temperature since one is guided by the extent of the visible ice ball. If a small portion of the vagina should become attached to the probe during the freezing process no serious sequelae result. However, if a rather large area of the vagina becomes attached to the probe tip, the tip should be defrosted and reapplied. Once the area or areas to be frozen have been adequately treated, the probe is defrosted and removed. The cervix should be carefully inspected to be certain that the ice ball has extended the necessary 4 to 5 mm onto normal-appearing epithelium. Only a freeze-thaw cycle is used if nitrous oxide is the refrigerant. If liquid Freon or carbon dioxide gas is used as the refrigerant, a freeze, partial thaw, and refreeze cycle should be employed to achieve satisfactory tissue necrosis.

Posttreatment side effects are usually few and not of a serious nature. A profuse watery discharge is noted for approximately 4 to 6 weeks following the cryosurgery. This is somewhat of a nuisance to the patient but in most instances presents little problem. Other complications such as occasional spotting and cervical stenosis have been reported. Subsequent infertility in patients who have received cryosurgery to the cervix has not been a frequently reported finding. The endocervical glands appear to regenerate, leaving in most instances a normal endocervical canal.

OTHER INFLAMMATORY LESIONS OF THE CERVIX

CERVICAL TUBERCULOSIS

Cervical tuberculosis represents a very small fraction of congenital tuberculosis. Stallworthy estimated that this entity occurs in only 1 percent of cases of congenital tuberculosis. Although the earlier literature contains some correlations between this entity and epidermoid carcinoma of the cervix, no clear etiological relationship has been established. On clinical inspection of the cervix it is often found to be markedly irregular and sometimes ulcerated; this can easily give the appearance of a malignant tumor. The diagnosis is easily made on biopsy. The typical microscopic lesions, including the tuberculous granuloma with epithelioid cells surrounded by lymphocytes and Langhans' giant cells with lttle central cavitation, are usually found.

CERVICAL SYPHILIS

Cervical chancre is second to vulva localization in the order of frequency. The lesion is often confused with the simple cervical erosion. The chancre usually presents in one of two forms: (1) an ulcer with an indurated base and elevated borders surrounded by a zone of edema, or (2) a simple nonindurated erosion covered by a gray membranous exudate. As on the vulva, it is painless and is often accompanied by only a slight amount of serosanguineous discharge. It is particularly obvious during pregnancy because its indurated aspect contrasts sharply with the soft consistency of the cervix. Dark-field investigation is indicated, of course, in all doubtful cases. The differential

diagnosis must distinguish among granuloma inguinale, acute gonorrhea, chancroid, and carcinoma.

HERPETIC LESIONS

The organism type 2 herpesvirus hominis, closely related to herpes labialis (type 1 herpes simplex), can cause a lesion of the cervix which is quite similar to the vulvar lesion called herpes progenitalis. The occurrence of these lesions on the cervix is considered to be a result of venereal transmission. The characteristic appearance is similar on the cervix to that of the vulva, with groups of multiple vesicles surrounded by a diffuse area of inflammation and edema. Occasionally they are associated with a burning sensation in the vaginal area, but this is difficult to analyze since they are often associated with vulvar lesions. These lesions may also appear as multiple small superficial ulcers with or without vesicles (Fig. 41-7). With the initial herpes infection there may be a prodromal period of several days with constitutional symptoms—fever, malaise, headache, etc. Cervical and vaginal

FIGURE 41–7 Herpetic ulcer on portio of the cervix.

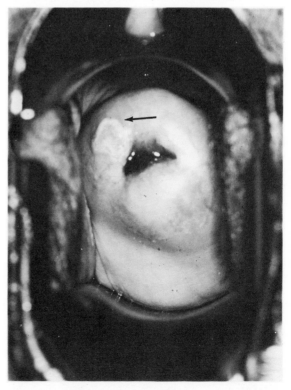

lesions are usually associated with discharge, occasional abnormal spotting, vaginal pain, and dyspareunia. Differential diagnosis will often include many of the other venereal diseases such as syphilis, tuberculosis, condylomata, and chancre. There is no specific treatment, but warm-water douches to eliminate some of the irritating discharge have proved to be helpful in some patients. The disease is usually short-lived, runs its course, and results in spontaneous healing of the lesions. An occasional patient will have recurrent episodes of these lesions and this may present a very troublesome situation.

CONDYLOMATA ACUMINATA

This is a warty growth which is frequently multiple and is believed to be caused by viral infection (Fig. 41-8). The cervix is far less common a site than the vulva or vagina. As with the other genital-tract condylomatas, pregnancy is likely to cause a marked stimulation of growth. These lesions are similar in their histologic architecture to other lesions called *squamous papilloma*. At times the lesions are confused or mistaken for carcinoma. However, their appearance is quite characteristic and the diagnosis is usually established by the clinician. A small biopsy is usually obtained for verification before medical treatment is begun. The satisfactory response to therapy with podophyllin (contraindicated during pregnancy) affords further confirmation of the diagnosis. Complete excision of the lesion is another acceptable means of therapy, provided an isolated or localized group of lesions is present.

FIGURE 41–8 Condylomata acuminata on lower lip of the cervix, viewed with colposcope.

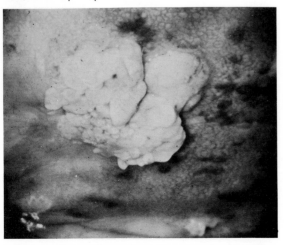

OTHER BENIGN LESIONS OF THE CERVIX

LEIOMYOMAS

Tumors composed principally of smooth muscle fibers are common in the uterus, but the cervix is rarely their primary site. Radman observed three cervical leiomyomas in a series of 1068 patients who were admitted to the hospital for definitive therapy. These tumors caused an irregular enlargement of the cervix and sometimes led to ulceration of the mucous membrane. Any leiomyomas of the body of the uterus may secondarily involve the cervix by extension or by prolapse into the cervical canal. Quite commonly myomas will present aborting through the cervical canal, associated with uterine contraction and a considerable amount of discomfort. If the diagnosis is to be made by biopsy, the specimen must be of sufficient depth to reveal the characteristic microscopic pattern. Superficial biopsies which involve only the mucosa will not lead to a definitive diagnosis.

The treatment is excision and usually connotes hysterectomy. A large cervical myoma or a large uterine myoma aborting through the cervix may present considerable technical difficulty for the surgeon. Often they become excessively large and occupy the entire pelvis, leaving little, if any, room for the operative procedure. It is often necessary to morcellate the myoma vaginally in order to achieve enough reduction in the size of the cervix to allow a reasonable hysterectomy. At times the cervical myoma will be on a relatively narrow stalk, and surgical excision above a heavy suture ligation or by electrocautery can be accomplished prior to beginning the abdominal procedure.

HEMANGIOMA

Hemangiomas are composed either of small vascular channels with narrow lumina, called *capillary hemangiomas,* or of distended closely grouped vessels, called *cavernous hemangiomas.* When the lesions are within the mucous membranes of the cervix, they appear as pink or red ill-defined areas. They are often asymptomatic but can cause hemorrhage. In a review by Marchant these lesions were said to be most often confused with endometriosis. Although biopsy often is associated with heavy bleeding, in many instances it is the only method of establishing the diagnosis. In addition to hemangiomas, neurofibroma and hemangioendotheliomas have been reported in the cervix. These rare tumors are indeed a curiosity and have no special clinical significance since they are usually asymptomatic. Treatment of all of these lesions is necessary only in case of annoying symptomatology or as a possible cause of infertility.

ENDOMETRIOSIS

Superficial endometriosis may readily be identified by examination. Gardner reported 40 cases seen in his own private practice in which the diagnosis had been made with a high accuracy prior to biopsy. The lesion usually presents as a slightly raised red area which does not fade when pressure is applied. Occasionally there will be a bluish discoloration along with the erythema. However, visible lesions such as this are a rare finding. In a high percentage of cases the lesion is associated with pelvic endometriosis. The treatment follows the same general outline as pelvic endometriosis (see Chap. 37).

VESTIGIAL MESONEPHRIC (WOLFFIAN) STRUCTURES AND ADENOSIS

The adult cervix often harbors remnants of the mesonephric ducts in the midlateral aspects of the connective-tissue body. A specimen of cervical conization is likely to contain the lateral area of the cervix where these structures occur, and in searching for other disease in the specimen one is apt to find ductal remnants. At times these present in a cystic or adenomatous form (Fig. 41-9), and in rare incidences they have constituted the source of adenocarcinoma.

The term *adenosis* is used to describe another adenomatous proliferation which takes place at times. In these instances there are many more gland-like spaces than can be accounted for by failure of involution and persistence of a fetal duct. Yet the lesion lacks the organization of a neoplasm which might be described as an adenoma. A considerable amount of evidence is now available which would suggest that adenosis is of Müllerian- and not Wolffian-duct origin. Indeed, the adenocarcinoma which may arise from these remnants is the so-called clear cell variety and has been correlated with mater-

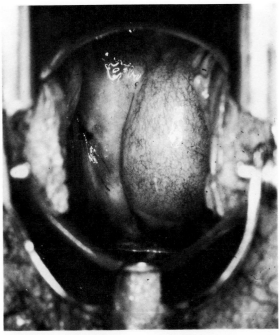

FIGURE 41-9 Mesonephric cyst of the left side of the cervix displacing cervical os into the right fornix.

nal ingestion of stilbestrol during the first and second trimesters of pregnancy.

LEUKOPLAKIA

Considerable divergence of opinion exists regarding the definition of cervical leukoplakia. The term is sometimes used loosely in connection with white or gray plaques which appear on the portio vaginalis as a result of keratinization and frequently accompany prolapse of the uterus. Leukoplakia of the cervix is, therefore, commonly regarded as a poorly defined entity which lacks any specific microscopic lesions. On the other hand, areas of hyperkeratotic thickening of the stratified squamous epithelium of the portio produce visible white patches which can be seen without concomitant prolapse of the cervix. These leukoplakial plaques are usually irregular, angular, and slightly raised from the surface (Fig. 41-10). They are often loosely attached at the base and vigorous wiping or scraping catches part or all of the white material. The area of leukoplakia is Schiller-positive.

Cytologic examination may reveal large aggregates of keratinized cells and numerous squames without nuclei. Excisional biopsy is warranted if the lesion is circumscribed. In view of the wide range of

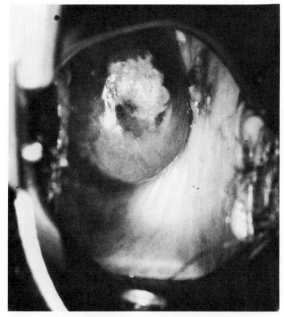

FIGURE 41-10   Leukoplakia on anterior lip of the cervix.

cellular activity associated with the lesion of clinical leukoplakia, it would be a mistake to make a prognostic conclusion that leukoplakia is precancerous and should be extirpated on sight. Henderson and Buck found coexisting carcinoma in 69 percent of their 23 patients with leukoplakia. However, this was an exceptionally high percentage, and in most series the incidence of concomitant carcinoma is considerably lower.

MALIGNANT LESIONS OF THE CERVIX

GENERAL REMARKS

Of all malignant diseases in women 25 percent arise in the genital tract, and half of these malignancies arise in the cervix. Next to cancer of the breast it is the most frequent cancer (preinvasive lesions included) to which womankind is subject. It is estimated 2 percent of women will be afflicted with cancer of the cervix before the age of 80. The unique accessibility of the uterus for cell and tissue study as well as for direct physical examination has led to the advances in diagnosis and treatment which have resulted in some of the best cure rates of any human

malignant neoplasm. The death rate for cancer of the cervix has fallen steadily over the past 40 years. The rate of 20 per 100,000 per year in 1930 has dropped to a rate of 8 per 100,000 per year in 1970. This decline has been secondary to diagnostic techniques such as the Papanicolaou smear and improved techniques of surgery and radiotheraphy. It is estimated that 30,000 to 40,000 cases of cervical cancer are discovered each year in the United States alone. In recent times, half this number have been diagnosed as carcinoma in situ. In spite of improved diagnostic and therapeutic modalities, the estimated death rate from cervical cancer remains at approximately 8000 cases per year in the United States.

Numerous epidemiologic studies reported in the literature have established a positive association between cancer of the cervix and multiple interdependent social factors. There is a greater incidence of cervical cancer observed among blacks and Mexican-Americans. This is undoubtedly related to their lower socioeconomic status. Increased occurrence of cancer of the cervix in multiparous women is probably related to other factors such as age at first marriage and age at first pregnancy. Combined with the high incidence of this disease in prostitutes, this information leads to a very firm conclusion that early age of first coitus and multiple sexual partners definitely increases the probability of developing this disease. Even socioeconomic status is interrelated, since the association has long been noted between relative poverty and early marriage and childbearing. The final common denominator appears to be not only the onset of regular sexual activity before the age of 20 but continued exposure to multiple sexual partners. Indeed, cervical cancer is very rare in celibate groups such as nuns. Many have labeled cancer of the cervix a "venereal disease."

The strikingly low incidence of cervical cancer in Jewish women requires explanation. Along with the observation that penile cancer is also extremely rare among Jews, this has led to the hypothesis that circumcision has a protective effect and that smegma of uncircumcised males plays a role in carcinogenesis. This association has been brought under considerable doubt by other studies among Moslems. Ritual circumcision is also practiced among this religious group, and study of comparable noncircumcised groups from the same countries and localities are inconclusive for substantiating smegma as a carcinogen.

Some epidemiologic features of cervical cancer suggest that a carcinogen, such as a virus, may be carried by the male; this carcinogen may be venereally transmitted to the female. Viruses are certainly known to produce malignancies in animals. It is possible that viruses also produce malignancies in humans. If a venereally transmitted virus is etiologically related to cervical cancer, it might be expected that the agent is a common inhabitant in the female genital tract. The number of viruses known to infect the genital tract of women is relatively small. Cytomegalovirus can be isolated from the cervix of some pregnant women, but there is no evidence supporting venereal transmission of this virus. Condyloma acuminatum is probably of viral etiology, but it has not been possible to isolate a virus from this lesion. On the other hand, type 2 herpesvirus is a common genital pathogen and this virus is venereally transmitted. The relationship of type 2 herpesvirus to cervical cancer is under active investigation. Rawls and his associates found neutralizing antibodies to type 2 herpesvirus in the sera of a significantly greater number of women with cervical cancer than in the sera of matched controls.

The age of patients with carcinoma in situ reproducibly is on the average 10 years less than the average age of patients with invasive cancer of the cervix. In most series, patients with carcinoma in situ have an average age of 35 and those patients with invasive disease, 45. There are, however, many exceptions, and in the past two decades an increasing number of patients in their late teens and early twenties have been reported with carcinoma in situ as well as invasive disease. Whether all invasive carcinomas begin as in situ lesions is unknown. Peterson reported that in one-third of 127 untreated patients, invasive carcinoma developed at the end of 9 years subsequent to in situ carcinoma. Masterson found that 28 percent of 25 untreated patients demonstrated invasive carcinoma at the end of 5 years.

EVALUATION OF THE ABNORMAL PAPANICOLAOU SMEAR

Results of recent studies on the origin and behavior of preinvasive cervical neoplasia as well as the ever-increasing number of young women presenting with this disease mandate a reevaluation of the commonly employed methods of evaluating the patient with an abnormal Pap test as well as treatment of these individuals if they should have preinvasive cervical neoplasia (dysplasia and carcinoma in situ). What is needed is an expeditious, safe, and economical method for evaluating the patient with the abnormal

Pap test, as well as managing those with preinvasive cervical neoplasia. As a result of multiple studies of dysplasia, the general consensus now prevails that cervical neoplasia is a spectrum of epithelial abnormalities ranging from dysplasia through carcinoma in situ to invasive cancer. The evaluation and treatment techniques to be presented here consider this spectrum of disease premise as valid.

The preferred outpatient method of evaluating a patient with an abnormal Pap test (suggestive of mild dysplasia or worse, or class III or worse) includes repeat cytology, gross examination of the cervix, Schiller staining, and cervical biopsies. If the biopsies show moderate dysplasia or worse, the patient is offered a cold-knife conization to rule out invasive cancer and to confirm the histologic and cytologic findings. If conization indeed shows severe dysplasia or carcinoma in situ, hysterectomy is generally carried out. Conization is considered therapeutic if moderate dysplasia or less is noted on the cone specimen or if the patient desires further pregnancies.

It is the opinion of some that the treatment plan outlined above may subject some women to unnecessary, expensive, and potentially hazardous procedures. This is certainly true *if office biopsy is not done*. Most of the physicians who follow this treatment plan are motivated by a desire to avoid inadequate therapy in a patient with invasive malignancy. Hysterectomy is strongly recommended in most cases of carcinoma in situ because of a possibility of residual disease after conization and the potential that more advanced cervical neoplasia will develop in the non-excised tissue.

A more conservative evaluation scheme and treatment plan for the patient with abnormal Pap test has been used in our clinic over the last decade (Fig. 41-11). Every step of the schema must be vigorously followed. If a step is left out, there is a possibility that invasive cancer could be missed, and indeed in the development of the scheme, when steps were occasionally eliminated, invasive carcinoma was missed.

Every patient must have repeat cytology since this provides valuable information regarding the type of abnormality. In taking the Pap test, every effort is made to sample the squamocolumnar junction where virtually all squamous-cell carcinoma will begin and reside. A thoroughly moistened cotton-tipped applicator or a disposable plastic or wooden spatula is used. The vaginal pool has a false-negative rate of 45 percent with carcinoma in situ, and 62 percent with cervical dysplasia, and is therefore ignored. A preferred technique is to use a saline-moistened, cotton-tipped applicator in the cervical canal and a spatula

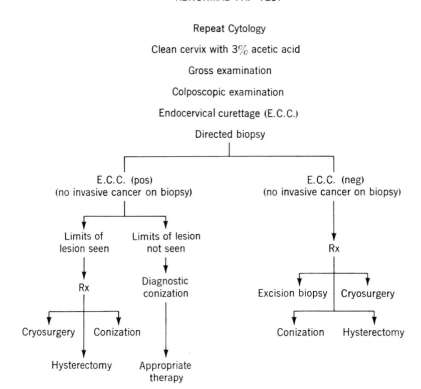

ABNORMAL PAP TEST

Repeat Cytology

Clean cervix with 3% acetic acid

Gross examination

Colposcopic examination

Endocervical curettage (E.C.C.)

Directed biopsy

FIGURE 41–11 A method of evaluating and managing patients with abnormal cytology.

on the portio. The endocervical sampling is useful in the detection of endometrial pathology as well. All samples from the cervix are placed on a single glass slide and then immediately dropped in fixative. The cervix is carefully inspected and suspicious areas are biopsied. Although the author prefers to inspect the cervix with a colposcope, the evaluation scheme can be followed quite adequately without it. The cervix must be carefully examined and the Schiller test employed. Biopsies should be taken from abnormal areas and from the endocervix. Carefully and thoroughly cleansing the cervix with 3% acetic acid helps to remove excess mucus and extenuates colposcopic patterns. The colposcope is focused on the cervix, and the transformation zone and squamocolumnar junction are examined. Endocervical curettage is performed prior to doing cervical biopsies, since bleeding from the latter will handicap the collection of material obtained by the curettage. Patients then have punch biopsies taken, if abnormal lesions are visible. Depending upon the results of the evaluation, patients are triaged for treatment.

Some mention should be given to the handling of the tissue specimens and the techniques of biopsy and curettage. Directed punch biopsy refers to a method by which with Schiller's test or colposcopy one can locate the most abnormal area and select this area for sampling with the appropriate biopsy instrument. In our clinic the Kevorkian-Younge punch biopsy instrument and the Kevorkian endocervical curette shown in Fig. 41-12 are best. The punch biopsy instrument has a square blade and is small in size. The rectangular design allows easy orientation of the cervix. The curette has a sharp small square jaw, without a basket, small enough to pass into almost all cervical canals.

The endocervical curettage is performed from the internal to the external os. The external os is the visible os that appears with the opening of the bivalve speculum. It is important in evaluating the patient with the abnormal Pap test that a speculum as large as the patient can tolerate be used. During the curettage, it is best first to curette the upper half of the canal and then to curette the lower half. Short firm motions in a

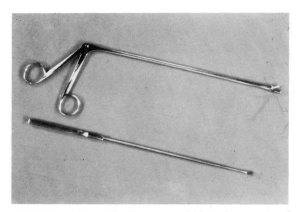

FIGURE 41–12 Kevorkian-Younge punch biopsy instrument and the Kevorkian endocervical curette.

circumferential pattern are the most satisfactory. Patients will experience some discomfort early in the cervical curettage, but rarely does one have to stop because of discomfort. Upon completion of the curettage all blood, mucus, and cellular debris must be collected and placed on a 2 × 2 absorbent paper towel. The material is then folded into a mound and, along with the absorbent paper towel, is placed into fixative. If any neoplastic tissue is found by the pathologist in the curettings, it is considered a *positive curettage*. After the curettage, directed punch biopsies are performed. The biopsy specimen is removed from the basket and is placed upon an absorbent towel so that the plane of the epithelium is perpendicular to the plane of the towel. Again, this will create a flat surface, thereby permitting a more accurate imbedding which reduces the problem of tangential sectioning. The biopsy specimen along with the towel is placed in the fixative. In most incidences, one to two biopsies are all that are necessary to properly evaluate the patient with the abnormal Pap test and a colposcopically visible cervical lesion.

The evaluation scheme permits a triage of patients based upon the endocervical curettage. If the curettage of the canal is negative and no evidence of invasive neoplastic tissue and only preinvasive cervical neoplasia are found under direct biopsy, the patient has been adequately evaluted and can be treated in a variety of ways. The type of treatment used for each patient will depend upon her age, desire for fertility, follow-up reliability, histologic appearance, and extent of the lesion. Cryosurgery can be performed in a number of patients who are good follow-up risks. Hysterectomy, either simple vaginal or abdominal, without preceding conization, is recommended to those patients who do not desire fertility.

No effort is made in the performance of the hysterectomy to excise the vaginal cuff unless there is evidence of abnormal epithelium extending onto the vagina, which occurs in less than 1 percent of the cases. A third possibility for treatment would be to perform a shallow conization or ring biopsy of the cervix. In every case these would be patients who had a negative endocervical curettage and in whom the upper limit of the abnormal area could be seen colposcopically.

The second major group of patients in the triage are those with positive endocervical curettage. Approximately 10 to 15 percent of patients with an abnormal Pap test will have a positive endocervical curettage. Patients with disease in the cervical canal are suspects for invasive carcinoma. From this group of patients two populations can be derived. In one repeat colposcopy and thorough use of the endocervical speculum or cotton-tipped applicator produce clear visualization of the upper limits of the disease. Since the curettage is performed from the internal to the external os, a lesion that extends only slightly into the canal will be picked up by the curette, resulting in a positive curettage. With the aid of a speculum it is possible to visualize up to 1½ cm of the canal. If, during this reevaluation, there is a reason to suspect there may be a skip lesion above the visible limits of the lesion, then a repeat curettage is performed. Patients in whom the upper limits of the disease can be seen clearly and in whom colposcopically directed biopsies have shown noninvasive lesions are treated by cryosurgery, conization, or primary hysterectomy.

Patients in whom the curettage is positive and in whom the upper limits of the lesion cannot be visualized must have a diagnostic conization to exclude or confirm invasive cancer (Fig. 41-11). With a diagnostic conization, ectocervical disease is disregarded since this area has already been evaluated by the colposcope and directed biopsies. The goal of the conization is to evaluate the endocervical canal so that patients can have appropriate treatment depending upon endocervical canal disease. If the cone is to be therapeutic, then all colposopically abnormal as well as Schiller-positive tissue of the ectocervix, and, if necessary, the vagina, is excised. In performance of the cone with high canal disease, as much of the canal as possible is removed, preferably up to the internal os. It is in this type of patient that complications occur and the procedure no doubt accounts for the 15 percent complication rate seen in this group of patients. If the patient shows invasive cancer on the cone biopsy, she will be treated with either irradiation or radical hysterectomy. If noninvasive disease is found, hysterectomy will be recommended unless the conization was to be therapeutic. Hysterectomy, which is usually carried out 24 hours after the conization, avoids the late complications of conizations. In over 90 percent of patients, conization completely excises the lesions.

One particular group of patients requires comment. These are the women who have persistently abnormal Pap tests but no disease in the endocervical canal or on the ectocervix. It is essential that a thorough inspection of the vulva and vagina be performed before admitting the patient to the hospital for surgical investigation. In nine patients, Townsend found that vulval and vaginal lesions (sometimes quite small) explained the source of a persistent abnormal Pap smear.

TECHNIQUE OF COLPOSCOPY

Colposcopy was introduced by Hans Hinselmann in 1925 (Hamburg, Germany) as a result of his efforts to devise a practical method for more minute and comprehensive examination of the cervix. At that time it was believed that cervical cancer began as miniature nodules and with increased magnification and illumination these nodules should be detectable. The meticulous examination of thousands of cases enabled him to clearly define the multiple physiologic and benign changes in the cervix as well as to correlate atypical changes with preinvasive and early invasive cancer. Unfortunately, Hinselmann was a clinician with little pathologic background, and this, in conjunction with the encumbrance of the tumor-nodule theory, led to the development of confusing concepts and terminology which initially produced a cumbersome, lengthy, and occasionally contradictory English translation.

Efforts were made to introduce colposcopy into the United States in the early 1930s as a means of early cervical-cancer detection. Primarily due to the awkward terminology, the method was generally ignored. With the introduction of cytology in the 1940s, the entire North American continent lost interest in colposcopy. The interest renewed in the 1950s and early 1960s, but progress was slow due to the competitive nature of cytologic examinations, which were more economical, certainly easier to learn, and had a lower false-negative rate. In recent years, colposcopy has gained considerable popularity and has been recognized as an adjunctive technique to cytology in the investigation of the epithelium. The popularity has been enhanced by the discovery of scientific bases for the morphologic changes and by the creation of a logical and simplified terminology.

The colposcope consists, in general, of a stereoscopic binocular microscope with low magnification. It is provided with a centered illuminating device and mounted on an adjustable stand with a transformer in the base. Various levels of magnification are available, the most practical being between 8 and 18×. A green filter is interposed between the light source and the tissue to accentuate the vascular patterns and color tone differences between normal and abnormal patterns. Interestingly, many instruments used in the operating theatres and offices of ophthalmologists, neurosurgeons, and otolaryngologists are essentially colposcopes. The examination of the epithelium of the female genital tract by colposcopy takes no more than a few minutes in the usual case.

Colposcopy is based upon study of the *transformation zone*. The transformation zone is simply that area of the cervix and/or vagina which was initially covered by columnar epithelium and, through a process referred to as *metaplasia,* has undergone replacement by squamous epithelium. The wide range and variation in the colposcopic features of this zone make up the science of colposcopy. The existence in this zone of variable vascular patterns, as well as the fate of residual columnar glands and clefts, determines the great variety of patterns. It had been generally believed that the cervix was normally covered by squamous epithelium and that the presence of endocervical columnar epithelium on the endocervix was an abnormal finding. Studies by Coppleson confirmed by others (Townsend) have established that columnar tissue initially exists on the ectocervix in at least 70 percent of young women and extends onto the vagina in an additional 5 percent of the female population. This process of transition from columnar to squamous epithelium, called metaplasia, probably occurs throughout an individual's lifetime. It has been suggested that this normal physiologic transformation zone is most active during three periods of a woman's life, i.e., fetal, adolescent, and during the first pregnancy. It is known that the process is enhanced by an acid pH environment and is considerably influenced by estrogen and progesterone levels.

The classification of colposcopic findings has been improved and simplified, facilitating the recognition of abnormal patterns: (1) white epithelium (Fig. 41–13), (2) mosaic structure (Fig. 41–14), (3) punctation (Fig. 41–15), and (4) leukoplakia (Fig. 41–16). Leukoplakia is generally reserved for the heavy, thick, white lesion that can frequently be seen with the na-

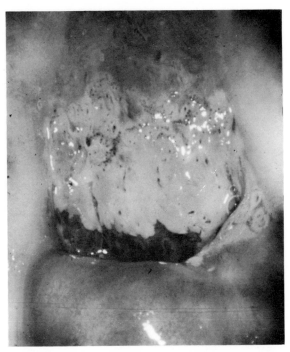

FIGURE 41–13 White epithelium as viewed with colposcope.

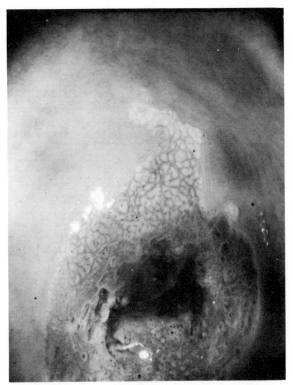

FIGURE 41–14 Mosaic pattern as viewed with colposcope.

ked eye. White epithelium, mosaic structure, and/or punctation herald atypical epithelium and provide the target for directed biopsies. Although the abnormal colposcopic patterns reflect cytologic and histologic alterations, they are not specific enough for final diagnosis and biopsy is necessary. The colposcope's greatest value is in directing the biopsy to the area which is most likely to yield the most significant histologic pattern.

In performing colposcopy, a standard procedure is followed. First, the cervix is sampled for cytology, then the cervix is cleansed with a 3% acetic acid to remove the excess mucus and cellular debris. The acetic acid also accentuates the difference between normal and abnormal colposcopic patterns. The colposcope is focused on the cervix and the transformation zone, including the squamocolumnar junction, and is inspected in a clockwise fashion. In most instances, the entire lesion can be outlined and the most atypical area selected for biopsy. If the lesion extends up the canal beyond the vision of the colposcopist, then, and only then, will the patient require a diagnostic conization to define the disease. An endocervical curettage is performed when the lesion extends up the canal. If invasive cancer is found at any time, plans for a cone biopsy are abandoned. The

plan of investigation which is outlined in Fig. 41–11 is based upon the assumption that there are no areas of intraepithelial neoplasia higher up in the canal, if the upper limits of the lesions can be seen colposcopically. In other words, intraepithelial neoplasia begins at the transformation zone and extends in continuity to other areas of the cervix, so that if the upper limits can be visualized, one can be assured that additional disease is not present higher in the canal. The colposcope only identifies a suspicion; final diagnosis must rest upon a tissue examination by a pathologist. Selected spot biopsies in the areas showing the atypical colposcopic patterns, under direct colposcopic guidance and in combination with cytologic testing, give the highest possible accuracy in the diagnosis and evaluation of the cervix. Probably of greatest value is the fact that in most instances a carefully chosen biopsy can establish and differentiate invasive cancer from intraepithelial neoplasia and thus can avoid the necessity of surgical conization of the cervix. This is especially valuable in young nulliparous women desirous of childbearing in whom cone biopsy of the cervix may result in problems of infertility. The avoidance of conization also is valu-

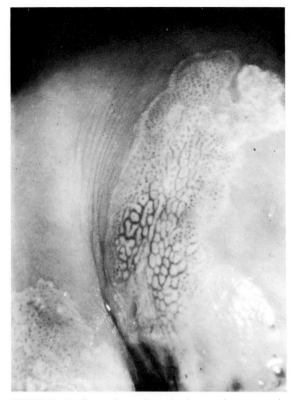

FIGURE 41–15 Punctation pattern clearly seen above a mosaic structure.

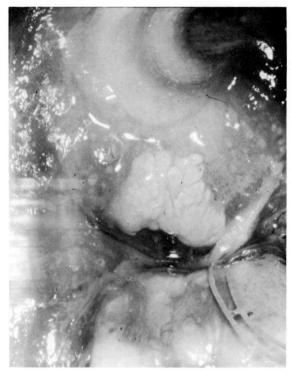

FIGURE 41–16 Clinical leukoplakia as seen with the colposcope.

able in reducing the risk to the patient from anesthesia, additional surgical procedure, and prolonged hospitalization.

ABNORMAL SMEAR IN PREGNANCY

The colposcopic evaluation of the cervix in the patient with an abnormal cervical smear has dramatically altered the management of the patient afflicted in pregnancy. The scheme outlined above is closely followed in pregnancy where the transformation zone is everted making visualization of the entire lesion almost a certainty. Cone biopsy in pregnancy is rarely indicated unless punch biopsy results suggest microinvasive cancer. This diagnosis must be confirmed by a cone biopsy to allow proper management. Patients with a firm diagnosis of preinvasive or microinvasive disease of the cervix should be allowed to deliver vaginally; further therapy can be tailored to their needs postpartum. The pregnant cervix is very vascular so that avoiding cone biopsy is in the best interests of the mother and fetus. *Small* biopsies are recommended of the *most* colposcopically abnormal

areas in an effort to minimize bleeding in the diagnostic evaluation.

CERVICAL DYSPLASIA AND CARCINOMA IN SITU

Dysplasia is a term which actually means "abnormality of development" and is used mainly with reference to atypical changes in the cervical epithelium. Dysplasia is similar to atypical hyperplasia, although it is not necessarily associated with increased thickness of the epithelium. It is characterized principally by atypia of the individual epithelial cells. Many pathologists divide cervical dysplasia into three subdivisions: mild, moderate, and severe. As one progresses up the spectrum from mild to severe, the likelihood of the lesion reverting back to normal epithelium becomes lessened and the progression to carcinoma in situ becomes more likely. All grades of dysplasia as well as carcinoma in situ will, of course, produce atypical colposcopic patterns. Interestingly, in most instances the cervix appears more normal to the naked eye.

Carcinoma in situ (preinvasive cancer) is a term applied to the lesion that has passed from the stage of hyperplasia of dysplasia to one of neoplasia. The development of the neoplasm involves loss of regulation of normal cell growth but the cells have not become invasive or produced metastases. The architecture of the epithelium is completely disrupted. The division into basal, parabasal, intermediate, and superficial cornified layers is impossible. There is complete absence of reasonable maturation. The entire thickness of the epithelium is occupied by a mass of cells of more or less the same type, irregularly distributed, without stratification, and with the polarity haphazard (Fig. 41–17). The nuclei are large and the nucleocytoplasmic ratio is increased. The nuclei vary in size and shape but are less irregular than in invasive cancer. The chromatin stains deeply and it is clumped or pyknotic. The fine granular appearance of the chromatin network is considerably altered. The nuclear membrane is accentuated and appears thickened, largely because of collections of chromatin within it. The nucleolus is prominent and large. Although there may be considerable involvement of endocervical glands with this process, the basement membrane is not violated and there is no invasion.

The relation of carcinoma in situ to invasive carcinoma has been the subject of many significant contributions in the field of gynecologic oncology. The cumulative information has been reviewed and summarized in several classic papers including those by Hertig and Gore, Friedell, and Fluhmann. The following observations support the belief that carcinoma in situ is a precursor of invasive cancer:

1. The highest incidence of carcinoma in situ occurs between the ages of 35 and 50, whereas the comparable range for invasive carcinoma is between 45 and 60 years of age. The distribution suggests that carcinoma in situ precedes invasive carcinoma.
2. The epidemiologic observation is that both carcinoma in situ and invasive carcinoma follow the same social patterns.
3. In several reported series where patients with carcinoma in situ received no major treatment, invasive carcinoma has occurred in a large percentage of the patients.
4. The two lesions are histologically quite similar and in many instances carcinoma in situ is often seen on the periphery of an invasive lesion.

Carcinoma in situ is usually asymptomatic, and on routine examination the lesion is frequently not

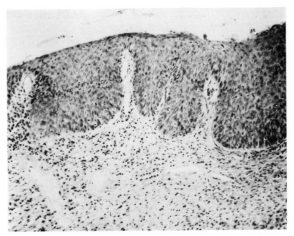

FIGURE 41–17 Carcinoma in situ of the cervix. Note complete loss of cellular polarity. All layers are pleomorphic.

observed. Recognition of the lesion is considerably assisted by the use of cytology and/or colposcopy. The mucous membrane sometimes bleeds easily on contact, and erosions or superficial defects of the ectocervix are relatively common in patients with carcinoma in situ, but these findings are not pathognomonic. The diagnosis must always be confirmed by histologic sections of a biopsy specimen.

In general, the treatment of carcinoma in situ of the cervix is based upon the reproductive requirements of the patient under consideration. Simple hysterectomy is generally preferred to radiotherapy since the morbidity is lower, preservation of normal tissue greater, preservation of ovarian function easier, and the problem of radiation resistance nonexistent. If the patient is still in her childbearing years with the family incomplete, excisional conization of the cervix can be utilized as a temporary treatment. This, in essence, is a coning excision of the transformation zone about the anatomic external os and the lower canal. This procedure can be utilized only with patients in whom the upper extent of the lesion has been visualized and invasive cancer has been ruled out. At our institution, this group of patients may undergo cryosurgery rather than excisional conization. In our hands, this procedure is as effective and carries considerably less morbidity and almost no chance of compromised fertility. The hazard lies in the fact that all of the diseased tissue is not removed for histologic study and thus colposcopically directed biopsies must be done by a very skilled colposcopist to minimize the chance of missing invasive cancer. The technique utilized for cryosurgery is identical to that previously described in this chapter for the treatment of chronic cervicitis.

One must be quite sure that the freeze ball extends at least 3 to 4 mm onto normal-appearing epithelium in order to be assured that the entire intraepithelial neoplastic lesion is destroyed. These patients must be followed with cytologic smears. The constant surveillance required when such conservative treatment is used makes it unjustifiable for a patient whose family is complete. Cryosurgery, of course, can also be used in the treatment of the varying degrees of cervical dysplasia.

MICROINVASIVE CARCINOMA OF THE CERVIX

The subject of microinvasive carcinoma of the cervix has presented itself over the past 10 years as a rather confusing dilemma. Contraindications and conflicts between the results of different investigators, incomplete information in the material presented, erratic interpretation of findings, and even erroneous use of the material can occur with such frequency as to confuse the most learned academician. A review of the literature shows that even the title of the subject itself has little accord among the various authors. *Microinvasive carcinoma* has been the most frequently used term, but the subject is considered under fourteen other headings. Some authors, seemingly unable to come to a decision, refer to the subject by several different terms in the same article. An attempt was made to eliminate some of the confusion in January 1971 when the committee of the International Federation of Gynecology and Obstetrics classified these lesions as stage IA and defined them as *early stromal invasion*. This definition is, of course, quite vague and others have specified that the depth of invasion should be no greater than 3 to 5 mm. Many authors have used the 3-mm rule and others have used the 5-mm rule. The Society of Gynecologic Oncology in January of 1973 accepted the following statement on microinvasion in cancer of the cervix uteri: (1) the cases of intraepithelial carcinoma with questionable invasion should be regarded as intraepithelial carcinoma; (2) a microinvasive lesion should be defined as one in which neoplastic epithelium invades the stroma in one or more places to a depth of 3 mm or less below the base of the epithelium and in which lymphatic or vascular involvement is not demonstrated. This definition was submitted to the executive board of the American College of Obstetricians and Gynecologists for consideration with the recommendation that it be approved and forwarded to the International Federation of Gynecology and Obstetrics.

At our institution, microinvasion has been defined as invasion to a depth of no more than 3 mm with no confluent tongues and no areas of lymphatic or vascular invasion. The bulk of the invasive process is probably the key to prognosticating the behavior of the disease. The physician should review the histologic section himself, and if indeed there are only scattered islands of invasion, the patient may be managed by simple hysterectomy. On the other hand, if one notes multiple confluent tongues of invasive disease, this patient should be considered at risk for lymphatic involvement and even though this is not seen on the microscopic sections, the patient should be treated with a radical hysterectomy. There are several prospective studies underway at this time including one by the Gynecologic Oncology group in which 25 member institutions are participating in an effort to clarify this dilemma. Creasman reported 1 patient of 19 who had invasion of 5 mm or less with a positive pelvic node, for an incidence of 5.2 percent. Others have reported an incidence of positive nodes in "microinvasion" of between 2 and 5 percent. These figures include of course those lesions with bulky invasion relative to the 5-mm depth.

INVASIVE CANCER OF THE CERVIX

The screening organization designed to reveal preinvasive cancer of the cervix has led to the discovery of patients with truly invasive but still limited invasion of the subepithelial tissues. When this invasion exceeds that of "early stromal invasion" (stage IA) but is still not clinically evident, it is called stage IB (occult cancer). These lesions and anything more advanced are considered truly invasive cancer of the cervix. A substantial and well-publicized screening program must make members of the public and the profession more aware of cancer as the possible cause of even minimal gynecologic symptoms. All public communication of an educative nature should emphasize the prevention and cure of cancer; a more hopeful and optimistic attitude would help to motivate patients and doctors alike to seek appropriate action. The need for early diagnosis rests upon the incontrovertible fact that definite cure, in actuarial terms, is readily achieved when cervical cancer is minimal, but is nearly impossible if the tumor is given time to grow and spread to the pelvic wall or into adjacent structures such as the bladder and rectum. The gradient of percentage curability from early invasive cancer to late and grossly invasive disease is such a steep one that even a moderate reduction in tumor size could not fail to create a substantial improvement in curability. It is true, of course, that like other cancers, some carcinomas of the cervix grow more rapidly than others. The basis for this differential in growth rate is still beyond our knowledge, but it is not beyond our capability to prevent undue growing time. Even the relatively slow-growing malignancy, if given enough time, will become incurable; and the most rapid-growing tumor, if diagnosed while of still moderate dimension, is definitely curable. The sooner all patients are detected and treated, the better the patient's chances of cure. The techniques of cytology and colposcopy have gifted the specialty of gynecology with the capability of eradicating cervical cancer. Every opportunity should be taken to disseminate modern concepts of cancer control to schools of nursing as well as other paramedical organizations. There is still a need for more coordinated effort in this field and the responsibility involves more than the physician alone.

The frequency with which invasive cancer of the cervix occurs is not known accurately, but the best incidence data would intimate a rate of approximately 8 per 100,000 per year. It appears to change from one locality to the other and it is noted to be less frequent in rural areas than in metropolitan areas. Cancer of the cervix is apparently less frequent in Norway and Sweden than in the United States. In underdeveloped areas of the world, cancer of the cervix looms larger in the cancer problem than in the United States and Western Europe. The development of carcinoma of the cervix in women who have never had sexual intercourse is so extremely rare as to be a medical curiosity; and only 10 to 12 percent of cases are encountered in women who have never been pregnant.

SYMPTOMS

A typical patient with clinically obvious cervical cancer is a multiparous woman between 45 and 55 years of age who married and delivered her first child at an early age, usually before the age of 20. Probably the first symptom of early cancer of the cervix is a thin, watery, blood-tinged vaginal discharge which frequently goes unrecognized by the patient. The classic symptom is often intermittent, painless, abnormal intermenstrual bleeding, initially only spotting occurring postcoitally or after douching. As the malignancy enlarges, the bleeding episodes become heavier, more frequent, and of longer duration. The patient may also describe what seems to her to be an increase in the amount and duration of her regular menstrual flow; ultimately the bleeding becomes essentially continuous. In the postmenopausal woman the bleeding is more likely to prompt early medical attention.

Late symptoms or more advanced symptoms of the disease include the development of pain referred to the flank or leg, which is usually secondary to the involvement of the ureters, pelvic wall, and/or sciatic-nerve routes. Some patients will complain of dysuria, hematuria, rectal bleeding, or obstipation due to bladder or rectal invasion. The appearance of persistent edema of one or both lower extremities as a result of lymphatic and venous blockage by extensive pelvic wall disease and distant metastatis are indeed a late manifestation of primary disease but a frequent manifestation of recurrent disease. Massive hemorrhage and development of uremia with profound inanition may also occur as preterminal events.

GROSS APPEARANCE

The clinical appearance of carcinoma of the cervix varies widely, depending on the nature of its growth pattern and the mode of regional involvement. There are essentially three categories of gross lesions. The exophytic lesion arising on the ectocervix often grows to form large friable polypoid masses (Fig. 41–18).

FIGURE 41–18 Large exophytic squamous-cell carcinoma of the cervix.

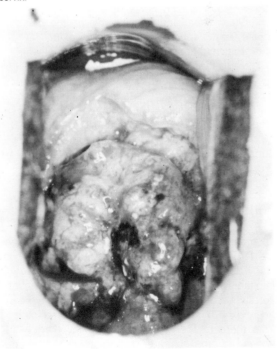

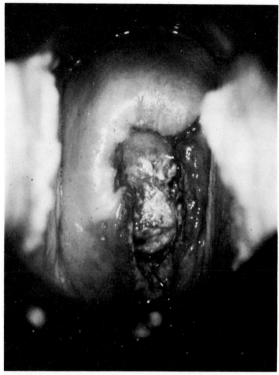

FIGURE 41–19 Ulcerative squamous-cell carcinoma of the cervix.

These exophytic lesions can also arise within the endocervical canal and usually enlarge the cervix to create the so-called "barrel-shaped lesion." A second gross manifestation of this lesion is that which is created by the infiltrating tumor, which tends to show very little visible ulceration and presents as a stony-hard cervix which regresses slowly under treatment with external radiation. The third type of lesion is the ulcerative tumor which can erode the entire cervix, replacing the cervix and upper vaginal vault by a large crater associated with infection and discharge (Fig. 41–19).

ROUTES OF SPREAD

The main routes of spread of carcinoma of the cervix are: (1) into the vaginal mucosa extending microscopically down beyond visible or palpable disease; (2) into the myometrium of the lower uterine segment and corpus, particularly with lesions originating in the endocervix; (3) into the paracervical lymphatics and from there to the most commonly involved lymph nodes, i.e., the obturator, hypogastric, and external iliac nodes; (4) direct extension into adjacent struc-

tures of parametria which may reach to the obturator fascia and the wall of the true pelvis. Extension of the disease to involve the bladder or rectum can result in the occurrence of a vesicovaginal or rectovaginal fistula.

The prevalence of lymph-node disease relates well to the stage of the malignancy in several anatomic studies. The prevalence rate of lymph-node involvement in stage I is between 15 and 20 percent. In stage II 25 to 40 percent are reported, while in stage III it is assumed that at least 50 percent have positive nodes. Variations are sometimes seen with different material. The best study of lymph-node involvement in cervical cancer was done by Henriksen. The nodal groups described by Henriksen were the following (see Fig. 41–20):

Primary Group

1. The parametrial nodes which are the small lymph nodes traversing the parametria.
2. The paracervical or ureteral nodes located above the uterine artery where it crosses the ureter.
3. The obturator or hypogastric nodes surrounding the obturator vessels and nerves.
4. The hypogastric nodes which course along the hypogastric vein near its junction with the external iliac vein.
5. The external iliac nodes which are a group of from 6 to 8 nodes which tend to be uniformly larger than the nodes of the other iliac groups.
6. The sacral nodes which are originally included in the secondary group of nodes.

Secondary Group

1. The common iliac nodes.
2. The inguinal nodes which consist of the deep and superficial femoral lymph nodes.
3. The periaortic nodes.

Henriksen plotted the percentage of nodal involvement both for treated and nontreated patients (Figs. 41–21 and 41–22, respectively). Distribution is as one would expect, with a great number of involved nodes found in the region of the cervix and a lower percentage of distant metastases. Although his series was an autopsy study, he found only 27 percent of the patients had metastasis above the aortic chain. Indeed, cervical cancer kills by local extension with ureteral obstruction in a high percentage of patients. Ninety-five percent of cervical cancers are of the squamous-cell variety, and the remaining 5 percent

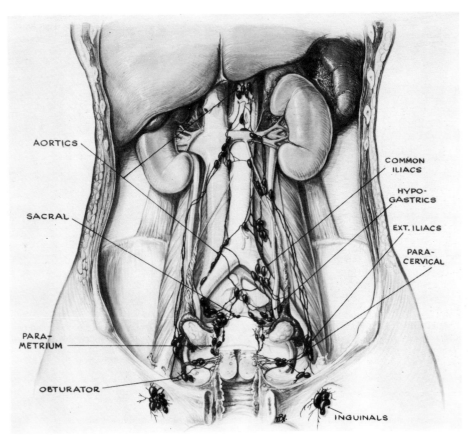

FIGURE 41–20 Lymph node chains draining the cervix. *(From E. Henriksen, Lymph nodes and lymph channels of pelvis, in Surgical Treatment of Cancer of the Cervix, N.Y.: Grune & Stratton, 1954. Courtesy of the author.)*

are primarily adenocarcinomas. The route of dissemination of the disease via lymphatics for practical purposes is identical for both histologic types. Adenocarcinoma of the cervix has a tendency to be of the infiltrating variety, with its origin in the endocervical canal causing the so-called "barrel-shaped lesion." Because of its mode of growth, these lesions often are quite bulky when they first present with symptoms.

STAGING (Fig. 41–23, Table 41–1)

The staging of cancer of the cervix is a clinical appraisal, ideally confirmed under anesthesia; it cannot be changed later if findings at operation or subsequent treatment reveal further advancement of the disease.

The following diagnostic aids are acceptable in arriving at a staging classification: physical examination, routine radiographs, colposcopy, cystoscopy, proctosigmoidoscopy, intravenous pyelogram, and barium studies of the lower colon and rectum. Other examinations such as lymphography, arteriography, venography, laparoscopy, and hysterography are not recommended for staging since they are not uniformly available from institution to institution. It is important to stress that staging is a means of communicating between one institution and another. Probably more important, however, staging is a means of evaluating the treatment plans utilized within one institution, and for these reasons the method of staging should remain fairly constant. Staging does not limit the treatment plan, and therapy can be tailored to the architecture of the malignancy in each individual patient. Unfortunately, clinical staging is only of rough value in prognosis since diseases of wide variability are often included under one subheading. This is particularly true in stage IB where a clinically obvious 0.5-cm lesion carries the same stage as a 6-cm lesion confined to the uterus.

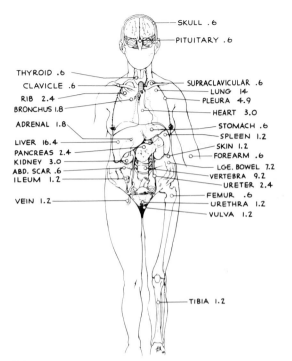

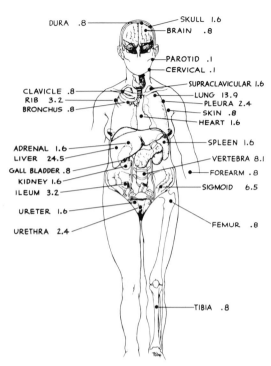

FIGURE 41–21 Metastatic sites of treated patients with cervical cancer. *(From E. Henriksen, Cancer of the cervix uteri. Radiology 54(6):803, 1950. Courtesy of the author.)*

FIGURE 41–22 Metastatic sites of untreated patients with cervical cancer. *(From E. Henriksen, Cancer of the cervix uteri. Radiology 54(6):803, 1950. Courtesy of the author.)*

FIGURE 41–23 FIGO staging and classification of cancer of the cervix.

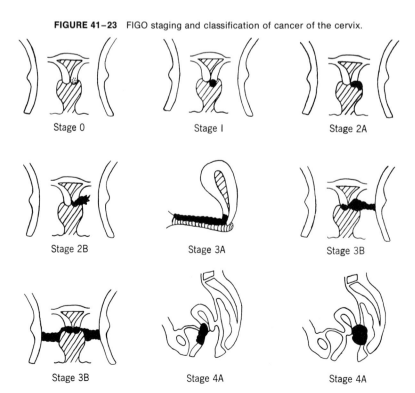

TABLE 41–1 Staging Classification
Nomenclature of the International Federation of Gynecology and Obstetrics (FIGO)

Stage 0
Carcinoma in situ, intraepithelial carcinoma.

Stage I
The carcinoma is strictly confined to the cervix (extension to the corpus should be disregarded).

Stage IA
Microinvasive carcinoma (early stromal invasion).

Stage IB
All other cases of stage I; occult cancer should be marked "occ".

Stage II
The carcinoma extends beyond the cervix but has not extended to the pelvic wall. The carcinoma involves the vagina, but not as far as the lower third.

Stage IIA
No obvious parametrial involvement.

Stage IIB
Obvious parametrial involvement.

Stage III
The carcinoma has extended to the pelvic wall. On rectal examination, there is no cancer-free space between the tumor and the pelvic wall. The tumor involves the lower third of the vagina. All cases with a hydronephrosis or nonfunctioning kidney are due to other causes.

Stage IIIA
No extension to the pelvic wall.

Stage IIIB
Extension to the pelvic wall and/or hydronephrosis or nonfunctioning kidney.

Stage IV
The carcinoma has extended beyond the true pelvis or has clinically involved the mucosa of the bladder or rectum. A bullous edema as such does not permit a case to be allotted to stage IV.

Stage IVA
Spread of the growth to adjacent organs.

Stage IVB
Spread to distant organs.

TREATMENT OF CERVICAL CANCER

Once the diagnosis of invasive cancer of the cervix is established, the question is how to best treat the patient. Specific therapeutic measures are usually gov-

erned by the age and general health of the patient, by the extent of the cancer, and by the presence and nature of any complicating abnormalities. It is thus essential to carry out a complete and careful investigation of the patient, and then a joint decision should be made by radiotherapist and gynecologist. The choice of treatment demands clinical judgment but, apart from the occasional patient for whom only symptomatic treatment may be deemed best, this choice lies between surgery and radiotherapy. In most institutions the initial method of treatment is radiotherapy, both by intracavitary radium and external x-ray therapy. The controversy between surgery and radiotherapy has been in existence for decades and essentially surrounds the treatment of stage I and stage IIA cervical cancer. For the most part, all stages above stage I and stage IIA are treated with radiotherapy. The 5-year survival figures from two large series, one treated with radiotherapy alone and the other with surgery, are included here. Currie reported the results of 552 radical operations for cancer of the cervix as follows:

Stage I	189 cases	86.3%
Stage IIA	103 cases	75.0%
Stage IIB	78 cases	58.9%
Other stages	41 cases	34.1%

Of 2000 patients treated at M. D. Anderson Hospital and Tumor Institute with radiotherapy, Fletcher reports the following results:

Stage I	91.5% 5-year cure
Stage IIA	83.5% 5-year cure
Stage IIB	66.5% 5-year cure
Stage IIIA	45.0% 5-year cure
Stage IIIB	36.0% 5-year cure
Stage IV	14.0% 5-year cure

In general it can be stated that comparable survivals are obtained by both treatment techniques. The advantage of radiotherapy is that it is applicable to virtually all patients, whereas radical surgery necessarily excludes certain medically inoperable patients. The selectivity of any surgical series along with the possible increase in morbidity must be kept in mind when selecting this treatment plan. In many institutions, surgery for stage I and stage IIA disease is reserved for young patients where preservation of ovarian function is desired. Other reasons for the selection of radical surgery over radiation include cervical cancer in pregnancy, concomitant inflammatory disease of the bowel, previous irradiation therapy for other disease, the presence of pelvic inflammatory disease or an adnexal neoplasm along with the malignancy, and lastly, patient preference.

Surgical Management

The renaissance of radical hysterectomy in this country was initiated by Joe V. Meigs at Harvard University in 1944, and shortly thereafter the radical hysterectomy with pelvic lymphadenectomy was adopted by many clinics in this country when dissatisfaction had been expressed over the limitations of radiotherapy. It was argued by some that many lesions were not radiosensitive and some patients had metastatic disease in regional lymph nodes which were alleged to be radioresistant. Radiation injuries had been reported, and one of the overriding points in favor of surgery was that gynecologists were surgeons rather than radiotherapists and felt more comfortable with this treatment modality. At the time of the popularization of this procedure, modern techniques of surgery, anesthesia, antibiotics, and electrolyte balance had emerged which reduced the enormous morbidity that once attended major operative procedures in the abdomen.

Radical hysterectomy is a procedure which must be performed by a skilled technician with sufficient experience to make the morbidity very acceptable (1 to 5 percent). The procedure involves removal of the uterus, the upper third of the vagina, the entire uterosacral and uterovesicle ligaments, and all of the parametrium on each side, along with a pelvic node dissection encompassing the four major pelvic lymph node chains: ureteral, obturator, hypogastric, and iliac. Metastatic lesions to the ovaries are, indeed, quite rare, and preservation of this structure is acceptable, especially in the young woman. The complexity of this procedure is supported by the observation that the tissues removed are in close proximity to many vital structures such as the bowel, the bladder, the ureters, and the great vessels of the pelvis. The object of the dissection is to preserve the bladder, rectum, and ureters, and to remove as much of the remaining tissue of the pelvis as is feasible without incurring a significant incidence of injury to these structures.

There is no doubt that in stage I as well as the more restricted of stage II cases, surgical removal of the disease is feasible. The addition of pelvic lymphadenectomy to the operative procedure met with considerable controversy in the early part of the century. Wertheim removed nodes only if they were enlarged and then not systematically. He believed that when accessible regional nodes were involved, the inaccessible distant nodes were also involved, and removals of suspicious nodes were more for prognostic than therapeutic value. He felt that node involvement

was a measure of the lethal quality of the tumor and not merely a mechanical extension of the disease. However, the operative procedure popularized by Meigs included a meticulous pelvic lymphadenectomy. Indeed, Meigs demonstrated a 42 percent 5-year survival in another series of patients with positive nodes. Lymphadenectomy now is an established part of the operative procedure for any patient with disease greater than stage IA. Indeed, there has been some interest in combining a radical vaginal operation with a retroperitoneal lymphadenectomy, and the results reported by Mitra, Navatril, and McCall are surprisingly good. The survival rate in patients with negative nodes is usually in the range of 90 percent or more.

The major complications of radical hysterectomy are the formation of ureteral fistulae and lymphocysts, pelvic infection, and hemorrhage. All these complications are preventable and the incidence is decreasing steadily. Ureteral fistulae are infrequent (0 to 5 percent) in the hands of modern technologists, primarily as a result of the improvement in techniques such as avoiding excess damage to the structure itself and preservation of alternate routes of blood supply. Retroperitoneal drainage of the lymphadenectomy sites via the use of suction catheters has considerably reduced the incidence of lymphocysts and pelvic infection. The use of electrocautery and hemoclips has assisted the surgeon immensely with hemostasis, and postoperative hemorrhage is rare. The wide spectrum of antibiotics available today is invaluable in the prevention of pelvic infection, which had contributed significantly to fistula formation as well as adhesions and bowel complications.

Radiotherapy for Cervical Cancer

Over the past two decades, radiotherapy has emerged as a notable alternative to radical surgery, primarily due to improvements in technique. The number of radiation-resistant lesions was discovered to be quite small, and radiation injury in the hands of a skilled radiotherapist is quite limited, especially with the moderate dosages used for early disease. A great deal of evidence has been recently presented which confirms the hypothesis that radiotherapy is able to destroy disease in the lymph nodes as well as the primary lesion. Over the past decade, radical hysterectomy has been reserved in many institutions for patients who are relatively young, lean, and in otherwise good health. In still other areas of the country, either radiotherapy or surgery has been utilized exclusively when the alternate modality is of limited availability.

Radiotherapy for cancer of the cervix was begun in 1903 in New York by Margaret Cleaves. Abbe in 1913 was able to report an 8-year cure. The Stockholm method was established in 1914, the Paris method by 1919, and the Manchester method in 1938. Radium was the first element used and it has always been the most important element in the radiotherapy of this lesion. External irradiation was used for treating the lymphatic drainage areas in the pelvis lateral to the cervix and the paracervical tissues.

Successful radiation therapy depends upon: (1) greater sensitivity to ionized irradiation of the cancer cell compared with the cells of normal tissue; (2) greater ability of normal tissue to recuperate following irradiation; (3) a patient in generally good physical condition.

The maximum effect of ionized irradiation on cancer is obtained in the presence of a good and intact circulation and adequate cellular oxygenation. The preparation of the patient for a radical course of irradiation therapy should be as careful as the preparation for radical surgery. The patient's general condition should be as well maintained as possible with a high-protein, high-vitamin, high-caloric diet. Excessive blood loss should be controlled and hemoglobin maintained well above 10 g.

Some consideration must be given to the tolerance of normal tissues of the pelvis which are likely to receive relatively high doses during the course of treatment of cervical malignancy. The vaginal mucosa in the area of the vault tolerates between 20,000 to 25,000 rads. The rectovaginal septum is said to tolerate approximately 6000 rads over 4 to 6 weeks without difficulty. The bladder mucosa can accept a maximum dose of 7000 rads. The colon will tolerate in the neighborhood of 4500 rads, and small-bowel loops, less tolerant, are said to have a maximum of between 4000 and 4200 rads. This, of course, pertains to small-bowel loops within the pelvis; the tolerance of the small bowel when the entire abdomen is irradiated is limited to 2500 rads. One of the basic principles of radiotherapy is implied here: the normal tissue tolerance of any organ is inversely related to the volume of the organ which is receiving irradiation.

External irradiation and intracavitary radium therapy must be used in various combinations. Treatment plans must be tailored for each patient and her particular lesion. The bulk of the cancer, not the stage, should be treated. Success in curing cancer of the cervix depends upon the ability of the therapy team to evaluate the lesion during treatment (as well as the geometry of the pelvis) and then make indicated changes in therapy as necessary. Intracavitary radium therapy is ideally suited to the treatment of early tumors. This is made possible by the accessibility of the portio of the cervix and the cervical canal. It is possible to place radium in close proximity to the lesion and thus deliver doses which approach 15,000 to 20,000 rads. The accessibility of the cervix is assisted by the particularly high tolerance of the normal cervical and vaginal tissue to irradiation. One thus has an ideal situation for the treatment of cancer in that there are accessible lesions that lie in a bed of normal tissue which is highly radioresistant.

Radium Therapy. Radium is the isotope that has been traditionally used in the treatment of cancer of the cervix. Its greatest value lies in the fact that its half-life is some 1620 years, and therefore it provides a very stable, durable element for therapy. In recent years, both cesium and cobalt have been used for intracavitary therapy. Cesium has a half-life of 30 years and with modern technology provides a very adequate substitute for radium. Four major techniques for the application of radium in the treatment of cervical cancer have found continuing favor among gynecologists. Three are intracavitary techniques utilizing specially designed applicators, and the fourth is the application of radium in the form of needles directly into the tumor. The variations which exist between the three techniques of intracavitary radium therapy are found in the Stockholm, Paris, and Manchester schools of treatment. The differences are largely in the number and length of time of applications, the size and placement of the vaginal colpostats, and the variations in radium loading. In this country, the tendency has been to use fixed radium applicators with the intrauterine tandem and vaginal colpostats originally attached to each other. Over the last two decades, a flexible afterloading system, Fletcher-Suit, has gained increasing popularity in that it provides flexibility and the safety of afterloading techniques (Fig. 41–25).

The Paris method originally utilized a daily insertion of 66.66 mg radium divided equally between the uterus and the vagina. The radium was allowed to remain in place for 12 to 14 hours and the period of treatment varied from 5 to 7 days. An essential feature of the Paris method and a part of the modification of this technique is the vaginal colpostat, consisting of two hollow corks that act as radium containers joined together by a steel spring which separates them into the lateral vaginal wall.

The Stockholm technique utilizes a tandem in the uterine cavity surrounded by a square radium plaque applied to the vaginal wall and portio vaginalis of the

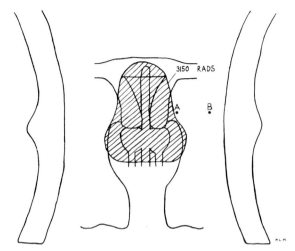

FIGURE 41-24 Isodose distribution around a Manchester-type radium system.

cervix. No radium is placed in the lower cervical canal, and vaginal sources are used to cover the cervical lesion. They are immobilized by packing and left in place for 12 to 36 hours. Two or three identical applications are made at weekly intervals.

The Manchester system is designed to yield constant isodose patterns regardless of the size of the uterus and vagina. The source placed in the neighborhood of the cervical canal is considered as the unit strength. The remaining sources in the corpus and vagina are applied as multiples of this unit and are selected and arranged to produce equivalent isodose curves in each case and an optimum dose at preselected points in the pelvis. The applicator is shaped to allow an isodose curve that delivers radiation to the cervix in a uniform amount. The Fletcher-Suit system mentioned above is a variation of the Manchester technique.

An effort is made in the two radium insertions to administer approximately 7000 rads to the paracervical tissues. The isodose distribution around a Manchester-type radium system is a pear-shaped structure, seen in Fig. 41-24. The maxima for a total dose delivered by the two radium insertions is a function of the sum dose to the bladder and rectum. The total dose received by the rectal mucosa from both radium applications usually ranges between 4000 and 6000 rads. The nearest bladder mucosa may receive between 5000 and 7000 rads. Where whole-pelvis irradiation is used, the radium dosage must be reduced in order to keep the total dose to the bladder and rectum within acceptable limits.

In conjunction with the development of a system of radium distribution, the British workers have defined two anatomical areas of the parametria where dose designation can be correlated with clinical effect. These are situated in the proximal parametria adjacent to the cervix at the level of the internal os and in a distal parametria in the area of the iliac lymph nodes. These are designated as point A and point B (Fig. 41-24). The description states that point A is located 2 cm from the midline of the cervical canal and 2 cm superior to the lateral vaginal fornix. The dose at point A is representative of the dose to the paracervical triangle that correlates well with the incidence of sequelae as well as the 5-year control rate in many studies. Point B is 3 cm lateral to point A. This point, together with the tissue superior to it, is of significance in considering the dose to the node-bearing tissue. It is clear from what has been said relative to points A and B that they can represent important points on a curve describing the dose gradient from the radium sources to the lateral pelvic wall. This gradient is different for the various techniques. In comparing the physical characteristics of radiotechniques, the ratio of the dose at point A over the dose at point B should assist in defining physical differences. The concepts of points A and B have been questioned by many authors including Fletcher. They remain as imaginary points but seem to provide a framework in which therapy can be planned. Again, the distribution of the disease must be the primary guide in planning therapy, and the total dose to either point A or point B is relative only to their position with regard to the disease distribution.

Whole pelvis irradiation is usually administered in conjunction with brachy therapy (e.g., intracavitary radium or cesium) in a dose range of 4000 to 5000 rads. Megavoltage machines such as cobalt, linear accelerators, and the betatron have the distinct advantage of giving greater homogeneity of dose in the pelvis. In addition, the hard, short rays of megavoltage pass through the skin without much absorption and cause very little injury, allowing virtually unlimited amounts of radiation to be delivered to pelvic depths with little, if any, skin irritation. Orthovoltage, because of its relatively long wavelength and low energy, has the disadvantage that doses to the skin are particularly high and, in delivering the required amount of radiation to the pelvis, temporary and permanent skin changes may be affected. Thus, for pelvic irradiation (Fig. 41-25), high-energy megavoltage equipment has definite advantages over orthovoltage and even low-energy megavoltage equipment.

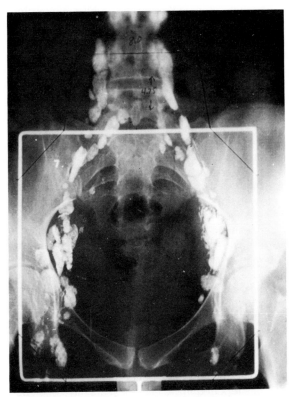

FIGURE 41–25 Pelvic field of external irradiation 16 × 16 cm in area. Patient has had a lymphangiogram and coverage of pelvic nodes is noted.

Complications of Radiation Therapy. Morbidity resulting from properly conducted radiation therapy of patients with carcinoma of the cervix is usually minimal. Frequent unfortunate misconceptions about the magnitude of this small radiation morbidity have several origins. Many have failed to distinguish that unnecessary adverse effects result from bad techniques which should not be extrapolated to the use of proper techniques. In addition, there has been a failure to recognize that a great deal of radiation morbidity is usually related to compromised treatment of patients with extensive tumor where surgery is not applicable. Results in these patients cannot be extrapolated to the use of optimum techniques in the treatment of patients with limited tumor. Also, it often is an unrecognized fact that a great deal of the morbidity attributed to irradiation results from uncontrolled tumor (i.e., rectovaginal-vesicovaginal fistula). As in the case of surgery, the treatment-related morbidity can be minimized by good application, but it cannot be eliminated.

The acute treatment complications which occur during or shortly following irradiation include irritation of the rectum, small bowel, and bladder, reactions in the skin folds, and mild bone-marrow suppression. Some of the transitory symptoms are tenesmus and the passage of mucus and even blood by rectum. The most frequent offending agent in producing proctitis is the vaginal radium, particularly if physical separation from the rectovaginal septum is less than adequate. Diarrhea and abdominal cramping characterize small-intestine irritation. Such morbidity is more frequent when a portion of intestine is fixed in the pelvis by previous surgical adhesions or other pathology. In this case, the usual offending agent is the external irradiation. In many patients, dysuria and frequency may result from bladder irritation secondary to localized high-irradiation dose from radium or combinations of external beam plus radium. This morbidity is more likely in patients with a preexisting abnormality such as infection and inadequate drainage with residual urine. Marked bone-marrow suppression is unusual, but a mild transitory depression of the circulating white cells and occasionally platelet levels is not uncommon. These changes are usually not severe enough to interfere with treatment. Anemia is not a consequence of properly conducted pelvic irradiation but is usually secondary to bleeding or infection, and should improve during the irradiation therapy.

Late radiation sequelae including damage to the rectum, bladder, and bone are less common. The symptoms of radiation proctitis may follow an asymptomatic interval of many months to years dating from treatment. The changes most often are localized to the anterior rectal wall at the site of maximum dosage from radium, and range from thickened fragile mucosa to thin atrophic mucosa or mucosal ulceration. These changes usually heal with conservative management. On occasion a diverting colostomy is necessary for either marked fibrosis of the rectal wall or excessive bleeding from the lower bowel. It is important that these stages be recognized and not confused with tumor, since diverting procedures are curative and result in the patient's returning to a state of well-being. Similarly, fibrostenotic changes in the sigmoid colon, cecum, and parts of the small intestine are occasionally seen as late complications of irradiation therapy. A typical patient with small-bowel injury presents with postprandial crampy abdominal pain and anorexia. All too often, these patients are classified as having recurrent disease and are allowed to waste away. Again, a diverting procedure with anastomosis of small bowel (proximal to the site of the injury) to the ascending colon usually results in adequate recovery of nutritional status for the patient.

The overall complication rate varies considerably depending on the total dose of irradiation used. In general, it can be said that the serious morbidity of pelvic irradiation is less than 5 percent if the external irradiation is below 5000 rads. Patients who receive more than 5000 rads of external irradiation are usually those individuals with advanced disease in whom radical radiation is a necessity. In these patients the serious complication rate approaches 10 to 20 percent.

SURVIVAL

Review of the annual reports on results of treatment of carcinoma of the uterus reveals a wide dispersion of 5-year recovery rates among several stages of carcinoma of the cervix. One can find data supporting any stand one wishes to take with regard to therapy. The overall cure rate in a cumulative series of 5228 patients (annual report, gynecologic cancer, FIGO) with stage I cancer of the cervix was 78.3 percent. The individual institutions reported 5-year cure rates from 69 to 90 percent with surgery alone and 60 to 93 percent with radiotherapy alone. Differences in results encountered may imply that one form of therapy has advantages over the other. However, in consideration of the rather wide dispersion of clinical variables, i.e., tumor size and volume, the patient's systemic condition and past history, which in fact may be unrelated to treatment, we must maintain collective open-mindedness with regard to forming definite opinions about the efficacy of individual therapeutic regimens. The best available figures for the two methods give results that are nearly indentical, and the presence of other factors affecting the samples being compared requires quite large differences to be significant. Individual physicians will probably continue to decide on the basis of their personal preferences and on comparison of complications and later disabilities.

EXENTERATION

Pelvic exenteration for recurrent squamous-cell carcinoma of the cervix limited to the central pelvis was introduced in 1948 by Brunschwig. Though this was initially conceived of as a palliative procedure, it is the opinion of most gynecologic oncologists today that exenterative procedures should not be undertaken unless there is a reasonably good chance of cure. The reason for this is the obvious extensive de-

formity of the patient that results and the decreasing but existent mortality. On the other hand, exenteration does provide an opportunity for salvage of patients who have failed to show improvement on irradiation therapy. It is particularly applicable to the patient who has a central recurrence without evidence of disseminated disease. Pelvic exenteration requires the removal of the bladder and/or rectum along with the uterus, entire vagina, entire parametria, uterosacral and uterovesical ligaments, and also often a portion of the levator muscles and vulva. Proof of the persistence of disease by biopsy is mandatory. All possible investigative studies should be done to rule out patients who have distant disease. If all of these studies are negative, exploratory laparotomy is appropriately undertaken for the purpose of proving operability. If the disease has not extended to the lateral pelvic sidewalls or beyond the pelvis, the patient may be indeed a candidate for pelvic exenteration. During the exploration, extensive search should be carried out to uncover metastasis in the upper abdomen, especially in the periaortic and lateral pelvic lymph nodes. Over the past decade, the operative mortality from this procedure has approached very reasonable levels, with some institutions reporting between 1 and 5 percent. Similarly, with better patient selection, the survivals reported in the last few years have been between 40 and 50 percent at 5 years. This reduced mortality and improved survival are due to the advances in anesthesia, antibiotics, fluid balance, and operative techniques. Patients in whom the bladder is excised will, of course, need construction of a urinary conduit either from ileum or sigmoid. Experience with this procedure has been perfected in several institutions and this, along with other technical advances, has improved the outlook for these patients.

CHEMOTHERAPY

Those patients with recurrent cancer of the cervix who are found to be inoperable become possible candidates for chemotherapy. Unfortunately, the results reported to date with various chemotherapeutic agents have not been promising. A wide variety of agents have been tried and disappointing activity has been noted. In many institutions, chemotherapy is reserved for those patients who are definitely symptomatic with severe pelvic pain; subjective responses are noted in some. All too often, recurrent cancer of the cervix is embedded in a thick bed of avascular fibrous tissue as a result of previous inflammation and irradiation therapy. The poor blood supply in this area creates a very unfavorable situation for effective chemotherapy. Distant metastases appear to respond in a much more gratifying manner, especially to multiple-drug chemotherapy.

CANCER OF THE CERVIX AND PREGNANCY

Carcinoma of the cervix complicates pregnancy in from 0.005 to 0.2 percent of cases, depending on which report is reviewed. The extent of the cancer and the duration of the pregnancy must be considered in the management of cervical cancer complicated by pregnancy. Despite many tales to the contrary, the effect of pregnancy on cancer of the cervix has never been demonstrated to be very great. Some people have suggested that the pregnancy accelerates the growth of tumor, but this has not been substantiated. Trauma at parturition may squeeze viable cells into vascular systems and thereby increase metastatic spread, but again this has not been documented in the literature. Metastases depend more upon the biologic quality of the tumor than on the pregnant state.

The treatment of cancer of the cervix in the pregnant uterus will depend on several factors including stage of disease, duration of pregnancy, religious conviction of patient and family, desire of the mother for child, and the background of the physician, as well as medical problems. During any trimester a radical surgical procedure is, or course, applicable to stage I and early stage II cases. Desire for preservation of the pregnancy often requires waiting several weeks for reasonable viability to be ensured. It is usually not recommended that patients in the first and early second trimester be allowed to continue the pregnancy.

Prior to 24 weeks' gestation, treatment with irradiation therapy can begin immediately after the diagnosis is made. The pregnancy is disregarded and whole-pelvis irradiation is begun. This usually will cause demise of the fetus and a resulting abortion by the fourth or fifth week of treatment. If abortion is not induced, excision of the cancer by means of an extended hysterectomy or surgical evacuation of the uterus is indicated. Once the uterus is evacuated, radium therapy can commence.

After the 24th week of gestation, therapy is usually delayed till viability is reached. Cesarean section can be carried out as soon as possible, consistent with pediatric and obstetric indications. If a radical hysterectomy with pelvic lymphadenectomy is not carried out at the time of cesarean section, whole-pelvis irradiation will begin immediately after the surgical wound has healed. These patients later can re-

ceive intracavitary radium upon completion of whole-pelvis irradiation. In general, those patients in whom cesarean section has been carried out can follow the same basic treatment plans used for cancer of the cervix in a nonpregnant patient.

ADENOCARCINOMAS OF THE CERVIX

There is a prevalent absence of information concerning the natural history, path of dissemination, and incidence of lymph-node metastasis in adenocarcinomas involving the cervix. Conflicting evidence exists in the literature, but in general it can be stated that this lesion behaves very similarly to its squamous-cell counterpart. The tendency of this lesion to infiltrate the cervix as an expanding endocervical lesion has been mentioned previously. It should be stated that the high central failure rate of this lesion previously noted in the literature is not likely to be due to radio-resistance but more appropriately results from the bulky barrel-shaped lesion which usually presents. Another basic principle of irradiation therapy lies in the fact that hypoxic cells are at least three times *less* radiosensitive when compared with tumor cells having normal oxygen tension. Considerable improvement in central control for these barrel-shaped lesions has been obtained by including hysterectomy in the treatment plan along with irradiation therapy. The dose of irradiation therapy to the midline must be reduced 20 percent in order to contribute safety to the operative procedure. In general, it can be said that patients with adenocarcinoma of the cervix should be treated no differently from those with squamous-cell carcinoma. Indeed, barrel-shaped lesions of squamous carcinoma origin should also have hysterectomy included in the control treatment plan.

SARCOMAS OF THE CERVIX

Isolated case reports of sarcomas arising in the cervix have been reviewed. Sarcoma botryoides is usually a malignancy arising in the vagina but it sometimes involves the cervix. Immature rhabdomyosarcoma of the cervix of the botryoid type has been reported in young women and successfully treated with radical hysterectomy. Lymphangiomas and lymphosarcomas of the reticulum-cell variety are also rarely seen. Identification of these lesions requires differentiation from anaplastic carcinoma, with which they may be readily confused. These lesions are usually metastatic and further investigation of the patient reveals multiple foci.

REFERENCES

Ashley DJB: The biological status of carcinoma in situ of the uterine cervix. *J Obstet Gynaecol Br Commonw* 73:372, 1966.

Badib AO et al.: Metastasis to organs in carcinoma of the uterine cervix: Influence of treatment on incidence and distribution. *Cancer* 21:434, 1968.

Barber HRK: Relative prognostic significance of preoperative and operative findings in pelvic exenteration. *Surg Clin North Am* 49:431, 1969.

———, Brunschwig A: Gynecologic cancer complicating pregnancy. *Am J Obstet Gynecol* 85:156, 1963.

Barron BA, Richart RM eds.: A statistical model of the natural history of cervical carcinoma based on a prospective study of 557 cases. *J Natl Cancer Inst* 41:1342–1353, 1968.

Bonfiglio M: The pathology of fracture of the femoral neck following irradiation. *Am J Roentgenol Radium Ther Nucl Med* 70:449, 1953.

Bosch A, Marcial VA: Carcinoma of the uterine cervix associated with pregnancy. *Am J Roentgenol Radium Ther Nucl Med* 96:92, 1966.

Brack CB et al.: Irradiation therapy for carcinoma of the cervix: Its effect on urinary tract. *Obstet Gynecol* 7:196, 1956.

Bricker EM, Modlin J: The role of pelvic evisceration in surgery. *Surgery* 30:76, 1951.

——— et al.: Results of pelvic exenteration. *Arch Sug* 73:661, 1956.

Brunschwig A: The surgical treatment of stage I cancer of the cervix. *Cancer* 13:34, 1960.

———: Surgical treatment of carcinoma of the cervix, recurrent after irradiation or combination of irradiation and surgery. *Am J Roentgenol Radium Ther Nucl Med* 99:365, 1967.

———, Pierce VK: Necropsy findings in patients with carcinoma of the cervix, implications for treatment. *Am J Obstet Gynecol* 56:1134, 1948.

Christopherson WM, Parker JE: A critical study of cervical biopsies including serial sectioning. *Cancer* 14:213, 1961.

Clayton RS: Carcinoma of the cervical uteri: Ten-year study with comparison of results of irradiation and radical surgery. *Radiology* 68:74, 1957.

Coppleson M et al.: *Colposcopy,* American Lecture Series, Springfield, Ill.: Charles C Thomas, 1971.

———, Reid B, with the assistance of E Pixley; with a foreword by J Stallworthy: *Preclinical Carcinoma of the Cervix Uteri; Its Nature, Origin, and Management,* New York: Pergamon Press, 1967.

———, ———: Editorial: The etiology of squamous carcinoma of the cervix. *Obstet Gynecol* 32:432, 1968.

Creadick RN: Carcinoma of the cervical stem. *Am J Obstet Gynecol* 75:565, 1958.

Creasman WT, Parker RT: Microinvasive carcinoma of the cervix. *Clin Obstet Gynecol* 16:261,1973.

Davajan V et al.: Spermatozoan transport in cervical mucus. *Obstet Gynecol Surv* 25:1–43, 1970.

Fletcher G: The role of supervoltage therapy. *Proceedings of the Conference on Research on Radiotherapy of Cancer,* New York: American Cancer Society, 1961.

Fletcher GH: External radiation therapy in cancer of the uterine cervix, in *New Concepts in Gynecological Oncology,* 1st ed., eds. Lewis, Wentz, and Jaffee, Philadelphia: F.A. Davis Co., 1966, p.11.

———: Results of radiotherapy of carcinoma of the uterine cervix. *Proc R Soc Med* 61:391, 1968.

——— et al.: A physical approach to the design of applicators in radium therapy of cancer of the cervix uteri. *Am J Roentgenol Radium Ther Nucl Med* 68:935, 1952.

Fluhmann CF: Carcinoma in situ and the transitional zone of the cervix uteri. *Obstet Gynecol,* 16:424, 1960.

———: *The cervix uteri and its diseases,* Philadelphia: Saunders, 1961.

———: Involvement of clefts and tunnels in carcinoma in situ of cervix uteri. *Am J Obstet Gynecol* 83:1410, 1962.

———: The squamocolumnar transitional zone of the cervix uteri. *Obstet Gynecol* 14:133, 1959.

———, Dickmann Z: The basic pattern of the glandular structures of the cervix uteri. *Obstet Gynecol* 11:543, 1958.

Friedell GM et al.: Carcinoma in situ of the uterine cervix, Springfield, Ill. Charles C Thomas, 1960.

Gagnon F: The lack of occurrence of cervical carcinoma in nuns. *Proc 2d Natl Cancer Conf* 1:625, 1952.

Gardner HL.: Cervical endometriosis, a lesion of increasing importance. *Am J Obstet Gynecol* 84:170, 1962.

Graham JB, Abab RS: Ureteral obstruction due to radiation. *Am J Obstet Gynecol* 99:409, 1967.

——— et al.: Recurrent cancer of the cervix uteri. *Surg Gynecol Obstet* 126:799, 1968.

Greiss FC et al.: Complications of intensive radiation therapy for cervical carcinoma: With emphasis on supervoltage radiation and supplemental radical pelvic operation. *Obst Gynecol* 18:417, 1961.

Gusberg SB, Marshall D: Intraepithelial carcinoma of

the cervix: A clinical reappraisal. *Obstet Gynecol* 19:713, 1962.

_____, Moore DB: Clinical pattern of intraepithelial cancer of the cervix and its pathological background. *Obstet Gynecol* 2:1, 1953.

_____, Rudolph J: Individualization of treatment for cancer of the cervix. *Proceedings of American College of Surgeons Meeting,* Munich, 1968. In press.

Gusberg SG, Corscaden JA: The pathology and treatment of adenocarcinoma of the cervix. *Cancer* 4:1066, 1951.

_____ et al.: The growth pattern of cervical cancer. *Obstet Gynecol* 2:557, 1953.

Helper TK et al.: Primary adenocarcinoma of the cervix. *Am J Obstet Gynecol* 63:800, 1952.

Henderson PH, Buck CE: Cervical leukoplakia. *Am J Obstet Gynecol* 82:887, 1961.

Henriksen E: The lymphatic spread of carcinoma of the cervix and of the body of the uterus: A study of 420 necropsies. *Am J Obstet Gynecol* 58:924, 1949.

_____: The dispersion of cancer of the cervix. *Radiology* 54:812, 1950.

_____: Pyometra associated with malignant lesions of the cervix and the uterus. *Am J Obstet Gynecol* 72:884, 1956.

_____: Distribution of metastases in stage I carcinoma of the cervix. *Am J Obstet Gynecol* 80:919, 1960.

Hertig AT, Gore H: *Atlas of Tumor Pathology, Fascicle 33 Tumors of the Female Sex Organs,* Part 2, Washington, D.C.: Armed Forces Institute of Pathology, 1960.

Hreshchyshyn MM, Sheehan FR: Lymphangiography in advanced gynecologic cancer. *Obstet Gynecol* 24:525, 1964.

_____, _____: Collateral lymphatics in patients with gynecologic cancer. *Am J Obstet Gynecol* 91:118, 1965.

Huffman JW: Mesonephric remnants in the cervix. *Am J Obstet Gynecol* 56:23, 1948.

Johnson LD et al.: Epidemiologic evidence for the spectrum of change from dysplasia through carcinoma in situ to invasive cancer. *Cancer* 22:901, 1968.

Keetel WC et al.: Management of recurrent carcinoma of the cervix. *Am J Obstet Gynecol* 102:671, 1968.

Kistner RW et al.: Cervical cancer in pregnancy: Review of the literature with presentation of thirty additional cases. *Obstet Gynecol* 9:554, 1957.

Kottmeier HL: Ten-year end results, radiological treatment of carcinoma of the cervix. *Acta Obstet Gynecol Scand* 41:195, 1962.

_____: Complications following radiation therapy in

carcinoma of the cervix and their treatment. *Am J Obstet Gynecol* 88:854, 1964.

Lewis GC et al.: Space dose relationships for points A and B in the radium therapy of cancer of the uterine cervix. *Am J Roentgenol Radium Ther Nucl Med* 83:432, 1960.

Liu W, Meigs JW: Radical hysterectomy and pelvic lymphadenectomy. *Am J Obstet Gynecol* 69:1, 1955.

Marchant PJ: Hemangioma of the cervix *Obstet Gynecol* 17:191, 1961.

Masterson JG: Analysis of untreated intraepithelial carcinoma of the cervix, in *Proceedings 3d National Cancer Conference,* Philadelphia: Lippincott, 1957.

McGee CT et al.: Mesonephric carcinoma of the cervix: Differentiation from endocervical adenocarcinoma. *Am J Obstet Gynecol* 84:358, 1962.

Mikuta JJ: Invasive carcinoma of the cervix in pregnancy. *South Med J* 60:843, 1967.

Mitra S: Cancer of the cervix: Prevalence, ethnology and treatment. *J Obstet Gynaecol India* 7:151, 1957.

Morton DG, Dignam W: The cause of death in patients treated for cervical cancer. *Am J Obstet Gynecol* 64:999, 1952.

Navratil E, Kastner H Unsere Erfahrungen mit 997 Amreichschen Operationen bei der Behandlung des invasiven Zervixkarzinoms. *Wien Med Wochenschr* 116:1012, 1966.

Ng AB, Reagan JW: Microinvasive carcinoma of the uterine cervix. *Am J Clin Pathol* 52:511, 1969.

Nolan JF et al.: A radium applicator for use in the treatment of cancer of the uterine cervix. *Am J Roentgenol Radium Ther Nucl Med* 79:36, 1958.

Novak ER, Woodruff JD: *Gynecologic and Obstetric Pathology,* Philadelphia: Saunders, 1972.

Ostergard DR, Morton DG: Multifocal carcinoma of the female genitals. *Am J Obstet Gynecol* 99:1006, 1968.

Parker RT et al.: Radical hysterectomy and pelvic lymphadenectomy with and without preoperative radiotherapy for cervical cancer. *Am J Obstet Gynecol* 99:933, 1967.

Peterson O: Spontaneous course of cervical precancerous conditions. *Am J Obstet Gynecol* 72:1063, 1956.

Radman HH: Myoma of the cervix. *Am J Obstet Gynecol* 82:361, 1961.

Rawls WE et al.: Herpes virus Type 2: Association with carcinoma of the cervix. *Science* 161:1255, 1968.

Reagan JW: Genesis of carcinoma of the uterine cervix. *Clin Obstet Gynecol* 10:883, 1967.

Richart RM: Natural history of cervical intraepithelial

neoplasia. *Clin Obstet Gynecol* 10:748, 1967.

Roddick JW Jr, Miller DH: Factors affecting the management of recurrent cervical carcinoma. *Am J Obstet Gynecol* 101:53, 1968.

Rutledge FN, Burns BC Jr: Pelvic exenteration. *Am J Obstet Gynecol* 91:692, 1965.

_____ et al.: Management of stage I and II adenocarcinomas of the uterine cervix on intact uterus. *Am J Roentgenol Radium Ther Nucl Med* 102:161, 1968.

_____, Fletcher GH: Transperitoneal pelvic lymphadenectomy following supervoltage irradiation for squamous cell carcinoma of the cervix. *Am J Obstet Gynecol* 76:321, 1958.

Sherman AI: *Cancer of the Female Reproductive Organs,* St. Louis: C.V. Mosby, 1963.

Song J: *The Human Uterus. Morphogenesis and Embryological Basis for Cancer,* Springfield, Ill.: Charles C Thomas, 1964.

Stallworthy J: Genital tuberculosis in the female. *J Obstet Gynaecol Br Commonw* 59:729–747, 1952.

_____: Radical surgery following radiation treatment for cervical carcinoma. *Ann R Coll Surg Engl* 34:161, 1964.

Stern E, Dixon WJ: Cancer of the cervix: A biometric approach to etiology. *Cancer* 14:153, 1961.

Stone et al.: Cervical carcinoma in pregnancy. *Am J Obstet Gynecol* 93:479, 1965

Townsend DE, Ostergard DR: Cryocauterization for preinvasive cervical neoplasia. *J Reprod Med* 6:171, 1971.

_____ et al.: Rationale evaluation and treatment of the patient with preinvasive cervical neoplasia. (Unpublished.)

Tredway DR et al.: Colposcopy and cryosurgery in cervical intraepithelial neoplasia. *Am J Obstet Gynecol* 114:1020, 1972.

Ulfelder H et al.: Invasive carcinoma of the cervix during pregnancy. *Am J Obstet Gynecol* 98:424 1967.

Wall JA et al.: Carcinoma of the cervix. *Am J Obstet Gynecol* 96:57, 1966.

White WC, Finn FW: The late complications following irradiation of pelvic viscera. *Am J Obstet Gynecol* 62:65, 1951.

42

The Uterus

SEYMOUR L. ROMNEY   WILLIAM B. OBER

The uterus is a target organ, a repository for pregnancy. In preparation for this major function, the endometrium undergoes cyclic changes and the entire organ undergoes a variety of adaptive responses, essential for normal intrauterine growth and the delivery of a normal baby. The endometrial changes reflect exquisite coordination of hypothalamic-pituitary and ovarian hormonal interactions, which are responsible for ovulation and the sequential changes of menstruation. Regularity of menstruation for women in the reproductive years is important to their physical and psychologic health and to their productive participation in daily activities (see Chap. 35). Irregular menstruation may be anovulatory, which may mean inability to become pregnant, or may be related to a disability. Amenorrhea is discussed in Chap. 20, infertility in Chap. 27. The kinds of bleeding abnormalities which may confront the patient and her physician are discussed in Chap. 20.

The principal problems of clinical gynecology center around abnormal bleeding, pelvic pain, or the presence of a pelvic mass. Abnormal bleeding may mean infection, infarction, a complication of pregnancy, or the presence of a benign or malignant neoplasm anywhere in the genital tract with special emphasis upon cervix, endometrium, or ovary.

Disorders of the uterus reflect intrinsic pathology in endometrium, myometrium, or in the myometrial or endometrial blood vessels. Uterine structures may also express primary pathology in ovary or fallopian tube of either an inflammatory or neoplastic nature. An endocrinopathy of pituitary, ovarian, or, less commonly, of adrenal or thyroid origin may also manifest itself as an endometrial disorder such as a menstrual irregularity, infertility, postmenopausal bleeding, mass, pain, or discharge (see Chaps. 20 to 24).

Hysterectomy is a common surgical procedure. It is often necessary to remove the uterus because of sepsis, uncontrollable bleeding, and benign or malignant neoplasm. Whenever laparotomy is performed and hysterectomy planned, an important decision is whether both ovaries and fallopian tubes should be removed. If pelvic inflammatory disease is the underlying pathology, bilateral salpingo-oophorectomy is in the patient's best interest regardless of age. The variables which require evaluation for elective oophorectomy are the extent and nature of pathology, the age, emotional stability, and general systemic health of the patient, and the ease or difficulty of the additional surgery. In the presence of normal ovaries, there has been less inclination recently to do bilateral oophorectomy as cancer prophylaxis. Carcinoma of the fallopian tube is rare.

In the absence of established organic disease, hysterectomy should not be performed. Surgeons have been criticized for removing the uterus without proper indication or for elective sterilization. Pelvic discomfort, backache, vaginal discharge, and generalized malaise may reflect an unhappy marital relationship, a bored, unhappy woman or fear of pregnancy. Hysterectomy is obviously not the solution for marital discord or an emotionally distressed woman. Although it solves the fear-of-pregnancy problem, removal of a normal uterus for this specific purpose imposes unnecessary surgical risk and eliminates any possibility for a future pregnancy. It is irrational to justify the removal of a normal uterus in view of the availability of other effective contraceptive measures (see Chap. 33). Depending upon the individual patient's educational, cultural, and emotional background, the response to hysterectomy when it is indicated is variable and is influenced by physician counseling. Many women need reassurance that the procedure will not affect their sexuality.

This chapter focuses upon the disorders of endometrium and myometrium. It includes a discussion of congenital malformations.

NORMAL UTERINE FUNCTION

EMBRYOLOGY AND MORPHOLOGY

The uterus is derived by the normal fusion of the Müllerian ducts which form the uterovaginal canal and fuse caudally with the urogenital sinus. All uterine elements are of mesenchymal origin. Müllerian duct epithelium forms the mucosal lining of the endometrial and endocervical glands. Mesenchymal condensations form the stromal components of endometrium, myometrium, and parametrium.

As a pear-shaped, hollow, muscular organ, the uterus exhibits a dome-shaped fundus which involves that part of the corpus above the insertion of the fallopian tubes. The corpus communicates with the cylindrical-shaped cervix, which inserts into the apex of the vagina. The endometrial cavity communicates with the peritoneum via the lumina of both fallopian tubes and with the endocervical canal below through the internal os. The cavity of the uterus has a depth of approximately 6 cm and a capacity of 4 to 8 mL.

The mucous membrane, which constitutes the endometrium, is soft and has a surface epithelium which is low columnar and contains glands of a simple tubular variety. The glands are embedded in a network of stromal cells that are, unless stimulated, the least specialized cells in the female genital tract. Under cyclic hormonal stimulation both glands and stroma undergo proliferative and secretory changes which result in an increase in thickness. Progressive growth of the endometrial layer requires that normal glands adapt to the spatial limitations of the endometrium. Thus, during the menstrual cycle, the glands become taller, coiled, and at times compressed. The unstimulated stroma is composed of small, round, or oval-shaped cells, predominantly occupied by nuclei of the same shape with very little cytoplasm. The stromal cells are supported by a fine fibrillary connective-tissue framework.

The uterus exhibits considerable physiologic mobility since it is influenced by its spatial orientation, the states of distention or collapse of the bladder or rectum, and the mobility and presence of loops of small bowel in the cul-de-sac. Its position is also influenced by the presence of pathology in its endometrial cavity, within its muscular walls or serosal surface, or in adjacent viscera, especially the fallopian tubes or ovaries.

Normally the uterus is anteverted, and its fundus is flexed anteriorly in relation to the long axis of the corpus; this is called anteflexion. The muscular wall of the uterus is covered by a serosa which is part of the pelvic peritoneum. Various peritoneal reflections—the round, broad, uterosacral, and the cardinal ligaments as well as the muscles and fascial supports of the pelvic diaphragm—maintain the position and mobility of the uterus. The disorders of the pelvic supporting structures are covered in Chap. 39. If the uterine size and shape are to be clinically estimated, the woman should empty her bladder before examination. The normal dimensions of the uterus in the nulliparous patient are approximately 7 to 9 cm in length, 6 to 7 cm in width, with an anteroposterior diameter of 4 cm.

BLOOD SUPPLY

Bilaterally paired uterine and ovarian arteries supply blood to the uterus. The uterine artery is present on both sides of the uterus, and its branches enter the myometrium at about the level of the internal os within the muscle layers just beneath the serosa; the uterine artery gives rise, at right angles, to branches termed arcuate branches. The latter give rise to myometrial radiate branches that penetrate the myometrium as medium-thick vessels then terminate in a straight vessel for the basal layer of endometrium and coiled arterioles. These extend through the inner myometrium and basal endometrium, eventually dividing as terminal capillaries in the superficial endometrium. Around the endometrial glands and within the stroma, capillary plexuses are formed. These plexuses and sinusoidal vascular lakes drain most of the endometrium (Schmidt-Matthiesen). The blood is returned to collecting veins in the myometrium and then to the main uterine veins at the lateral side of the uterus.

Under stimulation by progesterone in the late luteal phase, the coiled arterioles in the basal endometrium proliferate toward the surface and are known then as spiral arterioles. It is from these vessels that the early implanted conceptus must receive its supply of maternal blood. In contrast, the straight arteries terminate as capillaries in the basal layer. From these straight arteries, regeneration of the superficial layer begins. At times, some of the straight arteries may develop into coiled arteries but they may subsequently regress to again become straight arteries.

NERVE SUPPLY TO THE ENDOMETRIUM

The possibility that the sympathetic nervous system may innervate the endometrium is based on the clinical observation that significant uterine bleeding may occur after a severe emotional shock, fright, or anxiety. This type of bleeding may occur after menopause, following atrophy of the ovaries, or in patients in whom production of ovarian hormones ceases.

Several investigators have shown that the basal layer of endometrium contains nerve fibers, but none has been demonstrated in the upper portions of the superficial layer (Krantz). Neural elements originating in the myometrial nerve plexus extend into the basal layer as they accompany spiral arterioles, and they may proceed for a short distance to the functional layer. Some nerve fibers attach themselves to the basal arteries, but others not attached to arteries pass directly into the endometrium. In the myometrium the fibers are myelinated. However, in the endometrium, only nonmyelinated fibers are found. The nonmyelinated fibers decrease in size as they proceed into the endometrium and finally merge to form a plexus in the basal layer. The fibers may form either dense or loose networks and appear to intersect in all directions. The blood vessels and basal portions of the glands are enveloped by a fine network of nonmyelinated fibers. The nerve fibers do not terminate in the gland cells but come in contact with the outer cell surface. The close approximation of the nonmyelinated nerve fibers around the basal and coiled arteries suggests an anatomic arrangement which would allow for the constriction and relaxation of vessels and result in endometrial bleeding during periods of emotional stress or ill-defined autonomic or neuroendocrine phenomena.

PHYSIOLOGY OF THE ENDOMETRIUM

Predictable morphologic and physiologic changes occur during each menstrual cycle of the mature woman. The endometrium as a tissue shows greater variation in structure and growth within a relatively short period of time than any other tissue in the body. The descriptions in this section are mainly concerned with the superficial endometrium of the corpus and fundus of the uterus of the adult woman. The basal endometrium and that covering the lower uterine segment are relatively inert.

The endometrium undergoes rapid transition during the menstrual cycle. Early in the cycle it is thin and relatively inactive, but with estrogen stimulation it increases rapidly in size. During the latter portion of the cycle, glands and stroma increase in complexity under the influence of estrogen and then progesterone. Large quantities of uterine fluid are produced as the result of cellular changes during the midluteal stage of the cycle. At about this time spiral arterioles begin to develop. During this phase, the endometrial tissue is being primed in preparation for the implantation and nourishment of a conceptus.

The dynamic changes of the endometrium were first described less than a century ago. Hitschmann and Adler (1908) graphically illustrated the cyclic changes of the endometrium during the menstrual cycle. Schroder (1913) clarified the parallelism between the temporal and causal relationships of the ovarian and uterine cycles. Their descriptions have been of significance to generations of gynecologists and endocrinologists whose related studies have been based on theirs. In 1950, a well-illustrated description of the cyclic changes of the endometrium in the normal menstrual cycle was published (Noyes et al.).

The endometrium may conventionally be divided into two layers which differ in both morphology and function. The basal layer is nonfunctional and is also known as the lamina basalis. The superficial or functional layer, also known as the lamina functionalis, acts as the resting site for the implanting conceptus and has been known as the implantation layer. This layer of the mucosa forms the bulk of the decidua that develops after nidation. The basal layer, which remains inactive during the menstrual cycle, is contiguous with the superficial myometrium on one surface and the superficial endometrium on the other surface. It has an average thickness of 0.5 mm but may vary considerably in individuals, ranging from slightly less than 0.3 to 1.0 mm. The basal layer remains intact during menstruation, and reepithelialization of its surface begins as bleeding ceases. It is completely reepithelialized within 2 days after cessation of flow. The arterioles and venules grow from the basal layer. In contrast to the inactivity of the basal layer, the superficial layer undergoes continuous change. Throughout the menstrual cycle different phases merge imperceptibly into one another. The stroma consists of endometrial stromal cells, blood vessels, and intercellular connective tissue. Wandering cells, such as leukocytes, may be found in either the epithelial or stromal spaces. Nerves and lymphatics may be present in the stroma.

The superficial epithelium is composed of a single layer of cells which are continuous with the glandular epithelium. Although the cuboidal cells of the superficial epithelium merge with the glandular cells, the response of these two cell types to ovarian hormones is functionally different. For example, when the glandular epithelial cells develop sub- and supranuclear vacuoles in response to progesterone, the surface epithelial cells remain free of vacuoles. Following menstruation, the superficial epithelial cells are cuboidal, measuring approximately 6 mm in height, and during the late proliferative stage they attain a height of 16 to 20 mm.

The columnar cells of the glands produce glycogen, glycoproteins, and mucopolysaccharides. The amounts of glycogen and glycoprotein vary with the phase of the cycle, showing a distinct increase during the early and midluteal phases. Usually glycogen is absent from the basal layer of the endometrium. Small glycogen granules have been noted during the proliferative phase, and they appear to be more prominent toward the time of ovulation. The prominent glycogen deposits in the glandular cells noted after ovulation are present in such marked quantities as to suggest that they play an important role in the nutrition of preimplantation and the implanting of the conceptus.

The endometrial stroma consists of small specialized "naked nucleus" cells in an intercellular connective-tissue network. A reticular fiber system is present throughout both the basal and superficial layers. In the basal layer, the reticular fibers are compact and firmly anchored to the myometrium. In contrast, the fiber network of the superficial layer is subject to cyclic changes. The reticular fibers are in close contact with the cytoplasmic projections of the stromal cells. Some fibers penetrate into the basement membrane of the epithelial layer. The reticular layer is more compact just below the superficial epithelium and around the glandular epithelium and perivascular areas. When the stroma shows marked edema (during the preimplantation phase of the endometrium), the reticular fibers are torn apart in many places. This network appears to reinforce the individual stromal cells in preparation for the implantation of the embryo. During the late luteal phase, these stromal cells increase in volume and form predecidua which, if implantation takes place, develop into true decidua.

MENSTRUAL CYCLE

Menstruation is characterized by a succession of cycles from menarche to the menopause. The significant morphologic and physiologic changes occur in response to the secretion of hypothalamic, pituitary and ovarian hormones. The proliferative phase of endometrial development occurs in concert with the development of ovarian follicles and the secretion of estrogen and thus is called the follicular phase. The luteal phase of the endometrium occurs in response to circulating progesterone originating from the corpus luteum in the ovary. This phase has also been called the progestational phase. Either the term luteal or progestational phase is preferable to the use of the term "secretory phase," since intraglandular and intrauterine fluid is produced during both the follicular and luteal phases but is produced in significantly greater quantities during the luteal phase. The regression phase of the endometrium occurs late in the menstrual cycle, a few days prior to clinical onset of menstruation, and corresponds to regression of the corpus luteum. Throughout menstruation the endometrial tissues together with blood elements desquamate into the endometrial cavity.

FOLLICULAR OR PROLIFERATIVE PHASE

During the proliferative phase, the endometrium responds to stimulation by estrogens, primarily estradiol. Day-to-day changes are not sufficiently distinct to permit discrimination of more than broad subphases of growth. The proliferative phase is characterized by a marked increase in the number of glandular and stromal cells, and glandular and stromal mitoses are the hallmarks of estrogen stimulation. The glands gradually become coiled and the glandular epithelial cells often appear to be piled one on top of the other (termed pseudostratification). In the early part of the proliferative phase, the short, straight, narrow glands contain mitotic figures and the glands grow rapidly. The combined thickness of the superficial layer and the basal layer during the early proliferative phase is usually between 1 and 2 mm. During the latter part of the proliferative phase, the endometrial thickness reaches approximately 4 mm and occasionally may be as much as 7 mm. There is a steady growth of endometrium until the time of ovulation, which is followed by a second increase in thickness beginning on the 20th day and continuing until shortly before menstruation when regressive changes take place in the endometrium.

LUTEAL OR PROGESTATIONAL PHASE

During the early luteal phase, the glands increase in tortuosity and the lumina become distended. Approximately 36 to 48 hours after ovulation, subnuclear vacuoles appear in the glandular cells. The subnuclear vacuoles continue to increase and within a day or two migrate to a supranuclear position. The vacuoles then merge imperceptibly into the apical portion of the cytoplasm of the glandular cell, and products of secretion are discharged into gland lumina. At the time of implantation, the glands attain maximal tortuosity and luminal diameter, the result of increased glandular secretion. There is also marked edema of the stroma which disappears in several days to give way to a predecidual change of the stromal cells. At this time, the stromal cells show marked enlargement, cytoplasmic eosinophilia, and nuclear vesiculation. Shortly before the onset of menstruation, the stroma is compact, demonstrating a uniform confluent predecidual reaction throughout its superficial layers, and the glands maintain a secretory pattern and active secretion. Polymorphonuclear leukocytes begin to appear around small blood vessels and later become more prominent throughout the stroma. With the onset of menstruation, fibrin thrombi form in venules, and bleeding from small areas of necrosis occurs at different locations in the endometrium. These areas later enlarge and become confluent with other necrotic areas. In a sense, a menstrual endometrium shows the histopathology of infarction. The blood vessels are markedly distended and engorged with red blood cells, and there is increasing autolysis and dissolution of the endometrial glands and stroma. Eventually there is sloughing of tissue fragments into the endometrial cavity; usually only the basal layer of the endometrium remains. This portion of endometrium undergoes reepithelialization beginning in the necks of the glands. The process is usually completed by approximately the fifth day after the onset of bleeding.

The mitotic activity of the endometrium shows marked fluctuations during the menstrual cycle. The proliferative phase is characterized by a high frequency of mitoses in both the gland and stromal cells and also a high ribonucleic and desoxyribonucleic acid content. Mitoses are present in the stroma and in the epithelium as it regenerates after menstruation. The number of mitoses in glandular epithelium reaches a maximum around the time of ovulation, falling off rapidly during the early luteal phase, and mitotic figures are usually absent by cycle day 18. The various morphologic changes in the endometrium throughout the menstrual cycle are summarized in Fig. 42-1.

IMPLANTATION OF BLASTOCYST

The fertilized ovum enters the uterine cavity on about the third day after fertilization and continues cleavage during the time it is lying free in the uterine cavity. The zygote adheres to the viscid mucus in the endometrial cavity until the diminution of myometrial contractions resulting from progesterone allows the zygote to attach itself to the body of the uterine cavity. In the human an implant in the prepared endometrium occurs between the seventh and tenth days after ovulation, i.e., about the 21st to 24th day of the menstrual cycle.

During the time that the zygote is lying free in the uterine cavity, the glands continue maturation, showing maximal secretory activity by the sixth day after ovulation. At this time, the glands demonstrate secretion from the apical portion of the cell, as evidenced by budding of the cell membrane with release of a portion of the cytoplasm into the gland lumen. At the expected time of implantation of the blastocyst, stromal transformation allows the blastocyst to burrow into maternal tissues. Stromal edema is at its maximum around the sixth day post-ovulation, and as edema subsides, stromal cells enlarge, signaling the onset of predecidual change. At the time of implantation, the glands show maximal tortuosity and secretion, and the stroma is loose because of edema.

During this time, the spiral arterioles become increasingly prominent and proliferate toward the surface under the influence of progesterone. The predecidual response of the stromal cells is first seen in the periarteriolar zones, indicating that vascular diffusion of progesterone affects the closest stromal cells.

ONSET OF MENSES

If fertilization of the ovum does not take place, the stroma begins to show degeneration during the latter part of the luteal phase. There is concomitant migration of polymorphonuclear leukocytes into the stroma. The number of leukocytes progressively increases during the 2-day period prior to bleeding. Menses begin with fragmentation and autolysis but these phenomena do not occur uniformly throughout the endometrium and both sloughing and bleeding occur at varying times from varying sites. Necrosis begins with small areas that show tissue blanching with bleeding. Over the period of the next few hours, these areas enlarge and become confluent with other areas of bleeding and necrosis. Histologic examination of tissue at this time may show extremely variable patterns. Fragmentated glandular tissue and autolyzed stroma may be seen. If the endometrial tissue is examined within a few hours after the onset of flow, some of the stromal cell islands may show some evidence of the predecidual reaction. Endometrial biopsy is occasionally performed at this time.

An understanding of the events taking place at the time of menstruation was best acquired from classical experiments in which monkey endometrium was transplanted to the anterior chamber of the eye (Markee). The endometrial transplants developed cyclically and menstruation occurred at the time of the monkey's anticipated normal menstrual period. As the endometrium was observed in the anterior chamber prior to menstruation, the spiral arterioles underwent constriction that completely obstructed vascular flow and blanched the tissue. This period of arteriolar constriction was followed by arteriolar dilatation with a sudden burst of blood flow through the capillaries. With the blanching of endometrium, damage to the tissue occurred, resulting in later autolysis and necrosis. As the stroma collapsed, the spiral arterioles also buckled resulting in a partial obstruction of blood flow. Decreased oxygenation of the endometrial structures was postulated and degeneration of autolysis of the stroma ensued following blood stasis. The constriction of the spiral arterioles occurred from 4 to 24 hours before the time of visible bleeding. The pro-

Dating the Endrometrium

Approximate relationship of useful morphological factors

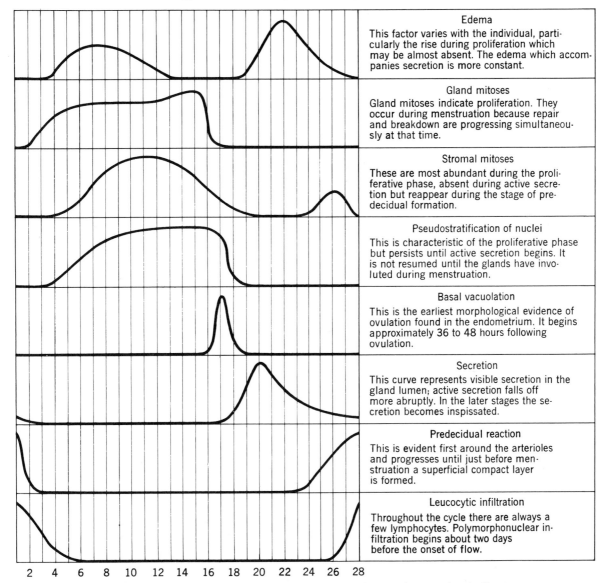

Edema
This factor varies with the individual, particularly the rise during proliferation which may be almost absent. The edema which accompanies secretion is more constant.

Gland mitoses
Gland mitoses indicate proliferation. They occur during menstruation because repair and breakdown are progressing simultaneously at that time.

Stromal mitoses
These are most abundant during the proliferative phase, absent during active secretion but reappear during the stage of predecidual formation.

Pseudostratification of nuclei
This is characteristic of the proliferative phase but persists until active secretion begins. It is not resumed until the glands have involuted during menstruation.

Basal vacuolation
This is the earliest morphological evidence of ovulation found in the endometrium. It begins approximately 36 to 48 hours following ovulation.

Secretion
This curve represents visible secretion in the gland lumen; active secretion falls off more abruptly. In the later stages the secretion becomes inspissated.

Predecidual reaction
This is evident first around the arterioles and progresses until just before menstruation a superficial compact layer is formed.

Leucocytic infiltration
Throughout the cycle there are always a few lymphocytes. Polymorphonuclear infiltration begins about two days before the onset of flow.

2 4 6 8 10 12 14 16 18 20 22 24 26 28

FIGURE 42–1 Sequential changes in the endometrium during the normal menstrual cycle. *(Courtesy of Dr. J.P.A. Latour.)*

cess usually began in one vessel and then developed in others, and the bleeding continued so long as there was arteriolar flow. As this process continued, numerous small hemorrhages became confluent, and the majority of the endometrial tissues disintegrated.

Myometrial and Vascular Responses

The main function of the smooth musculature which constitutes the uterine wall is to initiate and terminate parturition. The myometrial role in eliminating menstrual debris seems to be quite passive. If pathology exists in the endometrium, producing excessive bleeding, significant clots may develop which can provoke myometrial contractions in order to empty the cavity. During pregnancy the relatively simple blood supply and drainage of the myometrium undergo extensive structural modifications known as "vascular adaptation to pregnancy" (Ramsey). The stimulus for modification is increased uterine blood flow. Myometrial arteries dilate, become tortuous, and exhibit hyperplasia of the media as well as fibroblastic proliferation of the intima. The small-to-medium myometrial veins become distended to form small lakes, but the structure of their walls is not modified as much as those of the corresponding arteries. The blood vessels of the placental site develop from spiral arterioles which undergo incredible hypertrophy, and decidual transformation can extend to the intimal lining. Decidual veins become inordinately distended, and their walls become attenuated.

The physiology of uterine contractility and its pathophysiology are discussed in Chaps. 9 and 29. Important variables that regulate maintenance and termination of pregnancy have been and are being clarified. Maternal and fetal hormonal growth and intrauterine pressure relationships are involved. Such information has been useful in treating ineffectual labor. The data also constitute the base for examining the important problems of premature termination of pregnancy and prematurity.

DISORDERS OF THE ENDOMETRIUM

In the evaluation of disorders of the endometrium, the ability to easily obtain a tissue diagnosis by endometrial biopsy or dilatation and curettage is of inestimable value. Problems which may be related to hormonal imbalance, acute or chronic infection, retained products of conception, or the presence of a neoplasm can be diagnosed promptly and accurately.

VALUE OF DILATATION AND CURETTAGE, SUCTION CURETTAGE, AND ENDOMETRIAL BIOPSY

A sample of endometrial tissue can be obtained by biopsy, by dilatation and curettage, or by suction cu-

rettage. The latter is a simple procedure which often yields a good representative sample of tissue. Biopsy and suction curettage can be performed without anesthesia in the office or clinic as an ambulatory procedure. The only preparation necessary is to discuss the indication and procedure with the patient. She should be advised that she will have transient mild discomfort comparable to a menstrual cramp. Prior to the procedure an inquiry should be made as to the date and nature of the patient's last menses. Although an adequate specimen can often be obtained by biopsy curet or suction curettage, dilatation and curettage may be a hospital procedure requiring anesthesia in some instances. One advantage of the anesthesia is that pelvic relaxation is maximized, and a more satisfactory examination of pelvic organs can be made than in an office or clinic. The latter procedure is, diagnostic and often therapeutic.

The adequacy of estrogen priming of the endometrium may be evaluated by a biopsy during either the late proliferative phase (14 days after the last menstrual period) or by biopsy in the luteal phase. The diagnosis of an anovulatory cycle is suggested if mitotic activity and absence of anovulatory endometrial secretion are demonstrated in tissue obtained 23 or more days after the last menstrual period. The presence of a proliferative pattern alone, i.e., the presence of mitotic activity, is not sufficient to suggest that the ovarian follicle has failed to rupture. If mitotic activity is demonstrated without secretion, the inference is that the ovarian follicular phase is being prolonged; this should not be interpreted as evidence of anovulation. Full establishment of a justifiable diagnosis of anovulation requires an accurate clinical setting and appropriate endocrine testing. It has been shown that 92 percent of women studied had luteal phase endometrium by the 12th day preceding the next menses (Bergman, 1950). Duration of the luteal phase (postovulatory interval) usually remains constant around 14 days, plus or minus a day or two, where as the preovulatory or proliferative phase is much more variable (Hartman). Of interest is the observation that between 4 and 8 percent of women who menstruate with regularity may have anovulatory cycles. When endometrial biopsy was used in a group of college teachers and students to determine whether the patient ovulated, about 4 percent of the menstrual cycles were anovulatory; when the basal body temperature was used, 14 percent of the cycles were thought to be anovulatory. Anovulatory cycles occurred in a high percentage of instances during the 6 years following menarche and the 6 years preceding menopause.

The clinician may receive additional valuable data concerning a patient from a well-timed biopsy. The cumulative effects of estrogen alone or estrogen plus progesterone may best be evaluated by biopsy technique. Frequently, the reason for taking an endometrial biopsy, in addition to determining the presence or absence of ovulation, is to assess the action of estrogen and progesterone upon the development of glands and stroma. Quantitation of the glandular, stromal, and vascular responses and the correlation or lack of correlation of such responses to clinical problems are helpful in diagnosis and therapy. The optimum time for taking the endometrial biopsy is 12 to 14 days after presumed ovulation. Monitoring of basal body temperature is a valuable adjunct for timing the biopsy. The dip in the temperature curve may be used to estimate the time of ovulation. Should the basal body temperature be abnormal and the approximate time of ovulation unknown, it is then best to take the biopsy 20 to 28 days after the beginning of the last menstrual period. However, because the cycle may be either longer or shorter than 28 days, timing of the biopsy will not be optimum when this method is used. If the cycle is lengthened, there is a good possibility that the biopsy will be taken within the luteal phase and an estimate of both estrogen and progesterone effects may be determined.

A somewhat less-than-optimal time for taking the endometrial biopsy is at 5 to 6 days after presumed ovulation. This is just prior to the time of implantation of the blastocyst. A disadvantage of this timing is that the stromal predecidual reaction and arteriolar development are not present and may not be compared with the glandular changes. The advantage of a biopsy at this time is the elimination of the remote possibility of disturbing an implantation. There is no entirely safe time to obtain biopsy tissue unless the patient has used mechanical contraception, or has abstained from sexual intercourse during the cycle under study. Pathology which may be diagnosed during the proliferative phase includes chronic endometritis, neoplasia, adenomatous polyps, hyperplasia, or scar formation within the uterine cavity. These conditions may be detected during the late luteal phase as well. Tuberculosis of the endometrium may best be diagnosed during the late luteal phase when a relatively large amount of tissue is present and granulomas have had time to develop following previous sloughing.

Taking the biopsy at menses has been a popular practice because the possibility of interrupting a pregnancy is significantly decreased. It should be kept in mind that uterine bleeding or spotting simulating early menstrual bleeding may originate from a defect between the trophoblast and decidua. Spotting and superficial bleeding at the time of the first missed menstrual period are known as Hartman's placental sign.

Tissue taken in sufficient quantity from the body or fundus of the endometrium is quite representative of the remainder of the endometrial mucosa. However, a single specimen of endometrium removed by the biopsy curet from the anterior or posterior surface is representative of less than 1 percent of the total volume of endometrium. Therefore, in performing biopsy, many physicians perform multiple (three or four) strokes of the endometrial curet, involving both the anterior and posterior surfaces, in an attempt to sample three or four different locations of the endometrium.

Several additional factors may be responsible for inaccuracies in evaluating the endometrial biopsy. Submission of an endometrial biopsy to a pathologist requires that an adequate clinical history be supplied. A common error of endometrial biopsy evaluation can be made when the only tissue submitted is that obtained from the lower uterine segment. The endometrium from this area is significantly less responsive to hormonal stimulation than the tissue obtained from the corpus or fundus of the uterus. When only lower uterine segment fragments are present in the biopsy, it is best that the patient be rebiopsied and tissue obtained from the body of the uterus. An error in diagnosis can also occur when only tissue for the basal layer is present, and no representative tissue from the superficial layer of the corpus or fundus is in the specimen. This sampling difficulty commonly occurs following prolonged bleeding episodes when there is sloughing of the superficial layer. The basal layer in such circumstances shows a compact stroma and markedly tortuous glands. However, because the basal layer responds poorly to ovarian hormones, an accurate diagnosis cannot be made. A lesion which is microscopic and focal may be missed by the biopsy curet.

ENDOGENOUS HORMONAL RESPONSES

During the normal menstrual cycle the quantities and duration of action of the circulating ovarian hormones are reflected in the endometrium. In abnormal states, the endometrium responds to both the absolute amount of either estrogen and progesterone secreted and the ratio of these hormones to each other.

Three major patterns of endometrial development result from the presence or absence of ovarian steroids. A lack of estrogenic stimulation results in an atrophic endometrium. This type of endometrium is characteristic of the postmenopausal patient. Stimulation by estrogen alone results in proliferative changes which may result in a simple polyp or progress to simple cystic, or complex adenomatous hyperplasia, if estrogen stimulation is unopposed for several months to years. These morphologic changes depend upon the duration of stimulation, the biological activity of the estrogen molecules, and the threshold of tissue response. Sequential stimulation first by estrogen and later by progesterone synergistically produces a normal morphologic endometrial pattern if the amounts of available estrogen and progesterone correspond to those of the normal cycle and if the proper timing of progesterone stimulation is superimposed upon the estrogen-primed endometrium. Abnormalities in estrogen and progesterone secretion have been labeled inadequate luteal phase, inadequate secretory phase of the endometrium, secretory hypoplasia of endometrium, or underdeveloped endometrium. It is thought that progesterone neutralizes or eliminates an inhibitor of the normal glandular secretory processes. Progesterone also exerts a direct effect upon stromal cells producing, at first, edema which is then followed by a predecidual cellular response and accompanying vascular changes, especially proliferation of spiral arterioles.

Atypical secretory endometrium and endometrium out of phase with the luteinizing-hormone (LH) peak or presumed time of ovulation have been described (Strott et al.). In the experimental animal, it has been demonstrated that the effects of estrogen and progesterone are synergistic only when related to each other by a well-defined dose ratio. When this ratio is changed, the effect of each of the ovarian hormones is antagonized (Forbes). The characteristics of steroid antagonism have been previously summarized (Lerner). Inadequate luteal phase defect appears to be a syndrome consisting of an aberration in the estrogen-progesterone relationship and is not a specific deficiency of progesterone. In primates, the endometrial changes were shown to be dependent on the ratio of progesterone to estrogen as well as the absolute amounts of each hormone (Good, Moyer) (Fig. 42–2).

THE HYPERPLASIA PROBLEM

Estrogen stimulation, endogenous or exogenous, results in endometrial proliferation. If the stimulus is

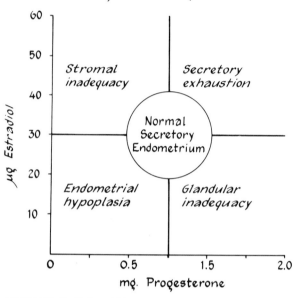

FIGURE 42–2 Endometrial secretory response to estrogen and progesterone. Normal secretory endometrium is produced when approximately 1 mg of progesterone is injected per day following a 2-week estrogen priming of 20 to 40 mg of estradiol per day. When both the estrogen and progesterone are less than these levels, the endometrium shows glandular and stromal hypoplasia. In those cases where the endometrium is primed with normal to high amounts of estrogen and the amount of progesterone is deficient, there is an adequate stromal maturation. When progesterone is present in normal to high quantities and follows a lower-than-normal amount of estrogen, the glands are inadequate although the stroma is well developed. When both estrogen and progesterone are present in higher-than-normal quantities, the stroma shows good maturation, and the glands show exhaustion of the secretory process. *(From Good, Moyer.)*

sustained and uninhibited, focal or diffuse hyperplasia may follow. Hyperplasia can thicken the entire mucosa or be intense at a focal site. Single polyps may be formed in the mucosa, or may assume a diffuse polypoid appearance. The induced hyperplasia produces only inconspicuous changes in the nonresponsive endocervix and cornifies the squamous epithelium of the exocervix. The common source of exogenous estrogen is prescribed medication, usually a nonsteroidal estrogen. But estrogen-enriched cosmetic creams, vaginal suppositories, and even digitalis preparations can and do produce endometrial hyperplasia. Sources for increased noncyclic production of estrogen include certain ovarian and adrenal tumors and altered pathways of steroid metabolism in certain anovulatory syndromes. Focal functional hyperplasias are seen in other receptor-tissue responses, specifically the breast and thyroid. Hyperadrenocorticism has on rare occasion also produced a hyperplastic endometrium.

ENDOMETRIAL POLYPS

The endometrium can be the site of localized hyperplasia without any apparent relation to a hormonal disturbance. If an excrescence occurs which progressively becomes sessile or pedunculated, that may then be called a polyp. The structure of these small benign tumors is simple. In general, polyps are not hormonally responsive and present a simple proliferative type of endometrium. Many benign polyps have a fibrous core in which thick-walled blood vessels are prominent. Bleeding, when it occurs, is usually from the infarcted tip of such polyps. Occasionally there is evidence of response to progesterone, and patches of both proliferative and secretory changes may be observed.

CYSTIC HYPERPLASIA

Cystic hyperplasia is the simplest pattern of the endometrial hyperplasias. It is most commonly seen at the two extremes of the childbearing ages but may occur at any age. During the postmenopausal years exogenous estrogen is the most common cause of cystic hyperplasia. The previously mentioned endocrine-secreting ovarian pathology may also be involved. When ovulation is uncertain and intermittent in either the postmenarchal or premenopausal patient, endogenous estrogen production without a balanced increment of essential progesterone may affect all the glandular, stromal, vascular, and superficial epithelial elements of the endometrium. Under such circumstances, the glands show marked pseudostratification and tortuosity in a nonuniform pattern. Some glands become cystic as a result of obstruction of their gland necks and the lack of elimination of secretory products. The irregularly enlarged cystic glands are lined by either tall cuboidal or columnar cells, which often exhibit less mitotic activity than the term hyperplasia suggests (Fig. 42–3).

COMPLEX ENDOMETRIAL HYPERPLASIAS

Comparable to the morphologic spectrum between anovulation and the milder forms of hyperplasia, a spectrum exists from hyperplasia to atypical hyperplasia (also known as adenomatous hyperplasia; see Fig. 42–4) to neoplasia. The concept of dysplasia of other epithelia involves an increase in cell numbers accompanied by qualitative atypia of cell character-

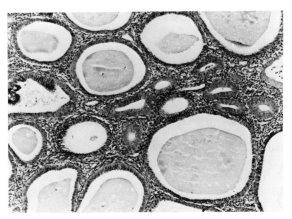

FIGURE 42–3 In cystic endometrial hyperplasia the glands are spherically dilated to varying degrees and lined by close-packed cells. H & E ×156.

istics resulting in a disturbed growth pattern. In an unspecified percentage of patients, this pattern may eventuate in neoplasia. The evidence is that, in any single patient, sequential progression through the various morphologic changes need not necessarily occur. Furthermore, it is impossible, at the present time, to predict prospectively whether a patient with a complex hyperplasia will develop a biologically aggressive tumor. Similar terminology has been applied to the squamous epithelium of the cervix, and such terms as atypia, dyskeratosis, and carcinoma in situ are familiar. Endometrial dysplasia is the term employed by some to describe disturbing degrees of atypia without committing themselves as to whether an autonomous and clinically significant tumor exists.

FIGURE 42–4 Endometrial carcinoma in situ. Glands are closely packed with some multilayered palisading of the epithelium and an alteration in cytoplasmic staining reaction. H & E ×156.

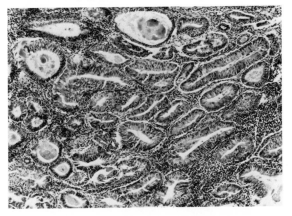

In some instances, adenocarcinoma in situ is used interchangeably to describe the most severe degrees of endometrial hyperplasia. It should be recognized that in many patients dysplastic changes have proved reversible.

The diagnosis of complex endometrial hyperplasia is made by microscopical examination of curettings and is based on such criteria as (1) excessive stratification of glandular epithelium; (2) budding, tufting, or epithelial bridging in individual glands; (3) the presence of epithelial cells with abundant eosinophilic cytoplasm (similar to oncocytes in other organs); and (4) the so-called "back to back" glandular pattern representing excessive glandular coiling and glandular crowding, and with compression and displacement of stroma.

Clinical Significance

The inability of pathologists to clarify the complex spectrum of histologic changes and their eventualities is the basis for the difficulties in treating patients with such lesions. The present state of the art is still based on Halban's doctrine of "Nicht Karzinom, aber besser heraus." This doctrine dates back to the 1920s and it is apparent that not much progress has been made since then. In practice this means that generally when a diagnosis of complex endometrial hyperplasia or its equivalent is established, it is reasonably sensible to remove the uterus.

Hysterectomy may be justified in women whose families are complete or in postmenopausal women, but this is not universally agreed. However, in younger women a single curettage may be curative as well as diagnostic. As a general rule, over 75 percent of women with microscopically diagnosed endometrial hyperplasia will have no further bleeding and will require no further treatment. It has been estimated that a woman with simple or cystic glandular hyperplasia has about a 2 percent chance of later developing endometrial adenocarcinoma, but a woman with so-called atypical adenomatous hyperplasia has about a 10 to 12 percent chance of developing endometrial adenocarcinoma. These figures do not take into account those cases in which the transformation from atypical to neoplastic glandular patterns can be interrupted and reversed by exogenous synthetic progestagens or antiestrogenic clomiphene citrate administration. It has been shown that women with persistent episodes of abnormal bleeding often progress through the complex hyperplasias to superficial and invasive adenocarcinoma. Although these studies are retrospective and do not necessarily reflect the usual mode of endometrial carcinogenesis, the value of the observations is that such sequences or progressive changes do occur in a small but significant number of women (Gusberg, Kaplan).

ENDOMETRIAL RESPONSES TO INFECTIOUS AGENTS AND FOREIGN BODIES

ACUTE ENDOMETRITIS

Infectious agents may enter the endometrial cavity by several routes. Bacteria, if present in sufficient numbers in the endometrial fluid and tissues, will cause an inflammatory cell reaction. The most common entry of bacteria is by instrumentation. Such operative procedures as the insertion of an intrauterine device, biopsy curet, or irrigation catheter potentially produce contamination. Tubal insufflation procedures or the insertion of gauze or radium into the uterine cavity may also introduce cervical mucus. Whenever the protective role and defense mechanisms of the cervical secretions are altered or destroyed, bacteria present in the vaginal and lower cervical secretions will enter the endometrial cavity. Procedures such as conization or cauterization of the cervix may temporarily eliminate the secretion of cervical mucus essential for protection against ascending nonpathogenic bacteria. Although cervical mucus normally protects against the migration of those organisms which constitute the vaginal flora, pathogens such as gonococci have the ability to overcome the usual bacteriostatic mechanisms of cervical mucus. When gonococci are present in cervical mucus, they can migrate to the endometrial cavity and thus gain entrance into the fallopian tubes, peritoneal cavity, and parametrium.

Under normal conditions, transient bacterial invaders are killed rapidly in the intrauterine cavity. However, when the bacteriostatic environment of the endometrium is altered, small numbers of nonpathogenic bacteria may multiply and produce a clinically symptomatic endometritis. This occurs most commonly after parturition when the endometrium is thin and quiescent. At that time, the tissues are not stimulated by estrogen, and there are additional alterations in the nature of uterine fluid secretion and the phagocytic system.

Bacteria may gain entrance to the endometrial cavity from the bloodstream or from drainage from a chronically infected fallopian tube. Patients with the latter condition may have constant leakage of purulent material into the endometrial cavity, which can result in severe inflammatory changes.

The infection of the uterine cavity from contaminated cervical mucus is usually short-lived. The most common bacteria found in cervical mucus are staphylococci, streptococci, diphtheroids, and the coliforms, including *Escherichia coli, Alcaligenes fecalis,* and *Pseudomonas.* A uterine infection may result from one or several organisms; a mixed infection can usually be identified several hours after the insertion of a foreign object.

A foreign object placed in the uterine cavity will produce a positive culture during the first 24 hours after insertion. Thereafter, the viable organisms are quickly eliminated in the majority of patients as the result of bactericidal substances found in the uterine secretions (Fig. 42–5). During the period from 24 hours to 7 days following the insertion of a foreign object, 80 percent of patients studied had negative endometrial cultures. By 45 days after insertion of a foreign body, all patients in this study had eliminated viable bacteria from the uterine cavity, and all endometrial cultures were negative (Mishell et al.).

The endometrial response following the introduction of a foreign body and cervical mucus bacteria is similar to the inflammatory responses in other tissues of the body (Moyer et al., 1970). During the first few hours, tissue edema occurs, followed by an influx of polymorphonuclear leukocytes. Several days after insertion, mononuclear cells, including macrophages and lymphocytes, migrate into the tissues although polymorphonuclear leukocytes remain the predominant inflammatory cell. Plasma cells mobilize in response to the bacterial products toward the end of the first week and usually persist for several months. In some patients histiocytes may remain as long as 5 or 6 months after the transient endometritis has been eliminated. The persistence of the imflammatory cells in the endometrium through several menstrual cycles is not surprising in view of the fact that the entire endometrium is not totally shed in each cycle. Even relatively inert polyethylene foreign bodies can elicit a low-grade chronic inflammatory response, and the longer the foreign body remains in loco, the greater will be the proportion of women with endometritis (Ober and Grady).

An intrauterine device produces an outpouring of uterine fluids and an increased migration of acute and chronic inflammatory cells into the tissues and uterine cavity (Moyer et al., 1972). Spermatozoa must be considered foreign bodies in the female genital tract since their protein composition differs from the maternal tissue (Moyer et al., 1970a). Phagocytosis of spermatozoa by polymorphonuclear and mononuclear cells is now a well-recognized entity. The normal defense mechanisms of the uterine cavity may be modified by the action of a sterile foreign body within the uterus as well as the presence or absence of ovarian hormones.

DIAGNOSIS AND TREATMENT

The presence of vaginal discharge, mucopurulent or purulent in nature, coming from the external cervical os, associated with crampy, lower abdominal pain and tenderness, as well as a febrile response constitutes the criterion for making a diagnosis of acute endometritis. In most instances, following simple operative procedures such as dilatation and curettage, cauterization, conization, insertion of an IUD or radium, the inflammatory response is minimal. In the event of a mild infection, establishing drainage in the endocervical canal in most instances controls the infection.

Should a severe or more virulent infection occur, the uterus on bimanual examination may be boggy and tender and there may be evidence of localized peritoneal irritation expressed by abdominal muscle spasm or rebound phenomenon. In the case of severe acute endometritis, the specific microorganism causing the infection should be identified by stain and culture. This should involve both aerobic and anaerobic culture. Establishing adequate drainage is the first

FIGURE 42–5 Relation of incidence of positive endometrial cultures to the duration of insertion of an IUD. During the first 24 hours after insertion, all the endometrial cultures were negative. From 24 hours to 7 days, 20 percent of the endometrial cultures were positive, and the remainder showed no growth of bacteria. From 7 to 45 days, 12 percent of the cultures were positive, and the remainder showed no growth. Cultures taken after 45 days showed no growth of bacteria. *(From Mishell et al.)*

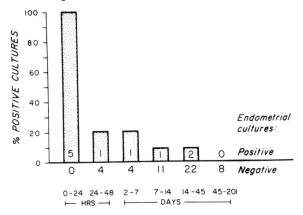

principle of therapy. Selection and implementation of an appropriate antibiotic regimen should be instituted as necessary. Severe staphylococcal infections should be treated for at least 6 weeks since they tend to persist and recur. Gram-negative bacilli are frequent contaminants in severe infection and require special attention. Should the infection persist and the tissue become more edematous and possibly necrotic, *Proteus* organisms and *Bacteroides* species may be secondary pathogens (see Chap. 11).

ENDOMETRIAL RESPONSE TO CONTRACEPTIVE STEROIDS

When synthetic progestagen-estrogen preparations are given to normal, cyclically ovulating, regularly menstruating females for contraceptive purposes, pituitary-gonadotropin secretion is inhibited, ovulation suppressed, and the endometrium responds in characteristic patterns. Endometrial morphology varies with dose and route of administration.

The commonest form of medication is the combined "pill" which is generally taken daily for 20 days starting on the fifth day of a cycle. Biopsies taken after 5 days of medication, i.e., on the tenth day of the cycle, show subnuclear secretory vacuoles in endometrial glands. This is an example of induced precocious secretion associated with estrogen priming and concomitant progestagen stimulation. The pattern of day 10 of such a cycle resembles that seen normally on day 16 or 17 of a nonmedicated cycle. As medication is continued, glandular secretion regresses, and the glands are exhausted by day 20 of the cycle. Depending on the amount of progestagen in the "pill," predecidual transformation of the stroma may or may not develop. If there is no predecidual response, the stroma appears loose, the nuclei naked and inert. In general, with combined cyclic regimens, the elongation and tortuosity of spiral arterioles are inhibited. Dilatation of venules seems to be related to the amount of estrogen in the preparation and the individual woman's sensitivity to it. When present, these irregular, dilated channels are prone to thrombosis, possibly because blood flow through them is slow. Such small thrombi in peripheral venules may produce local tissue infarction, accompanied by necrosis and sloughing, thereby yielding the clinical phenomenon known as "breakthrough bleeding." The mechanism is similar to that seen in estrogen-induced endometrial hyperplasia.

Biopsy of the endometrium at the end of the 20-day medication cycle reveals endometrial glands of small-caliber, tubular contour, showing no mitotic or secretory activity. They quite properly have been characterized as hyperinvoluted. In such biopsies on day 24 or 25 of the cycle, spiral arterioles are not seen as developed structures in the superficial third of the mucosa, though they may be detected in the resting phase, undeveloped, in deeper layers.

If combined progestagen-estrogen medication is given orally without cyclic interruption and in stepwise increments, as in the treatment of pelvic endometriosis, the effect on endometrial morphology is exaggerated. After 2 or 3 months the endometrial glands are small, often slitlike, and are lined by a low epithelium which is inactive. An intense pseudodecidual reaction is present diffusely in the stroma, almost indistinguishable from the decidua seen in early pregnancy. Spiral arterioles are almost entirely absent. Similar changes are seen in the epithelium and stroma of the "implants" or ectopic foci of endometrial tissue in the ovaries and pelvic soft tissue.

If continuous administration of synthetic progestagen is given at low dosage, 1 mg daily or less, as in attempts to control menopausal symptoms, the endometrium is seen as a thinned mucosa composed of small hyperinvoluted glands lined by low, inert epithelium, and there is a diffuse pseudodecidual reaction in the stroma. Spiral arterioles are inconspicuous. It takes 2 to 3 months of such a regimen to produce this alteration of endometrial morphology.

When synthetic progestagen is injected intramuscularly in therapeutic dosage for prolonged effects, the mucosa becomes thin and attenuated. Histopathologic examination of biopsies and hysterectomy specimens shows an atrophic endometrium with small, slitlike, inert glands, no vascular development, and a pseudodecidual reaction of low intensity, albeit rather diffuse.

When steroid medication is discontinued, recovery patterns may be irregular. Return to normal patterns usually requires two to three cycles after oral contraceptive steroids have been stopped, but the interval is usually prolonged and unpredictable after injectable steroids have been given. Patients with "postpill amenorrhea" also exhibit irregular patterns after steroid administration has been discontinued. Presumably, such patterns reflect incomplete return of normal hypothalamic-pituitary-gonadotropin-ovarian steroid cyclic secretion. A question which must be considered is whether many of such patients did not have abnormal pituitary-ovarian endocrine relationships before the medication was prescribed.

ENDOMETRIAL RESPONSE TO PREGNANCY (ARIAS-STELLA REACTION)

The response of the endometrium to both intrauterine and ectopic pregnancy may be utilized for diagnostic purposes. Both glandular and stromal elements respond to the secretions of the corpus luteum and trophoblast following implantation. When implantation of the blastocyst occurs, a gradual transition of luteal phase endometrium develops into a gestational endometrium. As pregnancy continues, a gradual transformation to the decidua vera of pregnancy takes place.

When the endometrium is stimulated by the impinging blastocyst, preimplantation endometrial changes do not regress but undergo further growth. The simultaneous growth of glands and stroma under the influence of estrogen and progesterone has been termed "gestational hyperplasia." As this growth occurs, the stromal cells are transformed into large polygonal decidual cells containing spherical and vesicular nuclei and an intensely eosinophilic cytoplasm. In those areas where the nuclei are markedly enlarged, with variation in size and hyperchromatic staining, the endometrial change is known as the Arias-Stella reaction (AS reaction).

The intensity of the endometrial changes produced by chorionic tissue does not appear to be related to the site of blastocyst implantation. The reaction may occur in isolated areas of the endometrium or may be widespread. When such changes are present, the endometrial glands and superficial epithelium are affected, and the intensity of the reaction may vary considerably. At times parallel changes may also be seen in the endocervical epithelium and in adenomyosis.

The incidence of these changes occurring during an ectopic pregnancy is important (Arias-Stella). In the series reported, 22 of 44 patients with an ectopic pregnancy had the AS reaction. If decidual changes and an AS reaction are seen without chorionic villi, the possibility of ectopic pregnancy must be seriously considered as well as intrauterine pregnancy.

Atypical endometrial changes have also been described in patients with either hydatidiform mole or choriocarcinoma. Large amounts of hormone from trophoblast and from luteinized ovarian tissue produce the same changes in the endometrium as those seen in an intrauterine or ectopic pregnancy. In a small number of patients receiving high doses of a synthetic progestational agent, atypical stromal decidual changes may be seen. In these patients, glandular components are not seen in the areas of atypism. It is the stroma that shows the atypical changes; this entity should not be confused with the AS reaction.

TUBERCULOSIS OF THE ENDOMETRIUM (see Chap. 44)

Tuberculosis of the endometrium is almost always secondary to or associated with tuberculosis of the fallopian tube. The disease is relatively uncommon in the United States. In India, 7.9 percent of women had the diagnosis made when studied in an infertility clinic (Malkani and Rajani), and in Israel, 5.3 percent of sterile women had endometrial tuberculosis (Sharman). Unsuspected endometrial tuberculosis in a group of women in Scotland was found to be slightly more than 5 percent (Sutherland). In 15 years of experience in Los Angeles, the prevalence of suspected and unsuspected endometrial tuberculosis was low. This included patients of different social and economic backgrounds attending public and private clinics for infertility and dysfunctional uterine bleeding. No more than two or three patients with endometrial tuberculosis are screened each year out of approximately a thousand endometrial biopsies. In those areas where pulmonary and gastrointestinal tuberculosis is high, the prevalence of endometrial disease is also high.

Diagnosis

The traditional methods of diagnosing endometrial tuberculosis are the use of endometrial biopsy and specific culture techniques for acid-fast organisms. Endometrial tissue containing noncaseating granulomas and destruction of the glands and stroma are highly suggestive of tuberculosis. Culture of the organisms gives definite proof of their presence. The endometrial tissue (usually menstrual tissue) is cultured on either Petragnani's or Dubos's medium which is selected for the specific growth of the acid-fast organisms, with inhibition of other nonspecific organisms. Inoculation of guinea pigs with menstrual blood may be used when other culture techniques fail to demonstrate organisms. The use of late luteal phase endometrium is also recommended both for culture and histologic examination because, given a cyclically menstruating patient, it takes over 3 weeks for visible granulomas to form and for sufficient multiplication of tubercle bacilli to make detection by culture feasible.

Both histologic examination of the endometrium

and culture for acid-fast bacilli should be used in patients suspected of having tuberculosis of the endometrium. The histologic diagnosis of endometrial tuberculosis was made in 90 percent of patients; the remaining 10 percent had only a positive culture but no tissue reaction (Govan). Not all patients with endometrial tuberculosis show histologic changes in the tissue. In another report, 722 endometrial specimens were positive for acid-fast organisms in culture. However, two patients had positive cultures and did not show evidence of histologic disease in the endometrium even though all the endometrial tissue was sectioned (Israel et al.).

In tuberculosis of the endometrium, the presence of caseation in the granulomas is not usually seen because of the periodic shedding of the endometrium. If menstruation occurs, calcification and fibrosis of the endometrium are rarely seen. The presence of multiple noncaseating granulomas is the typical histologic appearance of endometrial tuberculosis. These granulomas include Langhans' giant cells, epithelioid cells, and perifollicular lymphocytes. Plasma cells are rarely found among the lymphocytes in the granulomatous follicles, and acid-fast organisms are rarely detected in multiple sections of the endometrium. This is usually attributed to lack of caseated material where the majority of organisms are found. When the presence of a purulent exudate is found in the endometrial glands without noncaseating granulomas, the patient should be studied by culture techniques to rule out the presence of acid-fast organisms.

Treatment

The therapy for tuberculous endometritis is the same as that for pulmonary or renal tuberculosis. The disease should be controlled by appropriate chemotherapy for a period of stability extending over a period of 1 year. If stability is not achieved, relapse and recurrence frequently occur. Isoniazid is the mainstay of drug therapy and should be given with either ethambutol or rifampin (see Chap. 44).

ENDOMETRIAL RESPONSE TO TRAUMA (FRITSCH-ASHERMAN SYNDROME)

The presence of intrauterine adhesions was described almost 100 years ago in Germany when Fritsch described the syndrome of intrauterine adhesions and infertility. Approximately half a century later, 29 patients with traumatic amenorrhea were reported in the English literature (Asherman). Other synonyms for the Fritsch-Asherman syndrome include amenorrhea traumatica (atretica), intrauterine synechiae, endometrial sclerosis, traumatic intrauterine adhesions, or synechial postcurettage atresia of the endometrial cavity, the Asherman syndrome, and the Fritsch syndrome. The term "intrauterine adhesions" accurately describes the histopathology and the radiologic findings.

Clinically the syndrome may include infertility, amenorrhea and other menstrual abnormalities, or habitual abortion. The endometrial walls are either partially or completely adherent to each other following the formation of adhesions. As the cavity becomes reduced in size, the probability of a full-term pregnancy is lessened. If implantation of an embryo occurs, complications such as abortion, malpresentation, placenta accreta, or premature delivery may occur in the presence of the intrauterine adhesions.

Intrauterine adhesions result from traumatization of the endometrium and myometrium at a time when the tissues are susceptible to adhesion formation. A high rate of complications has been demonstrated when curettage is performed during the third or fourth postpartum week. Whenever a foreign instrument is inserted into the uterine cavity, bacteria are introduced; when combined with puerperal or postabortal curettage, these conditions provide an excellent medium for the development of adhesions. Adhesions have been described following the removal of hydatidiform moles and as the end result of endometrial tuberculosis. Enucleation of myomas and hysterotomies has also led to intrauterine adhesions. Caustic solutions produce chemical trauma when instilled into the uterus as abortifacients and have caused adhesions. The incidence of serious adhesions following a dilatation and curettage is relatively low, although adhesions have been described following such a procedure.

Menstrual irregularities combined with infertility are the most frequently reported symptoms. Adhesions in the lower uterine segment may cause complete obstruction to the flow of menstrual fluid. Complete adherence of the anterior and posterior walls of the uterus may produce the same end result. Partial adhesions of the uterine cavity may be responsible for a decrease in the amount of menstrual flow as well as infertility. Adhesions may mechanically obstruct the implantation of the blastocyst. When a pregnancy occurs, approximately one-third will end in abortion and another third will result in premature deliveries. Complications such as placenta accreta, placenta previa, and ectopic pregnancies have been described.

Diagnosis

A diagnosis of uterine adhesions may not be simple unless the entire cavity is obliterated or unless the clinician has a high degree of suspicion for this entity. If it is suspected, hysteroscopy is the most useful diagnostic tool. The detection of adhesions and the evaluation of their extent may be accurately made by the hysteroscope. Hysterography is the most commonly used diagnostic procedure. It is important that the procedure be performed by an experienced radiologist in order to eliminate artifacts. The adhesions may be either single or multiple and may be of variable size located anywhere within the uterine cavity. The diagnosis is suggested in patients in whom there is difficulty in sounding the endometrium or when the biopsy instrument encounters a gritty area. Histologically, the adhesions may be large areas of fibrous tissue or may include varying amounts of endometrial stroma surrounded by superficial epithelial cells. On rare occasions, the adhesions contain multiple calcific bodies. Uterine muscle may be found within the adhesions. Inflammatory cells, such as plasma cells, lymphocytes, and leukocytes, may be present. The prognosis of the syndrome usually varies with the severity of the disease. In one report, of the 57 patients studied, less than a third became pregnant, and there were only 10 living births (Bergman, 1961).

Treatment

Treatment consists of dilatation of the internal os of the cervix and the insertion of one or two intrauterine device(s) into the endometrial cavity. At the time of the dilatation, every effort should be made to eliminate synechiae which may exist. If pregnancy is desired, the patient should be advised to complete several menstrual cycles prior to attempting to conceive. Exogenous estrogen therapy has been employed by some. However, it does not appear to have a role in this entity inasmuch as endogenous hormone production is not impaired.

ATROPHIC ENDOMETRIUM

During those periods of life when the ovaries presumably produce little estrogen and no progesterone, the endometrium shows no evidence of proliferation of glands or stroma. In atrophic endometrium, the glands are composed of a single layer of quiescent cells which are devoid of mitoses and show minimal evidence of metabolic activity. The lumina are narrow and the glands lack tortuosity. The stroma is compact and composed of small, inactive spindle cells. There is a loose reticular network with edematous spaces between the cellular components.

Complete atrophy of the endometrium is commonly seen in the late postmenopausal or senescent female patient. In some patients with ovarian agenesis, there may be rare acystic follicles, and in these patients, the endometrium is atrophic. Pituitary dysfunction characterized by a deficiency of gonadotropins may result in several clinical syndromes, which are associated with either an atrophic endometrium or a proliferative pattern showing minimal growth (see Chap. 27). Simmonds' syndrome includes panhypopituitarism resulting from calcification, cystic degeneration, fibrosis of the pituitary gland, or a benign or malignant neoplasm. In both Chiari-Frommel syndrome and Sheehan's syndrome, there is gonadal failure. Lactation persists in the Chiari-Frommel syndrome and in this as well as other syndromes in which galactorrhea is a factor, many of the patients have elevated serum levels of prolactin, often from microadenomas in the adenohypophysis. Whether these lesions are true adenomas is not certain, but the endocrine effects rest on firm clinical and chemical ground. Not associated with parturition is the Argonez–del Castillo syndrome which results in infertility, amenorrhea, and lactation. Approximately 10 percent of the patients with pituitary dysfunction have endometrium which is atrophic. The remaining patients have a proliferative endometrium which borders on an atrophic endometrium showing only rudimentary growth.

ADENOCARCINOMA OF THE ENDOMETRIUM

An alarming increase in the incidence of endometrial carcinoma is being reported. The lesion is now more frequent than squamous carcinoma of the cervix. Whether this is in part because women are living longer and obtaining routine pelvic examination is conjectural. The fact that this carcinoma is being diagnosed with greater frequency is indicative of the usefulness of biopsy, cytology, and pelvic examination. The identification of cases of endometrial carcinoma is also a by-product of the effort to screen women with cytology against cervical neoplasms. In previous years, numbers of women never received the benefit of cytologic screening and pelvic examination. Still another consideration is greater physician awareness that postmenopausal bleeding is presumptively carcinoma until proved otherwise. Postmenopausal bleeding, by definition, constitutes any bleeding which occurs after menses have ceased for a period of 1 year.

It should also be mentioned that the apparent increased incidence of the tumor may reflect the concern that a spectrum of endometrial hyperplastic changes may be precursors of malignant states. This latter frame of reference may be responsible for a more aggressive approach by the gynecologist and the interpretation of endometrial lesions by the pathologist. It may be that some of the cases now being diagnosed as carcinoma reflect the pathologist's (and the gynecologist's) thinking that a malignancy cannot be overlooked or overdiagnosed. Thus the possibility that the neoplasm may be overdiagnosed is a reality that must be accepted until the histopathologic criteria and the biologic activity of premalignant and in situ carcinoma are better defined.

INCIDENCE

Carcinoma of the endometrium constitutes approximately 7 percent of all cancers in women. The reported yearly incidence of the disease is 20 per 100,000 women. It is unfortunate that in some institutions the distinction between carcinoma of the cervix and of the endometrium is not always clarified, and some of the reporting has been confused because hospital records simply note cancer of the uterus. Adenocarcinoma in situ and atypical hyperplastic lesions of the endometrium are not reportable diseases. The true incidence of the lesion is not accurately known.

AGE

Endometrial carcinoma is predominantly a postmenopausal lesion. Eighty-four percent of patients having the disease are at least 50 years of age or older. The mean age at detection is about 58 years. Carcinoma in situ of the endometrium is clinically seen at an average of 48 or 49 years, some 10 years before the average age when the peak incidence of the invasive stage is seen. In younger women, below 35 years of age, endometrial cancer has been observed in association with a number of ovarian disorders. Bona fide carcinoma has been detected in this group between 19 and 35 years of age (Sommers et al.). Approxi-

mately 0.4 percent of corpus carcinomas are in women less than 30 years of age (Christophersen et al.; Dockerty et al.). The age range extends from 16 to 88 years, with the average being 57 to 59 years of age (Hertig, Sommers).

ASSOCIATED DISEASES AND EPIDEMIOLOGY

There is a considerable body of literature which associates the triad of obesity, hypertension, and disturbed glucose tolerance (diabetes mellitus) with endometrial carcinoma. Arteriosclerotic heart disease and arthritis are also commonly cited as associated diseases, and an implied pathologic relationship to ovarian stromal hyperplasia and fibrocystic disease of the breast has also been reported. Most of these reports are poorly documented, anecdotal, and uncontrolled. There are no reliable figures on how many women in the age group over 55 are obese, hypertensive, etc., so that suitable controls are lacking. All the conditions cited are common so that the coincidence rate would be an appreciable one. The questions remain unanswered and the problems unresolved. Endometrial carcinoma is seen predominantly in middle-class groups. The women are frequently single or if married may have had difficulty in becoming pregnant. The best-controlled epidemiologic study (Wynder, 1966) found that only obesity was significantly correlated with endometrial cancer.

The associated ovarian pathology includes polycystic ovaries, sclerocystic ovaries, and ovarian thecomatosis. Patients with polycystic ovaries, obesity, and hirsutism, called the Stein-Leventhal syndrome, may be troublesome because many show progressively more severe endometrial atypia and hyperplasia from age 16 on. Such estrogenizing ovarian neoplasms as thecomas, granulosa-cell tumors, and occasionally cystadenofibromas have been reported in patients with endometrial carcinoma (Greene).

NATURAL HISTORY

Endometrial carcinoma is thought to be a slowgrowing neoplasm which usually develops over a relatively long period of time. It is sometimes characterized by precursor premalignant stages and ultimately a definite invasive lesion. The spectrum of atypical hyperplastic changes which constitutes the precursor abnormalities may or may not be seen in any given patient. Unfortunately, much of the data reflects retrospective analysis, and the current dilemma is that it is difficult to justify a prospective protocol in view of the stigmata associated with specific histologic lesions.

Despite the current emphasis on the histopathology of "precursors" of endometrial cancer, about 90 percent of such tumors seem to arise in an atrophic endometrium.

There is little evidence to implicate a virus as a primary etiologic factor responsible for malignant transformation and the development of endometrial cancer. It is more likely that carcinoma of the endometrium is triggered by a series of metabolic abnormalities associated with impaired glucose metabolism and pituitary hyperactivity superimposed upon a background of prolonged estrogen stimulation (Benjamin et al.). Conceivably the endometrial cell cannot function in the milieu developed by the metabolic abnormality. Prolonged sustained estrogen stimulation has been incriminated as a major factor in the development of endometrial carcinoma. However, estrogen values in urine or serum have been measured in only a few small series and the results are inconsistent. Studies of protein binding and estrogen receptor sites of hormonally sensitive cells are needed (Terenius et al.). Sustained estrogen stimulation is inhibited by progesterone, and progesterone is essential to the completion of the cell cycle. However, clarification of the role of progesterone in the differentiation of the endometrial cell is needed, and the estrogen-progesterone etiologic relationships, although circumstantial, are not established. Estrogen per se is not a carcinogen. In small doses, the steroid stimulates growth whereas in large doses, inhibition of cell growth occurs. Chromosomal studies have failed to reveal any karyotype which can be consistently identified with in situ or invasive endometrial carcinoma. Diploid and triploid cell lines and aneuploidy have been reported (Tseng and Jones). The recently developed "estrone hypothesis" argues that increased peripheral conversion of androstenedione to estrone, especially in fat depots, favors endometrial carcinogenesis. This hypothesis correlates well with the epidemiologic role of obesity, but it does not account for endometrial carcinoma in thin women, nor ought it be accepted as the only pathway for endocrine carcinogenesis.

The diagnosis of adenocarcinoma in situ of the endometrium is difficult and controversial. If diagnosed, the lesion average may be expected to progress irreversibly to invasive carcinoma, but it does so slowly and the patient may be carefully followed. One patient so diagnosed from curettings was followed through two successful pregnancies (Hertig et al.).

In complex hyperplasias, progression to carcinoma probably occurs in no more than 10 to 12 percent of the cases. Unfortunately, strict criteria for identifying benign hyperplasias and delineating such lesions from malignant transformation are not available. The diagnosis may depend upon subjective interpretation of histopathologic material which may not be specific and may be characterized unsatisfactorily as an atypia. For the patient and her physician, a nonspecific diagnosis confuses the therapy. However, the endometrium of some women so diagnosed has reverted to a normal pattern following treatment with long-acting progestagens.

In the early stages of endometrial carcinoma, enlargement of the corpus uteri is not a usual finding. The frequent association with leiomyomata has been previously mentioned and should be borne in mind when a distorted uterus is detected on pelvic examination. The corpus tumor generally grows slowly as an exophytic lesion along the endometrial surface and in about 60 percent of cases shows superficial encroachment on endometrial stroma. In some 25 percent of patients, infiltration of the inner half of the myometrium exists when the tumor is diagnosed; in about 10 percent of cases, deep penetration of the outer myometrium has occurred. In approximately 5 percent of patients, extrauterine extension exists when the patient is first seen.

Extension to the endocervix, significant penetration of the myometrium with invasion of lymphatic and vascular channels, serosal seeding, transfer of tumor cells via the lumen of the fallopian tube, and subsequent spillage into the peritoneal cavity may all occur and affect the anatomic distribution of the tumor. Ovarian involvement is not uncommon and may occur by several routes. The mechanism responsible for extrauterine dissemination is not clear. There has been speculation about the role of increased intrauterine pressure. The problem is made additionally complicated by the degree of differentiation inherent in the neoplasm. Lymphatic permeation in general occurs when the myometrium is invaded. Biologic aggressiveness and myometrial involvement have been correlated with the histologic grading of the tumor.

PATHOLOGY

The gross appearance of the tumor in the hysterectomy specimen varies from a localized polypoid nodule, flat or slightly elevated, to a diffuse involvement of the entire endometrial surface. In some instances, the lesion has been removed entirely by the diagnostic curettage or destroyed by the preoperative insertion of intracavitary radium. In such instances, careful search of the endometrial surface must be performed to establish where the site of the lesion may have been located. This may be a slightly depressed area

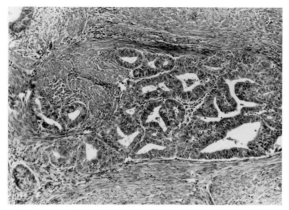

FIGURE 42–6 Invasive endometrial carcinoma shows glands within glands and an absence of stroma in a lesion which is penetrating the myometrium. H & E ×156.

or a superficially scarred area. This site should be carefully studied for residual tumor or even myometrial invasion.

In polypoid or diffuse lesions, ulceration, hemorrhage, and necrosis are helpful in distinguishing malignant from benign lesions with similar gross appearances. A large polypoid tumor can occasionally dilate the internal cervical os and protrude through the endocervical canal.

In curetted material, characteristically there is abundant polypoid, pale yellow-tan, cellular, friable tissue, which frequently contains foci of necrosis. Papillary fragments may be recognized grossly. All the curettings should be submitted for histologic examination because the carcinoma may be small or present along with benign endometrial lesions.

Microscopically, endometrial carcinoma is an adenocarcinoma which is usually well differentiated. Acinar structures composed of malignant cells with pseudostratification, nuclear hyperchromatism, atypism, and dyspolarity with relatively few atypical mitoses form the usual tumors. The microscopical diagnosis of endometrial adenocarcinoma is based on architecture rather than cellular changes. This is especially true in the usual case of a well differentiated adenocarcinoma which, as seen in curetted material, affords no clue as to its invasive potential (Fig. 42–6). Indeed, in most such cases, invasion of the myometrium is not demonstrable in hysterectomy specimens.

Histopathologic Diagnostic Complications

In practice, it is not uncommon to encounter a specimen with an unequivocal carcinoma in the endometrium and a solid adenocarcinoma of the ovary. The question usually posed is which is primary and which is metastatic? When clear-cut evidence is lacking, it is probably best to explain the case as a multiple primary tumor, i.e., Müllerian carcinogenesis in two separate loci, each field presumably responding to the same oncogenic stimulus.

Adenoacanthoma

Squamous metaplasia is a frequent microscopic finding in endometrial adenocarcinoma. It complicates the structure and is encountered to greater or lesser degree in as many as 35 percent of cases. In most instances, the squamous change is focal and often superficial. Usually, the pathologist does not bother to report minute deviations from the ordinary pattern. However, in about 5 percent of cases, the squamous element is prominent and occupies an apparent proportion of one or more histologic sections, hence the special term adenoacanthoma (Fig. 42–7). As a general rule, the more sections of an endometrial carcinoma one prepares and reviews, the more often one encounters this phenomenon. Cases have been reported in which metastatic foci contain both glandular and squamous elements, and in a rare instance only a neoplastic squamous element is seen. However, adenoacanthoma is of no special prognostic importance. Patients with squamous metaplasia in their endometrial carcinomas follow the same biologic patterns and have the same clinical characteristics, the same response to therapy, and the same prognosis as those in whom this epithelial change is absent. There is no reason to invoke the new term adenosquamous carcinoma, because the tumors so labeled are

FIGURE 42–7 Endometrial adenoacanthoma has nests of large, keratinized cells intermingled with the invasive glandular tumor. H & E ×156.

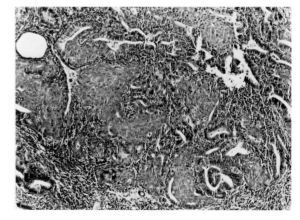

merely examples of poorly differentiated adenoacanthoma.

Histologic Grading

Broder in 1920 developed criteria for examining the histologic characteristics of epithelial tumors, with the objective of correlating their clinical aggressiveness and outcome. When his criteria are applied to endometrial carcinomas, grade I tumors are found to be composed of small to medium-sized, relatively uniform glands, linked by fairly regular columnar cells having normochromic nuclei and a low mitotic rate. Approximately 75 percent of endometrial carcinomas are grade I lesions and have a favorable prognosis. The fortunate clinical outcome is thought to be due to the slow rate of growth of the differentiated tumor and limited myometrial invasion. In grade I lesions, the anatomic extent of the neoplasm and its intrinsic histologic features seem closely related.

Grade II carcinomas show more variability in glandular patterns, more cellular atypia and pleomorphism, and a somewhat higher mitotic rate. Postsurgical examination of uteri having a grade II carcinoma often shows less invasion of the myometrium than in grade I and thus the prognosis is as favorable.

Grade III carcinomas are composed of poorly differentiated glands often containing areas of sheetlike growth and numerous mitoses. They are capable of rapid growth as well as diffuse and deeper invasion of the myometrium. Invasion of intramural veins and lymphatic channels is frequently seen. These factors combine to make for a relatively poor prognosis. Fortunately grade III lesions of the endometrium constitute less than 10 and probably as low as 5 percent of all endometrial adenocarcinomas.

CLINICAL STAGING

The practice of staging has as its objectives the evaluation of the anatomic extent of a tumor. As an arbitrary set of criteria, it provides guidance in clinical examination. Its limitations are that the biologic nature of the tumor in terms of differentiation, invasiveness, rate of growth, and metastatic patterns as well as, in some instances, accurate measure of tumor volume are difficult to assess. These deficiencies affect the ability to select therapeutic regimens which might be specific for a particular tumor. The advantages are that adherence to the staging criteria permits different institutions to compare experiences with specific focus on the efficacy of therapy.

The International Federation of Gynecology and Obstetrics (FIGO) has adopted the following classification for carcinoma of the corpus uteri:

Stage 0. Carcinoma in situ. Histologic findings suspicious of malignancy. Cases of stage 0 should not be included in any therapeutic statistics.

Stage I. The carcinoma is confined to the corpus.

Stage IA. The length of the uterine cavity is 8 cm or less.

Stage IB. The length of the uterine cavity is more than 8 cm.

Stage II. The carcinoma has involved the corpus and the cervix.

Stage III. The carcinoma has extended outside the uterus but not outside the true pelvis.

Stage IV. The carcinoma has extended outside the true pelvis or has obviously involved the mucosa of the bladder or rectum. A bullous edema as such does not permit allotment of a case to stage IV.

The stage I cases should be subgrouped with regard to the histologic type of the adenocarcinoma as follows:

G1. Highly differentiated adenomatous carcinomas.

G2. Differentiated adenomatous carcinomas with partly solid areas.

G3. Predominantly solid or undifferentiated carcinomas.

As a category, the stage I classification has not been clinically acceptable and effective mainly because tumor bulk and behavior cannot be precisely correlated. The principal reason that endometrial carcinoma has an overall 75 to 80 percent 5-year cure rate is that 75 to 85 percent of the cases are stage I, grade I lesions.

LYMPHATIC DRAINAGE AND INVOLVEMENT

Carcinoma of the endometrium may extend through the lymphatics of the upper broad ligament along the vessels within the infundibulopelvic ligament to the ovary and the lumbar paraaortic chain. Drainage from the midcorpus flows transversely through the broad ligaments to the iliac glands at the bifurcation of the common iliac arteries. The lower segment of the uterus drains to the external iliac group and also, via lymphatic channels, along the vessels which supply the cervix, to the internal iliac chain. There is free communication between the lymphatics of the corpus and the cervix. If tumor involves the endocervix, endometrial carcinoma can behave like a cervical neoplasm. Obturator node involvement and extension along the base of the broad ligaments to the pelvic sidewalls can occur and contribute to the widespread anatomic distribution of the cancer. Obstructive retrograde lymphatic flow causing periurethral metastases is an additional problem. Extensions to vaginal vault and vesicovaginal septum constitute major complications.

Pelvic lymph node involvement in endometrial cancer is of the order of 10 to 20 percent. Paraaortic nodal metastases are thought to be present in an equally high proportion of patients. With extensive penetration of the myometrium, positive regional node spread has been reported in 36.2 percent of cases (Lewis).

SYMPTOMS

The symptoms are not unlike those of cancer of the cervix. Abnormal bleeding or spotting is noted, which may be associated with a watery serous discharge. The bleeding is unpredictable and generally extends over a period of time. Brisk hemorrhage involving significant blood loss is not usually seen. The premenopausal woman reveals a progressive diminution in the duration of her menstrual flow or a gradual discontinuation of the regularity of her menstrual cycle. The interval between menses is prolonged, and the number of days of flow may be diminished. The overall picture is one of less and less regular bleeding. An irregular bleeding pattern in the perimenopausal patient is abnormal and requires investigation. All postmenopausal bleeding requires a specific acceptable explanation. Should the uterus be distorted by intrinsic endometrial drainage, secondary infection may occur and a bloody-purulent discharge or even a pyometra may intervene.

DIAGNOSIS

Approximately three-fourths of patients when seen have localized disease. The remainder have regional spread. The challenge upon seeing a woman suspected of having an endometrial cancer is to obtain a tissue diagnosis which explains abnormal uterine bleeding or discharge, a palpable pelvic mass, pelvic pain, or an abnormal cytologic report.

In most women with endometrial carcinoma, the uterus is not enlarged, is freely movable, and there are no adnexal masses. In a minority the uterus is globular, larger than normal, and softened, not unlike a pregnant uterus. The cervix may be soft and more easily dilatable. Sounding of all uteri should be cautiously performed if the uterus is to be biopsied, irrigated, or curetted. It is important to estimate the size of the uterus as determined by the length of the uterine cavity. (See Clinical Staging.) The hazard of perforation is real, and it is necessary to exercise great caution when curetting the endometrial cavity.

Endometrial carcinoma is sometimes discovered as an incidental finding after hysterectomy for submucous, obstructing leiomyomata. Adequate curettage in the presence of fibroids is more difficult and the possibility of a coexisting endometrial neoplasm should always be considered.

Pelvic examination should be carefully performed. In addition to examining the external genitalia, the vaginal mucosa should be inspected and a determination made whether atrophy or a good estrogen response exists. The ectocervical epithelium should be routinely inspected and repeat vaginal smears obtained from the posterior vaginal pool, the ectocervix, and the endocervical canal. Bimanual examination should determine the size and position of the uterus and a careful palpation should be made of the parametria. The ovaries should be carefully identified and an estimate made of their size and shape. The possible existence of an associated ovarian neoplasm, endocrine functioning or not, should be excluded. Rectovaginal examination of the cul-de-sac and the rectovaginal septum provides an additional opportunity to feel the parametria and the sidewalls of the pelvis. These features of the pelvic examination are essential to proper diagnosis and staging.

The diagnosis is established by curettage or endometrial biopsy. Cytologists of long-standing experience and special skill can make the diagnosis from cytograms obtained from the posterior vaginal fornix, direct endometrial cavity sampling, or by the jetwashing irrigation technique. In experienced cytology laboratories, endometrial carcinoma may be detected in 80 to 85 percent of cases. However, this is not the general experience. Routine cytologic screening of asymptomatic women rarely detects endometrial adenocarcinoma.

The accuracy of endometrial biopsy is significantly higher in lesions which are diffusely scattered throughout the endometrial cavity, compared with those whose distribution may be focal and limited. In the diagnosis of carcinoma of the endometrium, the accuracy ranged from 75 to 96 percent when a curet or cannula was used, when correlated with lesions in hysterectomy specimens. In a study of suction biopsy of 9489 endometrial biopsies, an accuracy of 92 percent in diagnosing endometrial cancer was reported (Nugent).

Initially there was an enthusiastic response to the use of the irrigation method. However, the claims for it have not been borne out in routine clinical practice. The irrigation method samples the superficial portions of the endometrium or the superficial epithelial cells. The irrigation of the cavity apparently works best when sufficient pressure is placed on the syringe so that a jet effect of the washing fluid dislodges small fragments of tissue, which are included in the specimen. Lesions situated beneath the superficial portion of endometrium may be entirely missed by this technique and therefore curettage or biopsy is preferred.

Fractional Curettage

Dilatation and curettage provides accurate information if a fractional curettage is performed. It is important to estimate the anatomic extent of the tumor since it is essential to know whether a lesion originating in the corpus has extended to and/or invaded the endocervix. The curettage should initially involve careful clockwise stroking of the endocervical mucosa; the curettings so obtained should be labeled endocervical curettings, in contrast to the tissue obtained from the endometrial cavity, and each should be submitted separately for pathologic examination. When initially examining the cavity with a curet after sounding the uterus, the operator should gently insert the instrument to the depth of the corpus and bring out a strip of the mucosa. By meticulously covering the interior surface of the cavity and bringing each stroke of the curet into the vagina, the location of the tumor may be identified and the regularity (or lack of regularity) of the cavity established. This information is useful for both the staging of the disease and the proper insertion of intracavity radium.

The gross appearance of the curettings is sufficiently characteristic in the presence of an overt cancer so that the diagnosis may be apparent. The tumor is friable, yellow-tan, and frequently has scattered foci of necrosis. By contrast, the curettings of endometrial hyperplasia are mucoid, smooth, soft, and resilient.

TREATMENT

The formulation of a plan of treatment depends upon (1) an accurate histopathologic diagnosis; (2) clarification of the anatomic localization of the tumor, i.e., its local, regional, or distant metastic spread; (3) pretreatment study to determine the general systemic condition of the patient and any specific local deleterious effects of the tumor, e.g., fistula or abscess formation; and (4) the selection of a mode of therapy best suited for the individual patient.

In deciding upon therapy, the cooperative efforts of gynecologist, pathologist, radiotherapist, and medical oncologist are desirable. For these reasons, institutions are creating tumor boards involving individuals preoccupied with the care of tumor patients. Such a group can coordinate their efforts and skills in the best interests of patient care. In such arrangements, the participation of the patient's own physician is to be encouraged and is essential to obtaining the patient's cooperation.

Determinants of Therapy

The size of the uterus, the degree of tumor differentiation, the invasion of the myometrium, and the question of involvement of the endocervix are four critical factors to be determined in the selection of therapy. There is an empirical correlation between these factors, i.e., an endometrial cavity more than 8.0 cm in length generally has (1) a larger, less well differentiated tumor and (2) this tumor is more prone to invade the myometrium, but the correlation is not absolute.

Size of Uterus. The external size and configuration of the uterus can be estimated by bimanual vaginal and rectovaginal examination. The presence or absence of serosal surface irregularities and adnexal or culde-sac masses should be determined. The length of the endometrial cavity is estimated by sounding the uterus. The latter should be cautiously performed because of the hazard of perforation. The presence of a pyometra may also be revealed by this maneuver.

Tumor Differentiation. Most tumors are well differentiated adenocarcinomas. However, within the same uterus, areas of endometrial atypia, carcinoma in situ, squamous metaplasia, and combinations of squamous and adenomatous, benign and malignant, elements may be found. It is thus important that an adequate and representative sample of tissue be submitted. Because of the spectrum of histopathology that may be encountered, a final diagnosis may be established only with difficulty. When the histopathologic diagnosis is not clear-cut, it is desirable that the opinons of a number of pathologists be obtained, particularly those having special competence in gynecologic pathology.

Invasion of the Myometrium. There is no way prior to therapy to determine specifically whether myometrial invasion exists. This can be established only after the uterus is removed and examined carefully for the original tumor site and for residual tumor. The fact that myometrial invasion cannot be estimated prior to treatment is a serious limitation of therapeutic protocols and to accurate projection of prognosis.

Endocervical Involvement. It makes little difference if a carcinoma invades the endocervix after having originated as a primary tumor of the cervix or as a primary tumor of the corpus. The important clinical fact is that both lesions behave comparably and treatment must be based on known patterns of tumor dissemination. Endocervical involvement for an endometrial carcinoma significantly changes the prognosis. Corpus and cervical carcinoma (stage II) is essentially treated as two carcinomas. The presence of cancer in the cervix increases the possibility of vaginal-vault metastases as well as parametrial and lymph node involvement. Fractional curettage and estimation of the size and configuration of the endocervix and of possible parametrial extension are the significant points in the selection of treatment.

Pretherapy Evaluation. A comprehensive history and physical examination with particular emphasis upon the cardiovascular, respiratory, and renal systems are essential. Monitoring of the patient's biochemical status and examination of the urine, including sediment and culture, should be completed. The values of blood urea nitrogen and 2-hour postprandial blood sugar determinations should be noted. A glucose tolerance test should be completed if indicated. The patient should additionally have the benefit of a search to identify the local limits or any metastatic spread of her primary disease. During the workup, it should be borne in mind that a patient with a cancer predisposition may develop more than one cancer. Other sites, particularly in the genitourinary tract as well as in the breasts, colon, and rectum, should be evaluated.

Mode of Therapy (see Chapter 47). Surgery is the treatment of choice in endometrial carcinoma. Adjuvant therapy includes irradiation and chemotherapy. Radiation therapy involves exposure of tumor tissue to radiation by x-ray, radium, radioactive cobalt, or other radioactive elements. Chemotherapy consists of the employment of hormones, antimetabolites, alkylating compounds, or cytotoxic agents. Some general guidelines have emerged which usually influence the selection of a specific modality. Personal preference, bias, competence, and the prevailing practices in any

given hospital community also are important considerations. The value of presenting a patient's problem to a tumor board is that errors of omission in pretherapy evaluation are by and large excluded. Furthermore, greater objectivity in selecting therapeutic modalities is more likely to be achieved, and those responsible for the implementation of therapy become determined to produce the best overall results. In general, it can be said that, where good results are obtained by surgery alone or in combination with preoperative or postoperative radiation, the nature and extent of the disease have been critical issues. If patients do not neglect abnormal bleeding, they will seek earlier care. In better than 75 percent of cases seen early, the tumor is limited to the endometrium. Instances have been noted where no tumor is present following hysterectomy. Curettage alone can produce a cure.

Surgery. Well-differentiated tumors in small uteri are adequately treated by total hysterectomy and bilateral salpingo-oophorectomy. Uteri having endometrial cavities which are larger than 8 cm or which have an undifferentiated endometrial lesion are optimally cared for with preoperative radiation followed by hysterectomy in 6 to 8 weeks. Where endocervical involvement is established (stage II), preoperative radiation therapy should be equivalent to that given a primary cervical carcinoma. Hysterectomy, following irradiation, should be restrained and of a simple type.

The role of radical hysterectomy with lymphadenectomy for stage II carcinoma is limited because of the lymphatic pattern of metastases to the aortic nodes. In isolated instances, where effective radiotherapy is precluded because of associated pelvic inflammatory disease or large leiomyomas, recourse to radical hysterectomy may be necessary. When advanced disease is present in the pelvis or if contiguous organs, i.e., bladder and rectum, are involved, the role of surgery may be limited to laparotomy for purposes of defining the anatomic extent of the disease. Selective lymph node biopsy may be performed merely for diagnostic purposes. Primary therapy in such cases is irradiation. Pelvic exenteration appears to have essentially no place in endometrial carcinoma, though conceivably a tumor established to be confined to the pelvis might be managed surgically, where other measures have failed. When surgery and radiation are combined, the therapeutic benefits of each appear to be achieved only if the methods are complementary. Excessive surgery superimposed on a patient who has had heavy radiation is a hazard.

In the presence of pyometra, the endometrial cavity should be drained, cultured, and treated with appropriate antibiotic(s) prior to the implementation of further therapy.

Combined Surgery and Radiotherapy. The rationale of radiotherapy, adjunctive to surgery, in cancer of the endometrium is based on (1) hysterectomy alone is accompanied by periurethral metastases and recurrence in the vaginal vault in 10 to 15 percent of cases in early stage I cancers (Way; Price et al.); (2) the presence of cancer in the cervix requires therapy to the parametrium and regional lymph nodes in fairly advanced but operable cancer; and (3) radiotherapy alone can effect a cure but yields far inferior results than when combined with surgery. In several studies, the 5-year survival rates reported were 20 and 74 percent (Sala and del Regato) and 54 and 90 percent, respectively, in stage I carcinoma. The principles of radiotherapy are discussed in Chap. 47.

The main objective of irradiation is to prevent vaginal-vault recurrence. For this purpose, local irradiation by intrauterine and intravaginal radioactive sources is sufficient. External radiotherapy in moderate doses is an alternative. Of particular concern are patients with (1) stage I disease with poorly differentiated carcinoma, (2) enlarged uteri with possibly myometrial invasion, and (3) stage II disease where the chance of dissemination beyond the body of the uterus, mainly to lymphatics, is greater. In such patients, the volume irradiated should cover the whole pelvis to include the uterus and the pelvic nodes with a fairly high dose.

Sequence of Therapy. Radiotherapy is preferably given preoperatively. The main advantage of preoperative irradiation is that the cells are better oxygenated (no elimination of blood supply or fibrosis caused by surgery) and thus are more radiosensitive. Additionally, cells implanted in the wound at the time of operation would be rendered nonviable by prior irradiation. Another possible advantage of preoperative irradiation is that an inoperable cancer may be converted to an operable one.

Surgery is usually performed, on the average, 6 (4 to 8) weeks after external radiotherapy with moderately high doses. This period is chosen because it represents the interval when the acute reaction has subsided and the chronic reaction (fibrosis) has not started.

Techniques

Intracavitary Irradiation. Heyman's packing technique is most widely known and applied for irradiating the uterine cavity. In the original procedure, the uterine cavity was packed with many radium capsules (Heyman et al.).

In the Manchester technique, the uterine cavity is irradiated by a central tandem source as in carcinoma of the cervix but is differentially loaded so that it is "hotter" near the fundal end. The vagina is irradiated by applying radium in the largest tolerated cylinder. Radium loaded in a colpostat, as in carcinoma of the cervix, is an alternative.

External Radiotherapy. High-energy source from a cobalt 60 unit or linear accelerator is used. If the dose delivered is 4000 rads (usually 200 rads daily), parallel opposing anterior and posterior fields are generally used. If a higher dose is to be delivered, then the exit dose with parallel opposing anteroposterior fields is usually high and unacceptable because of the subsequent cutaneous and subcutaneous fibrosis it may cause. In such cases more than two fields are used, generally two anterior oblique and two posterior oblique fields.

Fields should be sufficient to irradiate the whole pelvis.

Treatment Regimens. For stage I well-differentiated cancer with small or slightly enlarged uterus, external radiotherapy is given to the whole pelvis to a total dose of 4000 rads in 20 fractions in 4 weeks. The advantage of external irradiation is that such treatment can be done on an ambulatory basis and does not require either hospitalization or anesthesia. In very obese patients in whom poor depth dose from external irradiation is a problem, it is usually advisable to resort to the alternative method of internal irradiation. Heyman's packing is applied for a total dose of 3500 mg·h, followed in a 1-week interval by a vaginal cylinder to deliver a surface dose of 5000 rads. Hysterectomy is performed 6 weeks later.

Stage II and stage I poorly differentiated tumors or enlarged uteri of 6 to 8 weeks' size or more are treated with 2000 rads given to the whole pelvis by external radiotherapy in 10 fractions in 2 weeks. This is followed by two radium applications at a 1-week interval via tandem and colpostat, as in carcinoma of the cervix, using 5000 mg·h of radium. This is followed by another course of external radiotherapy to deliver 2000 rads in 2 weeks in 10 fractions with shielding of the midline. Hysterectomy is best performed 6 to 8 weeks later.

Radiation Only. Where contraindications to surgery exist, definitive radiotherapy can be given. In stage I well-differentiated cancer in a uterus less than 6 to 8 weeks in size, or in a uterine cavity that is very small, Heyman's packing or a differentially loaded tandem is used in two applications at 1- to 2-week intervals for a total dose of 6000 mg·h of radium. With each application, a vaginal colpostat is used for a surface dose of 4000 rads.

In a stage I lesion with poorly differentiated cancer and a uterus of 6 to 8 weeks' size or more, as well as in more advanced stages, external radiotherapy is used as previously described. Supplementing the external radiotherapy, two applications of Heyman's packing or differentially loaded tandem as well as two applications of colpostat are employed.

If radium cannot be applied because of a local uterovaginal condition or because the patient is a poor anesthetic risk, external radiotherapy can be given, for a total dose of 6000 rads in 30 fractions in 6 weeks.

Hormone Therapy. Progesterone therapy for patients with advanced or recurrent endometrial carcinomas has been an encouraging albeit poorly understood development. If unopposed estrogen is an underlying etiologic factor, then the progestational influence on an estrogen-primed hormonally dependent tumor would be expected to have therapeutic benefit. In clinical practice, this appears to be true in approximately 35 to 40 percent of patients. Unfortunately, the arrest and regression are temporary, and the mechanism of action is poorly understood. The favorable results are generally seen in younger patients, having well-differentiated and presumably slow-growing tumors and who thus present themselves with relatively late recurrences (Hustin). In the experience with intramuscular progesterone (medroxyprogesterone acetate) the drug was administered for a minimum of 4 to 5 weeks before any response was noted, and in some instances as many as 8 weeks were necessary (Reifenstein). Pulmonary metastases and extrapelvic lesions seemed to respond better than central recurrences. Unfortunately, where favorable responses have occurred, most of the regressions have lasted for only 1 to 2 years. Thereafter, the tumor apparently escapes and regains its biologic aggressiveness.

Several investigators favor the concept that progesterone acts cytolytically at the tumor-cell level. This has prompted intracavitary progesterone admin-

istration. In some instances, progesterone priming has been given prior to preoperative radiation therapy in an effort to enhance tumor susceptibility. These efforts support the thesis that the hormone produces a local cell response. Necrosis, prelethal glycogen accumulation, and an inflammatory cellular response occur. The reported cellular mobilization consisted of mature and immature lymphocytes and plasma cells. Such findings produce the provocative speculation that progesterone may enhance the host's immune response (Hustin).

More potent progestational agents are becoming available, including compounds which can be administered orally. This therapy remains an important palliative measure while providing the additional opportunity to acquire insight into the nature of tumor hormonal dependency. Other chemotherapeutic agents have not been particularly valuable in endometrial carcinoma. Whether combinations of agents will be more effective remains to be determined. Adriamycin and Cytoxan have shown some promise where progesterone has failed (see Chap. 48).

SURVIVAL AND END RESULTS

The factors influencing successful therapy and patient survival are:

1. The biologic nature and extent of the cancer
2. The accuracy of diagnosis
3. The selection of appropriate therapy
4. The nature of the patient and the ability to tolerate and respond to therapy
5. Successful follow-up

In endometrial carcinoma, better than 75 percent of patients when diagnosed have localized disease, and by and large the end results are good. As far as prognosis is concerned, the outlook for the patient with early endometrial carcinoma is more optimistic than in early cervical cancer. However, approximately 10 percent of patients have regional spread; in this group, there is a more pessimistic picture in terms of long-term survival (Fig. 42–8). Age is a factor, and both the observed and relative survival rates decrease as age increases. Beyond age 65, even among women who have localized disease, the age gradient appears to influence outcome. Whether this is a reflection of an altered tumor-host response is speculative. However, the salvage in elderly patients is not as good as that noted in women less than 60 years and the explanation is not available. Intercur-

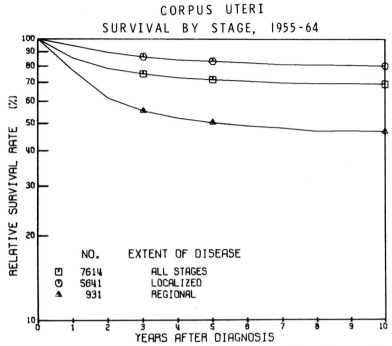

FIGURE 42–8 End results in endometrial carcinoma by stages, regardless of therapy. *(From End Results in Cancer.)*

rent disease as a cause of death has been excluded from the analysis (*End Results in Cancer,* 1972).

The overall salvage for all stages is approximately 55 percent. For stage I disease limited to the endometrium, the expectation is that the cure rate should be better than 90 percent. When the problems of the depth of the uterine cavity, the extent of myometrial invasion, the dedifferentiation of the tumor, and the possible extension to endocervix arise, the outcome is less certain. The present stage I 5-year survival rate is variously reported to be between 70 and 89 percent. Stage II survival reports range from 44 to 72 percent, and when significant myometrial penetration or endocervical involvement is present, the overall salvage approximates 50 percent. In far-advanced disease, stages III and IV, it is difficult to postulate cure rates as they may apply to any individual patient. The prognosis and the outlook are obviously guarded. If optimal therapy has been given, only the passage of time will clarify whether residual tumor exists or whether the patient's immune system will control isolated autonomous cancer cells. In small series, stages III and IV have been reported with salvage rates varying from 14 to 48 percent (stages III and IV combined), 18 to 38 percent for stage III, and 20 percent for stage IV by various investigators.

DISORDERS OF THE MYOMETRIUM

The constituent parts of the walls of the uterus are interwoven smooth-muscle fibers, blood vessels, connective tissue, nerve cells, and secretory elements. Collectively, they make up the myometrium, which is physiologically influenced by physical and hormonal factors. Estrogen and progesterone, acting synergistically, combine to stimulate hyperplasia and hypertrophy of the myometrium. The effects are most dramatically apparent during pregnancy. The capacity of the uterine wall to undergo hypertrophy and stretch and to contract effectively when fetal development is complete are essential features for successful parturition.

The main disorders of the myometrium include anatomic and pathologic deviations reflecting congenital malformations and the presence of benign and malignant neoplasms. Inflammatory responses and related pathology of the myometrium, i.e., abscesses, cysts, are not common and generally are secondary to disease of the endometrium, the adnexae, or diffuse intraperitoneal sepsis. The remainder of this chapter focuses upon disorders of the myometrium, and the discussion concludes with a description of subinvolution of the placental site, a vascular disorder seen in the puerperium.

CONGENITAL ANOMALIES

As a clinical entity, the diagnosis of uterine malformation is frequently made by a process of elimination. A malformation may be the explanation of a patient's problem involving menstruation, fertility, or ability to successfully conclude a pregnancy. It is possible for an anomalous uterine condition to remain undetected throughout a lifetime. A woman with a minor malformation can succeed in becoming pregnant without difficulty and carry a fetus uneventfully to viability. The true incidence of congenital anomalies or malformations is unknown. It is estimated that perhaps 1 in 300 women has some anomaly. Because of the close association in embryologic timing and the developmental events between the reproductive tract and the urinary tract, the finding of a defect in one system automatically requires investigation of a possible defect in the other.

EMBRYOLOGIC BACKGROUND

The specific cause or causes of uterine anomalies remains obscure. Some cases of uterine maldevelopment are presumed to be related to abnormal hormonal influences. The data in this connection are fragmentary and only now beginning to be elucidated. Müllerian duct fusion failures as well as defective canalization have features which are common to anomalies in other parts of the body. Fusion failure in facial clefts has been studied both in man and in mouse models and is assumed to represent an example of a multifactorial gene-environment interaction. This hypothetical explanation is thought to be operational in many human anomalies. The essential documentation which can contribute to establishing the importance of genetic predisposition is more difficult to obtain in uterine malformations because their presence is not detected at birth and may not be suspected until the active reproductive years when becoming pregnant or maintaining pregnancy may be a problem.

Between the sixth and ninth weeks of embryonic development, the two Müllerian (paramesonephric) ducts, which lie adjacent to the Wolffian (mesonephric) ducts, grow caudally. The Müllerian ducts develop as evaginations from the primitive coelom. As they extend caudally, the epithelium which lines these ducts becomes invested by subcoelomic mesenchymal cells that migrate caudally along with the epithelial component. Together, the epithelium and mesenchyme form what may be termed the Müllerian apparatus. The later differentiation of Müllerian epithelium into the mucosa of the endosalpinx, endometrium, endocervix, and the squamous lining of the ectocervix and upper portion of the vagina is matched by the maturation of the mesenchyme into endometrial stroma, myometrium, and the fibromuscular coats of the fallopian tube and cervix. The paired Müllerian ducts fuse and form the symmetrical uterine corpus and cervix but the fallopian tubes remain separate. In males, the Y chromosome and the production of a fetal testicular secretory product cause regression of the Müllerian ducts. In females, the Müllerian ducts continue their normal development and regression does not occur. A spectrum of uterine malformations may occur varying from complete absence of the uterus to partial or unilateral regression of uterine horns or to a multiplicity of fusion defects. The resulting defects may have major and minor functional clinical significance.

CLINICAL CLASSIFICATION

A classic paper by Jarcho in 1946 provided a classification and remains the basis for orientation in most clinical discussions. Recognizing that the anomalies represent either complete failure in development (agenesis), degrees of failure to fuse, or cavitation defects resulting in luminal problems, seven common types were proposed: (1) uterus didelphys, (2) uterus duplex bicornis bicollis vagina simplex, (3) uterus bicornis unicollis vagina simplex, (4) uterus septus, (5) uterus subseptus, (6) uterus arcuatus or cordiformis, and (7) uterus unicornis (Jarcho) (Fig. 42–9).

The uterus didelphys is comparatively rare and represents a complete duplication of vagina, cervix, and uterus. The patient's chances for obtaining a normal birth with this defect are greatly reduced. The endogenous vascular and muscular endowment of this abnormality is poor. Abortion and premature termination of pregnancy characterize reproductive performance. The bicornuate uterus bicollis essentially has two horns or two compartments, reflecting developmental arrest (Fig. 42–10). The vagina is generally normal. In bicornuate uterus unicollis, the separation of the horns is complete above the cervix, resulting from an incomplete absorption of the fundal portion. The uterus is prominently bicornuate. Nidation may occur in either or both horns. The major pregnancy

CONGENITAL MALFORMATION OF UTERUS

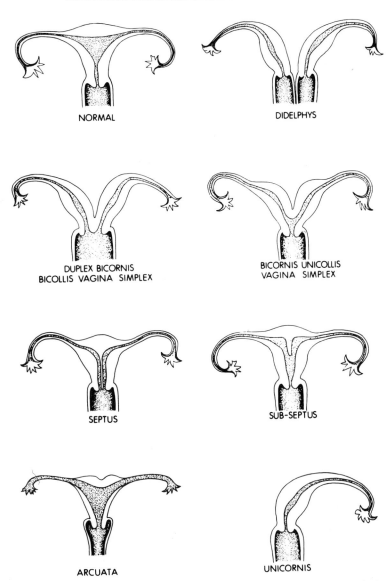

FIGURE 42–9 Types of uterine malformations. *(Drawn from the concepts of Jarcho.)*

complication is hemorrhage. Incarceration of one of the horns may occur during labor. A troublesome severe complication is intraperitoneal hemorrhage secondary to a rupture of an asymmetric essentially cornual pregnancy. The disaster of a cornual pregnancy is one of the most serious extrauterine pregnancy complications and has all the hazards of hemoperitoneum, hypovolemic shock, secondary sepsis, and death.

The septate uterus is noteworthy for its complete septum which divides the uterine cavity throughout its entire length. Should pregnancy occur, the nongravid portion may undergo myometrial hypertrophy and be responsible for obstructed labor and delivery. The correct diagnosis must be made early and the possibility of ineffectual labor anticipated. Leiomyoma, extrauterine pregnancy, and the possibility of an ovarian cyst should be considered in the differential diagno-

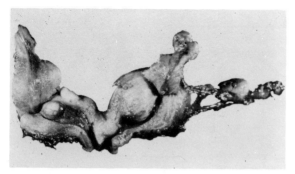

FIGURE 42–10 Bicornuate uterus with two separate compartments. A submucous fibroid is seen in one. The vagina was normal. *(Courtesy of Dr. Sheldon C. Sommers.)*

sis. The subseptate uterus generally does not cause dystocia. However, confronted with a persistent transverse lie or oblique fetal presentation, the physician should recognize that the underlying difficulty may be the distorted, obstructed uterine cavity. The arcuate uterus is a variation of the bicornuate defect and is frequently difficult to differentiate from the normal uterus. A depression in the uterine fundus is palpable on bimanual examination. On hysterography a complete or incomplete septum may be demonstrated. This is one of the more common uterine anomalies and may be associated with prematurity, postmaturity, prolonged first stage of labor, breech and transverse presentations, and retained placenta.

The uterus unicornis is a rare complication resulting from unilateral suppression of Müllerian duct fusion. It is generally not associated with any pregnancy complication and may be incidental finding during surgery or at autopsy examination. A periodic problem is the determination as to whether a uterus is small or infantile. This is a difficult diagnosis to make. In the presence of normal menstruation and ovulation, the diagnosis of an infantile uterus as a possible cause of infertility is hazardous and probably wrong. Small uteri undergo remarkable hypertrophy if implantation of a conceptus occurs. The size of the uterus is not likely to be a critical factor in a problem of female-male infertility.

CLINICAL MANIFESTATIONS AND DIAGNOSIS

The symptomatology associated with some uterine malformations may be totally absent or essentially negligible. In some instances the patient's presenting problem(s) may be related to difficulties in menstruation, coitus, ability to conceive or maintain an intrauterine gestation, or in having a normal labor and de-

livery. Dysmenorrhea and menorrhagia are common complaints. Hematocolpos and endometriosis may be associated problems. Among women with the problem of infertility, about 10 percent may have an underlying congenital malformation.

A history of repeated pregnancy losses and unusual endocrine or metabolic factors associated with familial or genetic aberrations complicating reproductive performance requires investigation for the possible existence of a uterine malformation. A minority of congenital anomalies of the uterus are associated with abnormal gonadal hormonal effects. Because the causes of aberrant developmental fusion of the Müllerian ducts are largely unknown and the general impression exists that genetic disorders may predispose to their development, it is important that a careful family history be obtained regarding possible hereditary influences. The true hermaphrodite can be assumed to represent an abnormality of genital-tract development related to abnormal fetal hormonal effects.

It can be anticipated that comprehensive evaluation of patients with genital-tract anomalies, including a careful family history, karyotyping, and selected maternal and fetal hormonal determinations, will contribute to a better understanding of the multifactorial variables influencing gene-environment interaction. Data of this sort hold promise of clarifying fusion failure or fetal environmental hormonal influences affecting genital-tract development. Hysterography, intravenous pyelography, and possibly hysteroscopy and angiography are important in establishing the specific nature of the abnormality.

TREATMENT

With the nature of the malformation established, therapy should be directed at the patient's defect only if it has been determined that the malformation is responsible for her disability. Clearly, the causes of habitual abortion, menorrhagia or dysmenorrhea, or pregnancy failure are multiple, and it is essential that the causal relationship with the patient's problem be established.

Where the defect causes a malformed uterine cavity and the history documents repeated pregnancy failure, surgical correction is necessary. In carefully selected patients, reduplicated, divided endometrial cavities have had septal and myometrial excisions resulting in the reconstruction of a single efficient uterus. The overall clinical results reported indicated an 85 percent postoperative success rate in bringing 128 women to term who previously had aborted or miscarried (70 percent) or had premature termination of pregnancy (15 percent) (Strassman).

BENIGN TUMORS

LEIOMYOMA (MYOMAS, FIBROIDS)

Leiomyomas are the most common benign tumors of women and occur more commonly in nulliparas. Whether this is a cause or effect is not clear. The incidence of leiomyomas is five times greater in blacks than in whites. There are suggestions that excessive estrogen stimulation is an important etiologic factor but conclusive evidence is lacking. For example, it has been noted that pregnancy, progesterone, and oral contraceptives may cause rapid enlargement of the tumor. Following completion of pregnancy, myomas regress. Infertility and spontaneous abortion are more common in individuals with leiomyomas but whether the myomas are etiologically responsible in specific instances is not established. Most investigators agree that leiomyomas tend to get smaller after the menopause. The complications associated with the tumor are also less frequent postmenopausally. Sarcomatous change is a rare complication, generally unanticipated, and occurs in about 1 in 200 to 1 in 500 leiomyomatous uteri.

Pathology

Grossly, leiomyomas resemble fibromas and are commonly called fibroids. The tumors usually form spherical nodules which on section are pearly white, exhibit a watered-silk texture to the cut surface, and are surrounded by a pseudocapsule of compressed myometrium. Leiomyomas may vary in size from seedlings, 1 mm in size to large masses weighing several kilograms. Solitary leiomyomas do occur, but in about 90 percent of cases they are multiple and distort the uterus asymmetrically. They may be submucous, intramural or subserosal in location or present in any combinations of these sites (Fig 42–11). Leiomyomas may also be found in the broad ligament, separate from the corpus uteri, and are called intraligamentous. Rarely, a solitary leiomyoma may develop in the round ligament. Their consistency is firm and extremely hard. The cut surface has a variable appearance sometimes pale pink or pure white. The homogeneous, compact surface may be interspersed with areas of degeneration. Compact fibrous bands may separate soft edematous regions, which are often streaked with hemorrhagic extravasations

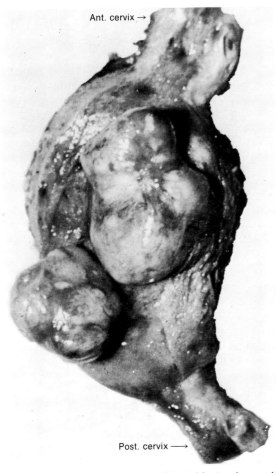

Ant. cervix →

Post. cervix →

FIGURE 42–11 Endometrial cavity distorted by two large submucous leiomyomas.

and contain cavities with cystic degeneration and necrosis. The characteristic microscopical picture of a leiomyoma is that of smooth interlacing muscle bundles, with varying amounts of connective tissue, running in all directions and giving a whorled appearance.

Natural History

The fate of leiomyomas in growth and development is determined principally by their imperfect vascularization, which controls their clinical manifestations. As the leiomyoma enlarges in loco, it compresses adjacent tissues and becomes more or less isolated by a pseudocapsule. Centers of proliferation may appear in it and contribute to the uneven, knobby appearance of the external surface. If growth compromises arterial blood supply, a variety of degenerative changes occur. These include (1) edema, (2) hyaline degeneration, (3) red degeneration, (4) hematoma formation, (5) necrosis, (6) cystic degeneration, (7) fatty degeneration, and (8) calcification.

With avascularity, groups of tumor cells become edematous and slowly die out, and their replacement involves an increased proportion of collagen. In certain cases, the tumor becomes hyaline and forms compact, poorly vascularized, relatively acellular nodules which calcify. In other sites, particulary in the center, collagen may liquefy and result in pseudocystic cavities. If blood vessels rupture, local hematomas are followed by necrosis and further cyst formation. These degenerative, edematous, and hemorrhagic softenings modify the gross appearance of the tumors and frequently raise the question of sarcomatous change. Red degeneration is seen mostly during pregnancy and the puerperium but can occur at other times. It is frequently associated with infarction of a leiomyoma. In association with necrosis, a myoma rarely contains fat, and calcification may occur in some phase of the degenerative process. Leiomyomas have been known occasionally to acquire a secondary blood supply from adherent omentum in a parasitic relationship.

Clinical Manifestations

Leiomyomas are most commonly discovered and diagnosed on routine pelvic examination. On such occasions, most fibroids are asymptomatic. Submucous leiomyomas can cause abnormal bleeding as a result of edema, congestion, and venous distention. Endometrial hyperplasia, carcinoma, pregnancy, and leiomyomas can all coexist. Necrosis and ulceration of the overlying endometrium rarely occur. A submucous leiomyoma may enlarge to a size where it distends the endometrial cavity. In such circumstances, the uterus responds as if a foreign body existed and painful contractions occur. The submucous leiomyoma may initiate cervical dilatation and be delivered into the vagina. Vascular compromise of any of the tumors, regardless of location, may result in degenerative changes which produce symptoms. Torsion of the pedicle of a subserous leiomyoma can produce acute infarction, with resulting manifestations of an abdominal emergency. Pain, tenderness, and occasionally evidence of peritoneal irritation may be noted.

The association of pregnancy and leiomyomas creates several important clinical correlations. Enlarging fibroids may mimic pregnancy, and the appearance of a mass may create confusion for patient and physician. Periodically, because the possibility of a coexisting pregnancy is overlooked, the diagnosis is established only in the hysterectomy specimen. During the reproductive years, the possibility of pregnancy should be considered in any differential diagnosis of a pelvic mass. Rapid growth frequently occurs during the gestational period, and otherwise asymptomatic leiomyomas may become symptomatic. This typically occurs in the middle trimester. Occasionally a low-lying intramural or intraligamentous subserosal leiomyoma in a pregnant woman may fill enough of the pelvis to obstruct labor.

Symptoms

The symptoms of fibroids are pain or discomfort due to size and compression, excessive flow at the time of menses, and/or irregular bleeding. Acute pain is occasionally encountered. Rectal or bladder complaints result from compression of these organs. Rapid enlargement of a pelvic tumor can occur. The patient may present with a history of involuntary infertility or repeat spontaneous abortion.

Differential Diagnosis

Pelvic examination frequently establishes the diagnosis. An enlarged uterus, distorted by multiple nodular masses, is most often a leiomyomatous uterus. Care should be taken to determine whether the masses are attached to the myometrium or whether independent adnexal masses coexist. If an ovarian neoplasm is present, its nature needs clarification. A hysterogram will provide information as to tubal patency as well as the possible distortion of the uterine cavity. Hysteroscopy may reveal submucous leiomyomas or the mucosal bulge of a leiomyoma that extends intramurally. In unusual circumstances, arteriography may be helpful in differentiating a uterine or an adnexal mass. Examination under anesthesia is frequently desirable especially if the clinical differentiation of other causes for uterine enlargement is difficult and can help to clarify the diagnosis.

The presence of a malignancy should be searched for in any patient having a uterus distorted by leiomyomas. Cervical or endometrial carcinoma and myomas can be found in the same uterus. Malignant change should be suspected if a myoma undergoes rapid enlargement, especially after the menopause, or if postmenopausal bleeding occurs in the presence of known myomas. Such cases may develop insidiously.

Treatment

Judicious observation is excellent treatment for asymptomatic myomas. Women can be reassured, observed periodically, and managed with routine care on into the menopause and postmenopausal periods.

If the presenting symptom is abnormal bleeding, the initial step in management is an adequate investigation to explain the bleeding. This is best accomplished by dilatation and curettage. When performing a diagnostic curettage, one should wait for the pathologic report before proceeding with a hysterectomy. The gross appearance of the endometrium may not reliably detect an endometrial carcinoma.

If the pathologic findings are within normal range, a reasonable period of observation may be planned to see whether the patient's menses improve. However, it is rare for a curettage to have much influence upon the menorrhagia due to submucous myomas. A follow-up period of 3 to 6 months generally provides the opportunity to determine whether the menstrual cycle returns to its usual character. In patients who are perimenopausal, malignancy must be ruled out. In patients with leiomyomas who have a demonstrated iron-deficiency anemia due to chronic blood loss, supplemental iron therapy is frequently effective. If the bleeding is of such magnitude as to require more expeditious therapy, transfusion may be an acceptable alternative. With adequate iron therapy, one may see a prompt response in the reticulocyte count and the hematocrit should be increasing at the end of 2 weeks. Treatment with progestins or androgenic substances may reduce the amount of bleeding, but these substances will not have a lasting effect. Coexisting polycythemia is a rare finding which disappears when the myoma is removed.

When a physician is confronted with a patient with leiomyomas in whom there is a prolonged history of infertility and an entirely negative male and female workup, a surgical effort to reconstruct the uterus is indicated. Multiple myomectomies should be completed, with the effort directed to restore a normal configuration to the endometrial cavity while not interfering with tubal patency and ovarian integrity.

In managing the pregnant patient with a previous history of multiple myomectomies, who successfully goes to term, the mode of delivery will depend upon the fetopelvic relationships, the nature of the cervix, and the extent of previous surgery. If the patient has a long-standing history of infertility and if the uterine cavity has been previously entered and reconstructed, the patient should be managed as if she had a previous cesarean section unless it can be anticipated that she will have a prompt, uneventful, normal labor and vaginal delivery.

Hysterectomy should be reserved for those symptomatic patients who cannot be managed with other, simpler methods or in whom the size of the tumor warrants removal. Hysterectomy would be the treatment of choice in a patient having persistent bleeding or tumors of 12-weeks' gestational size or more. This therapy would be additionally indicated in those women having symptomatic fibroids and who have no desire for future childbearing. If a period of more than 6 months has elapsed in the case of a patient who has recurrent, persistent menorrhagia after an initial dilatation and curettage, a repeat dilatation and curettage should be done prior to hysterectomy. Bilateral oophorectomy should not be incidental. The gonadal surgery should be resolved by an evaluation of the presence of pathology, the patient's age, emotional status, and her wishes.

ADENOMYOSIS (ADENOMYOMA)

Adenomyosis is a benign disorder of the uterus characterized by the presence of ectopic foci of endometrial glands and stroma in the myometrium. The ectopic foci must be separated from the basal endometrium. Pathologists have developed a rule-of-thumb guideline to distinguish between true downgrowth of basal endometrium and exaggerated interdigitation at the endometrial junction. The ectopic endometrium must be separated from the nearest visible, normally situated endometrium by one low-power microscopic field.

The ectopic foci of glands and stroma in the myometrium may be surrounded by local smooth-muscle proliferation. This lesion is termed adenomyoma. However, this is not a true neoplasm but a localized hyperplasia of smooth muscle surrounding the aberrant glands and stroma. Because the glands are derived from the basal, nonreactive segment of the endometrium, they do not respond to cyclic stimulation. This lack of response distinguishes these ectopic glandular and stromal foci from true endometriosis, with which it is often confused. Intramural bleeding is usually not encountered, and, though occasional secretory changes may be seen, the term endometriosis interna does not apply correctly to adenomyosis. Classic endometriosis (see Chap. 37) is not commonly found with adenomyosis.

Pathology

Random sampling of uteri removed for other causes often reveals scattered foci of adenomyosis. The abnormality is detected in approximately 20 percent of uteri. Usually such findings are incidental and have no clinical significance. The cut surface of the myometrium has a coarsely trabeculated appearance, and islands of ectopic glands and stroma may be visible as tiny, scattered, slightly depressed foci. Occasionally these sites are soft and cystic and the myometrium may give a moth-eaten appearance. Associated changes, which are periodically seen, include cystic hyperplasia, a progestational response coinciding with the end of the menstrual cycle, and decidual transformation during pregnancy.

In uteri containing both adenomyosis and endometrial carcinoma, if the islands of ectopic endometrium have also undergone neoplastic transformation in response to a carcinogenic stimulus, it may be difficult to distinguish between such transformation in the ectopic glandular component and true myometrial invasion.

Clinical Significance

Although the finding of adenomyosis as incidental histopathology in hysterectomy specimens has been stressed, as a symptomatic clinical entity, the condition may be underdiagnosed. The disease may be the explanation of progressive secondary dysmenorrhea seen in women during their late thirties and forties, who have heavy menstrual bleeding associated with generalized pelvic discomfort. In such patients, the uterus is often globular, firm, tender to palpation, and sometimes asymmetrically enlarged. The pelvic findings may be confused with an intramural leiomyoma. Myomas are more common and may also coexist with adenomyosis.

Heavy bleeding in this age group is sometimes associated with endometrial hyperplasia. The bleeding problem, if it exists, should be assessed in its own context. Adenomyosis as an indication for hysterectomy would represent an exclusion diagnosis after other, more commonly encountered significant pathology had been ruled in or out. As a preoperative indication for hysterectomy, the diagnosis can be made with greater frequency if the entity is kept in mind and patients examined and followed over a period of time. Adenomyosis obviously does not constitute a gynecologic emergency nor is it a life-threatening lesion, either as a result of any complication or its incidence of neoplastic transformation. Hysterec-

tomy should be selectively considered only for patients with significant symptoms and pelvic findings and in whom other major pathology has been excluded.

MALIGNANT TUMORS

Sarcoma

Sarcomas are not common tumors. They constitute perhaps 1 percent of all malignant tumors of the uterus. In addition to their rarity, they present unique clinical and pathologic problems. Careful study of these tumors furnishes special insights into basic tissue reactions of structures derived from the Müllerian ducts. For both clinical and histogenetic reasons, it is customary to divide uterine sarcomas into two major groups: (1) leiomyosarcoma and (2) mesenchymal sarcoma (mixed mesodermal tumor) (see Table 42–1).

Although benign uterine leiomyoma (fibromyoma, "fibroid") is the most common tumor of the human species, its malignant counterpart is distinctly uncommon. It occurs in two forms which are clinically and pathologically distinct: (1) diffuse leiomyosar-

TABLE 42–1 Classification of Mesenchymal Sarcomas of the Uterus

I Pure sarcomas
A Pure homologous
1 Endolymphatic stromal myosis (stromatous endometriosis)
2 Endometrial stromal sarcoma
3 Fibrosarcoma (fibromyxosarcoma)
4 Angiosarcoma
B Pure heterologous
1 Rhabdomyosarcoma (including most examples of sarcoma botryoides)
2 Chondrosarcoma
3 Osteosarcoma
4 Liposarcoma
II Mixed sarcomas
A Mixed homologous
1 Stromal sarcoma plus stromal myosis
2 Carcinoma plus stromal sarcoma
B Mixed heterologous
1 Stromal sarcoma plus mixtures of I.B.
2 Carcinoma plus mixtures of I.B.
III Sarcoma, not otherwise classified
IV Malignant lymphoma

Source: Modified from Kempson, Bari

coma and (2) leiomyosarcoma arising in a preexisting leiomyoma.

Diffuse Leiomyosarcoma

Clinical Manifestations. The usual clinical background for diffuse leiomyosarcoma is a short history of pelvic discomfort or other symptoms associated with a rapidly expanding pelvic mass, generally in a woman over 40 years old. Abnormal uterine bleeding or dysuria may be present but neither symptom is common. The clinical picture is nonspecific. Examination reveals an enlarged nodular uterus, often three or four times normal size. Indications for laparotomy are usually present, and exploration of the pelvis often reveals a multinodular uterus distorted by soft, fleshy tumors (Fig. 42–12). The gross features of malignant disease which are encountered include adherence to adjacent structures such as the pelvic parietes, bladder, or rectosigmoid, and metastatic deposits in the omentum. Hysterectomy may be difficult to accomplish.

Pathologic examination of the specimen often reveals multiple, irregular tumor masses involving the uterine corpus, with infiltration into the broad ligaments and other pelvic supporting tissues. The masses may be confluent and, on section, exhibit a fleshy tan color with occasional foci of hemorrhage and necrosis. Microscopical examination discloses the typical features of a malignant tumor of smooth-muscle origin. Local pelvic recurrence is usually prompt, and the clinical course may be short. Most patients die within a year as a result of both recurrent

FIGURE 42–12 Leiomyosarcoma. Uterus, tubes, and ovaries representing a multinodular, distorted mass.

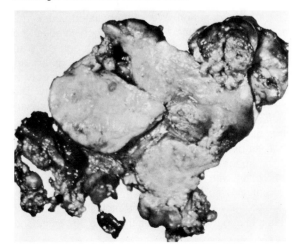

pelvic disease and secondary deposits in the lungs, liver, and other organs. Diffuse leiomyosarcoma does not respond appreciably to radiation therapy or chemotherapy.

Leiomyosarcoma in a Leiomyoma

Unlike diffuse leiomyosarcoma in which the ominous nature of the process is quite apparent, leiomyosarcoma arising in a preexisting leiomyoma is not usually diagnosed until careful histopathologic study has been made. The usual history is that a patient has had a hysterectomy for "fibroids," and the presence of malignant disease has not been suspected clinically. On pathologic examination, one of the multiple leiomyomas may appear different from the others. The cut surface does not show the usual pattern of interlacing bundles of smooth muscle but is rather homogeneous, often yellowish tan, and softer than the classic leiomyoma. Histopathologic examination reveals a smooth-muscle tumor of increased cellularity, and it is at this point that questions arise. The critical issue is the presence of increased mitotic figures. Occasional mitoses can be found in benign leiomyomas.

However, if mitotic figures are seen with ease and frequency in a cellular smooth-muscle tumor, the histopathologic diagnosis of leiomyosarcoma is usually warranted. Such tumors are often called "pathologist's cancer," because only a small proportion of them behave in a malignant fashion, i.e., recur locally or metastasize to distant sites. Nonetheless, smooth-muscle tumors with increased mitotic activity merit close scrutiny. Cases have been reported in which local pelvic recurrence has developed as late as 20 or 25 years after hysterectomy.

Histopathologic diagnosis is somewhat complicated by the question of symplastic giant cells, i.e., bizarre, multinucleated smooth-muscle cells. The atypical cells, alarming in appearance, may be found in smooth-muscle tumors undergoing ischemic change, in instances where growth has been stimulated by steroids (e.g., oral contraceptives), as well as in leiomyosarcomas. The presence or absence of mitotic figures rather than scattered multinucleated cells is the most reliable index of possible future malignant behavior.

Some degree of the complexity of the problem as well as its low numerical frequency can be found in a classic study of 1195 uterine smooth-muscle tumors (Przybora). Of these, 1090 (91.23 percent) were classified as leiomyoma simplex, and 66 (5.52 percent) as cellular leiomyoma; that is, 96.75 percent were clearly benign. In the remaining 39 cases (3.25 percent) 11 examples of "leiomyoma cum paratypia," 15 of "leiomyosarcoma in situ," 4 of "leiomyoma in sarcoma vertens," 7 of leiomyosarcoma fusocellulare, and 2 of leiomyosarcoma variocellulare were found. The 9 cases in the latter two categories were clearly malignant on histopathologic grounds, but the 30 cases in the other three categories were of borderline or questionable malignancy when judged on microscopical appearances. However, the 11 cases with "paratypia", i.e., with occasional bizarre cells, had a benign clinical course, and only 4 of the 15 patients diagnosed as having leiomyosarcoma in situ developed recurrent or metastatic disease. Thus, leiomyosarcoma very rarely develops in a preexisting leiomyoma, and the histopathologic grounds for making such a diagnosis remain imprecise. If any error is made, it is in the form of overdiagnosis, or else there is the possibility that the malignant process was fortunately resected in its entirety before it invaded beyond the benign leiomyoma in which it presumably arose.

Mesenchymal Sarcoma (Sarcoma Botryoides; Endolymphatic Stromal Myosis; Mixed Müllerian Tumor)

The various forms of neoplasm included under this heading are a special case of mesenchymoma (Stout). These tumors can be traced histogenetically to cells derived from the mesenchyme accompanying the Müllerian duct epithelium, a caudal proliferation of subcoelomic mesenchyme. Mesenchymal sarcomas of the female genital tract have been described at all ages from birth to senescence. The clinical and pathologic features, to some extent, depend upon both age and location.

Although exceptions have been noted, there is a tendency for these tumors to develop in infants, children, and young adults at the upper part of the vagina or the exocervix and present as complex, polypoid structures resembling a bunch of grapes, hence the term sarcoma botryoides. During the reproductive years in young women, mesenchymal sarcoma occurs more often in the cervix than in the corpus uteri. However, the proportion of this distribution is reversed after the menopause when the neoplasm tends to arise almost exclusively in the corpus.

In the adult, the cell of origin is the endometrial stromal cell or its congeners in the endocervical stroma. This is the least highly specialized cell in the female genital tract, and the complexity and variety of histologic patterns can be traced to variations of the pluripotency of this cell and the range of possible permutations and combinations of its transformation under special conditions. Any number of attempts have been made to classify these sarcomas, but in the long run they return to the descriptive analysis by Zenker in 1864. He described them as "pure," that is, composed of one cell type, or "mixed," composed of more than one cell type; and whether they contained only homologous elements, that is, direct derivatives of cells normally present in the uterus, or whether they contained heterologous elements, cells or tissues not normally indigenous to that organ (Zenker). Ober comprehensively reviewed the subject in 1959. A more recent classification combines simplicity with an emphasis on contemporary terminology (Table 42–1) (Kempson, Bari).

Clinical Manifestations. A majority of uterine mesenchymal sarcomas grow as polypoid, exophytic masses. This is certainly the characteristic feature of the botryoid growth in children, which enables a diagnosis to be made, or strongly suspected, on physical examination. In adults, it is not uncommon for such tumors to present as fleshy polypoid growths protruding through the cervical os. Vaginal spotting or bleeding may be an early symptom. When pelvic pain is due to uterine enlargement, the tumor is in an advanced state. Diagnosis of the malignant nature of the process is established by biopsy of accessible portions of the tumor. If the neoplasm has not extended downward far enough to become visible, curettage may be necessary. Finer classification of the tumor depends upon examination of carefully selected material from multiple sites and the application of special histopathologic staining methods.

In general, prognosis varies with the anatomic extent of tumor, resectability, and the degree of histologic differentiation. Well-differentiated, pure, homologous neoplasms which have not invaded the uterine wall very deeply have a better prognosis than poorly differentiated tumors with heterologous elements which have invaded the uterine wall deeply or diffusely and which seem to be growing rapidly. The best-differentiated form of uterine mesenchymal sarcoma is known as endolymphatic stromal myosis, stromatous endometriosis, and other synonyms. Despite its predilection for invading vascular and lymphatic spaces, it is slow-growing, composed of uniform cells with only rare mitoses. Following local extirpation of such primary uterine growths, pelvic recurrence may be quite late and metastasis to distant sites can occur after intervals from 5 to 30 years. One such case with histologically verified pulmonary metastases responded well to large doses of Depo-Provera; radiologically visible pulmonary deposits disappeared under treatment (Pellillo).

In general, however, well-differentiated mesenchymal sarcomas of the uterus are a minority in this family of tumors. The majority are poorly differentiated and invasive, and a high proportion of them contain such heterologous elements as striated muscle, cartilage, or bone. In such cases, the prognosis is usually unfavorable, most patients dying with recurrent or metastatic disease within 2 years. Neither radiotherapy nor chemotherapy exerts any appreciable effect on these poorly differentiated tumors. Between these extremes are a number of cases of moderately well-differentiated "pure, homologous" sarcomas derived from endometrial stroma and easily recognizable as such on microscopical examination. If such cases are recognized and hysterectomy performed before myometrial invasion is extensive, a guarded less unfavorable prognosis may be given. Taking the entire spectrum of mesenchymal sarcoma of the uterus together, the overall 5-year survival rate in most series is less than 20 percent. Exception must be made for series diluted by the inclusion of a large number of well-differentiated examples.

Carcinosarcoma

The most common form of mixed homologous mesenchymal sarcoma is the so-called carcinosarcoma, an admixture of neoplastic stromal and epithelial elements. The pathologist must guard against including in this category examples of undifferentiated carcinoma; the presence of a malignant stromal component must be demonstrated beyond doubt. In general, these are poorly differentiated, rapidly growing neoplasms which metastasize early. The metastases may be of either component or an admixture of both, but the presence of any metastasis is more decisive than its microscopical composition.

Retrospective analysis of series of mesenchymal uterine sarcomas usually reveals that a disproportionately high number of cases had received pelvic irradiation for benign disease at intervals of 10 to 25 years before the neoplasm became manifest. This is construed as evidence that a number of mesenchymal sarcomas have been radiation-induced. But an even greater proportion of such tumors have developed without antecedent irradiation. Clearly radiation is not the only possible element in the pathogenetic background.

SUBINVOLUTION OF THE PLACENTAL SITE: A VASCULAR DISORDER

The commonest cause of delayed postpartum bleeding is a lesion called subinvolution of the placental site. The lesion is vascular in nature, and it develops from unknown causes after either a term delivery or an abortion. The clinical entity is called delayed postpartum bleeding because, by arbitrary definition, it occurs following an interval of at least 1 week after delivery. Usually, the postpartum or postabortal course has been uneventful until suddenly there is a brisk flow of bright red blood from the uterus, unaccompanied by pain or other symptom. The hemorrhage may be brief and episodic, or it may continue until hospitalization. On examination, the uterus is found to be soft and boggy, and a variable amount of blood is frequently seen coming from a patulous, often bluish cervix. The patient is usually afebrile and clinically "well."

The clinical diagnosis generally considered is retained secundines, i.e., retention of some portion of the products of conception, and indeed such tissue may often be recovered when the patient is curetted. However, the vascular lesion is often present in the absence of retained secundines, and it is the vascular lesion which is microscopically distinctive and the cause of the bleeding.

In a reported series, 40 percent of the cases occurred between 1 and 4 weeks postpartum, 25 percent during the second, and 20 percent during the third postpartum month. Retained placental tissue was found in slightly over half the cases and was absent in slightly less than half. The presence of placental tissue is not necessarily a cause for the vascular lesion (Ober and Grady).

Myometrial contraction is probably the most effective hemostatic mechanism in biology. The anatomic distribution of smooth muscle about the uterine vasculature results in occlusion of uteroplacental blood vessels when postpartum contractions occur. In uterine atony, blood loss can be massive from failure of the uterine corpus to contract after expulsion of its contents, and a patient can almost exsanguinate in 15 minutes. The bleeding associated with abortion or term delivery is from the placental bed. Following primary hemostasis by uterine contraction, normally small and medium-sized blood vessels at the placental site undergo superficial thrombosis which seals them off. Whatever remains of decidua and tissue from the site of placental cleavage is passed physiologically as lochia. During the puerperium the endometrium regenerates, the superficial thrombi are resorbed, and the uterine blood vessels which have undergone considerable structural modification during pregnancy return to normal.

However, when subinvolution develops, the blood vessels do not return to normal even though the uterine mucosa may regenerate normally. During pregnancy, decidual transformation of the adventitia of the walls of both spiral arterioles and arteriae rectae occurs. Normally, decidua regresses by autolysis. However, abnormal regression may involve some form of hyalinization. If hyaline collars are formed around the circumference of these arterial channels, the vascular lumen is maintained in a rigid, dilated state, and the superficial thrombi do not resorb. In subinvolution, it is common for a medium-sized artery to be surrounded by a hyaline collar in which traces of decidual cells are seen. The lumen frequently contains an eccentric zone of partially organized thrombus, but alongside it is an open channel with liquid blood. Even if the tip of such vessels is sealed, the superficial thrombotic seal may give way, and a gush of arterial blood may be seen clinically. Parenthetically, postpartum or postabortal bleeding is bright red because of its arterial origin, in contrast to the dark purplish blood associated with bleeding from the distorted venules in hyperplastic or dysplastic endometria or the endometria associated with dysfunctional uterine bleeding.

Curettings from cases of delayed postpartum or postabortal bleeding are diagnosed by various terms in different laboratories. Almost invariably there is some necrotic tissue removed by the curet, which is accompanied by a modest inflammatory reaction. The latter is an exudation which is so universal that it must be considered physiologic. The terms postpartum endometritis or postabortal endometritis are often applied to such curettings. If any large fragments of decidua are removed by the curet, these, too, are accompanied by an inflammatory reaction, and "deciduitis" or retained decidua are commonly used terms. If a few fragments of chorionic villi are seen, or if a major portion of a cotyledon is detected, the specimen is properly labeled "retained placental tissue." However, when large fragments of placenta are retained, bleeding usually occurs in the first week of the puerperium. Another variant is the so-called placental polyp, which is really an example of focal placenta accreta. It is common to see a mixture of vessels, some of which have involuted normally and have tiny lumina admixed with dilated vessels, presumably in-

completely involuted with reference to the time interval following delivery. The former can serve as the microscopical controls for the latter.

In all these variations, the common denominator is failure of the placental-site blood vessels, specifically the spiral arterioles and arteriae rectae, to involute properly. In order to demonstrate the vascular pathology, it is often necessary to embed *all* the curetted material. Generally, the tendency is to look at endometrial glands and stroma or at decidua and chorionic villi, rather than at blood vessels. Since abnormal uterine bleeding is almost invariably associated with abnormal blood vessels, the blood vessels in the curettings from postpartum and postabortal patients should be focused upon. A greater awareness of the vascular nature of this disorder will result in an increased frequency of diagnosis of subinvolution.

Treatment consists of curettage followed by the administration of an oxytocic agent such as Ergotrate.

REFERENCES

Arias-Stella J: Atypical endometrial changes associated with the presence of chorionic tissue. *Arch Pathol* 58:112, 1954.

Asherman JG: Amenorrhea traumatica (atretica). *J Obstet Gynaecol Br Commonw* 55:23, 1948.

Benirschke K: The Uterus, in *Congenital Anomalies of the Uterus with Emphasis on Genetic Causes,* eds. HJ Norris et al., Baltimore: Williams & Wilkins, 1973.

Benjamin F et al.: Growth hormone secretion in patients with endometrial carcinoma. *N Engl J Med* 281:1448, 1969.

Bergman P: Sexual time, time of ovulation, and time of optimal fertility: studies on basal body temperature, endometrium and cervical mucus. *Acta Obstet Gynecol Scand* 29(Suppl 4):5, 1950.

————: Traumatic intra-uterine lesions. *Acta Obstet Gynecol Scand* 40(Suppl 4):1, 1961.

Christophersen WM et al.: Carcinoma of the endometrium: Study of changing rates over a 15 year period. *Cancer* 27:1005, 1971.

Dockerty MD et al.: Carcinoma of the corpus uterus in young women. *Am J Obstet Gynecol* 61:966, 1951.

End Results in Cancer, Report 4, DHEW Publ. NIH 73–272, 1972.

Forbes T: Synergisms and antagonisms of estrogens and progesterone in a mouse uterine bio-assay. *Endocrinology* 79:420, 1966.

Good RG, Moyer DL: Estrogen-progesterone relationships in the development of secretory endometrium. *Fertil Steril* 19:37, 1968.

Govan ADT: Tuberculous endometritis. *J Pathol* 83:363, 1962.

Greene JW Jr: Feminizing mesenchymomas (granulosa cell and theca cell tumors) with associated endometrial carcinoma. Review of the literature and a study of the material of the ovarian tumor registry. *Am J Obstet Gynecol* 74:31, 1957.

Gusberg SB, Kaplan AL: Precursors of corpus cancer IV. Adenomatous hyperplasia as stage 0 carcinoma of the endometrium. *Am J Obstet Gynecol* 87:662, 1963.

Hartman CG: *Science and the Safe Period.* Baltimore: William & Wilkins, 1962.

Hertig AT et al.: Genesis of endometrial carcinoma. III Carcinoma in situ. *Cancer* 2:964, 1949.

_____, Sommers SC: Genesis of endometrial cancer. I Study of prior biopsies. *Cancer* 2:946, 1949.

Heyman J et al.: Radiumhemmet experience with radiotherapy in cancer of corpus or uterus; classification, method of treatment and results. *Acta Radiol* 22:11–98, 1941.

Hitschmann F, Adler L: Der Bau der uteru Schleimhaut des geschlechtreifen Weibes mit besonderer Berucksichtigung der Menstruation. *Mschr. Geburtshilfe Gynakol* 27:1, 1908.

Hustin J.: Hormonal therapy of endometrial cancer: Effects of large doses given by parenteral or intracavity routes, in *Endometrial Cancer,* eds. MG Brush et al., London: Heinemann, 1973.

Israel SL et al.: Infrequency of unsuspected endometrial tuberculosis: A histologic and bacteriologic study. *JAMA* 183:149, 1963.

Jarcho J: Malformations of the uterus. *Am J Surg* 71: 106, 1946.

Kempson RL, Bari W: Uterine sarcomas: Classification, diagnosis, and prognosis. *Hum Pathol* 1:331, 1970.

Krantz KE: Innervation of the human uterus. *Ann NY Acad Sci* 75:770, 1958–59.

Lampe I: Endometrial carcinoma. *Am J Roentgenol Radium Ther Nucl Med* 90:1011, 1963.

Lees DH: An evaluation of the treatment in carcinoma of the body of the uterus. *J Obstet Gynaecol Br Commonw* 76:615, 1969.

Lerner LJ: Hormone antagonist: Inhibitors of specific activities of estrogen and androgen. *Recent Prog Horm Res* 20:435, 1964.

Lewis B: Nodule spread in relation to penetration and differentiation. *Proc R Soc Med* 64:406, 1971.

Malkani PK, Rajani CK: Pelvic tuberculosis and pregnancy. *Fertil Steril* 7:356, 1956.

Markee JE: Menstruation in intraocular endometrial transplants in the rhesus monkey. Pt I Observation of normal menstrual cycles. *Contrib Embryol* 28:219. 1940.

Mishell DR et al.: The intrauterine device. A bacteriologic study of the endometrial cavity. *Am J Obstet Gynecol* 96:119, 1966.

Moyer DL et al.: Investigations of intrauterine devices in *Macaca mulatta* monkeys. *Acta Endocrinol* 71 (Suppl 166):381, 1972.

_____ et al.: Reactions of human endometrium to the intrauterine device. 1. A correlation of the endometrial histology with the bacterial environment of the uterus following insertion of the IUD. *Am J Obstet Gynecol* 106:799, 1970.

_____ et al.: Sperm distribution and degradation in the human female reproductive tract. *Obstet Gynecol* 35:831, 1970a.

Noyes RW et al.: Dating the endometrial biopsy. *Fertil Steril* 1:3, 1950.

Nugent FB: Office suction biopsy of the endometrium. *Obstet Gynecol* 22:168, 1963.

Ober WB: Uterine sarcomas: Histogenesis and toxonomy. *Ann NY Acad Sci* 75:565, 1959.

_____, Grady HG: Subinvolution of the placental site. *Bull NY Acad Med* 37:713, 1961.

Pellillo D: Proliferative stromatosis of the uterus with pulmonary metastases: Remission following treatment with a long-acting synthetic progestin: A case report. *Obstet Gynecol* 31:33, 1968.

Price JJ et al.: Vaginal involvement in endometrial carcinoma. *Am J Obstet Gynecol* 91:1060, 1965.

Przybora LA: Leiomyosarcoma in situ of the uterus. *Cancer* 14:485, 1961.

Ramsey EM, Harris JWS: Comparison of uteroplacental vasculature and circulation in the Rhesus monkey and man. *Contrib Embryol* 38:59, 1966.

Reifenstein EC Jr: Hydroxyprogesterone caproate therapy in advanced endometrial carcinoma. *Cancer* 27:485, 1971.

Sala JM, del Regato JA: Treatment of carcinoma of the endometrium. *Radiology* 79:12, 1962.

Schmidt-Matthiesen H: Die Vaskularisierug des menschlichen Endometriums. *Arch Gynaekol* 196:575, 1962.

Schroder R: *Der normale menstruelle Cyklus der Uterusschleimhaut,* Berlin: Hirschwald, 1913.

Sharman A: Endometrial tuberculosis in sterility. *Fertil Steril* 3:144, 1952.

Sommers Sheldon C: The Uterus, in *Carcinoma of the Endometrium,* eds. HJ Norris, et al., Baltimore: Williams & Wilkins, 1973, chap. 14.

Sommers SC et al.: Genesis of endometrial carcinoma. II. Cases 19 to 35 years old. *Cancer* 2:957, 1949.

Stout AP: Mesenchymoma, the mixed tumor of mesenchymal derivatives. *Ann Surg* 127:278, 1948.

Strott CA et al.: The short luteal phase. *J Clin Endocrinol Metab* 30:246, 1970.

Strassman EO: Plastic unification of double uterus. *Am J Obstet Gynecol* 64:25, 1952.

Sutherland AM: Tuberculosis of the endometrium. *J Obstet Gynecol Br Commonw* 63:161, 1956.

Terenius L et al.: Binding of estradiol 17 beta to human cancer tissue of the female genital tract. *Cancer Res* 31:1895, 1971.

Tseng PY, Jones HW Jr: Chromosome constitution of carcinoma of the endometrium,. *Obstet Gynecol* 33:741, 1969.

Way SJ: Vaginal metastases of carcinoma of the body of the uterus. *J Obstet Gynaecol Br Commonw* 58:558, 1951.

Zenker FA: *Uber die Veränderungen der willkuhrlichen Muskeln in Typhus abdominalis: Nebst einem Excurs uber die pathologische Neubildung quergestreiften Muskelgewebes,* Leipzig: Vogel, 1864, pp. 84–86.

43

Gestational Trophoblastic Disease

MICHAEL L. BERMAN

UNIQUE FEATURES OF GESTATIONAL TROPHOBLASTIC DISEASE

HYDATIDIFORM MOLE
Pathologic features
Etiology
Diagnosis
Management
  Prophylactic chemotherapy
  Chorionic gonadotropin measurements
Prognosis
  Nonmetastatic tumor
  Low-risk metastatic tumor
  High-risk metastatic tumor

CHORIOADENOMA DESTRUENS

CHORIOCARCINOMA

The gestational trophoblastic diseases (GTD) consist of hydatidiform mole, chorioadenoma destruens, and choriocarcinoma. These pathologic entities result either from degenerative or neoplastic transformation of gestational trophoblastic elements. They are interrelated because hydatidiform mole invariably precedes chorioadenoma destruens. It precedes choriocarcinoma of gestational origin in 50 to 60 percent of instances. The diseases differ in their inherent biologic behavior. In approximately 90 percent of patients, hydatidiform mole regresses spontaneously after uterine evacuation. Chorioadenoma destruens characteristically is locally invasive with a limited tendency to metastasize. Choriocarcinoma usually grows rapidly and metastasizes early in the course of the disease.

UNIQUE FEATURES OF GESTATIONAL TROPHOBLASTIC DISEASE

Gestational trophoblastic disease is unique because of (1) its constant elaboration of human chorionic gonadotropin (HCG), (2) its exquisite responsiveness to chemotherapy, and (3) the presence of paternal transplantation antigens not found in the maternal host. The quantity of HCG secreted into the serum and excreted in the urine reflects the amount of functioning trophoblastic tissue, hence the amount of viable tumor. Specific sensitive assays for this hormone thus permit accurate monitoring of patients with GTD. Sequential measurements of HCG permit the clinician to determine (1) when therapy is indicated, (2) response to the therapy, and (3) follow-up status of patients after completion of therapy. The responsiveness of GTD to chemotherapy can be illustrated by comparing current survival rates with those of the era preceding effective antitumor agents. In 1961 Brewer reported that gestational choriocarcinoma, apparently confined to the uterus, was cured in only 40 percent of patients treated by hysterectomy. In contrast, trophoblastic disease, metastatic to lung or extrauterine sites in the pelvis, is now cured with chemotherapy in 90 to 95 percent of patients. The immunobiologic relationship between GTD and its host has attracted wide interest. Although many malignant neoplasms have been shown to contain tumor-associated antigens which can elicit an immune response, only the trophoblastic neoplasms of gestational origin also contain HLA antigens derived from the paternal genotype. It is possible, therefore, that the immunologic response mounted by the host against these tumors is different. The unique sensitivity to chemotherapy may represent synergistic action of a rejection phenomenon combined with the cytotoxic action of the drugs. Prior to the availability of effective chemotherapy, studies showed 2 to 6 percent of patients with metastatic choriocarcinoma lived 5 years, often with spontaneous regression of tumor. This fortunate but unusual occurrence can be explained entirely on an immunologic basis. Bagshawe has demonstrated that a marked mononuclear cell infiltration, usually considered a function of immunologic response, suggests a favorable prognosis in choriocarcinoma, while minimal or absent infiltration is associated with a poor prognosis.

The generic term GTD is preferable to hydatidiform mole, chorioadenoma destruens, or choriocarcinoma in the clinical setting since management of these neoplasms characteristically is determined by evaluation of HCG titers without precise knowledge of the histologic diagnosis. Criteria that appear to be more important than the histology in selecting a treatment regimen include (1) the presence or absence of metastases; and (2) when metastases are present, the specific sites of the metastases; duration of disease; and tumor volume as measured by quantitative determinations of HCG. Because of the important role of metastases in determining prognosis and treatment,

GTD is subdivided as metastatic (MTD) and nonmetastatic (NMTD) disease.

HYDATIDIFORM MOLE

PATHOLOGIC FEATURES

Hydatidiform mole is identified by characteristic gross and histologic changes in placental villi, usually without a coexisting fetus. The morphologic features common to this diagnosis include hydropic villi often measuring up to 1 cm in diameter, absence of fetal blood vessels, and varying degrees of hyperplasia of the cytotrophoblast and syncytiotrophoblast (Fig. 43–1). The etiology of these changes is unclear. Cytogenetic studies show that hydatidiform mole has a 46XX karyotype. Recent studies suggest that the total chromosomal content results from duplication of a paternal X-carrying haploid without any maternal contribution. The degree of hyperplasia and anaplasia of the trophoblast correlates with the risk of subsequent malignant sequelae; however, a mole with benign-appearing trophoblastic proliferation can undergo malignant change and, conversely, one with marked anaplasia and hyperplasia can regress spontaneously. Therefore, all patients with a histopathologic diagnosis of hydatidiform mole must be evaluated carefully and followed closely. It is unclear whether the morphologic changes seen are primarily degenerative, resulting from absent or inadequate fetal circulation, as advanced by Hertig, or neoplastic of low malignant potential, as suggested by Park. The hydatidiform mole diagnosis can be confused with the hydropic degenerative changes often seen with early spontaneous abortion, but the later is distinguished by the absence of associated trophoblastic hyperplasia. The importance of hydatidiform mole relates to the risk of subsequent malignant sequelae. Although only 10 to 20 percent of women with this diagnosis require treatment, approximately 85 to 90 percent of women needing chemotherapy for GTD had an antecedent molar gestation.

ETIOLOGY

The reported incidence of hydatidiform mole varies widely according to age, locale, and socioeconomic conditions. It occurs more often in older women, ten

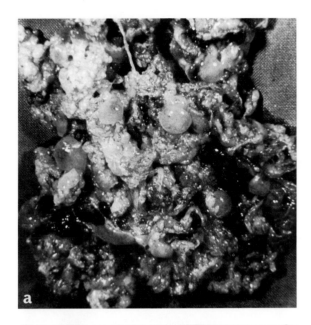

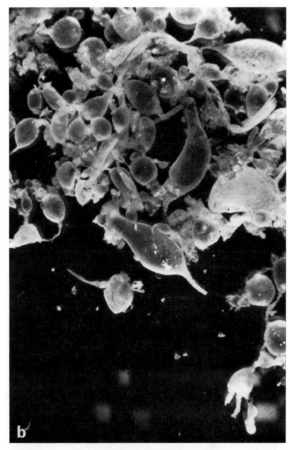

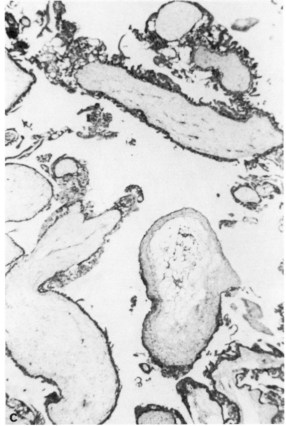

FIGURE 43–1 *A* and *B* Characteristic vesicular changes in a hydatidiform mole. *C* Hydropic avascular villi with focal hyperplasia of the trophoblast.

times more frequently in patients after age 45 than in those under age 40. It is the outcome of approximately 3000 pregnancies in the United States each year, an incidence estimated at 1 in 1500 pregnancies. In other developed nations, including Scandinavian countries and Australia, the incidence is similar to that reported in the United States. In less developed areas, including Mexico and Taiwan, the diagnosis is made 10 to 15 times more frequently. In the Philippines, the incidence in private patients is 1 in 2000; in a poorer clinic population, the occurrence is 10 times higher. The overall incidence in the Philippines during World War II, when there was widespread malnutrition in that country, was approximately 1 in 100 pregnancies. Li has reported that the incidence of gestational choriocarcinoma in Asians who immigrate to the United States falls to a level between that of the two geographic locales. These data

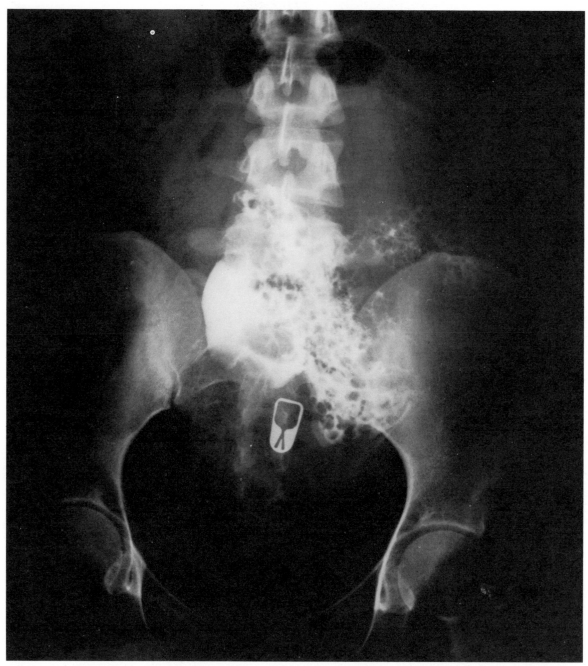

FIGURE 43-2 Amniography of hydatidiform mole with dye seen between hydropic villi. Note the absence of fetal outline *(By permission of Ballon et al.)*

suggest both nutritional and genetic factors in the etiology of the disease.

DIAGNOSIS

The diagnosis of hydatidiform mole should be considered in any patient with bleeding during the first two trimesters of pregnancy. Bleeding occurs in over 90 percent of molar pregnancies and can be intermittent or continuous, ranging from spotting to brisk hemorrhage. Because of the frequency and nonspecificity of bleeding in early pregnancy, additional findings usually are necessary to make this diagnosis. Disproportionate uterine growth is a common finding. Hypertension and proteinuria rarely encountered in the first two trimesters of pregnancy, are seen in 25 percent of patients with molar pregnancies, and hyperthyroidism is seen as a complication in about 5 percent. In 40 to 50 percent the diagnosis is confirmed by passage of characteristic clear grapelike vesicles. Symptoms commonly noted include intermittent low abdominal pain, excessive nausea and vomiting sometimes requiring hospitalization, and complaints indicating toxemia, such as visual disturbances, excessive weight gain, and edema.

Diagnostic studies can include abdominal roentgenogram, amniography, and ultrasonography. Abdominal roentgenograms are of value if the uterus extends above the umbilicus. Since coexisting fetus and mole gestations rarely occur, the hydatidiform mole diagnosis is unlikely if a fetal skeleton is visible; it is supported if a skeleton is not seen. The roentgenogram is less sensitive than either amniography or sonography, both of which are accurate in more than 90 percent of patients. With amniography, a dry amniotic tap suggests hydatidiform mole; the characteristic honeycomb appearance noted after injection of radiopaque dye is diagnostic (Fig. 43–2). In most centers, B-mode scanning, which has equal diagnostic accuracy, causes less discomfort, and carries no risk of radiation exposure or injury to a normal gestation, is preferred (Fig. 43–3). Sonography also can identify theca lutein cysts which result from ovarian hyperstimulation by HCG and which often coexist with GTD. HCG determinations are mandatory in following patients with GTD but are unreliable in diagnosing hydatidiform mole.

FIGURE 43–3 B-mode ultrasound scan of hydatidiform mole showing multiple homogeneous internal echoes and absent fetus.

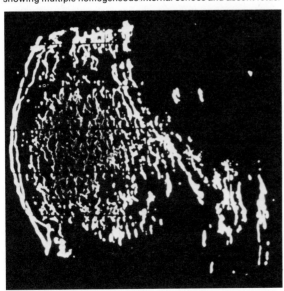

MANAGEMENT (Fig. 43–4)

Once the diagnosis is established, management should consist of uterine evacuation as promptly as practicable because malignant sequelae are markedly increased in untreated patients. The easiest and least morbid way to effect this is by suction curettage, even in the presence of marked uterine enlargement. Simultaneous administration of oxytocin and Ergotrate will minimize blood loss; however, because of the relative insensitivity of the uterus to oxytocics during the first two trimesters of pregnancy and the frequent brisk bleeding associated with uterine evacuation, blood should be available for immediate use. Oxytocin should be administered at a rate of 0.5 to 1 unit per minute during curettage and continued at 0.5 units per hour for 2 to 3 hours. Oxytocin administered prior to curettage appears to increase the risk of transport of molar tissue to the lungs, with subsequent respiratory embarrassment; it therefore should be given after the uterus is evacuated. The rapid rate of oxytocin infusion necessitates careful monitoring of urinary output since oxytocin's infrequent transient antidiuretic effect can cause congestive heart failure if excessive amounts of saline are administered, or can cause water intoxication if large volumes of salt-free fluids are given. If further childbearing is not desired, alternate initial management can consist of total abdominal hysterectomy. This operation minimizes the risk of malignant sequelae but does not eliminate it. The same careful follow-up must be carried out as for women treated initially with suction curettage.

PROPHYLACTIC CHEMOTHERAPY

Goldstein and Reid have advocated the use of one course of prophylactic chemotherapy in managing women at the time of uterine evacuation. They demonstrated an eightfold reduction in malignant sequelae using actinomycin D for 5 days, beginning 3 days prior to uterine evacuation. This regimen has not gained wide acceptance because 80 to 90 percent of women who would not require chemotherapy are exposed to the inherent risks of potent antitumor agents. Furthermore, the prognosis for cure of patients with malignant sequelae who have been under close scrutiny following uterine evacuation approaches 100 percent making routine prophylactic treatment of all patients seem unwarranted. In addition, Bagshawe found that prophylactic therapy can be associated with resistance to later multiple drug therapy if GTD persists.

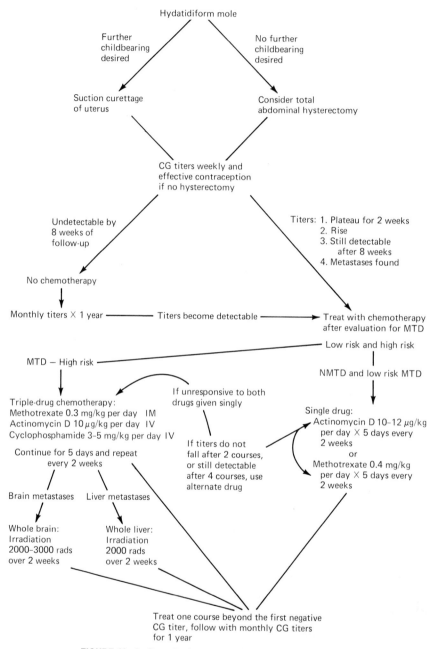

FIGURE 43–4 Steps in the management of hydatidiform mole.

CHORIONIC GONADOTROPIN MEASUREMENTS

Following uterine evacuation, patients should be monitored closely with quantitative HCG determinations. Because the biologic and immunologic properties of this double-chain (α and β) glycoprotein per-

mit bioassay, immunoassay, and radioimmunoassay (RIA), some confusion concerning sensitivity and specificity of the assays exists. The commonly performed pregnancy tests are examples of immunoassays using hemagglutination-inhibition and latex-fixation techniques. Although they are simple and inexpensive to perform, the relative insensitivity of the tests makes them of little value clinically in managing patients with GTD. These assays can detect a minimum of 750 IU of HCG per liter, but 25 percent of patients who require chemotherapy for NMTD will have titers below this level. Bioassay techniques are more sensitive, but are cumbersome and lack specificity because HCG and luteinizing hormone (LH) have similar biologic properties. The development of RIA provided a simple, highly sensitive technique for HCG measurement in small volumes of serum. Because of differences in the β chain of HCG and LH, Vaitukaitus et al. were able to develop an RIA which did not cross-react with LH. Radioimmunoassays currently available can measure as little as 0.003 to 0.005 IU of HCG per milliliter of serum and are highly specific, having minimal cross-reactivity with LH. These assays should be employed in managing all patients with GTD.

All patients under observation or treatment following evacuation of a hydatidiform mole must use an effective means of contraception since HCG from a subsequent gestation would be indistinguishable from that secreted by GTD. Birth control pills are preferred because of their efficacy, and are mandatory if an assay technique which does not distinguish HCG from LH is used. In this instance, the combination pills will suppress pituitary LH to undetectable levels. When birth control pills are used, they should not be started before the HCG titers become undetectable because the time interval from evacuation to unmeasurable titers is increased as is the incidence of patients requiring chemotherapy.

PROGNOSIS

Chorionic gonadotropin determinations should be performed weekly following evacuation of a hydatidiform mole. Delfs demonstrated that 80 percent of patients will have undetectable levels of HCG 8 weeks following uterine evacuation. Half of the remaining patients if followed without treatment will have undetectable titers within 6 months of follow-up. Of the final 10 percent of patients, approximately 8 percent will have chorioadenoma destruens and 2 percent will have choriocarcinoma. Because 50 percent of patients with detectable titers 8 weeks following evacuation will have malignant sequelae, chemotherapy usually is administered to these patients. Similarly, patients in whom titers of HCG rise or reach a plateau for 2 successive weeks following evacuation should be treated. A chest x-ray and pelvic examination should be performed at the time of diagnosis and monthly thereafter until the titers are undetectable. Any patient whose examination or chest x-ray demonstrates metastases should be treated immediately. Factors which increase the risk of malignant sequelae include age greater than 40 years, hyperplastic and anaplastic appearance of the trophoblastic tissue, uterine size larger than expected for the length of gestation, and presence of theca lutein cysts.

Any patient with GTD should undergo a careful evaluation before her physician institutes chemotherapy. Commonest sites of metastases are the lungs, vagina, and pelvis. Brain and liver metastases occur in 10 to 12 percent of patients. Therefore, studies performed should include a chest x-ray, liver function tests, liver scan, brain scan, and neurologic and pelvic examinations. If any metastases are found, a 24-hour urine collection must be obtained for quantitative HCG determination. Because chemotherapeutic agents used in managing GTD can cause bone-marrow depression, hepatotoxicity, or nephrotoxicity and are partially excreted by the kidneys, a complete blood count, blood urea nitrogen, serum creatinine, serum glutamic oxaloacetic transaminase (SGOT), and serum glutamic pyruvic transaminase (SGPT), should be obtained.

NONMETASTATIC TUMOR

If the evaluation for metastatic disease is negative, chemotherapy should consist of either actinomycin D or methotrexate. Both drugs can cause bone-marrow depression, stomatitis, ulcerations in the gastrointestinal tract, skin rash, nausea, vomiting, diarrhea, and alopecia. Actinomycin D often is employed as the drug of first choice because it does not cause the hepatic and neurologic damage sometimes seen with methotrexate. Moreover, it is not associated with the potentially fatal complications of methotrexate when administered to patients with impaired renal function. Actinomycin D must be given intravenously with great caution because extravasation will result in marked local tissue destruction. The recommended dosage of actinomycin D is 9 to 13 μg/kg per day intravenously for 5 days. This course should be repeated every 2 weeks until 3 successive weekly titers are undetectable. If there is no consistent decline and titers plateau or rise, indicating the need to change drugs, prompt intervention is necessary. Methotrexate is equally effective in treating GTD and can be used in lieu of actinomycin D. The recommended dosage of methotrexate is 0.4 mg/kg per day intramuscularly for

5 days, repeated as described for actinomycin D. Newer treatment regimens using higher doses of methotrexate with citrovorum, a specific antidote to the cytotoxic drug, are being investigated for the management of NMTD with the prospect for equal efficacy with minimal toxicity.

LOW-RISK METASTATIC TUMOR

When metastases are present, the treatment is determined by (1) the sites of metastases, (2) the duration of disease, as measured from the termination of the antecedent pregnancy, and (3) the tumor volume, as measured by the HCG titer. Patients with metastases confined to the pelvis or lungs, in whom the duration of disease is less than 4 months, and whose quantitative HCG in a 24-hour urine collection is less than 100,000 IU are characterized as "low risk" to fail single-drug chemotherapy. They are treated with actinomycin D or methotrexate as described above.

HIGH-RISK METASTATIC TUMOR

All other patients with MTD are "high risk" to fail single-drug chemotherapy and must be started initially on intensive triple-agent chemotherapy consisting of methotrexate, actinomycin D, and either cyclophosphamide or chlorambucil. The dosage of these drugs is as follows:

	Methotrexate	0.3 mg/kg IM
	Actinomycin D	10 μg/kg IV
or	{ Chlorambucil	0.2 mg/kg PO
	{ Cyclophosphamide	3 to 5 mg/kg IV

All drugs are administered daily for 5 days and are repeated every 2 weeks until 3 successive weekly HCG titers are undetectable. Chemotherapy is postponed if the neutrophil count is less than 1500 or the platelet count is less than 100,000 per cubic millimeter, and subsequently should be reinstituted at a lower dosage to permit an optimal treatment interval of 2 weeks. When metastases to brain or liver are present, adjunctive radiation therapy can improve survival; 2000 to 3000 rads should be delivered to the whole brain or 2000 rads to the liver, at a rate of 1000 rads per week. When high-risk patients are managed in this way, survival approaches 75 percent. However, if the patients are treated initially with a single drug, the survival rate is less than 25 percent even if more intensive therapy is administered later.

Other therapeutic measures which have been in-stituted include intrathecal methotrexate for resistant central-nervous-system metastases, or intraarterial infusion of methotrexate for resistant disease localized to the uterus. Surgery may be required to treat complications of disseminated disease, including small bowel obstruction and hemorrhage in the gastrointestinal tract or central nervous system. Since metastatic sites are sometimes more responsive to chemotherapy than the primary uterine tumor, hysterectomy may be indicated to cure disease in the pelvis. Thus far, most attempts at both specific and nonspecific, active and passive immunotherapy have been unsuccessful in treating GTD when it is resistant to conventional therapy. However, occasional responses to *Corynebacterium parvum* have been reported.

In patients under therapy whose HCG titers become undetectable, 90 percent will remain in complete remission; up to 10 percent will demonstrate a secondary rise in titers. Of the patients who relapse, most will have measurable HCG titers within 2 months of the initial negative titer; 1 to 2 percent will have a delay of up to 1 year. Therefore, all patients with GTD must be followed for 1 year following the initial undetectable HCG titer. Studies of the subsequent reproductive performance of patients with GTD have demonstrated high fertility, but there is a 4 percent risk of partial placenta accreta in patients who had prior chemotherapy. A reported 15 percent rate of subsequent abortion is similar to the rate in pregnancies without a history of antecedent GTD.

CHORIOADENOMA DESTRUENS

A more descriptive term in common use for chorioadenoma destruens is invasive mole. It is always preceded by a hydatidiform mole and is the outcome of approximately 8 to 10 percent of such pregnancies. Histologically it exhibits those features described for hydatidiform mole, but is distinguished by its invasion into the myometrium. Clinically it is characterized by uterine bleeding and often by abdominal pain. Uterine perforation can occur spontaneously from extensive myometrial penetration or can follow instrumentation at the time of curettage. This complication can result in death from exsanguination or sepsis in approximately 5 to 10 percent of patients. When perforation is recognized in association with chorioadenoma destruens, hysterectomy is indicated. Since

GTD confined to the uterus (NMTD) can represent either chorioadenoma destruens or choriocarcinoma, the histologic diagnosis can be made only by examining tissue following a hysterectomy or vigorous curettage in which both endometrium and myometrium are sampled. Therefore, in most instances, the histologic diagnosis of NMTD is uncertain when chemotherapy is instituted, and the term chorioadenoma destruens rarely has clinical applicability. In addition, because chorioadenoma destruens can metastasize, especially to vagina or lung, the definitive histologic diagnosis of MTD is not established in most instances.

CHORIOCARCINOMA

Choriocarcinoma is an aggressive malignant neoplasm which is usually fatal within 2 years if untreated. It can originate as a primary tumor of the gonad or arise in the trophoblastic elements of a gestation. Despite early and frequent metastases by the hematogenous route as well as rich vascular communication between the uterus and ovaries, metastases from gestational choriocarcinoma to the ovaries occur infrequently. Choriocarcinomas of ovarian or gestational origin are indistinguishable histologically and are characterized by extensive hemorrhage, necrosis, and exuberant growth of both syncytiotrophoblast and cytotrophoblast, and by the absence of villi. Grossly, these tumors are purplish because of rich vasculature and coexisting hemorrhage. They contain areas of necrosis because the rapidly dividing cells of the tumor outgrow their blood supply. Both tumors elaborate HCG and have similar patterns of metastases, commonly to the lungs and vagina, although nongestational choriocarcinoma is more likely to spread by the lymphatic and transperitoneal routes. Choriocarcinoma of gestational origin is more sensitive to antineoplastic agents, but aggressive chemotherapy can also cure patients with gonadal choriocarcinoma.

Choriocarcinoma of gestational origin is preceded by hydatidiform mole in approximately 50 percent of patients and by an abortion, ectopic pregnancy, or apparently normal gestation in the remainder. As with chorioadenoma destruens, when choriocarcinoma is preceded by a molar gestation, the histopathologic diagnosis usually is unknown, and again the terms NMTD and MTD have greater

clinical relevance. The prognosis for patients with choriocarcinoma following a nonmolar gestation appears to be worse than after hydatidiform mole, possibly because delayed diagnosis is more common and results in more advanced disease in the former group of patients. Choriocarcinoma should be suspected in any woman of childbearing age who has evidence of unexplained uterine bleeding following a gestation, metastatic cancer, or a cerebrovascular accident. It can be confirmed by the presence of measurable HCG in the absence of pregnancy. When the diagnosis is made, chemotherapy must be instituted immediately. The evaluation, chemotherapy, and follow-up of patients with choriocarcinoma following a nonmolar gestation are identical to procedures described above for GTD following a hydatidiform mole. Initial therapy consists of either actinomycin D or methotrexate alone, unless the high-risk factors discussed previously are present. Chemotherapy for patients with choriocarcinoma arising in the ovary should consist of triple therapy—actinomycin D, methotrexate, and cyclophosphamide.

REFERENCES

Bagshawe KD: Trophoblastic tumours and teratomas, in *Medical Oncology Medical Aspects of Malignant Disease,* Oxford: Blackwell Scien Pub, 1975, p. 453.

Ballon SC et al.: The unique aspects of gestational trophoblastic disease. *Obstet Gynecol Surv* 32: 405,1977.

Brewer JI et al.: Choriocarcinoma. *Am J Obstet Gynecol* 85:841, 1963.

Curry SL et al.: Hydatidiform mole—diagnosis, management and long-term follow-up of 347 patients. *Obstet Gynecol* 45:1, 1975.

Delfs E: Quantitative chorionic gonadotropin prognostic value in hydatidiform mole and chorionic epithelioma. *Obstet Gynecol* 9:1, 1957.

Goldstein DP, Reid DE: Recent developments in the management of molar pregnancy. *Clin Obstet Gynecol* 10:313,1967.

Hammond CB et al.: Treatment of metastatic trophoblastic disease; good and poor prognosis. *Am J Obstet Gynecol* 115:451, 1973

———, Lewis JL Jr: Gestational, trophoblastic neoplasms, in *Gynecology and Obstetrics,* vol. 1, New York: Harper & Row, 1972.

———, Parker, RT: Diagnosis and treatment of trophoblastic disease—a report from the Southeastern Regional Center. *Obstet Gynecol* 35:132, 1970.

Hertig AT, Edmonds HW: Genesis of hydatidiform mole. *Arch Pathol* 30:260, 1960.

Lewis JL Jr: Current status of treatment of gestational trophoblastic disease. *Cancer* 38:620, 1976.

_____ et al.: Treatment of trophoblastic disease. *Am J Obstet Gynecol* 96:710, 1966.

Li MC: Trophoblastic disease; natural history, diagnosis, treatment. *Ann Intern Med* 74:102, 1971.

Park WW: *Choriocarcinoma. A Study of Its Pathology,* Philadelphia: Davis, 1971.

Ross GT et al.: Chemotherapy of metastatic and nonmetastatic gestational trophoblastic neoplasms. *Texas Rep Biol Med* 24:326, 1966.

Vaitukaitus JL et al.: A radioimmunoassay which specifically measures human chorionic gonadotrophin in the presence of human luteinizing hormone. *Am J Obstet Gynecol* 113:751, 1972.

44

Fallopian Tubes

CARL J. PAUERSTEIN   RONALD S. GIBBS

NORMAL DEVELOPMENT

CONGENITAL ANOMALIES

INFLAMMATORY LESIONS
Pyogenic salpingitis (pelvic inflammatory disease)
Salpingitis isthmica nodosa
Granulomatous salpingitis
    Tuberculosis
    Leprosy
    Actinomycosis
    Bilharziasis (schistosomiasis)
    Oxyuriasis (Enterobius vermicularis)
    Sarcoidosis
    Foreign-body salpingitis

MALIGNANT TUMORS
Primary carcinoma of the fallopian tube
Carcinoma in situ
Carcinoma
Metastatic or combined malignancies
Other malignant tumors of the tube
    Mixed mesodermal tumors
    Sarcoma
    Trophoblastic tumors (hydatidiform mole and
    choriocarcinoma)

BENIGN TUMORS OF THE FALLOPIAN TUBE
Epithelial tumors

Endothelial or mesothelial tumors
Mesodermal tumors
Benign teratoma
Miscellaneous tumors

NORMAL DEVELOPMENT

The development of the Müllerian (paramesonephic) system is closely related to the Wolffian (mesonephric) system, which is in turn the successor to the pronephric duct. The undifferentiated gonad arises from the mesenchyme of the medial portion of the urogenital ridge. The pronephric tubules, which are connected to the pronephric duct by the fourth week of embryonic life, arise from the lateral portion of the urogenital ridge. By the sixth week, the Müllerian cleft appears between the gonadal and pronephric portions of the urogenital ridge. The Müllerian cleft is the open cranial extremity of what is destined to become the Müllerian duct, the precursor of the oviducts and uterus.

    The pronephric duct is completed by the end of the seventh week and is then called the mesonephric duct. The pronephric tubules have been replaced by the mesonephric tubules, which will degenerate when the mesonephros ceases to function as an excretory organ. Remnants of duct and tubules may persist in the paraovarian region of the adult. Immediately lateral to the mesonephric duct, the solid tip of the Müllerian cord begins to grow caudally, using the mesonephric duct as a guidon. The caudal tip of the Müllerian cord actually lies within the basement membrane of the mesonephric duct. The two become separate only after the Müllerian cord develops a lumen. The Müllerian cord crosses ventrally to lie medial to the Wolffian duct in the pelvis. The Müllerian ducts eventually reach the urogenital sinus, where their tips cause an elevation of the dorsal wall of the sinus (Müller's) tubercle. Each duct finally forms a tube, from the cranial ostium to Müller's tubercle, where it will later open into the urogenital sinus.

Experiments on infraprimates have shown that if embryos are castrated at the indifferent stage the mesonephric ducts disappear, and female internal ducts develop. A testis implanted in a female fetus causes regression of the Müllerian ducts and development of the Wolffian ducts. In contrast, a testosterone crystal will support Wolffian development but does not cause Müllerian regression. Thus, the inducing or organizing effect of the embryonic testis has two components: stimulation of the Wolffian ducts and inhibition of the Müllerian system. Testosterone can accomplish only the former. In the absence of fetal gonads, the genital primordia display their inherent female growth potential.

By the end of the third month, the mesonephric ducts in the female have largely disappeared. The medial walls of the right and left Müllerian ducts fuse. Fusion usually starts at Müller's tubercle and progresses cranially, ending at the junction of each duct with the round ligament. This process results in a single tube with two lumens. The median septum then disappears, completing the creation of the uterus simplex. Canalization may begin at any point along the fused ducts and can proceed in either direction. Fusion and canalization are complete by the 16th week. The muscular and connective-tissue layers of the oviduct begin to be sketched in mesenchymal concentrations during the third month. Marked growth occurs in the oviducts beginning at the 185-mm stage (about 16 weeks) and continuing until the 315-mm stage (about 20 weeks) is reached. By 4 to 5 months of embryonic life, characteristic arrangements can be clearly discerned. The differentiation of the ampulla, with its large lumen and complex plicae, occurs during the last trimester. The epithelium of the human oviduct is well developed at birth. Ciliated and secretory cells can be identified.

CONGENITAL ANOMALIES

Some, but not all, of the encountered congenital anomalies can be explained by referring to the sequence of normal development. Complete absence of the paramesonephric duct results in absence of the tubes, uterus, and upper vagina. This defect can occur in the presence of completely normal ovaries, as evidenced by normal secretion of luteinizing hormone, follicle-stimulating hormone, estrogen and progesterone in such women (Fraser et al.) Just as normal ovaries do not assure normal oviducts, neither do all castrates develop female internal ducts. A recent report concerned a patient with 46XX chromosome constitution. The patient displayed a Turner's syndrome phenotype. A rudimentary streak ovary and a fallopian tube were present on her left. On the right side, the ovary and tube were absent, as was the uterus. Since no testis was found, these findings are difficult to reconcile with our knowledge of embryogenesis (Wong et al.). Conversely, a recent report documented the presence of an oviduct on the same side as an ovotestis in a true hermaphrodite with a 46XX/46XY chromosome complement (Park et al.). This suggests that the ovotestis may behave like a normal ovary with regard to oviductal development. The other possibilities are that the testicular portion of the ovotestis was not functional, or that the ovotestis in aggregate had the effect of a streak gonad or functional castrate.

If development is arrested after formation of the Müllerian cleft and the cephalad portion of the Müllerian cord, formation of the oviducts, but not of the uterus or vagina, results. If only one Müllerian duct is arrested, the failure is usually complete, resulting in the uterus unicornis, an apparently normal uterus with only a single oviduct. In such conditions the kidney and ureter on the affected side may be missing.

Tubes with accessory ostia and multiple lumens have been described. The actual frequency of such abnormalities is unknown.

INFLAMMATORY LESIONS

PYOGENIC SALPINGITIS (PELVIC INFLAMMATORY DISEASE)

Salpingitis is a common and potentially serious infection, occurring an estimated 600,000 times per year in the United States. Physicians who treat women must be familiar with this condition and consider it in every female with lower abdominal pain.

Etiology and Pathogenesis

Recent investigations have improved our understanding of the bacteriology of acute salpingitis. Since Albert Neisser isolated the gonococcus, *Neisseria gonorrhoeae,* in 1879, this organism has traditionally been considered the causative organism in most cases of acute, pyogenic (nongranulomatous) salpingitis. However, it is now clear that acute salpingitis may be either gonococcal or nongonococcal. Each type accounts for approximately 50 percent of cases overall, with an apparently wide geographic variation.

In gonococcal salpingitis, *Neisseria gonorrhoeae* is, by definition, isolated from the cervix. In cultures of the peritoneal exudate of such patients (usually obtained by culdocentesis), a variety of observations have been made. Most recent investigators report *N. gonorrhoeae* (either in pure or mixed culture) in approximately half of the patients (Cunningham; Eschenbach; Monif). Others have found the gonococcus in the peritoneal exudate much less frequently and have reported mixed cultures of anaerobic and aerobic organisms (Chow). Further investigations are necessary to determine the exact role of the gonococcus.

In nongonococcal salpingitis, *N. gonorrhoeae* is not found either in the cervix or the peritoneal exudate. Rather, a variety of anaerobic and aerobic organisms are found. Bacteria commonly found in these specimens include *Bacteroides* species, aerobic and anaerobic streptococci, and *E. coli*. From other investigations it appears that *Chlamydia trachomatis* may also frequently be involved in acute salpingitis (Mardh et al.) The role of mycoplasma remains uncertain.

Chronic salpingitis is usually caused by mixed anaerobic and aerobic bacterial invaders. Early statements that most tubal abscesses were sterile reflected poor anaerobic technique.

In the mid-1970s, strains of penicillinase-producing *N. gonorrhoeae* (PPNG) were first isolated in the United States. Absolutely resistant to penicillin originally, these strains were traced to Southeast Asia and presently account for only a very small percentage of all gonococcal isolates in this country. Most isolates of PPNG have been from asymptomatic carriers, but some have been from patients with salpingitis or disseminated gonococcal disease. At the present time, PPNG has been susceptible to spectinomycin (Trob-

icin). Should these strains increase in frequency, major revisions in antibiotic strategies may be required.

The prevalence of gonorrhea is increasing, and the concept that gonorrhea is a disease solely of the lower socioeconomic classes is now untenable. Although the advent of chemotherapy has decreased the relative incidence of many of the sequelae of gonorrhea, the absolute increases of cases of gonorrhea have been so great that numbers of patients suffering complications of gonorrhea are now seen. In addition to salpingitis, disseminated gonococcal infection may include perihepatitis, carditis, meningitis, arthritis, and cutaneous lesions (Kraus).

Normally, the gonococcus remains localized in the endocervix by body defenses, and only 10 to 15 percent female gonococcal carriers develop acute salpingitis (Eschenbach and Holmes). If these localizing defenses are overcome by an alteration in the host-organism relationship, the gonococcus usually spreads contiguously along the mucosal surfaces. Less frequently, gonococci may spread by lymphatic or vascular channels, especially in pregnancy. The route of infection for nongonococcal salpingitis is uncertain, but most cases probably also arise from mucosal spread.

One of the most common alterations of the host-organism relationship is menstruation; 66 percent of all cases develop during or within 7 days of its onset. The intrauterine device (IUD) may also alter the host-organism relationship in favor of salpingitis (Gibbs). From recent indirect epidemiologic studies, it appears that IUD users are at an increased relative risk (calculated to be from four- to nine fold) for salpingitis. Other studies, however, have pointed out that the absolute risk of pelvic inflammatory disease in IUD users is still low (1 to 2.5 percent). Pregnancy has also been considered a predisposing cause to disseminated gonococcal disease (such as arthritis). However, salpingitis is extremely unusual during a gestation perhaps because the amniotic sac obstructs mucosal spread of the bacteria.

Clinical Diagnosis

The onset of symptoms of *acute salpingitis* usually coincides with the menses. Bilateral or diffuse pelvic pain and alteration of the menstrual flow are the initial complaints. Many patients note fever and chills and an increase in vaginal discharge. Other symptoms such as nausea, vomiting, anorexia, urinary frequency and dysuria occur in about 20 to 25 percent of patients (Jacobson and Westrom; Eschenbach and Holmes).

The patient with acute salpingitis usually does not appear toxic; mild degrees of pyrexia (100 to 102°F) are the rule. Bacteremic chills are rare. The abdomen is usually distended; bowel sounds are hyperactive, and point tenderness is not prevalent. Diffuse guarding over the hypochondria, often with rebound tenderness, is present. Pelvic examination may reveal Bartholin adenitis or a urethral discharge. However, these features, as well as cervical discharge and gross appearance of the cervix, are nonspecific findings. Motion of the cervix and uterus classically causes pain. Palpable masses or swellings may occur in up to 25 percent of patients despite the tenderness and guarding. The parametria are tender and edematous. Acute salpingitis is a bilateral condition in over 90 percent of cases. Unilateral symptoms should suggest other diseases in the differential diagnosis.

The clinical diagnosis of acute salpingitis is subject to considerable error. In one study, 814 patients were diagnosed as having acute salpingitis on the basis of acute abdominal pain and on two other of the following criteria: (1)discharge, (2) fever (only 41 percent had fever), (3) vomiting, (4) menstrual irregularities, (5) pelvic tenderness on bimanual examination, and (6) adnexal mass. The oviducts were visualized by laparoscopy, and salpingitis was diagnosed by the presence of oviductal hyperemia, edema, or a sticky exudate on the serosal surface and at the fimbriated ends when patent. The clinical diagnosis of acute salpingitis was visually verified in only 65 percent of cases overall; 12 percent had some other disease, and 23 percent had no pathology (Jacobson and Westrom).

In general, the more signs and symptoms a patient had, the better was the diagnostic accuracy. Thus in the patient with *bilateral* lower abdominal pain, fever, tender adnexal mass, and increased vaginal discharge, the diagnostic accuracy was 90 to 95 percent. Further, some cases of mild PID may have been missed by the laparoscopic criteria employed.

The patient with *chronic salpingitis* usually presents with complaints of lower abdominal pain, often without other symptoms. Physical findings may include lower abdominal and adnexal tenderness, perhaps with palpable masses.

At times, salpingitis may be clinically inapparent or may masquerade as other diseases. As many as 20 percent of cases of fever of unknown origin have been found at laparotomy to be due to chronic salpingitis (Barr et al.).

Among the entities confused with salpingitis are gastrointestinal problems such as appendicitis, diverticulitis, regional enteritis, ulcerative colitis, and spastic colon; other gynecologic diseases such as ectopic pregnancy, abortion, rupture of ovarian cysts, adnexal torsion, and endometriosis; and urinary-tract conditions, such as stones, pyelonephritis, and cystitis. Pain of pelvic origin emanates from the pelvic viscera and from any involvement of the parietal peritoneum. Thus, the differentiation of salpingeal pain from pain arising in other viscera becomes difficult, particularly when the peritoneum is also involved (Guerrero et al.).

Laboratory Diagnosis

The white blood count is elevated in only half of patients with acute salpingitis, and the erythrocyte sedimentation rate (ESR) may be abnormally high in 75 percent. An elevated ESR may persist for months. A urinalysis and abdominal radiograph may be helpful to rule out other diagnostic entities.

Bacteriologic Diagnosis

It is important to culture the endocervix for *N. gonorrhoeae,* but as this is a fastidious organism, special care is necessary. A swab should be obtained and immediately inoculated onto selected Thayer-Martin plates and placed in a candle jar. Alternatively, good results may also be obtained with transport media such as Transgrow bottles.

Yet, cervical cultures may be unreliable in proving the etiology of salpingitis. Because the gonococcus is so fastidious, cultures are falsely negative in about 15 to 20 percent of cases. In addition, most women who harbor endocervical gonococci are asymptomatic. Thus, a patient may be an incidental carrier of gonococci and have a completely different disorder as the cause of her acute symptoms.

Further, Gram's stain of the cervical exudate is of little value in identifying gonococci because of inherent false-negative and false-positive results and lack of experience of most physicians (Eschenbach et al.).

Culturing the endocervix for *organisms other than gonococci* is pointless in view of the poor correlation between their isolation in the cervix and in the peritoneal exudate (Chow).

A culdocentesis may be performed, especially if the diagnosis is uncertain or if a ruptured tuboovarian abscess is suspected. In acute salpingitis, a culdocentesis often yields a purulent or seropurulent fluid. In contrast to the endocervical sample, this specimen should be immediately examined by Gram's stain for bacteria and leukocytes. With proper handling, this specimen should then be sent for aerobic and anaerobic cultures. Nonclotting blood obtained upon culdocentesis is the hallmark of intraperitoneal hemorrhage, commonly from a ruptured ectopic pregnancy.

Laparoscopy and Laparotomy

Because of the error seen with clinical diagnosis of acute salpingitis, laparoscopy may be employed to establish the diagnosis. In Swedish studies, this technique has been remarkably free of complications (Jacobson and Westrom), and it should probably be employed more often.

At times, a patient with lower abdominal pain may undergo a laparotomy and then be found to have acute salpingitis. In this case, a specimen of the exudate should be obtained for Gram's stain and aerobic and anaerobic culture (with selective Thayer-Martin media). The abdomen should be closed and the patient treated with antibiotics. No further surgery is warranted.

Pathologic Diagnosis

The tube in acute gonococcal salpingitis is reddened, swollen, and edematous, usually with a purulent exudate dripping from the patent fimbriated end Histologic examination reveals vascular engorgement and edema of the plicae. Inflammatoy infiltrate of polymorphonuclear leukocytes and plasma cells involves the epithelium and lumen. The infiltrate sometimes also involves the stroma and muscular layers. Small patches of epithelial desquamation may be seen (Fig. 44–1). Alternatively, acute salpingitis

may result in an edematous tube, with absence of luminal exudate and minimal insult to the mucosa. Perisalpingitis, inflammation of the myosalpinx, and involvement of the mesosalpinx are common in such cases.

Chronic salpingitis presents as a spectrum, depending upon the degree of damage to the tubal mucosa and the amount of fluid accumulated. These entities include pyosalpinx, chronic endosalpingitis, follicular salpingitis, hydrosalpinx follicularis, hydrosalpinx simplex, and chronic interstitial salpingitis.

Pyosalpinx results from an acute infection superimposed upon a chronic salpingitis. The occluded abdominal ostium prevents drainage of the purulent exudate, which then accumulates in the lumen. The distended tube is usually adherent to the surrounding structures, due to associated perisalpingitis. If the tube becomes adherent to the ovary, a tuboovarian abscess may form.

Microscopic examination reveals purulent exudate in the lumen. The mucosal plicae are flattened and often agglutinated. The lamina propria is infiltrated with plasma cells, lymphocytes, and polymorphonuclear leukocytes. This infiltrate usually penetrates the markedly thickened tubal musculature with predominant perivascular concentrations. Resolution of the acute infection leaves the tubal plicae adherent to varying degrees. Extreme adherence divides the lumen into multiple smaller channels, giving an appearance termed *follicular salpingitis* (Fig. 44–2). Should this tube begin to be distended by fluid accumulation, the designation *hydrosalpinx follicularis*

FIGURE 44–1 Acute salpingitis. Inflammatory infiltrate of plicae and lumen.

FIGURE 44–2 Chronic salpingitis. Slightly dilated lumen surrounded by agglutinated folds and the resultant adenomatous pattern of follicular salpingitis.

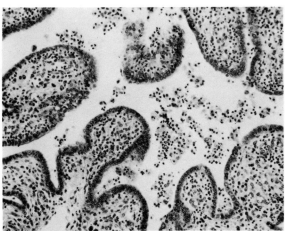

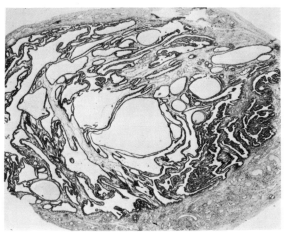

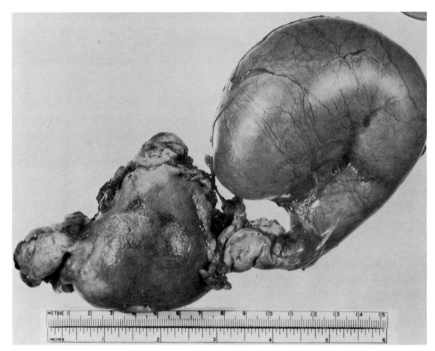

FIGURE 44–3 Hydrosalpinx. The ampullary portion of the oviduct is greatly dilated with fluid. The tube and ovary adhere to each other. The fimbriae and ostium cannot be identified.

is applied. In some instances, the distended lumen consists of a single cavity and is called *hydrosalpinx simplex* (Fig. 44–3). The epithelium in hydrosalpinx simplex is compressed, varying from a low cuboidal to an extremely flattened mesothelial type. Generally, one or several fronds of the mucosal folds protrude into the cavity, and on these the normal epithelial architecture including the cilia is remarkably well preserved.

In chronic interstitial salpingitis, the tube is enlarged due to thickening of the wall, rather than to the accumulation of intraluminal fluid. The distal end is usually clubbed, although some of the fimbriae may be preserved. Perisalpingitis causes adhesions to the pelvic peritoneum and surrounding structures. The inflammatory exudate, composed chiefly of lymphocytes and plasma cells, involves all the layers of the tube.

Treatment

Salpingitis may be treated on an in- or outpatient basis. If the patient is mildly ill and thus a candidate for outpatient treatment, her regimen should consist of bed rest, abstinence from coitus, adequate oral hydration, and antibiotics.

Acute gonococcal salpingitis may be treated with procaine penicillin, 4.8 million units intramuscularly with 1.0 g probenecid orally, followed by ampicillin 500 mg by mouth four times a day for 10 days. The procaine penicillin alone is adequate therapy for cervical gonorrhea only. For penicillin-allergic patients, tetracycline 1.5 g orally initially, followed by 500 mg orally four times a day for 10 days is recommended. Outpatient therapy for nongonococcal salpingitis is less well established. Since gonococcal salpingitis can never be ruled out with certainty in an emergency room setting (i.e., based upon Gram's stain), initial therapy ought to be effective against the gonococcus as well. In addition, recent trials have found that the penicillin-ampicillin or tetracycline regimen recommended for gonococcal disease is equally effective with nongonococcal (Cunningham et al.). It is necessary to see the patient within 7 days to ascertain the clinical response and to reculture for gonorrhea. If there is any worsening, the patient should be instructed to return immediately.

For more severely ill patients, inpatient treatment is indicated. Patients with these criteria are best treated in the hospital: (1) acute salpingitis with an adnexal mass; (2) acute salpingitis with marked symptoms or findings including high fever, nausea, vomiting or upper abdominal signs; or (3) an uncertain diagnosis.

Most of these patients will respond to medical management consisting of bed rest in semi-Fowler's position, correction of fluid and electrolyte imbalances, and antibiotics. Because of the wide spectrum of microorganisms which may cause salpingitis, the initial antibiotic selection should be effective against the gonococcus as well as the other pelvic pathogens. This area has not been well studied, but various regimens include intravenous ampicillin, intravenous tetracycline or doxycycline, and intravenous penicillin (20 million units per day) with an aminoglycoside (gentamicin or kanamycin). When a tuboovarian abscess is suspected or when there is failure of the above regimens, clindamycin or chloramphenicol should be employed because of the likelihood of *B. fragilis*.

Most women respond to this therapy, although several days may elapse before control is satisfactory. The best prognostic criteria are resolution of fever, tachycardia, and abdominal findings. The recommended therapy for gonococcal and presumably for nongonococcal PID is for continuation of antibiotics for 10 days. A bimanual examination should be performed to evaluate the patient for residual adnexal disease prior to discontinuing therapy. If a mass is detectable, we favor continuing antibiotics and re-evaluating.

Unfortunately, some cases of PID do not respond to antibiotic therapy since a patient may develop a tuboovarian or pelvic abscess. Such abscesses may "leak" or rupture. A "leaking" pyosalpinx may respond to intensive antibiotic therapy, but frank rupture is catastrophic. Rupture may be suspected if the abdominal findings persist or worsen, if the patient becomes lethargic, and if the pulse rate increases. Prior to 1947, ruptured adnexal abscesses with generalized peritonitis were treated with simple cul-de-sac or peritoneal drainage. The mortality in American clinics was 48 to 100 percent. Since the mid-1950s, therapy has included total extirpation of the uterus, tubes, and ovaries. The mortality rate promptly fell, especially when the operation was performed within the first 12 hours after rupture. More than 90 percent of patients are cured by extirpative operations (Altemeier et al.).

Unruptured tuboovarian abscess is generally treated initially with systemic antibiotics. Therapy is continued until the patient becomes afebrile. However, if the patient fails to respond to medical therapy, surgical intervention is indicated. If the pelvic abscess dissects down the rectovaginal septum to within a few centimeters of the introitus, drainage may be accomplished by colpotomy. Surgical treatment may vary from drainage only to removal of the involved side to removal of uterus, tubes, and ovaries (Fraser). The latter is usually the treatment of choice.

Other patients with chronic salpingitis do not suffer acute exacerbations, but complain of incapacitating chronic pelvic pain, abnormal uterine bleeding, and recurrent low-grade fevers. These women may be candidates for surgical treatment, depending upon the degree of incapacitation. Rarely, a patient may demonstrate other morbidity from chronic salpingitis, such as ureteric obstruction with hydronephrosis (Cox et al.). If surgical therapy is elected, the gynecologist should await a quiescent period in the illness. Bilateral cornual resection has been used successfully in the past to prevent acute exacerbations of chronic salpingitis, but modern gynecologists favor total abdominal hysterectomy and bilateral salpingo-oophorectomy, although some will attempt to conserve a normal-appearing ovary.

Prognosis

The prognosis for life with acute salpingitis is excellent. The prognosis for future well-being is less optimistic. Because many such patients are exposed repeatedly to venereal infection, it is difficult to decide whether subsequent exacerbations are due to recurrence or to reinfection. Acute salpingitis compromises future fertility. Swedish investigators have recently reported tubal obstruction in 12 percent of patients with one laparoscopically-proven infection, 35 percent of patients with two infections, and 75 percent of patients with three or more infections. It has previously been believed that gonococcal PID was more devastating to fertility than was nongonococcal disease. However, in Sweden, results to the contrary have been found in patients in whom the diagnosis was confirmed laparoscopically and microbiologically (Westrom).

As noted above, some patients with acute salpingitis develop chronic salpingitis, often complicated by recurrent acute exacerbations. These women endure several acute episodes of PID yearly, generally in relationship to menstruation and the proliferative phase of the cycle. While most of them respond satisfactorily to conservative measures and content themselves with intermittent freedom from acute pain, a small percentage are incapacitated. They are troubled with infertility and nonrhythmic uterine bleeding, and some develop life threatening complications that warrant surgical intervention.

SALPINGITIS ISTHMICA NODOSA

Although early writers were convinced that salpingitis isthmica nodosa occurred as an aftermath of acute salpingitis, this etiology is not universally accepted. It is quite possible that this lesion is more analogous to adenomyosis. Arguments advanced for and against various etiologies have no particular clinical pertinence.

About half of women with salpingitis isthmica nodosa are also infertile. The reasons for this association remain obscure. The lesion is generally asymptomatic and is not diagnosed on physical examination. Hysterosalpingography may reveal the typical honeycombed or stippled appearance caused by retention of opaque medium in the diverticula.

At operation, salpingitis isthmica nodosum is characterized by the presence of nodules involving the isthmic portion of the tube. These nodules impart a shotty feel to the isthmus. Microscopic examination discloses hypertrophy of the tubal musculature, with minimal scarring. The muscular layer is infiltrated with various-sized glandlike structures which extend to the serosal surface (Fig. 44–4). They are usually lined by typical tubal epithelium. These glandular spaces are true diverticula and connect with the tubal lumen.

GRANULOMATOUS SALPINGITIS

Although genital tuberculosis is the most important cause of granulomatous salpingitis in North America,

FIGURE 44–4 Salpingitis isthmica nodosa with adenomatous patterns throughout the wall of the tubule. No evidence of inflammatory infiltrate can be seen. *(From Woodruff and Pauerstein.)*

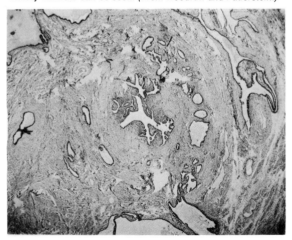

other entities can cause granulomatous reaction in the oviducts. These include leprosy, actinomycosis, bilharziasis, enterobiasis, sarcoidosis, and foreign-body reactions.

TUBERCULOSIS

Etiology and Pathogenesis

Genital tuberculosis is nearly always a manifestation of systemic tuberculosis. Primary genital tuberculosis is either nonexistent or extremely rare. For reasons not completely understood, menarche increases a girl's vulnerability to tuberculosis. This apparent activation of tuberculosis, manifested by greater morbidity and mortality in women than in men, persists until after the menopause. However, the incidence of genital tuberculosis in postmenopausal women may be increasing (Roberts).

Systemic tuberculosis passes through four stages. The first appears about 5 or 6 weeks after infection and is associated with the "primary complex." The next stage, which lasts approximately 3 months, includes miliary tuberculosis, tuberculous meningitis, and generalized tuberculosis. The third stage, pleuritic manifestations, occurs about 3 months after the primary infection and lasts about 4 months. The fourth stage exists until the primary complex has healed, or for roughly 3 years following the initial infection. Clinical and laboratory studies suggest that hematogenous dissemination of bacilli and implantation in the genital tract take place shortly after the primary infection is established. The closer to the menarche that the primary infection occurs, the greater the likelihood of genital tuberculosis developing. At menarche, the pelvic infection may become symptomatic because of systemic changes in the female organism. The latent period between primary genital infection and manifestation of genital tuberculosis averages about 10 years. In many women no overt clinical manifestations occur and genital tuberculosis remains latent, to become clinically symptomatic in later life or to be found in an otherwise asymptomatic patient during the course of an infertility study. It is, therefore, rational to treat every tuberculin-positive girl with specific chemotherapy for 1 year pre- and postmenarche as recommended by the American Academy of Pediatrics.

The prevalence of genital tuberculosis varies with geography and socioeconomic status. Older reports noted genital tuberculosis in 1 to 3 percent of female autopsies, and in up to 12 percent of autopsies on women with pulmonary tuberculosis. However, with the advent of chemotherapy, extragenital tuberculosis is decreasingly found at autopsies of women with pulmonary tuberculosis. As judged from extirpated oviducts and from endometrial biopsies, the incidence of genital tuberculosis among infertile women varies from less than 2 percent in America to almost 20 percent in India.

Clinical Diagnosis

The prominent historical findings in patients with genital tuberculosis are a family history of tuberculosis, past history of tuberculosis, history of infertility, amenorrhea, and pelvic pain. About 20 percent of patients who have genital tuberculosis have been exposed to a tuberculous member of their immediate family. Similarly, although pulmonary lesions are demonstrable in only one-third of patients with genital tuberculosis, a much higher percentage manifest either concurrent or historical extragenital tuberculosis. Particular attention should be directed to the association of urinary-tract tuberculosis and genital tuberculosis in the female. Of patients with genital tuberculosis 60 to 85 percent are infertile. Although the infertility may be related to abnormal ovarian function and systemic disease, it probably depends upon bilateral involvement of the fallopian tubes. A high percentage of Indian women suffering from genital tuberculosis complain of amenorrhea, but this is not true in the United States. Indeed, in America menstrual disorders are no more frequently associated with genital tuberculosis than with other gynecologic conditions. Although Schaeffer states that pelvic pain is the most common symptom of genital tuberculosis, and other authors recognize this complaint in a large number of their cases, at least half the patients with genital tuberculosis are free of pain. In fact, patients in whom infertility is the presenting symptom rarely have other symptoms or signs (Morris et al.).

The physical findings in tuberculous salpingitis are variable. Although as many as 50 percent of patients may present with adnexal masses, and shortening of the parametrium and vaginal vault has been described, there are no physical findings typical of genital tuberculosis. In many patients the pelvic examination is normal.

In summary, the "typical" patient with genital tuberculosis will be between 20 and 40 years of age, will likely present a history of extragenital tuberculosis, and will be infertile. In areas of the world where pulmonary tuberculosis is endemic, she will often complain of amenorrhea and abdominal pain. A palpable pelvic mass or a contracted left vaginal fornix

may be present. However, in many instances she will be asymptomatic and the pelvic organs will be normal to palpation.

Clinical examination may be supplemented by hysterosalpingography or laparoscopy. Salpingography causes few complications in patients with genital tuberculosis and may be helpful in suggesting the need for further evaluation of an infertile patient. The salpingographic changes are nonspecific. Histologic and bacteriologic diagnoses are necessary to establish a positive diagnosis of genital tuberculosis.

Palmer and Oliveira advocated the visual diagnosis of tuberculosis by laparoscopy. If the endometrial biopsy was negative and hysterosalpingograms suggested tuberculosis, but typical granulations were not seen, they biopsied the tubes at laparoscopy. Twenty-eight percent (27 biopsies) of a total of 99 tubal biopsies performed for suspected tuberculosis were unsatisfactory. Evidence of tuberculosis was found in 34 cases. They concluded that laparoscopy had a definite place in the diagnosis of latent genital tuberculosis.

Laboratory Diagnosis

Laboratory methods employed to establish the diagnosis of genital tuberculosis include pathologic examination of surgical material, bacteriologic examination of surgical material or menstrual discharge, and animal inoculations from the above materials.

Pathologic Diagnosis

The tuberculous fallopian tube is classically described as having a "tobacco pouch" appearance, with the tube enlarged and distended because of occlusion proximal to the everted, patent, fimbriated end. This "typical" gross pathologic appearance is seen in only a minority of cases. More commonly, the gross appearance is similar to that of chronic nontuberculous salpingitis. The interstitial and isthmic portions of the tube may be uninvolved. The abdominal ostium may be patent in as many as 50 percent of cases. If concomitant tuberculous peritonitis exists, the serosal surface of the tube and adjacent pelvic peritoneum may be studded with tubercles.

The microscopic diagnosis of tubal tuberculosis may be difficult. Many sections may reveal only nonspecific inflammatory change; however, thorough examination usually reveals tubercle formation. The epithelioid reaction is often more striking than the giant-cell formation. Other changes such as hyperplasia of the endosalpingeal folds and adenomatous hypertrophy of the tubal mucosa may suggest tuberculous salpingitis. Extreme adenomatous patterns resulting from agglutinations of the mucosal folds and associated epithelial hyperplasia may lead to the erroneous diagnosis of carcinoma (Puflett). Caseation is rarely seen. The presence of Schaumann bodies (birefringent rounded crystals, soluble in mineral acids, and easily disintegrated by microincineration) may support the diagnosis of tuberculous infection. Even in the absence of positive acid-fast smears most granulomatous lesions demonstrating these characteristic histologic criteria are usually due to tuberculous infection. However, unless tubercle bacilli are identified, a diagnosis of "granulomatous salpingitis" should be made because other conditions may cause similar histologic pictures.

Bacteriologic Diagnosis

The bacteriologic diagnosis of tuberculosis is more precise. Bacteriologic examination may be performed on tissues, on menstrual blood, and on fluids obtained by aspiration from the peritoneal cavity. Although various clinics have claimed superiority of one technique over another, there is little agreement. With careful bacteriologic study, including repeated cultures of menstrual blood and animal inoculations, a positive bacteriologic diagnosis should be obtained in about 75 percent of cases (Morris et al.; Woodruff and Pauerstein). Animal inoculation, cultures, and histologic examination are complementary, not competitive, techniques.

In summary, positive guinea pig inoculation or other bacteriologic demonstration of the Mycobacterium gives proof of tuberculosis. The classic histologic picture of granulomatous salpingitis, including gaint-cell formation with epithelioid reaction, is strongly suggestive of tuberculosis. Marked adenomatous reaction should increase the index of suspicion. Tubal biopsies taken under laparoscopic control may be utilized in cases with suggestive but unproven evidence of tuberculosis. Hysterosalpingography provides supportive but nonspecific information.

Treatment

The treatment of tuberculous salpingitis has changed with increased experience in the use of antibiotic and chemotherapeutic agents. Early in the use of such agents, both the appropriate combination of drugs and the duration of therapy were in question. It has now become apparent that longer periods of treatment will cure some patients in whom short-duration

therapy failed. All clinics agree that medical therapy plays a very important part in the attack on genital tuberculosis. Many clinics utilize surgical therapy in addition to medical treatment.

Most hospitals employ streptomycin, PAS (para-aminosalicylic acid), and INH (isonicotinic acid hydrazide) in some combination. A common method is to use streptomycin in a dose of 1 g twice weekly for the first 12 to 15 weeks in combination with PAS and INH. Therapy is continued with PAS and INH for at least 18 months. INH is generally given in a dose of 5 mg per kilogram of body weight, which approximates 300 to 400 mg daily, and PAS in a dose of 12 g daily. Some authorities treat tuberculous tubal occlusion with INH, PAS, and streptomycin combined with a daily dose of 25 to 30 mg of cortisone given intramuscularly. Patients are more apt to take their medicine faithfully if they are hospitalized for the first 6 weeks of treatment. In European clinics there has been a trend toward the use of topical therapy such as uterotubal or intraperitoneal instillation, parametrial infiltration, and vaginal aerosols with the addition of cortisone and/or trypsin to the chemotherapeutic agents.

Although few authorities advocate primary surgical removal of tuberculous adnexa, many experienced clinicians do think that surgery plays a role in the treatment of genital tuberculosis. Long-term drug therapy may eventually sterilize all endometria and oviducts. However, it is questionable whether several years of drug therapy are always preferable to a shorter course followed by surgery. Surgery should be considered in cases where pain or adnexal masses persist after a course of chemotherapy, in patients who will not continue long-term therapy and follow-up, and where malignancy is suspected. Surgery should not be performed without a preoperative course of drug therapy. If unsuspected genital tuberculosis is discovered at laparotomy for pelvic inflammatory disease or peritonitis, a small biopsy should be taken, the abdomen closed, and chemotherapy started (Schaefer). Antituberculous drugs should be given for at least 18 months after any operation for genital tuberculosis. Some authors have attempted tubal reconstructive surgery following adequate chemotherapy. The results have been discouraging. Because of the low success rate and the high risk of ectopic pregnancy, salpingoplasty is contraindicated when the tubes have been damaged by tuberculous salpingitis.

In summary, modern therapists agree that patients with genital tuberculosis should be given antibiotics and chemotherapy for a period of time. Those who favor surgical intervention operate after relatively short-term chemotherapy and then continue the medications for varying periods. It is likely that no patient should be operated upon electively prior to a minimum of 18 months of chemotherapy. At the end of that time, if the patient has residual masses or persistent pain, or reverts to positive endometrial histology or cultures, surgical intervention may be indicated. If surgery is undertaken it should consist of abdominal hysterectomy and bilateral salpingo-oophorectomy.

Prognosis

With appropriate chemotherapy and selected surgical intervention, the prognosis with regard to life and general well-being is good. However, the prognosis for reproductive function is poor. Patients with advanced genital tuberculosis should be considered permanently infertile, although term pregnancies may occur after adequate chemotherapy in patients with minimal tubal disease. Whereas the association of ectopic pregnancy with genital tuberculosis was rare prior to the advent of chemotherapy, an increasing number of ectopic gestations have been reported in treated patients.

LEPROSY

Leprous involvement of the female genitalia is uncommon, even in endemic areas. Gynecologic leprosy occurs in the ovary, cervix, myometrium, and tube, in that order of frequency. Involvement of the tube is unusual.

The histologic picture of leprosy may be nearly identical to that of tuberculosis. Langhans' giant cells and epithelioid cells may be prominent. The acid-fast stain is usually, although not invariably, positive in these lesions. It is often impossible to distinguish leprosy from tuberculosis by histopathologic examination (Woodruff and Pauerstein).

ACTINOMYCOSIS

More than 100 cases of actinomycosis of the fallopian tube have been reported. The causative agent belongs to the *Actinomycetales* group of fungi, as do the Mycobacteriaceae of tuberculosis and leprosy, and is named *Actinomyces,* or ray fungus, a term descriptive of its appearance in tissues and exudate. *A. israelii,* the organism pathogenic for man, is a normal and common inhabitant of the mouth and intestinal tract and becomes pathogenic when the environment is favorable, particulary if the oxygen supply to the

tissues is markedly diminished. Adnexal involvement is probably secondary to infection in the appendix or intestinal wall, although the lesion is seldom demonstrated in the bowel adjacent to the adnexal mass. Although the right tube should be more frequently involved, due to proximity to the appendix, nearly half the cases described in the literature are bilateral. Cases of tubal actinomycosis have been reported following abortion and other instrumentation. Ascending infection is also suggested by anecdotal cases of adnexal involvement which developed with an IUD in place (Gibbs).

Clinical Diagnosis

There is no typical clinical picture of oviductal actinomycosis. In the early stages the disease is confused with appendicitis and with other varieties of salpingitis. The most commonly affected group is age 20 to 40.

Pathologic Diagnosis

The gross appearance is that of a tuboovarian inflammatory mass. On cut section, cavities filled with necrotic material and pus give the involved tissue a honeycombed appearance in which yellowish granules may be found.

The microscopic pathology is similar to characteristic lesions elsewhere (Fig. 44–5). Bacteriologically, *Actinomyces* is nearly always found in mixed culture with other anaerobic or aerobic organisms.

FIGURE 44–5 Actinomycosis of tube with "sulfur" granule in lower right with surrounding inflammatory infiltrate and epithelioid reaction in lower left. *(From Woodruff and Pauerstein.)*

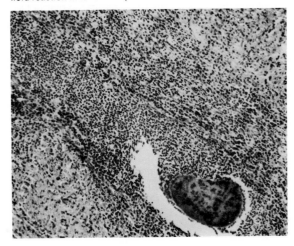

Treatment

Antimicrobial therapy in the form of large doses of penicillin should be continued for at least 5 weeks and may be necessary for as long as 3 years (Woodruff and Pauerstein).

BILHARZIASIS (SCHISTOSOMIASIS)

Tubal bilharziasis is rare and presents a difficult problem in diagnosis, because schistosomiasis and tuberculosis tend to be prevalent in the same geographic areas.

The preferential migration of the schistosome species explains the relative prevalence with which they cause involvement of the female genital tract. The female genital tract is involved in almost every case of *S. haematobium* in women. *S. mansoni* is less likely to involve female genital organs (Gelfand et al.), and *S. japonicum* involves the female genital tract only rarely.

Clinical Diagnosis

The clinical diagnosis of schistosomiasis of the fallopian tube is difficult. The reported range of ages is from 7 to 58. Most patients present with pain in the right lower quadrant and menorrhagia, and many complain of infertility. Even in endemic areas, this diagnosis is usually unsuspected.

Pathologic Diagnosis

When extruded into the tissue, the ova may cause a granulomatous reaction, with giant and epithelioid cells surrounded by fibroblasts and round cells. An eggshell or its fragments may be identified in the granuloma (Fig. 44–6). The reactions of the oviduct to schistosomes and their ova is quite variable (Bland and Gelfand; Coetzee and Jaffe).

OXYURIASIS (ENTEROBIUS VERMICULARIS)

Several cases of granulomatous salpingitis due to *Oxyuris* infestation have been reported. Current evidence suggests that the worm gains access to the peritoneal cavity by migrating through the vagina, cervix, uterus, and fallopian tube.

The pathologic findings are small pseudotubercles with granuloma formation, epithelioid cells, and multinucleated giant cells. Nodules may be scattered about the pelvic peritoneum, causing confusion with tuberculosis.

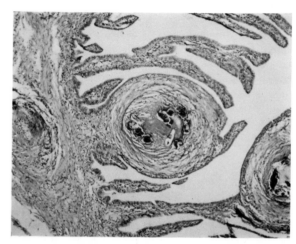

FIGURE 44–6 Schistosomiasis of tube with calcified shell fragments in mucosal folds but no associated tissue reaction. Tubercle-like reaction may be seen at the far left. *(From Woodruff and Pauerstein.)*

SARCOIDOSIS

Sarcoidosis may be a cause of granulomatous salpingitis. However, so few cases have actually been found that one need not seriously consider this diagnosis when granulomatous salpingitis is encountered, unless the patient is known to have sarcoidosis.

FOREIGN BODY SALPINGITIS

Among the foreign bodies causing granulomatous salpingitis are radiographic contrast media, mineral oil and other vaginal lubricants, starch and talc powder, suture materials and other foreign bodies introduced by operative procedures, and perhaps spermatozoa. Although oily radiographic contrast media are usually considered more likely than water-soluble agents to cause granulomatous salpingitis, granulomas are also produced by the latter. Bacteriologic confirmation is necessary before considering a granulomatous salpingitis to be of foreign-body origin even in the absence of caseation, fibrosis, or exudative disease.

Pathologic Diagnosis

The lesion may contain giant cells of either Langhans' or foreign-body type, in addition to epithelioid cells, lymphocytes, and plasma cells. Caseation is absent. Polarized light may reveal birefractile crystals if talc or other foreign crystals is the causative agent. The foreign material may be studied by determining the mineral-acid solubility of the crystals, or by microincineration and chemical analysis. Every effort must be made to rule out tuberculosis by careful bacteriologic studies.

MALIGNANT TUMORS

PRIMARY CARCINOMA OF THE FALLOPIAN TUBE

Primary carcinoma of the oviduct comprises 0.06 to 1.09 percent of all cancer of the female genital tract. Most clinics report incidences of 0.2 to 0.5 percent of female genital malignancy (Dodson et al.; Habibi; Momtazee and Kempson; Turunen). Since the first report in the American literature in 1897, a number of new cases have been added each year, so that more than 800 primary tubal malignancies are recorded (Woodruff and Pauerstein). The true incidence is difficult to assess, because in many cases both tube and ovary are involved, and it is difficult to decide which site is primary. Indeed, it is likely that many of these multiple lesions are the result of multicentric foci of origin (Woodruff and Julian). More than 90 percent of primary tubal malignancies are carcinomas. Mixed tumors, leiomyosarcomas, and trophoblastic tumors have been reported much less frequently.

CARCINOMA IN SITU

Carcinoma in situ has been occasionally discovered by cytologic study, but it is usually discovered at histologic study of tubes removed coincident to other surgery. It is difficult to differentiate invasive from preinvasive neoplasms in the oviduct. Invasion of the underlying stroma occurs late, and many frank neoplasms are thus technically still "intraepithelial." Some of the reported cases actually represent early papillary carcinomas, rather than carcinoma in situ, but others seem to be instances of focal epithelial anaplasia. Under normal circumstances, mitoses are extremely rare in tubal epithelium, although other hyperplastic changes such as pseudostratification and increased number of "indifferent cells" have been described. It is difficult to distinguish proliferation of the tubal epithelium that occurs in response to inflammation or to estrogen stimulation from true anaplasia. Recently, a heat artifact resembling carcinoma, caused by placing the

extirpated specimen on a radiator prior to fixation, was described. The heat caused nuclear elongation and hyperchromatism, and the epithelium displayed prominent papillary projections. However, no mitotic activity was present (Cornog et al.). One should be reluctant to make a diagnosis of carcinoma in situ of the tube in the absence of abnormal mitotic activity and individual cell anaplasia.

Cellular anaplasia in the tube may occur in association with ovarian malignancy, either as a superficial invasion from the nearby ovarian cancer or with multicentric foci of origin.

CARCINOMA

In spite of its rarity, primary carcinoma of the tube is clinically important, because of late diagnosis and poor salvage rates. The highest incidence of tubal cancer occurs in the fifth decade of life, with the extremes varying from 17 to 80 years. Infertility is commoner among patients afflicted with tubal carcinoma than in the general population. Preexisting tubal infection may play a role in both the infertility and the development of tubal malignancy (Turunen; Woodruff and Pauerstein).

Clinical Diagnosis

Tubal carcinoma usually produces no early symptoms. The diagnosis rarely is made prior to surgery. Most tubal cancers are diagnosed preoperatively as hydrosalpinges, pyosalpinges, tuboovarian inflammatory masses, myomata, or ovarian neoplasms. Among symptomatic patients, the commonest symptoms are vaginal discharge, irregular vaginal bleeding, and pain. The discharge is often yellow, but may become bloody at later stages of the disease. Episodic watery discharge has been reported, but is not frequent. Abnormal vaginal bleeding is commonly encountered, particularly in postmenopausal women (Momtazee and Kempson). Pain occurs in about half the patients, and may be crampy or intermittent. The classic triad of pain, discharge, and adnexal mass occurs in about 50 percent of patients (Boutselis and Thompson). The association of a serous, watery, or yellow discharge and an adnexal mass in the postmenopausal patient should alert the physician to the possibility of carcinoma of the oviduct. This suspicion is strengthened if the patient is nulliparous. Although adnexal masses in menopausal women always demand evaluation, the absence of a palpable mass does not rule out tubal carcinoma. Adnexal masses have not been detected prior to operation in as many as 50 percent of women who prove to have tubal carcinoma.

Hysterosalpingography, laparoscopy, and culdoscopy have all been utilized as aids to the clinical diagnosis of tubal malignancy. Hysterosalpingography is controversial. The tumor usually is well developed by the time a radiographic filling defect can be demonstrated, and some physicians express concern about the possibility of seeding the tumor by forcing dye through the tube. In spite of these objections, others consider this technique an important diagnostic aid. No extensive or methodical study of the diagnostic utility of culdoscopy or laparoscopy has been reported.

A number of cases have been reported in which tubal cancer was diagnosed by cytologic techniques. Unfortunately, many of the patients with positive cytology had palpable pelvic disease at the time of the study. Recent series report disappointingly low incidences of positive cytologic smears in women suffering from tubal carcinoma (Momtazee and Kempson; Turunen).

Pathology

The gross lesion often resembles a hydrosalpinx. In the early stages, the tubal wall is often uninvolved. When the hydrosalpinx is opened, the localized tumor mass may be identified. In more extensive cases the tubal lumen may be filled with tumor. The abdominal ostia are occluded in about 50 percent of cases. There is no predilection for involvement of either side. The tumors are bilateral in 15 to 30 percent of cases. Ascites is rarely encountered, and is a late finding (Turunen; Woodruff and Pauerstein).

Histologically, tubal carcinomas are primarily papillary. With more proliferation and agglutination of the papillary fronds, a papillary adenomatous pattern may occur. If the lesion is sufficiently anaplastic, alveoli interspersed with solid sheets of cells may be seen. The diagnosis of malignancy is based upon these architectural features, accompanied by abnormal nuclei, mitoses, hyperchromatism, and pleomorphism. By insisting on cellular evidence of anaplasia, confusion with the benign hyperplastic patterns seen in association with infections or hormonal stimulation can be avoided.

In addition to the usual papillary carcinoma, other varieties of primary tubal carcinoma have been seen. True adenocarcinoma can develop, but probably represents an endometrioid lesion. This speculation was lent credence by the occurrence of a tubal adenoacanthoma. The squamous element was dominant, and in spite of benign histologic appearance, was found in metastases in the ovary and bowel (Czernobilsky and Cornog). Squamous-cell (Anbrokh) and transitional-cell (Federman and Toker) carcinomas have also been reported. Although these may arise in Walthard's rests in tubal or paraovarian cysts (Anbrokh), typical squamous-cell carcinoma and carcinoma in situ can arise from the tubal mucosa (Woodruff and Pauerstein).

Primary tubal carcinoma spreads by direct extension rather than lymphatics until late in the course of the process. The local nodes, local peritoneum, ovary, bladder, rectum, and vagina are usually involved prior to the occurrence of extrapelvic spread.

Treatment

The primary treatment of carcinoma of the tube is total abdominal hysterectomy and bilateral salpingo-oophorectomy. More extensive procedures such as exenteration and regional lymph-node dissection have not been evaluated sufficiently to allow valid conclusions. As a rule, postoperative irradiation has been given regardless of the extent of the disease. It is difficult to evaluate the effectiveness of irradation because of the small numbers of cases reported in each series. Some authors state that postoperative radiation improved survival (Boutselis and Thompson; Turunen), but others do not think that radiation improved prognosis (Momtazee and Kempson). Intraperitoneal radioisotopes and chemotherapeutic agents have not been evaluated adequately in the treatment of tubal cancer. It seems wise to offer such adjuncts to patients with widespread disease, in view of early reports of promising results.

Prognosis

The 5-year survival rates vary from 0 to 44 percent. Recent series report higher salvages than did older series. Prognosis has been related to both histologic grade and stage of the lesion at the time of operation. Histologic grade seems to make little difference, except that tumors displaying solid sheets of malignant cells may have a worse prognosis than those displaying papillary or papillary-alveolar patterns. The clinical extent of the lesion at the time of operation definitely influences the prognosis. Bilateral tubal carcinoma is associated with a poorer prognosis than is unilateral disease. Presumably bilaterality occurs with more advanced disease (Schiller and Silverberg). The prognosis worsens if the disease has spread to other pelvic viscera, and is poorest if spread has occurred beyond the pelvis. Recent authors have suggested staging analogous either to FIGO staging for carcinoma of the ovary (Boutselis and Thompson; Dodson et al.) (Table 44-1), or to staging for cancers of other muscular-epithelial tubes, such as the colon. In this staging, stage I tumor is confined to the oviduct, and does not involve the serosa; stage II includes cases with serosal involvement; stage III cases display involvement of other reproductive organs and stage IV, spread beyond the pelvic organs (Momtazee and Kempson; Schiller and Silverberg). It is difficult to predict which classification will prove superior.

METASTATIC OR COMBINED MALIGNANCIES

Metastasis, or direct extension for lesions arising in adjacent organs, accounts for 80 to 90 percent of tubal malignancy. Metastatic lesions usually can be differentiated from primary carcinoma by the presence of subepithelial or myosalpingeal lymphatic invasion, or of external direct involvement of the serosa. However, alterations which apparently arise from the epithelial surface, or that are associated with detached intraluminal fragments of the neighboring ovarian lesion raise the possibilities of direct extension, implantation, or multiple primary sites of origin. When both tube and ovary are extensively involved, the salvage is poor, regardless of which was the original primary.

OTHER MALIGNANT TUMORS OF THE TUBE

MIXED MESODERMAL TUMORS

Only 14 primary cases of this lesion have been discovered in the tube (DeQueiroz and Roth; Woodruff and Pauerstein; Wu et al.). They represent about 4 percent of all mixed mesodermal tumors reported. The lesions present the same clinical appearance as primary tubal carcinoma.

Grossly, the appearance is indistinguishable from carcinoma. Slightly over one-third of the reported cases have been bilateral. These lesions show anaplastic change in both stromal and epithelial elements. Heterotopic formation of cartilage, bone, or striated muscle may be noted. Therapy is surgical. Adjunctive irradiation and chemotherapy, although probably of minimal value, may be employed in cases with extensive disease. The mean survival time has been 7 months after diagnosis; the longest survivor lived 15 months after diagnosis (DeQueiroz and Roth).

SARCOMA

Sarcoma of the oviduct is extremely rare. The prognosis is poor, similar to that of sarcoma elsewhere. The treatment is surgical. Adjunctive irradiation or chemotherapy has proved to be of little value in the treatment of uterine sarcoma, and the results would probably be similar for tubal lesions.

TROPHOBLASTIC TUMORS (HYDATIDIFORM MOLE AND CHORIOCARCINOMA)

Reports differ widely as to the frequency of trophoblastic tumors arising primarily in the fallopian tube. This variation in frequency may relate to inadequate study of ectopic trophoblast, or to biologic determinants. In any case, trophoblastic tumors of the oviduct are quite infrequent.

The microscopic appearance of primary tubal choriocarcinoma is similar to that in the endometrium. Although cases in which villi were present have been reported, the villous pattern is usually absent. Sheets

TABLE 44–1 Suggested Clinical and Operative Staging for Fallopian Tube Carcinoma

Stage I	Growth limited to the tube	
	Stage Ia:	Growth limited to one tube; no ascites
	Stage Ib:	Growth limited to both tubes; no ascites
	Stage Ic:	Growth limited to one or both tubes; ascites present with malignant cells in fluid
Stage II	Growth involving one or both tubes with pelvic extension	
	Stage IIa:	Extension and/or metastasis to the uterus or ovary
	Stage IIb:	Extension to other pelvic tissues
Stage III	Growth involving one or both tubes with widespread intraperitoneal metastasis to the abdomen (the omentum, the small intestine and its mesentery)	
Stage IV	Growth involving one or both tubes with distant metastasis outside the peritoneal cavity	

of syncytial and cytotrophoblastic cells invade and destroy the surrounding musculature.

The salvage rate prior to chemotherapy was very poor. With the advent of successful chemotherapy for gestational choriocarcinomas, one can anticipate improved salvage.

BENIGN TUMORS OF THE FALLOPIAN TUBE

The primary benign neoplasms of the fallopian tube are similar to those found in the uterus. True primary tubal neoplasms are uncommon. In addition to primary neoplasms, tumors of adjacent structures may involve the oviduct by extension. Most clinically apparent tubal masses are due to salpingitis or ectopic pregnancy. Cystic enlargements of the mesonephric tubules or the terminal portion of the paramesonephric duct may be discovered at pelvic examination or at laparotomy. These lesions are usually incidental findings, but hemorrhage or torsion may produce clinical symptoms, sometimes mimicking appendicitis or tubal pregnancy.

Woodruff has devised the following classification of primary benign neoplasms of the fallopian tube (Woodruff and Pauerstein):

Epithelial: papillomas, polyps, adenoma, endometriosis
Endothelial or *mesothelial:* lymphangioma, hemangioma, adenomatoid tumor, inclusion cysts
Mesodermal: leiomyoma (fibromyoma), lipoma, chondroma, osteoma
Teratoid: benign teratoma
Miscellaneous

EPITHELIAL TUMORS

Reports of primary benign papillomas of the fallopian tube have appeared sporadically since 1877. Recent studies confirm their existence and suggest an association of infertility with these lesions. Adenomatous reactions in the tube are often associated with inflammatory disease and especially with granulomatous salpingitis. Endometriosis may occur in the oviduct as in the uterus. Patterns suggestive of adenomyosis may be found in the intramural portion of the tube.

ENDOTHELIAL OR MESOTHELIAL TUMORS

About 25 cases of lymphangioma of the fallopian tube were recorded in the American literature during the first four decades of this century. It is probable that some cases called lymphangioma were actually adenomatoid tumors, as the two are sometimes difficult to differentiate. Hemangioma of the tube has also been reported. The sixth reported case was a typical cavernous hemangioma, found in the midportion of the oviduct (Ebrahimi and Okagaki).

The most common benign tubal neoplasm is the adenomatoid tumor. The lesions are usually asymptomatic discrete, firm, grayish-yellow, circumscribed nodules, rarely more than 1 to 2 cm in greatest dimension, but frequently occupying the entire thickness of the wall of the tube. They are also found on the serosal surfaces of the uterus and in the cul-de-sac. Although reported more frequently in the male than in the female, this may be due to the comparative ease of palpation of the lesion in the scrotum. The microscopic appearance may be confused with low-grade malignancy, but careful examination reveals absence of cellular anaplasia and good organization of the component cells (Fig. 44-7). Although these lesions have been said to recur locally, such cases probably represent new tumors or incomplete excision of the initial tumor. Various cells—endothelial, mesothelial and, epithelial (mesonephric and paramesonephric)—have been suggested as the origin of these lesions

FIGURE 44–7 High-power view of adenomatoid tumor showing good organization of cells and absence of individual cell anaplasia.

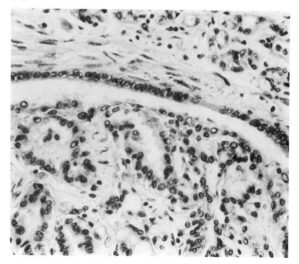

(Woodruff and Pauerstein). The mesothelial theory is supported by the presence of similar patterns in the peritoneum associated with infection, and by the continuity between the surface mesothelium and the lining of the tumor acini. Recent studies with the light and electron microscopes support the mesothelial origin of these tumors (Salazar et al.).

Peritoneal inclusion cysts, arising on the serosal surface of the tube and mesosalpinx, are common microscopic findings. Squamous metaplastic alterations occur in the lining epithelium. The resultant tiny solid nests of metaplastic cells, demonstrating the characteristic alignment of nuclear chromatin have been designated as Walthard's rests. As noted above, they may be involved in the histogenesis of some tubal carcinomas.

MESODERMAL TUMORS

Leiomyoma is rare in the tube. Only about 60 cases of tubal leiomyoma had been reported from 1818 to 1963 (Woodruff and Pauerstein). The majority of the reported cases occurred in the interstitial portion of the tube, the infundibulum and fimbriated end being only rarely involved. Histologically, tubal myomas resemble uterine myomas and may undergo the same degenerative processes. Instances of ectopic pregnancy have been recorded in which a tubal myoma was the obstructing factor; however, the evidence for a cause-and-effect relationship is circumstantial.

Lipomas, chondromas, and osteomas are rare, asymptomatic, and generally discovered in the course of pelvic surgery for other indications. These lesions are more clinical curiosities than of practical importance.

BENIGN TERATOMA

Benign teratoma of the uterine tube was first recorded in 1865. Another 43 cases had been reported as of 1972, and 8 of the 44 tumors were solid, but contained only mature elements and were uniformly benign. The age range was 21 to 60 years, but most of the women were in the fourth decade of life. A high percentage of patients have been nulliparous. There have been no diagnostic symptoms or signs. The tumors varied in diameter from 0.7 to 20 cm. Many of the lesions arose from a mucosal pedicle. Histologic examination revealed the same elements seen in benign teratomas of the ovary (Dowdeswell and Pratt; Mazzarella et al.).

MISCELLANEOUS TUMORS

These tumors include hilus-cell nests (Palomaki and Blair) a Sertoli-Leydig tumor, and xanthomas (Woodruff and Pauerstein); and recently a schwannoma (Okagaki and Richart) and a ganglioneuroma (Weber and Fazzini) of the oviduct have been reported. Such tumors are found incidentally in oviducts removed for other reasons and have little clinical importance.

REFERENCES

Acosta AA et al.: Intrauterine pregnancy and coexistent pelvic inflammatory disease. *Obstet Gynecol* 37:282, 1971.

Altemeier WA et al.: Intraabdominal sepsis. *Adv Surg* 5:281, 1971.

Anbrokh YM: Histological characteristics and questions concerning histogenesis of cancer of the fallopian tubes. *Neoplasma* 17:631, 1970.

———: Macroscopic characteristics of cancer of the fallopian tube. *Neoplasma* 17:557, 1970.

Barr J et al.: Diagnostic laparotomy in cases of obscure fever. *Acta Chir Scand* 138:153, 1972.

Bland KG, Gelfand M: The effects of schistosomiasis on the fallopian tubes in the African female. *J Obstet Gynaecol Br Commonw* 77:1024, 1970.

Boutselis JG, Thompson JN: Clinical aspects of primary carcinoma of the fallopian tube: A clinical study of 14 cases. *Am J Obstet Gynecol* 111:98, 1971.

Chow AW et al.: The bacteriology of acute pelvic inflammatory disease. *Am J Obstet Gynecol* 122:876, 1975.

Coetzee LF, Jaffee AA: Müllerian duct dysgenesis and bilharziasis; report of a case. *S Afr Med J* 45:447, 1971.

Cornog JL et al.: Heat artifact simulating adenocarcinoma of fallopian tube. *JAMA* 214:1118, 1970.

Cox BS et al.: Adnexal inflammation and ureteric obstruction. *J Obstet Gynaecol Br Commonw* 76:1117, 1969.

Cunningham FG et al.: Evaluation of tetracycline or penicillin and ampicillin for treatment of acute pelvic inflammatory disease. *N Eng J Med* 296:1380, 1977.

Czernobilsky B, Cornog JL: Squamous predominance in adenoacanthoma of adnexa. Report of a patient. *Obstet Gynecol* 37:555, 1971.

DeQueiroz AC, Roth LM: Malignant mixed Müllerian tumor of the fallopian tube. Report of a case. *Obstet Gynecol* 36:554, 1970.

Dodson MG et al.: Clinical aspects of fallopian tube carcinoma. *Obstet Gynecol* 36:935, 1970.

Dowdeswell RH, Pratt THR: Benign teratoma of fallopian tube. A case report. *Obstet Gynecol* 39:52, 1972.

Ebrahimi T, Okagaki T: Hemangioma of the fallopian tube. *Am J Obstet Gynecol* 115:864, 1973.

Elstein M: The effects of pelvic inflammation associated with the I.U.D. A salpingographic study. *Int J Fertil* 14:275, 1969.

Elston CW: Cellular reaction to choriocarcinoma. *J Pathol* 97:261, 1969.

Eschenbach DA et al.: Polymicrobial etiology of acute pelvic inflammatory disease. *N Eng J Med* 293:166, 1975.

Eschenbach DA, Holmes KK: Acute pelvic inflammatory disease: Current concepts of pathogenesis, etiology, and management. *Clin Obstet Gynecol* 18:35, 1975.

Federman Q, Toker C: Primary transitional cell tumor of the uterine adnexa. *Am J Obstet Gynecol* 115:863, 1973.

Fraser AC: Surgical treatment of acute pelvic sepsis. *J Obstet Gynaecol Br Commonw* 79:560, 1972.

Fraser IS et al.: Cyclical ovarian function in women with congenital absence of the uterus and vagina. *J Clin Endocrinol Metab* 36:634, 1973.

Friedman S: The treatment of tubal inflammatory disease. *S Afr Med J* 42:1199, 1968.

Gelfand M et al.: Distribution and extent of schistosomiasis in female pelvic organs, with special reference to the genital tract, as determined at autopsy. *Am J Trop Med Hyg* 20:846, 1971.

Gibbs RS: The IUD and PID: Is the contraceptive the culprit? *Contemporary Ob-Gyn* 11:163, 1978.

Guerrero WF et al.: Pelvic pain, gynecic and nongynecic; interpretation and management. *South Med J* 64:1043, 1971.

Habibi A: Cancer in Iran. Malignant tumors of the female genitalia. *Int Surg* 56:13, 1971.

Jacobson L, Westrom C: Objectivized diagnosis of acute pelvic inflammatory disease. *Am J Obstet Gynecol* 105:1088, 1969.

Kraus SJ: Complications of gonococcal infection *Med Clin North Am* 56:1115, 1972.

Mardh PA et al.: Chlamydia trachomatis infection in patients with acute salpingitis. *N Eng J Med* 296:1377, 1977.

Mardh PA, Westrom L: Antibodies to Mycoplasma hominis in patients with genital infections and in healthy controls. *Br J Vener Dis* 46:390, 1970.

————, ————: Tubal and cervical cultures in acute salpingitis with special reference to Mycoplasma hominis and T-strain Mycoplasmas. *Br J Vener Dis* 46:179, 1970.

Mazzarella P et al.: Teratoma of the uterine tube. A case report and review of the literature. *Obstet Gynecol* 39:381, 1972.

Momtazee S, Kempson RL: Primary adenocarcinoma of the fallopian tube. *Obstet Gynecol* 32:649, 1968.

Monif GR et al.: Cul-de-sac isolates from patients with endometritis-salpingitis-peritonitis and gonococcal endocervicitis. *Am J Obstet Gynecol* 26:158, 1976.

Morris CA et al.: Genital tract tuberculosis in subfertile women. *J Med Microbiol* 3:85, 1970.

Morris NF, Elstein M: Gonorrhea and the IUCD. *Br Med J* 4:828, 1968.

Okagaki T, Richart RM: Neurilemoma of the fallopian tube. *Am J Obstet Gynecol* 106:929, 1970.

Palmer R, Oliveira EM: Coelioscopy and per-coelioscopic biopsies in latent genital tuberculosis, in *Latent Female Genital Tuberculosis*, eds. ET Rippmann, RS Wenner, Basel: Karger, 1966.

Palomaki JF, Blair OM: Hilus cell rest of the fallopian tube. A case report. *Obstet Gynecol* 37:60, 1971.

Park I et al.: True hermaphroditism with 46XX/46XY chromosome complement. *Obstet Gynecol* 36:377, 1970.

Puflett D: Tuberculous salpingitis resembling adenocarcinoma. *Med J Aust* 2:149, 1972.

Ress E, Annels EH: Gonococcal salpingitis. *Br J Vener Dis* 45:205, 1969.

Roberts WH: Postmenopausal genital tuberculosis. *Br Med J* 2:526, 1972.

Salazar H et al.: Ultrastructure and observations on the histogenesis of mesotheliomas, "adenomatoid tumors", of the female genital tract. *Cancer* 29:141, 1972.

Schaefer G: Tuberculosis of the female genital tract. *Clin Obstet Gynecol* 13:965, 1970.

Schiller HM, Silverberg SG: Staging and prognosis in primary carcinoma of the fallopian tube. *Cancer* 28:389, 1971.

Taylor R: Mycoplasmas and the evidence for their pathogenicity in man. *Proc R Soc Med* 64:31, 1971.

Turunen A: Diagnosis and treatment of primary tubal carcinoma. *Int J Gynaecol Obstet* 7:294, 1969.

Weber DL, Fazzini E: Ganglioneuroma of the fallopian tube. A heretofore unreported finding. *Acta Neuropathol* 16:173, 1970.

Westrom L: Effect of acute pelvic inflammatory disease in fertility. *Am J Obstet Gynecol* 121:707, 1975.

Woodruff JD, Julian CG: Multiple malignancy in the

upper genital canal. *Am J Obstet Gynecol* 103:810, 1969.

———, Pauerstein CJ: *The Fallopian Tube,* Baltimore: Williams & Wilkins, 1969.

Wong SL et al.: The XX Turner phenotype with unilat-eral streak gonad and absent uterus. *Am J Dis Child* 122:449, 1971.

Wu JP et al.: Malignant mixed Müllerian tumor of the uterine tube. *Obstet Gynecol* 41:707, 1973.

45

Ovaries

C. PAUL MORROW   WILLIAM R. HART

The ovaries are paired organs of the female genital tract whose small size and relatively uncomplicated structure belie their complex functions. As the site of development and release of ova, they are indispensable for reproduction. The process of ovulation is inextricably linked with an intricate endocrine system that involves the hypothalamus and pituitary gland. While the ovaries serve as target organs for pituitary gonadotropin stimulation, the other female genitalia, particularly the endometrium, in turn respond to ovarian hormonal secretions.

Although mild disturbances of ovarian function are frequent, surprisingly few diseases afflict the ovaries. Congenital absence of an ovary and supernumerary and accessory ovaries occur, but they are clinical curiosities. More frequent are the anomalies of gonadal development found in various genetic disorders such as Turner's syndrome and other forms of gonadal dysgenesis (see Chap. 6).

Inflammations of the ovary are usually secondary to bacterial infections of the neighboring fallopian tube (see Chap. 44). Adhesions between the ovary and the tube and chronic perioophoritis are common components of so-called pelvic inflammatory disease. In some instances, a tuboovarian abscess results. Rarely, intrinsic inflammations occur in the absence of primary tubal disease as in mumps, oophoritis, or ovarian abscess following pelvic surgery.

From a clinical standpoint, however, an enlargement of the ovary constitutes one of the most important conditions in gynecology. An ovarian mass presents to the clinician a divirsified diagnostic problem with possible causes ranging from harmless functional cysts to some of the most ruthless cancers in human oncology. The clinician's principal responsibility is to determine the precise nature of the ovarian enlargement and the threat it presents to the patient's life and reproductive function. Of paramount importance, of course, is the differentiation between benign and malignant lesions. Yet, even this crucial diagnostic discrimination may be of secondary importance if torsion or rupture of the mass produces a surgical emergency. Only a sound knowledge of the clinical manifestations of an enlarged ovary coupled with a thorough understanding of the surgical and pathologic findings will reliably guide the physician to the proper diagnosis and management.

EMBRYOLOGY AND ANATOMY

In order to fully appreciate the pathogenesis of an enlarged ovary, a brief review of the embryologic development and anatomy of the ovary is essential. The morphologic components of the ovary, as well as those of its male counterpart, the testis, are histoge-netically derived from four different but intimately related embryologic elements: (1) primitive germ cells, (2) specialized gonadal stroma, (3) coelomic epithelium, and (4) nonspecific mesenchyme. The ovarian derivatives from these embryologic anlagen are listed in Table 45–1.

The primitive germ cells first appear in the endoderm of the yolk sac near the hindgut of the 3½- to 4-week embryo. Utilizing ameboid activity in response to unknown stimuli, they migrate through the mesentery of the gut to the genital ridge, an area of thickened mesoderm on the ventral border of the mesonephros, where the gonad is beginning to develop. The germ cells are concentrated in the gonad by 6 to 10 weeks of fetal life, and in this site they multiply and later differentiate to form oogonia in the ovary or spermatogonia in the testis. While as many as 4 to 6 million germ cells are found in the fetal ovary at the height of germ-cell proliferation, the majority degenerate so that only about 140,000 to 300,000 are present in each newborn ovary and about 10,500 at menarche. The gonad, however, is not the sole site of germ cells. They have been traced to extragonadal sites where they are believed to be the source of primary germ cell tumors that occasionally arise in the vagina, retroperitoneum, sacrococcygeal area, mediastinum, liver, and central nervous system.

The specialized gonadal stroma gives rise to the hormonally active tissues of the gonad. As early as 6 weeks of embryonic life, hydroxysteroid dehydrogenases that are utilized in steroid production are present

TABLE 45–1 Ovarian Derivatives of Embryologic Gonadal Elements

Embryologic element	Ovarian derivatives
Coelomic epithelium	Surface epithelium
	Epithelial inclusion cysts
	Rete ovarii (?)
Primitive germ cells	Oogonia
Specialized gonadal stroma	Granulosa cells
	Theca cells
	Cortical and medullary stromal cells
	Hilus cells
Nonspecific mesenchyme	Fibrous connective tissue
	Blood and lymphatic vessels
	Lymphoreticular tissue

in the genital ridge. Gonadal stroma consists of the specific sex mesenchyme of the genital ridge and epitheliallike structures referred to as *sex cords*. During the first 2 months of embryonic life, the gonads of the male and female are morphologically similar, and this early period of development is referred to as the *indifferent stage*. If the gonad is genetically destined to become a testis, the sex cords become very prominent in the 7- to 8-week male embryo. They envelop the germ cells and form Sertoli cells of the seminiferous tubules while the intervening sex mesenchyme gives rise to the interstitial or Leydig cells. Differentiation of the testis appears mainly to involve the medullary portion of the gonad.

In the fetal ovary, the sex cords do not become as well developed and are not easily distinguishable from the sex mesenchyme. Instead, growth of the ovary is characterized by a more or less diffuse proliferation of gonadal stromal cells and germ cells which later become aggregated into clusters. At about 20 weeks of fetal life, a single layer of cells differentiates from the specialized stroma and surrounds the germ cells to form primordial follicles. These cells are the progenitors of granulosa cells. By 28 weeks, theca forms around the primordial follicles, and secondary (graafian) follicles begin to develop. At about the same time, the characteristic wavy spindle-shaped cells of the specific ovarian stroma can be identified. In contrast to the testis, ovarian development predominantly affects the cortical region of the gonad. Thus, the specialized gonadal stroma of the ovary differentiates to form specific stroma of the cortex and medulla and the granulosa and theca cells of the follicle. The latter two cell types are homologous to the Sertoli and Leydig cells of the testis, respectively. It is likely that the Leydig-like cells (hilus cells) found intermingled with small nerves in the ovarian hilus also are derived from specialized gonadal stroma.

Coelomic epithelium comprises the surface of the genital ridge and contributes to the formation of the gonad. Downgrowths from the coelomic epithelium can be traced into the gonadal stroma, but embryologists disagree as to their role in the development of sex cords. Germ cells are not derived from coelomic epithelium, and thus "germinal" epithelium is an inappropriate, albeit popular, designation.

A layer of surface epithelium differentiates from the coelomic epithelium and becomes distinctly separated from the underlying ovarian cortex by formation of a thin tunica albuginea at about 36 weeks of fetal life. This modified mesothelium persists as a single layer of cuboidal or low columnar cells on the sur-

face of the ovary. In the fully developed ovary, and particularly in later adult life, invaginations of the cortical surface produce clefts and small inclusion cysts of surface epithelium. This process is analogous to the development of the paramesonephric (Müllerian) duct which forms by a similar invagination of coelomic epithelium just lateral to the genital ridge. The fallopian tubes, uterine corpus and cervix, and a portion of the vagina are derived from the paramesonephric ducts. In view of the common ancestry and close anatomic relationship of the ovarian coelomic epithelium and the paramesonephric ducts, it is not surprising that tubal-, endometrial-, and endocervical-like epithelia are found in cysts and neoplasms of the ovary. Lauchlan likened the potential of ovarian surface epithelium and epithelial inclusion cysts to a secondary Müllerian system.

The nonspecific and unspecialized mesenchyme of the gonad provides the supportive connective tissue and vascular framework of the ovary. It consists of fibrous connective tissue, blood and lymphatic vessels, and lymphoreticular tissue. These elements are not specific for the ovary, as they are basic components of all organs. Most of the medulla of the ovary consists of blood vessels and supportive tissues.

Rests of tissue from other organ systems frequently persist in connective tissue adjacent to the ovary. The mesonephric (Wolffian) ducts are vital for proper growth and differentiation of the paramesonephric ducts in the female, but they do not contribute directly to ovarian development. During involution of the mesonephric apparatus, small ductular remnants are incorporated in the mesovarium and mesosalpinx, where they may give rise to parovarian cysts or neoplasms.

Small, yellow nodules of accessory adrenal cortex (adrenals of Marchand), 1 to 3 mm in size, are not infrequent findings in the broad ligament and mesovarium and on at least one occasion have been identified within the parenchyma of a fetal ovary (Symonds, Driscoll). The proximity of the primitive gonad and adrenal cortex accounts for these adrenal rests which may function like normal suprarenal (adrenal) glands. Origin of some adrenocorticallike lipid-cell tumors from these rests has been postulated.

The ovary gradually increases in size during infancy and childhood. Partial development and atresia of follicles occur, and cystic follicles may be prominent in newborns as a result of placental gonadotropin stimulation. Ovulation and transformation of a follicle into a corpus luteum, however, await the onset of puberty and establishment of the cyclical hypothalamus-pituitary-ovary hormonal feedback system.

Each adult ovary is approximately 3½ by 2½ by ½ cm during the reproductive years. The ovary is attached to the uterus by the uteroovarian ligament, at the back of the broad ligament beneath the fallopian tube by the mesovarium, and to the pelvic wall by the infundibulopelvic or suspensory ligament which contains the ovarian blood vessels and major lymphatic channels. Its functional constituents include ovarian stroma, follicles, and corpora lutea, all of which diminish in quantity as the woman ages (Fig. 45–1). A follicle that becomes atretic and fibrotic is designated as a *corpus fibrosum* while a fibrotic, involuted corpus luteum is referred to as a *corpus albicans.*

After 35 to 40 years of cyclic ovarian function, the supply of ova is exhausted and ovulation ceases. The postmenopausal ovary shrinks into a small, firm structure. Consisting predominantly of corpora fibrosa and corpora albicantes, it is devoid of follicles and corpora lutea.

OVARIAN ENDOCRINOLOGY

The physiologic and functional capacities of the ovarian tissues are complex (Richardson). Potential steroidogenic elements of the ovary include the granulosa and theca cells of the follicle and corpus luteum, ovarian stromal cells, and hilus cells. The same types of steroids may be produced by the ovary as are manufactured by the testis and adrenal cortex.

Under normal circumstances, estrogen and progesterone are the major hormones of cycling ovaries. The former is a product of both the follicle and corpus luteum, while the latter is dependent upon ovulation and corpus luteum formation. It is thought that the theca cells are the main sources of steroid synthesis and that the granulosa cells are less complete manufacturers of sex hormones. In vitro incubation studies indicate that ovarian stroma is a potentially androgenic compartment.

Deranged hormonal biosynthesis is common in pathologic states of the ovary. A variety of androgens, including testosterone, may be produced by hyperplastic and neoplastic ovarian tissues. Rarely, corticosteroids apparently may be of ovarian origin. The clinical manifestations of aberrant steroid synthesis are those of hyperestrinism, defeminization, masculinization, and cushingoid effects. Identification of an endocrinopathy as being of adrenal or ovarian origin at times may be difficult. In such cases, the use of differential stimulation and suppression tests is sometimes clinically helpful (see Chap. 7). Nonsteroidal hormones such as chorionic gonadotropin, alpha-fetoprotein (AFP), and serotonin also can be produced by functioning ovarian neoplasms.

NONNEOPLASTIC LESIONS

FUNCTIONAL CYSTS

Cysts derived from the graafian follicle or corpus luteum undoubtedly are the most frequent cause of clinically detectable ovarian enlargement. They are

FIGURE 45–1 Adult ovary during reproductive years (photomicrograph). Several small cystic follicles and a mature, convoluted corpus luteum are apparent. H & E × 8.

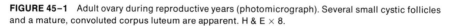
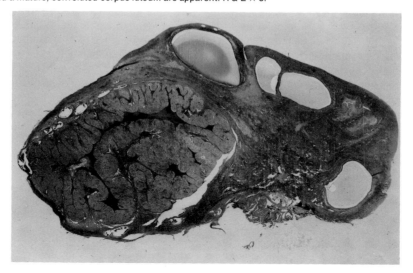

TABLE 45–2 Nonneoplastic Lesions of the Ovary and Mesovarium

1. Functional cysts
    a. Follicle cysts
    b. Corpus luteum cysts
    c. Theca lutein cysts
2. Sclerocystic disease
3. Parovarian cysts
4. Hyperplasias
    a. Pregnancy luteoma
    b. Hyperthecosis
    c. Cortical stromal hyperplasia
    d. Hilus-cell hyperplasia
5. Endometriosis
6. Massive edema

pathologic variants of the normal physiologic events that affect the follicular apparatus. They are not neoplastic and often are referred to as "functional" cysts. Included in this group are follicle cysts, corpus luteum cysts, and theca lutein cysts. These and other nonneoplastic lesions are listed in Table 45–2.

FOLLICLE CYSTS

In the course of normal development or involution of a graafian follicle, cystic dilatation is commonplace. Seldom, however, do cystic follicles achieve a diameter greater than 3 cm. When this size is exceeded, the designation of "follicle cyst" is rather arbitrarily applied. The pathogenesis of a follicle cyst is ill-understood but most likely involves subtle aberrations in the hormonal interactions among the hypothalamus, pituitary, and ovary.

Follicle cysts characteristically are less than 6 to 8 cm in diameter, although cysts up to 20 cm in size have been reported. Grossly, the cysts are unilocular, have thin walls with smooth outer and inner surfaces, and contain clear fluid which may be estrin-rich. Some examples are filled with bloody fluid because of intraluminal hemorrhage. Microscopic examination of the cyst wall reveals a compressed inner zone of granulosa cells and a peripheral theca layer which may be luteinized. In large or old lesions, definite granulosa and theca cells may be difficult to identify, and classification of the cyst may not be possible.

Follicular cysts may develop at any age prior to menopause. Most examples are clinically silent and spontaneously regress, their presence remaining unknown unless discovered by chance during a routine pelvic examination. Large cysts may produce mild pelvic discomfort, low-back pain, or deep dyspareunia. Some patients notice menstrual irregularities. Single-follicle cysts have been found in some children with the syndrome of pseudoprecocious puberty characterized by vaginal bleeding and breast development but without ovulation. Removal of the cyst has resulted in regression of the signs in some instances (Wieland et al.). Similar cysts, however, may be found in children with true sexual precocity and merely reflect premature gonadotropin stimulation. Acute abdominal pain producing a clinical picture similar to appendicitis may be produced by torsion of the cystic ovary.

CORPUS LUTEUM CYSTS

The corpus luteum also is commonly a cystic structure, especially during the early portion of pregnancy when it may become 5 to 6 cm in diameter. Excessive bleeding into the cavity of a corpus luteum or failure of the normal organization of the coagulum produced by ovulation results in a corpus luteum hematoma. Resorption of the blood may leave a corpus luteum cyst. Most hematomas and cysts of the corpus luteum are less than 8 cm in maximum dimension, but some may be larger than 10 cm in diameter. The distinction between a normal hemorrhagic cystic corpus luteum or a persistent corpus luteum and a corpus luteum cyst is not always clear-cut.

Gross examination reveals a unilocular smooth-walled cyst that has a distinct yellow color when the sectioned surface is viewed. Old or fresh blood may be in the lumen. Microscopically, the wall consists of the three layers of the normal corpus luteum which may be compressed and attenuated. The inner zone is made up of fibrous granulation tissue beneath which are layers of luteinized granulosa cells and luteinized theca cells in a convoluted or scalloped arrangement. Rarely, complete fibrosis of the wall results in a corpus albicans cyst.

Corpus luteum cysts are found only in ovulating women. They are less frequent than follicle cysts but are more apt to be symptomatic. Menses may be delayed and then followed by prolonged or irregular bleeding. Unilateral pelvic discomfort is a common accompaniment. These symptoms, coupled with the finding of a mildly tender adnexal mass on pelvic examination, frequently suggest the diagnosis of ectopic pregnancy. If rupture of the cyst occurs, massive intraperitoneal hemorrhage may result. The clinical picture of this acute surgical emergency precisely simulates a ruptured ectopic tubal pregnancy.

THECA LUTEIN CYSTS

Multiple atretic follicles with luteinization of the theca cells are designated as theca lutein cysts and are thought to result from excessive levels of human chorionic gonadotropin (HCG) or increased sensitivity to HCG. The role of pituitary gonadotropins and other factors remain to be elucidated. This condition also has been referred to as *hyperreactio luteinalis*.

Typically, theca lutein cysts are found with hydatidiform mole (one-third to one-half of cases) and choriocarcinoma, but occasionally they occur in patients with Rh sensitization, multiple gestation, toxemia, diabetes, and rarely in normal single pregnancy. Administration of gonadotropins or clomiphene to induce ovulation may produce follicle cysts, multiple corpora lutea, and, rarely, theca lutein cysts (overstimulation syndrome). Placental gonadotropin stimulation may be responsible for theca lutein cysts found in the ovaries of newborns.

Bilateral involvement is characteristic (Fig. 45–2). The ovaries contain multiple cysts and are enlarged. Some may exceed 25 cm in diameter. The histologic changes are merely an exaggeration of the follicular atresia and accompanying hyperplasia and luteinization of the perifollicular theca cells that normally occur in pregnancy.

The cysts may be associated with ascites, and occasionally torsion with rupture and hemorrhage occurs. An example of maternal virilization from excess ovarian androgen production has been recorded during a twin pregnancy complicated by theca lutein cysts (Judd et al.). In the absence of such complications, theca lutein cysts do not usually require special treatment as regression occurs following reduction of gonadotropin levels. Return to normal ovarian size, however, often lags behind the decline in gonadotropin levels following evacuation of a hydatidiform mole. Rarely, spontaneous regression may not occur and surgical resection is needed, as in the case reported by Barclay and associates.

MANAGEMENT

The major importance of functional cysts is the difficulty in clinically distinguishing them from true neoplasms. While the symptoms and physical findings are helpful, their rather fleeting existence is of prime importance. Tradition and clinical experience have taught that functional cysts usually persist for only a few days or weeks. Consequently, reexamination of the patient during a different phase of the menstrual cycle after an interval of 1 to 3 months has been common practice in evaluating cystic ovarian enlargements in young women.

Many gynecologists prescribe combination oral contraceptive pills to accelerate the involution of functional cysts. If these cysts are gonadotropin-dependent, the inhibitory effect of the contraceptive steroids on the release of gonadotropins from the pituitary should abbreviate their life-span, thereby hastening their identification as nonneoplastic "functional" cysts. Spanos studied 286 cases of unilateral, cystic adnexal masses in women of reproductive age. Steroid contraceptives were prescribed, and the women were reexamined in 6 weeks. The mass disappeared in 72 percent of patients during this interval. Of the 81 patients with a persistent mass, none was found to have a functional cyst at laparotomy (Table 45–3).

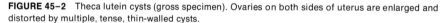

FIGURE 45–2   Theca lutein cysts (gross specimen). Ovaries on both sides of uterus are enlarged and distorted by multiple, tense, thin-walled cysts.

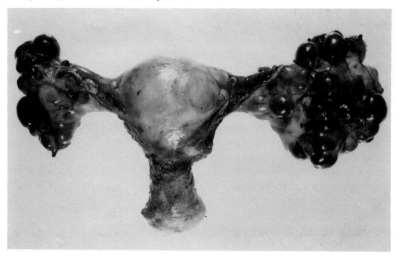

TABLE 45–3 Adnexal "Cysts" Persistent in 286 Patients Between the Ages of 16 and 48, Treated With Estrogen and Progesterone for 6 Weeks

Diagnosis	Number of patients
Nonneoplastic cysts	35
Functional	0
Endometriotic	28
Parovarian	4
Hydrosalpinx	3
Neoplasms	46
Dermoid	9
Epithelial, benign	32
Epithelial, malignant	4
Germinoma	1
Total	81

Source: Spanos.

The policy of delaying surgical intervention in women of reproductive age with an adnexal mass is valid provided the mass is unilateral, cystic, and 10 cm or less in diameter. Administration of oral contraceptives in an attempt to cause involution is theoretically sound. Exploratory laparotomy should be performed, however, if the mass persists for 6 weeks. If the patient has been taking oral contraceptives, the probability of a cyst being functional is remote.

The all too common practice of excising ovaries with small cysts found incidentally during an appendectomy or other unrelated surgical procedure on young women is to be condemned unless the cysts are clearly of neoplastic origin. Usually they are normal physiologic cystic follicles or corpora lutea. Microscopic examination of biopsy material by frozen-section technique should be performed if there is any doubt as to the nature of the cysts before the suspected ovary is removed.

SCLEROCYSTIC DISEASE

Sclerocystic ovaries are characteristically found in young women with the Stein-Leventhal syndrome of infertility, oligomenorrhea, and menstrual irregularities dating from the menarche. These patients are usually obese with varying degrees of hirsutism. Sclerocystic ovaries also may be associated with a clinical picture of menometrorrhagia due to endometrial hyperplasia, and some young women with sclerocystic ovaries develop adenocarcinoma of the endometrium. Deranged hypothalamic-pituitary-ovar-

ian hormonal function resulting in prolonged anovulation appears to be the common denominator of both the clinical and pathologic findings. The role of the adrenal gland in this disorder remains enigmatic (see Chap. 7).

Both ovaries are involved and usually are enlarged two- to threefold. The tunica albuginea is thickened and collagenized. Multiple subcapsular cystic follicles 1 to 2 cm in size dominate the gross appearance. Hyperplasia of cortical stroma and theca interna, which is often luteinized, is also an important histologic feature. Recent corpora lutea are absent or few. These morphologic changes indicate prolonged anovulation but otherwise are nonspecific. Identical histologic changes may be seen with adrenal virilism and other causes of anovulation.

Therapy is directed at initiating ovulation, either pharmacologically or by surgical wedge resections of the ovaries. When ovulation is not desirable, the cyclic administration of progestogens to prevent endometrial hyperplasia is recommended. Primary ovarian neoplasms have been found in patients with sclerocystic ovaries. In a histologic review of the ovaries in 241 examples of the Stein-Leventhal syndrome by Hutchison et al., 11 ovarian tumors (4.6 percent) were found. Almost half of these were benign cystic teratomas. Babaknia et al. reported 20 ovarian neoplasms incidentally discovered in 118 patients operated on for the Stein-Leventhal syndrome. Of the 20, 5 were stromal tumors, 6 were dermoids, and 4 were epithelial in type. It is unproved, however, that sclerocystic ovaries have an increased neoplastic potential.

PAROVARIAN CYSTS

Retention cysts may develop from embryologic remnants of the mesonephric or paramesonephric ducts in the mesovarium. Strictly speaking, these are not ovarian cysts but rather parovarian cysts of the broad ligament. They are considered here because clinically they may be impossible to distinguish from an ovarian cyst or neoplasm.

A parovarian cyst is easily recognizable at surgery by its anatomic position between the ovary and the fallopian tube. It may range in size from a few centimeters to more than 20 cm in diameter. They occur over a wide age range but the majority of large cysts (> 5 cm) occur in the third and fourth decades of life. In the large cysts, the tube is stretched over the superior pole of the cyst and the ovary is displaced inferiorly, but neither of these two organs contributes to formation of the cyst. The outer wall is smooth and covered by peritoneum of the broad ligament. Clear fluid fills the lumen. The smooth inner lining consists of a layer of benign columnar or cuboidal epithelial cells. A few small, inconspicuous papillae may be present. Bundles of smooth muscle usually are in the cyst wall. Rarely, a cystadenoma or carcinoma in the broad ligament appears to have arisen from a parovarian cyst (Genadry et al.). Excision of the cyst, with sparing of the ovary and tube if possible, is curative.

HYPERPLASIAS

PREGNANCY LUTEOMA

The "luteoma of pregnancy" is a nodular hyperplasia of lutein cells. First delineated by Sternberg in 1963, it occurs exclusively in pregnant women. Most patients are less than 30 years of age, and there is a tendency for the tumors to occur in multiparous black patients. Usually they are asymptomatic, and the luteoma is discovered incidentally at the time of cesarean section or postpartum tubal ligation. Maternal virilism occasionally occurs because of excessive androgen production by the lutein cells, and the fetus may also be virilized in such cases. An association between preexisting polycystic ovarian syndrome and luteoma of pregnancy has been proposed (Polansky et al.).

Pregnancy luteomas consist of soft reddish-brown, well-circumscribed nodules that average 6 cm in diameter but may reach sizes of 16 cm or more. Obstruction of the birth canal may result. Multiple nodules are found in half the patients, and bilaterality is observed in at least one-third of cases. The nodules spontaneously regress in the postpartum period but may recur in subsequent pregnancies.

Microscopically, the lesion consists of solid nodules of uniform, markedly luteinized cells. Norris and Taylor (1967) concluded that pregnancy luteomas are hyperplastic overgrowths of luteinized theca cells arising in the walls of theca lutein cysts. Others believe they are derived from luteinized stromal cells.

Since the lesion is multifocal, occurs only during pregnancy, and regresses postpartum, the pregnancy luteoma is best regarded as a gonadotropin-dependent pseudoneoplastic hyperplasia rather than a truly autonomous growth. The multinodularity, high incidence of bilaterality, and invariable association with pregnancy are important features in distinguishing this lesion from a lipid-cell neoplasm. When

doubt exists, frozen section examination should be made before excising the ovary.

HYPERTHECOSIS

Diffuse proliferation of ovarian stromal cells with multiple foci of luteinization has been variously termed *hyperthecosis, stromal thecosis,* or *thecomatosis.* Progressive virilism often characterizes the clinical picture. Onset unusually coincides with the menarche, and most patients are 20 to 30 years of age at the time of diagnosis. Menstrual irregularity is followed by oligo- or amenorrhea. Obesity, hypertension, and disturbances of glucose metabolism are frequently associated conditions, as are endometrial hyperplasia and adenocarcinoma. In some instances, the clinical and pathologic findings overlap with the Stein-Leventhal syndrome.

Both ovaries are involved and may be enlarged up to 7 to 8 cm in diameter. At times they are of normal size, causing clinical problems in differentiating this lesion from adrenal virilism. Generally, the ovaries are solid, but a few and sometimes several subcapsular cystic follicles may be present.

The clusters of vacuolated, lipid-containing luteinized cells are derived directly from ovarian stromal cells. Apparently, the hyperplastic stromal cells are the source of excessive androgenic steroid production. High levels of testosterone and androstenedione have been isolated from ovarian vein plasma. Urinary excretion of 17-ketosteroids is usually normal or slightly elevated. Ovarian wedge resection may be of therapeutic value, and hormonal therapy to induce ovulation has been advocated.

CORTICAL STROMAL HYPERPLASIA

This term refers to a nodular or diffuse thickening of ovarian stroma predominantly in the peripheral zone of the ovary. The significance of this lesion and the criteria for diagnosis have been debated. A relatively common condition, its peak incidence is between the ages of 55 and 70 years. Approximately one-third of patients in this age group have prominent ovarian stromal proliferation at autopsy.

A statistical relationship with a variety of diseases, including endometrial and breast carcinoma, uterine leiomyomas, and endometrial hyperplasia and polyps, has been reported. These associations suggest estrogenic stimulation. Others have not been able to substantiate this hypothesis and instead indicate that androgen hypersecretion is a more likely result. Bilateral ovarian involvement is typical, but not to the degree that palpable enlargement results.

HILUS-CELL HYPERPLASIA

Hilus cells resemble testicular Leydig cells and are a normal component of the ovary where they are found in the hilus in proximity to nerves. Crystals of Reinke can be found in their cytoplasm. They are often particularly prominent in the ovaries of postmenopausal women, in the newborn, and during pregnancy, suggesting a relationship with elevated gonadotropin levels. Several cases of hilus-cell hyperplasia associated with overt virilism have been recorded, but it also occurs in patients with no demonstrable clinical abnormality. When there is extensive overgrowth of hilus cells, distinction between nodular hyperplasia and a true neoplasm may be difficult, although the hyperplasia is more often bilateral. Ovarian size is usually not changed.

ENDOMETRIOSIS

About half the patients with endometriosis will have involvement of the ovaries, but in only 5 percent will there be a clinically detectable adnexal mass. An ovary enlarged by cystic endometriosis is commonly referred to as an *endometrioma*. While the etiology of endometriosis continues to be debated, few authorities have categorized cystic ovarian endometriosis as a neoplastic disease. A neoplasm may arise secondarily from endometriosis, but this is not a common event.

Endometriotic cysts are thought to result from cyclic hemorrhage involving foci of ovarian endometriosis. The progressive accumulation of old blood produces the classical "chocolate" cyst. These cysts are thin-walled, and minor degrees of leakage often occur, producing intermittent pain and inducing adhesion formation to surrounding structures.

On physical examination other findings consistent with endometriosis may be present such as uterosacral nodularity, retroversion of the uterus, and cul-de-sac tenderness. Endometriotic ovaries, which may reach 12 to 15 cm in diameter, are frequently tender to palpation. They are less inclined to undergo torsion and infarction than other ovarian cysts because of the frequency of adhesions to surrounding pelvic structures.

The management of a patient with endometriosis and an adnexal mass must be directed toward the ad-nexal mass. If uterosacral nodularity is present, avoidance of any delay in surgical exploration is even more urgent since the nodules may represent implants from ovarian carcinoma. The treatment of endometriosis is discussed in Chap. 37.

MASSIVE OVARIAN EDEMA

A rare cause of ovarian enlargement is massive interstitial edema. Eight cases have been reported and in seven the right ovary was involved. All patients have been between the ages of 13 and 33 years. Clinically, patients with massive ovarian edema may present with either acute abdominal pain or virilism. At surgical exploration, torsion of the involved adnexal structures has been discovered in some patients.

It has been hypothesized that partial torsion or kinking of the mesovarium, possibly recurrent, produces edema by interference with the lymphatic drainage and venous return. Chronic edema and mechanical stretching of ovarian stromal cells may result in stromal luteinization which is then responsible for androgen production and clinical virilism.

NEOPLASMS

CLASSIFICATION AND CLINICAL STAGING

The neoplastic lesions of the ovary constitute the most diverse group of tumors found in any organ of the human body. Because of their complexity, ovarian neoplasms have been classified according to a variety of schemes. Subdivisions based on gross appearance (cystic or solid) or hormonal effects (feminizing, masculinizing, or inert) have been popular. While these clinical and macroscopic features are useful in evaluating a particular ovarian tumor, a scheme based on the histogenesis of the ovary is more flexible and provides the physician with a rational approach that can be easily mastered. The classification presented in Table 45–4 is based on present-day knowledge of the histogenesis of the ovary. Similar classifications are in wide usage.

Ovarian neoplasms are first separated into primary and metastatic (secondary) tumors. Generally, such a separation is easily accomplished after care-

TABLE 45–4 Histogenetic Classification of Primary Ovarian Neoplasms

I. Coelomic epithelial origin
   A. "Common" epithelial tumors: benign, borderline, malignant
      1. Serous
      2. Mucinous
      3. Endometriod
      4. Mesonephroid (clear cell)
      5. Brenner (transitional cell)
   B. Undifferentiated carcinoma
   C. Carcinosarcoma and mixed mesodermal tumor
   D. Unclassified and miscellaneous tumors
II. Germ-cell origin
   A. Teratoma
      1. Mature teratoma
         a. Dermoid cyst
         b. Struma ovarii
         c. Neoplasms secondarily arising from teratomatous tissues (squamous carcinoma, carcinoid tumor, sarcoma, etc.)
      Immature teratoma
   B. Germinoma
   C. Endodermal sinus tumor
   D. Embryonal carcinoma
   E. Choriocarcinoma
   F. Mixed germ-cell tumors
   G. Gonadoblastoma*
III. Specialized gonadal stromal origin
   A. Granulosa-theca group
      1. Granulosa-cell tumor
      2. Thecoma
   B. Sertoli-Leydig group
      1. Sertoli-cell tumor
      2. Arrhenoblastoma (Sertoli-Leydig cell tumor)
      3. Leydig- and hilus-cell tumors
   C. Gynandroblastoma
   D. Lipid-cell tumors
   E. Unclassified gonadal stromal tumors
IV. Nonspecific mesenchymal origin
   A. Fibroma, angioma, leiomyoma, lipoma
   B. Lymphoma
   C. Sarcoma
   D. Miscellaneous tumors

*Combined germ-cell and specialized gonadal stromal elements.

TABLE 45–5 Relative Frequency of Ovarian Neoplasms According to Histogenetic Category

Histogenetic category	Percent
1. Primary neoplasms	
a. Coelomic epithelium	60–70
b. Germ cell	15–20
c. Specialized gonadal stroma	5–10
d. Nonspecific mesenchyme	5–10
2. Metastatic neoplasms*	5–10

*Excluding tumors found at autopsy in patients with widespread cancer or in palliative oophorectomy specimens from patients with metastatic breast carcinoma.

four major groups according to their presumed histogenesis from coelomic epithelium, primitive germ cells, specialized gonadal stroma, or nonspecific mesenchyme. While it is recognized that some neoplasms may have similar histologic appearances yet arise from different embryologic anlagen (e.g., mucinous tumors, lipid-cell tumors), each tumor is classified according to its most frequent origin. Conversely, a tumor may consist of a combination of tissues that originate from two different elements (e.g., gonadoblastoma) but be placed in the most closely related category.

By utilization of this histogenetic classification, the relative frequency of each group of ovarian tumors can be determined. About 60 to 70 percent of all ovarian neoplasms belong in the coelomic epithelium group, and 15 to 20 percent are of germ-cell origin. The specialized gonadal stroma and the nonspecific mesenchyme each accounts for 5 to 10 percent of tumors. Only about 5 to 10 percent are metastatic tumors, if those incidentally discovered at autopsy in patients with widespread cancer and in palliative oophorectomy specimens from patients with metastatic breast carcinoma are excluded.

Studies by Abell (1966) and others demonstrate that these relative percentages vary significantly with the age of the patient. In children and women less than 20 years of age, almost 60 percent of the tumors are of germ-cell origin, and before menarche germ-cell tumors account for 90 percent of all neoplasms. In contrast, coelomic epithelial tumors are rare in prepubertal girls. Over 80 percent of tumors occurring in postmenopausal women are of coelomic epithelial origin, while only 6 percent are germ-cell tumors, and these are almost invariably mature cystic teratomas (dermoids). Neoplasms derived from specialized gonadal stroma and nonspecific mesenchyme form a

ful clinical and pathologic examinations. Occasionally, however, an unequivocal distinction cannot be made initially, and only follow-up of the patient provides the answer.

The primary ovarian neoplasms are divided into

TABLE 45–6 Relationship of Age to Relative Frequency of Ovarian Neoplasms

Histogenetic category	Percent of category		
	Under 20 years	20 to 50 years	Over 50 years
Coelomic epithelium	29	71	81
Germ cell	59	14	6
Specialized gonadal stroma	8	5	4
Nonspecific mesenchyme	4	10	9
Totals	100	100	100

Source: Modified from Abell (1966).

relatively constant proportion at all ages, although distinct variations occur within each of these groups.

In addition to classifying ovarian neoplasms according to their histologic type and grade, categorizing malignant tumors into subgroups or stages which reflect the extent of tumor spread at the time of diagnosis is valuable. The system is purposely designed so that with each advance in stage there is a significant worsening of prognosis. In this manner, the clinician is provided with a rough guide to the prognosis of the individual patient. Treatment centers utilize the stage system to apportion their cases into relatively similar prognostic groups by means of which they can compare treatment results. A multitude of staging systems have been devised and utilized in the reporting of ovarian cancer. The very concept of staging, however, implies standardization, and only one staging system should be employed for reporting purposes. The International Federation of Obstetrics and Gynecology (Federation International de Gynecologie et Obstetrique, or FIGO) has adopted the stage grouping outlined in Table 45–7. Although primarily designed for epithelial ovarian cancers, it can and should be used in reporting all ovarian malignan-

TABLE 45–7 FIGO* Stage Grouping for Primary Carcinoma of the Ovary†

Stage I	Growth limited to the ovaries
Stage Ia	Growth limited to one ovary; no ascites
	(i) No tumor on the external surface; capsule intact
	(ii) Tumor present on the external surface and/or capsule ruptured
Stage Ib	Growth limited to both ovaries; no ascites
	(i) No tumor on the external surface; capsule intact
	(ii) Tumor present on the external surface and/or capsule ruptured
Stage Ic	Tumor either stage Ia or stage Ib, but with ascites‡ present or positive peritoneal washings
Stage II	Growth involving one or both ovaries with pelvic extension
Stage IIa	Extension and/or metastases to the uterus and/or tubes
Stage IIb	Extension to other pelvic tissues
Stage IIc	Tumor either stage IIa or stage IIb, but with ascites‡ present or positive peritoneal washings
Stage III	Growth involving one or both ovaries with intraperitoneal metastases outside the pelvis and/or positive retroperitoneal nodes
	Tumor limited to the true pelvis with histologically proven malignant extension to small bowel or omentum
Stage IV	Growth involving one or both ovaries with distant metastases. If pleural effusion is present, there must be positive cytology to allot a case to stage IV.
	Parenchymal liver metastasis equals stage IV.
Special category	Unexplored cases that are thought to be ovarian carcinoma

*Federation International de Gynecologie et Obstetrique.
†To be used from January 1, 1975.
‡Ascites is peritoneal effusion that in the opinion of the surgeon is pathologic and/or clearly exceeds normal amounts.

cies. According to the FIGO system, the stage of the cancer is assigned after the extent of spread is determined by the operative findings and pathologic examination of excised tissues. It is not strictly a clinical staging system, and thus it differs fundamentally from that used for cancers of the vulva, cervix, and endometrium.

The biologic potential of an ovarian neoplasm can be evaluated only after all these clinical and pathologic features are properly assessed. The prognosis of any patient with an ovarian cancer is determined by the histologic cell type, degree of differentiation (grade) of the tumor, and extent of its spread at the time of diagnosis (stage). Without knowledge of all these factors, a sound judgment of the malignant capabilities of an ovarian neoplasm cannot be made.

EPIDEMIOLOGY

Epidemiologic studies of ovarian tumors have focused almost exclusively on the malignant forms. This is understandable, even though benign ovarian neoplasms are four times more common, because the benign tumors are rarely a cause of death or permanent disability. By contrast, only 33 percent of all women diagnosed as having an ovarian cancer survive 5 years. The mortality rate from ovarian cancer in the United States has increased 250 percent since 1930. It now ranks as the fourth leading cause of death among cancers in women, surpassed only by cancer of the breast, colon, and lung. Approximately 17,000 new cases of ovarian cancer are diagnosed annually, while 10,800 women die of this malignancy each year. The risk of death from ovarian cancer in the State of New York has apparently surpassed the combined risk from cervical cancer and corpus cancer (Randall, 1970).

Ovarian cancer is predominantly a disease of perimenopausal and postmenopausal women with an average age at diagnosis of 52 years. Both the histologic type of neoplasms and the overall frequency of occurrence vary significantly with age. Prior to age 20, less than one case of ovarian cancer is diagnosed per 100,000 females per year. The occurrence rate increases to 27 at age 55 and continues rising thereafter, reaching about 75 cases per 100,000 females per year at age 75 (Table 45–8). The age-adjusted annual death rates on a worldwide basis range from a low of 2.0 per 100,000 population in Japan and Chile to 13 per 100,000 in the Scandinavian countries. In the United States the annual death rate due to

TABLE 45–8 Incidence Rates of Ovarian Cancer per 100,000 Women

Age, years	Oakland Kaiser Hospital (1958–1963)	New York (1960)
0–19	0	0.1
20–44	7.2	5.9
45–54	27.6	26.3
55–64	28.1	38.1
65–74	72.6	73.5
75 and over	158.0	131.0

Source: Bennington et al.

ovarian cancer for Caucasian women is 7 per 100,000, compared with 6 per 100,000 for non-Caucasians.

According to statistics of the American Cancer Society, the risk at birth of eventually developing ovarian cancer is 1.5 percent for white females and 0.9 percent for nonwhite females; the risk of eventually dying of ovarian cancer is 1.0 percent and 0.7 percent respectively. Reproductive experience appears to be more strongly associated with risk for ovarian malignancy than socioeconomic factors. Joly and associates noted that women with ovarian cancer consistently showed, in comparison with control women, fewer pregnancies, more miscarriages, more infertility, and a later age at first marriage. For the highest risk group, those who marry after age 20 and have fewer than three pregnancies, the risk ratio was as high as 4.5 depending upon the control group. Women with breast cancer may also be at high risk for the development of ovarian cancer and the cancer may have a familial association (Fraumeni, et al.).

Several familial aggregations of ovarian cancer suggestive of genetic predisposition have been described in the literature, but this apparently is a minor factor in the genesis of ovarian tumors. A familial occurrence has been reported for germinoma, arrhenoblastoma, mature cystic teratoma, and carcinomas. A genetic predisposition to the development of ovarian cancer, however, could not be confirmed by a study of identical twins (Harvald, Hauge). Ovarian tumors are common in certain genetic diseases. The reported incidence of ovarian tumors in women with the Peutz-Jeghers syndrome is approximately 5 percent. About 50 percent of these are gonadal stromal tumors of granulosa or Sertoli-cell type, a disproportionately high figure. Scully (1970c) has indicated that the "sex cord tumor with annular tubules" is a distinctive ovarian tumor of the Peutz-Jeghers syndrome, and its discovery may be the first clue to the diagnosis of the syndrome.

Patients with gonadal dysgenesis who have a Y sex chromosome have a predilection for developing an unusual gonadal tumor termed gonadoblastoma. Usually, these patients manifest the clinical features of pure or mixed gonadal dysgenesis or male pseudohermaphroditism. A malignant germ-cell neoplasm may arise from the germ-cell component of the gonadoblastoma.

DETECTION AND PREVENTION

Detection

The natural history of ovarian cancer mitigates against dramatic improvements in therapy. Like other visceral malignancies its early development often is cryptic; there are no warning signs or symptoms. Because of rapid growth and propensity for intraperitoneal spread, ovarian cancers are frequently massive and unresectable at the time of diagnosis. The hope of eradicating advanced malignancy by improvements in therapy is unlikely. A more reasonable prospect for enhancing the prognosis in ovarian cancer is earlier diagnosis. No feasible means of screening the entire at-risk population for this disease currently exists. Routine pelvic examination has been recommended as an immediately available avenue to earlier diagnosis. While the chance of detecting an ovarian cancer in this manner is remote, the yield can be increased by a more critical assessment of what constitutes a significant finding during a pelvic examination. Barber and Graber (1971) have pointed out that women who are more than 3 years postmenopausal with a palpable ovary undoubtedly have an ovarian neoplasm. Atrophy should have occurred to a sufficient degree by this time, making the ovaries no longer palpable. There is no role for "watchful expectancy" or delay under any other disguise in this age group. Immediate investigation of any pelvic lesion in a postmenopausal woman is mandatory. This dictum also applies to prepubertal girls. In the young woman, functional ovarian cysts are common, and an effort must be made to identify those patients with true neoplasms. The fact that an ovarian neoplasm in a young patient is probably benign is not justification for procrastination. It must be proved to be benign by surgical extirpation; delay is seldom in the interest of the patient.

Unfortunately, even the most scrupulous vigilance on the part of all physicians promises to add but a small increment to the detection rate of asymptomatic ovarian cancer. The greatest hope for early diagnosis lies in the discovery or development of a sufficiently sensitive and reliable cytologic, biochemical, or immunologic test which is suited to repetitive screening of the vast population at risk. The search for such a diagnostic laboratory test has resulted in a number of encouraging possibilities.

The unparalleled success of mass cytologic screening for carcinoma and related premalignant lesions of the uterine cervix has encouraged investigators to attempt to detect ovarian cancer by cytologic means. There is unequivocal evidence that well-established ovarian cancer sheds detectable cells. About 20 to 40 percent of patients with advanced, symptomatic ovarian cancer have malignant cells present in cervicovaginal smears. The exfoliated tumor cells usually arrive in the lower genital tract after transportation through the fallopian tube and endometrial cavity. In other instances, their presence in a cervicovaginal smear is indicative of metastasis to the uterus. Early detection of ovarian neoplasia, however, requires identification of tumors before symptoms develop. Rarely is an ovarian neoplasm initially detected in a cervicovaginal smear obtained during a routine pelvic examination.

Advanced carcinoma of the ovary often produces ascitic fluid which may then become a source of detectable tumor cells. Cytologic examinations of ascitic fluid obtained by paracentesis or cul-de-sac aspiration from patients with ovarian cancer have revealed malignant cells in over 85 percent of cases. Culdocentesis, which provides convenient access to the peritoneal cavity, has been advocated as a logical means to detect clinically occult ovarian cancers. Although early reports of this technique were encouraging, the overall results have been disappointing. The principal drawback to this method is that neoplastic cells are not exfoliated until relatively late in the disease after invasion of the cortex and extension onto the ovarian surface have occurred.

The initial clue to a functioning ovarian tumor may be provided by cytologic examination. The finding of a high "estrogen effect" in the cervicovaginal smear of a postmenopausal woman who is not receiving exogenous hormonal preparations is suggestive of an estrogen-secreting ovarian neoplasm, such as a granulosa tumor or thecoma.

The greatest prospect for developing a diagnostic screening test for ovarian cancer is in the field of tumor immunology. Tumor-specific and tumor-associated antigens have been identified for many human cancers including serous carcinoma of the ovary (Levi et al.). Serum radioimmunoassay of these tumor-associated antigens could prove to be sufficiently sensitive and specific to detect preclinical ovarian cancer. The prototype of tumor-associated antigens is the polypeptide hormone chorionic gonadotropin produced by trophoblastic tumors of gestational or germ-cell origin. The dependability of HCG assay is responsible in part for the high degree of success in the treatment of gestational choriocarcinoma. AFP has been identified in the serum of women with certain malignant germ-cell tumors (Masopust et al.). AFP determinations could prove suitable as a diagnostic test and therapeutic monitor for malignant germ-cell tumors.

Other serum factors may have abnormal values in patients with ovarian cancer including lactic dehydrogenase, haptoglobin, and fucose. The titer of these substances roughly reflects the size of the viable tumor-cell population. Whether such measurements will be of practical use has yet to be demonstrated.

Prevention

The only known method of preventing ovarian cancer is by surgical castration. Since the risk of any woman developing ovarian cancer during her lifetime is only about 1 percent, the probable benefit of ovariectomy to the individual is small. Operating solely for the purpose of cancer prophylaxis cannot be seriously considered, but routine oophorectomy at the time of pelvic surgery could reduce the occurrence of ovarian cancer. According to published series of ovarian cancer, 5 to 10 percent of cases occur in women who had previously undergone hysterectomy for benign disease (de Neef, Hollenbeck). There would seem to be no valid objection to preventive ovariectomy in postmenopausal women since the ovaries have neither a reproductive nor indispensable endocrine function at this time of life. Since the ovary is essential to conception, prophylactic oophorectomy during the reproductive years is reserved for patients undergoing hysterectomy for benign gynecologic disease. Most commonly the minimum age recommended for prophylactic oophorectomy falls within the fifth decade of life, although some recommendations extend down to age 35 years (Gibbs). The availability of medicinal estrogens has engendered the belief that the ovaries can be removed with impunity even in young women,

but this is speculative since only long-term follow-up of large numbers of patients and careful correlation of their general health status indices will decide the issue.

It has been suggested that hysterectomy compromises ovarian function by predisposing the ovary to a variety of diseases. While this would certainly strengthen the argument for routine oophorectomy, the contention is unproved. Paloucek found no evidence that hysterectomy or the indication for hysterectomy either increased or decreased the risk of developing an ovarian malignancy, nor did there seem to be any difference if one or both ovaries were preserved.

Grogan (1967a) rejected the idea that oophorectomy can be justified solely on the basis of preventing ovarian cancer, and he described a syndrome of pelvic pain, tenderness, dyspareunia, and adnexal mass in posthysterectomy patients due to multiple cystic, atretic, and/or hemorrhagic follicles with perioophoritis. These findings have suggested ovarian dysfunction after hysterectomy. However, several other investigations (Randall et al., 1957; TeLinde, Wharton; de Neef, Hollenbeck; Ranney) indicate that the function of preserved ovaries may be normal.

Until more explicit information becomes available regarding (1) deleterious effects of premature castration, (2) the value of exogenous estrogens, and (3) the hazards of the preserved ovary, the optimal age for routine oophorectomy during the reproductive years cannot be determined. The majority of women experience spontaneous ovarian failure after the age of 45 years. Oophorectomy prior to this time should be limited to women with specific indications such as a family history of ovarian cancer, previous surgery for an ovarian neoplasm, cancerphobia, and evidence of ovarian dysfunction or pelvic inflammatory disease.

CLINICAL MANIFESTATIONS

The clinical manifestations of ovarian tumors are in the main quite pedestrian. There exist, however, some remarkable, albeit unusual, manifestations of ovarian neoplasms. There are, of course, the clinical syndromes of pseudoprecocious puberty, postmenopausal refeminization, and virilization due to sex steroid production by functioning ovarian tumors. Autoimmune hemolytic anemia associated with mature cystic teratoma has been documented. Other endocrine disorders caused by ovarian tumors include hyperthyroidism and the carcinoid syndrome. Hypercalcemia has been observed in association with a variety of malignant ovarian tumors, and hypoglycemia has been reported in conjunction with serous carcinoma.

Symptoms

The early development of ovarian neoplasms, whether benign or malignant, is typically silent, As the mass enlarges, progressive compression of the surrounding pelvic organs produces such ordinary symptoms as urinary frequency, constipation, and a vague pelvic discomfort or feeling of heaviness. Dyspareunia is reported in some cases. When the diameter of the tumor reaches 12 to 15 cm, it begins to rise out of the pelvis which can no longer accommodate it. At this stage the patient is likely to notice abdominal enlargement. During the late reproductive years, the coincidental occurrence of menopausal amenorrhea and abdominal swelling may be misinterpreted as a pregnancy. Pain of various degrees is one of the most common presenting symptoms of ovarian tumors. Rapid enlargement of the ovary with capsular stretching, twisting, intracystic hemorrhage, and rupture are all mechanisms by which ovarian tumors produce pain. In childhood and during the early reproductive years, ovarian lesions frequently simulate acute appendicitis. Menstrual irregularities, more commonly associated with functional cysts, also may accompany true neoplasms.

Malignant ovarian tumors are seldom discovered in an asymptomatic patient, a fact which is attributable to their rapid growth. Abdominal pain and swelling are consistently the two most common complaints reported. In the presence of ascites or metastases to the upper abdomen, gastrointestinal symptoms such as bloating, heartburn, nausea, anorexia, and abdominal discomfort may predominate. It is understandable that the patient with ovarian carcinoma often seeks advice from an internist because her symptoms are suggestive of cholecystitis, peptic ulcer, and other gastrointestinal diseases. In the presence of clinically apparent ascites, this constellation of symptoms often leads to a tentative diagnosis of liver disease or upper abdominal cancer. Some women will have noticeable weight loss before reporting for medical care, apparently because of chronic anorexia and nausea. The relative frequency of the most common presenting complaints of women with ovarian cancer are listed in Table 45–9.

TABLE 45–9 Presenting Symptoms of Patients with Ovarian Cancer

Symptom	Percent
Abdominal swelling	70
Abdominal discomfort	50
Gastrointestinal	20
Urinary (frequency, etc.)	15
Abnormal bleeding	15
Weight loss	15
Asymptomatic	<2

Physical Findings

While ovarian neoplasms are often palpable abdominally, an adequate pelvic examination is usually the key to diagnosis. A small ovarian mass may be missed, especially in an obese patient. Usually the lower genital tract is normal in patients with an ovarian tumor, but the cervix and vagina may be displaced by extrinsic pressure. Bimanual palpation should delineate the ovarian mass. The uterus is often distinctly separate, but at times such a discrimination is not possible. Dermoids and endometriotic cysts tend to occupy the space anterior to the uterus, but most ovarian tumors lie posteriorly or have ascended into the abdomen. Generally speaking, most benign ovarian neoplasms are unilateral, cystic, and mobile, while malignancies are more likely to be at least partly solid, bilateral, and fixed. Ascites and even hydrothorax may accompany benign solid tumors (Meigs's syndrome) but are far more common with malignant growths.

An essential phase of the gynecologic examination is the rectovaginal bimanual palpation of the pelvic structures. This maneuver permits an evaluation of the posterior uterine surface, uterosacral ligaments, the pouch of Douglas, and the parametria. Small ovarian tumors, cul-de-sac nodularity, and disease in the rectovaginal septum may be detected in this manner; they might otherwise not be appreciated on physical examination.

The delineation of a large ovarian mass on abdominal examination is frequently a simple matter, particularly in the thin subject with a solid or semisolid tumor, but differentiation of ascites from a large ovarian cyst may be exceedingly difficult. A fluid wave can be elicited in either condition. With the patient supine, the tympanitic note of the small intestine should be central in a patient with ascites and lateral when the distention is secondary to a large mass.

Also, ascites will balloon an umbilical hernia sac but a mass will not.

It is imperative that the physical examination not be limited to the gynecologic evaluation. The peripheral areas bearing lymph nodes must be carefully palpated. The supraclavicular and inguinal nodes are frequent sites of metastases from ovarian cancer, and even the axillary nodes may be involved. The breast and rectum are more common sites for primary cancer in women than any of the genital organs, and they should always be examined. Especially in the patient with ascites, evidence of liver disease must be searched for as part of the physical examination.

DIAGNOSTIC STUDIES

In the effort to establish the presence of an ovarian neoplasm, several radiographic studies are needed.

FIGURE 45–3 Anterioposterior radiograph of the abdomen. Within the pelvis are two sets of calcified densities representing teeth within bilateral benign cystic teratomas (dermoids). *(Courtesy of Dr. J. Richmond, University of Southern California, Los Angeles.)*

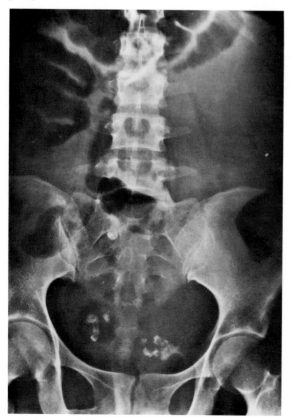

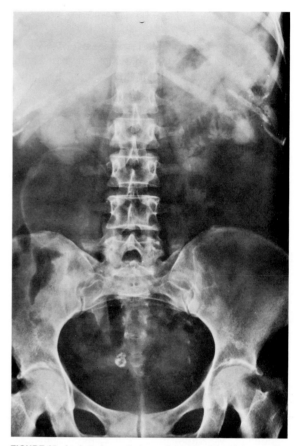

FIGURE 45–4 Anteriorposterior radiograph of the abdomen. The capsule or rim sign identifies the mass in the right lumbar region as a benign teratoma (dermoid). The interface between the cyst capsule and the relatively radiolucent sebaceous contents of the dermoid enhances the visibility of the capsule. The calcified density in the pelvis is in a uterine myoma. *(Courtesy of Dr. J. Richmond.)*

A plain film of the abdomen frequently provides clues to the presence and nature of a pelvic mass. Nearly one-half of ovarian dermoid cysts can be positively identified in this manner because of three characteristic radiographic features: (1) Calcifications due to tooth and bone formation (Fig. 45–3), (2) a radiolucent shadow cast by the lipidic fluid filling the cyst, and (3) the "capsule sign," a rim of radiodensity circumscribing the cyst (Fig. 45–4). Papillary serous tumors, benign and malignant, may contain sufficient calcification to be visible radiographically. The metastases from malignant serous tumors may similarly contain sufficient psammoma bodies to be visualized (Fig. 45–5). A mottled pattern of calcification also may be seen with gonadoblastoma. Numerous other causes of pelvic masses can have calcific densities,

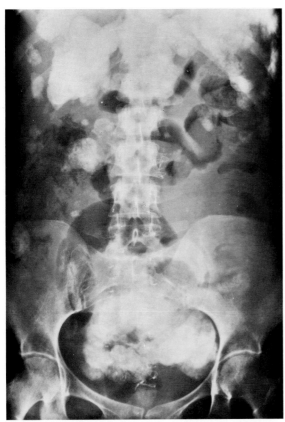

FIGURE 45–5 Anterioposterior radiograph of the abdomen. The extensive calcified densities are produced by psammoma bodies in a well-differentiated papillary serous carcinoma of the ovary. Both the unresectable primary tumor in the pelvis and abdominal metastases are visualized.

pecially valuable in identifying ovarian tumors during pregnancy. Ultrasound can detect clinically occult ascites and distinguish ascites from intracystic fluid. It has also been employed to follow the response of tumor masses and ascites during therapy, and to monitor the patient for recurrence after completion of treatment.

Laparoscopy has been suggested but never satisfactorily established as a modality useful in the evaluation of patients with ascites, ovarian cysts, or suspected pelvic malignancy. While the presence of an ovarian tumor may be verified at laparoscopy, visual examination alone is unreliable in determining whether a clinically significant ovarian cystic mass is functional or neoplastic. Aspiration of fluid from such ovarian cysts at laparoscopy must be condemned because of the risk of spilling malignant cells into the peritoneal cavity. Similarly, the laparoscopic biopsy of ovarian tumors, cystic or otherwise, is contraindicated. The laparoscope could be employed to clarify the clinical suspicion of a pelvic lesion. It might prove to be useful in selected patients with ovarian cancer to assess the extent of disease without laparotomy (Fig. 45–6), but its limitations must be recognized. Resectability may not be evaluable by laparoscopy, examination of the abdominal contents is limited, and the retroperitoneal space cannot be assessed. Culdoscopy and pelvic pneumography offer alternatives

including leiomyoma, intrauterine pregnancy, and lithopedion. Intravenous urography may be of great importance in evaluating the patient with a pelvic mass since it will identify the presence of ureteral obstruction and urinary tract anomalies, especially a pelvic kidney or duplicated ureter. X-ray contrast studies of the colon in conjunction with proctosigmoidoscopy are helpful in excluding the presence of primary neoplasms of this organ and may also define intrinsic inflammatory lesions which can be confused with ovarian tumors.

Ultrasound imaging is a well-established diagnostic technique in obstetrics and gynecology. Its role in the assessment of patients with ovarian neoplasia has not been defined, but there are many areas of promise. Ultrasound has the capability of localizing pelvic and intraabdominal masses, distinguishing cystic from solid tumors, and it may discriminate between uterine and adnexal masses. It seems es-

FIGURE 45–6 Laparascopic view of the right hemidiaphragm and surface of liver. The discrete nodules on the diaphragm are implants of ovarian carcinoma. The patient also had implants in pelvis and abdomen. (*Courtesy of C. Lacey, M.D., Chief of Gynecologic Oncology, Tulane University Medical School, New Orleans.*)

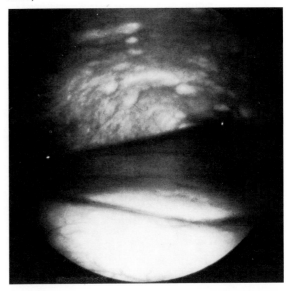

to laparoscopy in defining ovarian enlargement which is suspected but uncertain on pelvic examination.

Lymphangiography, venography, arteriography, and gallium scintigraphy have all been investigated as methods of evaluating pelvic masses and ovarian cancer, but none has an established role in this clinical problem.

COELOMIC EPITHELIAL NEOPLASMS

Tumors of coelomic epithelium arise from the epithelium of inclusion cysts that are common in the cortex of the adult ovary or, less often, directly from the surface epithelium. Rarely, origin from the rete ovarii is demonstrable. Histologically, most are composed of epithelium that resembles Müllerian epithelium of the endosalpinx, endometrium, or endocervix. Some examples simulate neoplasms of the colon, urinary bladder, and kidney. They are the most common type of primary ovarian tumor. At least 50 percent of all benign ovarian tumors and 85 percent of all malignant neoplasms are of epithelial origin.

Each tumor is classified according to its epithelial cell type into serous, mucinous, endometrioid, and mesonephroid, or Brenner groups. Often referred to as the "common" epithelial tumors, they are the most frequently encountered varieties. Each cell type can be categorized further as either benign, malignant, or borderline. Mixtures of different cell types often occur in the same neoplasm. In such cases, the tumor is classified according to the predominant cell type. The rare carcinosarcomas and mixed mesodermal tumors are also believed to arise from coelomic epithelium.

Epithelial ovarian tumors are notorious for the wide variations in degree of differentiation that can be found in different areas of the same tumor. Since the malignant potential is determined by the least differentiated portion, extensive sampling of the specimen by the pathologist is imperative for accurate diagnosis. This basic principle applies as well to all ovarian neoplasms. Particular attention should be given to papillary areas, nodular thickenings and roughened portions of a cyst wall, solid areas, and regions where hemorrhage or necrosis is conspicuous. These gross features are characteristic although not diagnostic of malignant neoplasms, and they serve as useful warnings to the informed surgeon as well as to the pathologist.

BENIGN EPITHELIAL NEOPLASMS

Considered in this group are cystadenomas and related tumors, and Brenner tumors.

Cystadenomas and Related Tumors

Most benign epithelial tumors are predominantly cystic and are diagnosed as cystadenomas. Some have a considerable connective tissue component in addition to epithelial cysts and are designated *adenofi-*

FIGURE 45–7 Papillary serous cystadenoma (gross specimen). Opened unilocular cyst has numerous small cauliflowerlike excrescences protruding from interior of otherwise smooth cyst wall. The cortical surface is uninvolved.

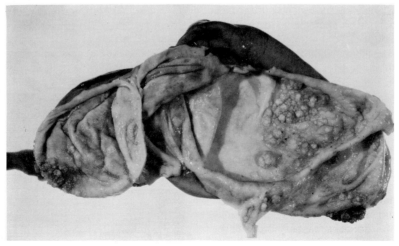

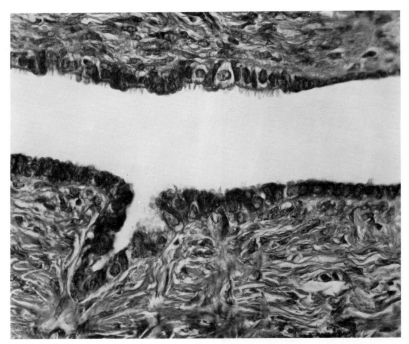

FIGURE 45–8 Papillary serous cystadenoma (photomicrograph). A single layer of cuboidal and co-lumnar cells covers fibrous connective tissue stalks of papillary projections. Cilia can be identified on several cells. H & E × 900.

bromas or *cystadenofibromas*. If the entire lesion is an exophytic growth on the cortical surface of the ovary, it is referred to as a *surface papilloma*. The character of the fluid within a cystadenoma often suggests the specific cell type but cannot be relied upon for diagnosis. Thin, watery fluid is typical of a serous cystadenoma, while viscid fluid usually indicates a mucinous lesion.

The majority of cystadenomas are of the serous type. They may be unilocular or multilocular. The cyst walls are smooth, but firm cauliflowerlike papillary projections sometimes protude into the lumen (Fig. 45–7). Papillations also may be located on the surface, but this finding is always worrisome since it is more typical of papillary serous cystadenocarcinomas. Bilaterality occurs in 15 to 20 percent of cases. Microscopically, the papillary serous cystadenoma is characterized by broad, fibrous connective tissue processes that are covered by a single layer of cuboidal or columnar cells. In many instances, ciliated epithelium with peg cells similar to fallopian tube epithelium is found (Fig. 45–8).

Mucinous cystadenomas are usually multiloculated and may reach gigantic proportions. Some of the largest tumors ever observed in human beings have been ovarian mucinous cystadenomas (Fig. 45–9). Papillary processes and surface involvement are unusual. Only about 5 percent are bilateral. The cysts are thin and smooth (Fig. 45–10) and contain mucoid fluid (Fig. 45–11). They usually are lined by a single layer of well-differentiated mucinous epithelium that is practically indistinguishable from that of the endocervix (Fig. 45–12). Other examples have goblet cells and more closely resemble intestinal epithelium. Argentaffin cells may also be identified. These latter features suggest that some mucinous cystadenomas are teratomatous in origin. About 5 percent of mucinous tumors are associated with either dermoid cysts or Brenner tumors. Ultrastructural studies have corroborated the impression that mucinous ovarian tumors are a heterogeneous group, possibly of diverse origin.

Intraoperative rupture of a mucinous cystadenoma with spillage of its contents into the peritoneal cavity is not as ominous as once thought. Such spillage does not appear to adversely affect the prognosis of patients with benign lesions, although implants of neoplastic epithelium may occasionally occur. However, mucinous ovarian tumors are often found in patients who have large pools of organizing mucus in their abdominal cavity and pelvis, a condition referred to as *pseudomyxoma peritonei*. Commonly, the epithelium of the mucinous ovarian tumor is well differentiated and is histologically benign.

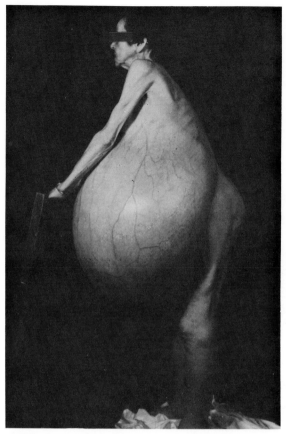

FIGURE 45-9 Clinical appearance of woman with massive abdominal distention due to a huge benign mucinous cystadenoma of the ovary.

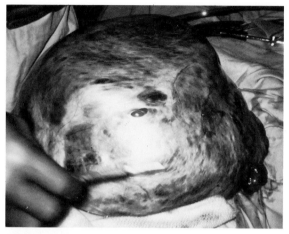

FIGURE 45-10 Large, mucinous cystadenoma just delivered through a vertical, midline abdominal incision. In two areas the capsule has been breached and portions of the multiloculated tumor are visible.

While circumstantial evidence suggests that pseudomyxoma may result from spontaneous, preoperative rupture of a benign or low-grade malignant mucinous tumor, the precise pathogenesis of this condition remains unclear. Mucoceles of the appendix and carcinomas of the colon may coexist with the ovarian tumor, and the primary source responsible for the pseudomyxoma may be difficult to determine. Regardless of cause, pseudomyxoma peritonei is a dangerous condition that may result in dense peritoneal adhesions, recurrent intestinal obstruction, inanition, and death.

FIGURE 45-11 Mucinous cystadenoma (gross specimen). Sectioned surface reveals multiple cysts of various sizes, several of which are still intact.

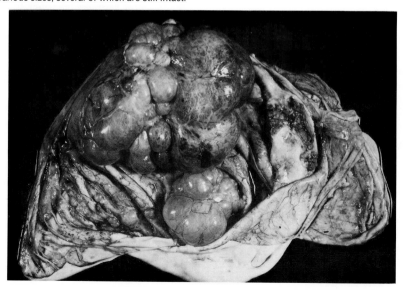

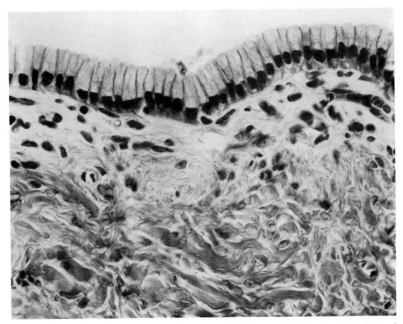

FIGURE 45–12 Mucinous cystadenoma (photomicrograph). Cyst wall is lined by single layer of well-differentiated mucinous epithelial cells similar to those of endocervical mucosa. H & E × 1000.

Some adenofibromas contain small cysts and glands lined by endometriumlike epithelium that is not surrounded by the typical cellular stroma of endometriosis. Squamous metaplasia may be prominent. Such examples should be classified as *endometrioid adenofibromas*. Mesonephroid adeno-fibromas are occasionally encountered, but their distinction from well-differentiated forms of clear-cell carcinoma can be difficult.

Brenner Tumors

Approximately 1 to 2 percent of ovarian neoplasms qualify for the eponymic designation of Brenner tumor. They are composed of nests of transitionallike epithelium embedded in abundant dense fibrous connective tissue (Fig. 45–13). Origins from numerous ovarian structures have been postulated, and Brenner believed it to be a variant of a granulosa tumor when he described it as *oophoroma folliculare*. Most modern investigators classify the Brenner tumor as arising from the coelomic epithelium which differentiates toward urinary tract (transitional) epithelium during neoplastic transformation.

Brenner tumors are usually incidentally discovered during surgery for other pelvic disorders. The mean age of patients at time of diagnosis is 45 to 50 years. None has been found in children. Their size varies, but about 50 percent are only of microscopic

dimensions. Associated mucinous cystadenomas are present in 10 percent of cases, and benign cystic teratomas are found in an additional 5 percent.

Patients are often asymptomatic, but those with larger tumors may have abdominal enlargement, pain, and menstrual irregularities. Endocrine disturbances suggestive of estrogen secretion by the tumor

FIGURE 45–13 Brenner tumor (photomicrograph). Nests of benign transitionallike epithelial cells are embedded in dense collagenous fibrous connective tissue. H & E × 400.

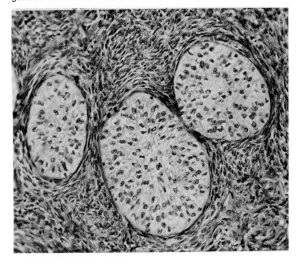

have occurred in several cases, and in vitro androgen synthesis also has been reported. Hormone production is believed to occur in the connective tissue stroma of the tumor which may be luteinized.

Grossly, Brenner tumors are solid masses that have a white or pale yellow sectioned surface which gives them an appearance similar to a fibroma or thecoma. Some examples are cystic. Bilaterality occurs in 6 to 7 percent of cases.

Over 99 percent are benign, both histologically and clinically. Recently, a number of proliferative Brenner tumors have been described. These resemble low-grade transitional cell neoplasms of the urinary bladder and are best regarded as borderline tumors. None has metastasized. A few Brenner tumors are malignant. In these, the epithelial element has undergone carcinomatous change, and behavior like other ovarian carcinomas is to be expected in such instances.

BORDERLINE TUMORS

Traditionally, the epithelial tumors have been sharply divided into either benign or malignant types, although the criteria for diagnosis have varied considerably among pathologists. About 15 percent, however, are intermediate in both their histologic appearance and clinical behavior between the innocuous cystadenoma and the frankly malignant cystadenocarcinoma. These borderline tumors were recognized by Taylor and his associates in the 1920s as low-grade malignancies, and others regarded them as semimalignant or questionably malignant tumors. In 1961 FIGO gave them official status in their classification of epithelial ovarian tumors by designating them as cystadenomas of low potential malignancy (Table 45–10). The World Health Organization also recognized the intermediate-grade tumors and referred to them as tumors of borderline malignancy or as carcinomas of low malignant potential (Serov et al.).

TABLE 45–10 FIGO* Histologic Classification of the Common Primary Epithelial Tumors of the Ovary

---

1. Benign cystadenomas
2. Cystadenomas with proliferative activity of the epithelial cells and nuclear abnormalities but with no infiltrative destructive growth (low potential malignancy)
3. Cystadenocarcinomas

---

*Federation International de Gynecologie et Obstetrique.

The borderline tumors are characterized by excessive proliferation of epithelial cells which display nuclear atypism. To qualify for the designation of borderline malignancy or carcinoma of low malignant potential, there must be no invasion of the ovarian stroma by the neoplastic cells. Furthermore, the cells should not display the degree of cytologic anaplasia of clearly malignant neoplasms (Hart). Most experience to date has been gained with the borderline tumors of serous and mucinous cell types.

Borderline serous tumors usually are cystic and have intraluminal papillae. Papillary excrescence also may involve the cortical surface as a result of direct neoplastic transformation of the surface epithelium. Occasionally the entire lesion consists of exophytic papillary surface tumor unassociated with internal cysts. Bilaterality has been reported in about 14 to 33 percent of cases and is believed to represent separate independent primary tumor development in most instances. Of greatest concern is the high incidence of extraovarian spread of borderline serous neoplasms. Extension beyond the ovaries has been found at the time of the initial operation in 20 to 46 percent of patients. Such spread typically appears as multiple superficial implantation "metastases" on the peritoneum, omentum, and serosal surfaces of pelvic organs. These are especially likely to develop when involvement of the external ovarian surface is prominent. Ascitic fluid often results, and it may contain papillary clusters of neoplastic cells. The presence of peritoneal implants does not alter the histologic diagnosis of borderline malignancy. Some implants presumably fail to proliferate and very rare instances of spontaneous regression have been cited. In spite of the frequency of spread beyond the ovary, the prognosis is highly favorable. Corrected 5-year survival rates of 92 to 100 percent have been reported and 10-year rates have ranged from about 75 to 90 percent. However, recurrent lesions within the pelvis or abdomen may develop after long latent intervals of up to 20 or even 50 years.

Mucinous cystadenomas of borderline malignancy have an even better prognosis than do serous tumors of similar type. The mucinous tumors are bilateral in only 10 percent or less of cases. Involvement of the ovarian cortical surface and widespread peritoneal implantation are infrequent, and most examples are classified as stage I. In a long-term follow-up study of stage I tumors, Hart and Norris reported corrected actuarial survival rates of 98 percent at 5 years and 96 percent at 10 years. Regardless of the diagnostic terminology used for these borderline tumors, their slow growth, indolent behavior, and favorable prognosis are recognized by most gynecologists and pathologists. They must be separated from the higher grades of carcinoma if meaningful data on prognosis and therapy are to be obtained.

MALIGNANT EPITHELIAL NEOPLASMS

A greater variety of malignant than benign tumors originate from derivatives of the coelomic epithelium. Typically, they appear as cystadenocarcinomas, although some have a predominantly solid configuration. Most can be readily classified according to cell type as mentioned previously. Some carcinomas of the ovary, however, are so poorly differentiated that the cell type cannot be determined. These undifferentiated carcinomas constitute from 5 to 15 percent of cases in large series. No useful purpose is served by forcing such a tumor into one of the other diagnostic categories. Their prognosis is dismal, as only 15 percent of patients survive 5 years. Survival rates of each histologic cell type correlate both with the degree of differentiation (grade) and the extent of spread (stage). Well-differentiated carcinomas of stage I have a favorable prognosis in all categories.

Serous Carcinoma

At least 35 percent of serous tumors are malignant, and they comprise approximately half of all ovarian adenocarcinomas (Table 45–11). Grossly, their cystic configuration is partially obliterated by solid overgrowths of tissue (Fig. 45–14). Papillary projections are bulky and soft because of the increased proliferation of epithelium at the expense of the connective tissue cores. Surface nodules and papillations are common, and their presence should always suggest the possibility of malignancy. The epithelium covering the papillary processes and lining the cysts is multilayered and dedifferentiated, and it infiltrates the ovarian stroma. Psammoma bodies are characteristic of serous tumors, although they are occasionally found in other tumors. They are more common in the

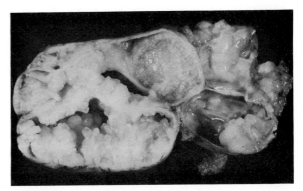

FIGURE 45–14 Papillary serous cystadenocarcinoma (gross specimen). Sectioned surface shows partial obliteration of cysts by solid papillary overgrowths. Involvement of the cortical surface by neoplasm is prominent.

well-differentiated papillary serous cystadenocarcinomas, but are also found in benign cystadenomas and epithelial inclusion cysts. Identification of psammoma bodies in biopsies from women with extensive peritoneal metastases is strong presumptive evidence that the primary tumor has arisen in the ovary and is of serous-cell type.

Bilaterality occurs in 35 to 50 percent of cases but may be found in two-thirds of cases when extensive peritoneal spread is present. Serous carcinoma spreads rapidly throughout the peritoneal cavity, and only 20 percent of patients have stage I neoplasms at the time of initial diagnosis (Table 45–12). Early peritoneal dissemination is related to involvement of the cortical surface which is so frequent in serous tumors. Prognosis is poor, with reported overall 5-year survival rates of only 15 to 30 percent (Table 45–13).

Mucinous Carcinoma

Mucinous cystadenocarcinomas account for about 15 percent of malignant epithelial tumors. In contrast to the serous neoplasms, only about 10 percent of all mucinous tumors are malignant. Their gross appear-

TABLE 45–11 Relative Frequency of Primary Carcinomas According to Epithelial Cell Type

Cell type	Percent
Serous	50
Mucinous	15
Endometrioid	20
Mesonephroid	5
Undifferentiated	10

TABLE 45–12 Incidence of Stage I Carcinomas in Each of the Epithelial Cell Types

Cell type	Percent stage I
Serous carcinoma	20
Mucinous carcinoma	50
Endometrioid carcinoma	48
Mesonephroid carcinoma	56
Undifferentiated carcinoma	25

Source: Aure et al. 1971a.

TABLE 45–13 Five-Year Survival Rates of Carcinomas According to Epithelial Cell Type

Cell type	5-year survival, percent
Serous carcinoma	15–30
Mucinous carcinoma	40–45
Endometrioid carcinoma	45–55
Mesonephroid carcinoma	40–45
Undifferentiated carcinoma	15

Source: Aure et al., 1971a; Santesson and Kottmeier.

ance often resembles a multiloculated mucinous cystadenoma, but usually areas of thickening or solid nodules are found. Papillations may protrude from the walls but are not as frequent as in serous carcinomas. Foci of hemorrhage and necrosis are common, but when extensive they should alert one to the possibility of a metastatic carcinoma of the colon masquerading as a primary ovarian mucinous cystadenocarcinoma. Many experienced surgeons and pathologists have made this error.

Mucinous carcinomas are unilateral in 90 percent of cases, and half of the tumors are stage I at the time of discovery. The absence of surface involvement, together with the high proportion of tumors confined to the ovary, is an important factor that contributes to the relatively favorable prognosis for patients with a mucinous carcinoma. Five-year survival rates of 40 to 45 percent can be expected.

Endometrioid Carcinoma

Although endometrium-like carcinomas have been recognized as a distinctive form of primary ovarian carcinoma since Sampson's description in 1925, it was not until the FIGO classification and the report of Long and Taylor in 1964 that the entity became widely recognized. In the past, endometrioid carcinomas were often referred to as *adenocanthoma* or *solid adenocarcinomas*. The term *endometrioid* does not imply an origin from endometriosis. While 9 percent of endometrioid carcinomas are accompanied by ovarian endometriosis (Aure et al., 1971d), few instances of actual malignant transformation from an endometriotic cyst have been documented. A variety of different cancers have originated from ovarian and extraovarian endometriosis including mesenchymal (i.e., endometrial stromal sarcoma) as well as epithelial lesions. These are not endometrioid carcinomas and should be considered separately.

Endometrioid carcinomas compose 15 to 25 per-

cent of all ovarian carcinomas. The relative proportion varies with the pathologist's zeal for observing microscopic features that are reminiscent of adenocarcinoma of the endometrium. Since primary carcinomas of the endometrium may have numerous appearances, there is a tendency to overutilize the endometrioid category. If it is restricted to tumors that mimic the most common pattern of endometrial adenocarcinoma, the endometrioid group is useful. Otherwise, it becomes a "wastebasket" of heterogeneous and unrelated tumors. Most investigators, therefore, include only well- or moderately differentiated adenocarcinomas and adenoacanthomatous carcinomas. This is not to deny that poorly differentiated endometrioid carcinomas occur, but their recognition and separation from nonspecific or undifferentiated carcinomas is difficult. The presence of squamous differentiation is heavily relied upon in such instances. About 30 percent of endometrioid carcinomas involve both ovaries, but a more accurate estimate of bilaterality is obtained if examples with extensive peritoneal spread are excluded. Thus, only 13 percent of tumors confined to the ovaries, uterus, and/or tubes (stages I to IIa) are bilateral, according to Kottmeier (1968a).

Adenocarcinoma of the endometrium occurs with ovarian endometrioid carcinoma in 15 to 30 percent of cases. This is in marked contrast to the overall 4 percent incidence found in patients with ovarian carcinoma of all histologic types. In the majority of instances, the synchronous ovarian and endometrial carcinomas are separate, independent, primary tumors and not metastases from one to the other. When the endometrial carcinoma is small and well differentiated, only superficially infiltrates the myometrium, and is accompanied by endometrial hyperplasia, then the accompanying ovarian tumor is practically certain to be a separate primary.

The prognosis of endometrioid carcinoma is relatively good with approximately 50 percent of patients surviving at least 5 years. As with mucinous carcinomas, about half are stage I lesions. Interestingly, the prognosis of those patients with an associated endometrial carcinoma is similar to those without such a lesion and exceeds the expected survival rates if either the ovarian or endometrial tumors represented a metastasis.

Clear-Cell (Mesonephroid) Carcinoma

Mesonephroid carcinoma accounts for 5 percent of ovarian carcinomas. Its histogenesis has been debated for decades. In 1939, Schiller described a group of unusual carcinomas that he named *meso-*

nephroma ovarii to indicate their histologic similarity and probable origin from remnants of the mesonephric apparatus. Teilum, in a series of studies in the 1950s, pointed out that Schiller had mistakenly combined two entirely different neoplasms in the mesonephroma category. Teilum separated the highly malignant carcinoma of germ-cell origin (endodermal sinus tumor) from the epithelial neoplasm currently called mesonephroid or clear-cell carcinoma of epithelial origin.

Histologically identical carcinomas also may originate in the vagina, cervix, endometrium, and broad ligament. The ovarian tumors are not known to be related to in utero exposure to diethylstilbestrol as are some of the cervicovaginal mesonephroid carcinomas. In contrast to the clear-cell carcinomas of the lower genital tract which are frequent in young women and children, practically all ovarian tumors of this type are found in women over 30 to 35 years of age, and the median age is about 50 years.

An important association with endometriosis has been established for mesonephroid carcinoma. Ovarian endometriosis has been identified in 24 percent of cases (Aure et al., 1971d). Its close relationship to endometrioid carcinoma as well as to endometriosis has been emphasized. The evidence indicates that mesonephroid carcinoma of the ovary arises from coelomic epithelial elements in most instances and from endometriosis, which also can be a derivative of coelomic epithelium according to the metaplastic theory of endometriosis, in some cases. While clear-cell carcinoma may originate from mesonephric structures in other sites, it has not been demonstrated in the ovary.

Bilaterality occurs in approximately 5 percent of cases. Grossly, the tumors may be cystic or solid. The microscopic pattern consists of variable mixtures of solid sheets of epithelium with clear cytoplasm and tubules or glands lined by clear and hobnail cells. Papillary areas are common. The prognosis is similar for mesonephroid and endometrioid carcinomas. Patients with stage I tumors (56 percent) have 5-year survival rates of 60 to 80 percent, while 40 to 45 percent of patients survive 5 years when all stages are considered.

Carcinosarcoma and Mixed Mesodermal Tumors

Rarely, ovarian tumors are composed of both malignant epithelial and mesenchymal tissues. These "mixed" cancers are referred to as *mixed mesodermal tumors* when the sarcomatous component contains heterologous elements that are foreign to the ovary such as chondro-, rhabdomyo-, or osteosarcoma. *Carcinosarcoma* is the term used when the sarcomatous portion does not contain such elements. Some prefer to regard all such mixed cancers as carcinosarcomas. Identical tumors more commonly originate in the uterus and rarely are primary in the fallopian tube.

Over 80 percent of the patients are older than 50 years of age, and about half are nulliparous. The tumors are large, bulky, and usually relatively solid. The median diameter is 15 cm. Metastases are frequently found at surgery. Few patients survive more than 1 or 2 years after diagnosis. According to Dehner et al., the median survival is 15 months for patients with a carcinosarcoma and only 6 months for those with a mixed mesodermal tumor.

MANAGEMENT OF OVARIAN NEOPLASIA

Preoperative Evaluation

The diagnosis and management of ovarian neoplasia, benign or malignant, ultimately are dependent upon surgical exploration. The preoperative workup must be tailored to the symptomatology, physical findings, and the patient's general medical condition. Table 45–14 lists some of the numerous conditions that may masquerade as an ovarian enlargement. The most common nongynecologic causes of an adnexal mass are appendiceal abscess, diverticulitis, and carcinoma of the rectosigmoid (White et al.; Kajanoja). Cervical cytology is of limited practical value in assessing a pelvic mass, but it should be performed to evaluate the cervix for neoplasia. The endometrium ought to be sampled to exclude the presence of carcinoma, especially in the patient with a history of abnormal bleeding or an enlarged uterus. While upper gastrointestinal symptoms in a patient with an adnexal tumor suggest ovarian cancer with abdominal metastases or ascites, the etiology may be unrelated to the pelvic mass, and investigative studies are necessary.

Symptoms referable to the colon are particularly important when the pelvic mass is fixed, irregular, or ill-defined, since inflammatory and neoplastic diseases of the colon are commonly confused with ovarian carcinoma, and vice versa. These conditions can usually be detected by obtaining a radiographic contrast examination of the colon. Intravenous urography provides the surgeon with valuable information about renal function,

TABLE 45–14 Nonovarian Causes of an Apparent Adnexal Mass

Neoplastic

Pedunculated uterine myoma
Round-ligament myoma
Tubal carcinoma
Carcinoma of sigmoid, cecum, appendix
Retroperitoneal neoplasm
Broad-ligament neoplasm

Nonneoplastic

Pelvic kidney
Tuboovarian abscess
Diverticulitis
Appendiceal abscess
Matted bowel and omentum
Peritoneal cyst
Stool in sigmoid
Full bladder
Urachal cyst
Anterior sacral meningocele
Pregnancy (intrauterine, tubal, abdominal)

TABLE 45–15 Frequent Gross Features of Benign and Malignant Ovarian Tumors

Benign	Malignant
Unilateral	Bilateral
Capsule intact	Capsule ruptured
Freely mobile	Adherent to adjacent organs
Smooth surface	Excrescences on surface
No ascitic fluid	Ascites, especially hemorrhagic
Smooth peritoneal surfaces	Peritoneal implants
Entire tumor viable	Areas of hemorrhage and necrosis
Cystic	Solid or semisolid
Smooth cyst lining	Extensive intracystic papillations
Uniform appearance	Variegated

urinary tract anomalies, and ureteral obstruction. The latter is of special importance when retroperitoneal dissection is contemplated. Liver function studies are essential in the evaluation of ascites, but paracentesis or cul-de-sac aspiration for cytology is seldom necessary if a pelvic mass is present.

Operative Management

All patients suspected of having an ovarian neoplasm, malignant or otherwise, should be subjected to laparotomy as soon as the diagnostic survey is completed. The type of abdominal incision selected must be suited to the physical findings and the range of operative procedures which might be necessitated by the different diagnostic possibilities. Since exfoliated malignant cells often are within the fluid of malignant ovarian cysts, the risk of contaminating the peritoneal cavity with cancer cells by unnecessarily decompressing or otherwise rupturing an ovarian cyst at surgery is contrary to the most fundamental principles of cancer surgery.

Frequently at the time of surgery, the preservation or sacrifice of the reproductive and endocrine functions of the genital tract depends upon recognition of the malignant potential of the ovarian neoplasm. While in most cases absolute identification of malignancy must await histopathologic examination, several gross features suggestive of malignancy may be observed at surgery (Table 45–15). No single finding

is absolutely diagnostic of malignancy, but hemorrhagic ascitic fluid, excrescences on the cortical surface (Fig. 45–15), and peritoneal implants are rarely found with benign tumors. Additional information can be obtained by sectioning the neoplasm after it has been removed. Areas of hemorrhage and necrosis, numerous intracystic papillations, friable tissue, and a mixture of cystic and solid areas all are suggestive of a malignant neoplasm. When a tumor is composed of one or more smooth-walled cysts devoid of papillary excrescences and has no solid or nodular areas, in all likelihood it is benign. The finding of hair, teeth,

FIGURE 45–15 Intraoperative view of ovarian carcinoma with extracystic or surface papillations. Portions of the tumor are cystic. Microscopic study confirmed its malignant nature.

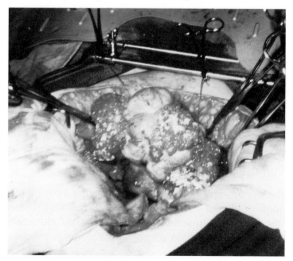

and sebaceous material in an ovarian cyst is evidence that the neoplasm is a cystic teratoma (dermoid cyst) which, with few exceptions, are benign.

MANAGEMENT OF BENIGN EPITHELIAL TUMORS

Surgical excision is adequate therapy for any benign ovarian neoplasm, but factors other than eradicating the tumor enter into the plan of therapy. In postmenopausal women, it is usual to remove the uterus and both adnexa. In the young woman, preservation of childbearing and hormonal functions of the reproductive tract is of major importance, and consequently conservative surgery is the rule. The risk of preserving the contralateral ovary has been studied by Randall et al. (1962). They followed 213 women having a unilateral oophorectomy for a benign serous or mucinous cystadenoma; 7.5 percent developed a neoplasm in the preserved ovary from 2 to 18 years after the initial operation. There did not seem to be any increase or decrease in the risk of the study group developing a benign or malignant ovarian tumor as compared with the general population.

Enucleation of a benign-appearing, unilateral cystic ovarian neoplasm is frequently recommended to conserve ovarian tissue. It is especially applicable to the young patient with bilateral benign cysts or when only a single ovary is present. There is some risk of subsequent development of another neoplasm in the same ovary. Surgical incision of the uninvolved ovary has been recommended to uncover an occult neoplasm. There is no doubt that an otherwise inapparent neoplasm can be discovered in this manner, but neither the discovery rate nor the morbidity to the bivalved ovary has been determined.

MANAGEMENT OF MALIGNANT EPITHELIAL NEOPLASMS

Growth Pattern

The epithelial ovarian malignancies initially grow locally, invading the capsule and mesovarium. Adjacent organs are involved by contiguous growth and lymphatic spread. Once the malignancy has reached the external surface of the capsule, cells and tissue particles are exfoliated into the peritoneal cavity where they are free to circulate and implant on any serosal surface. Local and regional lymphatic metastasis may involve the uterus, fallopian tubes, and the pelvic lymph nodes. Spread to the aortic nodes oc-

TABLE 45–16 Location of Metastases Noted at Operation and Autopsy in 86 Cases of Ovarian Carcinoma

Location	Number of cases	Percent
Peritoneum	75	87
Omentum	61	71
Opposite ovary	61	71
Uterus	16	19
Vagina	11	13
Lymph nodes		
Pelvic	69	80
Aortic	67	78
Mediastinal	43	50
Supraclavicular*		
Left	23	50
Right	21	46
Inguinal		
Left	37	43
Right	31	36
Axillary		
Left	25	29
Right	21	24
Pleura		
Left	25	29
Right	32	37
Lung	32	27
Liver	29	34
Bone	12	14
Spleen, kidney, adrenal, skin	5–7	6–8
Vulva, brain	1	1

*Examined in 46 cases only.
Source: Bergman.

curs via the lymphatic drainage of the infundibulopelvic ligament. Lymphatic involvement is extensive in fatal cases according to the autopsy data of Bergman (Table 45–16). In his study nearly 80 percent of patients dying of ovarian carcinoma had metastases to the pelvic and aortic nodes, and 50 percent had involvement of more distant nodal groups. Musumeci et al. have documented the high incidence of lymphatic metastasis in ovarian carcinoma at the time of diagnosis (Table 45–17). Clinically, hematogenous dissemination is the least apparent mode of spread for ovarian carcinoma, and parenchymal liver and lung metastases are noted only infrequently. It has been generally maintained that ovarian carcinoma remains confined to the abdomen and pelvis. According to Bergman's autopsy data, this concept is inaccurate. He found parenchymal liver and lung metastases in

TABLE 45–17 Incidence of Histologically Confirmed Pelvic-Aortic Lymph Node Metastasis in Ovarian Carcinoma

Stage	No. of cases	Positive	%
Ia	18	3	17
Ib	5	2	40
Ic	1	0	—
IIb	1	0	—
III	22	12	54
IV	3	3	100
Total	50	20	40

Source: Musumeci et al.

one-third of cases and bone involvement in 14 percent. The design of any treatment plan must take this spread pattern into account.

Factors in Management

The volume of tumor and extent of disease spread at the time of diagnosis are the most important variables influencing prognosis in epithelial ovarian cancer. Aure et al. (1971a) found that 43 percent of all cases were confined to the ovaries at the time of diagnosis (Table 45–18). If the borderline tumors (carcinomas of low potential malignancy) are excluded, the proportion of stage I cases drops to 37 percent. The 5-year survival rates for the true carcinomas were 63, 30, 12, and 8 percent for stages I, II, III, and IV, respectively. The stage Ia and Ib have survival rates of 70 and 45 percent, respectively. Survival in stage Ic was essentially the same as in stage Ib.

Accurate knowledge of the histologic type of

TABLE 45–18 Distribution of 990 Patients With Epithelial Ovarian Cancer by Stage

Stage	Percent
I	43
a	29
b	8
c	6
II	24
a	6
b	18
III	23
IV	10

Source: Aure et al. 1971a.

ovarian malignancy is indispensable in assessing the prognosis and planning the treatment. The biologic growth potential of borderline tumors is far more limited than for true carcinomas, and grade I carcinomas are less aggressive than the more undifferentiated forms. Stage for stage, the presence of ascites does not have any great effect on overall survival. The patient must always be considered in planning the treatment of ovarian carcinoma. The very elderly or severely debilitated often must be managed in a modified manner. Intercurrent illnesses as well as previous irradiation or chemotherapy and the patient's willingness to accept the risks, discomforts, and complications of treatment obviously are important.

Therapeutic Modalities

Surgery, radiotherapy, and chemotherapy all play an important role in the management of ovarian carcinoma. Each must be selectively incorporated into the treatment plan. Unfortunately, few controlled studies comparing different treatment methods have been reported, so any plan of management must be tentative. Therapy must be constantly reevaluated as new information develops.

Surgery

A meticulous search must be made for metastasis. This is of critical importance since the minimum scope of acceptable therapy must include all areas of known disease. There is no reasonable hope of cure if carcinoma resides outside the treatment field. The omentum, right hemidiaphragm, and all parietes must be carefully examined. Not only the location of peritoneal metastasis but also the size should be noted. If there is no gross evidence of disease extension outside the ovaries, washings are taken from the pelvis and abdomen for cytology, and a sample of the omentum is removed for pathologic examination. The aortic and pelvic nodes are palpated, and any suspicious lesion is biopsied. The general plan of surgical therapy is to excise the uterus, tubes, and ovaries and any other resectable tumor masses. The uterus may be involved with tumor by direct extension, retrograde lymphatic flow from the adnexa, serosal implants, or transtubal spread. In addition, the endometrium may contain a separate primary cancer. The high incidence of bilateral ovarian involvement generally necessitates removal of both adnexa. Ovarian preservation, with few exceptions, is unwarranted because of the incidence of occult tumor and the propensity for development of malignant disease in a normal ovary.

"Maximal surgical effort" espoused by Munnell (1968) to remove as much tumor as possible without risk of life-threatening complications seems to be valid. Aure et al. (1971a) found that patients with stage III resectable disease had a better prognosis than those with stage II tumors with residual unresectable disease. In 102 patients with stage II and III ovarian carcinoma, Griffiths (1975) found the most important prognostic factors were histologic grade and the diameter of the largest residual tumor mass. With masses under 1.6 cm, mean survival time was proportional to residual tumor size, ranging from 18 months (0.6 to 1.5 cm) to 39 months (no macroscopic residual tumor). Mean survival time with residual masses greater than 1.5 cm was only 12.7 months. Fine judgment is necessary in determining how great an effort should be made, but cases in which all visible disease can be removed, especially those without peritoneal implants, stand to gain the most by radical surgery. The therapeutic value of routine omentectomy in the management of epithelial ovarian carcinoma is unsettled, but excision is clearly indicated when this organ is involved by the malignancy. All too often the surgical phase of treatment for ovarian cancer, depending in part on the gynecologist's skill, is necessarily restricted to laparotomy and biopsy. In some cases, it may be impossible to determine the origin of the cancer. While the diagnosis may never be certain, it is helpful to identify and biopsy the ovaries whenever possible. It should be borne in mind that the extent of surgical management at the time of initial laparotomy is critical to the eventual survival of the patient.

Radiotherapy

There is general agreement that epithelial ovarian cancer is responsive but not sensitive to irradiation, although some believe mucinous tumors to be resistant (Rubin, 1962). A major shortcoming of this modality results from the usual spread pattern of ovarian cancer to involve the abdominal cavity. The primary treatment field should encompass this entire anatomic region. Although the pelvic tissues will tolerate doses in the range of 5000 rads in 5 weeks, the kidneys and liver will not, a fact which necessarily restricts the abdominal dose. Treatment of large volumes of tissue at one time is poorly tolerated, and so the rate at which the therapy proceeds must be reduced. To overcome such a problem, the abdomen

and pelvis may be treated separately by the open-field or the moving-strip technique. The latter permits a more favorable time-dose relationship (Delclos, Fletcher). The liver and kidneys still must be shielded.

While opinion strongly favors a beneficial role for radiotherapy in treating ovarian cancer (Perez, Bradfield), the best techniques and the precise indications for its use remain controversial. Munnell (1968) observed that postoperative irradiation for stages II and III improved survival over nonirradiated cases, but the differences may have been influenced by case selection. Radiation is most helpful in the management of patients whose disease is limited to the pelvis. Griffiths et al. (1972) collected a series of stage II cases; the 5-year survival rate obtained by surgery alone was 19 percent compared with 42 percent when irradiation was given postoperatively. Intraperitoneal radioactive colloidal gold (^{198}Au) has been widely used as a surgical adjunct in the management of resectable ovarian carcinoma (Müller). It is capable of delivering a higher dose of radiation to the peritoneal surfaces than can be achieved with external beam therapy. However, the superficial character of its irradiation restricts its usefulness to cases with microscopic residual disease. A major disadvantage is the difficulty in obtaining a uniform distribution of the colloid in the peritoneal cavity. Especially when adhesions are present, hot and cold spots may develop, the former predisposing to bowel complications and the latter to treatment failure. Recently, radioactive colloidal chromic phosphate (^{32}P) has been recommended for intraperitoneal therapy (Hester, White; Hilaris, Clark; Alderman et al.). Since ^{32}P is a pure beta-particle emitter, it poses less radiation hazard than radioactive gold which has some gamma radiation. The reports of Decker (1973) and Kolstad et al. have confirmed the therapeutic benefits of intraperitoneal gold. It is presumed that ^{32}P would be similarly effective.

Chemotherapy

Because ovarian carcinoma grows rapidly and disseminates early, at least within the abdominal cavity, most cases are unresectable at the time of diagnosis. With the very limited success achieved with radiotherapy, there was a need for a systemic approach to therapy. Fortunately, ovarian carcinoma has proved to be one of the most drug-sensitive solid tumors, and cytotoxic agents have become indispensable in its management. Initially drugs were used only in patients with far-advanced disease to palliate the dis-

TABLE 45–19   Reported Response Rates of Patients With Epithelial Ovarian Cancer (Stages III and IV) Treated With Chemotherapy

Drug	Schedule	Number of cases	Percent response
Melphalan*	0.2 mg/kg per day for 5 doses every 4 weeks	494	47
Chlorambucil†	0.2 mg/kg per day per os	280	50
Thiotepa‡	10 mg IV per day for 15 days	144	64
Cyclophosphamide§	50–150 mg per day per os or 200 mg IV per day for 10 days	126	49

*Smith and Rutledge. ‡Wallach et al.
†Masterson and Nelson. §Beck and Boyes.

comforts of large masses, bowel obstruction, and effusions. It is now clear that cytotoxic chemotherapy is capable of extending life in addition to relieving symptoms (Masterson, 1967; Smith et al., 1972). After two decades of experience, the nitrogen mustard group of alkylating agents remains the most active drug group against epithelial ovarian cancer (Table 45–19). The more commonly used are orally administered melphalan and chlorambucil; their adverse effects are limited almost exclusively to the bone marrow.

A number of new cytotoxic drugs have demonstrated activity against ovarian carcinoma. The most promising are doxorubicin (adriamycin) and cis-platinum. However because of dose-limiting toxicities, neither of these drugs is likely to emerge as a single-agent treatment for ovarian carcinoma. Progestins have been suggested as treatment for endometrioid ovarian carcinoma because of its histologic and histogenetic similarity to the hormone-sensitive uterine adenocarcinoma. Supportive clinical data are meager, however.

Combination drug therapy has proved superior to single-agent therapy for a number of malignant diseases. Reports suggesting that multiple-drug regimens may be superior to alkylating agent therapy in ovarian carcinoma are appearing with increasing frequency. Most of the regimens under evaluation employ various combinations of the drugs doxorubicin, cis-platinum, cyclophosphamide, and hexamethylmelamine (Parker et al.; Bruckner et al.; Young et al.; Smith et al.). (See Chap. 47.)

Combined Therapy

The responsiveness of ovarian epithelial carcinoma to irradiation and drug therapy has logically led to efforts to combine these two treatment types sequentially or concurrently. Griffiths et al., in a retrospective analysis of nonrandomized stage II and III patients, found that the radiation-plus-alkylating-agent group had a significantly better survival time than the radiation-only group. They recommended administering the chemotherapy after the radiation was completed because of problems with bone marrow depression which frequently required interruption of drug therapy when given concurrently with radiation. Decker et al. (1967a), reporting from the Mayo Clinic, observed a better survival slope for patients with advanced ovarian cancer receiving cyclophosphamide and radiotherapy than radiotherapy alone. The drug was given during radiotherapy and on a maintenance basis afterward. In a prospective randomized trial of stage I, II, and III patients, Bush and colleagues were unable to demonstrate any difference in survival for radiation therapy (pelvis and abdomen) compared with radiation therapy (pelvis only) and chlorambucil. Whether or not these modalities can be combined in a beneficial way, therefore, remains to be demonstrated.

Treatment

Postoperatively nearly every patient with epithelial ovarian carcinoma will require adjunctive irradiation or chemotherapy. An exception is the patient with a stage Ia borderline or well-differentiated tumor based on optimal surgical staging data. If the diagnosis of malignancy is discovered after unilateral salpingo-oophorectomy, removal of the residual ovary, tube, and uterus is advisable because they may contain microscopic disease or produce an independent primary tumor at a later time. The primary determinants of adjunctive postoperative therapy are the volume and location of residual disease. The effectiveness of irradiation is inherently dependent upon adequate oxygenation of tumor cells regardless of the natural radiosensitivity of the tumor tissue. Since the pool of hypoxic cells increases as the mass size of the tumor increases, the response to irradiation diminishes. Crowding and hypoxia probably become significant in tumor nodules of 1 to 2 cm in size. The limited dose of irradiation which can be administered to the abdomen will not eradicate disease of macroscopic dimensions. The pelvis, however, can be treated with a much heavier dose of radiation, but even in the pelvis there are practical limitations to the volume of tumor which can be managed radiotherapeutically. Whatever therapeutic combination is selected, it should encompass the entire peritoneal cavity. Pelvic radiation alone is inadequate adjuvant therapy for ovarian carcinoma.

The patient with no residual disease postoperatively can be properly managed by chemotherapy, intraperitoneal nuclide therapy, or pelvic-abdominal irradiation. Smith et al. (1975) reported equivalent survival results in a randomized trial of whole abdomen strip irradiation versus melphalan chemotherapy. In very early cases, however, the choice of melphalan for adjuvant therapy must be weighed against the apparent risk that the patient may subsequently develop leukemia (Reimer et al.). Women in the reproductive age group undergoing chemotherapy after conservative surgery for early ovarian cancer may continue to ovulate, and contraceptive measures should be prescribed. In resectable stage II and III disease, and also the stage I poorly differentiated tumors, a combination of radiotherapy followed by chemotherapy offers the maximum therapeutic effort which can be directed against this group of poor-prognosis malignancies. Residual disease confined to the pelvis is optimally treated by pelvic radiation and chemotherapy or pelvic and abdominal radiation.

The management of the patient with residual disease in the pelvis greater than 3 cm in diameter or with macroscopic disease outside the pelvis should be initiated with chemotherapy. This will include nearly 50 percent of all patients who have ovarian carcinoma. Drug therapy is continued as long as there is evidence of a beneficial effect. If no response is obtained after an adequate trial or if there is a response initially followed by disease progression, the therapy must be changed. Under these circumstances the feasibility of surgical excision and also irradiation should be reassessed. Occasionally the shrinkage of a tumor mass due to drug therapy will make an inoperable mass resectable or reduce its size enough that a good effect from radiotherapy can be anticipated.

The "Second Look" Operation

A small fraction of the patients treated with cytotoxic agents for advanced ovarian carcinoma will have a sustained response with all clinical evidence of disease having disappeared. The administration of alkylating agents indefinitely is not always possible because of the bone marrow toxicity. Even if it is well tolerated, continuing the chemotherapy is undesirable if it is unnecessary. At the M. D. Anderson Hospital, 103 patients were subjected to a "second look" operation after receiving melphalan for 1 year (Smith et al., 1976). Only patients having a complete or significant partial response were operated. Of these 103 cases, 23 were found to be free of disease and received no further therapy. Four of these patients have had recurrences, but they had not received a full year of chemotherapy. The place of second-look operations in the management of ovarian carcinoma remains to be defined. Certainly patients with stage I, well-differentiated carcinoma or borderline lesions should be excluded since their recurrence rate is low and the time of recurrence late.

Conservative Surgery in Ovarian Carcinoma

The occurrence of ovarian cancer in a young woman is a threat not only to her life but also to her reproductive faculties. In the more advanced stages and when the tumor is highly malignant, the danger to her life is so great that restricting therapy to a unilateral salpingo-oophorectomy in order to preserve the childbearing potential is not a reasonable alternative. However, the risk-to-benefit ratio of conservative surgery is considered acceptable when the tumor is a low-grade malignancy and confined to one ovary. Among the epithelial cancers, the borderline and grade I lesions, regardless of cell type, are suitable for conservative therapy. Certain germ-cell and stromal malignancies may also qualify for conservative therapy. The requirements for the conservative management of stage Ia ovarian cancer are outlined in Table 45–20.

There is an approximately 5 percent incidence of occult disease in the preserved ovary, but wedge biopsy will reduce the magnitude of this threat. The greatest danger in conservative therapy is the possibility that the disease has already produced microscopic metastases to the peritoneal surfaces.

TABLE 45–20 Requirements for Conservative Management in Patients With Ovarian Cancer

1. Stage I*a*
2. Favorable histologic type
   a. Borderline or well-differentiated epithelial ovarian carcinoma
   b. Pure germinoma; granulosa tumor; arrhenoblastoma
3. Young woman of low parity
4. Encapsulated and unruptured
5. No surface excrescences or adhesions
6. No invasion of capsule, mesovarium, or vessels
7. Negative peritoneal washings
8. Negative ovarian-wedge biopsy and omental biopsy
9. Close follow-up possible

Serous Effusions

Clinically apparent ascites is associated with ovarian carcinoma in about one-third of cases. Withdrawal of the abdominal fluid should be carried out to relieve respiratory embarrassment or pain (Fig. 45–16). Improved gastrointestinal function and relief of nausea, vomiting, and constipation also may occur following paracentesis. The concept of removing ascites preoperatively to avert the complications of sudden decompression of the abdomen at surgery is fallacious

FIGURE 45–16 A little-publicized complication of abdominal paracentesis in the presence of malignant ascites is seeding of the paracentesis track with cancer. The skin lesions in this picture developed after paracentesis for ovarian carcinoma.

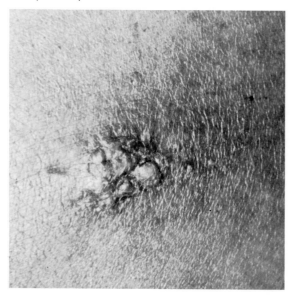

and may be harmful if the fluid reforms rapidly. There is no better way to do the initial paracentesis in patients with ovarian cancer than at surgery. If the patient proves to have a large malignant cyst rather than ascites, the cyst can be safely removed intact. If the tumor is resectable, the ascites will not reaccumulate postoperatively; when it is not resectable, the production of ascitic fluid will continue postoperatively and may be exceedingly rapid. Patients with unresectable ovarian cancer who did not have ascites preoperatively may develop it following surgery. An excessive production of intraperitoneal fluid postoperatively can result in fluid and electrolyte imbalance, hypovolemia, oliguria, and protein depletion.

Instillation of an antineoplastic agent into the peritoneal cavity at the time of exploratory laparotomy is not the optimal means of administering drugs to control ascites or treat cancer. They can be given more effectively and in a more controlled manner systemically. Other chemicals such as Atabrine and nitrogen mustard produce an adhesive serositis which may partly obliterate the peritoneal cavity, making further surgical intervention difficult if not impossible. When ascites reaccumulates following surgery, systemic chemotherapy is the treatment of choice. This is usually successful in controlling the ascites, one of the most sensitive indicators of tumor response. Irradiation is not recommended in the management of ascites, but intraperitoneal instillation of radioactive chromium phosphate or colloidal gold is frequently effective. Either can be used in concert with chemotherapy since there is no bone marrow or systemic toxicity. Pleural effusions unresponsive to chemotherapy are especially suitable to this mode of therapy. Intrapleural tetracyline or bleomycin is also effective (Paladine et al.).

GERM-CELL TUMORS

Germ-cell tumors constitute 15 to 20 percent of all primary ovarian tumors and are second to epithelial neoplasms in relative frequency. The same types of germ-cell tumors are found in the ovary as are encountered in the testis; however, there are important differences. Practically all testicular germ-cell tumors are malignant while the reverse is true in the ovary because of the relatively greater number of mature cystic teratomas in the female than in the male gonad. Identical germ-cell neoplasms arise in extragenital locations (see Embryology and Anatomy at the beginning of the chapter). In order of decreasing frequency, ovarian germ-cell tumors are subgrouped into teratoma, germinoma (dysgerminoma), endodermal sinus tumor, embryonal carcinoma, and choriocarcinoma. Mixtures of these types are not uncommon. Gonadoblastoma is considered here because of its close structural relationship and its propensity to give rise to germ-cell tumors.

TERATOMAS, MATURE AND IMMATURE

A teratoma is a neoplasm composed of tissues representative of at least two of the three embryonic germ layers (ectoderm, mesoderm, and endoderm). It is thought to be derived from germ cells. Sex chromatin has been consistently observed in ovarian teratomas, while testicular teratomas have been either chromatin-negative, -positive, or mixed. Origin from a displaced blastomere devoid of the normal organizing influences or an included monozygotic twin has been postulated for some teratomas. The mode of genesis may vary with the site of origin (Ashley).

The clinical behavior and metastatic potential of teratoma are not dependent upon whether it is solid or cystic. Rather, it is the degree of histologic differentiation or maturity that indicates if the tumor is benign or malignant. Benign teratomas usually are cystic, and malignant teratomas are typically more solid. Appropriate classification is based on a thorough microscopic evaluation. Teratomas that are composed entirely of mature tissues are benign regardless of whether they are cystic or solid. Those that are only partially differentiated may behave in a malignant fashion.

Mature "Solid" Teratoma

A rare variant of mature teratoma is the well-differentiated (grade O) solid teratoma. A teratoma composed entirely of mature adultlike structures and devoid of any other germ-cell tumor elements is benign regardless of whether it is predominantly cystic or solid.

Dermoid Cyst

Over 95 percent of ovarian teratomas are benign cystic neoplasms composed of mature tissues. *Dermoid cyst* is the popular name since the cyst is usually lined by skin. Dermoid cysts are one of the most common ovarian tumors, accounting for 5 to 20 percent of all ovarian neoplasms. Only the cystadenomas are more common. Mature cystic teratomas may occur at any age, but about 50 percent are discovered between the ages of 30 and 50 years. Up to 28 percent

have been found in postmenopausal women, and these account for almost all the germ-cell tumors in that age group. About half of the neoplasms in premenarchal girls are mature cystic teratomas. From 25 to 50 percent of mature cystic teratomas are discovered incidental to routine gynecologic examinations or radiographic studies or at the time of pelvic surgery for unrelated diseases.

Approximately 10 percent of dermoids are overtly bilateral at the time of discovery. They vary in size from less than 1 cm to over 20 cm, but 80 percent are 10 cm in diameter or smaller. Characteristically, the cysts are unilocular. The outer cortical surface of the ovary is smooth and uninvolved unless leakage has occurred. More than one dermoid may occur in the same ovary.

When the cyst is opened, the lumen is usually found to contain a yellow fatty liquid with tangled masses of hair. Other teratomas, particularly in children, contain clear fluid, like cerebrospinal fluid, secreted from teratomatous choroid plexus tissue. The cyst wall typically has one or more nodular thickenings known as the *dermoid process* or *Rokitansky's protuberance*. Hairs and often teeth protrude from this hillock, and it is within this area that the greatest variety of tissue types is found (Fig. 45–17). Ectodermal derivatives predominate with skin usually covering the greater part of the cyst wall (Fig. 45–18). Central-nervous-system elements are common. Thorough mi-

FIGURE 45–17 Mature cystic teratoma (dermoid cyst—gross specimen). Interior of cyst after evacuation of oily liquid contents reveals two well-formed teeth and a tangle of black hairs. Residual ovarian parenchyma is visible at the periphery.

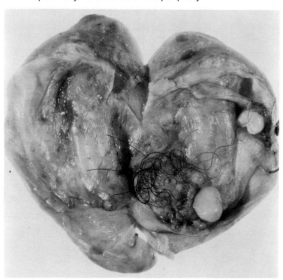

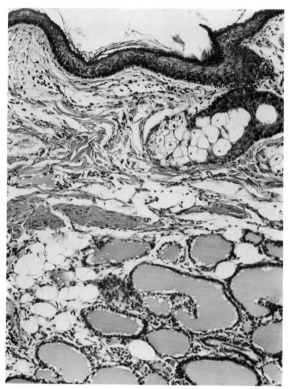

FIGURE 45-18 Mature cystic teratoma (photomicrograph). Section through Rokitansky's protuberance shows epidermis on surface with underlying sebaceous glands, adipose tissue, and colloid-filled thyroid follicles. All tissues are mature and are representative of the three embryonic germ layers. H & E × 250.

croscopic examination will reveal mesodermal and endodermal structures in most cases. Occasionally, a teratoma will form complex, well-organized structures resembling a head, extremities, or digits. These "fetiform" teratomas are curiosities that have fostered the belief that some teratomas are instances of an incorporated twin.

Several important complications may result from dermoids, the most frequent of which is torsion. When it is insufficient to produce infarction, torsion may cause inflammation and adhesions to surrounding structures, collateral circulation, and eventually hyalinization, calcification, or even a parasitic cyst. Infection of benign teratomas is reported to involve about 1 percent of cases in large series. Predisposing factors seem to be pregnancy, torsion, and transvaginal needling of the cyst.

Rupture of a dermoid cyst is a potentially serious complication because the sebaceous contents are ir-

ritating to the peritoneum, where they incite an intense granulomatous inflammatory reaction. Intraperitoneal rupture of a dermoid does not usually produce acute symptoms. The capsular rent is usually of small dimensions, permitting only a slow leakage of the contents. Symptoms appear over a period of months or years after the leak develops. These patients complain of progressive abdominal fullness, nausea, and diarrhea. Examination may reveal mild abdominal tenderness and low-grade fever (Kistner). At laparotomy multiple yellowish peritoneal nodules and adhesions suggestive of tuberculous peritonitis or carcinomatosis are found. The diagnosis may be resolved only after microscopic examination. Oily material may be present in the peritoneal fluid. The peritoneal cavity should be lavaged with copious amounts of saline. The condition was once considered to be fatal, but the outcome of reported cases in the past 40 years has been excellent.

A bizarre manifestation of the mature cystic teratoma is autoimmune hemolytic anemia. Although rare, this possibility should be considered in any woman with hemolytic anemia because of the excellent prognosis and crucial difference in management. Hemolytic anemia has also been reported in association with epithelial ovarian tumors.

Struma Ovarii

Another type of mature teratoma is struma ovarii. While thyroid tissue is found in 5 to 20 percent of teratomas, the designation of struma ovarii is reserved for those uncommon tumors in which it constitutes the major or sole tissue. Approximately 275 cases have been reported. Usually discovered in adult women, the mean age at time of diagnosis is 42 years. Struma ovarii is functional in approximately 10 to 15 percent of cases. Several patients have had evidence of hyperthyroidism, and some also have had a cervical goiter. Ascites occurs in a surprisingly high percentage of patients with struma ovarii, especially those with malignant struma, and occasionally pleural effusions also develop.

The gross and microscopic features of struma ovarii are identical to those of the normally situated thyroid gland. The entire gamut of pathologic thyroid patterns may be found. From 5 to 20 percent of ovarian strumas have areas of malignant change, usually papillary or follicular adenocarcinoma, but some are variants of carcinoid tumors (strumal carcinoid). The carcinomas have been of low-grade malignancy, but hematogenous spread to lungs, bone, and liver as well as peritoneal metastasis occur. Use of radioactive iodine isotopes may be of value in localizing and treating such metastases.

Malignant Neoplasms Arising Secondarily from Teratomatous Tissues

Malignant neoplasms may arise secondarily from any of the mature tissues in a teratoma but occur in only about 1 to 2 percent of cases at most. They do not differ in their histologic pattern from comparable tumors originating from the somatic tissues of the body. Over 90 percent are carcinomas, and the great majority are squamous carcinomas. Both in situ and infiltrative forms have been observed. A variety of other cancers including adenocarcinoma, sarcoma, and melanoma have been recorded.

The risk of malignancy in a dermoid cyst increases with age. Malignancy may be suspected at surgery if adhesions, thickened areas or solid nodules in the cyst wall, necrosis, or rupture are identified. Prognosis depends largely on the extent of spread.

Carcinoid Tumors. These tumors make up an increasing percentage of secondary neoplasms reported as arising in teratomas. The majority are discovered in postmenopausal women. Primary carcinoids are more frequent than carcinoids metastatic to the ovary from the gastrointestinal tract.

The *strumal carcinoid* is a rare variant that contains acinar structures resembling thyroid follicles. It may arise from parafollicular "C" cells of teratomatous thyroid tissue and be related to medullary thyroid carcinomas.

About one-third to one-half of primary ovarian carcinoids are associated with an unusual form of the carcinoid syndrome. In contrast to the situation with intestinal carcinoids, metastases are not required for production of the syndrome which includes cutaneous flushing, diarrhea, facial cyanosis, evidence of right-sided heart failure, and bronchospasm either in combination or alone. Secretion of serotonin (5-hydroxytryptamine), bradykinin, and possibly other hormones causes these symptoms, which disappear following removal of the ovarian tumor. The diagnosis can be substantiated preoperatively by measuring the urinary 5-hydroxyindoleacetic acid, a metabolite of serotonin.

Primary ovarian carcinoids are unilateral in contrast to metastatic carcinoids, which generally involve both ovaries. They appear as solid, firm, pale-yellow masses or as nodules in the wall of a dermoid cyst. However, some are pure carcinoids in which teratomatous elements are not demonstrable. Most are large tumors. Prognosis is excellent since only rare examples of metastasis from a primary ovarian carcinoid have been reported.

Immature Teratomas. About 1 percent of teratomas are composed entirely or in part of partially differentiated structures that resemble tissues of the developing embryo. Neuroectodermal derivatives are particularly common. Immature teratomas generally are more solid than mature teratomas, although cysts of diverse sizes are invariably present. Since some mature benign teratomas are also solid, the term *solid teratoma* should not be used interchangeably with *immature teratoma* or *malignant teratoma.*

Immature teratomas characteristically are found in children and young women. The peak incidence is in the second decade of life. No bona fide examples have occurred in postmenopausal women. Mixed mesodermal tumors and cancers arising in mature cystic teratomas, neoplasms which usually are found in older women, have been confused with immature teratomas.

Any teratoma that contains immature elements is potentially malignant. The likelihood of metastasis is directly proportional to the amount of immature tissue. Once extraovarian spread has occurred, survival is best correlated with the histologic grade of the metastases (Norris et al., 1976). None of the patients with mature glial implants reported by Robboy and Scully have died. Corrected actuarial survival rates were 63 percent at 5 years and 10 years in one large reported series (Norris et al., 1976). Serum gonadotropin and alpha-fetoprotein titers should be obtained to complement the histologic search for embryonal carcinoma and choriocarcinoma. The presence of these tissues worsens the prognosis.

GERMINOMA (DYSGERMINOMA)

The dysgerminoma has an identical appearance to the seminoma of the testis, and the term *germinoma* should be applied uniformly to tumors of this type irrespective of anatomic location or sex. Approximately 1 to 2 percent of ovarian tumors are germinomas. They occur predominantly in children and young women, and 80 percent are found in patients 30 years of age or younger. Only rarely is a germinoma discovered in a postmenopausal woman. It is the most common type of malignant neoplasm to arise in intersex states and is closely related to the gonadoblastoma.

Grossly, the germinoma is solid with a smooth, sometimes bosselated, capsular surface (Fig. 45–19).

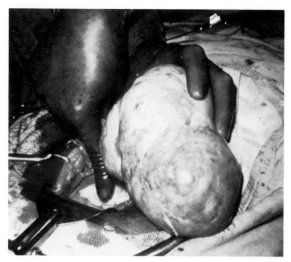

FIGURE 45–19 Typical gross appearance of ovarian (dys)germinoma as seen intraoperatively. This tumor proved to have foci of endodermal sinus tumor.

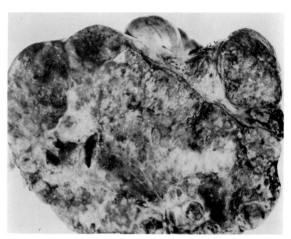

FIGURE 45–20 Endodermal sinus tumor (gross specimen). Variegated appearance is evident on cut surface. Areas of hemorrhage, necrosis, and cystic degeneration are prominent.

The cut surface is homogeneous tan-grey, and geographic areas of necrosis are common. The germinoma is composed exclusively of undifferentiated germ cells. Its stroma typically contains an infiltrate of lymphocytes or epithelioid granulomas. Areas of conspicuous hemorrhage, small cysts, or regions with different consistency suggest the presence of other germ-cell elements which coexist in 10 to 15 percent of cases. Usually germinoma is grossly confined to one ovary at the time of diagnosis. Bilaterality is reported in 10 percent of cases, and about one-fourth will have extraovarian spread. Involvement of the contralateral ovary may be clinically occult, requiring biopsy to adequately evaluate bilaterality. An important feature of this germ-cell malignancy is its proclivity for lymphatic metastases. Although it is capable of intraperitoneal spread in the manner of other ovarian tumors, the pelvic and paraaortic nodes seem to be more frequent targets for metastases. The prognosis in cases of pure germinoma confined to one ovary at the time of diagnosis is excellent with 5-year survival rates in the range of 90 to 95 percent.

ENDODERMAL SINUS TUMOR

The endodermal sinus tumor, or *yolk sac carcinoma,* is a highly aggressive malignant germ-cell tumor with several histologic subtypes. It was mistakenly combined with mesonephroid (clear-cell) carcinoma by Schiller. Teilum separated them and indicated that the germ-cell tumor had microscopic features that closely resembled the labyrinthine placenta of rodents. Subsequent studies showed a close relationship with the extraembryonal yolk sac of animals and humans, including the production and secretion of AFP. The endodermal sinus tumor is uncommon, but in one large study it accounted for about 20 percent of malignant germ-cell tumors of the ovary (Kurman, Norris). Most examples occur in children and young women and only rarely are they found after the age of 35 years.

At surgery, hemorrhagic peritoneal fluid is often present. The tumor is almost always unilateral and has a variegated appearance with prominent areas of hemorrhage, necrosis, and cystic degeneration (Fig. 45–20). Microscopically, the most characteristic pattern is a loose meshwork of malignant cells in which perivascular tufted structures protrude into narrow spaces analogous to endodermal sinuses. Prior to the chemotherapy era, patients had a very poor prognosis, as most tumors were fatal within months to a few years following operation.

EMBRYONAL CARCINOMA

The term embryonal carcinoma is restricted to those neoplasms resembling embryonal carcinoma of the adult testis. In pure form, such lesions are uncommon. Combinations with other germ-cell tumors are most frequently encountered. Embryonal carcinoma shares many clinical and pathologic features with the endodermal sinus tumor, including production of AFP by neoplastic cells.

Microscopically, the embryonal carcinoma consists of sheets of primitive cells. Glandlike clefts are often conspicuous. Of particular interest are small nests of syncytiotrophoblast cells which may be the source of elevated serum and urine levels of HCG. In such cases, patients may manifest hormonal aberrations such as pseudoprecocious puberty (Kurman, Norris). Without chemotherapy, the prognosis for patients with embryonal carcinoma is poor, although slightly better than that of the endodermal sinus tumor.

CHORIOCARCINOMA

Examples of primary choriocarcinoma of the ovary are very rare, and most occur as part of a mixed germ-cell tumor. As with many other varieties of malignant germ-cell tumors, they are lesions of children and young women. Production of chorionic gonadotropin by the trophoblastic tissue may produce pseudoprecocious puberty, and positive serologic tests for pregnancy may be found. Gestational choriocarcinoma is said to metastasize to the ovaries in 6 percent of fatal cases but should not cause a problem in differential diagnosis if the age of the patient, clinical history, and presence of teratomatous elements are evaluated. Theoretically, a primary gestational choriocarcinoma may develop from an ovarian ectopic pregnancy. This has rarely, if ever, occurred.

Histologically, choriocarcinomas of germ-cell origin are similar to those that arise from trophoblastic tissue of pregnancy (gestational choriocarcinoma). Syncytiotrophoblast and cytotrophoblastic cells are evident, but their presence may be overshadowed by extensive hemorrhagic necrosis so characteristic of choriocarcinoma.

The excellent therapeutic achievements of antineoplastic agents in gestational choriocarcinoma have not been realized in choriocarcinoma of germ-cell origin. It is postulated that gestational choriocarcinoma which develops from fetal tissue is more curable because it incites a more intense immunologic host response than nongestational choriocarcinoma. Poor results also may be related to the presence of endodermal sinus tumor or embryonal carcinoma. Nevertheless, several cases of prolonged remission induced by chemotherapeutic agents have been reported.

MIXED GERM-CELL TUMORS

Mixtures of teratoma, germinoma, endodermal sinus tumor, embryonal carcinoma, and choriocarcinoma in various combinations and proportions are found in approximately 10 to 15 percent of all ovarian germ-cell tumors. The term *teratocarcinoma* has been used for mixed teratoid malignancies but is an imprecise designation. The prognosis of a mixed germ-cell tumor is directly related to the behavior of its most malignant component. Consequently, any germ-cell tumor with significant areas of either endodermal sinus tumor, embryonal carcinoma, or choriocarcinoma must be considered highly malignant, as its potential for metastatic spread and response to therapy differ drastically from immature teratomas and germinomas.

GONADOBLASTOMA

In 1953, Scully first described the gonadoblastoma as a distinctive gonadal tumor composed of an intimate mixture of germ cells, sex-cord derivatives resembling immature granulosa and Sertoli cells, and in some instances luteinized stromal cells indistinguishable from Leydig cells. Since then over 70 cases have been reported. The gonadoblastoma has been encountered almost exclusively in abnormal individuals who can usually be classified as exhibiting pure gonadal dysgenesis, mixed gonadal dysgenesis, or male pseudohermaphroditism. Almost 90 percent of patients are sex chromatin–negative and the most common karyotypes are 46XY and 45XO/46XY mosaicism. The phenotype is female in 80 percent of cases. Ambiguous genitalia are common, and 60 percent of patients with a phenotypic female habitus show some evidence of masculine development.

Calcifications are common within the tumor and may be demonstrable on radiologic examination of the pelvis. The tumor often arises in a streak gonad or a dysgenetic undescended testis, but a few examples have been found in otherwise histologically normal ovaries. Gonadoblastomas are small, the largest only 8 cm in diameter. One-fourth of gonadoblastomas are identified only after microscopic examination of the gonad. Some investigators regard the gonadoblastoma as a gonadal malformation or hamartoma for these reasons, rather than a true neoplasm. Bilateral involvement is present in about one-third of cases.

The importance of the gonadoblastoma, in addition to its almost universal association with intersexuality, is its propensity to give rise to malignant germ-cell tumors. In about half the reported cases, there is an overgrowth of the germ-cell component which results in an invasive germinoma. The germinoma may completely obscure the gonadoblastoma, and the only indication of its origin in some cases is identification of residual calcific deposits in the neoplasm. Embryonal carcinomas, endodermal sinus tumors, choriocarcinomas, and teratomas have also been observed. Germ-cell neoplasms that develop in gonadoblastomas have the same behavior as those that arise de novo in otherwise normal ovaries (Hart, Burkons). While the gonadoblastoma itself is benign, the frequency with which malignant germ-cell neoplasms may arise from it justifies consideration of this curious "tumor" as a premalignant lesion. The marked tendency for the germ-cell component of the gonadoblastoma to develop into a malignant tumor, sometimes as early as the first decade in life, is sufficient reason for removing these tumors as soon as they are discovered. Bilateral excision of the gonads should be done except in the rare patient who has a normal ovary on the contralateral side. Because of its association with XY gonadal dysgenesis, any patient with a diagnosis of germinoma should be scrutinized for evidence of XY gonadal dysgenesis. A buccal smear or karyotype should be obtained.

MANAGEMENT OF GERM-CELL TUMORS

The principles developed for the management of epithelial ovarian neoplasms also are applicable to germ-cell tumors. The vast majority of germ-cell tumors are dermoids. Whether cystectomy or salpingo-oophorectomy is performed will depend upon the condition of the opposite adnexa and the surgeon's judgment regarding the salveagability of the involved ovary. Shelling out a dermoid does not always result in complete removal, and recurrences in the preserved ovary have been reported. Bivalving the apparently normal contralateral ovary in search of an occult dermoid is often recommended. Certainly if the ovary is enlarged or nodular to palpation, it needs to be opened. Doss and associates reported that no occult dermoids were found among 90 incised or excised normal-appearing contralateral ovaries. Randall et al. (1962) found that 6 percent of patients undergoing unilateral salpingo-oophorectomy for a benign cystic teratoma required surgery for a subsequent benign neoplasm in the preserved ovary, most of which were also dermoids.

Squamous carcinoma is the most common secondary malignancy encountered in dermoids, and the prognosis is largely contingent upon the extent of disease. If the cyst wall is intact, free of adhesions, and there is no evidence of extraovarian spread, surgical excision of the involved adnexa would be adequate therapy. However, this malignancy occurs almost exclusively in older women, and bilateral salpingo-oophorectomy with hysterectomy is indicated. In the presence of rupture, ascites, or other evidence of spread, pelvic and abdominal irradiation should be administered postoperatively. Prognosis in such cases is poor.

Primary ovarian carcinoids only rarely have been reported to metastasize. If a detailed search for evidence of extraovarian metastasis is negative, surgical excision would seem to be sufficient treatment. Periodic determinations of urinary 5-hydroxyindoleacetic acid (5-HIAA) are of limited value in the posttreatment surveillance of these cases. If there is unresectable or recurrent disease, chemotherapy is indicated, and 5-HIAA levels may serve as an indicator of therapeutic response. Both 5-fluorouracil and actinomycin D have demonstrated activity against this malignancy.

The prognosis for patients with immature teratoma of the ovary is dependent upon both the histologic grade and the surgical stage (Norris et al., 1976). Unilateral salpingo-oophorectomy is adequate therapy for stage I, grade I tumors. These neoplasms are rarely bilateral, although a benign cystic teratoma occasionally is present in the contralateral ovary. Adjunctive triple chemotherapy with vincristine, actinomycin D, and cyclophosphamide (VAC) may be useful for patients with stage I lesions of high histologic grade (grades II or III) and for those whose tumors have ruptured (Table 45–21). Postoperative VAC chemotherapy should be administered to all patients with definite evidence of metastases or tumor recurrence. The exception is the occasional patient whose implants are entirely mature (grade 0); in such cases, additional therapy probably is not required.

The germinoma does not qualify as a low-grade malignancy insofar as 20 percent of the cases confined to one ovary will experience recurrence, usually within 5 years after surgery. However, its extraordinary radiosensitivity permits the germinoma to be managed as a low-grade malignancy since most recurrences can be controlled with irradiation. The requirements for conservative therapy (i.e., unilateral salpingo-oophorectomy) are listed in Table 45–20. Sampling of the ipsilateral pelvic and aortic nodes will provide additional assurance that the disease is confined to the ovary because germinoma tends to disseminate via lymphatics earlier than do other ovarian cancers. The tumor must be examined for the presence of endodermal sinus tumor, embryonal carcinoma, or choriocarcinoma. Presence of these precludes conservative management. Serum HCG and AFP titers may help detect these tissues.

If not confined to one ovary, the treatment of choice in germinoma is total abdominal hysterectomy, bilateral salpingo-oophorectomy, and postoperative external irradiation to the pelvis and abdo-

TABLE 45–21 Combination Chemotherapy in Ovarian Cancer

Drug	Dosage	Schedule
Act-Fu-Cy		
Actinomycin D	0.01 mg/kg IV, not to exceed 0.5 mg per day	Daily for 5 days, repeated every 3–4 weeks
5-Fluorouracil	5 mg/kg IV	Daily for 5 days, repeated every 3–4 weeks
Cyclophosphamide	5 mg/kg IV	Daily for 5 days, repeated every 3–4 weeks
VAC		
Vincristine	1.5 mg/m² body surface area IV, not to exceed 2 mg per week	Weekly for 8–12 weeks
Actinomycin D	0.5 mg per day IV for 5 days	Every 4 weeks
Cyclophosphamide	5–7 mg/kg per day IV for 5 days	Every 4 weeks
MAC		
Methotrexate	0.75 mg/kg IV or IM, not to exceed 15 mg per day	Daily for 5 days every 2–3 weeks
Actinomycin D	0.010 mg/kg IV, not to exceed 0.5 mg per day	Daily for 5 days every 2–3 weeks
Chlorambucil*	0.2 mg/kg per os not to exceed 12 mg per day	Daily for 5 days every 2–3 weeks

Source: Modified from Smith et al. (1972) and Woodruff et al. (1968).
*Cyclophosphamide 5 mg/kg IV (maximum 250 mg) may be given daily instead of chlorambucil.

men. If there is evidence of aortic nodal disease, the irradiation should be extended to include the mediastinum and the supraclavicular nodes. Germinoma, like seminoma, is a very radiosensitive tumor, and the abdomen is able to tolerate therapeutic doses. Recurrence after conservative surgery is also managed with irradiation, but reexploration should be done first to (1) define the extent of disease, (2) excise bulky tumor masses, and (3) obtain adequate tissue for histologic examination. Apparently pure germinoma may recur occasionally as embryonal carcinoma or choriocarcinoma; either carries a much more grave prognosis and is treated with chemotherapy, not radiotherapy. The role of chemotherapy for germinoma has generally been limited to irradiation failures, but Hittle believes that radiotherapy is so poorly tolerated in children that adjunctive therapy with drugs is preferable to irradiation. He recommends the combination drug regimen of VAC. Obviously, treatment must be individualized and based on the age and reproductive history of the patient as well as the surgical stage of the tumor (Burkons, Hart).

On the other hand, endodermal sinus tumors and embryonal carcinomas of the ovary are extremely high-grade cancers with only occasional cures resulting from operation alone or in combination with radiation therapy. Few patients survive more than 2 years despite the fact that the tumors often appear to be grossly limited to one ovary at the time of operation. The prognosis for these patients has been improved by the use of postoperative combination chemotherapy (Smith et al., 1975). Using VAC following operation, Smith reported that all 7 patients with stage I disease were alive and well 4 to 47 months after treatment. Among the patients with more advanced disease, 8 of 13 patients in stages II to IV were well 3 to 78 months after beginning therapy. The addition of methotrexate has been suggested for those patients whose embryonal carcinoma contains syncytiotrophoblast cells or who have elevated levels of HCG in the serum (Kurman, Norris). Drug administration should begin about 1 week postoperatively and continue for 1 year. A second-look operation performed before discontinuing therapy provides the maximum assurance that no disease remains. Surveillance during and after chemotherapy by serial measurement of serum AFP and/or HCG may be helpful in assessing response to therapy and maintenance of remission (Talerman et al., 1978).

Primary ovarian choriocarcinoma occurs predominantly as one component of a mixed germ-cell tumor. When it coexists with endodermal sinus tumor or embryonal carcinoma, which is the characteristic case, the prognosis and treatment are determined by those elements. Therapy is specifically directed at the choriocarcinoma when it occurs in pure form or mixed with less malignant germ-cell elements such as germinoma. Teratomatous choriocarcinoma is not radiocurable but it does respond to combination chemotherapy which should begin in the immediate postoperative period. While ovarian choriocarcinoma does produce HCG, a very sensitive indicator of trophoblastic activity, delaying therapy until the presence of residual disease is proved by a rising gonadotropin titer may be harmful. Although the early experience with chemotherapy in ovarian choriocarcinoma indicated that it was not as susceptible to drug control as gestational choriocarcinoma, several cases with prolonged remission induced by the combination of methotrexate, actinomycin D, and chlorambucil (MAC) have been reported (Wider et al.; Goldstein, Piro; Smith et al., 1973). Treatment response is monitored by serial determination of HCG titers. It has been conventional in the management of gestational choriocarcinoma to discontinue therapy one to three drug cycles after a normal HCG titer has been achieved and maintained. This has proved inadequate for ovarian choriocarcinoma, and drug administration probably should be continued for 1 year after induction of remission. Because of the extreme sensitivity and reliability of gonadotropin assays in detecting small amounts of functioning trophoblastic tissue, there does not seem to be any role for a second-look operation in this disease.

A drug combination of *cis*-platinum, bleomycin, and vinblastine has been reported to be very active in testicular germ-cell tumors (Einhorn, Donohue). Its activity in ovarian germ-cell tumors has not been reported, but at least one ovarian choriocarcinoma patient is in remission after 1 year therapy with this regimen. She had failed MAC therapy (DePetrillo). It is anticipated that the combination will prove to be an important contribution to the management of ovarian germ-cell tumors.

GONADAL STROMAL TUMORS

About 5 to 10 percent of primary ovarian tumors originate from specialized gonadal stroma. Because of their capacity for hormone production and secretion, gonadal stromal tumors are frequently referred to as "functioning" tumors. In addition to estrogen and progesterone, which are normally synthesized by the ovary, various androgens, including testosterone, may be produced by cells of gonadal stromal tumors. Not all functioning tumors of the ovary are of gonadal stromal origin, however. The presence of other primary, and even metastatic, neoplasms may stimulate the nonneoplastic ovarian stroma to synthesize steroids.

Since the parenchyma of both the ovary and the testis is derived from gonadal stroma, it is not surprising that some ovarian neoplasms differentiate toward testicular structures. Teilum (1958) has emphasized that granulosa and Sertoli cells are homologous, as are theca and Leydig cells, and that homologous tumors may occur in both the ovary and the testis.

Gonadal stromal tumors are classified according to their differentiation toward elements resembling ovarian follicles, testicular tubules, Leydig cells, or adrenocortical cells. The majority are tumors of "female directed" cells that are classified in the granulosa-theca group. A smaller percentage belong in the Sertoli-Leydig category as they are tumors of "male directed" cells. The gynandroblastoma contains elements of both cell types. Lipid-cell tumors are composed of cells similar to Leydig (hilus) cells, adrenocortical cells, or both. About 10 to 15 percent do not demonstrate sufficient morphologic specificity to allow precise subdivision, and these are categorized as *unclassified gonadal stromal tumors*. While certain endocrinopathies are characteristic of specific tumor types, hormonal effects are not consistent and thus do not provide a reliable means of classification. A significant proportion of gonadal stromal tumors either are associated with seemingly paradoxical hormonal disturbances or are apparently hormonally inert.

GRANULOSA-THECA GROUP

This group of tumors consists of the granulosa tumor and the thecoma which occur with equal frequency. Together they represent the most common type of gonadal stromal tumors. They usually are estrogenic, and thus are sometimes referred to as *feminizing mesenchymomas*. While clinical effects of these two tumors often are identical and their histologic features overlap in many instances, it is essential to make the distinction between a granulosa tumor and a thecoma since the former is malignant and the latter is almost invariably benign.

Granulosa tumors may be discovered at any age including infancy, but about 50 percent of patients are postmenopausal. Five percent are found in prepubertal girls. The thecoma is especially likely to occur after the menopause and is rare in children.

The symptoms and signs of estrogen-producing granulosa and theca tumors depend to a certain degree upon the patient's age. The most dramatic clinical alterations occur in children who develop pseudoprecocious puberty in response to the estrogen stimulation. During the reproductive years menorrhagia and irregular bleeding are the most common symptoms, although amenorrhea may be experienced by some patients. In the postmenopausal group, resumption of vaginal bleeding, breast enlargement and tenderness, vaginal cornification, and other evidence of estrogen effect are the sequelae of estrogenic tumors. Rarely, virilization may be associated with a cystic granulosa-theca tumor in a young woman. Other common presenting complaints are abdominal swelling and pain. An unusual feature of granulosa tumors is their propensity to rupture and cause intraperitoneal hemorrhage which may be of major proportions. Hemoperitoneum has been observed in up to 5 percent of cases.

Adenocarcinoma of the endometrium is associated with a granulosa- or theca-cell tumor in approximately 15 percent of cases. An equal percentage have endometrial hyperplasia or polyps. The incidence of these proliferative endometrial lesions is increased twofold in postmenopausal women. This association is so prominent that any postmenopausal woman with recurrent endometrial hyperplasia who is not receiving exogenous estrogen should be suspected of harboring a functioning tumor in the granulosa-theca group.

Granulosa Tumor

This neoplasm is composed exclusively of granulosa cells or mixtures of granulosa and theca cells; the latter combination is often designated as a granulosa-theca cell tumor, but its behavior is the same as that of a pure granulosa tumor. It varies in size, averaging about 10 to 15 cm in diameter. Tumors less than 5 cm are found in 10 percent of patients, and such small masses may not be palpable during pelvic examination. Approximately 5 percent are bilateral.

Grossly, many forms are seen. Most characteristic are partially solid tumors with hemorrhagic areas or cystic degeneration (Fig. 45–21). The solid portions are pale yellow or grey. Other neoplasms are totally solid, while a few consist entirely of a single cyst or multiple thin-walled cysts and simulate a cystadenoma.

The microscopic pattern is also diverse. The cells are usually well differentiated and closely resemble granulosa cells of the graafian follicle. They may be arranged in sheets, columns, or cords, and combinations are frequent. The hallmark of the gran-

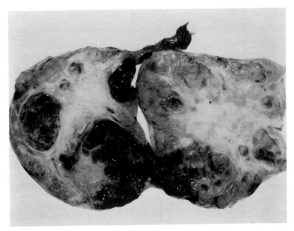

FIGURE 45–21 Granulosa tumor (gross specimen). Large foci of hemorrhage and cystic degeneration alternate with solid nodules of tissue protruding from cut surface. Central whitish areas indicate presence of thecal component.

ulosa tumor is the Call-Exner body, a small rosettelike structure of granulosa cells.

Metastases usually appear more than 5 years after treatment. It is not uncommon for recurrences to be detected 15 or 20 years after excision of the primary neoplasm. Thus, long-term follow-up of patients with a granulosa tumor is essential. Metastatic implants usually are found in the pelvis or abdomen. Lymphatic or hematogenous dissemination is uncommon, and distant metastases are rare. Prognosis is good, with corrected survival rates as high as 97 percent at 5 years and 93 percent at 10 years (Norris, Taylor 1968). Other studies have recorded mortality rates as high as 25 percent after 10 years.

Thecoma

A thecoma consists of interlacing bundles of plump, spindle-shaped mesenchymal cells that contain abundant neutral fat in their cytoplasm. Some degree of collagen production is invariably present. Less than 1 percent are bilateral, and recognition of this feature can be valuable in differential diagnosis. Thecomas are solid neoplasms, although foci of cystic degeneration are not rare. They are usually white, streaked with pale yellow because of their content of lipid. Differentiation from a fibroma or Brenner tumor is often not possible on gross examination alone. Edema is common, and calcific deposits or ossification may be prominent. Cortical stromal hyperplasia may be found in the same or opposite ovary, and many authorities believe thecomas develop from such hyperplastic areas. An association with uterine myomas, fibrocystic disease of the breast, and breast cancer has been reported. For all practical purposes, thecomas are benign. Documented examples of a malignant thecoma are rare. The majority of reported cases of metastasizing thecomas may be sarcomas of pelvic soft tissues that secondarily invaded the ovary or "sarcomatoid" granulosa tumors.

SERTOLI-LEYDIG GROUP

Neoplasms that appear to differentiate toward testicular structures are classified as Sertoli-Leydig tumors. Lesions in this group occur infrequently, representing less than 1 percent of all ovarian neoplasms. The most common type is the arrhenoblastoma which contains mixtures of Sertoli and Leydig cells and tissues similar to those of the fetal testis. Pure Sertoli-cell tumors analogous to those of the canine and human testis are rare. Leydig- and hilus-cell tumors are considered variants of lipid-cell tumors.

Arrhenoblastoma

The arrhenoblastoma, also referred to as Sertoli-Leydig cell tumor, is the prototype of the primary virilizing ovarian neoplasm. Yet, some may be associated with estrogenic manifestations, and about 15 percent are hormonally inert as determined by clinical examinations. The average patient's age at time of diagnosis is 30 to 35 years, and most of these tumors are discovered between ages of 20 and 40 years. They are rarely found in children.

Clinical hormonal effects are less age dependent in masculinizing tumors than in the estrogen-producing tumors, but the alterations are less obtrusive in the postmenopausal woman. During the reproductive years defeminization usually precedes virilization. This results in oligomenorrhea, which occurs in 70 percent of the cases, and atrophy of breast tissue. Virilization encompasses the positive changes which are more dependable clinical clues to excess androgen production. Hirsutism, especially of the face and trunk, acne, clitoromegaly, and hoarseness are reported most frequently, but increased muscle mass and temporal alopecia may occur also. Rapid onset of virilization is characteristic of a neoplastic etiology, but even in young women the symptoms and signs of an androgenic ovarian tumor may progress insidiously, thereby delaying chances for detection.

Less than 5 percent of arrhenoblastomas are bilateral. They range in size from less than 1 cm to more than 25 cm in diameter, with an average of 10 cm.

Grossly, their appearance is not unlike that of granulosa or other gonadal stromal tumors. Solid nodular areas with a yellow-orange or grey-brown color are common, and cystic areas may be found in 50 percent of cases.

Three histologic types were described in 1931 by Robert Meyer, who popularized the term *arrhenoblastoma*. Type I tumors *(tubular adenoma)* are well differentiated, composed predominantly of hollow tubules lined by Sertoli cells, and have few Leydig cells. Type II and III tumors are intermediate and poorly differentiated lesions, respectively, and are composed of mixtures of tubules, sex cord-like structures, mature Leydig cells, and abundant primitive mesenchyme. Combinations of these three types are common.

The diagnosis of a virilizing ovarian tumor is not difficult when the clinical evidence of excess androgen production is unequivocal and an adnexal mass is discovered on pelvic examination. In the absence of a palpable ovarian mass, the major problem is one of distinguishing between an ovarian and an adrenal source of androgen. Investigative studies designed to identify clinically occult neoplasms and steroidal hormone assays will usually identify the organ responsible for the virilization. An occult ovarian tumor can be delineated by culdoscopy, laparoscopy, or pelvic ultrasound while an adrenal mass may be revealed by an intravenous pyelogram or retroperitoneal air insufflation. Computerized tomography is also useful.

In the group of 29 patients with follow-up data accessioned at the Armed Forces Institute of Pathology, only one developed metastases (O'Hern, Neubecker). Intermediate and poorly differentiated tumors probably can be expected to behave like granulosa-cell tumors. Small, well-differentiated neoplasms usually have been benign.

Sertoli Tumors

Neoplasms composed entirely or predominantly of tubular structures resembling fetal seminiferous tubules are now classified as Sertoli tumors. Symptoms may be due to estrogen production, and the clinical manifestations are similar to those found in patients with granulosa-theca tumors. They have been discovered in young girls with pseudoprecocious puberty. Nodular lesions in the gonads of male pseudohermaphrodites with the testicular feminization syndrome have been regarded as *Sertoli adenomas,* but they more likely represent nodular hyperplasias or hamartomas rather than true neoplasms. Such gonads have been misinterpreted as arrhenoblastomas when the pathologist was not informed of the clinical findings.

The "sex cord tumors with annular tubules" described by Scully (1970c) that are often associated with the Peutz-Jeghers syndrome are small lesions that resemble miniature Sertoli tumors, although others resemble granulosa tumors. Rare examples of histologically malignant Sertoli-cell tumors have been reported.

GYNANDROBLASTOMA

Rarely a gonadal stromal tumor contains nests of unequivocal granulosa tumor with well-formed Call-Exner bodies together with hollow tubules and Leydig cells typical of a Sertoli-Leydig tumor. Such a lesion is appropriately designated a gynandroblastoma and may be associated with evidence of androgen or estrogen production. Unfortunately, this diagnosis has been overutilized by application to tumors that merely show variations of histologic pattern in an otherwise typical granulosa-theca or Sertoli-Leydig tumor. While too few examples that qualify as gynandroblastoma have been recorded to predict behavior, they should be regarded as low-grade malignancies similar to the individual components.

LIPID-CELL TUMORS

Neoplasms composed entirely of polygonal cells with considerable amounts of intracytoplasmic lipid are classified as lipid-cell tumors. Within this group are lesions that have been variously designated as hilus-cell tumors, Leydig-cell tumors, adrenal-rest tumors, stromal luteomas, and masculinovoblastomas either because of their topographic location within the ovary, microscopic likeness to Leydig and adrenocortical cells, or endocrine effects. Lipid-cell tumors have been regarded as a heterogeneous group of lutein-cell neoplasms of diverse origin by some investigators and as a specific histogenetic tumor type by others. Proponents of the former theory argue that while these tumors have histologic similarities, an origin from either hilus cells, ovarian stromal cells, or adrenocortical rests can be ascribed to individual tumors by morphologic and biochemical characteristics. The unitarian belief contends that all originate from the specialized ovarian stromal cells. Lipid-cell tumors are among the rarest functioning ovarian neoplasms. They usually are virilizing. About one-fourth, however, are associated with evidence of estrogenic activity. Obesity, impaired glucose tolerance, and hypertension are common, and a cushingoid syndrome may be found in 10 percent of patients. Hydroxycorticosteroids have been identified in tumor tissue in some instances. The clinical manifestations are easily mistaken for evidence of an adrenal disorder. Urinary levels of 17-ketosteroids are usually elevated and often exceed 30 mg per 24 hours, a level above which adrenal lesions are more common than ovarian lesions. Differential suppression and stimulation tests may be of particular value in such cases.

When crystals of Reinke are identified in the cells, the designation of hilus- or Leydig-cell tumor is preferred by some authorities. The crystals are globular protein inclusions that are normally found in mature Leydig cells of the testis and in hilus cells of the ovary. Crystal-positive lipid-cell tumors tend to occur in older, postmenopausal women and tend to be smaller (average size of 3 cm) than their crystal-negative counterparts. Thus, they may not be palpable and will remain undetected until the involved ovary is sectioned. Testosterone production may cause virilization without elevating the urinary 17-ketosteroids.

Lipid-cell tumors are unilateral and frequently are located in the medulla or hilar region of the ovary. They are lobulated solid masses of bright yellow-orange or tan-brown tissue because of their high lipid and lipochrome pigment content. The majority of lipid-cell tumors are histologically and clinically benign. Tumors that have spread to contiguous organs, or have microscopic cellular pleomorphism with high mitotic activity, should be considered malignant. However, a few large but histologically benign tumors have also been clinically malignant. All ovarian lipid-cell tumors with convincing crystals of Reinke (Leydig- or hilus-cell tumors) have been benign. Small neoplasms less than 8 cm in diameter, regardless of the presence or absence of Reinke crystals, probably can be expected to be benign.

TREATMENT OF GONADAL STROMAL TUMORS

Thecomas are benign and unilateral in nearly all cases, as are most lipid-cell tumors and Sertoli tumors. The granulosa-cell tumors and arrhenoblastomas are low-grade malignancies usually confined to one ovary at the time of diagnosis. If the peritoneal washings, omental biopsy, and wedge resection of the opposite ovary are normal, conservative surgery is sufficient therapy in the young woman, provided the tumor is intact (see Table 45–20). Following removal of an arrhenoblastoma, menses usually resume within

1 or 2 months, and the breasts rapidly return to normal. The acne is reversible, but the hirsutism, clitoromegaly, and hoarseness may be permanent or resolve very slowly. Fertility seems unimpaired. Patients whose disease is more advanced than stage Ia should have both adnexa and the uterus removed. Postoperatively, adjunctive external pelvic and abdominal irradiation is indicated. Occasionally, a lipid-cell tumor will have histologic evidence of malignancy necessitating removal of both ovaries, tubes, and the uterus followed by abdominal and pelvic irradiation. Patients with malignant stromal tumors should be followed with appropriate steroid assays.

TUMORS OF NONSPECIFIC MESENCHYME

Benign and malignant neoplasms that are not specific for the ovary include fibromas, angiomas, leiomyomas, lipomas, soft-tissue sarcomas, lymphomas, and other rare tumors. Their appearance and clinical behavior do not differ because they are located in the ovary. Of this group, fibromas and lymphomas are important.

FIBROMA

Ovarian fibromas are benign tumors that are composed of fibroblasts and abundant collagen. They are the most common tumor in this category. Some examples cannot be distinguished with certainty from collagenized thecomas. Perhaps some fibromas are nonfunctioning variants of thecoma.

The average age at time of discovery is 48 years. An enlarging abdomen due to ascites may be the initial finding. In 1937, Meigs and Cass reported the association of ascites, hydrothorax, and ovarian fibroma. Prior to that, patients with an ovarian mass, ascites, and pleural effusions were usually believed to have hopelessly disseminated ovarian cancer. The hydrothorax, often on the right side, and ascites of Meigs's syndrome are reversible following removal of the fibroma or other benign solid ovarian stromal neoplasm. Large tumors (over 10 cm in diameter) and those with "myxomatous" or edematous change are particularly likely to be associated with ascites (Samanth, Black), but less than 5 percent of fibromas are accompanied by Meigs's syndrome. Transudation of fluid from the tumor through the ovarian capsule and into the peritoneal cavity seems to be a reasonable explanation for the ascites. While torsion of the ovar-

ian pedicle could initiate this sequence, the pathogenesis of the ovarian edema remains obscure in most cases. Meigs demonstrated that India ink injected into the abdomen could be recovered from the pleural cavity, indicating that transportation of ascitic fluid through the diaphragm via small congenital defects or lymphatic channels could account for the accompanying hydrothorax.

About 10 percent of fibromas are bilateral. Their average diameter is 6 cm; less than 5 percent are larger than 20 cm. Grossly, the tumor is usually solid, grey-white, and firm except when edema is extensive. Calcification or ossification occurs in about 3 percent of tumors and may be detectable on pelvic radiographs.

LYMPHOMA

Ovarian enlargement may be the initial clinical manifestation of lymphoma. Whether it originates in the ovary, metastasizes to that organ, or is part of a multifocal systemic process cannot always be determined, but involvement of regional lymph nodes and/or other organs usually accompanies ovarian lymphoma.

Burkitt's lymphoma, a form of stem-cell lymphoma, has a predilection for developing in the ovary and other extralymph nodal sites, particularly the jawbones. Its occurrence in childhood and high incidence of bilaterality in the ovary have been found in the United States as well as in Africa, where it occurs with unusual frequency. Among disseminated malignancies, Burkitt's lymphoma is second only to gestational choriocarcinoma in its curability with chemotherapy. A 15 percent 5-year survival rate has been achieved using cyclophosphamide.

Other histologic types of lymphoma and leukemia may also present as an ovarian lesion. Hodgkin's disease is rare. Ovarian lymphomas are sometimes mistaken for granulosa tumors, germinomas, or undifferentiated carcinomas. A continual awareness of the possibility of ovarian lymphoma is the best means to avoid such an error.

METASTATIC OVARIAN TUMORS

Virchow has been quoted as saying that the organs which most frequently produce malignant neoplasms are seldom the site of metastases. This does not pertain to the ovary since ovarian metastases have been detected in up to 30 percent of autopsies performed on women with cancer. Spread to the ovaries is especially prevalent in patients with carcinoma of the breast. Microscopic examination of oophorectomy specimens performed for palliation of mammary carcinoma reveals metastases in 15 to 25 percent of cases. However, seldom do these metastases reach sufficient size to be clinically significant. Similarly, metastases from other genital organs rarely present as diagnostic problems. Only 5 to 10 percent of ovarian neoplasms encountered by a surgeon during investigation of a pelvic mass are metastases. When the ovary is the site of metastatic cancer, other metastases usually are present also. In 75 percent of cases, both ovaries are grossly involved by metastases. At least 85 percent of metastatic ovarian tumors are of gastrointestinal origin. Carcinomas of the stomach and colon are the prime sources of ovarian metastases. Carcinoid tumors of the ileum occasionally produce symptomatic ovarian metastases.

Krukenberg's Tumor

In 1896, E. F. Krukenberg described what he considered to be a primary mesenchymal tumor of the ovary and termed it *fibrosarcoma ovarii mucocellulare (carcinomatodes)*. Since that time the criteria for the diagnosis of Krukenberg's tumor and the implications of that designation have too often been clouded. If the use of the term *Krukenberg's tumor* is reserved for those ovarian tumors that contain large numbers of signet-ring adenocarcinoma cells within, and often partially obscured by, a cellular hyperplastic but non-neoplastic ovarian stroma, definite important and consistent clinicopathologic features become apparent (Fig. 45–22). For practical purposes, all so-defined Krukenberg's tumors represent metastases from another organ, primarily the stomach. A few examples of signet-ring adenocarcinomas metastatic to the ovary from other sites including the gallbladder, breast, and urinary bladder have been reported. The primary tumor may have been previously resected, but often it is clinically occult and is only discovered after the ovarian lesion is recognized as a Krukenberg's tumor.

Typically, Krukenberg's tumors are bilateral, solid masses that tend to retain the convolutions of the ovarian surface even though they may massively enlarge the organ. The cut surface usually appears edematous or gelatinous. Areas of hemorrhage and necrosis are variable. Occasionally, small cysts are found, but they do not approach the size of the cysts in cystadenocarcinomas or mucinous adenocarcinomas metastatic to the ovary from the large intestine.

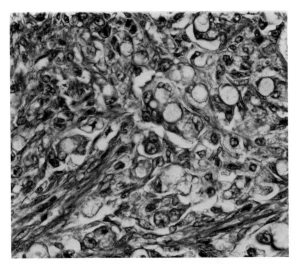

FIGURE 45–22 Krukenberg's tumor (photomicrograph). Signet-ring-shaped metastatic adenocarcinoma cells with large cytoplasmic vacuoles are intimately mixed with hyperplastic ovarian stromal cells. H & E × 1000.

Spread to the ovaries from the stomach probably results from retrograde lymphatic dissemination via the paraaortic chain. The average age of women with Krukenberg's tumors is 45 to 50 years, but considerably younger patients are often afflicted.

The existence of a primary Krukenberg's tumor of the ovary has been categorically denied by some authorities and championed by others. A few cases with the typical gross and microscopic features of a Krukenberg's tumor have been reported in which long-term survival has followed removal of the ovarian tumor or an autopsy failed to reveal another acceptable primary site. Nonetheless, a thorough and extensive evaluation of all patients with a Krukenberg's tumor is mandatory since a primary carcinoma will be present in the stomach or other glandular organ in practically every case.

Metastatic Carcinoma of the Colon

Ovaries with metastatic adenocarcinoma from the large intestine are more frequent than Krukenberg's tumors. Their gross and microscopic appearances may closely simulate a primary mucinous or endometrioid cystadenocarcinoma. Large areas of hemorrhage and necrosis are characteristic and can result in spontaneous rupture of the ovary. When these findings are encountered at surgery, the possibility of a metastatic tumor should be considered. The frequency with which carcinomas of the colon metastasize to the ovary and the large size that the metastases may attain have been put forth as arguments for combining "prophylactic" bilateral ovariectomy with resection of carcinoma of the colon in older women.

OVARIAN TUMORS WITH FUNCTIONING STROMA

Any type of ovarian neoplasm, benign or malignant, primary or metastatic, may induce the nonneoplastic ovarian stroma to become hyperplastic and luteinized. This is particularly apt to occur during pregnancy, probably related to the high levels of circulating chorionic gonadotropins. Usually these tumors are not associated with any noticeable hormonal disturbance, but a significant percentage have been hormonally functional. Apparently because of mechanical influence of the expanding tumor, the ovarian stromal cells may synthesize and secrete the same range of estrogenic, progestational, and androgenic steroids as does the graafian follicle, adrenal cortex, or testis. Virilism is the most striking disturbance, but evidence of hyperestrinism may predominate. Removal of the tumor eliminates the hormonal derangement. Unlike the situation with functioning tumors in which the neoplastic cells themselves are hormonally active, steroid secretion does not recur if metastases develop since ovarian stroma is no longer present. Tumors most often associated with functioning stroma include mucinous cystadenomas and cystadenocarcinomas, Brenner tumor, Krukenberg's tumor, and metastatic colonic carcinoma. Instances of dermoid cysts and embryonal carcinoma with functional stroma have also been recorded.

OVARIAN TUMORS IN PREGNANCY

An ovarian tumor is discovered approximately once in every 1000 consecutive pregnancies (see Chap. 28). This apparently coincidental occurrence is a threat to both maternal and fetal well-being because of complications relating to the tumor or resulting from therapeutic intervention. The probability of an ovarian tumor twisting on its vascular pedicle is increased during pregnancy, and it is especially prone to occur during labor or postpartum. Solid tumors are particularly susceptible to torsion, rupture, and hemorrhage, and such a sequence of events developing antepartum may clinically simulate abruptio placentae. Granulosa tumors are the most likely to hemorrhage, and they seem most disposed to do so in the immediate postpartum period. Maternal deaths have been reported from this complication.

Ovarian tumors in pregnancy may cause obstruction of labor. The mass becomes interposed between the presenting part and the pelvic floor, thereby preventing descent of the fetus. This situation leads to rupture of the tumor if the obstruction is not relieved by abdominal surgery.

Although functioning ovarian tumors frequently produce a state of infertility, they may rarely coexist with pregnancy. The estrogenic stromal neoplasms have been observed to cause recurrent spontaneous abortions. Maternal and fetal virilization have been reported with arrhenoblastomas, mucinous cystadenomas, Krukenberg's tumors, pregnancy luteomas, and theca lutein cysts.

About 12 percent of ovarian masses diagnosed during pregnancy are not neoplasms at all but are cystic corpora lutea of pregnancy (Chung, Birnbaum; White). These are invariably discovered and removed during the first half of pregnancy when the corpus luteum normally may achieve a size of 8 to 10 cm. Thus, the possibility that a cystic adnexal mass discovered during early pregnancy is a corpus luteum should always be considered.

Dermoid cysts and benign cystadenomas, especially the serous type (Fig. 45–23), account for over 90 percent of the neoplasms. Carcinomas and other malignant tumors compose only 3 to 6 percent of the neoplastic lesions. The incidence, stage, and histogenetic type do not seem, from the small number of cases available for analysis, to be different from what would be expected in a nonpregnant population of the same age range. Ovarian tumors may be obscured by the pregnant uterus during the second and third trimesters, causing delay in diagnosis, but this does not appear to be a major problem since most cases of the ovarian cancers coexisting with pregnancy are stage Ia. The risk to the fetus from ovarian cancer is primarily that of treatment, as metastasis to the placenta is exceptionally rare and spread to the fetus has not been documented (Rothman et al.).

The general plan of management of ovarian neoplasms during pregnancy is the same as in the nonpregnant patient, with some minor modifications. During the first trimester it is important to confirm the presence of an intrauterine pregnancy to avoid unnecessary delay in the investigation of an adnexal mass. Ultrasound, unlike diagnostic x-rays, can be utilized even during the first trimester of pregnancy to identify the gestational sac. When an adnexal mass discovered during the first trimester is unilateral, mobile, and cystic, operation should be delayed until the

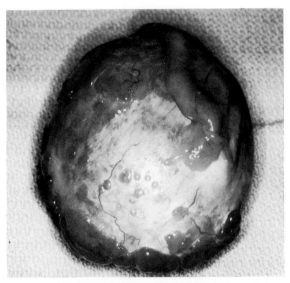

FIGURE 45-23 Benign serous cystoma 10 cm in diameter removed during the midtrimester of pregnancy. The fallopian tube is draped over the upper pole. There is extensive decidual reaction in the surface epithelium which should not be mistaken for tumor excrescences. The decidua is velvety in character and has a red color.

pregnancy enters the second trimester. At this time, the surgery is less likely to be followed by abortion. Furthermore, if the mass is a corpus luteum, it may regress during this short interval of observation. During the third trimester, surgery should be delayed until viability or term, depending on the age of gestation. If at term the tumor obstructs the birth canal, cesarean section and removal of the tumor may be indicated. Otherwise operation in the postpartum period may be more advantageous to the patient and the fetus. Ovarian cancer diagnosed during pregnancy is treated as in the nonpregnant patient.

OVARIAN TUMORS IN CHILDREN

Malignant diseases are the second leading cause of death in childhood and adolescence, exceeded in frequency only by accidents. A mere 3 percent of childhood malignancies are of genital-tract origin, but ovarian cancers account for two-thirds of these. By comparison, the ovary is the site for only 20 percent of genital-tract cancers in adults. Although ovarian neoplasms in the pediatric group are rare, they are of special importance because 50 percent are malignant.

The vast majority of abdominal masses in the newborn are renal in origin, but when the mass is ovarian, the most likely lesion is a functional or non-neoplastic cyst. These are predominantly follicular cysts, although theca lutein cysts also occur. Of 37 cases of ovarian masses in newborns reported by Carlson and Griscom, 8 were simple or serous cysts and 1 was a teratoma. Apparently none was malignant. Functional cysts in the neonate reflect the effect of intrauterine gonadotropin stimulation on the fetal ovary. The occurrence of functional cysts is rare after the first few weeks of life until after puberty, when approximately 20 percent of reported ovarian masses are functional cysts. Ovarian neoplasms are decidedly rare prior to puberty. Norris and Jensen reported on 353 cases in females less than 20 years of age (Table 45-22). Only 15 percent occurred in the 0 to 10-year age group, the majority of patients developing their tumor after the age of 15 years. The relative frequency of the various types of ovarian neoplasms is quite different during childhood and adolescence from that in adult life. Abell et al. found that 90 percent of the 35 ovarian neoplasms in their study group diagnosed prior to menarche were of germ-cell origin and half of them were malignant. The remaining benign germ-cell tumors were mature cystic teratomas.

Neoplasms of epithelial origin are exceedingly rare prior to puberty, and nearly all of them are benign. If the series of Norris and Jensen is combined with that of Abell and Holtz, 120 epithelial ovarian tumors accounted for only 22 percent of the neoplasms in females less than 20 years of age. One epithelial tumor occurred prior to 10 years of age and that was benign. Only 10 percent of the entire group of neoplasms were malignant including borderline lesions.

Stromal tumors compose about 15 percent of ovarian neoplasms reported in childhood and adolescence. This incidence is probably an exaggeration of their true occurrence rate. Their association with pseudoprecocious puberty and virilization makes them an object of special interest to clinicians and predisposes to overreporting. It is estimated that only 2 percent of all cases of precocious puberty are due to ovarian tumors. A few well-documented examples occurring secondary to follicular cysts have been reported in the literature, but pseudoprecocious puberty of ovarian origin is usually associated with true neoplasms, either granulosa-cell or Sertoli-cell tumors. Pseudopuberty rarely results from a choriocarcinoma. The granulosa tumors, like other nongerm-cell tumors in this age group, are less inclined to manifest malignant behavior than they are in older patients. Probably less than 5 percent of the childhood granulosa-cell tumors are malignant compared with a 10 to 20 percent malignancy rate in adults.

TABLE 45–22 Distribution of the 353 Cases of Ovarian Tumors of Childhood by Age of Patient

Type	Age of patient, years				Total no.
	0–9	5–9	10–14	15–19	
Germ cell					
Benign cystic teratoma	2	3	14	52	71
Solid teratoma, immature	0	3	11	8	22
Solid teratoma, mature	0	2	2	2	6
Mixed teratoma, germinoma, embryonal carcinoma, or choriocarcinoma	2	8	5	11	26
Germinoma (pure)	0	7	17	24	48
Embryonal carcinoma (predominating)	3	2	16	11	32
Subtotal	7	25	65	108	205
Epithelial					
Cystadenoma and adenofibroma	0	1	4	54	59
Borderline tumors	0	0	0	5	5
Cystadenocarcinoma	0	0	1	2	3
Subtotal	0	1	5	61	67
Stromal					
Fibrothecoma	2	2	1	18	23
Arrhenoblastoma	0	1	1	12	14
Granulosa	5	0	2	5	12
Nonspecific	2	5	2	4	13
Subtotal	9	8	6	39	62
Miscellaneous					
Malignant, unclassified	2	2	2	8	14
Germinoma arising in gonadoblastoma	0	0	1	1	2
Lymphoma	0	0	2	0	2
Lymphangioma	0	0	1	0	1
Subtotal	2	2	6	9	19
Total, all cases	18	36	82	217	353

Source: Modified from Norris and Jensen.

Thecomas and arrhenoblastomas are extremely rare before puberty.

Ovarian cysts and neoplasms are more inclined to undergo torsion in children and adolescents than in adults. The right side is involved in such accidents more often than the left, and frequently a diagnosis of acute appendicitis is suggested.

The management of gynecologic tumors in the pediatric age group poses some special problems. The incomplete physical and psychologic development of children makes them more vulnerable to permanent, crippling injuries from all modalities of cancer therapy. The immature tissues of the child are especially susceptible to irradiation injury. Damage to bone growth centers can produce significant deformities in long-term survivors. The liver, kidney, and small bowel of children are less tolerant to radiotherapy than in the adult, necessitating lower doses or a reduced dose rate when treating the abdomen or pelvis. Radiation enteritis is particularly dangerous in children because of the ease with which they develop fluid and electrolyte disturbances. Regarding chemotherapy, children tolerate a number of agents better than adults, but the synergistic effect of drugs used with irradiation, especially actinomycin D, may be seriously exaggerated in children.

The immediate and long-term effects of pelvic surgery are more predictable than with other treatment modes, and frequently sterilization is an inescapable side effect. The importance of reproductive integrity in the development of a young woman's self-image cannot be lightly regarded, but conservatism in cancer therapy is often not the best course. Any disease which threatens both the life of a girl and her sexual-reproductive faculties invariably produces an intensely emotional atmosphere. Assessment of the risks and benefits under these circumstances becomes even more difficult. Nevertheless, there should be no hesitation to remove or destroy the reproductive organs in the course of treating the cancer if there is a reasonable expectation that this therapy will contribute to a cure. In the face of disease which can only be palliated, the deleterious effects on the reproductive tract cannot be considered a major impediment to therapy.

REFERENCES

Abell MR: The nature and classification of ovarian neoplasms. *Can Med Assoc J* 94:1102, 1966.

_____ et al.: Ovarian neoplasms in childhood and adolescence, I. Tumors of germ cell origin. *Am J Obstet Gynecol* 92:1059, 1965.

_____, Holtz F: Ovarian neoplasms in childhood and adolescence, II. Tumors of non-germ cell origin. *Am J Obstet Gynecol* 93:850, 1965.

Acosta A et al.: Gynecologic cancer in children. *Am J Obstet Gynecol* 112:944, 1972.

_____ et al.: A proposed classification of pelvic endometriosis. *Obstet Gynecol* 42:19, 1973.

Aiman J et al.: Androgen and estrogen formation in women with ovarian hyperthecosis. *Obstet Gynecol* 51:1, 1978.

Alderman SJ et al.: Postoperative use of radioactive phosphorus in stage I ovarian carcinoma. *Obstet Gynecol* 49:659, 1977.

American Cancer Society: *Cancer facts and figures 1978.*

Anderson WR et al.: Granulosa-theca cell tumors: Clinical and pathologic study. *Am J Obstet Gynecol* 110:32, 1971.

Anikwue C et al.: Granulosa and theca cell tumors. *Obstet Gynecol* 51:214, 1978.

Arey LB: Origin and form of Brenner tumor. *Am J Obstet Gynecol* 81:743, 1961.

Arias-Bernal L, Jones HW: Chromosomes of a malignant ovarian teratoma. *Am J Obstet Gynecol* 100:785, 1968.

Asadourian LA, Taylor HB: Dysgerminoma: An analysis of 105 cases. *Obstet Gynecol* 33:370, 1969.

Ashley DJB: Origin of teratomas. *Cancer* 32:390, 1973.

Aure JC et al.: Clinical and histologic studies of ovar-ian carcinoma: Long-term followup of 990 cases. *Obstet Gynecol* 31:1, 1971a.

_____: Radioactive colloidal gold in the treatment of ovarian carcinoma. *Acta Radiol* 10:399, 1971b.

_____: Psammoma bodies in serous carcinoma of the ovary: A prognostic study. *Am J Obstet Gynecol* 109:113, 1971c.

_____: Carcinoma of the ovary and endometriosis. *Acta Obstet Gynecol* 50:63, 1971d.

Awais GM: Serum lactic dehydrogenase levels in the diagnosis and treatment of carcinoma of the ovary. *Am J Obstet Gynecol* 116:1053, 1973.

Azoury RS, Woodruff JD: Primary ovarian sarcomas: Report of 43 cases from the Emil Novak Ovarian Tumor Registry. *Obstet Gynecol* 37:920, 1971.

Babaknia A et al.: The Stein-Leventhal syndrome and coincidental ovarian tumors. *Obstet Gynecol* 47:223, 1976.

Bagley CM Jr. et al.: Treatment of ovarian carcinoma: Possibilities for progress. *N Engl J Med* 287:856, 1972.

_____ et al.: Ovarian carcinoma metastatic to the diaphragm—frequently undiagnosed at laparotomy. *Am J Obstet Gynecol* 116:397, 1973.

Baillie AH et al.: Histochemical evidence of steroid metabolism in the human genital ridge. *J Clin Endocrinol* 26:738, 1966.

Barber HRK, Graber EA: The PMPO syndrome (postmenopausal palpable ovary syndrome). *Obstet Gynecol* 38:921, 1971.

_____, _____: Gynecological tumors in childhood and adolescence. *Obstet Gynecol Surv* 28:357, 1973.

Barclay DL et al.: Hyperreactio luteinalis: Postpartum persistence. *Am J Obstet Gynecol* 105:642, 1969.

Bardin CW et al.: Studies of testosterone metabolism in a patient with masculinization due to stromal hyperthecosis. *N Engl J Med* 277:399, 1967.

Barlow JJ, Dillard PH: Serum protein-bound fucose in patients with gynecologic cancers. *Obstet Gynecol* 39:727, 1972.

_____ et al.: Adriamycin and bleomycin, alone and in combination, in gynecologic cancers. *Cancer* 32:735, 1973.

Barnès PH: Oophorectomy in primary carcinoma confined to one ovary. *Can Med Assoc J* 79:416, 1958.

Beck RE, Boyes DA: Treatment of 126 cases of advanced ovarian carcinoma with cyclophosphamide. *Can Med Assoc J* 98:539, 1968.

Bennington JL et al.: Incidence and relative frequency of benign and malignant ovarian neoplasms. *Obstet Gynecol* 32:627, 1968.

Bergman F: Carcinoma of the ovary: A clinicopathological study of 86 autopsied cases with special reference to mode of spread. *Acta Obstet Gynecol Scand* 45:211, 1966.

Blackwell WJ et al.: Dermoid cysts of the ovary, their clinical and pathologic significance. *Am J Obstet Gynecol* 51:151, 1946.

Boczkowski K et al.: Sibship occurrence of XY gonadal dysgenesis with dysgerminoma. *Am J Obstet Gynecol* 113:952, 1972.

Boivin Y, Richart RM: Hilus cell tumors of the ovary: A review with a report of 3 new cases. *Cancer* 18:231, 1965.

Boss JH et al.: Structural variations in the adult ovary: Clinical significance. *Obstet Gynecol* 25:747, 1965.

Breen JL, Neubecker RD: Ovarian malignancy in children with special reference to the germ cell tumors. *Ann NY Acad Sci* 142:208, 1962.

———, ———: Malignant teratoma of the ovary: An analysis of 17 cases. *Obstet Gynecol* 21:669, 1963.

Brody S: Clinical aspects of dysgerminoma of the ovary. *Acta Radiol* 56:209, 1961.

Bruckner HW et al.: Cis-platinum (DDP) for combination chemotherapy of ovarian carcinoma: Improved response rates and survival. *Cancer Letter* 5:5, 1978.

Burkons DM, Hart WR: Ovarian germinomas (dysgerminomas). *Obstet Gynecol* 51:221, 1978.

Burns BC Jr. et al.: Management of ovarian carcinoma: Surgery, irradiation and chemotherapy. *Am J Obstet Gynecol* 98:374, 1967.

Bush RS et al.: Treatment of epithelial carcinoma of the ovary: Operation, irradiation, and chemotherapy. *Am J Obstet Gynecol* 127:692, 1977.

Cariker M, Dockerty M: Mucinous cystadenomas and mucinous cystadenocarcinomas of the ovary: A clinical and pathological study of 335 cases. *Cancer* 7:302, 1954.

Carlson DH, Griscom NT: Ovarian cysts in the newborn. *Am J Roentgenol Radium Ther Nucl Med* 116:664, 1972.

Caspi E et al.: Ovarian lutein cysts in pregnancy. *Obstet Gynecol* 42:388, 1973.

Chalvardjian A, Scully RE: Sclerosing stromal tumors of the ovary. *Cancer* 31:664, 1973.

Chan LKC, Prathap K: Virilization in pregnancy associated with an ovarian mucinous cystadenoma. *Am J Obstet Gynecol* 108:946, 1970.

Chatterjee K, Heather JC: Carcinoid heart disease from primary ovarian carcinoid tumors. A case report and a review of the literature. *Am J Med* 45:643, 1968.

Chorlton I et al.: Malignant reticuloendothelial disease involving the ovary as a primary manifesta-

tion. A series of 19 lymphomas and 1 granulocytic sarcoma. *Cancer* 34:397, 1974.

Chung A, Birnbaum SJ: Ovarian cancer associated with pregnancy. *Obstet Gynecol* 41:211, 1973.

Cianfrani T: Neoplasms in apparently normal ovaries. *Am J Obstet Gynecol* 51:246, 1946.

Classification and staging of malignant tumours in the female pelvis. *Acta Obstet Gynecol Scand* 50:1, 1971.

Climie ARW, Heath LP: Malignant degeneration of benign cystic teratomas of the ovary: Review of the literature and report of a chondrosarcoma and carcinoid tumor. *Cancer* 22:824, 1968.

Cohen MH et al.: Burkitt's tumor in the United States. *Cancer* 23:1259, 1969.

Comparato M, Salgado C: Selective catheterization of the hypogastric artery: Its diagnostic value in gynecology. *Int J Obstet Gynecol* 10:108, 1972.

Corson SL, Bolognese RJ: Laparoscopic nuances. *Fertil Steril* 22:684, 1971.

Counseller VS et al.: Carcinoma of the ovary following hysterectomy. *Am J Obstet Gynecol* 69:538, 1955.

Creasman WT, Rutledge F: The prognostic value of peritoneal cytology in gynecologic malignant disease. *Am J Obstet Gynecol* 110:773, 1971.

——— et al.: Carcinoma of the ovary associated with pregnancy. *Obstet Gynecol* 38:111, 1971.

Cruikshank DP et al.: Differential adrenal and ovarian suppression: Diagnosis and treatment of androgenic disorders in women. *Obstet Gynecol* 38:724, 1971.

———, Buchsbaum, HJ: Effects of rapid paracentesis: Cardiovascular dynamics and body fluid composition. *JAMA* 225:1361, 1973.

Czernobilsky B, LaBarre GC: Carcinosarcoma and mixed mesodermal tumor of the ovary: A clinicopathologic analysis of 9 cases. *Obstet Gynecol* 31:21, 1968.

——— et al.: Clear-cell carcinoma of the ovary: A clinicopathologic analysis of pure and mixed forms and comparison with endometrioid carcinoma. *Cancer* 25:762, 1970.

——— et al.: Endometrioid carcinoma of the ovary: A clinicopathologic study of 75 cases. *Cancer* 26:1141, 1970.

Daane TA et al.: Ovarian lutein cysts associated with an otherwise normal pregnancy: Report of a case. *Obstet Gynecol* 34:655, 1969.

De Alvarez RR et al.: Virilizing lipoid tumors of the ovary. *Obstet Gynecol* 35:956, 1970.

De Bacalao EB, Dominguez I: Unilateral gonadoblastoma in a pregnant woman. *Am J Obstet Gynecol* 105:1279, 1969.

Decker DG et al.: Cyclophosphamide: Evaluation in recurrent and progressive ovarian cancer. *Am J Obstet Gynecol* 97:656, 1967a.

_____ et al.: Adjuvant therapy for advanced ovarian malignancy. *Am J Obstet Gynecol* 97:171, 1967b.

_____ et al.: Radiogold treatment of epithelial cancer of ovary: Late results. *Am J Obstet Gynecol* 115:751, 1973.

Dehner LP et al.: Carcinosarcomas and mixed mesodermal tumors of the ovary. *Cancer* 27:207, 1971.

Delclos L, Fletcher GH: Postoperative irradiation for ovarian carcinoma with the cobalt-60 moving strip technique. *Clin Obstet Gynecol* 12:993, 1969.

_____, Quinlan EJ: Malignant tumors of the ovary managed with postoperative megavoltage irradiation. *Radiology* 93:659, 1969.

DePetrillo, DA: Personal communication, 1979.

de Neef JC, Hollenbeck ZJR: The fate of ovaries preserved at the time of hysterectomy. *Am J Obstet Gynecol* 96:1088, 1966.

Dinnerstein AJ, O'Leary JA: Granulosa-theca cell tumors: A clinical review of 102 patients. *Obstet Gynecol* 31:654, 1968.

Dockerty MB: Primary and secondary ovarian adenoacanthoma. *Surg Gynecol Obstet* 99:392, 1954.

_____, Masson JC: Ovarian fibromas: A clinical and pathological study of 283 cases. *Am J Obstet Gynecol* 47:741, 1944.

Donald I: On launching a new diagnostic science. *Am J Obstet Gynecol* 103:609, 1969.

Doss N et al.: Covert bilaterality of mature ovarian teratomas. *Obstet Gynecol* 50:651, 1977.

Dunnihoo DR et al.: Hilar-cell tumors of the ovary: Report of two new cases and review of the world literature. *Obstet Gynecol* 27:703, 1966.

Einhorn LH, Donohue JP: Improved chemotherapy in disseminated testicular cancer. *J Urol* 117:65, 1977.

Emig OR et al.: Gynandroblastoma of the ovary: Review and report of a case. *Obstet Gynecol* 13:135, 1959.

Fathalla MF: Factors in the causation and incidence of ovarian cancer. *Obstet Gynecol Surv* 27:751, 1972.

Favara BE, Franciosi RA: Ovarian teratoma and neuroglial implants on the peritoneum. *Cancer* 31:678, 1973.

Feinberg R: Thecosis: A study of diffuse stromal thecosis of the ovary and superficial collagenization with follicular cysts (Stein-Leventhal ovary). *Obstet Gynecol* 21:687, 1963.

Felmus LB, Pedowitz P: Clinical malignancy of endocrine tumors of the ovary and dysgerminoma. *Obstet Gynecol* 29:344, 1967.

Fenn ME, Abell MR: Carcinosarcoma of the ovary. *Am J Obstet Gynecol* 110:1066, 1971.

Ferenczy A et al.: Para-endocrine hypercalcemia in ovarian neoplasms: Report of mesonephroma with hypercalcemia and review of literature. *Cancer* 27:427, 1971.

Fox H et al.: A clinicopathologic study of 92 uses of granulosa cell tumor of the ovary with special reference to the factors influencing prognosis. *Cancer* 35:231, 1975.

Fox LP, Stamm WJ: Krukenberg tumor complicating pregnancy: Report of a case with androgenic activity. *Am J Obstet Gynecol* 92:702, 1965.

Fraumeni JF et al.: Six families prone to ovarian cancer. *Cancer* 36:364, 1975.

Frei E: Selected considerations regarding chemotherapy as adjuvant in cancer treatment: A commentary. *Cancer Chemother Rep* 50:1, 1966.

Fuller ME: Oral contraceptive therapy for differentiating ovarian cysts. *Postgrad Med* 50:143, 1971.

Garcia-Bunuel R et al.: Luteomas of pregnancy. *Obstet Gynecol* 45:407, 1975.

Genadry R et al.: The origin and clinical behavior of the parovarian tumor. *Am J Obstet Gynecol* 129:873-880, 1977.

Gentil F, Junqueira AC (eds.): *Ovarian Cancer* U.I.C.C. Monograph Series, vol. 2, New York: Springer-Verlag, 1968.

Gibbs EK: Suggested prophylaxis for ovarian cancer. *Am J Obstet Gynecol* 111:756, 1971.

Gillibrand PN: Granulosa-theca cell tumors of the ovary associated with pregnancy: Case report and review of the literature. *Am J Obstet Gynecol* 94:1108, 1966.

Gillman J: The development of the gonads in man with a consideration of the role of fetal endocrines and the histogenesis of ovarian tumors. *Contrib Embryol Carneg Inst* 32:81, 1948.

Girouard DP et al.: Hyperreactio luteinalis: Review of the literature and report of 2 cases. *Obstet Gynecol* 23:513, 1964.

Goldberg BB et al.: Evaluation of ascites by ultrasound. *Radiology* 96:15, 1970.

Goldstein DJ, Lamb EJ: Arrhenoblastoma in first cousins: Report of 2 cases. *Obstet Gynecol* 35:444, 1970.

_____, Piro AJ: Combination chemotherapy in the treatment of germ cell tumors containing choriocarcinoma in males and females. *Surg Gynecol Obstet* 134:61, 1972.

Goldston WR et al.: Clinicopathologic studies in feminizing tumors of the ovary. *Am J Obstet Gynecol* 112:422, 1972.

———— et al.: A granulosa cell tumor in tissue culture. *Am J Obstet Gynecol* 114:652, 1972.

Graham J et al.: Prognostic significance of pleural effusion in ovarian cancer. *Am J Obstet Gynecol* 106:312, 1970.

———— et al.: Preclinical detection of ovarian cancer. *Cancer* 17:1414, 1964.

————, Graham RM: Ovarian cancer and asbestosis. *Environ Res* 1:115, 1967.

Gray LA, Barnes ML: Endometrioid carcinoma of the ovary. *Obstet Gynecol* 29:694, 1967.

Greenblatt RB et al.: Arrhenoblastoma: Three case reports. *Obstet Gynecol* 39:567, 1972.

Greene RR: Feminizing tumors of the ovary and carcinoma of the endometrium. *Obstet Gynecol Annu* 1973, p. 393.

Greenspan EM: Thio-tepa and methotrexate chemotherapy of advanced ovarian carcinoma. *Mt Sinai J Med NY* 32:52, 1968.

Griffiths CT et al.: Advanced ovarian cancer: Primary treatment with surgery, radiotherapy, and chemotherapy. *Cancer* 29:1, 1972.

————: Surgical resection of tumor bulk in the primary treatment of ovarian carcinoma. *Natl Cancer Inst Monogr* 42:101, 1975.

Groeber WR: Ovarian tumors during infancy and childhood. *Am J Obstet Gynecol* 86:1027, 1963.

Grogan RH: Reappraisal of residual ovaries. *Am J Obstet Gynecol* 97:124, 1967a.

————: Accidental rupture of malignant ovarian cysts during surgical removal. *Obstet Gynecol* 30:716, 1967b.

Gusberg SB, Kardon P: Proliferative endometrial response to theca-granulosa cell tumors. *Am J Obstet Gynecol* 111:633, 1971.

Hale RW: Krukenberg tumor of the ovaries: A review of 81 records. *Obstet Gynecol* 22:221, 1968.

Halpin TF, McCann TO: Dynamics of body fluids following the rapid removal of large volumes of ascites. *Am J Obstet Gynecol* 110:103, 1971.

Hart WR: Ovarian epithelial tumors of borderline malignancy (carcinomas of low malignant potential). *Hum Pathol* 8:541, 1977.

————, Burkons, DM: Germ cell neoplasms arising in gonadoblastomas. *Cancer* 43:669, 1979.

————, Norris HJ: Borderline and malignant mucinous tumors of the ovary: Histologic criteria and clinical behavior. *Cancer* 31:1031, 1973.

————, Regezi JA: Strumal carcinoid of the ovary. Ultrastructural observations and long-term follow-up study. *Am J Clin Pathol* 69:356, 1978.

Harvald B, Hauge M: Heredity of cancer elucidated by a study of unselected twins. *JAMA* 186:749, 1963.

Hay DM, Stewart DB: Primary ovarian choriocarcinoma *J Obstet Gynaecol Br Commonw* 76:941, 1969.

Henderson WJ et al.: Talc and carcinoma of the ovary and cervix. *J Obstet Gynaecol Br Commonw* 78:266, 1971.

Hester LL, White L: Radioactive colloidal chromic phosphate in the treatment of ovarian malignancies. *Am J Obstet Gynecol* 103:911, 1969.

Hilaris BS, Clark DGC: The value of postoperative intraperitoneal injection of radiocolloids in early cancer of the ovary. *Am J Radiol* 112:749, 1971.

Hill LM et al.: Ovarian surgery in pregnancy. *Am J Obstet Gynecol,* 122:565, 1975.

Hirabayashi K, Graham J: Genesis of ascites in ovarian cancer. *Am J Obstet Gynecol* 106:492, 1970.

Hittle RE (Associate radiologist, Head, Radiotherapy, Children's Hospital of Los Angeles): Personal communication, 1979.

Hughesdon PE: Thecal and allied reactions in epithelial ovarian tumors. *J Obstet Gynaec Br Commonw* 65:702, 1958.

————: Ovarian lipoid and theca cell tumors; their origins and interrelations. *Obstet Gynecol Surv* 21:245, 1966.

Huntington RW, Bullock WK: Yolk sac tumors of the ovary. *Cancer* 25:1357, 1970.

Hutchison JR et al.: The Stein-Leventhal syndrome and coincident ovarian neoplasms. *Obstet Gynecol* 28:700, 1966.

Izbicki R et al.: Pleural effusion in cancer patients: A prospective randomized study of pleural drainage with the addition of radioactive phosphorous to the pleural space vs. pleural drainage alone. *Cancer* 36:1511, 1975.

James DF et al.: Torsion of normal uterine adnexa in children: Report of three cases. *Obstet Gynecol* 35:226, 1970.

Janko AB, Sandberg EC: Histochemical evidence for the protein nature of the Reinke crystalloid. *Obstet Gynecol* 35:493, 1970.

Javert CT, Finn WF: Arrhenoblastoma: The incidence of malignancy and the relationship to pregnancy, to sterility, and to treatment. *Cancer* 4:60, 1951.

Jensen RD, Norris HJ: Epithelial tumors of the ovary. *Arch Pathol* 94:29, 1972.

Jewelewicz R et al.: Luteomas of pregnancy: A cause for maternal virilization. *Am J Obstet Gynecol* 109:24, 1971.

Johansson H: Clinical aspects of metastatic ovarian

cancer of extragenital origin. *Acta Obstet Gynecol Scand* 39:681, 1960.

Johnson CG: Discussion of paper by CL Randall and FP Paloucek, The frequency of oophorectomy at the time of hysterectomy. *Am J Obstet Gynecol* 100:716, 1968.

Joly DJ et al.: An epidemiologic study of the relationship of reproductive experience to cancer of the ovary. *Am J Epidemiol* 99:190, 1974.

Joshi VV: Primary Krukenberg tumor of ovary: Review of literature and case report. *Cancer* 22:1199, 1968.

Judd HL et al.: Maternal virilization developing during a twin pregnancy: Demonstration of excess ovarian androgen production associated with theca-lutein cysts. *N Engl J Med* 288:118, 1973.

Julian CG, Woodruff JD: The role of chemotherapy in the treatment of primary ovarian malignancy. *Obstet Gynecol Surv* 24:1307, 1969.

_____, _____: The biologic behavior of low-grade papillary serous carcinoma of the ovary. *Obstet Gynecol* 40:860, 1973.

Kajanoja P, Procope BJ: Nongenital pelvic tumors found at gynecologic operations. *Surg Gynecol Obstet* 140:605, 1975.

Kalstone CE et al.: Massive edema of the ovary simulating fibroma. *Obstet Gynecol* 34:564, 1969.

Kase N: Steroid synthesis in abnormal ovaries. II. Granulosa cell tumor. *Am J Obstet Gynecol* 90:1262, 1964.

_____, Conrad S: Steroid synthesis in abnormal ovaries. I. Arrhenoblastoma. *Am J Obstet Gynecol* 90:1251, 1964.

Kaslow RA et al.: Acute leukemia following cytotoxic chemotherapy. *JAMA* 219:75, 1972.

Keettel WC et al.: Prophylactic use of radioactive gold in the treatment of primary ovarian cancer. *AM J Obstet Gynecol* 94:766, 1966.

Kelley RR, Scully RE: Cancer developing in dermoid cysts of the ovary. *Cancer* 14:989, 1961.

Kempers RD et al.: Struma ovarii–ascitic, hyperthyroid, and asymptomatic syndromes. *Ann Intern Med* 72:883, 1970.

Kent SW, McKay DG: Primary cancer of the ovary: An analysis of 349 cases. *Am J Obstet Gynecol* 80:430, 1960.

Kistner RW: Intraperitoneal rupture of benign cystic teratomas: Review of the literature with a report of two cases. *Obstet Gynecol Surv* 7:603, 1952.

Koller O, Gjonnaess H: Dysgerminoma of the ovary: A clinical report of 20 cases. *Acta Obstet Gynecol Scand* 43:268, 1964.

Kolstad P et al.: Individualized treatment of ovarian cancer. *Am J Obstet Gynecol* 128:617, 1977.

Koss LG et al.: Pseudothecomas of ovaries: A syndrome of bilateral ovarian hypertrophy with diffuse luteinization, endometrial carcinoma, obesity, hirsutism, and diabetes mellitus: Report of 2 cases. *Cancer* 17:76, 1964.

_____ et al.: Masculinizing tumor of the ovary apparently with adrenocortical activity. *Cancer* 23:1345, 1969.

Kottmeier HL: The classification and treatment of ovarian tumors. *Acta Obstet Gynecol Scand* 31:313, 1952.

_____: *Carcinoma of the Female Genitalia,* Baltimore: Williams & Wilkins, 1953.

_____: Problems relating to classification and stage-grouping of malignant tumors in the female pelvis, in *Cancer of the Uterus and Ovary,* The University of Texas M.D. Anderson Hospital and Tumor Institute, Eleventh Annual Clinical Conference on Cancer, Chicago: Year Book, 1966, p. 17.

_____: Clinical staging in ovarian carcinoma, in *Ovarian Cancer,* vol. 11, eds. F Gentil, AC Junqueira, U.I.C.C. Monograph Series, New York: Springer-Verlag, 1968a, p. 146.

_____: Surgical management–conservative surgery, in *Ovarian Cancer,* vol. 11, eds. F Gentil, AC Junqueira, U.I.C.C. Monograph Series, New York: Springer-Verlag, 1968b, p. 157.

_____: Treatment of ovarian cancer with thiotepa. *Clin Obstet Gynecol* 11:428, 1968c.

Koven BJ et al.: Response to actinomycin D of malignant carcinoid arising in an ovarian teratoma. *Am J Obstet Gynecol* 101:267, 1968.

Kraus FT, Neubecker RD: Luteinization of the ovarian theca in infants and children. *Am J Clin Pathol* 37:389, 1962.

Krause DE, Stembridge VA: Luteomas of pregnancy *Am J Obstet Gynecol* 95:192, 1966.

Kurman RJ, Craig JM: Endometrioid and clear cell carcinoma of the ovary. *Cancer* 29:1653, 1972.

_____, Norris HJ: Malignant germ cell tumors of the ovary. *Hum Pathol* 8:551, 1977.

Langley FA et al.: An ultrastructural study of mucin secreting epithelia in ovarian neoplasms. *Acta Pathol Microbiol Scand* [Suppl. 233] 80:76, 1972.

Lauchlan SC: The secondary Müllerian system. *Obstet Gynecol Surv* 27:133, 1972.

Levi MM: Antigenicity of ovarian and cervical malignancies with a view toward possible immunodiagnosis. *Am J Obstet Gynecol* 109:689, 1971.

_____ et al.: Antigenicity of papillary serous cystadenocarcinoma tissue culture cells. *Am J Obstet Gynecol* 102:433, 1968.

Li FP et al.: Familial ovarian carcinoma. *JAMA* 214:1559, 1970.

Lomano JM et al.: Torsion of the uterine adnexa causing an acute abdomen. *Obstet Gynecol* 35:221, 1970.

Long ME, Taylor HC Jr.: Endometrioid carcinoma of the ovary. *Am J Obstet Gynecol* 90:936, 1964.

Luisi A: Metastatic ovarian tumors, in *Ovarian Cancer,* vol. 11, U.I.C.C. Monograph Series, Berlin: Springer-Verlag, 1968.

Lutwak-Mann C: The influence of nutrition on the ovary, in *The Ovary,* vol. 2, ed. S Zuckerman, New York: Academic, 1962, p. 291.

Lynch HT et al.: Familial association of carcinoma of the breast and ovary. *Surg Gynecol Obstet,* 138:717, 1974.

Lyon FA et al.: Granulosa-cell tumors of the ovary: Review of 23 cases. *Obstet Gynecol* 21:67, 1963.

McGowan L et al.: Cul-de-sac aspiration for diagnostic cytologic study. *Am J Obstet Gynecol* 96:413, 1966.

Malinak LR, Miller GV: Bilateral multicentric ovarian luteoma of pregnancy associated with masculinization of a female infant. *Am J Obstet Gynecol* 101:923, 1965.

Malkasian GD Jr, Symmonds RE: Treatment of the unilateral encapsulated ovarian disgerminoma. *Am J Obstet Gynecol* 90:379, 1964.

_____ et al.: Benign cystic teratomas. *Obstet Gynecol* 29:719, 1967.

_____ et al.: Observations on gynecologic malignancy treated with 5-fluorouracil. *Am J Obstet Gynecol* 100:1012, 1968.

_____ et al.: Medroxyprogesterone acetate for the treatment of metastatic and recurrent ovarian carcinoma. *Cancer Rep* 61:913, 1977.

Malloy JJ et al.: Papillary ovarian tumors. I. Benign tumors and serous mucinous cystadenocarcinomas. *Am J Obstet Gynecol* 93:867, 1965a.

_____ et al.: Papillary ovarian tumors II: Endometrioid cancers and mesonephroma ovarii. *Am J Obstet Gynecol* 93:880, 1965b.

Marshall JR: Ovarian enlargements in the first year of life: Review of 45 cases. *Ann Surg* 161:372, 1965.

Martin CB et al.: Diagnostic ultrasound in obstetrics and gynecology: Experience on a large clinical service. *Obstet Gynecol* 41:379, 1973.

Masopust J et al.: Occurrence of fetoprotein in patients with neoplasms and non-neoplastic disease. *Int J Cancer* 3:364, 1968.

Masterson JG: Discussion of paper by BC Burns Jr. et al., Management of ovarian carcinoma. *Am J Obstet Gynecol* 98:374, 1967.

_____, Nelson JH Jr.: The role of chemotherapy in the treatment of gynecologic malignancy. *Am J Obstet Gynecol* 93:1102, 1965.

Mattingly RF, Huang WY: Steroidogenesis of the menopausal and postmenopausal ovary. *Am J Obstet Gynecol* 103:679, 1969.

Meigs JV: Cancer of the ovary. *South Med J* 30:133, 1937.

_____, Cass JW: Fibroma of the ovary with ascites and hydrothorax with a report of 7 cases. *Am J Obstet Gynecol* 33:249, 1937.

Meyer RE: The pathology of some special ovarian tumors and their relationship to sex characteristics. *Am J Obstet Gynecol* 22:697, 1931.

Moench LM: A clinical study of 403 cases of adenocarcinoma of the ovary: Papillary cystadenoma, carcinomatous cystadenoma, and solid adenocarcinoma of the ovary. *Am J Obstet Gynecol* 26:22, 1933.

Moore DW, Langley II: Routine use of radiogold following operation for ovarian cancer. *Am J Obstet Gynecol* 98:624, 1967.

Moore JG et al.: Ovarian tumors in infancy, childhood, and adolescence. *Am J Obstet Gynecol* 99:913, 1967.

Morris JM, Scully RE: *Endocrine Pathology of the Ovary,* St. Louis: Mosby, 1958.

Mueller WK et al.: Serum haptoglobin in patients with ovarian malignancies. *Obstet Gynecol* 38:427, 1971.

Müller JH: Weitere entwicklung der therapie von peritonealcarzinosen bei ovarialcarzinom mit könstlicher radioaktivitat. *Gynaecologia* (Basel) 129:289, 1950.

Munnell EW: The changing prognosis and treatment in cancer of the ovary: A report of 235 patients with primary ovarian carcinoma 1952–1961. *Am J Obstet Gynecol* 100:790, 1968.

_____: Is conservative therapy ever justified in stage I(IA) cancer of the ovary? *Am J Obstet Gynecol* 103:641, 1969.

Musumeci R et al.: Lymphangiography in patients with ovarian epithelial cancer. *Cancer* 40:1444, 1977.

Nassar TR et al.: Massive edema of the ovary. A case report and a review of the literature. *Obstet Gynecol* 47:77s, 1976.

Neubecker RD, Breen JL: Embryonal carcinoma of the ovary. *Cancer* 15:546, 1962a.

_____, Breen JL: Gynandroblastoma: A report of five cases, with a discussion of the histogenesis and classification of ovarian tumors. *Am J Clin Pathol* 38:60, 1962b.

Nieminen V, Purola E: Stage and prognosis of ovarian cystadenocarcinomas. *Acta Obstet Gynecol Scand* 49:49, 1970.

Norris CC, Murphy DP: Malignant ovarian neoplasms: With a report of the end-results in a series of 93 cases. *Am J Obstet Gynecol* 23:833, 1933.

Norris HJ, Jensen RD: Relative frequency of ovarian neoplasms in children and adolescents. *Cancer* 30:713, 1972.

_____, Robinowitz M: Ovarian adenocarcinoma of mesonephric type. *Cancer* 28:1074, 1971.

_____, Taylor HB: Nodular theca-lutein hyperplasia of pregnancy (so-called "pregnancy luteoma"): A clinical and pathological study of 15 cases. *Am J Clin Pathol* 47:557, 1967.

_____: Prognosis of granulosa-theca tumors of the ovary. *Cancer* 21:255, 1968.

_____: Virilization associated with cystic granulosa tumors. *Obstet Gynecol* 34:629, 1969.

_____ et al.: Immature (malignant) teratoma of the ovary. A clinical and pathology study of 58 cases. *Cancer* 37:2359, 1976.

Novak ER et al.: Feminizing gonadal stromal tumors: Analysis of the granulosa-theca cell tumors of the Ovarian Tumor Registry. *Obstet Gynecol* 38:701, 1971.

_____, Mattingly RF: Hilus cell tumor of the ovary. *Obstet Gynecol* 15:425, 1960.

_____ et al.: Ovarian tumors in pregnancy. *Obstet Gynecol* 46:401, 1975.

O'Hern TM, Neubecker RD: Arrhenoblastoma. *Obstet Gynecol* 19:758, 1962.

O'Neill RT, Mikuta JJ: Hypoglycemia associated with serous cystadenocarcinoma of the ovary. *Obstet Gynecol* 35:287, 1970.

Ory H: Functional ovarian cysts and oral contraceptives. Negative association confirmed surgically. *JAMA* 228:68, 1974.

Osborn RH et al.: Androgen studies in a patient with lipoid-cell tumor of the ovary. *Obstet Gynecol* 33:666, 1969.

Paladine W et al.: Intracavitary bleomycin in the management of malignant effusions. *Cancer* 38:1903, 1976.

Paloucek FP: Quoted by CL Randall in *Gynecologic Oncology*, eds. HRK Barber, EA Graber, Baltimore: Williams & Wilkins, 1970, p. 211.

Parker LM et al.: Adriamycin-cyclophosphamide therapy in ovarian cancer. *Proc Am Assoc Cancer Res ASCO* 16:263, 1975.

Parker RT et al.: Cancer of the ovary: Survival studies based upon operative therapy, chemotherapy, and radiotherapy. *Am J Obstet Gynecol* 108:878, 1970.

Parrish HM et al.: Time interval from castration in premenopausal women to development of excessive coronary atherosclerosis. *Am J Obstet Gynecol* 90:155, 1967.

Pedowitz P et al.: Precocious pseudopuberty due to ovarian tumors. *Obstet Gynecol Surv* 10:633, 1955.

_____, O'Brien FB: Arrhenoblastoma of the ovary: Review of the literature and report of 2 cases. *Obstet Gynecol* 16:62, 1960.

Perez CA, Bradfield JS: Radiation therapy in the treatment of carcinoma of the ovary. *Cancer* 29:1027, 1972.

Peterson WF et al.: Benign cystic teratomas of the ovary: A clinico-statistical study of 1,007 cases with a review of the literature. *Am J Obstet Gynecol* 70:368, 1955.

_____: Solid histologically benign teratomas of the ovary. *Am J Obstet Gynecol* 72:1094, 1956.

_____: Malignant degeneration of benign cystic teratomas of the ovary. A collective review of the literature. *Obstet Gynecol Surv* 12:793, 1957.

Pinkerton JHM et al.: Development of the human ovary—a study using histochemical technics. *Obstet Gynecol* 18:152, 1961.

Piver MS: Radioactive colloids in the treatment of stage IA ovarian cancer. *Obstet Gynecol* 40:42, 1972.

Polansky S et al.: Virilization associated with bilateral luteomas of pregnancy. *Obstet Gynecol* 45:516, 1975.

Powell D et al.: Nonparathyroid humoral hypercalcemia in patients with neoplastic disease. *N Engl J Med* 289:176, 1973.

Pratt JH, Shamblin WR: Spontaneous rupture of endometrial cysts of the ovary presenting as an acute abdominal emergency. *Am J Obstet Gynecol* 108:56, 1970.

Printz JL et al.: The embryology of supernumerary ovaries. *Obstet Gynecol* 41:246, 1973.

Purola E: Serous papillary ovarian tumors: A study of 233 cases with special reference to the histological type of tumor and its influence in prognosis. *Acta Obstet Gynecol Scand* 42:7, 1963.

_____, Nieminen U: Does rupture of cystic carcinoma during operation influence the prognosis? *Ann Chir Gynaecol Fenn* 57:615, 1968.

Quer EA et al.: Ruptured dermoid cyst of the ovary simulating abdominal carcinomatosis. *Proc Staff Meet Mayo Clinic* 26:439, 1951.

Radisavljevic SV: The pathogenesis of ovarian inclusion cysts and cystomas. *Obstet Gynecol* 49:424, 1977.

Randall CL: Background of statistical data on ovarian

cancer, in *Gynecological Oncology,* eds. HRK Barber, EA Graber, Baltimore: Williams & Wilkins, 1970, p. 211.

———— et al.: Ovarian function after the menopause. *Am J Obstet Gynecol* 74:719, 1957.

———— et al.: Pathology in the preserved ovary after unilateral oophorectomy. *Am J Obstet Gynecol* 84:1233, 1962.

————, Gerhardt PR: The probability of the occurrence of the more common types of gynecologic malignancy. *Am J Obstet Gynecol* 68:1378, 1954.

————, Hall DW: Clinical considerations of benign ovarian cystomas. *Am J Obstet Gynecol* 62:806, 1951.

————, Paloucek FP: The frequency of oophorectomy at the time of hysterectomy. *Am J Obstet Gynecol* 100:716, 1968.

Ranney B: Endometriosis, II. Emergency operations due to hemoperitoneum. *Obstet Gynecol* 36:437, 1970.

————, Chastain D: Ovarian function, reproduction, and later operations following adnexal surgery. *Obstet Gynecol* 51:521, 1978.

Rashad MN et al.: Sex chromatin and chromosome analysis in ovarian teratomas. *Am J Obstet Gynecol* 96:461, 1966.

Reimer RR et al.: Acute leukemia after alkylating-agent therapy of ovarian cancer. *N Engl J Med* 297:177, 1977.

Rice BF et al.: Luteoma of pregnancy: Steroidogenic and morphologic considerations. *Am J Obstet Gynecol* 104:871, 1969.

Richardson GS: Ovarian physiology. *N Engl J Med* 274:1008, 1966a.

————: Ovarian physiology. *N Engl J Med* 274:1064, 1966b.

————: Ovarian physiology. *N Engl J Med* 274:1121, 1966c.

————: Ovarian physiology. *N Engl J Med* 274:1183, 1966d.

Robboy SJ, Scully RE: Ovarian teratoma with glial implants on the peritoneum: An analysis of 12 cases. *Hum Pathol* 1:643, 1970.

Roth LM: Massive ovarian edema with stromal luteinization. *Am J Clin Pathol* 55:757, 1971.

————, Sternberg WH: Proliferating Brenner tumor. *Cancer* 27:687, 1971.

Rothman LA et al.: Placental and fetal involvement by maternal malignancy: A report of rectal carcinoma and a review of the literature. *Am J Obstet Gynecol* 116:1023, 1973.

Rubin P: A critical analysis of current therapy of carcinoma of the ovary: Introduction to symposium. *Am J Roentgenol Radium Ther Nucl Med* 88:833, 1962.

———— et al.: Has postoperative irradiation proved itself? *Am J Roentgenol Radium Ther Nucl Med* 88:849, 1962.

Salerno LJ: Feminizing mesenchymomas of the ovary. *Am J Obstet Gynecol* 84:731, 1962.

Samanth KK, Black WC: Benign ovarian stromal tumors associated with free peritoneal fluid. *Am J Obstet Gynecol* 107:538, 1970.

Sampson JA: Endometrial carcinoma of ovary arising in endometrial tissue in that organ. *Arch Surg* 10:1, 1925.

Sandberg EC: The virilizing ovary, pt. 1: A histogenetic evaluation. *Obstet Gynecol Surv* 79:165, 1962.

Santesson L, Kottmeier HL: General classification of ovarian tumors, in *Ovarian Cancer*, vol. 2, eds. F Gentil, AC Junqueira, U.I.C.C. Monograph Series, New York: Springer-Verlag, 1968, p. 1.

————, Marrubini G: Clinical and pathological survey of ovarian embryonal carcinomas, including so-called "mesonephromas" (Schiller) or "mesoblastomas" (Teilum), treated at the Radiumhemmet. *Acta Obstet Gynecol Scand* 36:399, 1957.

Schellhas HF et al.: Germ Cell tumors associated with XY gonadal dysgenesis. *Am J Obstet Gynecol* 109:1197, 1971.

Schifrin BS et al.: Teen-age endometriosis. *Am J Obstet Gynecol* 116:973, 1973.

Schiller W: Mesonephroma ovarii. *Cancer* 35:1, 1939.

Schueller EF, Kirol PM: Prognosis in endometrial carcinoma of the ovary. *Obstet Gynecol* 27:850, 1966.

Scully RE: Gonadoblastoma: A gonadal tumor related to the dysgerminoma (seminoma) and capable of sex hormone production. *Cancer* 6:455, 1953.

————: Ovarian tumors of germ cell origin, in *Progress in Gynecology*, vol. 5, eds. SH Sturgis, ML Taymor, New York: Grune & Stratton, 1970a.

————: Recent progress in ovarian cancer. *Hum Pathol* 1:73, 1970b.

————: Sex cord tumor with annular tubules: A distinctive ovarian tumor of the Peutz-Jeghers syndrome. *Cancer* 25:1107, 1970c.

————: Gonadoblastoma. *Cancer* 25:1340, 1970d.

————: Ovarian tumors. A review. *Am J Pathol* 87:686, 1977.

————, Barlow JF: "Mesonephroma" of the ovary: Tumor of Müllerian nature related to the endometrioid carcinoma. *Cancer* 20:1405, 1967.

———— et al: The development of malignancy in endometriosis. *Clin Obstet Gynecol* 9:384, 1966.

————, Richardson GS: Luteinization of the stroma of metastatic cancer involving the ovary and its endocrine significance. *Cancer* 14:827, 1961.

Serov SF et al.: International Histological Classification of Tumours, no. 9. *Histological Typing of Ovarian Tumours,* Geneva: World Health Organization, 1973.

Serr DM et al.: Chromosomal studies in tumors of embryonic origin. *Obstet Gynecol* 33:324, 1969.

Shanks HGI: Pseudomyxoma peritonei. *J Obstet Gynaecol Br Commonw* 68:212, 1961.

Shettles LB: Recurrent theca lutein cysts. *Obstet Gynecol* 21:339, 1963.

Shuster M et al.: Carcinoid tumor metastasizing to the ovaries. *Obstet Gynecol* 36:515, 1970.

Silverman BB et al.: Multiple malignant tumors associated with primary carcinoma of the ovary. *Surg Gynecol Obstet* 134:244, 1972.

Simmons RL, Sciarra JJ: Treatment of late recurrent granulosa cell tumors of the ovary. *Surg Gynecol Obstet* 124:65, 1967.

Sjöstedt D, Wåhlén T: Prognosis of granulosa cell tumours. *Acta Obstet Gynecol Scand* [Suppl. 6] 40:1, 1961.

Skipper HE, et al.: On the criteria and kinetics associated with "curability" of experimental leukemia. *Cancer Chemother Rep* 35:1, 1964.

Smith CW, Foster CE: Surgical pathology of small ovarian cysts. *Am J Obstet Gynecol* 72:1255, 1956.

Smith JP et al.: Chemotherapy of ovarian cancer: New approaches to treatment. *Cancer* 30:1565, 1972.

_____ et al.: Malignant gynecologic tumors in children: Current approaches to treatment. *Am J Obstet Gynecol* 116:261, 1973.

_____, Rutledge F: Advances in chemotherapy for gynecologic cancer. *Cancer* 41:669, 1975.

_____, Chemotherapy in the treatment of cancer of the ovary. *Am J Obstet Gynecol* 107:691, 1970.

_____ et al.: Results of chemotherapy as an adjunct to surgery in patients with localized ovarian cancer. *Semin Oncol* 2:277, 1975.

_____ et al.: Second-look operation in ovarian carcinoma. Postchemotherapy. *Cancer* 38:1438, 1976.

Sobrinho LG et al.: Amenorrhea in patients with Hodgkin's disease treated with antineoplastic agents. *Am J Obstet Gynecol* 109:135, 1971.

Spadoni LR et al.: Virilization coexisting with Krukenberg tumor during pregnancy. *Am J Obstet Gynecol* 92:981, 1965.

Spanos WJ: Preoperative hormonal therapy of cystic adnexal masses. *Am J Obstet Gynecol* 116:551, 1973.

Speert H: The role of ionizing radiations in the causation of ovarian tumors. *Cancer* 5:478, 1952.

Stein IF, Leventhal ML: Amenorrhea associated with bilateral polycystic ovaries. *Am J Obstet Gynecol* 29:181, 1935.

Sternberg WH: The morphology, androgenic function, hyperplasia, and tumors of the human ovarian hilus cells. *Am J Pathol* 25:493, 1949.

_____: Nonfunctioning ovarian neoplasms, in *The Ovary,* eds. HG Grady, DE Smith, Baltimore: Wiliams & Wilkins, 1963.

_____, Barclay DL: Luteoma of pregnancy. *Am J Obstet Gynecol* 95:165, 1966.

_____, Gaskill CJ: Theca-cell tumors: With a report of twelve new cases and observations on the possible etiologic role of ovarian stromal hyperplasia. *Am J Obstet Gynecol* 59:575, 1950.

Stone ML et al.: Clinical applications of ultrasound in obstetrics and gynecology. *Am J Obstet Gynecol* 113:1046, 1972.

Symmonds RE, Tauxe WN: Gallium-67 scintigraphy of gynecologic tumors. *Am J Obstet Gynecol* 114:356, 1972.

Symonds DA, Driscoll SG: An adrenal cortical rest within the fetal ovary: Report of a case. *Am J Clin Pathol* 60:562, 1973.

Talerman A et al.: Dysgerminoma: Clinicopathologic study of 22 cases. *Obstet Gynecol* 41:137, 1973.

_____ et al.: Serum alpha-fetoprotein (AFP) in diagnosis and management of endodermal sinus (yolk sac) tumor and mixed germ cell tumor of the ovary. *Cancer* 41:272, 1978.

Taylor HB: Functioning ovarian tumors and related conditions, in *Pathology Annual* 1966, ed. SC Sommers, New York: Appleton-Century-Crofts, 1966, p. 148.

_____ et al.: Neoplasms of dysgenetic gonads. *Am J Obstet Gynecol* 96:816, 1966.

_____, Norris HJ: Lipid cell tumors of the ovary: An analysis of 30 cases. *Cancer* 20:1953, 1967.

Taylor HC Jr.: Malignant and semimalignant tumors of the ovary. *Surg Gynecol Obstet* 48:204, 1929.

_____: Studies in the clinical and biological evolution of adenocarcinoma of the ovary. *J Obstet Gynaecol Br Commonw* 66:827, 1959.

_____, Alsop WE: Spontaneous regression of peritoneal implantations from ovarian papillary cystadenoma. *Cancer* 16:1305, 1932.

_____, Long ME: Problems of cellular and tissue differentiation in papillary adenocarcinoma of the ovary. *Am J Obstet Gynecol* 70:753, 1955.

Teilum G: Histogenesis and classification of mesonephric tumors of female and male genital system and relationship to so-called benign adenomatoid tumours (mesotheliomas): Comparative histological study. *Acta Pathol Microbiol Scand* 34:431, 1954.

_____: Classification of testicular and ovarian androblastoma and Sertoli cell tumors. *Cancer* 11:769, 1958.

———: Endodermal sinus tumors of the ovary and testis: Comparative morphogenesis of the so-called mesonephroma ovarii (Schiller) and extra-embryonic (yolk sac allantoic) structures of the rat placenta. *Cancer* 12:1029, 1959.

———: Classification of endodermal sinus tumor (mesoblastoma vitellinum) and so-called "embryonal carcinoma" of the ovary. *Acta Pathol Microbiol Scand* 64:407, 1965.

Te Linde RW, Wharton LR: Ovarian function following pelvic operation: An experimental study on monkeys. *Am J Obstet Gynecol* 80:844, 1960.

Terz JJ et al.: Incidence of carcinoma in the retained ovary. *Am J Surg* 113:511, 1967.

Teter J: Prognosis, malignancy, and curability of the germ-cell tumor occurring in dysgenetic gonads. *Am J Obstet Gynecol* 108:894, 1970.

———, Boczkowski K: Occurrence of tumors in dysgenetic gonads. *Cancer* 20:1301, 1967.

Theiss EA et al.: Nuclear sex of testicular tumors and some related ovarian and extragonadal neoplasms. *Cancer* 13:323, 1960.

Thompson JP et al.: Ovarian and parovarian tumors in infants and children. *Am J Obstet Gynecol* 97:1059, 1967.

Thurlbeck WM, Scully RE: Solid teratoma of the ovary: A clinicopathological analysis of 9 cases. *Cancer* 13:804, 1960.

Turner HB et al.: Choriocarcinoma of the ovary. *Obstet Gynecol* 24:918, 1964.

Valdes-Dapena MA: The normal ovary of childhood. *Ann NY Acad Sci* 142:597, 1967.

van Wagemen G, Simpson ME: *Embryology of the Ovary and Testis Homo Sapiens and Macaca Mulatta,* New Haven: Yale, 1965.

Villasanta U, Bloedorn FG: Operation, external irradiation, radioactive isotopes, and chemotherapy in treatment of metastatic ovarian malignancies. *Am J Obstet Gynecol* 102:531, 1968.

Vogel EH: Anterior sacral meningocele as a gynecologic problem: Report of a case. *Obstet Gynecol* 36:766, 1970.

Wallach RC et al.: Thio-tepa chemotherapy for ovarian carcinoma: Influence of remission and toxicity on survival. *Obstet Gynecol* 35:278, 1970.

Walton PD et al.: The expanding role of diagnostic ultrasound in obstetrics and gynecology. *Surg Gynecol Obstet* 137:753, 1973.

Ward HWC: Progestogen therapy for ovarian carcinoma. *J Obstet Gynecol* 79:555, 1972.

Webb MJ et al.: Factors influencing survival in stage I ovarian cancer. *Am J Obstet Gynecol* 116:222, 1973.

White CA et al.: The importance of definitive recognition of intestinal disease from a suspected gynecologic process. *Am J Obstet Gynecol* 119:111, 1974.

White KC: Ovarian tumors in pregnancy: A private hospital ten year survey. *Am J Obstet Gynecol* 116:544, 1973.

Wider JA et al.: Sustained remissions after chemotherapy for primary ovarian cancers containing choriocarcinoma. *N Engl J Med* 280:1439, 1969.

Wieland RG et al.: Hormonal evaluation of premature menarche produced by a follicular cyst. *Am J Obstet Gynecol* 126:731, 1976.

———, O'Leary JA: Dysgerminoma: A clinical review. *Obstet Gynecol* 31:560, 1968.

Wilkinson EJ et al.: Alpha-fetoprotein and endodermal sinus tumor of the ovary. *Am J Obstet Gynecol* 116:711, 1973.

Williams TJ et al.: Management of unilateral and encapsulated ovarian cancer in young women. *Gynecol Onc* 1:143, 1973.

———, Dockerty MB: Status of the contralateral ovary in encapsulated low grade malignant tumors of the ovary. *Surg Gynecol Obstet* 143:763, 1976.

Wiltshaw E, Kroner T: Phase II study of *cis*-dichlorodiammineplatinum (II) (NSC-119875) in advanced adenocarcinoma of the ovary. *Cancer Treat Rep* 60:55, 1976.

Wisniewski M, Deppisch LM: Solid teratomas of ovary. *Cancer* 32:440, 1973.

Witschi E: Migration of the germ cells of human embryos from the yolk sac to the primitive gonadal folds. *Contrib Embryol Carneg Inst* 32:67, 1948.

Woll E et al.: The ovary in endometrial carcinoma. *Am J Obstet Gynecol* 56:617, 1948.

Woodruff JD: Papillary serous tumors of the ovary. *Am J Obstet Gynecol* 67:1112, 1954.

——— et al.: Mucinous tumors of the ovary. *Obstet Gynecol* 16:699, 1960.

——— et al.: Lymphoma of the ovary: A study of 35 cases from the Ovarian Tumor Registry of the American Gynecological Society. *Am J Obstet Gynecol* 85:912, 1963.

——— et al.: Ovarian struma. *Obstet Gynecol* 27:194, 1966.

——— et al.: Ovarian teratomas: Relationship of histologic and ontogenic factors to prognosis. *Am J Obstet Gynecol* 102:702, 1968.

——— et al.: Metastatic ovarian tumors. *Am J Obstet Gynecol* 107:202, 1970.

———, Julian CG: Histologic grading and morphologic changes of significance in the treatment of semi-malignant and malignant ovarian tumors. *Proc Natl Cancer Conf* 6:346, 1970.

_____, **Novak ER**: The Krukenberg tumor: Study of 48 cases from the Ovarian Tumor Registry. *Obstet Gynecol* 15:351, 1960.

Wynder EL et al.: Epidemiology of cancer of the ovary. *Cancer* 23:352, 1969.

Yin PH, Sommers SC: Some pathologic correlations of ovarian stromal hyperplasia. *J Clin Endocrinol* 21:472, 1961.

Young R et al.: Advanced ovarian adenocarcinoma: Melphalan (PAM) vs. combination chemotherapy (Hexa-CAF). *Cancer Letter* 5:6, 1978.

Younglai EV et al.: Arrhenoblastoma: In vivo and in vitro studies. *Am J Obstet Gynecol* 116:401, 1973.

Zourlas PA, Jones HW: Stein-Leventhal syndrome with masculinizing ovarian tumors: Report of 3 cases. *Obstet Gynecol* 34:861, 1969.

_____, **Jones HW Jr.**: The gynecologic aspects of adrenal tumors. *Obstet Gynecol* 41:234, 1973.

46

The Breast

GORDON K. JIMERSON

The mammary gland is a highly specialized variant of sweat gland and represents the distinguishing feature of a zoological class appropriately named mammals. These organs are normally present in pairs, with the number of such pairs generally correlated to the number of offspring arising in a usual pregnancy of the species studied. The human mammary gland is of ectodermal and mesodermal origin and appears along an ectodermal ridge (the mammary ridge) found in the embryo. Several papillae may be found on each ridge, which extends in the midclavicular line from the neck to the vulva, but only the papilla located in the fifth interspace persists and develops in the normal human being.

ANATOMY

The human female breast consists of a series of alveoli from which a ductal network extends to the nipple with interspersed fatty tissue and fibrous ligaments (Fig. 46–1). The alveoli are lined by cuboidal or low columnar cells that enlarge greatly and discharge their contents into the ductal system during lactation. Small groups of alveoli are found enmeshed in fatty tissue with such clusters representing lobules. The ducts from several lobules combine into a larger duct that terminates in the nipple. Each excretory duct, of which there are about twenty, with its secondary and tertiary ducts and accompanying alveoli represents a lobe. The breast is invested by fascia with a superficial layer just beneath the skin and a deep layer overlying the chest-wall muscles. Fibrous tissue processes, commonly referred to as Cooper's ligaments, are found extending from the deep fascia through the glandular and alveolar tissue and eventually fusing with the superficial fascia (Fig. 46–1).

The cutaneous nerve supply to the breast includes the third and fourth branches of the cervical plexus to the upper breast and the thoracic intercostal nerves to the lower breast. The chief external blood supply to the breast is from the perforating branches of the internal mammary artery. Additional arterial blood supply is derived from several branches of the axillary artery which are of importance primarily as anatomic landmarks to the surgeon and because of their intimate relationship to the lymphatics. The superficial veins of the breast drain into the internal mammary veins and the superficial veins of the lower neck, and the latter drain into the internal jugular vein. The deep breast tissue is served by veins emptying into the internal mammary, axillary, and intercostal veins. The communication of the intercostal veins with the vertebral plexus of veins is responsible for the frequency of vertebral metastasis. The lymphatic drainage of the breast has been extensively studied and the intricacy of this system is beyond the scope of this chapter, but in general the axillary lymphatic system provides the drainage for the lateral breast, and the internal mammary lymphatics receive the drainage from the medial breast. Intercommunications between these and other lymphatics exist, so simplistic explanations of metastatic routes are sometimes misleading.

PHYSIOLOGY

The recent isolation of human prolactin has allowed studies providing us with important new knowledge about normal and abnormal breast physiology. The information presently available seems best understood when divided into the useful, if somewhat artificial, categories of breast growth, milk secretion, and milk excretion.

BREAST GROWTH

Breast growth is largely dependent upon estrogen and progesterone. As indicated in studies utilizing oophorectomized animals, estrogen replacement stimulates ductal growth whereas progesterone is necessary for adequate alveolar growth. Additional hormonal input is necessary to obtain optimal breast

FIGURE 46–1 Normal breast anatomy with ductal and alveolar structures on left and fascial structures on right.

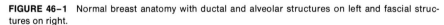

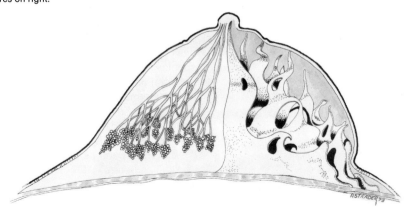

development. Data gathered from hypophysectomized and pancreatectomized experimental animal
models have revealed growth hormone, prolactin, insulin, cortisol, and thyroxine to be important in normal
breast development, though the precise role of each
of these hormones is yet to be defined (Fig. 46–2).
The rapid mammary growth during pregnancy is due
to ductal proliferation associated with increase in
number and size of the alveoli. This glandular tissue
displaces the connective-tissue stroma, so the total
increase in functional breast tissue is far greater than
outward measurements would imply. This growth in
preparation for milk production is largely secondary
to increased circulating levels of estrogen, progesterone, and prolactin. The precise role of placental lactogen in pregnancy-induced mammary growth is unknown.

MILK PRODUCTION

Milk production normally occurs only after parturition,
in spite of the fact that all hormonal components necessary for lactation are present in the prenatal period.

FIGURE 46–2 Factors influencing normal breast development
and function.

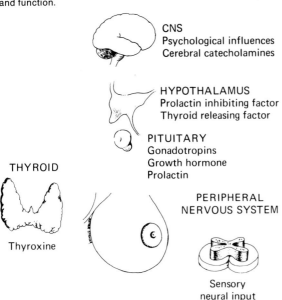

CNS
Psychological influences
Cerebral catecholamines

HYPOTHALAMUS
Prolactin inhibiting factor
Thyroid releasing factor

PITUITARY
Gonadotropins
Growth hormone
Prolactin

THYROID

Thyroxine

PERIPHERAL
NERVOUS SYSTEM

Sensory
neural input

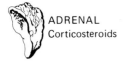

ADRENAL
Corticosteroids

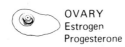

OVARY
Estrogen
Progesterone

The stimulation of prolactin release in pregnant patients, nontreated puerperal patients, and puerperal
patients treated with estradiol valerate and testosterone enanthate (Deladumone) is similar, but only the
untreated puerperal patients respond with milk production and engorged breasts, indicating that high
levels of sex steroids block the action of prolactin on
breast tissue. Thus with the rapid fall of estrogen and
progesterone at delivery, the blockade is lifted and
milk production is stimulated. The maintenance of elevated prolactin levels requires intermittent suckling
activity. Prolactin levels rise rapidly during suckling,
thus stimulating additional milk production or secretion. The afferent limb of this reflex is neural and the
efferent is hormonal. In the absence of suckling, prolactin levels return to the normal nonpregnant state
within 7 days after delivery.

MILK EXCRETION

Milk excretion occurs secondary to forces exerted on
alveoli and ducts by contracting myoepithelial cells
surrounding these structures. The intraductal pressure is increased in response to oxytocin, which is in
turn released by stimulation of afferent neural pathways during suckling. Suckling thus maintains milk
production by stimulating prolactin release and induces milk excretion by stimulating oxytocin release.

EXAMINATION OF THE BREAST

SELF-EXAMINATION

Early detection of breast cancer remains a primary
goal of efforts to improve survival rates in patients so
afflicted. The initial sign of breast cancer in the majority of cases is a palpable tumor discovered by the
patient. After discovery of the mass by the patient,
there is often a delay of several months. The causes
for patient delay are multiple but often involve fear
and anxiety. It is hoped that patient education, including the technique of self-breast examination, may
make patient delay a less common phenomenon.
There is some evidence that the patient-delay period
is shortening as a result of mass education.

Education of the patient should be a routine part
of the health care of women, and since gynecologists
play a central role in the delivery of primary health

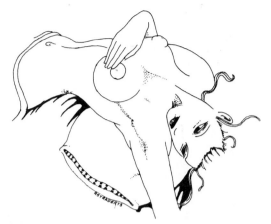

FIGURE 46-3 Self-examination of the medial breast.

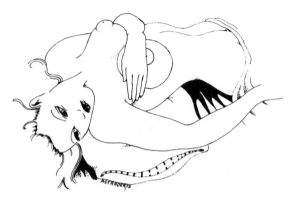

FIGURE 46-5 Self-examination of the axillary portion of the breast.

care to women, it is probable that they will be the primary source of education regarding breast disease. Each new patient should be provided basic information regarding breast disease and instructed in self-examination. Instruction in self-examination of the breast is only part of the educational process. The patient should also be told the purpose for such self-examination and be given the opportunity to ask questions.

Self-examination of the breast should be performed just after the cessation of menses in the premenopausal woman, as the estrogen stimulation is minimal at this time and there is less granularity and tenderness. In nonmenstruating women, self-examination should be recommended at the first of each month. If a definite time schedule is outlined and reinforced on subsequent office visits, the patient is more likely to comply. The exam should begin with elevation of the shoulder on the side to be examined. This shifts the breast medially, providing more balance and flattening of the breast on the chest wall. The me-

FIGURE 46-4 Self-examination of the lateral breast.

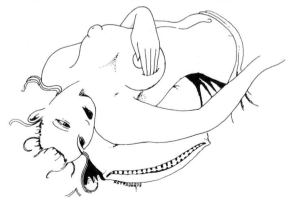

dial portion of the breast should be examined with the ipsilateral arm elevated (Fig. 46-3). The patient should be instructed to examine the breast in a meticulous and repetitive manner. After careful examination of the medial portion, the ipsilateral arm should be placed at the side and the outer half of the breast examined in the same careful manner (Fig. 46-4). Finally, the axilla should be examined because of the frequency of an axillary breast extension (Fig. 46-5). The patient should be instructed to report any suspicious finding immediately. In an effort to prevent cancerophobia, the patient should be reminded that most tumors are not malignant but all should be examined by a physician.

EXAMINATION BY THE PHYSICIAN

Most breast exams by gynecologists are performed as a part of preventive health care in patients without specific complaints. Data supporting the effectiveness of such screening are not entirely encouraging but indicate some progress in early detection and probably in long-term survival. Most available information is from cancer-detection clinics designed to find unsuspected cancers by periodic examination of apparently well individuals. Day reported the discovery of 31 breast carcinomas in asymptomatic patients during 43,411 examinations on 25,629 women over a 3-year period, representing an incidence of unsuspected cancer of 0.12 percent. Phillips and Miller reported a similar incidence (0.13 percent) during examination of 7767 women at the Cancer Prevention Center of Chicago. There is some evidence that asymptomatic breast carcinomas discovered by screening have a lower incidence of axillary node involvement, as Gilbertson reported only 19 percent of

47 women with asymptomatic breast cancer discovered by screening examination had axillary nodal involvement. Venet reported 30 percent axillary nodal involvement in patients with breast cancer discovered by screening versus 54 percent involvement in control patients. We would infer a greater cure rate in such patients, although solid long-term data are not yet available. It is also probable that periodic breast examination by the physician reinforces more frequent self-examination.

PHYSICAL EXAMINATION

Examination of the breast by palpation remains the single most significant aspect of the diagnosis of breast disease. Meticulous examination of the breast in patients with known or suspected breast disease is an obvious requirement for accurate diagnosis, but it is also important and far more difficult for the physician to be equally meticulous in the asymptomatic patient examined during the pressures of the usual busy practice. The breast exam should include palpation of the supraclavicular nodes and axilla, best accomplished while the patient is in a sitting position. The remainder of the exam should be done with the patient in a supine position and the ipsilateral shoulder elevated. Palpation of the breast should begin with the nipples and then proceed in an organized and meticulous fashion so as to include all the breast tissue. Any masses should be characterized as to size, shape, firmness, tenderness, fixation, and the degree of ease with which the margins can be identified. Symmetrical, well-defined, and cystic masses are more likely to be benign. Hard, irregular, fixed masses with ill-defined borders are more likely to be malignant. Often one is left with a questionable mass, a fullness, or a very prominent area of breast tissue. This disturbing "questionable" type of finding will be less commonly encountered if the exam is in the postmenstrual as opposed to the premenstrual or menstrual phase of the cycle. Most often when an area seems questionable after meticulous exam, it simply represents a prominent area of breast tissue. The thickening in the inframammary ridge at the lower edge of the breast is normal and should not be confused with disease. Mammography, thermography, and repeat examination during a more appropriate phase of the menstrual cycle are often helpful in patients with questionable findings.

Inspection of the breast will often give meaningful information such as skin retraction, local edema, erythema, obvious surface lesions, or distortion of the breast by tumors. Skin retraction is usually due to malignant disease with involvement and contraction of the fascial structures of the breast (Fig. 46–6). This dimpling may be apparent only with elevation of the arms, molding or manipulation of the breasts, or contraction of the pectoralis muscles. Carcinoma or chronic infectious disorders in the central portion of the breast may lead to nipple retraction. Nipple retraction of recent onset usually indicates serious breast pathology and should be differentiated from congenital or long-standing nipple retraction, which may be of no clinical significance. Edema of the breast often indicates malignancy with lymphatic obstruction, although it may be associated with local inflammatory lesions. Erythema of the skin overlying the breast is most often associated with infectious disease but may be seen with carcinoma, especially in the inflammatory type of carcinoma. Locally dilated vessels occasionally overlie both malignant and inflammatory lesions.

FIGURE 46–6 Skin retraction due to fascial involvement by cancer.

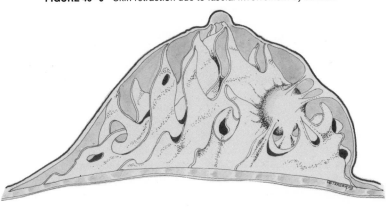

SYMPTOMS OF BREAST DISEASE

The most frequent complaints of the nonpuerperal woman related to her breast are pain and/or a mass. Breast pain which is cyclic in nature is usually of physiologic origin and unrelated to disease. Reassurance is often the only treatment needed for such cyclic discomfort. Cystic disease of the breast may also be associated with breast pain, and should be suspected when the pain is unilateral and confined to a specific area. Breast malignancy is usually painless except in advanced stages. The patient complaining of a breast tumor discovered on self-examination should be questioned regarding pain or tenderness, though the decision regarding biopsy will rest primarily with the physical characteristics of the mass.

Nipple discharge is a less common complaint but one that often distresses the patient and may be a sign of significant disease. Breast secretions may be obtained in many nonpuerperal women with vigorous manipulation of the breasts and are usually of no significance. Spontaneous breast secretions are, however, of importance and require evaluation. Breast secretion that is bilateral and has the gross appearance of milk frequently signifies abnormal physiology or systemic pathology and is discussed under the topic of inappropriate lactation. Abnormal breast discharge may be serous, grossly bloody, brown, or green, with the latter colors representing blood pigments. Though a bloody tinge to the drainage has been considered by many to indicate malignancy in a high percentage of cases, this is not substantiated in published data. Both serous and bloody breast discharge may be signs of either benign disease or malignancy and may go unexplained and resolve spontaneously. McPherson and MacKenzie found 12.5 percent of 72 patients with nipple discharge to have carcinoma of the breast, while Funderburk and Syphax found an 11.9 percent incidence of malignancy among 105 patients. Other breast diseases associated with nipple discharge include cystic disease, papillomas, and ductal ectasia. When no palpable tumor is present and a pressure point producing discharge cannot be identified, the patient should be followed closely with radiographic studies, cytologic smears, and frequent examinations.

RADIOGRAPHIC STUDIES

Injection of radiopaque dyes into the ducts has been utilized primarily in the investigation of serous or bloody drainage from the nipple. This requires cannulation of the duct from which the discharge appears and injection under gentle pressure of a water-miscible dye. The role of this procedure remains controversial. Funderburk states injection of dye is an essential procedure in the investigation of nipple discharge, but Haagensen states the procedure is of little benefit due to inconsistency and is contraindicated because of the possibility of dissemination of tumor during the injection. It is probable that this method is of value only in the hands of those with considerable experience with the methodology.

The technique of soft-tissue x-ray studies of the breast, mammography, has gained widespread acceptance over the past decade. The technique has three possible roles in the diagnosis of breast cancer. The first role is that of evaluation of breast lesions noted on physical examination. It should be clearly understood that *when breast biopsy is indicated by physical exam, it should be accomplished regardless of mammography interpretation,* as nearly 50 percent of clinically discovered breast carcinomas in asymptomatic patients may have negative mammography (Venet et al.). Thus, mammography is most helpful in the lesions or conditions (such as nipple discharge without a mass or pressure-point area) when observation is elected over biopsy. Mammography is very accurate when characteristic findings are present, such as increased density with typical stippling secondary to microcalcifications. When these findings are present in lesions which would otherwise be followed, immediate biopsy becomes mandatory. Mammographic study of breast lesions should increase the number of patients biopsied, not decrease it.

Mammography also is important in high-risk patients or patients where breast examination is difficult or confusing. Patients with prior breast cancer should have the remaining breast studied by mammography at regular intervals because of the increased incidence of breast cancer in the remaining breast. Other appropriate candidates under this category include patients with a family history of breast cancer, patients with diffuse cystic disease of the breasts, and patients over 50 with large breasts. Again it must be stressed that because of the relatively high number of breast cancers found by clinical exam and missed by mammography, physical examination of the breast should accompany mammography.

Although there is little question about the efficacy of mammography in the above patients, there continues to be considerable debate regarding mammography as a screening method in asymptomatic patients without high-risk factors. There is no question that mammography significantly increases the diagnosis of breast cancer in this group, as shown by Venet and Strax. With initial screening of over 20,000 women, they discovered 55 breast cancers, an incidence of 0.27 percent. This incidence is considerably higher than found by screening programs using only physical exam. With annual screenings the incidence remained as high as 0.15 percent, and an additional 77 malignancies were found in annual examinations after the initial screening. Of the 132 cancers detected on screening, 55 were diagnosed as a result of clinical findings only, 44 due to mammographic findings only, and 29 due to evidence of both exams. Thus one-third of the lesions would have been missed by clinical exam only. Of the 44 patients with radiographic evidence of a lesion, reexamination by the physician revealed only one-half of the lesions to be palpable even with prior knowledge of radiologic findings.

Nevertheless, the benefit/risk ratio of radiologic studies is not entirely clear. The number of lives saved by screening studies using mammography is probably less than 1 per 1000. The risks from radiation are considerably more difficult to document. It is commonly accepted, however, that even low dosages of radiation may be carcinogenic. While accurate figures are not available, it would seem prudent to restrict these studies to high-risk patients and patients over age 50 with large breasts.

Xeroradiography is the process of making x-ray images on a selenium plate. While better contrast may enhance the images with xeroradiography, there are no convincing studies showing greater reliability or accuracy. In at least one comparative study, mammography was clearly superior (Egan).

THERMOGRAPHY

Thermography is a technique by which infrared heat patterns of the skin are transmitted to film with interpretation dependent upon temperature differentials in the skin overlying the breast. Lilienfeld et al. found 226 of 305 thermographic examinations to be positive in patients with biopsy-proven malignancy. Unfortunately, others have been unable to achieve this degree of accuracy. Limitations include apparent inaccuracy (false negatives) in subclinical cancers and a high false-positive rate (Dodd). Thermography may prove to be an effective screening device for selection of patients in whom further evaluation is indicated. The expense of the equipment and the need for highly trained individuals for interpretation presently limit use of this methodology to cancer-detection centers.

OTHER TECHNIQUES

Cytologic studies can be obtained by direct aspiration of tumors, aspiration of fluid contents from cysts, or smears obtained from nipple secretions. The role of direct aspiration of breast lesions remains controversial. There is no convincing evidence of adverse effects though the incidence of false-negative reports is high enough to make biopsies necessary when indicated by clinical evaluation. It would seem that aspiration studies of solid breast lesions would be of value only in those lesions not suspicious enough to warrant biopsies, and the positive yield of nonsuspicious lesions is very low. Aspiration of cystic lesions rarely reveals malignant cells on cytologic examination; however, the ease and low cost of such studies would seem to make them worthwhile when breast biopsy is not planned. Cytologic smears of nipple discharge may be helpful when there is no palpable tumor. Masukawa found cytologic smears of nipple discharge to be positive in 6 of 16 patients with carcinoma of the breast. Thus, cytologic studies seem appropriate when clinical and radiologic examinations do not reveal a suspicious lesion in patients with abnormal nipple secretions.

Several other diagnostic techniques have been and/or are being evaluated. These include ultrasound mammometry, and radioisotope studies. At present the spatial resolution obtainable in ultrasonograms is inadequate for detection for subclinical cancers. Mammometry utilizes skin-contact thermometers for measuring breast temperature. Very few data are available as to the sensitivity and specificity of this methodology. The use of radioisotopes has been disappointing.

ABNORMAL DEVELOPMENT AND FUNCTION

PRECOCIOUS DEVELOPMENT

Precocious puberty is discussed in Chap. 17, and the present discussion is limited to precocious breast development in the absence of sexual maturation, properly known as *premature thelarche*. Most recorded cases of premature thelarche have been in female children under 2 years of age. Only about 200 cases have been recorded in the Western literature, though it is probably more common than this number would indicate. The diagnosis of premature thelarche should be made only after exogenous sources of estrogens and precocious puberty have been excluded. Of note is the absence of accelerated growth rate and advanced skeletal maturation as well as other signs of sexual maturation. Though sporadic cases of premature thelarche have been reported associated with central neurologic lesions, this association has not been established as a cause-and-effect relationship. Elevated serum estrogens have not been found in those patients where such studies are available, though several patients have had regression of breast growth after follicle cysts have been removed. This observation has led to the suggestion that transient elevation of serum estrogens associated with follicle cysts may be the etiology in many such patients. Another feasible explanation is increased end-organ sensitivity to minimal amounts of estrogen. Spontaneous regression of the precocious breast development is frequently seen and treatment should be limited to reassurance and periodic reexamination. Most patients will experience puberty at a normal age.

ANOMALOUS DEVELOPMENT

Amastia. Total absence of breast development may be unilateral or bilateral and is often associated with musculoskeletal anomalies, the most common of which is maldevelopment of the pectoralis muscles. Several families with apparent hereditary bilateral amastia have been reported. Insertion of prosthetic materials and nipple grafts using skin from the labia minora have resulted in satisfactory cosmetic appearance. *Athelia,* absence of the nipple in a normally situated breast, is extremely rare with no cases recorded in recent literature.

Asymmetry. Asymmetrical breast development is common and usually of little or no concern to the patient. Occasionally severe asymmetry is seen, requiring surgical intervention for cosmetic reasons. Augmentation mammoplasty, reduction mammoplasty, or a combination of the two procedures may yield satisfactory cosmetic results.

Accessory Breast Tissue. Accessory breast tissue is the most common form of anomalous development, occurring in 1 to 2 percent of females. Accessory breast tissue may consist of a nipple, areola, glandular tissue, or any combination of these elements. The most common forms are a nipple alone or a nipple, areola, and fatty pad (pseudomamma). Accessory breasts may occur along the embryologic milk line extending from the axilla to the vulva. They are usually located between the breast and the umbilicus with the most common location being beneath the breast. Occasionally more than one nipple is found on an otherwise normal breast (intraareolar polythelia). Even more rarely, accessory breasts are located outside the milk line in the acromial region, scapular region, or midline of the abdomen or thorax. Accessory breasts are usually of no clinical significance but may become symptomatically enlarged during pregnancy, and when glandular tissue is present in the absence of nipple elements they may be confused with lipomas or other solid tumors. Benign tumors, cystic tumors, and adenocarcinoma have been reported in accessory breast tissue. Accessory breasts have been described as being associated with a variety of systemic disorders including neurosis, peptic ulceration, cardiovascular disease, migraine headaches, and renal and gonadal hypoplasia (Brightmore). The significance, if any, of these findings remains unclear.

Hypoplasia. Failure of normal breast development or inadequate development at puberty may occur unilaterally, leading to asymmetrical breasts, or it may occur bilaterally. The cause of mammary hypoplasia may be hypoestrogenism or inadequate end-organ response.

Hypoplastic breast development accompanied by failure of other secondary sexual development is usually secondary to ovarian agenesis. The classical Turner syndrome consisting of XO sex-chromosomal complement, certain somatic changes, and sexual infantilism are features of ovarian agenesis. There is also a distinctive group of patients who begin puberty in a normal fashion and have one or more scanty menses after which they become hypoestrogenic. These patients have hypoplastic breasts and in our experience have a normal karyotype with a female sex-chromosomal complement, and hypoplastic ovaries with few, if any, primordial follicles. Less commonly, failure of pituitary-gonadotropin secretion (hypogonadotropic hypogonadism) is the cause of inadequate secondary sexual development. Following proper diagnosis, satisfactory breast development may be induced in hypoestrogenic patients by adequate exogenous estrogen therapy.

Hyperplasia. Massive breast hypertrophy is usually seen at puberty but may also occur during pregnancy. The breast may reach gigantic size, and spontaneous remission is rare. Endocrine studies have been normal, suggesting the basic etiology is an abnormal end-organ response. The size of the breasts is often such that they place great physical as well as psychological burden on the patient. Surgical correction usually consists of reduction mammoplasty with transplantation of the nipple. Not infrequently recurrence of the hypertrophy necessitates subcutaneous mastectomy with insertion of a prosthesis.

Although hypertrophy of the male breast is commonly seen secondary to systemic disease or exogenous medication, these associations are uncommon in women. Scott has reported a case of breast hypertrophy apparently associated with the use of Neo-Tizide and thiacetazone during therapy of tuberculosis, but other such cases have not been found in review of the literature. Exogenous estrogens will induce breast tenderness and mild enlargement in many patients, but this is rarely of clinical significance and is easily reversed by cessation of therapy. Rarely, a patient will develop rather massive breast hypertrophy while utilizing oral contraceptives, but a gradual and nearly complete return to normal after cessation of therapy may be expected.

Inappropriate Lactation

Inappropriate lactation is the spontaneous bilateral secretion of a milky fluid from the breast and is to be distinguished from unilateral or bilateral secretion of serous or bloody fluid. Secretion discovered with vigorous manipulation of the breast is commonly seen and of no significance. When the patient complains of secretions but examination does not reveal significant breast secretions, a simple request of the patient often results in an impressive demonstration of secretions by self-manipulation. Inappropriate lactation is often but not always associated with amenorrhea and hypoestrogenism. The multiplicity of conditions that may be associated with inappropriate lactation make an organized and systematic approach mandatory for appropriate evaluation (Table 46–1).

Drug therapy is a relatively common cause of inappropriate lactation and one which can be easily diagnosed and treated. Drugs associated with inappropriate lactation include the phenothiazines, the tricyclic tranquilizers, reserpine, and methyldopa. A common property of these drugs is the depletion of central nervous catecholamines, leading to a decreased secretion of prolactin-inhibiting factor and increase in serum prolactin. The administration and/or withdrawal of exogenous sex steroids, including oral contraceptives, has also been associated with inappropriate lactation. This seemingly paradoxical situation is due to the dual action of estrogen in which elevated levels induce prolactin secretion while blocking the action of prolactin on the breast.

Hypofunction or hyperfunction of both the thyroid and adrenal glands has also been associated with abnormal lactation. The association of thyroid disease with inappropriate lactation is more clearly understood with recent observations that thyroid-releasing factor acts directly on the pituitary, causing prolactin secretion.

Mechanical stimulation of the breast and/or chest wall may induce abnormal lactation through a neural reflex. Thoracic surgery, burns, suckling, manual stimulation, herpes zoster, and mastectomy are examples of this etiology. Spinal-cord lesions have also been associated with inappropriate lactation related to this neural reflex mechanism.

Central nervous lesions associated with lactation include trauma, tumors, pseudotumor cerebri, encephalitis, and pneumoencephalography. Presumably these lesions induce cerebral catecholamine changes leading to decreased prolactin-inhibiting factor secretion. Other lesions directly involving hypothalamus or pituitary-stalk section, may be associated with inappropriate lactation. The association of chromophobe adenomas with inappropriate lactation was first described by Forbes and subsequently has been named the Forbes-Albright syndrome. Destruction or division of the pituitary stalk interferes with hypothalamic inhibition of prolaction secretion, resulting in increased serum prolactin and often lactation.

TABLE 46–1 Inappropriate Lactation

Drug therapy	Hypothalamic–pituitary
Phenothiazines	disorders
Tricyclic	Tumors
tranquilizers	Forbes-Albright
Reserpine	syndrome
Methyldopa	Stalk section
Sex steroids	Sheehan's syndrome
Endocrine disorders	Empty sella
Castration	syndrome
Corpus luteum cysts	Central nervous system
Primary	Trauma
hypothyroidism	Tumors
Hyperthyroidism	Pseudotumor cerebri
Cushing's disease	Pneumoencephalo-
Adrenal insufficiency	gram
Neural–mechanical	Idiopathic
etiology	Chiari-Frommel
Herpes zoster	syndrome
Thoracotomy	Del Castillo
Chest-wall burns	syndrome
Mastectomy	Pseudocyesis
Suckling	Nonspecific
Manual stimulation	
Spinal-cord lesions	

Often investigation reveals none of the above factors leading to the diagnosis of idiopathic inappropriate lactation. Abnormal persistence of puerperal lactation was described first by Chiari and later by Frommel and is now referred to as Chiari-Frommel syndrome. The combination of inappropriate lactation, amenorrhea, and hypoestrogenism in the nonpuerperal patient and in the absence of any known etiology was described by del Castillo and is often referred to as the del Castillo syndrome. Young described a patient with episodes of persistent puerperal lactation with remission, followed by nonpuerperal lactation with remission, and finally the appearance of pituitary tumor 14 years after the initial episode of inappropriate lactation, thus emphasizing the importance of repeated evaluation in such patients. On occasion, inappropriate lactation is associated with a psychopathologic belief by the patient that she is pregnant (pseudocyesis). Finally, one is often presented with a patient with lactation not associated with menstrual disturbances or any of the above conditions. These patients often need only reassurance and periodic reexamination.

The therapy of abnormal lactation has long been fraught with frustration and lack of success. Recent reports using L-dopa and/or ergot alkaloids are encouraging, though further evaluation is needed. Oral administration of either L-dopa or ergocryptine markedly reduces serum prolactin levels and leads to cessation of lactation and return to menses in many patients. Unfortunately, cessation of therapy is usually associated with return of the symptoms.

INFECTIONS

The most common breast infections are puerperal mastitis and/or abscess. Other breast infections may be secondary to specific pathogens (tuberculosis, actinomycosis, etc.) or associated with ductal obstruction with secondary infection (recurrent subareolar abscesses, infected sebaceous cysts).

RECURRENT SUBAREOLAR ABSCESS

Subareolar abscess and fistula formation is usually a chronic recurring infection unrelated to pregnancy and is most commonly found in young women. Inverted nipple is frequently seen with this lesion, and it has been suggested that the chronic maceration leads to secondary infection (Caswell). Patey and others have provided convincing evidence showing lactiferous ductal squamous metaplasia, with obstruction, stasis, and secondary infection, is the most common etiology. The infection often involves only one duct, though several ducts may be diseased in chronic cases. The abscess frequently drains spontaneously, leaving a draining cutaneous fistula which may heal for a period of time only to be followed by recurrence of the abscess in most patients. Successful treatment requires excision of the diseased tissue. This is best accomplished after incision and drainage has induced a relatively quiescent state. Incision and drainage as the sole therapy is seldom successful, while excision of the diseased tissue is almost invariably successful.

INFECTED SEBACEOUS CYST

Sebaceous cysts are commonly found in the skin overlying the breast and on occasion may become infected. Infection is heralded by erythema, induration, and tenderness, with abscess formation. The superficial location of the sebaceous cyst usually allows differentiation from abscesses located in the breast tissue and inflammatory carcinoma. Local excision is the most successful form of therapy.

TUBERCULOSIS

Tuberculosis of the breast is an uncommon entity and the diagnosis is almost always first suspected when the biopsy specimen is examined by the pathologist. Most patients have coincident pulmonary or extramammary lymphatic involvement. Miller suggests the pathogenesis of mammary tuberculosis is retrograde extension via the lymphatics of the neck or axilla. Several reports have described patients with no evidence of extramammary tuberculosis. The treatment of mammary tuberculosis with chemotherapy is prolonged and often unsuccessful. Wilson and MacGregor have suggested simple mastectomy as the therapy of choice because of the difficulty encountered in eradicating mammary tuberculosis with chemotherapy.

OTHER INFECTIONS

Other less common infections of the breast include sarcoidosis, syphilis, hydatid disease, filariasis, blastomycosis, sporotrichosis, leprosy, and actinomycosis. The infrequency of these infections makes their diagnosis difficult and usually they are initially suspected at the time of histologic examination of a breast mass.

MAMMARY NECROSIS

The most common form of mammary necrosis is localized fat necrosis. Fat necrosis is typically found in large, pendulous breasts and often, though not always, a history of trauma can be elicited. Fat necrosis is characteristically located just below the skin and may be found in any sector of the breast. A tumor is palpable in virtually all patients and gross examination may reveal recent hemorrhage and indurated fat, cystic degeneration with a clear oily fluid, old blood, and in long-standing cases, calcification. Microscopic examination may reveal evidence of recent or old hemorrhage, vacuoles of various sizes, lipid-laden macrophages, chronic inflammatory cells, cholesterol crystals, and calcification.

The most common presenting symptom is a palpable mass. Ecchymosis, erythema of the overlying skin, and pain are common clinical features. The tumors tend to be firm, irregular, and fixed and are often associated with skin retraction, thus explaining the common clinical impression of malignancy. Mammography may reveal characteristic calcifications aiding in this diagnosis, but excisional biopsy is required to exclude malignancy.

Massive and diffuse breast necrosis, usually in both breasts, is a rare complication of anticoagulant therapy. The necrosis usually involves the most dependent portion of the breast but occasionally involves the entire breast with total gangrene. Extensive ecchymosis with pain is noted initially, followed by progressive necrosis. Discontinuation of the anticoagulants often does not result in improvement, and microscopic evidence ot necrotizing arteritis suggests an etiology more complex than simple hemorrhage and thrombosis.

MAMMARY DYSPLASIA

CYSTIC DISEASE

"Cystic disease of the breast" is the most appropriate and descriptive name for the common breast cysts found in the reproductive-age woman. When specific etiologic factors such as inspissated milk, cystic necrosis of carcinoma, ductal ectasia, fat necrosis, or intraductal papillomas are present, the associated disease process should be described and the process should not be classified as cystic disease. In the absence of these specific etiologic entities, the name "cystic disease of the breast" is preferred over the commonly used "chronic cystic mastitis" since inflammation plays no role in the etiology or clinical manifestation of cystic disease.

In a review of the literature, Davis et al. found the average incidence of unsuspected cystic disease in autopsy studies to be 58.5 percent, and 43 percent of the patients with cysts had bilateral involvement. This incidence reflects not only gross cystic lesions but lesions which are found only with microscopic studies. Clinically apparent cystic disease of the breast occurs most commonly in the fourth and fifth decade, as evidenced by Haagensen's report of 2017 women with cystic disease ranging in age from 25 to 59; 97 percent of the patients were between 30 and 54 years of age.

The etiology of cystic disease is unknown. It is almost always limited to women in the reproductive years and regresses after menopause, suggesting it is an estrogen-dependent disease. Haagensen found only 6 out of 2017 patients to be 55 years or older, and 4 of these were taking exogenous estrogen. Cystic disease has been induced in mice and rhesus monkeys by exogenous estrogen medication. Though these observations have caused concern regarding the possible induction of cystic disease by oral contraceptives and other oral estrogens, Sartwell reported that among 306 patients with cystic disease of the breast, fewer patients had utilized oral estrogens than their matched controls. Since the cysts are usually lined with epithelium, we may assume they are of ductal origin, and obstruction must play a role in their etiology. Accompanying histologic findings that may be associated with ductal obstruction are fibrosis, ductal hyperplasia, and ductal papillomatosis.

Grossly, the cysts are spherical and often bluish in color, explaining the descriptive term "blue-domed." The cysts tend to be thin-walled and the inner surface is smooth and glistening. The fluid is usually straw-colored, though on occasion greenish, brownish, or bloody fluid is seen. Microscopic examination usually reveals flattened or low cuboidal epithelium, but the epithelial lining is sometimes not apparent secondary to atrophy induced by pressure. There are often multiple microscopic cysts in the tissues surrounding larger cysts. Davis described hyperplasia of ductal epithelium in 30 percent of biopsies with cystic disease. Blunt-duct adenosis, a term describing the termination of ducts in microcysts rather than acini, apocrine metaplasia, and fibrosis are also common accompanying pathologic findings.

These cysts are often asymptomatic, though they may be painful and tender, especially in the premenstrual phase of the cycle. They may regress in size in the postmenstrual phase of the cycle. The cysts are usually firm, mobile, well defined, and often tender to palpation. Therapy remains controversial and some surgeons still favor excision to rule out coexistent carcinoma, while others (Haagenson; Devitt; Herrmann; Putzki) indicate coexistent malignancy is rare. Aspiration of the cysts affords rapid resolution with complications being rare. Putzki reported 526 successful aspirations of breast cysts with only one patient later developing carcinoma near the site of the original aspiration of straw-colored fluid. When bloody fluid was obtained, 4 of 15 patients had associated malignancy. Simple aspiration seems effective and safe if there is no residual mass and the fluid is not bloody. Hormonal therapy has met with mixed success. Ariel reported excellent symptomatic response in 50 percent of patients, utilizing moderate doses of norethynodrel combined with mestranol. The question of whether gynecologists should aspirate breast cysts or refer them to surgical colleagues seems moot to this observer: Breast-cyst aspiration, like other forms of therapy, should be accomplished by physicians familiar with the disease as well as with alternate methods of therapy and their advantages and disadvantages.

MAMMARY-DUCT ECTASIA

Ductal ectasia is most common in perimenopausal and menopausal women. The subareolar ducts are often palpable as rubbery lesions filled with a paste-like material. Microscopic examination reveals dilated ducts with desquamating secretory epithelium, necrotic debris, and chronic inflammatory cells. Symptoms associated with ductal ectasia include pain, nipple retraction, nipple discharge, and on occasion, enlarged regional lymph nodes. Excision of the palpably involved ducts and/or the area from which nipple discharge may be expressed is sufficient therapy. There is no known association with malignancy.

ADENOSIS

Adenosis of the breast is a condition in which proliferation of acinar and ductal epithelium is combined with varying degrees of intralobular fibrosis. This lesion is commonly associated with cystic disease but may present as a separate entity. Examination of autopsy material reveals adenosis to be a common finding, though it does not often produce clinical problems. It occurs in the same age group as cystic disease and tends to regress with menopause. When a tumor is formed, it is usually firm, irregular, and fixed, suggesting carcinoma to the clinician. When epithelial proliferation predominates, the microscopic picture is likewise easily confused with malignancy and this impression is further enhanced by occasional perineural extension of the disease. Because of these characteristics, unnecessary mastectomy has often resulted. Surgical excision of the palpable tumor is the only satisfactory therapy.

BENIGN TUMORS

FIBROADENOMA

Fibroadenomas are the most common benign breast tumors in women and account for the vast majority of breast tumors in females in the teens and early twenties. The tumors are typically rubbery in consistency, gray or tan in color, and are sharply delimited from the surrounding breast tissue. They are usually solitary but may be multiple and bilateral. Microscopically, they are composed of proliferating ductal epithelium and fibrous stroma. The stroma may be edematous and myxoid, and tumors present for many years often become hyalinized and/or calcified. Tumors containing only epithelial elements (adenomas) are rare and are usually seen in pregnancy.

Fibroadenomas usually present as asymptomatic, well-defined breast tumors in young women. They may enlarge rapidly and attain massive proportions shortly after puberty and during pregnancy. Simple excision is indicated for diagnosis and therapy.

INTRADUCTAL PAPILLOMA

Solitary intraductal papillomas are most commonly found in women near or shortly after menopause. Grossly, the tumors are usually 2 to 3 mm in diameter and easily missed by both the surgeon and pathologist unless meticulous inspection of the duct is accomplished. The most common location is in a major collection duct in the subareolar area. Microscopically, these tumors consist of a central fibrovascular stalk with delicate papillae covered by a double layer of cuboidal epithelium. Diffuse papillomatosis is occasionally seen, often in association with cystic disease of the breast. The microscopic differentiation from infiltrating ductal carcinoma is often difficult.

The presenting symptom of breast papilloma is almost always a serous or bloody nipple discharge. Haagensen reports 81 percent of 160 patients with proven intraductal papilloma had nipple discharge as the presenting symptom. Conversely, he found 69 percent of patients presenting with nipple discharge had an intraductal papilloma as the etiologic factor. The small size of the tumor precludes recognition by palpation in most patients, and the diagnosis often requires defining an area in the areolar region which produces nipple discharge in response to pressure and performing an excisional biopsy of this area. Occasionally the lesion which cannot be defined by a pressure point producing discharge may be located by cannulation of the duct from which the discharge exudes and injecting radiopaque dyes. Therapy for solitary intraductal papillomas is simple excision.

Multiple papillomas are far more difficult to manage and may be associated with apocrine-duct carcinoma. Repeat excision of palpable masses is required and meticulous microscopic examination is indicated to rule out associated malignancy.

OTHER BENIGN TUMORS

Any type of epidermoid or adnexal tumor may occur in the skin overlying the breasts. The most common are squamous papillomas, benign nevi, and seborrheic keratosis. Tumors of the adnexal structures of the skin are less common but of importance as they may be confused with tumors limited to the breasts.

Lipomas are the most common nonepithelial tumor of the breasts. They are usually solitary and asymptomatic. Lipomas are soft, mobile, and easily defined from the surrounding tissue by palpation. Despite these characteristic findings, excision and microscopic inspection are indicated to establish the diagnosis. Other benign tumors include leiomyomas, fibromas, neurofibromas, granular-cell tumors, hemangiomas, and lymphangiomas. The diagnosis and therapy of such tumors is of special interest only in that they may be confused with other breast tumors.

MALIGNANT TUMORS

PREVALENCE AND EPIDEMIOLOGY

Breast cancer is a major health problem by all standards of measurement. Approximately 25 percent of malignancies in women are breast cancers. Each year 70,000 new cases are diagnosed with an incidence rate of 65 per 100,000. The death rate from breast cancer is 22 per 100,000. Approximately 5 percent of women will develop breast cancer at some time during their life and nearly half of these will die of the disease. Though the most common age group seen with breast cancer is between 40 and 60 years, the risk to an individual patient continues to increase steadily with age.

With recent strides in screening programs, the identification of high-risk patients becomes especially important. There is voluminous literature dealing with epidemiologic data and considerable controversy persists. Nevertheless, the data seem to indicate certain consistent increased-risk factors, many of which are associated with reproductive function and suggest an important relationship between the endocrinologic factors of reproduction and breast cancer. The nulliparous patient has a twofold increased risk of breast cancer when compared with multiparous patients. Some studies indicate increasing parity through at least three pregnancies decreases the likelihood of breast cancer. The risk of breast cancer is three times higher in patients whose first pregnancy is after age 35 when compared with those who are pregnant by age 18. Patients undergoing oophorectomy before age 40 have been found to have a significantly decreased incidence of breast cancer. Women who experience menopause after age 50 have a 1.5-fold increased risk of breast cancer. The relationship of breast-feeding to breast-cancer risk seems so controversial as to be inconclusive to this author.

In addition to reproductive factors, there are genetic factors of importance, as illustrated by the increased risk in mothers, sisters, and daughters of patients with breast cancer. These relatives have a risk which is approximately double that of the general population. Finally, the patient who survives 3 or more years after mastectomy has approximately a 10 percent likelihood of developing cancer in the opposite breast.

Though additional data may show some of these factors to be more or less important than present data would indicate, the evidence is strong enough to warrant special efforts to identify and provide intensive screening of these high-risk groups.

NATURAL HISTORY

Since control of breast cancer is most likely to be accomplished if therapy precedes metastasis, early diagnosis and prompt therapy have been advocated to improve survival. Unfortunately, there is abundant evidence revealing early diagnosis coupled with prompt therapy is insufficient for control of the disease. Furthermore, delay in diagnosis and/or therapy is not always associated with failure. It has long been recognized that some patients with very small primary lesions treated promptly and appropriately may nevertheless have widespread metastasis and early death. Conversely, Vermund collected data from the literature revealing the 5-year survival from onset of symptoms in untreated patients with breast cancer to be 19 percent. Variable tumor-host interactions account for this apparent dichotomy. Devitt suggests metastatic nodal involvement is an expression, rather than the determinant, of poor prognosis. Indeed, the extreme viewpoint might suggest early diagnosis and type of therapy to be of little importance in prognosis of breast cancer. However, it would seem there must exist a certain time during which every tumor grows locally prior to metastasis. This assumption leads us to continue to strive for early diagnosis and therapy, at least until we are able to attain better understanding and control of host-tumor interactions.

MULTICENTRICITY

Carcinoma of the breast tends to be spatially and temporally multicentric. Qualheim studied multiple sections from 157 breast specimens from mastectomies for carcinoma and found 54 percent contained more than one focus of apparent primary malignancy. This observation is common to most pathologists who study multiple sections of breasts. This spatial multicentricity is one reason to remove all of the breast when treating malignancy.

Temporal multicentricity is best understood by studying the opposite breast in mastectomy patients. As is often true with paired organs, the breasts seem to respond as a single organ to carcinogenic stimuli. It is probable that most "recurrences" in the opposite breast represent new primary foci of malignancy. Moore quotes figures for "recurrence" in the second

breast ranging from 7 to 12 percent. Haagensen found the incidence of primary carcinoma in the remaining breast to be seven times that expected in the general population. The question of prophylactic mastectomy of the remaining breast has been seriously considered by some (Moore). Frequent and meticulous examination of the opposite breast by palpation and mammography is probably more important than examinations searching for recurrence or metastasis since a second primary lesion is more likely to be cured than a recurrence.

SIZE AND GROWTH RATE

The size of the primary breast cancer correlates less well than the presence or absence of metastasis. Because of this observation Haagensen has ignored size in his classification of breast cancer (Table 46-2). Haagensen reported the 10-year survival for stage A patients with primary tumors greater than 6 cm in diameter to be 65 percent as compared with 23 percent for stage C patients with tumors less than 6 cm in diameter.

The growth rate of a tumor more accurately reflects its biologic virulence and thereby the prognosis, but information on growth rate of primary tumors is usually lacking since prompt therapy is usually achieved. Measurements of growth rates of metastatic nodules are available and correlate well with prognosis, tumor-free interval prior to appearance of metastasis, and response to palliative therapy. Measurement of doubling time is a commonly used standard for growth rate. Collins measured the doubling time for pulmonary metastasis of breast cancer and found it to approximate 1 month in those

TABLE 46-2 Columbia Clinical Classification

A1 No clinically involved axillary nodes
  2 No grave signs as in clinical stage C
B1 Clinically involved axillary nodes less than 2.5 cm transverse diameter
  2 No grave signs as in clinical stage C
C Any of the five grave signs
  1 Edema of skin limited extent (less than one-third of skin involved)
  2 Ulceration of skin
  3 Solid fixation primary tumor to chest wall
  4 Axillary nodes 2.5 cm or more transverse diameter
  5 Fixation axillary nodes to overlying or surrounding tissues
D All more advanced cases

tumors studied. Assuming the doubling rate of metastasis to be similar to that of the primary tumor, he calculated a period to 2½ years necessary for a tumor to progress from one malignant cell to a tumor measuring 1 cm in diameter. Though considerable variation must occur in growth rates of different tumors, this observation emphasizes the relatively long period of existence before breast cancer attains an easily palpable size and supports efforts to find methods of diagnosis more sensitive than palpation.

LOCAL EXTENSION

A common growth pattern in breast cancer, as seen on microscopic examination, consists of fingerlike extensions of tumor extending through the breast tissue from the central tumor mass. These extensions may be in ducts, periductal lymphatics, other lymphatics, along fascial planes, or less commonly in blood vessels. Extension may involve the skin and be seen as satellite nodules around the primary tumor. Tumor emboli in lymphatic and blood vessels may be found a considerable distance from the primary tumor. This irregular growth pattern, with nonpalpable tumor extension and emboli, further emphasizes the need for total mastectomy as primary therapy.

METASTASIS

The lymphatic pathways involved by metastatic breast cancer have been extensively studied for many decades. From the plethora of studies several important facts are worthy of special consideration. The most common site of lymphatic metastasis is the axillary group of lymph nodes. These nodes are involved in approximately 50 percent of tumors located in the upper outer quadrant of the breast or the nipple, and in approximately 35 percent of tumors in other quadrants. The internal mammary lymph nodes are the next most commonly involved group. They are more often involved when the lesion is located in the medial aspect of the breast or in the nipple. Handley found 47 percent involvement of internal mammary nodes in nipple lesions, 31 percent in medial lesions, and 16 percent in lateral lesions. The third most commonly involved nodes are the supraclavicular group. Involvement of the supraclavicular nodes essentially never occurs in the absence of axillary involvement. Haagensen reviewed three separate series by Dahl-Iversen and reported 23 of 125 patients with axillary

metastasis had positive supraclavicular nodes. There were no patients in whom supraclavicular nodes were involved in the absence of axillary metastasis. Though surgical therapy of all three of these nodal groups has been utilized as part of primary therapy, the most commonly accepted operation includes excision of only the axillary group of nodes. This approach has resulted from a combination of low cure rates in the presence of involved supraclavicular and/or internal mammary nodes and the extensive surgery required to remove these nodes.

Death from breast cancer is secondary to distant metastases. Distant metastasis occurs primarily via the blood stream and usually, though not always, is preceded by regional lymphatic metastasis. Organs commonly involved, in order of frequency, include lungs, bone, liver, adrenals, brain, and ovaries. Virtually every tissue of the body may be involved by metastatic breast cancer. When distant metastases are present, therapy is of a palliative nature only.

HISTOLOGIC TYPES

DUCTAL CARCINOMA

More than 90 percent of breast cancer arises from ductal epithelium. There are many histologic types of ductal carcinoma, as indicated in Table 46–3. Survival rates vary somewhat according to histologic type, ranging from 83 percent 5-year survival with infiltrating papillary carcinoma to 54 percent survival with scirrhous carcinoma (McDivitt et al.). Scirrhous carcinoma accounts for approximately 80 percent of ductal breast carcinomas and 75 percent of all breast malignancy. The remainder of ductal carcinomas are considerably less common.

Paget's disease of the breast is relatively uncommon but merits special comment because of the unusual and distinctive clinical and microscopic findings. The most common symptoms are burning, pruritus, and nipple discharge. The nipple and areola

TABLE 46–3 Histologic Types of Breast Carcinoma

Ductal carcinoma
Papillary
Scirrhous
Comedocarcinoma
Colloid carcinoma
Medullary carcinoma
Paget's disease
Lobular carcinoma

characteristically have a striking eczematoid appearance with crusting and ulceration. The microscopic changes are equally striking with large, pale, anaplastic cells found in the epidermis of the nipple, areola, and large ducts. It is generally accepted that an underlying intraductal carcinoma is always present and the "Paget" cells are thought to represent intraepidermal extension. Diagnosis is easily confirmed by biopsy and therapy is identical to that used for other ductal carcinomas. The 5-year survival rate is approximately 50 percent.

LOBULAR CARCINOMA

Lobular carcinoma accounts for approximately 8 percent of breast cancer. In situ lobular carcinoma is occasionally seen with the terminal ductules and acini distended by small, round, malignant cells without any stromal invasion. The prognosis with infiltrating lobular carcinoma is similar to that of scirrhous carcinoma but of special note is the marked tendency for this tumor to be multicentric. Bilateral breast involvement is found in approximately 30 percent of cases.

CARCINOMA OF THE SKIN AND ACCESSORY GLANDS

Malignancies of the skin overlying the breast are uncommon. Tumors occasionally found include basalcell carcinoma, melanoma, and sweat-gland carcinoma. Diagnosis and therapy is similar to that utilized for these tumors when located elsewhere.

SARCOMA

Sarcomas account for about 1 percent of breast malignancies. The most common sarcoma is malignant cystosarcoma phyllodes. The adjective "malignant" is added because not all cystosarcoma phyllodes tumors are malignant. These tumors tend to be large and sharply circumscribed. Microscopically they are very similar to fibroadenomas but have a more cellular, hyperplastic stroma. The epithelial component is invariably benign and the classification as benign or malignant is dependent on stromal changes. The malignant stromal components may resemble fibrosarcoma or liposarcoma. Small foci of malignant cartilage, bone, and muscle have been described on rare occasions. Therapy for malignant cystosarcoma phyllodes should consist of total mastectomy. Axillary-node dissection is not indicated since metastasis tends to be blood-borne and axillary metastases are

rare. The prognosis is good unless evidence of distant metastasis is present.

Liposarcoma, fibrosarcoma, and angiosarcoma are occasionally seen in the breast. Other breast sarcomas are composed of a mixture of myxoid, fibrosarcomatous, and liposarcomatous elements. McDivitt classifies the latter tumors as stromal sarcomas and reports a 5-year survival of 60 percent.

DIAGNOSIS AND THERAPY

DIAGNOSIS

The diagnosis of breast cancer is discussed in detail under the topic of breast examination. Approximately 80 percent of breast cancers are initially discovered by the patient as a palpable tumor. Subclinical cancers discovered by radiographic techniques represent a growing minority of new cancers. Most of the remainder present with abnormal nipple discharge leading to discovery and biopsy of a mass or biopsy of a pressure point yielding the discharge. A tissue diagnosis must be established before initiating any therapy.

SURGERY

There remains considerable controversy regarding appropriate therapy for early breast cancer. Urban proposes extended radical mastectomy with excision of axillary and internal mammary nodes to ensure therapy to both sites of early regional metastasis. Crile suggests simple mastectomy in early lesion yields equal or superior cure rates and avoids theoretical interference with the host's immune response as might occur with lymphadenectomy. Nevertheless, the radical mastectomy with removal of both the pectoralis major and minor muscles has been the most widely accepted operation for many years. In support of this approach the following reasons have been given: (1) axillary nodes are most often the first site of metastasis; (2) histologic examination of the nodes may be used to judge the likelihood of other metastasis and as an aid in selecting adjuvant therapy; (3) occasional patients are cured following removal of positive axillary nodes. Recently, there has been a distinct trend toward avoiding removal of the pectoralis major muscle while removing the axillary nodes. This "modified radical" mastectomy seems to combine the advantages of the radical approach with the lower morbidity and superior cosmetic result of the simple mastectomy. In the absence of fixation to the underlying pectoralis fascia, preservation of the pectoralis major muscle seems in order.

Simple mastectomy combined with radiation therapy, chemotherapy, endocrine therapy, or endocrine ablation is often effective in obtaining palliation of advanced carcinoma. Removal or prevention of a large, ulcerated necrotic breast affords improvement of mental and physical well-being.

RADIATION THERAPY

Radiation therapy is curative in some cases of cancer of the breast for both the primary tumor and regional metastasis. It thus seems logical that maximum control would be accomplished by combining the two curative methods, radiation and surgery. Unfortunately most studies combining the two methods are inconclusive. Devitt and Beattie did observe a significant decrease in local recurrence and Guttman showed an apparently increased survival when radiation therapy was utilized in patients with regional metastasis or advanced lesions. There seems to be a general trend toward increased utilization of radiation therapy in combination with surgery, though the evidence would suggest this will not result in a remarkable increase in survival.

ENDOCRINE THERAPY

Bilateral oophorectomy for the control of metastatic breast cancer was first reported in 1896. Since that time several modes of endocrine therapy have been used with selection of the proper mode dependent upon arbitrary criteria. Endocrine ablation, used primarily in premenopausal women, has included bilateral oophorectomy, adrenalectomy, and hypophysectomy. Endocrine-additive therapy has included estrogens, androgen, progestins, and corticosteroids. Additive therapy has been used primarily in postmenopausal patients. While results from individual series vary somewhat, the average response rates for all types of endocrine therapy have been remarkably similar and in the range of 30 percent. The duration of the remissions are variable but often exceed 1 year. The recent development of estrogen-receptor (ER) assays has aided in selecting patients who are most likely to respond to endocrine therapy. Estrogen receptors are found in both premenopausal and postmenopausal patients in as many as 75 percent of cases. Estrogen receptors may be found in both primary and metastatic tumors. When ER assays are

positive, endocrine-ablation therapy and endocrine-additive therapy have both yielded response rates in the neighborhood of 55 percent. Patients with negative ER values respond in only about 8 percent of cases. Thus metastatic tumors that are not localized and do not lend themselves to radiation therapy should be assayed for ER values. If ER values are high, endocrine therapy is indicated. If estrogen receptors are not present, the patient should probably be treated with chemotherapy.

Other hormone receptors have been and are being identified. Included among them are receptors for androgens, progesterone, prolactins, growth hormone, and placental lactogen. Preliminary data suggest further evaluation of these receptors may aid in therapeutic decisions, though significant clinical data are lacking.

CHEMOTHERAPY

Many chemotherapeutic regimens have been attempted for palliative and adjuvant therapy. Most studies would indicate little if any benefit from adjuvant therapy, though Bonadonna et al. have reported data suggesting decreased recurrences in premenopausal patients treated with cyclophosphamide, methotrexate, and fluorouracil in conjunction with surgery. Most clinicians have not adopted routine use of adjuvant therapy at present. Treatment of metastatic disease has met with some success. The rate of objective remissions with fluorouracil has been approximately 35 percent while alkylating agents have yielded approximately 25 percent remission rates. Combination chemotherapy presently is yielding objective remission rates in the neighborhood of 50 percent. Unfortunately, remissions with chemotherapy rarely last for more than a few months.

REFERENCES

Ariel IM: Enovid therapy (norethynodrel with mestranol) for fibrocystic diseases. *Am J Obstet Gynecol* 117:453, 1973.

Bonadonna G et al.: The CMF program for operable breast cancer with positive axillary nodes: Updated analysis of disease-free interval, site of relapse and drug tolerance. *Cancer* 33:2904, 1977.

Capraro VJ et al.: Premature thelarche. *Obstet Gynecol Surv* 26:2, 1973.

Caswell HT, Mair WP: Chronic recurrent periareolar abscess secondary to inversion of the nipple. *Surg Gynecol Obstet* 128:597, 1969.

Collins VP et al.: Observation on growth rates of human tumors. *Am J Roentgenol Radium Ther Nucl Med* 76:988, 1956.

Cowie AT, Folley SJ: The mammary gland and lactation, in *Scientific Foundations of Obstetrics and Gynecology,* eds. EE Philipp et al., Philadelphia: FA Davis, 1970, p. 423.

Crile G: The smaller the cancer, the bigger the operation? *JAMA* 199:146, 1967.

Davis CEJ Jr et al.: Necrosis of the female breast complicating oral anticoagulant treatment. *Ann Surg* 175:647, 1972.

Davis HH et al.: Cystic disease of the breast: Relationship to carcinoma. *Cancer* 17:957, 1964.

Day E as quoted by Haagensen CD in *Disease of the Breast,* 2d ed, Philadelphia: Saunders, 1971, p. 99.

Devitt JE: Fibrocystic disease of the breast is not premalignant. *Surg Gynecol Obstet* 134:803, 1972.

———, Beattie WG: Rational treatment of carcinoma of the breast. *Ann Surg* 160:71, 1964.

Dodd GD: Present status of thermography, ultrasound and mammography in breast cancer detection. *Cancer* 39 (6 Suppl):2796, 1977.

Egan RL et al.: Conventional mammography, physical examination, thermography and xeroradiography in the detection of breast cancer. *Cancer* 39:1984, 1977.

Editorial: Hormone receptors and breast cancer. *Br Med J* 2:67, 1976.

Forbes AP et al.: Syndrome characterized by galactorrhea, amenorrhea and low urinary FSH, comparison with acromegaly and normal lactation. *J Clin Endocrinol Metab* 14:265, 1954.

Frantz VK et al.: Incidence of chronic cystic disease in so-called "normal breasts." *Cancer* 4:762, 1951.

Funderburk WW et al.: Contrast mammography in breast discharge. *Surg Gynecol Obstet* 119:276, 1964.

———, Syphax B: Evaluation of nipple discharge in benign and malignant disease. *Cancer* 24:1290, 1969.

Gilbertson VA: Detection of breast cancer in a specialized cancer detection center. *Cancer* 24:1192, 1969.

Gold MA: Causes of patients' delay in disease of the breast. *Cancer* 17:564, 1964.

Guttman RJ: Survival and results after 2 million volt irradiation in treatment of primary operable carcinoma of the breast with proved positive internal mammary nodes and/or highest axillary nodes. *Cancer* 15:383, 1962.

Haagensen CD: *Disease of the Breast,* 2d ed, Philadelphia: Saunders, 1971.

Hammerschlag CA et al.: Breast symptoms and patient delay: Psychological variables involved. *Cancer* 17:1480, 1964.

Handley RS as quoted by Haagensen CD in *Diseases of the Breast,* 2d ed., Philadelphia: Saunders, 1971, p. 424.

Herrmann JB: Mammary cancer subsequent to aspiration of cysts in the breast. *Ann Surg* 173:40, 1971.

Ho Yuen B et al.: Human prolactin: Secretion, regulation and pathophysiology. *Obstet Gynecol Surv* 28:527, 1973.

Lilienfeld AM et al.: An evaluation of thermography in the detection of breast cancer. *Cancer* 24:1206, 1969.

Masukawa T et al.: The cytologic examination of breast secretions. *Acta Cytol* 10:261, 1966.

McDivitt RW et al.: *Tumors of the Breast,* Washington: Armed Forces Institute of Pathology, 1968.

McGuire WL et al.: Estrogen receptors in human breast cancer: An overview, in *Estrogen Receptors in Human Breast Cancer,* eds. WL McGuire et al., New York: Raven Press, 1975.

McPherson, VA, MacKenzie WC: Lesions of the breast associated with nipple discharge. *Can J Surg* 5:6, 1962.

Moore FD et al.: Carcinoma of the breast: A decade of new results with old concepts. *N Engl J Med* 277:293, 1967.

Nyirjesy I: Galactorrhea without amenorrhea. *Obstet Gynecol* 32:52, 1968.

Patey DH, Thackeray AC: Pathology and treatment of mammary duct fistula. *Lancet* 2:871, 1958.

Putzki PS et al.: Aspiration of breast cysts: Method and results. *Med Ann DC* 39:149, 1970.

Qualheim RE, Gall EA: Breast carcinoma with multiple sites of origin. *Cancer* 10:460, 1957.

Ross WL: The magnitude of the breast cancer problem in the USA. *Cancer* 24:1106, 1969.

Scott EH: Hypertrophy of the breast, possibly related to medication: A case report. *S Afr Med J* 44:449, 1970.

Shapiro S et al.: Periodic breast cancer screening in reducing mortality from breast cancer. *JAMA* 215:1777, 1971.

Ship AG: Virginal and gravid mammary gigantism: Recurrence after reduction mammoplasty. *Br J Plast Surg* 24:396, 1971.

Strax P: The role of thermography as compared with mammography. *Int J Radiat Oncol Biol Phys* 2:751, 1977.

Urban JA: What is the rationale for an extended radical procedure in early cases? *JAMA* 199:152, 1967.

Venet L et al.: Adequacies and inadequacies of breast examinations by physicians in mass screening. *Cancer* 28:1546, 1971.

Vermund L.: Trends in radiotherapy of breast cancer, in *Proceedings of the Fifth National Cancer Conference,* Philadelphia: JB Lippincott, 1964, p. 183.

Wilson TS, MacGregor JW: Tuberculosis of the breast. *Can Med Assoc J* 89:1118, 1963.

Young RL et al.: Spectrum of nonpuerperal galactorrhea: Report of two cases evolving through the various syndromes. *J Clin Endocrinol Metab* 27:461, 1967.

Zajicek J et al.: Aspiration biopsy of mammary tumors in diagnosis and research: A critical review of 2,200 cases. *Acta Cytol* 11:169, 1967.

47

Principles of Cancer Therapy

INTRODUCTION

SEYMOUR L. ROMNEY   JOHN L. LEWIS, JR.

The goal of cancer care is to provide sufficient information and appropriate therapy so that the patient can look forward to survival, even cure, while maintaining a desired quality of life. Many unknown variables exist for all cancers. In addition, the tumor response to one modality or to combined modalities of therapy is sufficiently unpredictable that an accurate prognosis cannot be provided even in advanced, hopeless cases. Prognosis has been an educated guess based upon the accumulated experience of multiple institutions and the largely uncontrolled experiences of individuals. More recently, carefully designed protocols have been introduced to permit prospective, randomized clinical trials. From these it is hoped that a data base can be developed which, when subjected to careful statistical analysis, will make possible better predictions about therapeutic regimens.

Currently, the impressions concerning optimum therapy and survival come from the larger medical centers, reflecting their more extensive experience and their concentrations of personnel, physical facilities, and other resources. In these institutions individuals with special training and experience are focusing their efforts on the problems and the management of cancer patients. Unless a well-organized, structured effort is made to record the significant events, including complications, evidence of persisting or recurrent disease, and the patient's functional status, statistics and reports from institutions will have limited value.

Comprehensive cancer care is a multidisciplinary effort. The key role of the responsible gynecologist is to provide care and to coordinate the involvement of various professionals and agencies, such as the American Cancer Society, Cancer Care, the local Visiting Nurse Association, and other community resources.

The gynecologist has been conspicuous among medical specialists in orchestrating this kind of coordinated effort. Whether this is an outgrowth of the warm interpersonal relationship which has been traditional between the gynecologist and the patient or whether there is some other cause, it has become standard practice in caring for the woman with a cancer to mesh the efforts of specialists in pathology, radiation therapy, medical oncology, immunotherapy, and nursing care under the leadership of the gynecologist.

OVERVIEW

The delivery of a normal infant is one of life's exciting events. Today this event is often enhanced by the active participation of both parents during labor and birth. Advances in maternal, fetal, and perinatal medicine have made delivery markedly safer than formerly. Perhaps such satisfying medical experiences lead some individuals away from the care of patients with malignant disease, where less favorable outcomes are often likely.

Everyone who treats a patient who has cancer must develop a philosophy about how this serious disease should be managed over a period of time with respect to its treatment and the relationship with the patient.

The existence of a cancer becomes one of the greatest problems in the patient's life. Along with the emotional trauma created when the patient is required to accept the diagnosis and treatment, the malignancy and prognosis influence her life-style, family, and even the community. Rehabilitation involves use of community resources and not withdrawal from community life. Even the person cured of malignancy has less body integrity than before development of the tumor and requires an abundance of emotional support.

What the patient needs is holistic care, not simply concern with the lesion and its consequences. The health professionals involved must provide compassionate support of the patient's emotional and psychologic needs within the framework of an empirically sound plan for treatment.

Therapy of gynecologic malignancies must be tailored to the organ site, disease stage, prior therapy, and general health of the patient. In the early stages of localized disease, the therapy is intended to produce a cure. Successful surgery usually leaves the patient without one or more organs and often without other tissues as well. Radiation therapy leaves permanent effects on all treated tissues and occasionally brings about permanent damage. In both of these situations, the goal is to cure the patient without denying her the quality of life she requires.

Balancing the treatment against this requirement becomes much more problematic when the therapeutic goal is palliation rather than cure. In the view of some physicians, patients with advanced disease are better off not treated. In such circumstances each case requires individual assessment, and the major decision should be made by an informed patient. Some emotionally well-adjusted women are grateful for the opportunity to continue living, even with marked anatomic changes. Put another way, some women with a strong desire to live have a remarkable capability to adjust to physical alteration. Yet the more drastic operations should be considered only when a cure is possible. Then the physician's role should be to clarify all aspects and implications and not merely to convince the patient to go ahead.

The current state of the art in cancer care involves measured decisions as to which one or more of the current modalities of therapy to use. Surgery remains, by and large, the most effective treatment, the critical issue being whether the malignancy and its possible extensions and/or metastases can be totally excised in the operating room. In the preoperative evaluation of a patient, indications of surgical risks or likelihood of cure need to be assessed. If the cancer is responsive to radiotherapy with end results comparable to those of surgery, the preference of the patient should be influential. In young patients with localized cervical carcinoma, surgery is preferable because the ovaries can be retained and both radiation castration and radiation damage to the vagina can be avoided.

There is reason to question whether cancericidal doses are delivered to the center of large tumors. In any event, the shielding of vital viscera and bone marrow sites requires expert knowledge, and the delivery of full radiation doses must be tempered by knowledge that normal tissues may be damaged and long-term radiation complications may disable the patient over a period of time.

Chemotherapy is being vigorously pursued in a variety of clinical trials that seek to evaluate prospectively the effectiveness of single versus multiple agents. The hope is that some newly developed compounds will be tumor- and cell-cycle-specific. When tumor bulk and tumor cell populations have been significantly reduced, and when myelosuppression is not a constraint, encouraging results with chemotherapy are being recorded for many neoplasms, including ovarian carcinoma. Therapeutic regimens capable of producing significant remissions in otherwise hopeless clinical circumstances are now being offered to some patients.

If further progress is to be achieved in the care of cancer patients, there is need to take into account the views of multidisciplinary groups who have special interests, qualifications, and clinical experience. In accredited hospitals, this reality has resulted in the creation of tumor boards. Board recommendations are generated for patients having invasive disease. The advantages inherent in the tumor board's activities are that as a group they review history, pathology, and other laboratory findings, as well as the physical examination, in detail. Questions concerning degrees of tumor differentiation, extent of invasion, and presence of vascular or lymphatic metastases are discussed prior to therapy. The pros and cons of one mo-

dality versus another or the possible advantages of combined modality therapy are discussed prospectively. The recommendation for the individual patient is arrived at after a full resolution of pragmatic and theoretical questions.

THE EMOTIONAL PROBLEM

The revelation that a patient has an invasive malignancy, regardless of stage and organ, inevitably raises the possibility of a fatal outcome. Many patients have difficulty in accepting any diagnosis of cancer even if the lesion is limited and curable. Denial as a defense mechanism is frequently encountered, and in some instances hysteria may lead to complete amnesia regarding diagnostic examination, procedures, or discussions. In order to be effective in helping these patients communicate, the participating physician must be able to accept the malignant disease process as being as much a phase of living as the process of birth. Communications between doctor and patient at this time are often difficult because the information has come from the physician, and in the ancient tradition the patient often blames the physician as if this bearer of the news had created the disease. In making patients recognize and acknowledge their health problem, the physician is often automatically assigned responsibility for how bad patients feel.

The goal in communicating with a cancer patient is a spirit of openness and trust in which the physician can tell the patient the truth of her situation to the extent that she can accept it. At the same time, the reality of existing problems, whether they be complications of therapy, progression of disease, or possible terminal consequences, should be discussed. Whenever possible, a person close to the patient should also be acquainted with the facts. The language used must be understandable to all involved. Patients respond best to a sense that the physician is knowledgeable and straightforward and is prepared, given the possible occurrence of complications, to do whatever is necessary.

Understandably, one of the most common and perplexing problems surfaces in the question "What is the prognosis, Doctor?" There is a tendency to answer this question on the basis of reported statistics derived from large clinical studies. For example, if a patient has a stage I, grade I endometrial adenocarcinoma, one can say that the overall prognosis is better than 90 percent in the patient's favor. On the other hand, this is not what the individual is asking. The patient's concern is personal: What will happen to her? She will not get 90 percent better and 10 percent worse. She will either be one of the 90 percent who are cured or one of the 10 percent who die. In stage III ovarian carcinoma, the odds are approximately reversed. The patient with stage III ovarian cancer who is cured, however, is no more grateful than the patient who has endometrial cancer and is cured. It should be borne in mind that the patient whose disease is not controlled feels no better for having been one of a smaller percentage, the 10 percent whose endometrial cancer was not cured. Since we are unable by current technology to identify which patient in each group is going to be cured, a cautious optimistic approach seems appropriate for all patients until a recurrence or a complication, representing progression of the disease, indicates that further optimism is not justified for that individual. The saddest cancer patients for a gynecologist to care for are women who are cured of their disease but who have stopped living effectively because they assume that they are dying. Some of these patients remain miserable while they live out their full life-span, then die of other causes.

A constantly distressing challenge for the cancer therapist is the depressed patient. Depression often results from the conviction that the diagnosis of cancer is synonymous with impending and eventual death. Many patients with curable cancers are as depressed as patients with untreatable cancers. While death is the ultimate outcome for every human being, death from cancer is unlikely in a patient whose disease is detected early and treated appropriately. What many patients fear is that they have a disease which is not only serious and difficult to talk about, but is untreatable. It is essential that the involved professionals recognize the hopelessness and fear related to lack of understanding or orientation about the nature of the cancer, its state of progression, curability, and prognosis. It is commonly observed that the patient's fears are frequently far worse than the reality of the problem. Patients react less strongly to being told that they have a malignancy if at the same time they are advised that a definitive therapeutic regimen can be promptly implemented. There are a few situations where the patient should be confronted with the exact diagnosis and prognosis, but the decision to make such revelations should depend upon careful individual evaluation of a patient's personality, life-style, family support and unique circumstances.

THE PELVIC EXAMINATION AND DIAGNOSTIC AIDS

Were gynecologic malignancies detected in situ or in an early invasive stage, the cure rate for each would be above 90 percent. Failure to achieve such a cure rate can be attributed to (1) patient responsibility (2) physician responsibility, and (3) limitations in knowledge and/or technical skills. With the exception of the fallopian tubes and ovaries, all of the organs of the female reproductive tract are accessible to inspection, palpation, and/or biopsy and cytologic sampling by essentially noninvasive techniques.

A good number of women are reluctant and hesitant to have a pelvic vaginal examination. In addition, there is the distressing reality that many women, aware of a problem of abnormal vaginal bleeding, postcoital staining, unusual discharge, or pelvic pain, defer seeking an appointment for examination because of psychological denial or fear of learning the truth. The emotional element must be recognized. As for the physician, it is to be regretted that many times pelvic and rectal examinations are deferred for no justifiable reason. Failure to complete a pelvic examination only serves to introduce an element of delay in diagnosis and treatment. In some instances, vaginal creams, ointments, or occasionally hormone preparations are prescribed before a diagnosis has been established or before a neoplasm has been ruled out.

The accessibility of the female genital tract to direct examination has resulted in the introduction of a variety of special techniques for diagnostic purposes. In addition to the noninvasive evaluation of pelvic viscera by ultrasound scanning and computer axial tomography, the vulva, vagina, or cervix can be evaluated by the colposcope or colpomicroscope and directed biopsies can be obtained. The endocervix and endometrial cavity can be further evaluated by various aspiration and biopsy techniques, and also by hysteroscopy in conjunction with hysterography. The techniques of laparoscopy, culdoscopy, and colpotomy are used for inspection of the peritoneal cavity, the subdiaphragmatic spaces, and the cul-de-sac. Laparoscopy requires considerable experience and competence and its employment is not without risk, especially in patients who have had prior surgery and/or radiation therapy. Paracentesis, employed judiciously, can be invaluable in establishing a cytologic diagnosis. Peritoneal washings should be obtained at any laparotomy whenever there is a question of an ovarian neoplasm.

CANCER SCREENING

Detection of a cancer precursor or an early invasive lesion is the primary diagnostic goal in all neoplastic lesions. The patient who is to benefit from a personal, periodic health maintenance routine should receive a careful history and physical examination. The examination should (1) evaluate her general health status; (2) determine the existence of abnormal symptoms or signs; it should include (3) careful palpation of the breasts and abdomen; (4) inspection of the vulva, vagina, and cervix; (5) bimanual palpation of the pelvic structures; and (6) a combined rectovaginal examination, including a stool (hemoccult) guaiac analysis. If abnormal uterine bleeding is present in conjunction with abnormal cervicovaginal cytology, there should be a colposcopic examination and a directed biopsy ecto- or endocervix or endometrium.

A number of cancer screening programs have been developed for detecting asymptomatic lesions. Many routines have been explored at considerable personal, community, and governmental cost; some have focused upon specific organ sites. Unfortunately, the cost-effectiveness of these programs and their impact upon the incidence and mortality rates of various cancers are uncertain. It is a fact that it is difficult to evaluate the effectiveness of mammography, routine use of sigmoidoscopy and colonoscopy, and such radiologic investigations as chest x-rays, intravenous pyelograms, and barium enemas. More recently, the availability of computer axial tomography has introduced a new and costly technology without a realistic prospective appreciation of its capabilities.

Experiences with such screening activities point up the need for careful planning of randomized clinical trials for any screening routine. With such planning, the nature and frequency of routine usage and the success of the case finding can be expected to be established from a sound data base rather than from anecdotal experiences. The awkwardness of using such experiences as data is that once they have been reported and have gained reasonable public and professional acceptance, it becomes difficult to deny a patient a theoretically promising but unproven program. Ethical issues arise which are difficult to resolve.

The experience with the Pap smear is an important case in point. There can be little doubt that the availability of the Pap smear has been invaluable in improving the outlook for patients with cervical carcinoma. For more than 30 years, an annual Pap test screening policy has been offered to the public at considerable cost. However, there has been a steady annual decline in cervical cancer incidence and deaths. If a disease has a low prevalence, the yield from a screening effort will be low for a high effort (Foltz, Kelsey). Moreover, there is the risk that women identified by a positive test may not have the disease at all, yet will be subjected to further diagnostic and/or treatment procedures with accompanying costs and worry. In population groups rescreened for cervical cancer incurred 1 to 7 years previously, the prevalence rates for dysplasias, in situ carcinoma, invasive carcinoma (stage I), and invasive carcinoma (stages II to IV) were 2.4, 0.07, 0.09, and 0.0 respectively (Stern, Neely). However, the frequency of hysterectomy (nearly one-fifth of the women aged 40 to 49) has contributed to the difficulty of accurately estimating the mortality, incidence, and prevalence of the disease (Stern et al.; Cole).

The availability of the Pap smear and the motivation it gives women to seek an annual gynecologic checkup, even though they are asymptomatic, has the desirable effect of bringing presumably healthy women into the health care delivery system. It has led to earlier detection of other malignancies. However, determining the effectiveness of the existing technology in cancer screening and cancer control remains difficult (Kern, Zivolich; Evans et al.). When the realities of cost and cost-effectiveness, false-negative and false-positive cytologic interpretations, the pros and cons of surgical conization and cryosurgery, and the incidence and use of hysterectomy are assessed within the context of what is known about the natural history of uterine cervical carcinoma, there is reason to examine current practices critically. Foltz and Kelsey have reviewed the development and the rationale behind an annual Pap smear, which in some instances is mandated by state law. They contrast the practices and policies of the United States with those of Canada and Great Britain. The 1976 Walton Report, issued by a Canadian government task force, reviewed the Canadian experience with the Pap test in terms of its scientific effectiveness, availability, accuracy, and costs. In women who were identified to be at low risk if early Pap tests were negative, the task force recommended Pap tests at 3-year intervals until age 35, and thereafter at 5-year intervals to age 60. For high-risk women, i.e., those having low income, early onset of sexual activity, and multiple sexual partners, annual Pap smears were advised. It was noted that the high-risk women who stood to benefit most from regular Pap smear screening were frequently not being reached or were not availing themselves of this public health measure. In Great Britain, the question has focused on what women should receive the test and how frequently it should be used. The question of the value of cytologic screening per se has not been the issue. However, in the overall evaluation, the indications for hysterectomy, the high hysterectomy rates, the social and personal costs, as well as a perspective of the monetary costs, have all been examined. (Brindel et al.; Lyon, Gardner; Kinlen, Spriggs). Against this background a major question that worries all physicians responsible for the health care of women is why some women actively avoid obtaining a Pap smear or establishing a habit of periodic gynecologic examination. In many instances, it is obvious that this failure is not simply a result of lack of information because the availability of the Pap smear has been well publicized. Even many female scientists actively engaged in research of cervical neoplasia fail to obtain Pap smears.

Clearly the problem of cancer screening is extremely complex. It is too simplistic to assume that the availability of proven techniques, regardless of cost, is the answer to the early detection of a malignant neoplasm. A major emotional component plays an important role in patient compliance. The educational dimension must be carefully thought out and programmed in order to be understood and accepted by individuals of diverse cultural, ethnic, and socioeconomic backgrounds. It is also essential that before establishing programmatic screening routines and policies, which are costly, difficult to implement, and inevitably worrisome to the very individuals they are designed to help, carefully designed, randomized prospective clinical trials should be completed involving a full spectrum and adequate numbers of different population subgroups.

COLPOSCOPY

In recent years, the usefulness of colposcopy has been recognized. Its specific value when used in conjunction with careful exfoliative cytological studies has become more widely appreciated (Coppelson et al.). Advances in cytology are being pursued to establish criteria that will have predictive value which can be correlated with the histology of a cervical lesion. Cytologic diagnosis always requires tissue confirmation, which can usually be acquired with the help of colposcopy. Occasionally, in the presence of a visible cervical lesion, a Pap smear may be negative or

may show no evidence of malignant cells. An advanced cervical lesion may be covered by a necrotic slough and only inflammatory cells will be detected by the sampling technique.

Colposcopy is an effective technique for inspecting the surface of the ectocervix and the visible segment of the endocervix. Essentially, the technique permits precise evaluation of the squamous epithelium of the cervix and of the all-important transformation zone. The latter exists as a junctional area between the columnar epithelium of the endocervix and the squamous epithelium of the ectocervix. Its anatomic extent and histologic characteristics are variable for each individual. Columnar cells undergo squamous metaplasia at varying times during the life cycle of the female, particularly after an initial pregnancy. This junctional area is a vulnerable zone, thought to be a site of origin of cervical neoplasms, but subject to a variety of environmental, including hormonal, influences, as well as to bacterial, fungal, and viral infections.

Colposcopy brings the transformation zone into magnified focus revealing the nature of any surface lesions, the extent of metaplastic change, the opacity of surface epithelium to light transmission, and the possible associated abnormal vascular changes which identify precursor or neoplastic lesions. Aided by specific criteria, the colposcopist can complete colposcopically directed biopsies in obtaining a diagnosis of a visible lesion or a cytologic finding. Whenever the transformation zone cannot be totally visualized with a colposcope and especially when the upper limits appear to extend into the endocervical canal, the examination is incomplete. In such circumstances a careful endocervical curettage should always be performed (see Chap. 41).

The colposcope was popular in Europe in the early 1900s. At that time, it was used as a screening technique before George Papanicolaou's contributions to exfoliative cytology in the late 1920s. The major push for the popularization of colposcopy in this country came from investigators who felt that too many patients, screened with class II to III Pap smears, were being subjected to surgical conization of the cervix on the supposition that they might have an early neoplastic lesion. Colposcopy permits simple office biopsy as an initial and frequently the sole diagnostic requirement for instituting local proper therapy. Whether surgery, cautery, cryosurgery, application of caustics, use of the laser beam, or the initiation of a medical regimen is implemented depends upon the ability of the colposcopist to identify the nature of the lesion.

There is great variation in the colposcopic spectrum seen in early cervical neoplasia and there is also considerable variation in the histology of the lesion. It is not unusual to find an invasive squamous-cell cancer in the endocervix with coexisting carcinoma in situ and dysplasia extending onto the exocervix. The reliability of the colposcopically directed biopsy in detecting the worst area in a lesion is directly related to the experience and expertise of the colposcopist. The proponents of colposcopy have suggested that to attain and maintain efficiency, one must be in a position to evaluate a significant number of patients having abnormal cytology. In the United States, the use of the colposcope has produced a gratifying reduction in cold-knife conization, previously used as a combined diagnostic and therapeutic modality for women with abnormal Pap smears. Cold-knife conization has occasionally been misused in patients with mild or moderate dysplasia. Where the colposcopic approach and the office management of abnormal cytology are being utilized, it should be realized that patients may have unrecognized in situ or invasive lesions. In all instances, the endocervix must be carefully evaluated. Even if the entire transformation zone has been visualized some advocate a thorough endocervical curettage before therapy is initiated. The colposcope is thus useful in delineating the geography of cervical changes and the extent of tissue to be removed with conization. It can also determine whether the disease extends onto the vagina, and it has been invaluable in assessing patients with histories of prenatal exposure to diethylstilbestrol or with vulvar lesions.

THE IMPORTANCE OF PATHOLOGY

Proper therapy of a woman with a gynecologic malignancy requires the establishment of a definitive and accurate histologic diagnosis. To plan effective therapy, the extent to which the tumor involves the organ of primary origin, the cell type, the degree of differentiation and invasiveness, and the possible existence of vascular and lymphatic involvement must all be known. These factors may be determined in a biopsy, but the pathologist's contribution becomes even more important in the handling of the surgical specimen. As cancer therapy has become more sophisticated, particularly where it combines modalities of treatment, the identification of different subgroups of patients with a delineated stage of a disease rests largely upon the thoroughness and the competence of the pathologist. For example, in stage I adenocar-

cinoma of the endometrium, it is now clear that patients whose cancer is grade I (well differentiated) can be cured by a simple hysterectomy with removal of the adnexa as effectively as by any other means of treatment, including pre- or postoperative radiation therapy or radical surgery. However, the identical treatment given to a patient with a stage I adenocarcinoma determined to be Grade III (undifferentiated) will result in a reduction of survival by approximately 40 percent (Homesley et al.). Thus, the histopathologic diagnosis in combination with proper clinical staging alone, without the additional information of the degree of cell type differentiation, does not permit the planning of appropriate individualized therapy for a particular patient's tumor. If simple surgery alone is carried out, patients with undifferentiated lesions may have a decreased survival rate. Accordingly, if preoperative radiation therapy is given to all patients and then followed by surgery, individuals with well-differentiated lesions will have been exposed to radiation therapy unnecessarily.

Comparable and important reliance on the competence of the pathologist can be documented in every gynecologic tumor. In the vulva, the histologic differentiation between in situ lesions, which can be treated with local therapy, contrasted with invasive lesions, which require not only removal of the entire vulva but of the regional lymph nodes as well, is obviously important. On occasion, a more subtle determination is the identification of isolated Paget's cells at the margins of wide surgical specimens or the identification of underlying apocrine gland cancer below Paget's disease, requiring a totally different surgical approach. The role of the pathologist is critical in the interpretation of the spectrum of cervical intraepithelial lesions, and the initiation of specific therapy requires coordination with the delineated correct pathologic evaluation.

In probably no other organ of the body is the experience and knowledge of the pathologist more important than in evaluating lesions of the ovary. Even in the common epithelial tumors, there are five cell types, with three subcategories based on probability of malignant potential, namely (1) benign, (2) potentially malignant, and (3) malignant. When studying alternative forms of therapy for ovarian lesions, it is important not only to determine cell types, but also to estimate within the malignant group the histologic grade. Even in the same stage and with the same histologic type, the Decker report concerning the ovarian carcinoma experience at the Mayo Clinic showed that histologic grade is still very significant in determining response to all forms of therapy (Decker et al.).

STAGING AND TUMOR DIFFERENTIATION

Clinical staging requires determining the geographical distribution of a tumor. Since its histologic character must also be determined, a tissue diagnosis is needed.

The staging system for gynecologic malignancies has been proposed and is subject to revision by the International Federation of Gynecology and Obstetrics (FIGO). At this time, the system has virtual world-wide acceptance. Staging systems are important in order to plan and initiate therapy properly to determine prognosis, and to compare the effectiveness of various modes of treatment. Localized extension, the relationship to adjacent viscera, and possible regional or distant lymphatic or hematogenous metastatic pattern have to be clarified. An equally important consideration is the histologic determination of the degree of tumor differentiation. All of these factors influence decisions regarding choices of therapy. Although staging potentially serves the valuable purpose of identifying extent of tumor involvement, the tumor bulk volume is not accurately defined by any current criteria.

Other unknown variables determine therapeutic outcome, and it is apparent that tumor aggressiveness, tumor-host response, and optimum in vivo conditions for maximum radiotherapeutic effectiveness (tumor-tissue oxygen tension) are equally important factors. Histologic grading provides an approximation of the biologic aggressiveness of the tumor. The more differentiated tumors are slower growing; the undifferentiated, anaplastic cell types invade and metastasize more rapidly. In addition, unfortunately, a specific tumor and its biologic characteristics may not be accurately evaluated by any of the currently used criteria. The net effect is that in specific instances it is not possible to consistently relate therapeutic protocols to current staging classifications with their known limitations. This reality must be considered when therapeutic results are compared from one center to another. Because of these circumstances, the therapy of tumors must be individualized and based on a careful evaluation of as many factors as possible.

As technology changes it can be expected that the details of staging will be modified. The techniques employed in staging, in addition to inspection, palpation, and biopsy, should be commonly available in most hospitals. At this time the positive findings of such specialized techniques as ultrasonography, lymphangiography, angiography, computerized axial tomography, and invasive diagnostic techniques are not acceptable criteria in determining the staging in an individual patient.

Early in the history of the use of international staging systems in gynecologic cancer, the sole emphasis was on the comparison of outcomes of surgery and radiation therapy. This was particularly true in carcinoma of the cervix, where opinion was divided between the proponents of radiation therapy and those of radical surgery as to the better form of therapy for an individual patient. Since the patient treated with radiation therapy generally did not provide a surgical specimen for posttherapy study and the operative evaluation of the pelvis and peritoneal cavity could not be accomplished, comparison of results in patients treated with radiation versus those with surgery could only be made on the basis of the initial clinical findings. It is obvious that errors in staging will result from the limitations of the diagnostic techniques that can be used in any agreed-upon system.

In planning the individual patient's treatment and in arriving at a probable prognosis, the possibility that the disease may be more advanced than suspected clinically must be realistically and carefully determined. However, once established, the staging cannot be changed when end results are reported. Clearly, if carefully designed treatment protocols are to be evaluated and the overall approach to any cancer patient is to be objective and rational, the initial staging cannot be changed. Furthermore, provisions should be made for prospective randomized clinical trials whenever possible. At the present time, staging is a crude procedure for classifying and characterizing the biologic activity of a cancer; its eventual goal is to compare the value of various forms of treatment. As more emphasis is given to the importance of prospective clinical trials in all malignancies, other factors in addition to clinical stage will have to be taken into consideration. Patients with a specific stage of a disease who are entered into clinical trials must be stratified in order to determine the specific ultimate effectiveness of any therapeutic modality or combined modalities employed. Only in this fashion will statistical and clinical validity be established. However, regardless of the disease being evaluated and treated, the apparent anatomic distribution of the tumor prior to the onset of treatment remains a major consideration. Stratification factors for each cancer will vary and will involve such individual patient characteristics as age, race, parity, socioeconomic status, general health, and other unrelated disease aspects. Many specific considerations require evaluation in the ultimate decision as how best to treat an individual patient. These concern the neoplasm per se including cell type, histologic differentiation, past response to radiation or chemotherapy, indirect measurements of the host's immunologic competence and responsiveness to the tumor, as well as other still unknown variables including the nutritional status of the patient and the impact of the patient's emotional adjustment to the cancer.

DESIGNED TREATMENT

The therapy of a gynecologic malignancy involves a multidisciplinary effort with detailed planning, evaluation, and definitive implementation according to one of two plans. The first plan is that of *best available care standards* and consists of a proper workup to determine general health, operability, staging, pathologic evaluation, and implementation of therapy. Such an approach is considered standard operating practice in all accredited institutions and should characterize the programs of all hospitals in which gynecologic patients receive cancer care. The purpose of any defined plan is to be certain that clinically important details or procedures are not omitted and that the therapy instituted is based on established and accepted principles rather than on individual idiosyncrasies. Standard programs should be carefully discussed by all members of the staff prior to their acceptance, and then should be adhered to. The results of an institution's experience with accepted routines should be regularly evaluated by reviewing the end results recorded in the local tumor registry. If the overall results do not compare well with published reports, careful attention must be given to a review of procedural details or of the nature of complications associated with individual patients' problems. Less than optimum results may be obtained in advanced, complicated cases when therapy is initiated by a physician who only sees an occasional patient with a malignancy. Furthermore, in such instances, the chance for cure of a patient with an early lesion may be lost. In general, cancers that are not localized should be referred to specialized services or centers.

The second treatment regimen is the *experimental clinical trial*. Such programs must be carefully developed, with detailed consideration given to their safety, their potential benefits for the patient, and their possible adverse effects and complications. The justification for the clinical trial is that it assures the acquisition of a data base that permits evaluation of an effort to improve the results obtained with an existing standard program. The proposal must be based on reasonable evidence that the change from the standard plan is likely to improve the results. Informed

consent must be obtained from each patient. This comprises full indoctrination of each patient, along with assurance that the patient may elect to withdraw from the regimen at any time. Almost all investigational trials should be randomized in a prospective study against the best-known treatment for a particular stage of a specific neoplasm. Research approaches should not be carried out in all institutions but should be limited to those which, by their nature, have a large enough series of patients, as well as the facilities and personnel, to carry out the clinical trial in an expeditious manner. In the design of an experimental plan, all of the factors known to have an effect on prognosis of the neoplasm should be identified, then a program should be established which stratifies patients according to multiple variables. Consultation with a qualified epidemiologist and a biostatistician is desirable in the design and implementation of a new investigational proposal.

The morality of randomized clinical trials is based on acceptance of the fact that each treatment regimen represents therapy which is effective. Clearly, if one specific treatment plan is unequivocally better than another, there is no need for a study. However, therapeutic lore in cancer may be the result of single-arm studies, reported and supported by strong individuals, which have not necessarily been subjected to the scientific evaluation of a randomized clinical trial. Given a promising, scientifically sound therapeutic alternative, especially where the cancer patient is involved, the physician's obligation is to determine which of two or more forms of treatment is superior. This requires careful prospective planning and informed patient cooperation. In most instances, such a determination can only be made through randomized clinical trials. The difficulties of such clinical trials and the evaluation of their results require attention (Zelen). Occasionally a breakthrough occurs in which historical controls are appropriate. The first patients who received methotrexate for the treatment of gestational trophoblastic neoplasm were not randomized with those who received any other chemotherapeutic agent. Prior to that time, metastatic choriocarcinoma had a 95 percent mortality rate in one year following diagnosis.

DEBULKING AND OVARIAN CARCINOMA

A generalization in all cancer care is that the likelihood of a favorable result is inversely proportional to the amount of disease being treated. This dictum is true whether the modality employed is surgery, radiation, or chemotherapy. Experience related to the size of the lesion in cervical carcinoma is consistent with this rule, whether the lesion is treated by radiation therapy or by surgery. With chemotherapy, the dictum has clearly proved accurate for gestational trophoblastic disease, and it is presumed that other solid tumors also follow the rule.

In the great majority of patients with ovarian carcinoma, initial surgery cannot safely remove all of the disease. Thus, either radiation therapy or chemotherapy is utilized as an adjunct to treat the residual disease. Efforts to effectively decrease the persistent tumor burden as much as possible are justifiable. Although the operative process is characterized by the crude term "debulking," experience with advanced ovarian cancer indicates that the less tumor a patient has at the end of an operative procedure, the more likely she will be to obtain a beneficial response from subsequent therapy. The operating gynecologist should make every reasonable effort at the time of the initial surgery to remove the uterus, fallopian tubes, and both ovaries, and such obvious metastatic disease as is found in the cul-de-sac, omentum, retroperitoneal space, and other sites within the abdominal cavity. The entire subsequent clinical course is often determined by the completeness and aggressiveness of the initial surgery. However, aggressiveness in ovarian cancer does not imply the extirpative surgery comparable to other forms of cancer. Ovarian carcinoma is not a disease for exenterative surgery. Only rarely, unless obstruction is present, will a patient profit from resection of the intestine. The most common mistake in primary surgery is performing a laparotomy, establishing the diagnosis, removing easily mobilized tissue, and closing the abdomen. When this approach is taken for the patient with advanced ovarian carcinoma in the belief that systemic chemotherapy will adequately perfuse the residual tumor, it represents self-delusion. Laparotomy limited to biopsy may result in an undesirable delay; moreover, it may unnecessarily subject the patient to the risks of a second operation.

Subsequent surgery in advanced ovarian cancer is a difficult and complicated problem. Subsequent surgery often involves patients who have recurrent or progressive disease. The decision to operate depends largely upon the nature of the complication in relation to the patient's prognosis with her primary neoplasm. When operating for intestinal obstruction in an instance of progressive ovarian cancer, one should expect only 50 percent of women subsequently to leave the hospital. While it is possible to reestablish

gastrointestinal continuity and function in a high percentage of such women, failure of the tumor to respond to subsequent chemotherapy prevents the patient from leaving the hospital.

At the present time, an exploratory laparotomy to try to "debulk" recurrent disease can only be considered experimental. The difficult emotional decision which confronts the gynecologist in this situation is that the clinical course of advanced ovarian disease may involve progressive nonresectable growth of tumor, limited to the peritoneal cavity, in an otherwise alert, distressed patient. Given this set of circumstances in a patient whose disease has not responded to established chemotherapeutic protocols, the undertaking of additional surgery is difficult to justify.

"SECOND LOOK" AND OVARIAN CARCINOMA

Surgery remains the most important modality for treating ovarian cancer because the disease is extensive when first encountered. However, surgery alone is generally recognized as inadequate treatment. In isolated instances, stage I lesions are encountered which are histologically determined to be of low malignant potential. Occasionally, a small, encapsulated epithelial lesion is discovered in a young woman who wishes to retain reproductive capacity. In these special circumstances, surgery can be the sole modality employed. However blind, randomized studies show that survival rates are increased even in stage I disease by subsequent chemotherapy. Of equal significance is the fact that chemotherapy has as good a survival rate as does radiation therapy or radiation therapy plus chemotherapy in patients with advanced disease. Thus, the growing trend has been to give all patients chemotherapy subsequent to their initial surgery if measurable, residual disease is present. Inevitably, the question then becomes how long the patient should be maintained on chemotherapy.

In an effort to answer this critical question, various centers have embarked on programs involving exploratory laparotomies after various periods of clinical trials employing a number of chemotherapeutic protocols in order to determine whether the chemotherapy has been effective and can be stopped. The potential benefits of the information to be gained at laparotomy must be carefully weighed against the morbidity and complications of the procedure.

In ovarian cancer, a "second look" operation must be differentiated from procedures carried out to remove persistent tumor or to overcome complications such as intestinal obstruction. The technique involves a generous vertical incision, inspection and palpation of the diaphragm, liver, intraperitoneal organs, retroperitoneal nodes, particularly near the renal hila, and pelvic structures, with biopsies of any suspicious areas including all adhesions and known areas of previous tumor involvement. Cytologic washings should be taken from both peritoneal gutters and pelvis.

Some investigators have proposed laparoscopy instead of laparotomy for the second look. However, laparoscopic findings are trustworthy in this situation only if the presence of disease is confirmed. Negative laparoscopic procedure is an indication to proceed with laparotomy.

RECURRENT DISEASE

No condition presents a greater problem than a gynecologic malignancy in which initial therapy has failed. Because response rates for recurrent disease are so poor, it is critically important that optimum therapy be carried out initially. The treatment plans for recurrent disease are determined by the same factors as those considered in planning initial therapy. The general systemic medical evaluation of the patient is the background for focusing upon the organ of origin, cell type, geographical distribution, and individual characteristics of the tumor. However, in recurrent disease the options are more limited and often are related to the results and consequences of the prior therapy. For example, in a patient who has been irradiated for cervix cancer, reirradiation is not only ineffective but is extremely dangerous. In general, there is a tendency to use an alternative modality to the one used originally. In invasive cancer of the cervix treated by appropriate radiation therapy, should the modality unfortunately fail, it is rare for there to be central recurrence. Should the disease recur, it is generally found at the periphery or outside of the pelvis. In both these areas, exenterative surgery is limited in its application. On the other hand, if stage I cervical disease has been treated inappropriately by ineffective radiation therapy, such patients can sometimes be salvaged by a radical surgical procedure.

The problems of recurrent disease are formidable. Previous radical radiation therapy may be accompanied by severe side effects and complications, including depletion of bone marrow reserves of such magnitude that the possibility of an alternative chemotherapeutic clinical trial is limited. Radiation fibrosis in the pelvis may restrict pelvic perfusion and may also negate the possible trial of newly developed chemotherapeutic agents. In isolated instances, if a considerable period of time has elapsed, it may be possible for the radiotherapist to administer a palliative additional dose of radiotherapy. Such supplementary dosages are not employed with any enthusiasm since side effects and major complications including vesicovaginal or rectovaginal fistulas, radiation proctitis, colitis, enteritis, and cystitis may be encountered, accompanied by hemorrhage, tenesmus, and considerable morbidity.

The usefulness of chemotherapy in advanced and recurrent disease is currently being carefully evaluated. In general, newly available chemotherapeutic compounds have not been systematically and carefully studied in prospective randomized clinical trials. This area requires attention and cautious exploration. The compounds being employed are all associated with significant toxic side effects; thus considerable experience and knowledge of the pharmacokinetics of single or combined agent therapy is essential. This knowledge involves awareness of the myelosuppressive and immunosuppressive consequences of use of these agents and the recognition that patients will be susceptible to overwhelming infections. There is the need also to be aware of the fact that previously irradiated patients or those who have failed previous chemotherapy have limited bone marrow stores. The selection of any alternative regimen must consider the potential advantages compared to iatrogenic consequences, including the possible development of leukemia (Reimer et al.). (See section on chemotherapy later in this chapter.)

The initiation of a therapeutic protocol for recurrent disease requires a a careful assessment of quality of survival and quality of life.

HYPERALIMENTATION

Nutrition is being recognized as an increasingly important factor in the etiology, treatment, and rehabilitation of the cancer patient. It must be recognized, however, that interest in this fundamental subject has generally been focused on water and electrolyte balance, disturbances in carbohydrate metabolism, replacement of blood and blood fractionation products, and the maintenance of an adequate caloric intake. Unfortunately, the cancer patient is frequently beset with anorexia, nausea, vomiting, fatigue, and lassitude. The manifestations may be the result of the pathophysiologic consequences of the neoplasm and its complications or of iatrogenic adverse effects. For the patient, there is a disinterest in and/or an inability to consume balanced and essential nutrients and fluids. What frequently follows is a progressive negative nitrogen balance accompanied by weight loss and more anorexia. This results in a dehydrated, cachectic woman who is depressed, unable to eat, and who is often confined to a bed and chair existence. The intravenous administration of amino acids, as well as glucose, vitamins, and electrolytes, can promote the general well-being of the patient, and can promote wound healing and weight gain while countering the adverse effects of radiation and chemotherapy. Hyperalimentation should be employed aggressively and appropriately in the early stages of treatment and convalescence; it should not be an adjunctive routine in the terminal stages of the disease.

The nutrient regimen should be planned to provide a gradually increasing nutritional intake which can enhance the surgical recovery or the beneficial response to radiotherapy and chemotherapy. The caloric intake can be increased by progressively increasing the glucose concentration over a period of days from 5 to 10 to 15 and finally to 20 percent while monitoring the blood and urine sugar responses. Simultaneously, amino acids can be added to the glucose. Renal function involving blood urea nitrogen and creatinine levels, electrolytes, calcium, and phosphorus should be routinely followed. Patients have been maintained on adjunctive intravenous nutritional regimens over extended periods of time, averaging 20 to 25 days, with weight gains being noted in the order of 5 pounds. When practiced with sterile precautions, septic complications have not been a problem. Lanzotti et al. have reported a positive correlation between a good nutritional response to hyperalimentation and the favorably observed, measurable effects of chemotherapy. Intravenous hyperalimentation has proved to be a valuable adjunct in counteracting the effects of radiation enteritis and stomatitis and in restoring the general health status of debilitated patients. As a result, standard protocols and adequate tumor dose radiation have been made possible for these patients.

Concern has been expressed that renewed tumor growth could eventuate from systemic nutritional support. Such views have not been validated by experimental or clinical experiences. The interrelationships of cancer, nutrition, and immunity, and the interactions between tumor and host responses have not been extensively investigated. However, it is apparent that the nutritionally sound or replenished cancer patient is better able to respond to any therapeutic regimen, whether the single or the combined modalities.

THE PATIENT'S SUPPORT SYSTEM

The patient who has a cancer requires a personal support system. Despite the general impression that there is currently a greater public awareness of the growing incidence and consequences of the disease, there are still large gaps in the average person's understanding of what cancer is and of the reality that when detected early, it is often curable. What choices of treatment are available? What complications may occur related to the neoplasm or to the therapeutic efforts? What can be anticipated in the posttherapy period in terms of resumption of normal activities and the requirements of follow-up care? What are the residual limitations of surgery and for how long? What are the side effects, including the morbidity, of adjunctive radiation and/or chemotherapy? What are the realistic expectations of recurrence and complications? Is the goal of the therapeutic regimen palliation or cure? These are all valid questions for the responsible physician and the health professionals who constitute a cancer care team. Information should be provided to the patient and her family, and the opportunity should always exist for free communication about these questions and others which may arise. The cancer care team must act rationally in the face of strong emotions. Each member should be cautious about enthusiastic projections of therapeutic possibilities and prognosis. Promises or statements concerning the patient's prognosis should be restrained and should be determined by what can be accomplished within the framework of the patient's life-style and her family and community support.

The patient who learns she has a cancer is fearful, distraught, and frequently angry and hostile. In the past, the question has been raised as to whether the patient should be informed of her diagnosis. As the public has become better informed and as patient-physician relationships founded on mutual trust and confidence have increased, in most instances it is believed the diagnosis and the prognosis should be shared in understandable terms. When this is not done, the patient frequently learns her diagnosis from some casual inadvertent source. Information gained in this way jeopardizes patient compliance and the interpersonal support relationship.

The nature and extent of the patient's support system in the final analysis depends upon the extent and nature of the tumor and the availability of an effective therapeutic regimen. In self-contained, localized disease, for example, a well-differentiated carcinoma totally confined to the cervix without any evidence of vascular or lymphatic involvement or a well-differentiated endometrial carcinoma found in a small uterus, the choices of therapy and the effectiveness of any reasonable, time-proven protocol permit the cancer care team to look to the future with optimism. A hopeful attitude and the implementation of a routine of regular checkups will effectively motivate the patient and permit her to function normally. On the other hand, advanced or recurrent disease may be and often is punctuated by problems of pain, bleeding, urinary tract or other infections, nausea and vomiting, intestinal cramps, and the possibility of bowel obstruction. Patients confronted with these real or potential problems must recognize their limitations. However, they should be urged to be as active and involved as possible in daily routines which bring them into contact with family, friends, and the social community of their life-style. In effect, the support system should provide qualified cancer care encompassing factual information and the availability of comprehensive diagnostic and therapeutic regimens, combined with essential psychologic and emotional support. Clearly, the personnel requirements and the effectiveness and quality of care require coordination of the efforts of many individuals, i.e., physician, nurse, social worker, and laboratory technician, as well as representatives from such agencies as the American Cancer Society, Cancer Care, the local Visiting Nurse Association, and others who are prepared to participate as patient advocates. A cardinal rule which should always be observed is that if a support system exists, nothing should be done to jeopardize the patient's involvement and her confidence and reliance on it.

CHRONIC AND TERMINAL CARE

The nature of cancer, the emotional response it evokes in patients, families, friends, the community at large, and among health professionals all combine to make chronic and terminal care a challenging and demanding interdisciplinary effort. For the patient, living with the knowledge that palliation may be the reality and goal of whatever therapy is offered, there is a need for honest communication which will provide the patient and her family with some insight as to what may be anticipated. Such communication allows each patient to make adjustments and realistic plans

as to personal behavior, goals, routines, and daily activities. For families and friends, there is a need to be informed about the predictable and unpredictable events that may intervene in the course of the disease. Information concerning possible complications and the limitations of therapeutic efforts must be shared and is generally appreciated. Sensitivity to these issues is an essential prerequisite for the health professionals who care for cancer patients.

What are the ethical considerations in offering patients participation in a prospective clinical trial? What should be the management of the terminally ill patient? What does one tell the patient who asks how long she has to live? These are questions that inevitably arise and require answers. If patients are to be required to undergo combined regimens of extensive surgery, radiation therapy, and/or an extended period of chemotherapy, in most instances they should be fully informed in order to enlist their compliance (Strain) and cooperation. Compassion, gentleness, and the selection of appropriate, understandable words should characterize the physician's communication effort. The patient should sense that the physician will not only provide professional, technical competence, but also be aware personally and supportive of her emotional and psychologic needs. If the patient is capable and desirous of being fully informed, then the physician's responsibility is to the patient and every reasonable effort should be made clearly to answer her questions and to abide by her thinking in terms of maintaining her privacy and confidence. There are some patients who are unable to understand or are overcome by misinformation they have acquired about cancer. Such patients need time to cope with their disease. Responsible family members frequently request that the diagnosis be withheld from a patient, who they feel would be devastated by the information that she has a cancer. Since the patient will need all her family support, it is well to work with and through the family. It is a good idea to identify and establish a relationship with a single responsible family member who is kept fully informed.

THE HOSPICE CONCEPT

Dr. Cicely Saunders and her staff at St. Christopher's Hospice in London, England, deserve the credit for directing special attention to and implementing the needs of terminally ill patients. There is an expanding interest and an increase in the numbers of institutions in the United States dedicated to this movement of providing humane, comprehensive, and sympathetic care to the terminally ill. Dunphy has properly emphasized that hospice care is a concept, not a specially designated building with a specific programmatic orientation. The central focus is letting the patient know that she is not abandoned, that she and her family have an individually oriented backup support system, available 24 hours a day, which is capable of answering all questions and providing for her needs. This system includes relief of pain, nausea and vomiting; consultant oncologic, radiologic, and acute medical services; emotional, psychologic, and psychiatric support; and attention to human spiritual concerns designed to help the interaction between the patient, her family, and the group of concerned professionals and volunteers. It is debatable whether such a program requires an institutional setting or whether much of it can be accomplished at home. Obviously, considerable personal support and resources are needed if the patient is to successfully manage at home. There is little question that many individuals and many families derive mutual support and comfort from the knowledge that terminal days, including death, have been successfully managed at home.

DYING AND DEATH (THANATOLOGY)

Advances in medicine have served to focus society's attention on such issues as a legal definition of death, death with dignity, euthanasia, and other questions having theologic, philosophic, and ethical components. It is beyond the scope of this chapter to add to these debates other than to point to the need for interaction between the life sciences and the social sciences.

Cancer is not a unique terminal disease. Heart disease and chronic nephritis, for example, inevitably result in a patient's demise; yet with these diseases, there is frequently none of the hopelessness and despair which characterize the cancer patient. In part, this is because therapy has little to offer to some cancer patients. However, with the design and implementation of carefully designed prospective clinical trials involving combined modality treatment regimens and timed intervention of chemotherapy, radiation, and surgery, successful remissions are being recorded; individual patients are being provided with opportunities to accomplish personal goals and to function effectively socially.

The physician involved in the care of a dying patient has a responsibility to convey to the patient and her family an attitude of appropriate interest and professional competence. Both the patient and her family should be allowed to feel that every reasonable effort will be mobilized to keep the patient comfortable and capable of functioning in her own milieu. What does one tell the patient who asks how long she has to live? Honest, direct answers are always desirable and permit a supporting relationship to develop, but an honest answer to the above question may not be known. In part it will be determined by the patient's will to live, her ability to maintain an emotional equilibrium, and by her nutritional status.

Dr. Elisabeth Kübler-Ross has made an invaluable contribution to the care of the dying by stressing that dying is a part of living, an expression of our finiteness. She has been a proponent for opening up a dialogue between the patient and physician. She has provided considerable insight into the patient's thinking and feelings; at the same time, she has pointed out the frequent tendency on the part of the professionals, physicians, nurses, etc., to avoid, sometimes even unconsciously to neglect, talking to and providing emotional support to the dying patient. Her observations and writings stress five sequential stages which characterize the reactions of dying patients: (1) denial, (2) rage or anger, (3) bargaining, (4) depression, and (5) acceptance. The ability of the physician to recognize and respond to these manifestations can be mutually helpful in the otherwise potentially uncomfortable and difficult bedside visit.

The physician should prescribe and supervise useful therapy as long as there is the hope of helping the patient. The determination of the patient's status and the possible efficacy of therapeutic measures are questions which can be discussed with a patient who is responsible or with a patient advocate. Aggressive intervention which offers little to the patient is not justified.

SUMMARY OF CLINICAL THERAPEUTIC IMPLICATIONS

This section will provide a synopsis of the natural history of gynecologic malignancies and the essential points in diagnosis that influence prognosis and therapeutic decisions. Detailed discussions of specific neoplasms are presented in these chapters: The

Breast, Chap. 46; The Cervix, Chap. 41; Endometrium, in the The Uterus, Chap. 42; Fallopian Tubes, Chap. 44; Ovaries, Chap. 45; Gestational Trophoblastic Diseases, Chap. 43; Diseases of the Vulva and Vagina, Chap. 40.

CARCINOMA OF THE CERVIX (see Chap. 41)

Carcinoma of the cervix can appear at any age after puberty. The malignant lesion of sarcoma botyroides of the cervix is encountered prior to puberty. Current views hold that invasive carcinoma is preceded by sequential inflammatory, metaplastic, and dysplastic lesions. If undetected, the course may be progression to in situ disease and eventually to invasive carcinoma.

Colposcopic studies combined with careful pathologic correlations have provided important data on the spectrum of physiologic and pathologic conditions encountered clinically. Gradations of dysplasia can be detected in vivo and correlated with abnormal cytology. Severe dysplasia and carcinoma in situ are at times histologically almost indistinguishable. Degrees of dysplasia and carcinoma in situ are frequently noted in the same cervix. It is impossible to predict the biologic significance of the cellular atypia in any single case of dysplasia. Appropriate therapy can only be selected on the basis of individual evaluation. All the dysplasias and, in most instances, in situ cervical carcinoma are asymptomatic.

The progression to invasive carcinoma may express itself as an entity not clinically detectable (microinvasion or occult cancer) or as a gross lesion. The latter may appear as an exophytic, ulcerating, or infiltrating invasive lesion. In advanced cases, patients present with the problems of invasion to adjacent viscera, progressive extension of tumor throughout the pelvis, and evidence of lymphatic spread. The clinical features are uncontrolled hemorrhage, leakage of urine or feces, and persistent back pain, including radiation to a lower extremity if the sacral or obturator nerves are engulfed by tumor. Occasionally, lymph nodes are felt in the groin or a prominent left supraclavicular node may be noted (Virchow's or sentinel node). Such findings should alert the examiner to the possibility of a malignancy, perhaps primary, in the pelvis.

Squamous carcinomas can infiltrate the cervix progressively in a circular manner. Adenocarcinomas of the cervix initially form polypoid projections at the edge of the endocervical canal or the external os, or they may grow endophytically high in the endocervical canal. Such lesions invade the stroma of the endocervical canal in a circular fashion and give rise to the so-called barrel-shaped cervix. The tumor extension beyond the cervix is comparable for both the squamous and adenocarcinomas.

With respect to invasive cervical cancer, approximately 50 percent of cases are diagnosed when localized and more than one-third are discovered with regional node involvement. Unfortunately, since the period 1950 to 1959, there has been little improvement in the overall survival of patients with invasive carcinoma.

The accessibility of the cervix, the availability of cytology, colposcopy, and biopsy, and the growing knowledge of the transformation zone and the pathologic alterations which occur make cervical carcinoma a potentially preventable disease.

CARCINOMA OF THE ENDOMETRIUM (see also Chap. 42)

Unopposed endogenous or exogenous estrogen stimulation continues to be considered a prime etiologic factor in endometrial cancer. Hormonal imbalance expressed by anovulation, relative infertility, and abnormal uterine bleeding, premenopausally or perimenopausally, are associated with this neoplasm. Postmenopausal uterine bleeding, i.e., bleeding which occurs anytime after menses have ceased for 1 year, requires a diagnostic fractional curettage. A presumptive diagnosis of endometrial carcinoma should be investigated in every instance.

As a target organ, the endometrium responds with a spectrum of proliferative activity, resulting in a sometimes difficult-to-interpret variety of histologic patterns including cystic glandular hyperplasia, adenomatous hyperplasia, carcinoma in situ, and invasive carcinoma. When controversy or confusion exists in the histopathologic interpretation, consultation should be obtained prior to the initiation of therapy from qualified individuals having a special interest in gynecologic pathology. Some younger women have been empirically treated with large doses of progesterone. Some have been successfully induced to ovulate, with resumption of cyclic menstrual bleeding and a reversion to normal endometria. The triad of diabetes mellitus, hypertension, and obesity have frequently been clinically associated with endometrial carcinoma. Whether an endocrinopathy exists whose pathophysiology interrelates these frequently associated entities is not clear.

Carcinomas of the endometrium initially form small friable polypoid masses. Myometrial invasion does not occur early. When curettage is followed by prompt hysterectomy, it is often difficult to identify the tumor nidation site. In recent years, the advantages of preoperative irradiation have been recognized and the therapeutic use of surgery alone is reserved for patients with well-differentiated lesions. Most neoplasms are located in the fundus of the uterus (stage I). They infiltrate the surface of the endometrium, forming hyperplastic polypoid masses. Superficial infiltration is followed by myometrial invasion. The neoplasm can extend to the cervical canal and, if the endocervical stromal invasion occurs (stage II), the prognosis is more guarded.

The meshwork of adenomatous elements seen in endometrial carcinoma can be similar to that encountered in simple glandular and cystic hyperplasia. The diagnosis is sometimes difficult and only possible if adequate tissue is available to permit evaluation of the relationship of the various glandular components to one another. In superficial papillary projecting lesions, the glandular elements are closely packed, branched in all directions, and the intervening stroma is not abundant. The neoplasm is frequently infiltrated with inflammatory cells, particularly in areas which are ulcerated and necrotic. Macrophages and plasma cells are also present in the depth and zone of invasion.

If the tumor penetrates through the myometrium, it can involve adjacent pelvic viscera. One or both ovaries, the tubes, bladder, and rectum may have implants. Hematogenous spread is not usual, though hepatic, pulmonary, and brain metastases occur. Lymphatic extension occurs relatively early after myometrial invasion. Unfortunately, the lymph drainage from the uterine fundus is to the paraaortic region. This fact has limited the usefulness of radical hysterectomy and lymphadenectomy in the treatment of advanced stages of the disease. Several clinical protocols have been initiated to determine the usefulness of paraaortic radiation and/or chemotherapeutic adjunctive regimens. All such procedures have had considerable morbidity.

In carcinoma of the endometrium where localized disease has been diagnosed, the survival rate is about the same as in the 1950s. Where regional spread has been encountered, the survival rates are poor. The explanation is unknown.

CARCINOMA OF THE OVARY (see Chap. 45)

Nothing is known about the natural history of ovarian carcinoma that is useful in early detection of a lesion confined to the ovary. Most often ovarian metastases have occurred widely throughout the peritoneal cavity when first diagnosed. The unfortunate aspect of ovarian cancer is that at the time of diagnosis at least half the patients have distant metastases. It is essential that any persistent ovarian enlargement detected on examination in any age group be considered carcinoma until proved otherwise. Any solid or cystic tumor may be malignant, possibly malignant, or benign. In determining therapy, there is the need to clarify whether the tumor has its primary in an ovary or whether the gonadal involvement represents metastatic disease from another site.

Tumors of germ cell origin are generally encountered in childhood, early age, and the teenage period. Postmenopausal neoplasms are predominantly derived from celomic epithelium. The unusual tumors, such as the granulosa-cell carcinoma with its low malignancy, the benign Brenner tumor, the masculinizing arrhenoblastoma, and the dysgerminoma, are seen in the young.

The Diagnostic Problem

Clinically it may be impossible at surgery to determine whether the neoplasm is malignant or not. Frozen-section examination may not clarify the problem. Occasionally, microscopic examination of the permanent sections does not clarify the histology. A tumor which is not confined within the ovarian capsule and which has papillary excrescences poses a dilemma for the surgeon and the pathologist. Malignant disease is usually bilateral. Occasionally a borderline lesion with minimal proliferation of papillary epithelium and questionable invasion of stroma is encountered. In a young patient whose reproductive career is not completed, it is important to establish the histopathologic nature of a tumor. Consultation with a number of pathologists to clarify the histopathology may be necessary.

Cystic or Solid Tumors

Cystic tumors are the commonly encountered ovarian tumors. Cystadenomas are generally benign, though some have a malignant potential; they are either mucinous or serous. Clinically, the dermoid cyst is one of the common tumors seen in young women. The finding of an isolated calcified tooth on x-ray examination of the abdomen is pathognomonic. All solid tumors should be carefully evaluated for cul-de-sac, pelvic viscera, omental, or peritoneal spread.

Classification

In recent years therapy and prognosis have been assessed in relation to specifically identified morphologic types of ovarian tumors. It is anticipated that such studies will provide a clearer understanding of the natural history of the various forms of ovarian carcinoma (Scully). Benign, borderline, and malignant categories in a variety of epithelial neoplasms have been identified. Important considerations involving unilaterality or bilaterality of various tumors, as well as survival rates correlated with current therapeutic approaches, have been clarified. This information is necessary if the prognostic implications of therapeutic regimens are to be more critically analyzed.

The distinction between borderline tumor and true carcinoma is more meaningful from a prognostic viewpoint when applied to serous tumors than to any other category of ovarian cancer. Borderline serous cystadenomas have a 10-year survival rate of 76 percent, in contrast to a 13 percent survival for cases of serous carcinoma. Where borderline tumors were incompletely removed, the 10-year survival rate in patients treated with postoperative radiation was still as high as 74 percent (Santesson, Kottmeier). The important point is that borderline serous tumors appear to be slow-growing, and a rare spontaneous regression has even been reported. Histologic recognition of borderline versus malignant invasive mucinous tumors is more difficult than for serous tumors. While the histopathologic differentiation is difficult, the clinical importance is that the 10-year survival reported for the borderline mucinous cases is 68 percent, compared with 34 percent for the truly invasive tumors. In mucinous tumors, bilaterality is encountered in only about one-fifth of the cases, and extension to uterus and tubes has been reported in only 10 percent.

Metastatic Carcinoma

Most ovarian neoplasms are bilateral. The possibility that any ovarian neoplasm may be a secondary implant should also be recognized. Bilateral ovarian implantation of cancer cells from primary sites in the stomach, large bowel, breast, and uterus must be considered. Krukenberg's tumor represents such a secondary lesion. Hematogenous spread to the ovary from a primary thyroid tumor is a rare occurrence.

Major Problem

Ovarian lesions show symptoms or signs only in more advanced stages. When there has been extension and spillage of malignant cells to adjacent pelvic viscera or peritoneal surfaces, definitive therapy is difficult. Surgical excision is not possible and radiation and chemotherapy are uncertain. The data concerning carcinoma of the ovary make it the major problem in gynecologic oncology. At the present time, the patient who presents herself with ascites, multiple nodular pelvic masses, and symptomatology related to advance disease can be offered only palliation.

CARCINOMA OF THE VULVA AND VAGINA (see also Chap. 40)

It has been theorized for some time that malignant tumors of the vulva and vagina may represent a biologic expression in some patients of an inherent tendency to develop multicentric neoplasms of the anogenital tract (Newman, Cromer; Marcus). The embryologic derivation of vulva, perianal skin, vagina, and a transitional zone of ectocervix from the urogenital sinus has been the basis for this hypothesis. In establishing the diagnosis and planning the therapy for a primary carcinoma of either vulva or vagina, it is necessary to consider the possibility that the cervix, endometrium, or another genital tract site may be involved in an independent primary tumor. With respect to carcinomas of the genital tract, the possibility of multicentric origin of neoplasms is supported by the finding of transitional zones varying from normal to hyperplastic to malignant growth, and by the presence of uninvolved epithelium in an otherwise extensive neoplastic lesion.

Carcinoma of the vulva and vagina is generally considered to be a problem encountered in the seventh and eighth decades of life. Pruritus, bleeding, the palpation of a small lump, or the development of an ulcerated painful sore may bring the patient to the physician. However, single or multiple in situ lesions are observed in younger patients. In the vagina and vulva, the entire epithelium has a neoplastic potential. The existence of transitional zones makes it essential that the margins or periphery of resected specimens be examined for atypical epithelial or mucosal changes. Patients with suspicious and persistent lesions of the vulva, vagina, or perianal areas should have biopsy performed early.

Recent interest has focused upon the daughters of pregnant women who received stilbestrol therapy (Greenwald et al.). The detection of clear-cell carcinoma of the vagina and cervix in such females has focused attention on vaginal adenosis as a possible precancerous lesion. Careful annual examination including Pap smear colposcopy, and directed biopsy of suspicious lesions should be completed on patients with a maternal history of prenatal stilbestrol ingestion.

Melanomas of the skin of the vulva are included with other lesions at this site. Almost two-thirds of the vulvar carcinomas are diagnosed as localized, and about one-third are regional.

Surgery is the treatment of choice. Adjuvant therapies are rarely used for carcinoma of the vulva.

When the inguinal or femoral nodes are not involved, a 5-year survival rate of 70 to 80 percent has been achieved. When groin nodes are involved, the 5-year survival is 40 to 50 percent. When the deep pelvic lymph nodes are involved, the 5-year survival is 10 to 15 percent. Radiotherapy has had little curative value. It has been used postoperatively for palliation. Chemotherapy has offered little relief in advanced lesions. 5-fluorouracil has shown some promise.

Cancers of the vagina are the rarest of female genital malignancies. They are also among the rarest of all female cancers. The yearly incidence is estimated to be only five cancers per million women. Because of the small number of patients with this disease, the survival statistics may not be significant. Vaginal cancers are found predominantly in older women. Over half of the patients are 65 years of age or older at the time of diagnosis.

The reported experience since 1960 indicates that almost half of the vaginal cancers were diagnosed as localized. About one-third of the patients had regional disease; one-sixth were diagnosed with distant metastases. Survival rates for all patients have remained fairly stable since 1950. However, there is an indication of an increased survival for patients recently diagnosed with localized disease. Sixty-four percent of all patients treated had radiation alone. An additional 7 percent received some form of adjuvant therapy with radiation only (Asire, Shambaugh).

The results in general have been discouraging. Overall cure rates of 25 to 35 percent have been reported. Because neglected and advanced carcinomas frequently involve rectum and/or bladder and re-gional lymphatics, the prognosis is guarded whether the therapy consists of radiation or aggressive surgical intervention (Perez et al.).

TROPHOBLASTIC TUMORS (see Chap. 43)

Trophoblastic tumors are conveniently subdivided into two unequal groups, gestational and nongestational. Both types offer special problems in diagnosis and treatment. They have little in common beyond the presence of trophoblast, which elaborates gonadotrophic hormone. The traditional association of choriocarcinoma with hydatidiform mole rests on a numerical basis. In the United States and Great Britain, hydatidiform mole occurs in 1 out of 2000 pregnancies. Choriocarcinoma eventually appears in approximately 1.5 to 5.0 percent of these moles. By contrast, choriocarcinoma occurs following 1 out of 150,000 term deliveries. Comparable figures for choriocarcinoma after abortion not involving hydatidiform mole or after ectopic pregnancy are not reliable.

Gestational trophoblastic growths are unique because they derive from a tissue foreign to the host, originating from placental chorionic epithelium, which is a fetal tissue (Bagshawe). Normal, nonneoplastic trophoblast has special properties which may be either diminished or exaggerated under conditions of neoplasia. These conditions are related to the privileged immunologic position of the trophoblast, the ability to elaborate the polypeptide HCG (human chorionic gonadotropin), and early and widespread bloodstream dissemination.

Early and widespread hematogenous metastases are the general rule in choriocarcinoma. The lungs, liver, and brain are the most favored sites. Metastatic choriocarcinoma has been reported in every organ and tissue in the body except the sclera and articular cartilage, which are avascular. Peculiarly, gestational choriocarcinoma rarely metastasizes to the ovary despite the existence of venous anastomoses between uterus and ovary. Metastatic choriocarcinoma has been found in lymph nodes draining organs with secondary deposits; presumably these metastases are tertiary deposits. Occasional cases of postmolar choriocarcinoma have been reported without residual neoplasm in the uterus. The inference in these cases is that the molar products of conception were evacuated along with any existing neoplastic products. However, tumor embolization occurred prior to evacuation and such cells grew autonomously.

PRINCIPLES OF CANCER SURGERY

FELIX RUTLEDGE

The successful outcome of gynecologic cancers largely depends upon early detection. Less attention has been focused on the adequacy of the initial treatment, which in fact is the critically important issue. The physician who detects the disease and influences the patient's initial management has a responsibility which can literally make the difference between life and death. The multidisciplinary approach has been explicitly stressed in this chapter. Continuous follow-up care must be available and provided as an integrated component of any treatment protocol. If end results are to be carefully assessed and improved, persistent or early recurrent cancer must be promptly detected.

With greater understanding of the physiologic assessment of operative risks, the management of anesthesia and respiratory mechanisms, the microbiologic issues, and the control of sepsis, surgical intervention has remained the prime modality for en block excision and reduction of tumor cell volume, and whenever possible, of regional or distant metastases. While the basic goal is to dissect the cancer in its entirety without transecting the tumor, the reality in advanced cases is that the surgeon is frequently confronted with a challenge to safely reduce tumor population and volume in order to improve the efficacy of adjunctive therapy involving either radiation and/or chemotherapy. As the effectiveness of radiotherapy and chemotherapy, as well as their limitations, is better defined and appreciated, an emerging principle dominates the thinking of oncologists: utilizing the advantages of all or combinations of the available modalities whenever possible in the patient's best interest.

Since each of the modalities has advantages, risks, and complications, the treatment protocols which have evolved generally are designed to avoid predictable complications. Serious consequences occur if radical surgery and radical radiation are employed or if too aggressive chemotherapy is introduced after radical radiation. Impaired wound healing and sepsis, leaking intestinal anastomoses, bone marrow and peripherally expressed myelosuppression, the occurrence of hazardous fistulas, and an increased susceptibility to recurrent infections are iatrogenic developments which can contribute to the morbidity of the cancer patient.

ACUTE EMERGENCIES

Vaginal bleeding can be hemorrhagic but is rarely life-threatening except in the terminal stages of cancer. Bleeding vaginal lesions are usually controlled by vaginal pack. Occasionally bilateral hypogastric artery ligation may be necessary. Acute abdominal events such as rupture, torsion, or infarction of a germ-cell tumor of the ovary in children may force prompt laparotomy. Not infrequently ovarian cancer causes intestinal obstruction that requires prompt intervention. However, in general there is ample time for the physician to complete the diagnostic search and evaluation and to prepare the patient safely for optimal treatment.

FACTORS INFLUENCING SURGICAL TREATMENT

Location

The complexity of surgical treatment is affected by the location of the primary lesion along the genital tract. A lesion at either end of the tract, such as the vulva at the lower end or the ovary at the top, is suited for surgical excision because it is relatively distant from the rectum and the bladder. Moderately advanced cancers of the cervix and vagina are less likely to be resectable because they are close to the bladder and rectum, which may be injured during the surgery or through sacrifice of blood vessels or nerves. Furthermore, each may contain metastasis. For this situation irradiation methods may be chosen instead. Lesions of intermediate position, such as the endometrium or lower vaginal tract, may be resectable. However, irradiation is often given as a supplement to expand the range of the treatment.

Advancement of Growth

Treatment becomes more complex as the cancer spreads. This explains the wide range of operations that are acceptable, from cryoconization for cervical lesions and local excision for vulvar lesions to extended surgery for advanced carcinoma of the cervix and high-dosage irradiation for late-stage lesions which have spread.

Very early, "thin layer," shallow carcinomas covering a small area of the vulva, cervix, or endometrium may be treated by excision (vulvectomy or conventional hysterectomy). Healing will be prompt, the risk of complications minor, and the patient can be assured of a successful outcome. Carcinoma in situ or microinvasive carcinoma of the vulva, cervix, and endometrium all have these prospects. An ovarian carcinoma which is mobile and readily resectable, as well as endometrial cancer with favorable features, is also managed by conservative operation. A moderately advanced cancer at any site along the genital tract or in lymphatics or blood vessels to which it has spread may require both surgery and irradiation.

SURGICAL TREATMENT OF CARCINOMA OF THE CERVIX

Surgery may be the only treatment for cervical carcinoma or may be combined with irradiation in the following ways: (1) surgery may precede irradiation; (2) surgery may be carried out with irradiation as adjunctive treatment; or (3) surgery may follow irradiation.

Radical Hysterectomy

The hysterectomy for invasive cancer of the cervix must excise the paracervical, paravaginal tissues, and the upper one-third to one-half of the vagina. The position of the ureters along the cervix and the upper vagina limits the lateral boundary for excising the uterus to a line close to the cervix. The ureters must be moved laterally to avoid their injury by the dissection. The bladder and rectum are separated from the vagina below the midvagina. The cardinal and uterosacral ligaments are transected near the pelvic wall. The radical hysterectomy disrupts additional blood vessels and nerves to the ureters, bladder, and rectum. These consequences are noted by impaired function during the postoperative recovery.

The hazards of radical hysterectomy are intraoperative hemorrhage, postoperative sepsis, fistulation of urine or feces, and disturbed voiding. Recovery time is longer than from the conventional conservative hysterectomy.

Radical hysterectomy is an effective treatment for invasive carcinoma of the cervix, stages I and II. Its success has been defined and its limitations clarified by comparison with irradiation therapy. That radical hysterectomy has survived as a complete treatment for this disease affirms some advantages over irradiation therapy. These advantages are only evident when the operation is used properly.

Advantages of Radical Hysterectomy. Effective surgical excision has the following advantages: (1) There can be no recurrence of cancer in organs that are excised. (2) Ovaries need not be sacrificed and will continue to supply hormones, which benefit younger patients. (3) Information obtained at laparotomy provides a more certain prognosis than that obtained by alternative methods. There are also the gains from avoiding the shortcomings of irradiation therapy, such as (4) the radioresistance of some carcinomas, (5) the late-irradiation complications of the bladder and rectum, (6) the prolonged treatment, (7) the probability of activating chronic pelvic inflammatory disease, (8) the need to expose normal organs to irradiation, and (9) the need for prior removal of infected or cystic adnexa.

Disadvantages of Radical Hysterectomy. In performing radical hysterectomy, the following realities must be recognized: (1) Only some patients with carcinoma are suitable candidates for extended surgical treatment. (2) Radical hysterectomy is more hazardous, with a greater risk of death from an acute surgical complication. (3) The vagina is shortened. (4) There are more urinary and rectal fistulas after extended surgical treatment than after irradiation treatment. (5) Frequently there is need for postoperative x-ray therapy for metastases discovered at operation.

Indications for Radical Hysterectomy. For the early-stage carcinoma of the cervix the cure rate will be as good with radical hysterectomy as with irradiation therapy. Radical hysterectomy is preferred for the young patient since ovarian function can be conserved and the pliability of the vaginal canal maintained. In the properly selected, thin, healthy, and young patient, complications are infrequent. Yet for radical hysterectomy to provide 5-year survival results equal to radium and external therapy, the carcinoma must be small (stage I or IIA). With few exceptions, moderately advanced stage IIB cervical cancer is better treated by irradiation.

In addition to early-stage lesions, these other exceptional circumstances support a preference for radical hysterectomy: (1) Individuals with prior pelvic inflammatory disease are less suitable for irradiation therapy until the adnexa are removed. (2) If laparotomy is necessary, the surgeon may choose to complete the treatment by radical hysterectomy where cancer obstructs the proper application of a radium system and cannot be corrected by preliminary x-ray therapy. (3) A combination of carcinoma of the cervix and pregnancy may offer an opportunity to deliver the fetus by cesarean section followed by radical hysterectomy if the cancer is at a suitable stage. (4) Histologic types of tumors which have been identified as radioresistant should be considered for radical hysterectomy.

Radical hysterectomy may be suitable treatment and the preferred management for recurrent cancer of the cervix or a new growth in the area of a previously irradiated carcinoma of the cervix. A small proportion of patients with carcinoma of the cervix will have a localized central recurrence suitable for resection by radical hysterectomy. The hazards of the procedure under these conditions are considerably increased because of the diminished tolerance of the tissue and of its ability to heal due to prior irradiation treatment.

Thus, the role of the radical hysterectomy in gynecologic cancer is mainly that of treatment for early cancer of the cervix. To be suitable for this treatment, the carcinoma must be confined to the cervix or must have only minimal spread to the vagina and immediate vicinity of the cervix. A lesion which extends a distance into the parametrium and involves the ureter and base of the bladder cannot be resected by means of this operation. Proper selection of the stage of cervical cancer for radical operation strongly affects the percentage of cure. Therefore, thorough preoperative study of the disease must be completed.

Preirradiation Laparotomy

Laparotomy and definitive surgery are sometimes needed to prepare the carcinoma for primary irradiation. This preparation is essential where the infected adnexa must be removed prior to irradiation to avoid exacerbating an existing pelvic infection. Preirradiation surgery is also necessary (1) to establish renal competence when severe ureteral obstruction impairs renal function, or (2) if intestinal obstruction is present.

Occasionally preirradiation exploratory laparotomy is important to establish the extent of the disease, which may have extended or metastasized beyond reach of the clinical examination. When intrauterine pregnancy exists, surgery before irradiation is necessary to deliver a viable fetus. Surgery before irradiation should facilitate irradiation; thus the surgeon should take care not to create an impediment, such as to remove a receptacle for intracavitary radium, create a postoperative urinary or bowel fistula, or cause pelvic infection.

Combined or Adjunctive Therapy

The frequency with which both irradiation and surgery are used for the treatment of cancer of the cervix de-

pends on the philosophy of the physician in charge and the nature of the clinical problem. Patients cannot tolerate both radical surgery and high-dose irradiation without excessive complications. To maintain reasonable safety, either the dose of radiation or the extent of surgery must be reduced. It is our practice to reduce the latter rather than decrease the radiation dose. In patients requiring combination therapy, the disease is usually advanced and bulky and likely to have metastases; hence irradiation therapy has advantages. The extrafascial conservative hysterectomy is intended to complement the total irradiation of the residual viable cancer. Only a few of the patients treated for cancer of the cervix by irradiation will require combination therapy. Hysterectomy should not be routine after irradiation because for most patients the latter is sufficient. Furthermore, even with allowances made for healing impairment due to preoperative irradiation, still more complications should be expected. If the patients are properly selected and the surgery pursued to accomplish a cure not otherwise expected, the greater risk is acceptable.

SURGERY AS THE PRIMARY TREATMENT OF ENDOMETRIAL CARCINOMA

Total hysterectomy with bilateral salpingo-oophorectomy has proved successful in curing adenocarcinoma of the endometrium in the majority of patients and is thus the principal operation for it. Some patients benefit from preoperative intracavitary radium therapy and others from preoperative external radiotherapy of the pelvis. Selection of patients who would benefit from the additional irradiation has been a matter of debate over the past 20 years as varied clinical experience has been reported. Some physicians rarely employ preoperative radiation if the uterine size is small and the tumor thought to be limited to the corpus. Others design an individual treatment plan around features of the cancer that indicate possible myometrial invasion and hence likelihood of regional metastasis. A third school of thought believes in regularly treating endometrial cancer by both preoperative irradiation and hysterectomy.

Treatment of cancer of the corpus, like that of cervical cancer, is by operation alone in the patient for whom conditions are favorable, such as the existence of a small, confined lesion that has not deeply invaded or extended to the endocervix and that is less prone to metastasis to the vagina, parametrium, or regional nodes.

The following questions require attention in the pretreatment evaluation of the patient before a decision can be reached about employing irradiation:

1. Is the patient physically able to tolerate the operation? If not, irradiation must be employed although the cancer may be ideal for resection.
2. Is the cancer limited to the uterus? Although most patients have stage I cancer, spread to the cervix (stage II) is next most common. When this happens, conservative hysterectomy is no longer sufficient. As in the case of the squamous cancer of the cervix, conservative hysterectomy would not assure an adequate cancer-free margin around the tumor. Either radical hysterectomy or irradiation is needed to eliminate this portion of the cancer.
3. Has the cancer spread to the adnexa? Involvement of the regional pelvic structures (stage III) is a finding in about 10 percent of patients at the time of treatment. Most clinicians are then uncertain about the adequacy of conservative total hysterectomy and bilateral salpingo-oophorectomy and they supplement surgery with irradiation. The physician should search for pelvic masses, which may be metastases, and treat them preoperatively with x-rays. External irradiation postoperatively is common only because metastases are often discovered only during laparotomy.

    Metastases to regional pelvic organs which cannot be resected completely deserve postoperative irradiation. Adjuvant progestins can also be continued for extended periods after irradiation therapy.
4. What is the risk of metastasis to pelvic or aortic nodes? Before laparotomy, it is more difficult to detect metastasis in lymph nodes than metastasis in adnexa, as the former is usually not palpable. The information must be obtained indirectly or by predictions based on the size of the uterus and the histologic pattern.

Lymphangiography is still being tested as to accuracy. Sonography and computerized axial tomography, in experienced hands, have shown promise in detecting nodal involvement.

When lymph-node metastasis is expected, the standard operation is not adequate. For instance, when the fundus of the uterus is enlarged and/or the microscopic patterns of the endometrium are undifferentiated, surgery should be supplemented by external therapy or should include lymphadenectomy.

Radical hysterectomy for endometrial adenocarcinoma which has extended to the cervix is controversial. Yet it is assumed that the pattern of vascular spread and the influence upon contiguous organs are the same as if the lesion were primary in the cervix. Therefore, if surgery is advocated, the range of operations should be similar.

There has been much less experience with radical hysterectomy for stage II endometrial carcinoma because this lesion is less common than primary carcinoma of the cervix and the patients are usually older, obese, and less suited physically for extended hysterectomy. However, stage II corpus et collum of the endometrium is currently accepted as an indication for radical hysterectomy.

SURGICAL TREATMENT OF OVARIAN CANCER

Adjunctive external therapy and/or chemotherapy must be incorporated into carefully designed protocols if increased salvage is to be secured for patients with ovarian cancer. Since only about one-third of the patients are cured, a large part of the clinician's task concerns palliation. For this, surgery retains a role, although a smaller one than chemotherapy.

If surgery is to be effective, the cancer must be completely excised. To a lesser degree surgery can be useful even when complete resection is impossible by reducing the total tumor cell population and so enhancing the effect of irradiation therapy. To accomplish either end, the surgeon must be aware that, unlike other female genital cancers with a predictable direction of spread, ovarian cancer disseminates rapidly by (1) implantation about the peritoneal cavity and (2) the lymphatics. These facts should determine which areas are searched for metastasis, what tissues are excised for completeness, and where biopsies are needed to map the distribution of the cancer. The most effective surgeon will tenaciously dissect an apparently unresectable mass of ovarian cancer until it becomes clear it cannot be removed short of causing injury that would nullify the objective, for instance, uncontrollable hemorrhage, injury to bowel or urinary systems which would delay or exclude postoperative irradiation or chemotherapy, or entry into the bowel in a way that would risk peritoneal contamination and postoperative abscess.

Because ovarian cancer is so complex, the scope of the surgery cannot be predicted preoperatively nor can rigid dicta about minimal or maximal resection be adopted before laparotomy. However, for common ovarian epithelial cancer of Müllerian origin, certain guidelines are accepted:

1. Only in unusual circumstances can fertility be preserved. Both ovaries must be removed, the single exception being an intact, unilateral, nonadherent, nonmetastatic, mucinous ovarian cancer with well-differentiated microscopic pattern. Total abdominal hysterectomy with bilateral salpingo-oophorectomy is standard treatment.
2. Excision of an uninvolved omentum is debatable. The technical difficulty of complete removal, as well as the added hazard to the patient, leads some surgeons to favor partial removal. Yet this is of questionable value, and some gynecologists leave the uninvolved omentum intact. Nevertheless, the frequency of metastasis to the omentum supports regularly removing it, even when it is apparently uninvolved. Less controversial is complete removal when the omentum contains a metastasis.
3. Exenteration is not effective and has no place in this type of cancer.
4. Intestinal surgery, for instance resection of a loop of bowel, may be beneficial if it will complete the removal of a cancer or relieve intestinal obstruction.
5. An exploratory, "second look" laparotomy may be helpful after 12 to 18 months of good response to chemotherapy. Most tumors can be assessed accurately by clinical examination, sonography, or roentgenography. But when a tumor regresses so that it cannot be felt, or when it remains unchanged, questions arise that may be answered only by laparotomy. For instance, can chemotherapy be stopped, should the agent be changed, has the tumor become operable, or has the tumor become small enough for treatment by external therapy?

SURGERY FOR CARCINOMA OF THE VAGINA

Surgery is applicable for superficial lesions of the vagina at any level of the vaginal canal. A "radical hysterectomy" type of dissection is appropriate for invasive but still early lesions of the upper vagina. The lesions should be small, with a distribution equivalent to stage I or IIA cancer of the cervix. The depth of penetration should be the determining factor for lesions elsewhere along the vaginal tract. Location about the axis of the vagina is also important. Lesions immediately beneath the bladder or around the rectum are less suited to resection because a margin of tumor-free tissue is not available.

Exenteration may serve as primary treatment or as second choice after irradiation that fails to eradicate a carcinoma. If a surgical approach is selected, exenteration may be necessary for advanced tumors adherent to rectum and bladder. As exenteration carries a high risk and the prospect of marked disability even when successful, it is not justified if irradiation offers a reasonable chance for control.

For clear-cell carcinomas of the vagina, both surgery and irradiation are useful. As the majority of the lesions are in the upper one-third of the vagina, this type of carcinoma may be suitable for radical hysterectomy and lymphadenectomy. The upper half of the vagina must be included. More advanced lesions require exenteration if the bladder and/or rectum are involved. Irradiation is an alternative because clear-cell carcinoma is radiosensitive. Combining first irradiation and then a more limited surgery may also be advantageous. Larger lesions require more extensive treatment, such as exenteration. Often anterior exenteration will be sufficient. Plastic reconstruction of the vagina becomes part of the treatment.

SURGERY FOR CARCINOMA OF THE VULVA

Carcinoma of the vulva is eminently suitable for total excision. The vulva's anatomy, which guides the surgeon along planes and so assists adequate excision, the generally slow growth rate, and the predictable pathways of spread have all contributed to the 5-year cure rate of approximately 65 percent. A variety of operations are employed so that favorable results can be obtained for a range of patients, including the elderly and infirm.

Radical Vulvectomy and Bilateral Inguinal Lymphadenectomy

The standard operation for the majority of patients is radical vulvectomy and bilateral inguinal lymphadenectomy. It is appropriate for resectable lesions of all stages. However, clinical experience has led to the tentative conclusion that excellent results may be obtained with less extensive operations when the carcinoma is small and has not invaded deeply.

Radical Vulvectomy Without Inguinal Lymphadenectomy

For elderly, infirm patients who would fall in the high operative risk category for the more extended node dissection, the preferred operation is radical vulvectomy without inguinal lymphadenectomy. The operation is indicated if (1) the inguinal nodes are clinically negative and the primary carcinoma is less than 2 cm in diameter or (2) the primary lesion covers a larger area but is shallow.

To omit removing inguinal nodes is to balance the lower risk of operative mortality against the risk of recurrence in the retained nodes. Most recurrences are near the site of the primary tumor. The risk may be somewhat reduced by pre- or postoperative irradiation as a substitute for node removal. In view of satisfactory results obtained with the newer x-ray equipment, this approach promises to become more popular.

Radical Vulvectomy With Inguinal and Pelvic Lymphadenectomy

Metastasis to pelvic wall nodes is so infrequent that routine removal of the nodes is unwarranted. On the other hand, metastasis to the pelvic nodes without involvement of inguinal nodes seldom occurs; thus this first chain of inguinal nodes is studied carefully as a guide to the status of the deeper nodes.

Pelvic wall nodes should be removed if (1) the inguinal nodes appear positive on clinical examination or are proved positive by preoperative biopsy with histologic examination; (2) Cloquet's node demonstrates metastasis when removed and studied by frozen section at the time clinically normal inguinal nodes are removed; (3) the carcinoma discloses a histologic pattern of a melanoma or a Bartholin's gland tumor; or (4) the carcinoma (regardless of histologic type) originated on or spread to the clitoris or the vaginal mucosa.

The Operation

For invasive carcinoma, complete vulvectomy is superior to local excision because (1) multicentric development is frequent in vulvar cancer so that local excision runs an excessive risk of recurrence, and (2) the rich interconnection of lymphatics in the vulva

permits metastasis contralateral to the lesion. Hence, bilateral removal of the labia as well as the mons is essential.

In excising the vulva, the resection lines may vary from person to person depending on the location and size of the lesion and on the condition of the surrounding labial skin. Generally the labial-crural fold serves as the lateral boundary. Removal of the mons establishes the superior excision line. The size and position of the lesion determine the perineal boundary.

An en block resection of the fibroadipose node-bearing tissue in the groin often includes a bridge of overlying skin extending back to the vulva. The contents of the femoral triangle are removed and the femoral vein and artery stripped clean of node-bearing tissue. These vessels are then protected by transfer and reattachment of the superior end of the sartorius muscle. The reapproximated skin is tense and its survival precarious.

For the pelvic wall node dissection, the surgeon approaches the retroperitoneal area through an inguinal hernia type of incision. The node-containing tissue about the external and internal iliac vessels is excised to the level of the common iliac bifurcation.

Exenteration

About one-fourth of advanced lesions that invade the rectum or bladder are controlled by exenteration. Advanced and complicated carcinoma of the vulva that at first seems hopeless thus may warrant a trial of treatment. Extended operation supplemented by external therapy will usually be beneficial.

PELVIC EXENTERATION IN GYNECOLOGIC ONCOLOGY

Pelvic exenteration is an accepted treatment for cervical carcinoma too advanced for conventional treatment or recurrent after primary therapy. It is a formidable procedure and carries great risk because of the limited margin of safety. One error in management can eliminate the benefits. The risk can be justified only if there is a good chance for long-term control of the cancer.

Successful pelvic exenteration depends upon (1) careful selection of patients, (2) thorough preoperative study, (3) a definitive plan for resection and reconstruction, (4) skillful performance of the procedure, and (5) meticulous postoperative care and support of the patient.

The two basic criteria in patient selection are: (1) the tumor must be totally resectable, and (2) the patient must have an adequate physical and emotional reserve for recovery. Pelvic exenteration is contraindicated if the patient is elderly, obese, emotionally unstable or uncertain (or if her family is), has undergone excessive high-dose irradiation to the same area, or has systemic disease that makes her a poor operative risk. These are common criteria for undertaking any major surgery. For this radical, stressful procedure, however, they should be rigidly observed.

Pelvic exenteration is indicated if the cancer is too large to be removed by less radical procedures, if it involves the bladder and/or rectum but has not invaded the pelvic wall structures, and if has not rigidly attached itself to large pelvic wall vessels, nerves or fascia. Thus the first move in preoperative study is to assess resectability of the lesion.

The final decision must be made at laparotomy. Exenteration should be abandoned (1) if the cancer is found beyond the pelvic region; this finding carries a poor prognosis which is not altered by extending the dissection; (2) if the lesion does not allow a cancer-free margin; (3) if there are metastases to the small intestine or omentum which have become adherent within the pelvis—even if such foci are resectable; infiltration of these organs suggests probable metastasis along node groups that are not resectable, which would render the operation useless; (4) if there is a positive finding in bilateral pelvic wall nodes or large, adherent metastases in the pelvic nodes of one side; (5) if there is a positive finding in aortic nodes.

In reality, relatively few patients qualify for pelvic exenteration. It is unusual for any cancer center to perform more than 20 to 25 per year. It is also important for the physician to be aware of the operative hazards when counseling patients. Operative mortality was 20 percent in the early years of this procedure. This has declined to a very respectable 5 to 10 percent. Common postoperative complications follow from disruption of the gastrointestinal tract or reconstruction of the diversionary urinary tract. The fault is the large defect in the pelvic cavity resulting from removal of the bladder, rectum, vagina, uterus, tubes, ovaries, and pelvic wall lymph nodes. This large denuded cavity is then occupied by the small bowel. Adhesions associated with obstruction and leading to necrosis and fistula formation are frequent. As surgeons learn better how to deal with this pelvic defect, these complications will become less frequent.

The most common cause of failure is that the disease has spread beyond the field of resection. The massive, advanced cancers suited to the operation are also those most likely to recur within the pelvic area. In addition, patients who have undergone high-dosage irradiation, as many facing exenteration have, are more difficult to evaluate as prospects for resection and also experience a higher incidence of postoperative complication.

Exenteration may be used as the primary treatment for very advanced carcinomas of the pelvis, or for special tumors thought to be radioresistant. However, it is most often used in recurrent cancer after a tolerance dose of irradiation has been administered. The 5-year cure rate varies appreciably depending upon whether the operation was the primary treatment or a secondary one. The cure rate is better in the former case, as patients in the latter situation experience complications from the irradiation therapy. However, the 5-year cure rate of 30 percent for all patients undergoing this operation makes it an acceptable and reliable procedure in gynecologic oncology. When pelvic exenteration is employed for recurrent cancer of the cervix following primary irradiation therapy, the cure rate compares favorably with cure rates following operations upon lung and gastric cancer and primary resection of some of the lower GI tract tumors.

PRINCIPLES OF RADIATION THERAPY

J. TAYLOR WHARTON
GILBERT L. FLETCHER

BASIC PHYSICS

Both gamma rays and x-rays are photon irradiation produced by radioactive sources such as radioactive ^{60}Co or generators. The energy lost in the decay of radioactive nuclei appears as gamma rays. Generators accelerate electrons which may be used directly, or the electrons may strike a target and x-rays appear. The electrons may be accelerated in a circular fashion (betatron) or in a linear fashion (linear accelerator).

Photons interact with the atoms of the medium which they traverse by removing orbital electrons from the atom, producing ion pairs. The process is called *ionization*. The electron ejected from the atomic structure, called the *secondary electron*, dislodges in its path electrons from other atoms until all of its energy is used. The negatively charged electrons or electron clusters hit sensitive areas of the deoxyribonucleic acid (DNA) producing damage. The damage (due to single or multiple hits) may be lethal or sublethal depending on the dose per fraction and the dose rate. In addition, cells are damaged by free hydroxyl radicals produced as the ionization interacts with free molecular oxygen. These radicals disrupt molecular bonds and potentiate the lethal effect of photon irradiation. The oxygen tension with the tumor mass frequently assumes critical importance in the eradication attempt since it requires $2\frac{1}{2}$ times more irradiation to render a hypoxic cell nonviable.

The rate at which an ionizing particle loses energy along its path in the medium is termed linear energy transfer (LET). LET is measured by the number of ion pairs produced by irradiation per unit length traveled in the medium. The difference in LET for photons and electrons compared with heavy particles is well demonstrated in cloud chambers. With photon beam or electron beam (photon beams first make secondary electrons), one sees a sparse track in the cloud chamber—there is a low LET per unit length. Such particles as neutrons (a mass 1800 times greater than electrons), alpha particles, which are the nucleus of helium (a mass 4 times greater than the neutron), and, of course, heavier particles produce very dense tracks in the cloud chamber. When a strand of DNA is hit by low-LET irradiation, that single hit may produce only sublethal damage which can be repaired; when a strand of DNA is hit by the dense

track of high-LET irradiation, the damage is more often lethal and nonreparable.

Low-LET irradiation frequently has to rely on multiple hits, plus the indirect effect of hydroxyl radicals, to produce lethal damage to a cell. High-LET irradiation produces a cell kill by itself, no free oxygen is required, and it is effective on the anoxic cells of a tumor.

BIOLOGICAL ACTION OF RADIATION

The biological damage done to DNA by ionizing radiation may be severe enough to destroy the cell's ability to divide indefinitely. This cell is then classified as nonviable. In tissue culture, viability is the ability to produce a clone (Fig. 47–1). Following a given dose of irradiation, the percentage of cells destroyed is constant, regardless of the number of cells present (Table 47–1). This dose can be compared with an artillery unit shelling a city. Assume that a given dose of irradiation therapy is equivalent to a barrage consisting of a given number of shells, and that the cells in the tissue culture represent houses. Assume also that one hit is enough to destroy a house. The first barrage will destroy a number of the

FIGURE 47–1 Appearance of clones developing from normal and irradiated HeLa cells. *(1)* Colonies developing on a plate seeded with 200 S_3 HeLa cells and incubated 9 days in growth. *(2)* Colonies developing on a plate identical with that of *(1)* in every respect except that the plate was irradiated with 300 rads before incubation. *(From Puck et al.)*

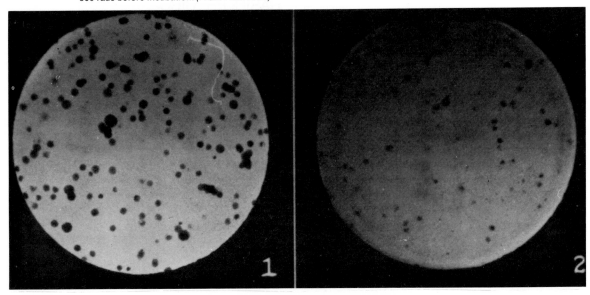

TABLE 47–1 Number of Cells Killed with Each 380-rad Radiation Dose Increment for Model Cell Population*

Accumulated dose, rads†	Radiation dose, increments of 380 rads	Number of viable cells irradiated	Number of cells killed	Number of cells surviving
380	380 × 1	10,000,000,000	9,000,000,000	1,000,000,000
760	380 × 2	1,000,000,000	900,000,000	100,000,000
1,140	380 × 3	100,000,000	90,000,000	10,000,000
1,520	380 × 4	10,000,000	9,000,000	1,000,000
1,900	380 × 5	1,000,000	900,000	100,000
2,280	380 × 6	100,000	90,000	10,000
2,660	380 × 7	10,000	9,000	1,000
3,040	380 × 8	1,000	900	100
3,420	380 × 9	100	90	10
3,800	380 × 10	10	9	1

*Initial population = 10^{10} viable cells; 90 percent of cells irradiated are killed by 380 rads; 10 percent of cells irradiated survive 380 rads.
†The total dose given at each level, i.e., 1 × 380 or 10 × 380, was given as a single treatment. There is no time elapsed between dose increments.
Source: Suite, in Fletcher, 1973.

houses in the target area. The next barrage with the same number of shells will destroy the same percent of the intact houses as did the first barrage. The following barrages will continue to destroy a constant percentage of the remaining intact houses. It is apparent that a town with a smaller number of houses can be destroyed with fewer barrages than can a town with a large number of houses. This is the same situation that exists in the tumor. A tumor consisting of 10^{10} cells will require more radiation to render all cells nonviable than does one consisting of 10^4 cells. These predictable results can be obtained only in the fixed environment of tissue culture. The experimental data can be represented by a mathematical formula (Suite, 1973).

In a human tumor population, the situation is not as well controlled and other variables play a role. The major variable is the presence of free oxygen. If cells are anoxic or deeply hypoxic, it takes more irradiation to render them nonviable. One can demonstrate that a small fraction of anoxic cells determines most of the irradiation dose required (Table 47–2). There is considerable evidence that it takes very few malignant clonogenic cells, possibly only one cell, for a tumor to stay active. Therefore, the control of a tumor can be achieved only by rendering nonviable all or nearly all malignant clonogenic cells. Considerably more radiation is required for control of large tumor masses because they contain more malignant cells and have a greater proportion of anoxic cells.

A microscopic aggregate of cancer cells or even clinical disease which is not microscopic can be con-

TABLE 47–2 Influence of Cell Number and Proportion of Anoxic Cells on Single Dose Necessary for Eradication of a Mammalian Cell Population (HeLa cells)

Oxic cells: A single dose of 380 rads kills 90 percent of the cell population.
Anoxic cells: A single dose of 380 × 2.5 = 950 rads kills 90 percent of the cell population.
    All cells oxic:
        10^9 cells (3-cm diameter): 380 rads kills 0 percent of $10^9 \rightarrow 10^8$ surviving cells.
        10^2 cells: 380 rads kills 90 percent of $10^2 \rightarrow 10^1$ surviving cells.
        10^9 cells: 380 × 9 = 3160 rads $\rightarrow$ 0 surviving cells.
    1/100 cells anoxic:
        Oxic cells 10^9 10^6 = 380 × 3 = 1140 rads
        Anoxic cells 10^6 = 950 × 6 = 5900 rads
                              7040 rads $\rightarrow$ 0 surviving cells

Source: Fletcher, 1974.

trolled with amounts of irradiation which do not exceed normal tissue tolerance. Considerable clinical data show that 5000 rads in 5 weeks given electively produces almost complete freedom of disease in lymphatics which have a known risk of containing occult deposits (subclinical disease). Such deposits later would show clinical metastases if unirradiated, as has been well documented in squamous-cell carcinoma of the upper respiratory and digestive tracts as well as in adenocarcinoma of the breast (Table 47–3). In contradistinction, to obtain 90 percent control of masses 3 to 5 cm in diameter, doses on the order of 7000 to 9000 rads are required.

Tumor-Mass Composition

A tumor mass has a mixed composition of clonogenic malignant cells, nonclonogenic malignant cells, and connective tissue, including the vascular system. The proportion of these components varies from tumor to tumor according to histology, growth pattern, and tissue invaded. For instance, an exophytic, friable mass on the exocervix is highly cellular and well vascular-

ized, whereas the same squamous-cell carcinoma in the cervix and lower uterine segment has more connective tissue and muscle component with hypoxic areas.

The measured growth of a tumor is a function of the length of the cell cycle (fast-dividing cells have a shorter cell cycle) and of the cell loss. Some cells become nonviable and therefore are lost to the proliferative capacity of the tumor. It is the balance of cell loss and cell population which determines the physical growth.

Regression Rate

Irradiation delivered either by external beam or by repeated intracavitary gamma-ray applications causes reduction in tumor size. Large lesions have multiple areas of focal necrosis, with hypoxic and anoxic cells present in the vicinity of these areas. As the mass shrinks, capillaries get closer to these areas, and eventually there should be a return of normal oxygenation throughout the tumor as it reaches a small size. In other words, protracted irradiation allows probable

TABLE 47–3 Probability of Control Correlated With Irradiation Dose and Volume of Cancer

Dosage, rads	Squamous-cell carcinoma of the upper respiratory and digestive tracts	Adenocarcinoma of the breast
5000*	>90% subclinical 60% T_1 lesions of nasopharynx ~50% 2- to 3-cm neck nodes	>90% subclinical
6000*	80–90% T_1 lesions of pharynx and larynx ~50% T_3 + T_4 lesions of tonsillar fossa	
7000*	~90% 1- to 3-cm neck nodes ~70% 3- to 5-cm neck nodes 80–90% T_2 lesions of tonsillar fossa and supraglottic larynx ~80% T_3 + T_4 lesions of tonsillar fossa	90% clinically positive axillary nodes 2.5–3 cm†
7000–8000 (8–9 wk)		65% 2- to 3-cm primary 30% > 5-cm primary
8000–9000 (8–10 wk)		56% > 5-cm primary
8000–10,000 (10–12 wk)		75% > 5- to 15-cm primary

*1000 rads per five fractions per week.
†The control rate is corrected for the percentage of nodes that would have been positive histologically if a dissection of the axilla had been done.
Source: Fletcher, Shukovsky. Used by permission.

reoxygenation of the hypoxic cells during regression.

The regression rate of a mass varies considerably, depending upon its composition. Exophytic, friable tumors shrink very rapidly by the sloughing process, whereas infiltrating tumors have a slower regression rate, and often at the end of treatment there is still a palpable mass.

The presence of a palpable mass should not be equated with the existence of malignant clonogenic cells. Irradiated cells may divide several times even though lethal damage has been done to their genetic material, and the daughter cells will produce aborted clones. There have been experimental studies showing that one cannot differentiate morphologically between tumor cells which are rendered nonviable and those which are still viable (Suite, 1964). In clinical practice, the presence of morphologically intact cells in a biopsy or surgical specimen taken within 2 to 3 months after irradiation does not mean that there are actually clonogenic malignant cells. This fact should be considered when evaluating a patient within this interval for residual disease.

Radiosensitivity

Radiobiological studies and clinical observations show no intrinsic difference in radiosensitivity between epithelial cancers of similar sizes. As previously indicated, microscopic foci of squamous carcinomas in the lymphatics of the neck can be controlled by 5000 rads in 5 weeks, as can microscopic foci of adenocarcinoma of the breast in the supraclavicular area.

The growth patterns of tumors have a bearing on the efficacy of control of irradiation. For instance, adenocarcinoma and squamous carcinoma of identical size on the exocervix are equally easily controlled by irradiation. As a rule, however, adenocarcinoma originates in the endocervix, grows silently, invades the myometrium, and reaches a barrel-shaped form. This growth pattern is often the reason for failure of irradiation. The growth pattern is also a cause of failure when squamous carcinoma is in the same location and of the same size.

Biological radioresistance must not be confused with inadequate irradiation. With applicators, because of the steep fall-off dose with intracavitary gamma-ray sources, underdosage can easily occur because of (1) a gap between the intrauterine and vaginal radium, (2) downward displacement of the radium system, (3) malposition of the colpostats, and (4) use of a vaginal cylinder instead of colpostats.

Tumor Control Versus Dose

The concept of an "all-or-none" tumor-control dose has dominated radiotherapy since the discovery of radium and x-rays. Clinical experience has shown this concept to be incorrect because higher doses are required to sterilize gross masses than to control subclinical aggregates of tumor cells. The radiobiology of this finding was discussed in the previous section. Furthermore, an increasing control rate with higher doses for similarly sized tumors places tumor control partially on a probabilistic basis. The dose-response curve has a sigmoid shape.

In 1944, Strandqvist showed a dose-response curve for carcinoma of the skin (Fig. 47–2). There is a similar curve for skin damage, demonstrating a fundamental principle in radiotherapy which relates tumor control to healing and damage of normal tissues. For instance, a 100 percent control can be obtained with lesser doses and a near-zero incidence of serious complications. The therapist who attempts 100 percent control for all patients may induce serious complications which will handicap a percentage of patients for the rest of their lives.

The risk of complications is to be gauged against the extensiveness of the disease. The therapy team readily accepts the risk of serious complications for a patient with an advanced cancer, but the risk is unacceptable for patients with small lesions.

CHARACTERISTICS OF IRRADIATION SOURCES

Intracavitary Gamma-Ray Sources

Dosimetry. The inverse-square law is all-important in the dosimetry of interstitial or intracavitary gamma-ray therapy. Figure 47–3 illustrates the influence of distance and diameter of applicators on depth doses from gamma-ray sources. It is readily apparent in examining the rapid fall-off from a source as distance increases that underirradiated areas are created by faulty positioning or ineffective arrangements of the gamma-ray sources due to technical error or poor anatomy.

The dose delivered to any point in the pelvis depends on (1) the amount of radium in each source; (2) the distance of each radium source to the point and the summation of the doses from multiple sources to that point; and (3) the time that the radium remains in place.

The contribution of the radium system to the re-

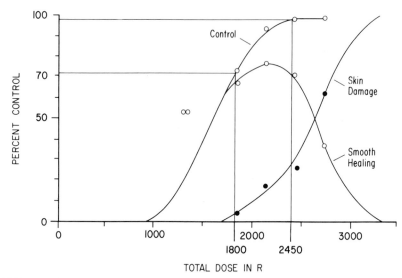

FIGURE 47–2 Curve of tumor control (1 year recurrence-free), curve of skin complications, and curve of smooth healing calculated by Strandqvist using the isoeffect equivalent single doses. *(From M Strandqvist.)*

gional nodes depends on (1) the total number of milligram hours of radium; (2) the respective loading of the uterine tandem and the colpostats; and (3) the location of the radium system in the pelvis.

Sources. There is no biological difference among the gamma rays of ^{226}Ra, ^{137}Cs, ^{60}Co, and ^{192}Ir. The ^{60}Co sources are impractical because of rapid decay (5.23 years half-life), but ^{137}Cs has a half-life of 30 years. The use of ^{192}Ir (half-life 74^{1}/$_2$ days) is only for interstitial irradiation. The iridium wires may be cut to any length and placed in hollow needles, a distinct advantage when a large area is to be irradiated. The ^{198}Au seeds are useful as interstitial sources for small implants. Removal of implanted gold seeds is not necessary because of their short half-life (2.694 days).

Applicators. Various applicators are needed to meet the different clinical situations. The Fletcher-Suit applicators are simple and effective to use (Fig. 47–4 A and B). They are loaded after the patient is brought back to the ward. Afterloading applicators allows their repositioning, if necessary, in the operating room—before the patient is awakened from anesthesia—without exposing the theater staff and technicians who take the films of the applications.

Tandems. A rigid metal afterloading tandem with an adjustable flange has the advantage of fixing the uterus in the center of the pelvis. This central location gives a higher dose to the external iliac, hypogastric, and lower common iliac nodes and spares the bladder and rectum.

Colpostats. Colpostats are used to treat the exocervix, the mucosa of the upper third of the vagina, and, to an extent, the paracervical areas and medial parametria. The largest colpostats possible, provided they fit in the lateral fornices, should be used for each application. This gives a better dose ratio between the mucosa and the lateral areas (Fig. 47–3).

EXTERNAL IRRADIATION

Energy Level

External irradiation can be delivered with energy levels varying from 3- to 35-MeV linear accelerators. The 4- to 6-MeV linear accelerators have beams almost identical to those of ^{60}Co teletherapy units. The maximum buildup at these energy levels is 0.5 to 1 cm beneath the skin surface, and the depth doses are

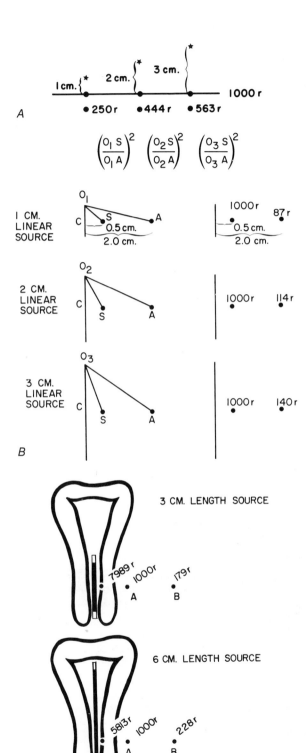

A

$$\left(\frac{O_1 S}{O_1 A}\right)^2 \quad \left(\frac{O_2 S}{O_2 A}\right)^2 \quad \left(\frac{O_3 S}{O_3 A}\right)^2$$

1 CM. LINEAR SOURCE

2 CM. LINEAR SOURCE

3 CM. LINEAR SOURCE

B

3 CM. LENGTH SOURCE

6 CM. LENGTH SOURCE

C

equal. Photon beams of 22 MeV or more have a greater depth dose than the 4- to 6-MeV linear accelerators, and since the maximum buildup is 4 cm from the skin surface, the subcutaneous tissues are spared as well as the skin (Fig. 47–5). This greater-depth dose is of particular advantage in patients with an anteroposterior diameter of 25 cm or more.

With an electron beam, energy is transferred at initial contact with the surface but there is a fast drop of dose after it passes a few centimeters below the skin surface. Therefore, the electron beam is used primarily to treat superficial lesions at or near the skin surface, extending no more than 2 or 3 cm beneath the skin. It may be useful in treatment of pelvic malignancies when disease is on the perineum, vulva, and groins. By and large, however, the electron beam plays a minor role in the treatment of gynecologic malignancies.

Planning of External Irradiation

Whole-pelvis irradiation is best given through parallel opposing portals or with a 25-MeV beam with the addition of lateral portals. The anterior and posterior portals are usually 15 by 15 cm. With a 25-MeV photon beam, 1000 rads a week is well tolerated; with the 3- to 6-MeV units, a lower weekly dosage of 850 to 900 rads is recommended. Both fields should be ir-

FIGURE 47–3 *A.* The inverse-square law applied to the design of radium applicators states that the dose delivered by a source of radium to a point varies inversely as the square of the distance from the source to that point. In this illustration, three points (*) 1, 2, and 3 cm represent the diameter of a radium applicator. The dose delivered to a point 1 cm below the vaginal mucosa is influenced as the treatment distance from this point increases. With the 1-cm applicator the two points are 1 cm apart; since the dose to the near point is 1000 rads the dose to the far point is $(1/2)^2$ or $1/4$ of 1000 = 250 rads. When the distance from the near point is increased from 1 to 2 cm, the dose to the point 1 cm below the vaginal mucosa (far point) is $(2/3)^2$ or $4/9$ of 1000 = 444 rads. With the 3-cm applicator the dose to the far point is $(3/4)^2$ or $9/16$ of 1000 = 563 rads.

B. Dose contribution from the center of the source C to point A is $(0.5/2)^2$ or $1/16$ of that to point S. As source length increases, OS/OA approaches unity. When this occurs, dose contribution from point O, the end of the source, to points A and S approaches equality: $(OS/OA)^2$ 1. The addition of nearly equal doses to points A and S, already connected by the steep dose gradient, produces a decrease of that gradient, i.e., an increase in the depth dose.

C. The dose at point A is kept at 1000 rads. As the length of the sources increases, the dose to the mucosa decreases and the dose at point B increases. In view of this, the linear source used in a uterine tandem should be as long as the anatomy permits. *(After Fletcher, 1971.)*

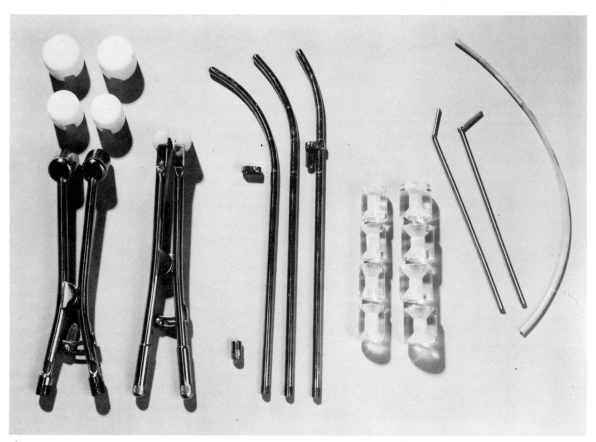

A

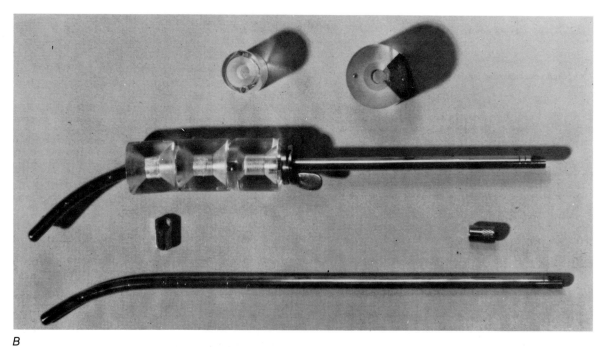

B

FIGURE 47–4 *A.* From left to right: After loading colpostats (2-cm diameter), and plastic jackets used to increase the size to medium (2.5-cm diameter) and large (3-cm diameter). Half cylinders (0.8 cm in radium for narrow vaults; maximum diameter with the afterloading tandem in between equals 3 cm), designed to have the vaginal sources perpendicular to the vaginal axis in order

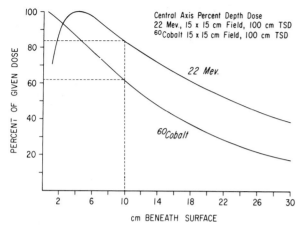

FIGURE 47–5 The maximum buildup of the ^{60}Co unit is 0.5 cm beneath the skin surface, whereas the maximum buildup for a 22-MeV betatron is near 5-cm depth. At 10-cm depth (midpelvis for a 20-cm anteriorposterior diameter) the depth with the 22-MeV betatron is 83 percent of the maximum dose, whereas it is only 61 percent with a ^{60}Co unit. (From Fletcher, 1973.)

radiated daily in order to cause less subcutaneous fibrosis. Doses in excess of 4000 rads given in 4 weeks at midplane of the pelvis with a ^{60}Co or 4-MeV unit may induce subcutaneous fibrosis since the subcutaneous dose may be up to 20 percent more than the midplane dose. Obese patients (anteroposterior diameter of 25 cm or more) pose a problem because higher given doses are necessary in order to deliver the required midplane dose.

Whole-pelvis irradiation is used for the following reasons:

1. To shrink bulky central disease. It is essential to produce regression of the central component with external irradiation so that the remaining viable cells in the tumor can be brought closer to the intracavity gamma-ray sources.
2. To treat lateral spread adequately, since the lateral parametrial area and regional lymphatics receive only a small dose from intracavity radium.

to minimize the dose to the bladder and rectum as compared to protruding sources with the axis parallel to the vaginal axis. The depth is not as good as with one 3-cm colpostat. Uterine afterloading tandems (the three most useful curvatures) with metal flange with "keel" (to stabilize the tandem by means of proper packing around it) and without (to be used with vaginal cylinders).

B. Sample of vaginal cylinders of different diameters and length to be used for the irradiation of a selected part or the whole of the vagina (A, from Fletcher et al., 1971; B, from Fletcher, 1973.)

3. To make up for a poor geometry of the radium system and ensure that the paracervical areas are adequately irradiated. The poor geometric shape may be the result of distortion caused by disease or of narrowness of the vaginal vault related to advanced age.

Transvaginal Therapy

One of the most important uses of transvaginal therapy is for hemostasis of cervical cancers. Two or three doses of 500 rads will usually stop bleeding of a fungating mass and will also help to initiate regression of the central mass. Transvaginal therapy has therapeutic use in treating carcinomas of the cervical stump when the endocervical canal is not long enough to hold at least two radium sources. Transvaginal irradiation is also used for small primary carcinomas or isolated metastases in the vagina.

Staging

The major shortcoming of the current staging system for carcinoma of the cervix is that it does not take tumor volume into consideration. This can be illustrated by examining stage I and stage II carcinomas of the cervix. Stage I lesions, as long as they are confined to the cervix, range from tiny invasive squamous-cell carcinoma to masses 6 cm in diameter. Stage II cases range from minimal paracervical infiltration to extension almost to both pelvic walls.

When squamous-cell carcinoma or adenocarcinoma originates within the endocervix, the cervix enlarges concentrically producing a barrel-shaped lesion, and disease spreads to the lower uterine segment and into the myometrium. This mode of spread is ignored in the FIGO staging system. Table 47–4 shows the size distribution of the lesions in FIGO stages I and II of endocervical carcinoma. Table 47–5 correlates survival rates with size of lesions with FIGO stages.

The FIGO staging system, which is designed for comparison of treatment modalities, should not be used in treatment planning for the individual patient. The protocols currently being used for cervix and endometrium at the M. D. Anderson Hospital and Tumor Institute are seen in Tables 47–6 and 47–7.

Care during and after Therapy

The night before the radium insertion a cleansing douche and enema are ordered. A general anesthetic is desirable for the placement unless only colpostats are inserted. The tandem and ovoids are packed with

TABLE 47–4 FIGO Staging Versus Size of Cervix in Lesions of the Endocervix (1955–1969; Analysis 1976)

Size, cm	Stage IB (257 patients)	Stage IIA (68 patients)	Stage IIB (206 patients)
<3	98	19	24
3–6	104	29	77
6–8	35	15	81
>8	5	1	10
Unknown	15	4	14

Source: W Wilson, personal communication.

TABLE 47–5 Five Year Survival Rates for Variable Size Lesions in Carcinoma of The Endocervix* (1955–1969; Analysis 1976)

	Stage IB (82%)		Stage IIA (74%)		Stage IIB (63%)	
No. of patients	202	40	48	16	91	91
Lesion size, cm	<6	>6	<6	<6	>6	>6
Survival rate, %	86	54	85	40	68	58
p	0.000		0.000		0.13	

*FIGO staging.
Source: W Wilson, personal communication.

TABLE 47–6 Squamous-Cell Carcinoma of the Cervix on Intact Uterus Maxima for Combining Whole-Pelvis Irradiation and Intracavity Radium Therapy

Stage	Whole pelvis	Maximum hours*	Maximum mg·h*	Parametrial
I (≤1 cm)		72 hours; after 2 weeks, 72 hours	10,000	
I (≥ 1 cm)	2000	72 hours; after 2 weeks, 72 hours	10,000 9,000	3000–4000 rads 1000–2000 rads
IIA	4000	48 hours; after 2 weeks, 48 hours‡	6,500	
IIB*	4000	48 hours; after 2 weeks, 48 hours	6,500	
IIIA	4000	48 hours; after 2 weeks, 48 hours	6,500	1000–1500 rads on side involved
	5000	72 or 48 hours; after 2 weeks, 24–48 hours	5,000	Possibly 1000 rads on side involved
IIIB	6000	72 hours	4,000	
IV	7000			

*Use whichever maximum occurs first, either the time or the mg·h.
†May be exceeded for unusual tumor size, then use three insertions, 2 weeks apart.
‡May use the longer time first if the vault size may not permit two colpostats for the second application.
§ If the status of central disease indicates it, the time may be increased beyond 72 hours or above 5000 mg. Then split into 48 hours-2 weeks-24 to 48 hours. Whole pelvis irradiation may be carried to 5000 rads if regression is slow.
*Note:*A tandem with a protruding source and a 3-cm diameter vaginal cylinder should have a 20-mg source in the cylinder with sources protruding. The loading is 15-10-20, 15-10-10-20, etc.
Source: Fletcher, Rutledge.

TABLE 47-7 Adenocarcinoma of the Endometrium, Technically and Medically Operable

Clinical situations	Treatment to uterus	Treatment to vagina
Small uterine cavity, well-differentiated tumor	Hysterectomy only	Wide vaginal cuff
Slightly enlarged uterine cavity, well-differentiated tumor	Radium: 1–72 hours tandem or 3000–3500 mg·h with packing Hysterectomy	Colpostats: 7000 rads surface dose, one application
Moderately enlarged uterine cavity (6- to 8-week size), well-differentiated tumor	Radium: 2000 mg·h, two treatments 3 weeks apart or 4000 rads whole pelvis and radium One Heyman packing, 2500 mg·h, or tandem 72 hours with 15- and 10-mg sources Hysterectomy	Colpostats: 4000 rads surface dose, 3 weeks apart; 4000 rads surface dose, one application
Large uterine cavity or anaplastic tumor	4000 rads whole pelvis and radium Heyman packing, 2500 mg·h, or tandem 72 hours with 15- and 10-mg sources Hysterectomy	Colpostats: 4000 rads surface dose, one application.

Source: Fletcher et al., 1970.

gauze soaked with 1:2000 benzalkonium chloride solution or impregnated with nitrofurazone. The degree of movement allowed each patient with intracavitary radium depends on the design of the radium applicator. With an afterloading system, the patient may rotate the thorax from side to side in order to eat and to take care of herself.

Medications for pain, nausea, and sleep contribute to the patient's comfort. Since a Foley catheter is inserted into the bladder, Azo Gantrisin (sulfisoxazole plus phenazopyridine hydrochloride) is often given as a urinary antiseptic. Antibiotics are not routinely used. If the patient has a temperature elevation while the radium is in place, antibiotics are given. Should the temperature not respond to antibiotic therapy or should the patient develop abdominal distention and manifestations of pelvic cellulitis, then the radium system is removed.

Causes of Failure

The possible causes of failure in the treatment of gynecologic malignancies are multiple. They include the following:

1. Primary (central) lesion.
   a. *Technical.* Improper placement of the radioactive sources, either from lack of experience or skill, creates areas receiving inadequate dosage. Faulty placement of the system can also result if the patient's vagina will not accept an effective radium system. Situations such as a short, scarred vaginal fornix resulting from prior obstetric laceration; a narrow vault due to age; or destruction of the cervix and fornix by cancer can make proper application difficult.
   b. *Bulky central disease.* A large volume of tumor can account for radiation failures. Recognition of the barrel-shaped lesions and adjunctive surgery have proved effective in managing this clinical situation (Fig. 47–6).
2. Regional spread.
   a. *Geographic miss.* This situation occurs when part of the tumor is not included in the radiation fields. A good example is treatment of a patient with a pelvic malignancy using the standard 15- by 15-cm pelvic portals when the patient has metastases to common iliac and aortic nodes which are clearly beyond the irradiated volume.
3. New primary.
   a. A new lesion in the vagina may develop many years following radiation therapy for a cervical cancer. There is a question as to whether this may be a recurrence or a new primary.

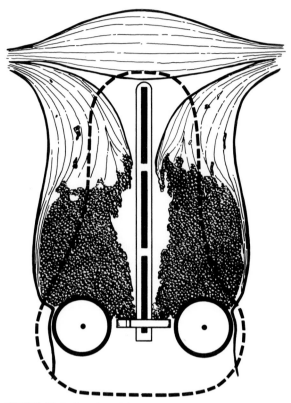

FIGURE 47–6 Invasion of the myometrium of the isthmus (barrel-shaped lesion). Tumor cells are too far from the radium sources for adequate contribution. Even after 4000 rads, shrinkage may not bring peripheral disease in close enough to the radium sources. *(From Fletcher, 1973.)*

SPECIAL SITUATIONS

Carcinoma in Situ and Microinvasive Carcinoma

If there is some medical contraindication to surgery so that a hysterectomy cannot be performed for carcinoma in situ or for microinvasive carcinoma, radium alone can be used. A single 72-hour tandem and ovoid insertion is recommended for carcinoma in situ. Microinvasive carcinoma is treated more comprehensively with two 48-hour systems spaced 2 weeks apart.

Conservative Extrafascial Hysterectomy

Lesions originating in the endocervix, either squamous-cell carcinomas or adenocarcinomas, invade the myometrium of the lower uterine segment, resulting

in a barrel-shaped palpatory finding on pelvic-rectal examination. These lesions can attain considerable dimensions, reaching from pelvic wall to pelvic wall, but without fixation. Even after external irradiation of 4000 rads, they can still be so large that despite the addition of intensified intracavitary x-ray therapy there is a significant incidence of central failures. The combination of 4000 rads to the whole pelvis alone with diminished intracavitary x-ray therapy followed by a conservative extrafascial hysterectomy is very effective in the larger lesions. Of 102 patients (92 with lesions larger than 5 cm) treated from 1970 through 1976, a few had pelvic recurrences (Table 47–8). Careful sharp-knife dissection and avoidance of excessive doses at the vaginal apex will eliminate almost all severe complications (Table 47–9) (O'Quinn et al.). Patients with unrecognized infected adnexa before irradiation and hysterectomy constitute the group most likely to experience postoperative complications. Dissection of chronically infected areas is difficult and is followed frequently by formation of adhesions.

Extended Field Technique

From 1961 through 1976, 247 patients with cancer of the uterine cervix were treated with field heights of more than 17.5 cm. During that period, 76 patients had a preirradiation therapy laparotomy and lymphadenectomy as part of an investigation of the potential value of the procedure.

In this series, survival rates were poor, and the incidence of distant metastases was high, as expected, since almost all patients had disease in the regional lymphatics. A similarly high incidence of distant metastases in patients with positive nodes in the lymphadenectomy specimen had been found in a previous analysis (El Senoussi et al.).

In the extended field experience, severe complications were frequent. Of the various parameters involved—i.e., height of the extended fields; dose to

TABLE 47–8 Failure Sites in 102 Patients (January 1970–October 1976; Analysis April 1978)

Central	1
Pelvis	3
Pelvis and distant	3
Distant only	10
Total	17

Source: O'Quinn et al. Used by permission.

TABLE 47–9 Significant Complications of Combined Treatment Correlated With Type of Surgical Procedure (January 1970–October 1976; Analysis March 1978)

Complication	Extrafascial hysterectomy (78 patients)	Extrafascial hysterectomy and lymphadenectomy (17 patients)	Preirradiation lymphadenectomy and hysterectomy (7 patients)
Severe vault necrosis	1*	0	1†
Bladder bleeding requiring irrigation	0	0	0
Fistula involving vagina	1*	0	1†
Small bowel obstruction	1‡	0	1†§
Obstruction related to sigmoiditis	0	0	1

*Same patient; vault necrosis healed and fistula developed 54 months after treatment.
†Same patient; time-related events.
‡Patient died 5 months later from a ruptured cerebral aneurysm.
§Relieved by lysis of adhesions.
Source: O'Quinn et al. Used by permission.

the extended fields; additional external irradiation boost doses; intracavitary radium therapy dose; and performance or omission of surgical procedures—most significant contributing parameter was found to be the dose to the extended fields (Table 47–10) (El Senoussi et al.).

A total dose of 4500 rads to the extended fields at a rate of 900 rads per week is all that can be safely given. Preirradiation laparotomy is no longer performed. In patients with positive lymph nodes and no massive parametrial disease, intracavitary x-ray therapy can be performed without diminution of dose. The

TABLE 47–10 Obstructing Sigmoiditis and Small Bowel Perforation or Obstruction Versus Doses of External Irradiation and Total Milligram-Hours (Uterine plus Vaginal)

External irradiation to extended fields, rads	External irradiation boost, rads	Milligram-hours				No. of patients	%
		≤4000	>4000, ≤5000	>5000, ≤6000	>6000		
4000	0–500		0/4	0/2	0/1	(1/11)	
	1000–1500		1/2				
	≥2000	0/1	0/1				
4500	0–500	0/3	0/14	3/18	0/1	(3/36)	8
	1000–1500	2/7	2/6	0/1		(4/14	28.5
	≥2000	4/12	0/1			(4/13)	30
5000	0–500	3/7	1/18	1/7		(5/32)	15.5
	1000–1500	3/13	5/13			(8/26)	30
	≥2000	6/31				(6/31)	19
5500	0–500	1/5	10/30	3/14	1/5	(15/54)	28
	1000–1500	6/30	0/3			(6/33)	18
	≥2000	1/2				(1/2)	50
6000	0–500						
	1000–1500	3/5				(3/5)	60
	≥2000						
Total						(56*/257)	22

*Twenty-seven patients with no surgery and 29 patients with surgery.
Source: El Senoussi et al. Used by permission.

policy of irradiating the next relay of noninvolved lymphatics is no longer followed. For instance, if external iliac nodes are positive, a field with a 2- to 3-cm margin beyond the positive node(s) is used, and then 1000 to 1500 rads is added with a 6- by 5-cm or 7- by 6-cm field.

The results of the study have served as a reminder that a very important factor in complications is the size of the volume irradiated.

Invasive Carcinoma Inadequately Treated by Simple Hysterectomy

If a patient has had a simple hysterectomy for any one of several reasons and invasive squamous carcinoma is found in the surgical specimen, postoperative radiotherapy is indicated. If the volume of cancer in the specimen is very small and is well confined within the surgical specimen, irradiation to only the vaginal vault with radium is adequate. If there has been a close cutthrough or absolute cutthrough, whole-pelvis irradiation followed by vaginal radium is employed.

Adenocarcinoma of the endometrium found unexpectedly in a postoperative specimen may also require additional therapy. If the carcinoma has invaded the myometrium to a depth equal to one-half its thickness, then 5000 rads whole-pelvis irradiation plus 3000 rads surface dose from a vaginal applicator to the vaginal apex are needed. Undifferentiated adenocarcinomas or cervical invasion demands equally aggressive treatment.

OTHER GYNECOLOGIC SITUATIONS

Vagina

Lesions of the upper third of the vagina behave similarly to cervical cancer, but lesions in the lower half of the vagina may metastasize to the groins.

Stage I squamous carcinoma of the vagina is highly curable with intracavitary or interstitial irradiation (Brown et al.). These lesions are limited to the vaginal mucosa, and if an exophytic component exists, transvaginal therapy or whole-pelvis irradiation is used first to reduce its volume so that an interstitial implant can be effectively used. Since these lesions have a low incidence of regional lymph-node involvement, the whole-pelvis irradiation, when indicated, is given through 12- by 12-cm or even 10- by 10-cm parallel opposing portals.

In stage II or stage III lesions, a 4000- to 5000-rad tumor dose is first given, with external irradiation followed by interstitial gamma-ray therapy. If the area to be irradiated is extensive, long ^{192}Ir needles should be used.

Primary adenocarcinoma of the vagina may also be treated with irradiation therapy. Patients with small superficial cancers limited to the vagina may be treated with interstitial gamma-ray therapy or with transvaginal cone, thus preserving child-bearing function. Pelvic lymphadenectomy prior to irradiation therapy may be useful in patient selection in that patients with no evidence of nodal disease would be best suited for conservative therapy. Larger, more extensive cancers or patients with positive nodes are treated with external therapy followed by interstitial and/or intracavitary sources (Wilson).

Ovary

Ovarian cancer is often a disease of the entire abdominal cavity and irradiation therapy must, when indicated, treat the whole abdomen. As a rule, the patient will tolerate only 3000 rads to the whole abdomen, and this requires 4 to 5 weeks for administration since nausea, vomiting, and diarrhea may be severe. One can then add 2000 rads to the pelvis. An alternative way to treat the entire abdomen is to employ the moving-strip technique (Fig. 47–7). This will give 2800 rads to each strip over a 12-day interval, a dose biologically equivalent to about 3500 rads given in 3½ weeks. An additional 2000 rads can be given to the pelvis in such situations.

These doses are obviously not enough to eradicate large masses of tumor, but higher doses exceed tolerance. Patients who have residual tumor greater than 2 cm in diameter after surgical exploration should be treated with chemotherapy. Patients with ascites, lesions metastatic to the liver, or implants on the peritoneal surface covering the kidneys are also candidates for chemotherapy, since doses above 3000 rads are definitely not tolerated by the kidney and also are dangerous for the liver (Wharton, 1973). Postoperative irradiation for patients with ovarian cancer is much more effective when only microscopic disease confined to the pelvis is left after surgical excision.

REACTIONS AND COMPLICATIONS OF IRRADIATION

Bladder Injury

Postirradiation cystitis and bladder ulcers are usually caused by high doses of irradiation delivered to the bladder floor. Dysuria is a frequent complaint. Antispasmodics are the treatment of choice and produce

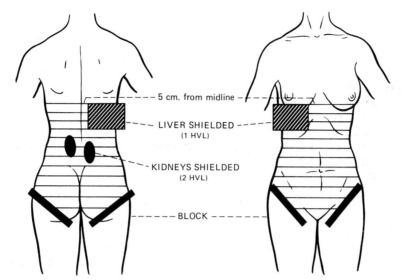

FIGURE 47–7 Volume covered with the megavoltage moving strip technique. (*From Delclos, Smith, in Fletcher, 1973.*)

symptomatic relief. Urine cultures should be checked routinely since infection may aggravate the problem.

Hematuria is one of the more troublesome problems and is due to rupture of telangiectatic vessels or to mucosa necrosis. Cystoscopic examination may show ulcerations and edema in the area of the trigone or thinning of the mucosa with prominent vessels. The treatment for hematuria is continuous irrigation through a three-way catheter with 0.5% acetic acid or 1:10,000 potassium permanganate solution. The flow rate should be rapid enough to prevent accumulation of clots in the bladder. The bladder distended by blood clots will not respond to irrigation. Fulguration has limited usefulness because the bleeding points are usually multifocal. A suprapubic cystostomy is useful in selected patients. Urinary diversion by ileal conduit is not always effective, and cystectomy has been associated with severe complications, even with death. Blood replacement and continuous irrigation constitute the treatment of choice.

Various and repeated biopsies of the bladder wall at the time of cystoscopy should be avoided because the injured tissue and its impaired healing ability will not tolerate additional trauma, and a vesicovaginal fistula may result. An isolated recurrence in the bladder base following completion of irradiation therapy is quite common.

Fistulas

Vesicovaginal and rectovaginal fistulas may develop following treatment for carcinoma of the cervix when there has been massive central disease or extensive vaginal involvement. Extensive fornix involvement weakens the vaginal wall and predisposes to the subsequent development of fistulas. Vaginal necrosis with fistula formation induced by a compact radium system is especially disturbing because the injury can be prevented by improved application.

Vesicovaginal and rectovaginal fistulas frequently occur together. When one appears, the other may develop within 1 or 2 months. Vaginal necrosis almost always precedes this development and should be treated vigorously with hydrogen peroxide douches (one part 3% hydrogen peroxide and three parts water) or 0.25% sodium hypochlorite douches if the fistulas are to be prevented. Fistulas may be precipitated by trauma or biopsy of the vaginal wall after full-dose irradiation therapy. Certainly suspicious areas warrant biopsy; however, additional trauma to the tissue by repeated biopsies precipitates a breakdown in the vesical or rectal wall septum.

The onset of a vaginal fistula usually occurs 6 to 24 months after treatment. An occasional patient will develop a fistula 10 years after treatment when systemic vascular disease further embarrasses the blood supply to the area.

The treatment of choice is usually urinary or fecal diversion. Occasionally a small fistula can be closed by colpocleisis (Latzko technique) or by utilizing the gracilis muscle or bulbocavernosus fat pad.

Sigmoiditis

The changes range from a temporary spasm of the sigmoid with some bleeding and intermittent periods of diarrhea to permanent narrowing with obstruction and necrosis. The changes, therefore, represent a spectrum of injury varying from transient reversible changes to surgical emergencies.

Sigmoiditis in its more serious form is a product of the megavoltage irradiation era. The injury is much more frequently encountered with whole-pelvis irradiation doses greater than 4000 rads or with 4000 rads and the radium system located in a retroposed position in the hollow of the sacrum. The management of the acute changes, which consist primarily of diarrhea with tenesmus and possibly bleeding, are controlled with antispasmodics (Lomotil), adequate hydration, low-residue diet, and topical treatment for the inflamed rectal area. The intermediate injury, consisting of bleeding, fecal impaction due to stricture, and pain, is managed with long-term use of stool softeners, proper diet, and patient education. Rarely will this injury require colostomy; with proper management, it is partially reversible. Colostomy is required in patients with obstruction or necrosis. Conservative management in this latter group of patients may result in a catastrophe since perforation may occur, bleeding may become excessive, and may not respond to supportive measures. Diversionary colostomy is the treatment of choice; surgical excision of the injured segment has no place in the treatment of this complication because irradiated tissues will not heal and low success rate or fatalities may result. Patients with severe sigmoiditis frequently have injury to an associated loop of the small bowel, usually the terminal ileum. Combination injuries such as these are not infrequent with extended-field therapy.

Small-Bowel Complications

The terminal small bowel may receive an excess amount of irradiation when the standard 15- by 15-cm or larger parallel opposing portal is used. The use of extended-field irradiation therapy to encompass a greater portion of the regional nodes has resulted in a marked increase in the incidence of small-bowel injuries, which are extremely difficult problems to manage.

Injury to the small bowel may occur during treatment; symptoms result because the rapidly proliferating epithelial lining of the ileum is compromised. This acute injury is reversible and requires cessation of therapy, tube suction, and intravenous fluids. This is adequate treatment since regeneration of the mucosa with increase in absorption capacity requires 14 to 21 days. These early injuries vary in severity. Some patients have, in addition to intractable diarrhea, ab-

dominal pain with guarding and symptoms of peritonitis. These patients should be managed conservatively unless the attending physician is convinced that a perforation or unrelated problem has developed. Radiation therapy is continued after the patient has resumed normal diet and bowel functions.

Of major clinical interest is the more extensive injury which is usually noted 6 to 18 months following therapy. Fibrosis of the muscular wall of the small bowel, especially the terminal ileum, results in narrowing of the lumen and permanent changes in the epithelial lining. The patient experiences weight loss, intermittent episodes of partial obstruction, nausea, vomiting, and there is a general failure to survive. The x-ray examinations, including a small-bowel series and barium enema study, all too frequently are normal, and therefore the diagnosis is delayed. The patient may also present with a picture of intestinal obstruction or a complication related to necrosis of the bowel wall. An enterovaginal or enterovesical fistula may occur. Fulminating peritonitis due to a perforation with resulting gram-negative septicemia also is a threat. Advanced small-bowel injuries are associated with a high mortality rate, and it is important that surgery be performed before these complications develop. At the time of exploratory laparotomy, the findings dictate the surgical procedure to be performed. Patients with segments of necrotic bowel require resection. Abscesses must be drained. The status of the tissues influences the operation. Removal of the injured segment is a tangible objective but not always an easy or safe procedure. The treatment of choice in our experience is by-pass of the injured intestine by means of side-to-side anastomosis of proximal healthy-appearing small bowel to the ascending or transverse colon. This relieves the obstruction with the least extensive surgery. Pelvic dissection should be kept to an absolute minimum.

Patients with enterovaginal fistulas should have the injured loop bypassed but isolated. The fecal stream is interrupted and the ends of the by-passed segment are attached to the skin to allow egress of secretions. As a rule, small-bowel fistulas due to irradiation injury will not heal with parenteral hyperalimentation, but the patient will benefit and be a better operative candidate.

Small-bowel injuries are more frequent in patients who have had previous pelvic surgery and/or infection. These cause loops of small bowel to become fixed in the pelvis where they receive an excessive dose. The total dose of external irradiation should never exceed 5000 rads in these patients.

PRINCIPLES OF CANCER CHEMOTHERAPY

STEVEN E. VOGL

RATIONALE

Chemotherapy represents an attempt to achieve selective destruction of neoplastic tissues, sparing host organs and their functions. In general, chemotherapeutic agents are given *systemically,* in contrast to the *regional* treatments for cancer represented by surgery and radiotherapy. It has been hoped that some unique characteristics of malignant neoplasms can be exploited so that only neoplastic cells will be damaged and killed by a chemotherapeutic agent. An obvious disease model for such an agent is pneumococcal pneumonia, where a selective inhibitor of bacterial cell wall synthesis (penicillin G) is highly lethal to the parasitic organism but has negligible toxicity for the human host.

Unfortunately, no vital difference similar to cell wall synthesis in the pneumococcus has been identified between neoplastic cells and normal cells. Since most neoplasms are derived from host tissues, and share the host genome, the differences that have been found have been largely quantitative rather than qualitative. Therefore, clinical chemotherapy has been forced to exploit relatively minor differences in drug sensitivity between neoplastic and normal tissues. These relatively minor differences vary among the different tumor types according to primary site and histologic appearance. Thus, single alkylating agents produce major objective remissions in advanced epithelial ovarian cancer in 35 to 50 percent of the patients (Young et al.), but similar doses of the same agents have minimal or no activity against sarcomas arising in the female pelvic organs or elsewhere. Even in a given tumor type at a given site, similar, relatively minor differences presumably account for the fact that excellent clinical remissions are obtained in some tumors but no effect is observed in others. Part of this heterogeneity may relate to variations in host drug metabolism (absorption, distribution, conjugation, anabolism, catabolism, and excretion). Since most chemotherapy is given at fixed doses (adjusted to body surface area) that will generally give acceptable toxicity, variations in the tolerance of the tissues of different hosts for drug toxicity does not have a major impact on reported response rates among various tumors.

Most of the anticancer drugs whose action is understood to any extent act in some way on cell proliferation. Rapid proliferation is not a unique characteristic of cancer cells, since normal intestinal mucosal crypt cells and normal bone marrow stem cells replicate faster than the vast majority of tumor cells. The degree of selectivity achieved in killing cells multiplying less rapidly than these critical host tissues may relate to the latter's greater capacity to recover from drug-induced injury when compared to the recovery of neoplastic cells. Thus, while 90 percent of cells of both tumor and marrow may be destroyed by a single dose of a drug like cyclophosphamide, the marrow population may recover in 3 weeks while the tumor may take 3 months to fully repopulate. Once marrow recovery has occurred, additional drug can be given, again reducing both tissues by 90 percent. The marrow would again repopulate in 3 weeks, but the cumulative cell kill in the tumor would be nearly 99 percent. It is this rationale which underlies the current practice of administering repeated courses of chemotherapy in doses which, while causing toxicity to normal tissues, allow recovery, so that more treatment can be sequentially administered.

The chemotherapeutic attack on cell proliferation may be directly on (1) DNA [alkylating agents, *cis*-diamminedichloroplatinum II (DDP), dactinoamycin, adriamycin, mitomycin C, bleomycin]; (2) on the enzyme DNA polymerase (cytosine arabinoside); (3) on nucleic acid function by the incorporation of false bases in essential cellular materials (6-thioguanine, 5-fluorouracil); (4) on enzymes that lead to the synthesis of DNA precursor compounds (methotrexate, which inhibits dihydrofolate reductase and therefore purine and thymidine synthesis; hydroxyurea, which inhibits ribonucleotide reductase; 5-fluorouracil, which inhibits thymidylate synthetase); or (5) on the mitotic spindle (vincristine, vinblastine, and the epipodophyllotoxins) (USA-USSR Monograph).

For a few of the agents, duration of exposure of cells in normal and neoplastic tissues is critical in determining efficacy and toxicity. Most such agents (including methotrexate, cytosine arabinoside, and hydroxyurea) affect only cells that are actively synthesizing DNA during exposure to the drug. Major differences in efficacy and toxicity with changes in schedule are not generally apparent for the remainder of clinically useful anticancer drugs.

Most chemotherapeutic agents are given at or very near a dose which causes major but reversible side effects, since tumor cell kill is generally proportional to dose. Small increments in dose at this critical level, however, can produce markedly enhanced toxicity with insignificant increases in antitumor efficacy. This has been well documented for 5-fluorouracil in colon cancer, and has also been shown for alkylating agents in the treatment of ovarian cancer (Young et al.).

PRINCIPLES OF DRUG DEVELOPMENT

Many of the most useful drugs in clinical cancer chemotherapy have resulted from careful development of chance observations. Alkylating agents were investigated after the observation of lymphopenia in normal men dying after accidental exposure to mustard gases during World War II. Folic acid antagonists (such as methotrexate and aminopterin) were synthesized after it was noted that folic acid could sometimes exacerbate the course of acute leukemia. *cis*-Diamminedichloroplatinum II (DDP) was investigated as a result of a chance observation that electrolysis products from a platinum electrode prevented normal proliferation of bacteria. Discovery of one active agent in the treatment of cancer in animals or men in general leads to the synthesis of a number of similar compounds which are then tested and compared in a variety of systems (USA-USSR Monograph).

A number of useful drugs for the treatment of cancer have come from rational synthesis of new agents in an effort to inhibit an essential metabolic pathway. A compound in which a fluorine atom is substituted for the methyl group in thymine, 5-fluorouracil, is the classic example of such a drug. The antifols, such as methotrexate, and the antipurines, such as 6-mercaptopurine, are other examples.

In addition to chance observation of activity and rational synthesis, a major program is now underway at the National Cancer Institute to *screen* random synthetic compounds for evidence of antitumor activity. The current screening system involves a transplantable leukemia in mice. Prolongation of life at a toxic but tolerable dose is the end point used. Evidence of activity in this system leads to testing in a number of tumor systems in animals, including mouse tumors which grow much more slowly than the leukemias and human tumors which have been carried in immunologically incompetent mice.

Should an agent, after being tested in these systems, be considered to have sufficient evidence of activity from human trials, toxicologic investigations are undertaken. These investigations involve very careful trials in at least two species (one small and one large; usually the mouse and the dog) in order to define minimally toxic, severely toxic, and lethal doses. Once the tests are completed and all tissues have been carefully examined for signs of acute and chronic toxicity, human studies may begin.

Initial human trials are generally performed in patients with far-advanced cancers for whom no treatment of established value is available. The application of *new* treatments is thus reasonable, since no previously available treatment has a reasonable chance of helping the patient. The initial trials generally start at one-third of a dose which produces mild toxicity in dogs. Doses are escalated after several patients are treated at each dose level until reproducible but reversible toxicity on normal tissues is produced. The goal of such a *phase I* study is to define a tolerable dose and the extent and pattern of toxicity in humans. While it is hoped that some patients will respond, a phase I study is not a test of efficacy, since the dose is being constantly changed.

Once a tolerable dose and schedule have been defined in phase I trials, *phase II* studies are undertaken in an attempt to define whether the agent is active for a given tumor type. Activity is generally defined as the production of complete remission (disappearance of all known evidence of disease), or partial remission (50 percent decrease in the estimated cross-sectional area of measurable lesions without the appearance of new lesions or deterioration in the general health of the patient). For most tumors, a complete plus partial response rate of greater than 20 percent in phase II studies is considered a significant finding that should lead to further use of the drug in that particular disease. A response rate of less than 10 percent in most tumors is considered evidence that the drug has little activity and that further trial is not justified. A response rate falling between 10 and 20 percent usually will lead to further clinical trials on a limited basis in an effort to further define the activity of the agent. In analyzing these phase II trials, it is essential that the choice of patients selected for treatment be carefully reviewed. It is clear that patients who have failed several trials of prior treatment (whether radiation, drugs, surgery, or all of these) will have a lower response rate, a shorter duration of remission, and a shorter survival than patients who are treated with an agent initially, prior to other interventions. For instance, DDP has a 37 percent response rate in advanced ovarian cancer if given as the first chemotherapeutic agent (Bruckner et al.), a 25 percent response rate if given after failure of only one prior chemotherapeutic regimen (Wiltshaw et al.), and a 5 percent response rate if given after failure of two prior chemotherapeutic programs (Piver et al.).

Once activity for an agent in a given tumor type is established, then it may be made available for general use. Further research into the utility of this drug may take the form of "head to head" comparison with known active agents, application to different groups of patients (such as those without prior therapy), use in combination with other modalities (such as after surgery or radiotherapy in groups of patients known to be at high risk of relapse), or concurrent administration with other known active agents.

COMBINATION CHEMOTHERAPY

Common current practice is to combine newly discovered active agents with already known active agents into *drug combinations*. It has been clearly established in clinical trials, first in choriocarcinoma, then acute lymphocytic leukemia in childhood, and also in Hodgkin's disease, that some agents when given singly lead to remissions but not cures. These same agents can, when combined, yield a very high remission rate and cure in a significant proportion of patients.

Ideally, the drugs chosen for combination regimens should demonstrate convergent antineoplastic activity against the tumor alone with divergent toxicities against host tissues, so that full doses of each agent can be given. Many combinations that fulfill these requirements have been devised for the treatment of lymphoma (cyclophosphamide, vincristine, and prednisone); cancer of the head and neck and cervix (methotrexate, bleomycin, and platinum); cancer of the cervix (mitomycin C, vincristine and bleomycin); and cancer of the testis (vinblastine, bleomycin, and DDP). In practice, it has turned out that the concurrent administration of agents with the same dose-limiting toxicity (bone marrow suppression) can be accomplished at nearly full doses with acceptable toxicity. Thus cyclophosphamide, methotrexate, and 5-fluorouracil all have dose-limiting myelosuppression, but the response rate in breast cancer to this combination is twice that achieved with an alkylating agent alone, and the clinical responses to the combination are of better quality and longer duration.

It is essential in the design of combination regimens that interactions which could enhance toxicity be avoided. Thus, one would not administer a nephrotoxic agent and follow it with a drug whose excretion is largely renal. Within limits of acceptable tox-

icity, efforts are made to administer each agent in an optimum dose and schedule. In some instances, this means the addition of an inactive agent to optimize the activity of a component of the combination (an example would be the addition of citrovorum rescue to high doses of methotrexate). Occasionally, combination regimens can produce synergistic activity against the tumor by a timed attack in which one drug holds cells in a particular phase of their growth and a second agent kills cells most efficiently in that phase. It is critical in the design of such timed attack protocols to ensure that tumor cell kill is enhanced and normal host cell kill is not enhanced.

Another rationale for combined chemotherapy is an attack on sequential steps in the same metabolic pathway.

Combination chemotherapy is generally administered in repeated courses. Single doses of one or many drugs are rarely curative (exceptions are in hydatidiform mole and early-stage Burkitt's lymphoma). While one dose or a single course may yield gratifying improvement in the clinical condition of a patient with a sensitive neoplasm, prolonged treatment is generally necessary to sequentially induce fractional kills of remaining tumor cells. For example, patients with Hodgkin's disease, histiocytic lymphoma, testicular cancer, and ovarian cancer can sometimes be cured by repeated cycles of active agents, singly or in combination. After a fixed period of treatment, those patients in complete remission may be taken off chemotherapy. Some of these patients will never have recurrences of their disease, and may be considered cured.

PRACTICAL GYNECOLOGIC CHEMOTHERAPY

Cancer chemotherapy remains a rapidly evolving discipline in which most regimens often yield major toxicity that is sometimes life-threatening. Since success has heretofore been relatively limited (most patients continue to die of their diseases in spite of the best available chemotherapy), new regimens are constantly being developed and tested. Because the field is changing so rapidly, and because the margin of safety with most chemotherapeutic regimens is so slim, chemotherapy should be given by experts well versed in the indications and side effects of the currently employed agents given singly, in combination, or together with surgery, irradiation, or other treatment modalities.

The goal of this section is not to give precise

TABLE 47–11 Active Drugs in Gynecologic Cancers

Choriocarcinoma
  Methotrexate*
  Actinomycin D*
  Cyclophosphamide and other alkylating agents
  Vinblastine
  6-Mercaptopurine
Ovarian cancer
  Cyclophosphamide and other alkylating agents
  Adriamycin
  Hexamethylmelamine
  cis-Diamminedichloroplatinum II
Cervical cancer
  cis-Diamminedichloroplatinum II
  Mitomycin C
Endometrial cancer
  Adriamycin
  ? 5-Fluorouracil
  ? Alkylating agents

*Preferred drugs.

doses and schedules for the treatment of various sorts of patients. Since gynecologists are called upon to participate in the care of patients receiving chemotherapy, this section will attempt to list the agents now in use for the treatment of gynecologic neoplasms and their major indications and toxicities (Table 47–11). The current indications for chemotherapeutic treatment for each gynecologic neoplasm are given in Chaps. 40 to 45.

Alkylating agents were the first clinically applied anticancer drugs. They act by cross-linking DNA and preventing its cellular function. The prototype drug in the group is nitrogen mustard. It is extremely caustic, must be given intravenously, and causes severe nausea and vomiting and alopecia, as well as bone marrow suppression. A congener, *melphalan* (L-phenylalanine mustard, Alkeran, L-PAM), because it is orally active and does not cause alopecia, nausea, or vomiting and can be given easily in intermittent courses, is now the preferred single agent in the treatment of ovarian cancer. Myelosuppression is the only significant side effect for the majority of patients treated with this drug.

Chlorambucil (Leukeran) is another orally active alkylating agent with minimal side effects aside from myelosuppression. *Cyclophosphamide* (Cytoxan) is an alkylating agent which can be given both orally and intravenously. In addition to myelosuppression, it can cause a chemical cystitis and frequently causes moderate degrees of alopecia. Cyclophosphamide has been the preferred alkylating agent for use in

combination chemotherapy regimens because it is believed to cause less cumulative damage to platelet production than other members of this group of drugs.

Alkylating agents are essential drugs in the chemotherapy of ovarian cancer. Some patients have been cured of this cancer by alkylating agents alone. Alkylating agents have established activity in cancer of the cervix and the endometrium. They have been used in combination regimens in the treatment of sarcomas, choriocarcinomas, and germ-cell tumors, but evidence of activity as single agents in these neoplasms is not firm.

The most important *antimetabolite* in the treatment of gynecologic neoplasms is methotrexate (amethopterin). This is an inhibitor of dihydrofolate reductase and thus deprives cells of active methyl groups necessary for thymidine, purine, and methionine synthesis. Methotrexate can be administered orally, intramuscularly, or intravenously. It causes no local toxicity at the site of administration, nor does it cause alopecia. The duration of effective exposure to methotrexate is critical in terms of toxicity. Prolonged exposure to even very low doses can result in profound toxicity and death. Dose-limiting side effects are myelosuppression, stomatitis, skin rash, and diarrhea. Methotrexate has some established activity against ovarian and cervical cancer, but its major impact in gynecologic practice has been in treating gestational trophoblastic disease, where it can be curative for many patients when given as a single agent.

5-Fluorouracil is an inhibitor of thymidylate synthetase and is incorporated into RNA (ribonucleic acid) as nonsense message. Toxicity includes myelosuppression, stomatitis, diarrhea, skin rash, and cerebellar ataxia. This agent has limited activity in ovarian cancer.

Among the *antitumor antibiotics, adriamycin* (Doxorubicin) is probably the most important. This drug has established activity in cancers of the ovary and cervix, and is the best single agent available for the chemotherapy of sarcomas. Adriamycin is profoundly myelosuppressive, causes severe alopecia even at low doses, and frequently causes mild degrees of nausea and vomiting. It must be given intravenously with great care, since paravenous infiltration of even a small amount can lead to severe and irreversible skin ulceration. Cumulative doses in excess of 500 mg/m² frequently result in a cardiomyopathy which can be fatal. Thus, careful limitation of total dose is essential.

The antibiotic *dactinomycin* (actinomycin C, Cosmegen) causes severe nausea and vomiting and myelosuppression. It is a drug with a high order of activity against gestational trophoblastic disease, where it can be curative, and has clear-cut activity against sarcomas in children and germ-cell tumors of the ovary. Its previous widespread use in the combination chemotherapy of ovarian cancer was not justified by objective phase II data supporting its activity as a single agent.

Bleomycin (Blenoxane) is a mixture of polypeptides which has shown some activity against squamous cancer of the uterine cervix. Bleomycin is not myelosuppressive, but causes acute febrile reactions which can occasionally be fatal. It sometimes causes thickening of the skin. Intersititial pulmonary fibrosis can occur from any dose of bleomycin, but is most common when cumulative doses in excess of 400 units have been administered. Bleomycin may be given intravenously or intramuscularly without risk of local toxicity at the site of administration.

Mitomycin C (Mutamycin) is an antibiotic with some activity against cancer of the uterine cervix. Major toxicity is myelosuppression, characteristically occurring 4 to 6 weeks after drug administration. Paravenous infiltration can cause severe local tissue necrosis.

Vincristine (Oncovin) and *vinblastine* (Velban) are alkaloid derivatives of the periwinkle plant which act against the mitotic spindle. The dose-limiting toxicity of vincristine is peripheral neuropathy and ileus, while that of vinblastine is marrow suppression. Since they are chemically similar, some overlap in toxicities is seen. Both agents must be administered intravenously, and both can cause local tissue necrosis of a moderate degree if paravenous infiltration occurs. Vincristine has some activity in cancer of the uterine cervix, in germ-cell tumors of the ovary, and has been used in combination regimens for the treatment of sarcomas without much evidence for activity as a single agent. The use of vinblastine in the treatment of gynecologic cancer has been limited to occasional employment as a second-line agent in the treatment of choriocarcinoma.

Hormonal agents are not widely used in the treatment of gynecologic cancer except for progestational drugs in the treatment of endometrial carcinoma with lung metastases. Minor activity has been reported for progestational agents in the treatment of advanced ovarian cancer. Progestational agents are without major side effects, and can be administered orally or intramuscularly.

cis-Diamminedichloroplatinum II (DDP), is an agent with clear-cut activity against ovarian cancer and cancer of the uterine cervix (Vogl et al.). Myelosuppression from DDP is mild, but dose-limiting nephrotoxicity has been observed. This can be greatly ameliorated by concomitant hydration and diuresis. DDP must be given intravenously, is not locally caustic, and causes severe nausea and vomiting, which can be protracted. It occasionally causes nerve deafness, and rarely leads to anaphylactic reactions. Because DDP is not myelosuppressive, it has been successfully combined with other agents in the chemotherapy of ovarian and cervical cancer.

Hexamethylolmelamine has clear-cut activity against ovarian cancer. It can be administered only orally. Dosages are generally limited by nausea and vomiting. Myelosuppression is mild, but peripheral neuropathy has been reported after prolonged treatment.

CANCER CHEMOTHERAPY DURING PREGNANCY

Special problems occur with regard to the treatment of patients with extragenital cancer who are coincidentally pregnant. There is only a limited amount of data on acute effects on the fetus. These include spontaneous abortion when a lesion incompatible with further fetal development is induced, and severe congenital malformations when a less severe lesion is produced. There are almost no data on later effects of cancer treatment during pregnancy. These could conceivably involve abnormalities of postnatal growth and organ function in lung, bone marrow, brain, liver, kidney, and the reproductive tract. It remains conceivable that prenatal exposure to carcinogenic drugs could lead to the development of malignant neoplasms in the offspring many years later. Because of the paucity of data on both acute and late effects on the fetus, any recommendation as to preferred courses of therapy during pregnancy must be considered tentative, and extreme caution remains necessary in administering any drug to the mother during any stage of pregnancy.

Given the unquantified, perhaps substantial, risks to the fetus, it would seem prudent to treat indolent diseases as little as possible during pregnancy, especially if the diseases cannot be cured. This would include asymptomatic or minimally symptomatic patients with multiple myeloma; nodular, lymphocytic, poorly differentiated lymphoma; and chronic myelogenous leukemia. When treatment of these is clearly required, it should be as limited as possible in scope and intensity, and be accomplished with an agent that has been determined to be least likely to cause fetal problems on the basis of available experience.

In situations where treatment of the maternal neoplasm is of no established value, or is of minor transient value to the mother, it should not be undertaken in the pregnant patient. This would include chemotherapy of advanced colon cancer and advanced non-small-cell carcinoma of the lung. Surgical treatment for cancer which is potentially curable by this modality should be pursued essentially unaltered by the fact of pregnancy, though pregnancy may be associated with increased virulence of some cancers, such as those arising in the breast.

In a situation in which a malignant neoplasm is likely to be rapidly fatal to the mother, thus representing a clear and present danger both to the mother and the fetus, the most effective therapy should be given to the mother immediately. Acute leukemia is such a situation (Nicholson, 1968a; Lilleyman et al.). One may be encouraged to aggressively treat pregnant patients with acute leukemia by reading reports of a normal fetus produced by mothers treated with cytosine arabinoside and 6-thioguanine in the 10th, 25th, and 26th weeks of their pregnancies (Lilleyman et al.; Raich et al.; Pawliger et al.). However, trisomy C has been demonstrated in a placenta delivered by a therapeutic abortion after the mother was treated at 20 weeks with these drugs (Maurer et al.). Disseminated symptomatic non-Hodgkin's lymphoma may also be a situation where systemic treatment is essential during pregnancy, though only 12 patients have been reported (Ortega). One patient was treated with combination chemotherapy through her second and third trimester and was in complete remission when a normal infant was delivered.

Some pregnant patients with Hodgkin's disease may have asymptomatic disease of limited extent which progresses slowly. Many of these patients can have therapy delayed until after the pregnancy is complete, or until very late in the pregnancy, if they are followed very closely for progression of disease or development of symptoms. Since most patients present with lymphadenopathy only above the diaphragm, those patients who need to be treated during pregnancy can often be treated by radiation only; and adjuvant chemotherapy, if planned, may be deferred until after delivery. The abdomen should be shielded when radiation is delivered during pregnancy to avoid external scatter of the beam. Any radiation delivered during pregnancy should be delivered with the highest energy apparatus available, greater than 22 MeV if possible, to minimize internal scatter to the fetus. The smallest field encompassing all known disease should be employed, to areas as far from the fetus as possible. Paradoxically, the large fetus whose organs are formed and who is not sensitive to the teratogenic effects of ionizing radiation, because of a higher position in the abdomen during growth, gets more radiation than the embryo. Thus the fundal dose from mantle radiotherapy (to nodes in the upper half of the torso) is calculated as 10 rads for the 16-week fetus, 30 rads for the 25-week fetus, and greater than 100 rads for the 30-week fetus when 6-MeV electrons are used (Thomas et al.).

Diagnostic x-rays should be minimized in the evaluation of pregnant patients with Hodgkin's disease, since each abdominal film gives the fetus a total body dose of approximately 1 rad. For the symptomatic patient with advanced progressive Hodgkin's disease in the second and third trimester, chemotherapy is needed and should be given in an optimum schedule in an effort to achieve cure of the mother.

If chemotherapeutic drugs must be given during pregnancy, most of those who are experienced in the field advocate abortion for women treated in the first trimester, based on reports of a high incidence of spontaneous abortion of severe fetal malformations in those mothers who received aminopterin or 6-mercaptopurine (Nicholson, 1968b). Cyclophosphamide administered in the first trimester has led to at least two malformed fetuses (Toledo et al.; Wells et al.). Two normal neonates have also been reported (Lergier et al.; Lacher et al.). Chlorambucil has led to at least one malformed fetus (Wells et al.). Surprisingly, the microtubular poison vinblastine has been given at least three times in the first trimester resulting in normal babies (Wells et al.; Lacher; Lacher et al.). Procarbazine, a very potent teratogenic and carcinogenic compound in the monkey, was given to one pregnant patient in the first trimester and a normal baby resulted (Wells et al.). No data are available on the administration of anthracyclines such as adriamycin and daunorubicin during pregnancy. Because definitive information is lacking on fetal outcome after maternal therapy with modern combination regimens, a full discussion of the issues with the patient is essential, offering the mother the option of therapeutic abortion. The latter should be especially strongly considered during the first trimester of pregnancy if chemotherapy is necessary.

REFERENCES

Overview

Brindle G et al.: Cervical smears: Are the right women being examined? *Br Med J* 1:1196–1197, 1976.

Candian Task Force: Cervical cancer screening

(Walton Report). *Can Med Assoc J* 114:1003–1033, 1976.

Cole P: Elective hysterectomy: Pro and con. *N Engl J Med* 295:264–266, 1976.

Coppelson M et al.: *Colposcopy: A Scientific and Practical Approach to the Cervix in Health and Disease,* Springfield, Ill.: Charles C Thomas, 1971.

Decker DG et al.: Grading of gynecologic malignancy: Epithelial ovarian cancer, in *Proceedings, Seventh National Cancer Conference,* Philadelphia and Toronto, 1973, pp. 223–231.

Dunphy JE: On caring for the patient with cancer. *N Engl J Med* 295:313–319, 1979.

Evans DMD et al.: Observer variation and quality control of cytodiagnosis. *J Clin Pathol* 27:945–950, 1974.

Foltz AM, Kelsey JL: The annual Pap test: A dubious policy success. *Milbank Mem Fund Q* 56:426–462, 1978.

Homesley HD et al.: Treatment of adenocarcinoma of the endometrium at Memorial-James Ewing hospitals, 1949–1965. *Obstet Gynecol* 47:100–105, 1976.

Kern WH, Zivolich MR: The accuracy and consistency of the cytologic classifications of squamous lesions of the uterine cervix. *Acta Cytol* 21:519–523, 1977

Kinlen LJ, Spriggs AI: Women with positive cervical smears but without surgical intervention. *Lancet* 2:463–465, 1978.

Kübler-Ross E: *Death: The Final Stage of Growth,* Englewood Cliffs, N.J.: Prentice-Hall, 1975.

——: *Questions and Answers on Death and Dying,* New York: Macmillan, 1974.

Lanzotti VJ et al.: Cancer chemotherapeutic response and intravenous hyperalimentation. *Cancer Chemother Rep* 59:437–439, 1975.

Lyon JL, Gardner JW: The rising frequency of hysterectomy: Its effect on uterine cancer rates. *Am J Epidemiol* 105:439–443, 1977.

Reimer RR et al.: Acute leukemia after alkylating agent therapy of ovarian cancer. *N Engl J Med* 297:177–181, 1977.

Saunders C: St. Christopher's Hospice. *Br J Soc Serv Rev,* November 10, 1967.

Stern E, Neely PM: Carcinoma and dysplasia of the cervix: A comparison of rates for new and returning population. *Acta Cytol* 7:357–361, 1963.

—— et al.: Pap testing and hysterectomy prevalence: A survey of comments with high and low cervical cancer rates. *Am J Epidemiol* 106:296–305, 1977.

Strain JJ: The Pharos of Alpha Omega Alpha. 41:27–32, 1978.

Zelen M: A new design for randomized clinical trials. *N Engl J Med* 300:1242–1245, 1979.

Clinical Therapeutic Implications

Ackerman LV, del Regato JA: *Cancer Diagnosis, Treatment and Prognosis,* 4th ed., St. Louis: Mosby, 1970.

Andrews JR: Combined cancer radiotherapy and chemotherapy: The relevance of cell population kinetics and pharmacodynamics. *Cancer Chemother Rep* 53:313, 1969.

Asire AJ, Shambaugh MA: *Cancers of the Female Genital Tract: End Results Report,* Cancer Patient Survival Report no. 5, NCT HEW, 1976, pp. 164–189.

Aurelian L: Virions and antigens of herpes virus type 2 in cervical carcinoma. *Cancer Res* 33:1539–1947, 1973.

Bagshawe KD: *Choriocarcinoma, The Clinical Biology of the Trophoblast and its Tumours,* London: E. Arnold, 1969.

Brown CR et al.: Irradiation of in situ and invasive squamous cell carcinoma of the vagina. *Cancer* 28:1278, 1971.

Cancer Committee (FIGO): Classification and staging of malignant tumors in the female pelvis. *Int J Gynaecol Obstet* 9:172, 1971.

Cole WH: *Chemotherapy of Cancer,* Philadelphia: Lea & Febiger, 1970.

Coppelson M et al.: *Colposcopy: A Scientific and Practical Approach to the Cervix in Health and Disease,* Springfield, Ill: Charles C Thomas, 1971.

Delclos L et al.: Tumors of the ovary, in *Textbook of Radiotherapy,* 2d ed., ed. GH Fletcher, Philadelphia: Lea & Febiger, 1973.

Durrance FY et al.: Computer calculation of dose contribution to regional lymphatics from gynecological radium insertions. *Radiology* 91:140, 1968.

El Senoussi MA et al.: Correlation of radiation and surgical parameters in complications in the extended field technique for carcinoma of the cervix. *Int J Radiat Biol* 5:927–934, 1979.

Fletcher GH: Clinical dose response curves of human malignant epithelial tumors. *Br J Radiol* 46:1, 1973.

——: Radiation therapy and subclinical disease, in *Neoplasms of the Head and Neck,* Chicago: Year Book, 1974.

——: *Textbook of Radiotherapy,* 2d ed., Philadelphia: Lea & Febiger, 1973.

—— et al.: Adenocarcinoma of the uterus, in *Frontiers of Radiation Therapy and Oncology,* vol. 5, Basel: S. Karger AG, 1970.

—— et al.: Carcinoma of the uterine cervix, in

Modern Radiotherapy, ed. TJ Deeley, London: Butterworths, 1971.

—— et al.: Radiotherapy of cancers of the cervix uteri, in *Carcinoma of the Uterine Cervix, Endometrium and Ovary,* Chicago: Year Book, 1962.

——, Shukovsky LJ: The interplay of radiocurability and tolerance in the irradiation of human cancers. *J Radiol Electrol Med Nucl* 56:383, 1975.

Folkman J: Tumor angiogenesis: Therapeutic implications. *N Engl J Med* 285:182–186, 1971.

Greenwald P et al.: Prenatal stilbestrol experience of mothers of young cancer patients. *Cancer* 31:568–572, 1973.

Hellstrom I et al.: Demonstration of cell mediated immunity to human neoplasms of various histological types. *Int J Cancer* 7:1, 1971.

Hryniuk WM, Bertino JR: Rationale for selection of chemotherapeutic agents. *Adv Intern Med* 15:267, 1969.

Janovski NA, Douglas CP: *Diseases of the Vulva,* New York: Harper & Row, 1972.

Lewis L Jr.: Chemotherapy of gestational choriocarcinoma. *Cancer* 30:44–48, 1972.

Marcus SL: Multiple squamous cell carcinomas involving the cervix, vagina and vulva. *Am J Obstet Gynecol* 80:802–812, 1960.

Nahmias AJ et al.: Antibodies to herpes virus hominis type 1 and 2 in humans: Women with cervical cancer. *Am J Epidemiol* 91:547–552, 1970.

Nelson AJ et al.: Indications for adjunctive, conservative extra fascial hysterectomy in selected cases of carcinoma of the uterine cervix. *Am J Roentgenol Radium Ther Nucl Med.* 123, 1:91–99, 1975.

Newman W, Cromer JK: The multicentric origin of carcinomas of the female genital tract. *Surg Gynecol Obstet* 108:273–281, 1959.

Nicholson HO: Cytotoxic drugs in pregnancy. *J Obstet Gynaecol Br Commonw* 75:307, 1968.

O'Quinn AG et al.: Guidelines for conservative hysterectomy after irradiation. *Gynecol Oncol* 9:68–79, 1980.

Perez CH et al.: Malignant tumor of the vagina. *Cancer* 31:36–44, 1973.

Puck TT, Marcus PI: Action of x-rays on mammalian cells. *J Exp Med* 103:653, 1956.

Rawls WE et al.: Herpes type 2 antibodies and carcinoma of the cervix. *Lancet* 2:1142–1143, 1970.

Royston I, Aurelian L: The association of genital herpes and cervical atypia and carcinoma in situ. *Am J Epidemiol* 91:531–538, 1970.

Rutledge FN et al.: Surgical procedures associated with radiation therapy for cervical cancer, in *Textbook of Radiotherapy,* 2d ed., ed. GH Fletcher, Philadelphia: Lea & Febiger, 1973.

Rutledge F et al.: Carcinoma of the vulva. *Am J Obstet Gynecol* 106:1117–1130, 1970.

Sabin AB: Viral carcinogenesis: Phenomena of special significance in the search for a viral etiology in human cancers. *Cancer Res* 28:1849–1858, 1968.

Santesson L, Kottmeier HL: General classification of ovarian tumors, in *Ovarian Cancer,* U.I.C.C. Monograph Series, vol. 2, eds. F Gentil, AC Junqueira, New York: Springer-Verlag, 1968.

Sartorelli AC, Creasey WA: Cancer chemotherapy. *Ann Rev Pharmacol* 9:51, 1969.

Scully RE: Recent progress in ovarian cancer. *Hum Pathol* 1:73–98, 1970.

Strandqvist M: Studien über die kumulative wirkung der rontgenstrahlen bei fraktionierung. *Acta Radiol* (Stockh), suppl 55, 1944, p. 257.

Suite HD: Radiation biology: A basis for radiotherapy, in *Textbook of Radiotherapy,* 2d ed., ed. GH Fletcher, Philadelphia: Lea & Febiger, 1973.

—— et al.: Intact tumor cells in irradiated tissues. *Arch Pathol* 78:648, 1964.

Vermund H, Gollin FF: Mechanisms of action of radiotherapy and chemotherapy adjuvants. *Cancer* 21:58, 1968.

Wharton JT et al.: Irradiation therapy for gynecologic malignancies, in *Davis' Obstetrics and Gynecology,* vol. 2, Hagerstown, Md.: Harper & Row, 1972.

—— et al.: Radiation hepatitis induced by abdominal irradiation with the cobalt 60 moving strip technique. *Am J Roentgenol Radium Ther Nucl Med* 117:73, 1973.

Williams DC (ed.): *Symposium on Endometrial Cancer,* London: Heinemann, 1971.

Wilson W: Personal communication.

Principles of Cancer Surgery

Boronow RE: Carcinoma of the corpus: Treatment at M. D. Anderson Hospital, in *Cancer of the Uterus and Ovary,* Chicago: Year Book, 1969, p. 35.

Fletcher GH, Rutledge FN: Overall results in radiotherapy for carcinoma of the cervix. *Am J Obstet Gynecol* 5:958, 1968.

Frick, HC et al.: Carcinoma of the endometrium. *Am J Obstet Gynecol* 115:663–675, 1973.

Graham J: The value of preoperative or postoperative treatment by radium for carcinoma of the uterine body. *Surg Gynecol Obstet* 132:855, 1971.

Gusberg SB, Yannopoulos D: Therapeutic decisions in corpus cancer. *Am J Obstet Gynecol* 88:157–162, 1964.

Herbst AL et al.: *N Engl J Med* 284:878, 1971.

McLennan CE: The argument against preoperative radium for endometrial cancer. *Trans Pacif Coast Obstet Gynecol Soc* 25:122, 1957.

Meigs JV: The Wertheim operation for carcinoma of the cervix. *Am J Obstet Gynecol* 49:542, 1945.

Morrow CP et al.: Current management of endometrial carcinoma. *Obstet Gynecol* 42:399–405, 1972.

Pack RC et al.: Treatment of stage I carcinoma of the cervix. *Obstet Gynecol* 41:117–122, 1973.

Rutledge FN: The role of surgical resection in the management of cervical carcinoma, in *Carcinoma of the Uterine Cervix, Endometrium and Ovary*, Chicago: Year Book, 1962, p. 149.

———, **Burns BC:** Pelvic exenteration. *Am J Obstet Gynecol* 91:692–708, 1965.

——— **et al.:** Pelvic Lymphadenectomy as adjunct to radiation therapy in treatment of cancer of the cervix. *Am J Roentgenol Radium Ther Nucl Med* 93:607, 1965.

———: Surgery versus x-ray for treatment in carcinoma of the cervix, in *Controversy in Obstetrics and Gynecology*, eds. D Reid, TC Barton, Philadelphia: Saunders, 1969, p. 397.

———: Carcinoma of the vulva. *Am J Obstet Gynecol* 106:1117–1130, 1970.

Smith JP, Rutledge FN: Chemotherapy in treatment of cancer of the ovary. *Am J Obstet Gynecol* 107:691–703, 1970.

——— **et al.:** Chemotherapy of ovarian cancer. New approaches to treatment. *Cancer* 30:1565–1571, 1972.

Stallworthy JA: Radical surgery following radiation treatment for cervical carcinoma. *Ann R Coll Surg Engl* 34:161–178, 1964.

———: Surgery of endometrial cancer in the Bonney tradition. *Ann R Coll Surg Engl* 48:293–305, 1971.

Principles of Cancer Chemotherapy

Bruckner HW et al.: Chemotherapy of ovarian cancer with adriamycin and cis-diamminedichloroplatinum (II). *Proc Am Soc Clin Onc* 17:287, 1976.

Piver MS et al.: Cis-dichlorodiammineplatinum (II) as third-line chemotherapy in advanced ovarian adenocarcinoma. *Cancer Treat Rep* 62:559, 1978.

USA–USSR Monograph: *Method of Development of New Anticancer Drugs*, Natl Cancer Inst Monogr 45, Bethesda, Md.: Department of Health, Education, and Welfare, 1978.

Vogl SE et al.: Ovarian cancer: Effective treatment of alkylating agent failures. JAMA 241:1908, 1979.

Wasserman TH, Carter SK: The integration of chemotherapy into combined modality treatment of solid tumors: VIII. Cervical cancer. *Cancer Treat Rev* 4:25, 1977.

Wiltshaw E et al.: Phase II study of cis-dichlorodiammineplatinum (II) (NSC-119875) in advanced adenocarcinoma of the ovary. *Cancer Treat Rep* 60:55, 1976.

Young, RC: Chemotherapy of ovarian cancer: Past and present. *Semin Oncol* 2:267, 195.

——— **et al.:** Chemotherapy of advanced ovarian carcinoma: A prospectively randomized comparison of phenylalanine mustard and high dose cyclophosphamide. *Gynecol Oncol* 2:489, 1974.

Cancer Chemotherapy During Pregnancy

Lacher Mortimer J: Use of vinblastine sulfate to treat Hodgkin's disease during pregnancy. *Ann Int Med* 61:113–115, 1964.

——— **et al.:** Cyclophosphamide and vinblastine sulfate in Hodgkin's disease during pregnancy. *JAMA,* 195:486–488, 1966.

Lergier Julio E et al.: Normal pregnancy in multiple myeloma treated with cyclophosphamide. *Cancer* 34:1018–1022, 1974.

Lilleyman JS et al.: Consequences of acute myelogenous leukemia in early pregnancy. *Cancer* 40:1300–1303, 1977.

Maurer LH et al.: Fetal group C trisomy after cytosine arabinoside and thioguanine. *Ann Int Med* 75:809–810, 1971.

Nicholson H Oliphant: Leukemia and pregnancy. *J Obstet Gynaec Br Commonw* 75:517–520, 1968a.

———: Cytotoxic drugs in pregnancy. *J Obstet Gynaec Br Commonw* 75:307–312, 1968b.

Ortega, Jesus: Multiple agent chemotherapy including bleomycin of non-Hodgkin's lymphoma during pregnancy. *Cancer* 40:2829–2835, 1977.

Pawliger DF et al.: Normal fetus after cytosine arabinoside therapy. *Ann Int Med* 74:1012, 1971.

Raich Peter C et al.: Treatment of acute leukemia during pregnancy. *Cancer* 36:861–862, 1975.

Thomas PRM et al.: The investigation and management of Hodgkin's disease in the pregnant patient. *Cancer* 38:1443–1451, 1976.

Toledo TM et al.: Fetal effects during cyclophosphamide and irradiation therapy. *Ann Int Med* 74:87–91, 1971.

Wells James H et al.: Procarbazine therapy for Hodgkin's disease in early pregnancy. *JAMA* 205:935–937, 1968.

48

Principles of Surgery

JOHN A. SCHILLING

INTRODUCTION

This chapter is about the operative and nonoperative
care of patients for whom a surgical procedure is, or
may be, the most specific treatment during the time-
course of a disease process. The author supports the
dictum that no surgical procedure is to be employed
if there is an equally good or better and safer non-

surgical modality of treatment. All surgical patients face the risks of their underlying pathology and of the accompanying metabolic and physiologic decrements. They also face the iatrogenic risks of diagnosis and of treatment. The counterpart of these risks is the potential benefit of treatment. There is, therefore, a mathematical trade-off of risks and benefits for each patient, and decisions should be based on judgment gained from statistically valid observations of groups of patients. Inherent in the principles of surgery is knowledge of these underlying risks and benefits. Patient management must be governed by that which produces the greatest benefit with the least risk. In addition, a specific diagnosis is imperative in planning surgical care; any exceptions to this should also be specific.

Three distinct periods occur in the time-course of all surgical patients: the preoperative, the operative, and the postoperative. It is impossible to approach these areas authoritatively in the space of one chapter, and it would be naive to attempt it. Two splendid, recently published textbooks of surgery do cover this body of knowledge (Sabiston; Schwartz), and they include many references to every aspect of the management of the surgical patient. Several recent manuals and symposia on special areas of care of the surgical patient also add to this body of knowledge. Their chapters, contributed by recognized authorities, will be referred to instead of articles in scientific journals. These volumes, appended as general references, are readily available. Their references can lead the reader, better than any casual perusal of journals, to specific publications in the library. Finally, there is an advantage in having an authoritative body of knowledge under one cover. The principles of surgery will be outlined in this chapter as they arise during the time-course of care of the surgical patient.

PREOPERATIVE CONSIDERATIONS

Surgical patients face stress and metabolic demands of the operative procedure with its possible complications and morbidity, their residual organ function supplied only by their endogenous stores of protein, fat, carbohydrates, water, and minerals (Dudrick, Rhoads; Moore; Polk; Shires et al., 1977, 1979). As the physiologic response to the underlying disease state and surgery is cellular, requiring energy, it is essential that organ function, body composition, fat, and protein stores be carefully evaluated. Organ system deficits must be assayed through history, physical examination, and appropriate laboratory study. Particularly important are the exact details of prior or concurrent treatment when it may have caused cellular suppression of vital organs. The most significant are bone marrow and reticuloendothelial depression from cancer chemotherapy or x-radiation. The blood supply of irradiated tissues may be reduced profoundly in the operative area. The use of other drugs such as aspirin, steroids, alcohol, and nicotine should be determined, as they can affect the blood-clotting mechanisms, suppress the bone marrow, and influence hepatic, renal, pancreatic, or cardiopulmonary function. In our drug-oriented society, which involves all ages, this is becoming a more frequent consideration. The iatrogenic influences of drugs and their interactions are complex and unpredictable, particularly when added to starvation, anesthesia, and surgery.

METABOLIC AND OPERATIVE RISK FACTORS

Metabolic disease states and *risk factors* must be considered. First in importance are *starvation* and malnutrition with cachexia (*Manual of Surgical Nutrition*), which may be masked by obesity. Prolonged steroid administration may result in unrecognized protein depletion and potassium deficiency. Partial intestinal obstruction, chronic diarrhea from any cause, and enteric fistulas can also cause extreme protein depletion with sodium and potassium deficiency. *Obesity* is the second major risk factor. Its deleterious influences (Jones) include an increase in postoperative complications of all types, most notably wound and pulmonary complications and thromboembolic phenomena. Protein depletion, erosion of the muscle mass, and suppression of organ function may be subtle accompaniments. *Sepsis* is third (*Manual on Control of Infection in Surgical Patients;* Altemeier, Alexander). Some place it ahead of all other risk factors. Sepsis precludes elective surgery because the incidence of postoperative septic wound complications is prohibitive. Organs with marginal function may decompensate as a result of sepsis, and aseptic shock is one of the most lethal of all surgical catastrophes. *Diabetes* (Davis) must be known and be under control. *Hepatic cirrhosis* (Orloff) and uremia (Powers) render the patient particularly vulnerable to complications during and after surgery. A recent *myocardial infarct* (Greenfield) prohibits surgery except in an emergency. *Chronic pulmonary disease* (Laver, Austen) and emphysema may make a surgical procedure untenable in the trade-off between treatment risk and benefit. *Agedness* (Greenfield) is associated with higher morbidity and mortality because of the patient's lack of immune responsiveness and reserve in the organ systems. *Atherosclerosis* (*Manual of Preoperative and Postoperative Care*) and diminished arterial blood supply to the tissues of the brain, heart, kidney, and viscera increase risks. *Immune suppression* (Alexander, Good) from drugs, x-ray, cancer chemotherapy, sepsis, starvation, age, or any other cause must be evaluated, particularly if there is a diminution of polymorphonuclear cells, antibacterial globulins, complement, and platelets.

Emotional instability is a more subtle risk factor. Psychologic evaluation is important in that it relates to age, maturity, and motivation, and provides an essential insight into the patient as a person as well as information about the patient's family, social surroundings, and occupation. This area, often neglected by the specialist, goes far beyond informed consent and, when properly used and understood, can help the patient cope with surgical stresses and can minimize the cerebrally induced adrenocortical stress response.

HISTORY AND PHYSICAL EXAMINATION; LABORATORY EVALUATION

In these preoperative evaluations in the office and at the hospital, most of the areas mentioned are covered by a careful patient *history* and *physical examination*. Routine *laboratory evaluation* should also be added and should include a urinalysis for cells, sugar, and protein; a stool examination for occult blood; a complete blood count, hematocrit, and smear; a roentgenogram of the chest; electrocardiogram; and a screening battery of blood chemistry determinations—BUN (blood urea nitrogen), bilirubin, creatinine, electrolytes, plasma proteins, blood sugar, and uric acid (Conn). If a patient is obviously depleted, showing evidence of starvation, weight loss, and sepsis, a skin test to determine anergy is important diagnostically and for monitoring preoperative repletion. Often overlooked is an evaluation of the patient's endogenous bacterial flora of the skin, in the nasopharynx, and in the intertriginous zones. They are a frequent source of

postoperative sepsis. Special studies of individual organ functions may be indicated, e.g., hepatic, cardiac, pulmonary, renal, gastrointestinal, immunologic, and vascular. Details of these studies are included in general references (Sabiston; Schwartz; *Manual of Preoperative and Postoperative Care*).

Particular emphasis must be placed on *bleeding and clotting mechanisms* in every surgical patient. Without intravascular platelet aggregation and thrombus formation, the surgical patient will bleed to death. History of excessive menstrual flow, extensive bruising, post-tooth-extraction bleeding, family history of bleeding, ecchymoses, purpuric spots, widespread lymph-node enlargement, splenomegaly, and hepatomegaly may suggest the necessity for a screening laboratory study. This should include a partial thromboplastic time, a Quick one-stage prothrombin time. For details of the evaluation and treatment of surgical bleeding, see both Schwartz and Silver.

SEPSIS

Next to bleeding complications, *sepsis* is foremost in the problems faced by the surgical patient (Sabiston; *Manual on Control of Infection in Surgical Patients*). Despite remarkable medical advances in this area, infections are still as great a problem today as in the past. Staphylococci and the gram-negative bacteria have risen in incidence and now lead streptococci and pneumococci. The hospital environment, through autoinfection, invasive diagnostic studies, long-term supportive procedures, needles, intravenous catheters, tracheostomies, and supportive pulmonary, respiratory, and anesthetic equipment, has contributed to contamination of patients with pathogenic bacteria, or has contaminated patients with opportunistic bacteria when their defenses are low. It is essential that every surgeon develop a septic conscience and be aware of the sources of bacterial contamination. Cultures of nasopharynges, intertriginous areas, urine, cervix, and vagina should be made when indicated. Appropriate antibiotic therapy, prophylactic antibiotics of broad spectrum 2 hours before surgery and continued for 2 to 3 days after surgery, may be indicated. In certain instances, mechanical and antibacterial colon preparation may be required. Since it is impossible to eliminate bacteria, it is important to be aware of all the ways to reduce the number to tolerable levels. Certainly included would be periodic monitoring of housekeeping and laundry methods, dietary preparation of food, guards against infections in participating personnel, sterilization procedures, handwashing and scrubbing methods, isolation techniques, and means of ventilation and recirculation of air.

Infections must be dealt with on an individual basis, and elective surgery should be postponed until all clinical signs of sepsis have subsided. Several weeks should then elapse to allow for more complete elimination of bacteria by the patient and for development or enhancement of the patient's immune cellular and humoral antibacterial mechanisms.

NUTRITION

The preoperative patient is usually starved (*Manual of Surgical Nutrition*) to some extent because of special gastrointestinal studies, blood chemistries, and anesthesia. When these decrements are subtracted from marginal reserves, they can adversely tip the balance; the patient then faces the operative procedure with significant protein depletion, which is always at the expense of an essential function, enzyme, or secretion. Clear liquids are essentially protein-free; thus, the addition of an *elemental diet* during this period with 50 to 100 g of protein and 150 g of carbohydrate will enable the patient to benefit from additional protein and the protein sparing effect of carbohydrates. Further, it can contribute to a large-bowel mechanical preparation.

When protein deficiency is severe, a prolonged period of preoperative repletion is imperative. This can now be achieved since the advent of total parenteral nutrition. Often its importance is unappreciated, or its need unrecognized. *Oral alimentation* causes the fewest complications. If this is not possible, nasopharyngeal gastric feeding through a small soft tube should be tried. Intravenous alimentation may be used initially if the former two routes cannot be employed, but its potential complications are too serious for routine use if an alternate, safer method is effective.

It is difficult to decide how long a patient should be alimented before surgery. During the time of repletion, the progress of the disease may force an assessment of the risks and benefits of total alimentation, and termination may be necessary before total repletion is possible. Therefore, a reasonable compromise would be to continue preoperative alimentation until the patient is in a positive nitrogen balance, is gaining weight, and is no longer anergic by skin test. The obese patient, conversely, may benefit from a significant weight loss. Again, this must be carefully supervised. Weeks and months may be involved, but the weight loss must not be at the expense of the protein-containing lean body mass. An exercise program and psychiatric counseling may be needed.

ANESTHESIA ISSUES

The surgeon should participate in the preoperative *selection of the anesthetic* (Brunner, Eckenhoff; Greene). The anesthesiologist should be aware of the condition of the patient, concurrent disease, prior or concurrent treatment, requirements of the procedure, special problems, and the psychologic makeup of the patient. The experience of the anesthesiologist, as well as that of the surgeon, has a bearing on the particular anesthetic selected. Choice of anesthetic for a given patient varies from local infiltration to regional block, epidural block, spinal, inhalation, or intravenous anesthesia with the addition of narcotics and relaxants. Anesthesia is a poison or depressant but its benefits are greater than the risks. The importance of its choice and the mutual relationship between anesthesiologist and surgeon in the operative and perioperative care of the surgical patient cannot be overemphasized.

Induction of anesthesia is a critical time for every patient. With the transient periods of hypoxia and hypercapnia during induction and the vagal stimulation from tracheal intubation, there is an increased risk of cardiac arrest. For this reason, the responsible surgeon, or an effective member of his team with the knowledge and ability to manage cardiac arrest if it occurs, should be present during this period (Greenfield). Problems of inadequate ventilation and oxygenation when the intratracheal tube has entered the esophagus or has slipped past the carina are subtle. Anesthesiologists occasionally overlook this cause of cardiac arrhythmia or arrest. Gas or air insufflated into the stomach during induction should be aspirated to minimize the problems of postoperative gastric dilatation or ileus.

WOUND PREPARATION

Preparation of the wound area (*Manual on Control of Infection in Surgical Patients*), perineum, groin, and vagina is usually a routine procedure in every operating room. It can become so routine that occasionally the individuals responsible become careless.

The practice of shaving the operative area the night before surgery is pernicious and should be avoided because of frequent macroscopic and microscopic cuts in the skin and the development of wound sepsis. The purpose of mechanical and chemical cleansing is to reduce the surface bacteria to as near zero as possible. Repeated washes of the operative area with hexachlorophene or Betadine reduce the number of bacteria and should be routine practice in the days before most procedures. Cultures should be made occasionally to check the effectiveness of the "prep." They might include the hands of the operating team.

There is divergence of opinion concerning the efficacy of *skin drapes* in wound protection from bacteria. Towels are ineffectual and rough. The plastic drapes are smooth, glistening, sterile, and impervious to moisture. On the other hand, sweat and moisture accumulate beneath their internal surface, with exuded endogenous bacteria. Further, unless the skin surface is dry on application, the drapes do not stick. The author prefers plastic drapes where they can be used effectively, particularly if small bowel is to be eviscerated or large areas need protection from moisture. For additional protection, eviscerated small bowel should be placed in a plastic bag to prevent drying and abrasion. Plastic ring protectors of the wound may be useful in certain circumstances and seem to reduce wound infections.

OPERATIVE CONSIDERATIONS

In the operating room and during the operation, the surgeon's attention should be devoted at all times to the technical procedure being performed (Postlethwait). It should not be diverted to prior considerations of the patient's body composition or organ function. Nor should it be diverted by postoperative commitments, office appointments, or intervening communications. The surgeon should have a complete knowledge of the procedures being employed as well as alternate procedures and their technical steps for unexpected circumstances. In addition to a precise knowledge of the anatomy of the particular operative area, its anomalies or variations from normal, the surgeon should be aware of all the complications that may arise from procedures in a specific anatomic area. Finally, the surgeon should be intellectually and technically prepared to deal with the technical accidents that can occur to adjacent blood vessels, ducts, and viscera. In the pelvis this means the ureters, large

and small bowel, urinary bladder, trigone, and the iliac arteries and veins and their branches. The surgeon must be able to manage cardiac arrest. In short, education, experience, and preoperative considerations must provide a conscious intellectual preparation for each operative procedure. It is equally essential that good assistance and consultation be available when needed. It is untenable, however, for the surgeon to substitute assistance or consultative help for inadequacy except at the resident educational level. Finally, the surgeon should never let personal ego or ignorance stand in the way of the best care for the patient.

The *selection of the proper surgical procedure* for the specific pathology, the patient, and the variable biologic circumstances is of primary importance. What is considered the proper procedure today may not be the proper one tomorrow. The surgeon who is unprepared intellectually and technically to exchange older choices for new and better procedures or techniques becomes antiquated quickly. Sometimes certain outmoded procedures may be superior under an unusual set of clinical circumstances, but this selection must be specific. Perhaps the most subtle problem here is the surgeon's routine employment of a particular procedure or technique without occasionally inquiring if there is a better way.

TECHNICAL ASPECTS

Half of all postoperative complications can be termed wound complications; about half of these are wound infections which include incisional wounds of extirpation and reconstruction (Schilling). The incidence of wound complications can be kept to a minimum by a number of technical considerations. First, *good anesthesia* and *relaxation* are imperative. In addition, capable *surgical assistants* must be found, and the surgeon should participate in their special training and experience. Third, an *adequate incision* must be made. Adequacy relates to length, position, muscle and fascial planes, underlying viscera, and, most important, to pathology. Good exposure is governed by these variables which usually simplify any surgical procedure, make it safer and easier, and reduce complications. An adequate incision minimizes retraction. Most incisions should lend themselves to appropriate extension. Incisions that are considered cosmetically superior but which limit exposure should be avoided.

Fourth, good overhead *lighting* and the appropriate use of lighted retractors and head lamps are essential. Transillumination may be extremely helpful, and optic loops with two or four magnifications provide precise visualization.

Fifth is the *availability of proper retractors and instruments* and the knowledge of how to use them. The surgeon is responsible for ascertaining their presence and their sterility. Sometimes a special instrument is not available because its routine supply by the operating room personnel is taken for granted.

The knowledge, as well as the presence, of *appropriate materials for sutures and ligatures* is another technical consideration. The selection of sizes and tensile strengths should be commensurate with the tissues in which they are to be placed and, in general, the materials used should only moderately exceed the holding strength of the tissues. Most of the absorbable suture material (chromic and plain gut) and the braided fibers (cotton and silk) used at the present time are structured from foreign protein and evoke a greater tissue reaction than the monofilaments of wire and plastic origin. Monofilament sutures are superior to others when bacterial wound contamination, or sepsis, is present. Nonabsorbable suture materials should not be placed through inaccessible mucosal surfaces where they cannot be removed and may persist as contaminated foreign material. Braided fibers may harbor bacteria in their interstices that will cause granulomas. An increasing number of synthetic, absorbable materials for sutures seem superior to the guts. It is important to select the proper suture material and to know its properties.

The seventh point is the *proper use of sutures and ligatures*. Sutures serve only to approximate and temporarily provide a tensile strength equal to that of the tissues in which they are placed. It is collagen that supplies the strength and permanence to the wound scar. The average surgeon tends to tie fascial sutures to the limits of their tensile strength, rather than tying them with tension just sufficient for approximation. If suture tension continuously exceeds 30 mmHg, ischemic necrosis can develop with the suture area, producing an excessive inflammatory response and a partial or complete dehiscence. Skin sutures are seldom tied too tightly because the inflammatory results can readily be seen by the surgeon, the patient, and the patient's family. The same inflammation occurs in the deeper planes, although it is invisible. When tension is excessive, the suture line should be protected by relaxing incisions, by retention sutures, or by reconstruction.

Another common abuse by surgeons is selecting suture material that is too large in diameter, creating an excessive inflammatory and encapsulating response which, in turn, leads to a higher incidence of wound infection and dehiscence. Thus, the combination of sutures that are too large, too tight, and too close together can cause a higher rate of dehiscence and infection, along with the pathologic production of collagen.

The last technical consideration is the surgeon's *ability to operate*. The expert surgeon is often denigrated as a technician, but it has been the author's observation that knowledgeable patients select competent technical surgeons whose expertise enhances and augments knowledge, experience, and surgical judgment. Basically involved is the application of Halsted's principles of surgery. These principles specify gentleness, asepsis, a good blood supply, avoidance of tension, hemostasis, careful approximation, and obliteration of dead spaces.

HALSTED'S PRINCIPLES OF SURGERY

GENTLENESS

Gentleness should characterize the many small and large traumas by hand and by instrument during surgery. They cannot be eliminated, but they can be minimized. Surgeons vary in their *dissection techniques*. A sharp, cold scalpel creates less cellular damage than do dissecting scissors. The moist, gloved hand may be the gentlest or the roughest blunt dissector. Cutting current, especially in the abdominal cavity, is dangerous and should not be used in this area as it may create excessive necrotic tissue; worse, like coagulating current, it can burn a hole into an adjacent bowel loop, which can be difficult to detect. Laser knives are too primitive in their development for routine clinical use. Whenever possible, gentle tension and a No. 15 Bard-Parker blade are preferred for dissection, along with soft brush or shavinglike strokes, rather than the spreading, blunt dissecting technique in which scissors and cutting crush and shear several cell layers. The latter method occasionally leads to the inadvertent total transection of a contiguous ureter, artery, or vein. Properly employed, particularly deep in the apices of body cavities or spaces, scissor dissection may be a safer and more effective technique than the scalpel. Blunt dissection with the back of a broad scalpel or moist fingers may effectively delineate the tissue planes. Blunt wiping with a small sponge on a hemostat is irritating to the tissues. This type of dissection might be of some advantage on fascial planes, but not around ducts, tubes, or blood vessels. The skilled surgeon is adept with all dissecting techniques and selects the method best suited to the circumstances encountered. Irrespective of method, the bulk of the dissecting forces should be applied to the tissue being extirpated, with minimal trauma to surrounding tissues.

Next is the *selection of properly sized forceps and hemostats*. Tissue that is clamped necrotizes. One cubic centimeter of necrotic tissue contains 100 million cells that must be lysed, absorbed, dispersed, phagocytosed, encapsulated, or calcified by the body's inflammatory defense mechanisms. The combination of necrotic tissue, a little blood, a silk suture, and a few bacteria is a perfect setting for the development of a wound infection. A hemostat too small for the area, which has to be reapplied repeatedly or which requires additional clamps, is more traumatic than a large hemostat. The use of hemostats to stabilize tissue planes should be minimized or eliminated. Hooks are often a better choice. When tissue is being divided between clamps for hemostatic reasons, the hemostats should be placed parallel and as close together as possible, permitting only a small cuff, as all tissue distal to the proximal edge of the clamps will become necrotic. This principle has to be sacrificed when the risk from slipping is greater than the risk of more dead tissue.

The principles set forth for the use of hemostats apply equally to *forceps and suturing*. The suture needle puncture is a wound through which a foreign body is placed. Obviously, the surgeon should select the smallest effective suture and a needle with an appropriate curve or cutting edge. Often this is not prospectively analyzed, and the surgeon can fall into a routine of using standard sutures and needles that are too large. To minimize turning, needle holders and their jaws should be matched to the size of the needle and its use. Small needle holders are irreparably damaged by large, heavy needles, and, conversely, small needles can be broken by large needle holders. These events can be catastrophic if they occur during suture ligature of a large vessel deep within a body cavity. Forceps stabilize tissue for suturing, but they create multiple miscroscopic wounds. If one doubts this, let him grasp his sclera with a pair of Adson forceps. However, plain forceps that slip are more traumatic than toothed forceps that do not slip. Sharp-pointed forceps can inadvertently perforate a viscus. Broad forceps can spread with less tissue trauma. Ophthalmic scleral forceps are ideal for some anastomoses. The trauma of forceps can be eliminated, or minimized, when only gentle counterpressure of the fingers or tissue resistance is used instead. These considerations are particularly important with tissue that has a poor blood supply or has been devitalized.

The *tying of sutures and ligatures* is usually routine. Just one faulty suture or ligature and its knot, however, can cause a fatal wound complication. The two-handed knot is usually better, more precise, and safer although slower than the one-handed knot, which unfortunately is often learned first by the junior surgeon or assistant. Occasionally a one-finger or instrument knot may be preferable. The surgeon should be able to lead with either hand when tying by any method. Irrespective of technique, the first throw maintains the desired approximation; the second throw holds the first one where it was placed; and the third throw holds the knot. With monofilaments, a double over-and-over first throw may be used with three instead of two additional throws. Care must be taken to ascertain that each throw is flat and square. If one end of the ligature or suture is continually kept taut in one hand, the square throws are often converted to half hitches, and the whole knot will slip, irrespective of the number of throws.

No matter what technique is used, knots in plastic monofilament sutures and ligatures are treacherous, and there must be conscious adherence to the foregoing techniques. Such attention is better than casually adding a half dozen or more "extra" throws, thus creating a painful knot or granuloma. Twisting wire is a pernicious expedient, leading to earlier fatigue and breakage of the wire suture and to sharp wire ends. Use of a flat square knot of two or three throws with individual clipping of each wire end, leaving them parallel, not perpendicular, to the curve of the suture, is best. In many places, clips are superior to all types of ligatures, provided the clip is sized correctly for its tissue requirements. In the deep body cavities, it is easier and safer to clip and divide small vessels than to isolate, ligate, and divide; or to clamp, divide, and ligate. Despite their visibility by x-ray, clips cause minimal tissue reaction. If irradiation is to be employed postoperatively, however, they should not be used except as markers. Further, computerized tomography may be invalidated by clips and wire sutures. Reoperation with dissection in a field of clips is often very difficult and hazardous.

Sponging is a far greater source of tissue trauma than is usually appreciated, especially when a wiping rather than a blotting technique is employed. Seldom does one wipe an eye when it tears. It is gently blotted once. Sometimes sponging can be a repetitive, nervous habit that is employed needlessly, or unconsciously, while the surgeon ponders the next move.

Another problem that can be subtly destructive is *drying* of tissue. Obviously, cells beneath the integument die if they desiccate, yet this effect is seldom routinely considered in operative technique. A nurse or assistant should be instructed to watch for drying tissues, because the surgeon understandably will forget when engrossed in the primary procedure. Such tissues should be kept moist with Ringer's solution. Plastic intestinal bags and moist laparotomy pads can be of assistance.

The expert *use of laparotomy pads* and sponges for packing viscera out of the field is an art that must be learned. Because the procedure adds to exposure and to protection of the abdominal wall and viscera, time should be spent in perfecting the packing of the field.

So many factors contribute to gentleness that it is essential for every surgeon to develop a "tissue conscience" with a histologic knowledge enabling visualization of the microscopic consequences of each technical maneuver. By training, experience, practice, postoperative critique, a record of complications, morbidity, and mortality, one can minimize tissue trauma and objectively evaluate operative technique.

ASEPSIS

Asepsis is the second Halsted principle of operative technique. Since every surgical wound is contaminated bacterially to some extent, asepsis can only be relative. The total concept of bacterial coexistence, the balance of host-defense mechanisms against bacterial numbers and virulence, and the environmental, bacterial, metabolic, and therapeutic factors that influence this balance must be appreciated. Every surgical procedure disturbs this balance and each wound, regardless of size, evokes a local and systemic inflammatory response. Normal tissue with normal cellular and humoral defense mechanisms will tolerate 10^5 bacteria per cubic centimeter. This tolerance is reduced by the existence or occurrence of risk factors such as malnutrition, pathogenicity, steroids, age, blood supply, immunosuppressive drugs, shock, malignancy, acidosis, hemorrhage, foreign bodies (sutures), necrotic tissue, and blood. It is important to minimize these risk factors where possible, or eliminate them. It is equally important to reduce the number of contaminating bacteria in the operative field, and to try to avoid accidentally entering the gut or spilling septic fluids. Such an event occurs in every surgeon's experience, and when it does, the contents should be aspirated immediately, the lacer-

ation repaired, and the area copiously irrigated to reduce bacteria to tolerable levels. Cultures should always be taken from the contaminated area. Depending on the pathology and potential procedure to be done, prophylactic antibiotics may be administered and continued 3 to 4 days postoperatively. Mechanical cleansing of the colon and administration of preoperative broad-spectrum intestinal antibiotics may be indicated to reduce the numbers of bacteria in the colon and the potential sepsis from an iatrogenic enterotomy or colotomy (Altemeier, Alexander; Cohn). Other sources of contamination, sometimes overlooked, include excessive talking, levity, numbers of people, and motion within the operating room, and these should be kept to a minimum. Finally, before wound closure, copious irrigation with Ringer's solution assists in removing and dispersing contaminating bacteria from all sources, including septic foci. Aspiration in the lumbar gutters and the pelvis to remove a possible collection of contaminated irrigating fluid, blood, or serum is often neglected.

GOOD BLOOD SUPPLY

Assurance of good *blood supply* to remaining tissue is the third Halsted principle. Tissues deprived of their blood supply before or during operation must be debrided as they will not heal but will become necrotic. It is far better to try to avoid damaging the blood supply by an exact knowledge of anatomy and with good dissecting technique. Judgmental problems of procedure arise when the remaining blood supply is marginal. Observation, color, peristalsis, period of blanching following pressure, fluorescin injection with ultraviolet lighting, and Doppler pulse measurement may assist in this evaluation. If there has been previous irradiation with reduction of blood supply and fibrosis, the bowel, ureters, bladder, and wound are particularly vulnerable, and the importance of every technical, metabolic, and prophylactic factor mentioned must be reemphasized (DeCosse). Injured avascular intestine cannot be repaired and must be resected or diverted. Occasionally, a planned second look in 36 to 48 hours is indicated to check the adequacy of a marginal blood supply. The sequelae of sepsis and intestinal fistulas from unappreciated avascularity and ischemic necrosis of the gut are catastrophic.

AVOIDANCE OF TENSION

The fourth principle is the *avoidance of tension* in reconstruction, approximation of tissue planes, and wound closure. When tension constantly exceeds 35 mmHg capillary pressure, ischemic necrosis of the area within the suture can result. Dehiscence of the suture line is an inevitable sequel. Ischemic tissues and irradiated tissues are especially vulnerable to tension.

HEMOSTASIS

The fifth principle is technical *hemostasis*. Intravascular coagulation and thrombus formation in small vessels are physiologic and occur spontaneously if clotting mechanisms are normal. Pressure, hemostats, sutures, ligatures, coagulation, apposition of layers, thrombin, free muscle, and avatin are all useful in securing hemostasis for bleeding from larger vessels or surface oozing. The use of coagulation current for bleeding points in the wounds of access is effective and reduces foreign ligature material in the wound. Deep coagulation is dangerous as a loop of bowel may be inadvertently touched. Coagulation of an artery that is too large can lead to delayed massive hemorrhage. Stainless steel clips are often superior and much easier to apply, with a minimum of foreign-body reaction. They are ideal in a septic field. Suture ligatures of nonabsorbable material should be used for the larger arteries. Often it is better and safer to divide a major artery between two properly separated suture ligatures than between two clamps placed too close together where there is risk of suture breakage or retraction during tying. In septic fields, coagulation for small bleeding vessels and ligature of larger vessels with monofilament ligatures or clips is superior, since it avoids the granulomas of silk or cotton as well as the premature enzymatic breakdown of the guts.

Major bleeding leads to one of the most serious operative complications, shock (MacLean; Shires, et al., 1979). Sooner or later, it happens to a patient of every surgeon, and all surgeons must be prepared to cope with this emergency. First, the bleeding area must be controlled by pressure of hand, fingers, clamp, or laparotomy pad. Next, extraneous instruments and sponges should be removed from the operative field, and appropriate instruments, hemostats, and suture-ligature materials should be obtained and made ready. Extra blood should be procured. If necessary, the incision should be extended to permit better visualization with room for extra hands and instruments. Important adjacent structures should be identified and their positions noted. With maximum lighting and retraction, the bleeding area should be approached slowly and a large clamp applied discreetly, or a finger substituted for a larger sponge. A rather gross suture ligature beneath a finger may be appropriate. Blind clamping, in general, is to be con-

demned. Suture ligatures of the figure-of-eight type should be applied to hemostats rather than ligatures. Proximal and distal control of a major artery or vein should be secured where possible while the rent is sutured. This is an area where generalities are inappropriate. The principles of exposure, relaxation, lighting, assistance, consultation, knowledge, experience, a calm temperament, and ingenuity are applicable. The ever-present threat of major, uncontrollable hemorrhage from surgery in the body cavities is perhaps the most potent of all the stimuli to the outstanding technical surgeon, and the greatest deterrent to the inept and untrained.

CAREFUL APPROXIMATION

The sixth principle is *careful approximation* of fascial planes, viscera, and epithelium. It decreases the magnitude of the wound-healing process, decreases inflammation and pathologic fibrosis, and prevents dehiscence and hernias. The choice of appropriate suture material and the importance of avoiding tension have been emphasized. Continuous sutures in general are to be condemned, in the author's opinion, as they can lead to ischemia of the wound edge, sepsis, and dehiscence. Retention sutures may be indicated in secondary closures, or in wounds where there is a marginal blood supply from previous irradiation. In general, the author prefers interrupted fascial sutures of 2-0/3-0 nylon, prolene, or wire. Often a few buried, interrupted stay sutures of 0 or 1 prolene may be used. These sutures should only approximate; they should not be too close together nor too far apart with gaping. They should be of an appropriate depth gauged to the tensile strength of the fascial plane and suture. Wound closure demands care and attention to details. Careless wound closure can lead to sepsis, dehiscence, fistulas, hernias, and intestinal obstruction with a prohibitive mortality rate, in some series 20 to 25 percent. The subcutaneous wound, if bacterially contaminated by septic pathology, should be left open initially and closed secondarily in 4 to 6 days.

OBLITERATION OF DEAD SPACES

The seventh Halsted principle is *obliteration of dead spaces* in the wounds of access, extirpation, and reconstruction. It is difficult to accomplish this with external positive pressure, though a large, bulky dressing can serve as a stent. Negative pressure applied to a soft rubber catheter in sterile spaces is far superior to external pressure and removes transudates of blood and serum. But *drains* introduce contaminating bacteria and sepsis, and if left in place too long, may lead to deep abscesses. Necrosis of blood vessels and intestine can result from the pressure of hard rubber or plastic drains. Drains in sterile spaces should be removed within 48 to 72 hours when their effective function has ceased. Conversely, a drain or catheter introduced into a septic cavity usually should be left in place many days. This keeps the cavity exteriorized, prevents the formation of another deep, closed abscess cavity, and allows it to contract. In general, drains should be placed dependently through a separate stab wound, and never through the primary incision. It should be remembered that drains are foreign bodies. They evoke an immediate fibrinous exteriorizing sealing reaction and often cease to function within 36 hours. To prevent this, they should be twisted, shortened, or disturbed a little once or twice a day, always keeping track of their location with a safety pin and a written note in the chart. The fibrin seal leads to a collagenic fibrotic reaction and sinus tract in a few days that can cause pathologic adhesions within the peritoneal cavity. These, in turn, can cause small-bowel obstruction. Certain sterile spaces can be obliterated more appropriately with buried sutures. When possible, this procedure reduces the septic risk of a drain.

In past decades and centuries, a surgeon was judged by the smallness of an incision and the brevity of operating time. But wounds heal from side to side, and there are fewer complications if there has been less retraction from a longer incision. *Haste* during the operation may lead to rough handling of tissues; or worse, it may lead to the faulty choice of procedure; or still worse, it may lead to technical errors with major intraoperative and postoperative complications. Technical surgery today should be deliberate and considered. Even so, there is no place for dillydallying or repetitive efforts, and there is a real clinical and economic premium on shorter operating times. But this reduction of operating time should be the by-product of experience, good anesthesia, good assistance, and teamwork. The final arbiter must be the quickest, most complete rehabilitation of the patient, the fewest complications, and lowest mortality rate at the least cost, not the anesthesiologist's or administration's emphasis only on time and cost-effectiveness, using for comparison a norm of dubious validity. Yet, 18 million operations are performed annually in this nation at the present time. A reduction of wound complications of 1 percent as a result of better education, training, and ability of surgeons would lead to an enormous reduction in patient morbidity, mortality, and suffering. The economic saving would approximate 2 billion dollars.

POSTOPERATIVE CONSIDERATIONS

With the last suture in place, the postoperative period begins. If the preoperative period was one of diagnosis, assessment, correction, and repletion, the postoperative period is one of critical observation, monitoring (Del Guercio; Siegel), diagnosis, and specific supportive, symptomatic, and prophylactic care. There are predictable local and systemic responses to the operation (Schenk; Moore; Gann; Madden; Peacock). These are fairly constant qualitatively, but they vary enormously quantitatively. Certain organ system problems or complications occur more frequently than others during each phase of the time-course of the postoperative period. Certain complications are uniquely related to a specific operation and its anatomic site; others are common to all operative procedures (Artz, Hardy; Hardy; Schwartz, 1979a). The surgeon making rounds is aware of the diagnosis, the preoperative metabolic state of the patient, the operative procedure, and the stage of convalescence. These variables should be integrated into the evaluation of the patient at any given point in time. Postoperative care (*Manual of Preoperative and Postoperative Care*) essentially is concerned with the prevention, diagnosis, and treatment of complications, one of the most serious of which is failure of individual rehabilitation, the worst of which is death. Each surgical complication becomes a separate entity with its own unique body of literature. The surgeon must know the etiology, diagnosis, and management of all postoperative complications. The acquisition of this knowledge is a lifelong pursuit as the surgeon strives to reduce morbidity and mortality to the ideal goal of zero.

PROBLEMS OF THE FIRST FEW HOURS

Most of the problems that arise in the first few postoperative hours relate to loss of airway, decreased cardiac output and perfusion, physical control of the semiconscious patient, and the sequelae of anesthetic paralysis and prolonged immobility.

INADEQUATE VENTILATION

Complications that relate to *inadequate ventilation* (Laver, Austen; Clowes, 1976a, 1976b) during the period of extubation are much more prolonged and subtle than those connected with intubation. Respiratory failure is a major cause of 25 to 50 percent of postoperative deaths, particularly in the aged. The array of drugs used in modern anesthesia often has unpredictable effects on the respiratory centers, their recovery or reversal, and the drive to breathe. The effects are further compounded by the idiosyncrasies of the patients, their metabolic status, the presence or absence of shock and hypotension, and postoperative drugs. Failure to recognize inadequate ventilation after extubation and a delay in mechanical support of ventilation or reintubation may lead rapidly to respiratory failure and to anoxic cardiac arrest with its catastrophic sequelae. Vomiting and aspiration may be independent or contributing events. Because of the presence of anesthesiologists and trained personnel in the recovery room, the incidence of such accidents is reduced, although the details of their prevention and care must never be taken for granted by the anesthesiologist or surgeon. The chance of such accidents decreases exponentially with time, but when they occur during or immediately after transfer to an intensive care unit, room, or ward, skilled personnel may be unavailable and the inadequate ventilation unrecognized. Each patient must be considered individually. Ventilatory volumes and measurements of P_{CO_2}, P_{O_2} and pH of the arterial blood should be obtained if there is suspicion of hypoventilation, shunting from atelectasis, abnormalities in ventilation/perfusion ratios, decreased perfusion, or a diffusion defect. Congestive failure, dyspnea, cyanosis, pulmonary edema, obstructive lung disease, a P_{O_2} less than normal (80 mmHg), and a P_{CO_2} greater than 50 mmHg should alert the observer to pulmonary insufficiency.

HYPOTENSION AND SHOCK

Hypotension and shock in the postoperative patient must be considered the result of hemorrhagic or hypovolemic shock until proved otherwise (Shires et al., 1979b; MacLean). However, there are several other serious causes of hypotension which may or may not be related. The first is cardiac failure from a myocardial infarct, arrhythmia, cardiac arrest, or hypokalemia. Electrolyte imbalance, hypoxia, hypercapnia, and a vagal stimulus in any combination can trigger a ventricular fibrillation in an otherwise normal heart. The second is an increase in volume of the vascular system from peripheral vasodilatation of spinal anesthesia or from central-nervous-system influences of general anesthesia. Third, septicemia or endotox-

emia may cause an early, profound hypotension in patients with sepsis from vasodilatation, increased capillary permeability, and capillovenous pooling. Fourth, anything that blocks venous return to the right or left heart, e.g., tension pneumothorax, or pulmonary embolism, will cause hypotension. Thus, anything that decreases cardiac output or blood volume, that dilates and increases the volume or permeability of the conduit system, that causes capillovenous pooling, or that decreases venous return to the heart is capable of producing shock and hypotension in the postoperative period. Specific and supportive treatment depends on accurate diagnosis. Monitoring of the cardiac rate, rhythm, and pattern by electrocardiography, cardiac output and pressures by a central venous or Swan-Ganz catheter, and the measurement of blood gases and serum electrolytes will assist in making an accurate diagnosis and serve as a baseline for management. Urinary output assists in evaluating tissue perfusion.

SEMICONSCIOUS PATIENT

The *semiconscious patient* has few inhibiting pain stimuli from motion, straining, or vomiting and at times may become violent. These patients must be protected from themselves, from falling, or more subtly from dehiscing their fascial planes, particularly after extubation. They should be flexed and on their side when straining or vomiting. Attendants should be instructed to listen and feel for bursting fascial sutures. If they are observed, it is best to reexplore the wound immediately.

PATCHY ATELECTASIS

The most subtle part of the early hours or first day or two of recovery are the *sequelae of immobility of partial neuromuscular paresis* from anesthesia and the operation. Most frequent is *patchy atelectasis*, its only sign depressed breath sounds. Fiberoptic bronchoscopy should be employed if atelectasis is major and does not respond to the simpler measure of deep breathing, coughing, and intratracheal catheterization. One of the most serious early sequelae of paresis is *venous stasis*, which when coupled with the intimal damage of abnormal positioning of the lower extremities and the hypercoagulability of the postoperative state, can set the stage for deep femoral vein thrombosis and later thromboembolism (Sabiston). Very early leg motion, dorsiflexion of the toes, coughing, and deep breathing are excellent prophylaxis for both atelectasis and venous stasis. The use of small amounts of heparin immediately before surgery and postoperatively may be indicated in those patients at special risk of thromboembolism from varicosities, obesity, agedness, heart disease, and extensive pelvic inflammatory pathology. Low-molecular-weight dextran seems to be equally effective and is accompanied by fewer wound complications. The prophylaxis of thromboembolism is a very important but controversial area.

INABILITY TO URINATE

Inability to urinate may lead to overdistention of the urinary bladder with such serious sequelae as mechanical disruptions of the operative area, a continual paresis of the bladder, incontinence, and urinary tract infection. If a patient cannot void spontaneously, and if a single catheterization is inadequate, then an indwelling urethral or occasionally a suprapubic catheter is indicated. Early oliguria or anuria with or without flank pain and peritoneal signs should raise the question of ureteral damage with immediate assessment by intravenous pyelography, renal scan, and retrograde catheterization with reexploration.

PARALYTIC ILEUS

Paralytic ileus to a greater or lesser degree accompanies every major operative procedure. Early mobilization, a judicious oral intake, and appropriate nasogastric suction usually suffice. However, one of the great dangers of a prolonged paralytic ileus is oversight of a mechanical obstruction. Any paralytic ileus that persists beyond 3 days postoperatively should be suspected of being a mechanical small-bowel obstruction until proved otherwise. Diagnostic and therapeutic steps should be planned accordingly. Postoperative acute appendicitis or cholecystitis may be masked by postoperative ileus, escape detection, and present as septic shock.

NEED FOR INTENSIVE CARE

Transfer to the *intensive care unit* (Schenk) may follow the recovery room period and should be available for patients who have organ system deficits, particularly in the cardiopulmonary and renal systems. Shock and sepsis can quickly and adversely tip the balance of chronic pulmonary or renal disease to acute respiratory failure (ARF) and renal failure of the high output or oliguric type. In circumstances such as these, monitoring of cardiac output, wedge pressures, blood gases, and electrolytes is essential for

therapeutic support (Del Guercio; Siegel). Though beyond the scope of this chapter, the specialized care that can be provided in modern intensive care units is one of the great resources that has been developed for the surgical patient in the last decade.

PROBLEMS OF THE SECOND TO FOURTH DAY

The second to fourth day postoperatively is the period when attention must be given to intravenous water and electrolyte administration, regulation of the internal environment, the question of renal failure (Powers), or respiratory failure (Laver, Austen), and to the febrile responses (Kinney, Caldwell) of the septic sequelae of atelectasis, urinary tract retention, and venous stasis. Early dialysis is recommended after the diagnosis of renal failure in the first postoperative days as it can minimize the cellular depression of uremia and its ramifications. Ordinarily, the maintenance of a constant internal environment poses no problem in the average patient. All intravenous fluids should contain 5% glucose to provide for the daily cerebral requirements of about 150 g of glucose administered evenly over a 24-hour period. Further, this has a major protein sparing effect. No nitrogen or fat need be supplied to the average uncomplicated patient; such patients have sufficient reserves for this relatively brief period of starvation and negative balance and can be spared the risks of intravenous alimentation. Oral intake can be started after the period of ileus has subsided. Mobilization, walking, leg exercises, breathing, and coughing are essential in this period. An overhead trapeze is an important adjunct to assist movement in bed, exercise, and stabilization of the shoulder girdle to extend deep breathing and coughing. Sitting in a chair for prolonged periods is hazardous since it promotes pelvic venous stasis. In the first few days after surgery, a chair can be used for brief rest periods after walking, standing, and breathing exercises. A transient elevation of temperature and pulse may be a warning of deep-vein thrombosis during this period.

PROBLEMS OF THE FOURTH TO EIGHTH DAY

SEPSIS

The fourth to the eighth day postoperatively is the period of the wound complications of *sepsis* and dehiscence (Schilling). Any elevation of temperature and pulse at this time should be considered an infection of superficial wound origin, or from deep within the body cavities or pelvis, until proved otherwise. It is also the turning point period described by Moore when patients begin to feel better psychologically, when appetite and peristalsis return, and when the wounds lose their acute pain and tenderness. A reversal of this normal progression, along with malaise and ileus, should lead to suspicion of sepsis. The abdomen may harbor a deep abscess, and ultrasound studies of the abdomen will be very helpful in identifying fluid and purulent collections. Wounds should be explored if they are red and indurated. The abdomen should be explored under antibiotic support if there is clinical, laboratory, x-ray, and ultrasound evidence of an abscess. An intraperitoneal phlegmon should not be reexplored but should be allowed to resolve or progress to an abscess.

DEHISCENCE

A transient burst of serosanguineous fluid on the patient's bed linen may be the only sign of *dehiscence*. Such patients should always be examined immediately, night or day. The wound should be palpated for lack of a healing ridge, and despite the comforting appearance of an intact skin suture line, preparations for exploration of the wound under general anesthesia should be made. There are exceptions to this basic rule, but they should be individualized. The risks of total visceral eventration, small-bowel obstruction, an overlooked abscess, or a late massive ventral hernia far outweigh the risks of an early exploration and reclosure of the wound. This is best accomplished with a single layer of large No. 2 through-and-through nylon or prolene retention sutures, care being taken to place them just external to the peritoneum, yet deep to the fascia. Wound dehiscence is frequently accompanied or preceded by intraabdominal sepsis and in a sense may be regarded as a symptom and sign of intraabdominal sepsis. Deep abscesses, if present, should be drained, but the drain should be brought out through a separate independent stab wound, never through the incision.

SMALL-BOWEL OBSTRUCTION

During this period, a mechanical *small-bowel obstruction* may occur from early inflammatory adhesions, a twist, or herniation of small bowel into a fascial dehiscence or peritoneal or mesenteric defect that was not securely closed. It may follow a prolonged paralytic ileus or a period of normal bowel function. Not an easy diagnosis to make, it should always be suspected when there is continued ileus or recurrent crampy abdominal pain and nausea. A dilute barium swallow and follow-through are extremely helpful in the differential diagnosis between paralytic and mechanical small-bowel obstruction. The obstruction is a lethal entity when unrecognized. When the diagnosis has been made, the patient should be reexplored immediately after there has been appropriate volume repletion, nasogastric intubation and aspiration, administration of prophylactic antibiotics, correction of acid-base imbalances, restoration of renal function, and pulmonary support. Long-tube nasogastric-enteric decompression may be elected under some circumstances.

PULMONARY EMBOLUS

Pneumonitis, cough, chest pain, and fever should raise the suspicion of a *pulmonary embolus* (Sabiston), which occurs with greatest frequency between the fourth to the eighth days postoperatively. It, too, may be masked by, or confused with, an atelectatic pneumonitis or cardiac arrhythmia. The details of the prevention, diagnosis, and management of this serious complication are contained in the references.

ENERGY EXHAUSTION

Ordinarily, a patient will be discharged within a few days postoperatively if convalescence has proceeded without incident. However, if there have been complications such as sepsis, dehiscence, intestinal obstruction with shock, or pulmonary embolus, the patient may be threatened by *energy exhaustion* and protein depletion. Cellular responses of the bone marrow and reticuloendothelial system and the production of antibodies, complement, and enzymes are suppressed. The patient is threatened by a further risk of sepsis from atelectasis and pneumonia when the energy reserves for the work of breathing dwindle. Doubling ventilatory volumes or airway resistance quintuples the work of breathing. When the work of breathing exceeds the energy equivalent of oxygen diffused across the pulmonary alveolar membranes, acute respiratory failure rapidly ensues. Now the benefits of intravenous alimentation exceed the risks in this complicated postoperative course. At this time attention should be focused on oral alimentation or intravenous alimentation with ventilatory assistance to reduce the caloric expenditure for the work of breathing. The details of these considerations are described completely in the chapters of both Dudrick and Moore (*Manual of Surgical Nutrition;* Dudrick, Rhoads; Moore). Intravenous alimentation provides exogenous protein and calories to give time for survival and recovery from underlying problems in which energy requirements exceed endogenous energy reserves.

This is also the period of late secondary organ failure, most frequently pulmonary and renal, but also cardiac and hepatic. The brain, too, shares metabolically in these derangements with accompanying lethargy, stupor, coma, and decreased levels of consciousness. These manifestations are accentuated if there is poor arterial perfusion of the brain. The management of certain organ failures is beyond the scope of this chapter, but is reviewed completely in the general and specific references.

PROBLEMS AFTER THE NINTH AND TENTH DAYS

After the ninth and tenth days, the patient usually will quickly replete the endogenous protein stores, restore muscle mass, and regain neuromuscular function by oral alimentation and increased motor activity. When the protein mass has been completely restored, the excess calories will be stored as fat, and the fat gain phase occurs. Negative calorie and nitrogen balances during this period can block, slow down, or prolong functional and psychiatric rehabilitation. Upon being discharged from the hospital, the patient is without the personal counsel, guidance, and stimulus of the physician and may fail to secure an adequate diet and exercise. Loss of motivation, lethargy, and weakness may result. If this period is ignored or prolonged, the patient may fail to rehabilitate or resume normal, fulfilling activities and employment.

LATER PROBLEMS

FIBROSIS

Finally, the wound complications of *pathologic fibrosis* may occur weeks, months, and even years after surgery. Complications include intestinal obstruction from adhesions; fibrotic narrowing of anastromoses of intestines, ureters, and fallopian tubes; development of pathologic contractures around body orifices or intertriginous areas; and ankylosing contractures around joints, joint capsules, and tendons which limit

motion. These examples, by no means complete, serve to emphasize the importance of prevention and early correction of such wound complications. Excessive fibrosis is enhanced by prolonged sepsis and inflammation from any cause, by x-radiation, and by excessive tension on suture lines. It can be minimized by careful surgical technique and skill. Reconstructive procedures can correct some of the debits of excessive fibrosis but can rarely restore function to normal.

HERNIA

Late hernias occur when there is partial wound dehiscence or prolonged excessive tension, pull, or strain. It should be routine practice to examine an incision 6 months after surgery to check for the presence of a potential hernia.

No effort has been made to review the early, intermediate, or late complications that are unique to gynecologic operative procedures, pathology, and anatomic location. These are reviewed in this volume and other specialty volumes. It is the author's opinion that anyone operating in the abdomen should be thoroughly familiar with small-bowel and colon surgery. The major surgical texts and their references should assist in providing this information.

CONCLUSION

This chapter would not be complete without a summary of the body's local (Schilling), systemic (Gann; Moore), and psychologic responses to surgery and wounding, which are integral to and superimposed on the disease process regardless of age or metabolic state of the patient. They are constant qualitatively although their extent and duration vary quantitatively.

LOCAL RESPONSE

The local response of the wound has four phases. First, the *wounding-injury phase* breaches cellular continuity with hemorrhage, intravascular coagulation, variable loss of specific organ function, and contamination with bacteria and foreign material. There is an afferent neural-endocrine-chemical stimulus from the wound. Following initial vasoconstriction, there is vasodilatation and increased permeability of the capillaries.

This ushers in the second or *inflammatory phase* when the wound tissue becomes wet with serum and plasma, which deliver antibacterial globulins with antibodies and complement to the bacterially contaminated wound. During this phase the wound tissue is infiltrated with polymorphonuclear cells, lymphocytes, and plasma cells. Under ordinary circumstances, this phase reaches its maximum by the end of 72 hours. The wound in this phase may be likened to an in vivo bacterial culture where bacterial multiplication is balanced and overridden by the body's humoral and cellular defense mechanisms. A proliferation of epithelial, endothelial, and fibroblastic cells becomes apparent at this time. Following the stimulus of the breach of continuity by the wounding agent, there is random migration of these proliferating cells.

They usher in the third or *proliferative phase,* characterized by granulation tissue formation, contraction, and collagen production by the fibroblasts. The progessively cross-linked collagen provides strength and permanence to the wound scar. The granulating surfaces of the wound become covered with epithelium and mucosa, sealing them from further bacterial invasion. No wound is healed completely until all epithelial and mucosal surfaces are covered. An open wound inhibits protein anabolism. In this phase, the wound may be likened to an in vivo tissue culture where the migrating cells are guided by the histologic fibrillar framework of the wound within and the physical forces without. Contact inhibition of like cells leads to an orderly sorting out of the enormous mixed cell population.

Remodeling, absorption, and redeposition of collagen characterize the *fourth phase.* This phase is profoundly influenced by function, tension, and sepsis, and can lead to the overproduction of collagen.

The *local wound complications* of the wound-injury phase are hemorrhage, hematoma formation, shock, and loss of the wounded organ's function. The complications of the inflammatory phase are sepsis and abscess formation. The most serious complication of the proliferative phase is dehiscence of the superficial wound of access, or the deep wounds of extirpation and reconstruction, including anastomoses and closure of hollow viscera. Finally, the complications of the remodeling phase are excessive scarring, narrowing, and occluding of involved hollow structures, the gut, the ureters, the fallopian tubes, arteries, and veins, with partial or complete obstruction, intestinal adhesions, keloid and pathologic contractures. These complications are outlined as they may extend, alter, reinitiate, or interrupt the normal progression of the biologic pattern of the systemic response to surgery which follows.

SYSTEMIC RESPONSE

This neuroendocrine response is evoked by pain and fear from the *wound injury* with secretion of ACTH (adrenocorticotropic hormone) and catecholamines. It is profoundly augmented by shock, hypoxia, acidosis, and sepsis. The catecholamine secretion of epinephrine and norepinephrine from the adrenal medulla causes increased heart rate, blood pressure, and cardiac output, with increased pulmonary ventilation, shunting of blood away from the gut and kidneys, and mobilization of hepatic glycogen. These catecholamines and shock are a further potent stimulus to ACTH production from the pituitary. They provide for the fight or flight mechanisms of survival in the animal kingdom. In man, kept alive by supportive measures, there may be an intense persistence of these catecholamine responses, which may lead to renal failure, pulmonary edema, and cardiac failure. *Aldosterone* and *antidiuretic hormones* are secreted in response to ACTH and to volume deficits from the adrenal cortex and posterior pituitary respectively, with resulting sodium and water retention and volume conservation.

In response to ACTH, *glucocorticoids* are also secreted by the adrenal cortex with a mobilization of protein and fat from endogenous stores for utilization as body fuels. The magnitude of these catabolic responses relates to the degree of injury and is enhanced by shock, sepsis, and acidosis. The end result is a major depletion of the body's protein and fat stores, with a shift to fat oxidation for most of the patient's energy requirements.

The catecholamines and the glucocorticoids stimulate cyclic *adenosine monophosphate* (AMP) which stimulates a variety of cells to perform synthetic or metabolic functions at an increased rate. They also stimulate the secretion of *glucagon,* which hastens the conversion of nitrogen compounds to glucose. *Insulin,* on the other hand, opposes the peripheral effects of glucagon since it hastens glucose oxidation and is the major anabolic hormone that favors entry of amino acids into cells with protein synthesis. Thus, early after injury, it is not surprising to find a pseudodiabetic state with apparent insulin resistance.

After a few days of uncomplicated convalescence, Moore's turning point is reached with reversal of these catabolic changes. There is diuresis of sodium and water, retention of potassium and nitrogen, and restoration of insulin to normal levels. Peristalsis and appetite return. The patient begins the *anabolic* phase with a positive nitrogen balance and with ultimate body cell mass repletion.

Following body cell mass repletion of nitrogen and protein, excess calories are stored as fat and the *fat gain phase* begins. There is no limit to this phase and hypertrophic obesity can result if calories are not controlled. These systemic responses to wounding and injury may be damped or minimized by expert surgical care, or they may be sustained, reinitiated, or magnified by complications of sepsis, shock, pulmonary embolism, and reoperation, leading to ultimate energy exhaustion.

PSYCHOLOGIC RESPONSE

These responses to surgery, wounding, and trauma also follow a predictable pattern. They vary widely and are difficult to quantitate, but certain important, often overlooked, generalizations may be made. Prior to surgery, a patient usually has *fear and anxiety* about the operation, the disease, the involuntary induction of coma, of not awakening, and apprehension over possible loss of function or deformity. This is particularly true in the woman when an operation on reproductive organs threatens her identity, sexuality, and ability to bear children. These fears must be appreciated and ameliorated by the surgeon in his professional relationship with the patient, through honest discussion, and by informed consent. Such reassurance can lessen the postoperative systemic neuroendocrine stress response.

The first day or two after surgery the patient is often *euphoric*, relieved to be alive, with pain and anxiety held in check by drugs. Postoperative pain and tenderness increase and reach their maximum in 48 to 72 hours. With the further discomfort of immobilization and a more complete psychologic awareness, the euphoric state may give way to *depression* and *apprehension*, a sense of impending disaster, and a fear that things may not turn out well after all. This feeling may be greater when there has been loss of an organ, such as a breast, or a diagnosis of cancer. It is accentuated by ileus and its accompanying crampy pain and distention. With the gradual resolution of problems of postoperative convalescence, the patient begins to think about going home, feels better, has "turned the corner" with a positive nitrogen and calorie balance, and develops a *sense of well-being*. These relatively predictable responses may be over-

ridden, extended, or altered by *special fears* of the disease, e.g., cancer. Another variable is the response to *sensory deprivation* and isolation in a room, or to *sleep deprivation* and *overstimulation* in an intensive care unit. When the patient has been discharged from the hospital, euphoria is often replaced by a profound depression as the patient must begin to look after herself and must assume household responsibilities which can be overwhelming. This feeling can be accentuated by a husband who is unattentive, unsympathetic, or overdemanding, and by children who are uncared for. The fear of *social isolation* or *rejection*, or the fear of or *desire for death* may further complicate this posthospital period. *Anorexia* with body cell mass depletion may recur; or more subtly, body cell mass repletion may be delayed with resulting *malaise, loss of motivation*, and *weakness*. Failure to manage these subtle areas of emotional response may lead to a breakdown of doctor-patient relationships, *failure of rehabilitation*, and to feelings by the patient of *anger* and of having been assaulted. Success in management leads more promptly to the gratifying total physical and psychologic rehabilitation of the patient.

The principles of surgery are, therefore, the rules that govern the conduct of the operative and nonoperative care of a surgical patient. They relate to the total time-course of the patient's disease and to operative care. Their application involves the specific details of relevant knowledge and judgment that have evolved to date.

REFERENCES

General

Alexander JW, Good RA: *Fundamentals of Clinical Immunology*, Philadelphia: Saunders, 1977.

Clowes GHA (ed.): Symposium on response to infection and injury, Part I. *Surg Clin North Am* 56:801, 1976a.

——— (ed.): Symposium on response to infection and injury, Part II. *Surg Clin North Am* 56:997, 1976b.

Greenfield LJ: Surgery in the aged, in *Major Problems in Clinical Surgery*, vol. 17, eds. JE Dunphy, PA Ebert, Philadelphia: Saunders, 1975.

Manual of Medical Care of the Surgical Patient, ed. S Papper, Boston: Little Brown, 1976.

Manual of Preoperative and Postoperative Care, Committee on Pre and Postoperative Care, American College of Surgeons, eds. JM Kinney et al., Philadelphia: Saunders, 1971.

Manual of Surgical Nutrition, Committee on Pre and Postoperative Care, American College of Surgeons, eds. WB Ballinger et al., Philadelphia: Saunders, 1975.

Manual on Control of Infection in Surgical Patients, Committee on Control of Surgical Infections of the Committee on Pre and Postoperative Care, American College of Surgeons, eds. WA Altemeier et al., Philadelphia: Lippincott, 1976.

Sabiston DC Jr. (ed.): *Davis-Christopher's Textbook of Surgery,* 11th ed., Philadelphia: Saunders, 1977.

Schwartz SI et al. (eds.): *Principles of Surgery,* 3d ed., New York: McGraw-Hill, 1979.

Artz CP, Hardy JD: *Management of Surgical Complications,* 3d ed., Philadelphia: Saunders, 1975.

Selected References

Altemeier WA, Alexander JW: Surgical infections and choice of antibiotics, in *Davis-Christopher's Textbook of Surgery,* 11th ed., ed. DC Sabiston Jr, Philadelphia: Saunders, 1977, p. 340.

Brunner EA, Eckenhoff JE: Anesthesia, in *Davis-Christopher's Textbook of Surgery,* 11th ed., ed. DC Sabiston Jr, Philadelphia: Saunders, 1977, p. 200.

Cohn I, Bornside GH: Infections, in *Principles of Surgery,* 3d ed., eds. SI Schwartz et al., New York: McGraw-Hill, 1979, p. 185.

Conn RB: Normal laboratory values of clinical importance, in *Davis-Christopher's Textbook of Surgery,* 11th ed., ed. DC Sabiston Jr, Philadelphia: Saunders, 1977, p. 2461.

Davis JH: Surgical aspects of diabetes mellitus, in *Davis-Christopher's Textbook of Surgery,* 11th ed., ed. DC Sabiston Jr, Philadelphia: Saunders, 1977, p. 178.

DeCosse JJ: Radiation injury to the intestine, in *Davis-Christopher's Textbook of Surgery,* 11th ed., ed. DC Sabiston Jr, Philadelphia: Saunders, 1977, p. 1057.

Del Guercio LRM: Physiologic monitoring of the surgical patient, in *Principles of Surgery,* 3d ed., eds. SI Schwartz et al., New York: McGraw-Hill, 1979, p. 525.

Dudrick SJ, Rhoads JE: Metabolism in surgical patients: Protein, carbohydrate, and fat utilization by oral and parenteral routes, in *Davis-Christopher's Textbook of Surgery,* 11th ed., ed. DC Sabiston Jr, Philadelphia: Saunders, 1977, p. 150.

Gann DS: Endocrine and metabolic responses to injury, in *Principles of Surgery,* 3d ed., eds. SI Schwartz et al., New York: McGraw-Hill, 1979, p. 1.

Greene NM: Anesthesia, in *Principles of Surgery,* 3d ed., eds. SI Schwartz et al., New York: McGraw-Hill, 1979, p. 475.

Greenfield LJ: Cardiac arrest, in *Davis-Christopher's Textbook of Surgery,* 11th ed., ed. DC Sabiston Jr, Philadelphia: Saunders, 1977, p. 2206.

Hardy JD: Surgical complications, in *Davis-Christopher's Textbook of Surgery,* 11th ed., ed. DC Sabiston Jr, Philadelphia: Saunders, 1977, p. 424.

Jones RS: The small intestine, in *Davis-Christopher's Textbook of Surgery,* 11th ed., ed. DC Sabiston Jr, Philadelphia: Saunders, 1977, p. 1033.

Kinney JM, Caldwell FT Jr: Fever: Etiology, physiologic and metabolic effects, and management in surgical patients, in *Davis-Christopher's Textbook of Surgery,* 11th ed., ed. DC Sabiston Jr, Philadelphia: Saunders, 1977, p. 185.

Laver MB, Austen WG: Lung function: Physiologic consideration applicable to surgery, in *Davis-Christopher's Textbook of Surgery,* 11th ed., ed. DC Sabiston Jr, Philadelphia: Saunders, 1977, p. 2019.

MacLean LD: Shock: Causes and management of circulatory collapse, in *Davis-Christopher's Textbook of Surgery,* 11th ed., ed. DC Sabiston Jr, Philadelphia: Saunders, 1977, p. 65.

Madden JW: Wound healing: Biologic and clinical features, in *Davis-Christopher's Textbook of Surgery,* 11th ed., ed. DC Sabiston Jr, Philadelphia: Saunders, 1977, p. 271.

Moore FD: Homeostasis: Bodily changes in trauma and surgery: The responses to injury in man as the basis for clinical management, in *Davis-Christopher's Textbook of Surgery,* 11th ed., ed. DC Sabiston Jr, Philadelphia: Saunders, 1977, p. 27.

Orloff MJ: The liver, in *Davis-Christopher's Textbook of Surgery,* 11th ed., ed. DC Sabiston Jr, Philadelphia: Saunders, 1977, p. 1149.

Peacock EE: Wound healing, in *Principles of Surgery,* 3d ed., eds. SI Schwartz et al., New York: McGraw-Hill, 1979, p. 303.

Polk HC Jr: Principles of preoperative preparation of the surgical patient, in *Davis-Christopher's Textbook of Surgery,* 11th ed., ed. DC Sabiston Jr, Philadelphia: Saunders, 1977, p. 119.

Postlethwait RW: Principles of operative surgery: Antisepsis, technique, sutures, and drains, in *Davis-Christopher's Textbook of Surgery,* 11th ed., ed. DC Sabiston Jr, Philadelphia: Saunders, 1977, p. 323.

Powers SR Jr: Acute postoperative renal failure: Prophylaxis and management, in *Davis-Christopher's Textbook of Surgery,* 11th ed., ed. DC Sabiston Jr, Philadelphia: Saunders, 1977, p. 443.

Christopher's Textbook of Surgery, 11th ed., ed. DC Sabiston Jr, Philadelphia: Saunders, 1977, p. 225.

Schilling JA: Wound healing. *Surg Clin North Am,* 56:859, 1976.

Schwartz SI: Complications, in *Principles of Surgery,* 3d ed., eds. SI Schwartz et al., New York: McGraw-Hill, 1979a, p. 495.

———: Hemostasis, surgical bleeding, and transfusion, in *Principles of Surgery,* 3d ed., eds. SI Schwartz et al., New York: McGraw-Hill, 1979b, p. 99.

Shires GT et al.: Fluid and electrolyte management of the surgical patient, in *Davis-Christopher's Textbook of Surgery,* 11th ed., ed. DC Sabiston Jr, Philadelphia: Saunders, 1977, p. 95.

——— et al.: Fluid, electrolyte, and nutritional management of the surgical patient, in *Principles of Surgery* 3d ed., eds. SI Schwartz et al., New York: McGraw-Hill, 1979a, p. 65.

——— et al.: Shock, in *Principles of Surgery* 3d ed., eds. SI Schwartz et al., New York: McGraw-Hill, 1979b, p. 135.

Siegel JH: Computers and mathematical techniques in surgery, in *Davis-Christopher's Textbook of Surgery,* 11th ed., ed. DC Sabiston Jr, Philadelphia: Saunders, 1977, p. 231.

Silver D: Blood transfusions and disorders of surgical bleeding, in *Davis-Christopher's Textbook of Surgery,* 11th ed., ed. DC Sabiston Jr, Philadelphia: Saunders, 1977, p. 131.

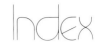